# Histology *for* Pathologists

*Second Edition*

# Histology *for* Pathologists

*Second Edition*

EDITOR

Stephen S. Sternberg, M.D.

*Attending Pathologist*
*Department of Pathology*
*Memorial Sloan-Kettering Cancer Center*
*New York, New York*

LIPPINCOTT WILLIAMS & WILKINS
A **Wolters Kluwer** Company
Philadelphia • Baltimore • New York • London
Buenos Aires • Hong Kong • Sydney • Tokyo

Acquisitions Editor: Vickie E. Thaw
Developmental Editor: Judith E. Hummel
Manufacturing Manager: Dennis Teston
Production Manager: Larry Bernstein
Production Editors: Linda B. Bass, Dee Josephson
Cover Designer: Karen Quigley
Indexer: Mary Kidd
Compositor: Maryland Composition
Produced by Phoenix Offset



Printed and bound in China

9 8 7 6 5 4 3

Library of Congress Cataloging-in-Publication Data

Histology for pathologists/edited by Stephen S. Sternberg.–2nd ed.
p. Cm.
Includes bibliographical references and index.
ISBN 0-397-51718-1
1. Histology. 2. Histology, Pathological. I. Sternberg, Stephen S.
[DNLM: 1. Histology. 2. Pathology. QS 504 H6765 1997]
QM551.H667 1997
611′.018-dc20
DNLM/DLC
For Library of Congress

# Contents

## Serous Membranes



## Central Nervous System



## Peripheral Nervous System



## Head and Neck



## Lungs



## Alimentary Canal

## Associated Intestinal Tract Organs



## Hematopoietic and Lymphoid System



## Heart and Blood Vessels



## Urinary Tract



## Female Genital System

## Male Genital System



## Endocrine System

# Contributing Authors

**Graziella M. Abu-Jawdeh, M.D.** *Department of Pathology, Beth Israel Hospital, Harvard Medical School, Boston, Massachusetts 02215*

**Karoly Balogh, M.D.** *Department of Pathology, West Campus, Beth Israel Deaconess Medical Center, One Deaconess Road, Boston, Massachusetts 02215*

**José Barreto, M.D.** *Department of Pathology, Hospital del Cáncer, Eligio Ayala 1068, Asunción, Paraguay*

**J. Bruce Beckwith, M.D.** *Professor of Pathology, Department of Pathology and Human Anatomy, Division of Pediatric Pathology, Loma Linda University, Loma Linda, California 92350*

**Kurt Benirschke, M.D.** *Professor Emeritus of Pathology and Reproductive Medicine, University of California, San Diego, University Medical Center, 200 West Arbor Drive, San Diego, California 92103-8321*

**Rex C. Bentley, M.D., Ph.D.** *Assistant Professor of Pathology, Duke University Medical Center, Box 3712, Durham, North Carolina 27710*

**Margaret E. Billingham, M.B., B.S., F.R.C.Path.** *Professor of Pathology Emerita, Department of Cardiothoracic Surgery, Stanford University Medical School, 300 Pasteur Drive, Stanford, California 94305-5247*

**Jacques Bosq, M.D.** *Assistant Professor of Pathology, Department of Histopathology "A", Institut Gustave-Roussy, 39 Rue Camille Desmoulins, 94805 Villejuif Cedex, France*

**John S. J. Brooks, M.D., M.R.C.Path.** *Professor and Chairman, Department of Pathology, Roswell Park Cancer Institute, Elm and Carlton Streets, Buffalo, New York 14263; Professor and Vice Chair, Department of Pathology, SUNY Buffalo Medical School*

**Peter G. Bullough, M.B., Ch.B.** *Professor of Pathology, Cornell University Medical College, Laboratory Medicine, The Hospital for Special Surgery, 535 East 70th Street, New York, New York 10021*

**Peter C. Burger, M.D.** *Professor of Pathology, Department of Pathology, The Johns Hopkins University School of Medicine, 600 N. Wolfe Street, Baltimore, Maryland 21287*

**Carmelo Caballero, M.D.** *Department of Pathology, Hospital del Cáncer, Eligio Ayala 1068, Asunción, Paraguay*

**Maria L. Carcangiu, M.D.** *Professor of Pathology, Obstetrics, and Gynecology, Department of Pathology, Yale University School of Medicine, P.O. Box 208070, New Haven, Connecticut 06520-8070*

**J. Aidan Carney, M.D., Ph.D., F.R.C.P.I.** *Department of Laboratory Medicine and Pathology, Mayo Clinic and Mayo Foundation, 200 First Street S.W., Rochester, Minnesota 55905*

**Darryl Carter, M.D.** *Professor of Pathology, Department of Pathology, Yale University School of Medicine, P.O. Box 208070, New Haven, Connecticut 06510-8070*

**Odile Casiraghi, M.D.** *Department of Histopathology "A", Institut Gustave-Roussy, Rue Camille Desmoulins, 94805 Villejuif Cedex, France*

**William L. Clapp, M.D.** *Assistant Professor of Pathology, Department of Pathology and Laboratory Medicine, University of Florida College of Medicine and VA Medical Center, P.O. Box 100275 JHMHC, Gainesville, Florida 32610*

**Philip B. Clement, M.D.** *Professor of Pathology, Department of Pathology, Vancouver Hospital and Health Sciences Center, University of British Columbia, 855 West 12th Avenue, Vancouver, British Columbia, V5Z 1M9, Canada*

**Thomas V. Colby, M.D.** *Professor of Pathology, Department of Pathology, Mayo Clinic Scottsdale, 13400 East Shea Blvd., Scottsdale, Arizona 85259*

**Julián Sánchez Conejo-Mir, M.D.** *Assistant Professor of Dermatology, Department of Dermatology, Virgen del Rocio University Hospital, Republica Argentina 22-B; Seville 41011 Spain*

**Byron P. Croker, M.D., Ph.D.** *Professor of Pathology and Laboratory Medicine and Chief, Pathology and Laboratory Service, VA Medical Center, University of Florida College of Medicine, 1601 SW Archer Road, Gainesville, Florida 32608*

**Antonio Cubilla, M.D.** *Department of Pathology, Hospital del Cáncer, Eligio Ayala 1068, Asunción, Paraguay*

**Margaret C. Cummings, M.B., B.S., F.R.C.P.A.** *Lecturer in Pathology, Department of Pathology, University of Queensland Medical School, Herston Road, Herston, Queensland, 4006 Australia*

**Yogeshwar Dayal, M.D.** *Professor of Pathology, Department of Pathology, Tufts University School of Medicine and the New England Medical Center, 750 Washington Street, Boston, Massachusetts 02111*

**Ronald A. DeLellis, M.D.** *Department of Pathology, Tufts University School of Medicine, and the New England Medical Center, 750 Washington Street, Boston, Massachusetts 02111*

**Franco G. DeNardi, M.D., F.R.C.P.(C).** *Assistant Professor, Anatomical Pathology Laboratory Medicine, Hamilton Civic Hospital, Henderson Division, McMaster University , 711 Concession Street, Hamilton, Ontario, L8V 1C3, Canada*

**Robert E. Fechner, M.D.** *Professor of Pathology, Department of Pathology, University of Virginia Health Sciences Center, Box 214, Charlottesville, Virginia 22908*

**Claus Fenger, M.D., Ph.D.** *Associate Professor of Pathology, Institute of Pathology, Odense University Hospital, Winsløwparken 15, DK-5000 Odense C, Denmark*

**Henry F. Frierson, Jr., M.D.** *Associate Professor of Pathology, Department of Pathology, University of Virginia Health Sciences Center, Box 214, Charlottesville, Virginia 22908*

**Gregory N. Fuller, M.D., Ph.D.** *Assistant Professor of Pathology (Neuropathology), Department of Pathology, M. D. Anderson Cancer Center, 1515 Holcombe Blvd., Houston, Texas 77030*

**Giulio Gabbiani, M.D., Ph.D.** *Professor of Pathology Department of Pathology, University of Geneva—CMU, 1 rue Michel-Servet, CH-1211 Geneva 4, Switzerland*

**Patrick J. Gallagher, M.D., Ph.D., F.R.C.Path.** *Reader in Pathology, Department of Pathology, Southampton University Hospital, Tremona Road, Southampton SO16 6YD, United Kingdom*

**A. Marion Gurley, M.B., Ch.B., F.I.A.C.** *Pathologist, c/o Dr. Colin Laverty and Associates, 18 Glen Street, Eastwood, NSW 2122 Australia*

**Rodger C. Haggitt, M.D.** *Department of Pathology, Division of Gastroenterology University of Washington, 1959 NE Pacific Street, P.O. Box 356100, Seattle, Washington 98195-6100*

**Nancy S. Hardt, M.D.** *Associate Professor, Department of Pathology and Laboratory Medicine and Obstetrics Gynecology, College of Medicine, University of Florida, P.O. Box 100275, Gainesville, Florida 32610-0275*

**Reid R. Heffner, Jr., M.D.** *Professor and Vice-Chairman, Department of Pathology, SUNY-Buffalo School of Medicine and Biomedical Sciences, 3435 Main Street, Buffalo, New York 14214*

**Michael R. Hendrickson, M.D.** *Professor of Pathology and Co-Director of Surgical Pathology, Pathology Department, Stanford University School of Medicine, 300 Pasteur Drive, Stanford, California 94305*

**E. Horvath, M.D.** *Department of Pathology, St. Michael's Hospital, Toronto, Ontario, M5B 1W8, Canada*

**Richard L. Kempson, M.D.** *Professor of Pathology and Co-Director of Surgical Pathology, Department of Pathology, Stanford University School of Medicine, 300 Pasteur Drive, Stanford, California 94305*

**David Klimstra, M.D.** *Department of Pathology, Memorial Sloan-Kettering Cancer Center, 1275 York Avenue, New York, New York 10021*

**Gordon K. Klintworth, M.D., Ph.D.** *Departments of Pathology and Ophthalmology, Duke University Medical Center, Box 3802, Durham, North Carolina 27710*

**K. Kovacs, M.D.** *Department of Pathology, St. Michael's Hospital, Toronto, Ontario, M5B 1W8, Canada*

**Douglas S. Levine, M.D.** *Associate Professor, Department of Medicine, Division of Gastroenterology, Box 356424, University of Washington, 1959 NE Pacific Street, Seattle, Washington 98195-6424*

**Steven H. Lewis, M.D.** *Clinical Associate Professor of Obstetrics, Gynecology and Pathology, The University of South Florida College of Medicine; Director of OB/GYN Pathology, Department of Gynecology, The Doctor's Clinic, 2300 5th Avenue, Vero Beach, Florida 32960*

**Fernando Martínez-Madrigal, M.D.** *Department of Pathology, Hospital General "Dr. Miguel Silva," Hospital General de Zona No. 1, IMSS and the Medical Faculty of the Universidad Michoacana de San Nicolas de Hidalgo, Morelia, Michoacán, Mexico*

**Kenneth S. McCarty, Jr., M.D., Ph.D.** *Professor of Pathology, Professor of Medicine, Department of Medicine, University of Pittsburgh, Magee-Women's Hospital, Department of Pathology, 200 Lothrop Street, Pittsburgh, Pennsylvania 15213*

**John Enright McNeal, M.D.** *Clinical Professor of Urology and Pathology, Department of Urology, Stanford University Medical School, 300 Pasteur Drive, Stanford, California 94305-5118*

**Chris J. L. M. Meijer, M.D., Ph.D.** *Professor of Pathology, Department of Pathology, Free University Hospital, de Boelelaan 1117, 1081 HV Amsterdam, The Netherlands*

**Leslie Michaels, M.D., F.R.C. Path, F.R.C.P.(C), D.Path.** *Professor Emeritus, Department of Histopathology, University College London Medical School, University Street, London WC1E 6JJ, United Kingdom*

**Stacy E. Mills, M.D.** *Professor of Pathology, Department of Pathology, University of Virginia Health Sciences Center, Jefferson Park Avenue, Charlottesville, Virginia 22908*

**Manju E. Nath, M.D.** *Assistant Professor of Pathology, Department of Pathology, University of Pittsburgh School of Medicine, Magee-Women's Hospital, 300 Halket Street, Pittsburgh, Pennsylvania 15213*

**Manuel Navarrete Ortega, M.D.** *Consultant of Dermatopathology, Department of Pathology, Hospital Universitario Virgen del Rocio, Avenida Manuel Siurot, Seville, 41013 Spain*

**Carlos Ortiz-Hidalgo, M.D.** *Department of Surgical Pathology, ABC Hospital, Calle Sur 136, Observatorio, Mexico City 01120, Mexico*

**Christopher N. Otis, M.D.** *Assistant Professor of Pathology, Tufts University School of Medicine, Director of Surgical Pathology, Department of Pathology, Bay State Medical Center, Springfield, Massachusetts 01199*

**David A. Owen, M.B., B.Ch., F.R.C.Pathol., F.R.C.P.(C)** *Professor of Pathology, Department of Pathology and Laboratory Science, University of British Columbia, 855 West 12th Avenue, Vancouver, British Columbia, V5G 1M9, Canada*

**P. J. Pernicone, M.D.** *Department of Pathology, Florida Hospital, 601 East Rollins Street, Orlando, Florida 32803*

**Patricia M. Perosio, M.D.** *Staff Pathologist, The Toledo Hospital, 2142 North Cove Blvd., Toledo, Ohio 43606*

**Robert E. Petras, M.D.** *Chairman, Department of Anatomic Pathology, Cleveland Clinic Foundation, 9500 Euclid Avenue, Cleveland, Ohio 44195*

**Glyn A. Porter, M.D., Ph.D.** *Department of Pathology, Northwestern University Medical School, Chicago, Illinois 60611*

**Robert H. Riddell, M.D., F.R.C.Path., F.R.C.P.(C)** *Department of Pathology, McMaster University Medical Center, 1200 Main Street West, Hamilton, Ontario L8N 3Z5, Canada*

**Victor E. Reuter, M.D.** *Associate Attending Pathologist, Department of Pathology, Memorial Sloan-Kettering Cancer Center, 1275 York Avenue, New York, New York 10021*

**Stanley J. Robboy, M.D.** *Professor of Pathology, Obstetrics and Gynecology, Department of Pathology (Box 3712), Duke University Medical Center, Durham, North Carolina 27710*

**Juan Rosai, M.D.** *Chairman, Department of Pathology, and James Ewing Alumni Chair in Pathology, Memorial Sloan-Kettering Cancer Center, 1275 York Avenue, New York, New York 10021*

**Sanford I. Roth, M.D.** *Department of Pathology, Northwestern Memorial Hospital, Superior Street and Fairbanks, Chicago, Illinois 60611*

**Bernd W. Scheithauer, M.D.** *Department of Laboratory Medicine and Pathology, Mayo Clinic, 200 First Street SW, Rochester, Minnesota 55905*

**Walter Schürch, M.D.** *Professor of Pathology, Department of Pathology, Hôtel-Dieu Hospital and University of Montreal, 3840 St. Urbain, Montreal, Quebec, H2W 1T8, Canada*

**Mark W. Scroggs, M.D.** *Departments of Pathology and Ophthalmology, Box 3802, Duke University Medical Center, Durham, North Carolina 27710*

**Thomas A. Seemayer, M.D.** *Professor of Pathology, Microbiology and Pediatrics, Department of Pathology and Microbiology, University of Nebraska Medical Center, 600 South 42nd Street, Omaha, Nebraska 68198-3139*

**Glenn H. Segal, D.O.** *Assistant Professor of Pathology, Department of Pathology, University of Utah Health Sciences Center, 50 North Medical Drive, Salt Lake City, Utah 84132*

**Saul Suster, M.D.** *Associate Clinical Professor of Pathology, University of Miami School of Medicine, and Director of Surgical Pathology, The Arkadi M. Rywlin Department of Pathology and Laboratory Medicine, Mount Sinai Medical Center of Greater Miami, 4300 Alton Road, Miami Beach, Florida 33140*

**Jan te Velde, M.D.** *Spaarne Ziekenhuis, Department of Pathology, P.O. Box 354, 2100 AJ Heemstede, The Netherlands*

**Swan N. Thung, M.D.** *Professor of Pathology, Department of Pathology, The Mount Sinai Medical Center, One Gustave L. Levy Place, New York, New York 10029*

**Arthur S. Tischler, M.D.** *Department of Pathology, Tufts University School of Medicine, New England Medical Center, 750 Washington Street, NEMC 802, Boston, Massachusetts 02111*

**Thomas D. Trainer, M.D.** *Professor of Pathology, Department of Pathology, University of Vermont College of Medicine, 111 Colchester Avenue, Burlington, Vermont 05401-1429*

**Lawrence D. True, M.D.** *Department of Pathology, University of Washington, Seattle, Washington 98195*

**Carlos D. Urmacher, M.D.** *Associate Professor of Pathology, Laboratories, North Shore University Hospital, 300 Community Drive, Manhasset, New York 11030*

**Paul van der Valk, M.D., Ph.D.** *Professor of Pathology, Department of Pathology, Academic Hospital, Free University, Postbus 7057, 1007 MB Amsterdam, The Netherlands*

**J. Han J. M. van Krieken, M.D.** *Attending Pathologist, Leiden University Hospital, Department of Pathology, Rijnsburgerweg 10, Building 1, P1–28, P.O. Box 9600, L1–Q, 2300 RC Leiden, The Netherlands*

**Neal I. Walker, B.Sc., M.D., B.S., F.R.C.P.A.** *Associate Professor of Pathology, Department of Pathology, University of Queensland, Herston Road, Herston, Queensland, 4006 Australia*

**Roy O. Weller, B.Sc., M.D., Ph.D., F.R.C.Path.** *Professor of Neuropathology, Department of Pathology (Neuropathology), Southampton University Hospital, Tremona Road, Southampton SO16 6YD, United Kingdom*

**Sunitha N. Wickramasinghe, Sc.D., Ph.D., F.R.C.P., F.R.C.Path.** *Professor of Haematology, Department of Haematology, Imperial College School of Medicine at St. Mary's, Norfolk Place, London W2 1PG, United Kingdom*

**Edward J. Wilkinson, M.D.** *Professor and Interim Chairman, Department of Pathology, Immunology and Laboratory Medicine, University of Florida, 1600 SW Archer Road, Gainesville, Florida 32610-0275*

**Clay M. Winterford, Ass. Dip. App. Sci.** *Department of Pathology, University of Queensland, Herston Medical School, Herston Road, Herston, Brisbane, Queensland, 4006 Australia*

# Preface to the First Edition

Histology textbooks exist in abundance. Some are classics of their kind and have gone through innumerable editions over many years. They have served pathologists well, for the most part, especially in terms of strict tissue and cell histology. There is, however, a borderline between histology and pathology in which information for the pathologist is often lacking.

With this textbook we made an attempt to fill the gap. The significance and function of many histological structures in terms of pathological interpretation is often absent or obscure. In particular, variations of the norm related to such variables as age, sex, and race are often not clarified in conventional textbooks. For example, the chapter on paraganglia notes that the connective tissue between the lobules in the carotid body increases with age. Another example related to age is in the pediatric kidney chapter where it is noted that the glomeruli of fetuses are disproportionately large, and are rarely seen in a state of histological "immaturity." While the chapter on the myofibroblast details the location, staining, ultrastructure, and cytoskeletal protein composition of this unusual cell, we also learn of its importance in the desmoplastic reaction in cancerous tissue, and most importantly, that it is not found in carcinomas which are still *in situ.*

Some gross observations occasionally will be found as lagniappe, such as the notation that in patients with congenital absence of a kidney, the ipsilateral adrenal will be round rather than angulated. Another example would be that there is a crease in the earlobe associated with coronary artery disease.

Variations in staining reactions are considered, such as the failure of Factor VIII to stain renal glomerular vessels. One finds that intestinal endocrine cells can be detected with hematoxylin and eosin (sic) stains by the infranuclear location of the granules. Uncommonly known fixation artifacts are uncovered, i.e. the prickle-cell layer (with so-called intercellular bridges) is actually a retraction artifact of the plasma membranes with the desmosomes remaining relatively fixed.

In most chapters "prepathological" considerations are emphasized, while in others the developed pathological alterations related to the norm represent the major thrust of the chapter.

Some comments will be perceived as gratuitous, such as the remark in the penis chapter to the effect that "the prepuce could be a mistake of nature." Furthermore, we learn that the "collagen fibers are wavy in the flaccid state and become straight during erection."

The pathology neophyte as well as the many esteemed and experienced pathologists will find helpful information in this book.

*Stephen S. Sternberg, M.D.*

# Preface

Our intention with this book, as noted in the first edition, was to bridge the gap between histology and pathology. Our success quickly became manifest with very favorable reviews, a reflection of the generally high quality of the writing. Indeed, that edition was the first-place winner in the Physicians Category in the 1992 American Medical Writers Association Medical Book Awards competition.

This new edition has revised chapters, some of which were completely rewritten, as well as new chapters. We have added, for example, a chapter on apoptosis (the lead chapter), which is a reflection of an extraordinary discovery made by light microscopy, without special stains, without immunohistochemistry, and without electron microscopy. This newly delineated type of necrosis has led, in effect, to a revolution in the interpretation of numerous physiological and pathological processes, many hitherto thought to be unrelated. Although this type of cell death occurs in normal tissues as well as pathological tissues, of major importance was the discovery that the treatment effects of cancer chemotherapy (and other types of chemotherapy) as well as cell death from ionizing radiation come about by apoptosis. (It is perhaps a little embarrassing for us as microscopists and pathologists to realize we have been observing these now easily recognizable apoptotic cells for many years, not understanding their uniqueness or significance. On the other hand, if it is any consolation, neither did Virchow, Morgagni, or Paget, among many others.)

In response to reviewers' comments we have added a chapter on joints, and altered a chapter to include paranasal sinuses and oral cavity structures not previously noted. We have also completely rearranged the chapters into logical, systemic groupings, and sought a standard format of presentation in each chapter.

A comment was made in one review about the disproportionate size of some chapters, in particular the one on the nail. We have chosen to retain the chapter as such in terms of length, realizing that, while the need to look up information on the nail rarely occurs, conventional texts are usually inadequate to provide particular details needed to answer obscure questions about the nail.

I am sure we have not as yet responded to all the necessary refinements, but most of our authors have fulfilled a major undertaking to provide the necessary revisions for this new edition.

*Stephen S. Sternberg, M.D.*

# Apoptosis

*Histology for Pathologists, second edition,*
Edited by Stephen S. Sternberg.
Lippincott-Raven Publishers, Philadelphia


# CHAPTER 1

# Apoptosis

Margaret C. Cummings, Clay M. Winterford, and Neal I. Walker



Over the past three decades, two fundamentally different forms of cell death, apoptosis and necrosis, have been defined in terms of morphology, biochemistry, and incidence. Apoptosis is a genetically determined, biologically meaningful, active process playing a role opposite to mitosis in tissue size regulation, shaping organs during mammalian morphogenesis, and removing cells that are immunologically reactive against self, infected or genetically damaged, whose continued existence pose a danger to the host. Necrosis, in contrast, is an accidental passive process resulting in progressive breakdown of ordered cell structure and function after irreversible damage caused by major environmental change such as sudden severe ischemia, extremes of temperature, and mechanical trauma.

By its nature, necrosis has no role in normal tissue physiology or development and will not be considered further. Detailed information on necrosis is available elsewhere (1–5). Apoptosis, on the other hand, is actively involved in many physiological and developmental processes. An account of its discovery, morphology, biochemistry, identification, and incidence follows.

## HISTORICAL PERSPECTIVE

Early evidence of the existence of two morphologically distinct types of cell death came from the studies of Australian pathologist, John Kerr, working under the supervision of Sir Roy Cameron at the University of London (6,7). Refining work on atrophy undertaken by the American pathologist, Peyton Rous, some 30 years before, he ligated portal vein branches to the left and median lobes of the rat liver. These lobes shrank over 1 to 2 weeks, while other lobes simultaneously underwent hyperplasia. In the atrophying lobes, patches of confluent necrosis occurred around terminal hepatic venules while periportal parenchyma, sustained by blood from the hepatic artery, survived. Individual hepatocytes outside the zone of necrosis, in the absence of inflammation, gave rise to small round cytoplasmic masses, some containing pyknotic chromatin, clearly a manifestation of cell death. Histochemistry for acid phosphatase activity showed that although lysosomes in necrotic cells had ruptured with dispersal of enzyme product in the cytoplasm, lysosomes in the small round cytoplasmic masses stained discretely, indicating the lysosomes were still intact. Identical bodies were found in the livers of normal rats.

Later, electron microscopic studies in Brisbane, Australia indicated the small round masses in the liver comprised membrane-bound cellular fragments containing crowded but structurally well-preserved organelles, sometimes with compacted chromatin, that were formed by the shrinkage and budding of hepatocytes (8). Kerr called the phenomenon "shrinkage necrosis," reflecting these morphological changes (6,8).

In 1972, Kerr accepted an invitation from British pathologist, the late Sir Alastair Currie, to continue his work in Aberdeen (7). Together with Currie's PhD student, Andrew

M.C. Cummings, C.M. Winterford, and N.I. Walker: Department of Pathology, University of Queensland Medical School, Herston, 4006, Queensland, Australia.

Wyllie, they realized the importance in cell kinetics and the broader significance of the process Kerr had described. This, with the distinctive morphology, and the inappropriateness of the term "necrosis" in describing cell death occurring under physiological conditions, led them to publish a seminal article in the *British Journal of Cancer* in 1972. There, they proposed the term "apoptosis" for this form of cell death, thereby emphasizing its opposite role to mitosis in the regulation of tissue size (9). Like mitosis, the term apoptosis is of Greek origin, and means falling off or dropping off as petals from a flower or leaves from a tree. It was proposed that apoptosis was a general mechanism for controlled cell deletion and that its morphological features indicated an active inherently programmed phenomenon.

Earlier, embryologists had recognized the role of this form of cell death during tissue morphogenesis, but had not appreciated its distinctness from necrosis or its wider biological implications (10, 11). Subsequently, apoptosis has been shown to occur in a wide range of circumstances (1,4,12). For over two decades, Kerr in Brisbane, Wyllie in Edinburgh, their colleagues and others have further defined the morphology, incidence, biochemistry, and genetics of apoptosis. Since the late 1980s, exploitation of molecular biological techniques, in particular, has led to rapid advances in knowledge of this process.

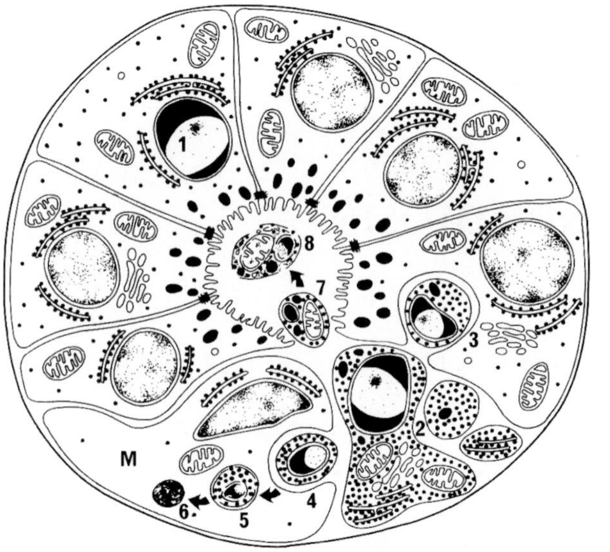


**FIG. 1.** Sequence of ultrastructural changes in apoptosis of glandular epithelial cells. The earliest change is segregation of the chromatin in sharply circumscribed masses that abut the nuclear envelope (**1**). Convolution of the nuclear and cell outlines precedes fragmentation of the nucleus and budding of the cell as a whole to produce membrane-bound apoptotic bodies of varying size and structure (**2**), which are phagocytosed by adjacent epithelial cells (**3**) and macrophages (**4**) and degraded within lysosomes (**5**). Finally, the bodies are reduced to unrecognizable residues (**6**). An occasional apoptotic body escapes phagocytosis and is shed into the gland lumen (**7**) where it undergoes degenerative changes similar to those occurring in necrosis (**8**). M = intraepithelial macrophage.

## MORPHOLOGY

Because the light microscopic manifestations of apoptosis are better appreciated with knowledge of the diagnostic ultrastructural appearances, the electron microscopic changes will be described first.

### Electron Microscopy

In the account that follows, detailed referencing of the individual events described will not be attempted. Instead, readers are referred to the many detailed illustrated reviews on which this account is based (1,3–5,13–15). An illustrative diagrammatic representation of the sequential, ultrastructural changes occurring during apoptosis of cells in glandular epithelium is shown in Figure 1.

In tissues, apoptosis affects cells asynchronously, typically in the absence of inflammatory change. The earliest event observed is condensation of chromatin to form sharply circumscribed, uniformly dense, finely granular crescentic or toroidal masses that abut the nuclear envelope (Figs. 1 and 2). The proportion of the nucleus occupied by condensed chromatin varies with cell type, being high in lymphoid cells and low in cells with little heterochromatin. Nuclear pores are seldom observed adjacent to the masses of condensed chromatin but are clearly visible in other parts of the envelope. Nucleolar changes also occur (13) but are only seen in some planes of section. The peripheral nucleolar chromatin forms aggregates of osmiophilic granules which separate from the fibrillar core and disperse to the center of the nucleus. The protein fibrillar core remains as a round or oval compact granular mass of different texture to the condensed nuclear chromatin, and is usually closely opposed to the inner surface of that chromatin (Fig. 2).

Simultaneously with the nuclear changes, apoptotic cells detach from neighboring cells or culture substrata, their desmosomes break down, and specialized surface structures such as microvilli disappear. Cell volume decreases, cell density increases, cytoplasmic organelles compact, and convolution of the cell and nuclear outline is usually evident (Figs. 1 and 3). The nucleus may split into several discrete fragments mostly bound by a double membrane, and in which segregation of the chromatin persists (Fig. 3). The size and chromatin content of individual fragments varies; condensed chromatin may occupy the whole cross-sectional area of a fragment or remain as a peripheral crescent. Nuclear convolution and fragmentation is limited in cells with high nuclear-to-cytoplasmic ratios such as thymocytes. Cytoplasmic changes at this time include aggregation of cytoskeletal filaments in arrays parallel to the cell surface, clumping of ribosomal particles in semicrystalline formations, and in secretory cells, rearrangement of rough endoplasmic reticulum (RER) to form a series of concentric

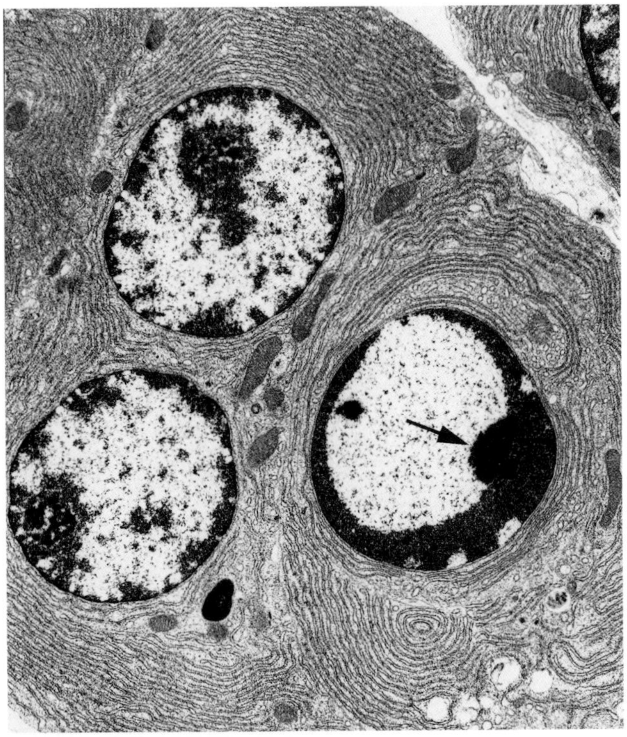

**FIG. 2.** Early apoptosis of acinar cell in rat pancreas after duct ligation. Note granular fibrillar core remnant of nucleolus adjacent condensed chromatin (*arrow*). Adjacent cells appear normal **(×6200)**.

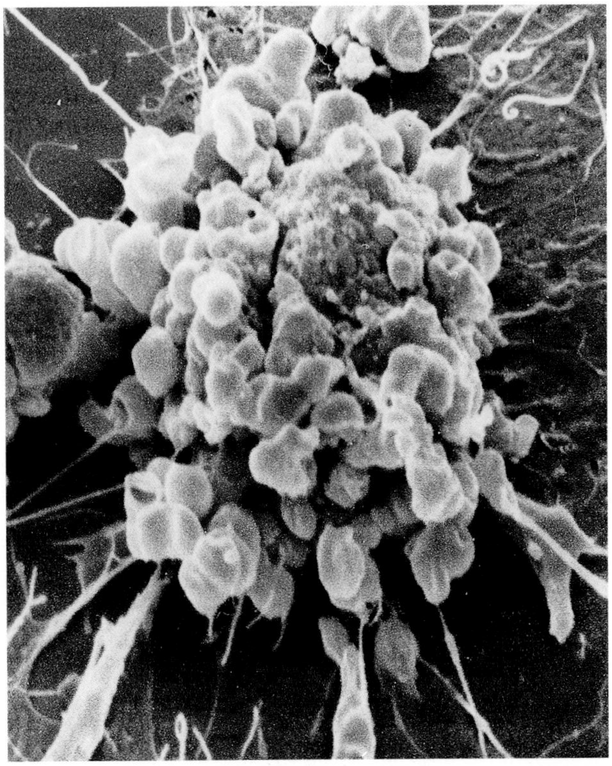

**FIG. 4.** Apoptotic HeLa cell after addition of actinomycin D (*15μ*g/ml) to culture medium **(SEM × 9000)**.

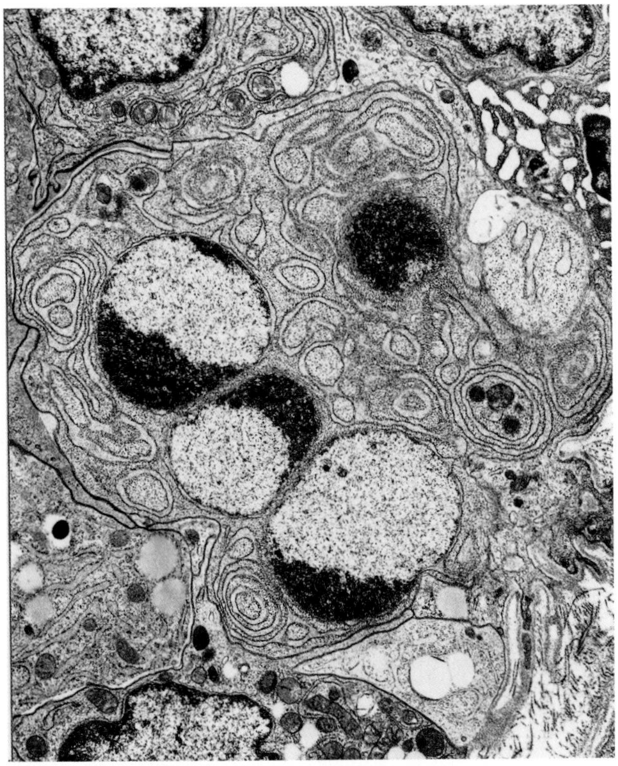

**FIG. 3.** Early apoptosis of rat prostatic epithelial cell after castration. Note irregular cell outline, basal position of cell in epithelium, segregated chromatin in nuclear fragments and whorling of endoplasmic reticulum **(×8200)**.

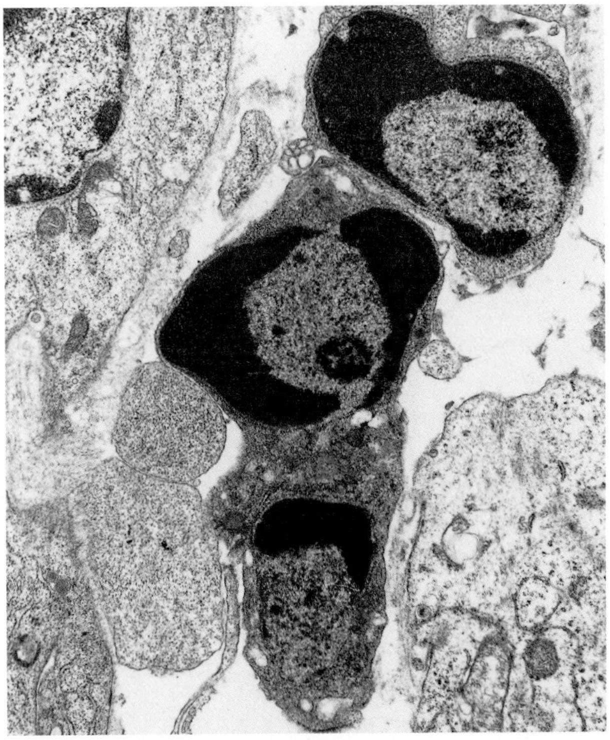

**FIG. 5.** Intact extracellular condensed apoptotic bodies, some containing characteristic nuclear fragments, derived from transplanted EMT 6 sarcoma cell after mild hyperthermic treatment **(×10,000)**.

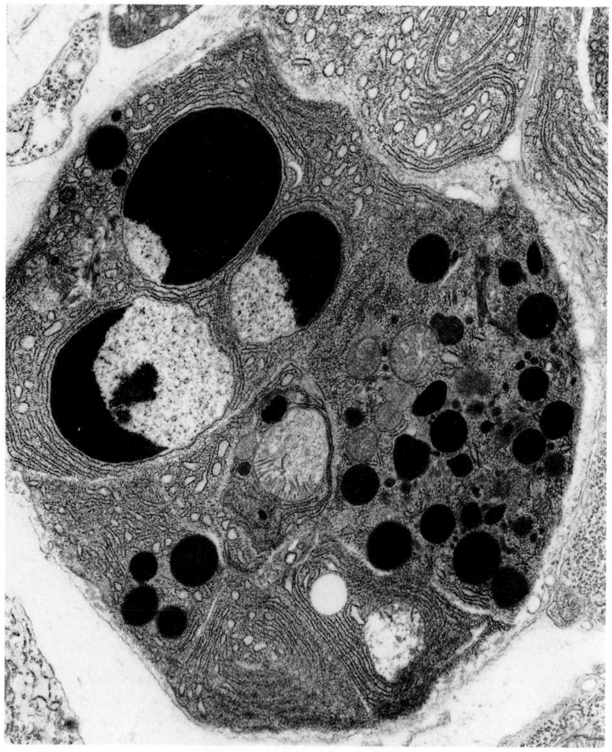

**FIG. 6.** Crowded condensed intraepithelial apoptotic bodies derived from rat pancreatic acinar cell after subcutaneous cerulein injections (*24 μg per kg, 8 hourly*) (Courtesy of L. Reid) **(×8,300)**.

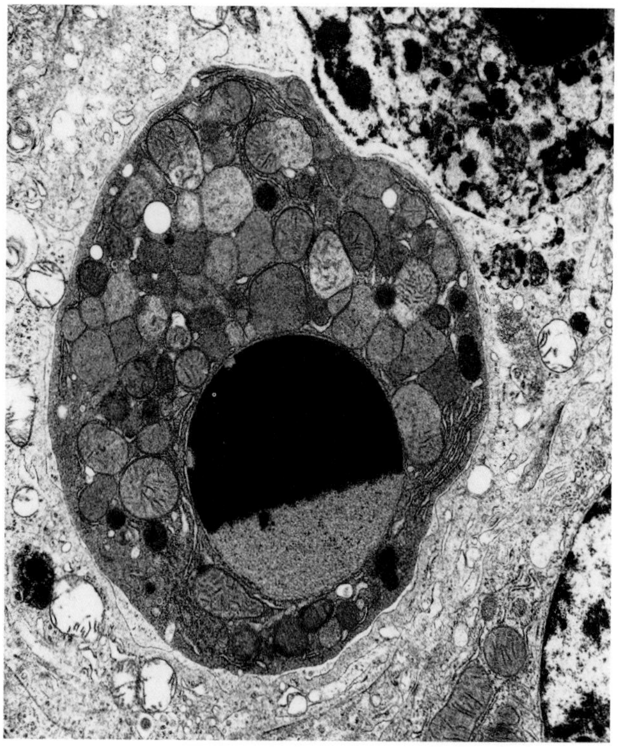

**FIG. 8.** Well-preserved hepatocyte-derived apoptotic body with condensed cytoplasm, crowded organelles, and characteristic nuclear fragment phagocytosed by Kupffer cell in rat liver after portal vein branch ligation. Note adjacent partly degraded apoptotic body **(×7700)**.

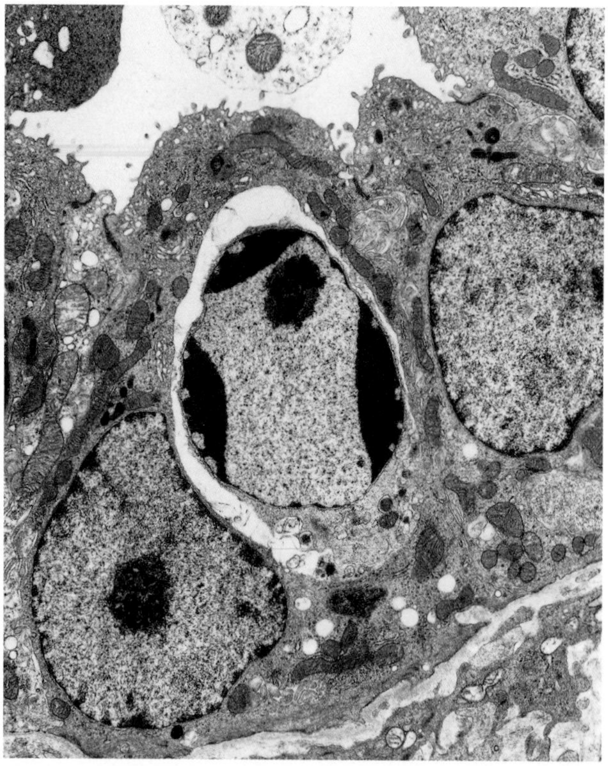

**FIG. 7.** Well-preserved large apoptotic body with characteristic nuclear fragment phagocytosed by a tubular epithelial cell in rat kidney after ureteric ligation **(×4500)**.

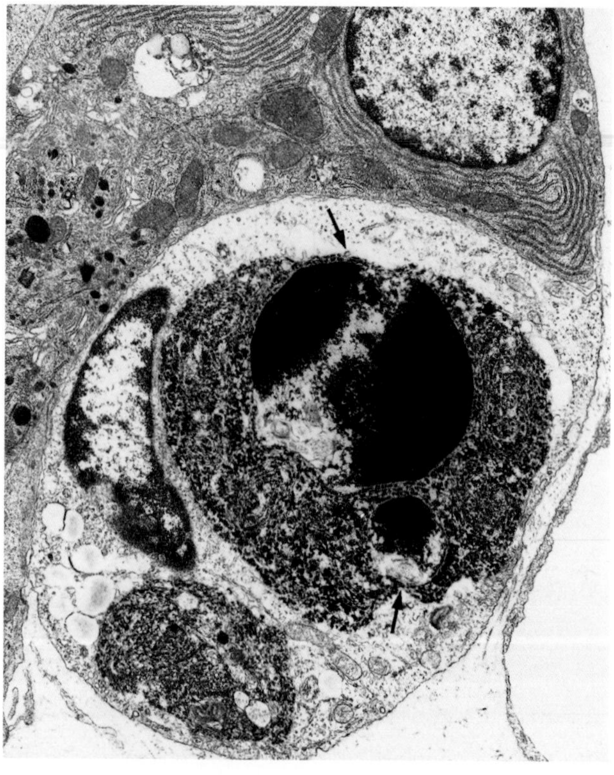

**FIG. 9.** Partly degraded apoptotic bodies, one with nuclear fragments (*arrows*), in intraepithelial macrophage in rat pancreas after duct ligation **(×7500)**.

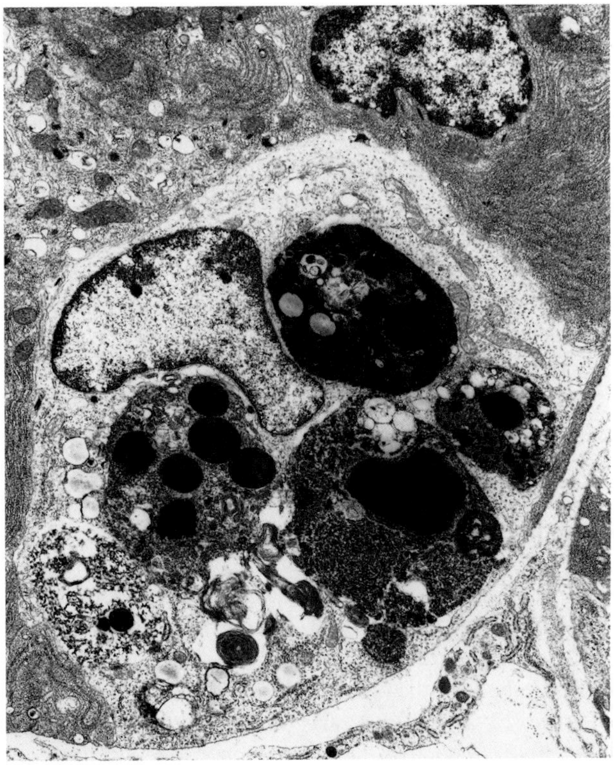

**FIG. 10.** Multiple partly degraded apoptotic bodies in intraepithelial macrophage in rat pancreas after duct ligation **(×6700)**.

whorls (16,17). Inconstantly, numerous clear vacuoles formed from smooth endoplasmic reticulum are found in the subplasmalemmal cytoplasm where they may fuse with the plasma membrane, discharge their fluid contents, and form surface craters seen by scanning electron microscopy (SEM) (13).

Closely associated with the nuclear and cytoplasmic changes described, cells with abundant cytoplasm form extensive surface blebs and protuberances best demonstrated by SEM (Fig. 4). The latter subsequently separate with sealing of the plasmalemma to form membrane-bound apoptotic bodies of varying size with condensed cytoplasm and crowded intact cytoplasmic organelles (Figs. 1, 5, and 6). The condensation varies between cells but is best seen in tissues where electron-dense apoptotic bodies stand out against unaffected neighboring cells (Figs. 5 and 6). The number of nuclear fragments in an apoptotic body varies and is not consistently related to its size (Fig. 6). In secretory cells, cell fragmentation appears to occur along planes separating areas of segregated concentrically arranged RER (Fig. 6)(16,17). Restriction of surface protuberance formation and budding to form apoptotic bodies is seen in cells with high nuclear-to-cytoplasmic ratio such as thymocytes and small lymphocytes, and in keratinocytes, myoepithelial cells, and adipocytes where abundant tonofilaments, myofilaments, and a large lipid droplet respectively cause splinting of the cytoplasm (18–20). When apoptosis occurs in tissues, the resulting apoptotic bodies are often squeezed along the intercellular spaces (Fig. 5); within epithelia, such movement may be resticted by the basement membrane (Fig. 6).

In vivo, apoptotic bodies are phagocytosed almost immediately after formation by adjacent epithelial cells (Figs. 1 and 7), mononuclear phagocytes (Figs. 1 and 8), or tumor cells. Intraepithelial macrophages, in particular, play an important role in the removal of apoptotic bodies formed in glandular epithelia (16,17, 19,21,22) where, during glandular atrophy and involution, their number increases through mononuclear phagocyte immigration and mitosis. Phagocytosed apoptotic bodies can be distinguished from autophagic vacuoles by their content of chromatin and organelles foreign to the ingesting cell and, in epithelial cells, by their large size (Figs. 1, 7–10). Once phagocytosed, apoptotic bodies are degraded by lysosomal enzymes derived from the ingesting cell (Figs. 1, 9 and 10). Early in this process, condensed chromatin in nuclear fragments increases in density and the sharp demarcation between electron-lucent and electron-dense areas is lost; the ribosomes become swollen and coarse, and the cytoplasmic and bounding membranes indistinct (Fig. 9)(16). When the apoptotic rate is high, phagocytes may contain large numbers of variably degraded apoptotic bodies (Fig. 10)(16,17). Eventually, they are reduced to residual bodies with granular and amorphous electron-dense material, lipid droplets, and myelin figures (Figs. 1 and 11). Rapid phagocytosis of apoptotic bodies prior to their secondary degeneration may explain the abscence of inflammation associated with apoptosis.

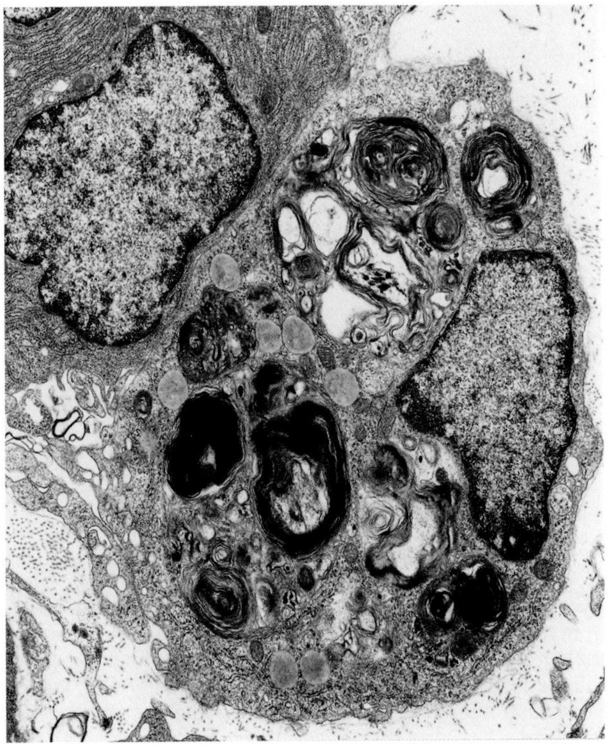

**FIG. 11.** Residual bodies in cytoplasm of intraepithelial macrophage in rat pancreas after duct ligation (×**7500**).

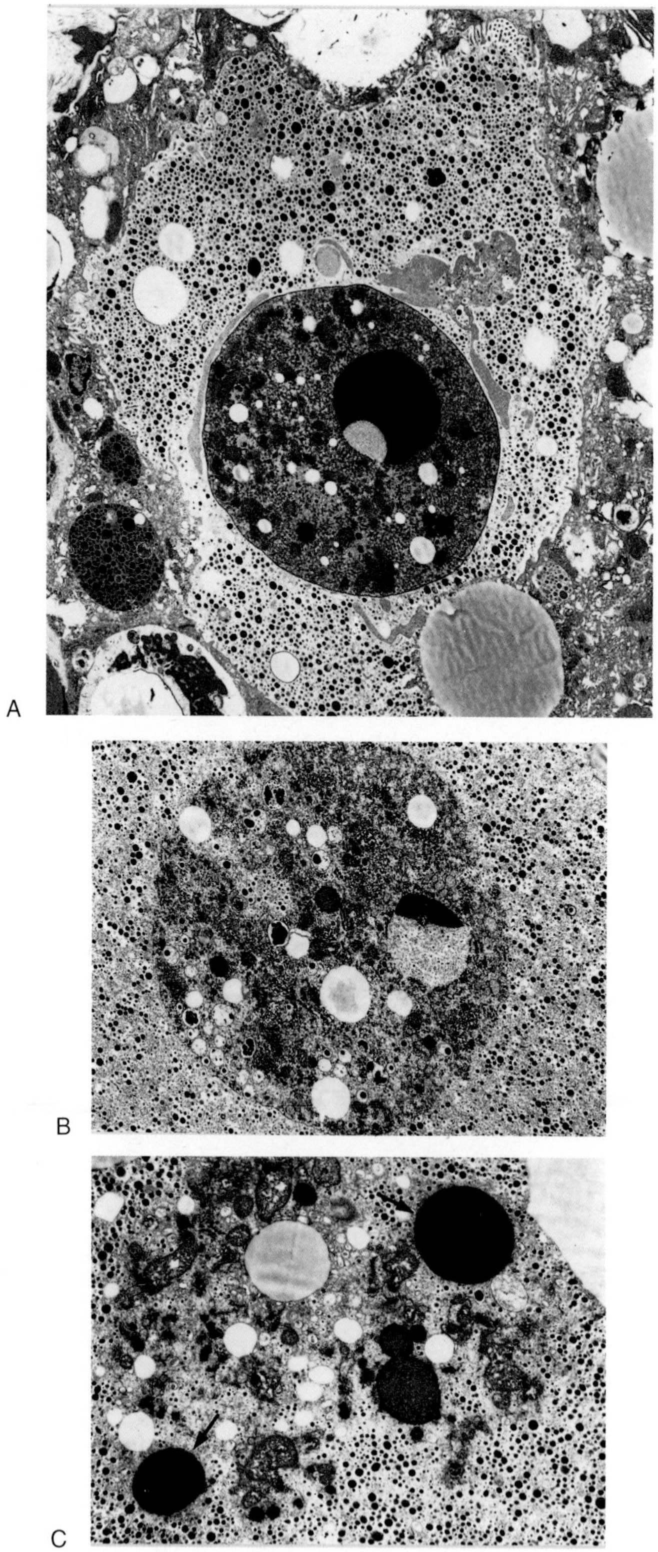

**FIG. 12.** Luminal apoptotic bodies in lactating mouse breast after weaning. (**A**), Intact apoptotic body with characteristic nuclear fragment. (**B**), Partly degraded apoptotic body with nuclear fragment showing decreased density and loss of membrane integrity. (**C**), Degraded apoptotic body showing membrane loss and dispersal of nuclear fragments (*arrows*) and organelles. (A) ×**3000**; (B) ×**3900**; (C) ×**5200**.

In luminal glandular epithelia, a variable proportion of apoptotic bodies are extruded into the gland lumen (Figs. 1 and 12). Such bodies and those that escape phagocytosis in culture lose their integrity after an hour or so, resulting in swelling, loss of density, membrane rupture (Figs. 1 and 12B), and organelle disruption and dispersal (Fig. 12C) referred to as secondary necrosis. Early on, the latter can be distinguished from necrosis ab initio by the small size, spheroid or ovoid shape, or characteristic pattern of chromatin condensation in nuclear fragments of apoptotic bodies; such differentiation in the later stages may be impossible. The initial integrity of the apoptotic bodies is shown by their capacity to exclude vital dyes, but this is lost once de generative changes supervene (23,24).

### Light Microscopy

By phase contrast microscopy, cells in culture undergoing apoptosis show an abrupt onset of cell shrinkage and surface convolution, resulting in protuberances that bud off to form apoptotic bodies; the whole process is completed in a few minutes (25–27). In contrast, the bodies formed during a short wave of apoptosis in vivo remain visible histologically for 3 to 4 hours (28). Thus, in tissues where apoptosis is occurring asynchronously, budding cells are rarely seen (Fig. 13) and apoptotic bodies in various stages of degeneration predominate. Under the usual conditions of fixation for light microscopy, it is possible that budding cells progress to apoptotic body formation before fixation is complete.

Histologically, apoptotic bodies appear as round or oval cytoplasmic masses with or without contained basophilic nuclear material (Fig. 13). Although most apoptotic bodies are eosinophilic, those derived from cells containing abundant ribosomes, such as pancreatic acinar cells, may be basophilic. Apoptotic bodies derived from cells in which budding is restricted appear slightly smaller than the cell of origin. Where extensive budding is possible, apoptotic bodies vary considerably in size (Fig. 13), the smallest being undetectable by light microscopy unless it contains at least one basophilic nuclear fragment. Those derived from cells with a high nuclear-to-cytoplasmic ratio appear as a mass of pyknotic chromatin surrounded by a narrow rim of cytoplasm. Other bodies comprise mostly cytoplasm with a variable content of smaller nuclear fragments (Fig. 13). The characteristic well-defined crescentic clumps of chromatin, seen in apoptotic nuclei and nuclear fragments ultrastructurally, are rarely seen in 5$\mu$ paraffin sections or smears (Fig. 13); instead, the chromatin appears as uniformly dense basophilic masses. In sections, apoptotic bodies often lie within clear spaces. Some of these represent bodies in pale staining macrophages; others may be extracellular, the space resulting from shrinkage artifact during tissue processing. Larger discrete apoptotic bodies have long been recognized in normal and pathological states in a variety of tissues under other

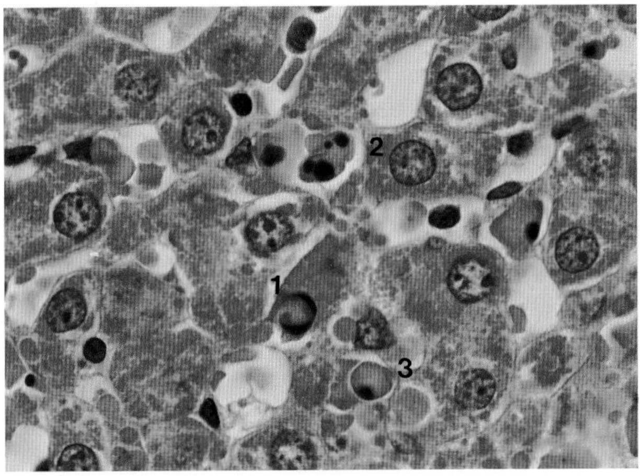


**FIG. 13.** Apoptotic cells and bodies in rat liver after portal vein branch ligation. Note apoptotic hepatocyte with characteristic crescentic chromatin clumps in nucleus (**1**), budding cell (**2**), and typical apoptotic body with basophilic chromatin dot (**3**). Also note numerous small inconspicuous phagocytosed apoptotic bodies without nuclear fragments in the background.

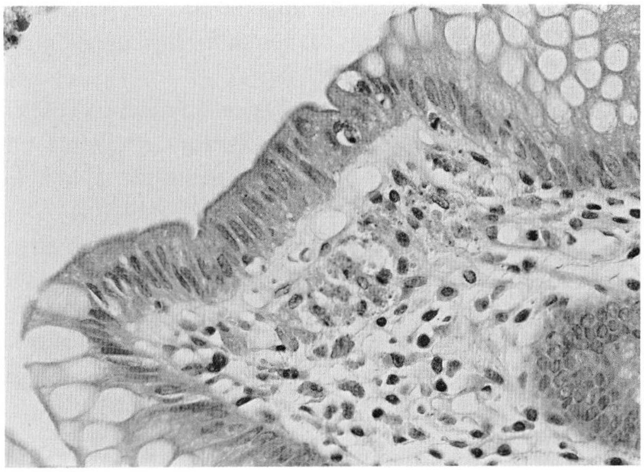

**FIG. 15.** Human colonic mucosa showing mild melanosis coli. Note apoptotic bodies in basal epithelium, band of variably degraded apoptotic bodies in superficial lamina propria and underlying pigmented macrophages.

names. These include Councilman bodies in liver (Fig. 13), karyolytic bodies in gut crypts, tingible bodies in germinal center macrophages of lymph nodes, and in skin, Civatte bodies in lichen planus and sunburn cells after ultraviolet irradiation.

Apoptotic bodies may also occur as dispersed clusters within a tissue (Fig. 14). These may result from fragmentation of single cells or, particularly larger aggregates—the gathering together of apoptotic bodies from several cells within a single phagocyte—typically a macrophage. When the number of apoptotic bodies formed over time is large, their degradation within macrophages results in lipofuscin pigment formation, best seen in melanosis coli (Fig. 15) (16,17,19,22). Phagocytosis of apoptotic bodies does not induce macrophages to incite an inflammatory response (29).

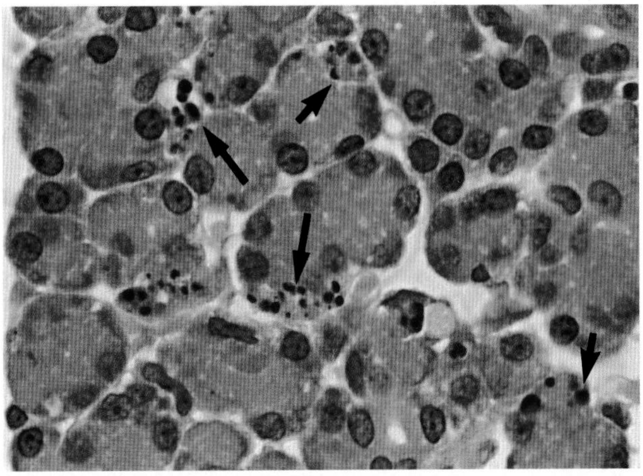

**FIG. 14.** Clusters of apoptotic bodies in rat parotid after duct ligation. Some small clusters may represent bodies derived from a single cell (*short arrows*). Larger clusters are likely to be phagocytosed apoptotic bodies within intraepithelial macrophages (*long arrows*).

The small size and short half-life of apoptotic bodies, the lack of inflammation, and the closing of ranks by residual cells as apoptotic cells are removed makes apoptosis relatively inconspicuous histologically, even when the rate of cell deletion is high. Even small increases in the proportion of apoptosis within a tissue can represent considerable cumulative cell loss. For example, an intravenous bolus of anti-CD4 antibody increases the apoptotic index in murine lymph nodes from 0.06 to 1.33%, sufficient to halve the total cell count of lymph nodes within 48 hours (30). Closure of ranks by residual cells results in coherent tissue shrinkage, usually with little disruption of the normal architecture. Thus, liver and adrenal glands on completion of induced atrophy appear structurally normal histologically (8, 31). In exocrine gland atrophy, however, there is orderly regression back to the underlying duct system (16,17,32,33); when complete, lipofuscin pigment in macrophages, and collapsed and folded basement membranes seen ultrastructurally, provide evidence of the cell loss that has occurred.

## BIOCHEMISTRY AND GENETIC REGULATION

Rapid nuclear DNA cleavage has long been regarded as the biochemical hallmark of apoptosis (34). Such DNA degradation takes place in two stages. The first, occurring rapidly and probably in all cells undergoing apoptosis, involves DNA cleavage into 200 to 300 kilobase pair fragments (35). Margination of chromatin against the nuclear envelope is the probable morphological correlate (36), and topoisomerase II has been suggested as a candidate nuclease (35,37). Later, double-stranded cleavage of internucleosomal DNA affects most, but not all, cells undergoing apoptosis (38). Candidate enzymes suggested for this second phase include DNAse I (39) and DNAse II (40).

Recent studies with cell-free systems, however, suggest that nuclease activation occurs downstream of cytoplasmic proteinase activity (41,42). Proteases implicated include interleukin-1$\beta$-converting enzyme (ICE) (43), Ich-1 (44), and the cytotoxic T-lymphocyte protease, Granzyme B. During cell death mediated by T-lymphocytes, Granzyme B, a serine protease, enters target cells through membrane pores formed by perforin, and initiates death of the target cell by apoptosis (45,46). Substrates of proteases identified include $\alpha$-fodrin, a major component of the cytoskeleton, disruption of which may be associated with cell blebbing (47), and lamin, a component of the nuclear lamina adjacent to the nuclear envelope (48, 49), the breakdown of which may facilitate nuclear fragmentation.

Another enzyme, tissue transglutaminase, activated in late apoptosis, produces highly cross-linked subplasmalemmal protein scaffolds that prevent release of potentially harmful intracellular enzymes from apoptotic bodies prior to their phagocytosis (50).

The rapid phagocytosis of apoptotic bodies by adjacent cells suggests there is activation of specific mechanisms promoting apoptotic body recognition. At least three potential pathways have been identified (51). Sialic acid loss from surface glycoproteins of apoptotic thymocytes results in exposure of side chain sugars that may be important in macrophage binding. Secondly, thrombospondin secreted by macrophages may form a bridge between apoptotic cells and the macrophage vitronectin-receptor integrin. Finally, increased phosphatidyl serine exposure on the surface of apoptotic lymphocytes may facilitate their recognition by macrophages.

The genetic regulation of apoptosis is, as yet, incompletely determined. Better-understood genes implicated in its control include c-myc, p53 and bcl-2. C-myc protein expression, tightly linked to cell proliferation and growth, is, paradoxically, also linked to apoptosis. Induction of apoptosis may be a normal function of c-myc which is suppressed by growth factors (52). With sufficient and appropriate growth factors present, apoptosis of cells expressing deregulated c-myc is blocked, and the cells proliferate. When insufficient growth factors are present, specifically IGF-2 for fibroblasts (53) and IL-3 for myeloid cells (54), the cells rapidly undergo apoptosis. C-myc expression, however, is not essential for apoptosis under all circumstances; it is not directly involved in apoptosis that can be modulated by the protein bcl-2 (55).

The p53 tumor suppressor gene, the most frequently mutated gene in human malignancies, is critically important in inducing apoptosis after DNA damage (56). Following ionizing radiation, p53 protein levels in the irradiated cells increase, producing cell cycle arrest, allowing time for DNA repair; if repair is not possible, damaged cells are deleted by apoptosis. The normal p53 protein has a very short half-life and is virtually undetectable in histological sections. In contrast, mutant p53, ineffective in inducing apoptosis, is readily detectable in about one half of the common carcinomas, including pancreas, breast, and colon, where it is often associated with a poor prognosis.

Bcl-2 is one of a family of genes involved in the regulation of apoptosis, promoting cell survival rather than cell death (57). Bcl-2 protein forms a heterodimer with the protein Bax such that Bcl-2-Bax inhibits apoptosis, whereas Bax-Bax homodimers favor it (58). Other Bcl-2 family members include Bcl-x, which exists as splice variants, Bcl-$x_L$ and Bcl-$x_S$—the former inhibiting, and the latter promoting apoptosis (59). Bcl-2 protein is readily detected immunohistochemically and certain cell types, particularly progenitor cells expressing the protein are resistent to apoptosis (60). Reactive germinal centers in lymph nodes, sites where apoptosis is prominent, are generally immunonegative for bcl-2 protein; follicular lymphomas, on the other hand, are usually positive. By promoting cell survival, bcl-2 facilitates acquisition of mutations and malignant transformation (61). Increased expression of bcl-2 in breast, lung, and colon cancers may reflect resistance of the tumor cells to apoptosis with implications for their responsiveness to treatment modalities.

## METHODS OF DETECTION

At present, morphological assessment is the only irrefutable means of identifying apoptosis, though a number of other techniques can assist. In the most frequently used of these, DNA agarose gel electrophoresis, apoptotic cells show a ladder pattern resulting from internucleosomal DNA

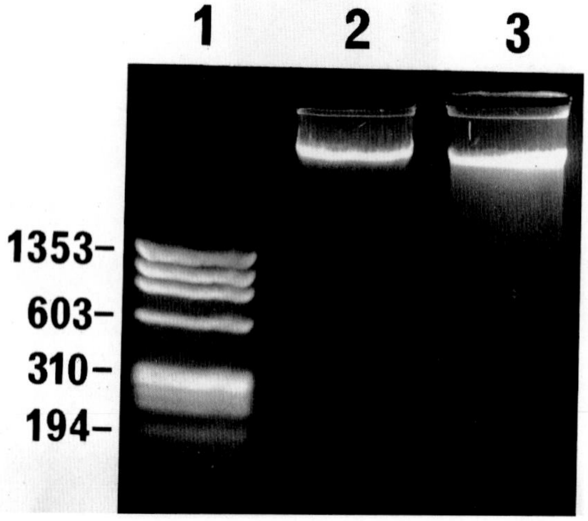


**FIG. 16.** Agarose gel electrophoresis of DNA extracted from normal and apoptotic cell populations. Lane 1, molecular weight markers (0 **x174** RF DNA-Hae III digest, New England Biolabs, Beverly, MA.) Lane 2, untreated normal human adipocytes in vitro showing only high-molecular weight DNA. Lane 3, apoptotic human adipocytes after mild hyperthermic treatment.

cleavage; this produces DNA fragments with molecular weights (MW) that are multiples of 180 base pairs (Fig. 16) (34). Pulse-field gel electrophoresis detects high MW DNA fragments produced earlier in DNA degradation that may be the only DNA cleavage products produced in some cells, but this is a complex technique and not suitable for routine use (62).

Apoptosis may also be detected by flow cytometry. With the altered DNA content of apoptotic cells, a sub $G1(A_0)$ peak is produced (63,64). The reduced size of apoptotic cells compared with normal cells alters their light-scattering properties, resulting in a reduction in forward light scatter (65). Distinction from necrosis is not always possible (66), although analysis of multiple parameters is helpful (67).

Finally, two procedures have been developed that allow in situ detection of apoptosis in formalin-fixed paraffin-embedded material. These are terminal deoxytransferase-mediated bio-dUTP nick end labeling (TUNEL) (68) and in situ end labeling (ISEL) (69) (Fig. 17). Both techniques rely on the presence of fragmented chromatin in apoptotic cells, the former using terminal transferase and the latter DNA polymerase, to incorporate biotinylated nucleotides at the DNA

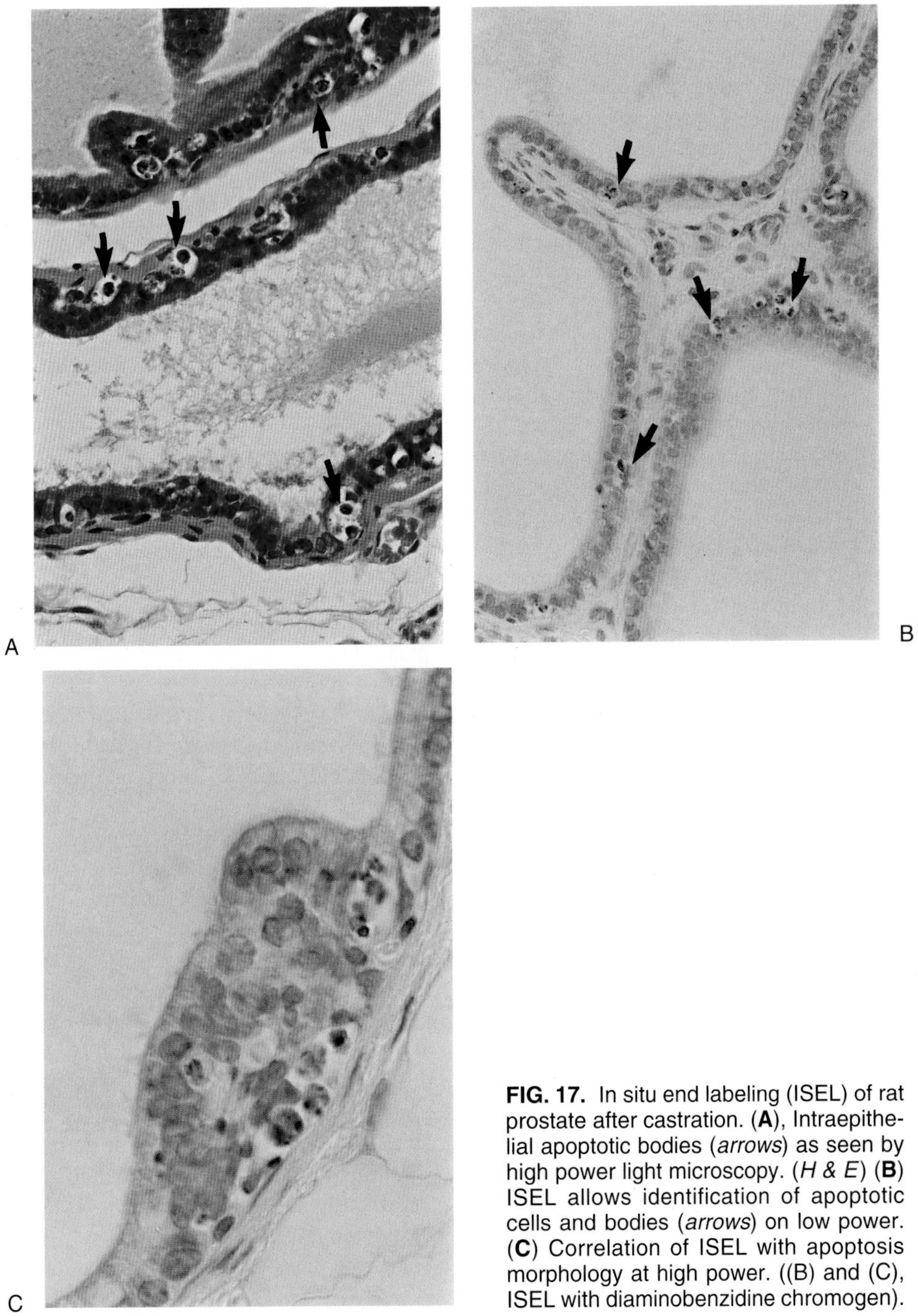


**FIG. 17.** In situ end labeling (ISEL) of rat prostate after castration. (**A**), Intraepithelial apoptotic bodies (*arrows*) as seen by high power light microscopy. (*H & E*) (**B**) ISEL allows identification of apoptotic cells and bodies (*arrows*) on low power. (**C**) Correlation of ISEL with apoptosis morphology at high power. ((B) and (C), ISEL with diaminobenzidine chromogen).

strand breaks. The labeled DNA is visualized immunohistochemically. Caution should be used when interpreting the results of end-labeling studies because DNA strand breaks may occur with necrosis and autolysis, as well as apoptosis, producing false-positive results (70,71).

## INCIDENCE

Apoptosis has a significant role in physiological and developmental process, but also accounts for cell death occurring under a variety of pathological circumstances (see 1,4,12,72,73). Hence, under normal conditions, it is involved in tissue homeostasis where a fine balance between cell proliferation and cell death is required, normal embryogenesis dependent on spatially and temporally regulated cell loss, deletion of self-reactive clones during development of the immune system, and involution of hormonally dependent tissues following falls in circulating levels of specific trophic hormones. Under pathological conditions, apoptosis accounts for regression of tissue hyperplasia, once the proximal stimulus to the hyperplasia is removed, and atrophy of exocrine glands and kidney, after duct and ureteric obstruction respectively. Whereas severe tissue injury produces necrosis, mild injury, for example, mild ischemia, and mild hyperthermia lead to cell loss through apoptosis. Spontaneous apoptosis in tumors may account for substantial cell loss and retardation of tumor growth whereas cells damaged by radiation, cancer therapeutic substances, chemical carcinogens, and certain types and quantities of toxins often undergo apoptosis. Finally, tissue injury in diseases of cellular immunity involves cell loss by apoptosis.

As this volume deals with histological rather than pathological appearances, the following account will mainly address normal processes, i.e. embryological development, cell turnover in adult tissues, and involution. Because induction of target cell apoptosis is a normal function of the body's immune cells, cell-mediated cell death will also be discussed.

### Normal Development

Many parallels can be drawn between developmental processes in lower species and mammals. Study of the finely regulated developmental death that occurs in the nematode, *Caenorhabditis elegans*, has provided insights into the genetic control of apoptosis in higher animals (74). For example, ICE and bcl-2 are the homologues of the *C. elegans* death-modulating genes, ced-3 and ced-9.

During metamorphosis, regression of larval organs in lower vertebrates, such as the loss of the tail as a tadpole matures into a frog (Fig. 18), occurs by morphologically typical apoptosis (75). Programmed cell death during the normal development of invertebrates, however, differs from classical apoptosis in a number of ways (78).

In vertebrates, apoptosis has been implicated in the development of most body systems (10), selected examples of which will be presented.

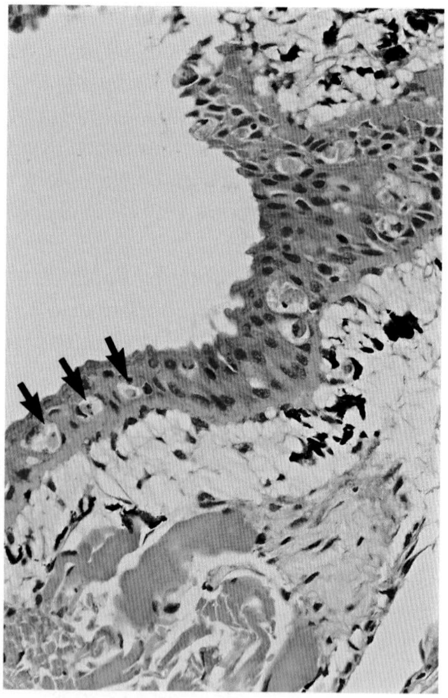

**FIG. 18.** Apoptosis in epithelium of tadpole tail (*arrows*) during amphibian metamorphosis. Although histologically inconspicuous, apoptosis of epithelial and striated muscle cells accounts for loss of the tail, approximately one-half the tadpole mass, over 2 to 3 days (76,77).

In 1966, Saunders showed the interdigital tissue of amniota embryos underwent extensive, but controlled, cell death allowing digits to emerge from the early hand- or footplate (11). Morphological studies of the regressing tissue showed apoptosis (Fig. 19), correlating with internucleosomal DNA fragmentation found on DNA gel electrophoresis (12,79). During fusion of the palatine shelves, redundant epithelium undergoes apoptosis as fusion progresses (Fig. 20) (12,80).

Cell death during the development of the vertebrate nervous system has been studied extensively. It takes the form of apoptosis and involves a range of cell types including astrocytes, oligodendrocytes, (81) and neurones. Up to 50% of neurones die soon after forming synaptic connections with their target cells, the cell death thought to reflect failure of neurones to receive specific survival factors from the target cells (82). In the developing human retina, apoptotic cell death is seen in the inner nuclear, ganglion cell, and subventricular layers where the apoptotic bodies are phagocytosed by retinal cells, rather than by infiltrating macrophages (83).

During intrauterine life, epithelial cells in the mammalian intestinal mucosa undergo apoptosis, allowing widening of the lumen and the formation of villi (84). Most apoptotic bodies are phagocytosed by surrounding epithelial cells, but

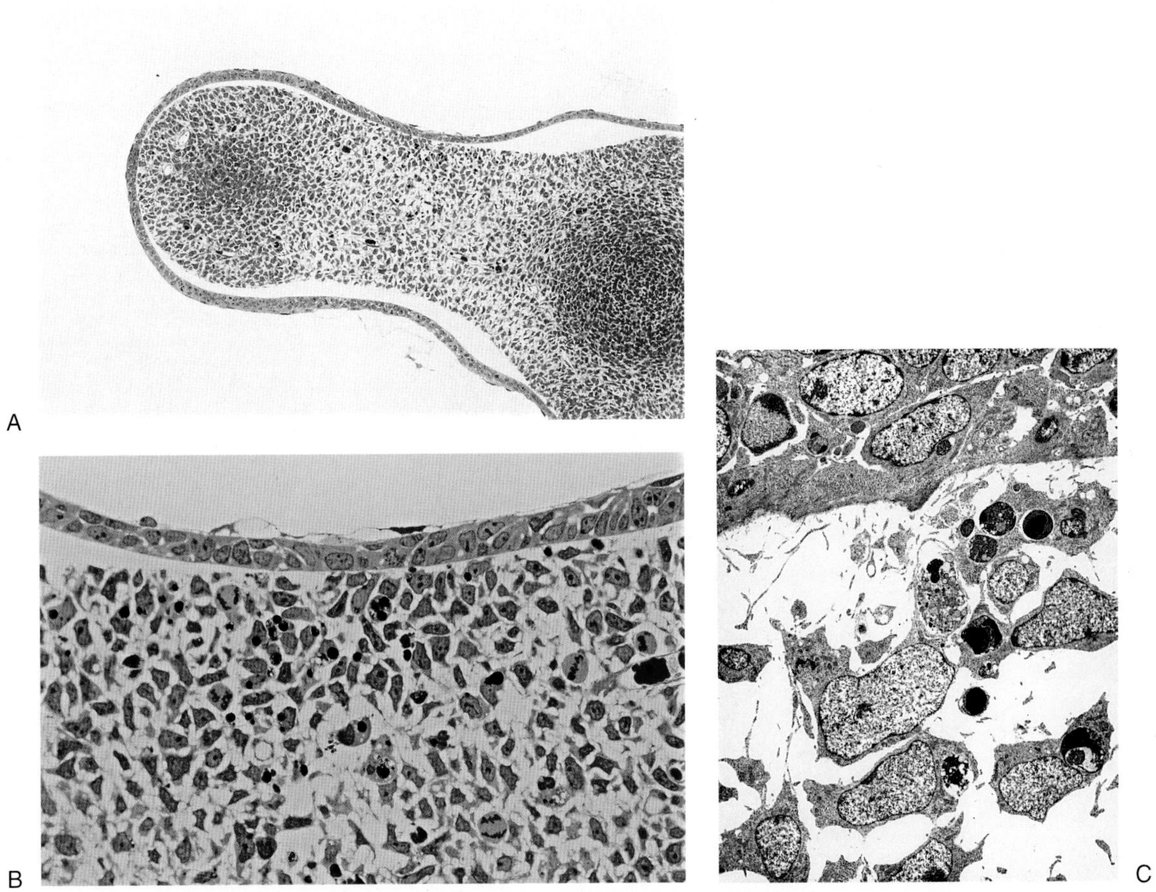


**FIG. 19.** Regression of interdigital web in 16½ day rat embryo forefoot. (**A**), Coronal section through forefoot showing developing digits (densely cellular foci) and interdigital web. (**B** and **C**) Leading edge of web showing (B) numerous stromal pyknotic apoptotic cells and bodies, and (C) apoptotic cells and bodies in epithelium and stroma (×**2000**). [(A) and (B), 1$\mu$m toluidine blue sections).]

some are shed into the lumen. In the normal developing rat kidney, metanephric mesenchymal cells are programmed for apoptosis, dying if they fail to receive survival signals from ureteric bud cells (85). Invasion of the mesenchyme by the ureteric bud, an outgrowth of the wolffian duct, blocks apoptosis and the mesenchyme converts to epithelium and differentiates.

Apoptosis plays a key role in both the development and maintenance of the immune system (86). In the developing thymus, engagement of the T cell receptor on immature T cells by self-antigen induces their death by apoptosis, self-reactive T cells, thus, being eliminated (87,88). Induction of tolerance in B cells probably also involves apoptosis, a similar process deleting autoreactive B cells (89).

### Atypical Apoptosis During Terminal Cell Differentiation

In some tissues, cells undergoing terminal differentiation exhibit some, but not all features of apoptosis. For example, normoblast nuclei undergo condensation in association with DNA cleavage to regularly sized fragments (90). The nucleus is displaced to one pole of the cell where it is covered by a thin rim of cytoplasm and plasma membrane (91). A cleavage furrow develops between the nucleated portion and the remainder of the cell, the nucleated portion alone being recognized and phagocytosed by macrophages, leaving behind an intact erythrocyte.

In the developing chicken lens, primary lens fiber cell nuclei undergo pyknosis and disappear after cleavage of DNA to form nucleosomal fragments, so that by birth the center of the lens comprises non-nucleated tissue (92). Both p53 and retinoblastoma proteins are essential for regulating fiber development so that apoptotic nuclear changes occur at the appropriate time and in the appopriate location (93).

A specialized form of apoptosis also occurs in the skin as keratinocytes in the granular layer undergo terminal differentiation to form squames. Here, cells with classical apoptotic nuclear morphology are observed and cleavage of their DNA to form nucleosomal-sized fragments can be

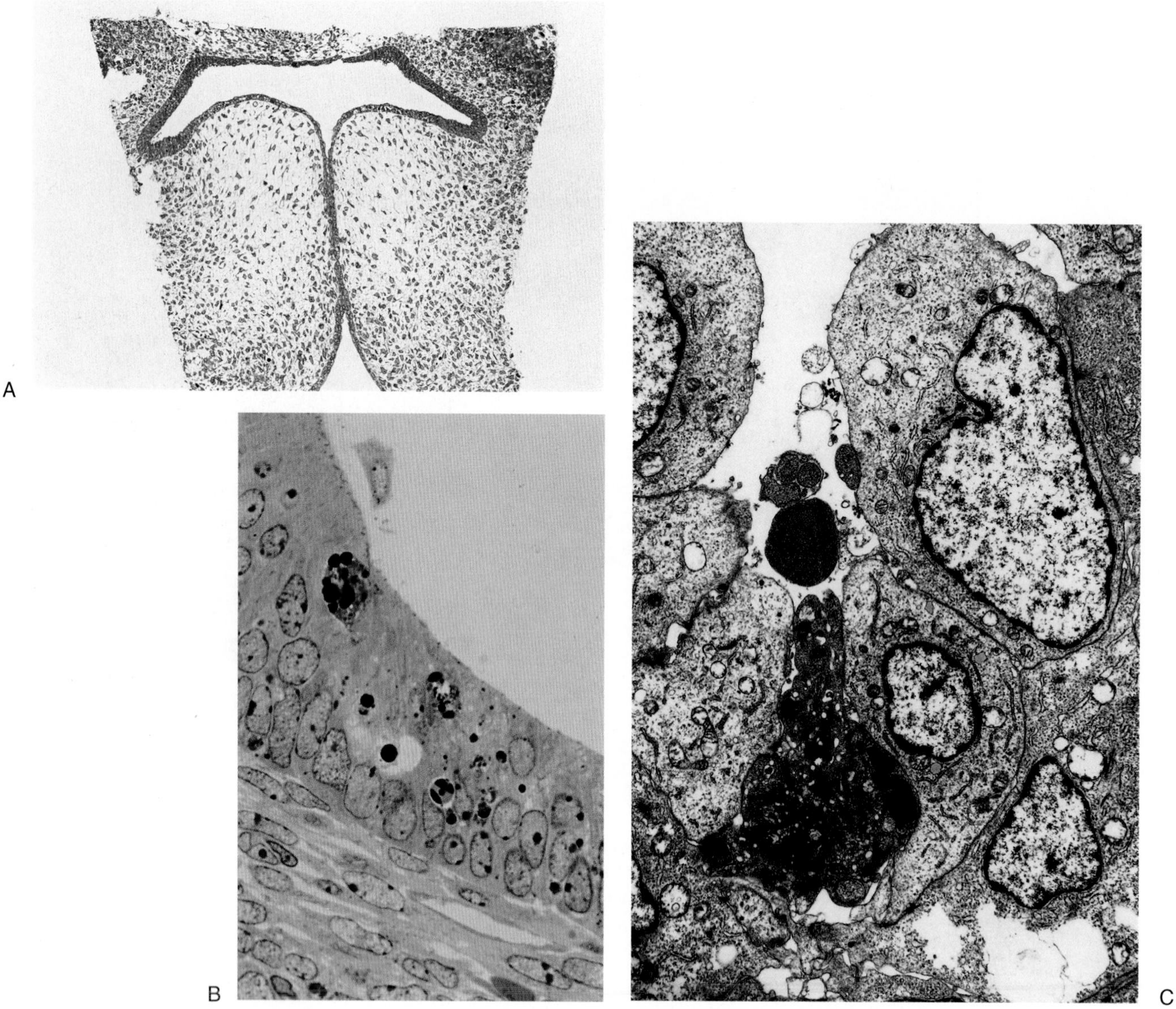

FIG. 20. Regression of epithelium during fusion of palatine processes in 16½ day rat embryo. (**A**), Apposition of epithelial linings of palatal shelves is seen centrally. (**B**), Apoptotic bodies in regressing epithelium. (**C**), Budding apoptotic epithelial cell where epithelia of the two shelves meet **(x5000)**. [(A) and (B), 1 $\mu$m toluidine blue sections.]

demonstrated (94). Budding and cellular fragmentation associated with normal apoptosis does not occur, the cell forming a flattened anucleate keratinocyte on the skin surface.

## Normal Cell Turnover in Adult Tissues

Spontaneous apoptotic deletion of cells is a consistent feature of slowly and rapidly proliferating mammalian cell populations (4). In tissues that predominantly comprise postmitotic cells, such as the brain and the heart, apoptosis is not normally identified.

In slowly proliferating tissues such as liver, prostate, pancreas, and parotid gland, small numbers of apoptotic bodies are found in the normal tissue (6,16,17,21). In the liver these are almost always found in zone 3, next to the terminal hepatic venule (95). In the adult rat adrenal gland, where maintenance of the inner two thirds of the adrenal cortex is finely regulated by serum ACTH levels, calculations suggest that, over time, the rate of apoptotic cell loss equals that of cell gain through mitosis (1). Apoptotic bodies are mostly seen in the zona reticularis (31). Positive 3′-OH nick end labeling indicative of apoptosis is also seen predominantly in the zona reticularis (96). Suppression of endogenous ACTH by corticosteroid administration produces greatly increased adrenocortical cell apoptosis in a similar distribution that is prevented by concomitant administration of exogenous ACTH (31).

In rapidly proliferating tissues, such as gastrointestinal epithelium, there are well-defined zones of both proliferation and apoptosis (97). In the small intestine, apoptotic cells are most frequently seen toward the tips of villi, though occasional apoptotic bodies are also identified close to the proliferative compartment within the intestinal crypts. Apoptotic bodies within the epithelium, and less frequently in the lamina propria, are also seen in the colon toward the top of crypts. Within the gut, luminal shedding has long been accepted as the predominant mechanism of epithelial cell loss, balancing the high levels of epithelial cell proliferation. Hall et al. have shown apoptosis to be a numerically more significant and, implicitly, a more energy-efficient route of cell disposal (97). Melanosis coli thus appears to result from an exaggeration of physiological cell death in colonic mucosa induced by the ingestion of anthraquinone derivatives (22).

In seminiferous tubules, loss of cells is effected by migration, terminal differentiation, and export as well as by apoptosis of developing spermatogonia; unusually, spontaneous death of spermatocytes and spermatids appears to involve classical necrosis (98).

In lymph nodes, there is a high death rate among germinal center centrocytes as they are selected for their ability to bind antigen (99). Those not selected undergo apoptosis and become the tingible bodies seen in germinal center macrophages (Figs. 21 and 22) (76,100).

After releasing most of their cytoplasm as platelets, megakaryocyte remnants in the bone marrow die by apoptosis (101). Senescent neutrophils also undergo apoptosis, such cells being recognized and phagocytosed by macrophages: thus preventing release of their lysosomal enzymes as they die, and augmentation of the inflammatory response (102). Apoptosis and ingestion by macrophages may also represent a mechanism whereby the tissue longevity and removal of eosinophils is controlled (103). Varying erythropoietin levels regulate the extent of apoptosis of late erythroid progenitors, thus controlling the size of the red blood cell pool (104,105).

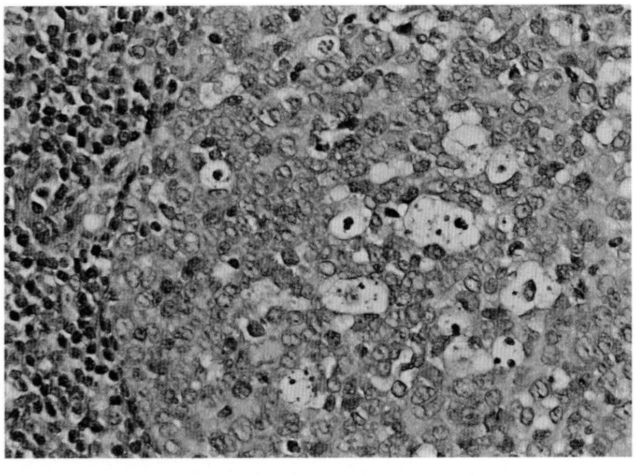

**FIG. 21.** Tingible body macrophages in germinal center of human lymph node.

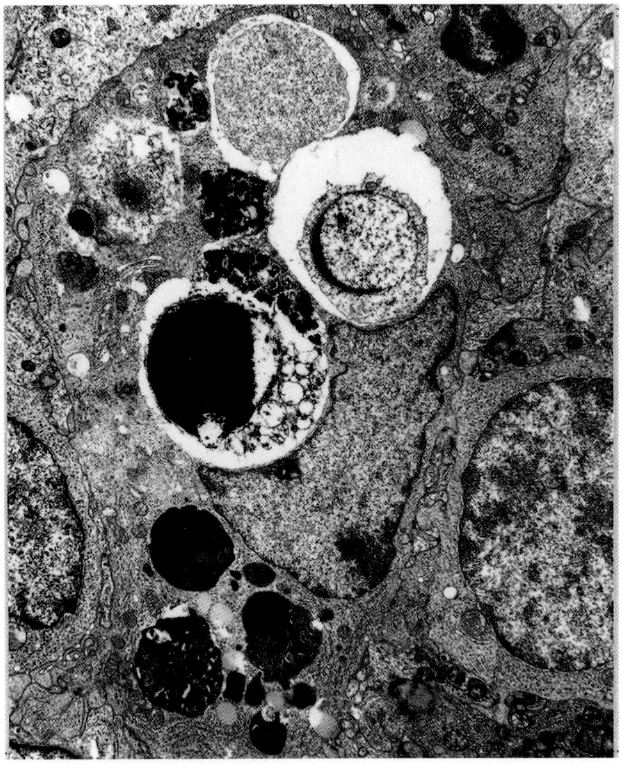

**FIG. 22.** Well-preserved and variably degraded apoptotic lymphocytes in cytoplasm of germinal center macrophage in normal guinea pig lymph node **(x4900)**.

### Cyclical Cell Loss In Adult Tissues

The size of many cell populations is under the control of growth factors or hormones, with cell deletion occurring when circulating levels of relevant factors fall. The cell loss invariably occurs by apoptosis.

In the normal adult human breast, mitosis of duct and ductular epithelial cells is maximal at day 25 of a 28-day menstrual cycle and apoptosis is maximal on day 28 (106). The apoptosis is evenly distributed throughout the breast, the apoptotic cells phagocytosed by neighboring epithelial and myoepithelial cells and intraepithelial macrophages, rather than shed into glandular lumens (Fig. 23) (107). The apoptotic peak correlates with a sharp decrease in immunostaining for bcl-2 protein of lobular epithelium at the end of the menstrual cycle (108).

Human endometrium shows increased loss of glandular epithelial cells by apoptosis in the late secretory, premenstrual, and menstrual phases (Fig. 24) (109). Apoptotic cells and bodies are seen in epithelial cells and macrophages within and beneath the epithelium, and rarely within gland lumens. Similar changes are seen in the hamster endometrium at estrus (110) and ewe endometrium at parturition (111). Uterine epithelial cells surrounding the blastocyst at the implantation sites of mice and rats also undergo apoptosis, bringing blastocyst into close association with endometrial stroma (112).

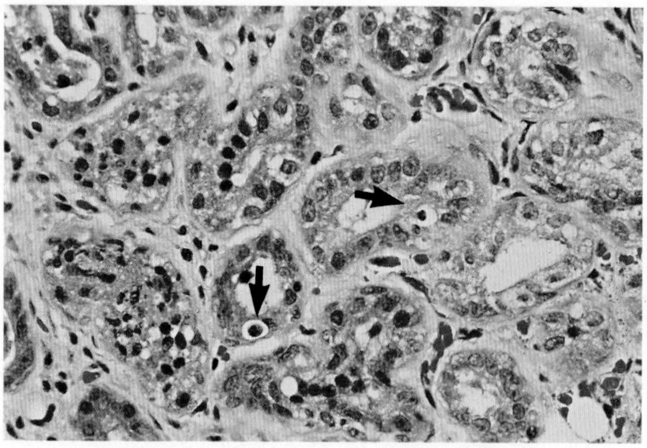

**FIG. 23.** Apoptosis of epithelial cells (*arrows*) in ductules of normal human breast.

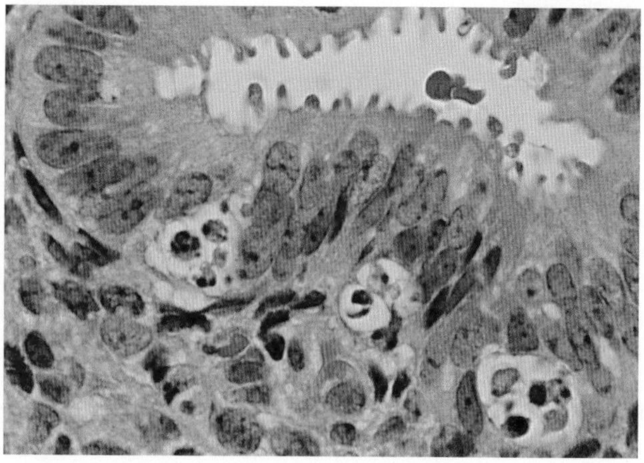

**FIG. 24.** Apoptotic bodies in intraepithelial macrophages in late secretory human endometrium.

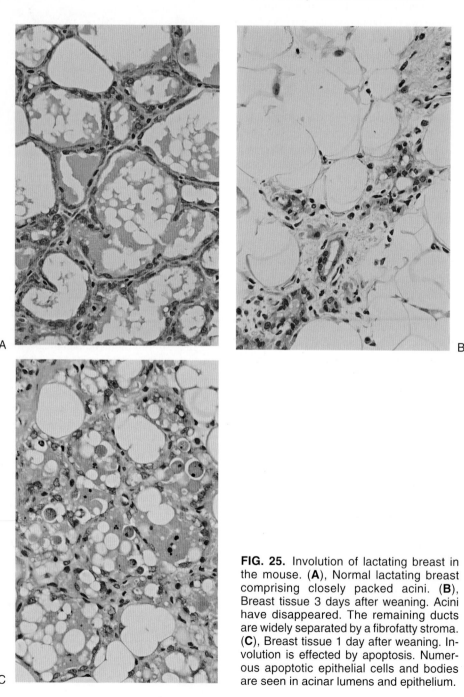

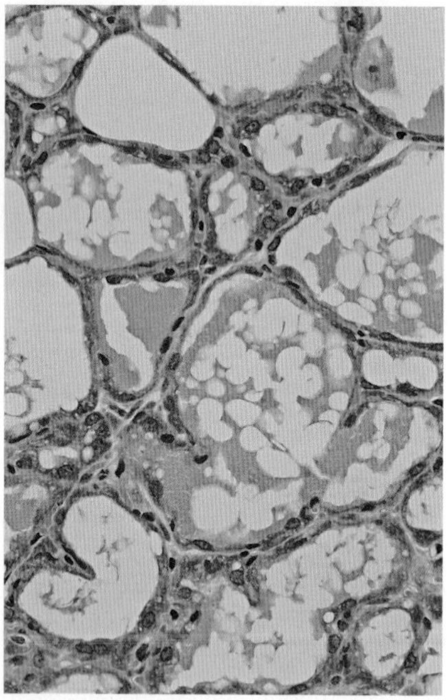

A

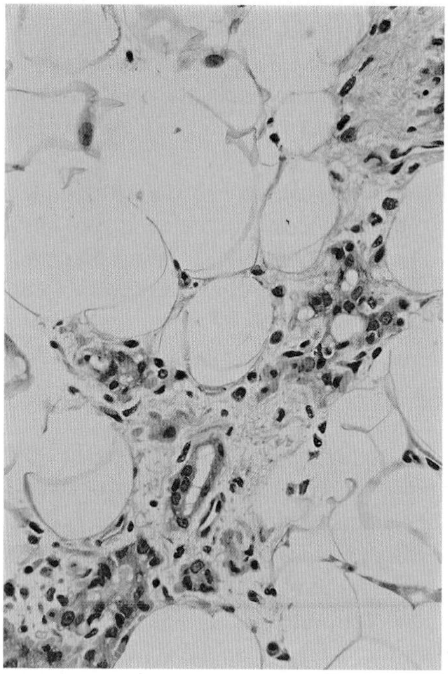

B

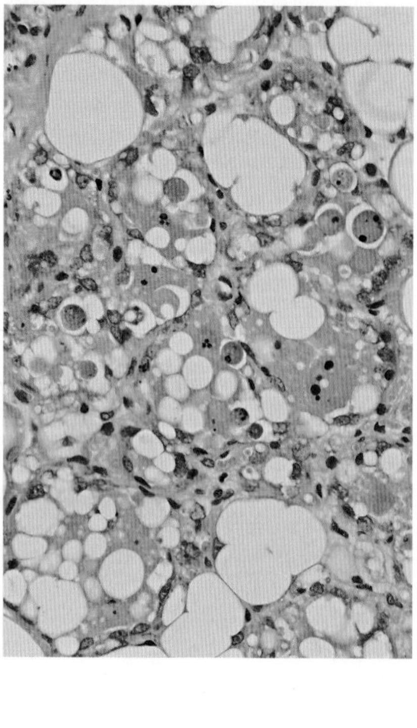

C

**FIG. 25.** Involution of lactating breast in the mouse. (**A**), Normal lactating breast comprising closely packed acini. (**B**), Breast tissue 3 days after weaning. Acini have disappeared. The remaining ducts are widely separated by a fibrofatty stroma. (**C**), Breast tissue 1 day after weaning. Involution is effected by apoptosis. Numerous apoptotic epithelial cells and bodies are seen in acinar lumens and epithelium.

### Involution

Involution of the neonatal rat adrenal cortex occurs synchronously with known falls in circulating ACTH in the neonatal period (113). In the first 3 to 5 days after birth, large numbers of apoptotic bodies are found in the inner adrenal cortex; subsequently, the number falls to low levels.

The lactating breast after weaning undergoes rapid involution (Fig. 25), presumably related to falls in circulating prolactin levels (19). In the mouse, initial involution proceeds rapidly, large numbers of apoptotic epithelial cells being shed into gland lumens (Figs. 12 and 25). Subsequently, there is more gradual regression to the resting state, apoptotic bodies derived from epithelial and myoepithelial cells mostly being phagocytosed by intraepithelial macrophages. In the rat, the changes are more gradual, and shedding of apoptotic cells into lumens is not prominent. In both animals, apoptosis of endothelial cells, resulting in regression of the capillary networks, accompanies the loss of glandular tissue. Internucleosomal DNA fragmentation characteristic of apoptosis accompanies involution in the mouse (114).

Greater than 99% of ovarian follicles present at birth undergo atresia (115). Using a 3′-end labeling technique, DNA fragmentation, charactertistic of apoptosis, is identified in atretic follicles of both chicken and porcine ovaries (116). In postovulatory follicles, there is fragmentation of DNA, whereas DNA from preovulatory follicles remains intact (116). In the former, granulosa cells undergo apoptosis whereas thecal cells are relatively spared; the theca interna is gradually absorbed into the ovarian stroma (117). In normal atresia of sheep ovarian follicles, however, theca interna cells die by apoptosis (118). In the regressing corpus luteum of sheep, endothelial cell apoptosis results in blood vessel depletion (119).

In other tissues, the stimulus to involution is unknown, but apoptosis remains the mechanism of cell loss. For example, spontaneous involution of hair follicles during catagen involves apoptosis of epithelial cells in the outer root sheath, apoptotic bodies being predominantly phagocytosed by adjacent epithelial cells (120). The resorption of tissues around erupting teeth also involves apoptosis (121).

Pathological atrophy is in many ways similar to involution, involving cell deletion by apoptosis. Thus, falls in circulating levels of trophic hormones following castration induce atrophy of the rat prostate (21). Exocrine gland atrophy after duct obstruction (16, 17), renal atrophy in experimental hydronephrosis, (122) and atrophy of liver (Fig. 13) and kidney caused by mild ischemia (8,123) similarly involve apoptosis. As in involution of the lactating breast and corpus luteum, apoptosis of endothelial cells may accompany the tissue atrophy (16,17).

### Cell-Mediated Immunity

Cell death induced by cytotoxic T cells, K cells, and natural killer cells takes the form of apoptosis (Fig. 26) (4,125). Such death is part of immune surveillance, transformed and virally infected cells, potentially dangerous to the host, being recognized and removed. Induction of apoptosis in target cells by specifically sensitized T-lymphocytes may involve activation of cytoplasmic proteases in the target cell by a number of mechanisms including engagement of the Fas receptor (also known as Apo 1 or CD95) (126). T cell-mediated apoptotic cell death is also involved in transplant rejection (127), graft-versus-host disease (Fig. 27) (128), and diseases where cell-mediated death of cells is likely to be important, i.e. acute and chronic hepatitis (129), primary biliary cirrhosis, (130) and lichen planus (131). Viral infection may also cause apoptosis through direct viral cytotoxicity, induction of tumor necrosis factor, or conflicting signals controlling cell growth (132). Inappropriate induction of $CD4^+$ T cell apoptosis by HIV may be relevant to the pathogenesis of AIDS (133,134).

## CONCLUSION

Apoptosis was first identified as a distinct form of cell death on the basis of its morphology. Subsequent studies of its incidence, biochemistry, and genetics have upheld predictions of its general role in controlled cell deletion and its

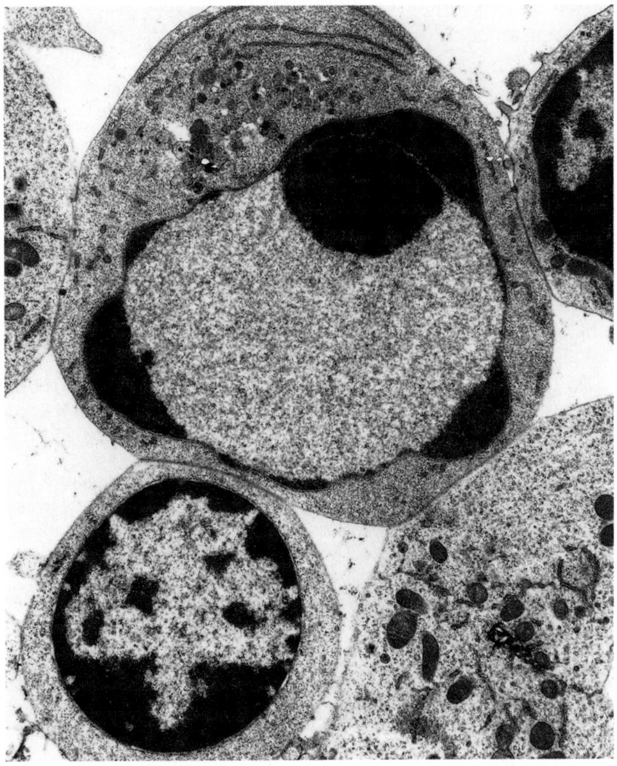

**FIG. 26.** Early apoptosis of mouse mastocytoma cell following incubation with specifically sensitized T-lymphocytes (124). Note large nucleolar remnant in apoptotic cell nucleus and close apposition of cell membranes of lymphocytes and mastocytoma cell.

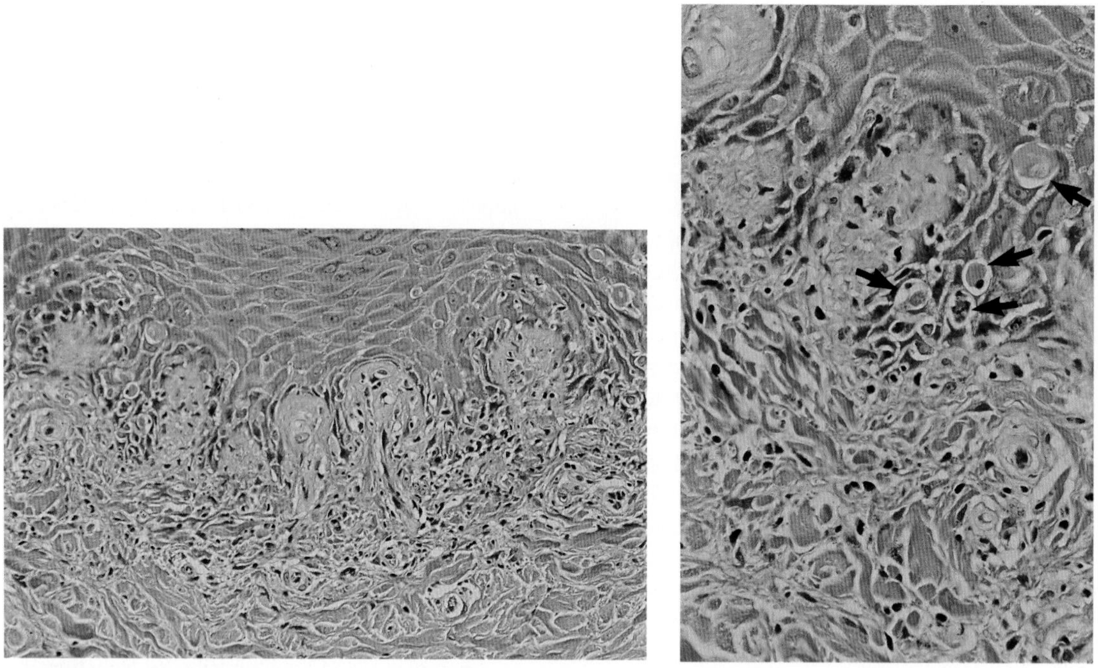

A B

**FIG. 27.** Apoptosis of keratinocytes in graft-versus-host disease in man. (**A**), Lichenoid infiltrate with apoptosis of basal keratinocytes (*arrows*) better seen at higher power (**B**).

genetically determined nature. As the genetic controls and biochemical mechanisms of apoptosis become better understood, development of therapeutic strategies that modulate its occurrence in disease processes can be expected (135).


## ACKNOWLEDGMENTS

This work was supported by research funds of The University of Queensland.


## REFERENCES


1. Wyllie AH, Kerr JFR, Currie AR. Cell death. The significance of apoptosis. *Int Rev Cytol* 1980;68:251–306.
2. Trump BF, Berezesky IK, Osornio-Vargas AR. Cell death and the disease process. The role of calcium. In: Bowen D, Lockshin RA, eds. *Cell death in biology and pathology*. London; Chapman and Hall, 1981;209–242.
3. Wyllie AH. Cell death. A new classification separating apoptosis from necrosis. In: Bowen D, Lockshin RA, eds. *Cell death in biology and pathology*. London; Chapman and Hall, 1981;9–34.
4. Walker NI, Harmon BV, Gobé GC, Kerr JFR. Patterns of cell death. *Methods Achiev Exp Pathol* 1988;13:18–54.
5. Kerr JFR, Gobé GC, Winterford CM, Harmon BV. Anatomical methods in cell death. *Methods Cell Biol* 1995;46:1–27.
6. Kerr JFR. A histochemical study of hypertrophy and ischaemic injury of rat liver with special reference to changes in lysosomes. *J Pathol Bacteriol* 1965;90:419–435.
7. Allen R. Who discovered cell suicide? *Medical Observer* Oct 13, 1995;59–60.
8. Kerr JFR. Shrinkage necrosis. A distinct mode of cellular death. *J Pathol* 1971;105:13–20.
9. Kerr JFR, Wyllie AH, Currie AR. Apoptosis. A basic biological phenomenon with wide-ranging implications in tissue kinetics. *Br J Cancer* 1972;26:239–257.
10. Glücksmann A. Cell deaths in normal vertebrate autogeny. *Biol Rev* 1951;26:59–86.
11. Saunders JW. Death in embryonic systems. *Science* 1966;154: 604–612.
12. Kerr JFR, Searle J, Harmon BV, Bishop CJ. Apoptosis. In: Potten CS, ed. *Perspectives on mammalian cell death*. Oxford; Oxford University Press, 1987;93–128.
13. Wyllie AH. Cell death. *Int Rev Cytol* 1987;Suppl 17:755–785.
14. Arends JA, Wyllie AH. Apoptosis. Mechanisms and roles in pathology. *Int Rev Exp Pathol* 1991;32:223–254.
15. Kerr JFR, Winterford CM, Harmon BV. Morphological criteria for identifying apoptosis. In: Celis JE, ed. *Cell biology. A laboratory handbook*. New York; Academic Press, 1994;319–329.
16. Walker NI. Ultrastructure of the rat pancreas after experimental duct ligation. I. The role of apoptosis and intraepithelial macrophages in acinar cell deletion. *Am J Pathol* 1987;126:439–451.
17. Walker NI, Gobé GC. Cell death and cell proliferation during atrophy of the rat parotid gland induced by duct obstruction. *J Pathol* 1987; 153:333–344.
18. Weedon D, Searle S, Kerr JFR. Apoptosis. Its nature and implications for dermatopathology. *Am J Dermatopathol* 1979;1:133–144.
19. Walker NI, Bennett RE, Kerr JFR. Cell death during involution of the lactating breast in mice and rats. *Am J Anat* 1989;185:19–32.
20. Prins JB, Walker NI, Winterford CM, Cameron DP. Apoptosis of human adipocytes in vitro. *Biochem Biophys Res Commun* 1994;201: 500–507.
21. Kerr JFR, Searle J. Deletion of cells by apoptosis during castration-induced involution of the rat prostate. *Virchows Arch [B] Cell Pathol* 1973;13:87–102.
22. Walker NI, Bennett RE, Axelsen RA. Melanosis coli. A consequence of anthraquinone-induced apoptosis of colonic epithelial cells. *Am J Pathol* 1988;131:465–476.
23. Sheridan JW, Bishop CJ, Simmons RJ. Biophysical and morphological correlates of kinetic change and death in a starved human melanoma cell line. *J Cell Sci* 1981;49:119–137.
24. Wyllie AH. The biology of cell death in tumours. *Anticancer Res* 1985;5:131–136.
25. Russell SW, Rosenau W, Lee JC. Cytolysis induced by human lymphotoxin. Cinemicrographic and electron microscopic observations. *Am J Pathol* 1972;69:103–118.
26. Sanderson CJ. The mechanism of T cell mediated cytotoxicity. II. Morphological studies of cell death by time-lapse microcinematography. *Proc R Soc Lond B Biol Sci* 1976;192:241–255.

27. Matter A. Microcinematographic and electron microscopic analysis of target cell lysis induced by cytotoxic T lymphocytes. *Immunology* 1979;36:179–190.
28. Bursch W, Paffe S, Putz B, Barthel G, Schulte-Hermann R. Determination of the length of the histological stages of apoptosis in normal liver and in altered hepatic foci of rats. *Carcinogenesis* 1990;11: 847–853.
29. Meagher LC, Savill JS, Baker A, Fuller RW, Haslett C. Phagocytosis of apoptotic neutrophils does not induce macrophage release of thromboxane $B_2$. *J Leukoc Biol* 1992;52:269–273.
30. Howie SE, Sommerfield AJ, Gray E, Harrison DJ. Peripheral T lymphocyte depletion by apoptosis after CD4 ligation in vivo. Selective loss of $CD44^-$ and activating memory T cells. *Clin Exp Immunol* 1994;95:195–200.
31. Wyllie AH, Kerr JFR, Macaskill IAM, Currie AR. Adrenocortical cell deletion. The role of ACTH. *J Pathol* 1973;111:85–94.
32. Walker NI, Winterford CM, Kerr JFR. Ultrastructure of the rat pancreas after experimental duct ligation. II. Duct and stromal cell proliferation, differentiation, and deletion. *Pancreas* 1992;7:420–434.
33. Walker NI, Winterford CM, Williamson RM, Kerr JFR. Ethionine-induced atrophy of rat pancreas involves apoptosis of acinar cells. *Pancreas* 1993;8:443–449.
34. Wyllie AH. Glucocorticoid-induced thymocyte apoptosis is associated with endogenous endonuclease activation. *Nature* 1980;284: 555–556.
35. Oberhammer F, Wilson JW, Dive C, et al. Apoptotic death in epithelial cells: Cleavage of DNA to 300 and/or 50 kb fragments prior to or in the absence of internucleosomal fragmentation. *EMBO J* 1993;12: 3679–3684.
36. Earnshaw WC. Nuclear changes in apoptosis. *Curr Opin Cell Biol* 1995;7:337–343.
37. Sun X-M, Cohen GM. $Mg^{2+}$-dependent cleavage of DNA into kilobase pair fragments is responsible for the initial degradation of DNA in apoptosis. *J Biol Chem* 1994;269:14857–14860.
38. Collins RJ, Harmon BV, Gobé GC, Kerr JFR. Internucleosomal DNA cleavage should not be the sole criterion for identifying apoptosis. *Int J Radiat Biol* 1992;61:451–453.
39. Peitsch MC, Polzar B, Stephan H, et al. Characterization of the endogenous deoxyribonuclease involved in nuclear DNA degradation during apoptosis (programmed cell death) *EMBO J* 1993;12:371–377.
40. Barry MA, Eastman A. Identification of deoxyribonuclease II as an endonuclease involved in apoptosis. *Arch Biochem Biophys* 1993;300: 440–450.
41. Wyllie AH. The genetic regulation of apopotosis. *Current Opin Genet Dev* 1995;5:97–104.
42. Martin SJ, Green DR. Protease activation during apoptosis: Death by a thousand cuts? *Cell* 1995;82:349–352.
43. Miura M, Zhu H, Rotello R, Hartwieg EA, Yuan J. Induction of apoptosis in fibroblasts by IL-1$\beta$-converting enzyme, a mammalian homolog of the *C. elegans* cell death gene *ced-3*. *Cell* 1993;75:653–660.
44. Wang L, Muira M, Bergeron L, Zhu H, Yuan J. *Ich*-1, and *Ice/ced*-3-related gene, encodes both positive and negative regulators of programmed cell death. *Cell* 1994;78:739–750.
45. Smyth MJ, Trapani JA. Granzymes: Exogenous proteinases that induce target cell apoptosis. *Immunol Today* 1995;16:202–206.
46. Shresta S, Heusel JW, MacIvor DM, Wesselschmidt RL, Russell JH, Ley TJ. Granzyme B plays a critical role in cytotoxic lymphocyte-induced apoptosis. *Immunol Rev* 1995;146:211–221.
47. Martin SJ, O'Brien GA, Nishioka WK et al. Proteolysis of fodrin (non-erythroid spectrin) during apoptosis. *J Biol Chem* 1995;270: 6425–6428.
48. Lazebnik YA, Takahashi A, Moir RD, et al. Studies of the lamin proteinase reveal multiple parallel biochemical pathways during apoptotic execution. *Proc Natl Acad Sci U S A* 1995;92:9042–9046.
49. Neamati N, Fernandez A, Wright S, Kiefer J, McConkey DJ. Degradation of Lamin $B_1$ precedes oligonucleosomal DNA fragmentation in apoptotic thymocytes and isolated thymocyte nuclei. *J Immunol* 1995; 154:3788–3795.
50. Fesus L, Thomazy V, Falus A. Induction and activation of tissue transglutaminase during programmed cell death. *FEBS Lett* 1987;224: 104–108.
51. Savill J, Fadok V, Henson P, Haslett C. Phagocyte recognition of cells undergoing apoptosis. *Immunol Today* 1993;14:131–136.
52. Evan G, Harrington E, Fanidi A, Land H, Amati B, Bennett M. Integrated control of cell proliferation and cell death by the c-*myc* oncogene. *Philos Trans R Soc Lond B Biol Sci* 1994;345:269–275.
53. Harrington EA, Bennett MR, Fanidi A, Evan GI. c-Myc-induced apoptosis in fibroblasts is inhibited by specific cytokines. *EMBO J* 1994;13:3286–3295.
54. Askew DS, Ashmun RA, Simmons BC, Cleveland JL. Constitutive c-*myc* expression in an IL-3 dependent myeloid cell line suppresses cell cycle arrest and accelerates apoptosis. *Oncogene* 1991;6:1915–1922.
55. Vaux DL, Weissman IL. Neither macromolecular synthesis nor myc is required for cell death via the mechanism that can be controlled by bcl-2. *Mol Cell Biol* 1993;13:7000–7005.
56. Hooper ML. The role of *p53* and *Rb-1* genes in cancer, development and apoptosis. *J Cell Sci* 1994;18:13–17.
57. Korsmeyer SJ. Regulators of cell death. *TIG* 1995;11:101–105.
58. Oltvai ZN, Millman CL, Korsmeyer SJ. Bcl-2 heterodimerizes in vivo with a conserved homolog, bax, that accelerates programmed cell death. *Cell* 1993;74:609–619.
59. Boise LH, González-Garcia M, Postema CE, et al. bcl-x, a bcl-2-related gene that functions as a dominant regulator of apoptotic cell death. *Cell* 1993;77:597–608.
60. Pezzella F, Gatter K. What is the value of bcl-2 protein detection for histopathologists? *Histopathology* 1995;26:89–93.
61. Vaux DL, Cory S, Adams JM. bcl-2 gene promotes haemopoietic cell survival and cooperates with c-myc to immortalize pre-B cells. *Nature* 1988;335:440–442.
62. Walker PR, Kokileva L, LeBlanc J, Sikorska M. Detection of the initial stages of DNA fragmentation in apoptosis. *Biotechniques* 1993; 15:1032–1040.
63. Tounekti O, Belehradek J Jr, Mir LM. Relationships between DNA fragmentation, chromatin condensation, and changes in flow cytometry profiles detected during apoptosis. *Exp Cell Res* 1995;217: 506–516.
64. Telford WG, King LE, Fraker PJ. Comparative evaluation of several DNA binding dyes in the detection of apoptosis-associated chromatin degradation by flow cytometry. *Cytometry* 1992;13:137–143.
65. Darzynkiewicz Z, Bruno S, Del Bino G, et al. Features of apoptotic cells measured by flow cytometry. *Cytometry* 1992;13:795–808.
66. Bryson GJ, Harmon BV, Collins RJ. A flow cytometric study of cell death. Failure of some models to correlate with morphological assessment. *Immunol Cell Biol* 1994;72:35–41.
67. Dive C, Gregory CD, Phipps DJ, Evans DL, Milner AE, Wyllie AH. Analysis and discrimination of necrosis and apoptosis (programmed cell death) by multiparameter flow cytometry. *Biochim Biophys Acta* 1992;1133:275–285.
68. Gavrieli Y, Sherman Y, Ben-Sasson SA. Identification of programmed cell death in situ via specific labeling of nuclear DNA fragmentation. *J Cell Biol* 1992;119:493–501.
69. Wijsman JH, Jonker RR, Keijzer R, Van De Velde CJH, Cornelisse CJ, Van Dierendonck JH. A new method to detect apoptosis in paraffin sections: in situ end-labeling of fragmented DNA. *J Histochem Cytochem* 1993;41:7–12.
70. Grasl-Kraupp B, Ruttkay-Nedecky B, Koudelka H, Bukowska K, Bursch W, Schulte-Hermann R. In situ detection of fragmented DNA (TUNEL assay) fails to discriminate among apoptosis, necrosis, and autolytic cell death: A cautionary note. *Hepatology* 1995;21: 1465–1468.
71. Ansari B, Coates PJ, Greenstein BD, Hall PA. In situ end-labelling detects DNA strand breaks in apoptosis and other physiological and pathological states. *J Pathol* 1993;170:1–8.
72. Kerr JFR, Harmon BV. Definition and incidence of apoptosis. An historical perspective. In: Tomei LD, Cope FO, eds. *Apoptosis: The molecular basis of cell death.* Cold Spring Harbor; Cold Spring Harbor Laboratory Press, 1991;5–29.
73. Kerr JFR, Winterford CM, Harmon BV. Apoptosis. Its significance in cancer and cancer therapy. *Cancer* 1994;73:2013–2026.
74. Yuan J, Horvitz HR. The *Caenorhabditis elegans* genes ced-3 and ced-4 act cell autonomously to cause programmed cell death. *Dev Biol* 1990;138:33–41.
75. Kerr JFR, Harmon B, Searle J. An electron-microscope study of cell deletion in the anuran tadpole tail during spontaneous metamorphosis with special reference to apoptosis of striated muscle fibres. *J Cell Sci* 1974;14:571–585.
76. Searle J, Kerr JFR, Bishop CJ. Necrosis and apoptosis. Distinct modes of cell death with fundamentally different significance. *Pathol Annu* 1982;17(2):229–259.

77. Kerr JFR, Bishop CJ, Searle J. Apoptosis. In: Anthony PP, McSween RNM, eds. *Recent advances in histopathology*. Edinburgh; Churchill Livingstone, 1984;12:1–15.
78. Lockshin RA, Zakeri Z. Programmed cell death and apoptosis. In: Tomei LD, Cope FO, eds. *Apoptosis. The molecular basis of cell death*. Cold Spring Harbor; Cold Spring Harbor Laboratory Press, 1991;47–60.
79. Garcia-Martinez V Macias D, Gañan Y, et al. Internucleosomal DNA fragmentation and programmed cell death (apoptosis) in the interdigital tissue of the embryonic chick leg bud. *J Cell Sci* 1993;106:201–208.
80. Farbman AI. Electron microscope study of palate fusion in mouse embryos. *Dev Biol* 1968;18:93–116.
81. Barres BA, Hart IK, Coles HSR, et al. Cell death and control of cell survival in the oligodendrocyte lineage. *Cell* 1992;70:31–46.
82. Raff MC, Barres BA, Burne JF, Coles HS, Ishizaki Y, Jacobson MD. Programmed cell death and the control of cell survival. Lessons from the nervous system. *Science* 1993;262:695–700.
83. Penfold PL, Provis JM. Cell death in the development of the human retina: Phagocytosis of pyknotic and apoptotic bodies by retinal cells. *Graefes Arch Clin Exp Ophthalmol* 1986;224:549–553.
84. Harmon B, Bell L, Williams L. An ultrastructural study on the meconium corpuscles in rat foetal intestinal epithelium with particular reference to apoptosis. *Anat Embryol (Berl)* 1984;169:119–124.
85. Koseki C, Herzlinger D, al-Awqati Q. Apoptosis in metanephric development. *J Cell Biol* 1992;119:1327–1333.
86. Williams GT. Apoptosis in the immune system. *J Pathol* 1994;173: 1–4.
87. Smith CA, Williams GT, Kingston R, Jenkinson EJ, Owen JJT. Antibodies to CS2/T-cell receptor complex induce death by apoptosis in immature T cells in thymic cultures. *Nature* 1989;337:181–184.
88. Murphy KM, Heimberger AB, Loh DY. Induction by antigen of intrathymic apoptosis of $CD4^+$ $CD8^+$ $TCR^{LO}$ thymocytes *in vivo*. *Science* 1990;250:1720–1723.
89. Carsetti R, Köhler G, Lamers MC. A role for immunoglobulin D. Interference with tolerance induction. *Eur J Immunol* 1993;23:168–178.
90. Williamson R. Properties of rapidly labelled deoxyribonucleic acid fragments isolated from the cytoplasm of primary cultures of embryonic mouse liver cells. *J Mol Biol* 1970;51:157–168.
91. Skutelsky E, Danon D. On the expulsion of the erythroid nucleus and its phagocytosis. *Anat Rec* 1972;173:123–126.
92. Appleby DW, Modak SP. DNA degradation in terminally differentiating lens fiber cells from chick embryos. *Proc Natl Acad Sci U S A* 1977;12:5579–5583.
93. Pan H, Griep AE. Altered cell cycle regulation in the lens of HPV-16 E6 or E7 transgenic mice. Implications for tumor suppressor gene function in development. *Genes Dev* 1994;8:1285–1299.
94. McCall CA, Cohen JJ. Programmed cell death in terminally differentiating keratinocytes. Role of endogenous endonuclease. *J Invest Dermatol* 1991;97:111–114.
95. Benedetti A, Jézéquel AM, Orlandi F. Preferential distribution of apoptotic bodies in acinar zone 3 of normal human and rat liver. *J Hepatol* 1988;7:319–324.
96. Sasano H, Imatani A, Shizawa S, Suzuki T, Nagura H. Cell proliferation and apoptosis in normal and pathologic human adrenal. *Mod Pathol* 1995;8:11–17.
97. Hall PA, Coates PJ, Ansari B, Hopwood D. Regulation of cell number in the mammalian gastrointestinal tract: The importance of apoptosis. *J Cell Sci* 1994;107:3569–3577.
98. Allan DJ, Harmon BV, Kerr JFR. Cell death in spermatogenesis. In: Potten CS, ed. *Perspectives on mammalian cell death*. Oxford; Oxford University Press, 1987;229–258.
99. MacLennan IC. Germinal centers. *Annu Rev Immunol* 1994;12: 117–139.
100. Liu Y-J, Joshua DE, Williams GT, Smith CA, Gordon J, MacLennan ICM. Mechanism of antigen-driven selection in germinal centres. *Nature* 1989;342:929–931.
101. Radley JM, Haller CJ. Fate of senescent megakaryocytes in the bone marrow. *Br J Haematol* 1983;53:277–287.
102. Savill J. Macrophage recognition of senescent neutrophils. *Clin Sci (Colch)* 1992;83:649–655.
103. Stern M, Meagher L, Savill J, Haslett C. Apoptosis in human eosinophils. Programmed cell death in the eosinophil leads to phagocytosis by macrophages and is modulated by IL-5. *J Immunol* 1992; 148:3543–3549.
104. Koury MJ, Bondurant MC. Erythropoietin retards DNA breakdown and prevents programmed death in erythroid progenitor cells. *Science* 1990;248:378–381.
105. Koury MJ. Programmed cell death (apoptosis) in hematopoiesis. *Exp Hematol* 1992;20:391–394.
106. Ferguson DJP, Anderson TJ. Morphological evaluation of cell turnover in relation to the menstrual cycle in the "resting" human breast. *Br J Cancer* 1981;44:177–181.
107. Ferguson DJP, Anderson TJ. Ultrastructural observations on cell death by apoptosis in the "resting" human breast. *Virchows Arch [Pathol Anat]* 1981;393:193–203.
108. Sabourin JC, Martin A, Baruch J, Truc JB, Gompel A, Poitout P. bcl-2 expression in normal breast tissue during the menstrual cycle. *Int J Cancer* 1994;59:1–6.
109. Hopwood D, Levison DA. Atrophy and apoptosis in the cyclical human endometrium. *J Pathol* 1976;119:159–166.
110. Sandow BA, West NB, Norman RL, Brenner RM. Hormonal control of apoptosis in hamster uterine luminal epithelium. *Am J Anat* 1979; 156:15–35.
111. O'Shea JD, Wright PJ. Involution and regeneration of the endometrium following parturition in the ewe. *Cell Tissue Res* 1984; 236:477–485.
112. Parr EL, Tung HN, Parr MB. Apoptosis as the mode of uterine epithelial cell death during embryo implantation in mice and rats. *Biol Reprod* 1987;36:211–225.
113. Wyllie AH, Kerr JFR, Currie AR. Cell death in the normal neonatal rat adrenal cortex. *J Pathol* 1973;111:255–261.
114. Strange R, Li F, Saurer S, Burkhard A, Friis RR. Apoptotic cell death and tissue remodelling during mouse mammary gland involution. *Development* 1992;115:49–58.
115. Hsueh AJW, Billig H, Tsafriri A. Ovarian follicle atresia. A hormonally controlled apoptotic process. *Endocr Rev* 1994;15:707–724.
116. Tilly J, Kowalski KI, Johnson AL, Hsueh AJW. Involvement of apoptosis in ovarian follicular atresia and postovulatory regression. *Endocrinology* 1991;129:2799–2801.
117. Hurwitz A, Adashi EY. Ovarian follicular atresia as an apoptotic process. In: Adashi EY, Leung PCK, eds. *The Ovary*. New York; Raven Press, 1993;473–485.
118. O'Shea JD, Hay MF, Cran DG. Ultrastructural changes in the theca interna during follicular atresia in sheep. *J Reprod Fertil* 1978;54: 183–187.
119. Azmi TI, O'Shea JD. Mechanism of deletion of endothelial cells during regression of the corpus luteum. *Lab Invest* 1984;51:206–217.
120. Weedon D, Strutton G. Apoptosis as the mechanism of the involution of hair follicles in catagen transformation. *Acta Derm Venereol (Stockh)* 1981;61:335–369.
121. Schellens JPM, Everts V, Beertsen W. Quantitative analysis of connective tissue resorption in the supra-alveolar region of the mouse incisor ligament. *J Periodontal Res* 1982;17:407–422.
122. Gobé GC, Axelsen RA. Genesis of renal tubular atrophy in experimental hydronephrosis in the rat. Role of apoptosis. *Lab Invest* 1987; 56:273–281.
123. Gobé GC, Axelsen RA, Searle JW. Cellular events in experimental unilateral ischemic renal atrophy and in regeneration after contralateral nephrectomy. *Lab Invest* 1990;63:770–779.
124. Don MM, Ablett G, Bishop CJ, et al. Death of cells by apoptosis following attachment of specifically allergized lymphocytes in vitro. *Aust J Exp Biol Med Sci* 1977;55:407–417.
125. Berke G. The binding and lysis of target cells by cytotoxic lymphocytes. Molecular and cellular aspects. *Annu Rev Immunol* 1994;12: 735–773.
126. Enari M, Hug H, Nagat S. Involvement of an ICE-like protease in Fas-mediated apoptosis. *Nature* 1995;375:78–81.
127. Krams SM, Egawa H, Quinn MB, Martinez OM. Apoptosis as a mechanism of cell death in a rat model of liver allograft rejection. *Transplant Proc* 1995;27:466–467
128. Ferrara JLM, Deeg HJ. Graft-versus-host disease. *N Engl J Med* 1991; 324:667–674.
129. Patel T, Gores GJ. Apoptosis and hepatobiliary disease. *Hepatology* 1995;21:1725–1741.
130. Nakanuma Y, Ohta G, Kono N. Kobayashi K, Kato Y. Electron mi-

croscopic observation of destruction of biliary epithelium in primary biliary cirrhosis. *Liver* 1983:3:238–248.
131. Paus R, Rosenbach T, Haas N, Czarnetzki BM. Patterns of cell death. The significance of apoptosis for dermatology. *Exp Dermatol* 1993; 2:3–11.
132. Shen Y, Shenk TE. Viruses and apoptosis. *Current Opin Genet Dev* 1995;5:105–111.
133. Ameisen JC, Estaquier J, Idziorek T. From AIDS to parasite infection. Pathogen-mediated subversion of programmed cell death as a mechanism for immune dysregulation. *Immunol Rev* 1994;142:9–51.
134. Laurent-Crawford AG, Krust B, Muller S, et al. The cytopathic effect of HIV is associated with apoptosis. *Virology* 1991;185:829–839.
135. Kerr JFR. Neglected opportunities in apoptosis research. *Trends Cell Biol* 1995;5:55–57.

# Cutaneous

*Histology for Pathologists, second edition,*
Edited by Stephen S. Sternberg.
Lippincott-Raven Publishers, Philadelphia
© 1997.

# CHAPTER 2

# Normal Skin

Carlos D. Urmacher



The skin is the largest organ of the body, covering its entire surface. The skin is divided into three layers: (a) epidermis; (b) dermis; and (c) the subcutaneous adipose tissue. Each layer has a complex structure and function (1–2) that varies according to age, gender, race, anatomic location, and structure. Functions of the skin are extremely diverse. It serves as a mechanical barrier and as an immunologic organ. It participates in electrolyte regulation and is an important organ of sensuality and psychological well-being. In addition, it is a vehicle that expresses not only primary diseases of the skin, but also of the internal organs. An understanding of the skin's normal histology is essential to the understanding of pathologic conditions.

## EMBRYOLOGY

### Epidermis

The ectoderm gives rise to the epithelial components of the skin. The mesoderm provides the mesenchymal elements of the dermis.

C. D. Urmacher: North Shore University Hospital, Manhasset, New York, 11020.

First, the embryo is covered by a single layer of ectodermal cells. By the sixth to eighth week of development a second layer, the periderm, is added. The surface of the periderm is covered by microvilli and is in contact with the amniotic fluid. The mitotic activity of the basal layer predominates over that of the periderm and soon the basal layer becomes the germinative layer. From this proliferating basal cell layer, rows of cells are added to form additional layers between the basal layer and the periderm. By week 23 keratinization has taken place in the upper stratum and the cells of the periderm have already been shed (3–5). In addition, by the end of the first trimester, the dermoepidermal junction with its components is ultrastructurally similar to that of mature skin (6). Thus, the characteristic neonatal epidermis is well developed by the 4th month.

Melanocytes, Merkel cells, and Langerhans' cells are seen in the epidermis of 8- to 10-week-old embryos. The precursor cells of melanocytes migrate from the neural crest to the dermis and then to the epidermis where they differentiate into melanocytes during the first 3 months of development. During this migration melanocytes can reside in other organs and tissues.

Langerhans' cells are derived from the bone marrow. The characteristic cytoplasmic marker, the Birbeck granule, is seen ultrastructurally in 10-week-old embryos (7), and the characteristic immunohistochemical markers are completed by week 12 of development.

The Merkel cells can also be seen in the epidermis of 8- to 10-week-old embryos. However, their origin is debatable. Some have suggested a neural crest derivation (8), whereas others suggest a process of differentiation from neighboring keratinocytes in the epidermis (9–12).

### Dermis

The dermis is derived from the primitive mesenchyme underlying the surface ectoderm. The papillary and reticular dermis are recognized by the 120th day of intrauterine life (13).

As described by Breathnach (13), three types of cells are recognized in 6- to 14-week-old embryos. Type 1 cells are stellate-dendritic cells with long slender processes. These are the most numerous primitive mesenchymal cells and probably give rise to the endothelial cells and the pericyte. Type 2 cells have less extensive cell processes; the nucleus is round, and the cytoplasm contains large vacuoles. They are clasified as phagocytic macrophages of yolk-sac origin.

Type 3 cells are round with little or no membrane extensions but they contain numerous vesicles, some with an internal content suggestive of secretory or granule formation. These cells could be melanoblasts on their way to the epidermis or they could be precursors to mast cells; Schwann cells associated with neuroaxons, but lacking basal lamina, are also identified during this period.

In weeks 14 to 21 of development, type III collagen fibers are abundantly present in the matrix. Eventually, they become type I collagen seen in adult skin. Fibroblasts are easily recognized as elongated spindle cells with abundant rough endoplasmic reticulum.

Also identified during this period are presumptive perineurial cells because of their association with the Schwann cell-axonal complex.

The type 2 mesenchymal cell is rarely seen after week 14 of development. However, another cell type with ultrastructural features of a histiocyte or free macrophage is frequently seen during this time.Also, well-formed mast cells are seen in the dermis.

Elastic fibers appear in the dermis during the 22nd week, and by week 32 a well-developed network is formed (5). After week 24, fat cells develop in the subcutaneous tissue from the primitive mesenchymal cells.

Initially, the dermis is organized into somites but soon this segmental organization stops and the dermis of the head and neck and extremities organize into dermatomes along the segmental nerves that are being formed (14).

### Epithelial Skin Appendages

The hair follicle originates from basal cells in the epidermis. In 10-week-old embryos, a group of mesenchymal cells of the developing dermis aggregate beneath a budding group of tightly packed basal cells (15). These epidermal cells grow both downward to the dermis as solid epithelial columns, and upward through the epidermis to form the opening of the hair canal. As the growing epithelial cells reach the subcutaneous fat, the lower portion becomes bulbous and partially encloses the mesenchymal cells descending with them, to form the dermal papillae of the hair follicle. The descending epidermal cells around the dermal papillae constitute the matrix cells from which the hair layers and the inner root sheath will develop. The outer root sheath derives from downward growth of the epidermis. The first hairs appear by the end of the third gestational month as lanugo hair around the eyebrows and upper lip. The lanugo hair is shed around the time of birth. The developing hair follicle gives rise to the sebaceous and apocrine glands.

The sebaceous glands originate as epithelial buds from the outer root sheath of the hair follicles and are developed at approximately the 13th to 15th gestational week (16). They respond to maternal hormones and are well formed at the time of birth.

The apocrine glands develop also as epithelial buds from the outer root sheath of the hair follicles in 5- to 6-month-old fetuses (14,15) and continue into late embryonic life as long as new hair follicles develop.

The eccrine glands develop from the fetal epidermis independent of the hair follicles (14). Initially, they are seen as regularly spaced undulations of the basal layer. At 14 to 15 weeks the tips of the primordial eccrine glands have reached the deep dermis, forming the eccrine coils (19). At the same time, the eccrine epithelium grows upward into the epidermis. The primordial eccrine epithelium acquires a lumen by the 7th to 8th fetal month and thus, the first eccrine unit is formed. Both ducts and secretory portions are lined by two layers of cells. The two layers in the secretory segment undergo further differentiation; the luminal cells into tall columnar secretory cells, and the basal layer into secretory cells or myoepithelial cells (5). The first glands are formed on the palms, soles, and digits by the 4th month, on the axillae in the 5th month, and finally on the rest of the hairy skin (18).

## PHYSIOLOGY

### Epidermis

The epidermis serves as a mechanical barrier against agents from within as well as from without. Langerhans' cells function as immunologic cells by recognizing antigens and presenting them to immunocompetent T-cell lymphocytes.

Melanocytes with their production of melanin are the natural protectors against the damaging effects of ultraviolet light.

The keratinocytes are responsible for the process of keratinization. The formation of keratin filaments, in association with desmosomes, hemidesmosomes, and basement membrane provides the structural integrity of the epidermis (20). Different types of keratin intermediate filaments are expressed in fetal and adult skin and this process is, in part, regulated by apoptosis.

### Apoptosis

Apoptosis or programmed cell death is the mechanism by which cells are deleted in normal tissues (21) and is the process responsible in establishing the final normal architecture of adult skin (22).

Terminal differentiation of the epidermis into a stratified squamous layer can be considered a specialized form of apoptosis (22).

Apoptosis also participates in the cycling of the hair follicle (23–25) and is the principal mechanism by which catagen hair is formed (26–28).

The bcl-2 proto-oncogen is a protein that blocks apoptosis or programmed cell death and is expressed in basal cell keratinocytes and in the dermal papillae, protecting the latter from apoptosis (26).

Apoptosis affects individual cells and not groups of cells as in necrosis (21). The basic morphologic changes include fragmentation of the nucleus, chromatin compaction, and budding of the cells to produce membrane-bound apoptotic bodies which are ingested by neighboring cells. No inflammation is seen with the process of apoptosis (21).

By light microscopy, apoptotic cells are seen as isolated cells with bright eosinophilic cytoplasms and with dark, pyknotic and fragmented nuclei (Fig. 1).

In routine hematoxilin-eosin (H&E)-stained sections, apoptotic bodies are seen in a large variety of inflammatory and neoplastic diseases such as graft-versus-host disease, lichen planus, erythema multiforme, squamous carcinomas, and malignant melanomas.

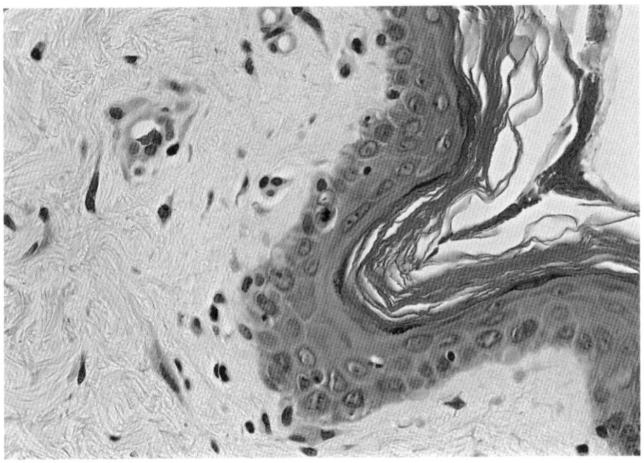

**FIG. 1.** Apoptotic cell in a case of erythema multiforme. Note eosinophilic cytoplasm and condensed nucleus..

### Eccrine and Apocrine Glands

The most important function of the eccrine glands is thermoregulation. The eccrine glands are the true sweat glands and their function begins in the neonatal period. Eccrine sweat is a colorless and odorless hypotonic solution composed predominately of water and the same electrolytes that are present in the plasma. The clear cell of the eccrine coil, responding predominately to cholinergic stimuli, and to a lesser degree to sympathetic stimulation (29–31), produces an isotonic sweat. When this reaches the duct, $Na+$ and $Cl-$ is reabsorbed, delivering a hypotonic solution to the surface.

The function of the dark cells is unknown. It has been suggested that they permit reabsorption of sodium, potassium, and chloride (15) and may contribute sialomucin (32) to the sweat.

In addition, the eccrine duct has the important function of delivering parenteral or orally administered drugs to the surface of the skin (33). Ductular epithelium also participates in the process of wound healing(14).

The major function of the myoepithelial cells is mechanical support against a high hydrostatic pressure.

Neither the composition nor the exact mode of secretion of the apocrine glands is known (15,17). In nonhuman mammals, apocrine glands are found over the entire skin surface; they are believed to serve as identifying or sexual organs (15). Apocrine secretion has a milky color and is sterile and odorless; however, when it reaches the surface of the skin the action of regional bacteria on the apocrine secretion causes the skin to become odorous (15).

Cystic fibrosis is (29,34) the best known of diseases affecting normal sweating. Few morphologic changes are seen in association with these diseases.

### Dermis

The dermis with its mesenchymal components provides the mechanical support, rigidity, and thickness to the skin. It also has immunologic functions because of its contents in dendritic cells and macrophages. Mast cells react to inflammatory processes and also participate in wound healing.

Blood vessels, in addition to providing nutrients to the skin, are also involved in thermoregulation, sharing this function with the sweat glands.

Small and large nerve plexuses participate in the innervation of the different cutaneous organs that are responsible in the detection of pain, pressure, and temperature variation.

## LIGHT MICROSCOPY

### Epidermis

The epidermis is a stratified squamous epithlium that constantly grows but maintains its normal thickness by the pro-

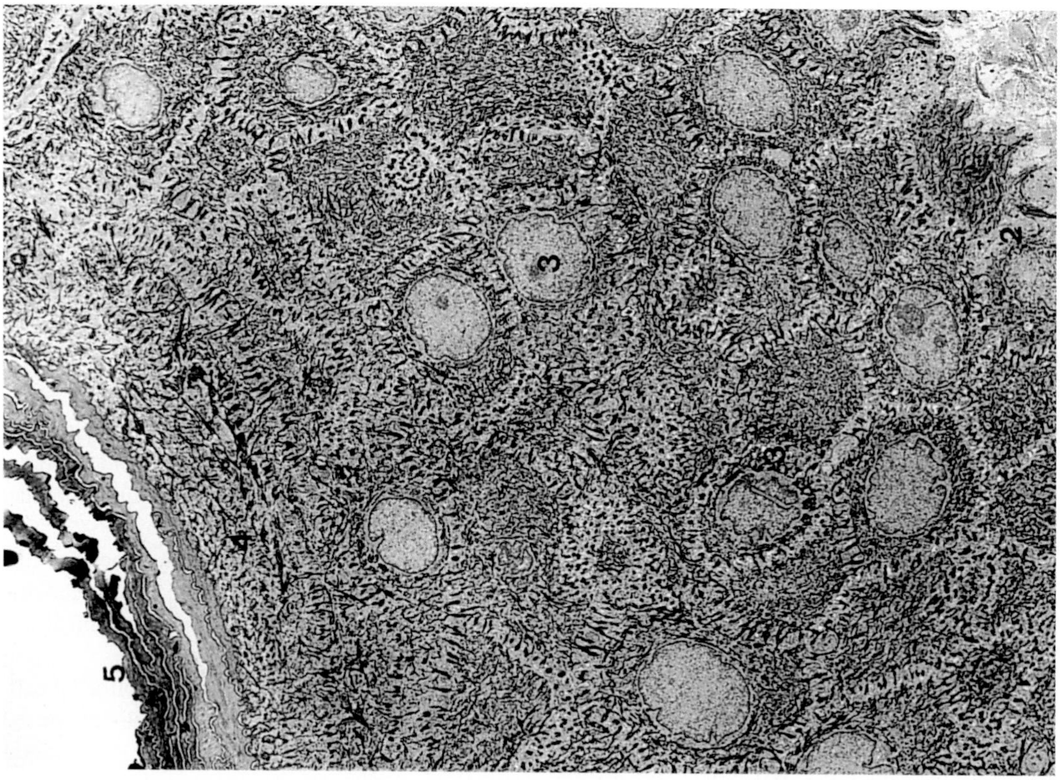


**FIG. 2.** Electron micrograph of normal epidermis and portion of papillary dermis (**x2,100**). 1 = papillary dermis, 2 = basal cells, 3 =squamous layer, 4 = granular layer, 5 = cornified layer.

cess of desquamation. The cells in the epidermis are: a) keratinocytes; b) melanocytes; c) Langerhans' cells; and d) Merkel cells. In addition, the epidermis also contains the openings for the eccrine ducts and hair follicles.

### *Keratinocytes*

The keratinocytes of the epidermis are orderly stratified into four layers: (a) the basal layer (stratum basale, germinatum); (b) the squamous layer (prickle cell or stratum spinosum); (c) the granular layer (stratum granulosum); and (d) the outermost layer, the cornified layer (stratum corneum, horny layer) (Fig. 2). In histologic sections the dermoepidermal junction has an irregular contour because of the upward extension of the papillary dermis to form the dermal papillae. The portion on the epidermis separating the dermal papillae are the rete ridges (Fig. 3).

### *Basal Layer*

Basal cells are the mitotically active cells that give rise to the other keratinocytes. In histologic sections, basal cells are seen as a single row of cells above the basement membrane that show some variation in size, shape, and melanin content. Basal cells are elongated or cuboidal, with melanin in their cytoplasms as a result of pigment transfer from neighboring melanocytes. The nucleus is round or oval with coarse chromatin and with an indistinct nucleolus. Basal cells are connected to each other and to keratinocytes by specialized regions located in plasma cell membranes known as desmosomes.

Dermatitis involving the basal layer produces vacuolar alteration of the basal cells which may progress to the forma-

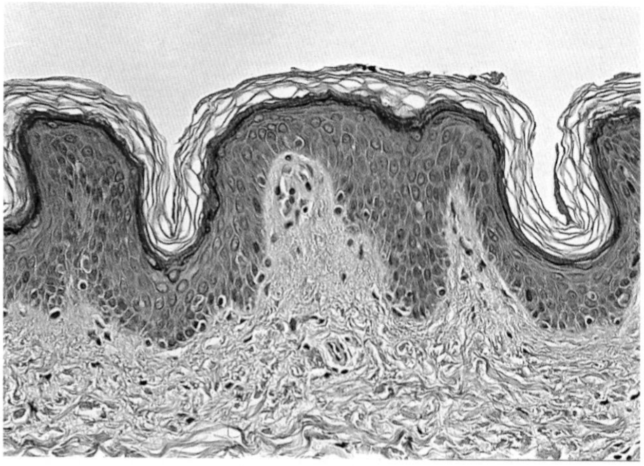

**FIG. 3.** Normal skin. Stratified epidermis. Note rete ridges. Papillary dermis is inmediately beneath the epidermis (*level II in melanoma staging*). Junction of papillary and reticular dermis (*level III*). Reticular dermis (*level IV*).

tion of subepidermal vesicles as seen in graft-versus-host disease, lupus erythematosus, and erythema multiforme.

### *Squamous Layer*

The squamous layer is also called the spinous or prickle cell layer because of the characteristic appearance by light microscopy of short projections extending from cell to cell. These projections are the result of retraction of the plasma membrane during tissue processing whereas the desmosomes remain relatively fixed.

Desmosomes are composed of a variety of polypeptides; the desmoplakins and the desmogleins. Antibodies to these desmosomes are used as additional markers for the study of neoplasms (35).

The squamous layer is composed of several layers of cells. The suprabasal keratinocytes are polyhedral, somewhat basophilic, and with a round nucleus. Again, melanin is seen scattered in many of these keratinocytes serving as natural protection against the damaging effects of sunlight. The more superficial cells are larger, flattened, eosinophilic, and oriented parallel to the surface. An intercellular space of constant dimensions (36) is present between each cell. The pemphigus antigen is localized in the cell membranes (37) or in the desmosomes of these cells (38).

In the interface between the squamous and granular layers, the keratinocytes contain lamellar granules composed of lipids and neutral sugars conjugated to proteins and lipids. They also contain acid hydrolases. These granules are not visible by light microscopy. Their function is to provide epidermal lipids, to increase the barrier properties of the cornified layer, and to aid in the desquamation process. This interface is also the site of synthesis and storage of cholesterol (36,39).

It is important to recognize that occasionally, cells with clear or pale cytoplasms are seen in the squamous layer. These cells must be distinguished from the neoplastic cells of Paget's disease. Benign clear cells have a pyknotic nucleus surrounded by a clear halo and a narrow rim of clear cytoplasm (Fig. 4). They lack the pleiomorphism, nuclear morphology, and intensity of chromatin staining of Paget's cells. These benign clear cells are often seen in the nipple epidermis (40) or in the epidermis at other sites often associated with benign papules. In the nipple, they have been considered to be nonneoplastic mammary elements (40). Those outside of the nipple are considered to be the result of either abnormal keratinization or aberrant derivatives of sweat gland epithelial cells (41,42). The immunohistochemical and mucin staining pattern of benign clear cells may resemble that of Paget's cells and, therefore, they must be distinguished on a morphologic basis from the neoplastic cells.

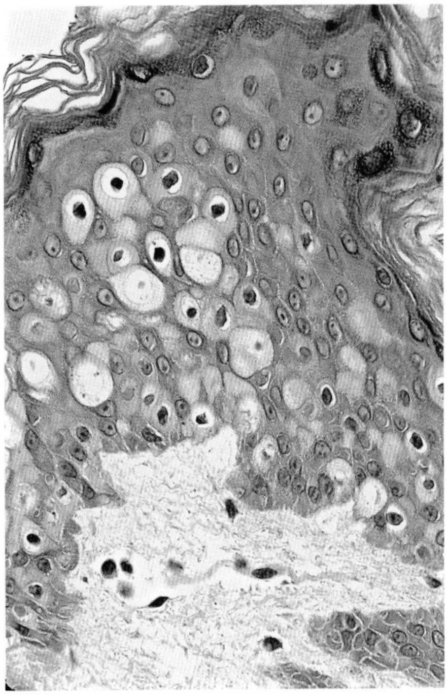

**FIG. 4.** Clear cells of the nipple epidermis.

Common inflammatory changes seen in the squamous layer are: (a) spongiosis: intercellular edema (e.g. contact dermatitis); (b) acanthosis : thickening of the epidermis (e.g. psoriasis); (c) atrophy: thinning of the epidermis (e.g. discoid lupus erythematosus); (d) acantholysis: detachment of keratinocytes because of changes involving the intercellular junctions (e.g. pemphigus); and (e) dyskeratosis: abnormal keratinization (e.g. squamous carcinoma).

### *Granular Layer*

The granular layer is composed of one to three layers of flattened cells containing intensely basophilic-stained granules known as the keratohyaline granules. Trichelemmal granules (hair follicles) are red in routine H&E-stained sections (H&E). These granules are histidine-rich and are the precursors to the protein filaggrin that promotes aggregation of keratin filaments in the cornified layer. The increase (e.g. lichen planus) or decrease (e.g. psoriasis) in the thickness of this layer can be used as a clue in the diagnosis of different pathologic entities.

### *Cornified Layer*

The cornified layer is composed of multiple layers of polyhedral cells that are arranged in a basket-weave pattern (Fig. 5). These cells are the most differentiated cells of the keratinizing system. They lose their nucleus and cytoplasmic organelles and are composed entirely of high-molecular-weight keratin filaments. These cells eventually shed from the surface of the skin. The process of keratinization takes 20 to 45 days.

In histologic sections taken from the skin of the palms and soles, it is possible to identify a homogeneous eosinophilic zone above the granular layer known as the *stratum lucidum*.

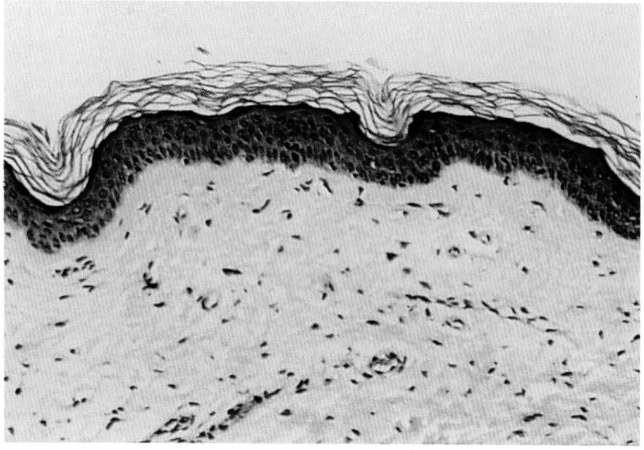

**FIG. 5.** Basket-weave pattern of the cornified layer (also in Fig. 3).

Common abnormalities of the cornified layer are: (a) hyperkeratosis (increased thickness of the cornified layer as seen in some cases of solar keratosis); (b) parakeratosis (the presence of nuclei in the cornified layer as seen focally in psoriasis); (c) presence of fungal forms (superficial dermatophytosis).

### *Basement Membrane Zone*

The basement membrane separates the epidermal basal layer from the dermis. It is seen by light microcopy as a continuous and thin periodic acid-Schiff (PAS)-stained layer (Fig. 6). As seen by electron microcopy, the basal cells are

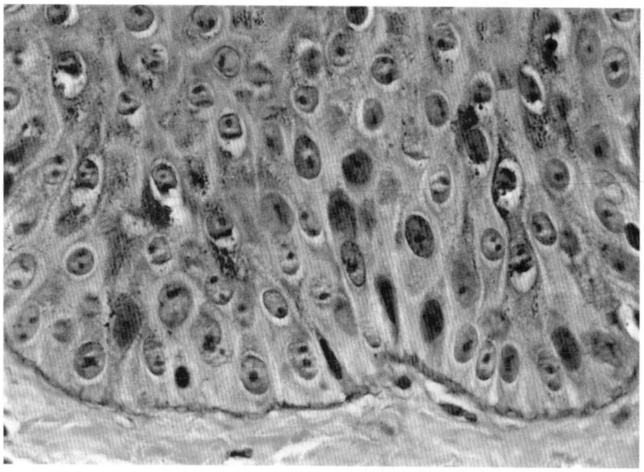

**FIG. 6.** PAS-positive basement membrane.

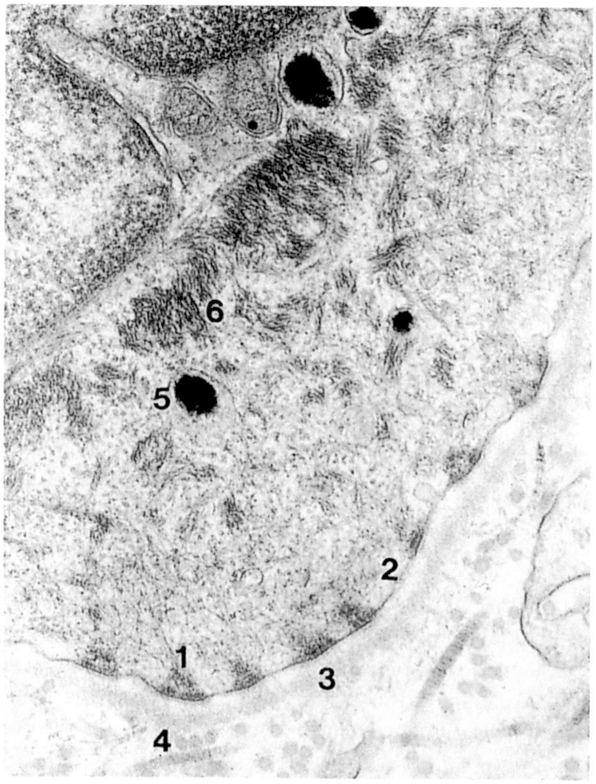


**FIG. 7.** Ultrastructure of basement membrane (**x37,800**). 1 = hemidesmosome, 2 = lamina lucida, 3 = lamina densa, 4 = lamina reticularis, 5 = melanin, 6 = tonofilaments.

attached to the basal lamina by hemidesmosomes (36). Ultrastructurally, the basal lamina is composed of four different regions (Fig. 7)(36,43). From the epidermis to the dermis, they are respectively: (a) the plasma membrane of the basal cells containing the hemidesmosomes and anchoring filaments; (b) the lamina lucida, an electron-lucent area composed of laminin (44) and bullous pemphigoid antigen (45,46), it is also the site of the blister in dermatitis herpetiformes (47); (c) the lamina densa, an electron-dense area composed of type IV collagen; and (d) the sublamina densa or pars fibroreticularis containing the structures that attach the basal lamina to the connective tissue of the dermis, namely extensions of the lamina densa and the anchoring fibrils (48), and the antigen to epidermolysis *bullosa acquisita* (47).

Inflammatory conditions of the basement membrane can be seen by light microscopy as thickening (discoid lupus erythematosus) or by the formation of subepidermal vesicles as in bullous pemphigoid.

### *Melanocytes*

Melanocytes are dendritic cells that derive from the neural crest. During migration from the neural crest melanocytes may localize in other epithelia. In the epidermis, the melanocytes are located in the basal layer and their dendritic processes extend in all directions. The dendritic nature of normal melanocytes is usually not seen in routine H&E-prepared histologic sections.

In H&E preparations, melanocytes are seen as cells in the basal layer and composed of elongated or ovoid nuclei surrounded by a clear space (Fig. 8). They are usually smaller than the neighboring basal keratinocytes. Melanocytes do not contain tonofilaments (17,32) and do not attach to basal cells. However, anchoring filaments extend from the plasma membrane of these melanocytes to the basalamina. In addition, melanocytes that are close to the basal lamina have structures resembling half-desmosomes.

Melanocytes produce and secrete melanin. Melanin can be red (pheomelanin) or yellow-black (eumelanin) (49,50). The most important function of melanin is to protect against the damaging effects of nonionizing ultraviolet irradiation.

Melanin is formed through a complex metabolic process in which tyrosinase is the main catabolic enzyme. The synthesis of melanin takes place in melanosomes, which in the early stages of development are membrane-limited vesicles, located in the Golgi-associated endoplasmic reticulum (32) or stage 1 melanosome. Stage 2 melanosomes contain numerous filaments with distinct periodicity. In stage 3, melanin deposits are prominent. In stage 4 the organelle is ellipsoidal, it is melanin-packed and with no recognized internal structure.

The developing melanosomes, with their content of melanin, are transferred to the neighboring basal cells and hair follicular cells. The mechanism of melanin transfer is a complex one, with the end result being phagocytosis of the tips of the melanocytic dendrites by the keratinocytes (Fig. 9) in a process called pigment donation (51).

The number of melanocytes in normal skin is constant in all races, the ratio being one melanocyte for every 4 to 10 basal keratinocytes (17,49). Thus, the color of the skin is determined by the number and size of melanosomes present both in keratinocytes and melanocytes, and not by the number of melanocytes. The number of melanocytes decreases

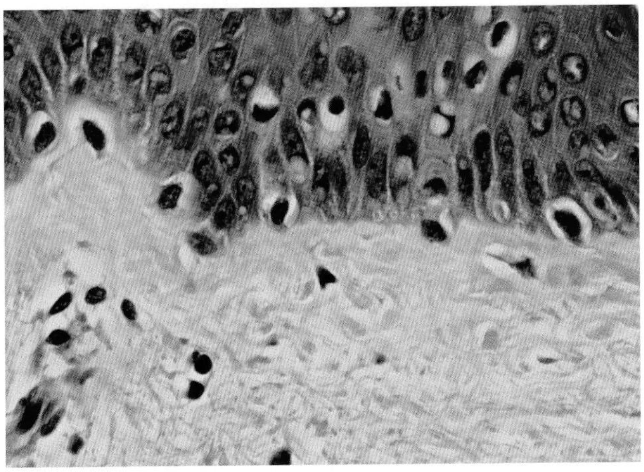

**FIG. 8.** Melanocytes in the basal layer, composed of ovoid nuclei within a clear space.

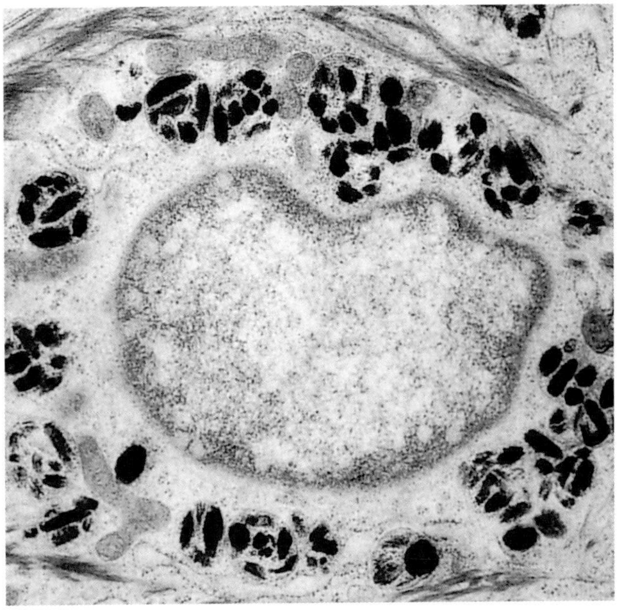

**FIG. 9.** Electron micrograph showing membrane-bound phagocytized melanin in keratinocyte (**x19,200**).

with age. As a result, the availability of melanin to keratinocytes diminishes, the skin becomes lighter, and the incidence of skin cancer increases.

Melanin is both argentaffin and argyrophilic. In addition, melanocytes and their dendritic processes are identified by the dopa reaction in histologic slides prepared from frozen sections and in paraffin-embedded sections with immunohistochemical reactions with S-100 protein. The latter is highly sensitive but is not specific for cells of melanocytic lineage. Under normal conditions, the melanoma-associated antigen HMB45 does not react with adult melanocytes (52). It is usully seen reacting with most melanoma cells, Spitz's nevus, the junctional component of nevi, and, at times, in dysplastic nevi.

A decrease or absent number of melanocytes is seen in vitiligo. In albinism, there is a defect in the synthesis of melanin but the number of melanocytes is normal in a skin biopsy. Melanocytic hyperplasia is seen in lentigos, benign and malignant melanocytic neoplasms, and as a reaction pattern in a variety of neoplastic and nonneoplastic conditions (e.g. dermatofibroma). In a freckle, there is an increase in pigment donation to adjacent keratinocytes, rather than melanocytic hyperplasia (51).

### *Langerhans' Cells*

Langerhans' cells (LC) are dendritic and are derived from precursor cells in the bone marrow. In the epidermis they are located in the mid-to-upper part of the squamous layer. In H&E-stained sections, LC can be suggested as they appear to lie within lacunae with darkly stained nuclei that at high magnification have a reniform shape (Fig. 10). As with the

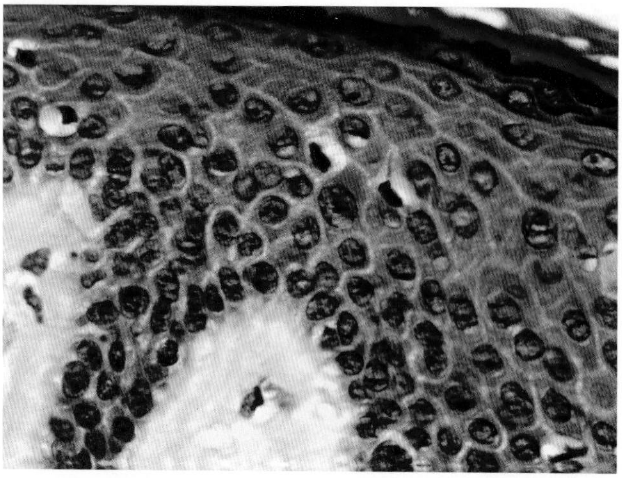

**FIG. 10.** H&E section of possible Langerhans' cells composed of elongated nuclei surrounded by a clear space in the mid-epidermis.

melanocyte, their dendritic nature cannot be seen in routine sections. LC can be detected in formalin-fixed, paraffin-embedded tissues using immunoreactivity for S-100 protein and, more specifically, the antibody to the CD1a antigen (Fig. 11). With these procedures the extensive dendritic nature of LC becomes evident.

By electron microscopy LC show no desmosomes, tonofilaments, or melanosomes. They contain small vesicles, multivesicular bodies, lysosomes, and the characteristic Birbeck granule (53), a rod-shape organelle measuring 15 to 50 nm long and 4 nm wide (Fig. 12). Birbeck granules have a centrally striated density and an occasional bulb at one end. Their function is not known.

LC are also present in other epithelia, lymphoid organs, and dermis and are increased in the skin in a variety of inflammatory conditions such as contact dermatitis, where they can be seen as minute nodular aggregates in the epidermis. Langerhans' cell granulomatosis is a reactive lesion most commonly seen in bones, but also appearing at other sites.

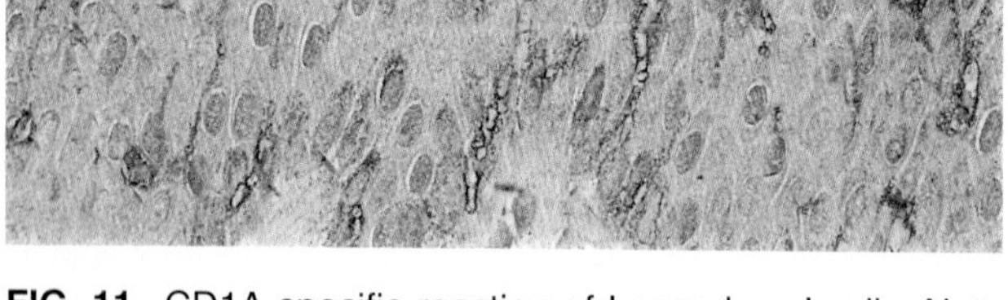

**FIG. 11.** CD1A specific reaction of Langerhans' cells. Note dendritic processes.

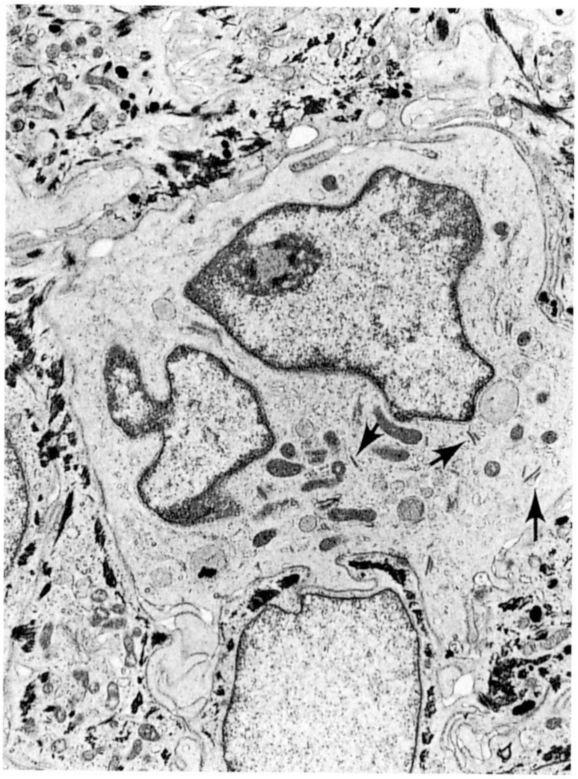

**FIG. 12.** Electron micrograph of a Langerhans' cell containig Birbeck granules (*arrows*) and multisegmented nucleus (**x8,000**).

### *Merkel Cells*

Merkel cells are considered to mediate tactile sensation. They are located in higher concentration in the glaborus skin of the digits, lips, and oral cavity (9), in the outer root sheath of hair follicles (54), and in the tactile hair discs (55).

Merkel cells are not seen in routine histologic preparations. Electron microscopy and immunostaining are required for their identification. By electron microscopy, Merkel cells are attached to adjacent keratinocytes by desmosomes. Merkel cells have scant cytoplasms, invaginated nuclei, a parallel array of cytokeratin filaments in the paranuclear zone, and the characteristic membrane-bound dense core granules that are often, but not always, related to unmyelinated neurites.

By immunostaining techniques normal and neoplastic Merkel cells may express neuron-specific enolase, bombesin, adrenocorticotrophic hormone, Leu-enkephalin, substance P, and vasoactive intestinal polypeptide (56–58). However, the expression of these substances in Merkel cells is heterogeneous and variable. Neurofilament expression is best seen on frozen sections as paranuclear balls (57,59). A

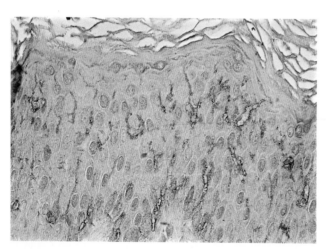

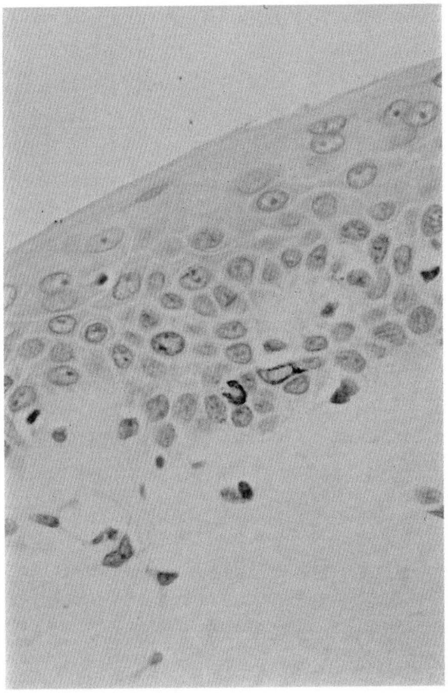

**FIG. 13.** Cytokeratin 20 staining a Merkel cell in the basal layer of the epidermis.

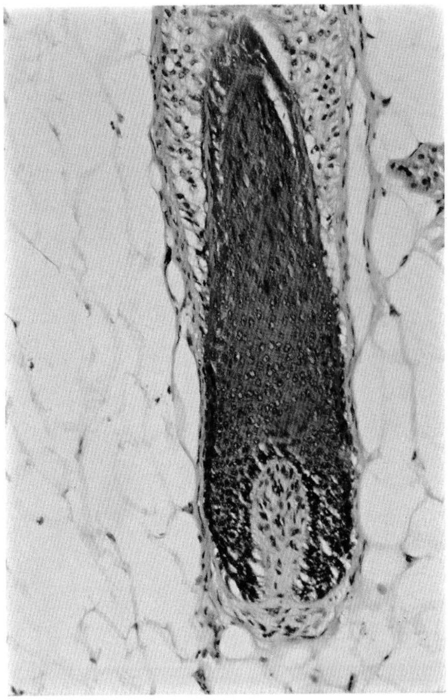

**FIG. 14.** Inferior segment of the hair follicle, showing the hair papilla.

constant pattern seen in Merkel cells is the presence of paranuclear aggregates of cytokeratins (10,58,59). The most specific cytokeratin is #20 (CK 20) because in addition to Merkel cells, they are expressed in simple epithelia and not in adjecent keratinocytes (60) (Fig. 13).

The importance of Merkel cells is their participation in neuroendocrine carcinomas.

### *Pilar Unit*

The pilar unit is composed of the hair follicle, sebaceous gland, arrector-pili muscle, and (when present) the apocrine gland.

#### *Hair Follicle*

The hair follicle is divided into three segments: (a) the infundibulum, which extends from the opening of the hair follicle in the epidermis to the opening of the sebaceous duct; (b) the isthmus, which extends from the opening of the sebaceous duct to the insertion of the arrector-pili muscle; and (c) the inferior segment, which extends to the base of the follicle. This segment is bulbous and encloses a vascularized component of the dermis referred to as the dermal papilla of the hair follicle (Fig. 14).

The microanatomy and function of the hair follicle is very complex.

The cells of the hair matrix differentiate along six cell lines (Fig. 15). Beginning from the innermost layer, the six cell lines are: (a) the hair medulla; (b) hair cortex; (c) hair cuticle; and (d) three layers of the inner root sheath, which are the cuticle of the inner root sheath, Huxley's layer, and Henle's layer.

The inner root sheath of the hair follicle is surrounded by a layer of clear cells, the outer root sheath (Fig. 16). These glycogen-rich cells are seen in some of the neoplasms with hair follicular differentiation (e.g. trichilemmoma). A PAS-positive basement membrane separates the outer root sheath from the surrounding connnective tissue.

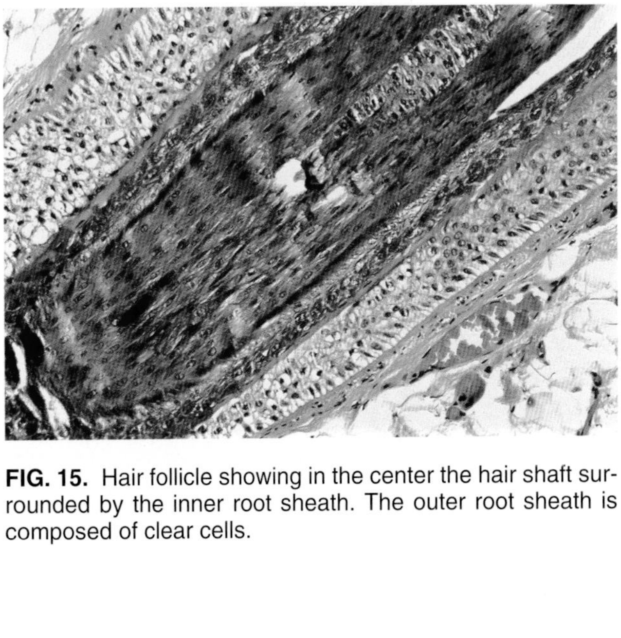

**FIG. 15.** Hair follicle showing in the center the hair shaft surrounded by the inner root sheath. The outer root sheath is composed of clear cells.

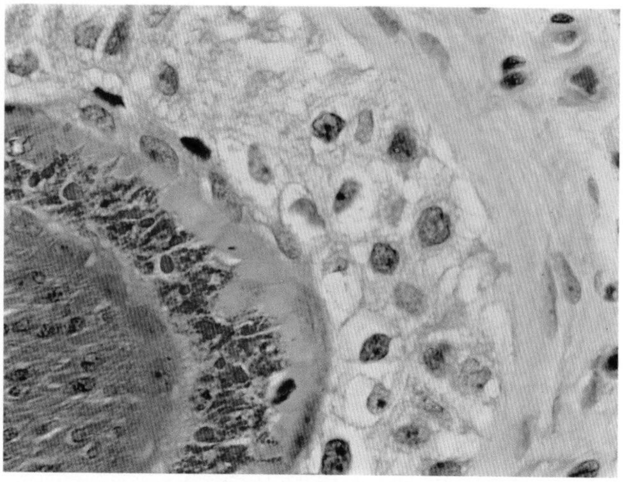

**FIG. 16.** Outer root sheath and Huxley's layer containing trichohyaline granules.

Dendritic melanocytes are present only in the upper half of the bulb, whereas inactive (amelanotic) melanocytes are present in the outer root sheath, These melanocytes can become active after injury, migrating into the regenerating epidermis (32).

At the level of the isthmus, the cells of the inner root sheath disentegrate and disappear whereas, the cells of the outer root sheath begin an abrupt sequence of keratinization. This process is called tricholemmal keratinization (61). Trichohyaline granules are red in routine H&E-stained sections as opposed to the blue granules of epidermal keratinization, also characteristic of the epithelium of the infundibulum of the hair follicle. The staining features of these granules permit neoplasms and cysts of either pilar or epidermal origin to be distinguised.

Under normal circumstances, microorganisms like *Staphylococcus epidermis*, yeasts of *Pityrosporum* (Fig. 17), and the *Demodex folliculorum* mite are encountered in the follicular infundibulum.

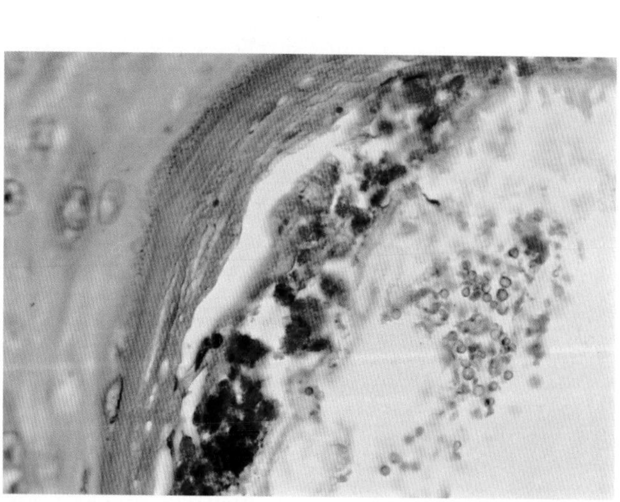

**FIG. 17.** Yeasts of *Pityrosporum* in the follicular infundibulum.

The mantle hair of Pinkus (62) is a hair follicle in which proliferation of basaloid epitheliod cells emanating from the infundibulum is seen. Sebaceous proliferation is present in these cords (Fig. 18). The significance of this hair follicle is not known.

The hair growth is cyclical. Three phases are recognized: (a) anagen, or growing phase; (b) catagen or involuting phase; and (c) telogen, the resting phase. The histologic features previously described correspond to the anagen hair.

During the catagen phase, mitosis and melanin synthesis ceases at the level of the hair bulb. The hair bulb is then replaced by a cornified sac formed by retraction of the outer root sheath around the hair bulb, and a club hair is formed. A thick glassy basement membrane surrrounds the hair follicle. Apoptosis of single cells in the outer root sheath is a characteristic finding during the catagen phase (28).

During telogen, the club hair and its cornified sac retract even further to the insertion of the arrector-pili muscle, leaving behind the dermal papillae, which is connected to the retracted hair follicle by a fibrous tract (Fig. 19) (15). When the cycle is complete a new anagen phase begins with the formation of new hair matrix.

The duration of the normal hair cycle varies. The anagen phase is measured in years for the scalp, but it is measured in shorter periods of time for the anagen cycle in other regions of the body. The length of the hair is also related to the amount of the anagen hair. More than 80% of hair present in normal scalp is anagen hair. The catagen phase takes 2 to 3 weeks and the telogen phase may last a few months.

The color of normal hair depends on the amount and distribution of melanin in the hair shaft (15). Fewer

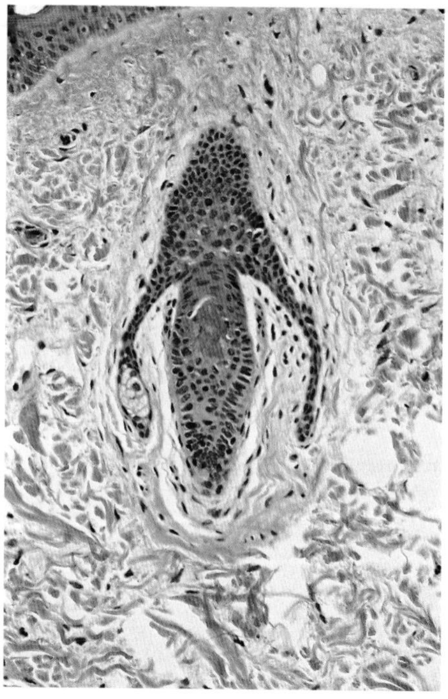

**FIG. 18.** Mantle hair of Pinkus with lateral extensions containing sebaceous cells.

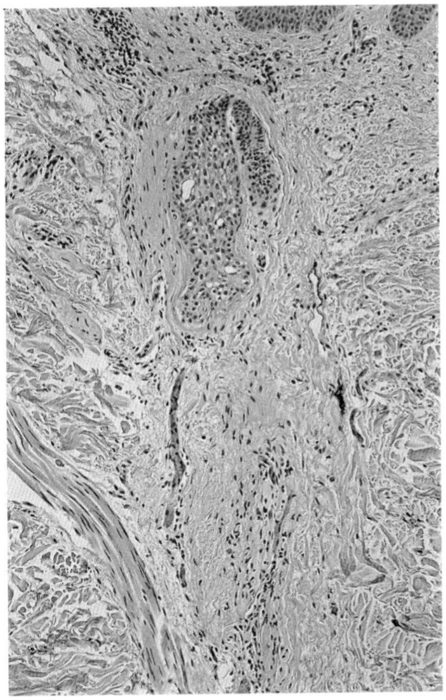

FIG. 19. Catagen-telogen hair follicle located entirely within the dermis.

melanosomes are produced in bulbar melanocytes of blond hair. A relative absence of melanin and fewer melanosomes are seen in gray hair. In red hair, the melanin has a different chemical composition and melanosomes are round, rather than ellipsoidal.

Another structure related to the pilar unit is the hair disc (Haarscheibe). This structure is usually not recognized on routine histologic sections. It is a touch receptor in close vicinity to hairs. The epidermis above this area has more Merkel cells in the basal layer and the dermal component is well vascularized, containing myelinated nerve fibers in contact with Merkel cells (14,55).

### *Sebaceous Glands*

The sebaceous glands are holocrine glands; their secretions are made of disintegrated cells. The palms and soles are the only regions devoid of sebaceous glands. Sebaceous glands are also seen in the buccal mucosa, vermilion of the lip (Fordyce), prepuce, labia minora, and, at times, in the parotid gland.

The sebaceous glands are lobulated structures composed of multiple acini in some locations like the head and neck; in other sites, such as the chest, they are composed of a single acinus. The periphery of the lobules contain the germinative cells, which are cuboidal or flat with large nucleoli and basophilic cytoplasms. As differentiation occurs lipid droplets accumulate in the cytoplasm until they fill the cell.

The more differentiated cells have a characteristic multivacuolated cytoplasm (Fig. 20). The nucleus is centrally lo-

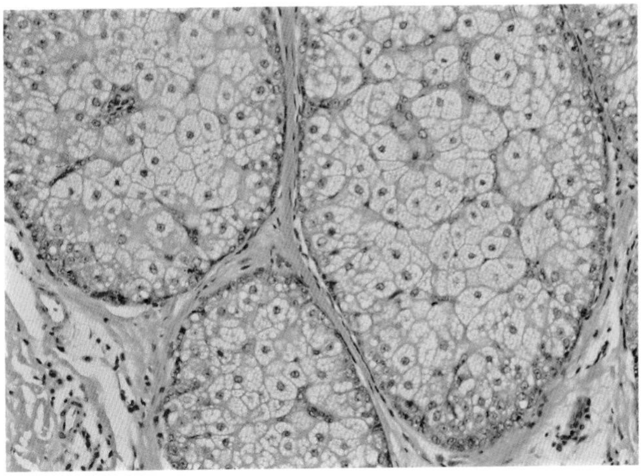

FIG. 20. Sebaceous glands with peripheral germinative cells and toward the center the differentiated vacuolated cells.

cated and scalloped due to the lipid imprints. The more differentiated cells disintegrate, discharging the cellular debris (sebum) into the excretory duct, which opens into the hair follicle in the lower portion of the infundibulum. The excretory duct is short, shared by several lobules, and lined by keratinized squamous epithelium.

### *Apocrine Glands*

The apocrine gland has a coiled secretory portion and an excretory (ductal) component. The secretory portion (Fig. 21) is much longer than its eccrine counterpart; it may reach 3 to 5 mm in diameter, compared to 0.3 to 0.4 mm for the eccrine gland (17). The secretory glands, which are located in the subcutaneous fat or in the deep dermis, are lined by one layer of cuboidal, columnar, or flat cells (luminal cells), and a layer of myoepithelial cells. The luminal cells are composed of eosinophilic cytoplasm, which may contain lipid, iron, lipofuscin, PAS-positive diastase-resistant granules (15), and a large nucleus located near the base of the cell. De-

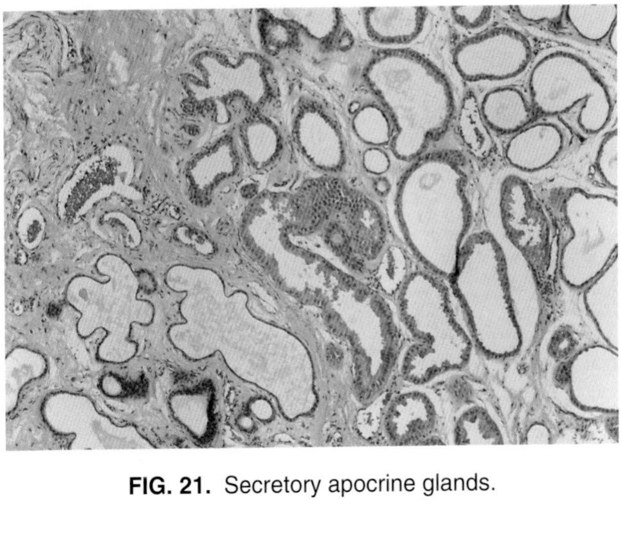

FIG. 21. Secretory apocrine glands.

tached fragments of apical cytoplasm are found in the lumen of these glands. In addition, a PAS-positive basement membrane surrounds the gland.

Histologically, the excretory (ductal) component of the apocrine gland has a double lining of cuboidal cells similar to the eccrine duct. Microvilli are identified on the surfaces of luminal cells and keratin filaments in their cytoplsms, the latter giving the hyaline appearance to the inner lining of the duct. No myoepithelial cells are identified in the excretory duct.

Apocrine glands are mostly located in the axilla, mammary region, anogenital area, eyelids (Moll), and ears (ceruminous) and their presence is characteristic in nevus sebaceous.

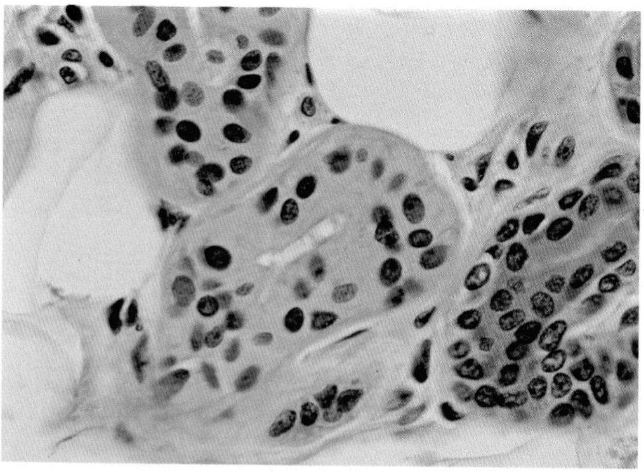

**FIG. 23.** Clear cells of the eccrine glands.

### *Eccrine Glands*

The eccrine glands are the true sweat glands responsible for thermoregulation. They are found in high concentration in palms, soles, the forehead, and axillae and have dual secretory and excretory properties.

The secretory portion of the eccrine gland is a convoluted tube located in the dermis, in the interface with the subcutaneous tissue and, rarely, within the subcutaneous tissue. In cross sections it appears that several glandular structures with a central lumen form the secretory coil. These are seen as lobular structures often surrounded by fat even when located within the dermis (Fig. 22).

Three cell types compose the eccrine coil: clear cells, dark cells, and myoepithelial cells. The clear cells are easily seen in routine sections (Fig. 23). They rest directly on the basement membrane and on the myoepithelial cells. Clear cells are composed of pale or finely granular cytoplasms with a round nucleus usually seen in the center of the cell. Deep invaginations of the luminal membranes of adjacent clear cells form intercellular canaliculi lined with microvilli (Fig. 24) (63). The intercellular canaliculi often persist in neoplasms derived from eccrine glands. The clear cells contain abundant mitochondria and variable amounts of glycogen.

The dark cells border the lumen of the glands. Electron microscopy shows that they contain abundant secretory granules that have glycogen-staining characteristics. They contain ribosomes and some fat. The dark cells are difficult to identify in routine H&E-stained sections; however, when acid-fast, PAS, or immunohistochemestry with S-100 protein are done, the granularity becomes apparent (Fig. 25)(14).

The myoepithelial cells are contractile spindle cells that surround the secretory coil (Fig. 26). In turn, they are surrounded by a PAS-positive basement membrane. Elastic fibers, fat, and small nerves are present in the adjacent stroma.

The excretory component of the eccrine gland is composed of three segments (a) a convoluted duct in close association with the secretory unit (Fig. 27); (b) a straight dermal component; and (c) a spiral intraepidermal portion, the

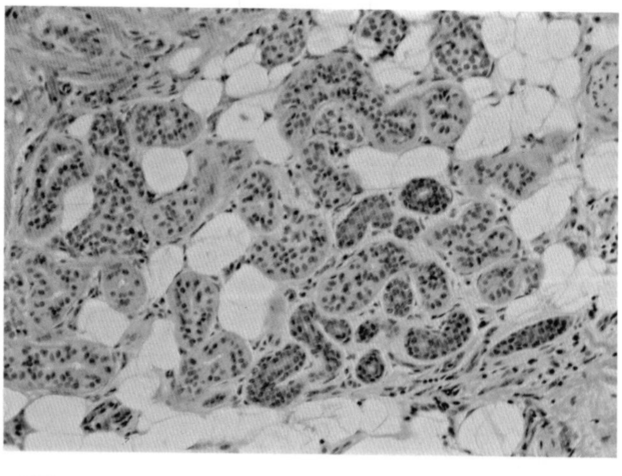

**FIG. 22.** Eccrine lobule containing fat, glands, and ducts.

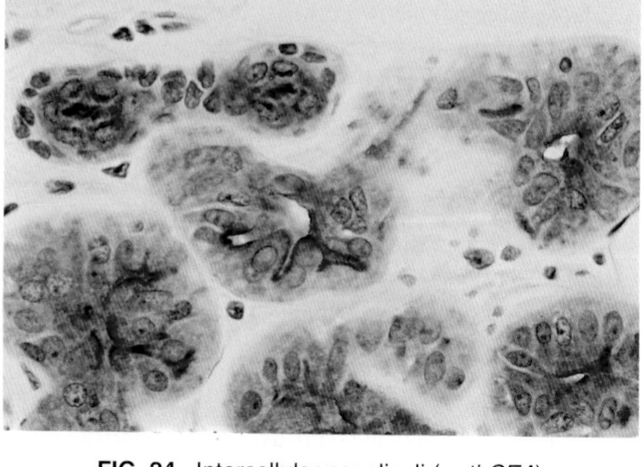

**FIG. 24.** Intercellular canaliculi (*anti-CEA*)

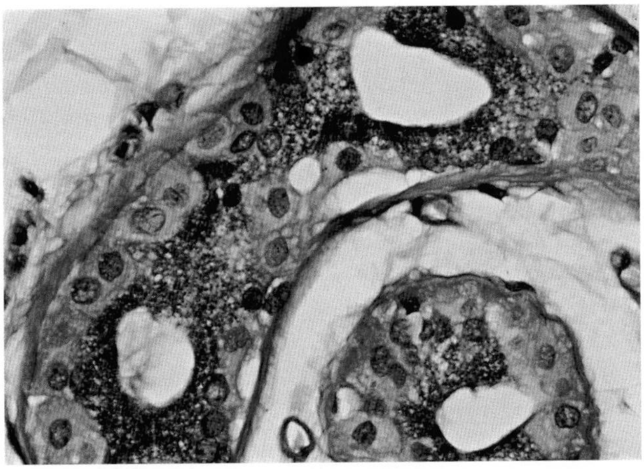

**FIG. 25.** Dark cells with granular cytoplasm (*acid-fast stain*).

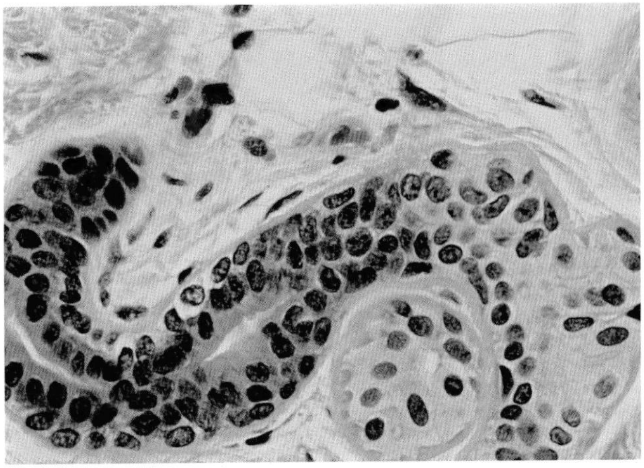

**FIG. 27.** Eccrine duct. Note abrupt transition from the secretory portion.

acrosyringium, which opens onto the surface (Fig. 28). The transition between the secretory and the excretory component is abrupt. Both convoluted and straight dermal ducts are histologically identical. They are narrow tubes with a slitlike lumina lined by a double layer of cuboidal cells. The adluminal cells have a more granular eosinophilic cytoplasm and a larger round nucleus than the peripheral row of cells. The peripheral cells are rich in mitochondria.

The luminal cells produce a layer of tonofilaments near the luminal membrane that are often referred to as "the cuticular border." This cuticular border often persists in eccrine neoplasms (e.g. *eccrine poroma*).

There are no myoepithelial cells. The intraepidermal segment of the duct consists of a single layer of luminal cells and two or three rows of concentrically arranged outer cells. The presence of keratohyaline granules indicates that they keratinize independently and at lower levels than surrounding keratinocytes (15,32). Melanin granules are absent.

The so-called "apoeccrine glands" of the human axillae (64) are composed of a dilated secretory portion which, by electron microscopy, is indistinguishable from the apocrine gland; however, they retain the intercellular canaliculi, as well as the dark cells of the eccrine glands. The duct does not open in the hair follicle but in the epidermis. These glands which develop from eccrine glands during puberty, account for as much as 45% of all axillary sweat glands in young persons.

## Dermis

The mesenchymal dermis is composed predominantely of type I collagen (65), a small amount of type III collagen, and elastic fibers. The dermis (Fig. 29) consists of two zones: the papillary dermis and the reticular dermis. The adventitial dermis (66) combines the papillary and the periadnexal dermis. These zones constitute important anatomic landmarks in the staging of malignant melanoma.

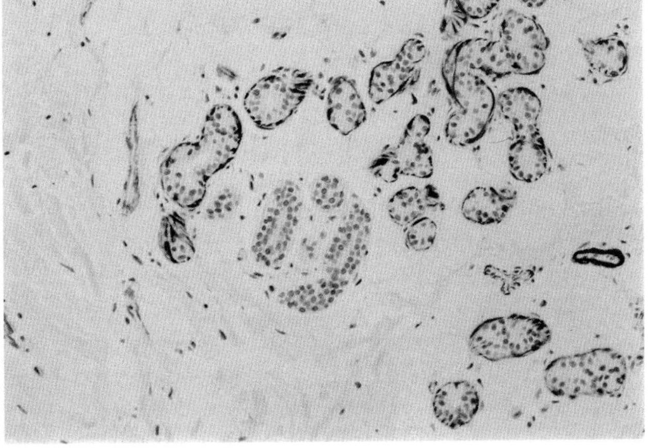

**FIG. 26.** Glands, but not the ducts are surrounded by myoepithelial cells (*anti-HHF35*).

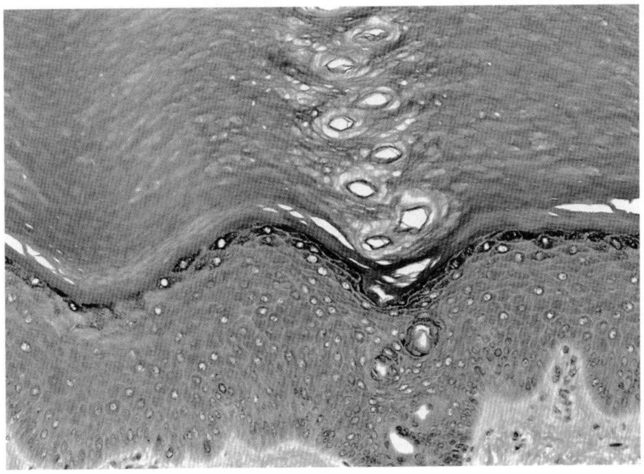

**FIG. 28.** Acrosyringium.

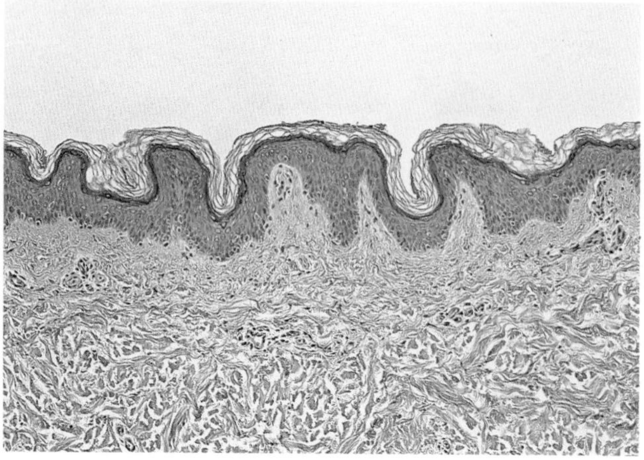

**FIG. 29.** Dermis with papillary and thick reticular dermis.

The papillary and periadnexal dermis can be recognized by their finely woven network of type I collagen mixed with some type III collagen and a delicate branching network of fine elastic fibers. The papillary dermis also contains abundant ground substance, the capillaries of the superficial plexuses and fibroblasts.

The reticular dermis is thicker than the papillary dermis and is composed of multiple layers of thick bundles of type I collagen, arranged parallel to the surface. These layers are built from overlapping plates of individual fibers of uniform size. The plates are oriented randomly in different directions (67). There are also thick, but fragmented elastic fibers which are detected with the appropiate stains (Fig. 30), some ground substance, and the vessels of the deep plexuses.

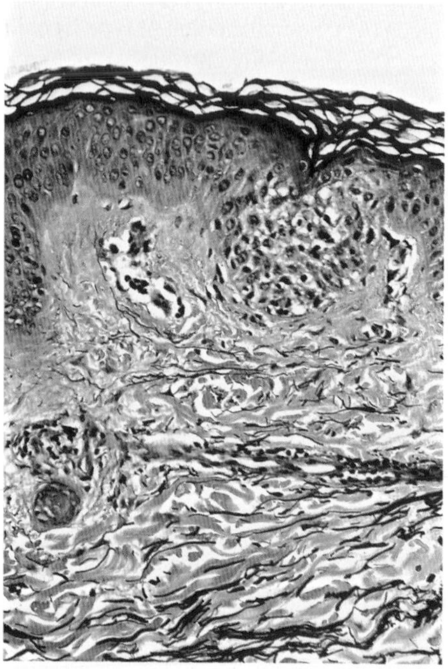

**FIG. 30.** Distribution of elastic fibers. Thin and branching in the papillary dermis, thick and fragmented in the reticular dermis.

Recent studies have shown that many, if not all, of the interstitial spindle cells of the dermis, seen in routine sections, have a dendritic appearance. Thus, the term dermal dendritic cells is being used for the interstitial cell of the collagenous dermis and subcutis (68).

The dermal dendrocyte has phagocytic function (68) and can be demonstrated immunohistochemically by using factor XIIIa (68,69).

The dermal connective tissue is embedded in a ground substance consisting mainly of nonsulfated acid mucopolysaccharides, predominantly hyaluronic acid, and to a lesser degree, chondroitin sulfate. In routine H&E-stained sections, ground substance is seen as empty spaces between collagen bundles. Special stains like colloidal iron and alcian blue are required for their visualization. In pathologic conditions such as lupus erythematosus, granuloma annulare, and dermal mucinosis the excessive amount of ground substance produced can be seen without the aid of special stains as strings of bluish material.

Besides fibroblasts or dendritic cells, the only other cells seen in the normal dermis are macrophages which become visible when pigment or other ingested material is present in the cytoplasm of the cell. There are also mast cells which are recognized by their darkly stained ovoid nucleus, granular cytoplasm, and their common perivascular location.

### Subcutaneous Tissue

The subcutaneous tissue is arranged into lobules of mature adipocytes. These lobules are separated by thin bands of dermal connective tissue that will constitute the interlobular septa (Fig. 31). Thus, inflammatory changes involving the subcutaneous tissue can be divided into septal panniculitis (e.g. erythema nodosum) and lobular panniculitis (e.g. panniculitis associated with pancreatitis) (15).

### Blood Vessels, Lymphatics, Nerves, and Muscle

The large arteries that supply the skin are located in the subcutaneous tissue, usually within the interlobular septa accompanied by larger veins. Smaller arteries, venules and capillaries constitute the main vasculature seen in the dermis and within the lobules of the subcutaneous fat.

A network of these smaller vessels are located in the deep reticular dermis (deep plexus) and in the papillary dermis (superficial plexus). Communicating vessels connect the two plexuses. This division of superficial and deep plexuses is important in the classification and recognition of many inflammatory diseases of the skin in which characteristic infiltrates are located around the superficial, deep or superificial, and deep plexuses.

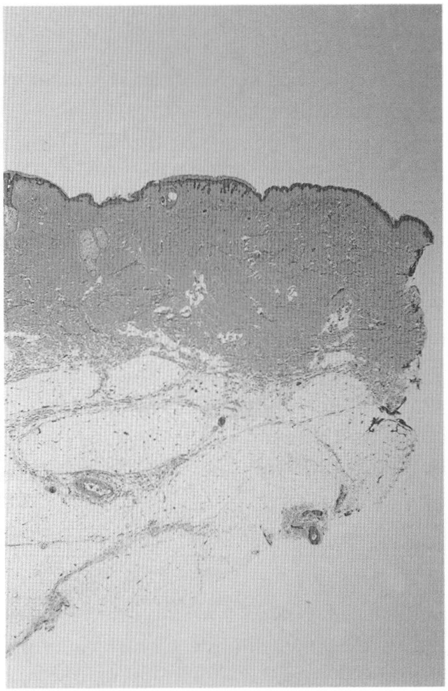

FIG. 31. Septa and lobules of subcutaneous fat.

Vasculitis is the inflammatory process that involves the blood vessels. It is important to remember that strict anatomic criteria are applied for the diagnosis of cutaneous vasculitis and they include: (a) the presence of inflammation within the vessel wall; and (b) the presence of thrombi within the lumina of these blood vessels. Inflammation within the wall (Fig. 32) may produce findings of fibrinoid necrosis and/or destruction of the blood vessel wall with extravasation of red blood cells into the adjacent tissues. Perivascular inflammation alone is not a sign of vasculitis.

In the acral skin there are arteriovenous anastomoses known as the Sucquet-Hoyer canals. They are surrounded by

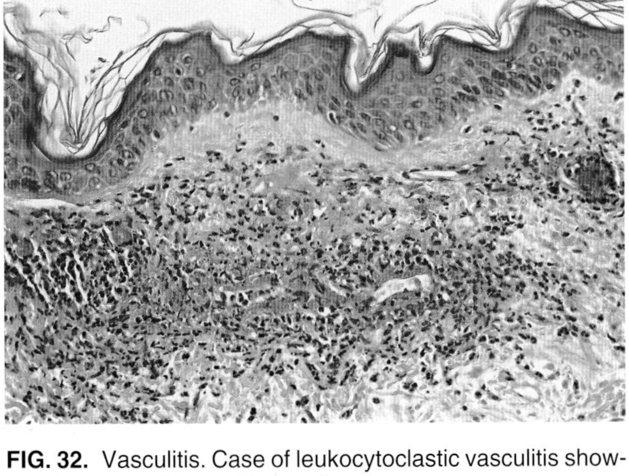

FIG. 32. Vasculitis. Case of leukocytoclastic vasculitis showing damage to the capillary wall.

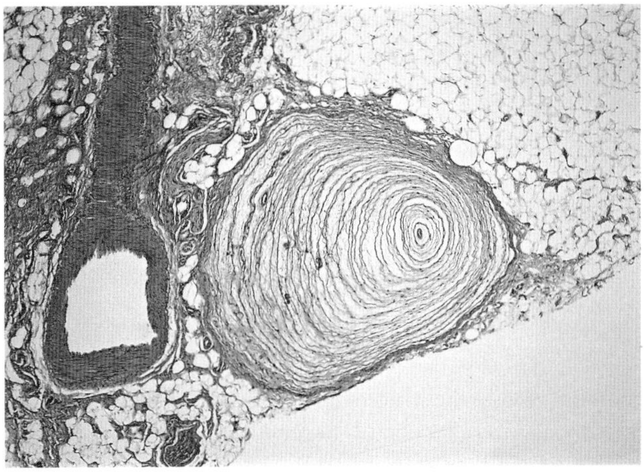

FIG. 33. Pacinian corpuscle.

a row of smooth muscle cells serving as sphincters. Each of these segments is known as glomus.

The lymphatics of the skin (70) accompany the venules and are also located in the deep and superficial plexuses. Unless valves are seen within these vessels, their recognition in routine sections is impossible. Under normal conditions they are surrounded by a cuff of elastic fibers.

Large nerve bundles are seen in the subcutaneous fat and in the deep reticular dermis; however, small nerve fibers are present throughout the skin reaching the papillary dermis. Depending on the anatomic site, concentric arrangement of cells forming nerve end organs are also seen in routine sections. In sections of the palms and soles, Meissner corpuscles are seen in the papillary dermis. In weight-bearing areas the Pacinian corpuscles are located in the deep dermis and subcutaneous fat (Fig. 33).

Smooth muscle is represented in the skin by the arrector pili muscle, which arises in the connective tissue of the dermis and inserts in the hair follicle below the sebaceous glands. Melanocytes of congenital nevi are often seen within the arrector pili muscle. Smooth muscle is also seen in the skin of external genitalia (dartos) and in the areolae.

Strands of striated muscle are found in the skin of the neck, face, and particularly the eyelids as muscles of expression.

## ANATOMIC DIFFERENCES WITH AGE

### Newborns and Children

The epidermis of newborns and children is usually of the same thickness as in adults, with the exception on the acral skin. There is a greater density of melanocytes and of Langerhans' cells.

The dermis is more cellular than in adults with a higher concentration of ground substance. The number of eccrine glands is higher at birth, while apocrine glands are not well developed until after puberty (71).

The sebaceous glands are developed in children but sebaceous secretion begins at puberty under the influence of androgen stimulation (72).

The adipocytes of the subcutaneous tissue in newborns and children are thin-walled and larger than the adult adipocytes.

### Elderly

In the elderly the histologic differences are mainly due to atrophy and to reduction of most cutaneous elements.

The thickness of the epidermis is probably the same; however, the cells are arranged haphazardly because of aberrant proliferation of the basal cell layer which may predispose to the development of neoplasms (73). There is a marked decrease in the number of melanocytes and, consequently, more exposure to the damaging effects of ultraviolet light. The number of aquired nevi also diminishes with age.

In addition, there is a decrease in the number of Langerhans' cells, which increases the damaging effects of contactants.

In the elderly, the dermis is thinned. The atrophy is the result of reduction of ground substance (73). The elastic fibers show structural and biochemical alterations that change the elasticity of the skin. The collagen bundles are thicker but stiffer. Fibroblasts, dendritic cells and mast cells are also reduced in number.

Because of the reduction in the number of capillaries of the superficial plexus, there is increased bruisability and decreased sweat with the consequent thermoregulatory problems.

Both eccrine and apocrine glands are also reduced in the elderly. However, sebaceous glands increase in size and manifest clinically as sebaceous hyperplasia.

With age, the number of hair follicles decreases and often, vellus hair will develop into terminal hairs in unusual sites such as the ear, nose, and nostrils resulting in possible cosmetic problems. Finally, there is marked atrophy of the subcutaneous tissue.

The pathologic hallmark of extrinsic aging is solar elastosis, whereas wrinkling is due to the intrinsic factors mentioned previously (74).

## STAINING METHODS

The majority of the skin lesions can be diagnosed with well-prepared H&E-stained sections. However, they will not provide an adequate answer in all cases. A comprehensive review of "special stains" is beyond the scope of this chapter because every case is different and may require a specific approach. The following are the most common stains used in our laboratory in the study of cutaneous tissues.

### Histochemical Stains:

1. PAS: to study the thickness of the basement membrane, for glycogen and fungal forms.
2. Gomori's methanamine silver: for fungal forms and cutaneous *Pneumocystis carinii*.
3. Ziehl-Nielsen and Fite stains: for acid-fast organisms.
4. Gram stains: for bacteria.
5. Steiner and Warthin-Starry stains: in cases of bacillary angiomatosis and for spirochetes.
6. Giemsa: for protozoan organisms and mast cells.
7. Mucicarmine: for mucin.
8. Alcian blue: for acid mucin.
9. Congo red: for amyloid.
10. Elastic Van Gieson (EVG): for elastic fibers.

### Immunofluorescence:

The specimens are received in saline-soaked gauze for direct immunofluorescence studies. Cryostat sections are prepared and antibodies against immunoglobulins A, G and M, as well as against fibrinogen and complement are routinely used.

### Immunohistochemical Stains:

Most of the time these stains are used in panels and not as single preparations. The most commonly used in our laboratory are:

1. Epithelial markers: Cytokeratins CAM 5.2 (Fig. 34), a combination of cytokeratins AE1/AE3 and carcinoembryonic antigen (CEA). They are used in the differential diagnosis of epithelial tumors and Paget's disease.
2. Melanocytic markers: S-100 protein and HMB45.
3. Mesenchymal markers:

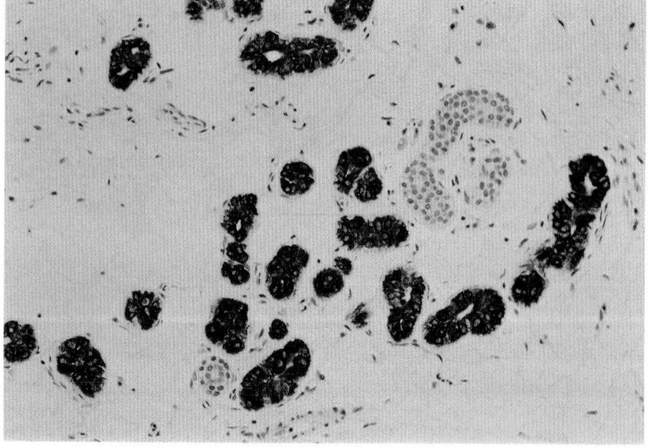

**FIG. 34.** CAM 5.2 immunostaining the secretory glands but not the ducts.

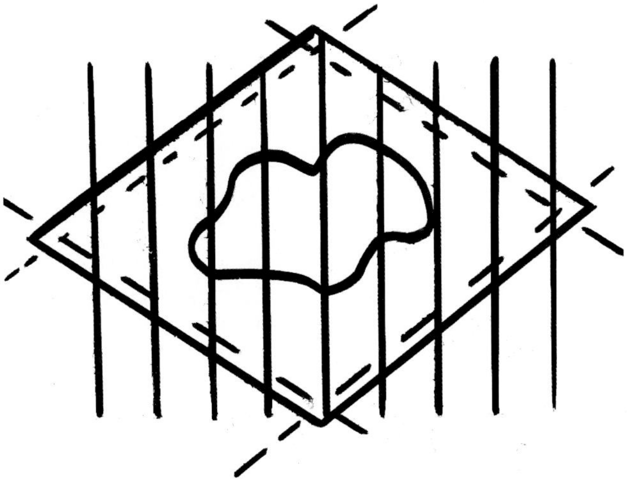

**FIG. 35.** The entire neoplasm in the center of the lesion is examined by bread-loafing the specimen; the deep margin is also evaluated. The lateral margins are included in each section submitted for histologic evaluation, or they can be submitted separately by cutting them along the depicted interrupted lines.

Vimentin and Factor XIII A (dendritic cells, macrophages).
S-100 protein for nerves, fat, and cartilage.
HHF35, smooth muscle actin and desmin for muscle differentiation.
Factor VIII-associated antigen, CD31, and CD34 in endothelial differentiation. CD34 in combination with Factor XIII A are useful markers in the diagnosis of dermatofibrosarcoma protuberans (75).

4. Lymphoid markers: CD40 (lymphocytes), CD45RO (T cell), CD20 (B cell), and CD30 (Ki-1). Others are added depending on each case.
5. Histiocytic markers: CD68 (KP-1) and lysozyme.
6. Langerhans' cells and Langerhans' cell granulomatosis: CD1A and S-100 protein.

## SPECIMEN HANDLING

Specimens needed for immunofluorescence, flow cytometry, molecular studies, and electron microscopy are sent fresh in saline-soaked gauze. If the specimens are excisional biopsies or larger surgical material, proper sharing of the specimen is done, always with consideration that histology has priority if no prior diagnosis exists for that particular patient.

"Punch" and "shave" biopsies are described grossly and embedded intact on "edge." Usually, five levels are cut.

Excisional biopsies and surgical specimens obtained for neoplasms are described grossly and the entire undersurface and sides of the specimen are inked prior to sectioning. The margins are evaluated by cutting along all margins or by entirely "bread loafing" the specimen. (Fig. 35). The entire neoplasm is evaluated also using the "bread-loafing" technique.

## ARTIFACTS

Poor histologic preparations can be the result of artifacts that will hamper the evaluation of a slide(s) by the pathologist. These artifacts can be the result of: (a) Poor or no fixation of the specimen prior to cutting. Solutions used are old, the fixation time is short, or the volume of fixative employed is not adequate. Ideally, the specimens must be properly fixed in solutions 15–20 times the volume of the specimen (76); (b) the lack of proper monitoring the different steps involved in the preparation of a slide such as cutting, temperature of the water bath, the freshness of the staining solutions employed, and other factors; (c) artifacts produce at the time of excision such as cautery (Fig. 36) and excessive squeezing of the specimen and, (d) artifacts produced characteristically by certain pathologic processes such as tissue holes in basal-cell carcinomas (Fig. 37) and, the lack of epidermis in sections from toxic epidermolytic necrolysis.

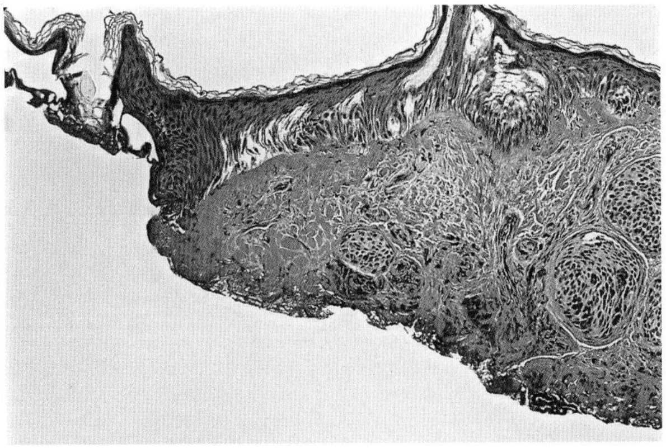

**FIG. 36.** Cautery effect in a melanocytic lesion of an adult patient, difficult to evaluate.

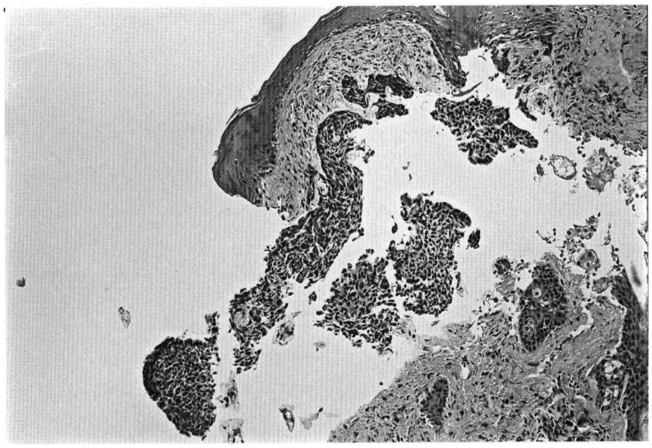

**FIG. 37.** Tissue defects in a basal cell carcinoma, which appear in the spaces after multiple sections were performed.

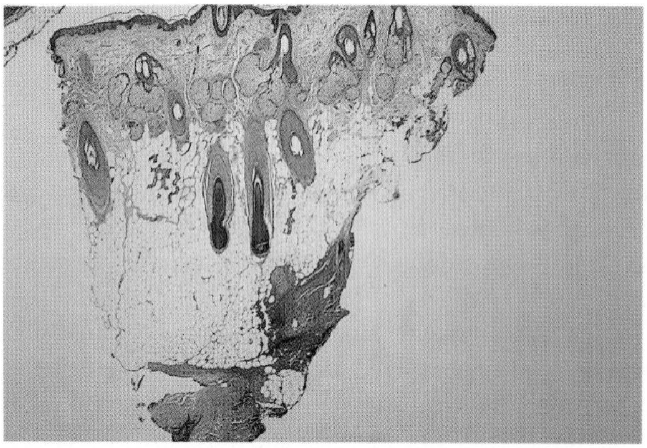

**FIG. 38.** Section of scalp showing hair follicles extending into the subcutaneous tissue.

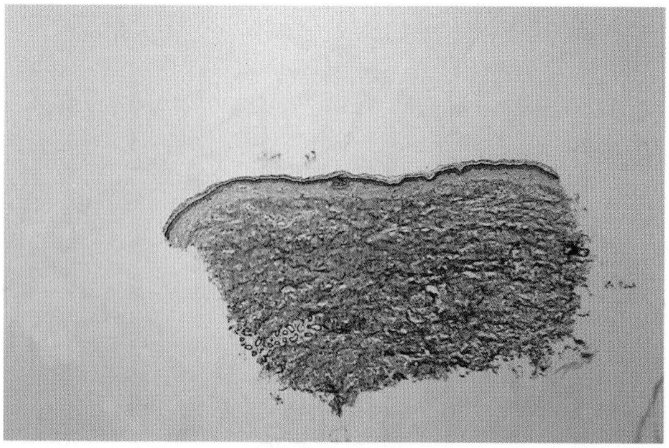

**FIG. 40.** Section of skin of the back showing the normal reticular dermis.

## HISTOLOGIC VARIATIONS ACCORDING TO ANATOMIC SITES

Regional variations of the normal histomorphology are important to recognize, so as not to interpret these variations as abnormal.

The normal scalp and other densely hair-containing regions show hair follicles extending through the dermis into the subcutaneous fat (Fig. 38). This is usually not seen in areas with less concentration of hair. Abundant vellous hair is seen in sections taken from the skin of the ear. The skin of the face shows characteristically numerous pilosebaceous units (Fig. 39), and large sebaceous glands are seen on the nose.

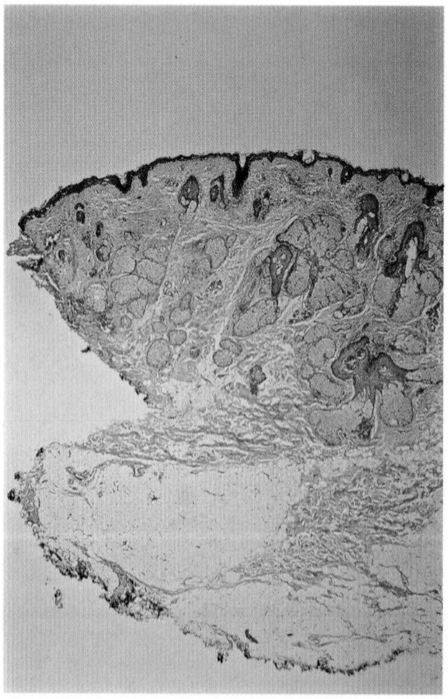

**FIG. 39.** Skin of face with pilosebaceous units.

The squamous layer of the eyelid epidermis is thin and composed of two to three layers of cells and basaloid epithelial buds. Modified apocrine glands (Moll's glands) and vellous hairs are seen in the dermis.

Sections taken from the skin of the trunk, especially the back, show a normally thick reticular dermis when compared to other sites (Fig. 40). Unawareness of this normal variation may lead to the erroneous diagnosis of processes producing thick collagen such as scleroderma.

The palms and soles show a thick and compact cornified layer with loss of the characteristic basket-weave pattern (Fig. 41). In addition, there are numerous eccrine units, nerve end organs, and glomus structures seen in the dermis. There are no pilosebaceous units.

Sections of the skin of the lower leg may show thicker blood vessels in the papillary dermis as a result of gravity and stasis (Fig. 42).

Muscle fibers are seen in the dermis of the skin of genitalia and areola.

Cutaneous-mucosal junctions may lack granular and

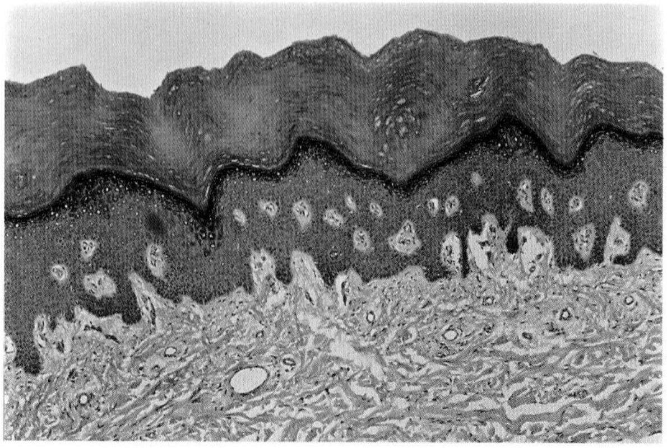

**FIG. 41.** Histologic section of the palm.

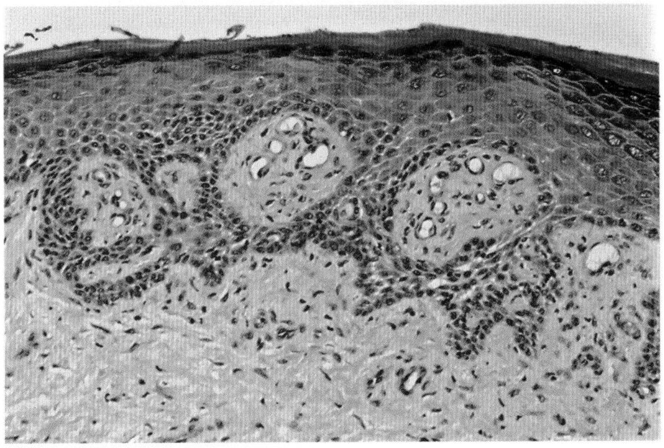

**FIG. 42.** Skin of the leg showing a proliferation of small thickened blood vessels secondary to stasis.

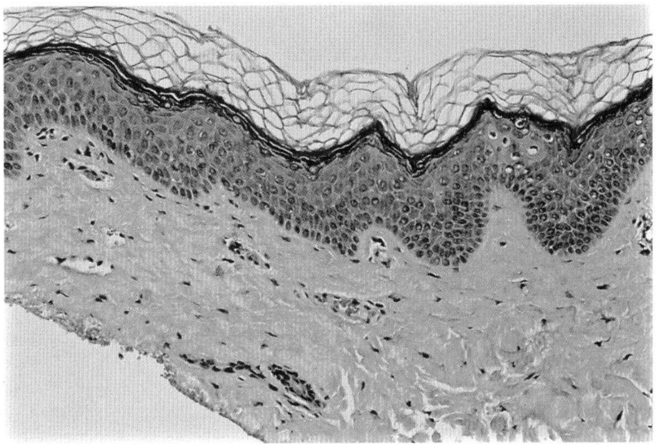

**FIG. 44.** Vitiligo. Note the absence of basal melanocytes.

cornified layers and the cells of the squamous layer are larger with a higher glycogen content.

## PATHOLOGIC CHANGES FOUND IN BIOPSIES INTERPRETED AS "NORMAL" SKIN

This refers to biopsies taken from clinically abnormal skin that histologically may be interpreted as normal because of the subtle changes present. The following are some examples.

Dermatophytosis is seen in the cornified layer (Fig. 43) of an otherwise normal skin.

A thick or absent granular layer may indicate an abnormal process of keratinization like psoriasis or an ichthyosiform dermatosis.

Vitiligo (Fig. 44) may give histologically the impression of normal skin unless one searches for melanocytes.

Lichen amyloidosis (Fig. 45) may be overlooked because the pink globules of amyloid seen in the papillary dermis can be mistaken for normal dermis.

Urticaria produces only edema, which in routine sections is seen as separation of collagen bundles in the dermis. Similar changes are seen in cases of dermal mucinosis in which deposition of mucinous material may not be obvious in routine sections.

The so-called "connective tissue nevi" with an overproduction of collagen, elastic fibers, and ground substance is another condition that can be erroneously interpreted as normal skin.

In telangiectasia macularis eruptiva pertans, a type of mast cell infiltrate of the skin, the changes can be quite subtle and are composed of dilated blood vessels in the upper dermis with a scant infiltrate of round cells. The infiltrate must be confirmed with appropiate stains for mast cells.

Trichotillomania is a hair-pulling habit resulting in areas of alopecia. Although histologic changes can be numerous (15), at times hair follicles devoid of hair are the only changes seen, which give an initial impression of normal skin in the biopsy material.

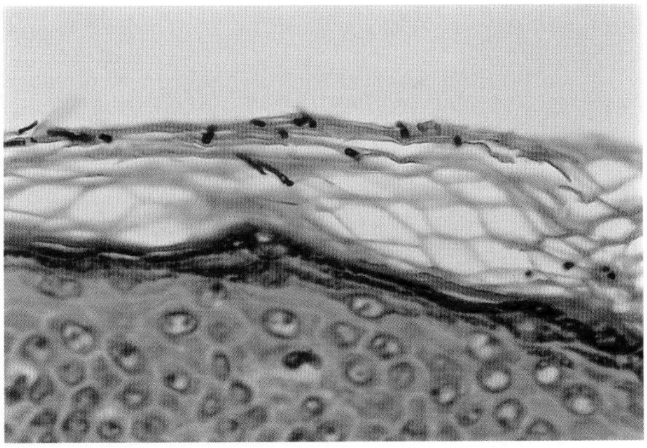

**FIG. 43.** Superficial dermatophytosis.

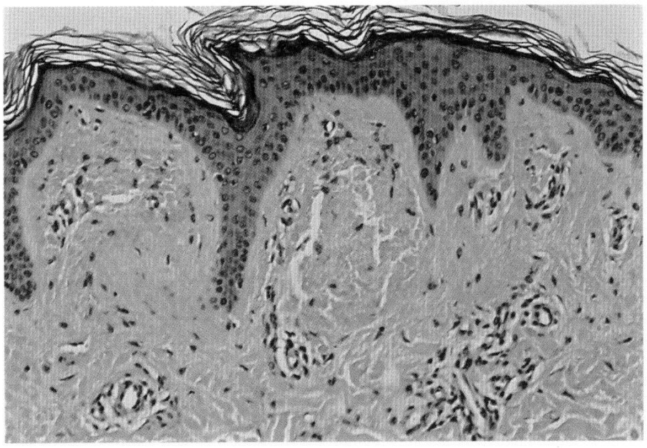

**FIG. 45.** Lichen amyloidosis composed of pink globules in the papillary dermis.

## REFERENCES


1. Montagna W, Parakkal PF. *The structure and function of the skin.* 3rd ed. New York; Academic Press, 1974.
2. Montagna W, Freedberg IM (eds). Cutaneous biology 1950-1975. *J Invest Dermatol* 1976;67:1–230.
3. Breathnach AS. Embryology of human skin. A review of ultrastructural studies. *J Invest Dermatol* 1971;57:133–143.
4. Holbrook KA, Odland GF. The fine structure of developing human epidermis: Light, scanning and transmission electron microscopy of the periderm. *J Invest Dermatol* 1975;65:16–38.
5. Lever WF, Schaumburg-Lever G. Embryology of the skin. In: Lever WF, Schaumburg-Lever G, eds. *Histopathology of the skin.* 6th ed. Philadelphia; JB Lippincott, 1983.
6. Smith LT, Sakai LY, Burgeson RE, Holbrook KA. Ontogeny of structural component at the dermal-epidermal junction in human embryonic and fetal skin: The appearance of anchoring fibrils and type VII collagen. *J Invest Dermatol* 1988;90:480–485.
7. Foster CA, Holbrook KA, Farr A. Ontogeny of Langerhans' cells in human embryonic and fetal skin: Expression of HLA-DR and OKT-6 determinants. *J Invest Dermatol* 1986;86:240–243.
8. Winkelmann RK, Breathnach AS. The Merkel cell. *J Invest Dermatol* 1973;60:2.
9. Gould VE, Moll R, Moll I, et al. Neuroendocrine (Merkel) cells of the skin: Hyperplasias, dysplasias and neoplasias. *Lab Invest* 1985; 52: 334–353.
10. Moll R, Moll I, Franke WW. Identification of Merkel cells in human skin by specific cytokeratin antibodies: Changes of cell density and distribution in fetal and adult plantar epidermis. *Differentiation* 1984;28: 136–154.
11. Ochiai T, Suzuki H. Fine structural and morphometric studies of the Merkel cell during fetal and post natal development. *J Invest Dermatol* 1981;77:437–443.
12. Moll I, Lane AT, Franke WW, Moll R. Intraepidermal formation of Merkel cells in xenografts of human fetal skin. *J Invest Dermatol* 1990; 94:359–364.
13. Breathnach AS. Development and differentiation of dermal cells in man. *J Invest Dermatol* 1978;71:2–8.
14. Mehregan AH, Hashimoto K, Mehregan DA and Mehregan DR. Normal structure of the skin. In: Mehregan AH, Hashimoto K, Mehregan DA, Mehregan DR, eds. Pinkus' *Guide to dermatohistopathology.* 6th ed. Norwalk; Appleton & Lange, 1995.
15. Ackerman AB. Skin, structure and function. In: Ackerman AB, ed. *Histologic diagnosis of inflammatory skin diseases.* Philadelphia; Lea & Febiger, 1978.
16. Downig DT, Stewart ME, Strauss JJ. Biology of sebaceous glands. In: Fitzpatrick TB, Eisen AZ, Wolff K, Freedberg IM, Austen KF, eds. *Dermatology in general medicine, vol 1.* 3rd ed. New York; McGraw-Hill, 1987;185–190.
17. Fawcett, Skin. In: Bloom, Fawcett, eds. *A textbook of histology.* 11th ed. Philadelphia; WB Saunders, 1986;543–578.
18. Montagna W. Embryology and anatomy of the cutaneous adnexa. *J Cutan Pathol* 1984;11:350–351.
19. Hashimoto K, Gross BG, Lever WF. The ultrastructure of the skin human embryos. I. The intraepidermal eccrine sweat duct. *J Invest Dermatol* 1965;45:139–151.
20. Smack DP, Korge BP, James WD: Keratin and Keratinization. *J Am Acad Dermatol* 1994;30:85–102.
21. Kerr JFR, Winterford CM, Harmon BV: Apoptosis. Its significance in cancer and cancer therapy. *Cancer* 1994;73:2013–2026.
22. Polakowska RH, Piacentini M, Bartlett R, et al. Apoptosis in human skin development: Morphogenesis, periderm, and stem cells. *Develop Dynamics* 1994;199:176–188.
23. Weedon D, Strutton G. Apoptosis as the mechanism of the involution of the hair follicles in catagen transformation. *Acta Derm Venereol (Stockh)* 1981;61:335–339.
24. McCall CA, Cohen JJ. Programmed cell death in terminally differentiating keratinocytes. *J Invest Dermatol* 1991;97:111–114.
25. Tamada Y, Takama H, Kitamura T, et al. Identification of programmed cell death in normal human skin tissues by using specific labeling of fragmented DNA. *Br J Dermatol* 1994;131:521–524.
26. Stenn KS, Lawrence L, Veis D, et al. Expression of the bcl-2 protooncogene in the cycling adult mouse hair follicle. *J Invest Dermatol* 1994;103:107–111.
27. Seiberg M, Marthinuss J, Stenn KS: Changes in expression of apoptósis-associated genes in skin mark early catagen. *J Invest Dermatol* 1995;104;78–82.
28. Weedon D, Strutton G. The recognition of early stages of catagen. *Am J Dermatopathol* 1984;6:553–555.
29. Sato K, Kang WH, Saga K, et al. Biology of sweat glands and their disorders. I. Normal sweat gland function. *J Am Acad Dermatol* 1989;20: 537–563.
30. Sato K, Sato F. Individual variations in structures and function of human eccrine sweat gland. *Am J Physiol* 1983;245;R203-R208.
31. Uno H. Sympathetic innervation of sweat glands and piloerector muscles of macaques and human beings. *J Invest Dermatol* 1977;69: 112–120.
32. Lever WF, Schaumburg-Lever G. Histology of the skin. In: Lever WF, Schaumburg-Lever G, eds. *Histopathology of the skin.* 6th ed. Philadelphia; JB Lippincott, 1983.
33. Sha VP, Epstein WL, Riegelman S. Role of sweat gland in accumulation or orally administered griseofulvin in skin. *J Clin Invest* 1974;53: 1673–1678.
34. Sato K, Kang WH, Saga K, et al. Biology of sweat glands and their disorders. II. Disorders of sweat gland function. *J Am Acad Dermatol* 1989;20:713–726.
35. Moll R, Cowin P, Kapprell HP, et al. Desmosomal proteins: New markers for identification and classification of tumors. *Lab Invest* 1986;54: 4–25.
36. Holbrook KA, Wolff K. The structure and development of skin. In: Fitzpatrick TB, Eisen AZ, Wolff K, Freedberg IM, Austen KF, eds. *Dermatology in general medicine.* 3rd ed. New York; McGraw-Hill, 1987.
37. Wolff K, Schreiner E. Pemphigus autoantibodies ultrastructural localization within the epidermis. *Nature* 1971;229:59.
38. Stanley JR, Klaus-Kouton V, Sampaio SAP. Antigen specificity of fogo salvagen autoantibodies is similar to North American pemphigus foliaceous and distinct from pemphigus vulgaris autoantibodies. *J Invest Dermatol* 1986;87:197–201.
39. Elias PM. Epidermal lipids, barrier function and desquamation. *J Invest Dermatol* 1983;80(suppl):44s–49s.
40. Toker C. Clear cells of the nipple epidermis. *Cancer* 1970; 25:601–610.
41. Kuo T-T, Chan HL, Hsueh S. Clear cell papulosis of the skin. A new entity with histogenetic implications for cutaneous Paget's disease. *Am J Surg Pathol* 1987;11:827–834.
42. Tschen JA, McGavran M, Kettler AH. Pagetoid dyskeratosis: A selective keratinocytic response. *J Am Acad Dermatol* 1988;19:891–894.
43. Katz SI. The epidermal basement membrane zone, structure, ontogeny and role in disease. *J Am Acad Dermatol* 1984;11:1025–1037.
44. Foidart JM, Bere EW, Yaar M, et al. Distribution and immunoelectronmicroscopic localization of laminin, a non-collagenous basement membrane glycoprotein. *Lab Invest* 1980;42:336–342.
45. Holubar K, Wolff K, Konrad K, et al. Ultrastructural localization of immunoglobulins in bullous pemphigoid skin. *J Invest Dermatol* 1975;64: 220–227.
46. Schaumburg-Lever G, Rule A, Scmidt-Ulbrich B, et al. Ultrastructural localization of in vivo bound immunoglobulins in bullous pemphigoid-a preliminary report. *J Invest Dermatol* 1975; 64:47–49.
47. Smith JB, Taylor TB, Zone JJ. The site of blister formation in dermatitis herpetiformes is within the lamina lucida. *J Am Acad Dermatol* 1992;27:209–213.
48. Leblond CP, Inoue S. Structure, composition and assembly of basement membrane. *Am J Anat* 1989;185:367–390.
49. Nordlund JJ, Sober AJ, Hansen TW. Periodic synopsis on pigmentation. *J Am Acad Dermatol* 1985;12:359–363.
50. Quevedo WC, Fitzpatrick TB, Szabo G, et al. Biology of the melanin pigmentary system. In: Fitzpatrick TB, Eisen AZ, Wolff K, Freedberg IM, Austen KF, eds. *Dermatology in general medicine,* vol I. 3rd ed. New York; McGraw-Hill, 1987.
51. Murphy GF: Structure, function and reaction patterns. In: Murphy GE, ed. *Dermatopathology.* Philadelphia; WB Saunders, 1995.
52. Gown AM, Vogel AM, Hoak D, et al. Monoclonal antibodies specific for melanocytic tumors distinguish subpopulations of melanocytes. *Am J Pathol* 1986;164:388–398.
53. Birbeck NS, Breathnach AS, Everall JD. An electron microscopic study of basal melanocytes and high-level clear cell (Langerhans' cell) in vitiligo. *J Invest Dermatol* 1961;37:51–64.
54. Santa Cruz DJ, Bauer EA. Merkel cells in the outer follicular sheath. *Ultrastruct Pathol* 1982;3:59–63.

55. Camisa C, Weissmann A. Friedrich Sigmund Merkel Part II. The cell. *Am J Dermatopathol* 1982;4:527–535.
56. Gu J, Polak JM, VanNoorden S, et al. Immunostaining of neuron specific enolase as a diagnostic tool for Merkel cell tumors. *Cancer* 1983; 52:1039–1043.
57. Leff EL, Brooks JSJ, Trojanowski JQ. Expression of neurofilament and neuron-specific enolase in small tumors of skin using immunohistochemestry. *Cancer* 1985;56:625–631.
58. Rosen ST, Gould VE, Salwen HR, et al. Establishment and characterization of a neuroendocrine skin carcinoma cell line. *Lab Invest* 1987; 56:302–311.
59. Van Muijen GNP, Ruiter DJ, Warnaar SO. Intermediate filaments in Merkel cell tumors. *Hum Pathol* 1985;16:590–595.
60. Wang NP, Zee S, Zarbo RJ et al. Coordinate expression of cytokeratins 7 and 20 defines unique subsets of carcinomas. *Appl Immunohistochem* 1995;3:99–107.
61. Headington JT. Transverse microscopic anatomy of the human scalp. A basis for a morphometric approach to disorders of the hair follicle. *Arch Dermatol* 1984;120:449–456.
62. Viragh PA. The mantle hair of Pinkus. A review on the occasion of its centennial. *Dermatology* 1995;191:82–87.
63. Baron DA, Briggman JV, Spicer SS. Tubulocisternal endoplasmic reticulum in human eccrine sweat glands. *Lab Invest* 1984;51:233–243.
64. Sato K, Leidal R, Sato F. Morphology and development of an apoeccrine sweat gland in human axillae. *Am J Physiol* 1987; 252:R166–R180.
65. Vitto J, Eisen AZ. Biology of the dermis. In: Fitzpatrick TB, Eisen AZ, Wolff K, Freedberg IM, Austen KF, eds. *Dermatology in general medicine,* vol I. 3rd ed. New York; McGraw-Hill, 1987.
66. Reed RJ, Ackerman AB. Pathology of the adventitial dermis. *Hum Pathol* 1973;4:207–217.
67. McNeal JE. Scleroderma and the structural basis of skin compliance. *Arch Dermatol* 1973;107:699–705.
68. Headington JT, Cerio R. Dendritic cells in the dermis. *Am J Dermatopathol* 1990;12:217–220.
69. Cerio R, Spaull J, Oliver GF, et al. A study of Factor XIIIA and MAC 387 immunolabeling in normal and pathological skin. *Am J Dermatopathol* 1990;12:221–233.
70. Ryan TJ, Mortimer PS, Jones RL. Lymphatics of the skin. Neglected but important. *Int J Dermatol* 1986;25:411–419.
71. Johnson BL, Honig PJ, Jaworsky C. In: Johnson BL, Honig PJ, Jaworsky C, eds. *Pediatric dermatopathology.* Newton; Butterworth-Heineman, 1994.
72. Pochi PE, Strauss JS, Downing DT. Age related changes in sebaceous gland activity. *J Invest Dermatol* 1979;73:108–111.
73. Patterson JAK. Structural and physiologic changes in the skin with age. In: Patterson JAK, ed. *Aging and clinical practice: skin disorders, diagnosis and treatment.* New York; Igaku-Shoin, 1989.
74. Rongioletti F, Rebora A: Fibroelastolytic patterns of intrinsic skin aging: Pseudoxanthoma elasticum-like papillary dermal elastolysis and white fibrous papulosis of the neck. *Dermatology* 1995; 191:19–24.
75. Altman DA, Nickoloff BJ, Fiveson DP. Differential expression of factor XIIIA and CD34 in cutaneous mesenchymal tumors. *J Cutan Pathol* 1993;20:154–158.
76. Mondragon G, Nygaard F. Routine and special procedures for processing biopsy specimens of lesions suspected to be malignant melanomas. *Am J Dermatopathol* 1981;3:265–272.

*Histology for Pathologists, second edition,*
Edited by Stephen S. Sternberg.
Lippincott-Raven Publishers, Philadelphia


# CHAPTER 3

# Nail

Julian Sánchez Conejo-Mir and Manuel Navarrete Ortega



The nail is a complex anatomical structure, often neglected in anatomic texts. It is important in certain animals for the prehension and capture of prey. In humans, the nail has a different function; it increases the fingertip's sensibility and serves as a skeleton for the distal zone of the finger.

Although most pathological specimens from the nail show well-known changes such as psoriasis, lichen planus, and the characteristic malignant tumors, a broad spectrum of other changes may be found. For the pathologist, knowledge of the normal histology and its more common variations is important in establishing a correct diagnosis.

Unfortunately, much of the literature on the nail can be troublesome and confusing because a great profusion of names and concepts exists and has changed over the years; also, many newer concepts of the embryology, physiology, immunohistochemistry, and nail growth mechanism find their way slowly into textbooks. This chapter emphasizes those observations and theories related to clinical pathology.

## HISTORY

Historical interest can be traced to the works of Galen in the second century (B.C.) when he noticed the nail's resemblance to hair structure. However, the real study of the nail begins at the end of the ninteenth century, mostly by Germans like Zander (1), Kolliker (2), and Unna (3). The first studies dealt with embryology and anatomy and their comparison to birds and primates (1,4,5). After the initial spark of interest, the nail literature was enriched by many authors, both on the embryology and the anatomy of the human nail (6,7). Due to the technical shortcomings of their time, the authors interpreted the nail plate as formed entirely by the matrix cells and concluded that other adjacent structures did not contribute in the formation of the plate.

During the 1950s, Lewis (8) challenged this view and published his idea of the "nail unit," consisting of a dorsal, intermediate, and ventral nail, with differentiation based on the use of a silver-proteinate stain. In 1963, Zaias (9) extended the concept of the "nail unit," including the proximal nail fold, the matrix, the nail bed, and the hyponychium, all contributing to the formation of the nail.

During the last 25 years, most studies on the nail have fundamentally tried to explain its biochemistry and physiology, with emphasis on analyzing nail growth; also considered were ultrastructure and, most recently, the immunohistochemistry of the nail. At the same time, new conditions, particularly tumors, unknown until a few years ago, have been described from the point of ungual structures, especially keratoacanthomas, merkelomas (Merkel cell tumors), and subungual Bowen's disease. In the last 5 years, however, publications have been very scarce following the great proliferation of papers in previous years.

J. S. Conejo-Mir: Department of Dermatology and Venereology, Virgen del Rocio University Hospital, Seville 41011, Spain.
M. Navarrete Ortega:Department of Pathology, Virgen del Rocio University Hospital, Seville 41011, Spain.

**TABLE 3-1.** *Comparison of the different stages of nail development with the epidermis of the embryo using scanning electron microscopy*

| Nail unit[a] | Embryonic/fetal skin[b] | Development |
|---|---|---|
| Plaque phase | Indifferent epithelium phase<br>Flattened surface phase<br>Elevated surface phase | 7–10 weeks |
| Fibrillar phase | Incipient bleb formation phase | 2.5–3 months |
| Granular phase | Single bleb formation phase | 3–4 months |
| Squamous phase | Complex bleb formation phase | 4–5 months |
| Definitive nail phase | Cornification phase | Up to 5 months |

[a] See ref. 13.
[b] See ref. 10.

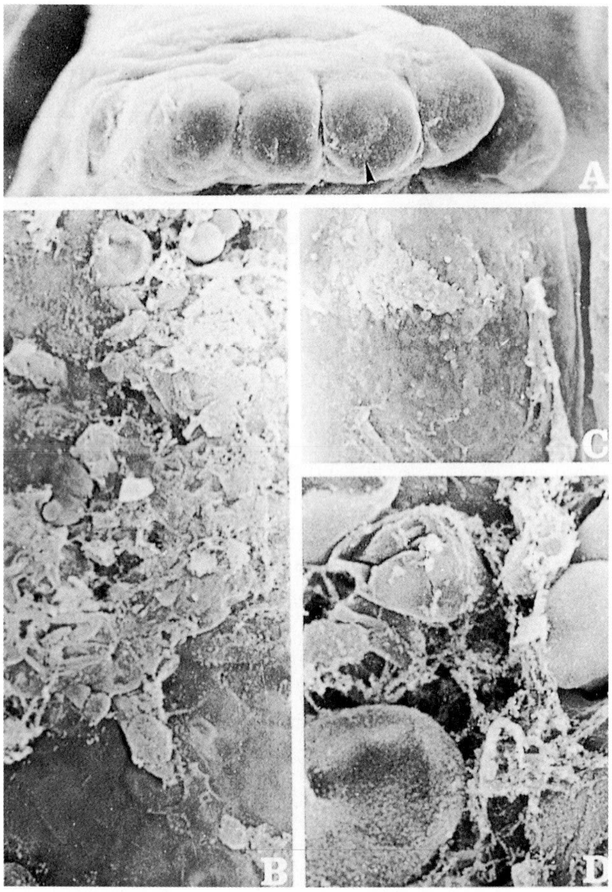


**FIG. 1.** Development of the human nail exhibited through scanning electron microscopy (13). Plaque phase: foot of 7-week-old human embryo. The fingers are already defined but have no interphalangeal folds (**A,** ×**50**). On the third toe, you can see distally poorly structured material accumulated (*arrow*), (**A,** ×**50**) that corresponds to apoptotic cells, which limits the future proximal nail fold (**B,** ×**500**) (**C,** ×**100**). Close-up view of the apoptotic cells: amorphous extracellular material appears with numerous vesicles of keratohyalin which are different phases of their evolution (**D,** ×**1,500**).

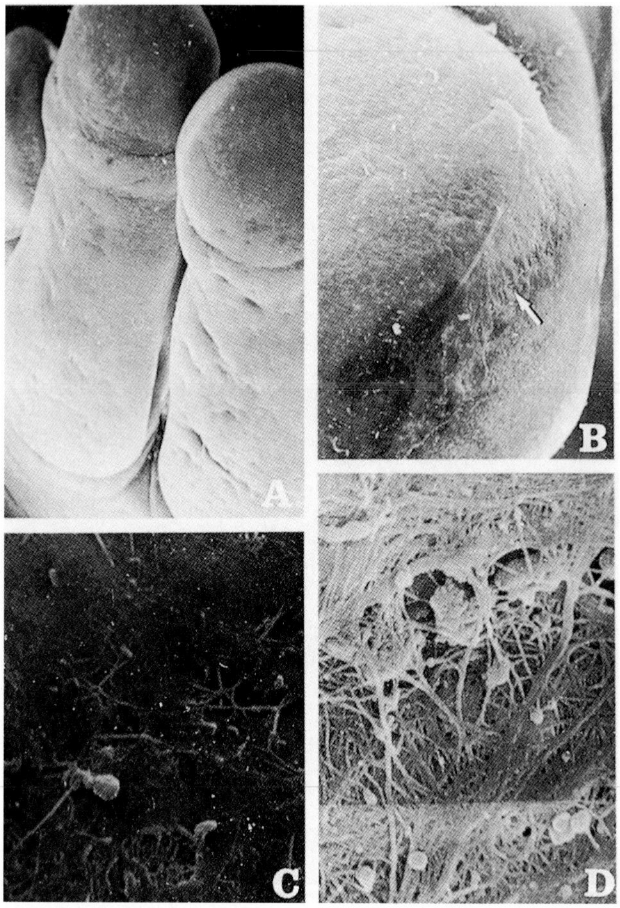


**FIG. 2.** Fibrillar phase: fingers of the hand of a 3-month-old embryo. The ungual region is perfectly delimited by the proximal nail fold (**A,** ×**40**). The ungual region is delimited by multiple fibrillar formations (**B,** ×**150**). Different morphology is seen in the nail bed surface (**C,** ×**2400**). Detail of the fibrillar attachment of the nail region to the neighboring tissue (**D,** ×**2400**).

Difficult biopsy access, as well as the complicated orientation and specimen handling, with the resulting difficulties of interpretation, are the main reasons why there are few histologic and histopathologic studies on the nail.

## EMBRYOLOGY

Wheareas the embryonic development of the fetal skin has been divided into eight stages, using scanning electron microscopy (10), the embryonic development of the nail shows only five stages (11,12): (a) plate phase; (b) fibrillar phase; (c) granular phase; (d) squamous phase; and (e) definitive nail phase or end phase (Table 1).

The earliest recognizable fingers are seen in 42- to 45-day-old embryos (16 mm crown-rump), while the toes lag somewhat and are seen at 52 to 54 days of age (18.5 mm) (13). Studies using optical microscopy showed that the ungual morphogenesis begins at the embryonal age of 10 weeks, with a smooth, shiny quadrangular surface delineated by continuous shallow grooves. This surface of the phalanx is the "primary nail base" of Zander (1) or "primary nail field" of Zaias (9), delimited proximally by a transversal groove: the proximal nail groove.

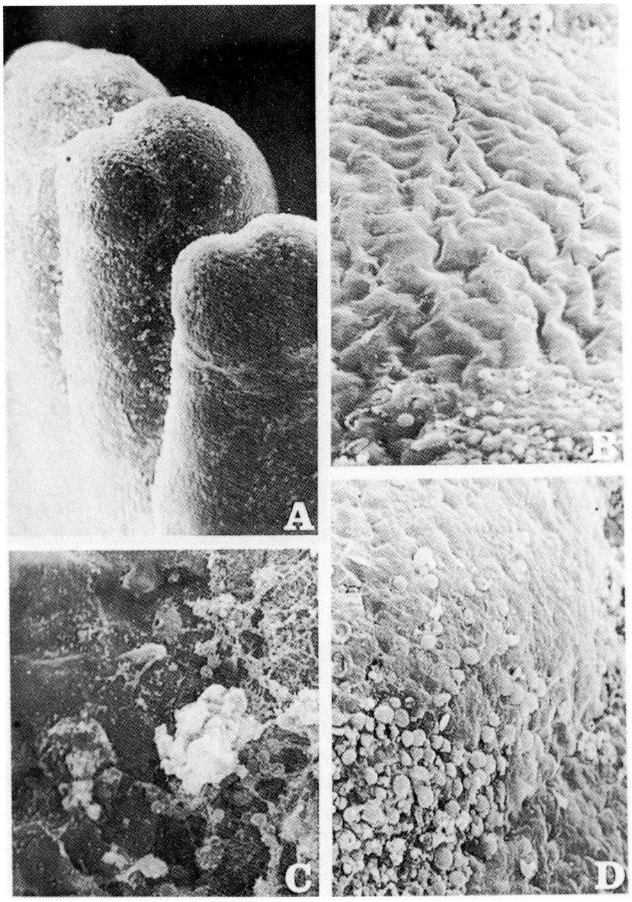


**FIG. 3.** Granular phase: fingers of the hand of 4.5-month-old embryo. All fingers show a granular aspect (**A, X40**). The nail bed has an undulating surface covered by keratin scales (**B, ×400**). The hyponychium zone is occupied by numerous keratohyalin vesicles (**C, ×400**) (**D, ×150**).

Studies we performed using scanning electron microscopy showed that the formation of the nail begins very early, at the embryonal age of 7 weeks, with an accumulation of strongly active cells, abundant mitosis, and cellular damage, followed by necrosis, with the presence of macrophages in the primary nail base (Fig. 1). This phenomenon, named apoptosis, occurs in all the epidermal accumulated cells following a transversal band in the dorsal area of the distal third of the fingers. Apoptosis of these epidermal cells is the most important step in the nail's development because it permits an immediate epidermal invagination identical to the one in the hair follicle except for one difference; in the hair follicle, the process starts at the age of 2.5 to 3 months. We observed apoptosis in nail development in this first phase only. Yet, the two processes are so identical that, sometimes, the layers of the nail have been compared with those of the hair follicle. The result is the formation of a transversal groove, which subsequently becomes the proximal nail fold.

An interesting feature of the first stages is the excessive size of the primitive nail plate (2.5 to 3 months), nearly occupying the total distal third part of the finger. This plate stays attached to its surroundings through some periungual-fixing filaments (Fig. 2). At the age of 11 weeks, all the folds are already formed, both proximal and lateral nail folds. The transversal distal fold, corresponding to the hyponychium, is completely keratinized at the age of 3.5 months (Fig. 3).

Afterward, the epidermal cells of the nail field suffer a process of keratin formation, different from the rest of the embryo. The result is a keratinized structure, covering the whole nail bed from the age of 14 weeks on, sometimes confused by some authors with a false nail (Fig. 4) (8,9). The production of the true nail plate starts from the matrix cells, located in the proximal nail groove and the most proximal portion of the nail bed. Its presence in the proximal fold is visible from the fifth month of intrauterine life on, the histochemical confirmation of its formation being the presence of sulfhydryl radicals (14).

From the fifth month on, the definitive nail plate starts to grow in a distal sense until it reaches the hyponychium at the time of birth. The growth mechanism of the definitive nail is discussed later in the section entitled "Nail Growth."

## GROSS ANATOMY

Various types of differently keratinizing epidermis make up the nail. What commonly is termed "the nail plate" is the horny end product of the most important epidermal component, the matrix. Usually, this nail plate is slightly convex or flat, rectangular, and of varying size between approximately 1 × 1 and 2 × 3 cm, depending on the finger (Figs. 5–7). In the hand, this is usually 25 to 50% of the dorsal surface of the fingertips, whereas in the big toe it occupies about 75%. The nail is translucent and becomes rosy from the underlying vascular network. In the proximal portion there is an arch

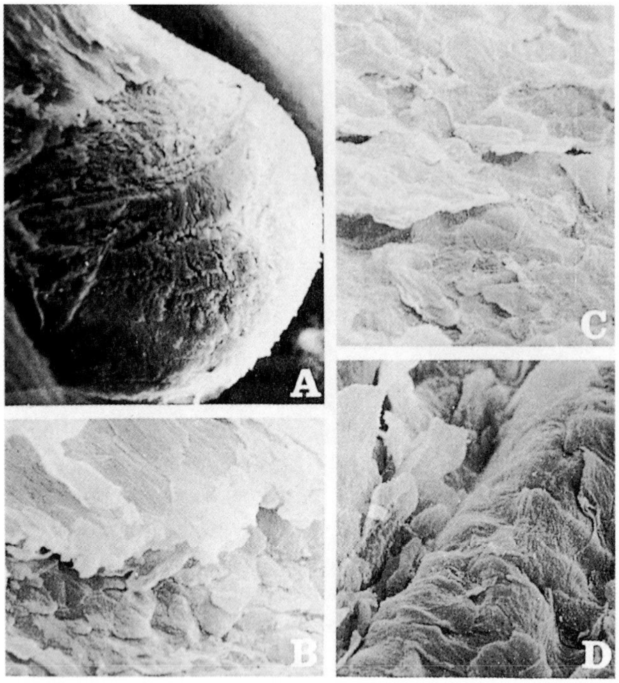


**FIG. 4.** Squamous phase: index finger of 5.5-month-old fetus (**A,** ×**200**). The keratinization process is complete in the nail bed surface, simulating a false nail (**C,** ×**500**). The cuticle (**B,** ×**500**) and hyponychium are also completely developed (**D,** ×**500**).

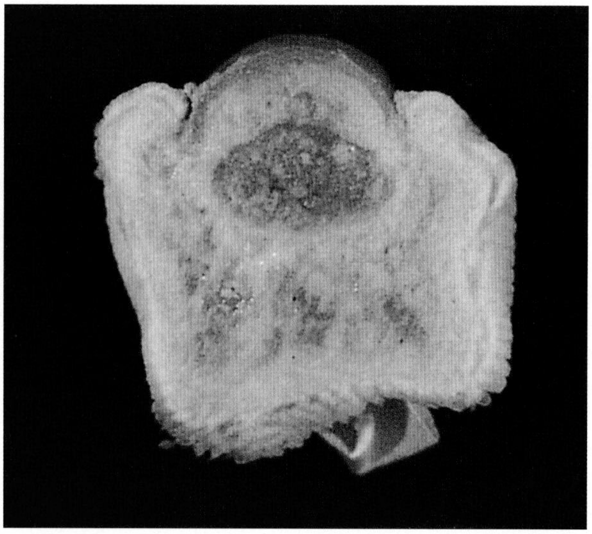

**FIG. 6.** Cross section of an adult finger. The nail plate lies on nail bed, and the lateral border is overlapped by lateral nail fold.

called the lunula. The thickness of the nail plate is 0.5 mm in women and 0.6 mm in men (15).

The nail plate is delimited by three folds: two lateral and one proximal (Fig. 8). If the nail plate is avulsed, the grooves become visible where the nail plate rested. These potential spaces are only real spaces in abnormal conditions of the nail, as in paronychia. In the lateral nail grooves the epidermal lining does not contribute to the formation of the nail plate, except in the most proximal portions where it becomes continuous with the epidermis of the proximal groove or matrix.

The proximal nail fold is the most important one, since, as we shall note later, its contribution to the formation of the nail plate is fundamental (16). This fold shows two portions: a dorsal portion, lodging the matrix, and a ventral portion. Twenty-five percent of the total surface of the nail plate is located under the ventral portion of the proximal nail fold.

A white crescent-shaped lunula can project from under the proximal nail fold. It is usual on the thumbs and common on

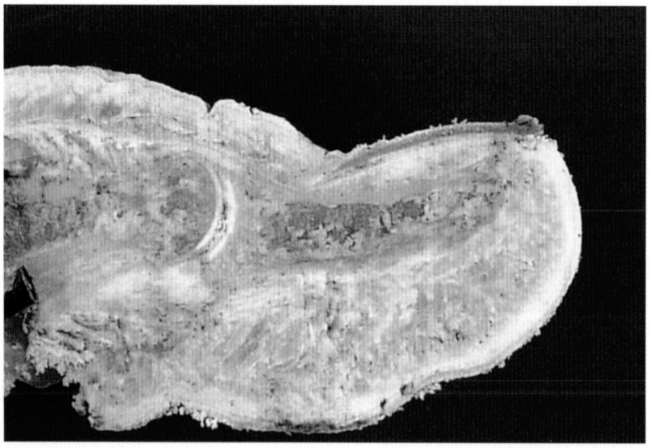

**FIG. 5.** Sagittal section of an adult thumb, in which it is possible to observe the relations of the nail unit with the adjacent tissues.

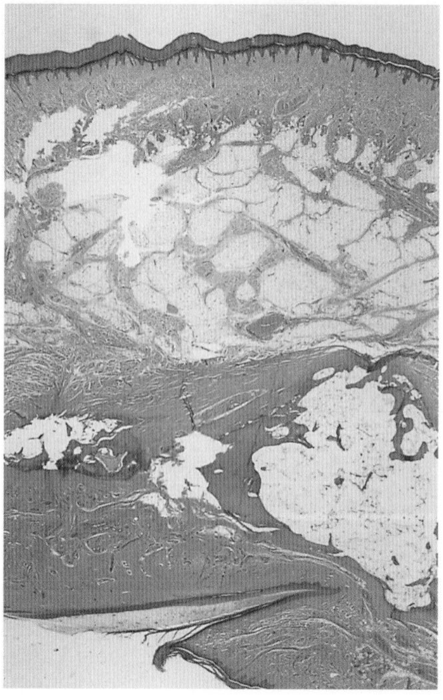

**FIG. 7.** Histological sagittal section of a finger (HE, **1**×)

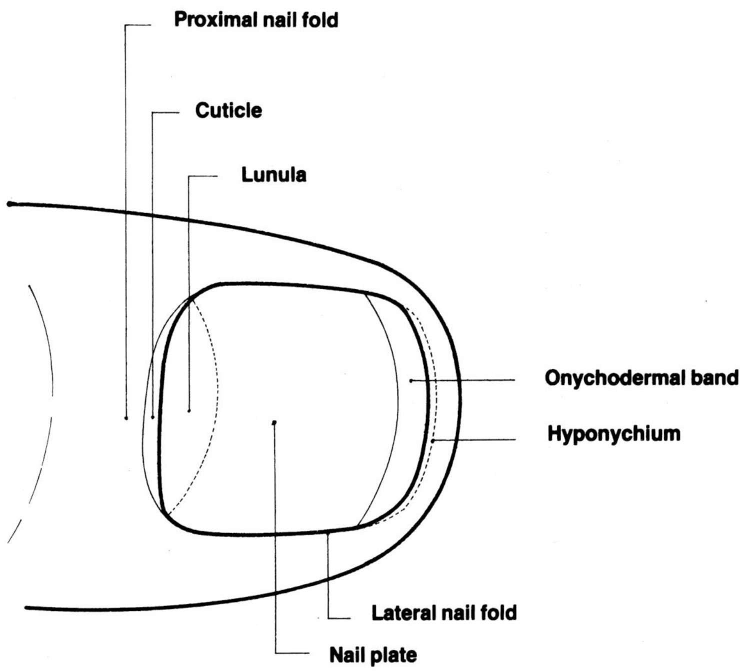


FIG. 8. Schematic diagram of the nail, including nomenclature.

other fingers and on large toenails. The lunula is the most distal portion of the matrix and determines the shape of the free edge of the nail plate. The color of the lunula is due, in part, to the effect of light scattered by the nucleated cells of the keratogenous zone of the matrix and, in part, to the thicker layer of epithelial cells making up the matrix (16,17).

At the point of separation of the nail plate and the nail bed, the subungual epidermis may be modified as the solehorn (18). In humans, this structure may only be vestigial: its original significance only being evident from comparative anatomical studies. However, in certain diseases, it could be the seat of distal subungual hyperkeratosis or parakeratosis, for example, in pachyonychia congenita and pityriasis rubra pilaris (19). The distal limit of the ungual layer is the hyponychium, determining the formation of the distal fold, a keratinized structure that continues until the fingertips. A subungual extension of the hyponichium and obliteration of the distal groove is named Pterygium inversum unguis (20). This term was coined because of the the similarity between the behavior of the hyponychium and the eponychium in classic cases of pterygium unguis.

On close examination, two further distal zones can often be identified: the distal yellow-whlte margin and, immediately proximal to this, the onychodermal band (21). This band is a barely perceptible narrow transverse band, 0.5 to 1.5 mm wide, that is more prominent in acrocyanosis. The exact anatomical basis for the onychodermal band is not known, but it appears to have a different blood supply from the main body of the nail bed (22). It is possible to explore it through a strong compression of the distal zone of the finger, leaving behind a white band. The band's color can occasionally be modified by diseases (19,23).

Recently, several studies have been published about the exploration of the nail apparatus. Although ultrasound transmission can be useful for studying the nail plate thickness (24), magnetic resonance imaging (MRI) permits the detection of subungual lesions smaller than 1 mm in diameter (25).

## MICROSCOPIC ANATOMY

### The Nail Plate

Microscopically, the nail plate consists of closely packed, adherent, interdigitating cells lacking nuclei or organelles (Fig. 9 and 10). Many intercellular links including tight, intermediate, and desmosomal junctions are present (26). The nail plate is made-up of three layers: a thin dorsal layer, a thick intermediate layer, and the ventral layer from the nail bed. The cells of the surface of the nail plate overlap, slanting from "proximal-dorsal to distal-volar." For this reason, the dorsal surface of the nail plate is smooth, whereas the palmar surface is irregular, showing longitudinal striations. This can also be observed with optical microscopy, as well

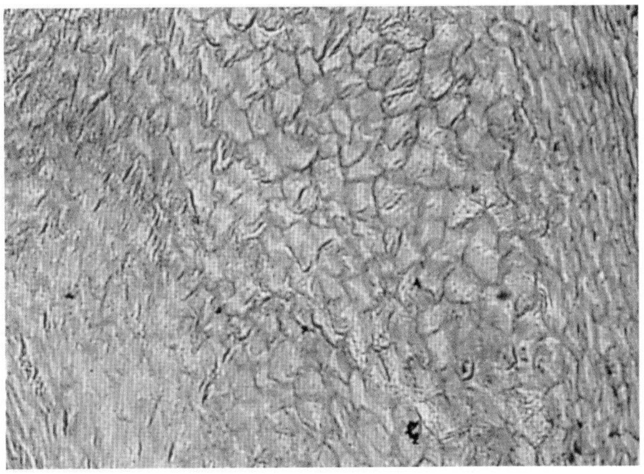

FIG. 9. Schematic diagram of a sagittal section through the nail unit.

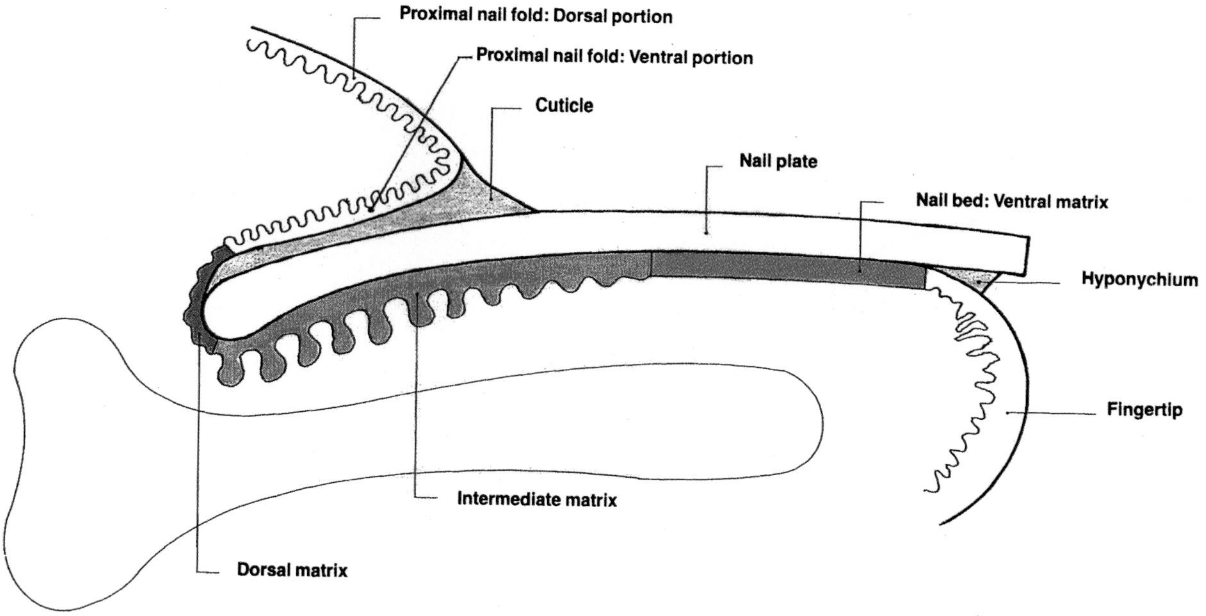


**FIG. 10.** Horizontal section of the dorsal nail plate. Corneocytes show a polydedral disposition, with rounded corners; the cells do not contain nuclei or elements (VVG stain, **X200**).

as with scanning electron microscopy (27). No keratohyalin granules were seen, but acidophilic masses, called pertinax bodies of Lewis and Montgomery (28), are occasionally seen in older age groups. Hamilton et al. (29) believed that the progressive increase in the thickness of the nail plate with age is attributable to the increasing size of the cells in the plate, consecutive to the frictional loss of nail; however, Johnson and Shuster (30), studied in 20 normal great toenails the determinant of final nail thickness and length at its point of detachment at the onychodermal band. They confirmed that the increase of nail thickness with age is independent of the frictional traumatisms on the plate.

Corneocytes of the human nail plate have been studied by German et al. (31). Corneocytes of the dorsal nail plates of normal nails are irregular and polyhedral, nonnucleated, and show distinctly irregular networks. These horny cells from nail plates increase in size with age: babies have small cells, adults have significantly larger cells, and aged subjects have significantly larger cells than the adults. These authors also commented that the faster-than-normal growing nail plates yield smaller cells; for example, corneocytes from psoriatic patients are smaller than normal. Corneocytes from slow-growing nails, such as from persons having lichen planus or dyskeratosis congenita, are larger than normal.

Frequent gap junctions were observed near the area where lamellar granules were discharging their contents, and it was suggested that a certain substance might be able to pass through the nail plate through such intercellular channels. Perhaps such channels explain the greater permeability of the nail plate to polar molecules compared with the permeability of the skin (32).

The biochemical composition of the nail plate has been widely studied. Calcium is an important component of the nail plate, found as the phosphate in hydroxyapatite crystals; it is intracelluiarly bound to phospholipids, particularly in the dorsal and ventral nail plate (33). Calcium concentration is approximately 0.1% of the weight, 10 times greater than in hair (34). However, some authors believe that the proportion of calcium in the nail contributes little to the hardness of the nail plate in men (19,35). Also, it is possible that calcium is not an intrinsic part of the nail but is incorporated from extrinsic sources, such as soaps; the nail is relatively porous and calcium could enter as ionic calcium or bound to fatty acids. Other metals such as copper, manganeso, zinc, and iron are also found in small quantities in the nail plate, although their function is still unknown (36).

The existence of sulfhydryl and disulfide groups has been demonstrated in the nail plate. During early embryonic life there is a very high concentration of the sulfhydryl groups (9), which decreases as the delivery date approaches and stabilizes at about the age of 3 years (14). These sulfurous radicals are formed at the expense of amino acids, such as cystine. Total sulfur concentration is similar in the dorsal and intermediate plate. The nail plate also contains glutamic acid, serine, and less tyrosine than hair (34,35,37,38).

In certain diseases, the quantity of various organic and metallic components of the nail plate can be increased. A brief listing is presented for reference: total nonprotein nitrogen, urea nitrogen, ammonia nitrogen, and uric acid in gout (39); creatinine in chronic renal failure (40); sodium in cystic fibrosis (41,42); calcium in older subjects (28,34); and copper in Wilson's disease (43).

An analysis of the keratin of the nail plate revealed the following (19,44): (a) alpha-fibrillar, low sulfur protein; (b) globular, high sulfur matrix protein; and (c) high glycine-tyrosine-rich matrix protein. All these fractions are also present in hair. The hardness of nail is due to the high sulfur matrix protein, contrasting with the relatively soft keratin of the epidermis. The cornified envelope of the epidermis is formed by several precursor proteins, including involucrin, keratolinin, loricrin, pancornulin, sciellin, 195-kD protein, keratin, and filiagrin. Baden and Kvedar (45) have demonstrated that in the nail, monoclonal antibodies show the presence of pancornulin in the nail fold and proximal matrix, while sciellin was detected in the nail fold, matrix, and bed. Similarly, in studies of the human nails (which contain hard keratins), the use of immunofluorescence, immunoblotting, and PCR have shown that trichohyalin, a 200-kDa protein of the inner root sheath and medulla, was present in the ventral matrix, but not in the nail bed; a few scattered cells stained for trichohyalin were observed within the nail plate (46).

Heid et al. (47) studied the keratin expression patterns observed in the human fetal nail matrix and revealed that the nail develops from both skin- and hair-type differentiating cells. Kitahara and Ogawa (48) demonstrated that AE13 antibody reacted with the dorsal nail matrix. As AE13 antibody recognized hard keratins which are characteristic of differentiation in hair, these results show that adult nail develops in such a way that hair-type differentiation is confined to the ventral nail matrix, supporting the Heid results (49,50).

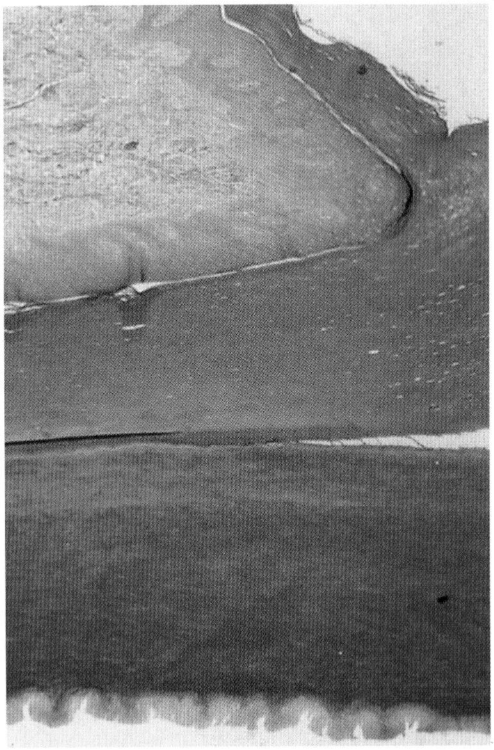

**FIG. 11.** Proximal nail fold with its two portions: dorsal portion, with identical histologic pattern to the skin of the dorsum of the distal digit; ventral portion, overlying the nail plate. Note the great thickness of the stratum corneum of this epithelium (MF stain, ×**63**).

### Proximal Nail Fold

The proximal nail fold is an invaginating, wedge-shaped fold of the skin on the dorsum of the distal digit, and the nail plate arises from under this fold (Fig. 11). The proximal nail fold consists of two layers of epidermis: the ventral portion overlying the newly formed nail plate, and the dorsal portion that forms the dorsum of the finger epidermis. The keratinization process in both portions does not differ from that of the epidermis elsewhere, possessing a granular layer that is absent in all parts of the nail matrix.

The dorsal portion of the proximal nail fold consists of a continuation of the epidermis and dermis of the dorsal digit with sweat glands, but no follicles or sebaceous glands. At the distal tip, a thick corneal layer called the cuticle shows on the dorsal surface of the nail plate (Fig. 12). Its function is the protection of the nail base, particularly the germinative matrix. Loss of the cuticle often allows acute and chronic inflammatory and infective processes to involve the nail matrix, leading to secondary nail plate dystrophies.

The ventral portion is thick-skinned, has no appendages, and is closely attached on the dorsal surface of the nail plate. The epithelium of the ventral surface of the proximal nail fold has been called the eponychium (9,17,19). Diseases that affect the ventral portion of the proximal nail fold can affect the newly formed nail plate. For this reason, some authors think that the proximal nail fold contributes to form the superficial layer of the nail plate. In particular, the apparition of pits and grooves (Beau's line) on the nail are due to parakeratotic and growth detection phenomena, respectively, in the ventral portion of the proximal nail fold.

### Matrix

The ventral surface of the proximal nail fold forms the roof of the proximal nail groove; the nail matrix forms its

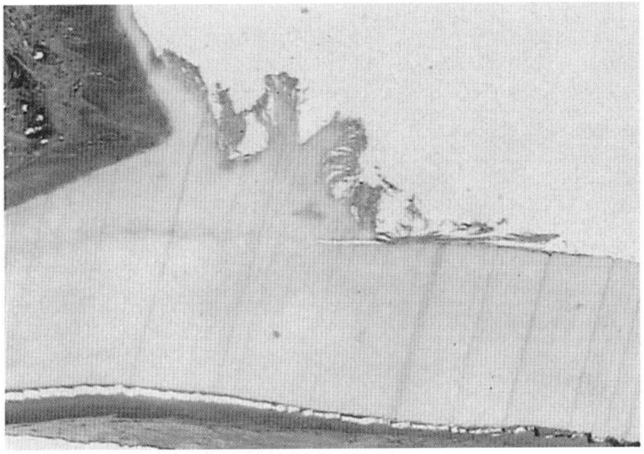

**FIG. 12.** Detail of the cuticle. At the distal tip, the proximal nail fold shows a thick corneal layer (cuticle) on the dorsal surface of the nail plate.

floor, and the nail plate lies between the two. The matrix is divided into three parts (8,9,19): dorsal, intermediate, and ventral. Of these, the dorsal and, above all, the intermediate portions play an important role in nail plate formation. In particular, the true matrix is the intermediate portion. For this reason, when we discuss the histology of the matrix, we are fundamentally referring to the intermediate portion. The ventral portion corresponds to the nail bed; the controversy about its participation in the formation of the definitive nail plate is discussed in "Nail Growth."

In the matrix area, we can observe epithelial cells, melanocytes, Merkel cells, and Langerhans' cells.

### *Epithelium Cells*

The matrix is an easily identified thick epithelium, situated immediately below the ventral portion of the proximal nail fold (Fig. 13). Its main feature is acanthosis, with between 8 and 15 mamelons (protuberances) (Fig. 14). Its undulation can only be seen for a few millimeters, flattening itself in the area corresponding to the nail bed. As in the epidermis of the skin, the matrix possesses a very active dividing basal layer of keratinoblasts, producing keratinocytes which differentiate, harden, die, and contribute to the nail plate (Fig. 15). The nail plate is formed by a process that involves flattening of the basal cells of the matrix, fragmentation of nuclei, and condensation of the cell cytoplasm to form horny flat cells. An important histologic feature is the lack of granular layer. Acanthosis and papillomatosis are only seen in the nail unit in the matrix and, distally, in the hyponychium (Table 2).

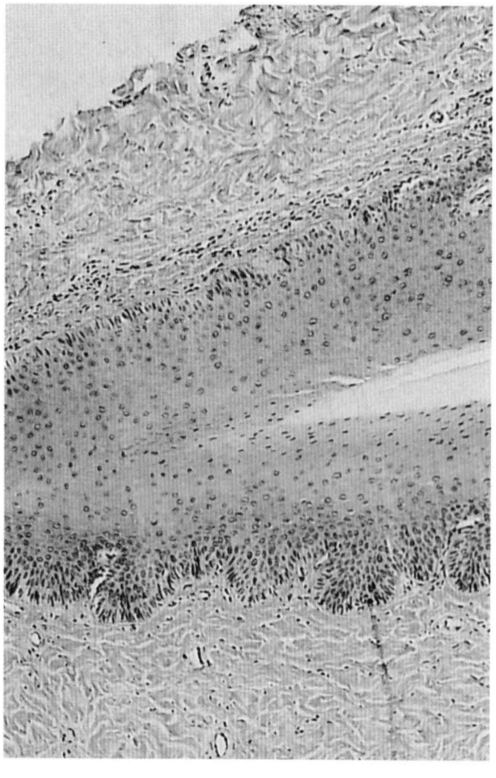

**FIG. 13.** Histologic appearance of the matrix angle, formed by the ventral portion of the nail fold and the dorsal and intermediate matrix.

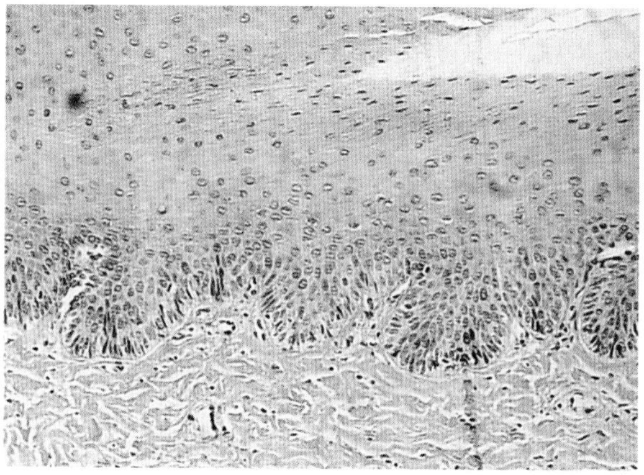

**FIG. 14.** Detail of matrix epithelium. This zone shows an acanthotic epithelium, with active keratinoblasts and scarce melanocytes.

Expression of integrins in the nail matrix have been studied by Cameli et al. (51). These authors found that alpha-2-beta-1 and alpha-3-beta-1 expression differ in nail matrix epithelium. In the nail matrix these integrins are not only expressed on the basal layer, but also on the fourth to fifth suprabasal layers, with suprabasal expression gradually decreasing from the distal to proximal matrix (Table 3). As in the normal human epidermis, alpha-1, alpha-4, and alpha-5 integrins subunits are not expressed in the nail matrix; in the same way, ICAM-1, the ligand of LFA1, was negative in the matrix cells. The expression of beta-1 subunits in the suprabasal layers of the nail matrix indicates a very strong cohesion between nail matrix cells, this probably revealing them to be an essential prerequisite for the development of a compact nail plate. Cultures of nail matrix cells may represent a useful model to study the biologic properties of nail structure (52).

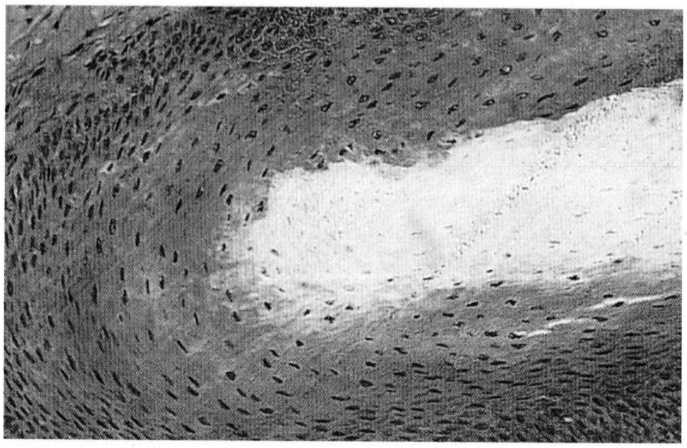

**FIG. 15.** Detail of the matrix zone, in which one can observe the abrupt keratinization.

**TABLE 3-2.** *Histologic characteristic features of each zone of the nail unit*

| Nail area | Epithelium | Granular layer | Horny end product |
|---|---|---|---|
| Proximal nail fold | Similar to normal skin or slightly acanthotic | Present | Cuticle |
| Matrix | Acanthotic | Absent | Nail plate |
| Nail bed | Flat | Absent | Lower layer of the nail plate |
| Hyponychium | Acanthotic | Present | Horny layer in the undersurface of the distal nail, similar to cuticle |

### *Melanocytes*

The nail matrix possesses melanocytes, just as the hair matrix does. The matrix of Caucasian patients contains sparse, poorly developed melanocytes (Fig. 16) (53). It is difficult to observe melanocytes in the proximal matrix zone using light microscopy, but their number is progressively increased distally. Nevertheless, the number of melanocytes is always less than in normal skin (53–57). There are distinct differences in the distribution of melanocytes in adult skin and nail matrix. Immunostaining of nail matrix melanocytes revealed that they are not singly interspersed between the keratinocytes of the basal layer, but that they are frequently arranged in small clusters among the suprabasal layers of the nail matrix (Figs. 17 and 18). A similar pattern of distribution of melanocytes has been described in fetal skin and in fetal skin equivalents, in which the melanocytes are grouped and localized both basally and suprabasally (58). The suprabasal location of nail matrix melanocytes may be a consequence of differences in the distribution of adhesion molecules in the nail epithelium.

Higashi and Saito (59) demonstrated that the number of melanocytes and the intensity of the dopa reaction in them were much greater in the distal than the proximal matrix. The melanocyte count in normal epidermis was reported to be 400 per 2.784 square mm (58,59), while the range was 208 to 576 in the distal areas of the intermediate nail matrix (59).

Ultraviolet rays and trauma are factors that could influence a more extensive distribution in the distal zone (57,59). In some races, i.e., Japanese, the matrix contains several hundred well-developed melanocytes per millimeter (59).

Pigment, therefore, arrives in the nail plate as in the keratinized cells of the stratum corneum and hair cortex (60). Nail pigmentation is most evident in African Americans in whom it is commonly seen as longitudinal linear streaks, although this anomalous distribution of pigmentation can also be seen in pathological states, such as subungual pigmented nevi and melanomas in the matrix zone (61). The location of melanocytes in the matrix is directly related to the location of pigmented bands, most of which originate in the distal matrix and do not cross the lunula (57). Longitudinal melanonychia in AIDS patients is a common finding. Although this nail pigmentary nail change can be related to the zidovudine oral treatment, in other cases it seems to be independent, associated with elevated levels of alpha-MSH (62).

Tosti el al. (63), have recently studied the melanocyte characterization of the normal nail matrix, using immunohistochemistry techniques. These authors found nail matrix melanocytes reacted with the antibodies anti-PEP-1, anti-Pep-8, and anti-TMP-1, which recognize the tyrosinase-related protein-1, the tyrosinase-related protein-2 (DOPA-chrometautomerase), and the tyrosinase-related protein encoded by pMT4 (Table 4). This confirms that, even if normally quiescent, nail matrix melanocytes possess the key enzymes responsible for the formation of melanin pigment.

### *Langerhans' and Merkel Cells*

Langerhans' and Merkel cells have also been identified in the matrix (54) although their signification is unknown. Studies of the Langerhans' cells in the nail matrix are almost absent. Nevertheless, interesting studies about the Merkel cells have been recently published. Moll and Moll (64) studied the Merkel cells (MCs) in ontogenesis of human nails, using immunohistochemical stains with cytokeratins 18 and

**TABLE 3-3.** *Integrin expression in human nail matrix*[a]

| | Alpha-1 | Alpha-2 | Alpha-3 | Alpha-4 | Alpha-5 | Alpha-6 | Alpha-v | Beta-1 | Beta-4 | ICAM-1 |
|---|---|---|---|---|---|---|---|---|---|---|
| Basal membrane zone | – | – | – | – | – | +++ | – | – | +++ | – |
| Basal layer | – | ++ | ++ | – | – | ++ | ++ | ++ | ++ | – |
| Suprabasal layer (Ventral matrix) | – | ++ | ++ | – | – | – | + | ++ | – | – |
| Suprabasal layers (Dorsal matrix) | – | + | + | – | – | – | + | + | – | – |
| Keratogenous zone | – | – | – | | – | – | – | – | – | – |

[a] Taken from ref. 51.

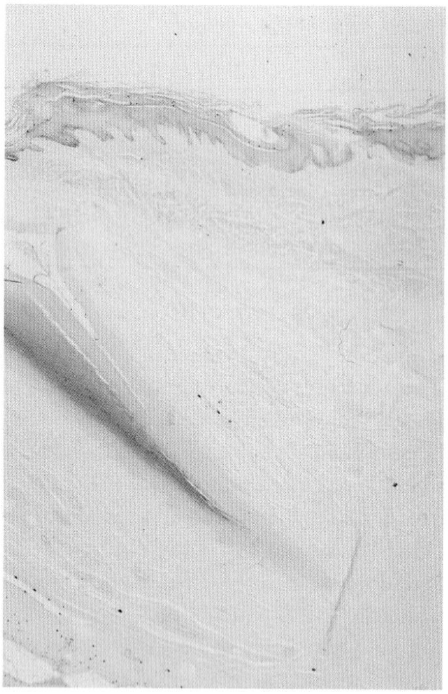

**FIG. 16.** Observe the notable hyperpigmentation of the basal layer in the pulp of the finger in contrast with the absence of pigmentation in the nail matrix (Fontana stain, **4x**).

20 in human fetuses of 9 to 22 weeks of life. These authors have concluded the number of MCs are detected very early (9 weeks) in the matrix primordium. However, MCs were found to decrease in number with aging of the fetuses: at 12 to 15 weeks, MCs were only seen in the proximal nail fold, and were essentially absent from the epithelium of the ventral matrix and nail bed in the adult. Lacour et al. (65), in a double indirect immunofluorescence and immunoelectron microscopy with the monoclonal antibody Troma-1, have only found MCs in the proximal nail fold of the adults, with a concentration greater than 50 MCs/mm2.

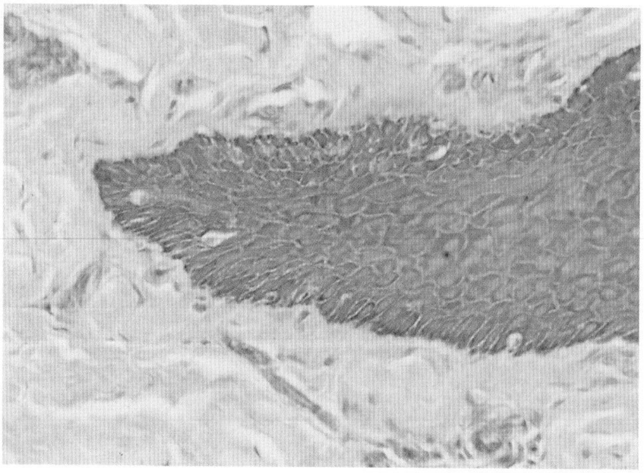

**FIG. 17.** Melanocytes of the nail matrix, not staining with cytokeratin antibody. Observe its scarce number in the nail matrix (Cytokeratin antibody, **10x**).

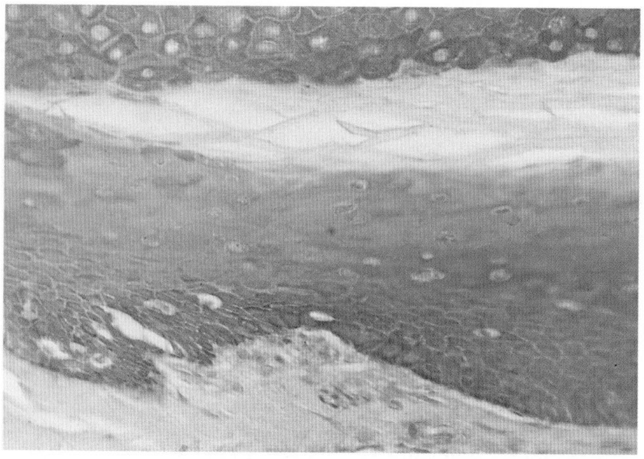

**FIG. 18.** Melanocytes of the lunula, not staining with cytokeratin antibody. Note its location in basal and suprabasal epithelial layers (Cytokeratin antibody, **20x**).

### *Lunula*

The intermediate matrix continues forward with a visible, white half-moon-shaped arca called the lunula. Although always present, it cannot be seen in some fingers but is most visible in the thumbs. The typical white color is related to some histologic features of this arca. Lewin (15) confirmed that the opacity of the proximal nail plate, the relative avascularity of the subepidermal layer, and the loose texture of the dermal collagen are responsable for its color. Samman (66,67) thought that it was a combination of incomplete keratinization in the nail plate and loose connective tissue in the underlying tissue. Zaias (68) believed that the nail plate would be thinner in the lunula because it coincides with the keratogenous zone, the zone of cytoplasmic condensation in the matrix just before cells form the nail plate. Other special histologic features of this zone of the matrix, including a different chemical composition of the nail plate and a different distribution of the dermal fibers, have been related to the typical white color of the lunula (69–71), although not one of these factors has been confirmed. We do not even know the exact function of the lunula.

### Nail Bed

The nail bed begins where the intermediate matrix ends, and some authors prefer to designate the ventral matrix as the site (19,72). A histologic appreciation of the end of the intermediate matrix and the beginning of the nail bed is very easy. The nail bed epidermal layer is usually a flat epithelium no more than three- or four-cells thick, without melanocytes (Figs. 19–21). The transition zone from living keratinocytes to dead ventral nail plate cells is abrupt, occurring in the space of one horizontal cell layer, very similar to what occurs in the Henle layer of the internal root sheath of the epidermis (71).

During its early development, the nail bed exhibits a ker-

**TABLE 3-4.** *Immunostaining of human nail melanocytes*[a]

| Antibody | Reactive to | Species | Nail matrix melanocytes |
|---|---|---|---|
| Anti-PEP1 | Tyrosinase-related protein-1 | Rabbit | + + |
| Anti-PEP8 | Tyrosinase-related protein-2 (DOPA-chrome tautomerasa) | Rabbit | + |
| HMB-45 | Glycoconjugate present in immature melanosomes | Mouse | + + |
| TMH-1 | Tyrosinase-related protein encoded by pMT4 | Mouse | + |

[a] Taken from ref. 63.

atinization process differing from the adult's, with a prominent granular layer at 17 to 20 weeks of development. However, after birth, the nail bed, like the matrix, keratinizes without a granular layer. It is less active than the matrix, with a longer turnover time than the matrix and skin (73). A thin parakeratotic keratin is produced, apparently dragged forward by the nail plate growing over it, rather than becoming incorporated into the nail.

In the nail bed, the dermis fits into the longitudinal and parallel nail bed ridges in tongue-and-groove fashion. The fine capillaries of the nail bed run in these parallel dermal ridges, and disruption of these accounts for the splinter hemorrhages commonly seen in normal and disease states (22). There is no fat tissue in the nail bed, although scattered dermal fat cells may be visible microscopically.

The nail bed epidermis moves distally toward the hyponychium. The cells that appear to be the germinative population lie near the lunula, so close together that they may be confused as belonging to one population. The distal movement from this position may also help explain why during development, the nail bed epidermis seems to lose keratohyaline granule layers from a proximal-to-distal direction concomitantly with the formation of the primitive nail plate (74).

The nail bed shows a granular layer in some pathologic states, in which the activity in the nail bed is greatly increased, such as occurs in onychogryphosis (75), pachyonychia congenita, and psoriasis (76); in these cases the horny cells produced push the nail plate upward and give it a claw-like appearance.

Histochemical studies of the nail bed prove the presence of bound phospholipids in the nail bed epidermis (Table 5). Bound cysteine can be detected in the transition zones (19,33); acid phosphatase and nonspecific esterase are absent in the dorsal and intermediate zones (77).

Immunohistochemical studies (78) have demonstrated that nail bed expressed all the target antigens found in the normal nonappendageal basement membrane. In particular, there was normal expression of the epidermal-associated antigens, the 220- and 180-kDa bullous pemphigoid antigens, and the alpha-6-beta-4 integrin. There was also normal expression of the lamina lucida antigens LH39, GB3, and laminin. Sinclair et al. (78) pointed out that the dermal-associated components, namely the 285-kDa linear IgA antigen, the extracellular matrix glycoproteins chondroitin sulphate, type VII collagen and its closely associated proteins, and the poorly characterized antigen for LH24 and LH39 were all normally expressed. All the former data were also found in the proximal nail fold, nail matrix, and hyponychium.

### Hyponychium

The most distal portion of the nail bed is the hyponychium, representing the union between the nail bed and the fingertips (Fig. 22); its histologic characteristics are rather

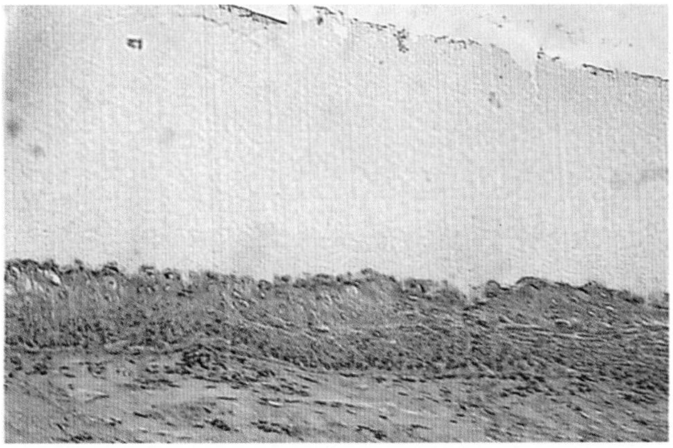

**FIG. 19.** Nail bed. Note the flat epithelium with an interdigitated upper zone.

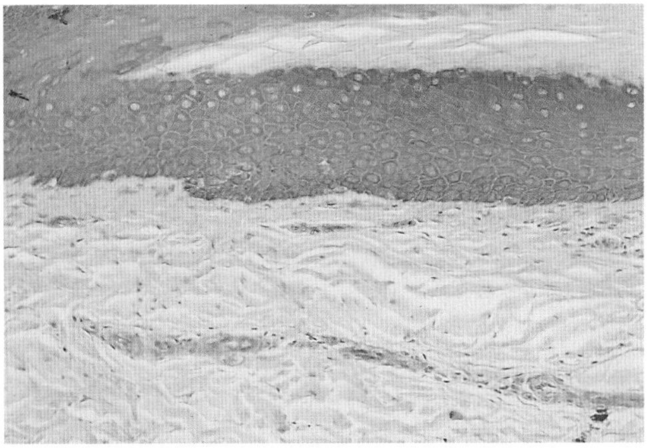

**FIG. 20.** Melanocytes are absent in the nail bed (Cytokeratin antibody stain, **10x**).

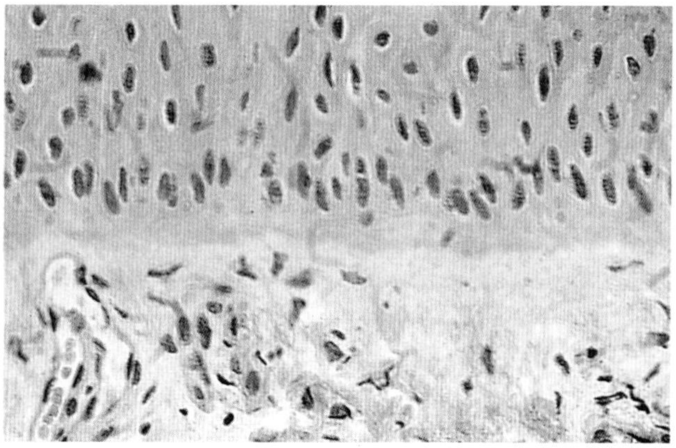

**FIG. 21.** Detail of the nail bed zone. The epithelium shows a few active keratinoblasts. In the upper dermis, it is possible to observe larger vessels than in the normal skin.

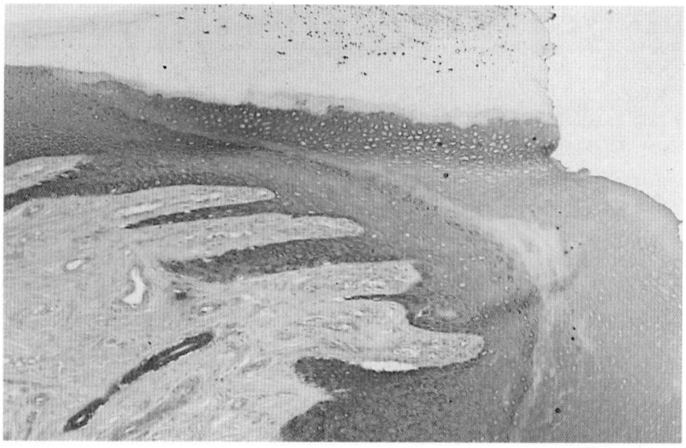

**FIG. 22.** Panoramic view of the hyponychio (Cytokeratin stain, **10x**).

peculiar. This transition zone presents a notable change of appearance after a few millimeters because the epithelium undergoes normal keratinization (Fig. 23). The result is marked acanthosis and papillomatosis with the crests oriented almost horizontally; this is associated with normal appendages (Fig. 24). An arca of abundant keratohyaline granules is present, and the horny layer produced tends to accumulate under the free edge of the nail plate, producing a keratin horn similar to the cuticle. The hyponychium is the first site of keratinization in the nail unit (8,9,11–13) and of all epidermis in the embryo (79). The function of this anatomical formation is to render the nail bed impermeable to protect it from external agents (80). If this structure fails, dermatophyte invasions wlll be frequent, producing onychomycosis (81).

Terry (21) describes an intermediate zone between the bed and the hyponychium, which he called the onychodermal band. Terry speculated that this area, normally from 0.5 to 1.5 mm wide, had a blood supply different from the remainder of the nail bed, a fact later confirmed by other authors (22). For this reason, the color is paler than the pink nail bed and has a slightly amber tinge with a translucent quality. The onychodermal band occasionally changes its color, especially in cirrhosis and other chronic diseases (19,23).

## Lateral Nail Folds

The lateral nail folds have a structure similar to the adjacent skin but are normally devoid of dermatoglyphic markings and pilosebaceous giands. Acanthosis and papillomatosis of the epithelium are present, similar to that of the hyponychium. Keratinization within the nail folds proceeds by keratohyalin formation in the granular layer (Fig. 25). The epidermis lining of these grooves does not contribute to the formation of the nail plate, except in the most proximal portions of the grooves, where it becomes continuous with the epidermis of the proximal nail fold or matrix.

When the lateral border of the nail plate pathologically breaks this fold, abundant granulation tissue forms, constituting the onychocryptosis, a frequent pathologic alteration of the great toenail.

**TABLE 3-5.** *Histochemistry of the nail*[a]

| | Matrix | | Nail bed | | Nail plate | | | Nail folds—hyponychium | | | |
|---|---|---|---|---|---|---|---|---|---|---|---|
| | Dorsal | Intermediate | Basal layer | Malpighian layer | Ventral | Intermediate | Dorsal | Basal layer | Malpighian layer | Keratinized layer | Dermis |
| Glycogen | − | − | − | ± | − | − | − | − | ± | − | |
| Mucopolysaccharide | + | + | ± | + | + + | − | + | ± | + | ± | + |
| Ribonucleic acid | + | + | + | + | − | − | − | + | + | − | |
| Sulfydryl groups | | | | | + + | + + | + | | + | + | |
| Acid phosphatase | + | | ± | ± | + | + + | − | + | + | + | |
| Alkaline phosphatase | − | | − | | − | − | − | | + | | + |
| Amylophosphorylase | + | + | + | − | − | − | | | | | |
| Cholinesterase | | | | | | | | | | | + |

[a] From ref. 20.

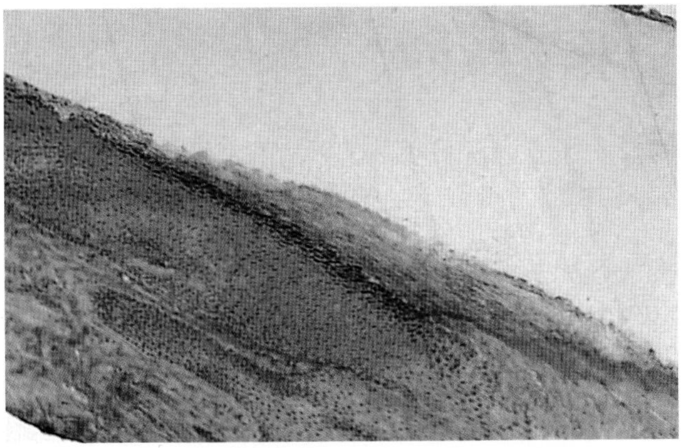

**FIG. 23.** Hyponychium zone. The most important feature of this zone is the great accumulation of keratin under the distal nail plate.

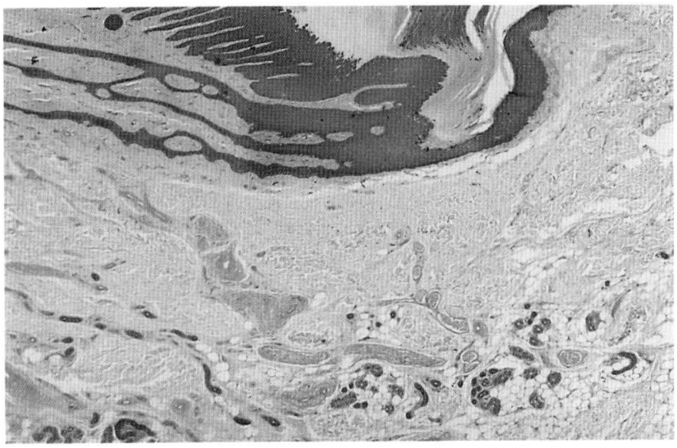

**FIG. 25.** Lateral nail fold. Observe its acantotic epithelial layer and the presence of eccrine glands in the middle dermis (Cytokeratin antibody, **4x**).

## ULTRASTRUCTURAL ANATOMY

Very few studies of the normal ultrastructural morphology of the nail exist (10–13,26,27,38,53–56,60,74), because of varied difficulties (54): (a) achieving proper fixation and adequate penetration of epoxy resin into the nail plate; (b) obtaining ultrathin sections; and (c) securing the high-voltage electron beam necessary to penetrate through extraordinarily hard tissue and availability of 100 to 200kV machines.

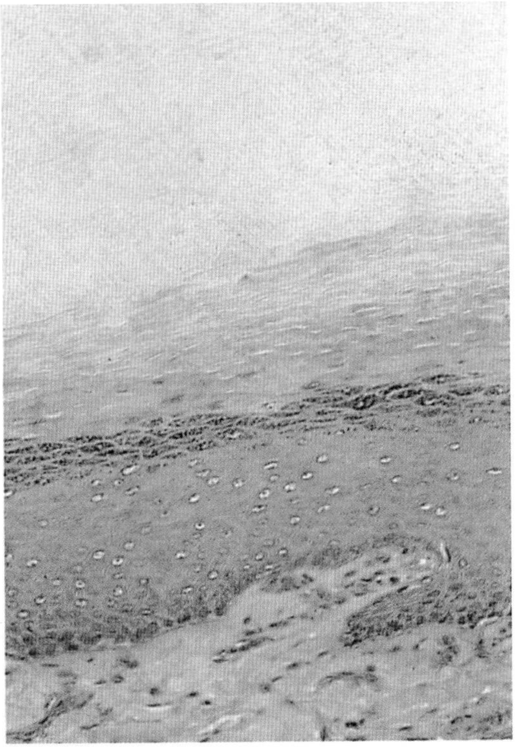

**FIG. 24.** Detail of the hyponychium zone. Note the great keratin layer under the nail plate and the visible granular layer. The epithelium shows an acanthotic aspect, with transversal papillae.

The proximal end of the human toenail is composed of several layers of epithelial cells. Hashimoto and coworkers (53–56) make the distinction between a proximal dorsal, apical, and ventral matrix, although noting that there are few differences between them. They found that the cells composing the proximal matrix were:

1. relatively small, elongated basal cells attached to the basal lamina
2. relatively large, round, or polygonal squamous cells filling the more central portion of the matrix
3. melanocytes
4. Langerhans' cells
5. Merkel cells.

Moreover, there exists a system of attachment to the dermis, showing the surface of the basal cell with frequent fingerlike elongations that interdigitate with the papillary dermis (Fig. 26). This results in the formation of numerous micropapillae, with bundles of very fine fibrils (11 to 12 mm). The subjacent dermis of the matrix zone shows poor vascularity and scarce collagen fibers, with abundant basic matrix.

The basal cells are very active, with frequent mitotic figures. They showed an elongated nucleus and cytoplasm with numerous, slender projections or villi intricately interdigitated with neighboring cells. Tonofibrils were also seen as a perinuclear ring with an interposition of the nuclear clear zone in which the majority of mitochondria, transferred melanosomes, and occasional centrioles are located. The suprabasal matrix cells are also round, with frequent mitotic figures. Generally, the long axes of these cells were oriented axiodistally, suggesting the direction of their migration. Large intercellular spaces were often seen between these suprabasal cells. The extensive interdigitation of the peripheral villi as seen in the basal cells disappeared and multiple desmosomal junctions alone connected these cells (Figs. 27 and 28).

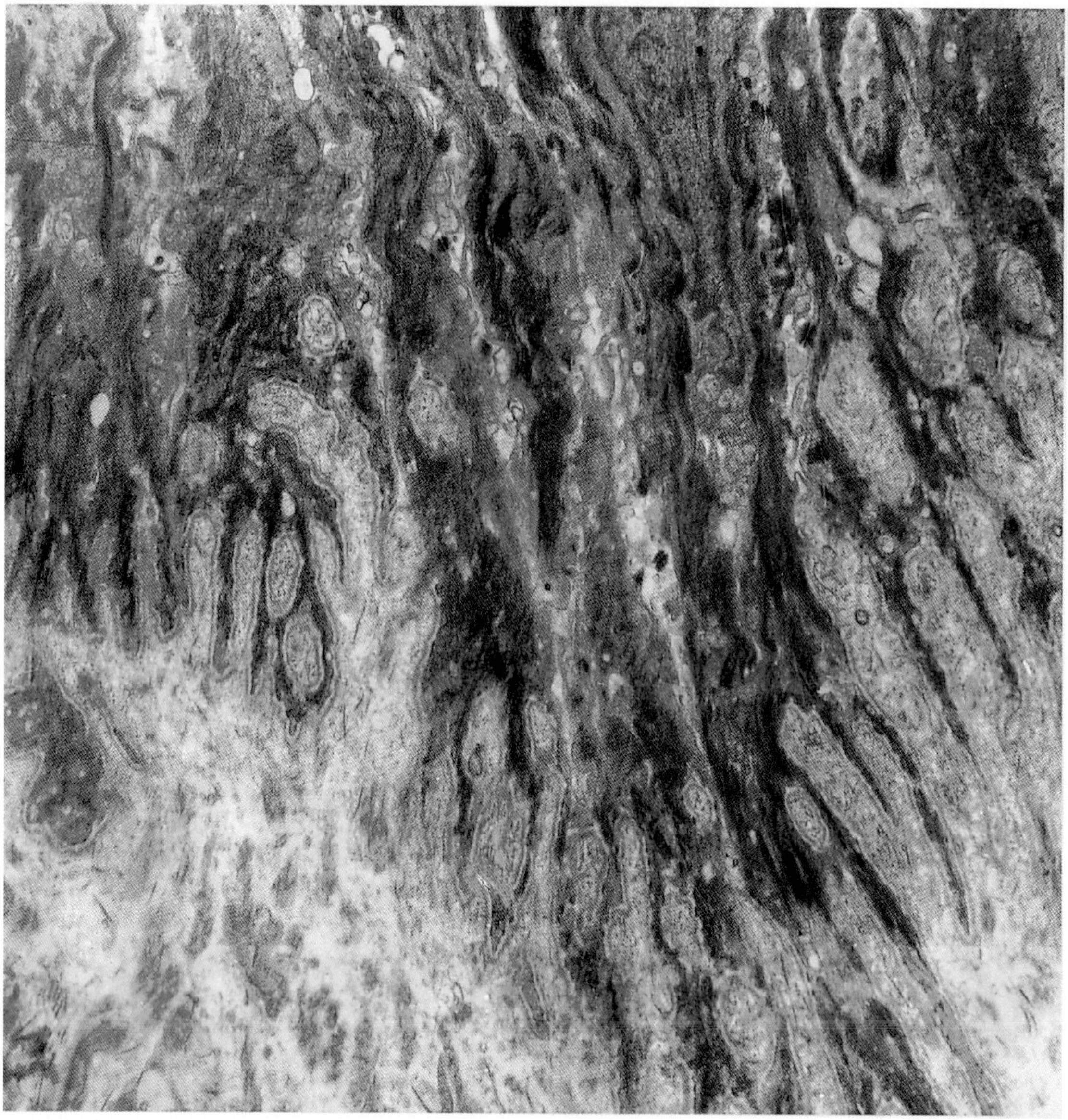

**FIG. 26.** Ultrastructural appearance of the dermoepidermal junction of the intermediate matrix. The basal layer shows an accentuated digitiform distribution, with multiple intermediate filaments (×**7000**).

Abundant desmosomes can be seen in the intermediate layers with high condensations of intermediate fibrils. The aspect of the intermediate layer of the nail matrix is similar to the upper layers of the normal epidermis (Fig. 29). The cells have lost their organelles, and their cytoplasm is nearly filled with tonofibrils. For this reason, the keratinization process is very abrupt, passing from three to four cellular lines to completely keratinized corneocytes.

### Dermis

The dermal component of the nail structures is a very specialized tissue, unique in that it is limited by the underlying phalanx and closely associated with its vasculature and nerve supply. There is no subcutaneous tissue, as previously noted.

Dermis, epithelium, and nail plate in the nail bed present special histologic features due to the great traction that is supported. The dermis is very thick with a dense collagen layer. These fibers are vertically situated in the proximal zone of the nail bed (Fig. 30) and inclined at 45° in the zone adjacent to the hyponychium (Fig. 31). Their mission is to attach the nail plate directly with the phalangeal periosteum. Conversely, the nail plate and nail bed are quite firmly attached to each other, more so than the nail plate to the matrix, and this seems to be accomplished by the striking, deep longitudinal ridges and furrows of the nail surface of the nail plate. The nail bed has a unique, longitudinal, tongue-and-groove spatial arrangement of papillary dermal papillae and epidermal rete ridges. This feature is easily observed in transverse sections, in which this arrangement is appreciated as a serrated interdigitation of the ventral surface of the nail, papillae, and rete. These furrows can be seen very well macroscopically just after avulsion of the nail plate, but they are also beautifully shown microscopically by scanning electron microscope (Figs. 32 and 33) (74).

There are few studies about the nerve supply of the nail. The matrix and nail bed present sparse nerve endings and few Vater-Pacini (82) and Meissner corpuscles (83). Intraepithelial nerve fibers were described at the beginning of this century (82), but other authors (84) were unable to confirm the description.

The hyponychium is the area with greater abundance of nerve endings of the nail, and with abundant Meissner and Merkel-Ranvier corpuscles, as in the lateral nail folds (84). This histologic feature gives the hyponychium an important role in the fine sensibility of the finger.

## Bone

The nail apparatus includes the subjacent bone. Although the bone has been ignored during the last years, a recent study of postamputational repair following digit-tip amputation revealed an unexpected correlation between nail regrowth and bone regrowth. In this way, Zhao and Neufeld (85) have studied this relationship, observing that in the absence of nail, bone did not regrow at distal levels, and conversely, when the nail was surgically retained, bone regrew from proximal levels.

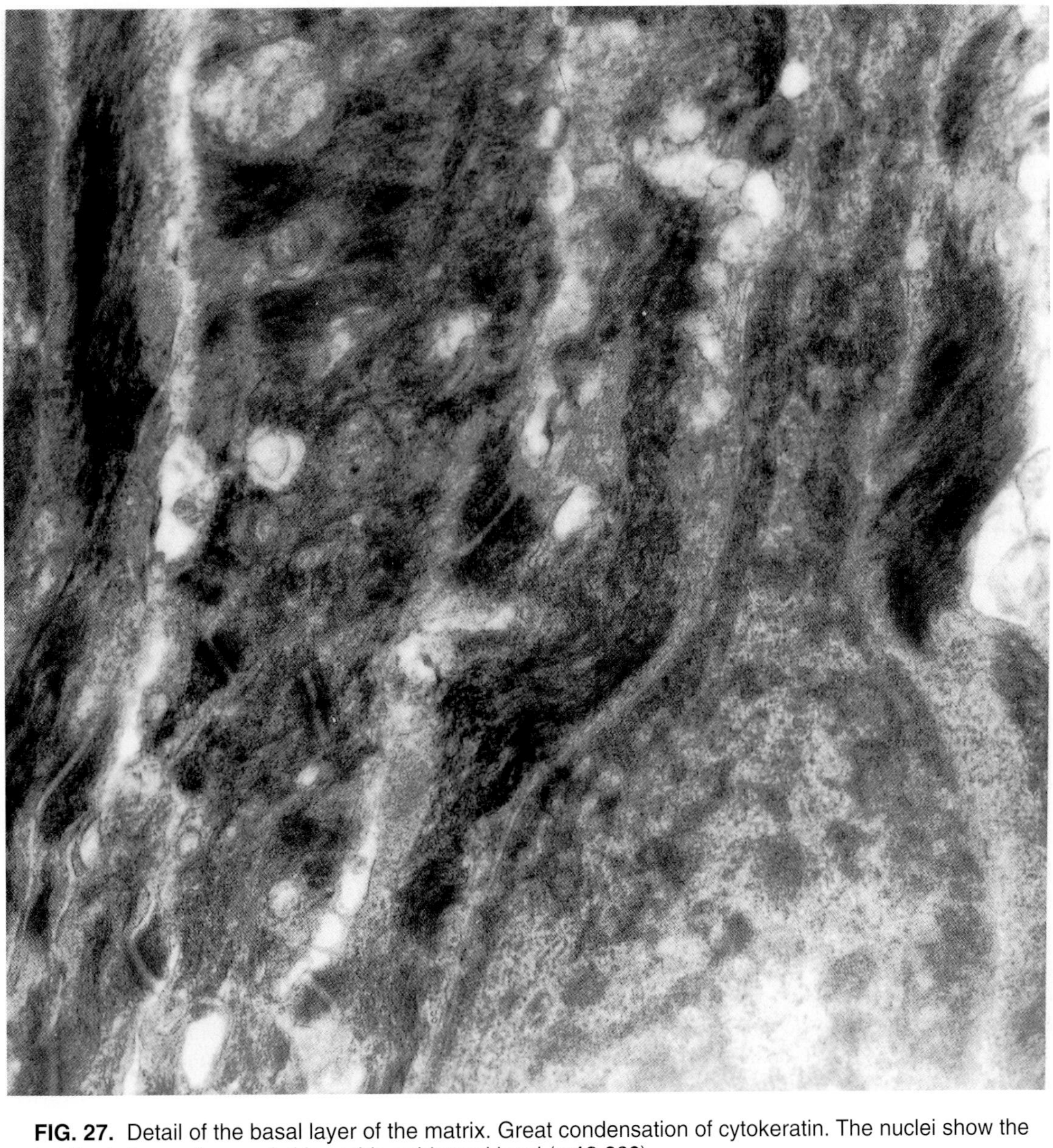

**FIG. 27.** Detail of the basal layer of the matrix. Great condensation of cytokeratin. The nuclei show the habitual shape of normal skin at this epidermal level (×**12,000**).

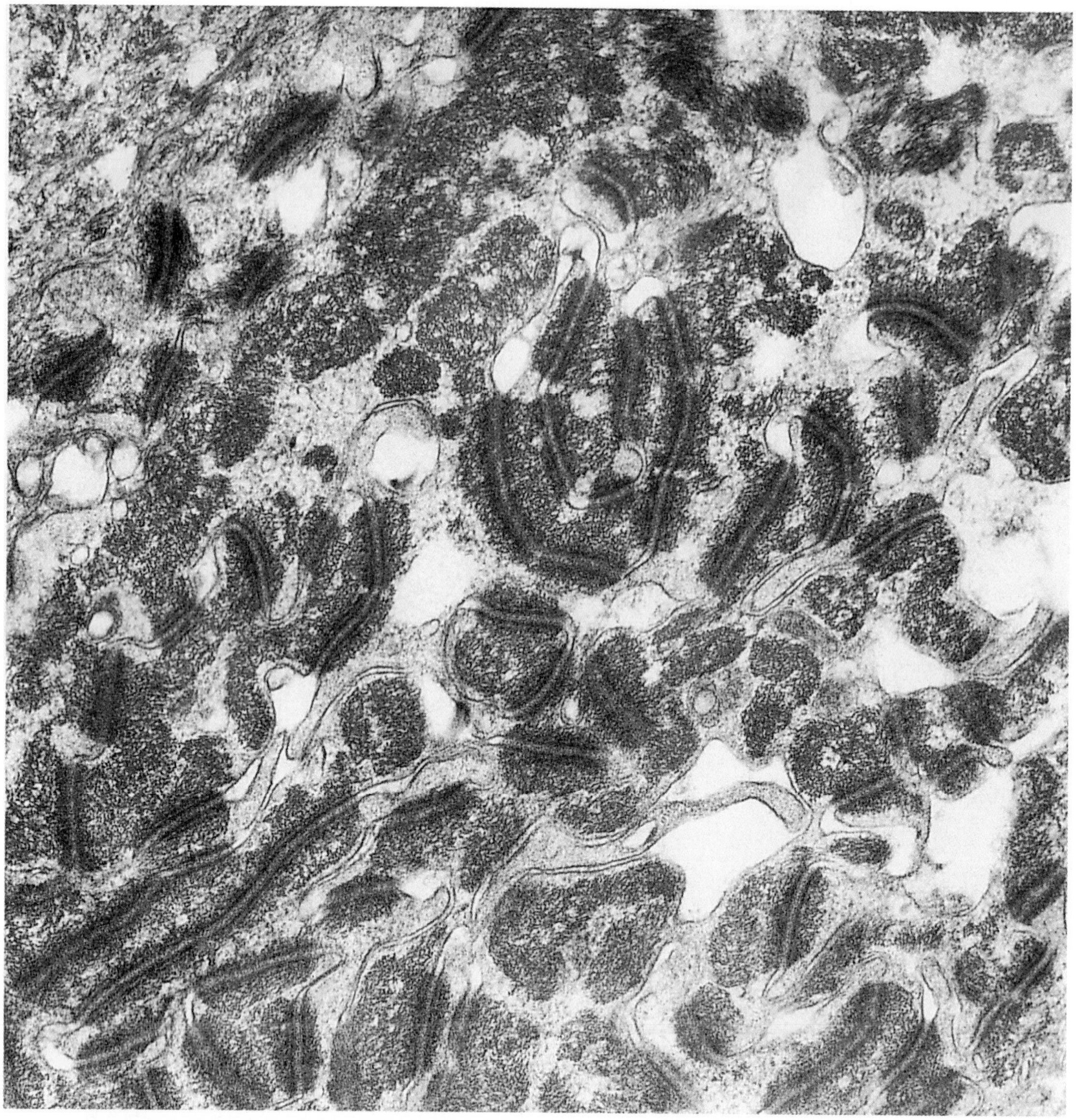

**FIG. 28.** Detail of the desmosomal junctions of the suprabasal layer. They are bigger and more abundant than in a normal epidermis (×**12,000**).

**Blood Supply**

The nail has a rich vascularization that deserves separate mention. The arterial blood supply of the nail bed and matrix is derived from paired digital arteries. The most important studies have been published by Flint in 1955 (86), Ryan in 1973 (87), and Smith et al. in 1991 (88) concluding that the main supply passes into the pulp space of the distal phalanx before reaching the dorsum of the digit. An accessory supply arises further back on the digit and does not enter the pulp space. The digital arterial system manifests three characteristic anatomic features: arched anastomotic arteries in the deep dermis; more superficial terminal arteries branching to supply the rete (89), and the great tortuosity of the arterial architecture subjacent to the nail apparatus (Fig. 34). The arteries possess inner longitudinal and outer circular coats of smooth muscle, but no internal elastic lamina (Fig. 35). The vasculature in the nail bed is unique in that it must supply a vascular structure between two hard surfaces, the nail plate and the bone.

The venous drainage is achieved by two veins, one on each side of the nail plate, in the proximal nail folds (89). The capillary network is easily seen in the proximal nail fold with a magnifying lens, and is seen in more detail with an ophthalmoscopic or capillary microscope. It is essentially the same as the network of the skin but the capillary loops are more horizontal and visible throughout their length. Certain diseases (e.g., connective tissue disorders, macroglobuline-

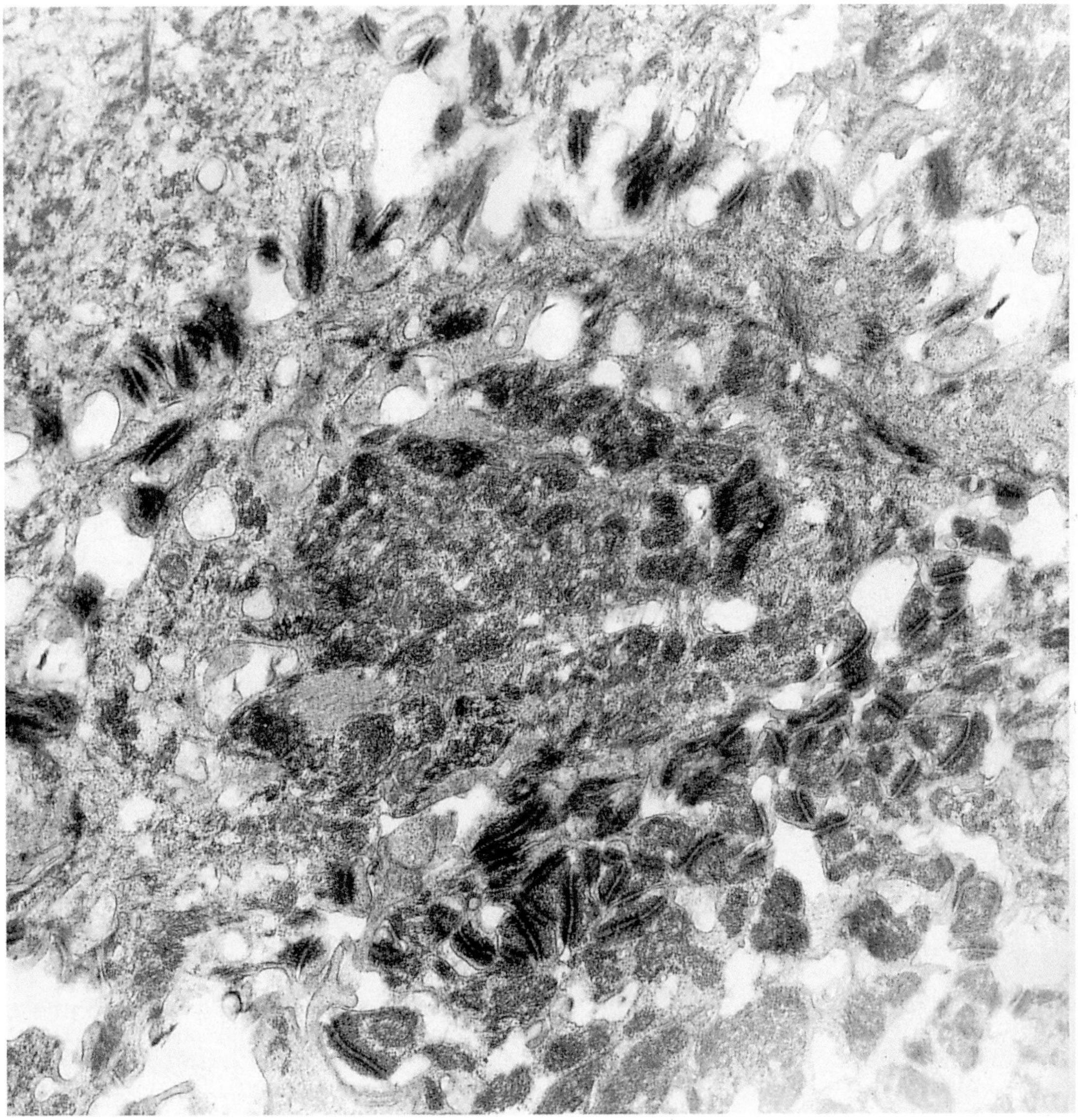

**FIG. 29**. Intermediate stratum of the matrix epithelium. The intermediate filaments of cytokeratin show a special disposition in the nail matrix (×**4400**).

mia, cryoglobulinemia, psoriasis) can modify its normal structure and a simple clinical examination can be very useful as an aid in diagnosis (90–93).

A special vascular formation is present in the distal zone of the nail bed: the glomus bodies. This vascular structure has the mission of regulating the peripheral temperature by means of arteriovenous shunts (94,95).

## NAIL GROWTH

The rate of growth of the nail plate has been studied extensively. Normal nail growth varies between 0.1 and 1.12 mm per day or 1.9 to 4.4 mm per month (96,97). This growth, however, is not the same in all fingers or toes. For example, fingernails grow faster than toenails. Whereas a normal fingernail grows out completely in approximately 6 months, a normal toenail takes 12 to 18 months to do the same (67), (although nails grow faster when regenerating after avulsion) (19).

Several physiological circumstances can cause variations in the nail growth (Table 6). Nail growth is quicker in males (19), during the day than during the night, during pregnancy (98), in persons who bite their nails (23), and in summer or warm climates (99). Conversely, nails grow more slowly in females, during the night, in toes, in winter, after age 20 (100), and during lactation (96).

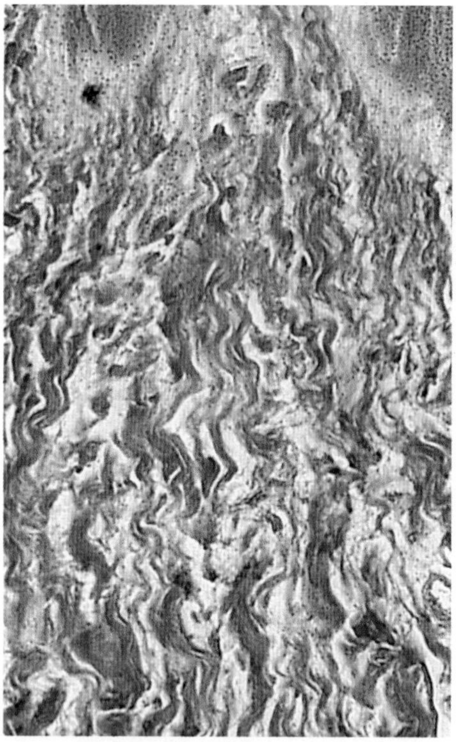

**FIG. 30**. Collagen fibers of the proximal nail bed. Observe the peculiar vertical disposition (reticulin stain, ×**400**).

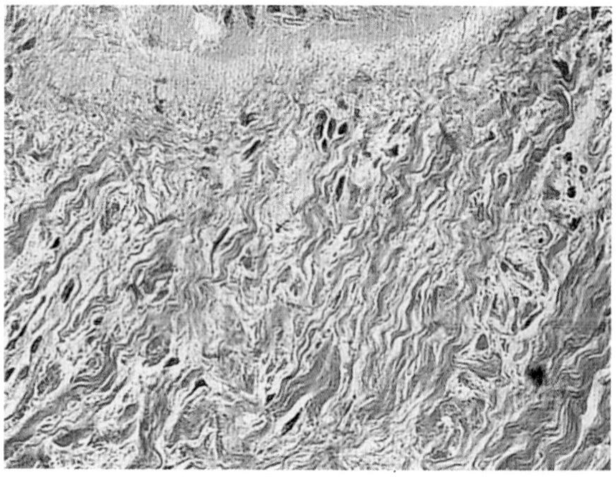

**FIG. 31.** Collagen fibers of the distal nail bed. Observe the pecular inclined disposition (VVG stain, ×**200**).

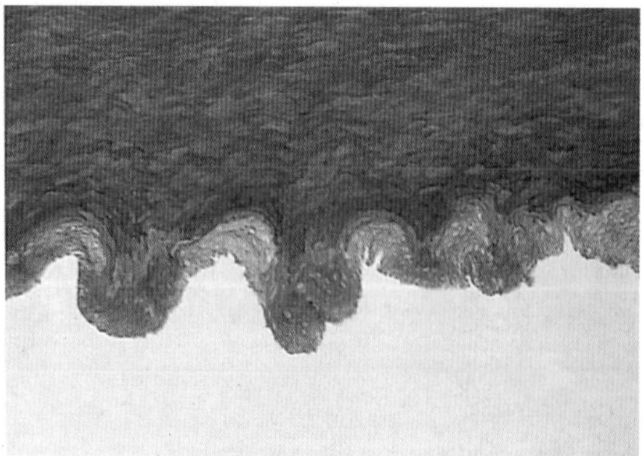

**FIG. 32.** Transverse section of the nail plate. Note the serrated lower surface of the nail plate (MF stain, ×**200**).

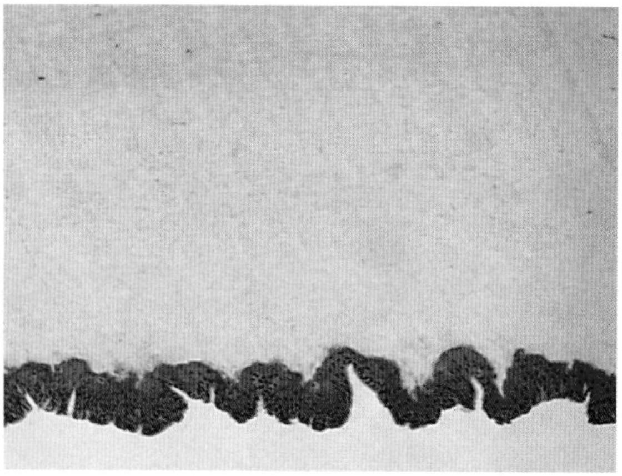

**FIG. 33.** Avulsed nail plate. Observe the sinusoidal form of the nail bed epithelium attached to the lower surface of the nail plate.

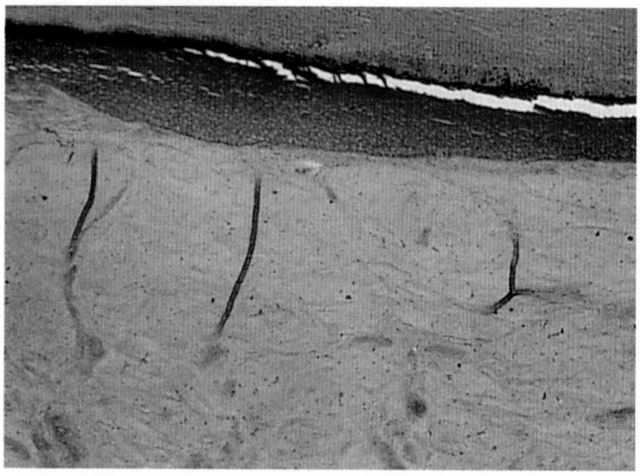

**FIG. 34.** Vascular system of the nail bed. This zone has a rich vascular supply, with numerous vertical arteries, branches of the arched arteries of the deep dermis (MF stain, ×**47**).

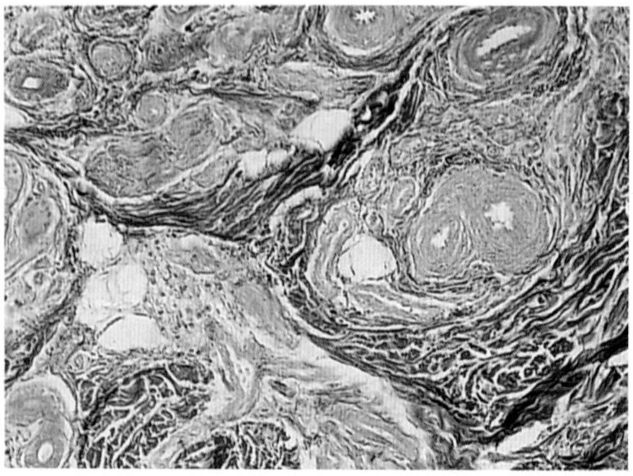

**FIG. 35.** Detail of the rich vascular supply of the nail bed (reticulin stain, ×**158**).

**TABLE 3-6.** *Physiological and pathological variations that influence nail growth*

| Physiological | | Pathological | |
|---|---|---|---|
| Increased | Decreased | Increased | Decreased |
| Men | Women | Psoriasis | Fever |
| Daytime | Night | Pityriasis rubra pilaris | Poor nutrition |
| Summer | Winter | Hyperthyroidism | Hypothyroidism |
| Pregnancy | First day of life | Etretinate | Kwashiorkor |
| Right hand | Left hand | L-Dopa treatment | Azathioprine |
| Youth | Old age | A-V shunts | Methotrexate |
| Nail biting | | Idiopathic onycholysis in women | Beau's lines |
| Avulsion | | | Denervation/immobilization |

Nail growth is also altered in several diseases (Table 6). Nails grow quicker with psoriasis (101), pityriasis rubra pilaris (80), etretinate treatment (102), and hyperthyroidism (19); nails grow slower in cases of immobilization or paralysis (103), local ischemic conditions (96), cytostatic therapy (19,67), denutrition (104), hypothyroidism (100), and yellow nail syndrome (105). In the case of a sudden decrease in nail growth, for example, in acute infections (97), a transverse band will appear afterward, depressed in the proximal line called Beau's line.

The rate of growth of the nail plate is determined by the turnover rate of the matrix cells. Shortly after death, matrix cells do not incorporate tritiated thymidine in their nuclei; the cells appear to be incapable of DNA synthesis and cell division, and, therefore, the nail does not grow (73). Previous reports of nail growth after death are, in fact, erroneous. Apparent growth, caused by severe postmortem drying and shrinking of the soft tissues around the nail plate, is what was observed (106).

The question of where the nail plate is formed is still controversial (107). The first theories at the beginning of the century pointed toward a complete formation by the matrix (108). Years later, Lewis (8), however, concluded that the nail plate was the product of three different matrices on the basis of staining of the nail plate with a silver-protein stain and the morphology of keratinizing cells. Lewis's hypothesis was supported by differential staining of the nail plate (8), by differential interference contrast microscopy (53–56), and by ultrastructural observation of keratohyalin granules in embryonic nail (53). Lewis's hypothesis, however, has been extensively reviewed. Zaias and Alvarez (73) used radioautography to show that the nail plate was formed exclusively by the matrix in normal conditions; Samman (109) and Norton (107) confirmed it by following the incorporation of H-labeled glycine and thymidine in human toenails; and Caputo and Dadati (26) reported that, ultrastructurally, the nail plate was a homogeneous structure with no evidence of formation from three different matrices. To add one final bit to the confusion, Samman (109) suggests that although under normal conditions the nail plate is made exclusively by the matrix, in certain pathologic conditions, the nail bed adds a ventral nail to the undersurface of the nail plate. Finally, Kato published a case with an ectopic nail at the palmar tip, with a vertical growth. In this case, the proximal nail fold promotes upward growth of the nail plate, in absence of a proper nail bed (110).

Some authors asked themselves why nail pitting appears in several pathologic situations, affecting the dorsal matrix, such as in psoriasis, if the dorsal matrix does not intervene in the formation of the nail (111). Thus, some authors have also suggested that a further contribution is made by the proximal hyponychial area (112).

All these theories concur that the dorsal, intermediale, and ventral matrices may contribute in the formation of the nail plate, but the nail is formed fundamentally by the intermediate matrix (Fig. 36). Johnson et al. (30,113) have shown that the 20% final nail mass contributed by the ventral nail of the bed is produced continuosly and equally along the length of the bed up to its point of separation at the onychodermal band.

These authors found that nail thickness increased from 43% of the final thickness over the midpoint of the lunula, to 81% at its distal margin, the remaining increase in thickness being formed by the nail bed (Table 7).

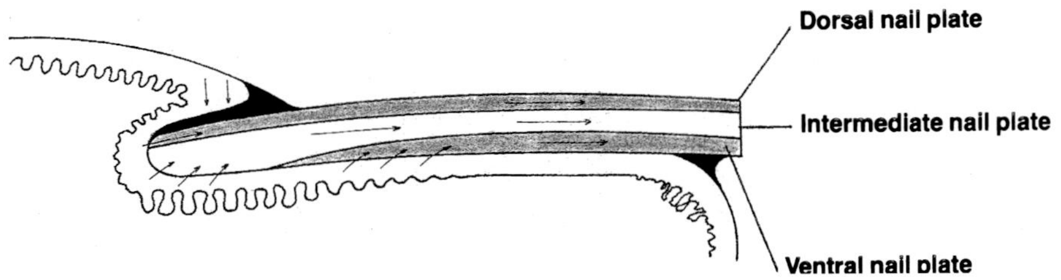


**FIG. 36.** Schematic diagram of nail growth.

**TABLE 3-7.** *Thickness and mass of the nail*[a]

| | Lunula | Nail bed | Distal portion |
|---|---|---|---|
| Thickness | 0.66 ± 0.09 mm (43%) | 1.24 ± 0.09 mm (81%) | 1.53 ± 10 mm (19%) |
| Mass | 52 ± 4 mg/cm$^2$ | 70 ± 5 mg/cm$^2$ | 87 ± 10 mg/cm$^2$ |

[a] Taken from refs. 30 and 113.

Therefore, a shortening of the matrix distal to proximal villi results in a thin nail plate top-to-bottom. Focal loss or scarring of the matrix will result in a linear absence of the nail plate with pterygium formation (20), and that complete loss of the matrix will cause a complete absence of the nail plate.

An important controversy is why nails grow out instead of up. Kligman postulated that the cul-de-sac of the proximal nail groove forced the cells of the matrix to grow out (114,115). To confirm his theory he transplanted nail matrix to the forearm, producing a vertical cylinder of hard keratin that had histologic characteristies of the nail. Hashimoto et al. (53) stated later that the long axis of matrix cells in embryonic nail was directed upward and distally.

Another important question is why the nail bed accompanies the nail plate in its growth. A well-known fact is that a hemorrhage, which occurs between the plate and bed, grows forward with the plate. If the plate merely moved over the bed, the blood would not move; therefore, the upper part of the bed must move out with the plate. Some authors, such as Krantz (116), Kligman (114,115), and Zaias (68), tried to study this phenomenon in an experimental way. Of all theories, the one by Zaias is most acceptable at present: he believes that the proximal nail bed moves out, either by pressure by advancing plate or because of trauma, but that the distal nail bed and hyponychium do not move. The question remains: If the nail bed contributes directly to the undersurface of the nail plate and the nail plate is firmly attached to the nail bed, how does the plate move out?. Today, the answer to this question and to those mentioned previously remains to be clarified.

## HANDLING AND PROCESSING OF THE NAIL

The major problem of the nail unit is the difficulty of tissue selection and the need for proper orientation of the specimen. These problems are the reason for the small number of histologic studies.

The first important point is how to take a biopsy of the nail unit (117–122). The best way of studying a biopsy of the nail is to ascertain that it includes the complete thickness of the nail unit, (which means nail plate, bed, and subjacent dermis); these can be sectioned transversely. If a punch biopsy is taken, it should be done by boring firmly through the nail plate and into the underlying tissue to obtain a specimen with the plate attached. If one wishes to eliminate the nail plate before taking the biopsy, special care has to be taken about nail avulsion, because if it has been avulsed without care, the epithelium of the bed or matrix may become separated, the undersurface may remain attached to the plate and distort the true histopathologic picture. The ideal biopsy technique for the nail is a longitudinal biopsy (121), which includes the hyponychium, the nail bed, and matrix with overlying plate, and the proximal nail fold and cuticle. The specimen may be taken from the center of the nail apparatus or from the lateral edge (119), or may be modified to provide elliptical excision of a tumor of the nail bed (121).

The second point is the orientation of the specimen for cutting. In all cases, the surgeon should alert the pathologist on the submission form as to the way the specimen was obtained, whether a particular orientation is needed, and whether a piece of the nail plate is included.

The third point is how to treat the specimen in the laboratory. If the nail plate is present in the specimen, it will be too hard for ready cutting with a microtome unless some method of softening is used. A special fixative of 5% trichloroacetic acid and 10% formalin will leave the plate softer (119). Alternatively, the specimen can be placed in distilled water for a few hours before placing in formalin (120).

In the coming years, complex studies by indirect immunofluorescence, immunoblotting, PCR, and monoclonal antibodies will be very useful to explain some of the controversial aspects formerly commented on in this chapter.

## REFERENCES

1. Zander R. Untersuchungen uber den Verhornungsprogress: 1. Die Histogenese des Nagels beim menschiichen Fetus. *Arch Anat Entwicklungsmech* 1886;273.
2. Kolliker A. Die entwicklung des menschlichen Nagels. *Z Wiss Zool* 1988;1:1–12.
3. Unna PG. Entwicklungsgeschichte und Anatomie. In: *Piemssens Handbook der speciellen Pathologie zínd Therapie, vol. 14.* Leipzig, 1883.
4. Boas JEV. Ein Beitrag zur Morphologie der Nagel, Kralien, Hufe and Klauen der Saugetiere. *Morphol Jahrb* 1883;9:390.
5. Henle J. *Das Wachstrum des menschlichen Nagels und des Pferderhiffs.* Gottingen, Dieterich, 1884.
6. Branca A. Notes sur la structure de l'ongle. *Ann Dermatol Syphiligr (Paris)* 1910;1:353–371.
7. Clark WE, Buxton LH. Studies in nail growth. *Br J Dermatol* 1938; 50:221.
8. Lewis BL. Microscopic studies of fetal and mature nail and surrounding soft tissues. *AMA Arch Dermatol Syphil* 1954;70:732.
9. Zaias N. Embryology of the human nail. *Arch Dermatol* 1963;87: 37–53.
10. Holbrook K.A, Odland GF. The fine structure of the developing human epidermis. *J Invest Dermatol* 1975;65:16–38.
11. Conejo-Mir JS, Ambrosiani J, Dorado M. Analisis de la morfogénesis ungueal. *Estudio con microscopio electronica de barrido en el embrion humano.* Barcelona: lsdin, 1985;1–8.

12. Conejo-Mir JS, Ambrosiani J, Dorado M, Camacho F, Genis BJM. Human nail development. *A scanning electron microscopy study.* Abstract book of the Meeting of the American Academy of Dermatopathology, Washington DC, 1988.
13. Suchard R. Des modifications des celluies de la matrice et du lit de l'ongle dans quelques cas pathologiques. *Arch Physiol (Paris)* 1882; 2:445.
14. Ogura R, Knox JM, Griffin AC, Kusuhara M. The concentration of sulphydryl and disulfide in human epidermis, hair and nail. *J Invest Dermatol* 1962;38:69–75.
15. Lewin K. The normal fingernail. *Br J Dermatol* 1965;77:421.
16. Pinkus F. The development of the integument. In: Kleibel F, Mali F, eds. *Manual of human embryology.* Philadelphia; Lippincott, 1910;chap 10.
17. Le Groos Clark WB. The problems of the claw in primates. *Proc Zool Soc* 1936;I:1–24.
18. Pinkus F. Der Nagel. In: *Jadassohns Handbuch, der Haut und Geschlechtskrankeilen.* Berlin; Springer-Verlag, 1927.
19. Baran R, Dawber RPR. *Diseases of the nail and their management.* Oxford; Blackwell Scientific, 1984;1–21.
20. Caputo R, Cappio F, Rigoni C, Scarabelli G, Toffolo P, Spinelli G, Crosti C. Pterygium inversum unguis. Report of 19 cases and review of the literature. *Arch Dermatol* 1993;129:1307–1309.
21. Terry RB. The onychodermal hand in health and discase. *Lancet* 1955;1:179–181.
22. Martin BF, Platts MM. A histological study of the nail region in normal human subjects and in those showing splinter hemorrhages of the nail. *J Anal* 1959;93:323–330.
23. Raffle EJ. Terry's nails. *Lancet* 1984;1:1131.
24. Finlay AY, Moseley H, Duggan TC. Ultrasound transmission time: an in vivo guide to nail thickness. *Br J Dermatol* 1987;117:765–770.
25. Goettman S, Drape JL, Lidy-Peretti I, et al. Magnetic resonance imaging: a new tool in the diagnosis of tumors of the nail apparatus. *Br J Dermatol* 1994,130:701–710.
26. Caputo R, Dadati E. Preliminary observations about the ultrastructure of the human nail plate treated with thioglycolic acid. *Arch Klin Exp Dermatol* 1968;231:344–354.
27. Forslind B, Thyresson N. On the structure of the normal nail. A scanning electron microscope study. *Arch Dermatol Forsch* 1975;251: 199–204.
28. Lewis BL, Montgomery H. The senile nail. *J Invest Dermatol* 1955; 24:11–18.
29. Hamilton JB, Tereda H, Mestier GE. Studies of growth through the lifespan in Japanese. Growth and size of nails and their relationship to age, sex, hereditary and other factors. *J Gerontol* 1955;10:401–415.
30. Johnson M, Shuster S. Determinants of nail thickness and length. *Br J Dermatol* 1994;130:195–198.
31. German H, Barran W, Plewig G. Morphology of corneocytes from human nail plates. *J Invest Dermatol* 1980;74:115–118.
32. Walters KA, Flynn GL, Marvel JR. Physicochemical characterization of the human nail. I. Pressure sealed apparatus for measuring nail plate permeabilities. *J Invest Dermatol* 1981;76:76–79.
33. Jarret A, Spearman RI. The histochemistry of the human nail. *Arch Dermatol* 1966;94:652–657.
34. Pautard FGE. Mineralization of keratin and its comparison with enamel matrix. *Nature* 1963;199:531–540.
35. Forslind B, Wroblewski R, Afzelius BA. Calcium and sulphur location in human nail. *J Invest Dermatol* 1976;67:273–290.
36. Zaias N. *The nail in health and disease.* Lancaster; MTP Press, 1980.
37. Dawber RPR. Industrial koilonychia. *Br J Dermatol* 1974;91:10–11.
38. Dawber RPR. The ultrastructure and growth of human nails. *Arch Dermatol Res* 1980;269:197–204.
39. Bolliger A, Gross R. Non-keratin of human toenails. *Aust J Exp Biol Med Sci* 1953;127–130.
40. Levitt JI. Creatinine concentraron of human fingernail and toenail clippings. Application in determining the duration of renal failure. *Ann Intern Med* 1966;64:312–327.
41. Goldblum RW, Derby S, Lerner AB. The metal content of skin, nails and hair. *J Invest Dermatol* 1953;20:13–18.
42. Kopito L, Mahmoodian A, Townley RRW, Khaw KT, Schwachman H. Studies in cystic fibrosis. *N Engl J Med* 1965;272:504–509.
43. Martin SM. Copper content of hair and nails of normal individuals and of patients with hepatolenticular degeneration. *Nature* 1964;202: 903–904.
44. Gillespie JM, Frenkel MJ. The diversity of keratins. *Comp Biochem Physiol* 1974;47B:339–349.
45. Baden H, Kvedar JC. Epithelial cornified envelope precursors are in the hair follicle and nail. *J Invest Dermatol* 1993;101:72S–74S.
46. O'Keefe EJ, Hamilton EH, Lee S-C, Steinert P. Trichohyalin: a structural protein of hair, tongue, nail and epidermis. *J Invest Dermatol* 1993;101:65S–71S.
47. Heid HW, Moll I, Franke WW: Pattern of expression of trichocytic and epithelial cytokeratins in mammalian tissues. *Differentiation* 1988;37:215–230.
48. Kitahara T, Ogawa H. The expression and characterization of human nail keratin. *J Dermatol Sci* 1991;2:402–406.
49. Kitahara T, Ogawa H. Cultured nail keratinocytes express hard keratins characteristic of nail and hair in vivo. *Arch Dermatol Res* 1992: 253–256.
50. Kitahara T, Ogawa H. Coexpression of keratins characteristics of skin and hair differentiation in nail cells. *J Invest Dermatol* 1993;100: 171–175.
51. Cameli N, Picardo M, Tosti A, Perrin C, Pisani A, Ortonne JP. Expression of integrins in human nail matrix. *Br J Dermatol* 1994;130: 583–588.
52. Picardo M, Tosti A, Marchese C, et al. Characterization of cultured nail matrix cells. *J Am Acad Dermatol* 1994;30:434–440.
53. Hashimoto K, Gross BG, Nelson R, Lever W. The ultrastructure of the skin of human embryos. III. The formation of the nail in 16-18 week old embryos. *J Invest Dermatol* 1966;47:205–217.
54. Hashimoto K. Ultrastructure of the human toenails. l. Proximal nail matrix. *J Invest Dermatol* 1971;56:235–246.
55. Hashimoto K. Ultrastructure of the human toenail. II. Keratinization and formation of the marginal band. *J Ultrastruct Res* 1971;36: 391–410.
56. Hashimoto K. Ultrastructure of the human toenail. Cell migration, keratinization and formation of the intercellular cement. *Arch Dermatol Forsch* 1971;240:1–22.
57. Higashi N. Melanocytes of nail matrix and nail pigmentation. *Arch Dermatol* 1968;97:570–574.
58. Scott GA, Haake AR. Keratinocytes regulate melanocyte number in human fetal and neonatal skin equivalents. *J Invest Dermatol* 1991;97: 776–781.
59. Higashi N, Saito T. Horizontal distribution of dopa-positive melanocytes in the nail matrix. *J Invest Dermatol* 1969;53:16–165.
60. Jimbrow K, Takahashi M, Sato S, Kukita A. Ultrastructural and cytochemical studies on melanogenesis in melanocytes of normal human hair matrix. *J Electron Microsc (Tokyo)* 1971;20:87–90.
61. Feibleman CE, Stoll H, Maize JC. Melanomas of the palm, sole and nail bed. *Cancer* 1980;46:2492–2504.
62. Gallais V, Lacour JP, Perrin C, et al. Acral pigmented macules and longitudinal melanonychia in AIDS patients. *Br J Dermatol* 1992; 126:387–391.
63. Tosti A, Cameli N, Piraccini BM, et al. Characterization of nail matrix melanocytes with anti-PEP1, antiPEP8, TMH-1 and HMB-45 antibodies. *J Am Acad Dermatol* 1994;31:193–196.
64. Moll I, Moll R. Merkel cells in ontogenesis of human nails. *Arch Dermatol Res* 1993;285:366–-371.
65. Lacour JP, Dubois D, Pisani A, Ortonne JP. Anatomical mapping of Merkel cells in normal human adult epidermis. *Br J Dermatol* 1991; 125:535–542.
66. Samman PD. The ventral nail. *Arch Dermatol* 1961;84:192–195.
67. Samman PD. *The nail in disease.* 3rd ed. London; Heinemann Medical Books, 1978.
68. Zaias N. The movement of the nail bed. *J Invest Dermatol* 1967;48: 402–403.
69. Achten G. L'ongle normal et pathologique. *Dermatologica* 1963;126: 229–245.
70. Baran R, Giovanni T. Les dyschromies ungueales. *Hospital (Paris)* 1969;57:101–107.
71. Burrows MT. The significance of the lunula of the nail. *Johns Hopkins Hosp Res* 1919;18:357–361.
72. Dawber RPR, Baran R. The nails. In: Rook A, Wilkinson DS, Ebling FJG, Champion RH, Burton JL, eds. *Textbook of dermatology.* Oxford; Blackwell Scientific, 1986;2039–2044.
73. Zaias N, Alvarez J. The formation of the nail plate. An autoradiographic study in squirrel monkeys. *J Invest Dermatol* 1968;51: 120–126.
74. Meyer JC, Grundmand HP. Scanning electron microscopic investigation of the healthy nail and its surrounding tissue. *J Cutan Pathol* 1984;11:74–79.

75. Kouskouski CE, Scher RK. Onychogryphosis. *J Dermatol Surg Oncol* 1982;8:138–140.
76. Omura EF. Histopathology of the nail. *Dermatol Clin* 1985;3: 531–541.
77. Sayag J, Jancovici E. Physiologie de I'ongle. In: Meynadier J, ed. *Precis de physiologie cutanee.* Paris; Editions de la Porte Verte, 1980; 121.
78. Sinclair RD, Wojnarowska F, Leigh IM, Dawber RP. The basement zone of the nail. *Br J Dermatol* 1994;131:499–505.
79. Holbrook K.A. Human epidermal embryogenesis. *Int J Dermatol* 1979;18:329–356.
80. Runne U, Orfanos CE. The human nail. Structure, growth and pathological changes. *Curr Probl Dermatol* 1981;9:102–149.
81. Zaias N. Onychomycosis. *Arch Dermatol* 1972;105:263–274.
82. Doigel AS. Die nerbenendigungen im nagelbett des Menschen. *Arch Mikros Anat* 1904;64:173–188.
83. Martino L. Sulia innervazione dell'apparato ungueale. *Boll Soc Ilal Biol Sper* 1942;1;7:488–489.
84. Winkelmann RK. *Nerve endings in normal and pathologic skin.* Springfield, IL; Charles C Thomas, 1960;100.
85. Zhao W, Neufeld DA.: Bone regrowth in young mice stimulated by nail organ. *J Exp Zool* 1995;271:155–159.
86. Flint MH. Some observations on the vascular supply of the nail bed and terminal segments of the finger. *Br J Plastic Surg* 1955;8: 186–189.
87. Ryan TJ. In: Jarret A, ed. *The physiology and pathophysiology of the skin, vol II.* London; Academic Press, 1973;612,658–659.
88. Smith DO, Oura C, Kimura C, Toshimori K. Artery anatomy and tortuosity in the distal finger. *J Hand Surg* 1991;16:297–302.
89. Hale AR, Burch GE. The arteriovenous anastomoses and blood vessels of the human finger. *Medicine* 1960;39:191–240.
90. Ross JB. Nail fold capillaroscopy. *J Invest Dermatol* 1966;47: 282–285.
91. Gilje O, Kierland R, Baldes EJ. Capillary microscopy in the diagnosis of dermatologic diseases. *J Invest Dermatol* 1974;22:199–206.
92. Kenik JG, Maricq HR, Bole GG. Blind evaluation of the diagnostic specificity of nail fold capillary microscopy in connective tissue diseases. *Arch Rheum* 1981;24:885–891.
93. Ohtsuka T, Yamakage A, Miyachi Y. Statistical definition of nailfold capillary pattern in patients with psoriasis. *Int J Dermatol* 1992;33: 779–782.
94. Mehregan AH. *Pinkus'guide to dermatohistopathology*. 4th ed. Norwalk CT; Appleton-Century-Crofts, 1986;563–564.
95. Goodman TF, Abele D-C. Multiple glomus tumors. A clinical and electron microscopic study. *Arch Dermatol* 1971;103:11–16.
96. Bean WB. Nail growth. 30 years of observation. *Arch Intern Med* 1974;134:497–502.
97. Sibinga MS. Observations on growth of fingernails in health and disease. *Pediatrics* 1959;24:225–233.
98. Halban J, Spitzer MZ. On the increased growth of nails in pregnancy. *Monatsschr Gerburtshilfe Gjnaekol* 1929;82:25.
99. Geoghegan B, Roberts DF, Sanford MR. A possible climatic effect on nail growth. *J Appl Physiol* 1958;13:135–137.
100. Orentreich N, Markofsky J, Vogelman JH. The effect of aging on the rate of linear nail growth. *J Invest Dermatol* 1979;56:61–68.
101. Landherr G, Braun-Falco O, Hofmann C, Plewig G, Galosl A. Fingernagelwachstum bei Psoriatikem unter puvatherapie. *Hautarzt* 1982; 33:210–213.
102. Baran R. Action therapeutique et complications due retinoique aromatique sur l'appareil ungueal. *Ann Dermatol Venereol* 1982;109: 367–371.
103. Fleckrnan P. Anatomy and physioiogy of the nail. *Dermatol Clin* 1985;3:373–381.
104. Babcock MJ. Methods of measuring fingernail growth rates in nutritional studies. *J Nutr* 1955;55:323–326.
105. Pavlidakey GP, Hashimoto K, Blurn D. Yellow nail syndrome. *J Am Acad Dermatol* 1984;11:509–512.
106. Zaias N. Nails. components, growth and composition of the nail. In: Demis J, Dobson RL, McGuire J, eds. *Clinical dermatology, vol. 1.* New York; Harper & Row, 1980; 31:1–6.
107. Norton LA. lncorporation of thymidine-methyl-H3 and glycine 2-H3 in the nail matrix and bed of humans. *J Invest Dermatol* 1971;56: 61–68.
108. Unna PG. Entwichtlunggsgeschichte und anatomy. In: *Ziemessens handbuch der speciaellen pathologie und therapie, vol IV.* Leipzig, 1883.
109. Samman PD. The human toe nail. Its genesis and blood supply. *Br J Dermatol* 1959;71:296–302.
110. Kato N. Ectopic nail at palmar tip. *J Cutan Pathol* 1992;19:445–447.
111. Lovy MR, Bluhm GB, Morales A. The occurrence of the nail pitting in Reiter's syndrome. *J Am Acad Dermatol* 1980;2:66–68.
112. Pinkus F. Nagels. In: Jadassohn J, ed. *Handbuch der halit und geschlechtskrankheiten.* Berlin; Springer, 1927;267.
113. Johnson M, Shuster S. Nail is produced by the normal nail bed: a controversy resolved. *Br J Dermatol* 1991;125:27–29.
114. Kligman AM. Nails. In: Pillsbury DM, Shelley WB, Kligman AM, eds. *Dermatology.* Philadelphia; WB Saunders, 1956;80–86.
115. Kligman AM. Why do nails grow out instead of up? *Arch Dermatol* 1961;84:181–183.
116. Krantz W. Beitrag zur anatomie des nagels. *Dermatol Z* 1932; 239–242.
117. Baran R, Sayag J. Nail biopsy. Why, when, where, how? *J Dermatol Surg Oncol* 1976;2:322–324.
118. Bennet RG. Technique of biopsy of nails. *J Dermatol Surg Oncol* 1976;2:325–326.
119. Stone OJ, Barr RJ, Herten RJ. Biopsy of the nail area. *Cutis* 1978; 21:257–260.
120. Scher RK. Biopsy of the matrix of a nail. *J Dermatol Surg* Oncol 1980;6:19–21.
121. Scher RK. Longitudinal resection of nails for purposes of biopsy and treatment. *J Dermatol Surg Oncol* 1980;6:805–807.
122. Rich P. Nail biopsy. Indications and methods. *J Dermatol Surg Oncol* 1993;19:499–500.

# Breast

*Histology for Pathologists, second edition,*
Edited by Stephen S. Sternberg.
Lippincott-Raven Publishers, Philadelphia


# CHAPTER 4

# Breast

Kenneth S. McCarty, Jr. and Manju Nath



Despite all the efforts expended in breast disease diagnosis, the detection of breast cancer begins with a palpable or mammographic abnormality, which leads to a biopsy. As a consequence, pathologists are presented with a spectrum of histologic pictures associated with clinical "findings" that often are physiologic variations of "normal" histology. The situation is made more complex by the fact that the mature breast, as does the uterine endometrium, responds to ovarian cycling. However, even though they are often cited for their similarities, there are many differences between these tissues and how they respond to hormonal and growth factor changes. Differences range from the epithelial/myoepithelial cell relationship and the epithelial stromal junction in the breast ductules/glands as contrasted to the glandular epithelial stromal contact in the endometrium, to the mitotic effect of progesterone on the epithelium of the estrogen-primed breast epithelium as contrasted to estrogen providing the major stimulus to proliferation in the endometrium.

The influence of sex steroid hormones, pituitary peptide hormones, and autocrine and paracrine effects result in breast tissues that undergo changes throughout a woman's lifetime. Structural and histologic parameters are set with infancy but are not fully expressed until puberty, and they are determined as much by the relative absence of testosterone and androgen as by the differentiating effect of progesterone in a properly estrogen-primed breast. Demonstrable changes occur in the epithelium, the myoepithelium, and the stroma with each menstrual cycle, pregnancy, and lactation. Menopause is associated with variable effects in different individuals and is confounded by differences in endogenous hormone levels from peripheral conversion of androstenedione, as well as by medications and hormonal agents which a woman may take. It is generally assumed that glandular involution follows menopause, but, clearly, differences exist among individuals with respect to the effect of menopausal reduction in estrogen/progesterone levels and cycling, and the transformation from a "dense" breast to the more fatty appearance of the menopausal breast. The transformation is effected through stromal changes, as well as epithelial changes. However, studies are underway to evaluate paracrine and autocrine effects and stromal-epithelial interaction under differing endocrine environments to understand the effects of the "menopause."

The breast has a broad range of what may be considered "normal" histology. It is an inherently nodular, glandular organ in which a given area may be sufficiently prominent to lead to a biopsy. Many of the histologic patterns seen in specimens submitted for pathologic examination are physiologic. As a result, it is important to consider the physiology and endocrinology of the human breast and the influence of such factors on the development and differentiation of the breast.

## EMBRYOLOGY

The early stages of mammary development are remarkably independent of sex steroid hormones, but at the 15th week of fetal development the breast tissue is transiently sensitive to testosterone. The target of the testosterone appears to be the mesenchyme. The breast mesenchyme condenses around the epithelial stalk, apparently stimulated by

K. S. McCarty, Jr. and M. Nath: Department of Pathology, University of Pittsburgh, Magee-Womens Hospital, Pittsburgh, PA 15213.

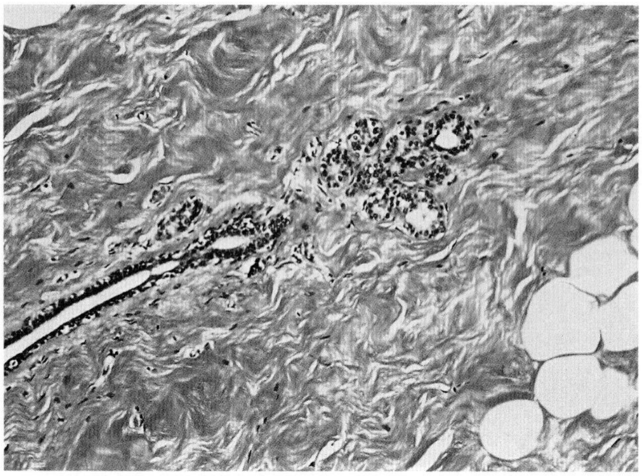

**FIG. 1.** Early pubertal breast tissue demonstrates ductal formation with minimal acinar formation. The presence of myoepithelial cells can be discerned, but as in breast tissue from the early follicular phase of the menstrual cycle, the distinction of epithelial and myoepithelial cells may be difficult.

testosterone, resulting in the subdermal isolation of the mammary bud and prevention of the development of the alveolar ductal system. If significant testosterone exposure does not occur, the epithelial sprouts begin to canalize, leading to the formation of milk ducts by weeks 20 to 32. The branching lobuloacinar development of the breast occurs between week 32 and 40 as a consequence of mesenchymal paracrine effects.

As the fetus matures, the fetal breast is effected by maternal and placental steroids, and under this influence, the monolayered acini become secretory. At birth there is withdrawal of the maternal sex steroids, and stimulation of prolactin leads to colostrum secretion which generally continues for 3 to 4 weeks. The sex of the infant does not influence this stage of development. As the interval from withdrawal of maternal steroids increases and fetal prolactin eventually declines, the gland is observed with a simple ductular organization which persists until puberty (Fig. 1).

## PHYSIOLOGY AND ENDOCRINOLOGY

After the reversion of the mammary gland to simple ductular organization in early infancy the subsequent development and differentiation of the breast depends on steroid and peptide hormones and growth factors (Table 1). The growth regulatory and differentiation mechanisms involved in breast development and maintenance involve systemic, local, cell surface, and intracellular controls (1). The local, cell surface, and intracellular controls serve to modulate the sex steroid and endocrine peptide hormones. Local factors include both growth factors and soluble regulatory molecules, whereas the cell surface interactions include the regulation of peptide hormone and other receptor molecules, adhesion (both cell-cell and cell-substrate) molecules, and transmembrane growth factors. At the intracellular level of differentiation regulation are the early signal transduction events, the late signal transduction events, the activation of early and intermediate response genes, "tumor" suppressor genes and cyclins, cyclin-dependent kinases, and their inhibitors. All of these levels of control are involved in the maintenance, growth, and function of the mammary gland. The development of the breast form (mound) at thelarche requires only the relative absence of testosterone. This is most dramatically shown in patients with testicular feminization. Once the breast is developed at puberty, the follicular, luteal, and menstrual phase of the mature menstrual cycle are associated with observed histologic changes (Table 2). Proliferation of

**TABLE 4-1.** *Major hormonal influences on the human breast*

| Hormone | Effects |
|---|---|
| Estrogen | Required for ductal growth during adolescence<br>Required for lobuloalveolar growth during pregnancy<br>Not necessary for maintenance of lactation or "secretion"<br>Required to prime progesterone receptor induction |
| Progesterone | Required for lobuloalveolar differentiation and growth<br>Not necessary for ductal formation<br>Probable mitogen in "normal" estrogen-primed breast |
| Testosterone | Causes mesenchymal destruction of mammary epithelium during critical period of testosterone sensitivity<br>Inhibits estrogen action, suppresses estrogen and progesterone receptor levels |
| Glucocorticoid | Required for maximal ductal growth<br>Nonessential but enhances lobuloalveolar growth during pregnancy |
| Insulin | Enhances protein synthesis of mammary epithelium<br>Enhances ductal alveolar growth<br>Required for secretory activity with glucocorticoid and prolactin<br>Associated with mitoses |
| Prolactin | Required for lactogenesis and maintenance of lactation<br>Stimulates epithelial growth after parturition |
| Human placental lactogen | Able to substitute for prolactin in epithelial growth and differentiation<br>Stimulates alveolar growth and lactogenesis in second half of pregnancy |
| Growth | Required for ductal growth in adolescence<br>May contribute to lobuloacinar growth during pregnancy |
| Thyroid | Increases epithelial secretory response to prolactin<br>Nonessential for ductal growth; may enhance glandular-acinar growth |

**TABLE 4-2.** *Morphologic criteria for menstrual phase assignment*

A. Early follicular
  1. Stroma: dense, cellular
  2. Lumen: tight
  3. Epithelium:
    a. Cell types: single predominant pale eosinophilic cell
    b. Orientation: no stratification apparent
    c. Secretion: none
B. Late follicular
  1. Stroma: dense, cellular-collagenous
  2. Lumen: defined
  3. Epithelium:
    a. Cell types:
      1) Luminal columnar basophilic cell
      2) Intermediate pale cell
      3) Basal clear cell with hyperchromatic nucleus (myoepithelial)
    b. Orientation: radial around lumen
    c. Secretion: none
C. Early luteal
  1. Stroma: loose, broken
  2. Lumen: open, slight secretion
  3. Epithelium:
    a. Cell types:
      1) Luminal basophilic cell
      2) Intermediate pale cell
      3) Prominent vacuolization of basal clear cell (myoepithelial)
    b. Orientation: radial around lumen
    c. Secretion: none
D. Late luteal
  1. Stroma: loose, edematous
  2. Lumen: open with secretion
  3. Epithelium:
    a. Cell types:
      1) Luminal basophilic cell
      2) Intermediate pale cell
  3) Prominent vacuolization of basal clear cell (myoepithelial)
    b. Orientation: radial around lumen
    c. Secretion: active apocrine secretion from luminal cell
E. Menstrual
  1. Stroma: dense, cellular
  2. Lumen: distended with secretion
  3. Epithelium:
    a. Cell types:
      1) Luminal basophilic cell with scant cytoplasm
      2) Extensive vacuolization of basal cells
    b. Orientation: radial around lumen
    c. Secretion: resorbing

the epithelium may be observed throughout the cycle, but it is principally observed in the luteal phase of the cycle as a consequence of progesterone effect on properly estrogen-primed tissue. This is in stark contrast to the endometrium, where estrogen exerts the dominant proliferative effect and occurs in the follicular phase of the menstrual cycle. Similar to its effects on the endometrium, progesterone has a differentiation effect on the breast, and three important changes occur: (a) the myoepithelial cells accumulate glycogen; (b) the epithelial cells develop more prominent nucleoli and secretion; and (c) the stroma changes with an increase in intralobular and interlobular edema. Several anovulatory menstrual cycles, followed by an ovulatory cycle, may be accompanied by an exaggerated progesterone effect on the breast. This increases accumulation of secretions and increases intralobular edema in a pattern that may be transiently "cystic." There is also alteration in the mononuclear cell infiltrate in the interstitium.

Knowledge of these changes helps in recognizing the normal variation associated with the menstrual cycle and helps to avoid overinterpretation of such "normal" cycling as "cystic change" or similar diagnoses. It should be particularly noted that the breast may demonstrate areas in which the local paracrine effects and stromal interactions dominate the systemic cycling of the sex steroids. Furthermore, breast tissues can convert androstenedione to estrone and other derivatives for which the breast stroma and epithelium have specific receptors and are responsive. Thus, local concentration of the steroids may provide the dominant influence on the tissue histology. The consequence of these local effects is that the breast, in contrast to the endometrium, does not show a uniform synchrony of lobes or lobules with the menstrual cycle, even when the cycle is regular. However, the patterns can be distinguished within each portion of the cycle.

## ADOLESCENCE

Puberty is associated with alterations in gonadotropin [follicle-stimulating hormone (FSH) and luteinizing hormone (LH) secretion], which stimulates ovarian primordial follicles to mature into graafian follicles. This is associated with the cyclic production of estrogens and significant levels of progesterone as the corpus luteum forms. This production of cyclic estrogen in the presence of growth hormone or prolactin restimulates breast ductal growth, which has been dormant since the first few weeks after birth. Neither sex steroid nor peptide hormone is effective alone, and more specifically, the ductal growth (as distinct from proliferation of the epithelium of the lobuloacinar units) is relatively independent of progesterone (1). The elongation of mammary ducts, thickening of ductal epithelium, and the early formation of lobular buds from terminal ductular elements is seen at early puberty. There is also an accompanying increase in the connective tissue density in the periductal regions, also the consequence of relative estrogen dominance. The pattern of stimulation of the connective tissue of the lobular unit is of note in view of the adolescent period being the time when fibroadenomas are most commonly noted (again occurring during the perimenopausal period when estrogen is relatively dominant over progesterone as ovulation fails). Stromal/ductal growth continues until a characteristic ductal spacing is reached, apparently governed by paracrine factors (1,2). Differentiation into lobuloacinar structures requires progesterone (2). Full pigmentation of the areolae and nip-

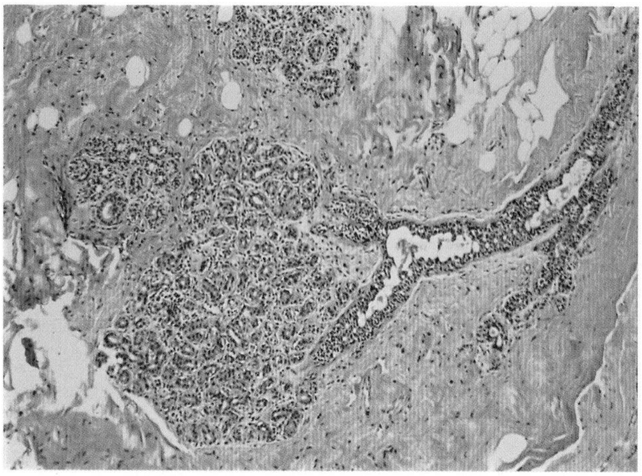

**FIG. 2.** Full lobule-acinar development after several cycles of estrogen priming and progesterone cycling. The ductal structure extends into the terminal acinar lobular unit. Such terminal lobular units occur along the course of the duct/ductule as well as in orientation shown in this example of a mature ductal acinar lobular unit

ples also occurs only when both female sex steroids are present, although this also requires pituitary peptide hormones. The different components of mammary ductal and alveolar formation are influenced by multiple hormones in differing combinations and exposure sequence (Table 1) (1). Cyclic progesterone following appropriate levels and duration of estrogen priming associated with a full ovulatory cycle, drive the development of the mammary lobuloacinar elements, as well as connective tissue growth (Fig. 2). This process of development usually continues, even without pregnancy, into the third decade of life. Each cycle is also associated with apoptotic events under the influence of an intricate balance of endocrine, autocrine, and paracrine growth factors (1).

## DEVELOPMENTAL ANOMALIES

Developmental abnormalities of the breast may occur even though there is no dysfunction of the breast epithelium resulting from a relative imbalance of sex steroid hormones, peptide hormones, or medications. This may occur in conjunction with various disease states. Functional breasts may fail to develop in Turner's syndrome, ovarian agenesis, congenital adrenal hyperplasia, and delayed menarche (3). Estrogen therapy and androgen suppression may result in the development of breast form, although full replacement with cyclic estrogen and progestins is required to produce a gland capable of responding to lactogenic stimuli. Precocious development of the female breast occurs in constitutional precocious puberty, a state of relative aberration of sex steroid levels or proportion in which no causative lesion is found (3). There are reported instances of aberrations in sex steroid secretion due to childhood ovarian tumors, lutein cysts, or lesions of the third ventricle associated with precocious hypertrophy of the female breast. Female breast hypertrophy is not uncommon during adolescence in girls with apparently normal hormonal function (3). Sometimes affecting one breast more than the other, the excessive growth is of the connective tissue and fat, not of the epithelial elements. If bothersome to the patient, the excessive tissue can be excised. In the male, adolescent pubescent gynecomastia will generally resolve with time and sexual maturity.

## THE MATURE BREAST

The "normal" mature female breast ranges from less than 30 grams to greater than 500 grams. Size and density of the breast is greatly influenced by the individual's body habitus because the breast is a major repository of fat (3). Mammary tissue extends variably into the axilla as the glandular tail of Spence.

Approximately three quarters of the breast is on the pectoralis major muscle (superior and medial portions). The lateral portion of the breast extends over the third and fourth digitation of the serratus anterior muscle. The inferior portion of the breast is partly over the serratus anterior muscle, external oblique muscle, and medially over the superior rectus muscle fascia.

The breast gland is typically composed of between 15 and 25 lobes, each emptying into a separate major duct terminating in the nipple (3). Each lobe is surrounded by connective tissue and is divided into many lobules. The lobule is the basic structural unit of the breast and is delimited by a somewhat thicker connective tissue envelope. The lobule is subdivided into 10 to 100 alveoli, which are enveloped by a true basement lamina. The basement membrane extends to invest the collecting duct.

The nipple is ectodermally derived. The skin of the nipple contains numerous sebaceous and apocrine glands. The 15 to 25 parenchymal milk ducts enter the base of the nipple, where they dilate to form the milk sinuses. Slightly below the nipple's surface, the sinuses terminate in cone-shaped ampullae. In the nonlactating breast these ampullae typically contain epithelial debris in their lumen. During lactation the ampullae function as milk repositories. The bulk of the nipple is comprised of circular and longitudinal smooth muscle fibers, with collagenous and elastic connective tissue intermeshed with the nipple's milk ducts (Figs. 3–5). Contraction of these muscle fibers results in local venous stasis, nipple erection, and emptying of the milk sinuses.

In the areolar region, Montgomery's glands are large glands with miniature milk ducts that open into Morgan's tubercles in the epidermis of the areola. Although sometimes described as sebaceous glands, they appear to represent modified eccrine glands. They enlarge and secrete with pregnancy and, unlike sebaceous glands, undergo involution postmenopausally (4). The areola, too, contains smooth mus-

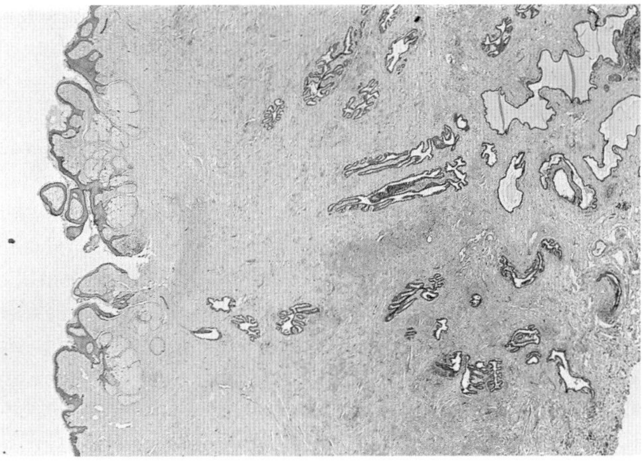

**FIG. 3.** Major ducts in proximity to the nipple epithelium. The major ducts of the 15 to 25 lobes collect at the nipple (5 ducts are seen in this section). The muscular nature of the periductal stroma is readily apparent. The ducts are obstructed by epithelial plugs in the non-nursing breast. The surface epithelium may invaginate down the most distal portions of the ducts.

cle fibers arranged circularly and radially. Hair follicles may be present but are usually at the perimeter of the areola.

The skin overlying the breast contains hair follicles, sebaceous glands, and eccrine sweat glands (5). Fibrous bands extend beneath the superficial and deep layers of the superficial fascia, continuous above with the cervical fascia and below with Cooper's superficial abdominal fascia. Fibrosis or displacement by mass may cause traction on these fibrous bands, resulting in skin dimpling or nipple retraction. The superficial layer of the superficial fascia is delicate, defining an avascular plane just below the dermis. The deep layer of the superficial fascia is more developed, lying partly on the pectoral fascia that covers the underlying pectoralis major muscle. Between these two fasciae there is a retromammary space filled with loose tissue that allows the breast to move freely over the chest wall. Projections of the deep layer of the

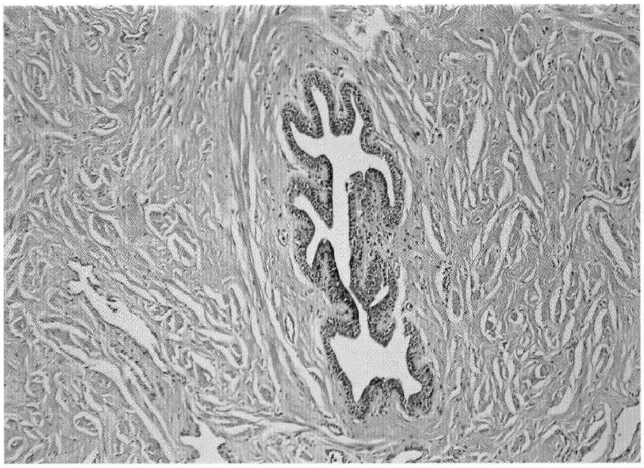

**FIG. 4.** Major duct in proximity to nipple. In addition to the epithelial myoepithelial two-layer pattern, investment with muscle tissue is characteristically seen.

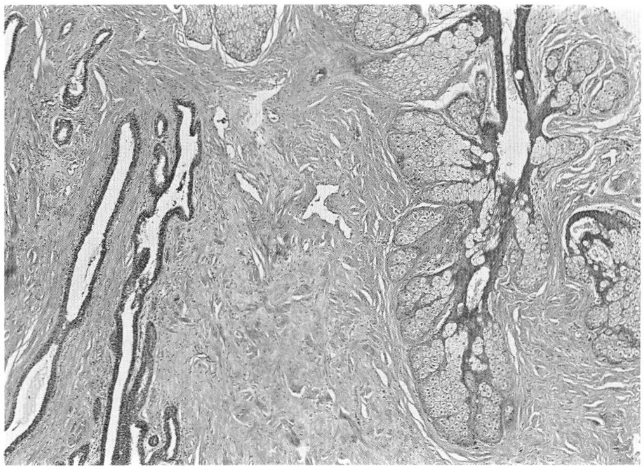

**FIG. 5.** In addition to the ductal elements, sebaceous glands of Montgomery are present in the subareolar tissue in proximity to the nipple.

superficial fascia cross this retromammary space, fuse with the pectoralis fascia, and form the posterior suspensory ligaments of the breast. Breast parenchyma may accompany these fibrous processes into the pectoralis major muscle itself (6). Therefore, complete removal of breast parenchyma necessitates excision of a portion of the muscle, as well.

The pectoralis fascia encases the pectoralis major, extends medially to the contralateral pectoral fascia, and continues cephalad with the deltoid and clavicular fasciae. Although it is common to consider the entire breast as lying on the pectoral fascia, only approximately one-half overlies this fascia, and the remainder lies on other muscles of the chest wall (3). These muscles include the serratus anterior, although the same deep fascia muscles blend them together. An axillary fascia encloses and separates the two pectoral muscles and forms a bridge from the deltoid and clavicle to the muscles of the chest wall. Its superficial layer invests the pectoralis major muscle guarding the nerves, vessels, and lymphatics of the axilla.

## BLOOD SUPPLY

Mammary venous drainage is divided into superficial and deep systems. The transverse veins (91%) run medially in the subcutaneous tissues, then deeply, to join perforating vessels that empty into the internal thoracic veins. Longitudinal vessels (9%) ascend to the suprasternal notch and empty into the superficial veins of the lower neck. The superficial veins may become clinically obvious in certain diseases of the breast, including some highly malignant and rapidly growing tumors. Thrombophlebitis of a superficial vein may resemble breast cancer by causing skin edema and retraction over a firm mass.

There are three groups of veins in the deep drainage system of the breast. The perforating branches of the internal thoracic vein are the largest and empty into the corresponding innominate veins. The axillary vein has many tributaries that drain the chest wall, pectoral muscles, and deep breast tissue. The third deep drainage system is posteriorly directed through the intercostal veins. These veins communicate with the vertebral veins and the azygos vein, which leads to the superior vena cava. All three of these venous pathways lead to the pulmonary capillary network and provide a route for metastatic carcinoma emboli to the lungs (3). The vertebral system of veins connected to the intercostal drainage at each vertebral segment provides an entirely different metastatic route. These veins form vertebral venous plexuses and provide a direct venous pathway for metastases to bones of the spine, pelvis, femur, shoulder girdle, humerus, and skull (3).

## LYMPHATIC DRAINAGE

The lymphatic drainage of the breast is of particular importance. Four principal lymphatic pathways drain the breast: cutaneous, axillary, internal thoracic, and posterior intercostal lymphatics (3,7). In a study involving injection of labeled colloidal particles, autoradiographs of breast specimens found no striking tendency for the material to migrate from any particular quadrant into lymph nodes. The mammary gland is associated with an average of 35 nodes. If a lymph node is blocked, as by cancer, retrograde lymph flow can occur, leading to greater dispersal through lymphatic channels in the gland and the surrounding tissues (7).

The cutaneous lymphatics consist of a superficial plexus without valves that sends branches around the dermal papillae and a perilobular deeper network with valves that follows the mammary ducts in the subareolar area of the breast (3). Most of the cutaneous lymphatics of the superior, medial, and inferior breast, including the subareolar plexus, drain laterally to the axilla. From the lower border of the breast, cutaneous lymph vessels may drain to the epigastric plexus in the rectus abdominous sheath (Gerota's pathway), and empty into the subdiaphragmatic and subperitoneal lymph plexuses. Flow can then continue to the lymphatic of the liver and intra-abdominal nodes, providing a route by which metastases from breast carcinoma can reach the liver.

The axilla receives most of the lymphatic flow from the breast, ranging from 75 [shown by autoradiographs of surgical specimens (8)] to 97% (demonstrated by postradical mastectomy with radioactive colloidal gold uptake studies (9)). There are six groups of axillary nodes, and they all lie beneath the costocoracoid fascia, which encloses them with the blood vessels and nerves of the axilla (3). The external mammary nodes lie beneath the lateral edge of the pectoralis major muscle adjacent to the lateral thoracic artery from the sixth to second rib. The scapular nodes are closely applied to the subscapular vessels and their thoracodorsal branches. The intercostobrachial and thoracodorsal nerves are also intimately associated with these nodes, necessitating their sacrifice in an axillary dissection. The nodes most easily palpated, the central nodes, lie embedded in the center of the axilla. They receive the greatest proportion of the axillary lymph flow and represent the group of nodes in which metastases are most often found. The interpectoral (Rotter's) nodes lie between the pectoralis major and minor muscles. If these nodes must be excised, removal of the pectoralis major is necessary (10). The axillary vein nodes lie on the lateral, caudad, and ventral aspects of the axillary vein, separated from it by a delicate layer of fascia. The subclavicular nodes are the most medial group, situated along the ventral and caudad aspects of the axillary vein. They extend from the origin of the thoracoacromial vein to the apex of the axilla and represent the highest point to which the surgeon can carry an axillary dissection. The lymphatic drainage from all the other groups of axillary nodes empties into these subclavicular nodes. One or more large lymphatic trunks arise from the plexus of lymphatic vessels and conduct the subclavicular lymph upward and medially to the junction of the jugular and subclavian veins. The subclavicular nodes are beyond "regional" nodes, and involvement by tumor is a grave sign (3).

The internal thoracic lymphatic route carries from 3 to 25% of breast lymph flow (8,9). The lymphatic vessels then turn inward and penetrate the pectoralis major and intercostal muscles to reach the internal mammary nodes. These nodes are interspersed along the course of the internal thoracic trunk lymphatic and number 3 to 4 per side of the sternal edge. The internal thoracic trunks eventually empty into the great veins in one of several ways: (a) via the thoracic duct on the left and right lymphatic duct; (b) via lower cervical nodes; or (c) directly into the jugular-subclavian confluence.

The posterior intercostal lymphatics empty into the posterior intercostal lymph nodes, which lie within the thorax in front of the junction of ribs and vertebrae.

## MICROSCOPIC ANATOMY OF THE BREAST PARENCHYMA

The breast consists of ducts, ductules, and lobuloacinar (lobular units, lobuloalveolar units) structures surrounded by basement membrane and collagenous stroma with fibroblasts, vessels, and fat. The immature mammary ductular and alveolar lining consists of a two-cell-layered basal cuboidal and low cylindrical surface epithelium (4). The cells of the duct epithelium, as opposed to the alveolar epithelial cells, contain few mitochondria and sparse endoplasmic reticulum. Under hormonal influence, especially sex steroids, the alveolar epithelium specializes into A, B, and myoepithelial cells. Columnar, basophilic, luminal A cells are rich in ribosomes and are actively involved in the process of secretion. B cells, thought to be the precursors of A and myoepithelial cells, are basal cells with clear cytoplasm and round nuclei. Myoepithelial cells are located in close contact with the plasma membrane of the alveolar epithelium and the lining epithelium of small ducts. They contain myofibrils and dense nuclei (Figs. 6 and 7); in the luteal phase of the cy-

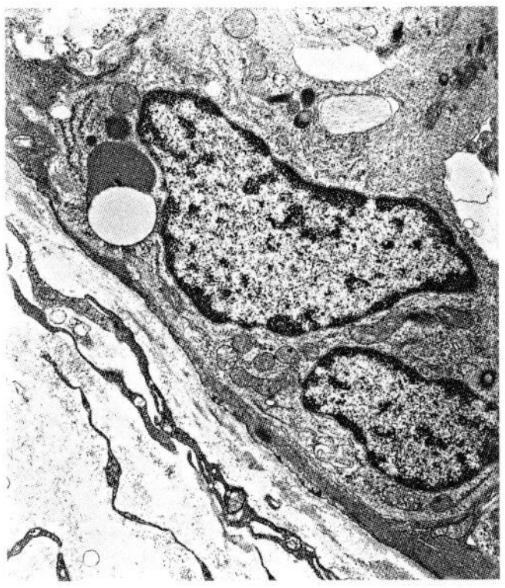

**FIG. 6.** Epithelial stromal junction consists of the epithelial cell, the myoepithelial cell, the lamina lucida, the basal lamina, and the delimiting fibroblast. All are contained in this electron micrograph. The myoepithelial cells contain contractile fiber bundles. Whereas, in general, a normal duct will have a continuous layer of myoepithelial cells, the cytoplasm may become quite attenuated in areas, and focal absence of this component is seen in late luteal breast tissue, rarely in early follicular tissue. The thin basal lamina is continuous around the acinar unit and along the ducts. Electron micrograph uriny1 acetate/osmium tetroxide stain.

cle there is glycogen accumulation which gives a cleared appearance in hematoxylin and eosin (H&E)-stained sections of tissues that have been fixed in formalin. As contractile ectodermal smooth muscle cells, myoepithelial cells of the breast are 10 to 20 times more sensitive to oxytocin than mesodermal myometrial cells (4). The myoepithelial cells do not appear to be innervated. Surrounding the epithelial elements is the epithelial stromal junction. This is composed of the plasma membranes of the epithelial and myoepithelial cells, a lamina lucida, a basal lamina, and delimiting fibroblasts (Fig. 6) (10).

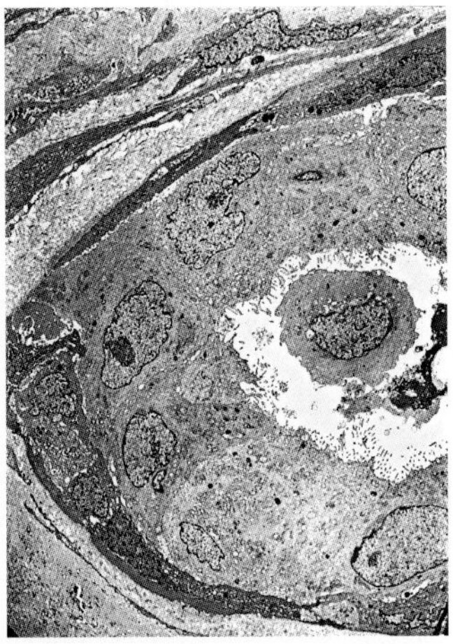

**FIG. 7.** Follicular phase acinar unit demonstrates a relatively tight lumen, epithelial cells surrounding the lumen, and the more electron-dense myoepithelial cells around the periphery of the acinus. External to this is the basal lamina and delimiting fibroblasts. Occasionally, shed epithelial cells are seen, as are apoptotic cell remnants. The relative absence of secretion is characteristic of the normal breast acinar epithelium in the follicular phase of the menstrual cycle. Electron micrograph: uranyl acetate/osmium tetroxide stain.

Changes occur in the mature breasts associated with the menstrual cycle, pregnancy and lactation, and menopause. An understanding of the normal changes in the breast is necessary to distinguish physiologic from pathologic states.

Breast size, density, and nodularity are correlated with the menstrual cycle. Magnetic resonance studies have shown variations of 25 to 30% in water content in the breast at different phases of the menstrual cycle. Glandular nodularity can be so marked during the premenstrual (postovulatory) phase of the cycle that it can be mistaken for clinically significant tumors of the breast. Biopsy should be withheld, however, until the breasts are reexamined near the midpoint of the next menstrual cycle, before ovulation, when physiologic nodularity is minimized. The histology of samples acquired during the late luteal phase of the menstrual cycle are often designated as showing cystic change as a result of physiologic variations in secretion.

Attempts to correlate cyclic physical and endocrine changes with histologic changes in the breast have produced conflicting reports. Although some authors maintain that the nongravid breast is essentially a resting gland (3), morphologic changes in the mammary epithelial and stromal components have been identified as they relate to specific pituitary-ovarian events in the menstrual cycle (11,12). Vogel et al. in our laboratory (12) described five phases of morphologic alterations in the breast associated with the menstrual cycle (Table 2). Although the designation of the first phase of the cycle (early follicular) as proliferative was in error (the mitotic count is greatest in the luteal phase), the remainder of the histologic characterizations of the cycle have stood the test of time. From days 3 to 7 of the menstrual cycle, the postmenstrual phase, the epithelium is oriented in acini lined by two- to three-cell layers with poorly defined lumina. The acinar epithelial cells are of one type, small and polygonal, with pale eosinophilic cytoplasm and a dark, centrally located nucleus. The lobules and their acini are relatively compact. The stroma is a dense cellular mantle with plump fibroblasts (Fig. 8). Maximal mitotic activity occurs in a later phase of the cycle, although some mitotic activity is seen throughout the cycle (11); apoptotic events are seen, as well.

The follicular phase occurs from days 8 through 14 of a normal 28-day cycle; at this time, three morphologically distinct cells become apparent (Table 2). The myoepithelial cells have clear cytoplasm and small, dense nuclei. The intermediate pale B cells of the first postmenstrual phase persist. The third type of cells, A cells, begin to border well-defined lumina and have basophilic cytoplasm and a dense basal nucleus. The basophilia of this cell correlates with increasing ribonucleic acid and ribosome content, observed by electron microscopy (Fig. 9) (13). The stroma remains dense, but is less cellular and has more eosinophilic collagen than in the postmenstrual phase.

The breast enters the luteal phase of the differentiation

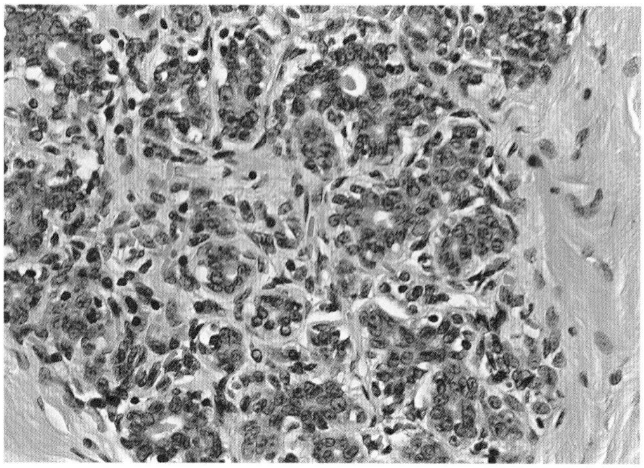

**FIG. 8.** Early follicular phase normal breast. The epithelium is oriented in acini lined by two- to three-cell layers with poorly defined lumina. The acinar epithelial cells are of one type, small and polygonal, with pale eosinophilic cytoplasm and a dark, centrally located nucleus. The lobules and their acini are relatively compact. The stroma is a dense cellular mantle with plump fibroblasts.

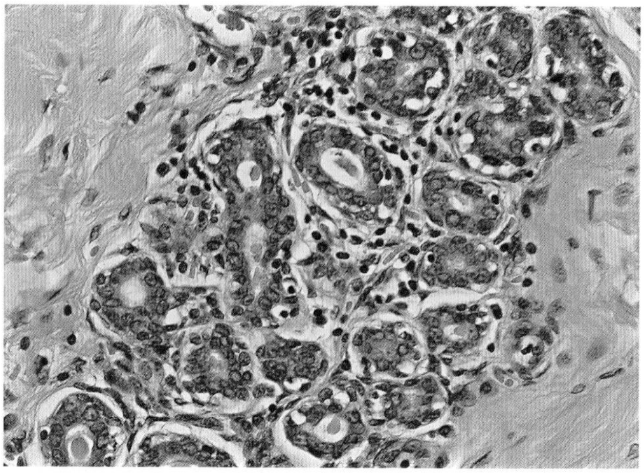

**FIG. 10.** Early luteal breast lobular unit. Vacuolization and ballooning of the basal cell layer is seen due to an increase in glycogen content of the myoepithelial cells. The lumina are enlarged over previous phases and contain eosinophilic secretory product.

with ovulation and increasing progesterone from days 15 through 20 of the normal cycle. The hallmark of this phase is vacuolization and ballooning of the basal cell layer due to an increase in glycogen content of the myoepithelial cells. The lumina are enlarged over previous phases and contain eosinophilic secretory product with early minimal evidence of active apical scouting. There is an overall increase in the size of lobules and the number of terminal duct structures (11). The stroma loosens and the basal lamina becomes less apparent (Fig. 10).

The secretory phase, days 21 through 27, is characterized by apocrine secretion from the luminal epithelial cells into dilated lumina. The apical budding also appears to be a progestational effect. Ultrastructurally, there is a marked increase in polysomes, rough endoplasmic reticulum, enlarging Golgi, and secretory vacuoles, supporting this phase as one of active protein synthesis and secretion (13). The maximum size of lobules and number of acini are expressed during this time (11). Another prominent feature of this phase is the onset of stromal edema. Large, congested venous spaces are present in the mantle tissue, as well (Figs. 11 and 12). As mentioned previously, peak mitotic activity is seen during this phase of the menstrual cycle (11,14). Such activity occurs shortly after the progesterone peak and second estradiol peak at cycle days 22 through 24, and is highly suggestive of a progestational effect or a combined estrogenic and progestational effect (11).

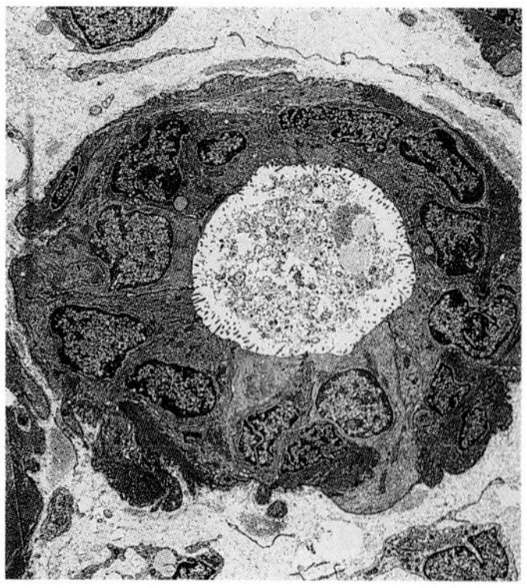

**FIG. 9.** Late follicular breast lobular unit. Three morphologically distinct cells become apparent. The myoepithelial cells have clear cytoplasm and small, dense nuclei. The intermediate pale B cells of the first postmenstrual phase persist. The third type of cells, A cells, begin to border well-defined lumina and have ribosome-rich cytoplasm and a dense basal nucleus. The stroma remains dense but is less cellular and has more mature collagen than in the early follicular phase.

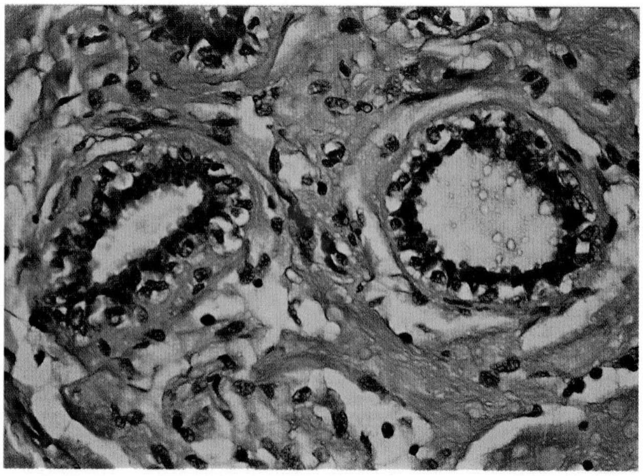

**FIG. 11.** Luteal phase acinar unit. Secretory phase acinar unit characterized by apocrine secretion from the luminal epithelial cells into dilated lumina. Stromal edema is also prominent. Large, congested venous spaces are present in the mantle tissue.

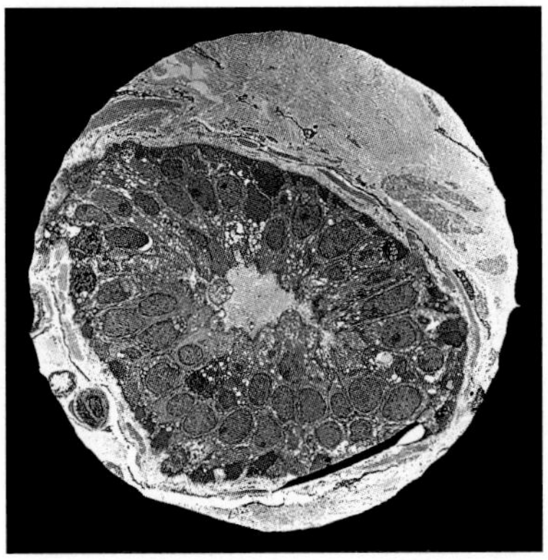

**FIG. 12.** Ultrastructure of luteal phase acinar unit. Increased polysomes, rough endoplasmic reticulum, enlarging Golgi, and secretory vacuoles are seen with active protein synthesis and secretion. The apocrine snouting is seen with inclusion of cell membrane in the process. Electron micrograph: urinal acetate/osmium tetroxide stain.

The menstrual phase, days 28 through 32, is associated with estrogen and progesterone withdrawal. Apocrine budding abates, but the acinar lumina remain distended with eosinophilic granular secretions. The luminal cells have scant basophilic cytoplasm, whereas the basal cells remain extensively ballooned with glycogen. The lobules are decreased in size and the acini slightly less numerous than in the previous phases (11). The stroma is again compact and cellular. As the tissue reenters the postmenstrual phase, the luminal cells become less basophilic, the vacuolization diminishes in the basal cells, acinar lumina become tighter, and the cycle is reinitiated. The breast volume is at a minimum 5 to 7 days after menstruation.

To understand the morphologic changes in the breast accompanying the menstrual cycle, many investigators have studied the receptors for estrogen and progesterone. An abundance of evidence for the presence of estrogen and progesterone receptors in breast carcinoma tissue exists, but there is controversy concerning sex steroid receptors in non-neoplastic breast tissues. Several studies have found low levels of estrogen receptor. The study of progesterone receptor is more limited. A few studies have evaluated whether receptor expression varies with the menstrual cycle. John Silva et al., also in our laboratory, (15) measured estrogen and progesterone receptors with biochemical assays in epithelial-enriched preparations obtained from normal premenopausal women. Maximum estrogen receptor values occur on days 5 to 8, with a small second peak on days 25 and 26; two peak values of progesterone receptor levels are noted on days 13 and 14 and 21 and 23. The estrogen receptor levels are sufficient to detect during the early follicular phase, and progesterone receptor levels are demonstrable during the later follicular phase of differentiation. The menstrual cycle variation may account for some of the discrepancies reported for estrogen and progesterone receptor levels in normal breast tissue. The development of highly specific monoclonal antibodies to estrogen and progesterone receptor has allowed study of menstrual cycle variation of receptor expression in intact tissue (16). These studies have confirmed estrogen receptor concentration to be greatest in the follicular phase, with a less distinct maximal period for progesterone receptor occuring later in this phase. Both estrogen and progesterone receptors localize to the nuclei of the epithelium, and no staining is seen in surrounding stroma or myoepithelium (17,18). Furthermore, estrogen and progesterone receptor localization is often heterogeneous between lobules but tends to be uniform within a lobule of a given specimen. This observation correlates with the variation in lobular architecture within any single breast reported in morphologic studies (11–13).

The functional significance of the cyclic alterations observed in stromal connective tissue is not well understood, and the suggestion of Dickson and Lippman that this may be reflective of paracrine effect is intriguing (1). Important interactions of collagen and mucopolysaccharide with glandular epithelium in embryonal morphogenesis are well recognized, and they are not restricted to the embryonic period (11). Cyclic stromal alterations could play a local role in cyclic epithelial changes and estrogen and progesterone receptor expression, and as mentioned earlier, these paracrine local effects may contribute to local intra-breast/lobe variation in histologic response of the lobule/lobular alveolar unit.

## PREGNANCY AND LACTATION

In pregnancy, mammary epithelial cell proliferation resumes and alveolar differentiation leads to remarkable increases in lobuloacinar structures at the expense of fibrofatty stroma. Stromal changes associated with epithelial growth include increased vascularization and fat cell depletion. The intensified lobuloacinar growth requires estrogen, progesterone, prolactin, and growth hormone, and is enhanced by adrenal corticosteroid and insulin (1). A definite enlargement of the breast with dilation of the superficial veins occurs from week 5 to week 8 of the pregnancy. At the same time, nipple and areolar pigment intensifies, and fibroblasts and inflammatory cells become prominent in the stroma. Colostrum begins to collect in the alveoli by the 3rd month.

With the onset of the second trimester, the mammary alveoli begin to appear monolayered with flattening, whereas the ducts maintain their two-cell layer configuration. Although the rate of mammary epithelial proliferation begins to decline around midpregnancy, the alveolar epithelium differentiates to assume a presecretory function requiring the presence of prolactin, human placental lactogen or growth hormone, insulin, and glucocorticoid (1). Secretory activity and protein synthetic apparatus, stimulated by insulin and glucocorticoid, appears within the epithelial cells. Rough endoplasmic reticulum appears basally and the Golgi apparatus becomes apical. Golgi vacuoles, cytoplasmic fat droplets, mitochondria, and microvilli all increase. From midpreg-

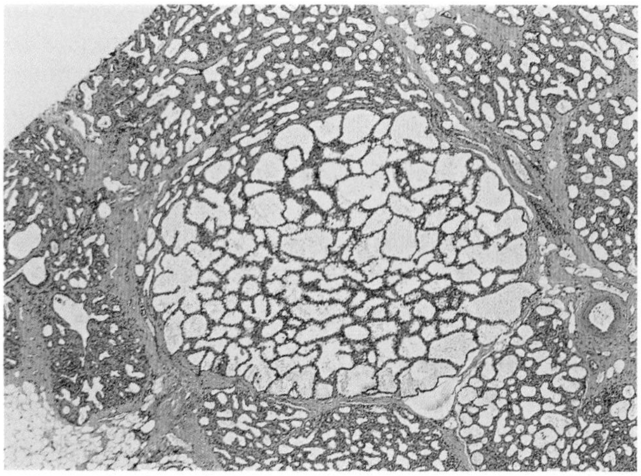

**FIG. 13.** Lactating lobular unit. The effective loss of the apex of the majority of cells is noted as a consequence of active apocrine secretory activity.

nancy on, alveolar mammary cells are actively synthesizing milk fat and proteins, but only small amounts are released into the acinar lumina. The continued increase in breast size during pregnancy is attributed to progressive dilation of mammary alveoli by continued secretion of colostrum and enhanced mammary vascularization. Fat and connective tissue are relatively decreased (Figs. 13 and 14) (4).

Prolactin secretion increases throughout pregnancy, but it appears that luteal and placental sex steroids (especially progesterone) antagonize the full secretory prolactin effect on mammary epithelium (1). The prolactin effect on mammary secretory cells is supported by glucocorticoid, growth hormone, insulin, and thyroid hormone. After postpartum withdrawal of sex steroids and placental lactogen, prolactin-induced lactation sets in. Presecretory mammary glandular cells are converted into actively milk-synthesizing and milk-releasing cells. Complex protein, milk fat, and lactose synthetic pathways are activated. Large fat vacuoles and Golgi vesicles containing lactose, protein, and water ascend to the secretory cell's apex. The epithelial cells release fat, lactose, and protein by apocrine secretion and lactose and protein by merocrine secretion. With synthesis and secretion, the cells alternate between columnar and cuboidal shape. Ions (primarily potassium, calcium, and chloride and, to a lesser extent, sodium, magnesium, and iron) enter the milk at the apical secretory cell membrane by diffusion and active transport (19). The final product of secretion and subsequent dilution from interstitial fluid is milk: fat and protein suspended in lactose solution. The concentration of fat, protein, and electrolytes may vary, but the lactose concentration remains constant as the major osmol-controlling factor from the volume of milk secreted (4). Approximately 1 to 2 ml of milk/g of breast tissue per day is produced.

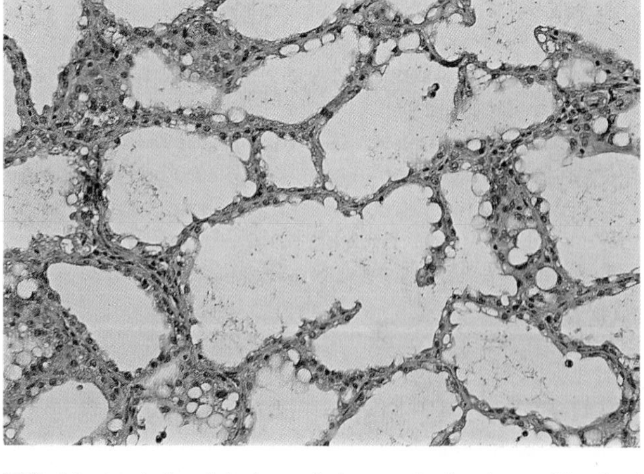

**FIG. 14.** Lactating lobular unit demonstrating loss of luminal (apical) aspect of cells through the apocrine secretory process.

Continued synthesis of milk is maintained during nursing because suckling releases both prolactin and adrenocorticotropic hormone. The stimulus of suckling or breast stimulation also releases oxytocin. This posterior pituitary hormone induces myoepithelial contraction and, thus, ejection of contents from alveoli and smaller ducts into lactiferous sinuses. The initial secretion, colostrum, contains nutritional elements as well as immunoglobulins, transferring passive immunity to the newborn. After the period of colostrum secretion, transitional milk (with a lower concentration of immunoglobulins and total protein) and then mature milk are elaborated.

Lactation is usually stopped approximately 4 to 6 months postpartum when secretory activities diminish. Cessation of lactation causes mammary involution, a process that encompasses nearly 3 months. Milk accumulates and distends alveoli, causing epithelial compression and eventual rupture of alveolar walls. Distended alveoli also lead to mammary capillary compression and resultant diminished nutrient, oxygen, prolactin, and oxytocin delivery. Milk secretion is greatly decreased. Epithelial cells degenerate, desquamate, and are phagocytized, reducing the number and size of glandular elements (4). The remaining alveolar lining returns to a nonsecretory two-cell-layered epithelium. As the lobuloacinar structures become smaller and fewer, the breast returns to a more ductular system. New connective tissue and fat are formed between the involuted mammary alveolar structures.

## MENOPAUSE

Just as there is variation in the hisotologic manifestations associated with development and menstrual cycling, the variation in the patterns of breast stroma, stromal epithelial proportions, and fat/collagen proportions seen in the menopause cover an equally broad range. Unlike postlactational mammary involution, in which there is principally a reduction of mammary alveoli, postmenopausal breast involution is generally characterized by regression of the parenchymal lobuloacinar structures. At menopause, ovarian

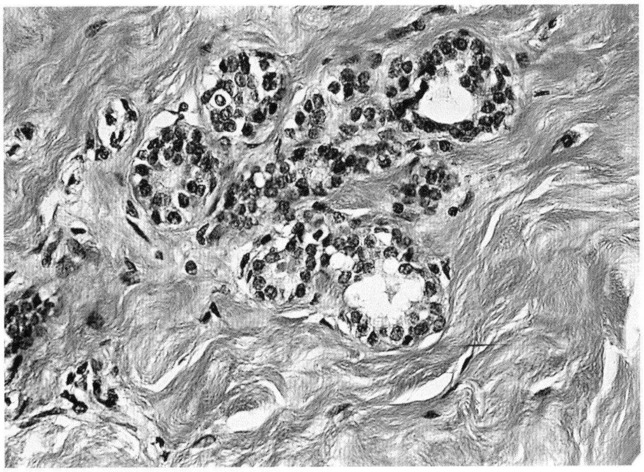

**FIG. 15.** Menopausal breast tissue. Marked variation occurs in the pattern of epithelium and stroma observed in the menopausal breast, paralleling the wide variation in postmenopausal hormonal levels. The relative dominance of adrenal-derived steroid effect is seen without estrogen-priming effect, resulting in a relatively atrophic pattern of lobular development despite maintenance of the epithelial integrity.

secretion of estrogen and progesterone declines, and ovarian secretion of androgens such as androstenedione, testosterone, and dihydroepiandrosterone becomes predominant. Specifically, the plasma levels of estrone, estradiol, estriol, and progesterone in postmenopausal women are 53%, 16%, 8%, and 30%, respectively, of those found at the midfollicular phase of cycling women, and 27%, 5%, 6%, and 10% of those found in women at midcycle (20). Plasma levels of testosterone, in contrast, are similar in premenopausal and postmenopausal women. The declining levels of estrogen and progesterone are associated with menopausal breast involution. In the climacteric phase, between 45 and 55 years of age, a moderate decrease in glandular epithelium with round-cell infiltration occurs. The postmenopausal phase, after approximately age 50, has a marked reduction of glandular tissue with an increase in fat deposition and relative predominance of connective tissue. Parenchymal vascularity and round-cell infiltration diminish. At the end stage of menopausal mammary involution only small islands of an epithelial ductular system embedded in dense, hyalinized fibrous tissue remain (Fig. 15). Although this glandular involution is striking, little is known about the factors responsible for this process. Immunohistochemistry is sometimes useful to appreciate the retention of the normal epithelial/myoepithelial relationship in breasts where regular hormonal cycling is altered (Fig. 16).

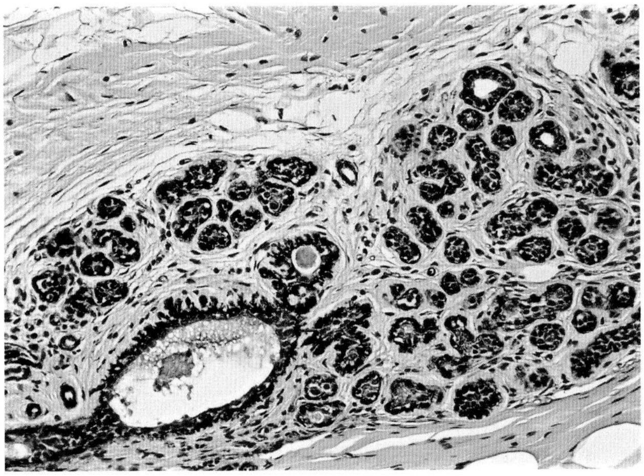

**FIG. 16.** Myoepithelial cell staining by immunohistochemistry using anti-actin antibodies. The presence of a myoepithelial cell layer may be useful in characterizing some difficult lesions often seen in breast biopsies of menopausal women (although sclerosing lesions are by no means limited to postmenopausal breasts). The use of immunohistochemistry to demonstrate actin is effective in demonstrating the myoepithelial cells.

## REFERENCES


1. Dickson, RB, Lippman, ME. Growth Factors in Breast Cancer. *Endocr Rev* 1995;16:559–589.
2. Topper YJ, Freeman CS. Multiple hormone interactions in the developmental biology of the mammary gland. *Physiol Rev* 1980;60: 1049–1106.
3. Haagensen DC. *Diseases of the breast*. 3rd ed. Philadelphia; WB Saunders, 1986.
4. Vorherr H. *The breast: morphology, physiology and lactation*. New York; Academic Press, 1974.
5. Osborne MP. Breast development and anatomy. In: Harris JR, Lippman ME, Morrow M, et al., eds. *Breast diseases*. Philadelphia; JB Lippincott, 1987.
6. Stiles HJ. Uber eine neue methode der mammaplastic. *Wien Med Wochenschr* 1936;86:100.
7. Edwards EA. Surgical anatomy of the breast. In: Goldwyn RM, ed. *Plastic and reconstructive surgery of the breast*. Boston; Little, Brown, 1976;37.
8. Turner-Warwick RT. The lymphatics of the breast. *Br J Surg* 1959;46: 574.
9. Hultborn KA, Larrsson LG, Ragnhult I. The lymph drainage from the breast to the axillary and parasternal lymph nodes, studied with the aid of colloidal au. *Acta Radiol* 1955;43:52.
10. McCarty KS Jr, Glaubitz LC, Thienemann M, et al. The breast: Anatomy and physiology. In: Georgiade NG, ed. *Aesthetic plastic surgery*. Philadelphia; WB Saunders, 1983:1.
11. Longacre TA, Bartow SA. A correlative morphologic study of human breast and endometrium in the menstrual cycle. *Am J Surg Pathol* 1986; 10:382–393.
12. Vogel PM, Georgiade NC, Fetter BF, et al. The correlation of histologic changes in the human breast with the menstrual cycle. *Am J Pathol* 1984;104:23–34.
13. Fanger H, Ree HJ. Cyclic changes of human mammary gland epithelium in relation to the menstrual cycle: An ultrastructural study. *Cancer* 1974;34:574.
14. Ferguson DJP, Anderson TJ. Morphological evaluation of cell turnover in relation to the menstrual cycle in the "resting" human breast. *Br J Cancer* 1981;44:177–181.
15. Silva JS, Georgiade GS, Dilley WG, et al. Menstrual cycle-dependent variations of breast cyst fluid proteins and sex steroid receptors in the normal human breast. *Cancer* 1981;51:1297–1302.
16. Greene GL, Press MF. Immunochemical evaluation of estrogen receptor and progesterone receptor in breast cancer. In: Ceriani R, ed. *Immunological approaches to the diagnosis and therapy of breast cancer*. New York; Plenum Press, 1987.
17. Fabris G, Marchetti E, Marzola A, et al. Pathophysiology of estrogen receptors in mammary tissue by monoclonal antibodies. *J Steroid Biochem Mol Biol* 1987;27:171–176.
18. Peterson OW, Hoyer PE, van Deeurs B. Frequency and distribution of estrogen receptor-positive cells in normal, nonlactating human breast tissue. *Cancer Res* 1987;47:5748–5751.

19. Linzell JL, Peaker M. Mechanism of milk secretion. *Physiol Rev* 1971; 51:564-597.
20. Vorherr H. *Breast cancer, epidemiology, endocrinology, biochemistry, and pathobiology*. Baltimore; Urban & Schwarzenberg, 1980.

## ADDITIONAL SOURCES

Cathcart EP, Gairns FW, and Garven HSD. The innervation of the human quiescent nipple, with notes on pigmentation, erection and hyperneury. *Trans R Soc Edinb Trans* 1948;61:699.

Cooper AP, *On the anatomy of the breast vol 2*. London: Longmans, 1840.

Courtiss EH, Goldwyn RM. Breast sensation before and after plastic surgery. *Plast Reconstr Surg* 1976;58:1–13.

Dabelow A. Die milchdruse. In: Bargmann W, ed. *Handbuch der mikroskopischen anatomie des menschen (haut aund sinnesorgane), vol 3, part 3*. Berlin: Springer-Verlag, 1957;277.

Goldwyn RM. *Plastic and reconstructive surgery of the breast*. Boston; Little, Brown, 1976;52.

Kuhns JG, Ackermann, DM. Microscopic anatomy of the breast. In: Donegan WL, Spratt JS eds. *Cancer of the Breast*. Philadelphia: WB Saunders, 1995;16.

Maliniac JW. *Breast deformities and their repair*. New York: Grune & Stratton, 1950.

Massopust LC, Gardner WD. Infrared photographic studies of the superficial thoracic veins in the female. *Surg Gynecol Obstet* 1950;91:717.

Spratt, JS, and Gordon, GR. Gross anatomy of the breast. In: Donegan WL, Spratt JS eds. *Cancer of the Breast*. Philadelphia: WB Saunders, 1995; 22.

Tavassoli, FA. Normal development and anatomy. In: Tavassoli, FA. *Pathology of the breast*. Norwalk: Appleton & Lange. 1992:1.

# Skeletal System

*Histology for Pathologists, second edition,*
Edited by Stephen S. Sternberg.
Lippincott-Raven Publishers, Philadelphia


# CHAPTER 5

# Bone

Glyn A. Porter, A. Marion Gurley, and Sanford I. Roth



Bones are the 206 individual organs that comprise the human skeletal system. They are composed of multiple tissues including bone (tissue), cartilage, fat, connective tissue, hematopoietic bone marrow, nerves, and vessels. The skeleton is divided into two regions: the axial skeleton, including the vertebrae, skull, ribs, sternum, and hyoid, and the peripheral skeleton, including the limbs and pelvis (Fig. 1). Bones are classified as to shape (tubular and flat, long and short), and as to the manner of their embryological development (membranous, if they are formed *de nova* from undifferentiated connective tissue, and enchondral, if their formation is preceded by a cartilaginous anlage). Though in the normal adult, membranous and enchondral bones are histologically indistinguishable, some tumors, such as enchondromas and osteochondromas, arise almost exclusively in enchondral bones. In prepubertal children and patients in whom growth continues due to endocrine abnormalities, the enchondral bones can be distinguished by the presence of the residua of the cartilage anlage, the regions of interstitial growth, and the epiphyseal growth plates (or physes) (see below).

The definition of bone tissue, the one we are primarily concerned with in this chapter, is that it is a hard, biphasic tissue composed of a mineralized organic (largely collagenous) matrix (1) and at least three identifiable specialized cell types. The biphasic structure provides bone with ideal hardness, flexibility, and tensile strength without its being excessively brittle.

Bones have three major functions: metabolic, mechanical, and hematopoietic. The metabolic function serves as a reservoir for calcium, phosphate, and other ions. Protection for the soft tissue organs and levers for muscle action comprise the mechanical functions. Lastly, the bones provide host sites for the hematopoietic tissue (the bone marrow). During the life of an individual, the bones are continuously growing or remodeling. This process alters their size and shape in response to various normal and pathologic, mechanical, and biochemical stimuli (2,3). Many pathologic alterations of bone are the result of the efforts of this organ system to fulfill its functions. The reactions of the bones teleologically respond to stimuli to preserve the functions in the order listed earlier. For comprehension of the histopathology of the bones, the pathologist must understand these processes, as well as the interrelationships of the embryology, macroscopic anatomy, histology, ultrastructure, biochemistry, and biophysics of bone, and their variations with age.

Bone tissue is classified on the basis of its gross and microscopic structure into compact bone, which constitutes the cortex, and cancellous bone, which forms the central regions of the bones (Figs. 2 and 3). On a histologic basis, the bone

G. A. Porter, Department of Pathology, Northwestern University Medical School, Chicago, Illinois 60611.

A. M. Gurley: Dr. Colin Laferty and Associates, Eastwood, NSW 2122, Australia.

S. I. Roth: Department of Pathology, Northwestern University Medical School, Chicago, Illinois 60611.

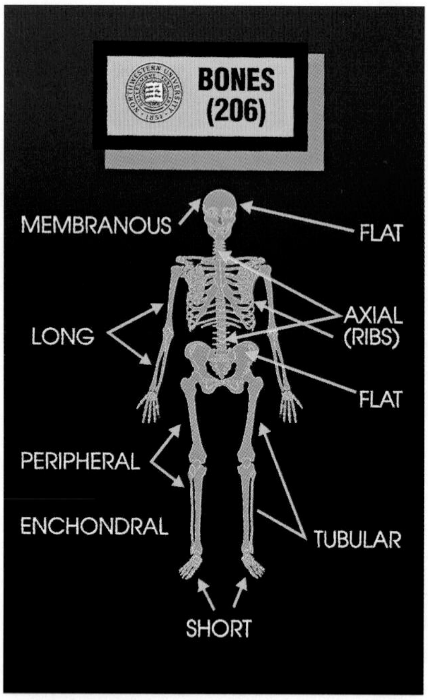


**FIG. 1.** Diagram of a stereotypical skeleton illustrating the classification of bones.

tissue is categorized according to its collagenous organization into woven and lamellar bone. In woven bone, the collagen is arranged in an irregular feltwork, while in lamellar bone the collagen consists of regularly arranged sheets. Woven bone is seen in areas of rapid bone growth, including the primary bone of the embryo, fracture callus, Codman's triangle (associated with periosteal elevation by tumors), and tumor bone. Lamellar bone is formed in regions of relatively slower growth, such as adult remodeling. In some conditions, such as healing aseptic necrosis, when healing is intermediate in rate, bone is formed with features intermediate between woven and lamellar bone.

The fibrous matrix of bone is predominantly type I collagen, with a closely associated mineral phase, hydroxyapatite [$Ca_{10}(PO4)_6(OH)_2$] (2,3). The mineral phase comprises 60%, the type I collagen 30%, and the type V collagen 1.5% of the total bone weight. In pathologic conditions, type III collagen may also be found (1). Trace amounts of collagens III, XI, and XIII, $\gamma$-glutamic acid-containing proteins, glycosaminoglycans, lipids, cells, and water are the remaining constituents of the bone (2).

Mineralization occurs by two mechanisms (3,4). In cartilage and woven bone, there are numerous small vesicles (matrix vesicles) that are derived from the chondroblasts and osteoblasts (3,4). The matrix vesicles, 2 to 4 $\mu$m in diameter, are the sites where small hydroxyapatite crystals are often seen early in the mineralization process. These initial crystals apparently serve as a nidus for the deposition of larger masses of crystals, deposited in and around the collagen fibers. Initiation of mineralization in woven bone also occurs within the collagen fibers (see below). The organization of woven bone is, thus, relatively irregular, with more than 50% of the mineral outside the collagen fibers. This organizational structure fosters rapid mineralization, formation, and resorption compared to that of lamellar bone. The mineral content of woven bone is higher and more rapidly deposited than that of lamellar bone. In addition, since the mineral and fibers are not well-organized, woven bone has a lower strength, less rigidity, and more flexibility than lamellar bone.

In lamellar bone, and to some extent in woven bone, initiation of mineralization begins almost exclusively within the collagen fibers. The mineral is regularly spaced along the fibers and is initially deposited at the ends of the collagen molecules, within the hole regions of the collagen fibers (4,5). There is some dispute as to the initial form of the mineral, but crystals of hydroxyapatite, as well as amorphous calcium phosphate and brushite, (4–7) are seen early in the process. The initiators, inhibitors, control mechanisms, and biochemistry of the mineralization process are still under debate (4,5); however, osteoblasts are a necessary component of this mineralization process. As mineralization progresses toward completion, crystals grow within the collagen fibers and also into the interstitium. In adult mammalian lamellar bone, at least 50% of the crystal is within the collagen fibers. Mineralization is slower in lamellar bone than in woven bone and continues long after the initial bone formation. Microradiographs of undemineralized sections reveal varying densities, with the oldest bone being most heavily mineralized (Fig. 4). Since the mineral and fibers are well-organized and closely associated, lamellar bone has greater rigidity and tensile strength, and less elasticity than woven bone.

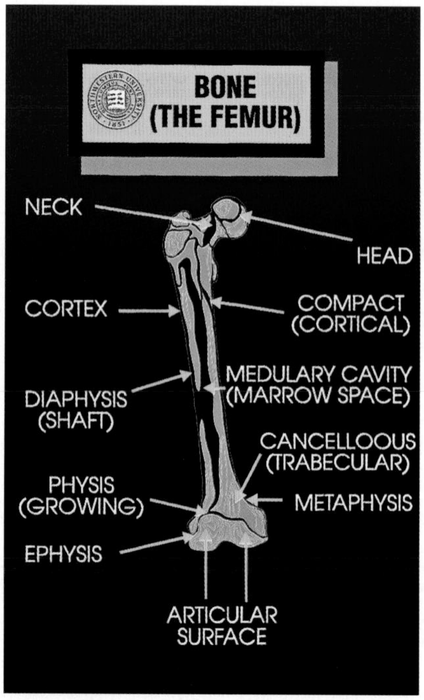


**FIG. 2.** Diagram of a femur illustrating the various gross regions of a stereotypical bone.

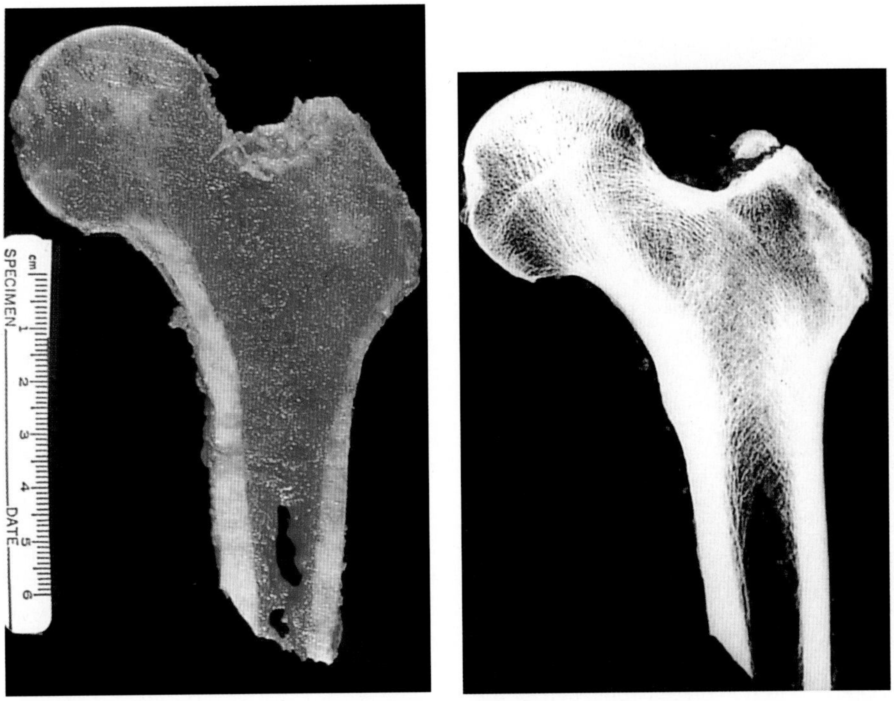


A B

**FIG. 3.** **A,** Section of the frontal plane of the femoral head, neck, and upper diaphysis. The compact bone of the cortex is thicker along the medial surface of the neck and diaphysis where there is a greater load bearing than it is along the lateral surface, as suggested by Wolff's law (61, 62). The subchondral plate under the articular cartilage is thinner where the weight load is perpendicular than it is along the medial surface of the head where the weight bearing is parallel to the cortex. The trabeculae of cancellous bone of the head also follow the lines of stress. The hematopoietic marrow is present between the trabeculae. The yellow areas of the head have only adipose tissue and no hematopoiesis. **B,** Roentgenograph of a section of the femoral head, in the frontal plane. The articular cartilage overlies the subchondral plate. The alignment of the trabeculae in the head and neck can be seen to follow the lines of stress; this is especially prominent from the subchondral plate to the medial compact cortex. The relative thickness of the cortices as seen in the gross photograph is easily seen. The trabeculum at right angles to the line of stress represents the remnant of the epiphyseal growth plate.

## GROSS ANATOMY

The mechanical functions of bones determine their gross appearance, as well as their microscopic form. The manner of bones' responses have been defined by Wolff's law (8,9): "every change in the form and function of bones, or in their functions alone, is followed by certain definite changes in their internal architecture and equally definite changes in their external conformation in accordance with mathematical laws." The bones are rigid, but not brittle, lightweight structures, of a relatively high tensile strength. On cross-section examination, most bones are reinforced, asymmetric, hollow, tubular structures or bilaminar plates, designed to provide a maximum strength-to-weight ratio. The cortex is a plate or tube, composed of compact sheets of cortical bone, strengthened by spicules or sheets of coarse cancellous bone. The size and thickness of the cortex and the arrangement of the spicules follow the lines of maximum force or stress, as predicted by Wolff's law (Figs. 3 and 5). Cross struts connect the trabeculae following the lines of stress for added support (Figs. 3 and 5). Growth, modeling, and remodeling after injury or in pathologic conditions is also influenced by this effect (8–10), even in the embryo (11). The inner, less dense portion of the bone is called the medulla and it contains the cancellous bone and the soft tissues, nerves, vessels, adipose tissue, and hematopoietic elements.

Cancellous bone is composed of fine or coarse sheets and

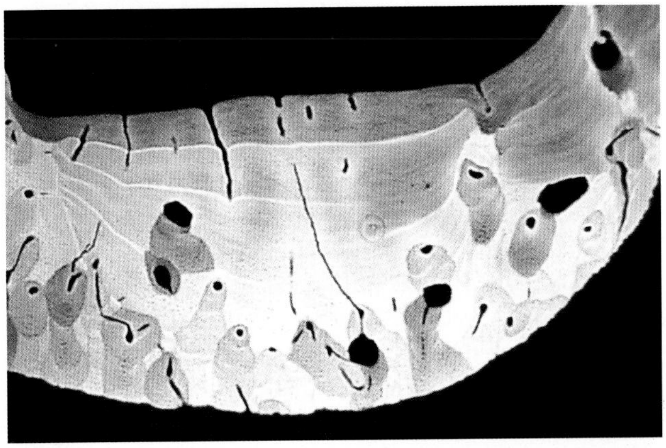

**FIG. 4.** Microradiograph of the cortex of a normal rib of a 2-month-old female. The longitudinal lamellae show various degrees of mineralization. The endosteal lamellae are the youngest and least radiodense. Vascular channels traverse the bone.

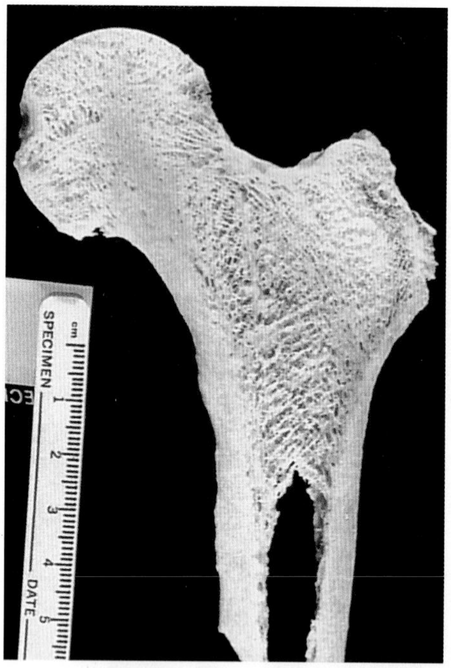


**FIG. 5.** Gross photograph of a macerated specimen of the bone seen in Fig. 3. Note that with the soft tissue removed the trabeculae following the stress lines are seen to be interconnected with cross struts for added support. The cortex and cancellous bone can clearly be seen.

spicules of bone, with greater or lesser amounts of intervening soft tissue (Figs. 3 and 5). Cancellous bone is found in the marrow space and the cortex of embryonic bone. It is woven or lamellar, depending on its rate of formation. Compact bone is dense bone composed of lamellae of bone with minimal soft tissue (usually not grossly visible).

The adult long bones contain three regions: a central shaft region (the diaphysis), an end region near the joint (the epiphysis), and a connecting region (the metaphysis) (Fig. 2). In growing bones the metaphysis is separated from the epiphysis by the epiphyseal growth plate (the physis) (3). Recognition of these regions is important in diagnoses of bone tumors, because various tumors tend to be localized to different regions of the long bone shafts.

The classic example used to illustrate these features is the femoral head. Its epiphysis is a ball-like structure (Figs. 2, 3, and 5), covered by an articular cartilage that fits into the socket of the ilium. The surface of the bone has several protuberances to serve as attachment sites for tendons and the joint capsule. The medullary cavity is filled with spicules of cancellous bone, which follow the lines of stress as prescribed by Wolff's law (8,9) (Figs. 3 and 5). The medial side of the cortex is thicker than the lateral, since this weight-bearing region is under higher stress. Under pathologic conditions, such as osteoarthritis, aseptic necrosis, or fractures, the angles of the stress change and the ensuing remodeling changes the macroscopic and microscopic structures of this region (10,11). In the absence of adequate calcium and/or phosphorus, such as in rickets or osteomalacia, the relatively rapid remodeling of the femoral head and neck results in alteration of the form of the bone. Loss of bone mass in the femoral neck with aging (osteoporosis), frequently results in fractures.

## HISTOLOGY

Woven or immature bone (Fig. 6) is seen in the embryo, growing prepubertal bone, malformed bone (such as in osteogenesis imperfecta), rickets, scurvy, fracture callus, or other sites of periosteal injury, and at sites of bone repair, such as the involucrum of osteomyelitis or the reaction to bone tumors (Codman's triangle). Woven bone is generally a fine cancellous or spongy bone, organized in trabeculae and spicules. The collagen fibers, which can be visualized with plane polarized light, are arranged in a meshwork or felt-like pattern (Fig. 7). The noncollagenous elements form a greater percentage of the matrix than found in mature bone. Mineralization is intense. The osteocytes are randomly and unevenly distributed within the trabeculae, with large spherical to plump spindle-shaped lacunae (Figs. 6 and 7), and their number is higher per unit volume than in lamellar bone.

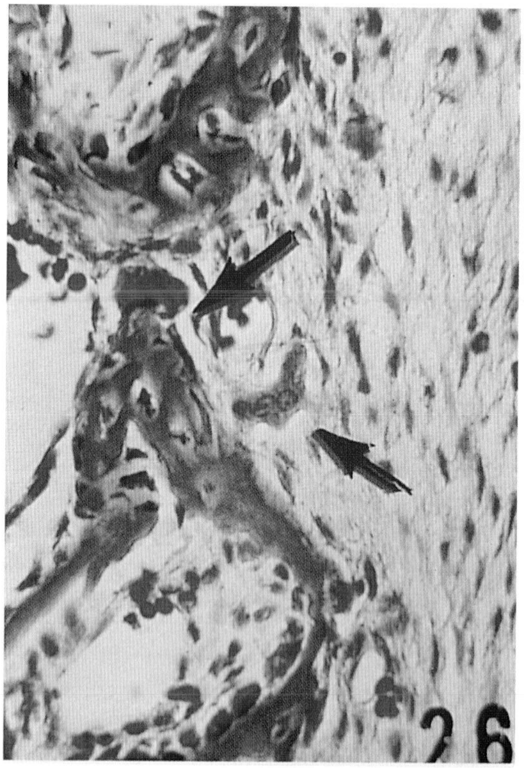

**FIG. 6.** Photomicrograph of woven bone from the skull of a fetus. The osteoblasts line the almost randomly organized trabeculae. The osteocytes are large and irregularly spaced. Prominent capillaries and undifferentiated mesenchymal cells are present between the trabeculae. Osteoclasts (*arrows*) are seen resorbing the trabeculae, indicating active resorption as well as formation. (*Trichrome stain.*) (This slide was prepared by M. J. Glimcher, M.D., S. I. Roth, M.D., and A. L. Schiller, M.D. as part of a course in the Pathophysiology of Bone for the Harvard Medical School, Boston MA.)

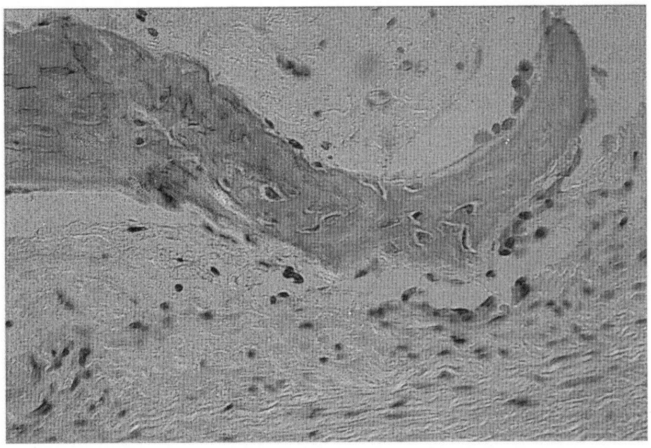

**FIG. 7.** Photomicrograph of woven bone from the skull of a second trimester fetus. The felt-like arrangement of the collagen fibers can be seen in this section. The collagen fibers of the bone are blue or yellow, depending on their direction with respect to the polarizing filter. The collagen fibers of the periosteum are all yellow and well aligned. Polarized light with one-quarter-wave retardant filter.

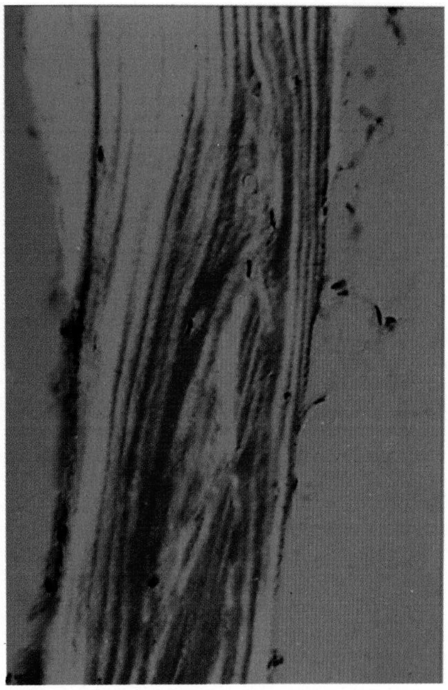

**FIG. 9.** Longitudinal section of trabecular lamellar bone. The lamellae parallel the long axis of the trabeculum. The osteocyte lacunae are spindle-shaped and parallel the lamellae. Polarized light with one-quarter-wave retardant filter.

Lamellar bone occurs whenever the rate of bone formation is relatively slow or when there is a preexisting lattice of either woven or lamellar bone. The collagen fibers are arrayed in parallel sheets and bundles. The lamellae are organized in several different patterns: circumferentially within compact or cortical bone (Fig. 8), longitudinally in the trabeculae of mature cancellous bone (Fig. 9), or concentrically around a central blood vessel in remodeled haversian bone (Figs. 10 and 11). The osteocytes are regularly dispersed within the bone and are small and spindle-shaped, with the long axes of the cells parallel to the collagen lamellae (Figs. 8–11). Long processes connect adjacent osteocytes through canaliculi across the lamellae (Fig. 12), but not across adjacent osteons.

Both lamellar and woven bone are covered in regions of active bone formation by a layer of unmineralized bone, called osteoid (Figs. 13 and 14). The width of this layer is dependent on the relative rate of bone formation and bone mineralization. The zone of mineralization can be identified by the administration of the fluorescent antibiotic tetracycline,

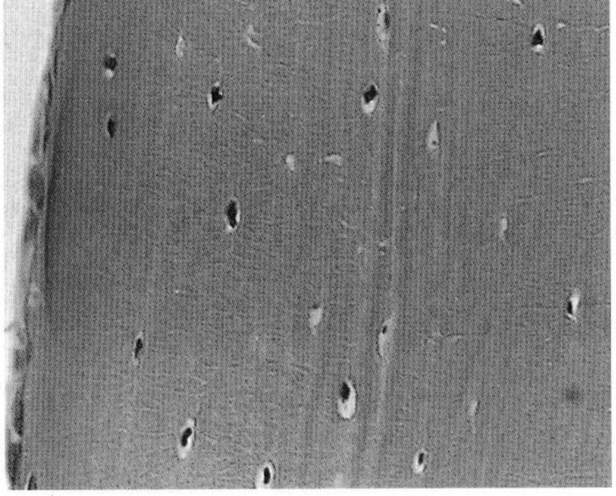

**FIG. 8.** Photomicrograph of a cross section of the cortex of a young long bone. The circumferential lamellae are visible. The osteocytes are small, regularly spaced, and spindle-shaped. Flattened, inactive resting osteoblasts are seen embedded in a thin fibrous layer on the endosteal surface.

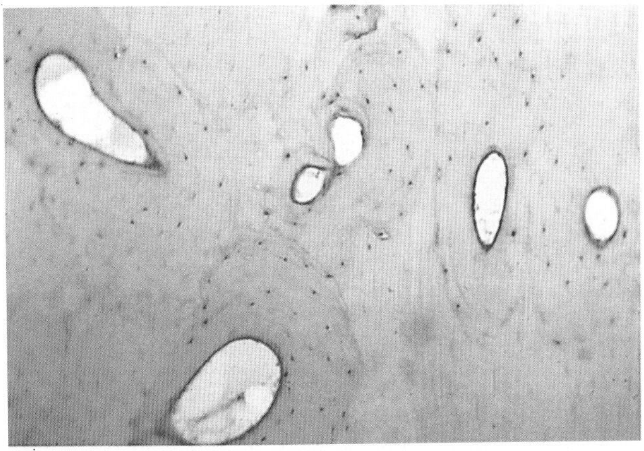

**FIG. 10.** Cross section of demineralized bone showing numerous haversian systems of varying ages. The newer systems have larger central canals. The cement lines are visible at the edge of each system. The osteocytes are aligned along the circumferential lamellae. Interstitial lamellae are present between the haversian systems.

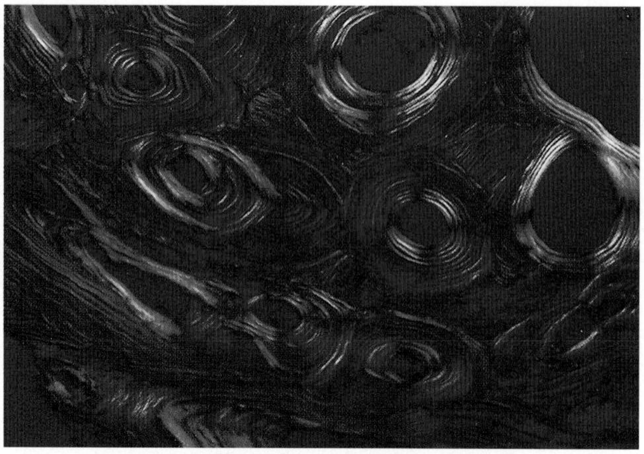

**FIG. 11.** Cross section of a normal cortical bone with numerous haversian systems. The concentric lamellae are clearly visible. There are several interstitial lamellae. Polarized light with one-quarter-wave retardant filter.

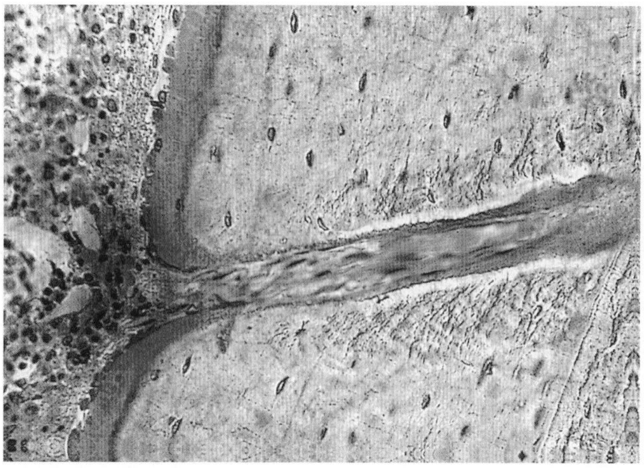

**FIG. 13.** A forming Volkmann's canal coursing through the cortex of the bone. The canal is angled with respect to the bone lamellae and is filled with connective tissue. No osteoblasts are seen within the canal. Osteoid and osteoblasts, indicating new bone formation, are present around the endosteal opening of the canal. The cortex shows circumferential lamellar bone with spindle-shaped regularly placed osteocytes. Undemineralized bone section.

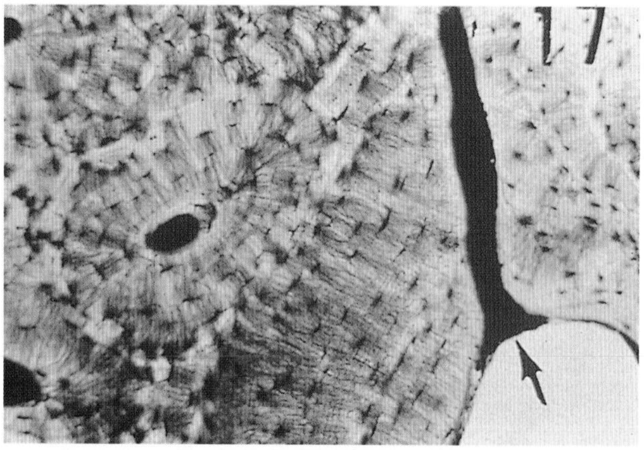

**FIG. 12.** Ground section of undemineralized compact, cortical lamellar bone. The dark areas represent soft tissue. A Volkmann's canal (*arrow*) is seen arising from the endosteum. Canaliculi are seen connecting adjacent lacunae. (*Unstained*) (This slide was prepared by M. J. Glimcher, M.D., S. I. Roth, M.D., and A. L. Schiller, M.D. as part of a course in the Pathophysiology of Bone for the Harvard Medical School, Boston MA.)

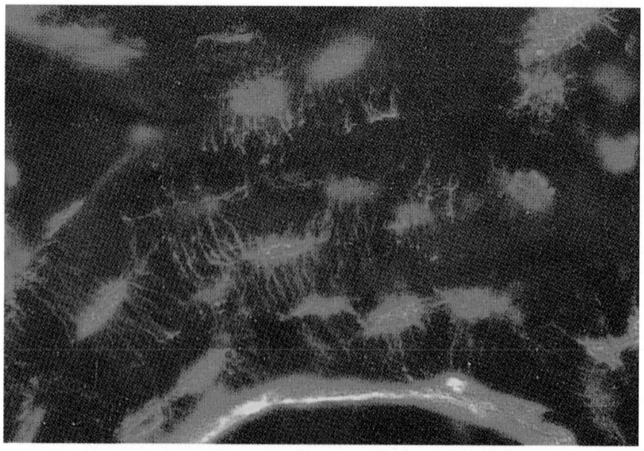

**FIG. 14.** An undemineralized section of cortical bone, stained in vivo, with tetracycline. A layer of tetracycline appears at the mineralization front where new bone is being formed. The osteocytes and their dendritic processes have also taken up the dye. (*Unstained, fluorescent light*.)

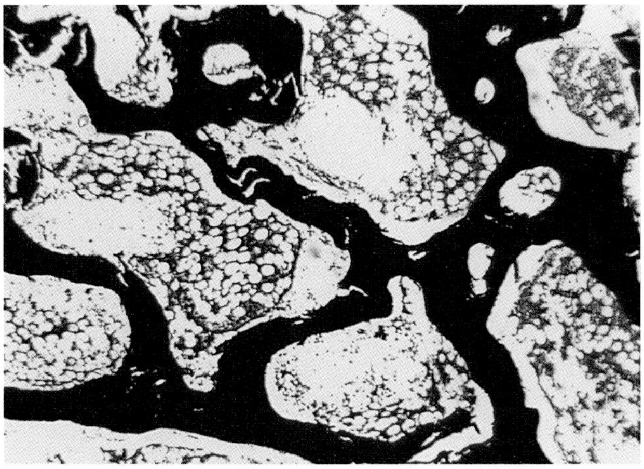

**FIG. 15.** Photomicrograph of normal cancellous bone. The mineral phase is black. Little osteoid is present. Undemineralized section. (*Von Kossa stain*)

which is bound to the bone at zones of mineralization (Fig. 14). In inactive regions, the bone is fully mineralized, there is minimal osteoid (Figs. 4 and 15), and the surface is covered by a layer of thin flattened cells.

### Cortical (Compact) Bone

The bone cortex, except in the region of the articular cartilage, is surrounded by the periosteum (Fig. 16), which consists of an outer fibrous layer and an inner cellular (cambium) layer of osteoprogenitor cells, fibroblasts, and osteoblasts. The cellularity of the cambium layer depends on the age and bone remodeling activity in the particular region. The collagen of the outer fibrous layer is continuous with that of the joint capsule, tendons, and muscle fascia. Where the tendons insert into the periosteum, collagen fibers (Sharpey's fibers) pass through the periosteum into the bone lamellae. The cortex is a dense or compact bone composed of longitudinal, circumferential, and concentric (haversian) lamellae, best demonstrated by their birefringence with plane polarized light (Figs. 9 and 11). The bundles of collagen in adjacent bone lamellae are parallel within each lamella and at varying angles to those in the adjacent lamellae.

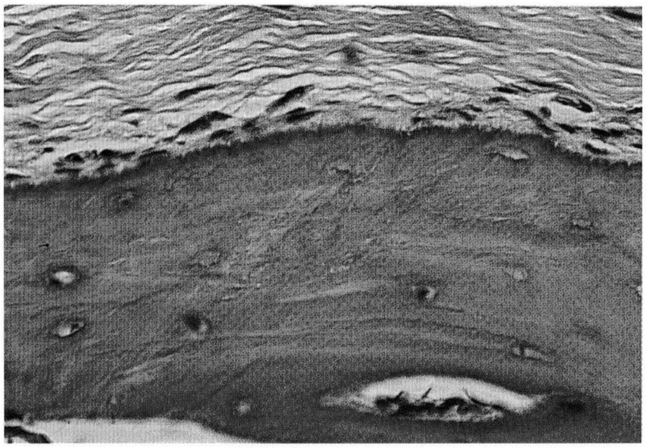

**FIG. 16.** Photomicrograph of the periosteum of a mature bone. The circumferential lamellae are seen. The cambium layer is composed of thin flattened cells. The overlying fibrous layer contains a few fibroblasts.

### Cancellous (Spongy) Bone

The centers of most adult bone are composed of sheets or struts (trabeculae) of mature lamellar bone. The lamellae parallel the long axis of the trabeculae (Fig. 9) and are laid down following the lines of stress as determined by Wolff's law. Small trabeculae are avascular, while larger ones may contain Haversian systems of concentric lamellar bone. Separating the bone from the marrow space is the endosteum, a layer composed of osteoclasts, macrophage-like cells, and active and inactive (Fig. 8) osteoblasts. In some areas, a thin, loose fibrous tissue is present around the cells of the endosteum (Fig. 8).

## CARTILAGE

Cartilage, like bone, is a specialized form of connective tissue composed of specialized cells, chondrocytes, and a largely avascular extracellular matrix of collagen fibers embedded in gel-like proteoglycan matrix. Cartilage is classified into three types: hyaline cartilage, elastic cartilage, and fibrocartilage (12–16). They differ not only in morphology, but in the relative amounts of collagens and elastic fibers in their extracellular matrix.

Hyaline cartilage is the most abundant form of cartilage. Developmentally, it forms the model (anlage) for the axial and appendicular skeleton which is replaced by bone (enchondral bone formation) (17). In the adult, hyaline cartilage is found at the ends of ribs, in the tracheal and bronchial rings, in the larynx, Meckel's cartilage, and the articular surfaces of the joints.

Embryologically, human cartilage develops from mesenchyme at about 5 weeks' gestational age. The mesenchyme condenses and the undifferentiated progenitor cells proliferate and change from a stellate to spherical shape. As the cells enlarge and differentiate into chondrocytes, they synthesize and secrete extracellular matrix which separates the cells from one another. The cells become more angulated and isolated in lacunae as differentiation continues. The mature chondrocytes of hyaline cartilage lie in a zone of finely textured matrix containing abundant ground substance intermixed with collagen fibers (12–16).

The chondrocytes are highly specialized cells responsible for the synthesis and maintenance of the extracellular matrix. They have a round-to-oval nucleus, cytoplasm that contains a juxtanuclear Golgi complex, mitochondria, and variable amounts of glycogen. When the cells are actively producing matrix (chondroblasts), as in new or regenerating cartilage, the Golgi and rough endoplasmic reticulum become more prominent, giving the cytoplasm a more basophilic-staining characteristic.

The matrix in which the cells are embedded is also highly specialized and locally variable. The primary fibers are a network of type II collagen (13,14,16). However, attached to the large type II collagen fibers are minor collagens, types I, III, V, VI, IX, X, and XI, which provide for flexible spacing of the fibers.

The other main proteins of the cartilage extracellular matrix, providing about 10% of the overall net weight, are the proteoglycans. The proteoglycans are primarily of the large aggregating type such as "aggregan" found in hyaline cartilage (15). The nonaggregating proteoglycans form a lesser component of the stroma. The composition and size of the proteoglycan aggregates and collagen fibers in the matrix are not uniform. The proteoglycan concentrations are lowest and the collagen fibers largest in the middle and outer zones furthest from the chondrocytes (the "interterritorial" matrix), while the highest concentrations and smallest collagen fibers are nearest the chondrocytes in the "territorial" matrix (Figs. 17 and 18) (16). Such variability in distribution, architecture, and organization of the proteoglycans serves to maintain a highly nondiffusible negative charge. The higher concentration of chondroitin sulfate near the lacunae causes an increased basophilia (staining with hematoxylin) and alcian blue staining in the territorial matrix. The variability in composition gives the cartilage the ability to function as a hydrated gel which can withstand and absorb compressive forces.

The proteoglycans consist of core proteins with complex carbohydrates, glycosaminoglycans, radiating from them. The proteoglycans are predominately chondroitin sulfate and keratan sulfate. In normal cartilage, the components of the extracellular matrix are degraded by proteolytic enzymes synthesized by the chondrocytes. The rate of degradation is determined by the balance between the enzyme synthesis and activation (18). Under normal conditions, chondrocytes rarely divide, and the cell population tends to decrease with age. Consequently, the presence of mitoses is often a histopathologic criteria used in the diagnoses of chondroid neoplasms.

Water and inorganic salts comprise approximately 80% of the extracellular matrix, giving cartilage its resilience and lubricating capabilities (19). It is also this high degree of hydration that causes the artifactual separation of the chondrocyte cell membrane from the wall of the surrounding lacunae during the dehydration processes used in preparing tissues for histologic examination (20).

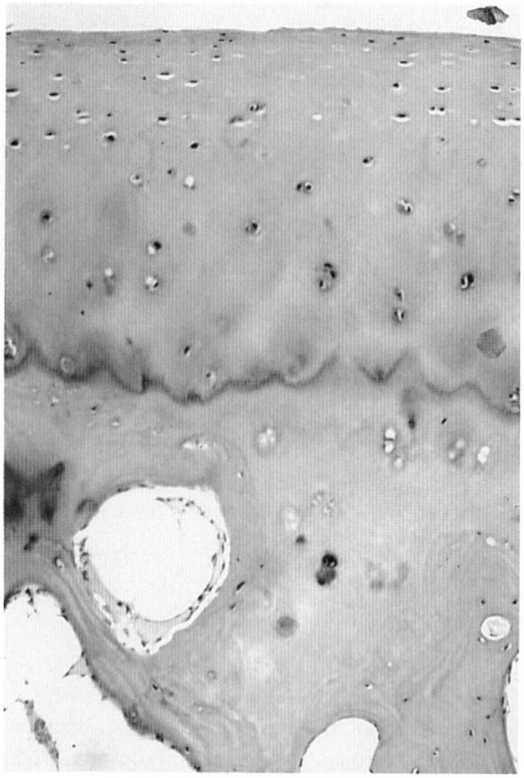

**FIG. 17.** A longitudinal section through the articular cartilage. The surface is smooth and regular. The chondrocytes nearer the articular surface are smaller and less dense than those deeper in the cartilage. The tide mark separates the articular nonmineralized cartilage above from the mineralized cartilage below. Beneath the mineralized cartilage is the lamellar bone of the subchondral plate, the remnant of the secondary center of ossification.

### Articular Cartilage

The articular cartilage is a highly ordered form of hyaline cartilage that covers the bony surfaces of the articular joints (Figs. 17 and 18). It is a weight-bearing structure that permits the smooth, even movement of one bone upon another. Articular cartilage is divided into three unmineralized zones and one mineralized zone (zone IV) separated by the tide mark (Figs. 17 and 18) (16). The mineralized region serves primarily to transfer the load bearing to the subchondral bone plate and the underlying bony trabeculae. The regions of the unmineralized portion are a superficial tangential zone (I), a transitional or intermediate zone (II), and a deep radial zone (III) (16). The chondrocytes are embedded in lacunae in the matrix. In zone I chondrocytes are small, angulated, and oriented parallel to the articular surface. Zone II chondrocytes are larger, spherical, and randomly oriented. In zone III the chondrocytes are oriented in columns. The matrix between the chondrocytes is composed of 68 to 78% water, 13.5 to 18% type II collagen, 7 to 10% proteoglycans, and 1.5% other collagens, largely types IX, X, and XI. The collagen fibers are arranged in statistical arcades (Benninghoff arcades), perpendicular to the surface between the chondro-

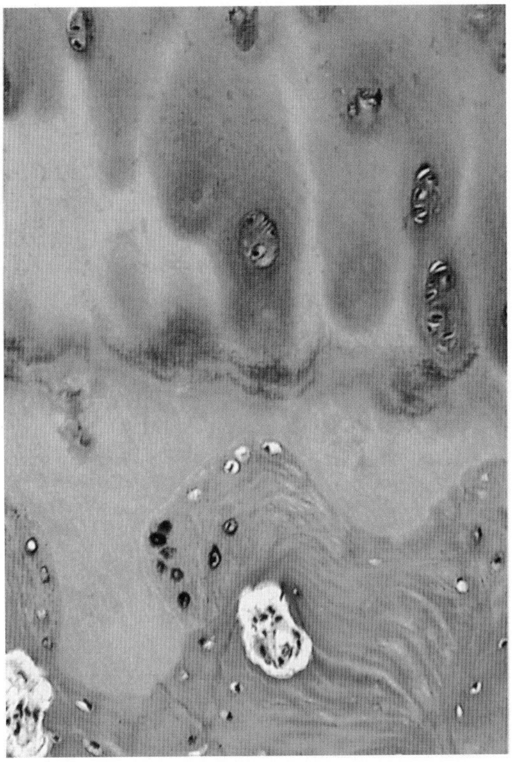

**FIG. 18.** Section of the articular cartilage in the region of the tide mark. The intense staining of the territorial matrix is seen in the cells of zone III, which form column-like regions. The underlying mineralized zone IV and the subchondral plate are seen.

cyte columns in zone III, and parallel to the articular surface in zone I (Fig. 19). Between the larger collagen fibers forming the arcades are a meshwork of smaller collagen fibers and the proteoglycan molecules. The matrix is divided into two poorly demarcated regions: the territorial and the interterritorial (Figs. 17 and 18). The former surrounds the chondrocytes and has smaller collagen fibers and an increased proteoglycan content compared to the interterritorial matrix (16).

The earliest recognizable histologic change in osteoarthritis is a fraying of the superficial cartilaginous matrix of zone I along the lines of the Benninghoff arcades. Structural alterations of aging in the articular cartilage, such as decreased numbers of chondrocytes, often leads to osteoarthritis (21). The decreased ability of the chondrocytes to keep pace with the wear-and-tear breakdown of the proteoglycans, and the subsequent changes in water-binding capacity, are thought to be important in the pathogenesis of osteoarthritis. In rheumatoid and other inflammatory arthritides, proteases are released by the chondrocytes, monocytic inflammatory cells, and pannus cells in response to interleukin-I (IL-I) and tumor necrosis factor-$\alpha$ (TNF-$\alpha$). In such cases, the core proteins of the proteoglycans are degraded more rapidly than they are produced (21).

### Elastic Cartilage

Elastic cartilage is found in the pinna of the external ear, the walls of the external auditory and eustachian canal, and the epiglottis. Grossly, elastic cartilage is opaque yellow, compared to the blue opalescence of fresh hyaline cartilage. Histologically, the cells are spherical and in single cells or isogenic groups, separated by extracellular matrix. The extracellular matrix is unique in the expression of elastin fibers which form an extremely dense network.

### Fibrocartilage

Fibrocartilage is found in intervertebral discs, the symphysis pubis, as well as in the regions of attachment of some

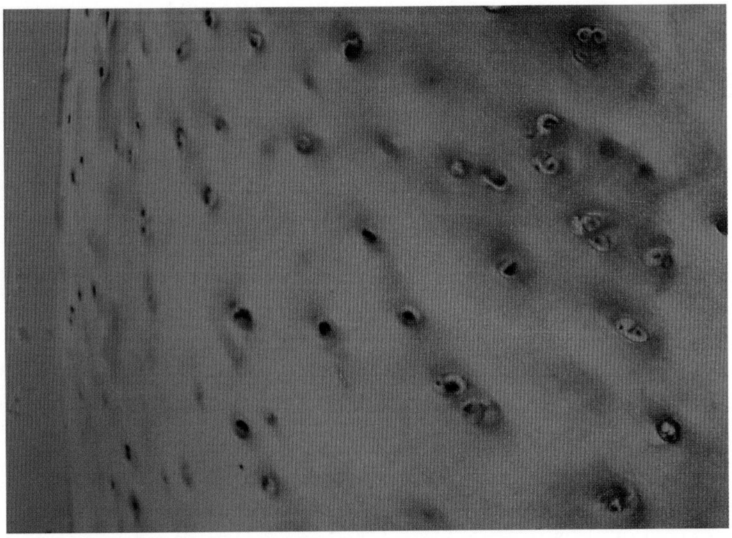

**FIG. 19.** Section of articular cartilage. The surface collagen bundles in zone I are parallel to the articular surface. The polarized light does not show the perpendicular bundles in the deeper layers, zones II and III. Polarized light, with one-quarter-wave retardant filter.

tendons to bones. Functionally, fibrocartilage serves as a transition from cartilage to dense connective tissue (tendon). Histologically, the typical chondrocytes are found singly, in pairs, or lined up in rows among abundant fibrous elements. The extracellular matrix contains large numbers of thick bundles of type I collagen fibers immediately surrounding the chondrocytes.

## BONE CELLS

### Osteoprogenitor Cells

The osteoprogenitor cells are undifferentiated primitive mesenchymal cells of the fibroblastic-colony-forming units (F-CFU)(23–25), which presumably are able to modulate to osteoblasts, chondroblasts, or fibroblasts depending on the nature and degree of the stimulus (22). They are thought to be located in the perivascular connective tissue, the cambium layer of the periosteum, and the bone marrow (23,24). Because bone can be formed in ectopic sites, such as the skin, under experimental and pathologic conditions, osteoprogenitor cells presumably are present in these sites. These cells cannot be demonstrated in ordinary histologic sections. Friedenstein has shown the presence of undifferentiated cells in the marrow, capable of forming bone when injected into ectopic sites (25,26), whereas undifferentiated cells from other sites, such as the skin, require osteostimulants to modulate to osteoblasts.

### Osteoblasts

The osteoblasts derived from the osteoprogenitor cells, are the cells responsible for the production of the collagen that forms the unmineralized bone (osteoid), and are principally responsible for bone mineralization (5,24,27). These cells cover the bone-forming surface. During bone formation, the active osteoblasts consist of a row of columnar cells with amphophilic to basophilic cytoplasm and eccentrically located nuclei, often with a prominent nucleolus (Fig. 20). There is often a perinuclear halo. In regions of very active bone formation, such as fracture callus or other reactive new bone in response to tumors or infections (involucrum), the cells may form a stratified layer and appear to be piled-up on the surface of the bone. Cellular and nuclear pleomorphism under these conditions may cause some alarm to an observer not accustomed to seeing these changes. The osteoblasts are 50 to 80 $\mu$m in height. Histochemical and biochemical studies reveal the presence of alkaline phosphatase in the cell cytoplasm and parathyroid hormone (PTH) receptors on their surfaces (28–30). Osteoblasts are the first cells to respond to PTH. They are postulated to activate bone resorption via paracrine or autocrine secretion of one of a number of factors in response to the PTH stimulation (23). The ultrastructure of these cells reveals an extensive, granular, endoplasmic reticulum, a large prominent Golgi apparatus (accounting for the perinuclear halo seen with the light microscope), and numerous mitochondria and lysosomes (2,24). The cytoplasmic surface demonstrates multiple processes in contact with adjacent osteoblasts and osteocytes. The connections between the cells are formed by nexus (gap) junctions. The osteoblasts synthesize type I collagen and glycosaminoglycans, and liberate calcium and phosphate ions to form the bone mineral. The inactive osteoblasts are flattened cells covering the resting bone surface, which appear spindle-shaped in histologic sections (Fig. 8). Ultrastructurally, these cells resemble inactive fibroblasts (24). The osteoblasts respond to mechanical stimuli to mediate the changes in bone growth, size, and shape. As osteoid deposition occurs, the osteoblast modulates to an osteocyte as it is surrounded by osteoid matrix and bone (Fig. 20).

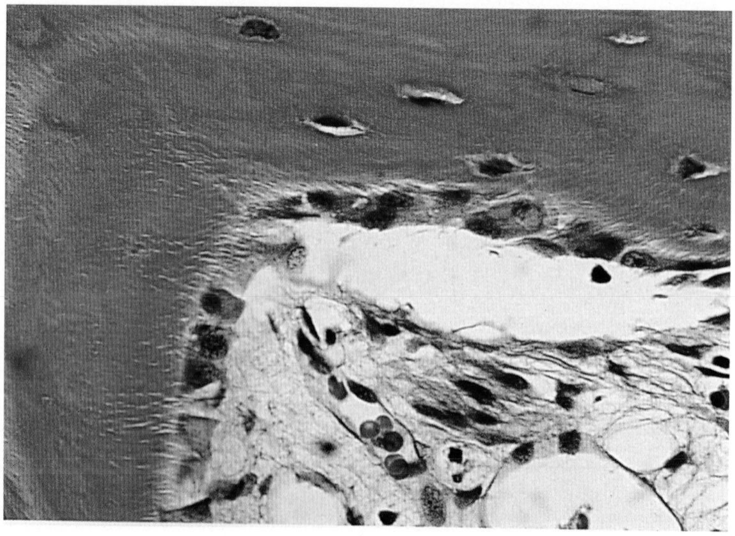

**FIG. 20.** Section of lamellar bone with active bone formation. The osteoblasts form a columnar layer on the surface of the bone. The unmineralized osteoid is seen as a pale pink layer between the darker bone and the osteoblasts. Near the right the osteoblasts are flatter, inactive, and are being incorporated into the bone as osteocytes. The osteocytes in the lamellar bone are spindle-shaped and regular.

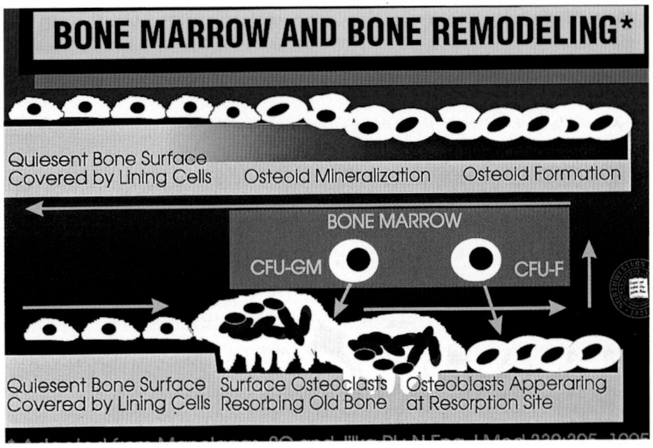


**FIG. 22.** A Howship's lacuna with two osteoclasts on the surface of a trabeculum of lamellar bone. Capillaries and a loose vascular connective tissue fill the marrow space.

### Osteocytes

When completely surrounded by osteoid or bone matrix, the osteoblast becomes an osteocyte, the cell responsible for the maintenance of the bone. These cells are responsible for the exchange of ions with the bone matrix and the extracellular spaces. Under certain conditions they are felt to be involved with the rapid release of calcium and phosphorus from the mineralized bone by a process termed "osteocytic osteolysis" (31). The main body of the osteocyte is located in small soft tissue areas of the mineralized bone, the lacuna. In specially prepared preparations, such as for electron microscopy in which cell shrinkage is minimized, it can be seen that the wall of the osteocyte is in close relationship to the mineralized bone matrix adjacent to the lacuna. The size, shape, and organization of the osteocytes and their lacunae vary with the type of bone (see below). In woven bone, they are randomly distributed throughout the matrix, are large and spherical, or plump spindles (Fig. 6), while in lamellar bone they are relatively rarer, smaller and spindle-shaped, and evenly distributed along the bone lamellae (Figs. 6, 12, 13, and 20). Long dendritic processes of the osteocytes extend through the canaliculi of the bone (Figs. 12 and 14), often crossing the lamellae but not the cement lines, and connect via gap or nexus junctions with the processes of adjacent osteocytes and osteoblasts.

### Osteoclasts

Osteoclasts are multinucleated cells largely responsible for bone resorption (Figs. 8, 21, and 22). These cells are derived from mononuclear, hematopoietic progenitor cells, granulocytic-macrophage colony-forming units (GM-CFU) and macrophage colony-forming units (M-CFU) (22,26, 32–42). These progenitor cells are felt by most workers to be related to the monocyte/macrophage cell lineages (34), though others (33) feel that this issue is not settled and that there may even be a stem cell committed to osteoclast formation that is entirely separate from the hematopoietic cell lines. Osteoclasts are thought to arise primarily by fusion of the progenitor cells from the GM- or M-CFUs, and are felt to have an ongoing ability to acquire and shed nuclei (42). It is clear that the number and activity of the osteoclasts are increased by PTH and decreased by calcitonin; they have calcitonin receptors, but not PTH or vitamin D receptors. Thus, their stimulation is felt to be the result of a reaction to paracrine and, possibly, autocrine factors secreted by osteoblasts or the osteoclast monocytic precursors, which do have PTH receptors (28–30,41). Lymphokines, osteoclast-activating factors, leukotrienes, and prostaglandins are among the factors that have been suggested as the messengers for osteoclast stimulation (23–25,33,34,41). Under normal conditions, the osteoclasts are directly apposed to the bone surface that is to be resorbed. After a period of bone resorption, they are found in small hollows on the bone surface, named Howship's lacunae (Fig. 21). The cells are 40 to 100 $\mu$m in diameter with an average of 10 to 15 nuclei, though the number may range from 2 to as many as 100. The cells are highly polarized with the nuclei congregating away from the resorbing bone surface. The cell cytoplasm is generally amphophilic with numerous small vacuoles and clear areas in routine histologic preparations. A clear zone is located between the nuclei and the bone matrix at the edge of the Howship's lacunae, with clear amphophilic cytoplasm and smooth cytoplasmic borders that closely follow the contour of the underlying bone matrix. Ultrastructurally, this region is poor in organelles, except for actin filaments (24,40). This region is believed to play a role in sealing the osteoclast to the bone matrix. In contrast to the smooth contour of the cell membrane away from the resorbing surface, the resorbing surface is composed of numerous fingerlike projections of cytoplasm, pointing toward the bone surface. The cell membrane in this region is further specialized by the pres-

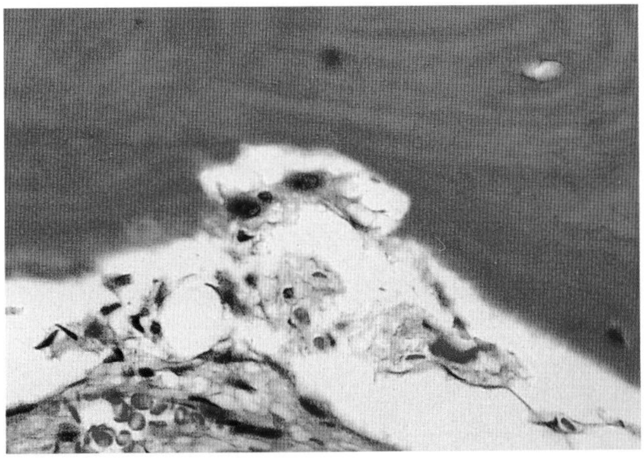

**FIG. 21.** Diagram illustrating the continuous process of bone remodeling. Autocrine factors from the PTH-stimulated surface inactive osteoblasts result in formation of osteoclasts (from the granulocytic-macrophage colony-forming units (GM-CFU), leading to bone resorption. This leads to replacement of the resorbed bone with osteoid and new bone by osteoblasts derived from the fibroblast colony-forming units (F-CFU).

ence of small surface spikes. The cell cytoplasm between the ruffled border and the nucleus contains many lysosomes and is rich in tartrate-resistant acid phosphatase and carbonic anhydrase. The Golgi is abundant and interspersed between the nuclei.

Though the precise processes involved in bone resorption have not been fully established, a great deal of information is available. Resorption of mineralized bone, as with cartilage, is more efficient than unmineralized bone. Focal or partial demineralization of the collagen fibers appears to be an early step in the process. It has been suggested that digestion of the noncollagenous matrix then follows, and, lastly, the collagen fibers themselves are degraded. Mononuclear phagocytes are thought to assist in the resorptive process.

## REMODELING

Throughout life, bone undergoes continuous remodeling in three processes (41,43). In adults, growth in size and changes in shape are largely accomplished by bone resorption and formation on the endosteal and periosteal surface of the compact bone (Fig. 21) and the endosteal surfaces of trabecular bone. Increases in this appositional process under the influence of excess hormone stimulus, such as in acromegaly, result in thickening and widening of the bones. Decreases in the resorptive process, such as in osteopetrosis and hypothyroidism, also result in thickened cortices. In contrast, increased rates of bone resorption relative to formation, such as in hyperthyroidism and some forms of osteoporosis, result in thin, delicate cortical and trabecular bone. The third form of bone remodeling that takes place in the cortex or compact bone of older children and adults is the formation of haversian systems (34). Remodeling requires three phases: activation, bone resorption, and bone formation (44). The replacement of compact lamellar bone begins with local activation of osteoclasts at the endosteal, or, rarely, periosteal surface of the cortical bone. This proceeds at an angle across the bone lamellae, forming a canal containing an arteriole or small artery. The area surrounding the large vessel is accompanied by F-CFU progenitor cells which form a loose connective tissue around the vessel. The leading edge of this canal during active resorption is lined by osteoclasts and is called a "cutting cone" (Fig. 23). Following the osteoclasts are osteoblasts that form new osteoid and bone along the wall of the cutting cone, narrowing its width. When the vessel and canal are large, the canal does and does not completely refill with bone, and the remnant forms a canal, called Volkmann's canal (Figs. 12 and 13). As the vessel divides into smaller and smaller vessels ending as capillaries, they turn and grow in a longitudinal direction within the compact bone, paralleling the long axis of the bone. The leading edge of this cone is formed by osteoclasts (Figs. 23–25). The void left behind is filled with a central capillary, pericytes, loose connective tissue, macrophages, mesenchymal cells, and undifferentiated osteoprogenitor cells. The mononuclear macrophages are generally found on the bone surface between the osteoclasts and the osteoblasts, where they may serve a role in final removal of bone debris. The osteoprogenitor cells modulate to form osteoblasts, which surround the central core of the defect. The osteoblasts (Figs. 24 and 26) lay down successive concentric, circumferential lamellae of bone until only the central vessel with a small region of connective tissue remains. After the connective tissue around the capillary is replaced by bone, additional bone formation ceases. The longitudinal array of concentric lamellae, with a central capillary formed by this remodeling process, is referred to as a haversian system or an osteon (Figs. 11 and 12). The dendrites of the osteocytes in each haversian system are confined to that system and connect only with the processes of the same system (Fig. 12). During the active phase of haversian remodeling, the cells, osteoclasts, macrophages, preosteoblasts, osteoblasts, and osteocytes are arranged into a so-called "bone remodeling unit" (10,45).

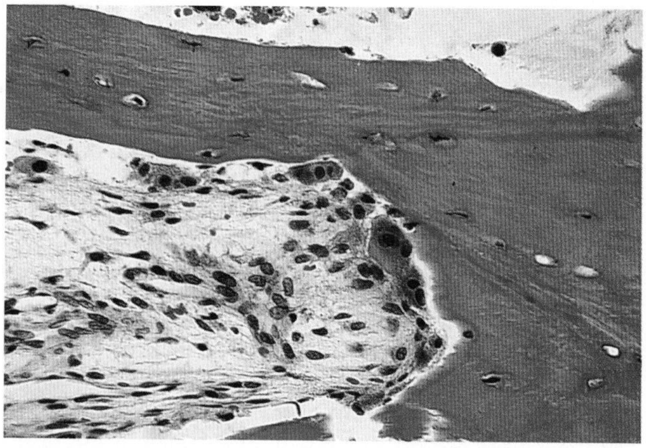

**FIG. 23.** The head of a cutting cone in lamellar bone. The osteoclasts form the leading edge of the bone resorption. Just behind the osteoclasts are mononuclear macrophages, followed by tall columnar osteoblasts. The cutting cone is filled with a vascular loose connective tissue.

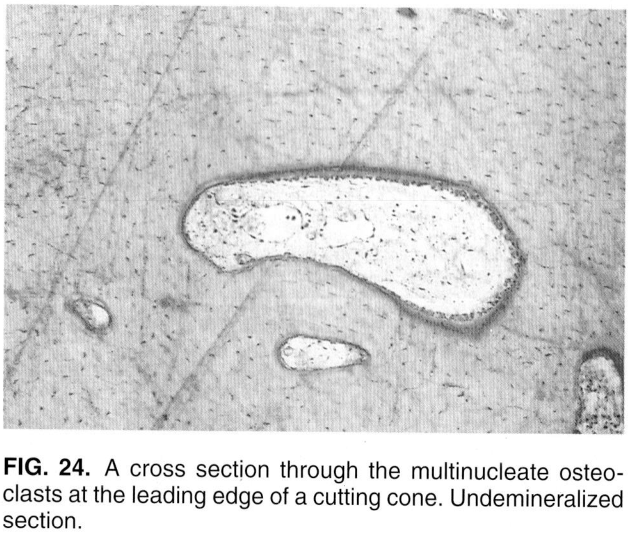

**FIG. 24.** A cross section through the multinucleate osteoclasts at the leading edge of a cutting cone. Undemineralized section.

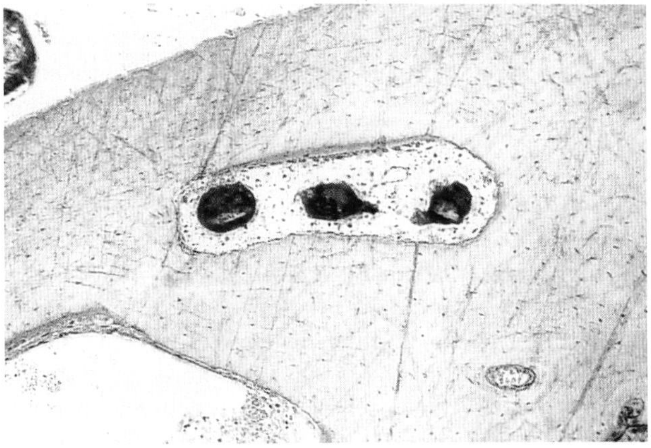

**FIG. 25.** An eccentric section of a cutting cone. The osteoclasts are not visible. The osteoblasts line the surface of the bone, separated by a pale layer of osteoid. The center of the cone is filled with a vascular loose connective tissue. Undemineralized section.

On the outer surface of the osteon, where bone resorption ceases and formation first begins, there is an intensely basophilic area in routine demineralized preparations (Fig. 10), stained with hematoxylin and eosin (H&E) (the cement or reversal line). Little is known about this area, but recent studies have indicated that it is poor in collagen, has less mineral than the surrounding bone matrix, has an increased Ca/P ratio compared to hydroxyapatite, and a higher sulfur content than the surrounding bone matrix (45,46). Schaffler et al. (47) have suggested that the cement line represents a residuum of mineralized "ground substance" from the initial reversal phase of formation of a secondary osteon. As the remodeling process proceeds during life, osteons overlap. The osteocytes of small areas of lamellar (both haversian and nonhaversian) bone are cut off from their nutrient supply and adjacent osteocytes, resulting in their necrosis. These dead osteocytes are resorbed, leaving empty lacunae, similar to the empty lacunae seen in aseptic necrosis of bone. These small areas of dead bone are referred to as interstitial lamellae (Figs. 10 and 11).

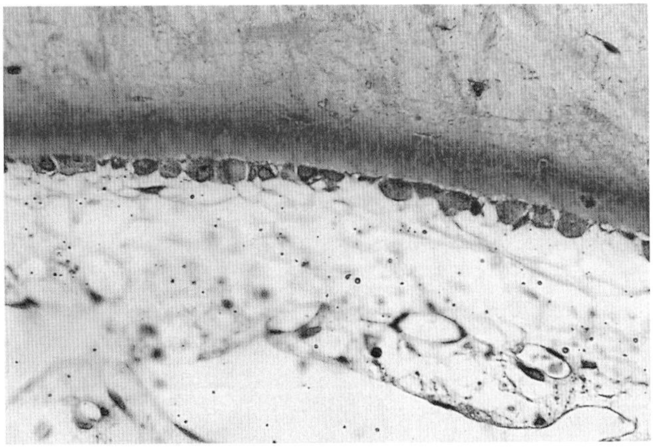

**FIG. 26.** A longitudinal section of the osteoblastic portion of a cutting cone. The tall columnar osteoblasts are separated from the bone by a layer of unmineralized osteoid. The vascular stroma is at the bottom of the micrograph. Undemineralized section.

Studies have demonstrated that the number of osteons in long bones is related to age (47,48) and the stress and weight that the bone is subjected to over its lifetime (47). The percentage of haversian to interstitial bone has been used in anthropologic studies (48). Remodeling of cancellous bone occurs largely at the trabecular surface by resorption and longitudinal new bone formation. In larger trabeculae of the long bones or vertebrae, haversian remodeling may be seen.

In Paget's disease, the rapid bone resorption and formation, unrelated to normal remodeling pressures, leave a mosaic pattern of interstitial lamellae and cement lines. This mosaic pattern can be demonstrated by the use of polarized light. As the lesion proceeds toward the sclerotic phase, there are increased numbers of these mosaic trabeculae in the cancellous bone and cortical bone.

Where bone remodeling is the result of injury, such as aseptic necrosis, cancellous bone is often incorporated in newly formed lamellae, while dead compact cortical bone requires resorption before the new lamellae are laid down (49–51).

## MORPHOMETRY

Evaluation of bone biopsies for metabolic bone disease is best done on specially prepared, plastic-embedded sections that have not been demineralized. Morphometry is a method for the quantitative evaluation of the amount of bone, bone density and mineralization, and the rates of bone formation and resorption (10,32,52,53) on this type of section. It provides a valuable adjunct to the histologic diagnosis of metabolic bone disease and in determining the effects of therapy. It is extremely useful in experimental and clinical studies of metabolic effects on bone. When coupled with tetracycline labeling of the mineralization fronts, one can measure the width of osteoid seams and evaluate the bone formation rate (32,53). A complete discussion of morphometry is beyond the scope of this chapter; however, a few remarks concerning this technique are worth considering. For the interested reader, several recent complete discussions of this subject are available (32,52–59).

Undemineralized sections embedded in plastic are used for evaluation. The patients are prelabeled with tetracycline at two defined times prior to the biopsy. Several factors can be assessed morphometrically (57): the total amount or percentage of bone in the biopsy (and the relative proportions of cancellous and compact bone); the amount or percentage of the bone surface on which new bone is being formed; the amount or width of the osteoid in these areas; with double tetracycline labeling, the rate of bone formation (as measured by the distances between the two tetracycline labels to define the amount of osteoid being deposited per unit time);

and the amount or percentage of the bone being resorbed. These studies are most useful in evaluating metabolic bone diseases such as osteoporosis, osteomalacia, rickets, and renal osteodystrophy. They can measure the changes in these diseases with time, and have been used extensively to correlate with radiologic evaluations of bone mineral density. They have proved very valuable in evaluating the results of therapeutic interventions.

Several cautions must be raised about the use of these techniques in evaluating human disease. The methodologies are not trivial: they require a bone biopsy, expensive equipment, skilled technicians, careful statistical evaluation, and an experienced morphometrist. Most of the studies are limited to evaluation of one site, the iliac crest, which may or may not be representative of the entire skeleton. There are wide variations in the normal values with respect to age, sex, endocrine status, other diseases, therapy, and so on. For these reasons, morphometric studies should be considered like any other laboratory test, with regard to its sensitivity and specificity, something that has not been widely done. Diagnoses should be made only after careful correlation with the clinical history, signs and symptoms, radiologic examinations, and histopathologic evaluation of the biopsy specimen; not solely on the morphometric data.

## EMBRYOLOGY

### Membranous Bone Growth

The flat bones of the skull and face, the frontal, parietal, occipital, and temporal bones, form by intramembranous ossification (3). Undifferentiated mesenchymal (osteoprogenitor) cells of the vascularized connective tissue aggregate at the sites where the new bone trabeculae are to be formed. These cells modulate into osteoblasts, which lay down the collagen fibers of the osteoid (Figs. 6 and 7). This collagen is deposited as a mat of interlacing fibers, thus forming trabeculae of woven bone. The osteoid is then mineralized into bone. Growth of membranous bone occurs radially by periosteal apposition of new bone, and endosteal resorption along the medullary cavity of the outer cortical table. Periosteal resorption and endosteal formation permit growth of the inner table. As the bones mature, the growth rate slows and the new bone takes on a lamellar character. In the adult, haversian remodeling occurs in the cortex of the skull bones.

Between the mineralized spicules of bone is a highly vascularized loose connective tissue, which is replaced by adipose and hematopoietic tissue. A chondroid bone has been described in the flat bones of the skull. This tissue contains both type I and type II collagens and has a histology intermediate between cartilage and bone. Chondroid bone is usually mineralized and apparently forms a scaffolding on which lamellar bone is deposited, though it is not replaced by bone, as occurs in enchondral bone formation (see below). It has been reported to be involved with suture growth and closure.

### Enchondral Bone Growth

Growth of the bones of the axial and radial skeleton requires a marked increase in length, as well as in the diameter, size, and shape. Since bone has a rigid structure, it cannot grow interstitially. Bone can grow only by the apposition of new bone on its surface. Although appositional growth is adequate for areas of slow expansion, such as the skull or in the adult, in other locations such as the long bones of the extremities, the vertebrae, and the ribs, apposition is insufficient for the increase in length required by the organism during prenatal life and childhood. In contrast, cartilage can grow interstitially; that is, it can add new cells within its volume and it can increase its volume by elaborating extracellular matrix, thus, expanding both its length and diameter. Consequently, long bone growth in embryos and prepubertal children occurs by replacement of cartilage with bone, and the majority of the increase in bone length occurs within a cartilage primordium; that is, enchondral growth.

The bone anlage begins as a condensation of the primitive cells of the mesenchyme at the site of the new bone. The exact timing varies from bone to bone, but the process begins prior to 40 days development. The condensed mesenchymal cells modulate to chondrocytes. This avascular cartilaginous anlage has the crude shape of the adult bone (Fig. 27). At the ends of the anlage there is poor separation from the neighboring bone anlagen. In the region between the neighboring anlagen, the primitive mesenchyme displays a further condensation and breakdown forming the joint space (Figs. 27 and 28). The shaft of the bone is surrounded by undifferenti-

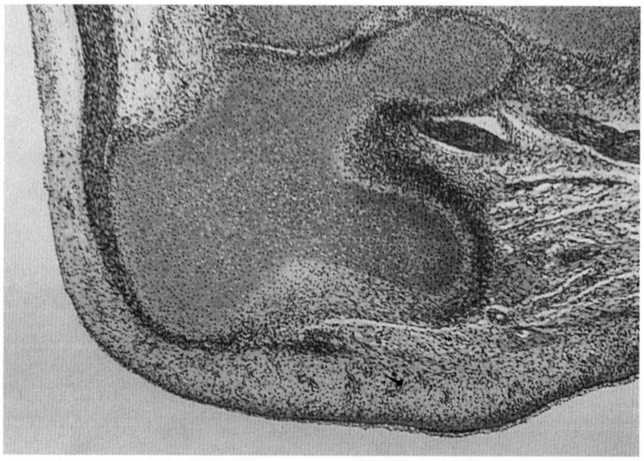

**FIG. 27.** Photomicrograph of an anterior-posterior section through the cartilage anlage of the os calcis. The anlage forms the approximate shape of the adult bone. The lower end of the tibia, the tibial-calcaneal joint, and the anlage of the achilles tendon are visible.

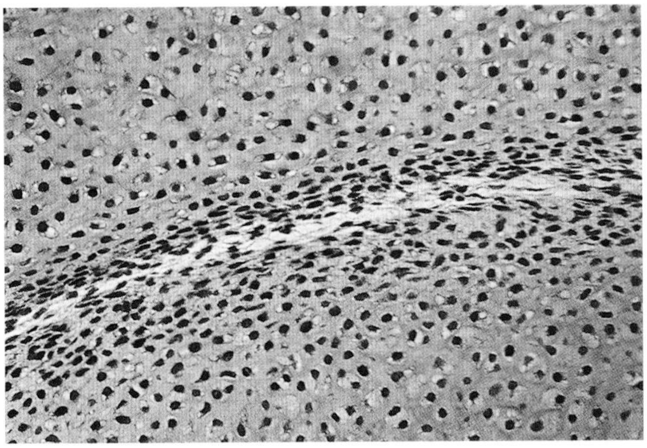

**FIG. 28.** Photomicrograph of the tibia-tarsal joint in an embryo, demonstrating early differentiation of the articular cartilage and breakdown of the mesenchymal cell forming the joint space. The chondrocytes fill their lacunae and there is no matrix resorption.

ated mesenchyme, which modulates into a perichondrium (Figs. 29–31) and subsequently into a periosteum (see below).

Growth occurs interstitially by proliferation of the chondrocytes and by accumulation of extracellular matrix (largely type II collagen with accompanying type IX, X, XI, and XIII collagens and proteoglycans) (3). The shaft of the anlage is generally cylindrical, and in the chick, Caplan and Pechak (60) believe that the shaft is clearly separated from

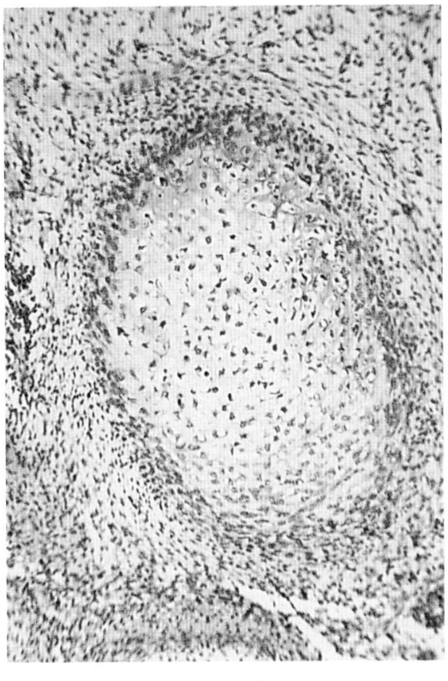

**FIG. 29.** Cross section of the cartilage anlage of the femur in an embryo. The chondrocytes are regular with little hypertrophy. The perichondrium is composed of undifferentiated spindle cells. The cells of this layer have little cytoplasm or intervening stroma. New chondrocytes appear to be added from the perichondrium.

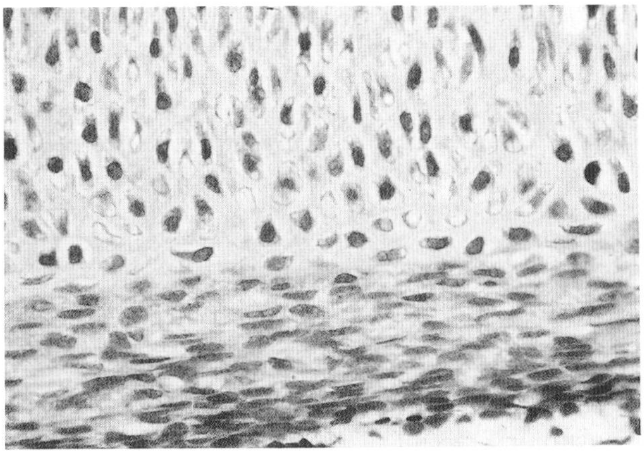

**FIG. 30.** Longitudinal section of the shaft of the femoral anlage in an embryo. The cells of the periosteum have not yet begun to modulate into columnar osteoblasts, and no osteoid is seen between the spindle-shaped cells of the periosteum and the center of the cartilaginous anlage. The cells of the perichondrium appear to be maturing with the addition of new matrix. The cartilage cells fill their lacunae and show little hypertrophy or matrix resorption.

the adjacent mesenchyme by a well-developed layer (referred to as the stacked cell layer) and a network of capillaries. This region is not nearly as well developed in human bones, and it is possible that additional chondrocytes are added to the bone surface from the perichondrium (Figs. 30

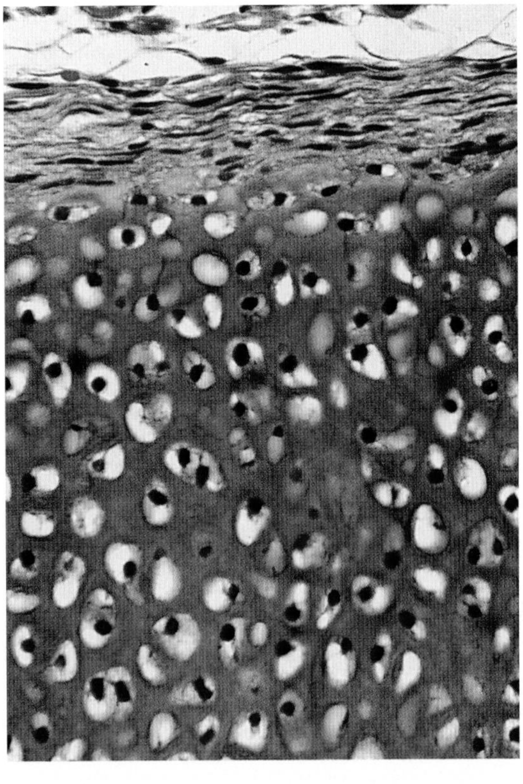

**FIG. 31.** Section of the center of the diaphysis of an embryonic femur. The cartilage cells show early hypertrophy with loss of matrix. The perichondrial cells have become more spindle-shaped with early vascularization and some fibrous matrix between the cells.

and 31) prior to formation of the primary center of ossification (see below). As the interstitial growth of the cartilage anlage continues, three events occur at very nearly the same time in an individual bone, though Caplan and Pechak (60) believe that the order is as follows:

1. Around the center of the cartilaginous shaft, the cells of the mesenchyme (the stacked cell layer of the chick) modulate to form osteoblasts, which deposit a collar of an unmineralized, feltwork of type I collagen (woven bone or osteoid). This osteoid collar (Figs. 32–36) is called the primary center of ossification and delimits the diaphysis. The osteoid then mineralizes. In the chick, the stacked cell layer is clearly delineated from the cartilage cells and modulates into the periosteum. In mammalian and human embryos, this delineation is not nearly as distinct, and the periosteum is not recognized until osteoid is deposited.
2. The chondrocytes in the center of the anlage begin to hypertrophy and swell, resorbing the adjacent intercellular matrix (Figs. 33–36). The hypertrophy is accompanied by an increase in type X collagen (61). The residual matrix becomes mineralized, largely via the matrix vesicles, though some initiation may occur in the collagen.
3. A capillary network forms from the periosteal capillaries (Figs. 36 and 37) and penetrates among the hypertrophied cartilage cells of the diaphysis accompanied by pericytes, hematopoietic elements, and other primitive mesenchymal cells, including the osteoprogenitor cells. The periosteal capillary network eventually evolves into the nutrient artery.

After completion of the collar of the primary center of ossification, no further interstitial growth can occur within its subtended volume. Continued growth in the diameter and shape of the diaphysis is the result of asymmetric subperiosteal appositional growth, identical to that which occurs in the membrane bones of the skull (Figs. 6, 7, and 37). At the same time, to preclude a massive increase in cortical thickness, the cortex is resorbed by osteoclasts along the endosteal surface. Under conditions, such as hypothyroidism or osteopetrosis, where there is a defect in osteoclastic resorption of bone, the cortex shows immense thickening.

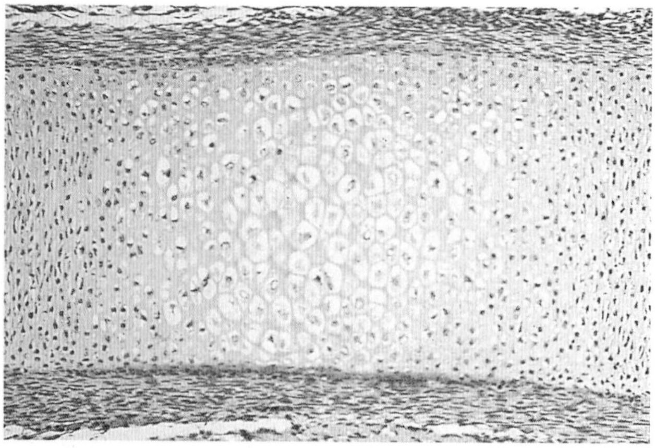

**FIG. 33.** Longitudinal section of the primary center of ossification in an embryonic femur. The cellular layer of the periosteum is modulating into osteoblasts, which have formed a layer of pink osteoid. The outer spindle cells of the periosteum are oriented longitudinally along the femoral shaft. The underlying chondrocytes show hypertrophy and matrix resorption. Compare the size of the lacunae with those in Fig. 27.

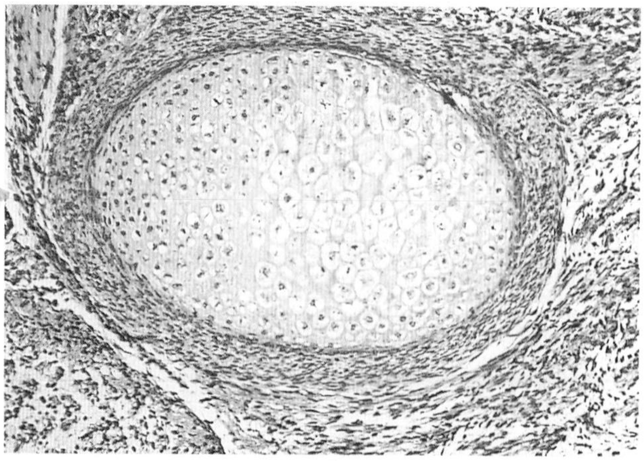

**FIG. 32.** Cross section of the diaphysis of an embryonic femur. The collar-like primary center of ossification is between the hypertrophying chondrocytes and the periosteal cells.

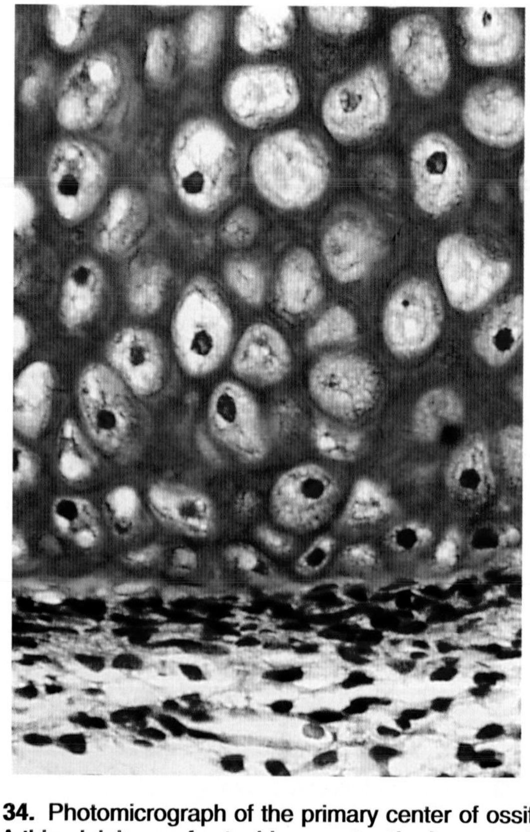

**FIG. 34. Photomicrograph of the primary center of ossification. A thin pink layer of osteoid separates the hypertrophied** chondrocytes from the perichondrial osteoblasts. The fibrous layer of the periosteum consists of a vascular loose connective tissue.

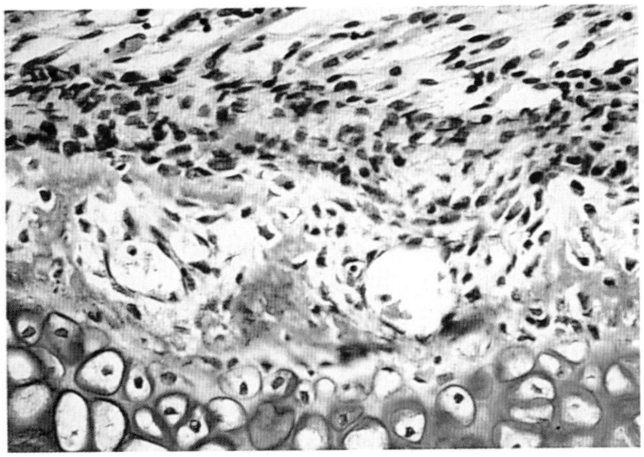

**FIG. 35.** Photomicrograph of the primary center of ossification with capillary proliferation indicating the early formation of the nutrient artery. Between these capillaries new bone is being formed: trabecular membranous woven bone in the cambium layer or the periosteum. The outer fibrous layer of the periosteum is more cellular than in the adult.

The chondrocytes within the primary center of ossification become increasingly hypertrophied, accompanied by deposition of type X collagen and mineralization of the matrix between the chondrocytes (61–63). The horizontally arranged matrix is resorbed, and capillaries, derived from the primary nutrient artery, invade the chondrocyte canals accompanied by pericytes, hematopoietic cells, and osteoprogenitor cells. These cells modulate to osteoblasts (24). The struts of longitudinally arranged cartilage matrix are coated with thin layers of osteoid. These primary trabeculae (bony trabeculae with central cartilaginous cores) are gradually removed by osteoclasts, leaving behind a cavity filled with loose connective, adipose, and hematopoietic tissue. This process begins with the cartilage cells nearest the center of the shaft and progresses toward the metaphysis. The carti-

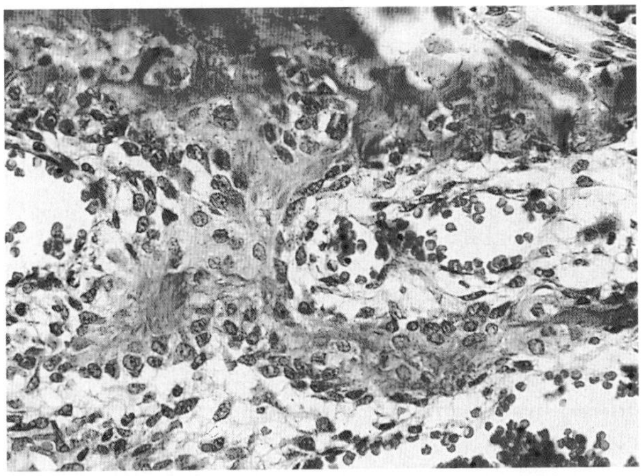

**FIG. 36.** Photomicrograph of the primary center of ossification in the humerus of a fetus. The cambium layer of the periosteum contains numerous osteoblasts forming multiple trabeculae of woven bone, the primitive cortex. Capillaries and undifferentiated mesenchymal cells fill the region between the trabeculae.

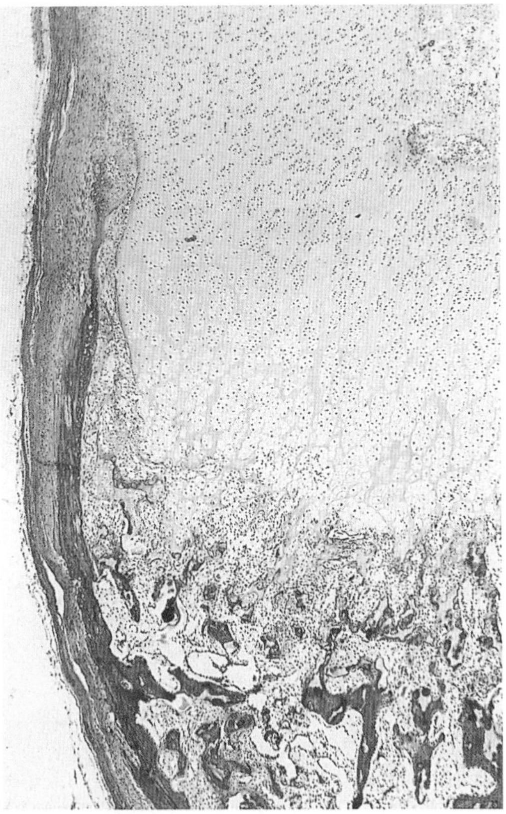

**FIG. 37.** Photomicrograph of the epiphyseal growth plate of the costochondral junction from a 2-month-old male. The growth plate is surrounded by the ring of Ranvier. No secondary center is present. Primary trabeculae with central cartilaginous cores are seen in the metaphysis and upper diaphysis.

lage cells and matrix do not move, but mature in the position they occupied when the primary center of ossification was formed.

When all the cartilage within the central space surrounded by the primary center of ossification has been supplanted by bone spicules, and the enchondral replacement of cartilage has reached the level of the diaphyseal-epiphyseal junction, the area of further lengthening of the bone and maturation occurs in a cylinder of cartilage at each end of the bone called the epiphyseal growth plate or physis. The structure of the physis is regular and composed of a cylinder of progressive cartilage maturation and replacement by bone (Figs. 37–39). Though the process is continuous and is identical to that described previously, this cylinder has arbitrarily been divided into five regions of progressive cartilage maturation: (a) a thin region of resting chondrocytes nearest the end of the bone; (b) a region of proliferating chondrocytes; (c) a region of chondrocyte hypertrophy, where additional matrix is deposited between the chondrocytes, which line up in columns or rows (Fig. 38); (d) a region of provisional mineralization of the cartilaginous matrix; and (e) a region of disappearance of the chondrocytes, resorption of the horizontal (but not the longitudinal) cartilage matrix, and application of osteoid on the bone struts (the zone of provisional

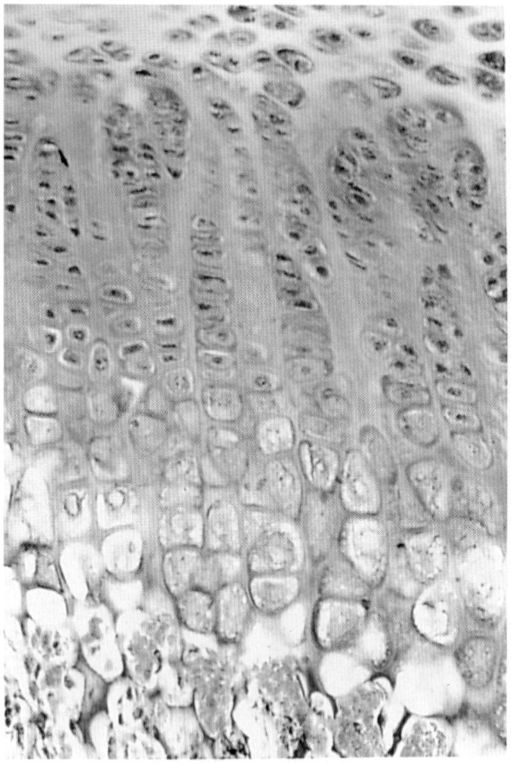

**FIG. 38.** Photomicrograph of a maturing epiphyseal growth plate, showing the proliferating zone (*top*), the hypertrophied zone and zone of provisional mineralization of the cartilage (since this specimen was demineralized, these two zones are indistinguishable), and the zone of provisional ossification. There are prominent capillaries between the vertical columns of the primary trabeculae. (This slide was prepared by M. J. Glimcher, M.D., S. I. Roth, M.D., and A. L. Schiller, M.D. as part of a course in the Pathophysiology of Bone for the Harvard Medical School, Boston MA.)

ossification) (Fig. 39). The areas between the primary trabeculae and the columns of chondrocytes are filled with a capillary loop and undifferentiated mesenchymal cells. The organization of the cartilage struts is determined by the columnar arrangement of the chondrocytes in the hypertrophied zone, and in diseases (rickets) where mineralization of the cartilage is impaired or where the formation of matrix is limited (scurvy), the organization of the primary trabeculae is chaotic. Furthermore, if cartilage mineralization is impaired, such as in renal osteodystrophy, removal of the cartilage is handicapped and often, large malformed masses of unmineralized cartilage are seen. All longitudinal growth of the bone occurs in the regions of cartilage proliferation and early maturation. After the maximum matrix has been formed, no additional longitudinal growth is possible. Pins placed in the bone straddling the proliferative and maturing zones will spread apart during growth, whereas pins placed in the bone central to these areas will maintain a constant distance between themselves. The hemispherical growth of the epiphysis (see below) causes the proliferative region of the physis to be wider than the diaphysis. This wider area is connected to the narrower diaphysis by a collar of membrane bone called the ring of Ranvier (Figs. 37 and 40) (64). Interstitial growth in length and diameter can continue in the cartilaginous epiphysis, and, thus, the epiphysis and physis have a greater diameter than the diaphysis. The reduction of this diameter to that of the shaft occurs at the metaphysis, so that in contrast to the diaphysis, bone resorption occurs on the periosteal surface and bone formation on the endosteal surface. This process is called funnelization.

In most long bones, a secondary center of ossification occurs in the epiphysis (Figs. 41 and 42). The maturation and replacement of the cartilage anlage in this secondary center are identical to that which occur in the diaphysis and the epiphyseal growth plate, except that the maturation proceeds from the center centrifugally, toward the periphery. This means that the growing area of the secondary center is, at first, a sphere. When the process reaches the growth area of the epiphyseal growth plate, the two proliferative zones merge. As maturation of the secondary center occurs in the cells adjacent to the proliferative zone, a plate of bone forms separating the secondary center from the epiphyseal growth

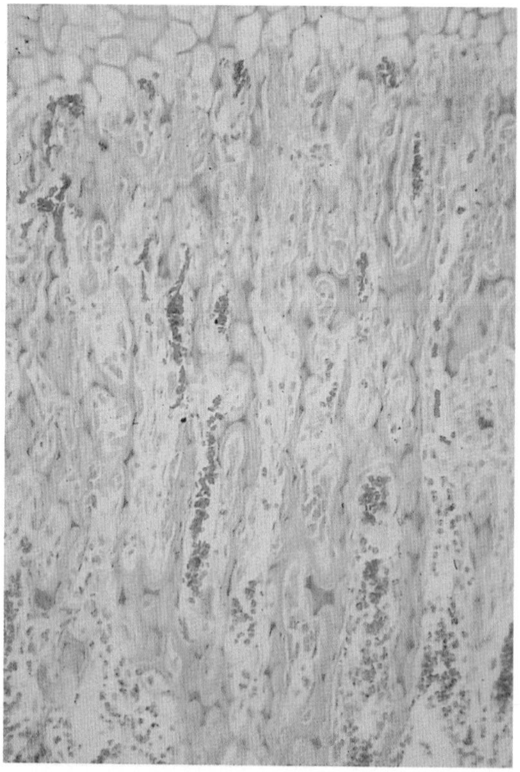

**FIG. 39.** Longitudinal section of the epiphyseal growth plate, showing the zone of provisional mineralization of the cartilage (*orange*). The cartilage struts are being covered by a thin layer of osteoid (*green*) in the zone of provisional ossification. Capillaries with numerous erythrocytes are present between the primary bone trabeculae. (*Goldner's stain.*) (This slide was prepared by M. J. Glimcher, M.D., S. I. Roth, M.D., and A. L. Schiller, M.D. as part of a course in the Pathophysiology of Bone for the Harvard Medical School, Boston MA.)

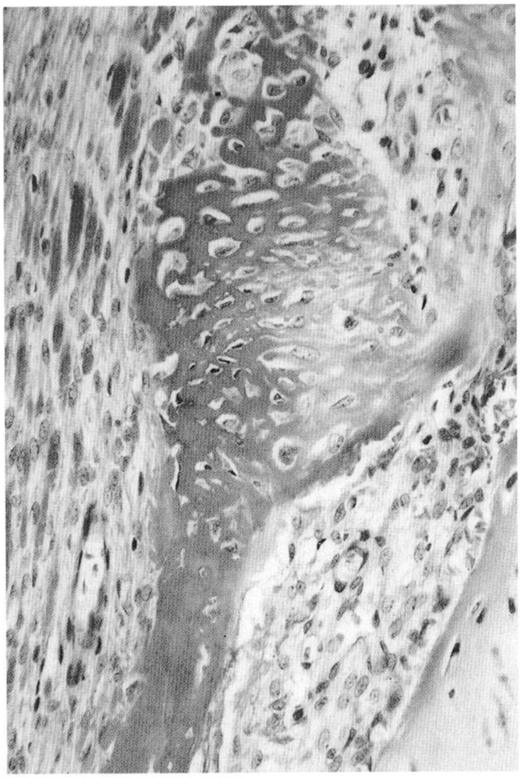

**FIG. 40.** Photomicrograph of the ring of Ranvier. The membrane bone is forming in the perichondrium of the epiphyseal growth plate.

plate, permitting only radial outward growth of the secondary center. This permits an increase in the size of the epiphysis, a process called hemispherization. The peripheral growth zone also supplies cartilage for the overlying articular cartilage.

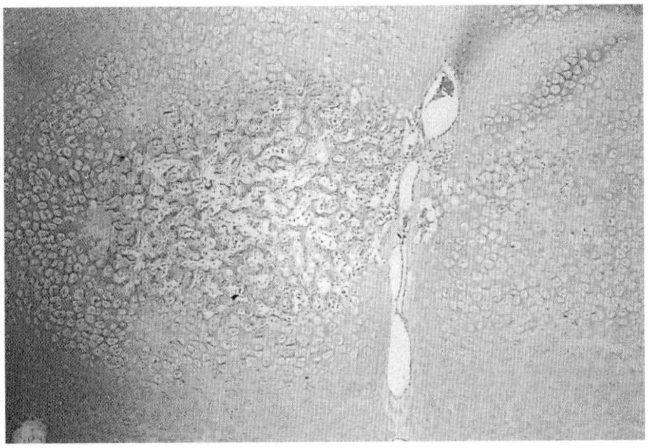

**FIG. 41.** Photomicrograph of the secondary center of ossification of the femoral head. The nutrient vessels from the ligamentum teres is seen. Osteoid (*green*) is seen on the cartilage trabeculae (*orange*) in the spherical center. (*Goldner's stain.*)

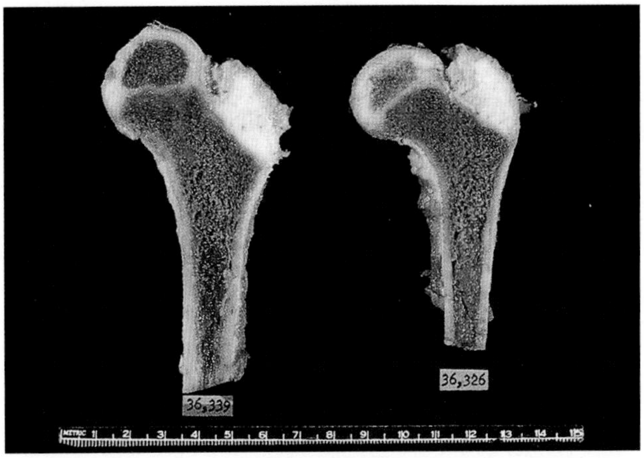


**FIG. 42.** Gross photograph of the femoral heads of 3.5-year-old male. The secondary centers of ossification in the femoral heads are separated from the primary centers by the epiphyseal growth plates (*the physes*). The secondary center of ossification of the greater trochanter has not as yet formed. The metaphyses and diaphyses resemble their adult shape.

Changes in the shape of the bones are brought about during growth, as determined by Wolff's law (8,9). Remodeling of the primary trabeculae occurs by osteoclastic removal and replacement with new secondary trabeculae. Complete osteoclastic resorption of the trabeculae allows formation of the medullary cavity, largely free of spicules of cancellous bone in the mid-diaphysis, which fills with the hematopoietic marrow. In the diaphysis, there is an asymmetric subperiosteal appositional addition of bone and endosteal resorption of cortex to maintain a proper, tubular shape. The secondary trabeculae are lamellar, and the appositionally applied cortical bone is composed of longitudinal lamellae. Mechanical forces exerted by muscle attachments alter the rate of these processes in various areas of the bone, thus, altering the final shape of the bone. In addition, the final shape of the bone is related to the relative rates of growth of the epiphyseal growth plates at each end of the bone and of subperiosteal growth.

Enchondral growth continues at the epiphyseal growth plate under the influence of several hormones: growth hormone, somatomedins, thyroid hormone, parathyroid hormone, androgens, estrogens, and adrenal cortical hormones,until puberty. At that time, the growth plate closes (Fig. 43) and all additional bone growth is appositional (3,24). At puberty, low doses of androgens and estrogens cause an increase in the rate of proliferation of the cells in both the proliferating zone of the growth plates and the secondary centers of ossification. This is accompanied by an increase in the rate of cartilage maturation and formation of the primary trabeculae. These effects result in the so-called "growth spurt" seen at puberty.

With increasing levels of estrogens and androgens, and a falling off of the growth hormone and somatomedin levels, cartilage proliferation decreases while maturation and bone formation proceed. This leads to a decreasing width of the

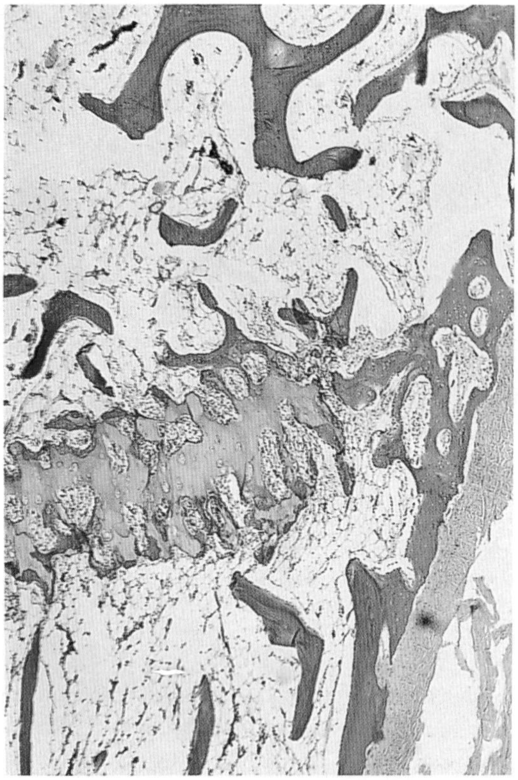

**FIG. 43.** Photomicrograph of a closing epiphyseal growth plate in a 16-year-old boy. The periphery of the plate has been bridged by bone connecting the diaphysis and the secondary center of ossification. Cellular proliferation in the physis has ceased while the maturation process continues.

growth plate and eventually to ossification of the entire growth plate, including the zone of proliferation. Bone at this time traverses the entire epiphyseal growth plate from the metaphysis to the epiphysis, and the growth plate is said to be closed. No residua of the growth plate remains, and no additional interstitial growth of the bone is possible. In adult life, additional bone growth is slow, subperiosteal appositional growth. With the closure of the epiphyseal growth plates, growth of the secondary centers of ossification also ceases. Proliferation of the cartilage cells terminates and their maturation continues until only the articular cartilage remains, above a plate of mature lamellar bone—the subchondral plate. A small amount of growth cartilage with mineralized matrix remains, separated from the articular cartilage by a thin zone of intense mineralization called the tide mark (Figs. 17 and 18). Reactivation of this growth cartilage and an increase in appositional subperiosteal growth occur in adult onset acromegaly, under the influence of increased levels of growth hormone.

## ACKNOWLEDGMENT

The authors thank Dr. Arthur Veis for reviewing the manuscript for this chapter, which appeared in the first edition of this book.

## REFERENCES

1. Veis A, Sabsay B. The collagen of mineralized matrices. In: Peck WA, ed. *Bone and mineral research/6*. Amsterdam; Elsevier, 1988;1–63.
2. Robey PG, Bianco P, Termine JD. The cellular biology and molecular biochemistry of bone formation. In: Coe FL, Favus MJ, eds. *Disorders of bone and mineral metabolism*. New York; Raven Press, 1992; 241–263.
3. Howell DS, Dean DD. The biology, chemistry and biochemistry of the mammalian growth plate. In: Coe FL, Favus MJ, eds. *Disorders of bone and mineral metabolism*. New York; Raven Press, 1992;313–353.
4. Glimcher MJ. Mechanism of calcification: role of collagen fibrils and collagen-phosphoprotein complexes in vitro and in vivo. *Anat Rec* 1989;224:139–153.
5. Glimcher MJ. The nature of the mineral component and the mechanism of calcification. In: Coe FL, Favus MJ, eds. *Disorders of bone and mineral metabolism*. New York; Raven Press, 1992;265–286.
6. Posner AS. Bone mineral and the mineralization process. In: Peck WA, ed. *Bone and mineral research/6*. Amsterdam; Elsevier, 1988;65–116.
7. Posner AS. The mineral of bone. *Clin Orthop* 1985;200:87–99.
8. Wolff J. *The law of bone remodeling*. Berlin: Springer-Verlag, 1986. Furlong, Maquet P, translator. Das Gesetz der Transformation der Knochen. Originally published by Berlin; Verlag von August Hirschwald, 1892.
9. Wolff J. Die Lehre von den funktionellen Knochengestalt. *Arch Pathol Anat* 1899;155:256–315.
10. Frost HM. Mechanical determinants of bone modeling. *Metab Bone Dis Relat Res* 1982;4:217–229.
11. Roth SI, Jimenez JF, Husted S, Seibert JJ, Haynes DW. The histopathology of camptomelia (bent limbs). A dyschondrogenesis. *Clin Orthop* 1982;167:152–159.
12. Ghadially FN. Fine structure of joints: In: Sokoloff L, ed. *The joints and synovial fluid*. New York; Academic Press, 1978;105–176.
13. LeGuellec D, Mallein-Gerin F, Treilleux J, Bonaventure J, Peysson P, Herbage D. Localization of the expression of Type I, I and II collagen genes in human normal and hypochondrogenesis cartilage canals. *Histochem J* 1994;26:695–704.
14. Eyre DR, Wu JJ, Woods PE. The cartilage collagens:structural and metabolic studies. *J Rheumatol* 1991;18(Suppl 27):49–51.
15. Roughley PJ, Lee ER. Cartilage proteoglycans:structure and potential functions. *Microsc Res Tech* 1994;28:385–397.
16. Poole CA, Flint MH, Beaumont BW. Morphological and function interrelationships of articular cartilage matrices. *J Anat* 1984;1:113–138.
17. Recker RR. Embryology, anatomy and microstructure of bone. In: Coe FL, Favus MJ, eds. *Disorders of bone and mineral metabolism*. New York; Raven Press, 1992;219–240.
18. Shay AK, Bliven ML, Scampoli DN, Otterness IG, Milici AJ. Effects of exercise on synovium and cartilage from normal and inflamed knees. *Rheumatol Int* 1995;14:183–189.
19. Mow VC, Settan LA, Ratcliffe A, et al. Structure and function relationships of articular cartilage and the effect of joint instability and trauma on cartilage functions.In: Brandt KD, ed. *Cartilage changes in osteoarthritis*. Indianapolis; University Press, 1990;22–42.
20. Davies DV, Barnett CH, Cochrane W, Palfrey AJ. Electron microscopy of articular cartilage in your adult rabbit. *Ann Rheum Dis* 1962;21: 11–22.
21. Pelletier JP, Roughley P, DiBattista JA, Martel-Pelletier JL. Are cytokines involved in osteoarthritis pathophysiology? *Semin Arthritis Rheum* 1991;20(Suppl 2);12–25.
22. Jotereau FV, LeDouarin NM. The developmental relationship between osteocytes and osteoclasts: a study using the quail-chick nuclear marker in endochondral ossification. *Dev Biol* 1978;63:253–265.
23. Manolagas SC, Jilka RL. Bone marrow cytokines and bone remodeling. Emerging insights into the pathophysiology of osteoporosis. *New Engl J Med* 1995:332:305–311.
24. Marks SC Jr, Popoff SN. Bone cell biology: the regulation of development, structure, and function in the skeleton. *Am J Anat* 1988;183:1–44.
25. Friedenstein AJ. Stromal mechanisms of bone marrow: cloning in vitro and retransplantation in vivo. In: Thienfelder S, ed. *Immunobiology of bone marrow transplantation*. Berlin; Springer-Verlag, 1980;19–29.
26. Friedenstein AJ. Determined and inducible osteogenic precursor cells. In: *Hard tissue growth, repair and remineralization*. Amsterdam; Elsevier-Excerpta Medica, 1973;169–185. Ciba Foundation Symposium 11.

27. LeBlond CP. Synthesis and secretion of collagen by cells of connective tissue, bone, and dentin. *Anat Rec* 1989;224:123–138.
28. Jilka RL. Are osteoblastic cells required for the control of osteoclastic activity by parathyroid hormone? *Bone Mineral* 1986;1:261–266.
29. Marks SC Jr. Osteoclast biology: lessons from mammalian mutations. *Am J Med Genet* 1989;43:43–54.
30. Rouleau MF, Mitchell J, Goltzman D. In vivo distribution of parathyroid hormone receptors in bone: evidence that a predominant osseous target cell is not the mature osteoblast. *Endocrinology* 1988;123:187–191.
31. Bélanger LF. Osteocytic osteolysis. *Calcif Tissue Res* 1969;4:1–12.
32. Fallon MD, Teitelbaum SL. The interpretation of fluorescent tetracycline markers in the diagnosis of metabolic bone diseases. *Hum Pathol* 1982;13:416–417.
33. Chambers TJ. The origin of the osteoclast. In: Peck WA, ed. *Bone and mineral research/6.* Amsterdam; Elsevier, 1989;1–25.
34. Mundy GR, Roodman DG. Osteoclast ontogeny and function. In: Peck WA, ed. *Bone and mineral research/5.* Amsterdam; Elsevier, 1987;209–279.
35. Walker DG. Congenital osteopetrosis in mice cured by parabiotic union with normal siblings. *Endocrinology* 1972;91:916–920.
36. Walker DG. Osteopetrosis cured by temporary parabiosis. *Science* 1973;180:875.
37. Walker DG. Bone resorption restored in osteopetrotic mice by transplants of normal bone marrow and spleen cells. *Science* 1975;190:784–785.
38. Walker DG. Spleen cells transmit osteopetrosis in mice. *Science* 1975;190:785–787.
39. Walker DG. Control of bone resorption by hematopoietic tissue. The induction and reversal of congenital osteopetrosis in mice through the use of bone marrow and splenic transplants. *J Exp Med* 1975;142:651–653.
40. Raisz LG. Mechanisms and regulation of bone resorption by osteoclastic cells. In: Coe FL, Favus MJ, eds. *Disorders of bone and mineral metabolism.* New York; Raven Press, 1992;287–311.
41. Dempster DW. Bone remodeling. In: Coe FL, Favus MJ, eds. *Disorders of bone and mineral metabolism.* New York; Raven Press, 1992;355–380.
42. Stout SD, Teitelbaum SL. Histomorphometric determination of formation rate or archaeological bone. *Calcif Tissue Res* 1976;21:163–169.
43. Canalis E, McCarthy T, Centrell M. The regulation of bone formation by local growth factors. In: Peck WA, ed. *Bone and mineral research/6.* Amsterdam; Elsevier, 1989;27–56.
44. Eriksen EF. Normal and pathological remodeling of human trabecular bone: three dimensional reconstruction of the remodeling sequence in normal and in metabolic bone disease. *Endocr Rev* 1986;7:379–408.
45. Huffer WE. Morphology and biochemistry of bone remodeling: possible control by vitamin D, parathyroid hormone, and other substances. *Lab Invest* 1988;59:418–442.
46. Burr DB, Martin RB. Errors in bone remodeling: toward a unified theory of metabolic bone disease. *Am J Anat* 1989;186:186–216.
47. Schaffler MB, Burr DB, Frederickson RG. Morphology of the osteonal cement line in human bone. *Anat Rec* 1987;217:223–228.
48. Ortner DJ. Aging effects on osteon remodeling. *Calcif Tissue Res* 1975;18:27–36.
49. Putschar WGJ. General pathology of the musculo-skeletal system. In: Buchner F, Letterer E, Roulet F, eds. *Handbuch der Allgemeinen Pathologie.* Berlin; Springer-Verlag, 1960;3:363–488.
50. Glimcher MJ, Kenzora JE. The biology of osteonecrosis of the human femoral head and its clinical implications: I. Tissue biology. *Clin Orthop* 1979;138:284–309.
51. Glimcher MJ, Kenzora JE. The biology of osteonecrosis of the human femoral head and its clinical implications: II. The pathological changes in the femoral head as an organ and in the hip joint. *Clin Orthop* 1979;139:283–312.
52. Glimcher MJ, Kenzora JE. The biology of osteonecrosis of the human femoral head and its clinical implications. III. Discussion of the etiology and genesis of the pathological sequelae; comments on treatment. *Clin Orthop* 1979;138:284–309.
53. Vedi S, Compston JE, Webb A, Tighe JR. Histomorphometric analysis of dynamic parameters of trabecular bone formation in the iliac crest of normal British subjects. *Metab Bone Dis Relat Res* 1983;5:69–74.
54. Frost HM. Tetracycline based histological analysis of bone remodeling. *Calcif Tissue Res* 1969;3:211–237.
55. Jaworski ZFG. Volume 2: bone histomorphometry: outline of theory and practice. In: Simmons OJ, Kunin AS, eds. *Skeletal research*, vol 2. New York; Academic Press, 1983;237–276.
56. Jee WSS, Parfitt AM. *Bone histomorphometry.* Third international workshop. Paris; Armour-Montagu, 1981.
57. Parfitt AM, Drezner MK, Glorieux FH, Kanis JA, Malluche H, Meuneir PJ, Ott SM, Recker RR. Bone histomorphometry: standardization of nomenclature, symbols and units. *J Bone Min Res* 1987;2:595–610.
58. Recker R, ed. *Bone histomorphometry: techniques and interpretations.* Boca Raton; CRC Press, 1983.
59. Eriksen EF, Steinche T, Mosekilde L, Melsen F. Histomorphometric analysis of bone in metabolic bone disease. *Endocrinol Metab Clin North Am* 1989;18:919–954.
60. Caplan AI, Pechak DG. The cellular and molecular embryology of bone formation. In: Peck WA, ed. *Bone and mineral research/6.* Amsterdam: Elsevier, 1988;117–183.
61. Linsenmayer TF, Eavy RD, Schmid TM. Type X collagen: a hypertrophic cartilage-specific molecule. *Pathol Immunopathol Res* 1988;7:14–19.
62. Poole AR, Matsui Y, Hinek A, Lee ER. Cartilage macromolecules and the calcification of cartilage matrix. *Anat Rec* 1989;224:167–179.
63. Poole AR, Pidoux I. Immunoelectron microscopic studies of type X collagen in enchondral ossification. *J Cell Biol* 1989;109:2547–2554.
64. Shapiro F, Holtrop ME, Glimcher MJ. Organization and cellular biology of the perichondrial ossification groove of Ranvier. A morphological study in rabbits. *J Bone Joint Surg Am* 1977;59A:703–723.

*Histology for Pathologists, second edition,*
Edited by Stephen S. Sternberg.
Lippincott-Raven Publishers, Philadelphia


# CHAPTER 6

# Joints

Peter G. Bullough



## THE NORMAL JOINT

The ends of contiguous bones, together with their soft tissue components (cartilage, ligaments, and synovium), constitute a functioning unit: the joint. Of the three types of joints, the most common is the diarthrodial joint, a cavitated movable connecting unit between two bones. Hyaline cartilage (articular cartilage) covers the articulating surfaces of the diarthrodial joints, with the exception of the sternoclavicular and temporomandibular joints, which are covered by fibrocartilage.

The second type of joint is the amphiarthrodial joint, typified by the intervertebral disc and characterized by limited mobility.

The third and final type of joint is the fibrous synarthrosis, such as the skull sutures, which are nonmovable joints.

### Diarthrodial Joint

Perhaps it is not inappropriate to begin by stating what the function of a joint is. Histology (the tissues) can only make sense when we have an understanding of both the function and dysfunction (i.e., the pathology) of the joint.

Normal joint function is characterized by the maintenance of stability during use, freedom of the opposed articular surfaces to move painlessly over each other within the required range of motion, and correct distribution of load across joint tissues. (Without proper loading, the tissues could be damaged by overloading or they could become atrophied because of disuse.)

Conversely, joint dysfunction is characterized clinically by instability, loss of motion, and maldistribution of load and pain, i.e., loss of normal function.

The three interdependent aspects of joint function depend on three features of anatomy: the shape (morphology), the mechanical properties of the extracellular matrices of the tissues that go to make up the joint, and the pericapsular structures.

#### *The Shape*

Perhaps the most obvious feature of any joint is the shape of its articulating surfaces. In general, one surface is convex, and the other concave. The convex or "male" side of the articulation usually has a larger surface than the concave or "female" side. These complementary shapes permit the normal range of motion, and provide stability and equitable loading during use, as well.

In some joints, (for example, the hip and the ankle) the articular surfaces appear at first sight to fit exactly (they appear congruent) (1). However, in other joints (such as the knee and finger joints) it is readily apparent that the surfaces are incongruent.

Congruence in all positions of the joint would necessitate that all joint surfaces were perfectly spherical or cylindrical, which they obviously are not. Therefore, no joint can be congruent in all positions (though in every joint there is usually a position in which it is most congruent) (2). In some joints, of which the knee is a notable example, the gross incongruencies of the opposed surfaces are partially compensated for by the interposed, pliable intra-articular fibrocartilaginous

Peter G. Bullough: Departments of Pathology and Laboratory Medicine, Cornell University Medical College, The Hospital for Special Surgery, New York, NY.

menisci (3). These latter structures constitute an important component contributing to joint morphology and function, and cannot be removed without significant consequences.

In many joints, perhaps most, the initial, limited, contact between the opposed articular surfaces seems to be at the periphery of the joint. However, because the tissues that make up the articulating surfaces undergo elastic deformation under load (particularly the cartilage but also the bone), as the load increases the surfaces come into increasing contact, thereby distributing the load more equitably. Both the incongruence and the deformation of the joint space under load, together with the movement of the joint, provide circulation and mixing of the synovial fluid, which, because the articular cartilage has no blood supply, are essential to the metabolism of the chondrocytes (Fig. 1).

### *The Mechanical Properties of the Extracellular Matrices*

In 1743 William Hunter (4) noted that: "The articulating cartilages are most happily contrived to all purposes of motion in those parts. By their uniform surface, they move upon one another with ease; by their soft, smooth and slippery surface, mutual abrasion is prevented; by their flexibility, the contiguous surfaces are constantly adapted to each other and the friction diffused equally over the whole; by their elasticity, the violence of any shock, which may happen in running, jumping, etc. is broken and gradually spent; which must have been extremely pernicious, if the hard surfaces of bones had been immediately contiguous."

The mechanical properties of articular cartilage, and of all other connective tissues, are determined by the extracellular matrices. In each of the different connective tissues, as well as in each particular structure, the matrices have a unique composition and structural organization, which provide mechanical function at that locus. Disturbances in the structure and/or composition of the extracellular matrix of articular cartilage, therefore, result in joint dysfunction; since the joint includes the bone beneath the cartilage, as well as the ligaments and tendons, alterations in the mechanical properties of bone or disruption of the ligaments could have equally disastrous effects on joint function. Clearly, some knowledge of the matrix components is necessary for an understanding of connective tissue diseases.

The connective tissue matrices are both synthesized and broken down by their intrinsic cells (e.g., fibroblasts, osteoblasts, osteoclasts, chondrocytes). In maintaining the physicochemical and mechanical properties of tissues, the metabolism of these cells must be subject to highly sensitive feedback systems involving both local and systemic factors.

Collagen fibers, the principal extracellular components of connective tissues, are made up of bundles of fibrils, which in turn, are composed of stacked molecules formed from polypeptide chains arranged in a helical pattern. Fourteen different types of collagen molecule are now known and these vary both in size and configuration (5). Many of these different collagens are aligned in a staggered array to form collagen fibrils. Type I collagen is the most common form of collagen and the major collagen found in skin, fascia, tendon, and bone. There are also nonfiber–forming collagens that may have varying functions, such as binding sites for other matrix components (type IX) or to facilitate calcification (type X) (6), or to limit growth of individual matrix constituents.

Hyaline cartilage has a unique type of collagen, type II, which is structurally characterized by three triple helical alpha-1 (II) chains. The type II fibrillar network gives articular cartilage its tensile strength and is essential for maintaining the tissue's volume and shape (7).

The fibrillar collagens are designed to provide tensile strength. However, the connective tissues are also subjected to compression. In bone, the compressive load is resisted by hydroxyapatite. In cartilage, the filler between the collagen fibers, which provides the compressive strength of cartilage as well as its viscoelastic properties, is composed of large negatively charged macromolecular aggregates (8). Proteoglycans (PGs) are a group of heterogeneous molecules consisting of protein chains and attached carbohydrates that have a sticky gellike quality. The major PG in cartilage is aggrecan, containing a protein core of Mr 215000 to which

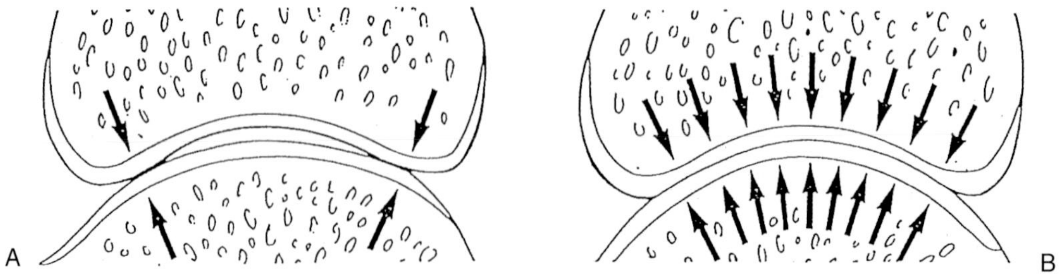


**FIG. 1. A,** Light load: At rest and under light load, limited contact at the joint periphery assures access for synovial fluid to the joint space. **B,** Increased load: With increasing load, deformation of the bone and cartilage allow for increased contact of the cartilage surfaces. Cyclical loading provides for circulation of the synovial fluid in the joint and between the articular surfaces to provide the metabolism of the cartilage.

carbohydrate side chains (keratan and chondroitin sulfate) are attached. The core protein, which contains three globular domains, interacts with hyaluronic acid, and this interaction is stabilized by link protein. As many as 200 aggrecan molecules bind to one hyaluronic acid chain (Mr 1-2 $\times 10^6$) to form an aggregate (Mr 5 $\times 10^7$ to 5 $\times 10^8$) (hence the name "aggrecan").

Proteoglycans are highly charged molecules that attract water and swell considerably. However, within cartilage the expansion of the PGs is restricted to approximately 20% of the maximum possible by the collagen network, creating a swelling pressure within cartilage tissue. When cartilage is loaded, some water is extruded and PGs are further compressed. Removal of the load permits the imbibing of water into the tissue together with essential nutrients until the swelling pressure of the PGs is again balanced by the tensile resistance of the collagen network. Aggrecan shows an age-related decrease in size and an enrichment in keratan sulfate relative to chondroitin sulfate; these changes may relate to the observed age-dependent change in the stiffness and water content of the cartilage.

In addition to aggrecan, cartilage contains other PGs containing dermatan sulfate (biglycan and decorin) (9). These PGs are present in low concentrations and show increasing concentration with age, especially in superficial layers. They appear to inhibit processes involved in tissue repair and may have a role in preventing joint adhesions.

#### *Capsular and Pericapsular Tissues*

A consideration of functional joint anatomy must include the capsule of the joint and its synovial lining and the ligamentous conjoining of the articulating surfaces, as well as the neuromuscular control of joint motion. Through the perception of touch, temperature, pain, and position, sensory feedbacks monitor our movements. Correct joint function is, thus, dependent on intact ligaments, muscles, and nerves. As recognized by Charcot, a breakdown of neuromuscular coordination can lead to profound arthritis (10).

### Amphiarthrodial Joint

The intervertebral disc can be divided into two components: the outermost fibrous ring (annulus fibrosus) and the innermost gelatinous core (nucleus pulposus).

The annulus, when viewed from above, is seen to contain fibrous tissue layers arranged in concentric circles (Fig. 2). Each layer extends obliquely from vertebral body to vertebral body, with the fibers of one layer running in a direction opposite to that of the adjacent layer. This arrangement of alternating layers provides motion that is universal in direction, but restricted in degree. The fibers of the annulus are attached by Sharpey's fibers to the bony endplates of the adjacent vertebral bodies. The fibrous lamellae are stronger and more numerous in the anterior and lateral aspects of the disc than in the posterior aspect, where they are sparser and thinner. The anterior anulus is, therefore, almost twice the thickness of the posterior anulus. This variation probably reflects the protection offered by the posterior elements of the vertebral bodies.

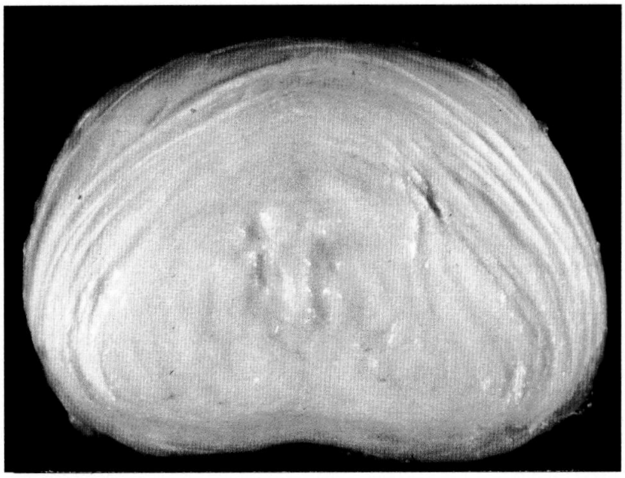

**FIG. 2.** Photograph of an intervertebral disc seen from above. Note the layers of circumferential fibers that make up the anulus fibrosus and the well-demarcated bulging central mass of the nucleus pulposus. Note also the marked variation in the width of the anulus from anterior (*top*) to posterior (*bottom*).

The nucleus pulposus typically occupies an eccentric position within the disc space, usually being closer to the posterior margin. The tissue of the nucleus is separated from that of the bone above and below by a clearly defined layer of hyaline cartilage extending to the inner margins of the insertion of the annulus (Fig. 3).

On microscopic examination the nucleus pulposus shows a varying number of stellate, and fusiform cells can be observed suspended in a loose fibromyxoid matrix.

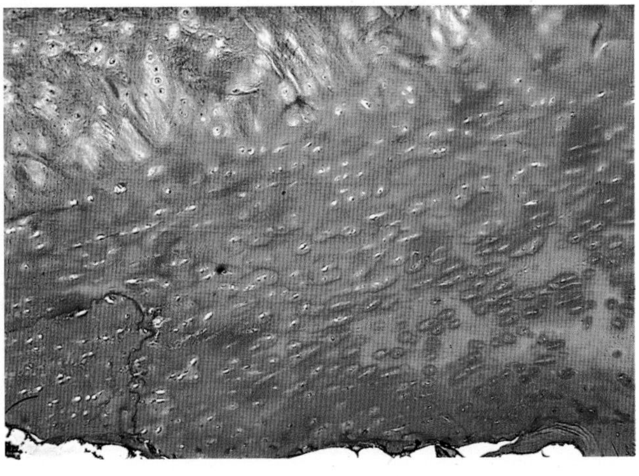

**FIG. 3.** The nucleus pulposus of the disc is separated from the bone by a dense layer of hyaline cartilage as demonstrated in this photomicrograph (**H&E stain, × 4 objective**).

Because no blood vessels are present in adult disc tissue, nutrients must travel by diffusion from capillary beds at the disc margins. The restricted flow of nutrients to the nucleus and inner annulus may contribute to or even underlie disc degeneration in the adult.

It should be noted that disc height, in general, is not the same in all segments of the spine, the cervical and thoracic discs being flatter than those of the lumbar region. Disc height also varies from front to back, relative to the curvature of the spine and with age, becoming thinner in older individuals.

## THE NORMAL JOINT TISSUES

### Articular Cartilage

#### *Morphology*

The articular ends of the bones are covered by hyaline cartilage, which is a nerveless, bloodless, firm and yet pliable tissue. Hyaline cartilage deforms under pressure but recovers its original shape on removal of pressure (11). In growing children, cartilage is the precursor of the bony skeleton and is also the means by which the bones increase in length through the medium of the growth plate. In young people hyaline cartilage is translucent and bluish-white, and in older individuals it is opaque and slightly yellowish (Fig. 4) (12).

This change with age in the appearance of the articular cartilage is also seen in other connective tissues and is probably related to a number of factors: dehydration of the tissues with age, increased numbers of cross linkages in the collagen, and the accumulation of pigment or structural alterations in the collagenous tissues of older individuals.

Articular cartilage is characterized on microscopic examination by its abundant glassy (hyaline) extracellular matrix with isolated, sparse cells located in well-defined spaces (lacunae). It is often described as having four layers or zones: the superficial, intermediate, deep, and calcified layers. In the superficial layers the cells are flat. In the intermediate zone the cells have a tendency to form radial groups which apparently follow the pattern of collagen disposition. And in the calcified zone, i.e., the zone adjacent to the bone, the cells are apparently nonviable and the matrix is heavily calcified (Fig. 5).

Within the calcified bone matrix the cells are connected with one another by means of cytoplasmic processes that run through the osteocytic canaliculi. No such syncytial arrangement is present within the cartilage, and the chondrocytes are dependent on the diffusion of solutes through the extracellular matrix for their metabolism; hence, the cells within the calcified layer of the cartilage appear mostly nonviable. The calcified matrix of this deepest zone of the articular cartilage effectively blocks the passage of solutes from the subchondral bone into the articular cartilage that is, thus, dependent on the diffusion of nutrient and the exchange of metabolites from the synovial fluid through the articular surface (13).

That some very precisely organized fibrous system exists within normal articular cartilage is readily demonstrable by the simple expedient of pricking the articular surface with a pin. A split results, and if the pricking is repeated all over the surface, a pattern of split lines is revealed, which, for each joint, is constant from individual to individual (Fig. 6). If the fissures reflect the internal fiber arrangement of the carti-

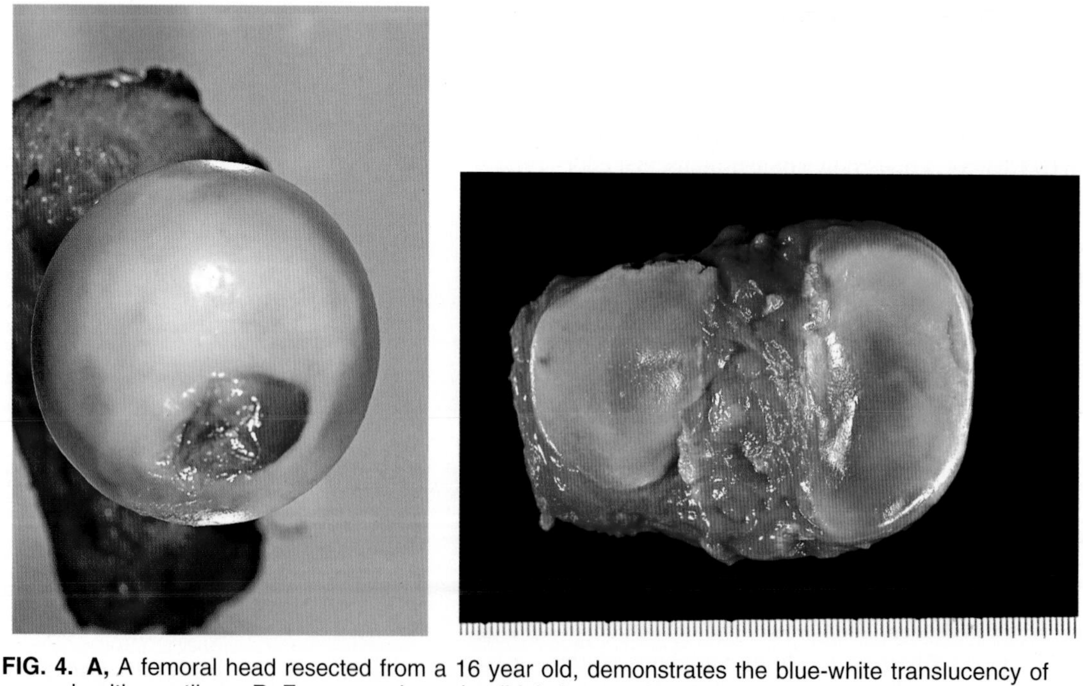

A B

**FIG. 4. A,** A femoral head resected from a 16 year old, demonstrates the blue-white translucency of young healthy cartilage. **B,** For comparison, the tibial plateau of a 50 year old. The cartilage is smooth and healthy in appearance but is more yellowish and opaque in quality than that of the 16 year old.

A 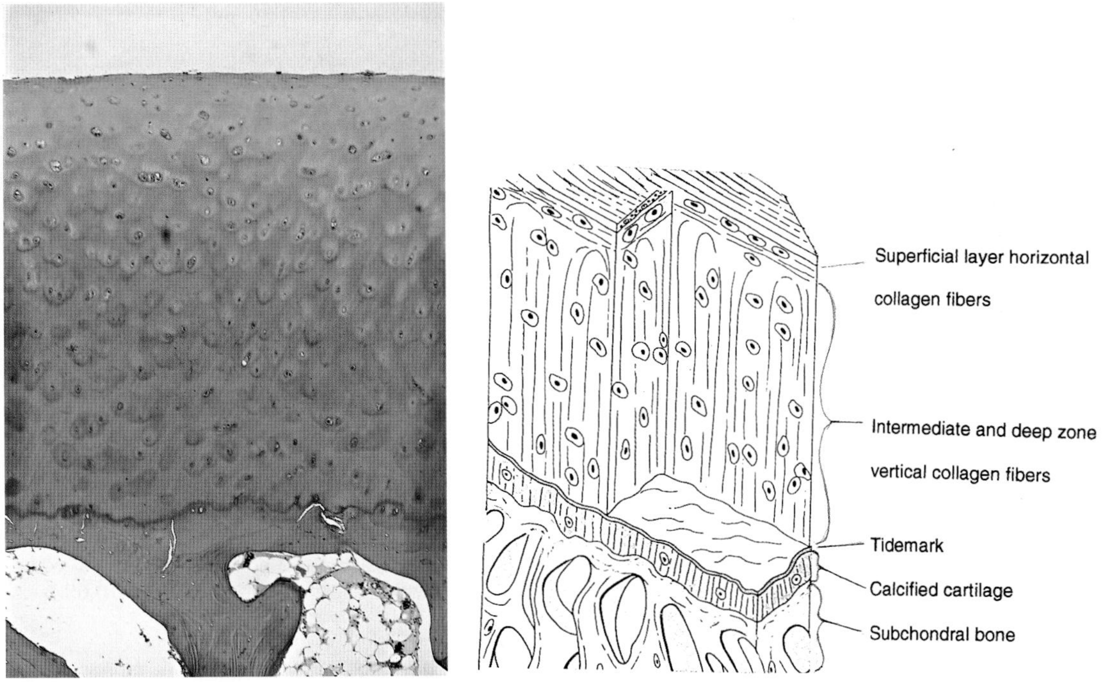 B


**FIG. 5. A,** Photomicrograph of normal articular cartilage obtained from the femoral condyle of a middle-aged individual (**H&E stain, × 4 objective**). **B,** Diagrammatic representation of articular cartilage.

lage, then at the articular surface the fibers run parallel to the surface and in the general direction of the split line.

If the superficial layer of the cartilage is pared away and the exposed surface pricked, instead of fissures appearing only small round holes appear. If the cut edge of the cartilage is pricked, a vertical split line is produced and this occurs in all planes of section (Fig. 7). These experiments indicate that in the deeper layers of the cartilage the fibers are predominantly vertical (14).

A combination of polarizing microscopy, transmission electron microscopy, and scanning electron microscopy confirm Benninghoff's proposal that the principal orientation of collagen fibers in articular cartilage is vertical through most of its thickness and horizontal at the surface (Fig. 8) (15).

Electron microscopic studies show that in the surface layer of normal articular cartilage, the collagen fibers are closely packed, of fine diameter, and mostly oriented parallel to the joint surface (Fig. 9). The collagen content of cartilage progressively diminishes from the superficial to the deep layer. In deep layers, collagen fibers are more widely separated, thicker in diameter, and are vertically aligned in such a fashion as to form a web of arch-shaped structures (Fig. 10) (16). The fibers are continuous with those in the calcified layer of cartilage, but not with underlying subchondral bone. The precise organization of collagen, as has been

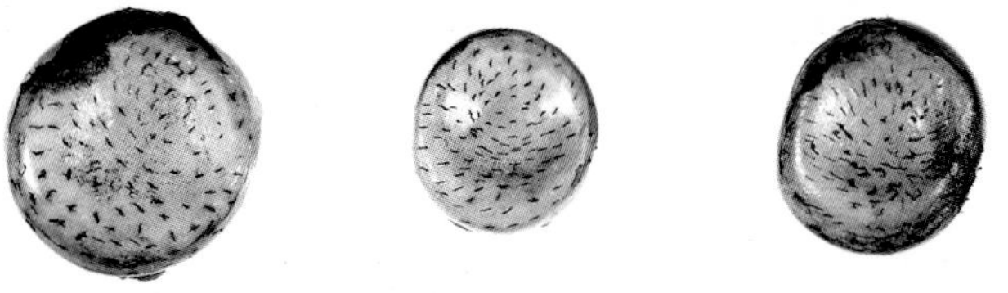

**FIG. 6.** Photograph of the articular surfaces of the radial heads after the surfaces have been pricked with a pin whose tip had been dipped in India ink. Note the resulting pattern of split lines which is unique for each joint in the body. Note that in the same joint it is similar from individual to individual.

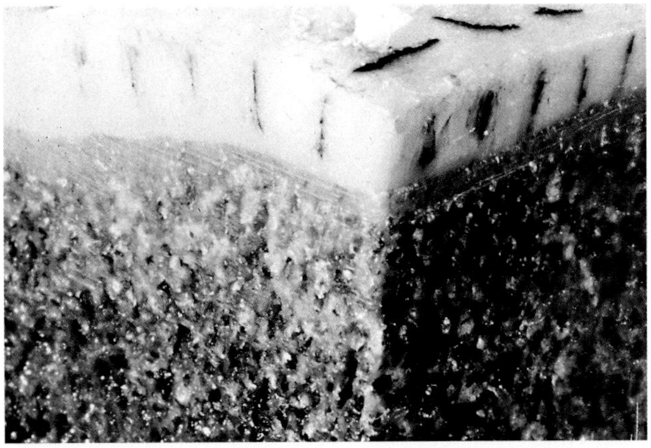

**FIG. 7.** A photograph of a portion of articular cartilage which has been sectioned vertically to show the cut edge and the underlying bone. The direction of pin pricks made on the surface can be seen and additional pin pricks have been made on the cut edge, all of which result in vertical splits.

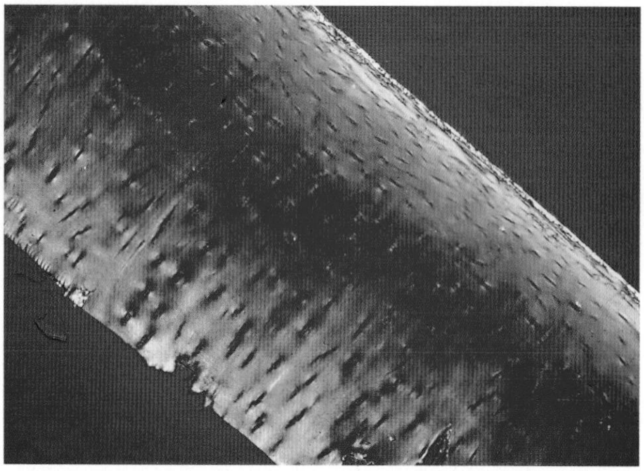

**FIG. 8.** In this polarized photomicrograph, the surface collagen fibers can be visualized as blue, the deeper collagen fibers (which are perpendicular) as yellow. Collagen cannot be seen in the intermediate area because the fibers in this zone are decussating as in the model of Benninghoff's arcade shown in Fig. 5B (**x 4 objective**).

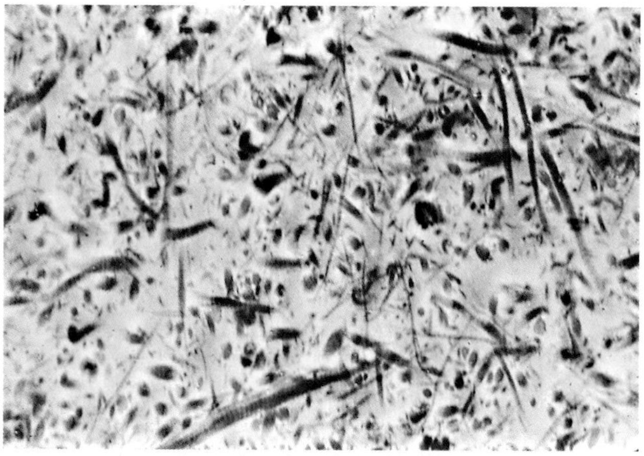

**FIG. 10.** Transmission electron micrograph at approximately the same magnification as Fig. 9 taken from tissue obtained from the midzone of the cartilage and cut randomly, demonstrates variable fiber thickness and more widely separated fibers than are seen at the surface (**x 10,000**).

described here in the cartilage, and in the anulus of the intervertebral disc, is also present in all the connective tissues of the body (for example, Langer's lines in the skin); in all of these locations, it serves a mechanical function.

For example, the menisci of the knee are composed mainly of collagen, although some PG is also present. Microscopic examination of carefully oriented sections has shown that the principal orientation of the collagen fibers in the menisci is circumferential, designed to withstand the circumferential tension within the meniscus during normal loading of the knee joint. The few small radially disposed fibers probably act as ties to resist any longitudinal splitting of the menisci that might result from undue compression (Fig. 11) (17).

The distribution of PGs in the cartilage matrix is also related to the mechanical requirements. It varies markedly from joint to joint, geographically within a single articular cartilage, and also varies according to age. (In general, PG distribution is more evenly diffuse in children than in adults.) The surface layers of the cartilage contain much less PG than the deeper layers. In the deeper layers, there is a higher concentration of staining with safranin O and toluidine blue around the cells (the pericellular matrix) than between the cells (the intercellular matrix) (18).

Besides the PG aggregates, the articular cartilage also contains other extracellular matrix proteins. Chondrocalcin (type X collagen) is a protein probably involved in the calcification process. Anchorin (type IX collagen) is a protein on the surface of chondrocytes involved in binding of these

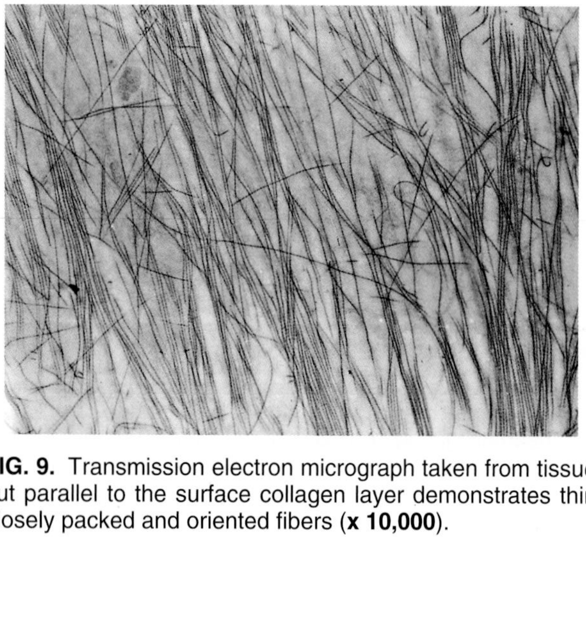

**FIG. 9.** Transmission electron micrograph taken from tissue cut parallel to the surface collagen layer demonstrates thin closely packed and oriented fibers (**x 10,000**).

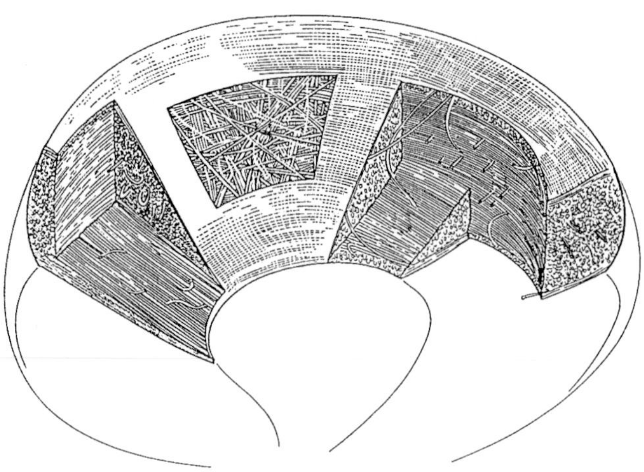

**FIG. 11.** A drawing to illustrate the distribution of collagen fibers in the meniscus. The majority of the fibers are circumferentially distributed to resist the tension generated in the meniscus when the knee is under compressive load. The radially distributed fibers are most obvious on the tibial surface of the meniscus. [Modified from Bullough et al.(17), with permission.]

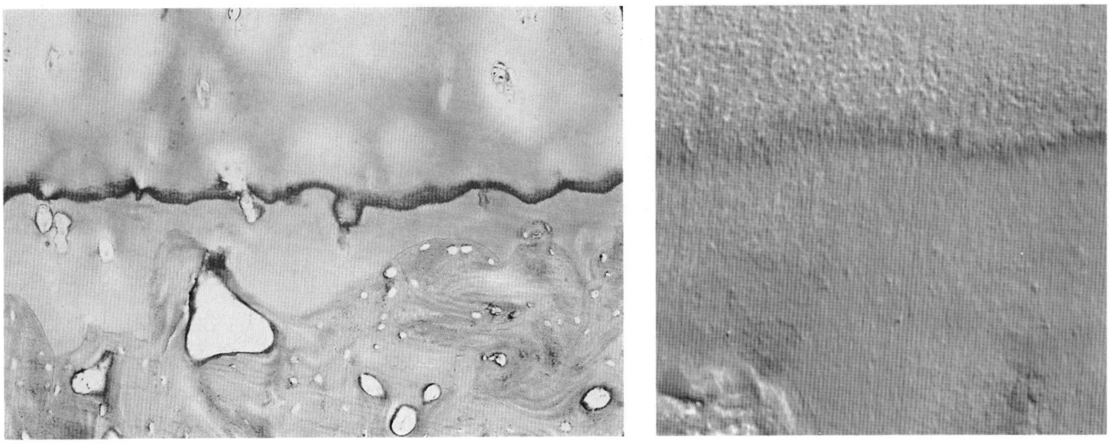

A B

**FIG. 12. A,** Photomicrograph of the deep and calcified layers of the articular cartilage. The deep layer is separated from the calcified layer by a deeply basophilic line referred to as the Tidemark which represents the mineralizing front (**H&E stain, × 4 objective**). **B,** A higher power of the tidemark viewed by Nomarski microscopy. The mineralizing front should probably not be regarded as a static phenomenon but rather as a zone in dynamic equilibrium, with those mediators favoring mineralization being in balance with antagonists of mineralization (**H&E stain, × 25 objective**).

cells to extracellular matrix components, possibly transmitting altered stress on type II fibers to chondrocytes. Fibronectin, thrombomodulin, cartilage oligomeric, and high Mr matrix protein are all found in cartilage, but their precise functions are not yet known.

In histologic sections stained with hematoxylin and eosin (H&E), the junction between the calcified cartilage and the noncalcified cartilage is marked by a basophilic line known as the tidemark (Fig. 12). This basophilic line is not seen in the developing skeleton, but is clearly visible in the adult. In older individuals (over age 60), replication of the tidemark is frequently evident and may be marked in osteoarthritic joints. (Fig. 13). Mechanical failure in the cartilage rarely, if ever, gives rise to the separation of bone and cartilage. However, when such failure occurs, it is seen as a horizontal cleft at the tidemark. Presumably, failure occurs at the tidemark because of the considerable change in the rigidity of the cartilage at this junction.

At its base, adult articular cartilage is bordered by the subchondral bone plate. The cartilage tissue is keyed into the irregular surface of the underlying bone, somewhat like a jigsaw puzzle. Because the cartilage adjacent to the bone is calcified and has a rigidity similar to that of bone, the keying is rigid (Fig. 14). The insertions of ligaments and tendons are also calcified and their insertions into the bone are effected by a similar keying. Because the insertions of ligament and tendons into the bone are generally studied in dry bone specimens the bone markings we see are, in fact, the calcified

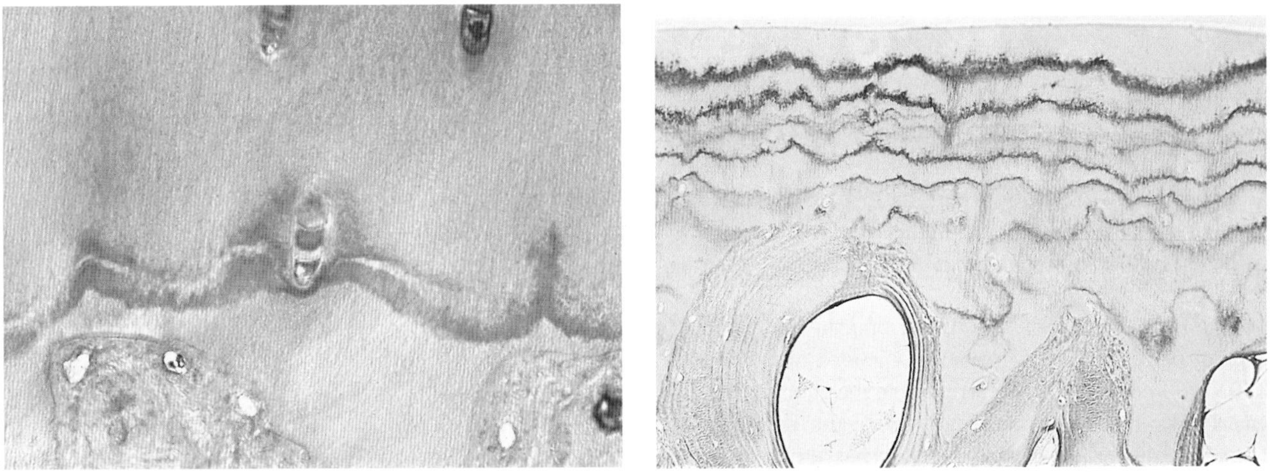

A B

**FIG. 13. A,** The mineralization front is almost certainly under cellular control and in this photomicrograph demonstrating accelerated mineralization with a replicated tidemark, a chondrocyte is seen caught up in the tidemark (**H&E stain, × 25 objective**). **B,** In normal cartilage in most areas only one tidemark is observed; however, in an early stage of osteoarthritis, multiple tidemarks indicating rapid advance of the mineralization front can often be seen (**H&E stain, × 10 objective**).

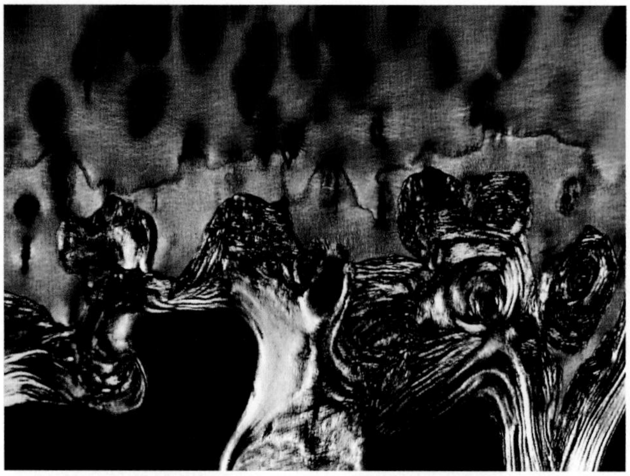

**FIG. 14.** In this photomicrograph taken with polarized light, the irregularity of the interface between the subchondral bone and the overlying calcified cartilage is obvious. The functional keying of the bone and cartilage depends on their having equal rigidity which is the reason for the calcified layer (× **4 objective**).

portion of the ligament or tendon. Because the sites of such insertions are approximately the same from individual to individual, there is a tendency to think of them as static structures. However, in the child, because growth is taking place continuously and in the adult, bone turnover is taking place slowly but continuously, it follows that the insertions of ligaments and tendons must be a dynamic process. Morphology always needs time to be put into the equation.

The chondrocytes embedded in the cartilage matrix are responsible for synthesis and maintenance of the tissue. They vary in size, shape, and number of cells per unit volume of tissue both from the superficial to the deep layers and in different anatomic locations (19). Generally, cells at the cartilage surface are flatter, smaller, and oriented parallel to the cartilage surface. They also have a greater density than the cells deeper in the matrix (20). In the middle zones, chondrocytes are more spherical, and arranged in columns. This vertical arrangement of cells probably reflects some interaction with collagen fibers. The highly organized arrangement of collagen fibers in cartilage suggests the possibility of movement of chondrocytes within the matrix substance as the collagen is being laid down, in the same way the precise organization of a spider web requires the movement of the spider.

Chondrocytes are immediately surrounded by a specialized matrix, distinctly different from the bulk of extracellular matrix. Forming a layer surrounding the chondrocytes is a matrix rich in proteoglycans and some hyaluronic acid, but relatively little collagen. Around this is a basketlike structure composed of cross-linked fibrillar collagen encapsulating the cell or sometimes groups of cells; this provides a protective framework. Collagen type VI is found in this region.

Mitochondria are sparse in chondrocytes, probably relating to their comparatively low rates of oxygen consumption. Cells in the deeper uncalcified zone have the most prominent endoplasmic reticulum and Golgi apparatus indicating active protein synthesis, as well as sulfation of proteoglycan carbohydrate side chains. The cell membrane shows numerous short as well as some longer, branched cytoplasmic processes, but they make no connection with the processes of other chondrocytes. In the extracellular matrix adjacent to the cells of adult articular cartilage, as in the hypertrophic zone of the growth plate, small membrane-bound vesicles are visible. These may play an important role in calcification of cartilage matrix (21).

An interesting ultrastructural feature of chondrocytes is a nonmotile monocilium which may have a mechanotransductory function in regulation of matrix synthesis (22). This monocilium has been more frequently observed in young cartilage and reactive or reparative cartilage (23).

In addition to hyaline cartilage, (of which articular cartilage is composed), two other forms of cartilage can be histologically recognized. Fibrocartilage is a tissue in which the matrix contains a high proportion of type I collagen, the fibers of which are usually visible by transmitted light microscopy, but in addition contains PG aggregates. Fibrocartilage may be found in the menisci of the knee, the anulus fibrosus, at the insertions of ligaments and tendons into the bone, and on the inner side of tendons as they angle around pulleys, e.g., at the malleoli. The second type of nonhyaline cartilage, elastic cartilage, in which the matrix contains a high proportion of elastin, is found in the ligamentum flavum, external ear, and epiglottis (Fig. 15). Elastin, compared to collagen, has much greater elasticity, particularly through the medium of the yellow ligaments making the flexion of the spinal canal possible.

Both the fibrocartilage and elastic cartilage incorporate the term "cartilage" because the cells are rounded and lie in

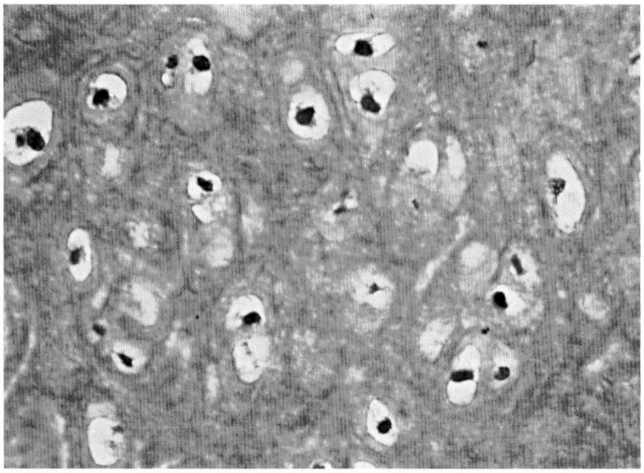

**FIG. 15.** Photomicrograph of ear cartilage. Although the cells resemble those seen in hyaline cartilage, the matrix contains many elastic fibers which appear bright red in this section (**phloxine and tartrazine stain, × 25 objective**).

tissue cells, including fat cells, fibroblast
mast cells (mast cells are omnipresent in
Sections of synovial membrane reveal, alo
the synovial cavity, a single row or someti
of closely packed cells with large elliptica

Electron microscopic studies have reve
types of synovial cells that have been desi
as Types A and B. (Many cells have feat
and have been called intermediate.) The
(Type A) has many of the features of a
there is good evidence that it is structu
phagocytic functions. The more common
richly endowed with rough endoplasmic
Golgi systems, and often show pinocytotic
synovial intima contains 25% Type A and
(Fig. 19) (34).

The synovial membrane has three princ
cretion of synovial fluid hyaluronate (B ce
of waste material derived from the vario
the joint (A cells); and regulation of the
lutes, electrolytes, and proteins from the c
synovial fluid, thus, providing the metabo
the joint chondrocytes and possibly also p
tory mechanism for maintenance of the n
role of various mediators.

In addition to lining the joints, synovia
the subcutaneous and subtendinous sacs
which permit freedom of movement over a
the structures adjacent to the bursae. Sy
also lines the sheaths that form around t
they pass under ligamentous bands or thr
tunnels.

**Ligaments and Tendon**

Ligaments, structures that join toget
bones, are formed mainly of collagen. Th

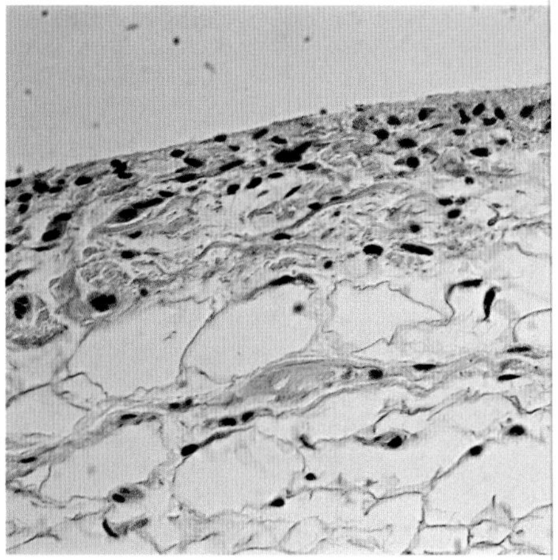

**FIG. 18.** Photomicrograph of normal syno
fat-to-fibrous tissue varies, depending on th
cation within the joint (**H&E, × 10 objectiv**

lacunae, which gives them a superficial resemblance to the cells of hyaline cartilage. However, the mechanical functions of these tissues are very different from those of hyaline cartilage. Hyaline cartilage is mainly subject to and resists compressive forces, whereas both fibrocartilage and elastic cartilage function principally as resisters of tension, with, however, some element of compression as occurs for example at the pulleys and the insertions of tendons.

***Physiology***

Wolff's law states that both bone density and bone architecture correlate with the magnitude and direction of applied load. At the articular end of a bone, this implies that the subchondral bone trabeculae must also undergo a self-regulated modeling which maintains a joint shape capable of optimal load distribution. In other words, the shape of bones, including their articular ends, reflects a dynamic state that incorporates a feedback dependent on mechanical stress. The question then arises: what is the mechanism for articular modeling?

An important process for both growth and bone modeling is endochondral ossification. This is exemplified in the epiphyseal growth plate where calcified cartilage is invaded by blood vessels from the subchondral bone and is then replaced by bone tissue synthesized by osteoblasts lying close to the blood vessels. Studies of adult joints have shown that replacement of the calcified layer of articular cartilage by bone tissue involves a similar process. Blood vessels from the subchondral bone penetrate the calcified cartilage. Alongside the channels created by this process, new bone is laid down, slowly replacing the calicified cartilage with new subchondral bone (Fig. 16).

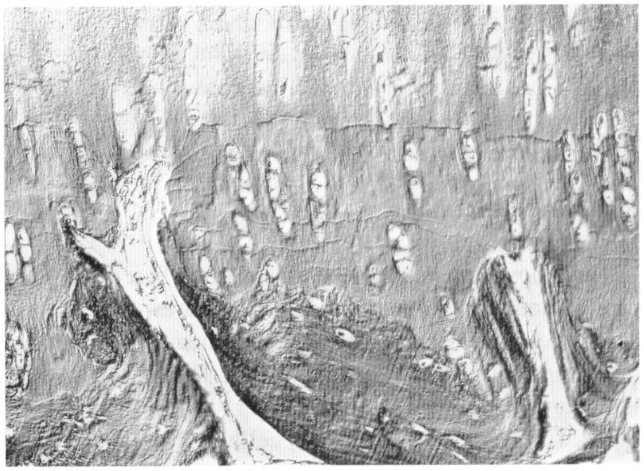

**FIG. 16.** In this photomicrograph two vessels can be seen which have extended into the calcified layer of cartilage. Around the circumference of each of these vessels a thin layer of lamellar bone can be appreciated. By this means (*endochondral ossification*) the articular bone end is continuously modeled (**H&E stain, × 10 objective**).

Replacement of the calcified layer of cartilage by new subchondral bone might be expected to result in thinning and eventual disappearance of the calcified cartilage layer. However, histologic study of articular cartilage from subjects of various ages shows that this does not happen. Calcified cartilage remains at the same thickness throughout life because the calcification front (tidemark) continues to advance into the noncalcified cartilage at a slow rate; this is in equilibrium with the rate of absorption of the calcified cartilage from the subchondral bone (24). Therefore, it can be postulated that articular cartilage is not a static tissue, as it was long believed to be. The extracellular matrix and the chondrocytes are replaced throughout life, and through this mechanism the joint undergoes continuous modeling. It seems likely that programmed cell death (apoptosis) plays an important role in this process in a similar way to that which Mitrovic (25) demonstrated in joint formation during limb development (26).

Heterogeneity of cartilage tissue, including both morphological and biochemical variations, can be observed within different regions of a normal weight-bearing joint. For example, there is a variation in stiffness in different areas of the femoral head which has been related both to PG content and to the amount of water held by the tissue (27).

Another example of normal geographic variation can be observed in the tibial plateau of humans as well as other animals, where there are distinct morphological differences between articular cartilage that is covered, and cartilage that is not covered by the meniscus (28). These differences consist of a rough surface and soft matrix in the uncovered area as compared to the smooth, firm areas covered by the meniscus. In adult human knee joints at autopsy, it has been found that articular cartilage not covered by meniscus always showed matrix softening and superficial fibrillation (29). The morphological and biochemical findings in these two distinct articular areas as studied in the adult dog are summarized in Figure 17.

It has been postulated that these naturally occurring variations in matrix structure and mechanical properties are related to joint loading. In the normally functioning knee, load is transmitted through the meniscus and onto the tibial cartilage underlying the meniscus, whereas the exposed cartilage, that which is not covered by the meniscus, remains relatively unloaded. Similar areas of possible disuse atrophy, have been described around the rim of the radial head, in the roof of the acetabulum, and on the perifoveal and inferomedial aspects of the femoral head (30).

The extracellular matrix of the cartilage and of the other connective tissues is synthesized by their intrinsic cells under the control of both local and systemic factors. Both in vivo and in vitro studies have demonstrated that changes in the immediate environment of the joint lead to alterations of the cartilage matrix. Thus, immobilization or unloading of a joint results in decreased synthesis of glycosaminoglycans (31). Conversely, exercise appears to increase synthesis (32). These experimentally induced variations are in agreement

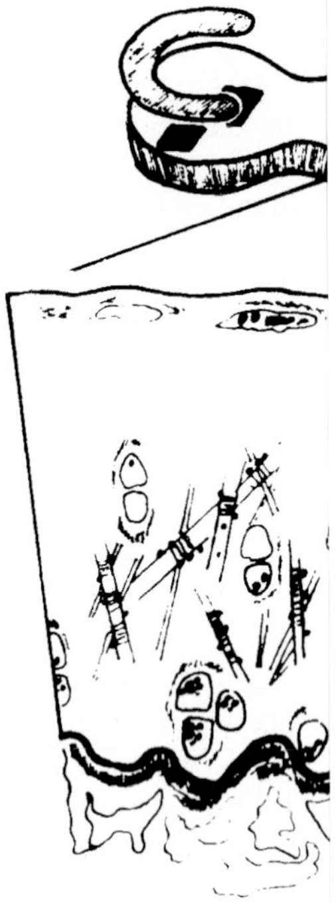

**FIG. 17.** A diagram to i
cartilage under the men
**Left:** In the covered a
dense layer; the chondr
cumulation in all three l
there are increased nur
sections collagen appe
binding of proteoglycan
The tidemark is irregula
**Right:** In the uncover
the chondrocytes are ro
pears in wavy aggregat
glycan to the collagen fi
matrix. The tidemark is
In both the covered a
same amount of DNA p
mission.]

with naturally observed topograp
which have been ascribed to norma
loading that affect the joints. In ge
levels of mechanical stress (i.e.,
range) are associated with enhan
whereas stress within the physiolo
with increased anabolic activity. Un
physiologic stress, the chondrocyte
other words, there is a window of ph
below which, the chondrocytes cann
functional matrix.

Although a number of substances
the transduction of mechanical stim
the exact mechanism still remains u



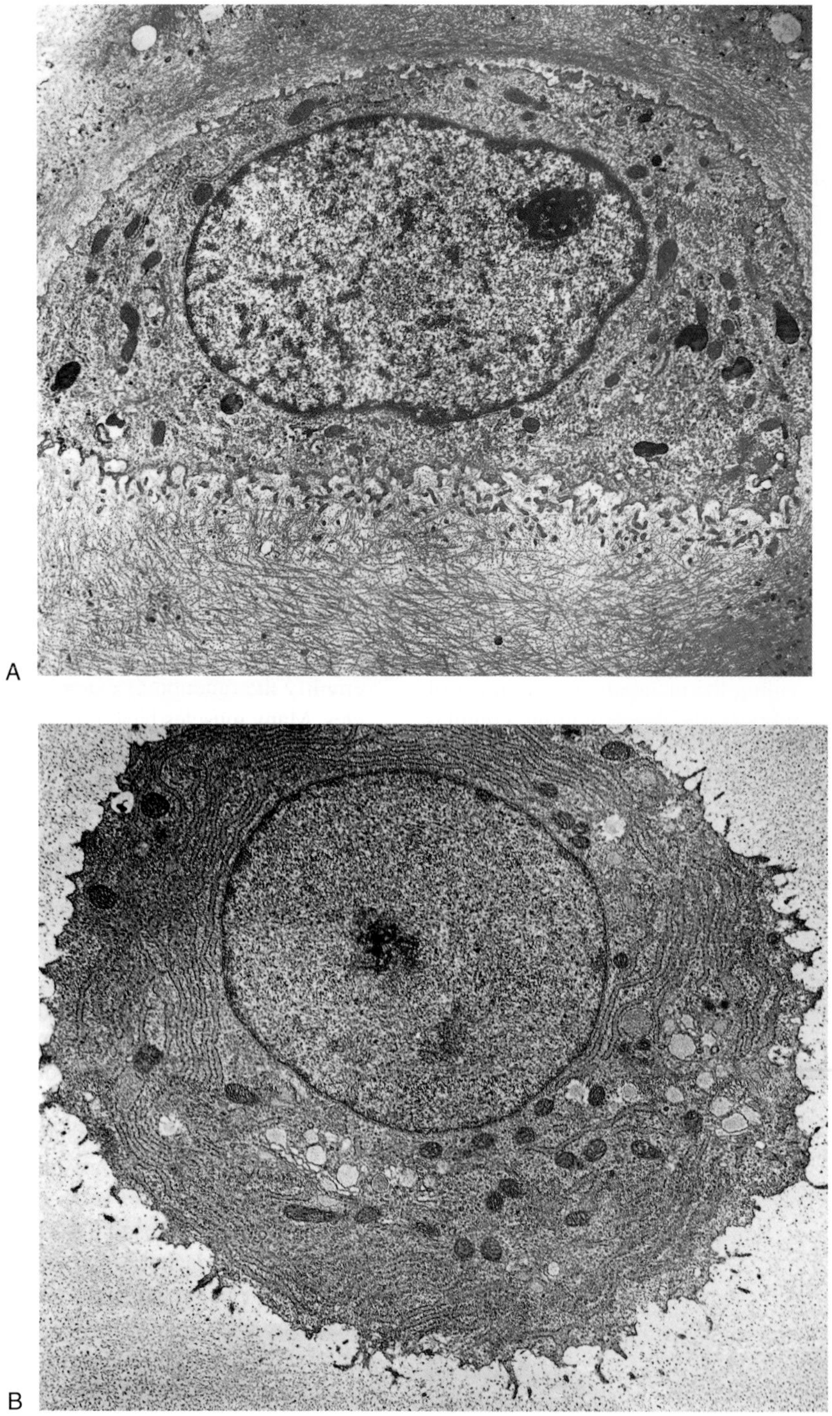


**FIG. 19.** Electron photomicrographs to illustrate the typical appearance of chondrocytes at the surface, midzone, and deep zone of the articular cartilage **(A)**. At the surface, the cell typically shows more cell processes on the inferior surface. The Golgi and endoplasmic reticulum are less well developed than in the midzone **(B)**. In the deep zone **(C)** the cells are degenerate with disaggregated chromatin in the nucleus and vacuolization and fragmentation of the cytoplasm (**(A)**, **(B)**, and **(C) approximately** × **10,000**).

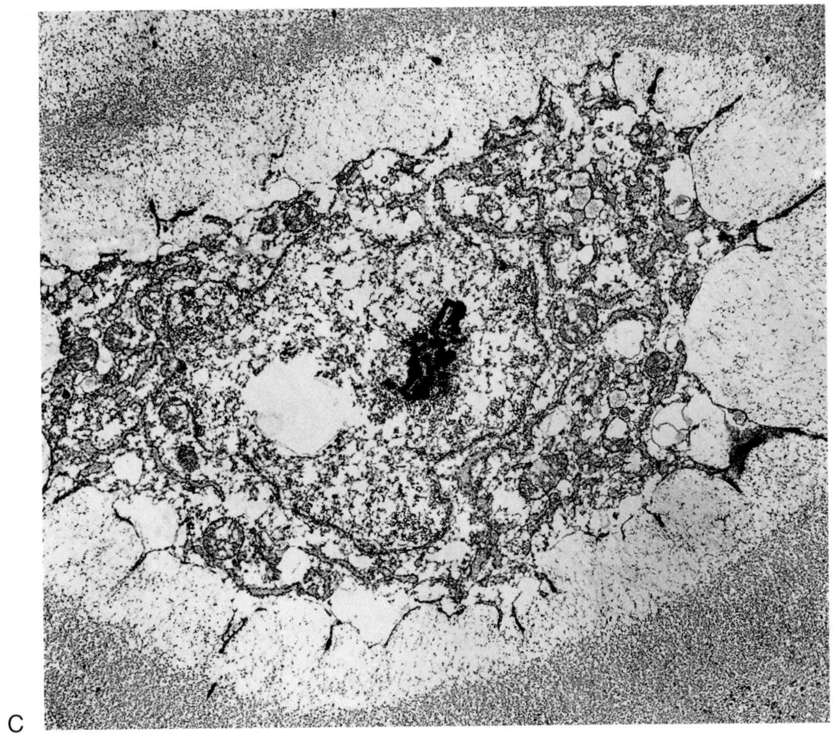

FIG. 19. *Continued.*

## THE ARTHRITIC JOINT

Clinical arthritis is the consequence of a breakdown in the joint's normal function; that is, a loss of capacity for the articulating surfaces to move over one another easily, loss of joint stability, and, almost always, pain. The loss of freedom of motion may be associated with a change in joint shape (resulting in severe incongruities), or a change in the tissue matrices themselves which, in turn, affects their mechanical properties. Instability may result from alterations in ligamentous support and neuromuscular control. Pain may have a variety of sources. It may originate in the bone, as a result

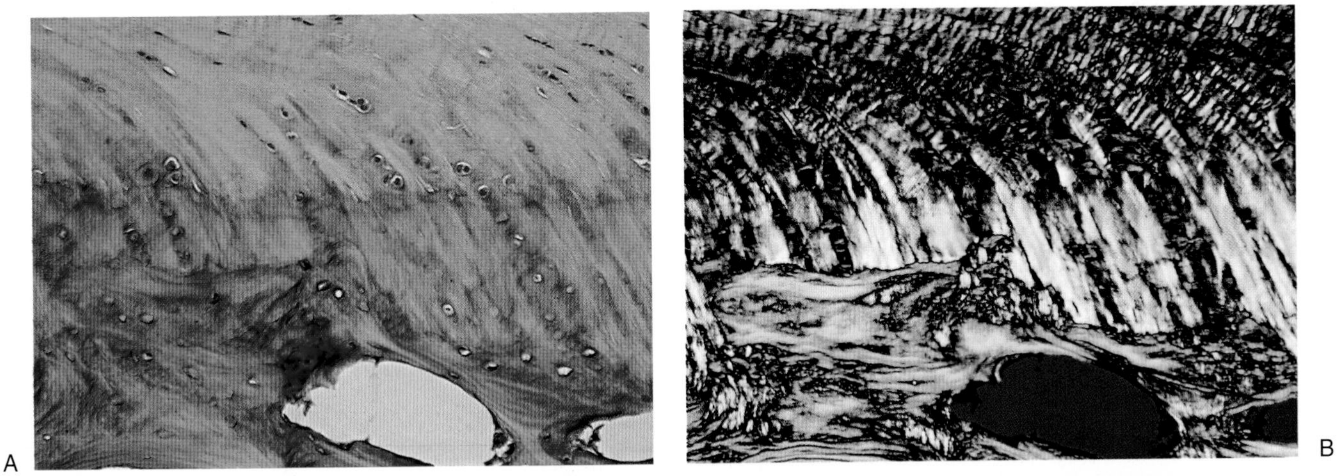

**FIG. 20. A,** Photomicrograph of a ligamentous insertion (**H&E stain, × 10 objective, transmitted white light**). **B,** Polarized light. The portion of the ligament that interfaces with the bone is calcified and the edge of the calcified portion of the ligament is marked by a basophilic line (*Tidemark*) which represents the mineralization front. Note the similarity with the bone cartilage interface illustrated in Fig. 14. **C,** A higher-powered view to demonstrate the rounded cells lying in lacunae, which are seen at the insertion site of both ligaments and tendons (fibrocartilaginous metaplasia) (**H&E stain, × 25 objective**). (*continued*)

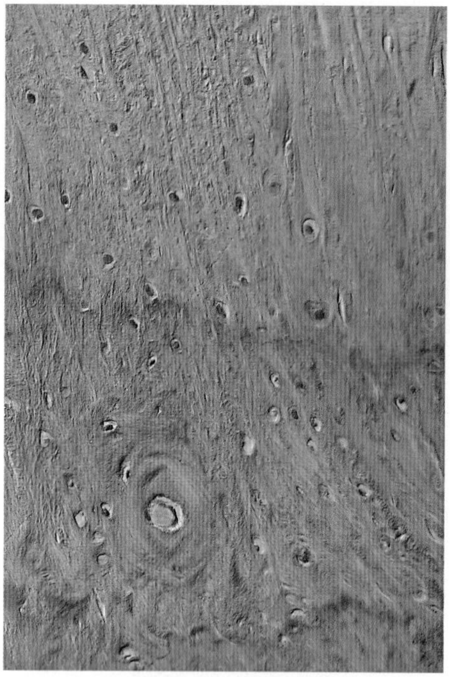

C

FIG. 20. *(continued)*

of maldistribution of load, in the synovium, as a result of reactive synovitis, or in the muscle as a consequence of reflex spasm.

Malfunction of a joint can be caused by acute or chronic injuries that produce either:

- Anatomic alterations in the shape of the articulating surfaces, e.g., a fracture, Paget's disease or acromegaly (37).
- Loss of integrity of the cartilage matrix or support structures around the joint, e.g., by enzymatic destruction in inflammatory arthritis.
- Alterations in the mechanical properties of the tissue matrices making up the joint, e.g., ochronosis.

During the past century, on the basis of their characteristic individual clinical presentations and their morbid anatomy, several types of arthritis have been well delineated. These include: (a) the infectious arthritides, both granulomatous and pyogenic; (b) metabolic arthritis (e.g., gout and ochronosis); and (c) the arthritis that complicates many cases of aseptic subchondral bone necrosis (38). The various "rheumatic syndromes" have been classified according to their clinical and immunologic characteristics; histologically, these inflammatory arthritides show a destructive pattern but are difficult to differentiate from each other solely by microscopic examination.

Even when these various etiologies have been considered, there remains an enormous number of cases of arthritis affecting especially certain small joints of the hands and feet and some larger joints, of which the hip and knee are particularly commonly involved. These cases, which run a chronic course, are essentially noninflammatory and usually occur in older individuals. The clinical presentation and morbid anatomy in these cases are similar enough for all of them to be classified under the general appellation of "osteoarthritis." In the majority of cases the etiology is, at best, unclear.

### Alteration in Shape

A change in joint shape, resulting from cartilage and bone loss, is characteristic of most forms of arthritis. In the inflammatory arthritides it is tissue loss from destruction. In osteoarthritis, however, although bone and cartilage loss play an important part in the process, it is the addition of new bone and cartilage in the form of osteophytes, particularly at the joint periphery and sometimes beneath the articular surface, that forms one of the characteristic features of the disease.

Conversely, a change in joint shape, either sudden, as with a fracture, or gradual, as in acromegaly or other metabolic disturbances such as Paget's disease, may play an important role in the etiology of arthritis. In other words, a change in the

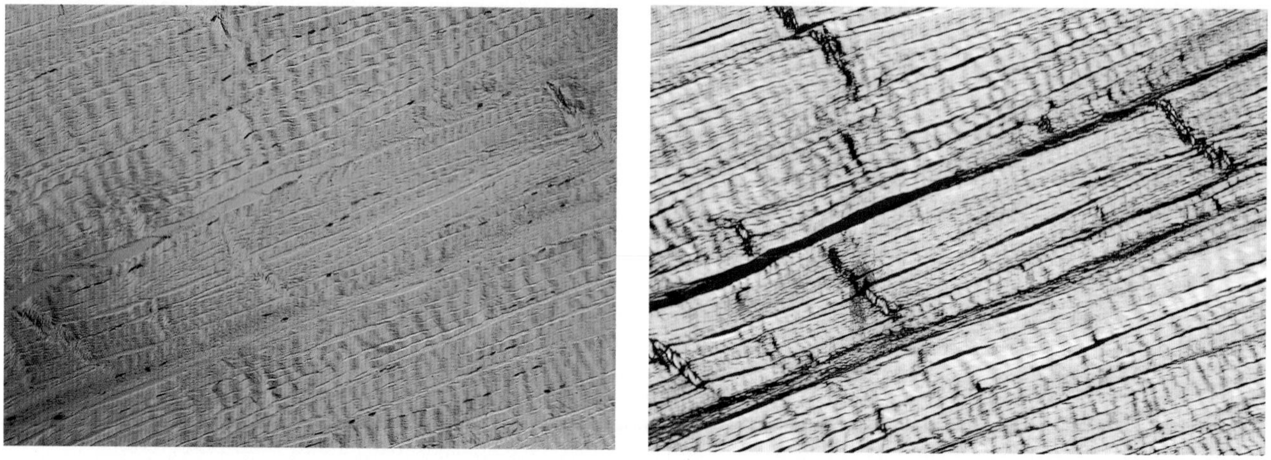

A B

**FIG. 21. (A and B),** Photomicrograph of a tendon in both transmitted white light and polarized light demonstrates the scant and elongated fibroblasts lying between the dense parallel collagen bundles characteristic of tendon (**H&E stain, × 4 objective**).

shape of the joint is an expected result of arthritis but, importantly, a change in shape may also be the cause of arthritis.

### Alteration in Tissues

Regardless of the cause, joint injury is characterized by certain basic cellular and tissue responses. There is usually macroscopic and microscopic evidence of both degeneration and of repair and there are alterations both in the cells and in the extracellular matrix. (In the extracellular matrix the changes may result from direct physical injury, from alteration in the cellular synthesis of the matrix, or from enzymatic breakdown.)

In vascularized tissues, injury is followed by an acute and then by a chronic inflammatory response. As a result, the necrotic injured tissue is removed and replaced by proliferative vascular tissue (granulation tissue). The inflammatory response results in "repair" of injured tissue by fibrous scar. Independently of scarring, a second mode of repair involves regeneration of tissue similar to that which was injured originally. In nonvascularized tissue, such as cartilage, an inflammatory response and subsequent scarring cannot occur, but this does not preclude tissue regeneration. (Note that cartilage injury always eventually invokes an inflammatory response, since some vascularized tissues, i.e., bone and/or synovium, are inevitably involved.)

#### *Cartilage*

Macroscopic evidence of injury to cartilage is evident only in the extracellular matrix, mainly the collagenous component. One of the earliest findings is a disruption of the collagen fibers at the surface which, instead of being smooth, becomes rough and/or eroded: a condition generally referred to as fibrillation (39). The incidence and severity of fibrillation is generally age-related and presents, in particular, joints in specific areas (40).

Three patterns of macroscopic alteration involving the cartilage surface and, to a variable degree, the underlying cartilage tissue, can be identified: fibrillation, (generally age related); erosion (ulceration); and cracking (probably trauma related).

The term "fibrillation" is used to describe replacement of the normally smooth, shiny surface by a surface similar to cut velvet. This type of transformation can be observed both on very thick cartilage, such as the patella, and on very thin cartilage, such as that found in the interphalangeal joints. The "pile" of the fibrillated area may be short or shaggy. The junction between the fibrillated area and the adjacent normal-appearing cartilage is usually well defined and generally distinct (Fig. 22).

There appear to be two patterns of fibrillation. Well-defined areas of fibrillation affect particular locations in certain joints and are present in everyone from an early age (41). It is suggested that these areas may be related to underloading of the cartilage. In osteoarthritic joints, there are areas of fibrillation which appear in different areas of the joint than those previously alluded to, and which appear to be secondary to mechanical erosion of the cartilage surface. The microscopic characterization of these two distinct types of fibrillation is incomplete, but perhaps the latter is distinguished by deeper clefts and a greater tendency to form cartilage clones (see following).

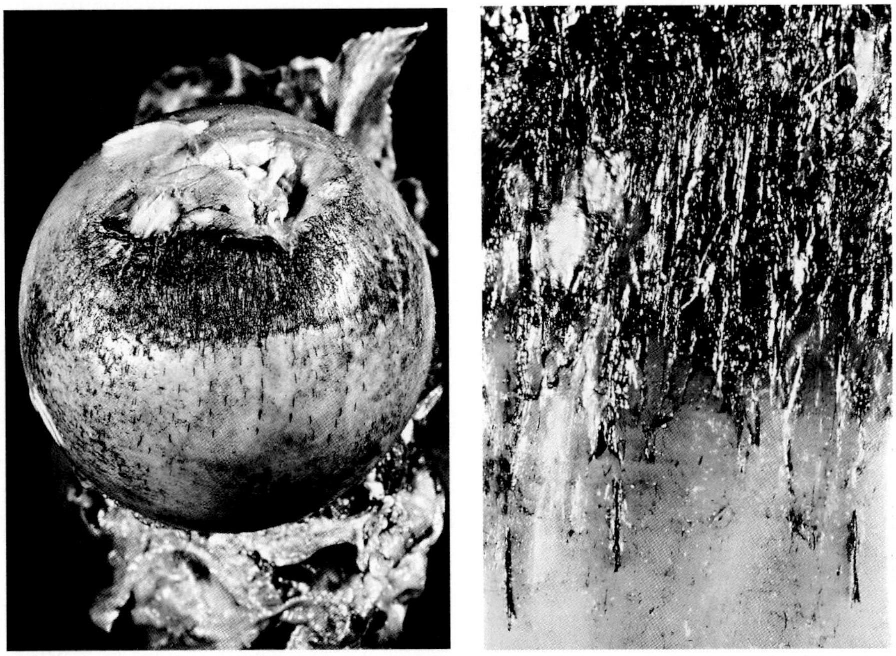

A B

**FIG. 22. A,** Photograph to demonstrate superficial fibrillation of the cartilage on the femoral head in the perifoveal region. The fibrillated cartilage has been highlighted by India ink. **B,** In a close-up photograph the pin splits in the cartilage seem to follow the orientation of the collagen fibers in the fibrillated area.

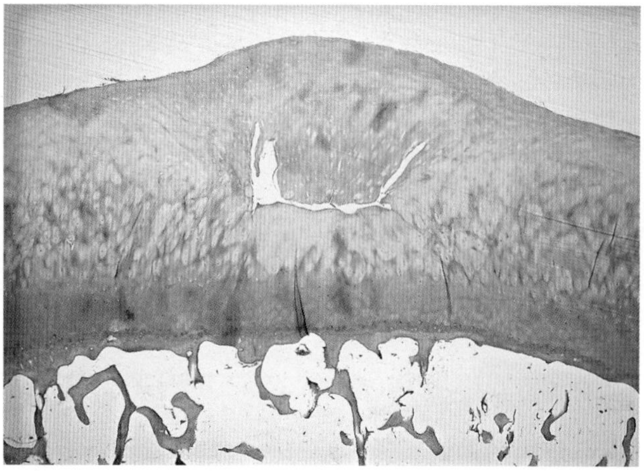

**FIG. 23.** Photomicrograph to demonstrate deep cracking of the cartilage matrix. The lesion shown is characteristic of a blisterlike lesion which is seen in many cases of chondromalacia patellae (**H&E stain, × 4 objective**).

Cartilage erosion, or solution of the surface, is characteristic of progressive degenerative changes in the joint. The base of the erosion appears initially to be either contoured or smooth. Tissue damage may eventually be so extensive as to completely denude the bone surface of its covering cartilage layer (eburnation).

The last form of structural lesion in this group, which is distinctly less common than either fibrillation or ulceration, is cracking of the cartilage. These cracks extend deep into the cartilage vertically, and, microscopically, often have a deep horizontal component. Perhaps these result from severe impact loading (Fig. 23).

In considering the pathogenesis of these three histologic types of cartilage matrix damage, it is important to recognize that in the early stages of osteoarthritis, they may affect the opposed articular surfaces in different areas and to different degrees. This is in marked contrast to eburnation, in which both of the opposed surfaces are affected. It, therefore, appears that in many cases fibrillation and other cartilage alteration cannot be ascribed simply to abrasion.

An increase in the ratio of water to PG in the cartilage matrix leads to softening of the cartilage (chondromalacia). Chondromalacia and fibrillation usually occur together, but chondromalacia may be present before there is any obvious gross evidence of fibrillation.

Injury at a cellular level may be recognizable only under a microscope. Necrosis can be identified when only the ghost outlines of the chondrocytes remain. This ghosting, usually scattered but focal in distribution, is a common finding in arthritis. Less often, all of the chondrocytes are seen to be necrotic (Fig. 24).

Just as the effect of injury to the articular cartilage is reflected by the histologic response of both matrix and cells, so too is the effect of subsequent cartilage regeneration. Within the preexisting cartilage matrix there is focal cell proliferation with clumps, or clones, of chondrocytes and, when the tissue is stained with toluidine blue, there is often intense metachromasia of the matrix around these clumps of proliferating chondrocytes—evidence of increased PG synthesis. This process can be thought of as "intrinsic" repair (Fig. 25) (42).

In a damaged joint, repair by new cartilage (extrinsic cartilage repair) may be initiated from either or both of two possible sites: either in the joint margin or in the subchondral bone. Extrinsic repair of cartilage, which develops from the joint margin, can be seen as a cellular layer of cartilage extending over, and sometimes dissecting into, the existing cartilage. This extrinsically repaired cartilage is usually much

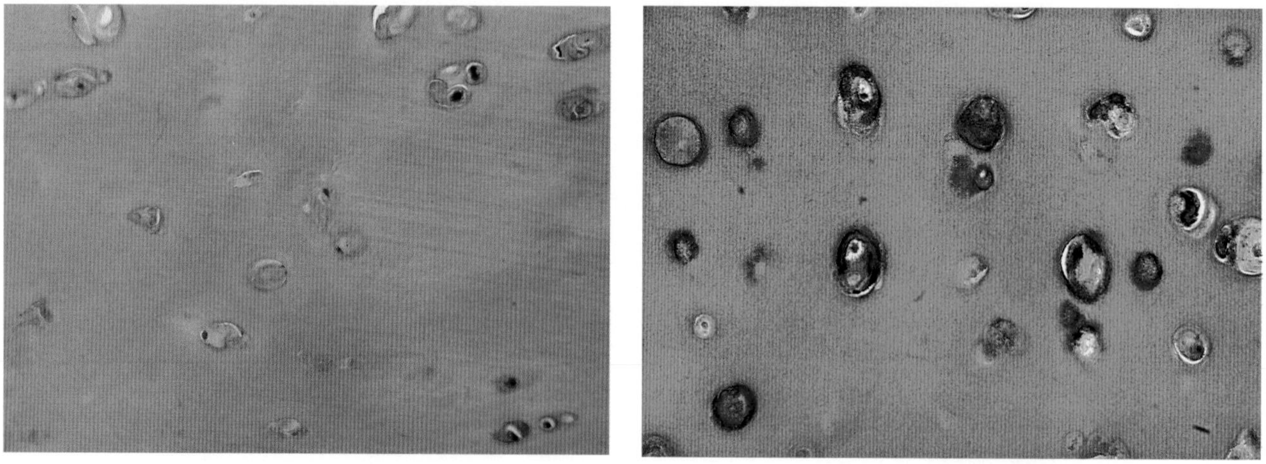

A B

**FIG. 24. A,** A photomicrograph to demonstrate focal chondrocyte necrosis. In cases of degenerative arthritis focal areas of necrosis, such as those seen here, are common. Rarely, the necrosis is extensive. In inflammatory arthritis chondrocyte necrosis is also common and often associated with an irregular lysis of the matrix around the necrotic cells so-called Weichselbaum's lacunae (**H&E stain, × 10 objective**). **B,** Photomicrograph to demonstrate necrotic focal calcification around chondrocytes in the deep zone of the cartilage (**H&E stain, × 25 objective**).

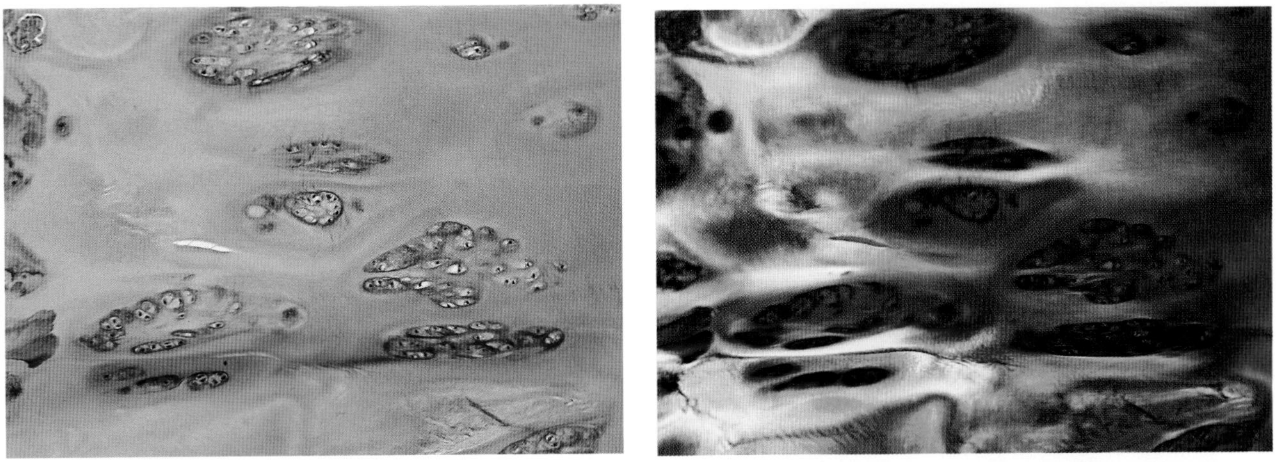

A B

**FIG. 25. A,** Photomicrograph to demonstrate clones of regenerating chondrocytes. Note the basophilia around the clones which corresponds to increased proteoglycan synthesis by the cells (**H&E stain, × 10 objective**). **B,** When examined by polarized light, it can be seen that the proliferating clones are displacing the existing collagen matrix.

more cellular than the preexisting articular cartilage, and the chondrocytes are evenly distributed throughout the matrix (Fig. 26).

On microscopic examination, this type of repair cartilage can easily be overlooked. However, examination under polarized light will clearly demonstrate the discontinuity between the collagen network of the repair cartilage and that of the preexisting cartilage (Fig. 27).

In arthritic joints in which loss of the articular cartilage has denuded the underlying bone, and especially in cases of osteoarthritis, there are frequently small pits in the bone surface, from which small nodules of firm white tissue protrude. On microscopic examination these nodules have the appearance of fibrocartilage and arise in the marrow spaces of the subchondral bone. They may extend over the previously denuded surface to form a more or less continuous layer of repair tissue. Most cases of osteoarthritis reveal both intrinsic and extrinsic repair of cartilage.

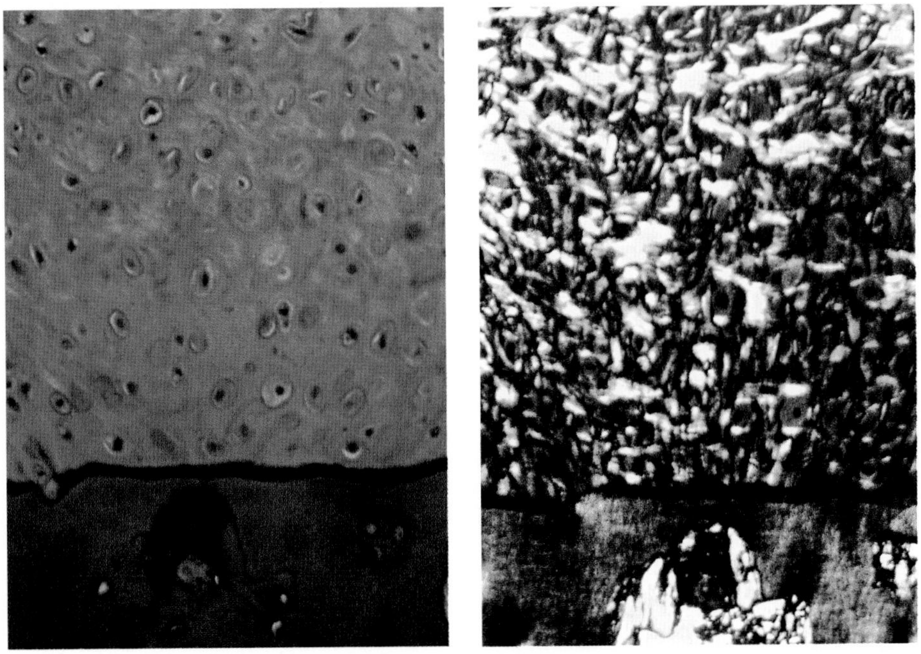

A B

**FIG. 26. A,** A section through the articular surface of an arthritic joint demonstrates extrinsic reparative fibrocartilage, which extends to the tidemark of the original articular hyaline cartilage (**H&E stain, × 10 objective**). **B,** The same field photographed with polarized light shows the discontinuity of the collagen between the calcified zone and the reparative cartilage previously.

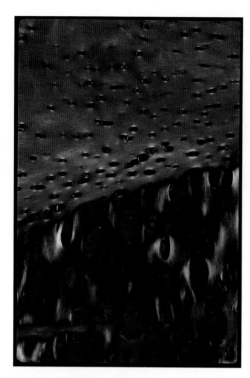

FIG. 27. In this photomicrograph taken with polarized light, a well-demarcated layer of cellular cartilage can be seen extending over the surface of previously eroded articular cartilage (× **10 objective**).

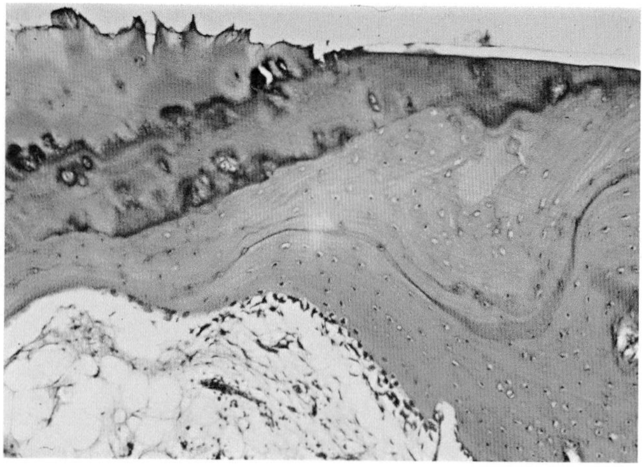

FIG. 28. Photomicrograph of the edge of an eburnated area of bone in a case of osteoarthritis. There is a very prominent layer of osteoblasts covering the sclerotic bone which underlies the area denuded of cartilage (**H&E stain,** × **4 objective**).

### *Bone*

Arthritis is a disease that affects not only the articular cartilage but also the underlying bone and the structures around the joint.

As the articular cartilage is eroded from the articular surface, the underlying bone is subjected to increasingly localized overloading. In subarticular bone that has been, thus, denuded, there is proliferation of osteoblasts and formation of new bone, which occurs both on the surfaces of existing intact trabeculae and around microfractures (Fig. 28) (43). In radiographs of arthritic joints, this new bone appears as increased density or sclerosis.

A further result of increased local stress is that the surface bone is likely to undergo focal pressure necrosis. (This superficial necrosis is different both in its etiology and pathogenesis from that associated with "primary" subchondral avascular necrosis, which itself leads to secondary osteoarthritis. However, in clinical practice differentiation between the two may be difficult, especially in the late stages of primary subchondral avascular necrosis) (44).

Subarticular cysts are usually seen only where the overlying cartilage is absent. Such cysts are common in cases of osteoarthritis, and are believed to result from transmission of interarticular pressure through defects in the articulating bony surface into the marrow spaces of the subchondral bone (45). The cysts increase in size until the pressure within them is equal to the intra-articular pressure. Cysts may also occur because of focal tissue necrosis (46). (In cases of arthritis due to rheumatoid disease or gout, periarticular radiologic "cysts" may be associated with erosion of the marginal subchondral bone by the diseased synovium.)

Separated fragments of bone and cartilage from a damaged joint surface may become incorporated into the synovial membrane and digested, or may remain free as loose bodies in the joint cavity. Under certain circumstances, proliferation of cartilage cells occurs on the surface of these loose bodies and, consequently, they grow larger. As they grow, their centers become necrotic and calcified. In histologic sections it is possible to visualize periodic extension of this central calcification in the form of concentric rings which increase in number as the loose body grows larger. Sometimes the bodies reattach to the synovial membrane, in which case they are invaded by blood vessels. Endochondral ossification then occurs and the loose bodies again develop a viable bony core.

There is some degree of loose body formation in many cases of arthritis. Occasionally, in cases of osteoarthritis, the loose bodies are so numerous that they must be distinguished from those that occur in primary synovial chondromatosis (47).

### *Ligaments*

Microscopic evidence both of lacerations and of repair by scar tissue is common in the ligamentous and capsular tissue around an arthritic joint. These changes are readily recognized by the use of polarized microscopy where the alterations in the organization of the collagen is made very clear (Fig. 29). Whether these preceded the arthritic process or whether they are a consequence of it cannot usually be determined by microscopic examination.

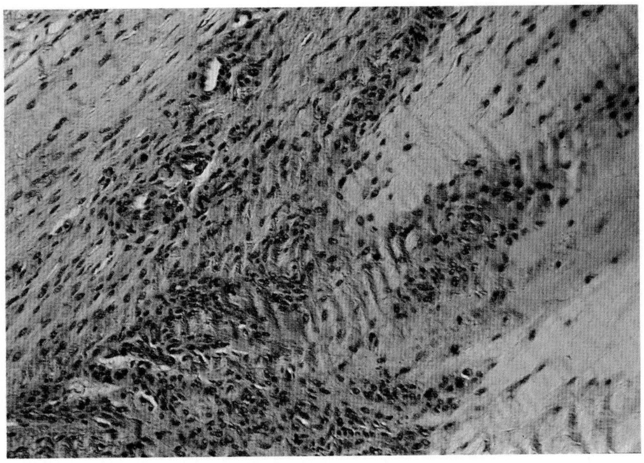

**FIG. 29.** Photomicrograph to demonstrate an area in a ligament where a laceration has occurred. The well-oriented collagen of the lacerated ligament is clearly demarcated from the resultant defect which can be seen to have been filled with a vascularized cellular fibrous scar tissue (**H&E stain, × 10 objective**).

### *Synovial Membrane*

Even when cases of arthritis that have a primary synovial etiology have been excluded, microscopic examination of the synovium still demonstrates some degree of synovitis.

Injury and breakdown of cartilage and bone result in increased amounts of breakdown product and particulate debris within the joint cavity. This is removed from the synovial fluid by phagocytic cells (the "A" cells) of the synovial membrane. In consequence, the membrane becomes both hypertrophic and hyperplastic. In addition, the breakdown products of cartilage and bone matrix evoke an inflammatory response (Fig. 30).

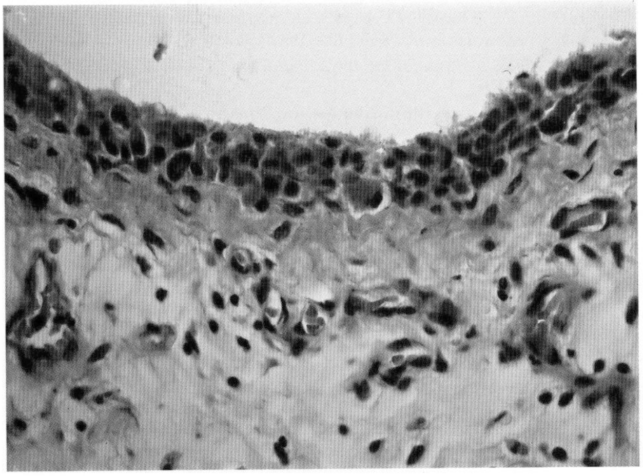

**FIG. 30.** Photomicrograph of the synovium removed from the joint of a patient with a moderate degree of osteoarthritis reveals not only a hypertrophy of the synovial lining cells, but also hyperplasia that has resulted in a piling-up of the synoviocytes. In the subsynovial tissue there is increased vascularity and a mild chronic inflammatory infiltrate (**H&E stain, × 25 objective**).

For this reason some degree of chronic inflammation can be expected in the synovial membrane of arthritic joints, even when the injury has been purely a mechanical one. Inflammation is especially prominent where there has been rapid breakdown of the articular components as evidenced by the presence in the synovium of bone and cartilage detritus. Histologic studies have shown that there may be a similarity between the degree of inflammatory response as seen in some cases of severe osteoarthritis and that of rheumatoid arthritis (48). However, in osteoarthritis the synovial inflammation is likely to be the result of cartilage breakdown, whereas in rheumatoid arthritis the synovial inflammation is the cause of the cartilage breakdown.

Extension of the hyperplastic synovium onto the articular surface of the joint (i.e., a pannus) is a common finding even in osteoarthritis, particularly in the hip (Fig. 31). However, the extent and the aggressiveness of this pannus with respect to the underlying cartilage destruction is much less marked in osteoarthritis than in rheumatoid arthritis.

Under normal conditions, the synovial membrane is responsible for the nutrition of articular cartilage. In this regard, it might be expected that the chronically inflamed and scarred synovial membrane of an arthritic joint would function less effectively than that of a normal joint. Disturbance in synovial nutrient function, as well as increased enzymatic activity, may very well contribute to the chronicity of the arthritic process. The hypertrophied and hyperplastic synovium is also likely to be traumatized as it extends into the joint cavity. Evidence of bleeding into the joint, with subsequent hemosiderin staining of the synovial membrane, is a common histologic finding, and may occasionally be marked. When this is the case, and despite their similar color, the orange-brown staining of the fine villous synovium seen at operation should not be confused with the swollen papillary synovium of pigmented villonodular synovitis.

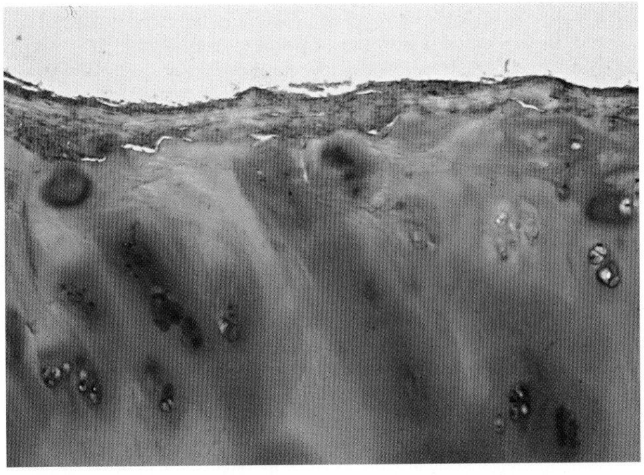

**FIG. 31.** Photomicrograph of a portion of the articular surface of a femoral head in a case of osteoarthritis, demonstrating a fibrous pannus extending over the articular surface ( **H&E stain, × 10 objective**).

### Synovial Fluid

Normal synovial fluid, a dialysate of plasma to which hyaluronic acid produced by the "B" cells of the synovial lining is added, is viscous, pale yellow, and clear. Even in large joints the volume is small.

Examination of synovial fluid is extremely helpful in the diagnosis of arthritis for determining both the cause and the stage of the disease. Whatever the cause of arthritis, the synovial fluid is altered.

In cases of inflammatory arthritis there is an increased volume of synovial fluid whereas the amount of hyaluronic acid is markedly diminished. This leads to a typical decrease in viscosity. However, in degenerate forms of arthritis the amount of hyaluronic acid is increased, resulting in an extremely viscous fluid. Often, there is also an increase in volume, although not to the same degree as that which is seen in the inflammatory arthritides.

## REFERENCES


1. Hammond BT, Charnley J. The sphericity of the femoral head. *J Med Biol Eng* 1967;5:445.
2. Bullough PG, Goodfellow J, O Connor JJ. The relationship between degenerative changes and local bearing in the human hip. *J Bone Joint Surg Br* 1973;55:746.
3. Bullough PG, Walker PS. The distribution of load through the knee joint and its possible significance to the observed patterns of articular cartilage breakdown. *Bull Hosp Jt Dis* 1977;37:110.
4. Hunter W: Of the structure and diseases of articulating cartilages. *Phil Trans*:1743, 267.
5. Van Der Rest M, Garrone R. Collagen family of proteins. *FASEB J*1991:2814.
6. Mayne R, Irwin MH. Collagen types in cartilage. In Kuettner KE, Schleyerbach R, Hascall VC (eds): *Articular cartilage biochemistry.* New York; Raven Press, 1986;23.
7. Eyre DR, Wu JJ, Woods P. Cartilage-specific collagens-structural studies. In Kuettner K, Schleyerbach R, Peyron JG, et al. (eds): *Articular cartilage and osteoarthritis.* New York; Raven Press, 1992.
8. Rosenberg LC, Buckwalter JA. Cartilage proteoglycans. In Kuettner KE, Schleyerbach R, Hascall VC (eds): *Articular cartilage biochemistry.* New York; Raven Press, 1986;39.
9. Bianco P, Fisher LW, Young MF. Expression and localization of two small proteoglycans biglycan and decorin in developing skeletal and non-skeletal tissue. *J Histochem Cytochem* 1990;38:1549.
10. Moskowitz RW. Experimental models of osteoarthritis. In: Moskowitz P, Howell H, Goldberg C, Mankin H (eds): *Osteoarthritis, Diagnosis and Medical/Surgical Management. Vol. 6.* Philadelphia; WB Saunders, 1992;109.
11. Kempson GE. Mechanical properties of articular cartilage. In: Freeman MAR, ed. *Adult articular cartilage.* London: Pitman Medical, 1973.
12. van der Korst JK, Sokoloff L, Miller EJ. Senescent pigmentation of cartilage and degenerative joint disease. *Archs Path* 1968;86:40.
13. Maroudas A, Bullough PG, Swanson SAV, Freeman MAR. The permeability of articular cartilage. *J Bone Joint Surg Br* 1968;50:166.
14. Bullough PG, Goodfellow JW. The significance of the fine structure of articular cartilage. *J Bone Joint Surg Br* 1968;50(4):852.
15. Benninghoff A. Form und Bau der Gelenkknorpel in ihren Beziehungen zur Function. II. Der Aufbau des Gelenkknorpels in seinen Beziehungen zur Function. *Z Zellforsch mikrosk Anat* 1925;2:783.
16. Muir H, Bullough P, Maroudas A. The distribution of collagen in human articular cartilage with some of its physiological implications. *J Bone Joint Surg Br* 1970;52:554.
17. Bullough PG, Munuera L, Murphy J, Weinstein A. The strength of the menisci of the knee as it relates to their fine structure. *J Bone Joint Surg Br* 1970;52:564.
18. Maroudas A, Evans H, Almeida L. Cartilage of the hip joint; topographical variation of glycosaminoglycan content in normal and fibrillated tissue. *Ann Rheum Dis* 1973;32:1.1
19. Stockwell RA, Meachim G. The chondrocytes. In: Freeman, MAR. ed. *Adult articular cartilage.* London; Pitman Medical, 1973.
20. Stockwell RA. The interrelationship of cell density and cartilage thickness in mammalian articular cartilage. *J Anat* 1971;109:411.
21. Anderson HC. Calcification processes. *Pathol Annu* 1980;15(2):45.
22. Wilsman NJ. Cilia of adult canine articular chondrocytes. *J Ultrastruct Mol Struct Res* 1978;64:270.
23. Stockwell RA. The ultrastructure of cartilage canals and the surrounding cartilage in the sheep fetus. *J Anat* 1971;109:397.
24. Boskey AL, Bullough PG, Dmitrovsky E. The biochemistry of the mineralization front. *Metab Bone Dis Rel Res* 1980;2S:61.
25. Mitrovic D. Régression des fentes articulaires normalement constituées chez l embryon de poulet paralysé. *C R Acad Sci III* 1972; 274:288.
26. Mori C, Nakamura N, Kimura S, et al. Programmed cell death in the interdigital tissue of the fetal mouse limb is apoptosis with DNA fragmentation. *Anat Rec* 1995;242:103.
27. Kempson GE. Mechanical properties of human articular cartilage. [PhD Thesis], University of London, 1970.
28. Bullough PG, Yawitz PS, Tafra L, et al. Topographical variations in the morphology and biochemistry of adult canine tibial plateau articular cartilage. *J Orthop Res* 1985;3:1.
29. Bennett GA, Waine H, Bauer W. *Changes in the knee joint at various ages, with particular reference to the nature and development of degenerative joint disease.* The Commonwealth Fund, New York, 1942.
30. Goodfellow JW, Bullough PG. The pattern of ageing of the articular cartilage of the elbow joint. *J Bone Joint Surg Br* 1967;49:175.
31. Palmoski MJ, Brandt KD. Effects of static and cyclic compressive loading on articular cartilage plugs in vitro. *Arthritis Rheum* 1984;27:675.
32. Palmoski MJ, Perricone E, Brandt KD. Development and reversal of a proteoglycan aggregation defect in normal canine knee cartilage after immobilization. *Arthritis Rheum* 1979;22:508.
33. Henderson B, Pettipher R. The synovial lining cell: biology and pathbiology. *Semin Arthritis Rheum* 1985;1:1.
34. Barland P, Novikoff AB, Hamerman D. Electron microscopy of human synovial membrane. *J Cell Biol* 1962;14:207.
35. Cooper RR, Misol SS. Tendon and ligament insertion. *J Bone Joint Surg* 1970;52A:1.
36. Lundborg G, Myrhage R. The vascularization and structure of the human digital tendon sheath as related to flexor tendon function. *Scand J Plast Reconstr Surg* 1977;11:195.
37. Johansen NA. Endocrine arthropathies. *Clin Rheum Dis* 1985; II(2):297.
38. Bullough PG, DiCarlo EF. Subchondral avascular necrosis: A common cause of arthritis. *Ann Rheum Dis* 1990;49:412.
39. Collins DH. *The pathology of articular and spinal diseases.* London; Arnold, 1949.
40. Heine J. Über die Arthritis deformans. *Virchows Arch path Anat Physiol* 1926;260:521.
41. Bennet GA, Waine H, Bauer W. *Changes in the knee joint at various ages.* New York; Commonwealth Fund, 1942.
42. Nakata K, Bullough PG. The injury and repair of human articular cartilage: A morphological study of 192 cases of osteoarthritis. *Jpn Orthop Assoc* 1986;60:763.
43. Christensen SB. Osteoarthrosis: Changes in bone, cartilage and synovial membrane in relation to bone scintigraphy. *Acta Orthop Scand Suppl* 1985;214(56):1.
44. Franchi A, Bullough PG. Secondary avascular necrosis in coxarthrosis; a morphologic study. *J Rheumatol* 1992;19:1263.
45. Landells JW. The bone cysts of osteoarthritis. *J Bone Joint Surg Br* 1953;35:643.
46. Rhaney K, Lamb DW. The cysts of osteoarthritis of the hip. A radiological and pathological study. *J Bone Joint Surg Br* 1955;37:663.
47. Villacin AB, Brigham LN, Bullough PG. Primary and secondary synovial chondrometaplasia. *Hum Pathol* 1979;10:439.
48. Ito S, Bullough PG. Synovial and osseous inflammation in degenerative joint disease and rheumatoid arthritis of the hip. Histometric Study. *Proceedings of the 25th Annual ORS.* 1979;199.

# Soft Tissues

*Histology for Pathologists, second edition,*
Edited by Stephen S. Sternberg.
Lippincott-Raven Publishers, Philadelphia
© 1997.

# CHAPTER 7

# Myofibroblast

Walter Schürch, Thomas A. Seemayer, and Giulio Gabbiani



## DISCOVERY OF THE MYOFIBROBLAST

The myofibroblast was discovered in electron micrographs from contracting (healing) experimental granulation tissue (1). Soon thereafter, its biochemical, pharmacological and immunohistochemical features were delineated (2–5). Since these early days, the list of pathologic conditions in which this cell has been identified has grown considerably (6–8). Looking back, it is somewhat surprising that such a pivotal element of diverse processes should not have been defined earlier (9).

The road to discovery stems from human interest in the process of wound healing as traced from the time of fossils to the ancient world (10). Indeed, the fate of civilization rested on the ability of people to recover from wounds inflicted through battle or disease. In more recent times, Carrel and Hartmann hypothesized that contractile forces were present in granulating wounds (11). For years it was believed, even taught, that collagen was the element essential for wound contraction. Dogma changed (slowly) with two reports in the mid-1950s. In one, experiments established that wound contraction was normal in guinea pigs rendered scorbutic (12). In the other, fibroblasts, under appropriate conditions, could be induced to contract in vitro (13). These findings cast doubt on the contractility of collagen and suggested that cells were central to tissue contraction.

In 1967, Majno and Levanthal performed experiments that established that histamine caused postcapillary venular interendothelial gaps that brought about vascular leakage (14). In electron micrographs, such endothelial cells were shrunken and distorted with notched nuclei. On this basis, he reasoned that gap formation might be produced by active endothelial contraction (14). This suggestion, made before the establishment of the concept that nonmuscle cells contain contractile proteins, was not easily accepted initially; in turn, it stimulated work based on the possibility that endothelial and other mesenchymal cells could exert contractile activities. A few years later, the ultrastructural observation was made that the cytoplasm of granulation tissue fibroblasts was loaded with bundles and aggregates of microfilaments (1), a feature typical of smooth muscle cells. On this basis, the possibility that these modified fibroblastic cells were responsible for granulation tissue contraction was relatively easy to suggest (1), but not so easy to be accepted (15). Further experiments, employing pharmacological agents known to affect cellular contraction/relaxation, established that granulating wounds indeed contained contractile cells, and the term myofibroblast was proposed (2). Subsequently, myofibroblasts were found to be capable of being decorated by hu-

W. Schürch: Department of Pathology, Hôtel-Dieu Hospital and University of Montreal, Montreal, Quebec, Canada.

T. A. Seemayer: Department of Pathology and Microbiology, University of Nebraska Medical Center, Omaha, NB 68198.

G. Gabbiani: Department of Pathology, University of Geneva—CMU, 1211 Geneva 4, Switzerland.

man smooth muscle antibodies (4); these were then shown to be specifically directed against actin (5). Shortly thereafter, myofibroblasts were identified within nodules of Dupuytren's disease (16) and in human granulation tissue (17), and shown to transmit their contractile forces from cell-to-cell through intermediate (adherens) junctions and from cell-to-stroma by means of microtendons: the whole being synchronized by intercellular gap junctions (18). The microtendon, an apparatus connecting myofibroblasts to the surrounding extracellular matrix, was named "fibronexus" (19).

In the late 1970s Tremblay (20) described the presence of myofibroblasts in the stroma of mammary carcinomas. The neoplasms in which these myofibroblasts had been noted were firm and retracted, unassociated with an inflammatory infiltrate. Because myofibroblasts are normally not present in mammary stroma, it was suggested that they contributed to the retraction phenomena and desmoplasia which characterized these neoplasms (20). It was then reasoned that such contractile cells might be contained in diverse carcinomas characterized by retraction and desmoplasia. Accordingly, a series of invasive and metastatic carcinomas was examined ultrastructurally. Myofibroblasts were present in the stroma of each and were particularly numerous in those that were hard, sclerotic, and retracted (21). Within several years, the spatial distribution of such cells within invasive and metastatic carcinomas was described (22,23), and it was proposed that similarities between the process of wound healing and the stromal response to neoplastic invasion might exist (22).

In the following years detailed studies of intermediate filament proteins and actin isoforms of myofibroblasts in various settings and conditions were performed; this led to the finding that myofibroblasts from diverse pathologic settings were heterogeneous in their content of intermediate filaments and actin isoforms (24,25). The presence of $\alpha$-smooth muscle actin, the actin isoform characteristic of vascular smooth muscle cells, was suggested as the main marker of the myofibroblastic phenotype (25). In these works it was shown that there is a correlation between the phenotypic modulation of myofibroblasts and the clinical behavior of lesions containing these cells. In particular, it was shown that myofibroblasts in granulation tissue of normally healing wounds express $\alpha$-smooth muscle actin only temporarily (25), whereas myofibroblasts with a smooth muscle phenotype persist in hypertrophic scars, fibrocontractive diseases, quasineoplastic proliferative conditions, and within the stroma of certain neoplasms (24,26).

More recently, it was shown that several extracellular matrix components (27) and cytokines (28–30) are capable of modulating the expression of $\alpha$-smooth muscle actin in fibroblastic cells, thereby furnishing the first hints on the mechanisms controlling the modulations of the myofibroblastic phenotype. It also became clear that $\alpha$-smooth muscle actin-expressing myofibroblasts were responsible for collagen synthesis during fibrotic phenomena (31). The possibility that myofibroblasts arise from specialized mesenchymal cells such as perisinusoidal stellate cells of the liver (32) and mesangial cells of the glomerulus (33) was also demonstrated. Finally, it was shown that myofibroblasts undergo apoptosis during the transition between granulation tissue and scar tissue (34).

In 1996, some 25 years after the initial discovery and 4 decades after the quest began, the myofibroblast is recognized as a pivotal element in normal and abnormal wound healing, in reactive proliferative conditions, and within the stroma of certain neoplasms. The sections that follow more fully characterize the myofibroblast, describe the settings in which it is found, and relate recent studies that provide further insight into the biology of this unique cell.

## CHARACTERIZATION OF THE MYOFIBROBLAST

### Ultrastructural

As initially described in granulation tissue and nodules of Dupuytren's disease (1,16) myofibroblasts share morphologic features in common with fibroblasts and smooth muscle cells.

Fibroblasts of adult animals and humans display a slender fusiform and smooth, contoured nucleus, a well-developed Golgi area, and numerous often dilated cisternae of rough endoplasmic reticulum, scattered mitochondria, and microfilaments, sometimes arranged in discrete bundles beneath the plasma membrane. Cell contours are generally smooth or display a few short cytoplasmic extensions. Plasmalemmal attachment plaques, dense patches or dense bands (35,36), basal lamina, pinocytotic vesicles, intercellular junctions, and cell-to-stroma attachment sites are absent.

Smooth muscle cells are enveloped by a continuous basal lamina. Their plasma membrane reveals numerous plasmalemmal attachment plaques or so-called membrane-associated dense bodies, dense plaques, dense patches, or dense bands (36), and numerous pinocytotic vesicles. Intercellular gap junctions and adherens junctions are present (37). The cytoplasm is laden with bundles of microfilaments, usually disposed parallel to the long axis of the cell, among which numerous dense bodies are interspersed. These are electron-dense structures scattered within the cytoplasm of smooth muscle cells. The material of the dense bodies appears similar to the one forming the dense bands, which are attached to the cell membrane in certain vascular smooth muscle cells. Some dense bodies are in continuity with dense bands. Dense bodies and dense bands probably correspond to Z-lines of striated muscle fibers. In both structures $\alpha$-actinin has been demonstrated by immunohistochemical techniques (38,39). Force transmission from the contractile apparatus to the cell membrane in smooth muscle cells occurs via the insertion of bundles of actin filaments into the dense bands (35). Transmission of the contractile force occurs also across cell membranes of smooth muscle cells and from cell membranes to the stroma. Although it seems clear that the traction generated by the myofilaments is transmitted to the dense bands, the exact mechanism of the transmission of the traction across the cell membrane is not fully understood. The fibronectin receptor as a transmembrane receptor glycoprotein complex (40–43) has extracellular binding sites for fibronectin (44), suggesting specific interactions between cytoplasmic actin filaments and extracellular fibronectin fibers across the plasma membrane at cell-to-matrix attachment sites. A close association between bundles of cytoplasmic actin filaments (stress fibers) and bundles of extracellular fibronectin fibrils has been observed in transformed fibroblasts and in myofibroblasts of granulation tissue in vivo; it was named fibronexus, an apparatus specialized for increased cell-to-matrix connection (45,46). Contractile forces from cell to cell are transmitted through adherens or intermediate junctions, which are symmetrical structures formed by two dense bands that match each other in adjacent smooth muscle cells (35). Nuclei are elongated, with blunt ends, and are deformed by shallow invaginations. In contrast to fibroblasts, the Golgi area and the rough endoplasmic reticulum are poorly developed.

Myofibroblasts disclose irregular, often stellate cellular outlines with numerous and long cytoplasmic extensions, and are connected by intermediate or adherens and by gap junctions, the latter considered as low-resistance pathways for intercellular communications (18). In addition, myofibroblasts are partly enveloped by a basal lamina, reveal plasmalemmal attachment plaques, dense patches or dense bands, and pinocytotic vesicles. They are also connected to the extracellular matrix by cell-to-stroma attachment sites through the fibronexus, which is a transmembrane complex of intracellular microfilament bundles in apparent continuity with extracellular fibronectin fibers (Fig. 1) (19,46). These cell-to-stroma attachment sites are well developed and numerous in myofibroblasts compared to their attenuated appearance in smooth muscle cells. At the surface of myofibroblasts three types of fibronexus are observed: (a) plaquelike; (b) tracklike; and (c) tandem associations (46). Within the cytoplasm, myofibroblasts contain numerous bundles of microfilaments (stress fibers) usually arranged parallel to the long axis of the cell, among which are interspersed numerous dense bodies (Fig. 1A). As in vascular smooth muscle cells, these structures may be in continuity with dense bands or plasmalemmal attachment plaques. Rough endoplasmic reticulum and Golgi area are well developed. The nucleus, finally, displays deep indentations (Fig. 1A), an ultrastructural feature that has been correlated with cellular contraction in several systems (47–50). Several nuclear bodies are usually present and nucleoli are conspicuous.

### Histologic

Although morphologically best defined with the electron microscope, myofibroblasts disclose several typical histologic traits that allow their recognition in routine paraffin sections. They are usually large, spindle shaped, often stellate (spiderlike) with several long cytoplasmic extensions, and distinct fibrillar and acidophilic cytoplasm with cable-like condensations (stress fibers) running through the subplasmalemmal cytoplasm parallel to the long axis (Fig. 2). Their nuclei often are indented or reveal strangulations of nuclear segments, a feature reflecting cellular contraction. The chromatin is finely granular, regularly dispersed, and nucleoli are conspicuous (Fig. 2). Well-differentiated myofibroblasts with the previously mentioned traits are observed in poorly collagenized and edematous areas of the various settings in which they have been described. In heavily collagenized zones, myofibroblasts are difficult to recognize with the light microscope since they correspond ultrastructurally to poorly developed myofibroblasts or to fibroblasts.

### Biochemical

Myofibroblasts possess not only contractile forces but also synthetic properties. Four major groups of macromolecules comprise the extracellular matrix: (a) the collagens; (b) the glycoproteins (e.g. fibronectins, laminins, tenascin); (c) the proteoglycans (e.g. aggrecan, synchrons, perlecan, decorin); and (d) the elastins with their associated proteins (51). Myofibroblasts possess synthetic properties for several of the extracellular matrix components, among them collagens of type I, III, IV and V (31, 52–54), glycoproteins (55) and proteoglycans, i.e., fibronectin, laminin, and tenascin (56). In addition, liver myofibroblasts from the murine schistosomiasis model secrete lysyloxidase, an enzyme that initiates the first step in the cross-linking of collagen and elastin, a crucial function for the stabilization of the extracellular matrix (57,58). Concerning collagen synthesis in granulating wounds, the collagen initially produced is type III. This form of collagen imparts a measure of plasticity to the wound in the early phase of healing. When granulation tissue is resorbed following wound closure, myofibroblasts disappear through the process of apoptosis (see below), and the more rigid type I collagen is biochemically identified (53,54). In similar fashion, the proliferative cellular phase of palmar fibromatosis and the young edematous mesenchyme of areas corresponding to early stromal invasion of breast carcinomas, both rich in myofibroblasts, contain increased amounts of type III collagen (26,59,60). Increased amounts of type V collagen are biochemically identified in desmoplastic human breast carcinomas, apparently also produced by myofibroblasts (54).

### Pharmacological

Strips of granulation tissue exposed in vitro to a variety of pharmacological agents, contract and relax in a manner analogous to smooth muscle. Prostaglandin $F_1$, bradykinin, serotonin, angiotensin, norepinephrine, epinephrine, and vasopressin initiate contraction. The intensity of the response depends on the origin, age, and initial degree of contraction of the granulation tissue tested. Prostaglandin $E_1$ and $E_2$ and

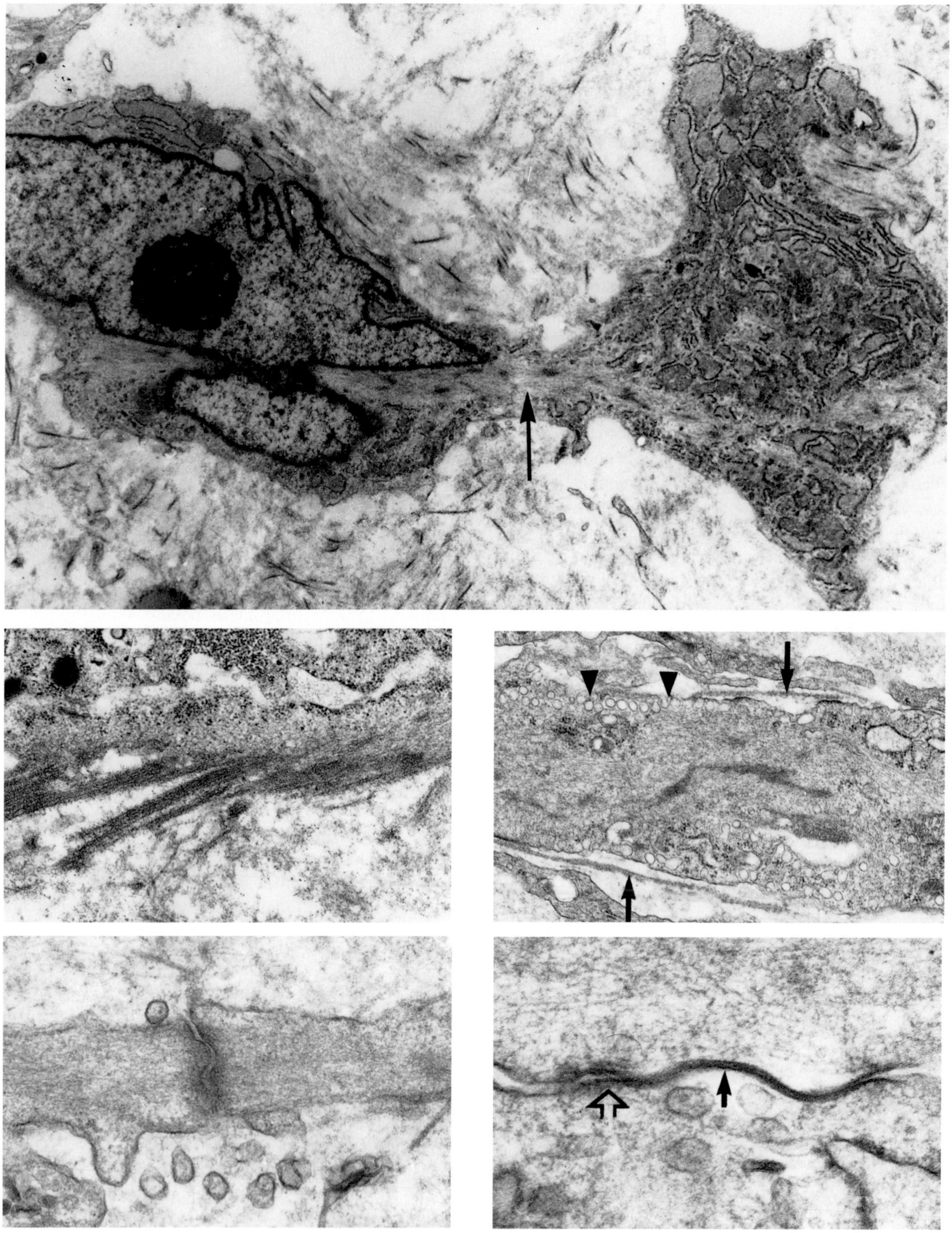

**FIG. 1.** Ultrastructural characterization of the myofibroblast. **A,** Typical myofibroblast with irregular shape and cytoplasmic extensions, well-developed rough endoplasmic reticulum, and bundle of cytoplasmic microfilaments (*arrow*) with numerous dense bodies running through the cytoplasm (stress fiber) and giving rise to a strangulation of a nuclear segment. **B,** Microtendons in apparent continuity with bundles of cytoplasmic microfilaments (cell-to-stroma attachment sites, i.e., fibronexus). **C,** Fragments of basal lamina (*arrows*), pinocytotic vesicles (*arrowheads*), and plasmalemmal attachment plaques. **D,** Intermediate or adherens junction between two cytoplasmic extensions of myofibroblasts. **E,** Gap junction (arrow), followed by intermediate junction (open arrow) joining two myofibroblasts. (Uranyl acetate and lead citrate: A, ×**9900**; B, ×**25,000**; C, ×**18,200**; D, ×**39,000**; E, ×**78,000.**)

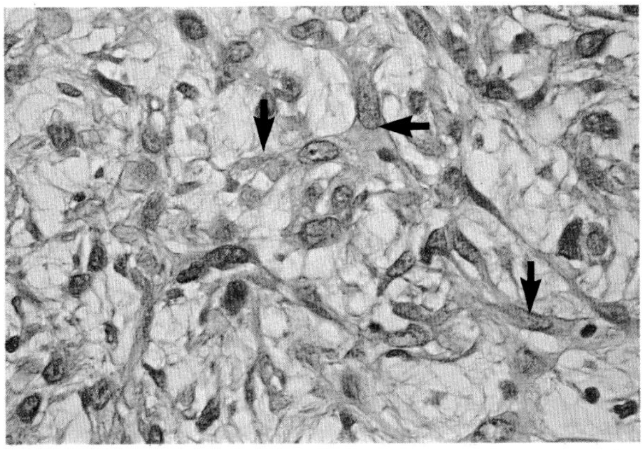

**FIG. 2.** Histological aspect of myofibroblasts from exudativo-productive layer of human granulation tissue, approximately 15 days old. Myofibroblasts disclose stellate, spiderlike shapes with long cytoplasmic extensions and distinct fibrillar cytoplasm with cablelike (*arrows*) subplasmalemmal condensations (stress fibers). (Hematoxylin-phloxine-saffron.)

papaverine induce relaxation in tissue submitted to contract (2,3,17). Cytochalasin B abolishes the contraction of granulation tissue, probably as a result of microfilament disruption (61). Trocinate ($\beta$-diethylaminoethylphenylthioacetate), another inhibitor of smooth muscle contraction, has been reported to decrease contraction when applied topically on rabbit wounds (62). Strips of cirrhotic liver, when exposed to smooth muscle stimulating agents, contract significantly when compared to strips of normal liver (63). A marked myofibroblastic fibrosis is also produced in lungs of bleomycin-injected rats, and when strips of these fibrotic lungs are exposed to acetylcholine, epinephrine, and a $K^+$depolarizing solution, the force developed is approximately twice that of normal lung tissue strips (64). The relative reactivity to various stimulating agents of myofibroblasts from diverse sources varies: thus, acetylcholine causes contraction of strips of fibrotic lungs but not of granulation tissue from a skin wound or a granuloma pouch; serotonin induces retraction of the granuloma pouch but not strips from a skin wound (3). In addition to this heterogeneity in the pharmacological reactivity of granulation tissue strips from various sources, there are also differences between the response of strips of granulation tissue and strips of smooth muscle; the former reach their peak contraction slower and maintain it for a longer period than the latter. Whereas the various enumerated agents were shown to reveal their activity on granulation tissue in vitro, the exact mechanism leading to myofibroblast contraction in vivo remains to be elucidated.

Endothelin-1 (an acid 21 amino acid peptide) was originally isolated from the conditioned medium of cultured porcine endothelial cells and shown to be the most potent vasopressor substance yet characterized (65). Endothelin-1 may be an endogenous modulator of myofibroblast-mediated granulation tissue contraction because it causes reversible and concentration-dependent contraction of granulation tissue, the 21-day granulation tissue being the most responsive. This response can be inhibited by calcium antagonists (66,67). The vasopressor effect of endothelin-1 possibly is controlled and mediated through the action of cytokines, among others, transforming growth factor-$\beta$ (68,69), which, in turn, is able to induce $\alpha$-smooth muscle actin expression in fibroblasts and myofibroblasts (for details, see below).

### In Vitro Culture Studies

Fibroblasts in culture rapidly develop the ability to attach to the wall of the container and move across its surface. Such adherence and mobility are attributed to the development of a system of microfilaments called stress fibers (70). These may measure up to 2$\mu$m in diameter and may branch or radiate from focal points (71). Microfilament constituting stress fibers are mainly composed of actin, including $\alpha$-smooth muscle actin, as shown by immunofluorescence and immunoelectron microscopy with specific antibodies (72–74). Several studies have shown that stress fibers also contain actin-associated proteins such as myosin, tropomyosin, alpha-actinin, and filamin (7). In addition to stress fibers, cultured fibroblasts develop gap junction (75), analogous to that observed between myofibroblasts in vivo (18). In primary passaged fibroblastic populations, the presence of $\alpha$-smooth muscle actin has been reported (74,76,77). Controversy, however, persists concerning whether these $\alpha$-smooth muscle actin-expressing cells are derived from smooth muscle cells and/or pericytes present in the tissues from which cultures were established, or represent a true feature of fibroblastic cultures.

In order to address this issue, fibroblast cultures from various species, including human, were established, using cloning and subcloning techniques; in all of these conditions, a certain percentage of cells was positive for $\alpha$-smooth muscle actin (78). It is very probable that $\alpha$-smooth muscle actin expression in cultured fibroblasts represents a feature of fibroblastic cultures themselves, which may be related to functions exerted by fibroblasts under particular environmental conditions in vivo. This assumption is supported by the observation that $\alpha$-smooth muscle actin is expressed by fibroblasts cultured from organs (lens cells, mammary gland, perisinusoidal cells of liver, and glomerular mesangial cells), where, normally, stromal cells expressing this protein do not occur (79–82), but which may contain stromal cells expressing $\alpha$-smooth muscle actin in pathologic conditions. Cultured fibroblasts may express different phenotypic features and a whole spectrum of differentiation steps has been described (83). Moreover, the concept of fibroblast heterogeneity in vivo is now also well established (for review see Schmitt-Gräff et al.(8).

Cytoskeletal proteins such as desmin and smooth muscle myosin heavy chains are also variably expressed by cultured fibroblasts derived from different organs or pathologic tissues. The expression of desmin and smooth muscle myosin heavy chains, however, is generally low, and in several populations these proteins are not expressed (78).

The forces generated by cultured fibroblasts are traction,

rather than contraction forces, as shown by experiments in which fibroblasts distorted a sheet of silicon on which they were grown (84). Several observations suggest that stress fibers are probably the force-generating elements in wound contraction, since they contract upon addition of adenosine triphosphate on glycerinated fibroblasts (13,85,86), and microinjection experiments revealed that they were functionally analogous to skeletal muscle fibers (86,87). When myofibroblasts from various sources (granulating wounds, Dupuytren's disease, and breast cancer) are cultured, they maintain their morphology in vitro but grow significantly slower than fibroblasts (88). If the growth rate and the actin concentration of cultured fibroblasts from normal dermis and myofibroblasts of human granulation tissue are compared, myofibroblasts grow slower than fibroblasts and contain a significant higher concentration of actin (89). Thus, myofibroblasts disclose many features of cultured fibroblasts (90).

The function of stress fibers is presently not known. In analogy to in vitro situations, stress fibers could play a role in cell-to-substrate adhesion, because they are well developed and well dispersed in stationary cultured fibroblasts, and relatively decreased in motile and transformed cells (91,92). Myofibroblasts maintain, under culture conditions, their unique features: that is, their resemblance to fibroblasts and smooth muscle cells. When placed in culture, myofibroblasts from skin wound granulation tissue maintain biologic features different from those of dermal fibroblasts (93). Similarly, fibroblastic cells cultured from Dupuytren's nodules maintain biologic features different from those of normal dermis or fascial fibroblasts, yet similar to those of neoplastic or embryonic fibroblasts (94). Wound-healing fibroblasts were shown to develop greater contractile properties than dermal fibroblasts (95).

Several in vitro models have been developed to study the dynamics of wound contraction using fibroblasts cultured in collagen or fibrin matrices (for review see Grinnell (96). In floating collagen matrices, fibroblasts develop stellate morphology with long processes and a cytoskeletal meshwork. In contrast, fibroblastic cells in anchored collagen matrices become bipolar, and orient along lines of tension. These cells develop then prominent stress fibers and cell-to-stroma attachment sites (fibronexus), and resemble myofibroblasts. This indicates that fibroblasts are able to contract a tissue matrix in vitro without differentiating into myofibroblasts, and that the appearance of myofibroblasts correlates with the appearance of stress within the matrix. Fibroblasts in floating versus anchored collagen matrices also show differences in cell proliferation and DNA synthesis. After contraction of floating collagen matrices there is a marked decline in cellular DNA synthesis; the cells become arrested, and cell regression begins. In contrast, fibroblastic cells in anchored matrices continue to proliferate and to synthesize DNA. Furthermore, and taking into account that the tension forces developed in a restrained collagen lattice by myofibroblasts obtained from human skin granulation tissue explants are more intense than those exerted by human dermis fibroblasts (95), it is very likely that inherent mechanical forces within granulation tissue can regulate cell proliferation and extracellular matrix organization (96).

## TISSUE DISTRIBUTION OF MYOFIBROBLASTS

For a better understanding and a more comprehensive appreciation of the various settings in which myofibroblasts occur, a detailed description of cytoskeletal proteins of muscular tissues, particularly smooth muscle cells, is presented.

Cytoskeletal proteins have been used extensively for studying differentiation of muscular tissues (97). They have proved to be reliable markers of adaptation to physiologic and pathologic conditions (98). Desmin is a general muscle-differentiation marker that appears early in embryogenesis. This intermediate filament protein, however, does not permit one to distinguish between different muscle types (7,99). Moreover, desmin is present in stromal cells of several organs, which traditionally were considered fibroblastic in nature (74). When smooth muscle cells are cultured, desmin disappears (100). Smooth muscle myosin is a precise marker of smooth muscle differentiation. This contractile protein, however, disappears rapidly from smooth muscle cells in several conditions in vivo and also early in culture (100, 101). These findings suggest that smooth muscle myosin is a more reliable marker of smooth muscle differentiation than smooth muscle origin.

Vascular smooth muscle cells are heterogeneous with respect to their intermediate filament proteins. Most contain vimentin as their sole detectable intermediate filament; a lesser proportion also express desmin (102–106). In contrast, parenchymal smooth muscle cells of the respiratory, gastrointestinal, and genitourinary tracts represent a homogeneous cell population in which desmin is almost the exclusive intermediate filament protein (107–109). With regard to actin expression, at least six isoforms are found in mammals (76,110,111): two nonmuscle actins ($\beta$ and $\gamma$), the so-called cytoplasmic actins, two smooth muscle actins ($\alpha$ and $\gamma$), and two sarcomeric actins ($\alpha$-cardiac and $\alpha$-skeletal). Two-dimensional gel electrophoresis resolves only three isoforms: $\beta$ and $\gamma$ (nonmuscle and muscle actins) and the $\alpha$-actins (smooth, striated skeletal, and striated cardiac). The biochemical identification of the six actin isoforms requires chemical analysis of the amino-terminal tryptic peptide of actin in cellular extracts (111). Vascular smooth muscle cells are characterized by a predominance of the $\alpha$-smooth muscle actin isoform. In contrast, parenchymal smooth muscle cells contain large amounts of the $\gamma$-smooth muscle actin isoform (76,103,110–112). The pattern of $\alpha$-, $\beta$-, and $\gamma$-actin isoform expression varies in smooth muscle tissues of adult mammals (112). This pattern varies also during non-neoplastic pathologic conditions such as atheromatosis (113, 114), but changes only slightly in uterine leiomyomas, compared with normal myometrium (112). During the early months of life, 50% of cells in the aortic media lack α-smooth muscle actin, whereas α-smooth muscle actin-negative cells constitute less than 1% in the adult. These findings demonstrate that, at least in vessels, differentiation of smooth muscle cells is completed after birth (99). These observations collectively suggest that the pattern of α-actin isoform expression and, particularly, the expression of α-smooth muscle actin in vascular smooth muscle cells is related to the degree of smooth muscle differentiation.

Pericytes resemble vascular smooth muscle cells (115). As early as 1923 Zimmermann showed, in a meticulously executed treatise, that pre-and postcapillary pericytes are connected to vascular smooth muscle cells (116). In 1991 (117), a very elegant study showed that pre-and postcapillary pericytes indeed expressed α-smooth muscle actin, whereas the midcapillary pericytes did not reveal this actin isoform. Pericytes were also shown to resemble vascular smooth muscle cells by their intermediate filament expression. Both cell types express vimentin or vimentin and desmin (118). In addition, the intermediate filament composition of pericytes discloses species and tissue differences similar to those observed in vascular smooth muscle cells (102–105).

Myofibroblasts as observed in normal tissue, granulation tissue, and pathologic tissue disclose various cytoskeletal phenotypes: phenotype V represented by cells expressing only vimentin; phenotype VA, represented by cells positive for vimentin and α-smooth muscle actin; phenotype VAD represented by cells expressing vimentin, α-smooth muscle actin and desmin; phenotyope VD represented by cells positive for vimentin and desmin; and, phenotype VA(D)M representing myofibroblasts reactive for vimentin, α-smooth muscle actin, and smooth muscle myosin heavy chains with and without desmin.

## Normal Tissue

Myofibroblasts were described in normal human and animal tissues on the basis of ultrastructural and/or immunohistochemical evidence of smooth muscle differentiation. The normal settings in which myofibroblasts were observed include the external theca of the rat ovarian follicle (119), developing human palatal mucosa (120), rat, rabbit, and human intestinal mucosa (121–123), rat and mouse adrenal gland capsule (124), human lamb and monkey pulmonary and alveolar septa (125), rat testicular stroma (74), rat testicular capsule (126), human theca externa of the ovary (127), Wharton's jelly of human umbilical cord (128), bovine endometrial caruncle (129), and periodontal ligament of the mouse (130) and rat (131), where they provide forces necessary for tooth eruption. Stromal cells with myoid features were also identified in rat and human lymph nodes and in the human spleen (132). Another group of stromal cells with myoid features include hepatic perisinusoidal cells (133), those in the human uterine submucosa (134), and human bone marrow (135), glomerular mesangial cells of mouse, rat, and human (136), and, perhaps, pre-and postcapillary pericytes (115,117).

Immunohistochemical studies disclosed heterogeneous cytoskeletal phenotypes among all these stromal cells ("myofibroblasts") in terms of intermediate filament protein, smooth muscle actin, and smooth muscle myosin expression, the most frequent phenotype being VD and VA(D)M followed by VA and VAD phenotypes (137,138). This cytoskeletal heterogeneity could reflect different functional needs, since all of these stromal cells seem to participate in visceral contraction or extracellular matrix remodeling, a view supported by the observation that stromal cells with myoid features are generally present in organs requiring contraction or high degrees of remodeling (139). Another interpretation recently advanced, proposes that most examples of spindle cells in normal tissues, cited in the literature as being myofibroblasts, might be closer to pericytes or smooth muscle cells (140), or simply represent stromal cells with myoid features of variable degrees according to functional demands.

## Granulation Tissue

Granulation tissue consists of several layers of fibroblastic cells separated by a collagenous matrix containing capillary buds and inflammatory cells. According to the relative predominance of each constituent, four layers are classically distinguished: (a) alterative; (b) exudative; (c) exudativo-productive; and (d) cicatrizing (Fig. 3A). Granulation tissue fibroblasts characteristically disclose ultrastructural features of myofibroblasts. In fact, they were first described within this tissue (1,2). They are most numerous and best developed within the exudativo-productive layer and become progressively replaced toward the deepest cicatrizing layer by fibroblasts. The orientation of the myofibroblasts varies in the different layers. In the exudative layer, the long axis is perpendicular to the surface, whereas in the exudativo-productive and cicatrizing layer, the long axis is parallel to the surface (Fig. 3B); this indicates that the modulation of the orientation of myofibroblasts serves to transmit contractile forces in order to effect wound closure. When the collagenous matrix is analyzed, type III collagen predominates. When granulation tissue is resorbed following wound closure, myofibroblasts disappear (25,53,141) and the more rigid type I collagen is identified (52).

Analysis of cytoskeletal proteins by immunohistochemical methods reveals that myofibroblasts from normal healing wounds never express desmin or smooth muscle myosin heavy chains during the process of wound closure in the experimental animal (25). Smooth muscle differentiation in early granulation tissue is absent, and myofibroblasts are often poorly developed and correspond to V cells (Fig. 4). Smooth muscle differentiation of myofibroblasts, however, becomes temporarily apparent because myofibroblasts express α-smooth muscle actin (VA cells) (Fig. 5A,B) in increasing amounts from the 8th to the 15th day; this protein is located within bundles of microfilaments (stress fibers) as il-

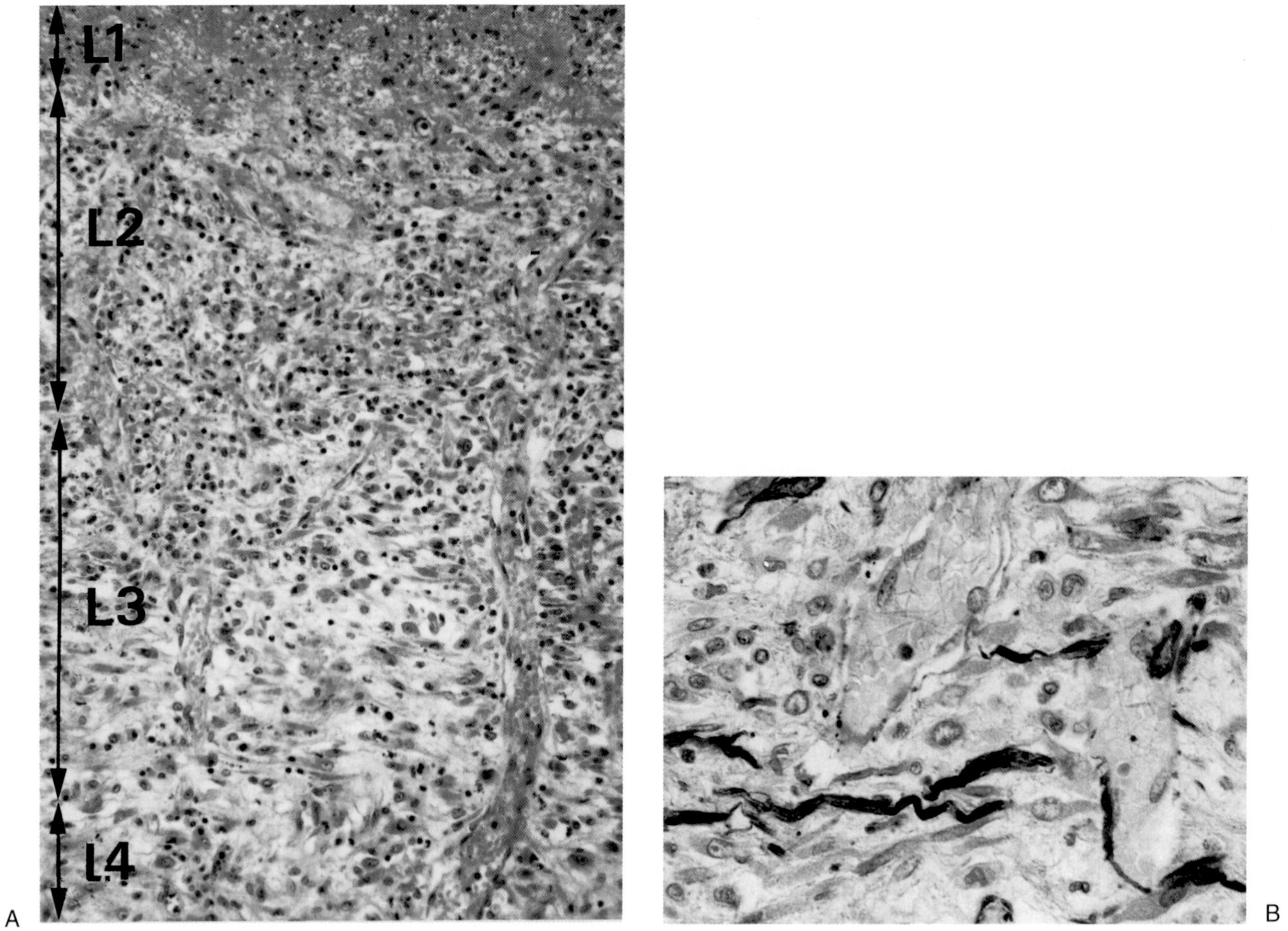


**FIG. 3.** Human granulation tissue, approximately 10 days old. **A,** The four layers (*L1-L4*) are clearly discernible: L1, alterative; L2, exudative; L3, exudativo–productive; L4, cicatrizing. (Hematoxylin-phloxine-saffron.) **B,** Several fibroblastic cells (myofibroblasts) from the exudativo-productive layer (*L3*) reveal intense immunostaining for $\alpha$-smooth muscle actin. (Avidin-biotin-complex-peroxidase.) Note that fibroblastic cells change their orientation within the different layers. In the exudative layer their long axis is perpendicular to the surface, whereas in the exudativo-productive layer their long axis is oriented parallel to the surface, which indicates that the modulation of cellular orientation serves to transmit contractile forces to effect wound closure.

lustrated by immunoelectron microscopic techniques (Fig. 5C,D). This actin isoform disappears progressively from myofibroblasts and is not detectable after the 30th day by immunohistochemical and immunoelectron microscopic methods. These results clearly indicate that granulation tissue myofibroblasts acquire, temporarily, a VA phenotype.

The study of the ontogenesis of wound healing reveals that many species possess the unique ability to heal wounds without scarring (142–147). Recently, Estes et al. (148), examining fetal wounds in the lamb, clearly showed that there are differences between early and late gestational wound healing: early gestational wounds (75 days; term 145 days) healed without scarring, i.e., by reparation of the epidermis, reconstitution of epidermal appendages, and restoration of the dermal collagenous network. In contrast, late gestational wounds (100 and 120 days) healed with scarring through formation of granulation tissue containing myofibroblasts.

### Pathologic Tissue

Upon analysis of the many pathologic conditions in which myofibroblasts have been described, three fundamental processes emerge: (a) responses to injury and repair phenomena or situations related to inflammation and tissue remodeling; (b) quasineoplastic proliferative conditions; and (c) stromal response to neoplasia (6,149). This concept enunciated some 15 years ago, appears to be valid today.

#### *Responses to Injury and Repair Phenomena*

These responses comprise human and experimental liver cirrhosis (150–152), tenosynovitis (153), radiation-induced pseudosarcoma of skin (154), burn contracture (155), ischemic contractures of intrinsic muscles of the hand (156), renal interstitial fibrosis during obstructive nephropathy (157), pulmonary sarcoidosis (158), giant cell granuloma of

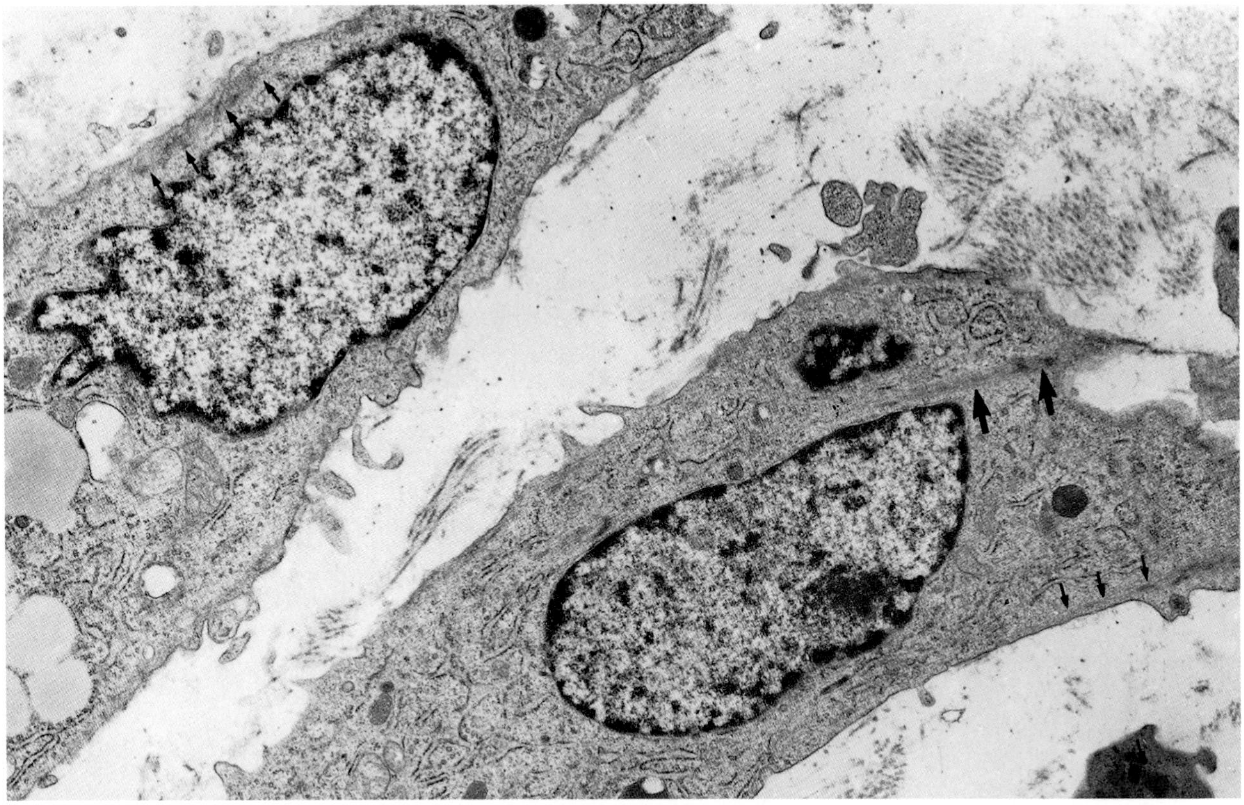

**FIG. 4.** Human granulation tissue, approximately 5 days old, composed of V-type myofibroblasts. These cells disclose subplasmalemmal bundles of microfilaments with few dense bodies (*small arrows*) and also intracytoplasmic bundles of microfilaments with dense bodies (*large arrows*), corresponding to stress fibers in formation. (Uranyl acetate and lead citrate, **×12,500**.)

jaws (159), schistosomal liver fibrosis (160), regenerating tendon (161), fibrous capsule around silicon mammary implants (162,163), nodular hyperplasia of the liver (164), ganglia of soft issue (165); hypertrophic scars (166), cataract (167); bleomycin-induced interstitial fibrosis of the lung in the rat (168), fibrous heart plaque in the carcinoid syndrome (169), atherosclerotic lesions in humans and experimental animals (170–173), localized and systemic scleroderma (174), and experimental hydronephrosis (175). A recent report also proposed that a reactive myofibroblastic proliferation with increased deposition/formation of extracellular matrix might be responsible for the progressive and irreversible obstruction of airways in chronic asthma (176). When cytoskeletal proteins of these conditions are analyzed, most reactive cells correspond to the VA, some to the VAD, and rarely to the VD and VA(D)M phenotype (137,141).

In abnormally healing wounds, (that is, hypertrophic scars and keloids), one observes several important differences. Hypertrophic scars always exhibit nodular structures in which fibroblastic cells, small vessels, and fine, randomly organized collagen fibers are present. Within these nodules numerous myofibroblasts of the VA phenotype are identified, and, in lesser numbers, myofibroblasts of the VAD phenotype (Fig. 6). Exceptionally, myofibroblasts of the VA(D)M phenotype are observed. Keloids that contain large thick bands of closely packed collagen fibers and only rarely nodular structures contain very limited numbers or no VA cells (177,178). VAD cells are not observed within keloids (177).

### *Quasineoplastic Proliferative Conditions*

This group embodies the poorly understood, but very important and frequent, soft tissue proliferations included under the broad heading of fibromatoses, as well as many other soft tissue proliferations, often mimicking sarcomas, which share a predominant myofibroblastic composition and a variable proliferative potential, yet do not disseminate or metastasize (6,149). Myofibroblasts constitute the principal cellular components of superficial and deep musculoaponeurotic fibromatoses (179). Superficial(fascial) fibromatoses include palmar fibromatosis (Dupuytren's disease) (16,59, 180–182), plantar fibromatosis (Ledderhose's disease)(16), penile fibromatosis (Peyronie's disease) (183), and knuckle pads (184). Deep musculoaponeurotic fibromatoses comprise extra-abdominal, abdominal, and intra-abdominal variants, collectively also named desmoid tumors (179). To this group belong the infantile fibromatoses (185). Other soft tis-

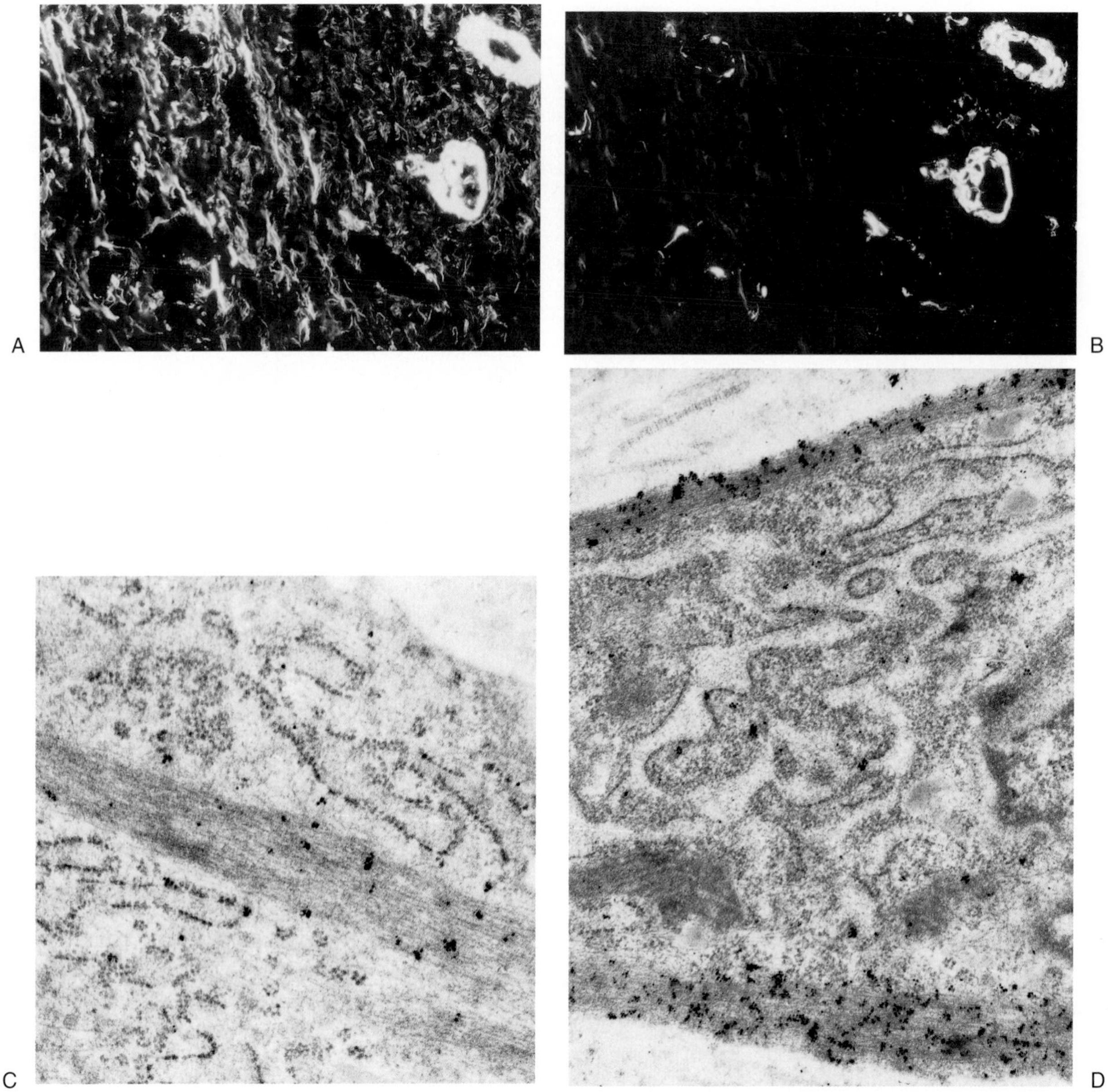


**FIG. 5.** Experimental granulation tissue from the rat, 15 days old. **A, B,** Double immunofluorescent staining for $\alpha$-smooth muscle actin (A) and desmin (B). Fibroblastic cells reveal intense staining for $\alpha$-smooth muscle actin (A) but are negative for desmin (B) Vascular smooth muscle cells are stained by both anti-$\alpha$-smooth muscle actin and anti-desmin A and B. **C, D,** Immunoelectron microscopic localization of $\alpha$-smooth muscle actin within intracytoplasmic bundles of microfilaments, that is, stress fibers (C), and in subplasmalemmal bundles of microfilaments (D). (C, **×31,000**; D, **×28,400.)**

sue proliferations predominantly composed of myofibroblasts are nodular fasciitis (186), proliferative fasciitis (187), proliferative myositis (188), giant fibroma of oral mucosa (189), dermatofibroma (190), elastofibroma (191), plasma cell granuloma of the lung (192), digital fibroma of infancy (193), and juvenile nasopharyngeal angiofibroma (194). Myofibroblasts are also present in cardiac myxomas (195) and in uterine plexiform tumors (196).

### *Dupuytren's Disease*

Among quasineoplastic proliferations, Dupuytren's-type fibromatosis has been studied extensively by morphologic, immunohistochemical, and biochemical techniques (24,26, 197,198). Cytoskeletal proteins have been widely used as markers of differentiation for neoplastic and quasineoplastic proliferations, as well as markers of adaptation to physiolog-

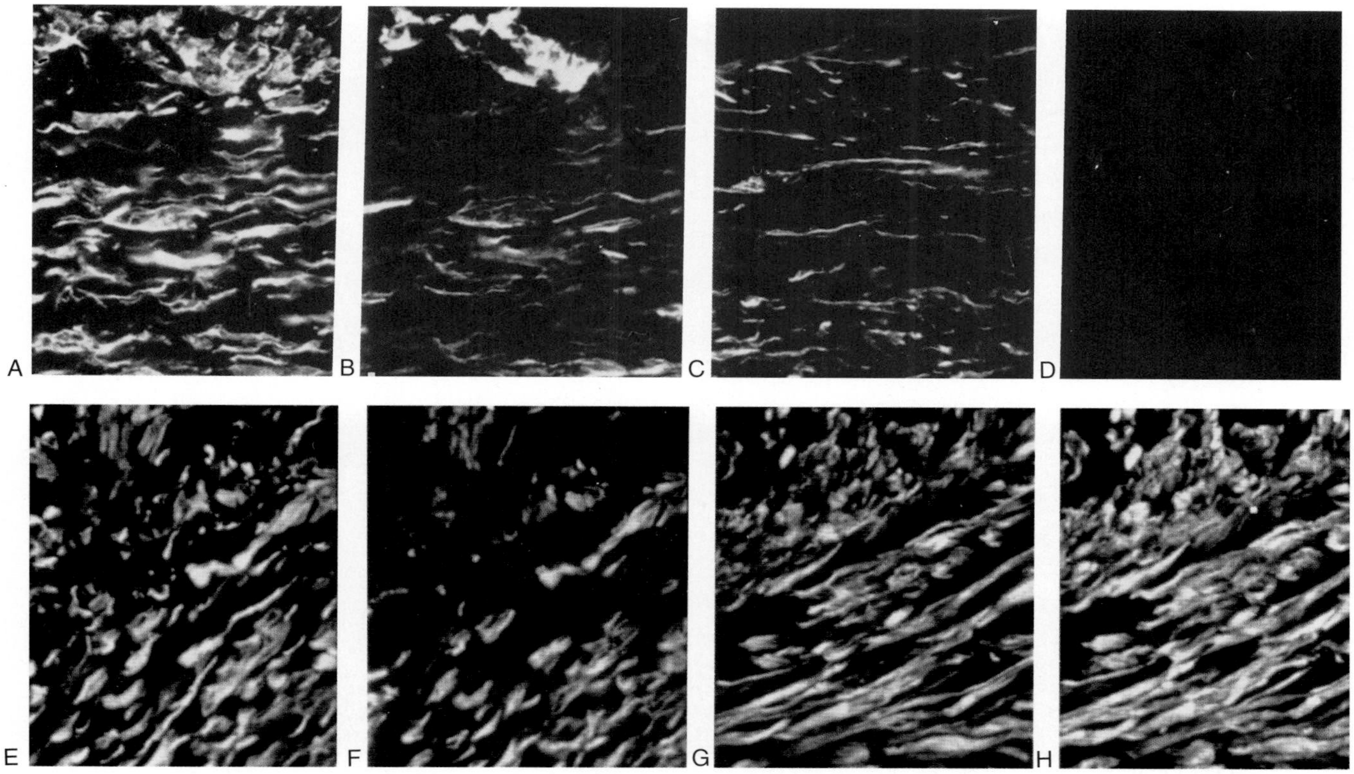


**FIG. 6.** Double immunofluorescent staining of two hypertrophic scars (**A-D;E-H**), one occurring at the site of smallpox vaccination (E-H), with anti-vimentin (A and E) and anti-$\alpha$-smooth muscle actin (B and F) and with anti-$\alpha$-smooth muscle actin (C and G) and anti-desmin (D and H). One hypertrophic scar (A-D) contains V and VA cells, and the other from the site of smallpox vaccination (E-H) contains mainly VAD cells. Note that most small blood vessels are positive for anti-vimentin and anti-$\alpha$-smooth muscle actin.

ical situations, particularly for muscular and related tissue proliferations (24,26,98).

According to Luck (199), the nodules of Dupuytren's disease are assigned to three different phases, depending on the histologic pattern of each lesion: (a) proliferative phase; (b) involutional phase; and (c) residual phase (Fig. 7). Patients with Dupuytren's disease often present multiple nodules showing considerable variation in their histologic appearance. The classification is, therefore, based on the predominant histologic pattern (61,200).

Proliferative phase nodules reveal on routine histology sections high cellular density, decreasing from the center to the periphery (Fig. 7A). They are well vascularized and display a poorly collagenized appearance. Ultrastructurally, they are composed of large myofibroblasts with numerous and long cytoplasmic extensions, joined by numerous gap and adherens junctions (Fig. 8A and inset). Their plasma membrane displays focal deposition of basal lamina, plasmalemmal attachment plaques, and pinocytotic vesicles, as well as cell-to-stroma attachment sites in the form of fibronexus (46). The cytoplasm features a well-developed granular endoplasmic reticulum and Golgi apparatus and numerous stress fibers, usually oriented parallel to the long axis of the cell (Fig. 8A). The nucleus is typically indented and often contains one or several nuclear bodies. The extracellular matrix is composed of a few mature collagen fibers (64 nm periodicity) admixed with indistinct granular and basal lamina-like material (Fig. 8A).

Involutional phase nodules also feature high cellularity, but individual cells are smaller than in proliferative phase nodules and tend to be aligned in the same direction (Fig. 7B,C). Ultrastructurally, these nodules are composed of myofibroblasts that are also connected by gap and adherens junctions. These intercellular junctions, however, seem to be less numerous than in proliferative phase nodules. The most striking difference with proliferative phase nodules is the increased amount of collagen. Individual myofibroblasts are enveloped by thick bundles of mature collagen fibers. By

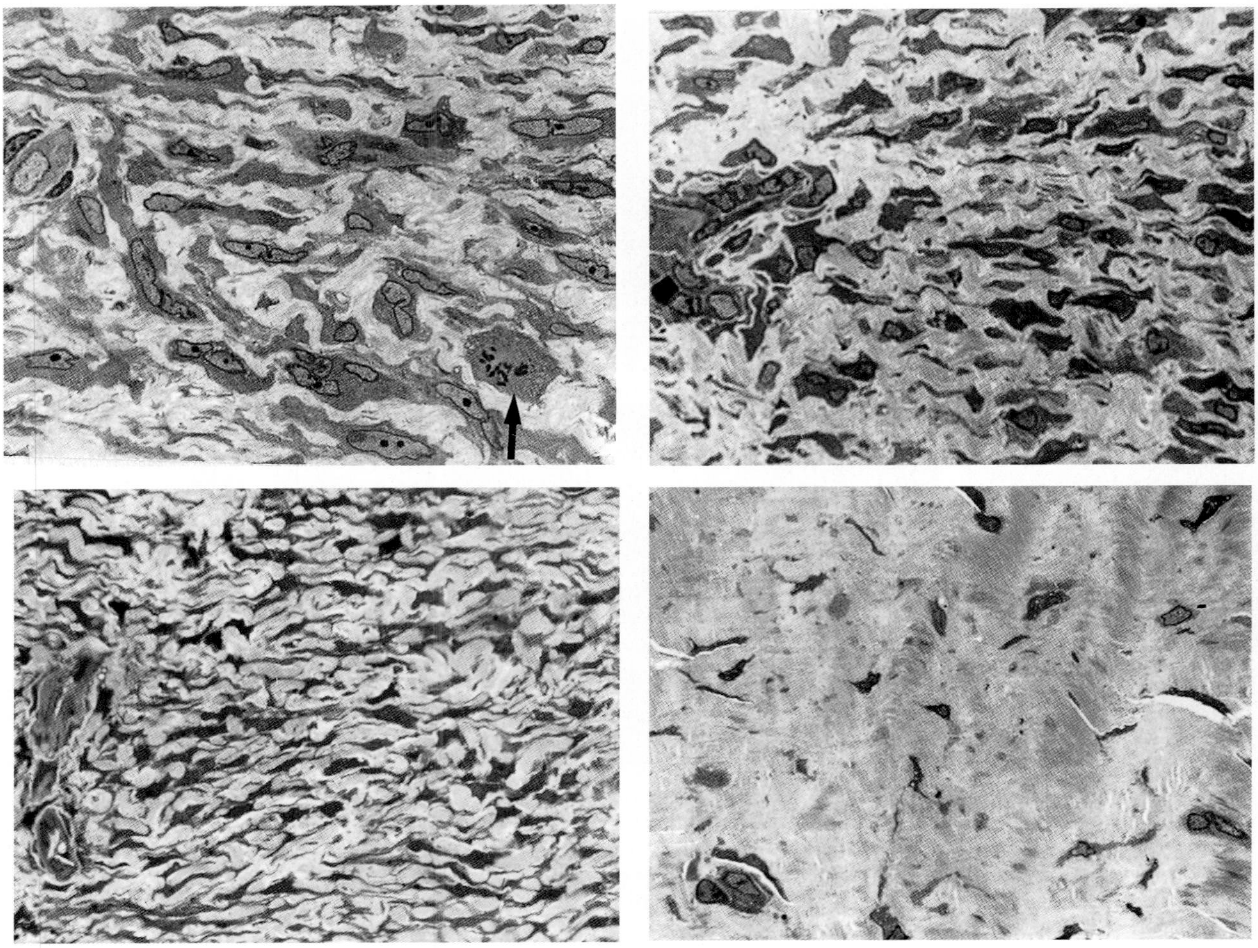


**FIG. 7.** Dupuytren's disease: toluidine blue-stained semithin sections. **A,** Proliferative phase nodule illustrating large elongated cells with numerous cytoplasmic extensions and indented nuclei, some of them in division (*arrow*). **B, C,** Involutional phase nodule composed of aligned spindle cells which display fewer and shorter cytoplasmic extensions than in (A) and which are also smaller in size. **D,** Residual phase nodule showing slender spindle cells in a poorly vascularized and intensely collagenous matrix.

immunoelectron microscopic techniques, $\alpha$-smooth muscle actin is localized within bundles of microfilaments of myofibroblasts of proliferative and involutional phase nodules.

Residual phase nodules are hypocellular, and the slender and aligned cells are surrounded by thick bands of collagen, giving them a tendonlike appearance (Fig. 7D). By ultrastructure, these nodules are composed of mature fibroblasts (Fig. 9A), some containing discrete subplasmalemmal bundles of microfilaments without dense bodies. The fibroblasts are connected by occasional poorly developed adherens-type junctions (Fig. 9A, inset), but gap junctions are no longer observed. The slender fibroblasts show smooth, contoured nuclei and are embedded in a dense collagenous matrix formed by thick bands of tightly packed collagen fibers. In conclusion, significant ultrastructural differences exist between proliferative, involutional, and residual phase nodules in Dupuytren's disease in relation to the cells, intercellular junctions, and extracellular matrix composition.

When the collagenous matrix of Dupuytren's disease is analyzed by immunohistochemical techniques, proliferative phase nodules reveal a predominance of type III collagen, whereas in the residual fibroblastic phase, type I collagen predominates (59). Differences between proliferative and residual phase nodules concern also the vascularization. In proliferative phase nodules, capillaries are numerous and feature, ultrastructurally, large and prominent pericytes displaying distinct smooth muscle differentiation, whereas in residual phase nodules, capillaries are few in number and are surrounded by small and inconspicuous pericytes devoid of a well-developed microfilamentous apparatus (26). Analogous to wound healing, the cicatrizing process within proliferative and involutional phase nodules is centripetal, being completed within residual phase nodules.

When immunohistochemical techniques are employed to study the different phases of Dupuytren's disease, the following results are obtained. Cells of proliferative phase nod-

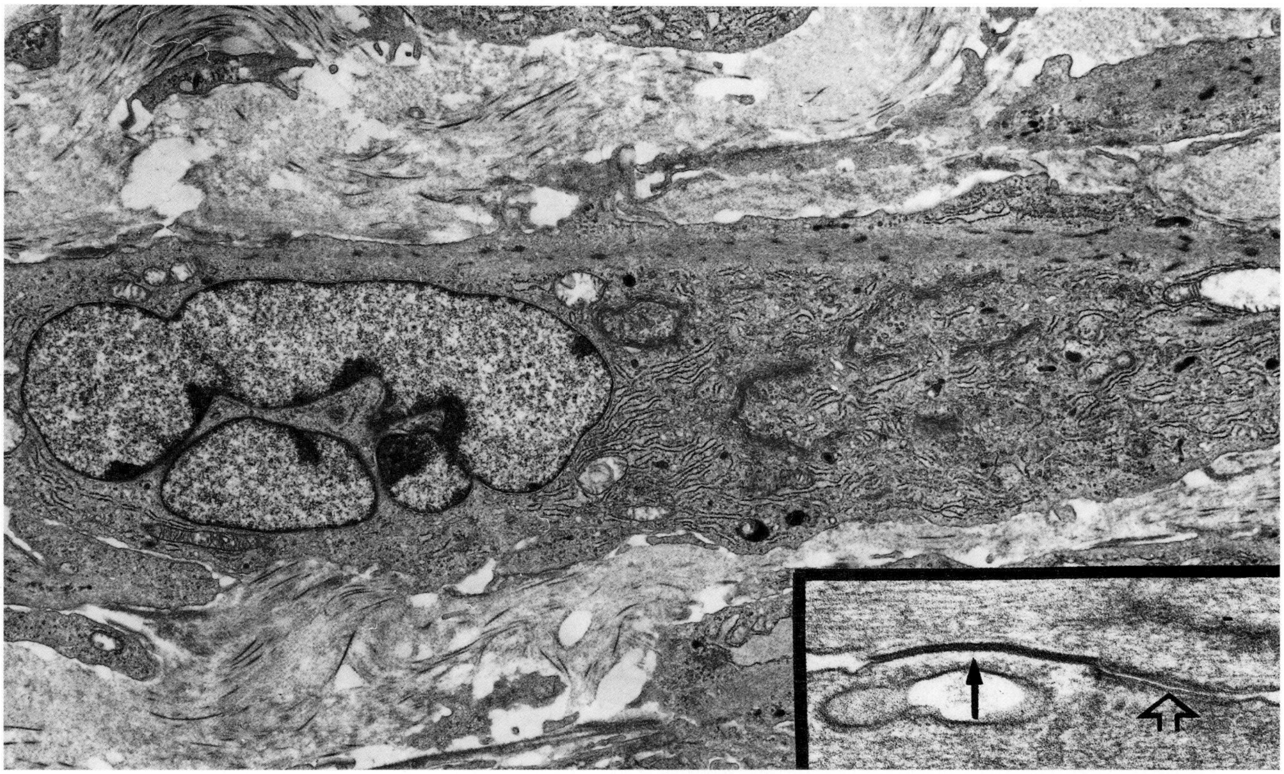

A

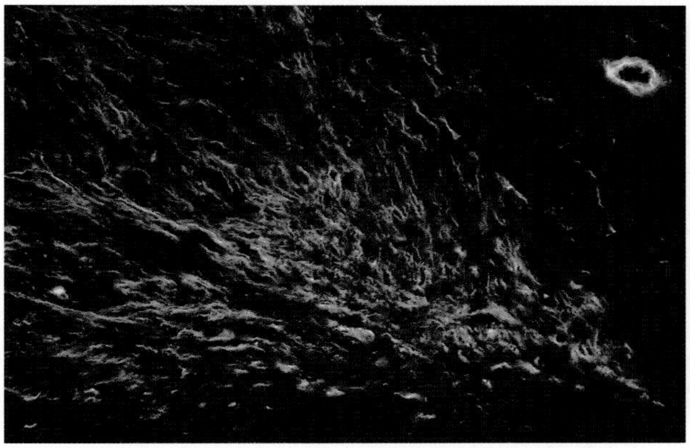

B

C

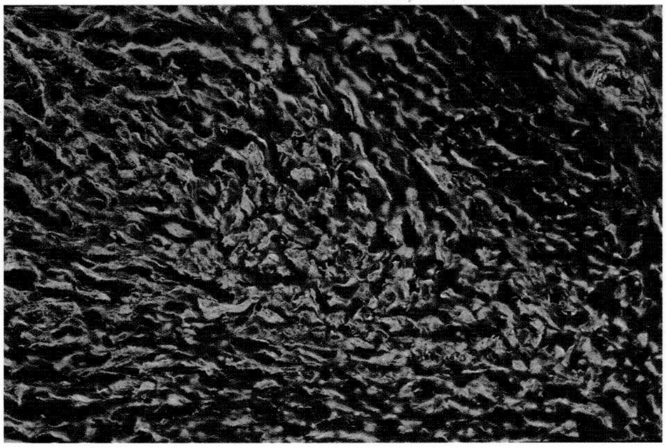

D

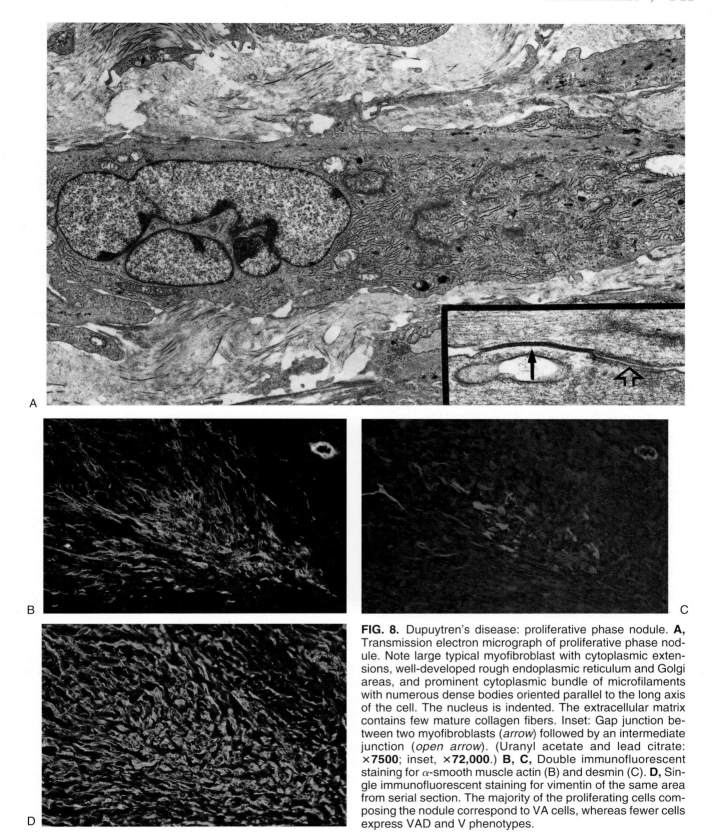

**FIG. 8.** Dupuytren's disease: proliferative phase nodule. **A,** Transmission electron micrograph of proliferative phase nodule. Note large typical myofibroblast with cytoplasmic extensions, well-developed rough endoplasmic reticulum and Golgi areas, and prominent cytoplasmic bundle of microfilaments with numerous dense bodies oriented parallel to the long axis of the cell. The nucleus is indented. The extracellular matrix contains few mature collagen fibers. Inset: Gap junction between two myofibroblasts (*arrow*) followed by an intermediate junction (*open arrow*). (Uranyl acetate and lead citrate: **×7500**; inset, **×72,000**.) **B, C,** Double immunofluorescent staining for $\alpha$-smooth muscle actin (B) and desmin (C). **D,** Single immunofluorescent staining for vimentin of the same area from serial section. The majority of the proliferating cells composing the nodule correspond to VA cells, whereas fewer cells express VAD and V phenotypes.

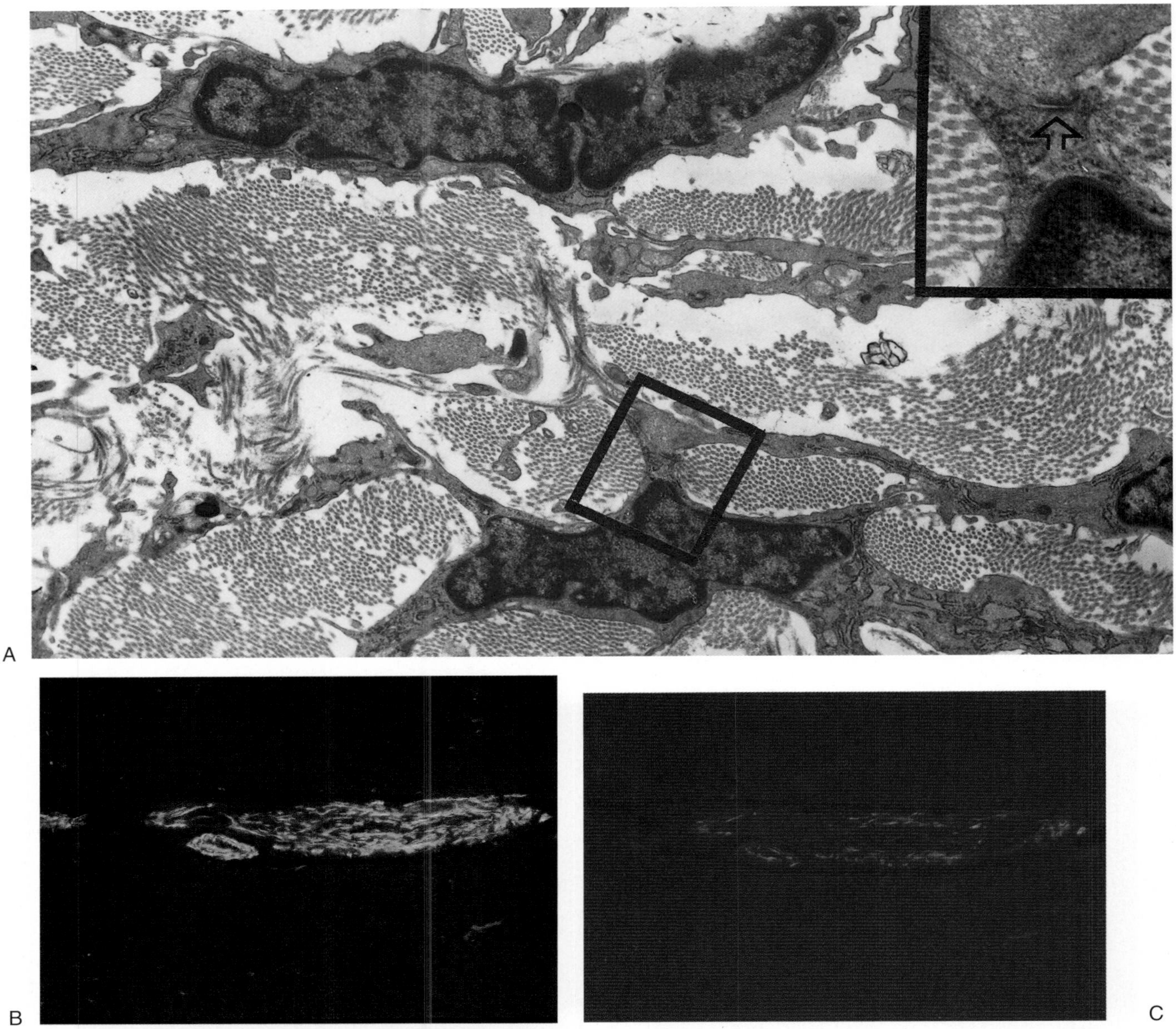


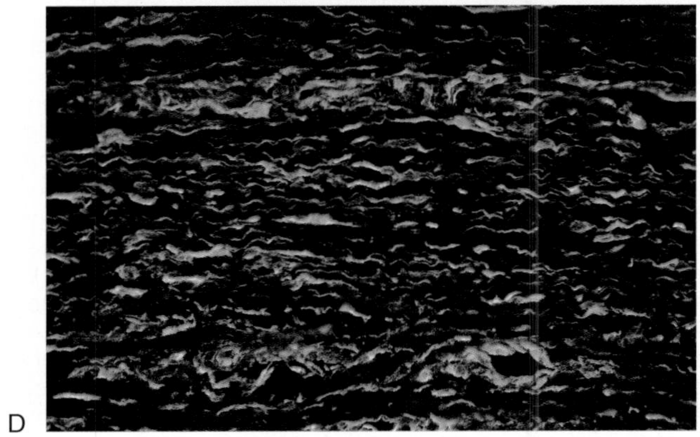


**FIG. 9.** Dupuytren's disease: residual phase nodule. **A,** Transmission electron micrograph illustrating slender fibroblasts with smooth contoured nuclei embedded in a dense collagenous matrix and joined by poorly differentiated junction (*open arrow, inset*). (Uranyl acetate and lead citrate: ×**12,150**; inset, ×**40,500**.) (From ref. 27.) **B, C,** Double immunofluorescent staining for $\alpha$-smooth muscle actin (B) and desmin (C). **D,** Single immunofluorescent staining for vimentin of the same area from serial section. Cells composing the residual phase nodule correspond to V cells. A few isolated cells only express VAD or VA phenotypes.

ules always express vimentin, which is associated in approximately 80% of the cells with $\alpha$-smooth muscle actin (74), and in about 20 to 40% with desmin when double-labeling immunofluorescence techniques are performed (Fig. 8B–D). Rarely, isolated cells positive for vimentin, $\alpha$-smooth muscle actin, and smooth muscle myosin heavy chains with or without desmin are present (VA(D)M-phenotype)(138). In involutional phase nodules desmin-positive cells are less numerous or even absent, whereas $\alpha$-smooth muscle actin-positive cells are still present, albeit in lesser numbers. In residual phase nodules a few or no $\alpha$-smooth muscle actin-positive cells persist, and the remaining slender cells express only vimentin (Fig. 9B–D). According to these results the cells constituting the nodules of Dupuytren's disease express different cytoskeletal phenotypes: (a) phenotype V; (b) phenotype VAD; (c) phenotype VA; and (d) phenotype VD. In most proliferative phase nodules of Dupuytren's disease and also in the cellular areas of musculoaponeurotic fibromatoses, the number of VA cells exceeds considerably the number of VAD and VD cells (24). At the interphase of proliferative and sclerotic, heavily collagenized areas of these conditions, the number of VAD and VD cells decreases progressively and is replaced by an almost pure population of V cells (24,26,198). Despite their heterogeneity in intermediate filament proteins and actin isoforms, myofibroblasts from Dupuytren's disease (100,197) express usually only non-muscle myosins. Exceptionally, isolated cells expressing smooth muscle myosin heavy chains (VA(D)M-phenotypes are observed (138). In these tissues, the extracellular matrix around myofibroblasts is strongly stained with antibodies to antifibronectin, but not for laminin (197,201).

#### *Other Quasineoplastic Proliferative Conditions*

A heterogeneous cytoskeletal composition is also observed in myofibroblasts of dermatofibromas, which reveal at least three cytoskeletal phenotypes: VA, VAD, and V cells with a predominance of VA cells in cellular dermatofibromas and an almost exclusive composition of V cells in fibrous dermatofibromas (202). Whether myofibroblasts of the VA(D)M phenotype exist has not yet been determined. By ultrastructure, cellular dermatofibromas are composed of well-developed myofibroblasts, joined by gap and intermediate junctions, admixed with variable numbers of fibroblasts and macrophages. Fibrous dermatofibromas, in contrast, are composed almost exclusively of fibroblasts and contain some poorly developed myofibroblasts. This heterogeneous cellular and cytoskeletal phenotypic composition permits one to distinguish this lesion from dermatofibrosarcoma protuberans, which represents a pure fibroblastic neoplasm, both at the ultrastructural level and with regard to the cytoskeletal phenotype (202). Furthermore, the heterogeneous cytoskeletal composition of dermatofibroma identifies this lesion definitively as a quasineoplastic, reactive proliferative condition, whereas dermatofibrosarcoma protuberans represents a fibroblastic neoplasm (202).

Nodular and proliferative fasciitis are predominantly composed of myofibroblasts with similar cytoskeletal phenotypes, which are VA and rare VAD cells, the latter more prominent in the proliferative variant (Fig. 10). Infantile myofibromatosis reveals a predominance of VA cells with limited numbers of VAD cells. By ultrastructure, in contrast to other fibromatoses, smooth muscle differentiation appears to be more prominent than in conventional fibromatoses, although typical myofibroblasts are numerous, a feature that justifies the term "infantile myofibromatosis." Furthermore, massive apoptosis has been documented in infantile myofibromatosis and proposed as a putative mechanism of regression of this proliferative myofibroblastic lesion (203), (for apoptosis, see below).

#### *Stromal Response to Neoplasia*

Many invasive and metastatic carcinomas are characterized by hard consistency and retraction, and are often fixed to adjacent tissues. Typical examples are invasive ductal mammary carcinomas, associated with skin and or nipple retraction (Fig. 11A), annular stenosing colon carcinomas (Fig. 11B), gastric linitis plastica, the so-called "frozen pelvis" in advanced gynecological carcinomas, and metastatic carcinomas to lymph nodes that are fixed to surrounding tissues and the overlying skin. The hard consistency and the retraction phenomena are due to the desmoplastic stromal reaction. Myofibroblasts are particularly numerous within the stroma of primary invasive and metastatic carcinomas (6, 20–23,204), and the retraction associated with such carcinomas is attributed to the contractile forces generated by stromal myofibroblasts. Myofibroblasts are not observed in the stroma contiguous to in situ carcinomas (Figs. 12 and 13) (6,23), suggesting that invasion beyond the basal lamina is required to evoke a myofibroblastic stromal reaction. These cells are notably absent or equivocally present within carcinomas lacking significant stromal desmoplasia (Fig. 14) (23).

Myofibroblasts are not uniformly distributed within desmoplastic carcinomas. When their spatial relation to other components of breast carcinomas is analyzed, they are most numerous within the young mesenchymal stroma, areas corresponding to early stromal invasion, or, more consistently, in the peripheral invasive cellular front of mammary carcinomas (Fig. 15A–F, and 16A) (23). In the central sclerotic area of such neoplasms, myofibroblasts are poorly developed or absent, this, possibly, a reflection of apoptosis (Figs. 15G,H and 16B) (23). Similarly, myofibroblasts are numerous in the cellular, edematous, and poorly collagenized stroma of other invasive and metastatic carcinomas (23). Three types of myofibroblastic stromal reactions are observed within ductal-infiltrating mammary carcinomas: (a) precocious (Figs. 15A,B), myofibroblasts precede the carcinoma cells by some distance into adjacent tissue; (b) synchronous (Figs. 15C,D), myofibroblasts appear spatially among the carcinoma cells; and (c) late (Figs. 15E,F), myofibroblasts are identified central to the periph-

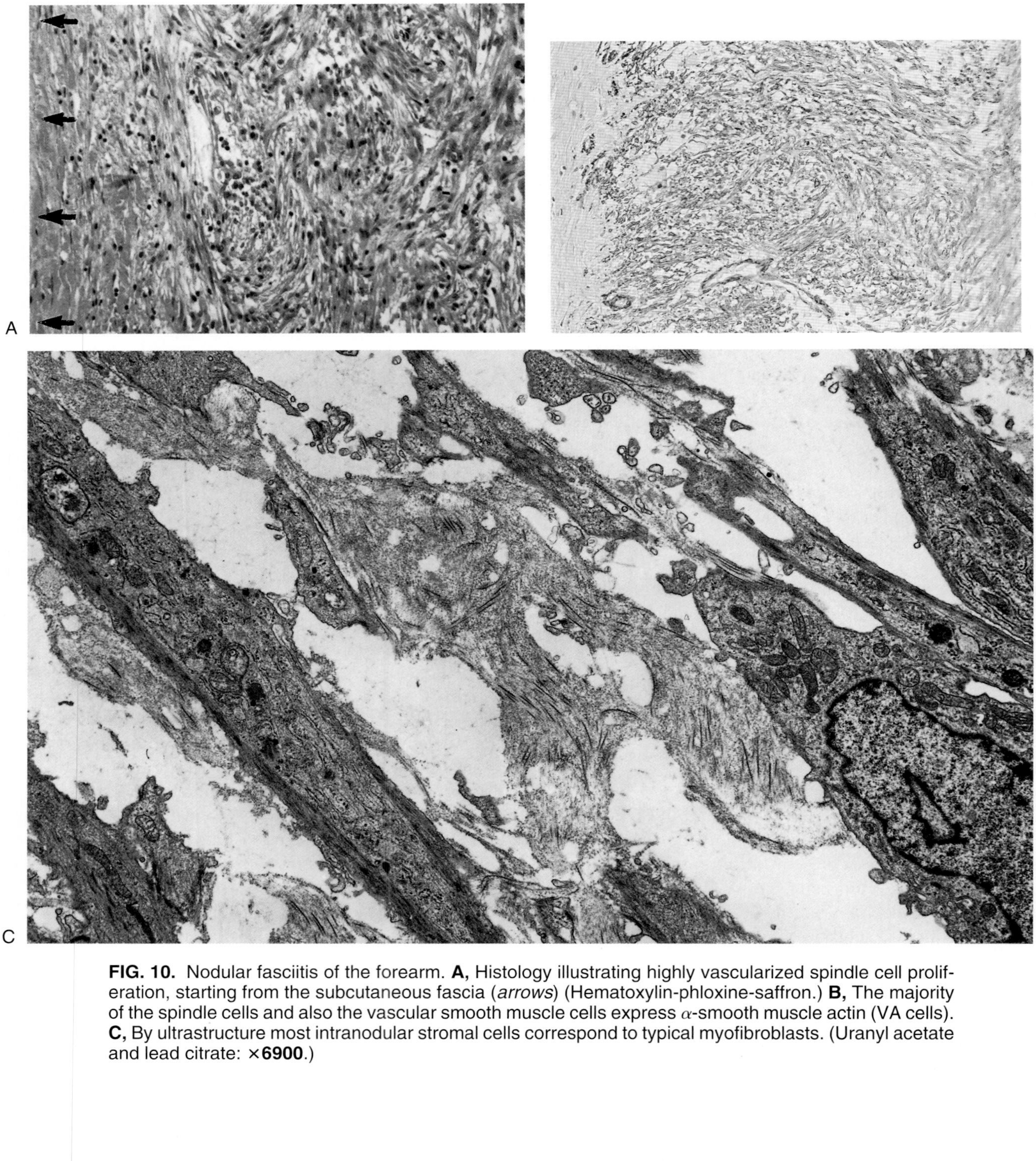

**FIG. 10.** Nodular fasciitis of the forearm. **A,** Histology illustrating highly vascularized spindle cell proliferation, starting from the subcutaneous fascia (*arrows*) (Hematoxylin-phloxine-saffron.) **B,** The majority of the spindle cells and also the vascular smooth muscle cells express $\alpha$-smooth muscle actin (VA cells). **C,** By ultrastructure most intranodular stromal cells correspond to typical myofibroblasts. (Uranyl acetate and lead citrate: ×**6900**.)

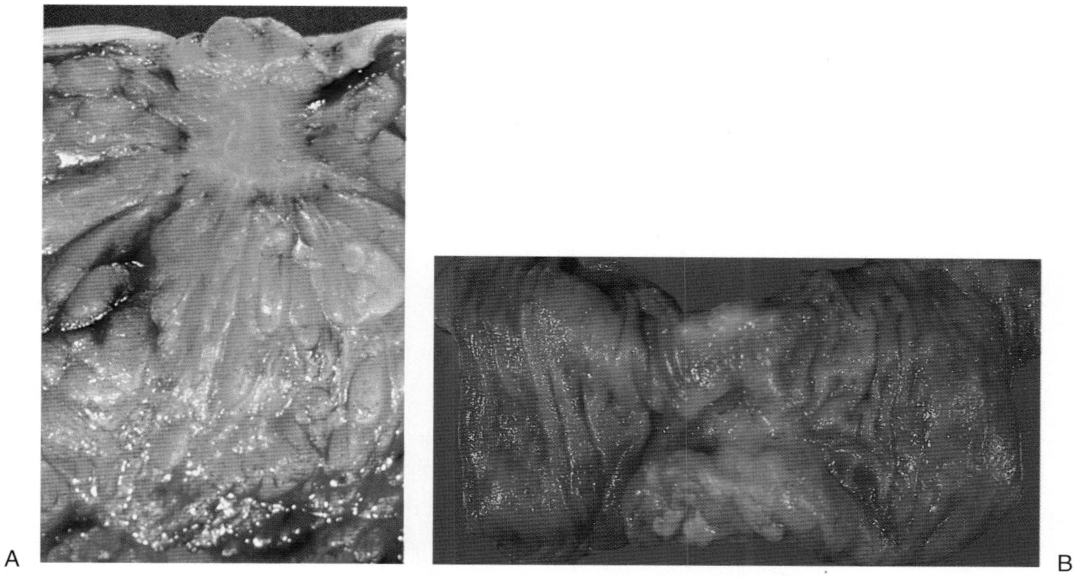

FIG. 11. Gross appearance of infiltrating ductal carcinoma of the breast and of infiltrating colon carcinoma. **A,** Note irregular stellate shape of the carcinoma, retraction of the cut surface, and retraction of the nipple. **B,** The colon carcinoma shows a circular and annular stenosis. The carcinoma was invading the pericolic fatty tissue.

eral invasive cellular front of the carcinoma cells (23). The three types of myofibroblastic stromal reactions (precocious, synchronous and late) are observed in different areas of the invading front of most infiltrating ductal carcinomas of the breast, the synchronous stromal reaction being usually predominant (23). When the collagenous matrix is analyzed, increased amounts of type III collagen are present within the young mesenchyme, areas with numerous myofibroblasts. In contrast, type I collagen is most prominent within the central sclerotic zone of breast carcinomas (62), areas in which myofibroblasts are replaced by fibroblasts (Figs. 16B) (22,23).

Many pulmonary carcinomas, especially peripheral adenocarcinomas, are associated with some degree of scarring and are often associated with pleural retraction. If this process is pronounced, the term *scar carcinoma* is applied to these neoplasms. In 1962, Carroll (205) reported that the presence of elastic fibers and anthracotic pigment in scars suggested that they had been present prior to the development of the neoplasm. The more recent literature suggests

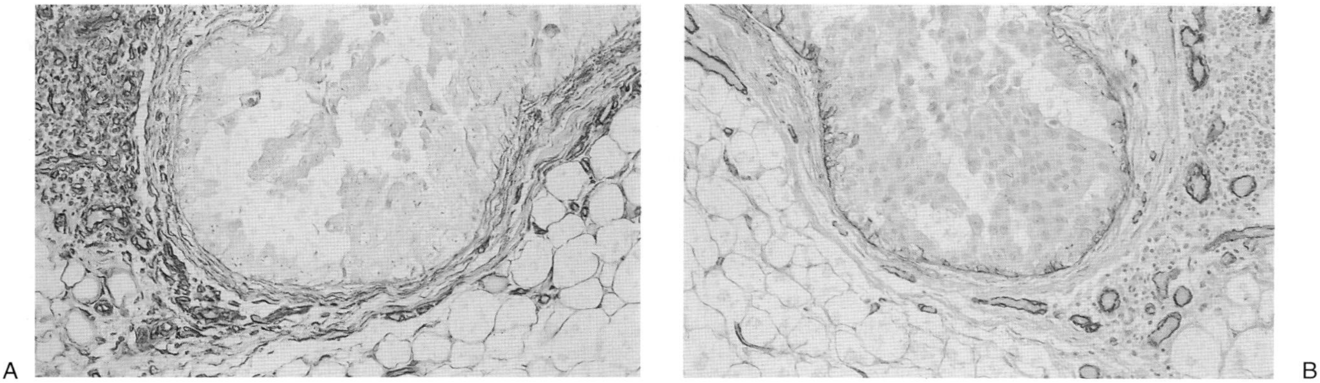

FIG. 12. Histological aspect of ductal in situ carcinoma of the breast. **A,** The periductal stromal cells are numerous and disclose intense immunostaining for vimentin. **B,** Same area as in (A). Periductal stromal cells lack significant immunostaining for $\alpha$-smooth muscle actin. A continuous flattened layer of myoepithelial cells and vascular smooth muscle cells of periductal stromal vessels are stained with this antibody. (Avidin-biotin-complex-peroxidase.)

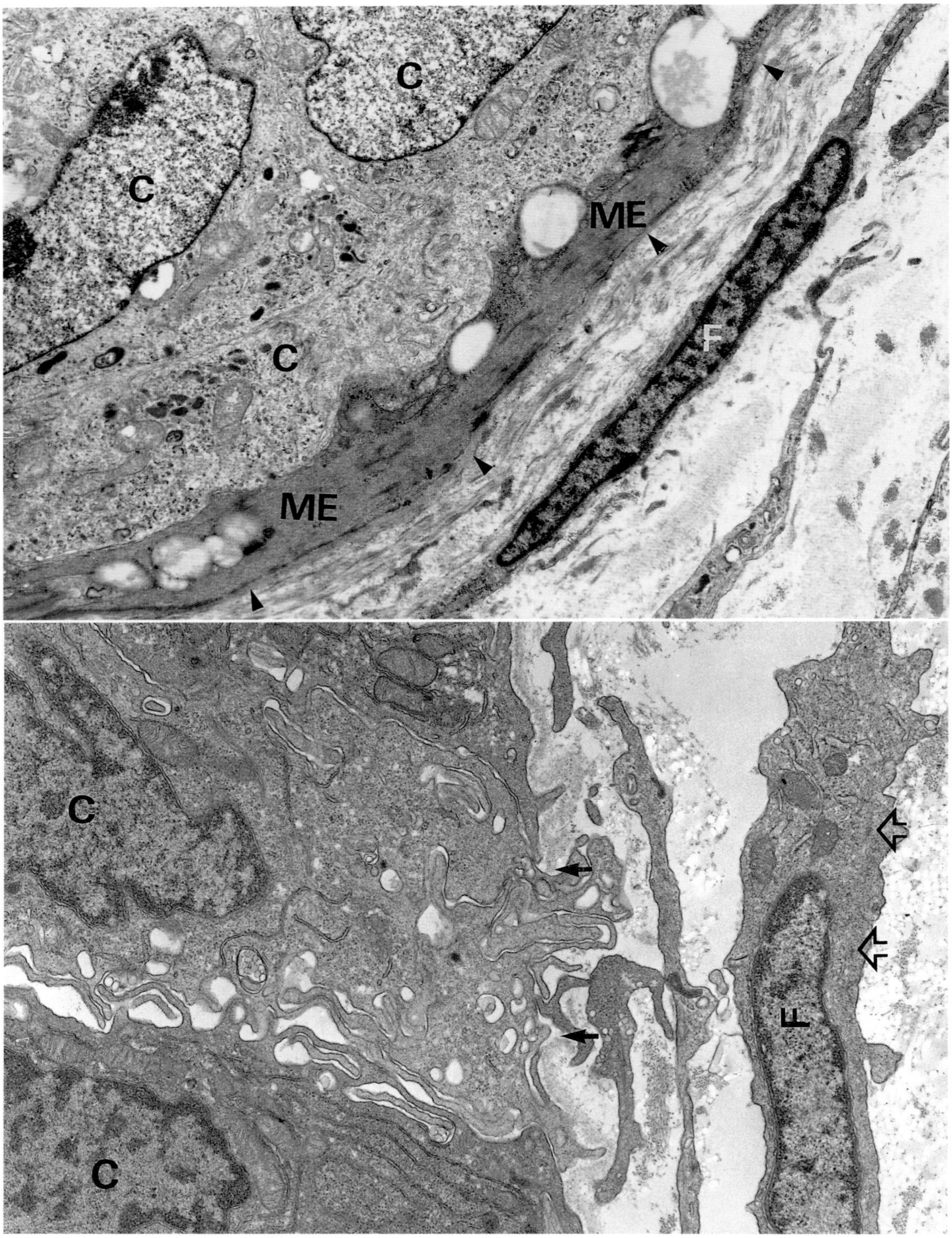


A

B

**FIG. 13.** Ultrastructural aspect of ductal in situ carcinoma of the breast. **A,** A continuous layer of myoepithelial cells (ME) and a continuous basal lamina (*arrowheads*) separate the carcinoma cells (C) from the surrounding stroma. The stromal fibroblast (F) discloses smooth cellular and nuclear contours; the cytoplasm is scant and devoid of bundles of microfilaments. **B,** Ultramicroinvasive ductal in situ carcinoma. A carcinoma cell (C) protrudes with a cytoplasmic extension into the periductal stroma through a gap within the basal lamina (*arrows*). The periductal fibroblast reveals abundant cytoplasm and discloses aggregates of microfilaments with attenuated dense bodies (*open arrows*). (Uranyl acetate and lead citrate: A, ×**11,250**; B, ×**13,500**.)

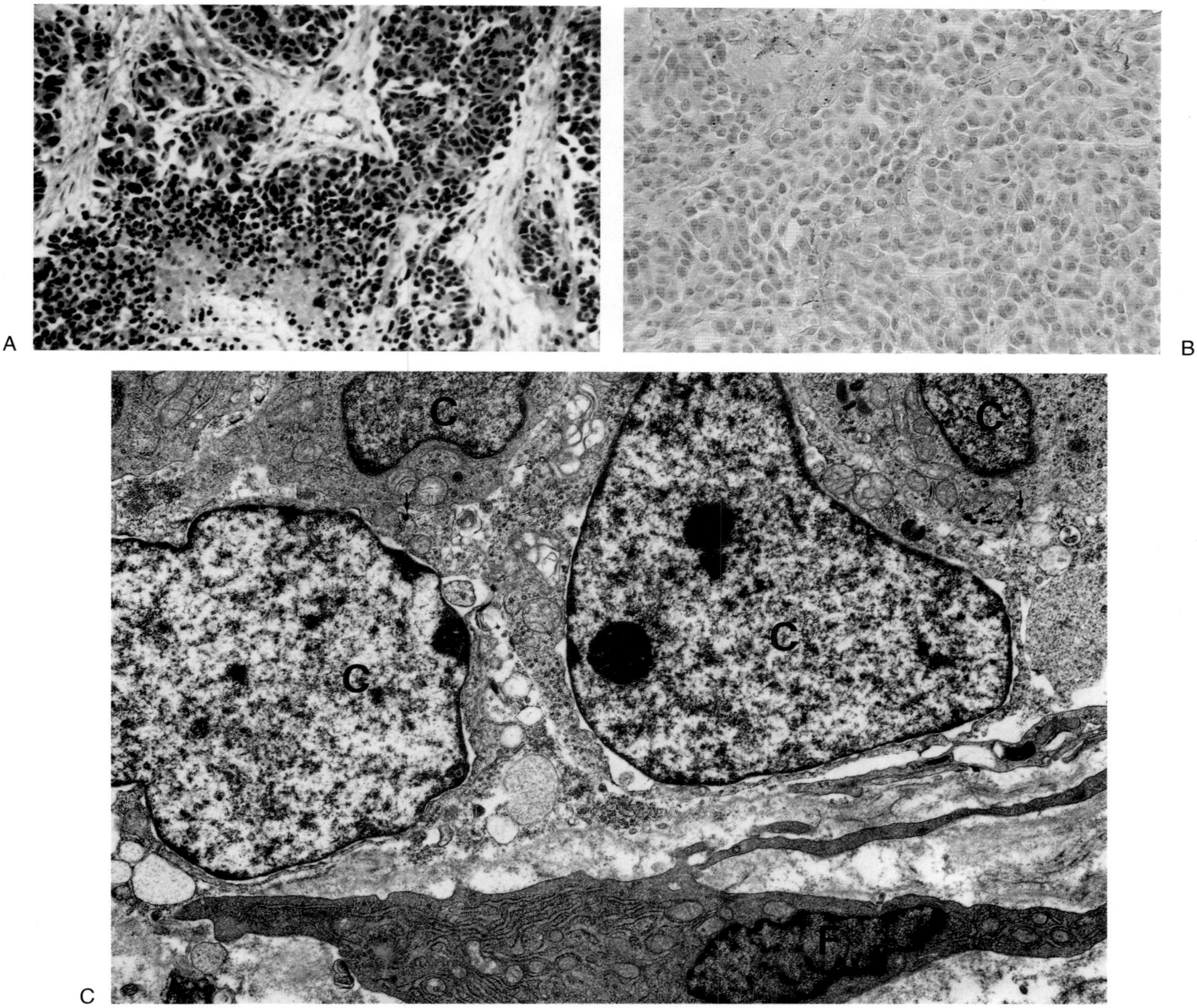


**FIG. 14.** Oat-cell carcinoma of the lung. **A,** Histological aspect illustrating clusters of small neoplastic cells separated by small connective tissue septa. (Hematoxylin-phloxine-saffron.) **B,** Stromal cells reveal no significant staining for $\alpha$-smooth muscle actin. (Avidin-biotin-complex-peroxidase.) **C,** Transmission electron micrograph illustrating neoplastic cells (C) with scattered electron-dense neurosecretory-type granules (arrows) in close vicinity of a fibroblast (F), with a smooth, contoured nucleus, that is devoid of microfilaments. (Uranyl acetate and lead citrate: ×**10,300**.)

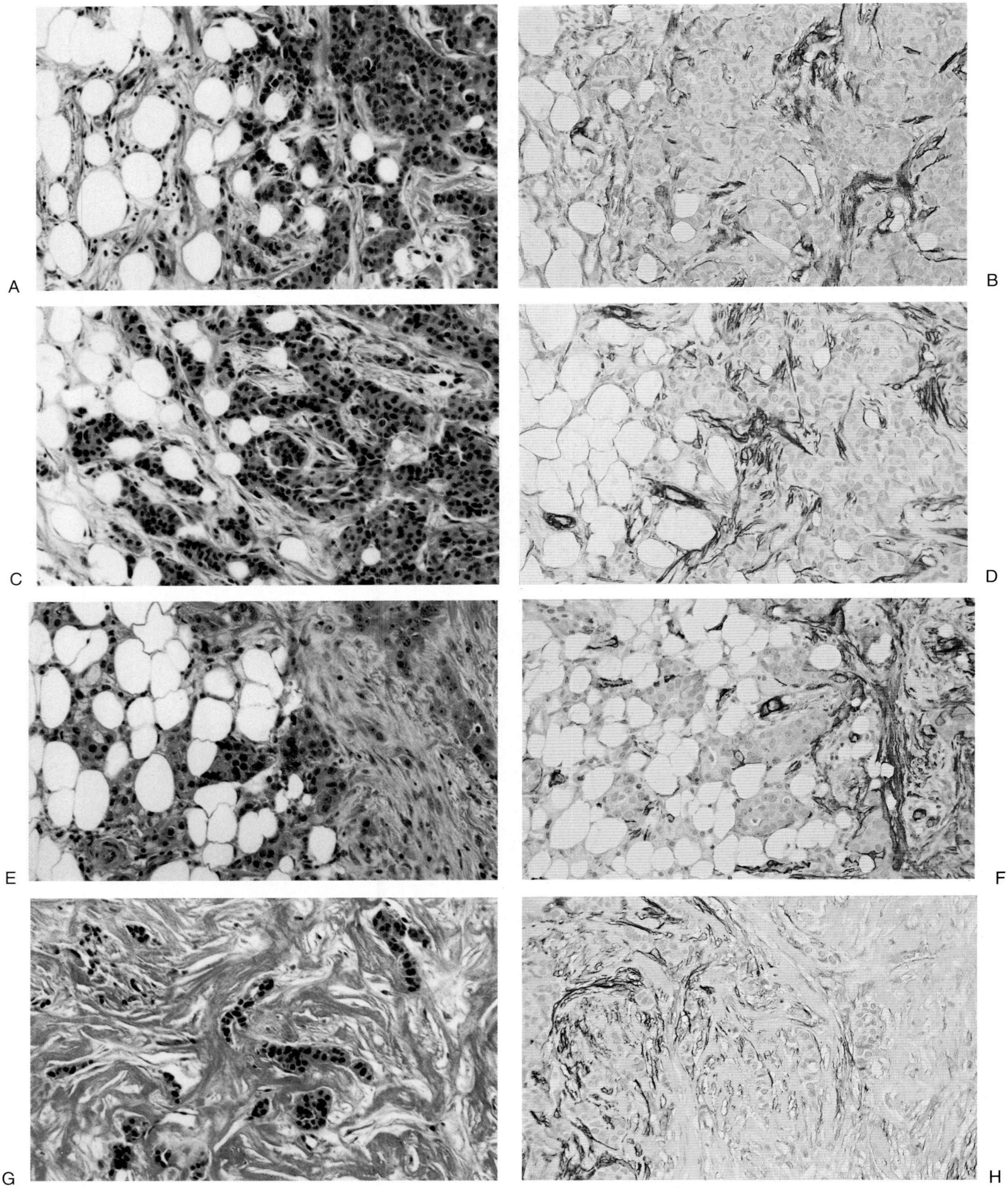

**FIG. 15.** Ductal-infiltrating carcinoma of the breast with stromal desmoplasia. **A, B,** Precocious stromal reaction; that is, stromal cells precede carcinoma cells by some distance into the adjacent fatty tissue. The majority of these stromal cells reveal immunostaining for $\alpha$-smooth muscle actin (B). **C, D,** Synchronous stromal reaction; that is, stromal cells appear spatially among the carcinoma cells. Most of these stromal cells express immunostaining for $\alpha$-smooth muscle actin (D).

that scarring represents a desmoplastic stromal reaction in response to neoplastic invasion, rather than a preexistent condition. In favor of this latter interpretation is the presence of increased amounts of type III collagen within pulmonary carcinomas with marked scarring (206). A predominance of type III collagen is also found in early invasive zones of mammary carcinomas (60). In addition, the majority of stromal cells in scar carcinomas of the lung reveal by ultrastructure, typical features of myofibroblasts (207), suggesting that pulmonary carcinomas with scarring are neoplasms with a desmoplastic stromal reaction, analogous to many invasive and metastatic carcinomas elsewhere (Fig. 17).

Analysis of cytoskeletal proteins, including intermediate filaments, actin isoforms, and smooth muscle myosin heavy chains, reveals phenotypic heterogeneity of stromal cells in invasive and metastatic carcinomas. Areas with numerous myofibroblasts, corresponding to early stromal invasion of breast carcinomas, contain a predominance of VA cells admixed with variable numbers of VAD, VA(D)M and V cells (Fig. 18), suggesting that certain stromal cells undergo definitive smooth muscle metaplasia (VA(D)M-cells). On the contrary, sclerotic areas disclose numerous V cells with occasional VA cells. VAD and VA(D)M cells are not observed (Results not shown).

Myofibroblasts have also been described in sarcomas where they generally constitute a small fraction of the cell population (208–210). They were identified in all cases of malignant fibrous histiocytomas and well-differentiated sclerosing liposarcomas (210). Though most numerous in areas of desmoplasia (Fig. 19), in no instance did myofibroblasts constitute the dominant cellular constituent of either neoplasm (210). Myofibroblasts have been identified with lesser frequency, and in smaller numbers in fibrosarcoma, synovial sarcoma, malignant hemangiopericytoma, and neuroblastoma. No myofibroblasts or equivocal forms were observed in a wide assortment of diverse sarcomas in which desmoplasia was not a feature.

Myofibroblasts were also identified in nodular sclerosing Hodgkin's disease; that is, at the nodule-stromal interphase, which is usually heavily collagenized (211). These areas contain numerous VA and V cells with very occasional VAD cells (Fig. 20).

### *Neoplasms of Myofibroblasts*

Finally, several reports describe myofibroblastic tumors, some considered sarcomas (212–214),others as benign myofibroblastomas (215–217), although the existence of such neoplasms has been questioned (6). Myofibroblasts generally signal a host response, whether to inflammation, injury, or neoplasia. Thus, according to this definition, a proliferative condition composed of myofibroblasts might belong to the group of quasineoplastic proliferative conditions, rather than the category of true neoplasms. Most of the conditions identified as myofibroblastic sarcomas lack the typical morphologic and cytoskeletal features of myofibroblasts as described originally (1,3,19,24,25) or were not sufficiently characterized. A sarcoma composed entirely or partially of cells disclosing some degree of morphologic and immunohistochemical features of myofibroblastic differentiation, but lacking the typical traits of myofibroblasts, as defined initially (1,3) could well belong to the group of myogenic sarcomas (218–220). It has to be kept in mind that the appearance and disappearance of myofibroblasts is mediated through a complex mechanism that implies changes within the microenvironment (growth factors and cytokines), and, that myofibroblasts above all, represent terminally differentiated cells which disappear through apoptosis. Thus, in our opinion, sarcomas of myofibroblasts have yet to be unequivocally demonstrated.

## THE ROLE OF CYTOKINES IN CONDITIONS ASSOCIATED WITH MYOFIBROBLAST PROLIFERATION

In the first edition of this book, this subject was not addressed because little was known about the process. Since then, a sizeable body of data has accumulated so that some discussion is appropriate. Since the myofibroblast was discovered in granulation tissue, it is not surprising that this model has served as the one best able to address the role of cytokines in the induction of the myofibroblast phenotype in reactive processes related to wound healing.

Utilizing the subcutaneously implanted mini-osmotic pump, this model allows for the direct introduction of diverse cytokines into wounds, followed by detailed morphologic (histologic and ultrastructural), immunohistochemical, and molecular analyses of the granulating wounds. Employing diverse cytokines in this perfusion model, it was shown that granulocyte macrophage colony stimulating factor (GM-CSF), tumor necrosis factor-alpha (TNF-$\alpha$), interleukin-1-$\alpha$ (IL-1-$\alpha$), transforming growth factor-beta (TGF-$\beta$), and platelet-derived growth factor (PDGF) affected fibroblast accumulation, neovascularization, and a modest

**FIG. 15.** *Continued.* **E, F,** Late stromal reaction; that is, stromal cells appear central to the peripheral invasive front of carcinoma cells and express immunostaining for $\alpha$-smooth muscle actin (F).**G, H,** Central sclerotic area of ductal-infiltrating carcinoma) Clusters of carcinoma cells are surrounded by thick bands of collagen (G). At the border of the invasive cellular front of the carcinoma a decrease of the immunostaining of the stromal cells toward the central area (left to right side) is observed. (A, C, E, and G, Hematoxylin–phloxine–saffron; B, D, F, and H, Avidin–biotin–complex–peroxidase.)

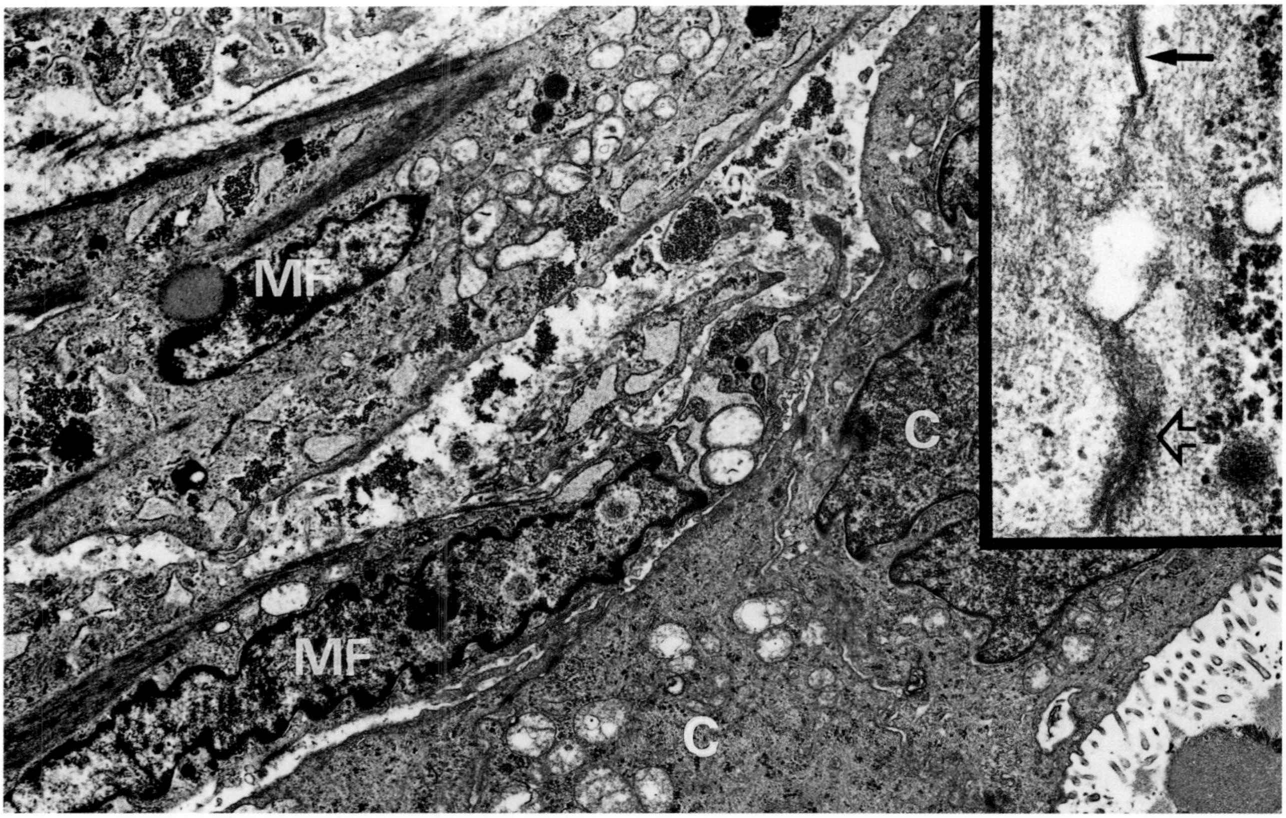


A

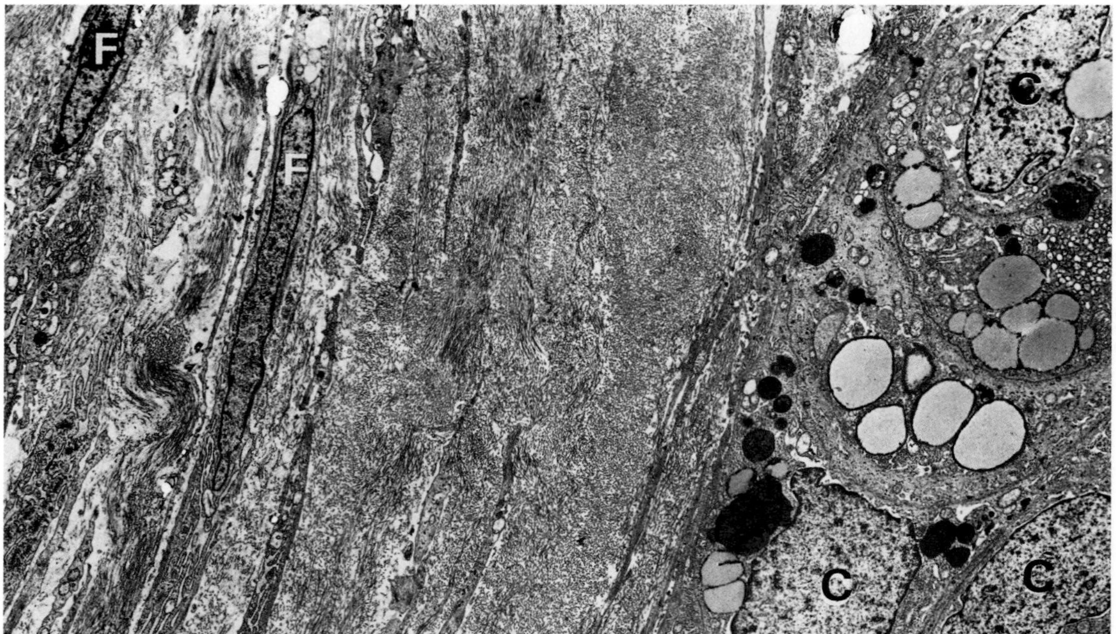


B

**FIG. 16.** Ultrastructural aspect of ductal-infiltrating carcinoma of the breast. **A,** Peripheral invasive cellular front revealing numerous typical stromal myofibroblasts (MF) with notched nuclei and bundles of cytoplasmic microfilaments with dense bodies around neoplastic cells (C) around an acinus. Stromal myofibroblasts are joined by gap (arrow) and intermediate junctions (open arrow). **B,** Central sclerotic area illustrating stromal cells (F) with smooth contoured nuclei devoid of abundant cytoplasmic microfilaments and separated by thick bands of mature collagen around clusters of carcinoma cells (C). (Uranyl acetate and lead citrate: A, ×**8400**; inset, ×**60,000;** B, ×**5000**.)

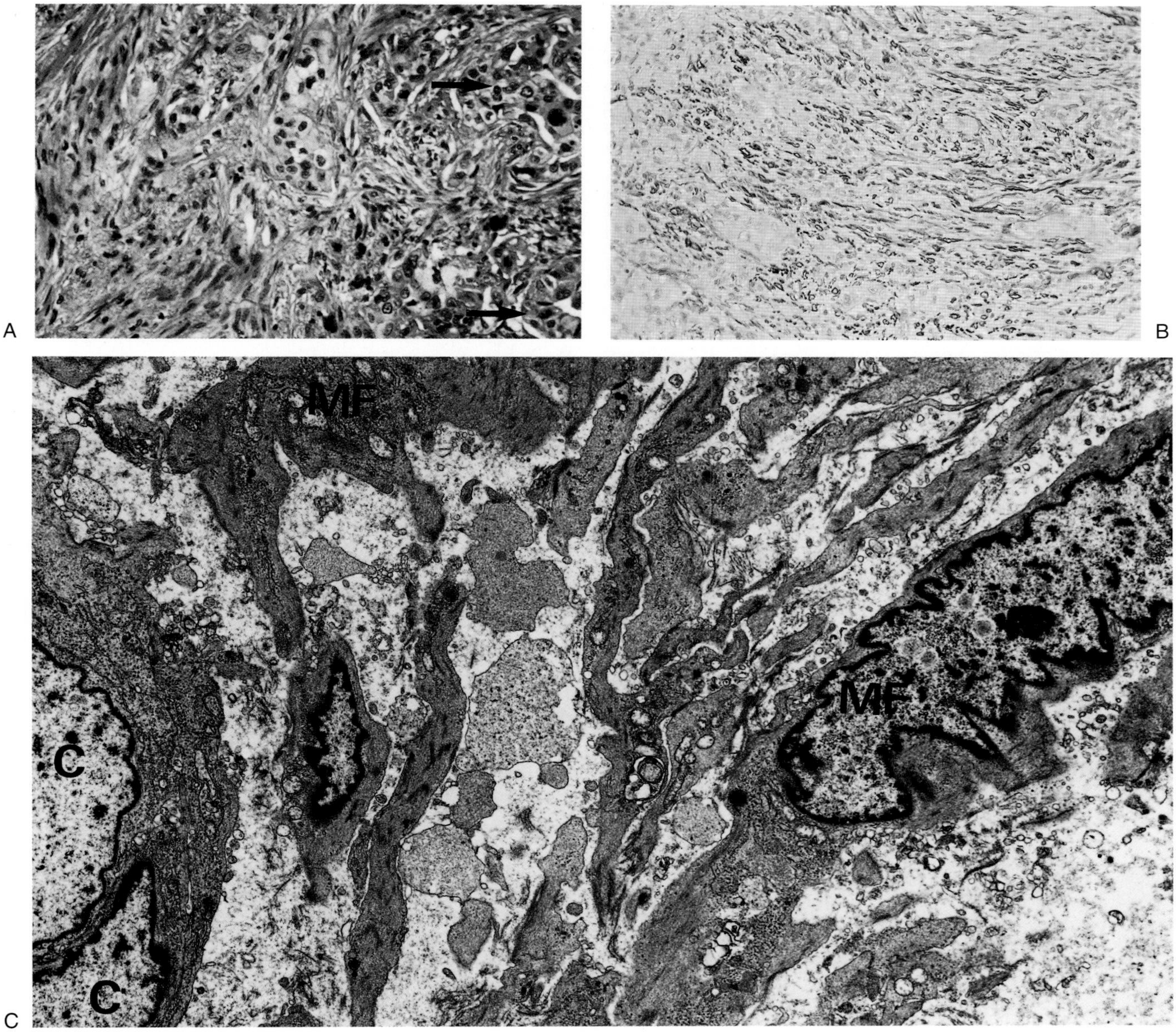


**FIG. 17.** Pulmonary "scar carcinoma." **A,** Histological aspect illustrating several neoplastic glands (*arrows*) at the border of the central desmoplastic area (Hematoxylin-phloxine-saffron.) **B,** The stromal cells are immunoreactive for anti-α-smooth muscle actin. **C,** Transmission electron micrograph illustrating several typical stromal myofibroblasts (MF) in a poorly collagenized matrix, surrounding clusters of neoplastic cells (C). (Uranyl acetate and lead citrate: ×**6900**.)

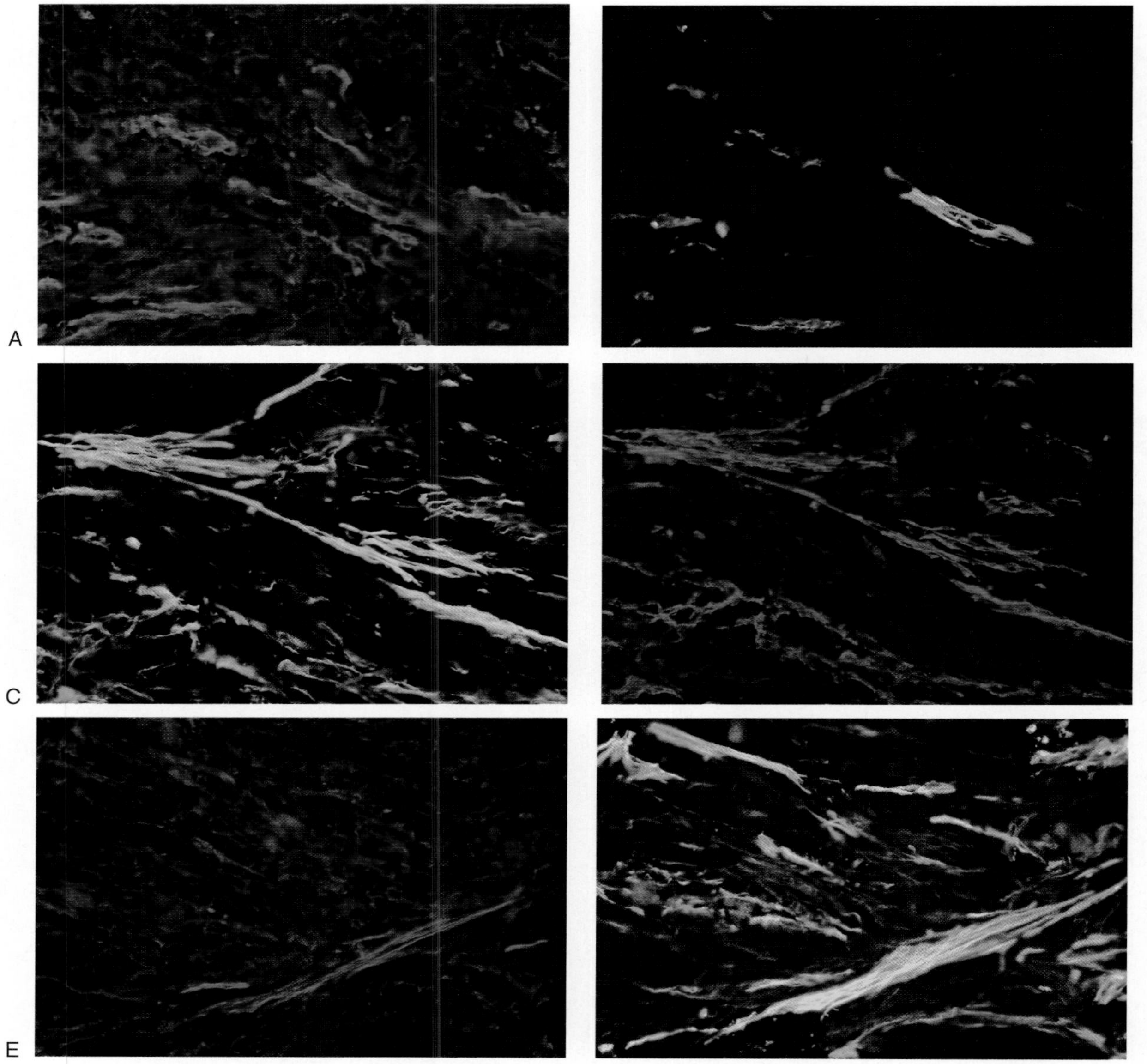

FIG. 18. Peripheral invasive cellular front of ductal breast carcinoma revealing V, VA, VAD, and VA(D)M myofibroblasts. **A and B,** Double immunofluorescent staining for $\alpha$-smooth muscle actin (A) and desmin (B): Stromal cells expressing $\alpha$-smooth muscle actin (VA-cells) are more numerous than those expressing $\alpha$-smooth muscle actin and desmin (VAD-cells). **C and D,** Double immunofluorescent staining for $\alpha$-smooth muscle actin (C) and smooth muscle myosin heavy chain (D): Stromal cells expressing $\alpha$-smooth muscle actin (VA-cells) are slightly more numerous than those expressing in addition smooth muscle myosin heavy chain (VAM-cells). **E and F,** Double immunofluorescent staining for desmin (E) and myosin heavy chain (F): Stromal cells expressing smooth muscle myosin heavy chain (VM–cells) are far more numerous than those that express in addition desmin (VDM-cells). In conclusion, the peripheral invasive front of ductal feast carcinomas contains predominantly VA-cells, followed by VA (D) M-cells.

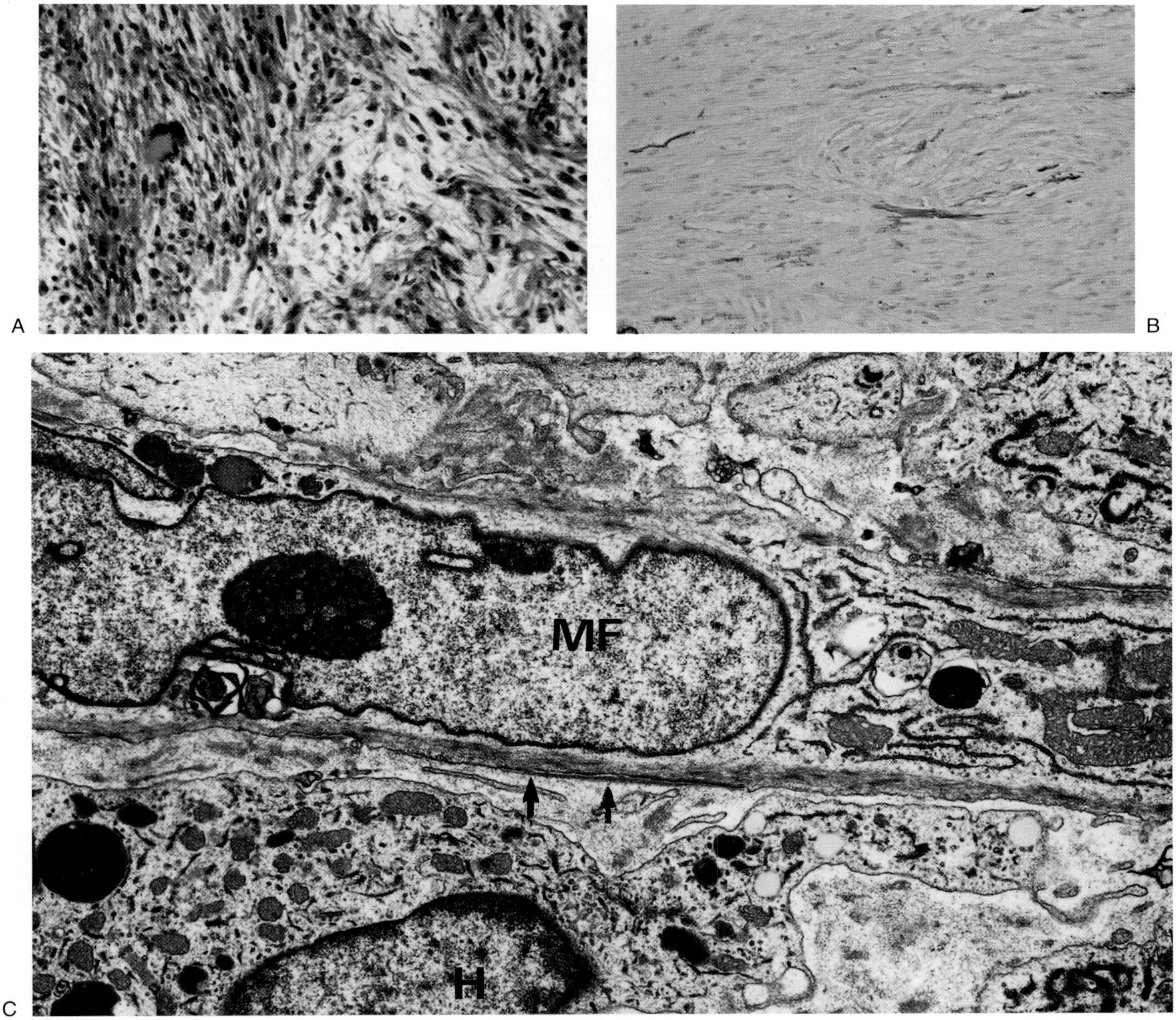


**FIG. 19.** Malignant fibrous histiocytoma (storiform-pleomorphic type). **A,** Histological aspect illustrating spindle cell tumor with storiform pattern and isolated pleomorphic cells. (Hematoxylin-phloxine-saffron.) **B,** Few spindle cells disclose immunostaining for $\alpha$-smooth muscle actin. (Avidin-biotin-complex-peroxidase.) **C,** Transmission electron micrograph illustrating a typical myofibroblast (MF), with cytoplasmic bundle of microfilaments, that is partly enveloped by a basal lamina (*arrows*). (Uranyl acetate and lead citrate: ×**25,000**.)

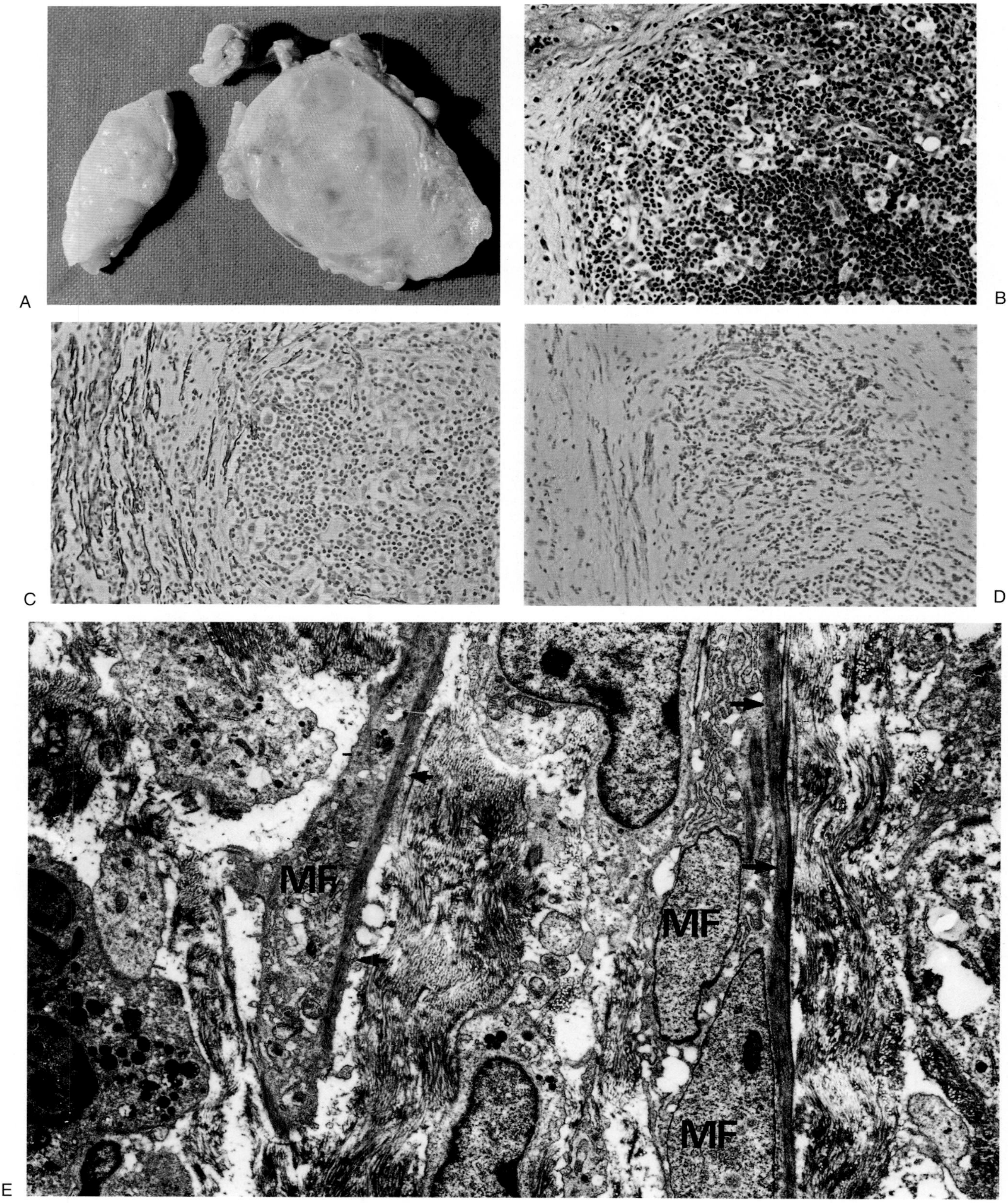
A
B
C
D
E
MF
MF
MF

mononuclear cell infiltrate. Yet among these, only GM-CSF induced a myofibroblast phenotype as reflected by the expression of $\alpha$-smooth muscle actin in the fibroblastic cell population (30). The same experiments showed that interferon-$\gamma$ (INF-$\gamma$) and interleukin-2 (IL-2) favored the ingress of macrophages into the wound. It was shown in subsequent experiments that the macrophage was critical to the induction of the myofibroblast phenotype, as GM-CSF, but not TNF-$\alpha$ or PDGF, stimulated an ingress and accumulation of macrophages into such wounds prior to the fibroblastic expression of $\alpha$-smooth muscle actin (29). About this time it was also shown that heparin, more specifically its nonanticoagulant derivates, induced fibroblasts toward a myofibroblast phenotype, both in the mini-osmotic pump model and in vitro in fibroblast cultures (27).

Subsequently, possibly the most significant fibrogenic cytokine, TGF-$\beta$1, was shown to induce $\alpha$-smooth muscle expression in granulating wounds and in quiescent growing fibroblasts (28). These series of experiments established clearly that, at least in healing wounds, the cellular phenotypes of the participants are modulated by proteins produced locally, and not by genetic factors. Additionally, they revealed that fibroblasts are a heterogeneous population of cells which can be up-regulated by the likes of GM-CSF or TGF-$\beta$1, or down-regulated by INF-$\gamma$ (78). This subject, along with potential therapeutic implications, is reviewed in several publications (8,137,221).

Further evidence of the role of PDGF-BB and TGF-$\beta$1 in the fibrogenic process of wound healing comes from experiments showing that the former cytokine-induced macrophage influx into wounds and that TGF-$\beta$1 promotes fibrosis (222). Furthermore, it was shown that the extracellular matrix regulates expression of the TGF-$\beta$1 gene, and it was also proposed that there is a feedback loop whereby TGF-$\beta$1-induced synthesis of basement membrane components (probably produced by myofibroblasts) is repressed once a functional basement membrane is present (223). Whereas TGF-$\beta$1 synthesis may play a major role regulating in vivo extracellular matrix synthesis and cell-to-extracellular matrix interactions, TGF-$\beta$2 may be more important in morphogenesis (223).

These collected studies, particularly in relation to the key participant, TGF-$\beta$1, in fibrogenic states, are the subject of several interesting reviews (224–228).

In addition, gene knockout technology has come to address this issue with the creation of a TGF-$\beta$1 knockout mouse, which features a florid inflammatory state, a not-unexpected finding because, among its many functions, the protein is a potent anti-inflammatory (229). Moreover, the tight-skin (Tsk) murine mutation is under study as a model for scleroderma (230), a condition in which there are compelling reasons to implicate TGF-$\beta$1 in this fibrosing condition.

Since the discovery that myofibroblasts were an element in the stromal response to mammary (20,21) and diverse carcinomas characterized by desmoplasia (22), we have followed events describing these epithelial-stromal interactions. From these, one learns that the interphase of stroma with diverse invasive carcinomas is also the site of an "internet" of sorts. Such cancers secrete TGF-$\beta$1 and PDGF, which result in the synthesis by stromal fibroblasts and myofibroblasts of tenascin (231), stromelysin-3 (232), a urokinase-type plasminogen activator (233), and insulin-like growth factor-2 (234). Paradoxically, as several of these agents elaborate stromal digestive enzymes (metalloproteinases), one would posit why such a mechanism were in place, because it would facilitate collagen digestion and, hence, stromal invasion by the tumor. Some of these issues were reviewed by Rønnov-Jessen and Petersen (235) and Rønnov-Jessen et al. (236).

The myofibroblast response in granulation tissue and invasive (primary and metastatic) carcinomas has only recently been the subject of serious investigations. At this writing, the role of the myofibroblast in affecting wound healing/closure is beyond dispute. In regard to invasive carcinomas, the relevance of the myofibroblastic response is far from resolved, especially because these stromal modulations appear to be associated with the emergence of a stromal cell that facilitates invasion by the neoplastic cells. To our knowledge, there are no studies describing cytokine interactions in the quasineoplastic fibroblastic conditions of fasciitis, fibromatosis, or desmoid tumors.

Many years ago Carrel prophesied the existence of substances capable of affecting cell proliferation and modulating wound healing and tissue regeneration (237). This prophecy has now become the cornerstone of an important aspect of all biology because cytokines (cellular products) have become fertile tools of investigation. Moreover, the development of agents to negate their nefarious effects has become the subject of hot pursuit by diverse scientists and biotechnology companies.

**FIG. 20.** Nodular sclerosing Hodgkin's disease. **A,** Gross aspect of cut surface from lymph node, illustrating nodules surrounded by thick connective tissue septa ("lymph node cirrhosis"). (Courtesy of Dr. Roger Gareau, Department of Pathology, Hôtel-Dieu Hospital, University of Montreal, Montreal, Quebec Canada.) **B,** Histological aspect illustrating nodules of atypical lymphoid cells, among them many lacunar cells, surrounded by a dense collagenous capsule containing numerous spindle cells. (Hematoxylin-phloxine-saffron.) **C,** Several spindle cells around the nodule reveal immunostaining for $\alpha$–smooth muscle actin (VA cells). **D,** Few spindle cells are immunoreactive for desmin (VAD cells). All internodular stromal cells are positive for anti-vimentin (results not shown). **E,** Transmission electron micrograph from internodular stroma illustrating numerous typical myofibroblasts (MF) with bundles of cytoplasmic microfilaments and dense bodies (*arrows*). (Uranyl acetate and lead citrate: ×**5000**.)

## CELLULAR DERIVATION OF MYOFIBROBLASTS AND THEIR RELATION TO THE FIBROBLAST AND THE VASCULAR SMOOTH MUSCLE CELL AND THE PERICYTE

Considering the many conditions in which myofibroblasts occur, their heterogeneous cytoskeletal composition and the various functions attributed to them, it seems, at first glance, difficult to assume a common origin for these cells. Cohnheim (238), introducing the vascular theory, proposed that leucocytes are transformed into fibroblasts during the process of wound healing. Several subsequent studies, however, provided substantial evidence that blood cells are not able to transform into fibroblasts, and, that granulation tissue fibroblasts arise instead from local connective tissue cells (239–242). Among connective tissue cells that could transform into myofibroblasts, any mesenchymal cell is a potential candidate: foremost is the fibroblast, followed by the pericyte and the smooth muscle cell (243). With the accumulated knowledge of cytoskeletal proteins and actin isoforms in these three cell types, both in vivo and in vitro, all of these cells could be considered possible progenitors of myofibroblasts.

Granulation tissue fibroblasts are most likely derived from local fibroblasts (25,201,244). Within experimental and human granulation tissues, myofibroblasts express temporarily markers of smooth muscle differentiation,($\alpha$-smooth muscle actin), which disappear after wound closure (25). This suggests that differentiation of myofibroblasts toward smooth muscle cells is only partial, at least during normal wound healing, because myofibroblasts in this condition never express desmin or smooth muscle myosin heavy chain isoforms. Recently, the cytoskeletal features of myofibroblasts during wound healing, Dupuytren's disease, and the stroma of mammary carcinomas were investigated. In these three conditions, myofibroblasts disclosed a progressive differentiation toward the smooth muscle phenotype (138). Whereas myofibroblasts during wound healing express only $\alpha$-smooth muscle actin, myofibroblasts in Dupuytren's disease express smooth muscle myosin heavy chains, at least in some cases. An important proportion of myofibroblasts within the stroma of all cases of mammary carcinomas express, in addition to $\alpha$-smooth muscle actin, desmin and smooth muscle myosin heavy chain isoforms. This suggests that fibroblastic cells are capable of differentiating into smooth muscle cells.

Ultrastructural data provide evidence that during pathologic or culture conditions, fibroblasts and smooth muscle cells acquire morphologic features resembling those of myofibroblasts (113,245–249), thereby suggesting that both cell types might be progenitors of myofibroblasts. Indeed, an extensive study on the modulation of mesenchymal cells within the mammary gland stroma when placed in culture in a microenvironment mimicking conditions observed in in vivo situations, indicates that although most myofibroblasts are derived from fibroblasts, a certain proportion of them are derived from vascular smooth muscle cells, and only a low proportion from pericytes (236). With the caution that it is difficult to extrapolate data from in vitro to in vivo situations, this work supports the concept of a heterogeneous origin of myofibroblastic cells.

A vascular origin of the myofibroblast was also proposed on the basis of morphologic observations. It was suggested that desmin-positive cells migrate from the wall of vessels to the tissue (198). A possible source of myofibroblasts expressing vimentin and desmin also are the stromal cells positive for desmin, but negative for $\alpha$-smooth muscle actin in various organs (99,132,133,250).

The possibility that myofibroblasts arise from specialized mesenchymal cells of certain organs has found a convincing confirmation in recent years. An abundant clinical and experimental literature has shown that during the onset of experimental and human hepatic fibrosis and cirrhosis, perisinusoidal stellate cells of the liver are the most likely source of myofibroblastic cells (32,251–253). The conditions allowing the modulation of perisinusoidal stellate cells into myofibroblasts have been studied and both extracellular matrix components, as well as cytokines, have been suggested as possible initiators (254–258). Similarly, glomerular mesangial cells have been shown to acquire myofibroblastic features, including the expression of $\alpha$-smooth muscle actin and collagen during several experimental and human pathologic situations (33,175,259,260). Septal fibroblastic cells in the lungs, which under normal conditions possess contractile features without expressing $\alpha$-smooth muscle actin (261), acquire the expression of this protein upon pathologic stimuli such as bleomycin treatment (262), and quickly express collagen I mRNA (31).

Thus, it appears that several cells including fibroblasts, smooth muscle cells, and specialized local mesenchymal cells can modulate (upon appropriate stimulation) into a myofibroblastic phenotype. The issue, as yet unresolved, relates to the stimuli which regulate this modulation. Several recent studies point to TGF-$\beta$1 as the main factor responsible for this change (28,263,264). This appears relatively well established, at least for fibroblastic cells (258,263), and has also been suggested for mesangial cells (33,226). It has been also shown in experimental animals that the topical application of GM-CSF is capable of stimulating the development of an abundant granulation tissue rich in $\alpha$-smooth muscle actin-positive myofibroblasts (29,30); this action is, however, indirect and could be mediated by TGF-$\beta$.

One could suggest, as previously proposed (98), that fibroblasts, myofibroblasts, vascular smooth muscle cells, pericytes, and other specialized mesenchymal cells with various myoid features, represent cellular isoforms of a common ancestor cell. The degree of differentiation toward the smooth muscle phenotype would thus, depend on microenvironmental factors.

From these considerations, it appears clear that our knowledge of the mechanisms of myofibroblastic modulation is better defined. Although we can not reach a definitive conclusion regarding their cellular derivation in each instance, the most probable situation is that myofibroblasts arise from several cells among which fibroblasts predominate. The interpretation that these cells represent isoformic transitions of a common ancestor cell, which develop in response to a functional demand or a change within the microenvironment, seems, at the present time, plausible.

## THE FINITE LIFE SPAN OF THE MYOFIBROBLAST AND THE ROLE OF APOPTOSIS

Granulation tissue formation involves replication and migration of fibroblasts from normal tissues, to the area of inflammation and the modulation of at least a proportion of them to the myofibroblastic phenotype. Angiogenesis takes place in a coordinated way and granulation tissue acquires its typical features. When the wound closes, a gradual evolution toward scar tissue takes place that involves disappearance of vascular cells and myofibroblasts with a proportional increase of extracellular matrix components. This phenomenon, which ends with the establishment of a scar, is more or less rapid according to the species, the location of granulation tissue, and the type of inflammation (7). When granulation tissue cells are not eliminated there is a development of pathologic scarring, i.e., hypertrophic scars and keloids, which are distinct clinical and pathologic conditions (178), both characterized by a relative high degree of cellularity.

Recently, using several morphologic and biochemical techniques, it has been shown that the reduction in cell number observed during the transition between granulation tissue and scar is achieved to a great extent through apoptosis (Fig. 21) (34); whether apoptosis or perhaps the lack of apoptosis plays a role in the establishment of hypertrophic scar and keloid remains, however, to be explored. It appears that apoptosis of granulation tissue cells takes place essentially after wound closure and affects target cells consecutively, rather than producing a simple wave of cell disappearance. This observation is in line with gradual resorption of granulation tissue after wound closure and with the observation that dead cells are digested by macrophages and surrounding cells. It appears that granulation tissue cell apoptosis can be accelerated significantly by the application of a viable cutaneous flap (265). This observation underlines the importance of cell communication between normal connective tissue and granulation tissue. These reports suggest that, at least during normal wound healing, the process of myofibroblast differentiation generally ends with cell death; thus, myofibroblasts can be considered terminally differentiated cells.

The question that remains to be answered is the stimulus that leads to apoptosis during wound healing. Recently gene products regulating cell death have been identified (266–271). In fibroblasts, the c-myc protein (272) and interleukin-1-B-converting enzyme, the mammalian homologue of the *Caenorhabditis elegans* gene ced-3 (273), have been shown to induce apoptosis. In turn, it has been shown that the bcl-2 protein is capable of blocking apoptosis (274); however, fibroblasts lack bcl-2 expression as assessed by antibody staining. A possible mechanism for apoptosis induction could be via the direct action and/or withdrawal of cytokines or growth factors (275–277). Several factors have been shown to increase the rate of wound healing including PDGF (278), TGF-$\beta$ (278–281), and tumor necrosis factor (282). These factors may be present in the normal healing wound, released by platelets and inflammatory cells (283). It is probable that, as the wound resolves, there is a decrease in the level of these factors. A possible explanation for the death of at least a subpopulation of myofibroblasts and vascular cells could be that they are growth-factor dependent. Alternatively, factors selectively causing the death of myofibroblastic and vascular cells could be liberated after epithelization has been completed. Additional work is necessary to identify these hypothetical factors, but it appears that apoptosis is the mechanism through which vascular and myofibroblastic cells are gradually eliminated from normally healing granulation tissue.

## CONCLUDING REMARKS

For this second edition, every section has been updated. In addition, several new topics have been added to reflect recent developments.

Since the myofibroblast was discovered in granulating wounds, one is left fascinated with recent studies that better account for events in this most basic process. It appears that resting fibroblasts are triggered, through the effects of cytokines released at the wound site, to assume a myofibroblastic phenotype to effect wound closure. As this approaches completion, genes that encode for apoptotic proteins are expressed to initiate myofibroblastic cell death; the formerly cellular wound is then converted into a poorly cellular scar. Commensurate with this, there is a shift from collagen type III gene expression/deposition to type I gene expression, resulting in the deposition of type I collagen that provides strength to the developing scar. Furthermore, cytokines stimulate extracellular matrix synthesis, and, in turn, are repressed once wound closure is completed, and a functional basement membrane is present, suggesting the existence of a feedback loop (223). It is possible that deviations from this finely orchestrated process contribute to the development of hypertrophic scars and keloids.

Regarding the diverse assortment of quasineoplastic myofibroblastic proliferative processes, the underlying cellular/molecular mechanisms central to their pathogenesis remain essentially unexplored.

Turning to the myofibroblastic response associated with diverse invasive and metastatic carcinomas, it was originally proposed that this represented an expression of host response to the cancer. The hypothesis appears valid today, although one could posit whether this is beneficial since many of these

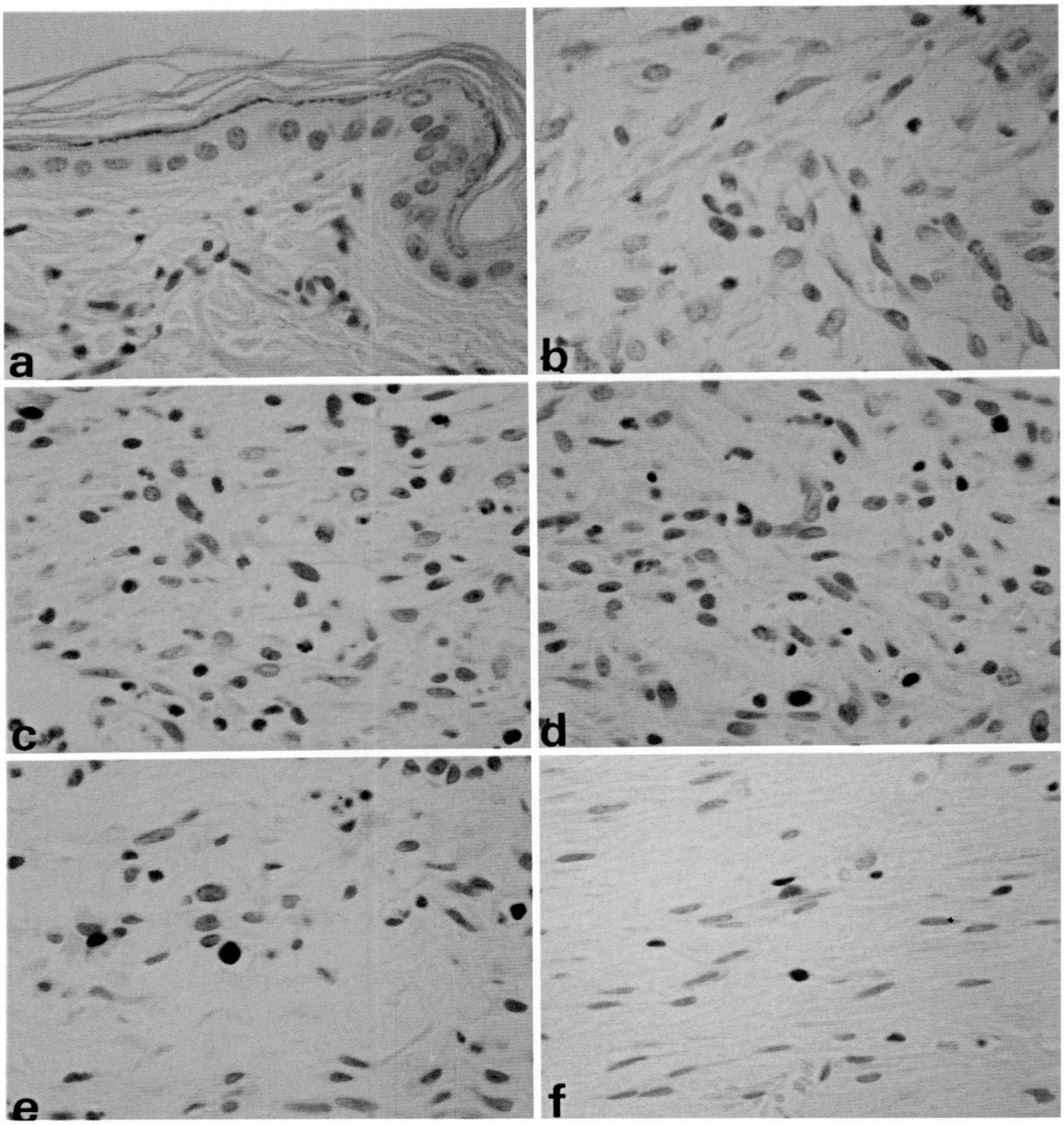


**FIG. 21.** Identification of apoptotic cells in rat tissues by in situ end labeling of fragmented DNA. **A,** Normal rat skin, no apoptotic cells are detected. **B,** 12-day-old wound tissue, **C,** 16-day–old wound tissue, **D,** 20-day-old wound tissue, **E,** 25-day-old wound tissue, and **F,** 30-day-old wound tissue. At 12 days, when $\alpha$-smooth muscle actin expression is maximal, there is no positive staining for apoptotic cells, after which the number of labeled cells increases with a maximum at 20 days (D) and decreases thereafter. (A-D, ×**1000**.)

cancers, despite the attending desmoplasia, continue to exact lives. Yet, death, in these settings, stems largely from the ability of the neoplastic cell to enter vascular channels and disseminate. It remains likely that these myofibroblasts, while affecting contraction and elaborating collagens and other extracellular matrix components, also release enzymes that allow for tissue/vascular invasion. Clearly, future studies of human cancer should be focused not only on the neoplastic cell, but on the regulation of the extracellular matrix synthesis and the cell-to-extracellular matrix interactions, i.e., to the stroma that attempts to contain it.

Some 15 years ago (22), we proposed that similarities might exist between the process of wound healing and the stromal response to neoplastic invasion. This assumption may also be extended to quasineoplastic proliferative conditions, e.g., Dupuytren's disease. During normal wound healing and within nodules of Dupuytren's disease and possibly other quasineoplastic proliferations, the myofibroblastic/fibroblastic reaction appears to be centripetal (Fig. 22A), whereas within neoplastic invasion this reaction is centrifugal (Fig. 22B), indicating that cancers are wounds that do not heal (284). The underlying cellular/molecular mechanisms explaining these fundamental differences, including the presence, delay, or absence of apoptosis, remain to be explored.

Finally, we conclude this chapter with a most intriguing report uncovered in our literature search of TGF-$\beta$. It would appear that fetal skin wounds heal without scarring and that such wounds, apart from that contained in platelets, are devoid of TGF-$\beta$ (285). Once again, one is reminded of the lessons to be learned by study of the events of early life.


## ACKNOWLEDGMENTS

This work was supported in part by the Cancer Research Society Inc. Montreal, Canada, the Swiss National Science Foundation (Grant No. 31-40372-94), and The Macdonald Stewart Foundation, Montreal, whose benefactors, Mrs. Liliane Stewart and the late David M. Stewart, have generously supported the Department of Pathology of the Hôtel-Dieu Hospital of Montreal over many years. We thank Mr. Som Chatterjee and Ms. Myrielle Vermette for skillful technical assistance and Ms. Louise Gendron and Mr. Gaston Lambert for the photographic work. We thank also the publishers of Laboratory Investigation (Fig. 6), Surgery Gynecology and Obstetrics (Figs. 13A and 16A, inset), Virchows Arch A (Figs. 1A and 18A,B), Churchill Livingstone, London (Figs. 7 and 9A), and The American Journal of Pathology (Fig. 21) for the permission to reproduce the above indicated photographic material.


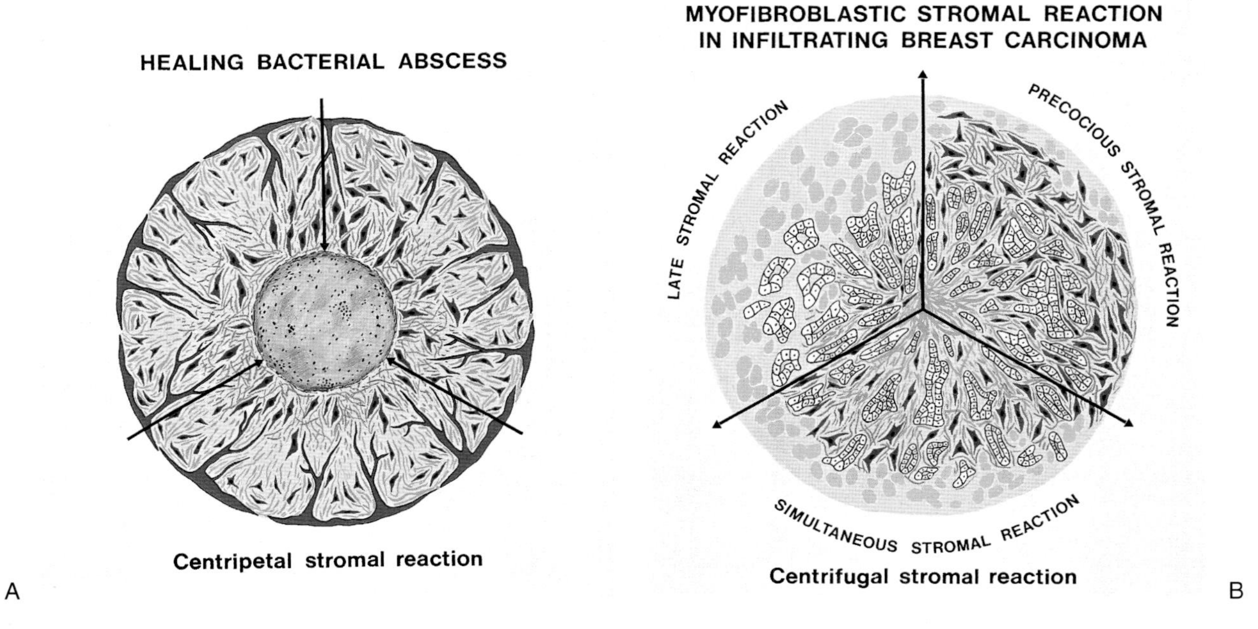


**FIG. 22.** Schematic illustration of stromal reaction in healing bacterial abscess **(A)** and in infiltrating ductal breast carcinoma **(B)**. In the healing bacterial abscess the cicatrizing layer is in the periphery, and the two layers containing myofibroblasts (exudutaivo-productive and exudative respectively) are developing toward the center (A). In infiltrating ductal breast carcinomas the cicatrizing area is in the center, and myofibroblasts develop variably in the peripheral invasive cellular front of the carcinoma, i.e. precocious (preceding invasive carcinoma cells), simultaneous (developing among invasive carcinoma cells), and late (appearing behind invasive carcinoma cells). Compared to normal wound healing with centripetal stromal reaction (B), invasive ductal breast carcinomas display a centrifugal stromal reaction, indicating that cancers are wounds that do not heal.

## REFERENCES


1. Gabbiani G, Ryan GB, Majno G. Presence of modified fibroblasts in granulation tissue and their possible role in wound contraction. *Experientia* 1971;27:549–550.
2. Majno G, Gabbiani G, Hirschel BJ, Ryan GB, Statkov PR. Contraction of granulation tissue in vitro: similarity to smooth muscle. *Science* 1971;173:548–550.
3. Gabbiani G, Hirschel BJ, Ryan GB, Statkov PR, Majno G. Granulation tissue as a contractile organ. A study of structure and function. *J Exp Med* 1972;135:719–734.
4. Hirschel BJ, Gabbiani G, Ryan GB, Majno G. Fibroblasts of granulation tissue: immunofluorescent staining with antismooth muscle serum. *Proc Soc Exp Biol Med* 1971;138:466–469.
5. Gabbiani G, Ryan GB, Lamelin JP, Vasalli P, Majno G, Bouvier CA, Cruchaud A, Lüscher EF. Human smooth muscle autoantibody. Its identification as antiactin autoantibody and a study of its binding to "nonmuscular" cells. *Am J Pathol* 1973;72:473–488.
6. Seemayer TA, Lagacé R, Schürch W, Thelmo WL. The myofibroblast: biologic pathologic and theoretical considerations. *Pathol Annu* 1980;15:443–470.
7. Skalli O, Gabbiani G. The biology of the myofibroblast: relationship to wound contraction and fibrocontractive diseases. In: Clark RAF, Henson PM, eds. *Molecular and cellular biology of wound repair.* New York: Plenum Press, 1988;373–402.
8. Schmitt-Gräff A, Desmoulière A, Gabbiani G. Heterogeneity of myofibroblast phenotypic features: an example of fibroblastic cell plasticity. *Virchows Archiv* 1994;425:3–24.
9. Majno G. The story of the myofibroblast. *Am J Surg Pathol* 1979; 3:535–542.
10. Majno G. *The healing hand: man and wound in the ancient world.* Cambridge: Harvard University Press, 1975.
11. Carrel A, Hartmann A. Cicatrization of wounds. I. The relation between the size and the rate of its cicatrization. *J Exp Med* 1916;24:429–450.
12. Abercrombie, M, Flint MH, James DW. Wound contraction in relation to collagen formation in scorbutic guinea pigs. *J Embryol Exp Morphol* 1956;4:167–175.
13. Hoffmann-Beerling H. Adenosintriphosphat als Betriebsstoff von Zellbewegungen. *Biochim Biophys Acta* 1954;14:182–194.
14. Majno G, Leventhal M. Pathogenesis of histamine-type vascular leakage. *Lancet* 1967;2:99–100.
15. Gabbiani G. Curr Contents 1988; 31(30), July 24:16.
16. Gabbiani G, Majno G. Dupuytren's contracture: fibroblast contraction? An ultrastructural study. *Am J Pathol* 1972;66:131–146.
17. Ryan GB, Cliff WJ, Gabbiani G, Irlé C, Montandon D, Statkov PR, Majno G. Myofibroblasts in human granulation tissue. *Hum Pathol* 1974;5:55–67,
18. Gabbiani G, Chaponnier C, Hüttner I. Cytoplasmic filaments and gap junctions in epithelial cells and myofibroblasts during wound healing. *J Cell Biol* 1978;76:561–568.
19. Singer II, Kawka DW, Kazazis DM, Clark RA. In vivo co-distribution of fibronectin and actin fibers in granulation tissue: immunofluorescence and electron microscope studies of the fibronexus at the myofibroblast surface. *J Cell Biol* 1984;98:2091–2106.
20. Tremblay G. Stromal aspects of breast carcinoma. *Exp Mol Pathol* 1979;31:248–260.
21. Seemayer TA, Lagacé R, Schürch W, Tremblay G. Myofibroblasts in the stroma of invasive and metastatic carcinoma: a possible host response to neoplasia. *Am J Surg Pathol* 1979;3:525–533.
22. Schürch W, Seemayer TA, Lagacé R. Stromal myofibroblasts in primary invasive and metastatic carcinomas. A combined immunological, light and electron microscopic study. *Virchows Arch A* 1981;391: 125–139.
23. Schürch W, Lagacé R, Seemayer TA. Myofibroblastic stromal reaction in retracted scirrhous carcinomas of the breast. *Surg Gynecol Obstet* 1982;154:351–358.
24. Skalli O, Schürch W, Seemayer TA, Lagacé R, Montandon D, Pittet B, Gabbiani G. Myofibroblasts from diverse pathologic settings are heterogeneous in their content of actin isoforms and intermediate filament proteins. *Lab Invest* 1989;60:275–285.
25. Darby I, Skalli O, Gabbiani G. $\alpha$-Smooth muscle actin is transiently expressed by myofibroblasts during experimental wound healing. *Lab Invest* 1990;63:21–29.
26. Schürch W, Skalli O, Gabbiani G. Cellular biology of Dupuytren's disease. In: McFarland RM, McGrouther DA, Flint MH, eds. *Dupuytren's disease*. London: Churchill Livingstone, 1990.
27. Desmoulière A, Rubbbia-Brandt L, Grau G, Gabbiani G. Heparin induced smooth muscle actin expression in cultured fibroblasts and in granulation tissue myofibroblasts. *Lab Invest* 1992;67:716–726.
28. Desmoulière A, Geinoz A Gabbiani F, Gabbiani G. Transforming growth factor-$\beta$1 induces alpha-smooth muscle actin expression in granulation tissue myofibroblasts and in quiescent and growing cultured fibroblasts. *J Cell Biol* 1993;122:103–111.
29. Vyalov S, Desmoulière A, Gabbiani G. GM-CSF-induced granulation tissue formation: relationships between macrophage and myofibroblast accumulation. *Virchows Archiv B* 1993;63:231–239.
30. Rubbia-Brandt L, Sappino AP, Gabbiani G. Locally applied GM-CSF induces the accumulation of $\alpha$-smooth muscle actin containing myofibroblasts. *Virchows Archiv B*;1991;60:73–82.
31. Zhang K, Rekhter MD, Gordon D, Phan SH. Myofibroblasts and their role in lung collagen gene expression during pulmonary fibrosis. A combined immunohistochemical and in situ hybridization study.*Am J Pathol* 1994;145:114–125.
32. Friedman SL. The cellular basis of hepatic fibrosis. Mechanisms and treatment strategies. *New Engl J Med* 1993;328:1828–1835.
33. Johnson RJ, Iida H, Alpers CE, Majesky MW, Schwartz SM, Pritzl P, Gordon K, Gown AM. Expression of smooth muscle phenotype by rat mesangial cells in immune complex nephritis. Alpha-smooth muscle actin is a marker of mesangial cell proliferation. *J Clin Invest* 1991; 87:847–858.
34. Desmoulière A, Redard M, Darby I, Gabbiani G. Apoptosis mediates the decrease in cellularity during the transition between granulation tissue and scar. *Am J Pathol* 1995;146:56–66.
35. Gabella G. Structural apparatus for force transmission in smooth muscles. *Physiol Rev* 1984;64:455–477..
36. Somlyo AV. Ultrastructure of vascular smooth muscle. In: Bohr DF, Somlyo AV, Sparks HV, eds. *Handbook of physiology, section 2: The cardiovascular system, Vol II: vascular smooth muscle.* Bethesda; American Physiological Society, 1980;33–67.
37. Hüttner I, Kocher O, Gabbiani G. Endothelial and smooth muscle cells. In: Camilleri JP, Berry CL, Fiessinger JN, Bariety J, eds. *Diseases of the arterial wall.* New York: Springer-Verlag, 1989; 3–41.
38. Schollmeyer JE, Goll DE, Robson RM, et al. Localization of alpha actinin and tropomyosin in different muscles. *J Cell Biol* 1973; 59: 306(abst).
39. Schollmeyer JE, Furcht LT, Goll DE, et al. Localization of contractile proteins in smooth muscle cells and in normal and transformed fibroblasts. In: Goldman R, Pollard T, Rosenbaum J, eds. *Cell motility, vol A.* Cold Spring Harbor, NY: Cold Spring Harbor Laboratory, 1976:306–361.
40. Brown PJ, Juliano RL. Expression and function of a putative cell surface receptor for fibronectin in hamster and human cell lines. *J Cell Biol* 1986;103:1595–1603.
41. Hasegawa T, Hasegawa E, Chen WT. Characterization of a membrane-associated glycoprotein complex implicated in cell adhesion to fibronectin. *J Cell Biochem* 1985;28:307–318.
42. Knudsen KA, Horwitz AF, Buck CA. A monoclonal antibody identifies a glycoprotein complex involved in cell-substratum adhesion. *Exp Cell Res* 1985;157:218–226.
43. Rogalski AA, Singer SJ. An integral glycoprotein associated with the membrane attachment sites of actin microfilaments. *J Cell Biol* 1985; 101:785–801.
44. Horwitz A, Duggan K, Buck C, Beckerle MC, Burridge K. Interaction of plasma membrane fibronectin receptor with talin: a transmembrane linkage. *Nature* 1986;320;531–533.
45. Hynes RO, Yamada KM. Fibronectins: multifunctional modular glycoproteins. *J Cell Biol* 1982;95:369–377.
46. Singer II. The fibronexus: a transmembrane association of fibronectin-containing fibers and bundles of 5nm microfilaments in hamster and human fibroblasts. *Cell* 1979;16:675–685.
47. Bloom S, Cancilla PA. Conformational changes in myocardial nuclei of rats. *Circ Res* 1969;24:189–196.
48. Franke WW, Schinko W. Nuclear shape in muscle cells. *J Cell Biol* 1969;42:326–331.
49. Lane BP. Alterations in the cytologic detail of intestinal smooth muscle cells in various stages of contraction. *J Cell Biol* 1965;27:199–213.
50. Majno G, Shea SM, Leventhal M. Endothelial contraction induced by histamine-type mediators. An electron microscopic study. *J Cell Biol* 1969;42:647–672.

51. Clément B, Loréal O, Guiouzo A. Fibrogénèse hépatique. Editions techniques. Encycl. Méd. Chir.(Paris., Hépatologie, 7-005-A-35, 1995.
52. Gabbiani G, LeLous M, Bailey AJ, Bazin S, Delaunay A. Collagen and myofibroblasts of granulation tissue. A chemical, ultrastuctural and immunologic study. *Virchows Arch B* 1976;21:133–145.
53. Rudolph R, Guber S, Suzuki M, Woodward M. The life cycle of the myofibroblast. *Surg Gynecol Obstet* 1977;145:389–394.
54. Barsky SH, Rao CN, Grotendorst GR, Liotta LA.Increased content of type V collagen in desmoplasia of human breast carcinoma. *Am J Pathol*;1982:108: 276–283.
55. Gressner AM, Bachem MG. Cellular sources of noncollagenous matrix proteins : role of fat-storing cells in fibrogenesis. *Semin Liver Dis* 1990;10:30–46.
56. Berndt A, Kosmehl H, Katenkamp D, Tauchmann V. Appearance of the myofibroblastic phenotype in Dupuytren's disease is associated with fibronectin, laminin, collagen type IV and tenascin extracellular matrix. *Pathobiology* 1994;92:55–58.
57. Sommer P, Gleyzal C, Raccurt M, Delbourg M, Serrar M, Joazeiro P, Peyrol S, Kagan H, Trackman PC, Grimaud JA. Transient expression of lysil oxidase by liver myofibroblasts in murine schistosomiasis. *Lab Invest* 1993;69:460–470.
58. Jourdan-Le Saux C, Gleyzal C, Garnier JM, Peraldi M, Sommer P, Grimaud JA. Lysyl oxidase cDNA of myofibroblast from mouse fibrotic liver. *Biochem Biophys Res Commun* 1994;199:587–592.
59. Meister P, Gokel JM, Remberger K. Palmar fibromatosis-Dupuytren's contracture: A comparison of light, electron and immunofluorescence microscopic findings. *Pathol Res Pract* 1979;164: 402–412.
60. Lagacé R, Grimaud JA, Schürch W, Seemayer TA. Myofibroblastic stromal reaction in carcinoma of the breast and variations of collagenous matrix and structural glycoproteins. *Virchows Arch A* 1985; 408:49–59.
61. Wessels NK, Spooner BS, Ash JF, Bradley MO, Luduena MA,Taylor EL, Wrenn JT, Yamada KM. Microfilaments in cellular and developmental processes. *Science* 1971;117:135–143.
62. Madden JW, Morton D, Peacock EE. Contraction of experimental wounds. I. Inhibiting wound contraction by using a topical smooth muscle antagonist. *Surgery* 1974;76:8–15.
63. Irlé C, Kocher O, Gabbiani G. Contractility of myofibroblasts during experimental liver cirrhosis. *J Submicrosc Cytol Pathol* 1980;12: 209–217.
64. Evans JN, Kelley J, Low RB, Adler KB. Increased contractility of isolated lung parenchyma in an animal model of pulmonary fibrosis induced by bleomycin. *Am Rev Respir Dis* 1982;125:89–94.
65. Yanagisawa M, Kurihara H, Kimura S, Tomobe Y, Kobayashi M, Mitsui Y,Yazaki Y, Goto K, Masaki T. A novel potent vasoconstrictor peptide produced by vascular endothelial cells. *Nature* 1988;332: 411–415.
66. Appleton I, Tomlinson A, Chandler CL, Willoughby DA. Effect of endothelin-1 on croton oil-induced granulation tissue in the rat. A pharmacologic and immunohistochemical study. *Lab Invest* 1992;67: 703–710.
67. Thiemermann C, Corder R. Is endothelin-1 the regulator of myofibroblast contraction during wound healing? *Lab Invest* 1992;67: 677–679.
68. Kurihara H, Yoshizumi M, Sugiyama T, Takaku F, Yanagisawa M, Masaki T, Hamaoki M, Kato H,Yazaki Y. TGF $\beta$ stimulates the expression of ET-1 mRNA by vascular endothelial cells. *Biochem Biophys Res Commun* 1989;159:1435–1440.
69. Hahn AW, Resink TJ, Kern F, Bühler FR. Effects of endothelin-1 on vascular smooth muscle cell phenotypic differentiation. *J Cardiovasc Pharmacol* 1992;20(Suppl 12):533–536.
70. Buckley IK, Porter KR. Cytoplasmic fibrils in living cultured cells. A light and electron microscope study. *Protoplasma* 1967;64:349–380.
71. Goldman RD. The use of heavy meromyosin binding as an ultrastructural cytochemical method for localizing and determining the possible functions of actin-like microfilaments in nonmuscle cells. *J Histochem Cytochem* 1975;23:529–542.
72. Goldman RD, Lazarides E, Pollack R, Weber K. The distribution of actin in nonmuscle cells. The use of actin antibody in the localization of actin within the microfilament bundles of mouse 3T3 cells. *Exp Cell Res* 1975;90:333–344.
73. Willingham MC, Yamada SS, Davies PJ, Rutherford AV, Gallo MG, Pastan I. Intracellular localization of actin in cultured fibroblasts by electron microscopic immunochemistry. *J Histochem Cytochem* 1981; 29:17–37.
74. Skalli O, Ropraz P, Trzeciak A, Benzonana G, Gillessen B, Gabbiani G. A monoclonal antibody against $\alpha$-smooth muscle actin; a new probe for smooth muscle differentiation. *J Cell Biol* 1986;103: 2787–2796.
75. Bellows CG, Melcher AH, Aubin JE. Contraction and organization of collagen gels by cell cultured from periodontal ligament, gingiva and bone suggest functional differences between cell types. *J Cell Biol* 1981;211:1052–1054.
76. Vandekerckhove J, Weber K. At least six different actins are expressed in a higher mammal: An analysis based on the amino acid sequence of the amino-terminal tryptic peptide. *J Mol Biol* 1978;126: 783–802.
77. Leavitt J, Gunning P, Kedes L, Jariwalla R. Smooth muscle $\alpha$-actin is a transformation-sensitive marker for mouse NIH 3t3 and rat-2 cells. *Nature* 1985;316:840–842.
78. Desmoulière A, Rubbia-Brandt L, Abdiu A, Walz T, Macieira-Coelho A, Gabbiani G. $\alpha$-Smooth muscle actin is expressed in a subpopulation of cultured and cloned fibroblasts and is modulated by $\gamma$-interferon. *Exp Cell Res* 1992;201:64–73.
79. Schmitt-Gräff A, Pau H, Spahr R, Piper, HM, Skalli O, Gabbiani G. Appearance of $\alpha$-smooth muscle actin in human eye lens cells of anterior capsular cataract and in cultured bovine lens-forming cells. *Differentiation* 1990;43:115–122.
80. Rønnov-Jessen L, van Deurs B, Celis JE, Petersen OW. Smooth muscle differentiation in cultured human breast gland stromal cells. *Lab Invest* 1990;63:532–543.
81. Rockey DC, Friedman SL. Cytoskeleton of liver perisinusoidal cells (lipocytes in normal and pathological conditions. *Cell Motil Cytoskeleton* 1992;22:227–234.
82. Elger M, Drenckhahn D, Nobiling R, Mundel P, Kriz W. Cultured rat mesangial cells contain smooth muscle $\alpha$-actin not found in vivo. *Am J Pathol* 1993;142:497–509.
83. Bayreuther K, Rodemann HP, Hommel R, Dittmann K Albiez M, Francz PI. Human skin fibroblasts in vitro differentiate along a terminal cell lineage. *Proc Natl Acad Sci U S A* 1988;85:5112–5116.
84. Harris AK, Stopack D, Wild P. Fibroblast traction as a mechanism for collagen morphogenesis. *Nature* 1981;290;249–251.
85. Isenberg G, Rathke PC, Hülsmann N, Franke WW, Wohlfarth-Bottermann KE. Cytoplasmic actomyosin fibrils in tissue culture cells. Direct proof of contractility by visualization of ATP-induced contraction in fibrils isolated by laser microbeam dissection. *Cell Tissue Res* 1976; 166:427–443.
86. Kreis TE, Birchmeier W. Stress fiber sarcomeres of fibroblasts are contractile. *Cell* 1980;22:555–561.
87. Burridge K. Are stress fibres contractile? *Nature* 1981;294: 691–692.
88. Vande Berg JS, Rudolph R, Woodward M. Comparative growth dynamics and morphology between cultured myofibroblasts from granulating wounds and dermal fibroblasts. *Am J Pathol* 1984;114: 187–200.
89. Vande Berg JS, Rudolph R, Poolman WL, Disharoon DR. Comparative growth dynamics and actin concentration between cultured human myofibroblasts from granulating wounds and dermal fibroblasts from normal skin. *Lab Invest* 1989;61:532–538.
90. Gabbiani G, Majno G, Ryan GB. The myofibroblast as a contractile cell. In Pikkarainen J, Kulonen K, eds. *Biology of the fibroblast.* New York: Academic Press, 1973:139–154.
91. Herman IM, Crisona NJ, Pollard DT. Relation between cell activity and the distribution of cytoplasmic actin and myosin. *J Cell Biol* 1981; 90:84–91.
92. Hynes RO, Destree AT, Wagner DD. Relationships between microfilaments, cell-substratum adhesion, and fibronectin. *Cold Spring Harbor Symp Quant Biol* 1982;46:659–670.
93. Vande Berg JS, Rudolph R, Woodward M. Growth dynamics of cultured myofibroblasts from human breast cancer and nonmalignant contracting tissues. *Plast Reconstr Surg* 1984;73:605–618.
94. Azzarone B, Failly-Crepin C, Daya-Grosjean L, Chaponnier C, Gabbiani G. Abnormal behavior of cultured fibroblasts from nodule and nonaffected aponeurosis of Dupuytren's disease. *J Cell Physiol* 1983; 117:353–361.
95. Germain L, Jean A, Auger FA, Garrel DR. Human wound healing fibroblasts have greater contractile properties than dermal fibroblasts. *J Surg Res* 1994;57:268–273.
96. Grinnell F. Mini-review on the cellular mechanisms of disease. Fibroblasts, myofibroblasts, and wound contraction. *J Cell Biol* 1994;124: 401–404.

97. Caplan AI; Fiszman MY, Eppenberger HM. Molecular and cell isofoms during development. *Science* 1983;221:921–927.
98. Rungger-Brändle E, Gabbiani G. The role of cytoskeletal and cytocontractile elements in pathologic processes. *Am J Pathol* 1983;110: 361–392.
99. Skalli O, Bloom WS, Ropraz P, Azzarone B, Gabbiani G. Cytoskeletal remodeling of rat aortic smooth muscle cells in vitro relationships to culture conditions and analogies to in vivo situations. *J Submicrosc Cytoskeleton* 1986;18:481–493.
100. Benzonana G, Skalli O, Gabbiani G. Correlation between the distribution of smooth muscle or non muscle myosins and α-smooth muscle actin in normal and pathological soft tissues. *Cell Motil Cytoskel* 1988;11:260–274.
101. Larson DM, Fujiwara K, Alexander RW, Gimbrone MA Jr. Myosin in cultured vascular smooth muscle cells: immunofluorescence and immunochemical studies of alterations in antigenic expression. *J Cell Biol* 1984;99:1582–1589.
102. Schmid E, Osborn M, Rungger-Brändle E, Gabbiani G, Weber K, Franke WW. Distribution of vimentin and desmin filaments in smooth muscle tissue of mammalian and avian aorta. *Exp Cell Res* 1982;137: 329–340.
103. Gabbiani G, Schmid E, Winter S, Chaponnier C, de Chastonay C, Vandekerckhove J, Weber K, Franke WW. Vascular smooth muscle cells differ from other smooth muscle cells: predominance of vimentin filaments and a specific α-type actin. *Proc Natl Acad Sci U S A* 1981; 78:298–302.
104. Frank ED, Warren L. Aortic smooth muscle cells contain vimentin instead of desmin. *Proc Natl Acad Sci U S A* 1981;78:3020–3024.
105. Osborn M, Caselitz J, Puschel K, Weber K. Intermediate filament expression in human vascular smooth muscle and in arteriosclerotic plaques. *Virchows Arch A* 1987;411:449–458.
106. Travo P, Weber K, Osborn M. Co-existence of vimentin and desmin type intermediate filaments in a subpopulation of adult vascular smooth muscle cells growing in primary culture. *Exp Cell Res* 1982;139:87–94.
107. Schmid E, Tapscott S, Bennett GS, Croop J, Fellini SA, Holtzer H, Franke WW. Differential location of different types of intermediate sized filaments in various tissues of the chicken embryo. *Differentiation* 1979;15:27–40.
108. Lazarides E. Intermediate filaments as mechanical integrators of cellular space. *Nature* 1980;283:249–256.
109. Franke WW, Schmid E, Freudenstein C, Appelhans B, Osborn M, Weber K, Keenan TW. Intermediate-sized filaments of the prekeratin type in myoepithelial cells. *J Cell Biol* 1980;84;633–654.
110. Vandekerckhove J, Weber K. The complete amino acid sequence of actins from bovine aorta, bovine heart, bovine fast skeletal muscle and rabbit slow skeletal muscle. *Differentiation* 1979;14:123–133.
111. Vandekerckhove J, Weber K. Actin typing on total cellular extracts. A highly sensitive protein chemical procedure able to distinguish different actins. *Eur J Biochem* 1981;113:595–603.
112. Skalli O, Vandekerckhove J, Gabbiani G. Actin isoform pattern as a marker of normal or pathological smooth muscle and fibroblastic tissues. *Differentiation* 1987;33:232–238.
113. Kocher O, Skalli O, Bloom WS, Gabbiani G. Cytoskeleton of rat aortic smooth muscle cells. Normal conditions and experimental intimal thickening. *Lab Invest* 1984;50:645–652.
114. Gabbiani G, Kocher O, Bloom WS, Vanderkerckhove J, Weber K. Actin expression in smooth muscle cells of rat aortic intimal thickening, human atheromatous plaque, and cultured rat aortic media. *J Clin Invest* 1984;73:148–152.
115. Skalli O, Pelte MF, Peclet MC, Gabbiani G, Gugliotta P, Bussolati G, Ravazzola M, Orci L. α-Smooth muscle actin, a differentiation marker of smooth muscle cells is present in microfilamentous bundles of pericytes. *J Histochem Cytochem* 1989;37: 315–321.
116. Zimmermann KW. Der feine Bau der Blutcapillaren. *Z Anat Entwicklungsgesch* 1923;68:3–109.
117. Nehls V, Drenkhahn D. Heterogeneity of microvascular pericytes for smooth muscle type alpha-actin. *J Cell Biol* 1991;113: 147–154.
118. Fujimoto T, Singer SJ. Immunocytochemical studies of desmin and vimentin in pericapillary cells of chicken. *J Histochem Cytochem* 1987;35:1105–1115.
119. O'Shea. JD. An ultrastructural study of smooth muscle-like cells in the theca externa of ovarian follicles of the rat. *Anat Rec (Basel)* 1970; 167:127–131.
120. Boya J, Carbonell AL, Martinez A. Myofibroblats in human palatal mucosa. *Acta Anat* 1988;131:161–165.
121. Güldner FH, Wolff JR, Keyserling DG. Fibroblasts as a part of the contractile system in duodenal villi of rat. *Z Zellforsch Mikrosk Anat* 1972;135:349–360.
122. Kaye GI, Lane N, Pascal PR. Colonic pericryptal fibroblast sheath: replication, migration and cytodifferentiation of a mesenchymal cell system in adult tissue. II. Fine structural aspects of normal rabbit and human colon. *Gastroenterology* 1968;54:852–865.
123. Sappino AP, Dietrich PY, Skalli O, Widgren S, Gabbiani G. Colonic pericryptal fibroblasts. Differentiation pattern in embryogenesis and phenotypic modulation in epithelial proliferative lesions. *Virchows Arch A* 1989;415:551–557.
124. Bressler RS. Myoid cells in the capsule of the adrenal gland and in monolayers derived from cultured adrenal capsules. *Anat Rec* 1973; 177:525–531.
125. Kapanci Y, Assimacopoulos A, Irlé C, Zwahlen A, Gabbiani G. "Contractile interstitial cells" in pulmonary septa: A possible regulator of ventilation-perfusion ratio? Ultastructural, immunofluorescence, and in vitro studies. *J Cell Biol* 1974;60:375–392.
126. Gorgas K, Böck P. Myofibroblasts in the rat testicular capsule. *Cell Tissue Res* 1974;154:533–541.
127. Czernobilsky B, Shezen E, Lifschitz-Mercer B, Fogel M, Luzon A, Jacob N, Skalli O, Gabbiani G. Alpha smooth muscle actin (α-SM actin. in normal human ovaries, in ovarian stromal hyperplasia and in ovarian neoplasms. *Virchows Arch B* 1989;57:55–61.
128. Parry EW. Some electron microscope observations on the mesenchymal structures of full-term umbilical cord. *J Anat* 1970;107: 505–518.
129. Tabone E, Andujar MB, DeBarros SS, Dos Santos MN, Barros CL, Graca DL. Myofibroblast-like cells in non-pathologic bovine endometrial caruncle. *Cell Biol Int Rep* 1983;7:395–400.
130. Beertesen W, Events V, van den Hoof A. Fine structure of fibroblasts in the periodontal ligament of the rat incisor and their possible role in tooth eruption. *Arch Oral Biol* 1974;19:1097–1098.
131. Beertsen W. Migration of fibroblasts in the periodontal ligament of the mouse incisor as revealed by autoradiography. *Arch Oral Biol* 1975; 20:659–666.
132. Toccanier-Pelte MF, Skalli O, Kapanci Y, Gabbiani G. Characterization of stromal cells with myoid features in lymph nodes and spleen in normal and pathologic conditions. *Am J Pathol* 1987;129: 109–118.
133. Yokoi Y, Namihisa T, Kuroda H, Komatsu I, Miyasaki A, Watanabe S. Usui K. Immunocytochemical detection of desmin in fat-storing cells (Ito cells) *Hepatology* 1984;4:709–714.
134. Glasser SR, Julian J. Intermediate filament protein as a marker of uterine stromal cell decidualization. *Biol Reprod* 1986;35: 463–474.
135. Charbord P, Lerat H, Newton I, Tamayo E, Gown AM, Singer JW, Herye P. The cytoskeleton of stromal cells from human bone marrow cultures resembles that of cultured smooth muscle cells. *Exp Hematol* 1990;118:276–282.
136. Becker CG. Demonstration of actomyosin in mesangial cells of the renal glomerulus. *Am J Pathol* 1972;66:97–110.
137. Desmoulière A, Gabbiani G. Modulation of fibroblastic cytoskeletal features during pathological situations: The role of extracellular matrix and cytokines *Cell Motil Cytoskeleton* 1994;29: 195–203.
138. Chiavegato A, Bochaton-Piallat ML, D'Amore E, Sartore S, Gabbiani G. Expression of myosin heavy chain isoforms in mammary epithelial cells and in myofibroblasts from different fibrotic settings during neoplasia. *Virchows Arch* 1995;426:77–86.
139. Sappino AP, Schürch W, Gabbiani G. Differentiation repertoire of fibroblastic cells: Expression of cytoskeletal proteins as markers of phenotypic modulations. *Lab Invest* 1990;63:144–161.
140. Eyden BP, Ponting H, Davies H Bartley C, Torgersen E. Defining the myofibroblast: normal tissues, with special reference to the stromal cells of Wharton's jelly in human umbilical cord. *J Submicrosc Cytol Pathol* 1994;26:347–355.
141. Desmouliére A, Gabbiani G. The role of the myofibroblast in wound healing and fibrocontractive diseases. In: Clark RAF, ed. *The molecular and cellular biology of wound repair*, 2nd ed. New York: Plenum Press, 1996:391–423.
142. Burrington JD. Wound healing in the fetal lamb. *J Pediatr Surg* 1971; 6:523–528.
143. Goss AN. Intra–uterine healing of fetal rat oral mucosal, skin and cartilage wounds. *J Oral Pathol* 1977;6:35–43.
144. Adzick NS, Harrison MR, Glick PL, Beckstead JH, Villa RL, Scheuenstuhl H, Goodson WH. Comparison of fetal newborn, and adult wound healing by histologic, enzyme-histochemical, and hydroxyproline determinations. *J Pediatr Surg* 1985;20:315–319.

145. Rowsell AR. The intra–uterine healing of foetal muscle wounds: Experimental study in the rat. *Br J Plast Surg* 1986;37:635–642.
146. Krummel TM, Nelson JM, Diegelmann RF, Lindblad WJ, Salzberg AM, Greenfield LJ, Cohen IK. Fetal response to injury in the rabbit. *J Pediatr Surg* 1987;22:640–644.
147. Adzick NS, Longaker MT. Scarless fetal wound healing: Therapeutic implications. *Ann Surg 1992 215*:3–7.
148. Estes JM, Vande Berg JS, Adzick NS, MacGillivray TE, Desmoulière A, Gabbiani G. Phenotypical and functional features of myofibroblasts in sheep fetal wounds. *Differentiation* 1994;56:173–181.
149. Seemayer TA Schürch W, Lagacé R. Myofibroblasts in human pathology. *Hum Pathol* 1972;12:491–492.
150. Bhathal PS. Presence of modified fibroblasts in cirrhotic livers in man. *Pathology* 1972;4:139–144.
151. Irlé C, Kocher O, Gabbiani G. Contractility of myofibroblasts during experimental liver cirrhosis. *J Submicrosc Cytol Pathol* 1980;12:209–217.
152. Rudolph R, McLure WJ, Woodward M. Contractile fibroblasts in chronic alcoholic liver cirrhosis. *Gastroenterology* 1979;76:704–709.
153. Madden JW. On "the contractile fibroblast." *Plast Recontstr Surg* 1973;52:291–292.
154. Woyke S, Domagala W, Olszewski W, Korabiec M. Pseudosarcoma of the skin. An electron microscopic study and comparison with fine structure of the spindle–cell variant of squamous cell carcinoma. *Cancer* 1974;33:970–980.
155. Larson DL, Abston S, Willis B, Linares H, Dobrowsky M. Evans EB, Lewis SR. Contracture and scar formation in the burn patient. *Clin Plast Surg* 1974;1:653–656.
156. Madden JW, Carlson EC, Hines J. Presence of modified fibroblasts in ischemic contracture of the intrinsic musculature of the hand. *Surg Gynecol Obstet* 1975;140:509–516.
157. Nagle RB, Kneiser MR, Bulger RE, Benditt EP. Induction of smooth muscle characteristics in renal interstitial fibroblasts during obstructive nephropathy. *Lab Invest* 1973;29:422–427.
158. Judd PA, Finnegan P, Curran RC. Pulmonary sarcoidosis: a clinico–pathological study. *J Pathol* 1975;115:191–198.
159. El–Labban NG, Lee KW. Myofibroblasts in central giant cell granuloma of the jaws: an ultrastructural study. *Histopathology* 1983; 7:907–918.
160. Grimaud JA, Borojevi CR. Myofibroblasts in hepatic schistosomal fibrosis. *Experientia* 1977;33:890–892.
161. Postacchini F, Natali PG, Accinni L, Ippolito E, De Martino C. Contractile filaments in cells of regenerating tendon. *Experientia* 1977;33: 957–959.
162. Rudolph R, Woodward M. Spatial orientation of microtubules in contractile fibroblasts in vivo. *Anat Rec* 1978;191:169–181.
163. Ziman OA, Robles JM, Lee JC. The fibrous capsule around mammary implants: an investigation. *Aesthetic Plast Surg* 1978;2: 217–134.
164. Callea F, Mebis J, Desmet VJ. Myofibroblasts in focal nodular hyperplasia of the liver. *Virchows Arch A* 1982;396:155–166.
165. Ghadially FN, Mehta PN. Multifunctional mesenchymal cells resembling smooth muscle cells in ganglia of the wrist. *Ann Rheum Dis* 1971;30:31–42.
166. Baur PS, Larson DL, Stacey TR. The observation of myofibroblasts in hypertrophic scars. *Surg Gynecol Obstet* 1975;141: 22–26.
167. Novotny GE, Pau H. Myofibroblast–like cells in human anterior capsular cataract. *Virchows Arch A* 1984;404:393–401.
168. Woodcock–Mitchell J, Adler KB, Low RB. Immunohistochemical identification of cell types in normal and in bleomycin– induced fibrotic rat lung: cellular origin of interstitial cells. *Am Rev Respir Dis* 1984;130:910–916.
169. Lagacé R, Delage C, Boutet M. Light and electron microscopic study of cellular proliferation in carcinoid heart disease. *Recent Adv Stud Cardiac Struct Metab* 1975;10:605–616.
170. Thomas WA, Jones R, Scotte RF, Morrison E, Goodale F. Imai H. Production of early atherosclerotic lesions in rats characterized by proliferation of "modified smooth muscle cells." *Exp Mol Pathol* 1963;2(suppl 1):40–61.
171. Flora G, Dahl E, Nelson E. Electron microsocopic observations on human intracranial arteries. Changes seen with aging and atherosclerosis. *Arch Neurol* 1967;17:162–173.
172. Wissler RW. The arterial medial cell, smooth muscle or multifunctional mesenchyme? *Circulation* 1967;36:1–4.
173. Gabbiani G, Badonnel MC. Contractile apparatus in aortic endothelium of hypertensive rat. *Recent Adv Cardiac Struct Metab* 1975; 10: 591–601.
174. Sappino AP, Massouyé I, Saurat JH, Gabbiani G. Smooth muscle differentiation in scleroderma fibroblastic cells. *Am J Pathol* 1990; 137: 585–591.
175. Diamond JR, van Goor H, Ding G, Engelmyer E. Myofibroblasts in experimental hydronephrosis. *Am J Pathol* 1995;146:121–129.
176. Gabbrielli S, DiLollo S, Stanflin N, Romagnoli P. Myofibroblast and elastic and collagen fiber hyperplasia in the bronchial mucosa: a possible basis for the progressive irreversibility of airway obstruction in chronic asthma. *Pathologica* 1994;86:157–160.
177. Schürch W, Seemayer TA, Gabbiani G. In: Sternberg SS, ed. *Histology for Pathologists*. New York: Raven Press, 1992;109–144.
178. Ehrlich HP, Desmoulière A, Diegelmann RF, Cohen IK, Compton CC, Garner WL, Kapanci Y, Gabbiani G. Morphological and immunohistochemical differences between keloid and hypertrophic scar. *Am J Pathol* 1994;145:105–113.
179. Enzinger FM, Weiss SW. *Soft tissue tumors*. 3rd ed. St Louis: CV Mosby, 1994:201–229.
180. Chiu HF, McFarlane RM. Pathogenesis of Dupuytren's contracture: A correlative clinical-pathological study. *J Hand Surg* (Am)1978; 3:1–10.
181. Navas-Palacios JJ. The fibomatoses. An ultrastructural study of 31 cases. *Pathol Res Pract* 1983;176:158–175.
182. Ushijama M, Tsuneyoshi M, Enjoji M. Dupuytren type fibromatoses. A clinicopathologic study of 62 cases. *Acta Pathol Jpn* 1984;34: 991–1001.
183. Ariyan S, Enrique R, Krizek TJ. Wound contraction and fibrocontractive disorders. *Arch Surg* 1978;113:1034–1046.
184. Allen PW. The fibromatoses: a clinocopathologic classification based on 140 cases. *Am J Surg Pathol* 1977;1:255–270.
185. Chung EB, Enzinger FM. Infantile myofibromatosis. A review of 59 cases with localized and generalized involvement. *Cancer* 1981; 48: 1807–1818.
186. Wirman JA. Nodular fasciitis, a lesion of myofibroblasts. An ultrastructural study. *Cancer* 1976;38:2378–2389.
187. Chung EB, Enzinger FM. Proliferative fasciitis. *Cancer* 1975; 36: 1450–1458.
188. Povysil C, Matejovsky Z. Ultrastructural evidence of myofibroblasts in pseudomalignant myositis ossificans. *Virchows Arch A* 1979;381: 189–203.
189. Weathers DR, Campbell WG. Ultrastructure of the giant–cell fibroma of the oral mucosa. *Oral Surg* 1974;38:550–561.
190. Stiller D, Katenkamp D. Cellular features in desmoid fibromatosis and well–differentiated fibrosarcomas. An electron microscopic study. *Virchows Arch A* 1975;369:155–164.
191. Ramos CV, Gillespie W, Narconis RJ. Elastofibroma. A pseudotumor of myofibroblasts. *Arch Pathol Lab Med* 1978;102:538–540.
192. Buell R, Wang NS, Seemayer TA, Ahmed MN. Endobronchial plasma cell granuloma. A light and electron microscopic study. *Hum Pathol* 1976;7:411–426.
193. Bhawan J, Bacchetta C, Joris I, Majno G. A myofibroblastic tumor. Infantile digital fibroma(recurrent digital fibrous tumor of childhood). *Am J Pathol* 1979;94:19–36.
194. Taxy JB. Juvenile nasopharyngeal angiofibroma. An ultrastructural study. *Cancer* 1977;39:1044–1054.
195. Ferrans VJ, Roberts WC. Structural features of cardiac myxomas. Histology, histochemistry and electron microscopy. *Human Pathol* 1973; 4:111–146.
196. Fisher ER, Paulson JD, Gregorio RM. The myofibroblastic nature of the uterine plexiform tumor. *Arch Pathol Lab Med* 1978;102: 477–480.
197. Tomasek JJ, Schultz RJ, Episalla CW, Newman SA. The cytoskeleton and extracellular matrix of the Dupuytren's disease "myofibroblast": an immunofluorescence study of a non-muscle cell type. *J Hand Surg(Am)* 1986;11A:365–371.
198. Shum DT, McFarlane RM. Histogenesis of Dupuytren's disease; an immunohistochemical study of 30 cases. *J Hand Surg(Am)* 1988;13A: 61–67.
199. Luck JV. Dupuyten's contracture. A new concept of the pathogenesis correlated with surgical management. *J Bone Joint Surg(Am)* 1959;41: 635–664.
200. Iwasaki H, Müller H, Stutte HJ, Brennscheidt U. Palmar fibromatosis (Dupuytren's contracture). Ultrastructural and enzyme histochemical study of 43 cases. *Virchows Arch A* 1984;404:41–53.
201. Eddy RJ, Petro JA, Tomasek JJ. Evidence for the nonmuscle nature of the "myofibroblast"of granulation tissue and hypertrophic scar. An immunofluorescence study. *Am J Pathol* 1988;130:252–260.

202. Matte C, Cadotte M, Schürch W. Intermediate filament proteins and actin isoforms of dermatofibrosarcoma protuberans and dermatofibroma. *Lab Invest* 1990;62(1):64A(abst. 373).
203. Fukusawa Y, Ishikura H, Takada A, Yokoyama S, Imamura M, Yoshiki T, Sato H. Massive apoptosis in infantile myofibromatosis. A putative mechanism of tumor regression. *Am J Pathol* 1994;144: 480–485.
204. Ohtani H, Sasano N. Myofibroblasts and myoepithelial cells in human breast carcinoma. An ultrastructural study. *Virchows Arch A* 1980; 385:247–261.
205. Carroll R. Influence of lung scars on primary lung cancer. *J Bacteriol* 1962;83:293–297.
206. Madri JA, Carter D. Scar cancers of the lung: origin and significance. *Hum Pathol* 1984;15:625–631.
207. Barsky SH, Huang SJ, Bhuta S. The extracellular matrix of pulmonary scar carcinomas is suggestive of a desmoplastic origin. *Am J Pathol* 1986;124:412–419.
208. Gabbiani G, Kaye GI, Lattes R, Majno G. Synovial sarcoma. Electron microscopic study of a typical case. *Cancer* 1971;28:1031–1039.
209. Gabbiani G, Fu YS, Kaye GI,Lattes R, Majno G. Epitheloid sarcoma. A light and electron microscopic study suggesting a synovial origin. *Cancer* 1972;30:486–499.
210. Lagacé R, Schürch W, Seemayer TA. Myofibroblasts in soft tissue sarcomas. *Virchows Arch A* 1980;389:1–11.
211. Seemayer TA, Lagacé R, Schürch W. On the pathogenesis of sclerosis and nodularity in nodular sclerosing Hodgkin's disease. *Virchows Arch A* 1980;385:283–291.
212. Churg AM, Kahn LB. Myofibroblats and related cells in malignant fibrous histiocytic tumors. *Hum Pathol* 1977;8:205–218.
213. D'Andiran G, Gabbiani G. A metastasizing sarcoma of the pleura composed of myofibroblasts. In: Fenoglio CM, Wolff M, eds. *Progress in surgical pathology*. New York: Masson, 1980; 31–40.
214. Ghadially FN, McNaughton JD, Lalonde JM. Myofibroblastoma: a tumor of myofibroblasts. *J Submicrosc Cytol Pathol* 1983;15: 1055–1063.
215. Wargotz ES, Weiss SW, Norris HJ. Myofibroblastoma of the breast: sixteen cases of a distinctive benign mesenchymal tumor. *Am J Surg Pathol* 1987;11:493–502.
216. Weiss SW, Gnepp DR, Bratthauer GL. Palisaded myofibroblastoma: a benign mesenchymal tumor of lymph node. *Am J Surg Pathol* 1989; 13:341–346.
217. Suster S, Rosai J. Intranodal hemorrhagic spindle cell tumor with"amianthoid" fibers: report of six cases with a distinctive mesenchymal neoplasm of the inguinal region that simulates Kaposi's sarcoma. *Am J Surg Pathol* 1989;13:347–357.
218. Schürch W, Skalli O, Seemayer TA, Gabbiani G. Intermediate filament proteins and actin isoforms as markers for soft tissue tumor differentiation and origin. I. Smooth muscle tumors. *Am J Pathol* 1987; 128:91–103.
219. Schürch W, Skalli O, Lagacé R, Seemayer TA, Gabbiani G. Intermediate filament proteins and actin isoforms as markers for soft tissue tumor differentiation and origin. III. Hemangiopericytomas and glomus tumors. *Am J Pathol* 1990;136:771–786.
220. Schürch W, Bégin LR, Seemayer TA, Lagacé R, Boivin JC, Lamoureux C, Bluteau P, Pich J, Gabbiani G. Pleomorphic soft tissue myogenic sarcomas of adulthood. A reappraisal in the mid-1990s. *Am J Surg Pathol* 1996; 20:131–137.
221. Gabbiani G. Modulation of fibroblastic cytoskeletal features during wound healing, fibrosis. *Path Res Pract* 1994;190:851–853.
222. Pierce GF, Vande Berg J, Rudolph R, Tarpley J, Mustoe TA. Platelet–derived growth factor–BB, transforming growth factor Beta–1 selectively modulate glycosaminoglycans, collagen, myofibroblasts in excisional wounds. *Am J Pathol* 1991;130:629–646.
223. Streuli CH, Schmidhauser C, Kobrin M, Bissell MJ, Derynck R. Extracellular matrix regulates expression of the TGF–$\beta$1 gene. *J Cell Biol* 1993;120:253–260.
224. Deuel TF, Kawahara RS, Mustoe TA. Pierce AF. Growth factors and, wound healing: platelet–derived growth factor as a model cytokine. *Annu Rev Med* 1991;42:567–584.
225. Kovacs EJ. Fibrogenic cytokines: the role of immuno mediators in the development of scar tissue. *Immunol Today* 1991;12: 17–23.
226. Border WA, Ruoslahti E. Transfoming growth factor-$\beta$ in disease: the dark side of tissue repair. *J Clin Invest* 1992;90:1–7.
227. Sporn MB, Roberts AB. Transforming growth factor-$\beta$: recent progress, new challenges. *J Cell Biol* 1992;119:1017–1021.
228. Border WA, Noble NA. Transforming growth factor $\beta$ in tissue fibrosis. *N Engl J Med* 1994;331:1286–1292.
229. Kulkarni AB, Karlsson S. Transforming growth factor $\beta$1 knockout mice: A mutation in one cytokine gene causes a dramatic inflammatory disease. *Am J Pathol* 1993;143:3–9.
230. Pablos JL, Everett ET, Harley R, LeRoy EC, Norris JS. Transforming growth factor–$\beta$1, and collagen gene expession during postnatal skin development and fibrosis in the tight-skin mouse. *Lab Invest* 1995;72: 670–678.
231. Mackie EJ, Chiquet–Ehrismann R, Pearson CA, Inaguma Y, Taya K, Kawarada Y, Sakakura T. Tenascin is a stromal marker for epithelial malignancy in the mammary gland. *Proc Natl Acad Sci U S A* 1987; 84:4621–4625.
232. Basset P, Bellocq JP, Wolf C, Stoll I, Hutin P, Limacher JM, Podhajcer OL, Chenard MP, Rio MC, Chambon P. A novel metalloproteinase gene specifically expressed in stromal cells of breast carcinomas. *Nature* 1990;348:699–704.
233. Pyke C, Kristensen P, Ralfkiaer E, Grøndahl–Hansen J, Ericksen J, Blasi F, Danø K. Urokinase-type plasminogen activator is expressed in stromal cells and its receptor in cancer cells at invasive foci in human colon adenocarcinomas. *Am J Pathol* 1991;138: 1059–1067.
234. Cullen KJ, Smith HS, Hill S, Rosen N, Lippman ME. Growth factor messenger RNA expression by human breast fibroblasts from benign and malignant lesions. *Cancer Res* 1991;51:4978–4985.
235. Rønnov-Jessen L, Petersen OW. Induction of alpha smooth muscle actin by transforming growth factor-$\beta$1 in quiescent human breast gland fibroblasts. *Lab Invest* 1993;68:696–707.
236. Rønnov-Jessen L, Petersen OW, Koteliansky VE, Bissell MJ. The origin of the myofibroblasts in breast cancer: recapitulation of tumor environment in culture unravels diversity and implicates converted fibroblasts and recruited smooth muscle cells. *J Clin Invest* 1995;95: 859–873.
237. Carrel A. Growth promoting function of leucocytes. *J Exp Med* 1922; 36:385–397.
238. Cohnheim J. Ueber Entzündung und Eiterung. *Virchows Arch A* 1867; 40:1–9.
239. Arey LB. Wound healing. *Physiol Rev* 1936;16:327–406.
240. Grillo HC. Derivation of fibroblasts in healing wound. *Arch Surg* 1964;88:218–224.
241. Allgöwer M. *The cellular basis of wound repair*. Springfield, IL: Charles C Thomas, 1967.
242. Ross R, Everett NB, Tyler R. Wound healing and collagen formation. VI. The origin of the wound fibroblast studied in parabiosis. *J Cell Biol* 1970;44:645–654.
243. Crocker DJ, Murad TM, Geer JC. Role of the pericyte in wound healing. An ultrastructural study. *Exp Mol Pathol* 1970;13:51–65.
244. Oda G, Gown AM, Vande Berg JS, Stern R. The fibroblast-like nature of myofibroblasts. *Exp Mol Pathol* 1988;49:316–329.
245. Chamley JH, Campbell GR, McConnell JD, Gröschel-Stewart U. Comparison of vascular smooth muscle cells from adult human monkey and rabbit in primary culture and subculture. *Cell Tissue Res* 1977;177: 503–522.
246. Moss NS, Benditt EP. Spontaneous and experimentally induced arterial lesions. I. An ultrastructural survey of the normal chicken aorta. *Lab Invest* 1970;22:166–183.
247. Mosse PR, Campbell GR, Wang ZL, Campbell JH. Smooth muscle phenotypic expression in human carotid arteries. I. Comparison of cells from diffuse intimal thickenings adjacent to atheromatous plaques with those of the media. *Lab Invest* 1985;53:556–562.
248. Olivetti G, Anversa P, Melissari M, Loud AV. Morphometric study of early postnatal development of the thoracic aorta in the rat. *Circ Res* 1980;47:417–424.
249. Poole JC, Cromwell SB, Benditt EP. Behavior of smooth muscle cells and formation of extracellular structures in the reaction of arterial walls to injury. *Am J Pathol* 1971;62:391–414.
250. Franke WW, Moll R. Cytoskeletal components of lymphoid organs. I. Synthesis of cytokeratin 8 and 18 and desmin in subpopulations of extrafollicular reticulum cells of human lymph nodes, tonsils and spleen. *Differentiation* 1987;36:145–163.
251. Ramadori G, Veit T, Schwogler S, Dienes HP, Knittel T, Rieder H, Meyer zum Buschenfelde KH. Expression of the gene of the $\alpha$-smooth muscle actin isoform in rat liver and in rat fat-storing (ITO) cells. *Virchows Arch B* 1990;59:349–357.
252. Schmitt-Gräff A, Krüger S, Bochard F, Gabbiani G, Denk H. Modulation of alpha smooth muscle actin and desmin expression in perisi-

nusoidal cells of normal and diseased human livers. *Am J Pathol* 1991; 138:1233–1242.
253. Blazejewski S, Preaux AM, Mallat A, Brocheriou I, Mavier P, Dhumeaux D, Hartmann D, Schuppan D, Rosenbaum J. Human myofibroblastlike cells obtained by outgrowth are representative of the fibrogenic cells in the liver. *Hepatology* 1995;22:788–797.
254. Milani S, Herbst H, Schuppan D, Riecken EO, Stein H. Cellular localization of laminin gene transcripts in normal and fibrotic human liver. *Am J Pathol* 1989;134:1175–1182.
255. Milani S, Herbst H, Schuppan D, Surrenti C, Riecken EO, Stein H. Cellular localization of type I, III, and IV procollagen gene transcripts in normal and fibrotic human liver. *Am J Pathol* 1990;137: 59–70.
256. Takahara T, Nakayama Y, Itoh H, Miyabayashi C, Watanabe A, Sasaki H, Inoue K. Extracellular matrix formation in piecemeal necrosis: immunoelectron microscopic study. *Liver* 1992;12:368–380.
257. Nagy P, Schaff Z, Lapis K. Immunohistochemical detection of transforming growth factor $\beta 1$ in fibrotic liver diseases. *Hepatology* 1991; 14:269–273.
258. Friedman SL, Yamasaki G, Wong L. Modulation of transforming growth factor $\beta$ receptors of rat lipocytes during the hepatic wound healing response: enhanced binding and reduced gene expression accompany cellular activation in culture and in vivo. *J Biol Chem* 1994; 269:10551–10558.
259. Goumenos DS, Brown CB, Shortland J, El Nahas AM. Myofibroblasts predictors of progression of mesangial IgA nephropathy? *Nephrol Dial Transplant* 1994;9:1418–1425.
260. Boukhalfa G, Desmoulière A, Rondeau E, Gabbiani G, Sraer JD. Relationship between $\alpha$-smooth muscle actin expression and fibrotic changes in the human kidney. *Exp Nephrol* 1996; 4:241–247.
261. Kapanci Y, Ribaux C, Chaponnier C, Gabbiani G. Cytoskeletal features of alveolar myofibroblasts and pericytes in normal human and rat lung. *J Histochem Cytochem* 1992;40:1955–1963.
262. Vyalov SL, Gabbiani G, Kapanci Y. Rat alveolar myofibroblasts acquire $\alpha$-smooth muscle actin expression during bleomycin-induced pulmonary fibrosis. *Am J Pathol* 1993;143:1754–1765.
263. Roberts AB, Sporn MB, Assoian RK, Smith JM, Roche NS, Wakefield LM, Heine UI, Liotta LA,Falanga V, Kehrl JH, Fauci AS. Transforming growth factor type beta: rapid induction of fibrosis and angiogenesis in vivo and stimulation of collagen formation in vitro. *Proc Natl Acad Sci U S A* 1986;83:4167–4171.
264. Ignotz RA, Massagué J. Transforming growth factor-$\beta$ stimulates the expression of fibronectin and collagen and their incorporation into the extracellular matrix. *J Biol Chem* 1986;261: 4337–4345.
265. Garbin S, Pittet B Montandon D, Gabbiani G, Desmoulière A. Covering by a flap induces apoptosis of granulation tissue myofibroblasts and vascular cells. *Wound Rep Reg* 1996; 4:244–256.
266. Evans VG. Multiple pathways to apoptosis. *Cell Biol Int* 1993;17: 461–476.
267. Lee S, Christakos S, Small MB. Apoptosis and signal transduction: clues to a molecular mechanism. *Current Opin Cell Biol* 1993; 5:286–291.
268. Schwartzman RA, Cidlowski JA. Apoptosis: the biochemistry and molecular biology of programmed cell death. *Endocr Rev* 1993;14: 133–151.
269. White E. Death defying acts: a meeting review on apoptosis: genetic controls on cell death. *Genes Dev* 1993;7:2277–2284.
270. Williams GT, Smith CA. Molecular regulation of apoptosis. *Cell* 1993;74:777–779.
271. Martin SJ, Green DR, Cotter TG. Dicing with death: dissecting the components of the apoptosis machinery. *Trends Biochem Sci* 1994;19: 26–30.
272. Evan GI, Wyllie AH, Gilbert CS, Littlewood TD, Land H, Brooks M, Waters CM, Penn LZ, Hancock DC. Induction of apoptosis in fibroblasts by c-Myc protein. *Cell* 1992;69:119–128.
273. Miura M, Zhu H, Rotello R, Hartwieg EA, Yuan J. Induction of apoptosis in fibroblasts by IL-1$\beta$ converting enzyme, a mammalian homolog of the *C. elegans* cell death gene ced-3. *Cell* 1993;75: 653–660.
274. Reed JC. Bcl-2 and the regulation of programmed cell death. *J Cell Biol* 1994;124:1–6.
275. Laster SM, Wood JG, Gooding LR. Tumor necrosis factor can induce both apoptotic and necrotic forms of cell lysis. *J Immunol* 1988;141; 2629–2634.
276. Robaye B, Mosselmans R, Fiers W, Dumont JE, Galand P. Tumor necrosis factor induces apoptosis (programmed cell death) in normal endothelial cells in vitro. *Am J Pathol* 1991;138:447–453.
277. Moulton BC. Transforming growth factor-$\beta$ stimulates endometrial stromal apoptosis in vitro. *Endocrinology* 1994;134: 1055–1060.
278. Pierce GF, Mustoe TA, Senior RM, Reed J, Griffin GL, Thomason A, Deuel TF. In vivo incisional wound healing augmented by platelet-derived growth factor and recombinant c-sis gene homodimeric proteins. *J Exp Med* 1988;167:974–987.
279. Mustoe TA Pierce GF, Thomason A, Gramates P, Sporn MB, Deuel TF. Accelerated healing of incisional wounds in rats induced by transforming growth factor-$\beta$. *Science* 1987;237:1333–1336.
280. Beck LS, DeGuzman L, Lee WP, Xu Y, Siegel MW, Amento EP. One systemic administration of transforming growth factor-$\beta 1$ reverses age/or glucocorticoid-impaired wound healing. *J Clin Invest* 1993;92: 2841–2849.
281. Schultz GS, White M, Mitchell, R, Brown G, Lynch J, Twardzik DR, Todaro GJ. Epithelial wound healing enhanced by transforming growth factor-$\alpha$ and vaccinia growth factor. *Science* 1987;235: 350–352.
282. Mooney DP, O'Reilly M, Gamelli RL. Tumor necrosis factor and wound healing. *Ann Surg* 1990;211:124–129.
283. Martin P, Hopkinson-Woolley J, McCluskey J. Growth factors and cutaneous wound repair. *Prog Growth Factor Res* 1992;4:25–44.
284. Dvorak HF. Tumors: wounds that do not heal. Similarities between tumor stroma generation and wound healing. *New Engl J Med* 1986;15: 1650–1659.
285. Whitby DJ, Ferguson MW. Immunohistochemical localization of growth factors in fetal wound healing. *Dev Biol* 1991;147:207–215.

*Histology for Pathologists, second edition,*
Edited by Stephen S. Sternberg.
Lippincott-Raven Publishers, Philadelphia


CHAPTER 8

# Adipose Tissue

John S. J. Brooks and Patricia M. Perosio



In compiling this chapter, our intention was to provide practicing surgical pathologists with both a description of normal and abnormal adipose tissue and a reference source. We were inclusive in our approach and considered all bodily lesions containing mature fat appropriate for discussion regardless of site. The section on development should provide a deeper understanding for the diagnostician and a starting point for the researcher. Collected and detailed as a group are the fatty infiltrations of organs, the inflammations affecting fat, the hamartomas and mesenchymomas, and the lipomas and variants thereof. Up-to-date definitions are provided where necessary. Importantly, we have also summarized clinical and genetic syndromes in which fat cells may participate. Unusual but distinctive histologies are enumerated such as may occur in starvation, pancreatic fat necrosis, and true lipodystrophy. All topics are well referenced, hopefully providing the reader with a valuable resource. In short, we have attempted to describe as many lesions as possible, not just primary fatty entities, but also anything extraneous within adipose tissue or confused with it.

J. S. J. Brooks: Department of Pathology, Roswell Park Cancer Institute, Buffalo, NY 14263.
P.M. Perosio: Department of Pathology, The Toledo Hospital, Toledo, OH 43606.

## WHITE FAT

### Prenatal Development

The morphology of developing adipose tissue has been studied in detail. By examining serial sections obtained from 805 human fetuses of various ages, Poissonnet et al. have determined that prior to the second trimester of pregnancy, adipose tissue primordia cannot be identified by light microscopy (1). After 14 weeks' gestation, aggregates of mesenchymal cells are seen condensed around proliferating primitive blood vessels. They refer to these findings as stage II in the development of adipose tissue (Fig. 1). Prior to this time, future adipose tissue is characterized by loose, spindle cells and ground substance (stage I). Later on, capillaries continue to proliferate into a rich network, around which preadipocytes become stellate and organized into a mesenchymal lobule (stage III). These preadipocytes do not contain lipid. With further development, fine lipid vacuoles characteristic of stage IV, accumulate within cytoplasm (Fig. 2). Continued proliferation of the components of the lobule results in the formation of densely packed aggregates of vacuolated fat cells with a rich capillary vascular network. Finally, condensation of perilobular mesenchyme at the periphery of the lobule results in formation of fibrous interlobular septa in stage V. This process occurs over the 10-week period between the 14- and 24-week gestation period. From approximately 24 to 29 weeks, the number of fat lobules is relatively constant. Continued growth occurs mainly due to proliferation of capillaries and adipocytes, causing an increase in the size of the fat lobules (Fig. 2).

The same sequence of development of adipose tissue occurs at all sites throughout the body (2). The earliest white fat lobules appear first in the face, neck, breast, and abdominal wall at 14 weeks' gestation. By 15 weeks they are also evident over the back and shoulders. Development in the upper and lower extremities and anterior chest begins around the 16th week. By the end of the 23rd week, a layer of subcutaneous fat completely covers the extremities.

There is a very close association of adipocyte development and angiogenesis. Fat appears first in well-vascularized regions such as the shoulder joint, before differentiation can be identified in the less well supplied adjacent subcutaneous tissue. There is also an important physiologic significance to this close anatomic relationship. Lipoprotein lipase, the hormone responsible for transfer of triglyceride from circulating lipoproteins to adipose tissue, is synthesized by adipocytes and transferred to the luminal surface of the capillary endothelium (3). Thus, this close spatial relationship provides efficient transfer of enzyme and lipid.

Because of this close developmental association of capillaries and adipocytes, some have proposed that the adipocyte precursor or preadipocyte actually is derived from endothelial cells (4). Others have felt the preadipocyte may be a perivascular reticulum cell, perivascular fibroblast-like cell, or undifferentiated mesenchymal cell. The presumptive

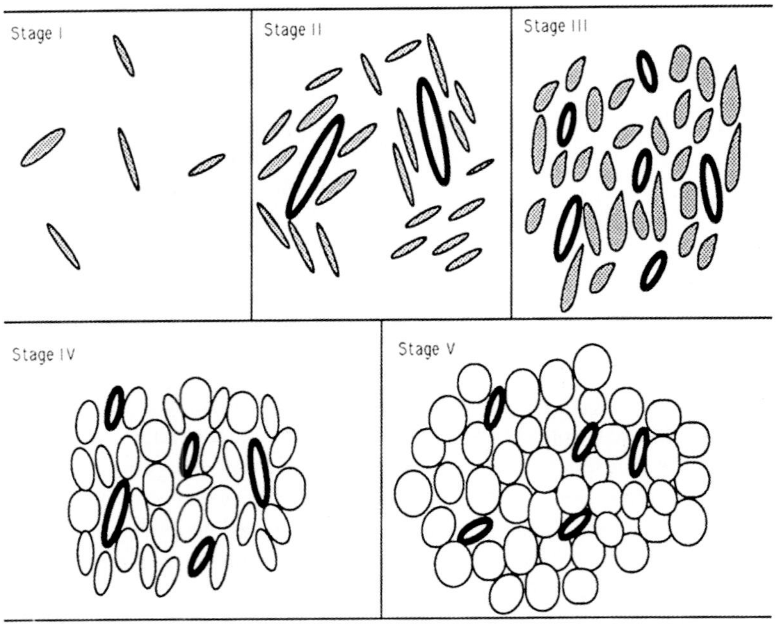


**FIG. 1.** Stage I: Stellate cells (stippled) embedded in amorphous ground substance. Stage II: As angiogenesis begins, mesenchymal cells (*stippled*) condense around the blood vessels (*bold ovals*). Stage III: A rich capillary network develops from each vessel, forming a glomerulus-like network around which each lobule forms. The preadipocytes become more stellate. Stage IV: With accumulation of lipid, these adipocytes, with multiple small lipid droplets, become closely packed around the capillaries. Stage V: Further accumulation of lipid with many unilocular cells (*clear circles*) is evident. The perilobular mesenchyme condenses into interlobular septa at this stage.

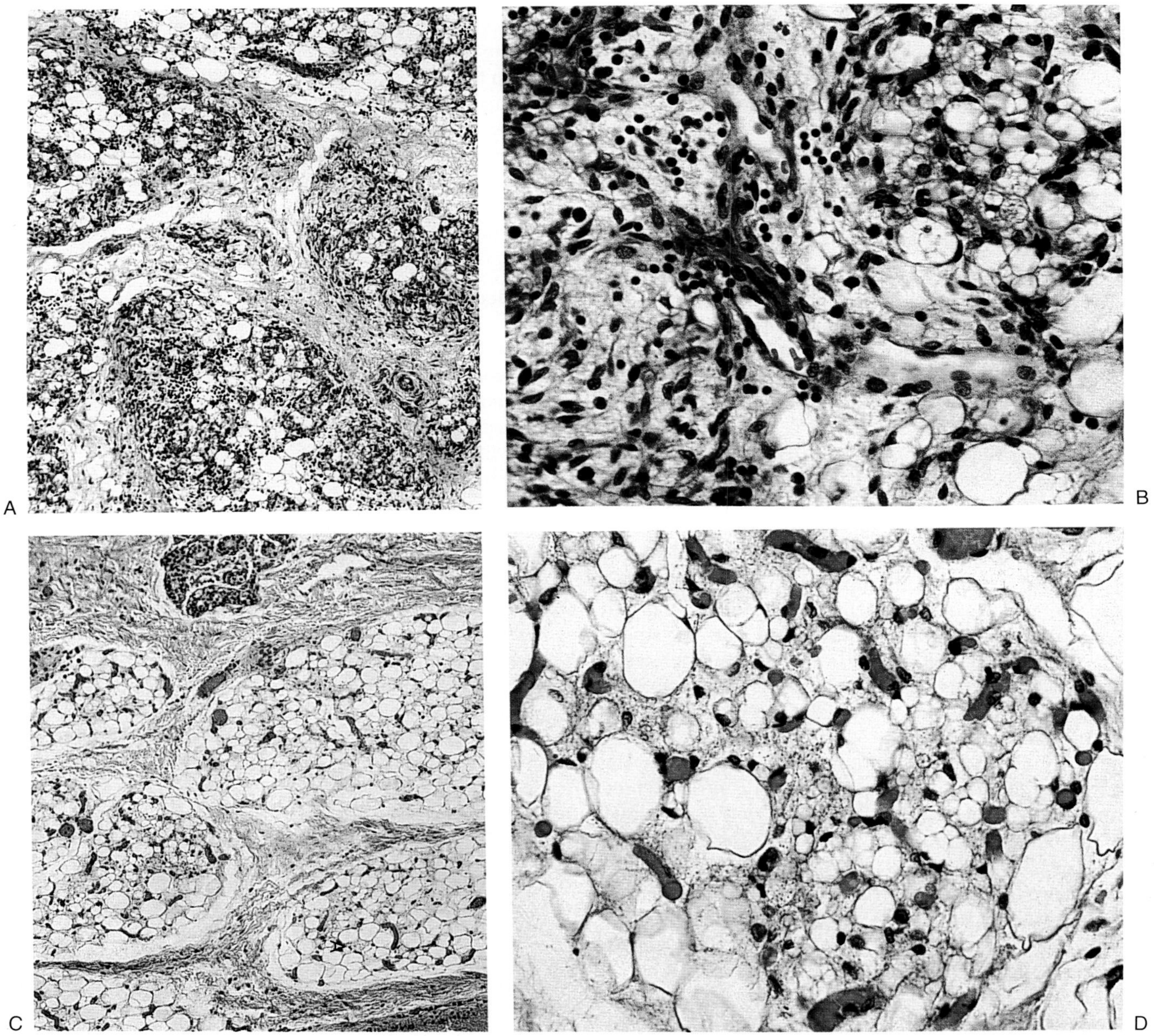

**FIG. 2.** Fetal fat. Fat lobules from a 25 week fetus with a myxoid quality and prominent vasculature (**A**). At high power, both univacuolated and multivacuolated cells are noted together with small capillaries (**B**). By 37 weeks, the lobules are more developed (**C**) and many of the cells are univacuolated (**D**).

adipocyte precursor has been characterized ultrastructurally in the newborn rat (5). The preadipocyte is a spindle cell with 4 to 5 cytoplasmic extensions along its long axis and abundant rough endoplasmic reticulum (ER). Lipid accumulates first as small droplets adjacent to the nucleus. As more lipid appears, it coalesces into a single large vacuole and the cell takes on an oval, and, finally, a round shape. The amount of rough ER decreases as the cell matures. Although cell shape and abundance of rough ER were taken as supportive evidence for the common origin of the preadipocyte and the fibroblast, which has a similar ultrastructural appearance, these similarities may have been a coincidence. The immature adipocyte needs to synthesize and excrete lipoprotein lipase—thus the abundant rough ER. Fibroblasts synthesizing and secreting procollagen would be expected to have a similar array of organelles.

As the preadipocyte accumulates lipid to become an adipocyte, both multilocular and unilocular adipocytes can be seen. Multilocular adipocytes predominate at first. With further lipid accumulation, more cells assume the unilocular appearance characteristic of mature adipocytes. Thus, attempts to differentiate brown from white adipocyte tissue at the light microscopic level, which rely on the presence of multivacuolated cells to characterize and identify brown fat, are not reliable. Reliance on ultrastructural and biochemical differences helps to distinguish between these different forms of adipose tissue.

### Molecular Biology

Through work on the adipocytic neoplasm known as myxoid liposarcoma (MLS), at least one gene involved in adipocytic differentiation has been identified. The translocation t(12;16)(q13;p11) of that tumor disrupts the normal function of the CHOP gene found at 12q13. First, the CHOP gene was shown to be rearranged in nearly all MLS (6) and, subsequently, the actual breakpoint was cloned (7,8). The CHOP gene, also known as GADD153, encodes a member of the CCAAT/enhancer binding (C/EBP) protein family and has a DNA binding domain. It appears to be involved in normal adipocyte differentiation because the protein it produces may be a dominant inhibitor of other C/EBP transcription factors known to be important in cell proliferation (9). Members of this C/EBP group are highly expressed in fat and are involved in the differentiation of fibroblasts into adipocytes and in the growth arrest of terminally differentiated adipocytes (6). CHOP itself is induced in the differentiation of 3T3-L1 cells to adipocytes. In the neoplasm, the translocation results in a fusion gene involving CHOP and TLS (translocated in liposarcoma), an RNA binding gene with much similarity structurally and functionally to the EWS gene of Ewing's sarcoma. Presumably, the lack of the normal inhibitory function of an intact CHOP gene allows the fatty tumor to proliferate unchecked. The use of both Southern blots and fluorescent in situ hybridation techniques detecting the rearranged gene will have usefulness in the diagnosis of fatty tumors. Likewise, when it becomes commercially available, antibody to the CHOP protein might be used immunohistochemically to detect such tumors.

Apoptosis or programmed cell death probably occurs in adipocytic tissues, but studies localizing the bcl-2 gene protein in human fetal tissues fail to mention its detection in fat (10).

### Postnatal Development

At birth, the average-size infant has approximately 5 billion adipocytes (11). This represents only 16% of the total number of adipocytes in adults. Adipose tissue continues to grow in parallel with general growth throughout the first 10 years of life. Fat cells enlarge significantly during the first six months of life without much increase in cell number (12). Until puberty, the cell size remains fairly constant while the number of adipocytes progressively increases. At puberty, there is a substantial increase in adipocyte size and number (12). Although at the end of puberty, the total number of adipocytes is similar to the adult, new adipocytes may continue to form throughout life (13). Studies on adult rats have shown that overfeeding results in proliferation of adipocyte precursors and development of new fat cells (14). De novo adipocyte formation can be triggered by overdistension of existing fat cells and the mass of stored triglycerides (15). Loss of fat cells may also occur and has been shown in overweight women following several years of strict dietary restriction (16).

### Gender Differences

The differences in body fat content noted between men and women begins in early childhood. Young girls are fatter than boys. Studies on fetuses, however, have not noted differences in the pattern of distribution or quantity of fat in prenatal life (1). The distribution of adipose tissue, however, even in prenatal life is not homogeneous throughout the body. Gender differences in the distribution of adipose tissue following puberty are well known and thought to be related to steroid hormone secretion (12). In humans, estrogens and progesterone induce an increase in trochanteric fat. The localization of more fat in the lower body in women results in the so-called gyneoid habitus. These same deposits are reduced by androgens in men, resulting in an android distribution of fat. The percentage of body fat also differs in men and women. Males reach a peak in body fat content during early adolescence, whereas women continue to accumulate fat relative to body weight throughout the teen years.

### Functions

White adipose tissue serves several functions. Fat provides thermal insulation and mechanical protection for underlying tissues. Its main role, however, is in the uptake, synthesis, and storage of lipid and release of free fatty acids in response to various neural and hormonal stimuli. Briefly, triglycerides circulate in the blood in the form of chylomicrons from the intestine and very low density lipoproteins from the liver (17). Lipoprotein lipase present on the luminal surface of endothelial cells hydrolyzes the triglyceride to release free fatty acids. This enzyme is synthesized by adipocytes and transferred to the endothelial cells. Most of the free fatty acids are taken up by the fat cells and reesterified to glycerol phosphate within the adipocyte to form triacylglycerol, which is then stored within the cell's lipid droplet. The fat is mobilized through the action of hormone-sensitive lipase, which hydrolyzes stored triglycerides. The released free fatty acids may be reesterified or released to the circulation and bound to albumin for transfer to other cells. Adipose tissue also has an endocrine function and is active in the conversion of androstenedione to estrone, the major source of estrogen in men and postmenopausal women. The aromatase action, however, has been localized through cell culture studies predominantly to the stromal cell fraction of adipose tissue, and not the adipocyte (18).

**Regulation**

Various factors regulate these processes. Adipocyte lipoprotein lipase (LPL) levels increase in obesity and decrease with fasting and diabetes (18). Insulin inhibits the action of hormone-sensitive lipase and, thereby, blocks release of free fatty acid. It also serves to promote adipocyte uptake of glucose, the precursor of the glycerol phosphate needed for triglyceride synthesis. Adipocytes are also richly supplied with $\alpha$- and $\beta$-adrenoreceptors. The $\beta1$ agonists enhance lipolysis while $\alpha2$ agonists inhibit it. Both act through a cyclic AMP second messenger. There are regional differences in the number of adrenergic receptors. In some women, the gluteal fat has the predominance of $\alpha2$ receptors. Thus, although body weight reduction occurs, little fat is lost from these regions (17). Regional differences in LPL levels also occur in women. Gluteal fat in premenopausal women tends to have high LPL levels, and these regions contain larger fat cells. Such regional differences disappear after menopause and are not present in obese men (19,20). Both enzyme levels and adrenergic receptors may, therefore, play a role in the regional differences in fat distribution and the development of gyneoid and android patterns of obesity. Such differences in LPL activity between pre- and postmenopausal women suggest that the sex steroids in women play a role in regulating LPL activity, particularly in the gluteal region. Rat studies have shown that it is actually progesterone that exerts this effect. Estrogens are needed probably to facilitate receptor-mediated transport of progesterone into the adipocyte nucleus (21).

In addition to adipocyte function, fat-cell size and number are also regulated. Numerous studies have been done in rats to identify mitotically active cells within fat using tritiated thymidine incorporation as a marker for cell division in adipose tissue. Mature lipid-laden adipocytes are generally considered to be incapable of cell differentiation due to the absence of mitotic figures seen histologically in normal adipose tissue. Sampling fat from rat injected with tritiated thymidine at 1 day and 3 days of age, which are then sacrificed at various times up to 5 months of age, has shown that the number of labeled cells in subcutaneous fat initially rises due to cell proliferation. The concentration of radioactivity then falls probably due to a dilutional effect resulting from continued cell division (21). This study, however, failed to distinguish adipocyte from stromal labeling. Similar studies had been performed on rats in which the subcutaneous tissue is separated into stromal and adipose components. In one study, the specific radioactivity of the adipocyte fraction did not increase until 2 to 5 days after injection (22). Thus, they concluded that DNA synthesis occurs in nonlipid-laden cells or preadipocytes. As these cells accumulate lipid, labeled cells are detected within the adipocyte fraction.

The factors that regulate adipocyte division have been studied in culture systems and in animal models. Growth hormone stimulates DNA synthesis in adipose tissue and abolishes the inhibitory effect of fasting on cell division (4). Insulin and glucocorticoids also stimulate DNA synthesis in cultured human adipocytes. These effects are enhanced on cells obtained from obese, as compared to lean people. Insulin not only increases DNA synthesis in adipocyte precursors but also enhances lipid accumulation and conversion to mature adipocytes. Estradiol-17$\beta$ has also been shown to stimulate division of cultured preadipocytes obtained from both men and women. Progesterone acts in vitro to stimulate both preadipocyte division and LPL activity (23). This dual role facilitates triglyceride accumulation in women. Prostaglandins, thyroid hormone, cytokines, and poorly defined pituitary and serum factors have also been demonstrated to influence preadipocyte differentiation in culture (18).

Adipose tissue grown in culture also secretes several proteins and potential regulators (18). Adipose tissue is a source of apolipoprotein E, angiotensin, and insulin-like growth factor I. Several less well characterized products are also synthesized and secreted. Adipsin, a serine protease, is also made by cultured adipocytes and may be active in local regulation of adipocyte growth and metabolism. Indeed, very low levels of adipsin are expressed in several animal models of genetic obesity (18). It is possible that the tendency toward obesity in these rodents is related to loss of this regulatory function.

**Gross**

Fatty tissue is typically a homogeneous, bright cadmium-like yellow, with a glistening and greasy surface texture and finely divided by faint septa. Any variation in color indicates a pathologic process: white to white/yellow in fat necrosis, paler yellows in many lipomas, reddish tinge to orange/yellow in angiolipoma, definite gray/white to whitish streaks in spindle cell lipoma, and white/yellow to white nodules in liposarcoma.

**Histology**

Microscopically, a mature white fat cell is spherical and measures up to 120 $\mu$m in diameter (24). The cytoplasm is compressed at the perimeter of the cell and only a thin rim of cell membrane is evident on hematoxylin-eosin (H&E)-stained sections. Periodic acid-Schiff (PAS) and reticulin stains highlight the adipocyte basement membrane (Fig. 3). The cytoplasm is displaced by a single lipid vacuole and the cells are fairly uniform in size (Fig. 4). The nucleus, although oval, is thin and small with finely distributed chromatin; when seen in profile, a central minute clear vacuole may be seen within the nucleus (Fig. 4). Normal subcutaneous fat is finely divided into ill-defined lobules by thin bands of collagen (Fig. 5).

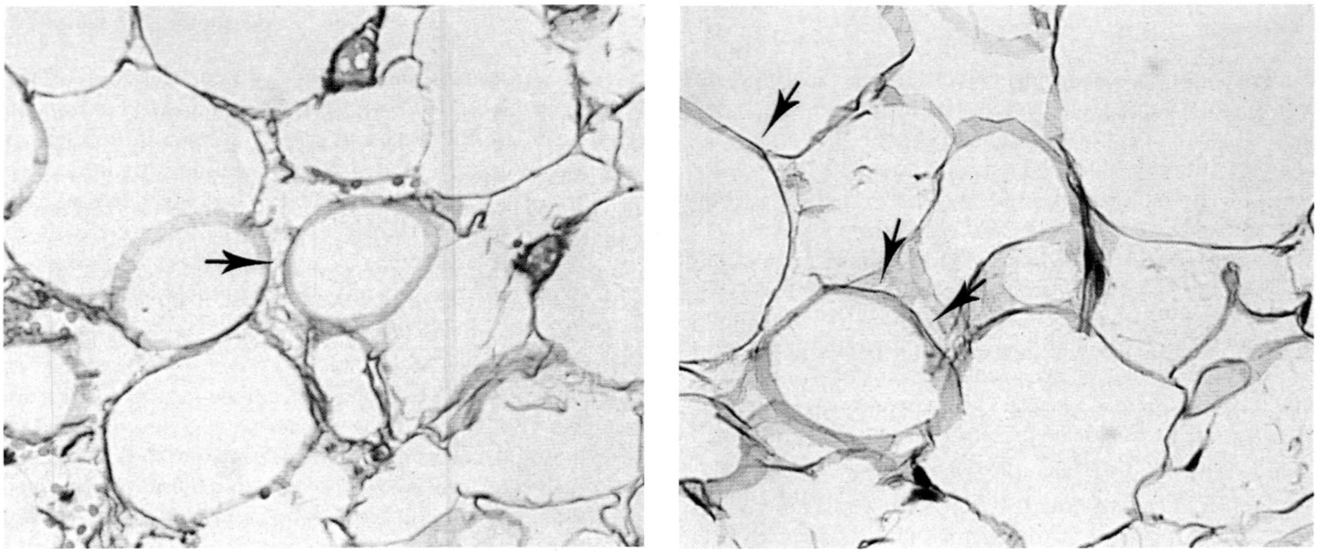

**FIG. 3.** Normal adult adipocyte. On a reticulin stain (**A**), each adipocyte is outlined by reticulin (*arrow*), which is present outside the cytoplasm; the same is true on PAS stain (**B**), where the basement membrane is highlighted *(arrows)* and encompasses the pale residue of cytoplasm remaining after fixation and embedding.

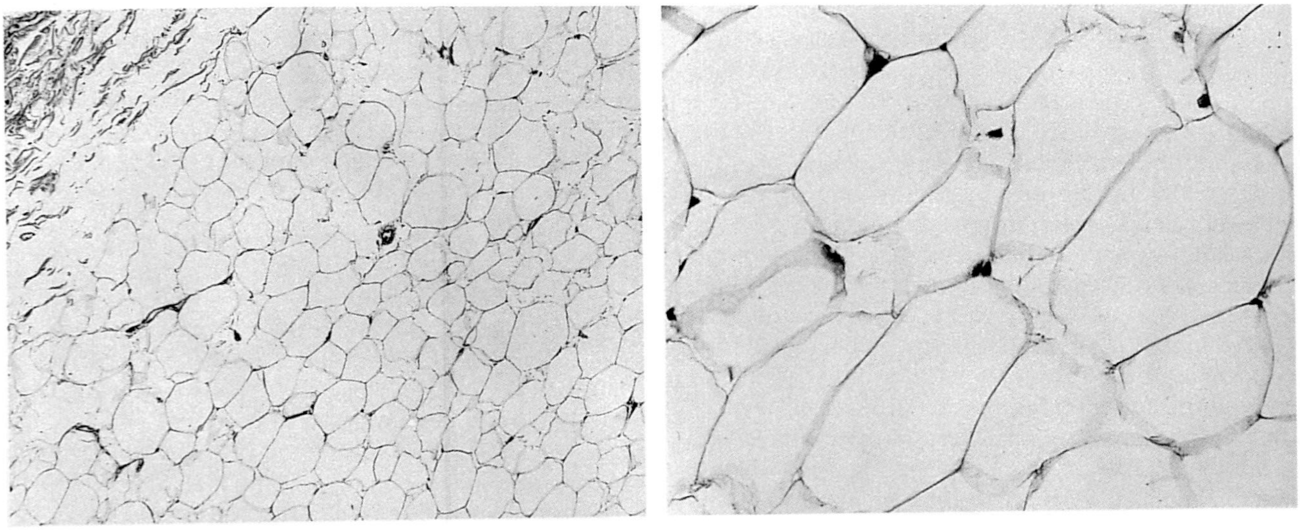

A B

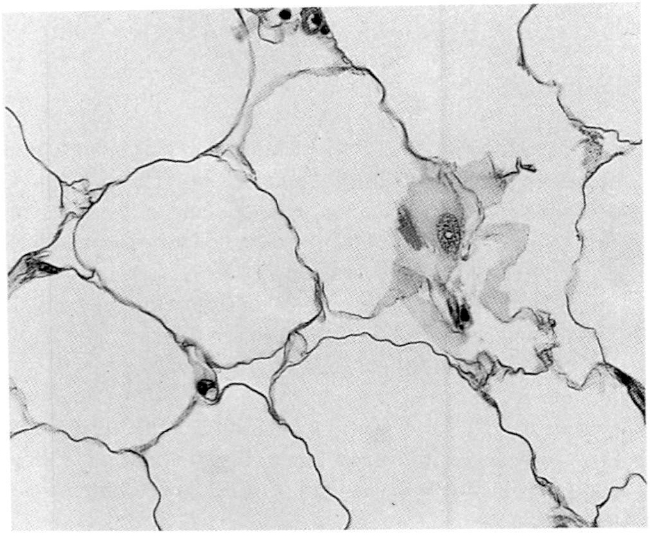

C

**FIG. 4.** At medium power the size of subcutaneous adipocytes appears relatively uniform (**A**); at high power, pale areas represent portions of basement membrane and cytoplasm cut on the bias (**B**). Nuclei of capillary endothelial cells are present at intersections between multiple cells. In contrast to other nuclei, an ideal section of an adipocyte nucleus (**C**) shows a pale character due to its thin nature and the common central vacuole or "Locherne." The wrinkled cell outlines are an artifact occasionally seen, the result of improper fixation.

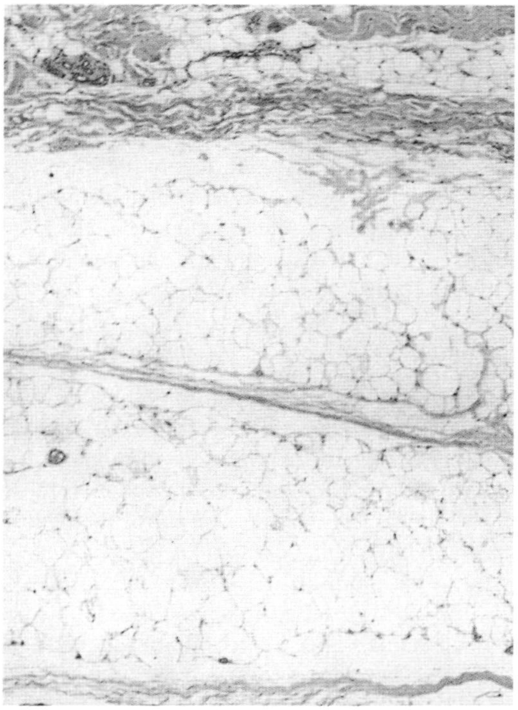

**FIG. 5.** Adult subcutaneous fat lobule with associated microvasculature; note the thin and delicate fibrous tissue septa.

### Ultrastructure

The ultrastructure of developing adipocytes has previously been discussed. In brief, a spindle shape with abundant endoplasmic reticulin and small spherical mitochondria characterizes preadipocytes (24). Lipid accumulates as small perinuclear inclusions that coalesce to form larger lipid droplets. The mitochondria become filamentous and the endoplasmic reticulum less prominent. In a mature adipocyte, the nucleus is flattened against the cytoplasmic membrane by a large lipid droplet. There is only a thin, tenuous rim of cytoplasm that surrounds it. Pinocytotic vesicles are seen in variable numbers but are very numerous following periods of starvation. Adjacent to the cell membrane are deposits of basement membrane. Capillaries are closely opposed to the adipocyte basement membrane. Only rarely have nerves been identified adjacent to white fat cells, although they may be seen in intercellular collagenous septa.

## BROWN FAT

### Prenatal Development

The development of brown adipose tissue has been studied in animal models. The brown adipocyte precursors are spindled cells closely related to a network of capillaries (25). As the cells and vessels proliferate, they are organized into lobules by connective tissue septa. As the cells accumulate lipid, they initially are unilocular. However, with further lipid accumulation, multiple cytoplasmic lipid vacuoles appear. As in white fat, the close association of developing adipocytes and blood vessels has led some to speculate that adipocytes actually develop from endothelial cells. Although similar ultrastructural features are cited as supportive evidence of theory, more recent investigations have attributed these similarities to a common origin from undifferentiated mesenchyme. In fact, ultrastructural and biochemical studies that have examined developing brown adipose tissue have shown that unique features such as large mitochondria and a unique mitochondrial protein are found early in development and distinguish brown from white fat.

Fetal necropsy studies have identified lobules of developing brown fat in the human fetus (26). The largest of these are from the posterior cervical, axillary, suprailiac, and perirenal regions. Those in the neck and axilla are closely associated with the major blood vessels of these regions in such a way that they extend along the course of the cervical blood vessels into the root of the neck. The suprailiac collections lie deep to the abdominal muscles, yet superficial to the peritoneum, and invest the anterior abdominal wall to the diaphragm. Intermediate-sized brown fat pads are seen in the interscapular paralateral trapezius and deltoid regions. Small collections are evident in the intercostal area. In this study, no difference was noted in distribution between the sexes or among the races. The amount of brown fat increases in proportion to growth throughout life. Deposits are well established by the fifth month of gestation.

### Postnatal Development

The presence of brown fat beyond the neonatal period in humans has been debated. An autopsy study by Heaton, however, has identified lobules of brown fat throughout life to the eighth decade (27). Brown fat is most widely distributed in young children and over the next several decades gradually disappears from most sites. In children under age 10, identifiable deposits of brown fat were identified in the interscapular region, around the neck vessels and muscles, around the structures of the mediastinum, and adjacent to the lung hila. Intra-abdominal and retroperitoneal deposits were noted around the kidneys, pancreas, spleen, mesocolon, and omentum, as well as in the anterior abdominal wall. The extremities were not sampled. Although brown fat disappeared from most areas, it was found to persist around the kidneys, adrenals, and aorta and within the mediastinum and neck throughout adult life. As in fetal life, no difference in distribution based on gender was noted.

### Function

The main function of brown adipose tissue is heat production. It has been estimated that the maximal aerobic capacity per gram of tissue is almost 10 times that of skeletal muscle (28). It has been estimated that even in humans, the small quantities of brown fat present are capable of raising heat production by over 20% (29). The production of heat is closely related to the active sympathetic innervation of brown fat and stimulation by norepinephrine. Release of norepinephrine results in the production of cyclic adenosine monophosphate (AMP) and lipolysis to release free fatty acids (30). These undergo oxidation within the mitochondria to produce ATP. Brown fat mitochondria contain a unique uncoupling protein, also known as thermogenin, which uncouples the oxidation of fatty acids from generation of adenosine triphosphate (ATP) (31,32). The resultant energy is dissipated as heat. In small rodents and hibernating animals, brown fat is activated by cold temperatures to produce heat, resulting in what is known as nonshivering thermogenesis. Teleologically, this would be useful in those at risk for hypothermia. Thus, neonates, unable to alter the external environment in order to maintain body temperature, would be expected to have relatively more active brown fat than adults. In addition, brown fat accumulation and activation may play a role in weight regulation. Experimentally overfed rats show a compensatory increase in brown fat activation in metabolic rate minimizing weight gain (33). Many types of obesity in laboratory mice and rats are related to defective regulation of brown adipose tissue, including that seen in ob/ob mice (34). In contrast, exaggerated leanness may be associated with excessive brown adipose tissue responsiveness to external factors such as sympathetic stimulation. Although brown adipose tissue is present in humans, its role in weight regulation, obesity, and thermal regulation in adults remains controversial (35). Increased amounts of periadrenal brown fat in malnourished people at autopsy suggest a compensatory increase in nonshivering thermogenesis to maintain body temperature in those with diminished subcutaneous fat and cachexia (36).

## Regulation

Unlike white fat, brown fat is highly innervated and regulated by sympathetic stimulation. Nerves enter each lobe and branch within the interlobular septa, running along the vessels to terminate on the fat cells (37). Brown fat cells have numerous $\beta1$- and $\beta2$-adrenoreceptors that regulate lipolysis and thermogenesis (30). The $\alpha$-adrenoreceptors, although present, probably do not act directly in heat production. Norepinephrine also may act to increase the number and character of brown fat cells. Using continuous infusions of norepinephrine, Mory et al. have shown that such chronic sympathetic stimulation results in increased cellularity, increased protein content, and increased mitochondrial density in brown fat (38). Because of this close association of sympathetic activity and brown fat activity, several investigators have used pheochromocytoma as a model to study brown fat activities in humans. These studies have provided evidence supportive of early autopsy studies. Functional brown adipose tissue was identified in adults with pheochromocytomas that had similar biochemical features to the better-characterized brown adipose tissue of rodents (39).

Hormones also play a role in brown fat regulation, although minor in comparison to the sympathetic system. Thyroid hormone, although active in regulating metabolic rate, has little importance in diet-induced or nonshivering thermogenesis (30). Insulin stimulates glucose intake into brown adipose tissue. Both cortisol and gonadal steroid hormones inhibit thermogenesis, thus, promoting energy conservation.

## Histology

The term *brown fat* was applied to this tissue because of its characteristic gross appearance. It is incorrect to refer to it as "fetal" fat because it is present throughout life. The abundant vascularity and numerous mitochondria within the cells impart a characteristic reddish-brown color to the tissue. Brown fat has a glandular lobulated appearance. This is in contrast to the more diffuse growth pattern of white fat. Histologically, brown fat is organized into lobules of cells that are made up of adipocytes, capillaries, nerves, and connective tissue. These are surrounded by a thin, fibrous capsule containing blood vessels, nerves, and scattered white adipose cells (40). The cells are polygonal in shape, with a mixture of multivacuolated and univacuolated cells (Fig. 6). The occurrence of both cell types is emphasized, and their presence in developing white fat initially confused studies on its origin. The multivacuolated cell, characteristic of brown fat, has a highly granular cytoplasm with numerous lipid inclusions. Its granular appearance is due to the numerous mitochondria necessary for thermogenesis. The nucleus is

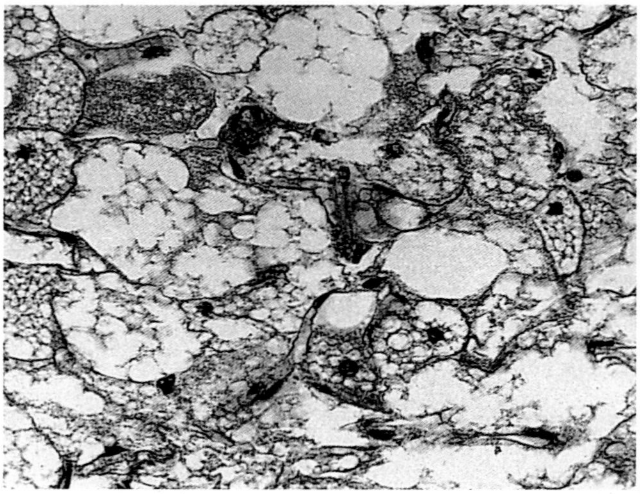

**FIG. 6.** Normal adult brown fat. Nearly all cells have centrally placed nuclei and multivacuolated cytoplasm. Rare cells (*top left*) are nonvacuolated. An arborizing thin capillary network is noted.

spherical and often centrally located, although a large lipid inclusion may displace it toward the periphery of the cell, although rarely to the extreme perimeter as in white fat. Small nucleoli are common. The unilobular cells are indistinguishable histologically from the mature signet-ring cell-type white adipocytes, but are different ultrastructurally. On average, the size of the brown fat cells is smaller than white adipocytes, approximately 25 to 40 $\mu$m. In animals that hibernate, marked seasonal variation in cell size has been noted. Both exposure to cold and starvation result in lipid depletion, causing reduction in cell size and wrinkling of the cell membrane.

Brown adipose cells are surrounded by a network of collagen fibers that contain numerous minute nerve axons and blood vessels. Nonmyelinated axons terminate on the fat cells, providing an avenue for direct sympathetic regulation. The vascularity is quite prominent with numerous capillaries coursing between the adipocytes. It is estimated in rats that the vascularity of brown fat is 4 to 6 times greater than that of white fat (40).

## HISTOCHEMISTRY

### Enzyme Histochemistry

In development, enzyme histochemistry within developing adipocytes is related to the stage of adipocyte differentiation. In fact, in some systems such as the rat, it is clear that enzymatic differentiation of adipocytes precedes morphologic differentiation (41,42). In regions destined to become adipose tissue, undifferentiated morphology is initially present without a capillary bed and without any enzymatic capacity. Subsequently, immature cells or what can be termed "preadipocytes" exist in the form of spindle cells within an area containing a capillary bed. These cells lack any lipid or a basal lamina and have a large complement of enzymatic activity; but they lack the capability to release fat due to the absence of esterase (lipase). In mature lobules, adipocytes in the form of rounded cells now contain lipid, a basal lamina, and a well-developed capillary bed; the entire complement of enzymatic activity is present, including NADH-tetrazolium reductase, ADPH-tetrazolium reductase, and glucose 6-phosphate dehydrogenase (G6PDH). Malate dehydrogenase (NADP) activity is acquired only by late-stage adipocytes (41). Hausman and Thomas (41) demonstrated the presence of such enzymatic differentiation before the assumption of an obviously rounded cell shape consistent with an adipocyte.

Lipoprotein lipase is an enzyme found at high concentration in fatty tissues. It is involved in the transport of serum triglycerides into adipocytes in the form of fatty acids. However, it can be found in other tissues such as skeletal muscles (43,44) and cardiac muscle (45), where it may be localized to endothelial cells. Concentration in fat is directly related to the serum insulin concentration.

### Lipid Histochemistry

Lipids in adipose tissue are generally identified using various stains, such as oil red O and Sudan IV (46–52). It should be noted that lipids are lost in formaldehyde after prolonged fixation, and, thus, cases to be tested using frozen cryostat sections of fixed material should be obtained as soon as possible. Of the two time-honored lipid stains mentioned, oil red O gives the more intense stain and is more rapid to perform. Sudan Black B may stain nonlipid substances nonspecifically, such as coagulated proteins. As a rule, neutral fats are detected using these fat stains. However, a differential staining pattern between neutral fats and fatty acid components and phospholipids can be obtained with the Nile blue sulfate stain (53); with this stain, neutral fat stains pink to red and fatty acids and phospholipids stain bluish. The lipid composition of fatty tissues may also be investigated using new techniques such as the hot-stage polarizing-light microscopic method (54).

The normal composition of lipid in white adipose tissue consists of 99% triglyceride in the form of neutral fat, and less than 1% in the form of phospholipid, cholesterol, and fatty acids (53). In less-differentiated adipocytes, such as those found in liposarcomas, there is a shift away from neutral fat to phospholipids and cholesterol (53). Unfortunately, lipid stains appear to have little use in the everyday examination of adipocyte lesions. The droplets seen on the stains may represent nonspecific staining, and a variety of other mesenchymal lesions may contain lipid (51). An exception is the distinction between lesions with artificial vacuoles such as epithelioid smooth muscle lesions, which are negative with fat stains.

#### *Intracellular Lipid in Nonadipocytes*

Lipid may accumulate in a variety of other cell types and in nonadipocytic tumors.

#### *Steatosis*

According to *Stedman's Medical Dictionary* (55), steatosis has two main meanings: adiposis and fatty degeneration (e.g., steatosis cordis = fatty degeneration of heart). These terms (and the terms used in a variety of pathology texts) are unclear and the distinction between intracellular lipid accumulation and adipocyte infiltration of organs is not made. When nonadipocytes store lipid intracellularly, the phrase "lipid accumulation" is accurate; in the liver, the term "steatosis" is used and, in major pathology texts (56,57), the term appears to be applied solely to the hepatocyte. However, intracytoplasmic lipid can be found within other solid organs, such as the heart [in the myocardial fibers in hypoxia (56)] and the kidney [in the renal tubule in diabetes, poisonings, Reye's syndrome (58)]. Theoretically, there is no rea-

**TABLE 8-1.** *Oil red O-positive carcinomas*[a]

| | |
|---|---|
| Squamous cell carcinoma | Ovarian carcinoma |
| Gastric carcinoma | Breast carcinoma |
| Lung carcinomas | Prostatic carcinoma |
| Renal cell carcinoma | Thyroid carcinoma |
| Lymphoma, large cell | Myeloma |

[a] From ref. 61. For the majority, a high percentage of the tumors listed showed a positive reaction.

son why these processes cannot be referred to as myocardial or renal tubular "steatosis." Regardless, in referring to intracellular lipid accumulation, terms such as "lipid accumulation" or "steatosis" are preferable to unclear and archaic designations, such as "adiposis" or "fatty degeneration." Discussion of adipocyte infiltration of organs is found later.

Lipid accumulation may occur in the placenta after prolonged parenteral nutrition; there, it takes the form of foamy vacuoles within the syncytial and Hofbauer cells of the chorionic villi (59).

Aside from adipocytes, lipid in the form of cholesterol and cholesterol esters may be identified in cells with a steroid-producing function in organs such as the adrenal, ovary, and testis (and tumors thereof). In addition, other types of lipid are found within a variety of tumors. In practice, it is generally thought that a lipid stain (e.g., oil red O) can aid in the differential diagnosis of certain tumors. For example, it is well known that renal-cell carcinomas typically contain lipid (60) and most pathologists have the impression that many other tumors do not. However, it is clear from studies 2 decades ago (61) that fat stains are positive in the majority of cancers (Table 1). Thus, there are problems with the use of the fat stain in the diagnosis of carcinoma and caution should be exercised in interpretation. Furthermore, although some clear cell lesions in the differential diagnosis of renal cancer contain glycogen (benign sugar tumor of lung) (62), others such as xanthoma of bone (63) contain lipid and a fat stain is of no assistance.

## IMMUNOHISTOCHEMISTRY

Currently, there is no commercially available specific immunohistochemical marker for adipose tissue. However, an adipocyte lipid-binding protein, p422 or aP2, is a protein expressed exclusively in preadipocytes late in adipogenesis. Preliminary studies with an antibody to aP2 demonstrate that it stains only lipoblasts and brown fat cells and is capable of identifying liposarcomas selectively (64). This may be quite useful diagnostically in the future.

Adipocytes and tumors thereof stain positively for vimentin and, in our experience, adipocytic tumors have been negative for cytokeratin, desmin, and muscle-specific actin. In 1983, Michetti et al. (65) were the first to describe S-100 immunoreactivity in adipocytes, specifically of rat origin. The S-100 protein was extracted and shown to be identical to that found in the rat brain. Ultrastructurally, S-100 reactivity was widely dispersed within adipocyte cytoplasm, but was not found within mitochondria, lipid droplets, or most of the endoplasmic reticulum. In a similar ultrastructural study, Haimoto et al. (66) identified S-100 protein in the plasma membranes, in membranes of microvesicles, and within polysomes. The Golgi apparatus was negative for this marker, although some reactivity was found within the rough endoplasmic reticulum. During the process of lipolysis in fat cells, Haimoto et al. (66) noted a change in the distribution of S-100 antigen and suggested that S-100 protein molecules interact with free fatty acids, indicating that this protein may act as a carrier protein for free fatty acids.

S-100 protein is a highly acidic calcium-binding protein of molecular weight 21,000. It consists of two polypeptide chains ($\alpha$ and $\beta$) and may occur as dimers in three ways: S-

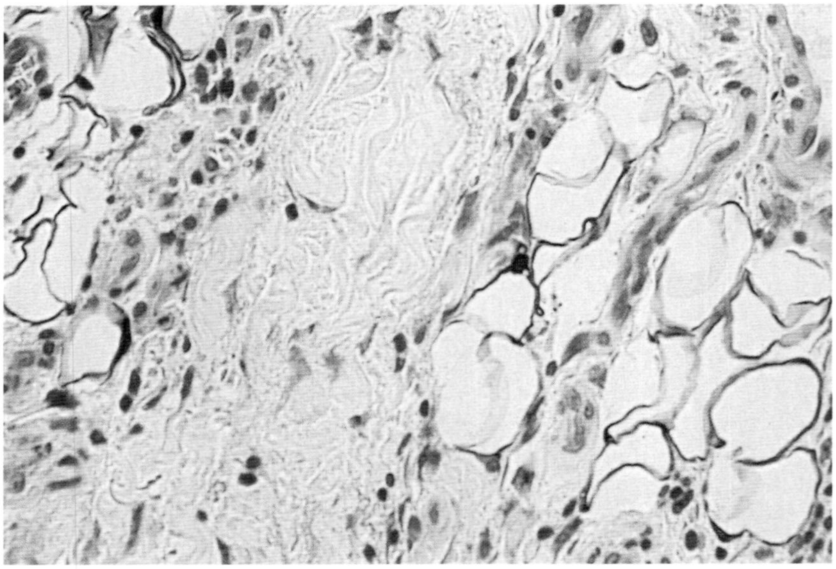

**FIG. 7.** S-100 immunohistochemistry. Reactivity is seen both in the nuclei and in the cytoplasm surrounding the lipid droplets. Such S-100-positive results appear to vary considerably from case to case, probably reflecting fixation differences.

100a ($\alpha$, $\beta$), S-100b ($\beta$, $\beta$), or S-100ao ($\alpha$, $\alpha$) (67). When fat cells have been analyzed, they have been shown to contain only S-100b ($\beta$ form), like Schwann cells (67,68). In the routine practice of immunohistochemistry, adipose tissue reacts in a variable fashion (Fig. 7), accounting for some negative reactions observed by Kahn et al. (69). Although lipomas and liposarcomas are reported to be frequently positive with S-100 (70–73), in our experience, this has not been true. Regardless of fixation with formalin or Bouin's solution, very few liposarcomas have exhibited S-100 immunoreactivity.

Adipocytic lesions do not stain with antibodies to neuron-specific enolase (74).

### Obesity

Human obesity is thought to be approximately 60% genetic in origin, with multiple genetic and environmental factors involved (75). The role of brown adipose tissue (BAT) was briefly alluded to earlier, and new research continues to underscore its importance. For example, in transgenic mice engineered to lack BAT, obesity develops routinely (76). In mice, the genetics of obesity are more clear than in humans. A team at the Rockefeller University led by Dr. Friedman first reported the identification of the "ob" mouse gene, and showed mutations of it are associated with the development of obesity (77). These same researchers have located the human counterpart (OB gene) (77) and mapped its location to chromosome 7 (78). The human protein produced by this gene has 84% homology with the mouse protein, appears to be a hormone secreted by adipose tissue, and likely functions as part of a pathway to regulate body fat. If, indeed, a defective hormone is responsible for some forms of obesity, then there is an immediate therapy available in the form of fully intact native hormone. In 1995, several research groups (79–81) have shown that injection of the ob protein into mice causes the animals to lose weight and maintain their weight loss. Even obesity due to a nongenetic defect like excess diet fat is corrected by the ob protein, now called "leptin."

Finally, the receptor for this protein has been identified recently and shown to be nonfunctional in obese animals (82). Clearly, there have been major advances constituting a breakthrough in obesity research and the fruits of this research should affect human therapy soon.

## ADIPOCYTE LESIONS

### Terminology

In contrast to other human tissue cell types, the terms "hypertrophy" and "hyperplasia" are not usually applied to the adipocyte. It is stressed here, however, that adipocyte hypertrophy (or increased fat cell size) is a recognized phenomenon and is found, for example, in obesity. Enlarged or hypertrophic fat cells (>120 $\mu$m or so) can also be identified in neoplasia (lipoma and liposarcoma) where cells appear to have 3 or 4 times the normal diameter (e.g., >300 $\mu$m). Hyperplasia (or an increased number of adipocytes), in contrast to widespread belief, is a definite occurrence. Again, it is common in obese patients, but it may also be seen in organ-based infiltrations; these are a type of site-specific adipocyte hyperplastic processes. Mature adipocytes are incapable of regeneration and new fat cells are added through in situ mesenchymal cell differentiation recruited from primitive perivascular cells. No disease or change involving adipocytes can appropriately be termed a degeneration (as mentioned earlier), other than liquefaction with necrosis. Atrophy of adipocytes may be seen in malnutrition, starvation, or as the effect of chemotherapy (see following). The appearance of mature fat cells in unusual places as small foci is termed "metaplasia" and is discussed later. Localized new growths of either pure adipocytes or mixtures of adipocytes in other tissue constitute neoplasia and are presumably clonal entities.

### Degeneration

In the condition sclerema adiposum neonatorum, the subcutaneous fat is grossly and microscopically abnormal. Rubbery plaques are due to fat necrosis and degenerative individual fat cells with intracellular needle-shaped crystals (83). This fat crystallization is brown and can be highlighted by polarization. Such crystals apparently may also be identified in up to 30% of stillbirths as a general degeneration following intrauterine demise (83). In another disease, Neu Laxova syndrome, a defect in lipid metabolism causes a lard like appearance to the adipose tissue and is lethal.

### Atrophy

The changes in fat lobules during starvation or malnutrition are particularly noticeable in the subcutaneous region or the omentum. Individual fat cells are reduced in size and fat content, and those without much lipid take on a rounded or epithelioid appearance (84). In the extreme, lobules of these epithelioid cells can simulate tumor nodules histologically (Fig. 8). The cytoplasm is variable in amount, being eosinophilic or granular with or without small lipid vacuoles of differing size, depending on the severity of the malnutrition. Some cells have a multivacuolated appearance. The intervening region between cells is constituted by homogeneous eosinophilic or amphophilic myxoid ground substance (Fig. 8): probably an extract of serum, although stimulation of proteoglycan matrix by the process of starvation (85) is possible. As part of this involution process, lipofuscin is deposited within the shrinking cells (Fig. 8). Importantly, each lobule retains its overall oval shape, although markedly reduced in size and considerably separated from other lobules (Fig. 8). In extreme cachexia, only streaks of tissue remain.

Nearly identical changes can also be seen in the white adipose tissue of fasted animals. As the cells gradually lose their

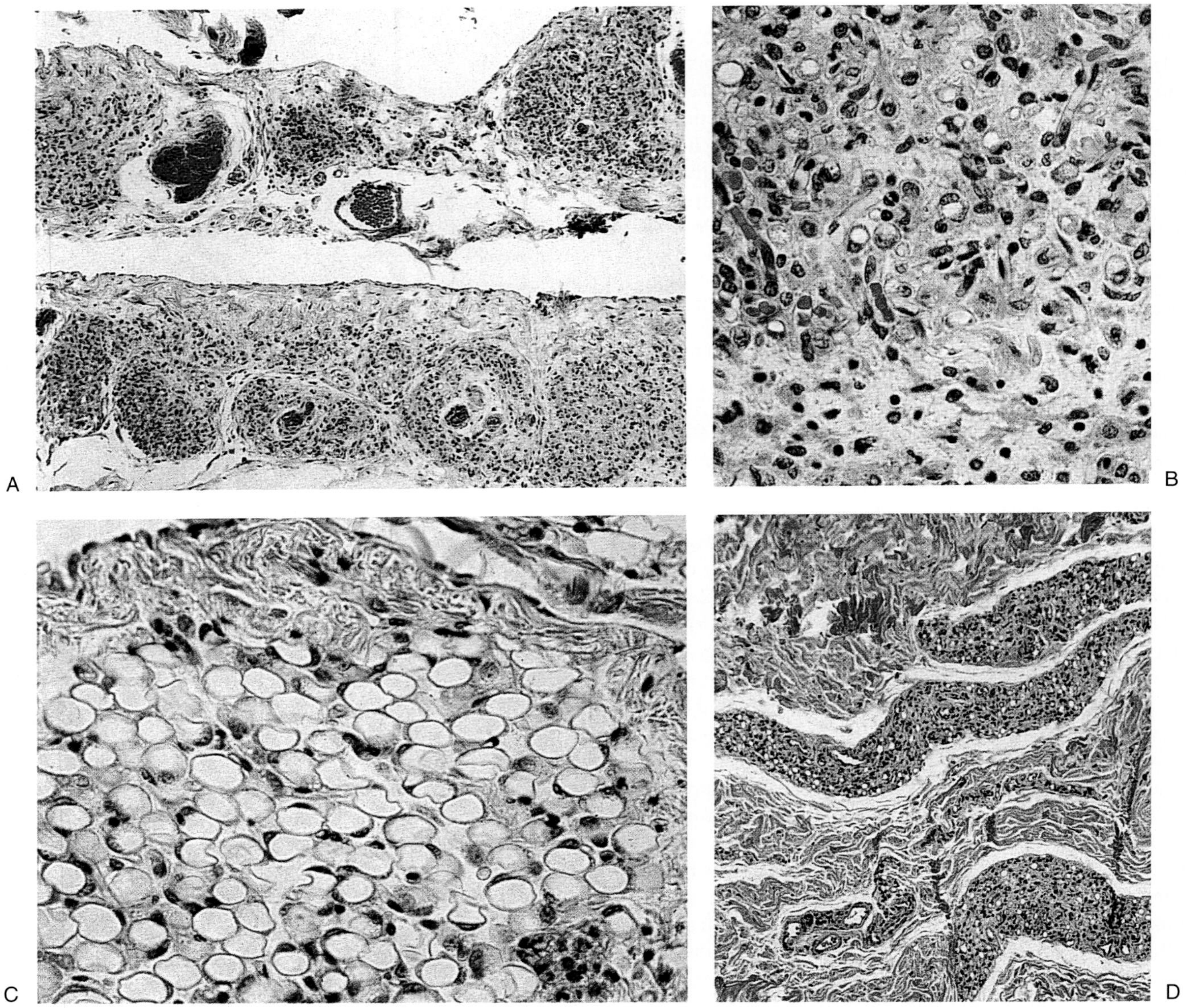


**FIG. 8.** The extreme atrophy seen here in the omentum of a patient with anorexia nervosa (**A**) may mimic tumor deposits; at high power (**B**), shrunken eosinophilic cells are seen with occasional vacuoles and lipofuscin pigment. In less severe starvation (**C**), these omental adipocytes are well recognized, although much smaller than normal size; again, note the presence of pigment. In the skin (**D**), severe cachexia secondary to a cancer resulted in marked involution of the cutaneous fat lobules, which appear only as elongated streaks.

lipid, the single lipid droplet breaks up into multiple vacuoles. Gradually, all lipid disappears. These cells become small and ovoid in shape, sometimes measuring only 15 $\mu$m in diameter (86). There is an apparent expansion of pericellular collagen in such a way that these cells appear as clusters of mesenchymal cells in fibrous stroma. Ultrastructurally, multiple pinocytotic vesicles are seen clustered along the entire cell membrane (40). Lipid is not seen within these vesicles and their significance is unknown.

In the bone marrow, chemotherapy causes changes referred to as "serous atrophy" or "gelatinous transformation" (87,88). The majority of the fat cells have been destroyed, leaving scattered adipocytes of varying size remaining. No lobular appearance is present in the marrow, but the interstitial compartment is composed of the same eosinophilic myxoid substance described previously, again probably consisting of serum fluid and proteins. Droplets of lipid scattered about are also found and, upon regeneration, may appear as foci of lipogranulomas.

Although the microscopic features of the starvation effect on human brown fat have not been described, animals maintained on a dextrose–thiamine diet are known to show distinct morphologic changes in brown fat (24). The mitochondria are disrupted and large irregular electron-dense inclusions are seen within the mitochondrial matrix. The cristae may assume a mosaic pattern with compartmentalization of the material. These cells revert to normal after 24 hours of a normal diet. Similar changes in white fat mitochondria have not been seen with starvation, suggesting that the active mitochondria of brown fat are particularly labile and sensitive to dietary changes.

### Ischemia

Little is written about the effect of ischemia on the adipocyte. We have observed changes in the subcutaneous fat of legs removed for atherosclerotic vascular disease. They consist of accentuation of the lobular architecture by thickening of the fibrous septa; wider and more myxoid in quality, the septa are edematous and also contain scattered inflammatory cells (Fig. 9). Actual necrosis was not observed.

### Metaplasia

As surgical pathologists, we most frequently encounter adipocytic metaplasia in cardiac valves (Fig. 10), usually calcified. There is little in the literature or textbooks on this phenomenon. The emergence of mature adipose tissue seems to parallel the appearance of osteoblasts forming bone within the calcific deposits. Once adipose tissue is present, bone marrow precursors may become resident, presumably from circulating cells, and cause hematopoiesis. Metaplasia is not limited to this site and may be encountered in calcified large vessels or elsewhere, such as in laryngeal cartilage undergoing ossification. We have even seen it in small ossified bronchioles. A similar phenomenon of hematopoiesis without adipose tissue and bone has been reported within acoustic neuromas (89).

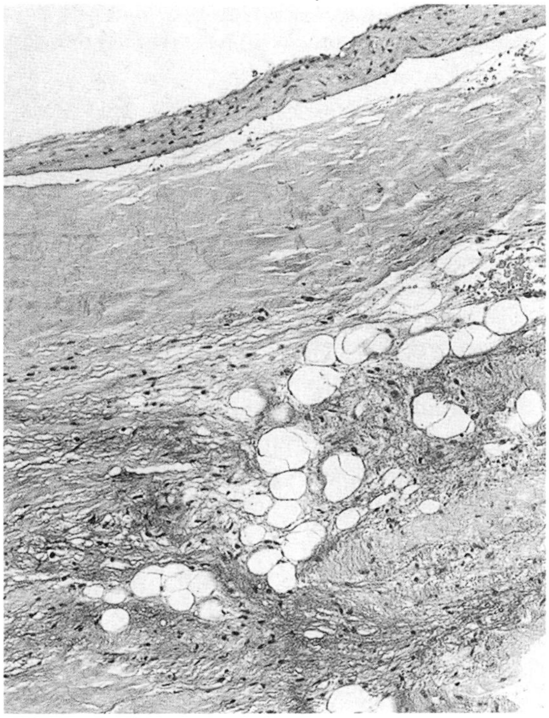

**FIG. 10.** Fatty metaplasia of cardiac valve. Mature adipocytes are found in a myxoid background but are more commonly seen in association with calcification or ossification.

## LIPODYSTROPHY

Although there are several different entities referred to in the past under this name, some (idiopathic intestinal lipodystrophy = Whipple's disease) are infectious and others (mesenteric lipodystrophy, see following) are inflammatory disorders without fundamental changes in the fat cells them-

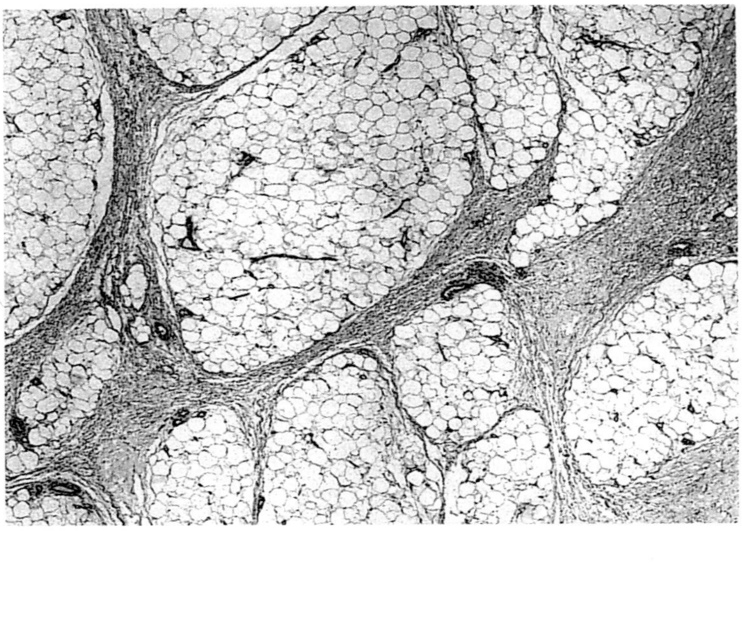

**FIG. 9.** Accentuated fat lobules in ischemia of the lower extremity. Loose myxoid connective tissue widens the septa between lobules; edema and a mild inflammatory infiltrate are present.

selves. The one example of a true lipodystrophy is called membranous lipodystrophy, a relatively new clinical entity characterized by abnormal fat cells, bone cysts with pathologic fractures, and leukodystrophy of the brain (90–92). The marrow fat is particularly effected (90), but the "membranocystic" lesions are also present to a lesser degree in the subcutaneous adipose tissue (92). The characteristic and pathognomonic finding is the highly shrivelled undulating outline of individual fat cell membranes, giving them hyaline eosinophilic convolutions or "arabesque profiles." Multiple small cysts are found, apparently formed by fusion of ruptured adipocytes. Young adults are affected in Japan and Finland primarily, but five cases have been seen in the United States (91). Its etiology and pathogenesis are unknown; it is probably related to an enzyme deficiency (90). A secondary form of membranous lipodystrophy has been described in association with lupus erythematosus and morphea profunda (93). Interestingly, the membranous changes in fat characteristic of lipodystrophy can also be seen in normal fat affected by radiation therapy (94).

## ADIPOCYTES IN ORGANS

### Fatty Infiltration

As distinct from lipid accumulation or steatosis (see previously), fatty infiltration is defined as the presence of mature adipose tissue in sites not normally containing fat. This is a disorder or condition relating to adipocyte cell growth and, therefore, the term "fatty degeneration" is a misnomer and incorrect. In some situations, such as within extremity muscle groups, the process of fatty infiltration is often related to atrophy of the involved site (95). This association between fatty infiltration and atrophy or involution is also

**TABLE 8-2.** *Syndromes associated with fatty processes*[a]

| Syndrome | Description |
|---|---|
| Diffuse mammary steatonecrosis | Fat necrosis with infarction and lipogranulomatous reaction; found in patients with large pendulous breasts (84) |
| Acute pancreatitis | Disseminated focal areas of fat necrosis in the subcutis; may also occur with pancreatic carcinoma (84) |
| Retractile mesenteritis | Fibrosis and retraction of mesentary with distortion of intestinal loops; the outcome of mesentary panniculitis/isolated mesenteric lipodystrophy (84,130) |
| Weber-Christian disease (avoid term) | Historic term for a clinical syndrome with chronic inflammation, fat necrosis, and scattered acute inflammatory cells in the subcutis—"nonsuppurative panniculitis" with recurrent lesions and febrile illness; this is now known to be due to a variety of separate diseases and is a term to be avoided (120,121) |
| Berardinelli's lipodystrophy | A minor part of a complex disorder including gigantism, hyperlipidemia, fatty cirrhosis of liver, muscular hypertrophy, and hyperpigmentation; familial (84) |
| Dercum's disease | Multiple lipomas with pain and tenderness (66,84,136,162) |
| Fröhlich's syndrome | Sexual infantilism with obesity and symmetrical or asymmetrical lipomas (a form of hypopituitarism) |
| Madelung's disease | Symmetrical lipomatosis; associated with alcohol intake (162,215–219) |
| Gardner's syndrome | Familial intestinal polyposis; subcutaneous lipomas may occur (237,238) |
| Multiple endocrine adenopathy I (MEA 1) | Subcutaneous lipomas occur (239); a case of liposarcoma reported (240) |
| Schwachman's syndrome | Lipomatous atrophy of the pancreas with prominent lipomatosis, maldigestion, neutropenia, and growth retardation (99) |
| Trite's syndrome | A combination of thymolipoma, thyrolipoma, and pharyngeal lipoma (187) |
| Carney's syndrome | Pulmonary hamartomas (which often contain fat), gastric smooth muscle tumors, and paraganglioma (244,245) |
| Tubulous sclerosis | Angiomyolipomas of kidney, other tumors, and hamartomas; occasionally diffuse lipomatosis (242) |
| Beckwith's hemihypertrophy | Congenital asymmetry, some with associated Wilm's tumor, occasional benign mesenchymoma with adipose tissue (164) |
| Familial multiple lipomas | Multiple subcutaneous lipomas (250) |
| Bannayan's syndrome | Autosomal dominant disorder with macrocephaly, lipomas, hemangiomas, and intracranial tumors (241) |
| Laurence-Moon-Biedl syndrome | Congenital optic nerve atrophy, polydactyly, mental defect, and occasional adrenal lipomas (249) |
| Carpal tunnel syndrome | Occasionally caused by tendon sheath lipoma (246) |
| Fishman's syndrome | Encephalocraniocutaneous lipomatosis (233,234) |
| Goldenhar-Gorlin syndrome | Oculoauriculo-vertebral dysplasia with CNS lipomas (248) |
| Cowden's disease | GI polyposis with orocutaneous hamartomas; angiolipomas have been observed (242) |
| Spinal epidural lipomatosis | Fatty infiltration of epidural space (226–229); occasionally secondary to steroids (229) |
| Membranous lipodystrophy | Abnormal subcutaneous and bony fat with bone cysts, pathologic fractures, and leukodystropy of brain (90–92) |

[a] References given in parentheses.

noted in other organs (thymus (96), bone marrow (97), and kidney (98)), and apparently signifies the propensity for adipocytes to fill a vacuum, in a sense, left by atrophic processes (84). Whatever the stimulus may be, the adipocytes probably arise from pleuripotent mesenchymal cells adjacent to blood vessels (84). The reversal of this relationship is found in the parathyroid gland where there is an inverse relationship between parenchymal cells and adipocytes, to the point where no adipocytes are present in complete parathyroid hyperplasia.

Nonatrophic organs can also accumulate fat cells ("lipomatosis"), and the classic examples are the heart and pancreas (56). In these locations, no parenchymal damage is discerned and the process is a type of "accidental lipogenesis" (84). In the case of the pancreas, normal parenchymal histology and function are present even though the pancreas may be nearly invisible grossly (56,99). This type of pancreatic lipomatosis is correlated with age and obesity and also occurs in diabetics (99). The amount of pancreatic tissue is thought to be either completely normal (56) or partially depleted (99). However, true pancreatic atrophy with resultant lipomatosis also exists as a rare condition known as Schwachman's disease (99) (see Table 2). Fatty infiltration of the heart is most often an innocuous condition with no effect on the myocardial fiber or cardiac function (56). However, there are rare exceptions in which severe adipocity has resulted in cardiac rupture (84). Another clinically important lesion is termed "lipomatous hypertrophy of the interatrial septum" (100), a focal enlargement that may cause sudden death, arrhymias, or congestive failure (101,102). Be mindful that the occasional appearance of fat in endocardial biopsies in no way indicates cardiac perforation (103).

Isolated fat cells can be found within lymph nodes in childhood, but enlarged nodes with prominent fatty infiltration mainly occur in adults, particularly in obesity (104). Common in the abdomen and retroperitoneum, such "lipolymph nodes" can be mistaken for lipomas (104) or be interpreted as positive in a lymphangiogram for lymphoma or Hodgkin's disease (*personal observation*), mimicking lymphoma relapse (105). Rarely, a lipoma or angiomyolipoma occurs in the liver (106), but those lesions should not be confused with the hepatic pseudolipoma (107). This pseudolipoma is often found as a bulge on the surface of the liver and probably represents capture of previously detached appendices epiploicae. In the mouth, fat is one of the components contributing to macroglossia in certain conditions (108).

The Ito cells of the liver are fat-containing cells along the sinuses and are a variation on normal histology (109); they may become prominent in the condition known as lipopeliosis (110) and involved in the benign neoplasm called spongiotic pericytoma (111).

## FAT BIOPSY FOR AMYLOID

It is becoming increasingly popular to perform a subcutaneous fat biopsy for the diagnosis of amyloidosis. In such instances, the Congo red stain may reveal amyloid around blood vessels and, occasionally, between adipocytes (112–114). This procedure is at least as sensitive as the rectal biopsy (114), can identify up to 84% of cases (113), can be combined with other studies to determine amyloid type (112), and is a safe and innocuous way to make the diagnosis (113).

Biopsy analysis of adipose tissue may become important in the future, to assess a given individual's storage content of toxic chemicals. A variety of industrial and environmental hydrocarbons are stored predominantly in fat, and subcutaneous adipose tissue deposits may be analyzed and results correlated with the development of diseases such as neoplasia.

## INFLAMMATIONS

### Fat Necrosis

Three histologically distinct types of fat necrosis exist: the ordinary variety secondary to trauma and other inflammation, that associated with pancreatitis, and infarction of fat. Histologically, ordinary fat necrosis is typified by the presence of epithelioid histiocytes, foamy macrophages, and giant cells in adipose tissue, often surrounding and isolating individual adipocytes (Fig. 11). Lymphocytes and plasma cells are also found in small numbers. Occasionally, unusual crystalloids may be seen (115). Fat cells become destroyed and the released lipid may fuse to result in a single droplet larger than the average cell, or in minute droplets. This process may resolve with mild fibrosis or, if extensive, may cause cyst formation with eventual dense fibrosis and even calcification at the periphery. Such cysts with central liquefaction may be located on the buttocks and be the final result of trauma, secondary to an injection. Just beneath the cyst wall, necrotic outlines of adipocytes are usually present, signifying the origin of the end-stage cyst in fat necrosis.

An unusual type of fat necrosis forming cystic spaces has been designated "membranous fat necrosis" by Poppiti et al. (116). In this example, actual cysts are formed containing pseudopapillary structures and central debris. Although the fat cell outlines are normal in appearance, the formation of these cysts resembles that seen in membranous lipodystrophy. Membranous fat necrosis can also occur secondary to radiation therapy (94).

Fat necrosis secondary to acute pancreatitis is histologically distinctive (Fig. 12). Rather than consisting of a histiocytic infiltrate, the pancreatic fat necrosis is accompanied by an infiltrate of neutrophils predominantly, and liquefaction of fat is apparent (117,118). In the center of the lesion, the infarctlike outlines of fat cells can be seen, and fat cell membranes are ruptured, releasing their contents into a central eosinophilic or basophilic material. The entire region is bordered by an acute inflammatory infiltrate. The process is thought to be secondary to the action of pancreatic lipolytic enzymes in the serum acting on susceptible foci.

Another disorder that often manifests itself as skin and

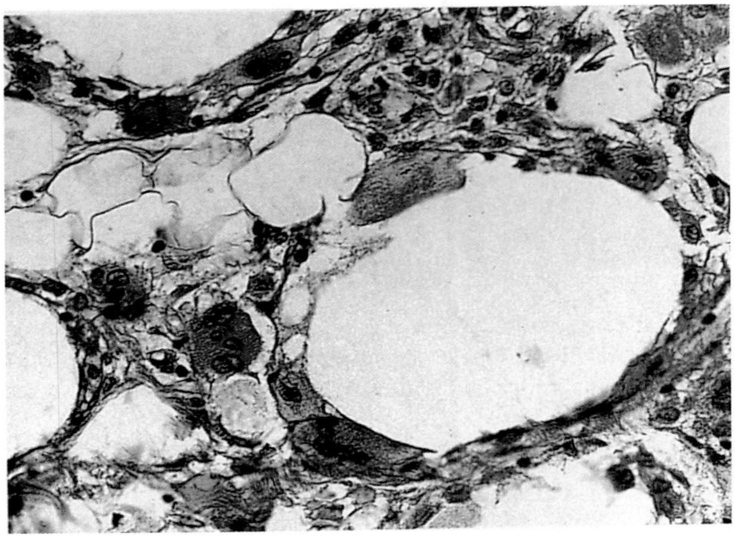

**FIG. 11.** Fat necrosis, ordinary type. Multinucleated histiocytic giant cells surround a large lipid vacuole formed by fusion of destroyed adipocytes. Scattered lymphocytes and monocytes occupy expanded spaces between cells at top.

subcutaneous fat necrosis is called calciphylaxis; here, the characteristic vascular necrosis with calcium precipitation will aid in the diagnosis (119).

The infarction type of fat necrosis, in which eosinophilic outlines of fat cells without nuclei or inflammation are present histologically, may be seen in lipomas and in detached peritoneal tissue originating from appendices epiploicae. The lipomas containing infarction may be pedunculated with twisting, causing compromise of blood flow.

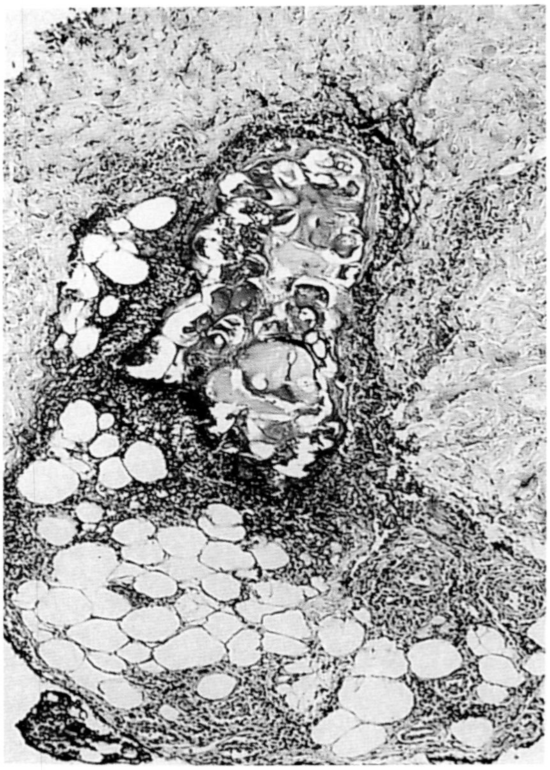

**FIG. 12.** Fat necrosis, pancreatic type. In contrast to regular fat necrosis, numerous neutrophils are found, together with central liquefaction. The central material may give either an eosinophilic or basophilic appearance, and disrupted cell membranes can be appreciated.

## Panniculitis

Numerous diseases and conditions may cause an inflammatory infiltrate of the subcutaneous adipose tissue, namely, a panniculitis; readers are referred to a variety of textbooks on skin pathology for an in-depth enumeration of these. Only a few relevant points are made here. First, the condition called Weber-Christian disease, or febrile nodular nonsuppurative panniculitis of the subcutaneous fat, was described early in this century and is consistently referred to in discussions of this topic. However, it became clear in the 1960s and 1970s that this disease was not a clinically distinct entity, but rather had many separate etiologies including steroid withdrawal, diabetes mellitus, tuberculosis, pancreatic disease, and systemic lupus erythematosus (120). Thus, it is generally agreed today that Weber-Christian "disease" was a clinical description of a presentation for numerous diseases, and is a term to be avoided (121).

Panniculitis, as a rule, can be divided into those that are septal and those that involve the lobules of adipose tissue (121). The character of the infiltrate is important and note should be made of the presence of eosinophils (122), neutrophils and granulomas (123), histiocytes with lymphophagocytosis (124), or other specific changes (125). Autoimmune diseases such as scleroderma (126) and lupus (127) may be causative, indicating the importance of historical detail. Unusual causes, such as $\alpha$-1-antitrypsin deficiency (121), have a characteristic histology, as does pancreatic fat necrosis (described elsewhere). Even withdrawal from steroids may cause a panniculitis (128).

## Mesenteritis

Inflammation of the mesenteric fat is a recognizable clinical entity that has more recently been termed "mesenteric panniculitis" to signify the active inflammatory stage and "retractile mesenteritis" to signify the fibrotic stage (129). Other terms complicate the literature, but it is generally held that they all refer to the same disease process and spectrum: liposclerotic mesenteritis, sclerosing mesenteritis, mesenteric lipodystrophy (ML), and Weber–Christian disease of the mesentery [see recent review by Kelly and Hwang (130)].

The process consists of a chronic inflammatory infiltrate of lymphocytes, plasma cells, and foamy histiocytes and giant cells, along with recognizable fat necrosis, edema, and a variable amount of fibrosis and calcification. Myofibroblasts proliferate and are directly involved in the pathogenesis of the retractile disease (130). While it most often thickens the mesentery (type 1 ML), it can appear as a single tumefaction at the mesenteric base (type 2 ML) or as multiple discrete nodules (type 3 ML) (131). Other space-occupying lesions, such as inflammatory pseudotumors, xanthogranulomatosis (see following) and fibromatosis, are in the differential diagnosis (105). Affected patients are usually middle-aged, predominantly males, and they complain of vague abdominal discomfort and weight loss, with over one-half presenting with fever. Nearly one half of them are, oddly enough, asymptomatic (130). Rare cases have been fatal, but the prognosis is generally excellent. Mass lesions regress within 2 years in about two thirds of the patients and any pain disappears in three quarters of them (129). Steroids are commonly given to treat the disease, but it is unclear whether the course of the disease or the progression to fibrosis is changed (129).

Retroperitoneal xanthogranulomatosis can be due to a primary inflammatory process of the kidney or it can represent involvement of the retroperitoneum by the mesenteritis. Many foamy histiocytes and lymphocytes are seen. Rarely it can be associated with Erdheim-Chester disease (multisystem fibroxanthomas with bone pain and sclerotic bone lesions) (132).

### Lipogranuloma

Small collections of epithelioid histiocytes with lipid droplets are commonly encountered in lymph nodes, draining the GI tract, (mesenteric, porta hepatis, retroperitoneal) and in the liver, spleen, and bone marrow. They do not imply a pancreatitis (in which necrosis should be present) or other pathologic process, and are completely incidental.

## TUMORS AND TUMORLIKE LESIONS

### Brown Fat Lesions

#### *Hibernoma*

The only pathologic lesion of brown fat known to date is the hibernoma, the neoplastic counterpart given its name by Gery (133). Although many of the cells in the hibernoma are multivacuolated, some cells lack vacuoles completely and are eosinophilic and granular in appearance. Both of these cell types have a centrally placed nucleus. Importantly, univacuolated cells with peripherally placed nuclei resembling white adipocytes can be identified, as they can in normal brown fat (133,134). The red-brown color of a hibernoma is the result of the increased vascularity in numerous mitochondria. The ultrastructure of hibernoma is similar to brown fat (135) and, indeed, when cellular organelles are compared, the ultrastructure suggested to a number of authors (133,134) is that brown fat and white fat are two distinct tissues, with different ultrastructural features.

Concerning location, many hibernomas arise in sites corresponding to the distribution of normal brown fat-interscapular area, neck, mediastinum, and axilla (133); other cases have been reported in the abdominal wall, thigh, and popliteal space (133): sites considered devoid of brown fat (136). Generally medium-sized tumors (5 to 10 cm), hibernomas may obtain a huge dimension [23 cm (137)] and are often present for years prior to excision. The tumors typically occur in young adults with a median age of 26 years, much younger than patients with ordinary lipoma (136). Interestingly, endocrine activity has been noted within these tumors, with steroid hormones (including cortisol and testosterone) detected (138). Hibernomas do not recur, but whether malignant hibernomas exist has been a controversial topic. A case having atypical mitoses and bizarre nuclei was reported by Enterline et al. (139), and a similar case with ultrastructural features was documented by Teplitz et al. (140).

### White Fat Lesions

#### *Adipose Tissue within Nonfatty Lesions*

Almost any malignant tumor may invade and incorporate mature fat cells. Occasionally, however, the presence of fat cells within mesenchymal proliferation can be confusing. For example, nodular fasciitis may incorporate individual fat cells that can appear smaller than normal, mimicking lipoblasts (136). Likewise, a very prominent component of adipose tissue accompanies intramuscular angiomatosis and lymphangiomatosis of the extremities (136). Benign teratomas of the ovary (141) and lung (142,143) occasionally contain mature adipose tissue as an incidental finding. So-called fibrous polyps of the esophagus (144) also contain adipose tissue. Other nonlipomatous tumors that may contain fat include the pleomorphic adenoma of the salivary gland and the benign spindle cell breast tumor described by Toker et al. (145). This lesion may be what has been described recently as a myofibroblastoma (146) with the incorporation of adipose tissue.

Perhaps by a process of cellular metaplasia, fat may also be found occasionally in the endometrium (147) or in epithelial tumors of various types (see following).

### *Ectopic Adipose Tissue*

Ectopic fat either in cardiac valves or within organs was discussed earlier under Metaplasia and Fatty Infiltration. Oddly enough, ectopic fat may occur in the dermis where it causes a pedunculated appearance; this has been termed "nevus lipomatosis superficialis" or, more recently, "pedunculated lipofibroma" (148).

### *Hamartomas Containing Fat Cells*

Many of us are aware that the benign pulmonary "chondroma" or "hamartoma" may contain fat (142). In fact, approximately 75% of these lesions do (149), and the presence of such a tissue foreign to the lung parenchyma supports the concept that these lesions are benign mesenchymomas (142,149). Occasionally, the lipomatous component may be so dominant as to suggest a lipoma (149,150).

Amazingly, adipose tissue can be a component of many other unusual lesions. It may be coupled with vascular, fibrous, and myofibroblastic components in multiple congenital mesenchymal hamartomas [multiple sites (151)]; with undifferentiated spindle cells and fibroblasts in the fibrous hamartoma of infancy [mainly in shoulder and axillary regions (152–154)]; with fibrous tissue and mature nerve in the sometimes congenital fibrolipomatous hamartoma of nerve with or without macrodactyly [palm, wrist, or fingers (155–157)]; or with smooth muscle and vessels in the angiomyolipoma (158,159). These hamartomatous lesions of tuberous sclerosis will be discussed further. In another oddity, adipose tissue is one component of human tails and pseudotails (160) along with skin and other tissues.

### *Mesenchymomas*

Adipose tissue is a nearly constant component of benign mesenchymomas—growth that should be redefined as having more than two mesenchymal elements. LeBer and Stout (161) required the presence of at least two different mesenchymal elements to make a diagnosis of mesenchymoma. However, we believe the trend has evolved in favor of more than two elements, and those lesions with only two elements currently appear to be designated separately as "chondrolipoma," "fibrolipoma," and so on (136,162). This seems appropriate since the secondary element, usually in a lipoma, is frequently a very focal finding (as it may be in a liposarcoma). Thus, aside from lesions with focal "metaplasia," lesions with three or more elements can be designated true mesenchymomas. For instance, a description of a trigeminal neurilemmoma (163) was really a mesenchymoma with cartilage, bone, hemangioma, schwannoma, and adipose tissue. Also, a thoracic tumor with smooth muscle, angiomatoid spaces, fibrous tissue, and adipose tissue is another mesenchymoma, reported in association with hemihypertrophy (164). Angiomyolipoma is another example of a benign mesenchymoma and is frequently found in the kidney where approximately 40% are associated with tuberous sclerosis (159). Although the fat seen here is practically always mature, rarely lipoblast-like cells may be seen in these (136,165). Angiomyolipomas have also been reported in other sites, such as lymph nodes (166).

### *Lipomas*

The distinction between adipose tissue lobules and true lipoma occasionally arises in the practice of surgical pathology, necessitating a strict definition of lipoma. Although lipoma is well described in two major texts (136,162), definitions are concise without detail. Lipoma is herein defined as a superficial or deep-circumscribed and expansile benign neoplasm composed of mature adipose tissue, which is commonly (but need not be) encapsulated. Such a definition emphasizes its well-differentiated and clonal nature (see following) and serves to distinguish most lipomas from normal fat and prominent posttraumatic skin folds or "fat fractures" (167). As Allen emphasizes, the capsule may be quite thin and poorly defined (162). Nonetheless, it is a crucial requirement for superficial tumors; deep lesions, on the contrary, are often nonencapsulated. When a subcutaneous lipoma is excised in a piecemeal fashion, the lesion may be diagnosed by noting the presence of portions of capsular fibrous tissue in the form of a circular arc of collagen of varying width at the edge of tissue fragments. In the absence of a clear-cut capsule or fragments thereof, a diagnosis of a superficial lipoma cannot be made.

Clinically, the majority of lipomas seen in surgical pathology are subcutaneous tumors typically in the middle-aged to elderly patient. Males and females are probably equally affected, and there are no racial differences. Most tumors are located on the trunk or upper extremities; if other sites are encountered, consideration should be given to one of the lipoma subtypes (e.g., forearm for angiolipoma, neck for spindle and pleomorphic types). Lipomas probably outnumber all other soft tissue tumors combined (136). Interesting facts about lipomas include (a) a nearly static size after the initial growth period (136); (b) the relative rarity of lesions on the hands, feet, face, and lower leg despite the presence of fat (136); (c) hardness after the application of ice, a diagnostic sign (136); (d) the lack of size reduction in starvation (136,162); (e) a definite, but low, recurrence rate [1 to 4% (136,162)]; (f) an unknown etiology; (g) a possible relation to potassium intake (168); and (h) a possible association with an increased incidence of cancer [46% (169)].

Many lesions of the subcutaneous region come to surgical pathology labeled as lipomas and, not uncommonly, a portion of these actually turn out to be something else, frequently more interesting.

When one views normal fat histologically, the size of fat cells appears to vary somewhat due to the sectioning plane; however, the variation is relatively small (80 to 120 $\mu$m, *personal observation*; refer to Fig. 4). In lipomas [including atypical lipoma (170)], there is a tendency for cell size to vary more widely with larger cells (e.g., >300 $\mu$m) being apparent. Practically, this means that a medium-power view will often disclose a two- to fivefold size range (Fig. 13). Normal fat has a netlike structure of fibrous tissue, wherein such dispersed fibrous bands or septa dissect the adipose tissue randomly. The fibrous tissue is thicker in quality in bodily regions exposed to pressure, such as the hands, feet, and buttocks (84). This netlike fibrous tissue arrangement is recapitulated within lipomas (Fig. 14), particularly at the periphery where small lobules are often found. A high degree of vascularity is a feature associated with lipogenic malignancy, but we should be aware that this refers to a visible network of capillaries, often in strings and branching arrays. However, normal adipose tissue and lipomas are likewise highly vascular, except the capillary vascular bed is more difficult to visualize. A PAS stain of a lipoma, for example, can highlight the minute, but diffuse, capillaries, particularly at the junctions between cells, where they are made more difficult to see due to compression. A delicate reticulin network is also present in lipomas, contributed to by the basement membranes of both lipocytes and capillaries; each lipocyte is completely encircled by reticulin in a manner similar to normal fat cells (Fig. 3). Normally, lipomas have a low degree of cellularity and no nuclear atypia; the presence of either is cause for concern. Sometimes increased cellularity is due to a diffuse low-grade form of fat necrosis (Fig. 15). The ultrastructure of lipoma recapitulates that of its normal counterpart (171).

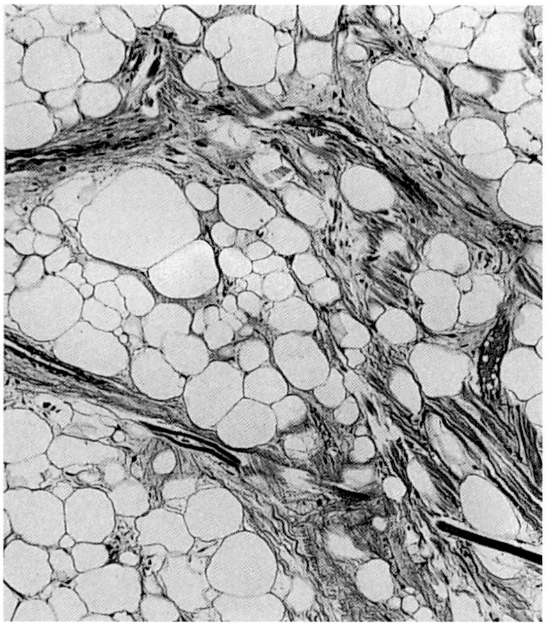

**FIG. 13.** Variation in fat cell size in spindle cell lipoma. Some adipocytes are three to five times the size of a normal adipocyte; compare with Fig. 4. Increased numbers of spindle cells together with collagen bands characterize this lipoma subtype, although the size variation seems to be present in all unusual types of lipoma.

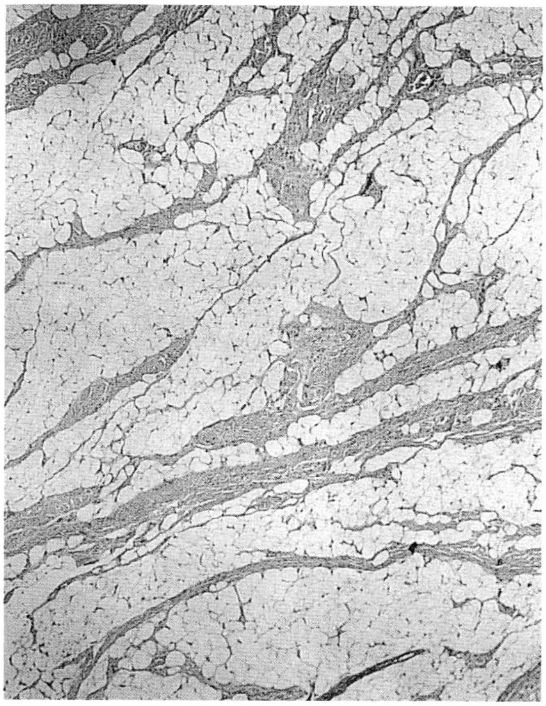

**FIG. 14.** Lipoma with accentuated lobulation. In certain sites such as the buttock, foot, and hand (*depicted here*), thick fibrous septa are noted throughout; these correspond to the thicker septa within the normal adipose tissue in these regions.

### *Myxoid Change*

In rare lipomas, the mature fat cells are separated by varying amounts of a loose basophilic ground substance, probably proteoglycan (Fig. 16). When prominent, the lesion may be designated a "myxolipoma" or "myxoid lipoma" (136,162). The myxoid quality often raises the possibility of a myxoid liposarcoma. However, these areas contain only widely scattered bland cells and are never hypercellular. Furthermore, the plexiform capillary network so typical of the malignant tumor is absent, as are lipoblasts. As Enzinger and Weiss (136) observed, rare cells may be vacuolated, but contain bluish mucoid material.

### *Intramuscular Lipoma*

Deep lipomas may be either intermuscular or intramuscular, with the latter unencapsulated tumors being the more common. Intramuscular lipomas (172), also known as infiltrating lipomas, involve the large muscles of the extremities (particularly the thigh, shoulder, and upper arm) or the paraspinal muscles. For extremity lesions, an inapparent mass may become visible upon voluntary contraction. Microscopically, the lipocytes are typically mature and mitoses or atypical nuclei are not found. Muscle fibers are widely dispersed throughout the lesion (Fig. 17). Any unusual fea-

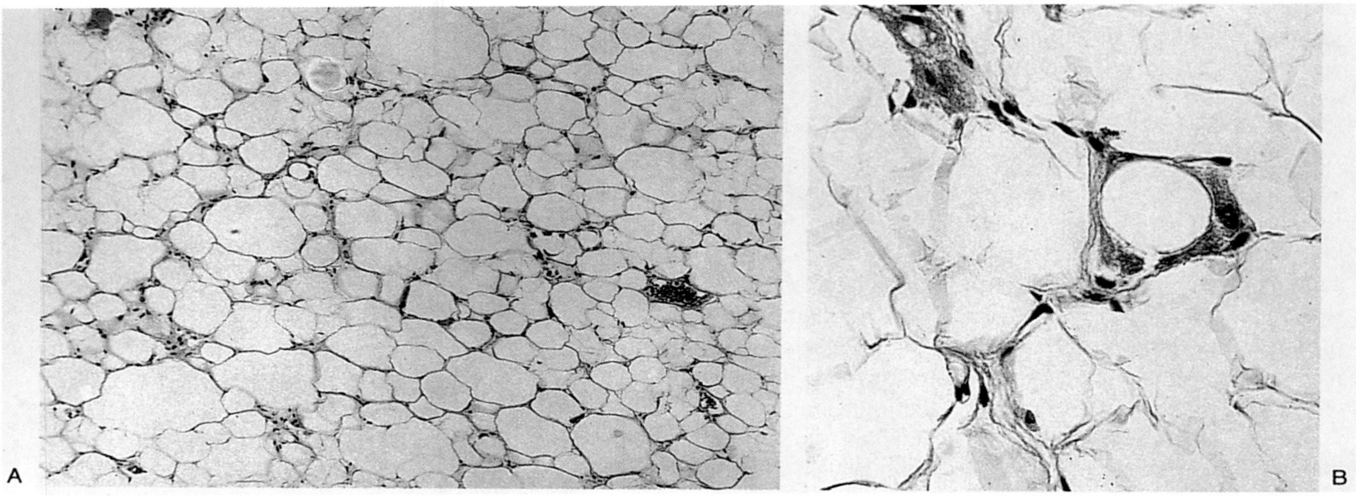

**FIG. 15.** Lipoma. In some tumors an increased cellularity at medium power (**A**) may cause concern, but it is frequently due to a mild but diffuse fat necrosis. The lipocytes are falsely enlarged by the histiocytes without much other inflammation (**B**).

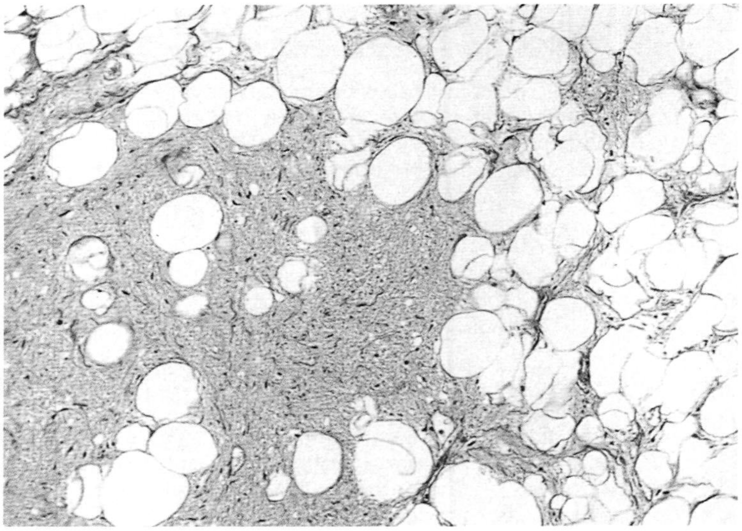

**FIG. 16.** Lipoma with myxoid change. Features that differentiate this from myxoid liposarcoma are the lack of branching capillary vessels and significant cellularity in the myxoid component.

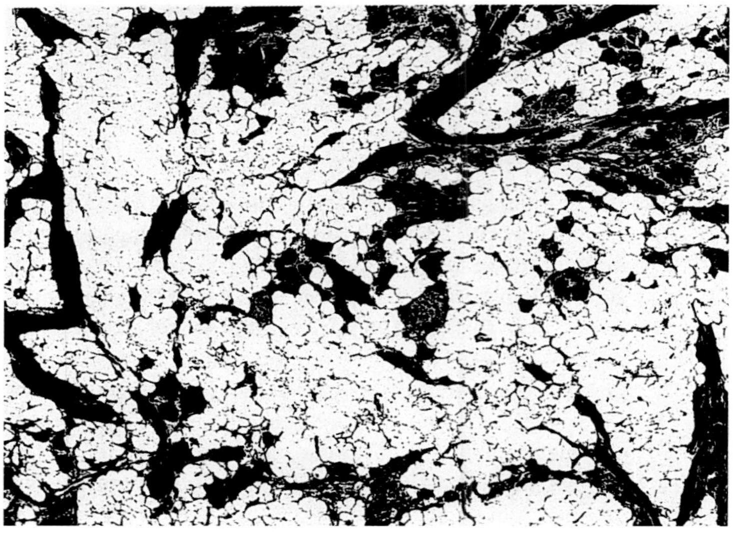

**FIG. 17.** Lipoma, intramuscular type. The light fat cells proliferate between dark individual skeletal muscle fibers in this commonly unencapsulated tumor (*trichrome stain*).

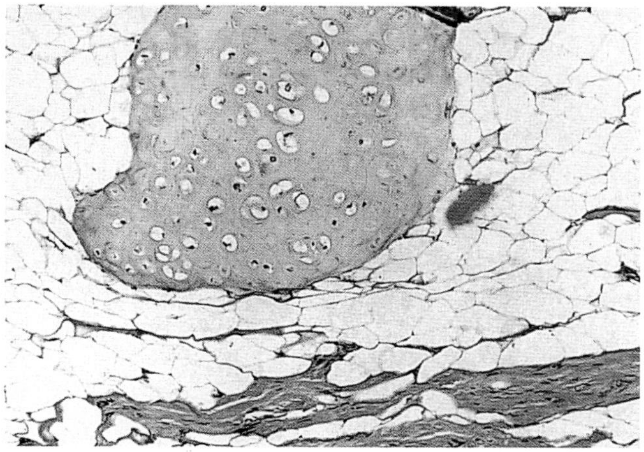

**FIG. 18.** Chondrolipoma. Small nodules of mature cartilage are present, often very focally; this combination alone should not be labeled a mesenchymoma.

tures should raise the suspicion of a well-differentiated liposarcoma (173). Often, intramuscular lipomas extend beyond the muscle fascia to involve the intervening connective tissue space. Therefore, it is often difficult to completely excise such lesions and the recurrence rate is higher than that for ordinary subcutaneous lipoma. This has been particularly true for paraspinal intramuscular lipomas.

Intramuscular angiolipomas are lesions considered to be intramuscular hemangiomas with a variable fat content (136).

Lipoma arborescens is a special type of lipoma occurring in a joint: it has a characteristic villiform gross appearance and the patients typically have a highly painful knee (162). The mere presence of adipose tissue on a synovial biopsy is not synonymous with this entity.

### *Other Elements in Lipomas*

Aside from the ordinary lipoma, extraneous elements of various types can be associated with an adipose tissue benign proliferation, including combinations with epithelial or other mesenchymal components.

### *Mesenchymal Components*

Perhaps the most common mesenchymal component associated with the lipoma is, as surgical pathologists are aware, benign cartilaginous metaplasia (Fig. 18). So-called chondrolipomas may occur in almost any site of the body, including the breast (174) and mediastinum (175). Although the term *benign mesenchymoma* has been applied to such lesions, the chondroid metaplasia is practically always an extremely minor component in the form of very small isolated islands of cartilage; therefore, the designation of mesenchymoma appears to be an exaggeration (as it is when cartilaginous metaplasia occurs in liposarcoma). Allen also prefers to avoid the term *mesenchymoma* (176).

Lipochondromatosis is a recently reported entity that involves the tendons and synovium of the ankle region as a mass lesion (177). Rarely benign osteoid is also found in lipomas, either solely or coupled with cartilage (178). Some of these osteolipomas are in contact with periosteum and may be termed "periosteal lipoma" (178). Smooth muscle lesions, particularly of the uterus, may be combined with adipose tissue to produce "lipoleiomyomas" (179) and "lipoleiomyomatosis" (180). Prominent blood vessels are a frequent component of superficial small subcutaneous tumors called "angiolipomas" (136). These lesions are interesting, as they may be multiple, cause pain due to frequent microthrombi, and give rise to the differential diagnosis of Kaposi's sarcoma when the angiomatoid component completely overcomes the lipocytic component (Fig. 19). These fat-poor variants are designated cellular angiolipomas (181). In such instances, the diagnosis is made by finding rare-to-scattered mature fat cells, usually at the periphery of the lesion.

Some lipomas contain an increased content of fibrous tissue. These usually superficial tumors have been called "fibrolipomas." However, it is likely that the amount of fibrous tissue in a lipoma is directly related to its anatomic site of origin (Fig. 14). Dense thicker fibrous tissue is typically found in lipomas of the pressure-bearing regions of the body such as the hands, feet, and buttocks; the lobular architecture accentuated by such fibrous bands may be apparent grossly.

### *Epithelial Components*

In some superficial lipomas, eccrine glands may be incorporated into the lesion. Eccrine glands may be found at the junction of dermal collagen; the subcutaneous fat and lipomas arising in this region can cause displacement of these glands, well within the substance of the lipoma. This phenomenon has been noted in locations such as the hand and buttock (*personal observation*).

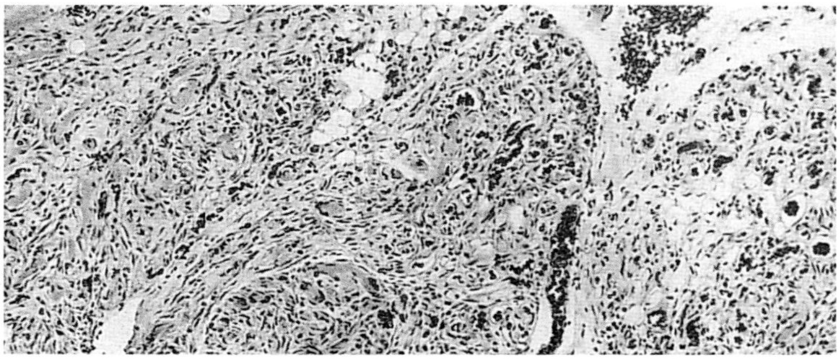

**FIG. 19.** Angiolipoma. In this unusual example, the rarity of adipocytes (*top middle*) makes the tumor resemble a deep Kaposi's-like lesion; the location, circumscription, frequent microthrombi (*center*), and isolated islands of fat cells at the periphery aid in the diagnosis.

Adipose tissue may accompany adenomas (i.e., "lipoadenomas") of the thyroid (182) and parathyroid (183). Aside from lipoadenomas, other lesions of the thyroid gland may contain fat—including colloid nodules, lymphocytic thyroiditis, and papillary carcinomas (184,185). Another unusual phenomenon is the formation of the "thymolipoma" (186). As listed in Table 2, an unusual lipomatous syndrome is described consisting of thyrolipoma, thymolipoma, and pharyngeal lipoma (187).

### *Lymphocytes in Lipomas*

Occasionally, one may observe a dense perivascular lymphocytic infiltrate in scattered vessels within and outside ordinary lipomas. Although not generally described, the authors have observed this phenomenon several times and investigated the patients; they have not exhibited evidence of chronic lymphocytic leukemia or autoimmune disease. Perhaps this may represent a localized host reaction to the proliferation.

## Special Lipoma Types

In the spindle cell (188–190) and pleomorphic (191,192) lipomas, the fat cells appear variable in size at low power. In spindle cell lipoma (Fig. 13), the spindle cell content may vary from scanty to abundant and the nuclei of the spindle cells are wavy, resembling nerve sheath lesions. Dense fibrous tissue is also found sometimes with a keloidal quality. Similar cells may be seen in pleomorphic lipoma, which has, in addition, characteristic floret tumor giant cells (Fig. 20). Both of these lesions are encapsulated and have characteristic locations commonly limited to the head and neck of elderly males. They may be related entities (193).

The chondroid lipoma is a well-circumscribed lesion with two elements: mature adipose tissue and focal or promine areas containing strands and nests of eosinophilic vacuolated cells resembling chondroblasts or lipoblasts. A hyalinised myxoid matrix is also seen. This tumor is S-100 protein, vimentin, and CD68-positive, and may be cytokeratin-positive. It occurs mainly in women in the superficial soft tissues or skeletal muscle of extremities and head and neck. While worrisome in appearance, the lesion does not recur or metastasize (194,195).

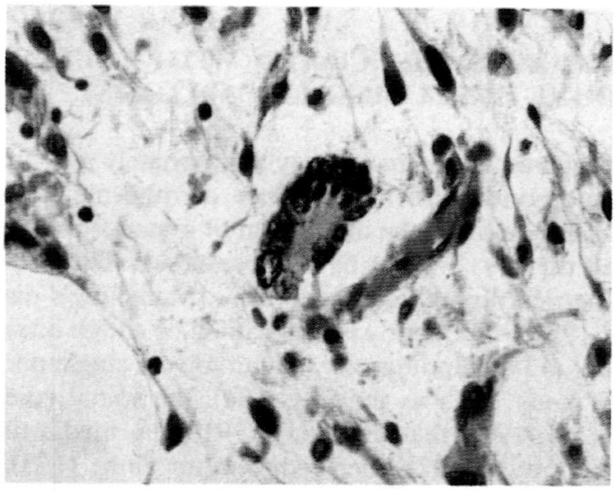

**FIG. 20.** Floret cell. The wreath of nuclei at the periphery characterizes this cell, which is classically present in pleomorphic lipoma but may occur in some liposarcomas.

Finally, an unusual fatty tumor of the mediastinum with elastic tissue has been described as elastofibrolipoma (196).

## Lipoblastoma

Frequently a congenital lesion, the lipoblastoma (197–203) is a benign solitary proliferation of fat, retaining the lobular architecture of developing fetal white adipose tissue. Nearly 90% of these superficial lesions occur before the age of 3 (136). Interestingly, lesions tend to mature with the age of the patient. Tumors may be predominantly myxoid with spindle cells, predominantly lipocytic, or mixed; all types have a prominent capillary bed and are often encapsulated. When mature fat cells are present, they are typically in the central portion of the lobules, in turn surrounded by collagen. In contrast, the presence of maturing adipocytes in myxoid liposarcoma is frequently found at the periphery of the lobule (202). Thus, while these tumors bear a resemblance to myxoid liposarcoma, there are clear differences, and the lobular accentuation with collagen is quite typical (Fig. 21), as is the age at presentation. Rare cells resembling brown fat or hibernoma cells have been identified in lipoblastoma (201). If these lesions are single, they should be termed "lipoblastoma" (198) and not "lipoblastomatosis" (200,203); that was the original designation given appropriately by Vellios et al. in 1958 for a diffuse form (197).

### *Lipoblastomatosis*

Lipoblastomatosis is the proper designation for the less common diffuse form of lipoblastoma. About one third of the patients have diffuse tumors, which (in contrast to the solitary form) are usually deeply situated, more poorly circumscribed, infiltrating muscle, and have a higher tendency to recur (198).

## CYTOGENETICS OF LIPOMAS

Chromosomal karyotypes of lipomas have been studied (204–211) and reveal nonrandom changes involving chromosomes 3 and 12, indicative of clonality. The balanced translocation t(3,12) is a common finding (206, 207) with breakpoints described at probably identical locations — q27;q13 (205) and q28;q14 (204). The breakpoint on chromosome 12 is very close to the one described in the t(12;16) translocation in myxoid liposarcomas (206). This balanced translocation involving chromosome 12 is seen in roughly

A

B

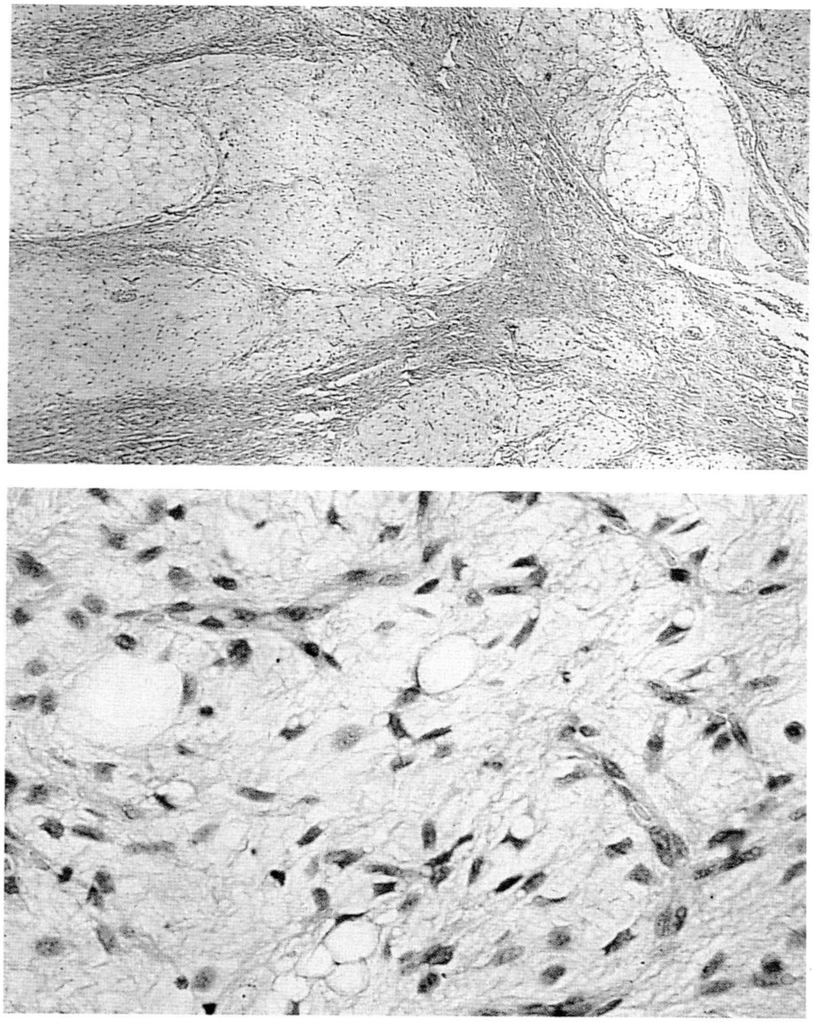

**FIG. 21.** Lipoblastoma. At low power (**A**), a distinctly lobulated appearance can be observed. In some lobules, differentiation has started in the center. Within the myxoid lobules, small lipoblasts and spindle cells are found (**B**). The spindle cells are similar to those in developing fat (see Fig. 2B).

50% of lipomas (207) and may involve other chromosomes such as 21 and 7 (207). Another one third of lipomas show a ring chromosome (207) originally described by Heim et al. (208) as a possible rearrangement of chromosome 3; this may be a marker for lipogenic tumors. Rarely, chromosome 6 has shown an abnormality (211). Interestingly, subgroups of lipomas may show different cytogenic changes (209).

Likewise, clonal chromosomal changes are notes in lipoblastoma with the abnormality at 8q11-q13 (212).

## SYNDROMES ASSOCIATED WITH FATTY LESIONS (INCLUDING LIPOMATOSIS)

The word *lipomatosis* may appropriately refer to two separate conditions: the presence of multiple subcutaneous lipomas and the infiltration of organs or sites such as the pelvis (213,214) by adipose tissue. The bilateral multiple symmetrical lipomatosis (MSL) syndrome [Madelung's disease (215–219)] is said to be frequently accompanied by a high intake of alcohol (162). However, there is increasing evidence that there is no association of MSL with alcohol abuse (220), that there may be a constitutional mitochondrial dysfunction (221), that mitochondral DNA may be abnormal (222), that patients have plasma lipid anomalies (223), and that the cells involved may be distorted brown fat cells supportive of a neoplastic nature to MSL (224).

Lipomatosis may involve a single portion of the body, such as the face (225), the spinal epidural area (226–229), the mesentery (230), the mediastinum and abdomen (231), the mediastinum alone (232), the brain (233, 234), and the kidney (235), as well as subcutaneous tissue (236). Syndromes relating to many of these are delineated in Table 2.

Lipomas, either as single or multiple tumors, may be part of a variety of syndromes (see Table 2), some of which are autosomal dominant [Gardner's syndrome (237,238), MEA type 1 (239,240), Bannayan's syndrome (241), or tuberous sclerosis (242)]. Pathologists may find it interesting to note that lipomatous lesions may also occur in Cowden's disease (243), Beckwith's hemihypertrophy (162), and as fat within a pulmonary "hamartoma" in Carney's syndrome (244,245).

Furthermore, adipose tissue lesions may be found in asso-

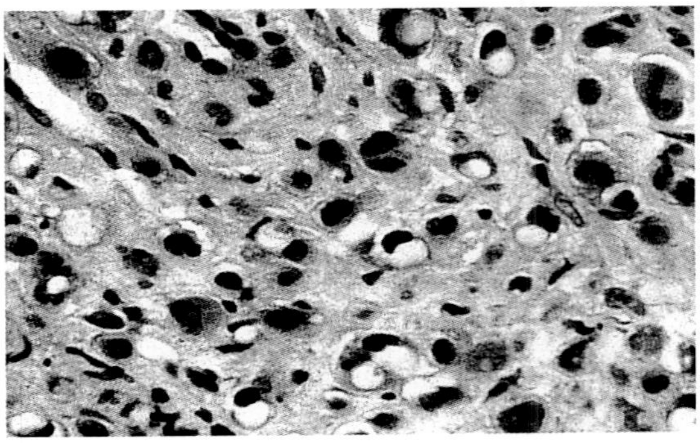

**FIG. 22.** Adipocyte mimic. Subcutaneous metastases from either signet-ring carcinoma or melanoma (*seen here*) may rarely imitate a lipocytic tumor.

ciation with other clinical syndromes, as well (246,247,251). The listing in Table 2 is meant to be as complete as possible for informational purposes. The lipodystrophies (membranous and intestinal or mesenteric) were discussed earlier.

## MIMICS OF FAT CELLS

### Mature Fat Cells

Pathologists visualize adipocytes as clear cells or "white holes" on routine sections. Therefore, other cells or processes with this white hole appearance may be confused with them. Some lesions are fairly obvious—like the vacuolated lymphadenopathy of lymphangiogram effect. Dilated superficial lymphatics if closely clustered, as they may be in a nasal polyp, remind one of adipocytes at medium power. The submucosal cystic spaces of pneumatosis cystoides intestinalis (252) are composed of gas with a lining of inflammatory cells, histiocytes, and giant cells. Cysts very similar in histology are occasionally noted within ovarian teratomas; here, it is probably a reaction to internal rupture. Likewise, small gaseous cysts without any lining in the intestinal mucosa truly mimic lipocytes in an entity termed *pseudolipomatosis* (252). Although not mentioned in placental texts, we have frequently observed a presumed artifact of chorionic villi giving them a pseudolipomatous appearance. Lipid-filled sinusoidal Ito cells in the liver simulate small adipocytes in vitamin A toxicity (253).

### Lipoblasts

The response to the lipidlike substance silicone after the rupture of a breast implant can cause concern: when the response to the silicone is marked with sheets of histiocytes containing a single dominant vacuole, the cells resemble lipoblasts and the lesion may be mistaken for liposarcoma.

Tumors with vacuoles also cause the pathologist to consider a lipocytic origin. Metastases to the skin or subcutaneous region of signet-ring carcinoma or signet-ring melanoma (254) (Fig. 22) may resemble lipoblasts, and other helpful features such as nesting or spindling are not always present. Lymphomas of both B- and T-cell origin exhibiting a vacuolated or signet-ring appearance have recently been described (255–259), may mimic liposarcoma (259), and

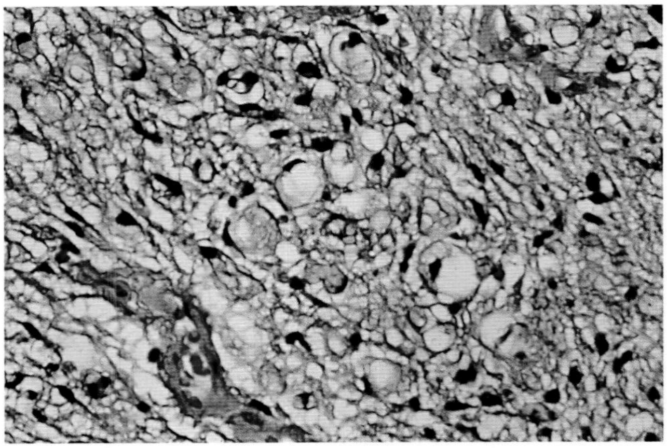

**FIG. 23.** Lipoblast mimic. In fibrohistiocytic tumors like myxoid dermatofibrosarcoma and myxoid malignant fibrous histiocytoma, cells with a vacuolated appearance may be confused with lipoblasts; however, the vacuole contains a wispy bluish coloration due to the presence of proteoglycan matrix.

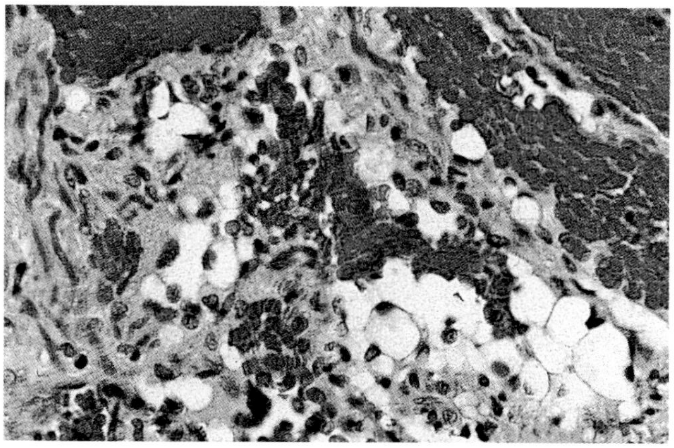

**FIG. 24.** Adipocyte mimic. Large vacuolated cells can be found in the spindle cell hemangioendothelioma, but they are endothelial in origin and often line vascular spaces as seen here.

should be in the differential diagnosis of cutaneous, nodal, or retroperitoneal tumors.

Mesenchymal tumors such as epithelioid smooth muscle lesions and fibrohistiocytic neoplasms (Fig. 23) can be vacuolated as well, due to an artifact and proteoglycan material, respectively. These two tumor groups, particularly in the form of GI stromal malignancies (leiomyosarcomas) and myxoid malignant fibrous histiocytoma, probably account for the largest number of lesions mistaken for liposarcoma. In the GI tumors, the perinuclear vacuole coupled with a cellular epithelioid morphology can closely mimic the round cell or cellular myxoid liposarcoma. In myxoid fibrohistiocytic tumors of various types, vacuolated cells superficially simulate the lipolast but closer inspection reveals a delicate basophilic substance in the cytoplasm, apparently due to matrix production by the tumor cells (Fig. 23). Unusual paragangliomas with vacuoles (260,261) may also be puzzling. Other lesions most often simulating lipocytes are those of endothelial origin because a true and often large vacuole is produced. Such cells may be identified in the histiocytoid hemangioma (262), in other epithelioid angiomas (263,264), in the spindle cell hemangioendothelioma (Fig. 24) (265), in epithelioid hemangioendothelioma (266), and in some poorly differentiated angiosarcomas (Fig. 25). In contrast to most large lipoblasts, the large vacuoles in endothelial tumors show a central septation. Chordomas, particularly with a sacral presentation, may be confused with a lipocytic tumor due to the prominent vacuolization of the physaliferous cells.

The best defense against a misdiagnosis of another tumor as a lipocytic one is strict adherence to the definition of a lipoblast: a cell, occasionally large but usually small, with a vacuole or vacuoles indenting the nucleus. The requirement for nuclear indentation assures an intracellular/cytoplasmic location for the vacuole and also excludes the semicircular nuclei around small vascular channels. Extracellular vacuoles are a common phenomenon, particularly in lesions with areas of mucoid matrix, and are often mistaken for a true intracellular finding; however, the nucleus is never affected since the substance is noncytoplasmic.

True liposarcomatous differentiation may be rarely identified in nonfatty malignancies such as medulloblastoma (267), cystosarcoma phyllodes (268), and even mesothelioma (269).

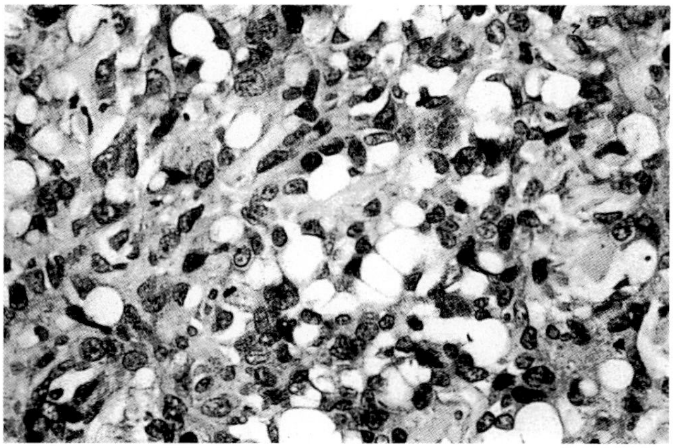

**FIG. 25.** Adipocyte mimic. In some poorly differentiated angiosarcomas, vacuolated endothelial cells also resemble fat cells; however, note the presence of occasional septated vacuoles (*center*), a feature typical for proliferating endothelial cells and unlike adipocytes.

## REFERENCES


1. Poissonnet CM, Burdi AR, Bookstein FL. Growth and development of human adipose tissue during early gestation. *Early Hum Dev* 1983; 8:1–11.
2. Poissonnet CM, Burdi AR, Garn JM. The chronology of adipose tissue appearance and distribution in the human fetus. *Early Hum Dev* 1984;10:1–11.
3. Robinson DS. In: Florkin M, Stotz EH, eds. *Comparative biochemistry*. Amsterdam; Elsevier, 1970;18:51–116.
4. Hausman GJ, Champion DR, Martin RJ. Search for the adipocyte precursor cell and factors that promote its differentiation. *J Lipid Res* 1980;21:657–670.
5. Napolitano L. The differentiation of white adipose cells: an electron microscope study. *J Cell Biol* 1963;18:663–679.
6. Aman P, Ron D, Mandahl N, Fioretos T, Heim S, Arheden K, Willen H, Rydholm A, Mitelman F. Rearrangement of the transcription factor gene CHOP in myxoid liposarcomas with t(12;16)(q13;p11). *Genes Chrom Cancer* 1992;5:278–285.
7. Crozat A, Aman P, Mandahl F, Ron D. Fusion of CHOP to a novel RNA-binding protein in human myxoid liposarcoma. *Nature* 1993; 363: 640–644.
8. Rabitts TH, Forster A, Larson R, Nathan P. Fusion of the dominant negative transcription regulator CHOP with a novel gene FUS by translocation t(12;16) in malignant liposarcoma. *Nature Genet* 1993; 4:175–180.
9. Ladanyi M. The emerging molecular genetics of sarcoma translocations. *Diag Molec Pathol* 1995;4:162–1173.
10. LeBrun DP, Warnke RA, Cleary ML. Expression of bcl-2 in fetal tissues suggests a role in morphogenesis. *Am J Pathol* 1993;142: 743–753.
11. Martin RJ, Ramsay T, Hausman GJ. Adipocyte development. *Pediatr Ann* 1984;13:448–453.
12. Poissonnet CM, LaVelle M, Bordi AR. Growth and development of adipose tissue. *J Pediatr* 1988;113:1–9.
13. Hirsch J, Batchelor B. Adipose tissue cellularity in human obesity. *Clin Endocrinol Metab* 1976;5:299–311.
14. Faust IM. Factors which affect adipocyte formation in the rat. In: Bjorntorp P, Cairella M, Howard AN, eds. *Recent advances in obesity research III. Proceedings of the 3rd International Congress on Obesity.* London: John Libbey, 1981:52–57.
15. Bjorntorp P. Adipocyte precursor cells. In: Bjorntorp P, Cairella M, Howard AN, eds. *Recent advances in obesity research III. Proceedings of the 3rd International Congress on Obesity.* London: John Libbey, 1981:58–69.
16. Sjostrom L, William-Olsson T. Prospective studies on adipose tissue development in man. *Int J Obes* 1981;5:597–604.
17. Kolata G. Why do people get fat? *Science* 1985;227:1327–1328.
18. Hirsch J, Fried SK, Edens NK, Leibel RL. The fat cell. *Med Clin North Am* 1989;73:83–96.
19. Rebuffe-Scrive M, Enk L, Crona N, et al. Fat cell metabolism in different regions in women. *J Clin Invest* 1985;75:1973–1976.
20. Fried SK, Kral JB. Sex differences in regional distribution of fat-cell size and lipoprotein lipase activity in morbidly obese patients. *Int J Obes* 1987;11:129–140.
21. Hillman B, Hellerstrom C. Cell renewal in the white and brown fat of the rat. *Acta Pathol Microbiol Scand* 1961;51:347–353.
22. Hollenberg CH, Vost A. Regulation of DNA synthesis in fat cells and stromal elements from rat adipose tissue. *J Clin Invest* 1968;47: 2485–2498.
23. Bjorntorp P. Fat cell distribution and metabolism. *Ann NY Acad Sci* 1987;499:66–72.
24. Napolitano L. The fine structure of adipose tissues. In: Reynold AE, Cahill GF, eds. *Handbook of physiology, Section 5: adipose tissue.* Washington DC: American Physical Society, 1965:109–123.
25. Nnodim JO. Development of adipose tissue. *Anat Rec* 1987;219: 331–337.
26. Merklin RJ. Growth and development of human fetal brown fat. *Anat Rec* 1978;178:637–646.
27. Heaton JM. The distribution of brown adipose tissue in the human. *J Anat* 1972;112:35–39.
28. Girardier L. Brown fat: an energy dissipating tissue. In: Girardier L, Stock MJ, eds. *Mammalian thermogenesis.* London; Chapman and Hall, 1983:50–98.
29. Rothwell NJ, Stock MJ. Brown adipose tissue. In: Baker PF, ed. *Recent advances in physiology*. Edinburgh; Churchill Livingstone, 1984: 349–384.
30. Rothwell NJ, Stock MJ. Whither brown fat? *Biosci Rep* 1986;6:3–18.
31. Bouillaud F, Combes-George M, Ricquier D. Mitochondria of adult human brown adipose tissue contain a 32,000-Mr uncoupling protein. *Biosci Rep* 1983;3:775–780.
32. Cunningham S, Leslie P, Hopwood D. The characterization and energetic potential of brown adipose tissue in man. *Clin Sci* 1985;69: 343–348.
33. Rothwell NJ, Stock MJ. A role for brown adipose tissue in diet-induced thermogenesis. *Nature* 1979;281:1–35.
34. Himms-Hagen J. Brown adipose tissue thermogenesis: interdisciplinary studies. *FASEB J* 4;2890-2898.
35. Blaza S. Brown adipose tissue in man: a review. *J R Soc Med* 1983; 76:213–216.
36. Santos GC, Araujo MR, Silveira TC, Soares FA. Accumulation of brown adipose tissue and nutritional status: a prospective study of 366 consecutive autopsies. *Arch Pathol Lab Med* 1992;116:1152–1154.
37. Cottle WH. The innervation of brown adipose tissue. In: Lindberg O, ed. *Brown adipose tissue*. New York; Elsevier, 1970:155–178.
38. Mory G, Bouillaud F, Combes-George M, Ricquier D. Noradrenaline controls the concentration of the uncoupling protein in brown adipose tissue. *FEBS Lett* 1981;166:393–396.
39. Ricquier D, Nechad M, Mory G. Ultrastructural and biochemical characterization of human brown adipose tissue in pheochromocytoma. *J Clin Endocrinol Metab* 1982;54:803–807.
40. Afzelius BA. Brown adipose tissue: its gross anatomy, histology, and cytology. In: Lindberg O, ed. *Histochemistry*
41. Pearse AG, *Histochemistry. Theoretical and Applied*, vol 2, 3rd ed. Baltimore: Williams and Wilkins, 1972.
42. Hausman GJ. Anatomical and enzyme histochemical differentiation of adipose tissue. *Int J Obes* 1985;9(1):1–6.
43. Lithell J, Boberg J, Hellsing K, Lundqvist G, Vessby B. Lipoprotein-lipase activity in human skeletal muscle and adipose tissue in the fasting and the fed states. *Atherosclerosis* 1978;30:89–94.
44. Lithell H, Hellsing K, Lundqvist G, Malmberg P. Lipoprotein-lipase activity of human skeletal-muscle and adipose tissue after intensive physical exercise. *Acta Physiol Scand* 1979;105:312–315.
45. Fielding CJ, Havel RJ. Lipoprotein lipase. *Arch Pathol Lab Med* 1977; 101:225–229.
46. Zugibe FT. *Diagnostic histochemistry.* St. Louis: CV Mosby, 1970.
47. Pearse AG. *Volume 2: Histochemistry: theoretical and applied. 3rd ed.* Baltimore; Williams & Wilkins, 1972.
48. Pearse AG. *Volume 2: Histochemistry: theoretical and applied. 3rd ed.* Baltimore; Williams & Wilkins, 1972.
49. Sheehan DC, Hrapshack BB. *Theory and practice of histotechnology.* St. Louis; CV Mosby, 1973.
50. Filipe MI, Lake BD, eds. *Histochemistry in pathology*. Edinburgh; Churchill Livingstone, 1983.
51. Spicer SS, ed. *Histochemistry in pathologic diagnosis*. New York; Marcel Dekker, 1987.
52. Hausman GJ. Techniques for studying adipocytes. *Stain Technol* 1981;56(3):149–154.
53. Popper H, Knipping G. A histochemical and biochemical study of a liposarcoma with several aspects on the development of fat synthesis. *Pathol Res Pract* 1981;171:373–380.
54. Waugh DA, Small DM. Methods in laboratory investigation. Identification and detection of in situ cellular and regional differences of lipid composition and class in lipid-rich tissue using hot stage polarizing light microscopy. *Lab Invest* 1984;51(6):702–714.
55. *Stedman's medical dictionary. 21st ed.* Baltimore; Williams & Wilkins, 1970.
56. Robbins SL, Cotran RS, Kumar V. *The pathologic basis of disease. 3rd ed.* Philadelphia; WB Saunders, 1984.
57. Rubin E, Farber JL. *Pathology*. Philadelphia; Lippincott, 1988.
58. Heptinstall RH. *Pathology of the kidney. 2nd ed.* Boston; Little, Brown, 1974.
59. Jasnosz KM, Pickeral JJ, Graner S. Fat deposits in the placenta following maternal total parenteral nutrition with intravenous lipid emulsion. *Arch Pathol Lab Med* 1995;119:555–557.
60. Bennington JL. Cancer of the kidney: etiology, epidemiology, and pathology. *Cancer* 1973;32:1017–1029.
61. Elizalde N, Korman A, Korman S. Cytochemical studies of glycogen, neutral mucopolysaccharides, and fat in malignant tissues. *Cancer* 1968;21:1061–1068.

62. Andrion A, Mazzucco G, Gugliotta P, Monga G. Benign clear cell ("sugar") tumor of the lung: a light microscopic, histochemical, and ultrastructural study with a review of the literature. *Cancer* 1985;56: 2657–2663.
63. Bertoni F, Unni KK, McLeod RA, Sim FH. Xanthoma of bone. *Am J Clin Pathol* 1988;90:377–384.
64. Bennett JH, Shousha S, Puddle B, Athanasou NA: Immunohistochemical identification of tumours of adipocytic differentiation using an antibody to aP2 protein. *J Clin Pathol* 1995; 48:950–954.
65. Michetti F, Dell'Anna E, Tiberio G, Cocchia D. Immunochemical and immunocytochemical study of S-100 protein in rat adipocytes. *Brain Res* 1983;262:352–356.
66. Haimoto H, Kato K, Suzuki F, Nagura H. The ultrastructural changes of S-100 protein localization during lipolysis in adipocytes. An immunoelectron-microscopic study. *Am J Pathol* 1985;121:185–191.
67. Takahashi K, Isobe T, Ohtusuki Y, Akagi T, Sonobe H, Okuyama T. Immunochemical study on the distribution of alpha and beta subunits of S100 protein in human neoplasms and normal tissues. *Virchows Arch [Cell Pathol]* 1984;45:385–396.
68. Nakazato Y, Ishida Y, Takahashi K, Suzuki K. Immunohistochemical distribution of S-100 protein and glial fibrillary acidic protein in normal and neoplastic salivary glands. *Virchows Arch [A]* 1985;405: 299–310.
69. Kahn HJ, Marks A, Thom H, Baumal R. Role of antibody to S100 protein in diagnostic pathology. *Am J Clin Pathol* 1983;79:341–347.
70. Nakajima T, Watanabe S, Sato Y, Kameya T, Hirota T, Shimosato Y. An immunoperoxidase study of S100 protein distribution in normal and neoplastic tissues. *Am J Surg Pathol* 1982;6:715–727.
71. Cocchia D, Lauriola L, Stolfi V, Tallini G, Michetti F. S-100 antigen labels neoplastic cells in liposarcoma and cartilaginous tumours. *Virchows Arch [A]* 1983;402:139–145.
72. Weiss SW, Langloss JM, Enzinger FM. Value of S-100 protein in the diagnosis of soft tissue tumors with particular reference to benign and malignant Schwann cell tumors. *Lab Invest* 1983;49(3):299–308.
73. Hashimoto H, Daimaru Y, Enjoji M. S100 protein distribution in liposarcoma. An immunoperoxidase study with special reference to the distinction of liposarcoma from myxoid malignant fibrous histiocytoma. *Virchows Arch [A]* 1984;405:1–10.
74. Haimoto H, Takahashi Y, Koshikawa T, Nagura H, Kato K. Immunohistochemical localization of γ-enolase in normal human tissues other than nervous and neuroendocrine tissues. *Lab Invest* 1985; 52(3):257–263.
75. Stunkard AJ, Wadden TA, eds. *Obesity: theory and therapy. 2nd ed.* New York; Raven Press, 1993.
76. Lowell BB, Susulic VS, Hamann A, Lawitts JA, Himms-Hagen J, Boyer BB, Kozak LP, Flier JS. Development of obesity in transgenic mice after ablation of brown adipose tissue. *Nature* 1993;366: 740–742.
77. Zhang Y, Proenca R, Maffei M, Barone M, Leopold L, Friedman JM. Positional cloning of the mouse obese gene and its human homologue. *Nature* 1994;372:425–432.
78. Green ED, Maffei M, Braden VV, Proenca R, DeSilva U, Zhang Y, Chua SC, Leibel RL, Weissenbach J, Friedman JM. The human obese (OB) gene: RNA expression pattern and mapping on the physical, cytogenetic, and genetic maps of chromosome 7. *Genome Research* 1995;5:5–12.
79. Pelleymounter MA, Cullen MJ, Baker MB, Hecht R, Winters D, Boone T, Collins F. Effects of the obese gene product on body weight regulation in ob/ob mice. *Science* 1995;269:540–543.
80. Halaas JL, Gajiwala KS, Maffei M, Cohen SL, Chait BT, Rabinowitz D, Lallone RL, Burley SK, Friedman JM. Weight-reducing effects of the plasma protein encoded by the obese gene. *Science* 1995; 269: 543–546.
81. Campfield LA, Smith FJ, Guisez Y, Devos R, Burn P. Recombinant mouse OB protein: evidence for a peripheral signal linking adiposity and central neural networks. *Science* 1995;269:546–549.
82. Chua SC, Chung WK, Wu-Peng S, Zhang Y, Liu SM, Tartaglia L, Leibel RL. Phenotypes of mouse diabetes and rat fatty due to mutations in the OB (Leptin) receptor. *Science* 1996;271:994–996.
83. Raife T, Landas SK. Intracellular crystalline material in visceral adipose tissue: a common autopsy finding. *Am J Clin Pathol* 1990;94: 511(abst).
84. Tedeschi CG. Pathologic anatomy of adipose tissue. In: Renold AE, Cahill GF, eds. *Handbook of physiology, section 5: adipose tissue.* Baltimore; Waverly Press, 1965:chap 14.
85. Manthorpe R, Melin G, Kofod B, Lorenzen I. Effect of glucocorticoid on connective tissue of aorta and skin in rabbits. *Acta Endocrinol* 1974;77:310–318.
86. Napolitano LM. Observations on the fine structure of adipose cells. *Ann NY Acad Sci* 1965;131:34–42.
87. Seaman JP, Kjeldsberg CR, Linker A. Gelatinous transformation of the bone marrow. *Hum Pathol* 1978;9:685–692.
88. Wittels B. Bone marrow biopsy changes following chemotherapy for acute leukemia. *Am J Surg Pathol* 1980;4:135–142.
89. Gruskin P, Canberry JN. Pathology of acoustic neuromas. In: House WF, Leutje CM, eds. *Acoustic Tumors.* Baltimore: University Park Press, 1979; 85–148.
90. Wood C. Membranous lipodystrophy of bone. *Arch Pathol Lab Med* 1978;102:22–27.
91. Bird TD, Koerker RM, Leaird BJ, Vluk BW, Thorning DR. Lipomembranous polycystic osteodysplasia (brain, bone and fat disease): a genetic cause of presenile dementia. *Neurology* 1983;33: 81–86.
92. Kitajima I, Suganuma T, Murata F, Nagamatsu K. Ultrastructural demonstration of Maclura pomifera agglutinin binding sites in the membranocystic lesions of membranous lipodystrophy (Nasu–Hakola disease). *Virchows Arch [A]* 1988; 413:475–483.
93. Chun SI, Chung K-Y: Membranous lipodystrophy: Secondary type. *J Am Acad Dermatol* 1994;31:601–605.
94. Coyne JD, Parkinson D, Baildam AD. Membranous fat necrosis of the breast. *Histopathol* 1996;28:61—64.
95. Adams RD. *Diseases of muscle: a study in pathology. 3rd ed.* New York; Harper & Row, 1975.
96. Rosai J, Levine GD. *Tumors of the thymus, fasc 13, second series of Atlas of tumor pathology.* Bethesda: Armed Forces Institute of Pathology, 1975.
97. Rywlin AM. *Histopathology of the bone marrow.* Boston: Little, Brown, 1976:19.
98. Ackerman LV, Rosai J. *Surgical pathology. 5th ed.* St Louis; CV-Mosby, 1974:649.
99. Seifert G. Lipomatous atrophy and other forms. In: Kloppel G, Heitz PU, eds. *Pancreatic pathology.* New York: Churchill Livingstone, 1984:chap 3.
100. Heggtveit HA, Fenoglio JJ, McAllister HA. Lipomatous hypertrophy of the interatrial septum: An assessment of 41 cases. *Lab Invest* 1976; 34:318.
101. McAllister HA, Fenoglio JJ. *Tumors of the cardiovascular system.* Armed Forces Institute of Pathology: Washington D.C. 1978; 44–46.
102. Rokey R, Mulvagh SL, Cheirif J, Mattox KL, Johnston DL. Lipomatous encasement and compression of the heart: antemortem diagnosis by cardiac nuclear magnetic resonance imaging and catheterization. *Am Heart J* 1989;117:952–953.
103. Waller BF. *Pathology of the heart and great vessels.* New York; Churchill Livingstone, 1988.
104. Symmers WSC. The lymphoreticular system. In: Symmers WSC, ed. *Systemic pathology*, Vol. 2. New York: Churchill Livingstone, 1978: chap 9.
105. Smith T. Fatty replacement of lymph nodes mimicking lymphoma relapse. *Cancer* 1986;58:2686–2688.
106. Takayasu K, Shima Y, Muramatsu Y, Moriyama N, Yamada T, Makuuchi M, Hirohashi S. Imaging characteristics of large lipoma and angiomyolipoma of the liver. Case reports. *Cancer* 1987;59:916–921.
107. Pounder DJ. Hepatic pseudolipoma. *Pathology* 1983;15:83–84.
108. Shafer WG, Hine MK, Levy BM. *A textbook of oral pathology. 4th ed.* WB Saunders: Philadelphia, 1983,24—25.
109. Ramadori G: The stellate cell (Ito-cell, fat-storing cell, lipocyte, perisinusoidal cell) of the liver. New insights into pathophysiology of an intriguing cell. *Virchows Arch [*B] 1991;61:147–158.
110. Cha I, Bass N, Ferrell LD: Lipopeliosis: An immunohistochemical and clinicopathologic study of five cases. *Am J Surg Pathol* 1994;18: 789–795.
111. Stroebel P, Mayer F, Zerban H, Bannasch P: Spongiotic pericytoma: A benign neoplasm deriving from the perisinusoidal (Ito) cells in rat liver. *Am J Pathol* 1995;146:903–913.
112. Orfila C, Giraud P, Modesto A, Suc JM. Abdominal fat tissue aspirate in human amyloidosis: light, electron, and immunofluorescence microscopic studies. *Hum Pathol* 1986;17:366–369.
113. Duston MA, Skinner M, Shirahama T, Cohen AS. Diagnosis of amyloidosis by abdominal fat aspiration: analysis of four years experience. *Am J Med* 1987;82:412–414.

114. Gertz MA, Li CY, Shirahama T, Kyle RA. Utility of subcutaneous fat aspiration for the diagnosis of systemic amyloidosis (immunoglobin light chain). *Arch Int Med* 1988;148:929–933.
115. Keen CE, Buk SJA, Brady K, Levison DA: Fat necrosis presenting as obscure abdominal mass: Birefringent saponified fatty acid crystalloids as a clue to diagnosis. *J Clin Pathol* 1994;47:1028–1031.
116. Poppiti RJ, Margulies M, Cabello B, Rywlin AM. Membranous fat necrosis. *Am J Surg Pathol* 1986;10:62–69.
117. Bennett RG, Petrozzi JW. Nodular subcutaneous fat necrosis: a manifestation of silent pancreatitis. *Arch Dermatol* 1975;111:896–898.
118. Hughes PS, Apisarnthanarax P, Mullins F. Subcutaneous fat necrosis associated with pancreatic disease. Arch Pathol Lab Med 1975; III:506–510.
119. Fischer AH, Morris DJ. Pathogenesis of calciphylaxis: study of three cases and literature review. *Hum Pathol* 1995;26:1055–1064.
120. MacDonald A, Feiwel M. A review of the concept of Weber–Christian panniculitis with a report of 5 cases. *Br J Dermatol* 1968;809: 355–361.
121. Solomon AR, Sanchez RL. Non-neoplastic diseases of the skin. In: Sternberg SS, ed. *Diagnostic surgical pathology*. New York: Raven Press, 1989:50–58.
122. Winkelmann RK, Frigas E. Eosinophilic panniculitis: a clinicopathologic study. *J Cutan Pathol* 1986;13:1–12.
123. Blaustein A, Moreno A, Noguera J, de Moragas JM. Septal granulomatous panniculitis in Sweet's syndrome: report of two cases. *Arch Dermatol* 1985;121:785–788.
124. Suster S, Cartagena N, Cabello SO, Inchausti B, Robinson MJ. Histiocytic lymphophagocytic panniculitis: an unusual extranodal presentation of sinus histiocytosis with massive lymphadenopathy (Rosai–Dorfman disease). *Arch Dermatol* 1988;124:1246–1249.
125. Alegre VA, Winkelmann RK, Aliaga A. Lipomembranous changes in chronic panniculitis. *J Am Acad Dermatol* 1988;19:39–46.
126. Vincent F, Prokopetz R, Miller RA. Plasma cell panniculitis: a unique clinical and pathologic presentation of linear scleroderma. *J Am Acad Dermatol* 1989;21:357–360.
127. Izumi AK, Takiguchi P. Lupus erythematosus panniculitis. *Arch Dermatol* 1983;119:61–64.
128. Silverman RA, Newman AJ, LeVine MJ, Kaplan B. Poststeroid panniculitis: a case report. *Pediatr Dermatol* 1988;5:92–93.
129. Sleisenger MH, Fordtran JS. *Gastrointestinal disease: pathophysiology diagnosis and management. 3rd ed.* Philadelphia: WB Saunders, 1983.
130. Kelly JK, Hwang W-S. Idiopathic retractile (sclerosing) mesenteritis and its differential diagnosis. *Am J Surg Pathol* 1989;13(6):513–521.
131. Scully RE, Galdabini JJ, McNeely BU. Lipodystrophy of mesentery (case 30-1976). *N Engl J Med* 1976;295:214–218.
132. Eble JN, Rosenberg AE, Young RH. Retroperitoneal xanthogranulomatosis in a patient with Erdheim-Chester disease. *Am J Surg Pathol* 1994;18:843–848.
133. Seemayer TA, Knaack J, Wang N-S, Ahmed MN. On the ultrastructure of hibernoma. *Cancer* 1975;36:1785–1793.
134. Dardick I. Hibernoma: a possible model of brown fat histogenesis. *Hum Pathol* 1978;9(3):321–329.
135. Gaffney EF, Hargreaves HK, Semple E, Vellios F. Hibernoma: distinctive light and electron microscopic features and relationship to brown adipose tissue. *Hum Pathol* 1983;14:677–687.
136. Enzinger FM, Weiss SW. *Soft tissue tumors. 2nd ed.* St. Louis: CV Mosby, 1988.
137. Rigor VU, Goldstone SE, Jones J, Bernstein R, Gold MS, Weiner S. Hibernoma. A case report and discussion of a rare tumor. *Cancer* 1986;57:2207–2211.
138. Allegra SR, Gmuer C, O'Leary GP. Endocrine activity in a large hibernoma. *Hum Pathol* 1983;14:1044–1052.
139. Enterline HT, Lowry LD, Richman AV. Does malignant hibernoma exist? *Am J Surg Pathol* 1979;3:265–271.
140. Teplitz C, Farrugia R, Glicksman AS. Malignant hibernoma does exist. *Lab Invest* 1980;42:59A.
141. Talerman A. Germ cell tumors of the ovary. In: Kurman R., ed. *Blaustein's pathology of the female genital tract,* 3rd ed. New York: Springer-Verlag, 1987:689.
142. Dail DH. Uncommon tumors. In: Dale DH, Hammar SP, eds. *Pulmonary pathology*. New York: Springer-Verlag, 1988:920–924.
143. Ali MY, Wong PK. Intrapulmonary teratoma. *Thorax* 1964;19: 228–235.
144. Lee RG. Esophagus. In: Sternberg SS, ed. *Diagnostic surgical pathology*. New York; Raven Press, 1989:928.
145. Toker C, Tang C-K, Whitely JF, Berkheiser SW, Rachman R. Benign spindle cell breast tumor. *Cancer* 1981;48:1615–1622.
146. Wargotz ES, Weiss SW, Norris HJ. Myofibroblastoma of the breast: sixteen cases of a distinctive benign mesenchymal tumor. *Am J Surg Pathol* 1987;11:493–502.
147. Nogales FF, Pavcovich M, Medina MT, Palomino M. Fatty change in the endometrium. *Histopathol* 1992;20:362–363.
148. Nogita T, Wong TY, Hidano A, Mihm MC, Kawashima M. Pedunculated lipofibroma: a clinicopathologic study of thirty-two cases supporting a simplified nomenclature. *J Am Acad Dermatol* 1994; 31: 235–240.
149. Tomashefski JF. Benign endobronchial mesenchymal tumors: their relationship to parenchymal pulmonary hamartomas. *Am J Surg Pathol* 1982;6:531–540.
150. Palvio D, Egeblad K, Paulsen SM. Atypical lipomatous hamartoma of the lung. *Virchows Arch [A]* 1985;405:253–261.
151. Benjamin SP, Mercer RD, Hawk WA. Myofibroblastic contraction in spontaneous regression of multiple congenital mesenchymal hamartomas. *Cancer* 1977;40:2343–2352.
152. Enzinger FM. Fibrous hamartoma of infancy. *Cancer* 1965;18: 241–248.
153. Reye RD. A consideration of certain subdermal "fibromatous tumours" of infancy. *J Pathol* 1956;72:149–154.
154. Fletcher CDM, Powell G, Van Noorden S, McKee PH. Fibrous hamartoma of infancy: a histochemical and immunohistochemical study. *Histopathology* 1988;12:65–74.
155. Silverman TA. Fibrolipomatous hamartoma of nerve: a clinocopatholigic analysis of 26 cases. *Am J Surg Pathol* 1985; 9:7–14.
156. Silverman TA, Enzinger FM. Fibrolipomatous hamartoma of nerve: a clinicopathologic analysis of 26 cases. *Am J Surg Pathol* 1985;9:7–14.
157. Aymard B, Bowman-Ferrand F, Vernhes L, Floquet A, Floquet J, Morel O, Merle M, Delagoutte JP. Hamartome lipofibromateux des nerfs peripheriques. Etude anatomo-clinique de 5 cas dont 2 avec etude ultrastructurale. *Ann Pathol* 1987;7(4-5):320–324.
158. Price EB, Mostofi FK. Symptomatic angiomyolipoma of the kidney. *Cancer* 1965;18:761–774.
159. McCullough DL, Scott R, Seybold HM. Angiomyolipoma (hamartoma: review of the literature and report on 7 cases). *J Urol* 1971;105: 32–44.
160. Dao AH, Netsky NG. Human tails and pseudotails. *Hum Pathol* 1984; 15:449–453.
161. LeBer MS, Stout AP. Benign mesenchymomas in children. *Cancer* 1962;15:598–605.
162. Allen P. *Tumors and proliferations of adipose tissue*. New York; Masson, 1981.
163. Kasantikul V, Brown WJ, Netsky MG. Mesenchymal differentiation in trigeminal neurilemmoma. *Cancer* 1982;50:1568–1571.
164. Majeski JA, Paxton ES, Wirman JA, Schrieber JT. A thoracic benign mesenchymoma in association with hemihypertrophy. *Am J Clin Pathol* 1981;76(6):827–832.
165. Rosai J. Case presentation at the European Society of Pathology meeting in Porto, Portugal, Sept 1989.
166. Brecher ME, Gill WB, Straus FH. Angiolipoma with regional lymph node involvement and long term follow-up study. *Hum Pathol* 1986; 17:962–963.
167. Meggitt BF, Wilson JN. The battered buttock syndrome—fat fractures: a report on a group of traumatic lipomata. *Br J Surg* 1972; 59:165–169.
168. Wilson JE. Lipomas and potassium intake. *Ann Intern Med* 1989;110: 750–751.
169. Solvonuk PF, Taylor GP, Hancock R, Wood WS, Frohlich J. Correlation of morphologic and biochemical observations in human lipomas. *Lab Invest* 1984;51(4):469–474.
170. Azumi N, Curtis J, Kempson R, Hendrickson M. Atypical and malignant neoplasms showing lipomatous differentiation: a study of 111 cases. *Am J Surg Pathol* 1987;11:161–183.
171. Fu YS, Parker FG, Kaye GI, Lattes R. Ultrastructure of benign and malignant adipose tissue tumors. *Pathol Ann* 1980;15(Pt 1):67.
172. Kindbloom L, Angervall L, Stener B, Wickbom I. Intermuscular and intramuscular lipomas and hibernomas. A clinical, roentgenologic, histologic and prognostic study of 46 cases. *Cancer* 1974;43:754–762.
173. Evans H, Soule E, Winkelman R. Atypical lipoma, atypical intramuscular lipoma and well-differentiated retroperitoneal liposarcoma. *Cancer* 1979;43:574–584.

174. Marsh WL Jr, Lucas JG, Olsen J. Chondrolipoma of the breast. *Arch Pathol Lab Med* 1989;113:369–371.
175. Lim YC. Mediastinal chondrolipoma. *Am J Surg Pathol* 1980; 4:407–409.
176. Allen P. Letter to the case. *Pathol Res Pract* 1989;184:444–445.
177. Hayden JW, Abellera RM. Tenosynovial lipochondromatosis of the flexor hallucis, common toe flexor, and posterior tibial tendons. *Clin Orthop* 1989;245:220–222.
178. Katzer B. Histopathology of rare chondroosteoblastic metaplasia in benign lipomas. *Pathol Res Pract* 1989;184:437–443.
179. Honore LH. Uterine fibrolipoleiomyoma: report of a case with discussion of histogenesis. *Am J Obstet Gynecol* 1978;13:635–638.
180. Brescia RJ, Tazelaar HD, Hobbs J, Miller A. Intravascular lipoleiomyomatosis: a report of two cases. *Hum Pathol* 1989;20:252–256.
181. Hunt SJ, Santa Cruz DJ, Barr RJ: Cellular angiolipoma. Am J *Surg Pathol* 1990;14:75–81.
182. DeRienzo D, Truong L. Thyroid neoplasms containing mature fat: a report of two cases and review of the literature. *Mod Pathol* 1989; 2(5):506.
183. Perosio P, Brooks JJ, LiVolsi VA. Orbital brown tumor as the initial manifestation of a parathyroid lipoadenoma. *Surg Pathol* 1988;1:1–6.
184. Gnepp DR, Ogorzalek JM, Heffess CA. Fat-containing lesions of the thyroid gland. *Am J Surg Pathol* 1989;13(7):605–612.
185. Bruno J, Ciancia EM, Pingitore R. Thyroid papillary adenocarcinoma; lipomatous-type. *Virchows Arch [A]* 1989;414:371–373.
186. Otto HF, Loning T, Lachenmayer L, Janzen RW, Gurtler KF, Fischer K. Thymolipoma in association with myasthenia gravis. *Cancer* 1982; 50:1623–1628.
187. Trites AEW. Thyrolipoma, thymolipoma and pharyngeal lipoma: a syndrome. *Can Med Assoc J* 1966; 95:1251–1259.
188. Enzinger F, Harvey D. Spindle cell lipoma. *Cancer* 1975;36: 1852–1859.
189. Angervall L, Dahl I, Kindbloom LG, Save-Soderbergh J. Spindle cell lipoma. *Acta Pathol Microbiol Scand* 1976;84:477–487.
190. Fletcher C, Martin-Bates E. Spindle cell lipoma: a clinicopathological study with some original observations. *Histopathol* 1987;11:803–817.
191. Shmookler B, Enzinger F. Pleomorphic lipoma: a benign tumor simulating liposarcoma: a clinicopathologic analysis of 48 cases. *Cancer* 1981;47:126-133.
192. Azzopardi J, Iocco J, Salm R. Pleomorphic lipoma: A tumour simulating liposarcoma.*Histopathol* 1983;7:511–523.
193. Beham A, Schmid C, Hödl S, Fletcher CDM: Spindle cell and pleomorphic lipoma: An immunohistochemical study and histogenetic analysis. *J Pathol* 1989;158:219–222.
194. Meis JM, Enzinger FM. Chondroid lipoma. A unique tumor simulating liposarcoma and myxoid chondrosarcoma. *Am J Surg Pathol* 1993;17:1103–1112.
195. Kindblom L-G, Meis-Kindblom JM: Chondroid lipoma: An ultrastructural and immunohistochemical analysis with further observations regarding its differentiation. *Hum Pathol* 1995;26:706–715.
196. De Nictolis M, Goteri G, Campanati G, Prat J: Elastofibrolipoma of the mediastinum: A previously undescribed benign tumor containing abnormal elastic fibers. *Am J Surg Pathol* 1995;19: 364–367.
197. Vellios F, Baez J, Schumacker H. Lipoblastomatosis: A tumor of fetal fat different from hibernoma. *Am J Pathol* 1958;34:1149–1158.
198. Chung E, Enzinger F. Benign lipoblastomatosis: an analysis of 35 cases. *Cancer* 1973;32:482–492.
199. Bolen JW, Thorning D. Benign lipoblastoma and myxoid liposarcoma: a comparative light- and electron-microscopic study. *Am J Surg Pathol* 1980;4:163–174.
200. Greco MA, Garcia RL, Vuletin JC. Benign lipoblastomatosis. Ultrastructure and histogenesis. *Cancer* 1980;45:511–515.
201. Chaudhuri B, Ronan SG, Ghosh L. Benign lipoblastoma. Report of a case. *Cancer* 1980;46:611–614.
202. Hanada M, Tokuda R, Ohnishi Y, Takami M, Takahashi T, Kimura M. Benign lipoblastoma and liposarcoma in children. *Acta Pathol Jpn* 1986;36(4):605–612.
203. Dudgeon DL, Haller JA Jr. Pediatric lipoblastomatosis:Two unusual cases. *Surgery* 1984; 95(3):371–373.
204. Turc-Carel C, Dal Cin P, Rao U, Karakousis C, Sandberg A. Cytogenetic studies of adipose tumors: I. A benign lipoma with reciprocal translocation t(3;12) (q28;q14). *Can Genet Cytogenet* 1986;23: 283–290.
205. Heim S, Mandahl N, Kristoffersson U, Mitelman F, Rydholm A, Willen H. Reciprocal translocation t(3;12) (q27;q13) in lipoma. *Can Genet Cytogenet* 1986;23:301–304.
206. Sandberg AA, Turc-Carel C. The cytogenetics of solid tumor. Relation to diagnosis, classification and pathology. *Cancer* 1987;59: 387–395.
207. Heim S, Mitelman F. *Cancer cytogenetics*. New York; Alan R. Liss, 1987:240–241.
208. Heim S, Mandahl N, Kristoffersson U, Mitelman F, Rooser B, Rydholm A, Willen H. Marker ring chromosome—a new cytogenetic abnormality characterizing lipogenic tumors? *Can Genet Cytogenet* 1987;24:319–326.
209. Heim S, Mandahl N, Rydholm A, Willen H, Mitelman F. Different karyotypic features characterize different clinicopathologic subgroups of benign lipogenic tumors. *Int J Cancer* 1988;42:863–867.
210. Turc-Carel C, Dal Cin P, Boghosian L, Leong SPL, Sandberg AA. Breakpoints in benign lipoma may be at 12q13 or 12q14. *Can Genet Cytogenet* 1988;36:131–135.
211. Sait SNJ, Dal Cin P, Sandberg AA, et al. Involvement of 6p in benign lipomas: A new cytogenetic entity. *Can Genet Cytogenet* 1989; 37:281–283.
212. Dal Cin P, Sciot R, De Wever I, Van Damme B, Van Den Berghe H: New discriminative chromosomal marker in adipose tissue tumors: The chromosome 8q11-q13 region in lipoblastoma. *Cancer Genet Cytogenet* 1994;78:232–235.
213. Bechtold R, Shaff MI. Pelvic lipomatosis with ureteral encasement and recurrent thrombophlebitis. *South Med J* 1983;76:1030–1032.
214. Henriksson L, Liljeholm H, Lonnerholm T. Pelvic lipomatosis causing constriction of the lower urinary tract and the rectum: Case report. *Scand J Urol Nephrol* 1984;18:249–252.
215. Shugar MA, Gavron JP. Benign symmetrical lipomatosis (Madelung's disease). *Otolaryngol Head Neck Surg* 1985;93:109–112.
216. Keller SM, Waxman JS, Kim US. Benign symmetrical lipomatosis. *South Med J* 1986;79:1428–1429.
217. Cinti S, Enzi G, Cigolini M, Bosello O. Ultrastructural features of cultured mature adipocyte precursors from adipose tissue in multiple symmetric lipomatosis. *Ultrastruct Pathol* 1983;5:145–152.
218. Enzi G. Multiple symmetric lipomatosis: an updated clinical report. *Medicine (Baltimore)* 1984;63:56–64.
219. Pollock M, Nicholson GI, Nukada H, Cameron S, Frankish P. Neuropathy in multiple symmetric lipomatosis: Madelung's disease. *Brain* 1988;111:1157–1171.
220. Boozan JA, Maves MD, Schuller DE: Surgical management of massive benign symmetric lipomatosis. *Laryngoscope* 1992;102:94–99.
221. Berkovic SF, Andermann F, Shoubridge EA, Carpenter S, Robitaille Y, Andermann E, Melmed C, Karpati G: Mitochondrial dysfunction in multiple symmetrical lipomatosis. *Ann Neurol* 1991; 29:566–569.
222. Klopstock T, Naumann M, Schalke B, Bischof F, Seibel P, Kottlors M, Eckert P, Reiners K, Toyka KV, Reichmann H: Multiple symmetric lipomatosis: Abnormalities in complex IV and multiple deletions in mitochondrial DNA. *Neurology* 1994;44:862–866.
223. Deiana L, Pes GM, Carru C, Campus GV, Tidore MGB, Cherchi GM: Extremely high HDL levels in a patient with multiple symmetric lipomatosis. *Clin Chim Acta* 1993;223:143–147.
224. Zancanaro C, Sbarbati A, Morroni M, Carraro R, Cigolini M, Enzi G, Cinti S: Multiple symmetric lipomatosis: Ultrastructural investigation of the tissue and preadipocytes in primary culture. *Lab Invest* 1990;63: 253–258.
225. DeRosa G, Cozzolino A, Guarino M, Giardino C. Congenital infiltrating lipomatosis of the face: Report of cases and review of the literature. *Oral Maxillofac Surg* 1987;12:879–883.
226. Quint DJ, Boulos RS, Sanders WP, Mehta BA, Patel SC, Tiel RL. Epidural lipomatosis. *Radiology* 1988;169:485–490.
227. Vazquez L, Ellis A, Saint-Genez D, Patino J, Nogues M. Epidural lipomatosis after renal transplantation—complete recovery without surgery. *Transplantation* 1988;46:773–774.
228. Doppman JL. Epidural lipomatosis. *Radiology* 1989;171:581–582.
229. Kaplan JG, Barasch E, Hirschfeld A, Ross L, Einberg K, Gordon M. Spinal epidural lipomatosis: A serious complication of iatrogenic Cushing's syndrome. *Neurology* 1989;39:1031–1034.
230. Siskind BN, Weiner FR, Frank M, Weiner SN, Bernstein RG, Luftschein S. Steroid-induced mesenteric lipomatosis. *Comput Radiol* 1984;8:175–177.
231. Enzi G, Digito M, Marin R, Carraro R, Baritussio A, Manzato E. Mediastino-abdominal lipomatosis: deep accumulation of fat mimicking a respiratory disease and ascites. Clinical aspects and metabolic studies in vitro. *Q J Med* 1984;53:453–463.

232. Shukla LW, Katz JA, Wagner ML. Mediastinal lipomatosis: a complication of high dose steroid therapy in children. *Pediatr Radiol* 1988;19:57–58.
233. Al-Mefty O, Fox JL, Sakati N, Bashir R, Probst F. The multiple manifestations of the encephalocraniocutaneous lipomatosis syndrome. *Childs Nerv Syst* 1987;3:132–134.
234. Brumback RA, Leech RW. Fishman's syndrome (encephalocraniocutaneous lipomatosis): a field defect of ectomesoderm. *J Child Neurol* 1987;2:168–169.
235. Arora PK. Re: Non-operative diagnosis of renal sinus lipomatosis simulating tumour of the renal pelvis [letter]. *Br J Urol* 1989;63:445.
236. Rubinstein A, Goor Y, Gazit E, Cabili S. Non-symmetric subcutaneous lipomatosis associated with familial combined hyperlipidaemia. *Br J Dermatol* 1989;120:689–694.
237. Scully RE, Galdabini JJ, McNeely BU. Case 53-1976 (Gardner's syndrome). *N Engl J Med* 1976;295:1526–1532.
238. Scully RE, Galdabini JJ, McNeely BU. Case 47-1978 (Gardner's syndrome). *N Engl J Med* 1976;299:1237–1244.
239. Snyder N III, Scurry MT, Diess WP Jr. Five families with multiple lipomas in endocrine adenomatosis. *Ann Intern Med* 1972;76:53–58.
240. Johnson GJ, Summerskill WHJ, Anderson VE, Keating FR Jr. Clinical and genetic investigation of a large kindred with multiple endocrine adenomatosis. *N Engl J Med* 1967;277(6):1379–1385.
241. Higginbottom MC, Schultz P. The Bannayan syndrome: an autosomal dominant disorder consisting of macrocephali, lipomas, hemangiomas, and a risk for intracranial tumors. *Pediatrics* 1982;69:632.
242. Klein JA, Barr RJ. Diffuse lipomatosis and tuberous sclerosis. *Arch Dermatol* 1986;122:1298–1302.
243. Weinstock JV, Kawanishi H. Gastrointestinal polyposis with orocutaneous hamartomas (Cowden's disease). *Gastroenterology* 1978;74: 890–895.
244. Carney JA. The triad of gastric epithelioid leiomyosarcoma, functioning extra-adrenal paraganglioma, and pulmonary chondroma. *Cancer* 1979;43:374–382.
245. Carney J. The triad of gastric epithelioid leiomyosarcoma, pulmonary chondroma, and functioning extra-adrenal paraganglioma: a five-year review. *Medicine* 1983;62(3):159–169.
246. Kremchek TE, Kremchek EJ. Carpal tunnel syndrome caused by flexor tendon sheath lipoma. *Orthop Rev* 1988;17:1083–1085.
247. Juhlin L, Strand A, Johnsen B. A syndrome with painful lipomas, familial dysarthria, abnormal eye-movements and clumsiness. *Acta Med Scand* 1987;221:215–218.
248. Aleksic S, Budzilovich G, Greco MA, et al. Intracranial lipomas, hydrocephalus and other CNS anomalies in oculoauriculo-vertebral dysplasia (Goldenhar–Gorlin syndrome). *Childs Brain* 1984;11:285–297.
249. Oochi N, Rikitake O, Maeda T, Yamaguchi M. A case of Laurence–Moon–Biedl syndrome associated with bilateral adrenal lipomas and renal abnormalities. *Nippon Naika Gakkai Zasshi* 1984;73: 89–93.
250. Humphrey AA, Kinsley PC. Familial multiple lipomas: report of a family. *Arch Dermatol* 1938;37:30.
251. Temtamy SA, Rogers JG. Macrodactyly, hemihypertrophy, and connective tissue nevi: report of a new syndrome and review of the literature. J Pediatr 1976; 89:924–927.
252. Petras RE. Non-eoplastic diseases. In: Sternberg SS, ed. *Diagnostic surgical pathology*. New York: Raven Press, 1989:1004–1005.
253. Russell RM, Boyer JL, Bagheri SA, Hruban Z. Hepatic injury from chronic hypervitaminosis A resulting in portal hypertension and ascites. *N Engl J Med* 1974;291:435–440.
254. Sheibani K, Battifora H. Signet-ring cell melanoma. A rare morphologic variant of malignant melanoma. *Am J Surg Pathol* 1988;12: 28–34.
255. Iossifides I, Mackay B, Butler JJ. Signet-ring cell lymphoma. *Ultrastruct Pathol* 1980;1:511–517.
256. Hanna W, Kahn HJ, From L. Signet ring lymphoma of the skin: ultrastructural and immunohistochemical features. *J Am Acad Dermatol* 1986;14:344–350.
257. Cross PA, Eyden BP, Harris M. Signet ring cell lymphoma of T cell type. *J Clin Pathol* 1989;42:239–245.
258. Uccini S, Pescarmona E, Ruco LP, Baroni CD, Monarca B, Modesti A. Immunohistochemical characterization of a B-cell signet ring cell lymphoma. Report of a case. *Pathol Res Pract* 1988;183:497–504.
259. Mathur DR, Ramdeo IN, Sharma SP, Singh H. Signet ring cell lymphoma simulating liposarcoma—a case report with brief review of literature. *Ind J Cancer* 1988;25:52–55.
260. Jacobs DM, Waisman J. Cervical paraganglioma with intranuclear vacuoles in a fine needle aspirate. *Acta Cytol* 1987;31:29–32.
261. Spagnolo DV, Paradinas FJ. Laryngeal neuroendocrine tumour with features of a paraganglioma, intracytoplasmic lumina and acinar formation. *Histopathology* 1985;9:117–131.
262. Rosai J, Gold J, Landy R. The histiocytoid hemangiomas: a unifying concept embracing several previously described entities of skin, soft tissue, large vessels, bone, and heart. *Hum Pathol* 1979; 10(6):707–730.
263. Barnes L, Koss W, Nieland M. Angiolymphoid hyperplasia with eosinophilia: a disease that may be confused with malignancy. *Head Neck Surg* 1980;2:425–434.
264. Kung I, Gibson J, Bannatyne P. Kimura's disease: a clinico-pathological study of 21 cases and its distinction from angiolymphoid hyperplasia with eosinophilia. *Pathology* 1984;16:39–44.
265. Weiss SW, Enzinger FM. Spindle cell hemangioendothelioma. A low-grade angiosarcoma resembling a cavernous hemangioma and Kaposi's sarcoma. *Am J Surg Pathol* 1986;10:521–530.
266. Weiss S, Enzinger F. Epithelioid hemangioendothelioma. A vascular tumor often mistaken for a carcinoma. *Cancer* 1982;50:970–981.
267. Chimelli L, Hahn MD, Budka H: Lipomatous differentiation in a medulloblastoma. *Acta Neuropathol (Berl)* 1991;81:471–473.
268. Powell CM, Rosen PP. Adipose differentiation in cystosarcoma phyllodes: a study of 14 cases. *Am J Surg Pathol* 1994;18:720–727.
269. Krishna J, Haqqani MT: Liposarcomatous differentiation in diffuse pleural mesothelioma. *Thorax* 1993;48:409–410.

*Histology for Pathologists, second edition,*
Edited by Stephen S. Sternberg.
Lippincott-Raven Publishers, Philadelphia


# CHAPTER 9

# Skeletal Muscle

Reid R. Heffner, Jr.



## EMBRYOLOGY

Skeletal muscle develops embryologically from somatic mesodermal tissue. The paraxial mesoderm is first apparent on day 17 and is the origin of the somites that are completely formed by day 30. At this time, a series of 42 to 44 pairs of rounded somites can be found adjacent to the notochord in the midline. By the 4th week, the mesodermal somites separate into the dermatomes and segmental myotomes. The latter give rise to the muscles of the body wall. The dorsal division of myotomes, the epimeres, represent the origin of the back muscles, while the ventral division hypomeres differentiate into the lateral and ventral muscles of the body wall including the intercostals, abdominal obliques, and strap muscles of the neck. The muscles of the extremities arise from the limb buds which form from the lateral plate mesoderm that is also the origin of the bone, tendon, ligaments, and blood vessels. In the human embryo, the mesenchyme of the limb buds appears at about the 4th week of gestation and is subject to induction by the somites. At the end of the 8th week, the primordia of individual muscles can be appreciated. Muscle tissue is not derived directly from the lateral plate mesoderm as previously thought, but from somitic mesoderm which invades the limb bud in week 5 (1). Differentiation of the limb musculature follows a cephalocaudad and proximal to distal progression. In each limb the somitic mesenchyme subdivides into a dorsal and ventral mass with respect to the skeletal elements. The extensor, abductor, and supinator muscles are derived from the dorsal mass, whereas the flexor, adductor, and pronator muscles originate from the ventral mass (2).

The most immature muscle cells are myoblasts. These are small, round, mononucleate cells with prominent nucleoli and evidence of mitotic activity. Myoblast cytoplasm contains no microscopically detectable filaments, but ribosomes can be identified. Masses of proliferating myoblasts represent the source of myotubes, the next step in myogenesis (3). Myotubes appear to arise as a result of fusion of the more primitive myoblasts (4). Myoblast fusion has been shown to depend on a plasma membrane glycoprotein with a molecular weight of 38 kDa (5). This surface marker presumably allows fusing myoblasts to recognize each other. The 38 kda membrane protein is also found on immature myotubes and satellite cells. Ultrastructurally, myoblasts are seen to have contact with each other through filopodia. Adjacent myoblasts are often joined by gap junctions (6). Fusing myoblasts become longitudinally oriented, a process that requires fibronectin (7). At this stage of myogenesis, groups of primitive muscle cells including myoblasts and myotubes are enclosed by a common basement membrane. In each cluster there is usually one larger primary myotube. Between groups of cells are aggregates of interstitial cells (8).

Myotubes differ from myoblasts by the presence of multiple nuclei and cytoplasmic filaments. Filaments first form at the peripheral portions of the sarcoplasm and consist of 10 nm fibroblast-like fibrils that disappear during maturation (9). Immunohistochemical techniques also demonstrate the presence of desmin and vimentin within myotubes. More mature secondary myotubes have a larger diameter, increased numbers of nuclei that are central in cross sections,

R. R. Heffner, Jr.: Department of Pathology and Neurology, SUNY-Buffalo School of Medicine and Biomedical Sciences, Buffalo, NY 14214.

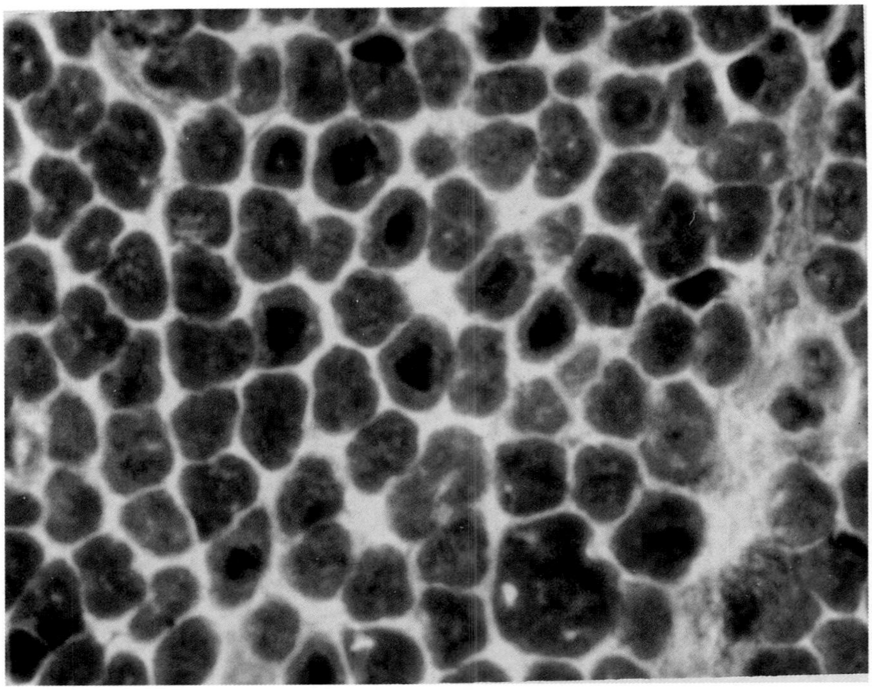

**FIG. 1.** Myotube stage of muscle development. Myotubes typically have large central nuclei (Trichrome).

and more prominent myofilaments (Fig. 1). These cells also begin to show evidence of contractile activity. Secondary myotubes eventually give rise to muscle fibers. As they approach this stage of development, secondary myotubes cease fusing and develop acetylcholine receptor protein on the cell surface. At first, receptor protein is diffusely distributed on the cell surface, but it later becomes focused into so-called "hot spots" where motor end-plates will develop (10).

Muscle fibers differ from myotubes in that their nuclei are peripheral and their filaments are organized into sarcomeres. Muscle fibers also develop a sarcotubular system and, in time, they become innervated. Immature muscle fibers often acquire multiple innervation sites, all but one of which eventually disappears.

The number of myotubes continues to decline after the twenty-first week of gestation so that at the time of birth myotubes are no longer conspicuous histologically. As myotubes become fewer in number, the muscle fibers undergo histochemical differentiation which begins in the fifth month of development. Between 15 and 20 weeks of gestation, a primitive progenitor of the checkerboard pattern emerges, in which all myotubes and myofibers have high adenosine triphosphatase (ATPase) and oxidative enzyme activity (11). By 20 weeks gestation, approximately 10% of fibers are larger in diameter with both high oxidatative enzyme activity and reduced ATPase activity. These fibers which are basophilic in hematoxylin-eosin (H&E) stains are the so-called Wohlfart B fibers and are the earliest example of type 1 fibers to be detected in developing muscle (12). The remaining 90% of fibers (Wohlfart type A) correspond to type 2 fibers with enhanced ATPase activity. Although type 2A and 2B fibers are not yet visible, a few type 2C fibers that stain dark in both acid and alkaline ATPase reactions are apparent. These fibers typically immunostain with antibodies to both fast and slow myosin. The more mature checkerboard histochemical pattern, which is stimulated by the innervation of fibers, is almost completed between 26 and 30 weeks of gestation (13). At birth the histochemical mosaic begins to resemble that of mature adult muscle (Fig. 2). Approximately 80% of fibers are clearly identified as type 1 or type 2. The remaining 20% are undifferentiated fibers which have both abundant oxidative enzyme activity and stain darkly in routine ATPase reactions. A few Wohlfart type B fibers remain at birth. Type 2C fibers are not encountered.

## POSTNATAL AND DEVELOPMENTAL CHANGES

During the prenatal period and after birth in childhood, muscle fibers continue to increase in length until full growth is attained. Muscle fibers lengthen in response to growth of the skeleton by virtue of two fundamental changes in the sarcomeres. Existing sarcomeres lengthen, producing longitudinal fiber growth (14). This mechanism may account for up to a 25% increase in fiber length and indicates that there is a relative excess of sarcomeres that may elongate during periods of rapid growth of the skeleton. Muscle fibers also undergo real longitudinal growth with the addition of new sarcomeres, which involves the synthesis of contractile proteins (15). New sarcomeres are known to be added at the end of fibers, usually at the myotendinous junctions (16). There is also evidence to suggest that new sarcomeres are not only added at the end of fibers, but within internal segments, as

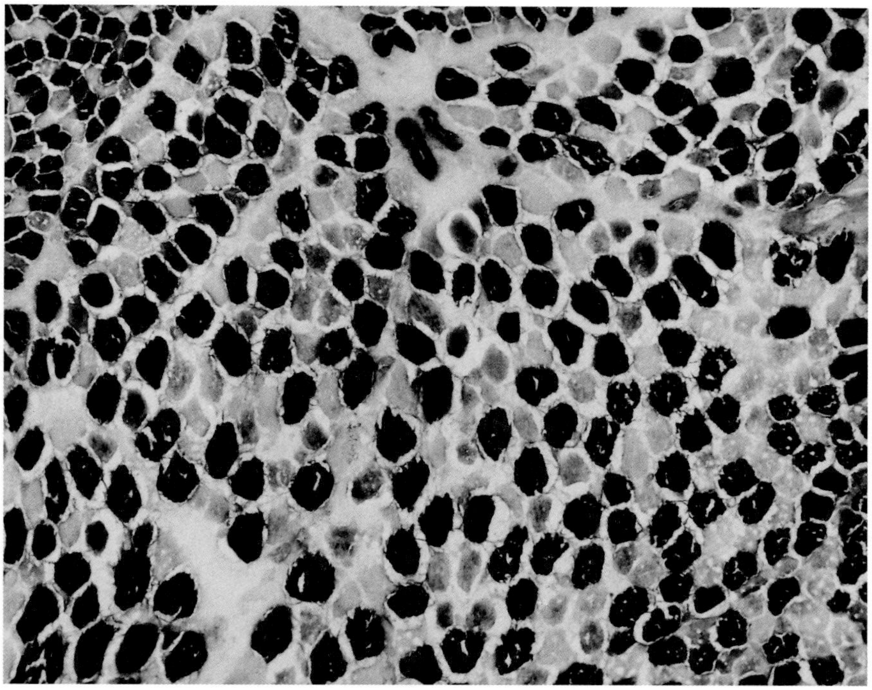

**FIG. 2.** Newborn muscle. Checkerboard pattern with type 1 and type 2 fibers is seen (ATPase, pH 9.4).

well. Whether the actual number of muscle fibers is augmented after birth is the subject of a current debate. Until recently the myofiber population was thought to be relatively stable after birth and throughout adult life (17). The studies of Adams and DeReuck (18) and others, however, seem to suggest a gradual rise in the number of fibers between birth and the end of the fifth decade. In some muscles, the total increase in fibers may reach 80 to 100% of the neonatal level. The mechanism accounting for an increase in the fiber population probably involves a population of dividing stem cells which, subsequently, undergo fusion to produce new mature fibers. A major aspect of growth of muscle fibers after birth relates to an increase in transverse dimension. In general, between birth and adulthood, there is a fivefold increase in

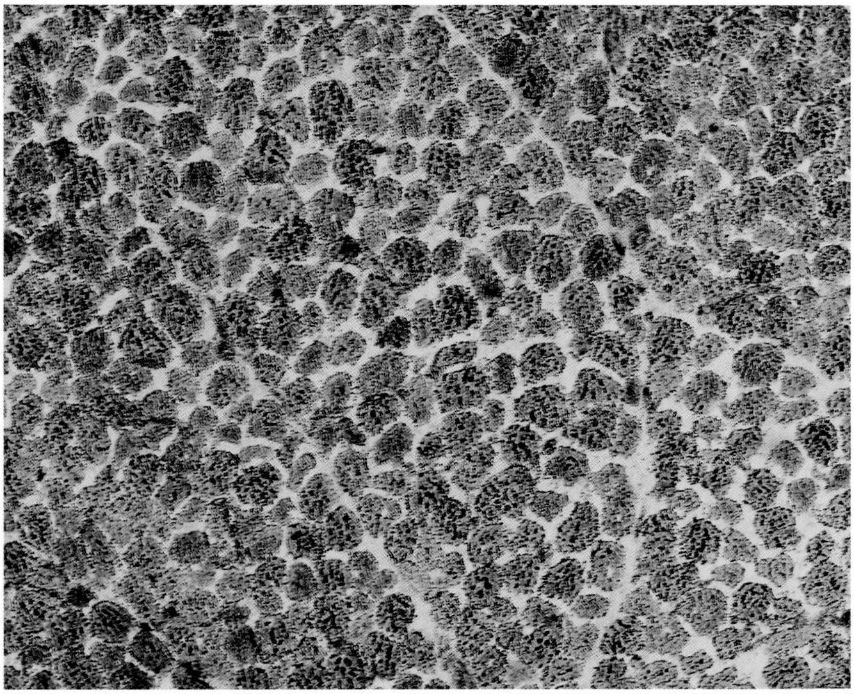

**FIG. 3.** Newborn muscle. Indistinct fiber typing is evident in oxidative-enzyme reactions (NADH-TR).

muscle fiber diameters (19). For example, in the leg muscles the average diameter of mature fibers is 45 $\mu$m compared to 7 $\mu$m at birth. The enlargement in fiber diameters does not proceed at an even rate from birth to early adulthood when fibers obtain a maximum diameter. Instead, fiber diameters increase at a relatively slow rate until puberty, when a burst of growth occurs. As an example, in the gastrocnemius, fibers more than triple in size from age 12 (average 19 $\mu$m) to age 21(average 62 $\mu$m).

A major revision in the histochemical profile of muscle occurs after birth. In the term infant, a checkerboard staining pattern is clearly evident in alkaline ATPase reactions. However, fiber typing is often not distinct in oxidative enzyme reactions (Fig. 3). The emergence of type 1, 2A, and 2B fibers in oxidative preparations occurs during infancy. Undifferentiated fibers having both abundant oxidative enzyme and ATPase activity represent approximately 20% of fibers at birth. These gradually differentiate into type 1 and type 2 fibers during the first year of life. The fate of Wohlfart B fibers comprising about 1% of myofibers at birth is unknown. They are not seen in biopsies of children past the age of 12 months.

The connective tissue elements of muscle are much more prominent at birth, particularly the perimysial components. Immediately after birth the perimysium may account for up to 20% of the cross-sectional area of muscle tissue. During early childhood, the perimysium and other connective tissue components rapidly shrink to less than 5% of the cross-sectional area, in part, because of the enlargement of the muscle fibers. In the immediate postnatal period, blood vessels, especially arteries, appear excessively thickened due to the presence of abundant smooth muscle elements. Expansion of the luminal diameter of blood vessels in the first year of life gives the vascular elements an adult appearance. The non-contractile-supporting connective tissue contains abundant collagen and scattered fibroblasts. Foci of hematopoiesis remain after birth, containing stem cells, erythroblasts, and myelocytes. These foci are more likely to be seen in the distal muscles of the extremities. They disappear within 1 month after birth.

## APOPTOSIS

Our scientific knowledge regarding apoptosis and skeletal muscle is in the formative stages. Most of the medical literature deals with either apoptosis as it pertains to the development of muscle, or as it relates to selected pathologic conditions.

During embryologic life, both neurons and skeletal muscle are effected by the process of apoptosis. A great deal more is known about programmed cell death in nerve cells, including motor neurons, than in muscle. A review of the earlier literature discussing natural neuronal death has been published by Hamburger (20). A recent article by Sohal addresses the subject of embryonic development of motor neurons and muscles culminating in the establishment of mature nerve-muscle relationships (21). A detailed discussion regarding apoptosis and motor neurons is well beyond the scope of this chapter, but a few comments are appropriate. In chick embryos, naturally occurring motor neuron death appears to be regulated by skeletal muscle. A muscle extract, which is an acidic 10-30 kDa protein, has been shown to extend neuron survival in vivo (22). Fibroblast growth factor (FGF-5) represents a survival factor for rat motor neurons in culture (23). Protease nexin I (PNI), a serine protease inhibitor, has been proposed as a neurotrophic agent. Experimentally, PNI rescues spinal motor neurons from programmed cell death in chicks (24).

Of interest are a number of publications which describe the developmentally programmed cell death of abdominal intersegmental muscles in the tobacco hawkmoth, Manduca sexta. The intersegmental muscles are important in the emergence behavior of the adult moth before they subsequently undergo apoptosis during the following 30 hours. It is now clear that apoptosis is regulated by declining titres of the insect molting hormone, 20-hydroxyecdysone, which signals the onset of apoptosis in the abdominal intersegmental muscles (25). This hormonally regulated event is at least, in part, subject to the polyubiquitin gene that causes the accumulation of ubiquitin polypeptide during this process (26). In the chick embryo, programmed cell death clearly occurs as the myofibers are developing. The large diameter primary myotubes are preferentially affected. The cytological features suggesting apoptosis include misshapen nuclei and irregular chromatin condensations along the nuclear envelope (27). It has been shown that in rat embryos, macrophages play an important role in the removal of necrotic fibers (28). In human fetal muscle, the programmed degeneration of both primary and mature myotubes occurs between 10 and 16 weeks of gestation (29).

A body of information regarding apoptosis and muscle disease is beginning to accumulate. For example, in the mdx mouse, dystrophin-deficient fibers undergo necrosis (30). Electron microscopic studies and assays for terminal deoxynucleotidyl transferase in prenecrotic and necrotic fibers indicate that apoptosis precedes necrotic change in mdx muscle. Recent studies also implicate an apoptotic process in gamma ray-induced cell death of muscle (31).

## ANATOMY

There are 434 voluntary muscles in the human body (32). They comprise 25% of the total body weight at birth and 40 to 50% of the total weight in adults. Not surprisingly, a greater muscle mass is encountered in males as opposed to females. Individual muscles vary greatly in size. For example, the smallest muscle in the body, the stapedius, measures only 2 mm in length. On the other hand, the sartorius (61 cm) and other large muscles of the extremities measure up to 2 feet in length. Skeletal muscles are composed of varying numbers of muscle fibers (i.e. 10,000 in lumbricalis and 1,000,000 in gastrocnemius) (33). These are connected at both ends to tendons or the epimysium. Because the fibers work in conjunction with each other, they are aligned in the same direction. Few skeletal muscles are modeled after the lumbricals, where all the fibers are arranged in a fusiform structure which tapers at either end at the site of tendinous insertion (34). The more familiar unit is a parallelogram composed of muscle fibers which insert at both ends on a flat tendon composed of dense collagen. In a parallel muscle, the fascicles are parallel to the longitudinal axis of the muscle, as in the thyrohyoid. In oblique muscles, a tendon typically runs within the muscle or on its surface and the muscle fibers insert obliquely on the tendon. Oblique muscles are most often pennate or featherlike. Some are bipennate, much like a feather in which there is a central shaft from which a series of barbs radiate on either side. Such muscles have a central tendinous structure from which two sets of parallel muscle fibers radiate (i.e. peroneus longus). Other muscles are simple pennate in which only one set of parallel muscle fibers attaches obliquely on a shaftlike tendon (i.e. extensor digitorum longus). Muscles are designated as complex pennate when the muscle consists of multiple parallelograms attaching to several tendons in the muscle mass. Not all skeletal muscles follow precisely the model of parallel or pennate design. They may be triangular, like the pectoralis minor, or spiral in structure like the forearm supinators. Although most muscles are attached to and are involved in moving bony skeletal structures, some voluntary muscles, such as those of the larynx and esophagus, do not have attachments to bone.

The blood supply to individual skeletal muscles has not been extensively studied and is, therefore, incompletely understood. It is known that the arterial supply to muscles varies somewhat with the individual. In general, the skeletal muscles are subserved by several, rather than a single artery, which renders them rather resistant to ischemia from an embolus or from disease of a single vessel. Much of our understanding regarding the pattern of vascularization in human muscle is derived from studies performed by Blomfield (35). The vascular supply to skeletal muscle falls into one of five categories:

1. The blood supply is derived from a single nutrient artery which divides in a longitudinal fashion within the muscle itself. The gastrocnemius is an example of such a system.
2. The muscle is supplied by several separate arteries entering the muscle along its length. Anastomoses are formed within the muscle between the territories of each artery. This pattern is typical of the soleus.
3. The blood supply arises from a single main artery that enters the belly of the muscle and, subsequently, forms a radiating pattern of collaterals, as in the biceps brachii.
4. In muscles like the tibialias anterior, a pattern of anastomosing arcades are derived from a series of penetrating arteries. This vascular pattern is considered to be the most efficient form of vascularization.
5. A less efficient form of the anastomosing arcade pattern is the rectangular pattern of anastomoses formed by a series of penetrating arteries. This so-called quadrilateral pattern is seen in the extensor hallucis longus muscle.

Once a main artery enters the muscle substance, it branches into a number of primary intramuscular arteries which ramify in the epimysium and perimysium. The primary arteries with a diameter which ranges from 80 to 360 μm give rise to numerous secondary arterioles which run parallel to the direction of the muscle fibers. The secondary arterioles often connect to primary arteries, forming artery-to-artery anastomoses. The secondary arterioles which range in diameter from 50 to 100 μm typically have a thin adventitia composed of fibroblasts and collagen. The smooth muscle coat is much thinner than that of the primary arteries, usually 2 to 3 layers. The internal elastica is prominent and continuous. The secondary arterioles branch to form terminal arterioles which measure 15 to 50 μm in diameter. Their smooth muscle coat is usually only one layer of cells. The internal elastica becomes discontinuous and is lost in smaller vessels. The distal portions of the terminal arterioles have precapillary sphincters that are formed from the smooth muscle cells of the media. These sphincters are found in blood vessels with an inner diameter of less than 15 μm. Footlike processes between the smooth muscle cells and the endothelium may be seen in the region of the sphincters. As in other tissues, the arterioles end in an elaborate system of capillaries.

As opposed to most other organs, in muscle a relatively small number of capillaries are open at rest (36). During muscle activity there is a considerable increase in the number of open capillaries. A marked difference in capillary density is observed in different muscles as well as in trained versus untrained subjects. Studies of capillary density reveal that the average single muscle fiber is surrounded by 1.7 capillaries (37). Capillary density may also be expressed as the number of capillaries per fiber, which, on average, in cross sections is 0.7. The density of capillaries also reflects oxygen consumption within muscle. Therefore, increased numbers of capillaries are evident where larger numbers of type 1 fibers are present. This phenomenon is less evident in humans than in animals such as the cat where muscles are composed chiefly or totally of one fiber type. Thus, in the cat soleus muscle composed almost entirely of type 1 fibers, the density of capillaries is 1600 per $mm^2$. In the gastrocnemius, a muscle with far fewer type 1 fibers, the capillary density is 600 per $mm^2$ (38). The capillaries within skeletal muscle travel primarily in a longitudinal direction, although they are frequently linked by short transverse branches. Ultrastructurally, capillaries are composed of endothelial cells surrounded by a basement lamina. Occasional pericytes are encountered outside the basement membrane. Endothelial cells typically contain numerous pinocytotic vesicles. Where endothelial cells are joined, they lack tight junctions. Hence the capillary endothelium is freely permeable to tracers such as

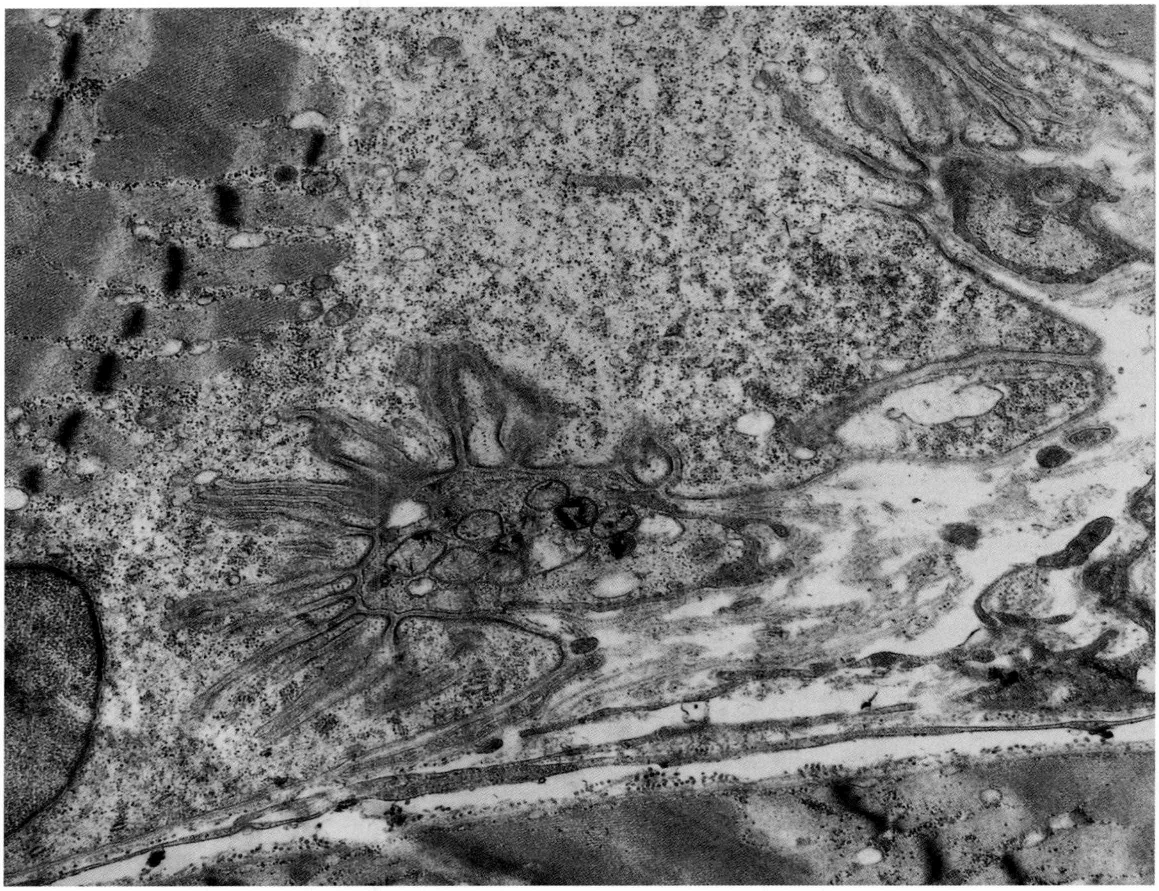

**FIG. 4.** Motor end-plate. Ultrastructurally the MEP consists of a terminal axon and a postsynaptic region formed by a specialized portion of the muscle fiber. The surface of the fiber is undulating representing the postjunctional folds (EM).

horseradish peroxidase. The capillary pericytes are essentially smooth muscle cells that contain large numbers of filaments. The pericytes are innervated by small diameter unmyelinated nerve fibers. The basement membrane, which lies between the endothelium and pericytes, measures 20 to 30 nm, although some thickening and reduplication of the basal lamina occurs in older patients.

The nerve supply to individual skeletal muscles often enters the surface of the muscle at the belly, accompanied by one or more major penetrating arteries. Within the main nerve trunk are myelinated and unmyelinated axons. Contributions to the nerve are made from myelinated efferent motor fibers that innervate the muscle fibers, somatic afferent sensory fibers from muscle spindles, Golgi tendon organs, pacinian corpuscles, and unmyelinated autonomic efferent fibers. At least 50% of the fibers are sensory in function. The motor fibers that innervate the myofibers demonstrate a bimodal size distribution. The large diameter $\alpha$ fibers innervate fast motor units whereas the $\beta$ fibers are distributed to slow motor units and some intrafusal fibers of the muscle spindle. The very small diameter $\gamma$ fibers supply the remainder of the muscle spindle fibers. The large motor fibers are relatively uniform in diameter, measuring between 10 and 15 $\mu$m. The small motor fibers vary from 2 to 7 $\mu$m in size.

As the distal motor axon approaches the muscle fiber, it is transformed into the terminal axon which represents the proximal portion of the neuromuscular junction or motor end-plate (MEP). The neuromuscular junction which measures about 50 $\mu$m in diameter is composed of the presynaptic (PRS) portion or terminal axon and the postsynaptic (POS) portion that is formed by a unique region in the muscle fiber (Fig. 4). The PRS and POS domains are separated by a specialized intercellular space, 50 nm wide, the synaptic cleft. The myelinated motor nerve terminates at the PRS region as an unmyelinated axonal segment which is enveloped by the teloglia, the distal projections of Schwann cells. The terminal axon and teloglia are covered by a layer of endoneurium, the sheath of Henle, which becomes continuous with the endomysium of the muscle fiber in the area of MEP. Numerous synaptic vesicles, each 45 to 50 nm in diameter, are found in the terminal axon. The vesicles are most plentiful around thickened zones of increased electron density at the presynaptic membrane. Studies utilizing freeze fracture electron microscopy have demonstrated that parallel pairs of double rows of intramembranous particles, measuring 10 nm in di-

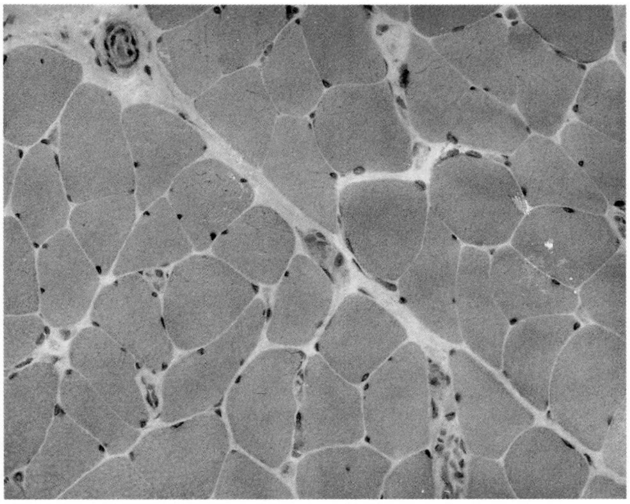

**FIG. 5.** Cross section of muscle. The sarcoplasm is textured and the sarcolemmal nuclei are peripheral in location (H&E).

ameter, are located at these electron-dense zones (39). The particles are considered to represent voltage-sensitive calcium channels known as active zones. At the POS region of the muscle fiber, the cell surface is elevated to form the hillock of Doyere or sole plate. Within the sole plate, the sarcoplasm is granular and a cluster of sarcolemmal nuclei is often seen. Nuclei in this location are plump and vesicular. The terminal axon ramifies in the sole plate as a series of branches called telodendria which indent the surface of the fiber, producing gutters or troughs. The surface of the fiber at the MEP is undulating and redundant, creating the complex of postjunctional folds which can be demonstrated by supravital staining as the subneural apparatus of Couteaux.

The spaces between the folds denote the secondary synaptic clefts. As a result of the formation of these clefts, the surface area of the POS membrane is increased approximately 10 times the surface area of the PRS. The POS membrane of the folds is thicker and more densely stained at the crests than in the depths of the clefts. By electron microscopy, the juxtaneural membrane at the crests of the folds contains irregularly spaced densities measuring 11 to 14 nm in diameter. In freeze fracture preparations, on the P face of the membrane the crests are studded with rows of particles that are similar in size to these densities (approximately 10 nm) (40). These large intramembranous particles are considered to represent the acetylcholine receptor, a pentameric 275 kDa glycoprotein (41).

## LIGHT MICROSCOPY

Familiarity with the normal structure of skeletal muscle provides a useful background for the pathologist in the evaluation of muscle biopsies. Other sources offering a more comprehensive discussion of the light microscopy, histochemistry, and electron microscopy of normal muscle than is possible here are found in the references (42–52). The muscle fiber is a multinucleated, syncytial-like unit shaped like a long, narrow cylinder. The normal adult myocyte is not perfectly round but is polygonal, producing a multifaceted profile in cross section. The nuclei are usually located subsarcolemmally, numbering four to six per cell when sectioned transversely. For each mm of fiber length, there are approximately 30 nuclei (53). In routine sections, the sarcolemmal nuclei are slender and flat with an orientation that is parallel to the long axis of the fiber. These nuclei measure 5 to 12 $\mu$m in length and 1 to 3 $\mu$m in width. Their chromatin is fine and

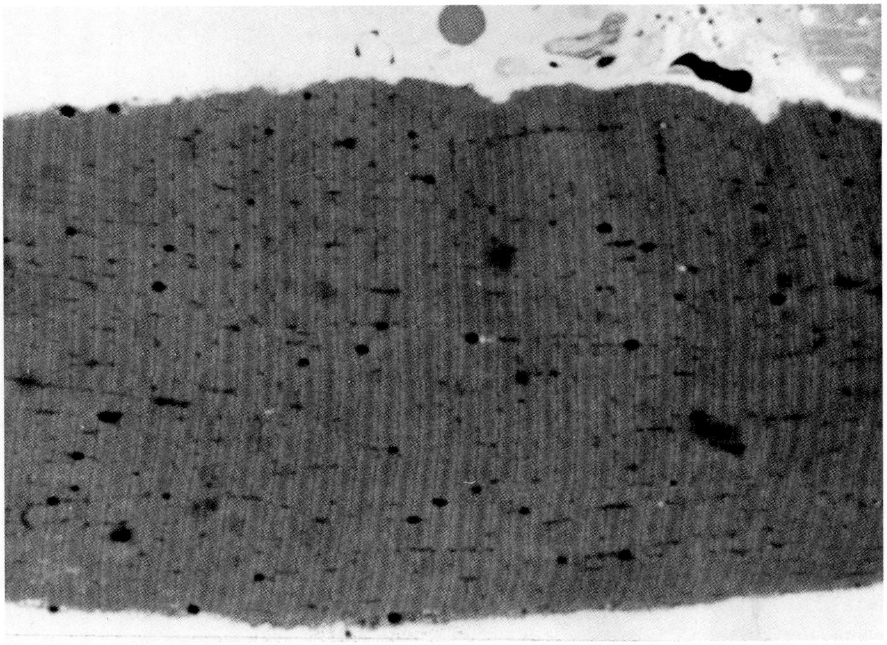

**FIG. 6.** Resin section. Sarcomere pattern is shown in longitudinal section (Toluidine blue).

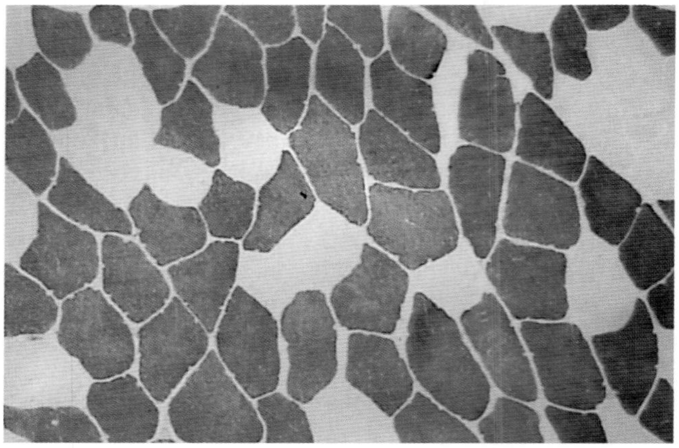

**FIG. 7.** Normal muscle. In the standard ATPase reaction, type 1 fibers are light and type 2 fibers are dark (ATPase, pH 9.4).

dustlike. The nucleoli are small and not visible in many fibers. In paraffin sections stained with H&E, the sarcoplasm is light pink and textured in cross sections (Fig. 5). The cross-striations must be viewed in longitudinal sections and are difficult to see in any detail without special stains. They are best demonstrated in periodic acid-Schiff (PAS) and PTAH stains or in resin-embedded material where alternating dark and light bands are evident (Fig. 6). The diameter of fibers is determined by several factors (see Gender, Training, and Aging).

Proximal muscles, where power rather than finely coordinated movement is required, have a fiber population with a larger mean diameter (85 to 90 $\mu$m) whereas those of smaller, distal, and ocular muscles are composed of thinner fibers (20 $\mu$m). Fiber size in males exceeds that in females, probably, in part, because of androgenic hormonal influences and more strenuous physical demands. In both genders, exercise promotes fiber hypertrophy. Muscle fibers are smaller in children and in the elderly than in young active adults, although comprehensive normative data at these ages are not easy to find (54–56).

Red muscle, having a larger mitochondrial content and higher capillary density, depends on aerobic respiration and is designed for postural function or sustained activity. The color of red muscles is actually due to relatively greater myoglobin content than white muscles which contain fewer mitochondria but abundant glycogen, rendering it better suited to anaerobic respiration and to sudden and intermittent contraction. In vertebrates, particularly in birds, red (i.e., soleus) can easily be distinguished from white (i.e., pectoralis) muscles upon external inspection, since an entire muscle in such species may be composed of either red or white fibers. Human muscles, on the other hand, contain both fiber types, which typically assume a mixed mosaic arrangement reminiscent of a checkerboard. Depending on anatomic location and function, the proportion of type 1 and type 2 fibers varies, but a typical muscle contains approximately twice as many type 2 fibers (60 to 65%) as type 1 fibers (35 to 40%). The demonstration of the histochemical properties of the muscle fibers comprising a biopsy, which is known as fiber typing, is accomplished by applying histochemical techniques. Fiber typing is not possible in routine H&E-stained slides and is only appreciated in using histoenzymatic reactions performed on frozen sections. In our laboratory, two complementary histochemical procedures are employed for the detection of fiber types. The most reliable method for this purpose is the myofibrillar ATPase reaction. By changing the pH during the procedure, a spectrum of staining reactions can be produced. In the standard or alkaline ATPase reaction, which is conducted at a pH of 9.4, two fiber types are seen. Type 2 fibers are dark in staining intensity, whereas type 1 fibers are pale (Fig. 7). Fibers of intermediate staining intensity are not observed in the alkaline incubation. If the pH of the incubating solution is brought into the acidic range (pH 4.6) in what is sometimes known as the reverse ATPase reaction, two populations of type 2 fibers emerge. Type 2A fibers are virtually unstained and type 2B fibers are intermediately stained, while type 1 fibers are extremely dark. All the oxidative enzyme reactions, like the NADH-TR used in our laboratory, merely reflect the mitochondrial content of the muscle fibers. Intensely stained fibers are designated as oxidative (Type 1) and lighter fibers as type 2 (Fig. 8). Most oxidative enzyme reactions further subdivide type 2 fibers into two categories. Type 2B fibers are poorly stained in contrast to type 2A fibers, which exhibit a staining intensity that is intermediate between type 1 and 2B. Although all muscle fibers contain glycogen and the companion enzyme phosphorylase, they are more abundant in type 2 (glycolytic) fibers. The PAS stain, a crude method of detecting glycogen, and the histochemical reaction for phosphorylase, can be used as a means of fiber typing. However, staining with these techniques is insufficiently reliable for fiber typing. We only use the phosphorylase reaction to investigate possible cases of enzyme deficiency (McArdle's disease).

Striated muscles are partitioned into fascicles, each of which is invested by a connective tissue sheath known as the perimysium. Within this sheath, the intramuscular nerves,

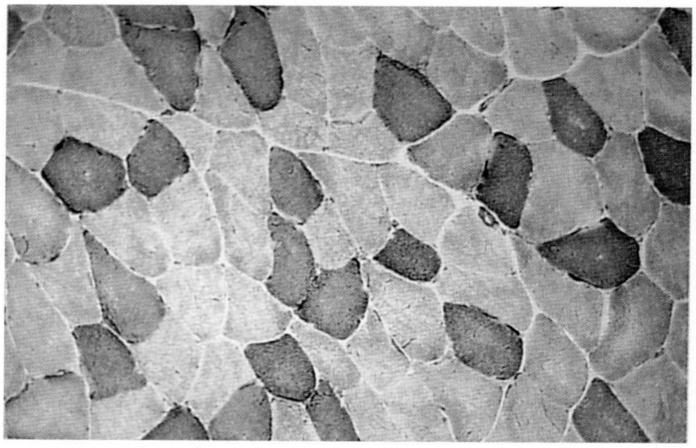

**FIG. 8.** Normal muscle. In oxidative-enzyme reactions, Type 1 fibers are very dark and type 2 fibers are intermediate or light in staining intensity (NADH-TR).

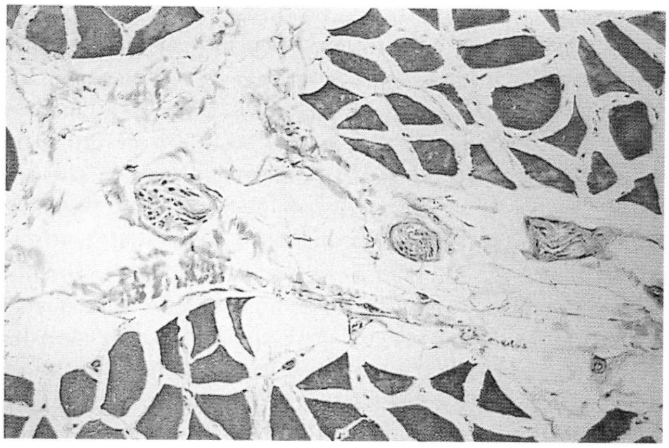

**FIG. 9.** Intramuscular nerves. Several twigs contain axons surrounded by red-staining myelin sheaths (Trichrome).

primary arteries, secondary arterioles and veins travel throughout the muscle. At the innervation zone in the belly of the muscle, intramuscular nerve bundles or twigs are especially numerous (Fig. 9). Up to 10 myelinated nerve fibers may be present in an individual twig that is surrounded by a thin mantle of perineurial connective tissue. The myelinated nerve fibers are perhaps best demonstrated in trichrome-stained sections in which the bright red-colored myelin sheaths resemble doughnuts surrounding the unstained axons. Tangential sections of twigs may be mistaken for areas of focal fibrosis or abnormal vascular structures. The perimysium is a framework that lends stability to the fascicles, in part, by its attachment to the epimysium. The epimysium forms septa that sequester groups of fascicles, as well as the fascia that encircles the entire muscle and merges with the dense collagenous connective tissue of the tendons. Within each fascicle the perimysium gives way to a normally unobtrusive network, the endomysium. Each muscle fiber may appear to be partly or completely invested by endomysium, a mesenchymal matrix composed of collagen, elastic, and reticulin fibers that support the preterminal arterioles and capillary blood supply to the fascicles. At the interface between muscle and either fascia or tendon, the muscle fibers become variable in size and internal nuclei are more abundant. As they attach to the tendon or fascia, the fibers are separated by dense collagenous trabeculae (Fig. 10). Because the normal histology of these regions may be misinterpreted as evidence of pathologic change, the muscle biopsy should be obtained from the belly of the muscle, avoiding the tendinous insertions. A deep, rather than a superficial biopsy is preferred to avoid the fascia.

Several specialized structures are found within the connective tissue-supporting framework. Muscle spindles, first described by Hassal and later by Kolliker were once considered to be a pathologic finding (57). Spindles are now known to be mechanoreceptors that sense the length and tension of skeletal muscle, governing integrated muscle activity. Although they are encountered in virtually all muscles, they are more frequently detected in smaller muscles devoted to finely coordinated activities such as those of the hand. They are more numerous in distal than in girdle muscles. Quantitative studies have shown that 70 to 100 muscle spindles may be located in an individual muscle. Muscle spindles tend to lie in the deeper portions of the muscle, particularly in the muscle belly. They are often found where type 1 fibers are more plentiful. As the name implies, muscle spindles are fusiform in shape with a swollen center and tapering ends. They measure 3 to 4 mm in length and 200 $\mu$m in diameter. A thin fibrous capsule represents the outer boundaries of the muscle spindle. The capsule is an extension of the perimysium where spindles are usually located. In certain muscles such as those of the eye, face, and mouth the capsule merges with the perimysium and is somewhat indistinct. The capsule is composed of ten to fifteen layers of flattened pavement cells that are specialized fibroblasts. The pavement cells are tightly adherent and separated only by thin layers of delicate collagen fibrils. The pavement cells are epithelial-like in that each is surrounded by a basement membrane. As one proceeds from the equatorial region of the spindle toward the poles, the number of layers of pavement cells progressively diminishes. Within the capsule are three to fifteen intrafusal fibers in the typical muscle spindle (Fig. 11).

Generally, the number of intrafusal fibers is less in small muscles than in larger axial muscles. Two distinct populations of intrafusal fibers are found, both of which are smaller in diameter than the extrafusal fibers. The larger bag fibers, usually one to three in number per spindle, measure about 20 $\mu$m in diameter. The chain fibers number two to seven per spindle with a diameter of 10 $\mu$m or less. The bag fibers are longer, sometimes extending beyond the polar ends of the capsule. They measure 4 to 8 mm in length. The chain fibers are shorter, measuring 2 to 4 mm. The bag fibers are recognized in the equatorial region of the spindle by the presence of large aggregations of nuclei. Away from the equatorial re-

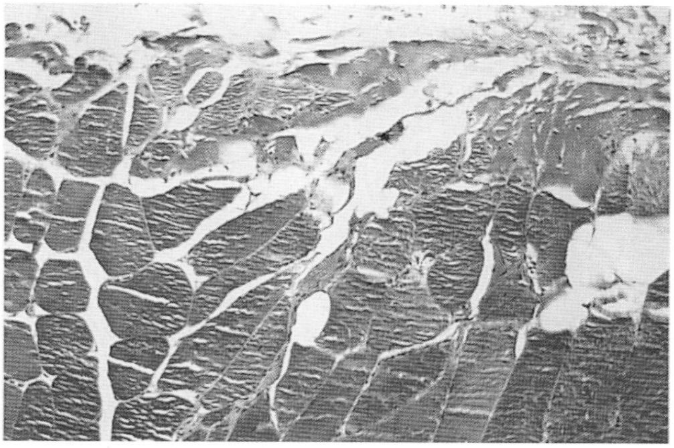

**FIG. 10.** Tendinous insertion. At the interface, the muscle fibers normally vary in size and are partly surrounded by connective tissue (Trichrome).

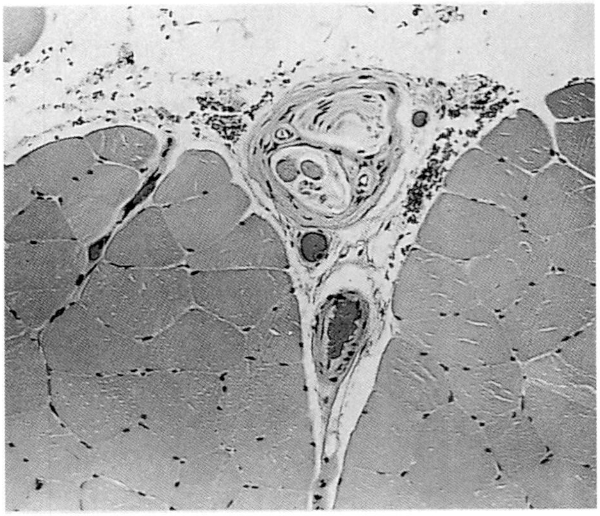

**FIG. 11.** Muscle spindle. A fibrous capsule encloses a nerve twig and several intrafusal fibers which are normally smaller than the extrafusal fibers.

gion, the nuclei remain internal or central in the bag fibers, but are far less numerous. The smaller chain fibers are distinguished by a row of central nuclei that extends along the length of the fiber. In histochemical stains, there are two types of bag fibers. Bag 1 fibers reveal considerable oxidative enzyme activity and are pale in ATPase reactions. On the other hand, bag 2 fibers, which also have high oxidative enzyme activity, reveal intermediate staining in ATPase reactions. Chain fibers, although they possess high oxidative enzyme activity, stain darkly in ATPase reactions and are considered by many to be type 2 fibers (58). The innervation of muscle spindles, which is both motor and sensory, is complex and will only be summarized here (59). The intrafusal efferent fibers are derived from branches of $\beta$ and $\gamma$ efferent axons. The $\beta$ axons appear to terminate primarily on nuclear bag fibers. The $\gamma$ fibers supply both nuclear bag and chain intrafusal fibers. It is not uncommon for intrafusal fibers to have polyneural innervation. Two types of sensory innervation are seen in the muscle spindle. The larger diameter group Ia afferents emanate from the equator. They originate as the annulospiral endings, a series of neural coils and spirals that attach to the nuclear bag and chain fibers. Smaller diameter group II afferent fibers come from the paraequatorial regions of the spindle and are associated mainly with the so-called flower spray endings of Ruffini. The majority of these endings project from the nuclear chain fibers. The secondary or flower spray endings consist of a branching network that enwraps the intrafusal fiber between its polar and equatorial regions.

The Golgi tendon organ is an encapsulated sensory nerve terminal which is located at the junction of muscle with tendon or aponeuroses. The location of these structures allows them to sense changes in muscle tension. They have an inhibitory function in the event of strong muscle contraction. These fusiform structures measure about 1.5 mm in length and 120 $\mu$m in diameter. They consist of one or more fascicles of collagen fibrils which are attached to tendon or aponeurosis and enveloped by a multilamellar capsule (Fig. 12). Each structure is connected to 20 to 30 muscle fibers. The Golgi tendon organ is innervated by a myelinated Ib afferent axon measuring 7 to 15 $\mu$m in diameter. The afferent nerve typically divides and arborizes around the individual collagen bundles.

Pacinian corpuscles are distributed widely in the subcutaneous tissues of the body, although they may also be encountered within the muscular fascial planes and adjacent to tendons or aponeuroses. They are seldom seen within mus-

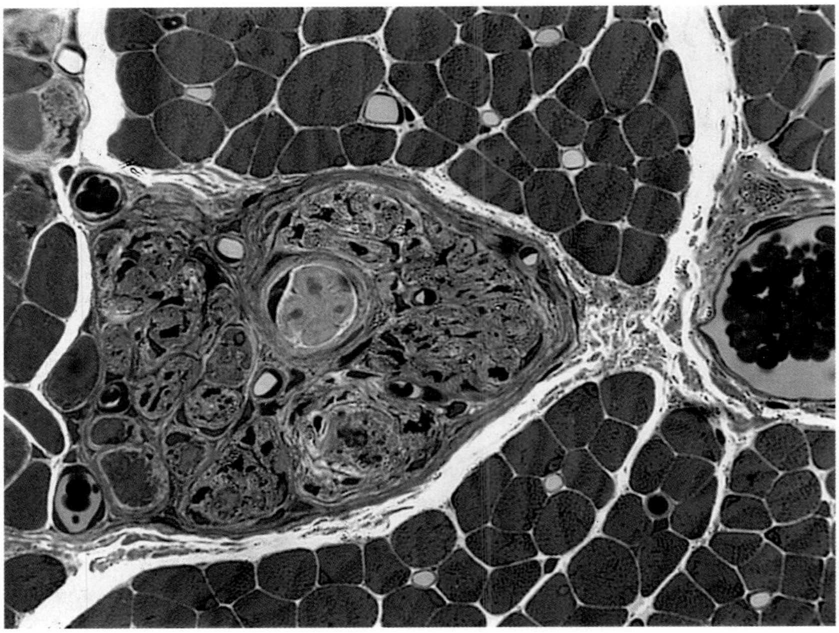

**FIG. 12.** Golgi tendon organ. Fascicles of collagen surrounded by several nerve bundles (Resin section, toluidine blue).

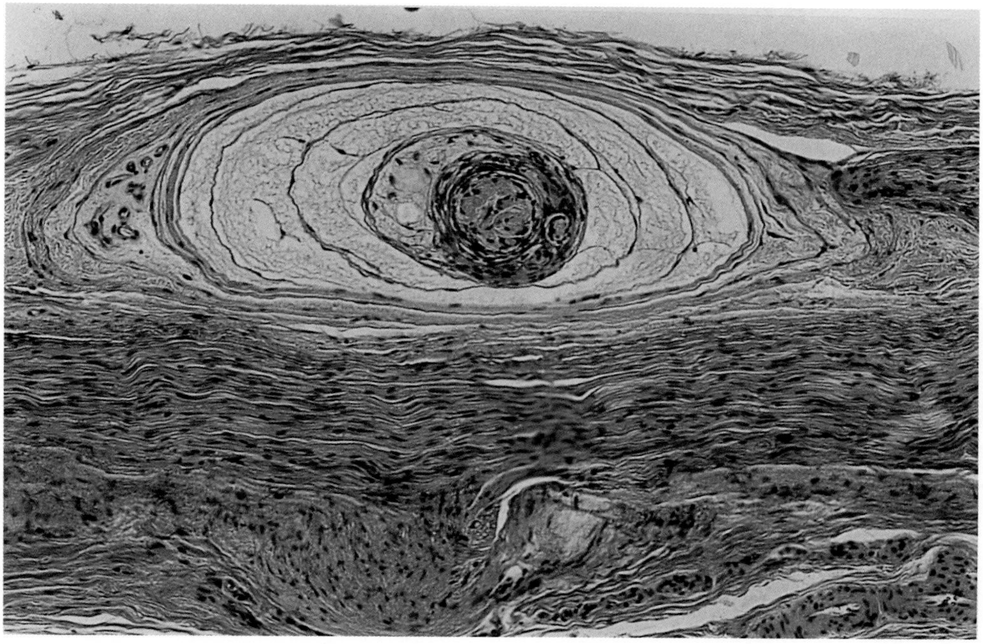

**FIG. 13.** Pacinian corpuscle. A central nerve terminal is surrounded by a capsule composed of concentric layers of cells (H&E).

cle tissue itself. In the center of the pacinian corpuscle is a central rodlike nerve terminal innervated by fast conducting group I or II afferent axons. The central axon is surrounded by a capsule composed of concentric layers of cells (Fig. 13). The elongated cells forming the capsule are surrounded by basal lamina and separated by fine collagen fibrils. Pacinian corpuscles are receptor organs which are sensitive to vibration.

## ULTRASTRUCTURE

The ultrastructural examination of skeletal muscle is conventionally performed on sections oriented longitudinally, wherein deviations from the orderly striated architecture are more easily detected than in cross sections. The sarcoplasm of each muscle fiber is divided into multiple parallel subunits, the myofibrils, which are minute, cylindroid contractile structures measuring approximately 1 $\mu$m in diameter. Myofibrils are segmented into a series of identical sarcomeres that are equal in length, whether the muscle is contracted or at rest, and are aligned in register with the sarcomeres of surrounding myofibrils. The unique periodicity of the fine structure of the muscle fiber is a function of the regimentation of this contractile system. The rectangular banding pattern within each sarcomere is produced by the arrangement of the filaments (Fig. 14). The Z band, which forms the lateral boundaries of the sarcomere, is an electron-dense, bar-shaped structure, oriented perpendicular to the long axis of the myofibril. The distance between consecutive Z bands represents the sarcomere length, an average of 2.5 to 3.0 $\mu$m. The I bands are the most electron-lucent portions of the sarcomere and stand in dramatic contrast to the dark Z bands that bisect them. The I bands are shorter in length than the moderately dense A bands located at the center of the sarcomeres. Within each sarcomere are stacks of parallel filaments that under the electron microscope appear to be of two types. The thicker filaments measuring 15 nm in diameter are principally composed of myosin. The thinner filaments containing chiefly actin are 8 nm in diameter. The thin filaments are attached to the Z band and extend across the I band, where only thin filaments are found. They penetrate the A band in which alternating thick and thin filaments are visualized. Thick filaments on the other hand, are restricted to the A band region of the sarcomere and determine its length.

The sarcoplasmic organelles are more concentrated around the sarcolemmal nuclei and between the myofibrils. The mitochondria are somewhat variable in shape and size, although the majority are oval or elliptical in configuration and 1.0 $\mu$m in greatest dimension. They are most easily recognized adjacent to the Z bands where their long axes are parallel to those of the myofibrils. Both mitochondria and lipid vacuoles are more conspicuous in oxidative fibers.

Glycogen, composed of granules with a diameter of 150 to 300 A, is more abundant in glycolytic fibers, particularly in the I band region of the sarcomere. The sarcoplasmic reticulum (SR) and the transverse (T) tubules together comprise the sarcotubular complex. The SR, which is analogous to the endoplasmic reticulum of other cells, is an elaborate system of tubules that, by branching in all directions, surrounds the myofibrils. In contrast to the SR, which has no communica-

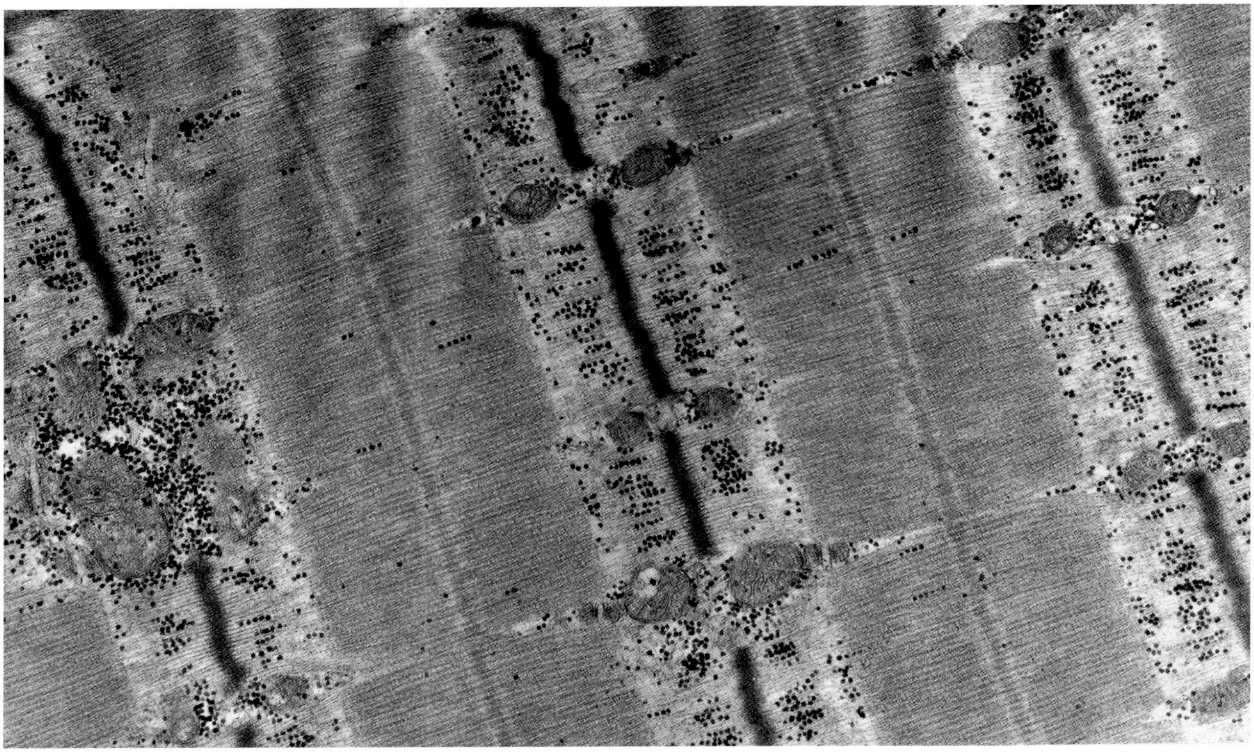

**FIG. 14.** Ultrastructurally the several myofibrils can be seen in register. Each is composed of a series of sarcomeres which contain A,I, and Z band regions (EM).

tion with the extracellular space, the T tubules arise as invaginations from the cell membrane. They are observed at regular intervals along the length of the fiber, particularly at the junction of the A and I bands. The T tubules encircle the myofibrils and are disposed in a predominantly transverse direction. Branches of the sarcotubular complex join together as triads at the A-I band junctions. Here, pairs of terminal cisterns derived from the SR are positioned on either side of a central T tubule. In this location, the SR tubules appear as hollow, membrane-bound profiles whereas the T tubules are somewhat more electron dense.

Satellite cells are a population of myoblastic stem cells which are a source of nuclei during muscle growth, particularly hypertrophy. Satellite cells also have the capacity to synthesize new muscle after myocyte injury. These primitive, indeterminate cells can, under appropriate circumstances, be transformed into blastic elements that serve as an important source of fiber regeneration. Satellite cells represent approximately 10% of the myonuclei seen in cross sections of muscle. There is a decline in the number of satellite cells as a result of the aging process so that they constitute only 2 to 3% of myofiber nuclei in older individuals. Satellite cells are small, mononuclear, fusiform cells which are situated beneath the basement membrane of neighboring muscle fibers (60). They cannot be reliably distinguished from the muscle fiber nuclei under the light microscope. Satellite cells are not randomly distributed along the length of the muscle fiber and are more numerous in certain locations, such as the sole plates of the neuromuscular junction and the polar regions of the muscle spindles. Ultrastructurally, the nuclei of satellite cells differ somewhat from the nuclei of muscle fibers. They are more elongated, their nuclear chromatin is peripherally dense, and nucleoli are lacking. The satellite cell nuclei are usually asymmetrical within the cytoplasm which contains only a few filaments without evidence of sarcomere formation (Fig. 15). The sarcoplasm also contains free ribosomes, microtubules, and centrioles which may be associated with cilia. Where the cell membranes of the satellite cell and muscle fiber are opposed, numerous pinocytotic vesicles are seen.

## SPECIAL TECHNIQUES

Perhaps more than any other tissue, skeletal muscle in humans has been studied using a wide variety of specialized techniques, in part, because human muscle biopsies are frequently collected in such a way as to make both fresh, unfixed tissue and material for special studies available. In addition to routine histochemical methods which are focused primarily on the identification of fiber types, a number of other histochemical procedures have been employed for the study of both normal and abnormal skeletal muscle. An array of histochemical techniques has been developed to pro-

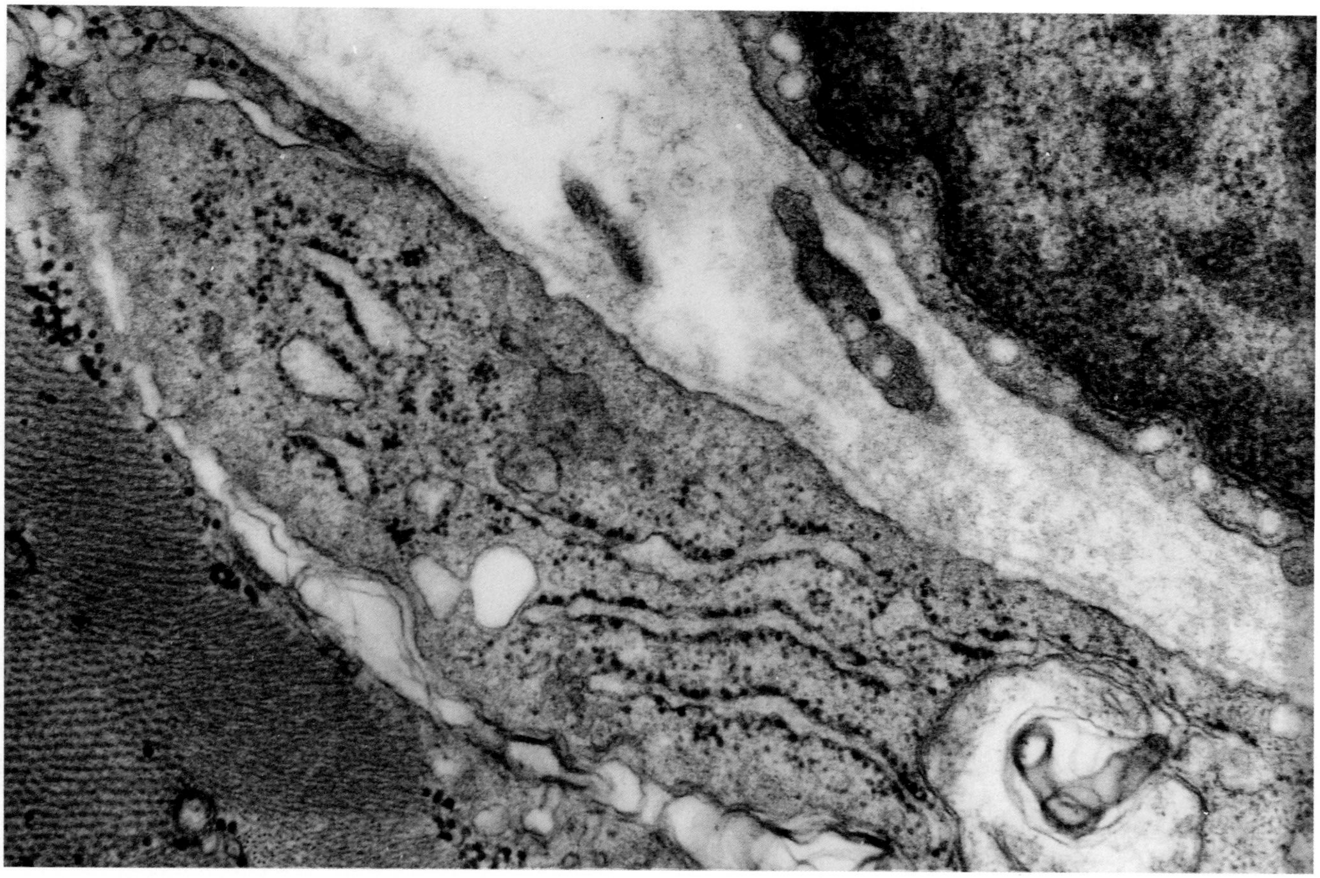

**FIG. 15.** Satellite cell. There is no evidence of sarcomere formation in this primitive cell located beneath the basement membrane of the muscle fiber (EM).

vide greater understanding of muscle metabolism (42, 44,45,50). Among these are histochemical techniques to identify various enzymes involved in glycogen metabolism and glycolysis. Familiar examples are histochemical stains for phosphorylase and phosphofructokinase. Other histochemical procedures have been developed to study mitochondrial function. The most widely used is the histochemical stain for cytochrome oxidase. In the workup of human disease, histochemical analysis of muscle tissue can be supplemented by biochemical analysis, specifically when histochemical techniques are unavailable. It is also best, whenever possible, to confirm histochemical findings with biochemical studies. Biochemical analysis has been particularly useful in the study of mitochondrial disease, examining such parameters as the respiratory chain. Molecular techniques are being used with increasing frequency in elucidating normal muscle development, as well as muscle disease. A number of abnormal conditions can now be diagnosed using molecular strategies. These include Duchenne dystrophy and other dystrophinopathies (61), and certain mitochondrial disorders in which there is a defect in the mitochondrial genome (62).

Several techniques have been adapted for the study of intramuscular blood vessels. For example, capillaries are particularly well seen in histochemical procedures for alkaline phosphatase. Capillaries are also nicely demonstrated in immunohistochemical stains for factor VIII (Fig. 16).

Immunohistochemistry is an emerging field in pathology

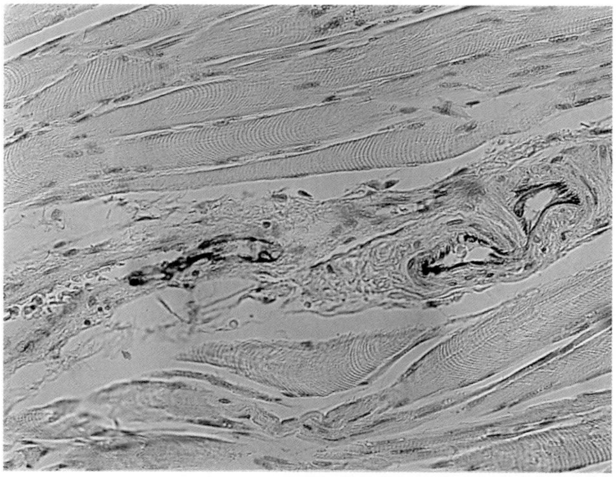

**FIG. 16.** Intramuscular blood vessels. The endothelium is darkly stained (Immunostain for factor VIII).

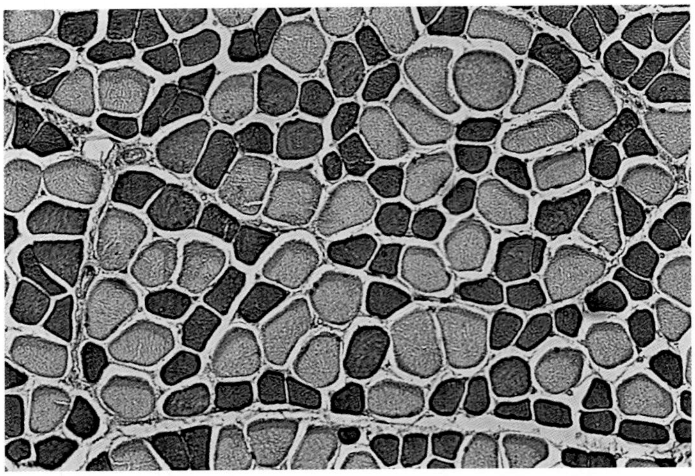

**FIG. 17.** Checkerboard pattern is seen with dark type 2 fibers and pale type 1 fibers (Immunostain for fast myosin).

which has begun to find a niche in the study of muscle. As already described, muscle fiber typing can be done in frozen sections using histochemical stains such as ATPase. Antibodies to fast and slow myosins are now available for the identification of type 1 and type 2 muscle fibers in fixed tissue (Fig. 17) (63). It is also possible to subdivide type 2 fibers into types 2A and 2B using myosin antibodies. Fibers undergoing regeneration can be detected by immunohistochemical methods. Regenerating fibers contain fetal myosins and react using antibodies to vimentin and desmin. Recently, visualization of the membrane-associated protein, dystrophin, has become practical (Fig. 18). Antibodies to dystrophin, as well as to some of the dystrophin-associated glycoproteins, permit the diagnosis of Duchenne dystrophy and selected other dystrophinopathies (64).

The nerve supply to muscle, including the intramuscular nerve twigs and motor end-plates, cannot be adequately studied in routine samples. The anatomical location of nerve endings and end-plates is variable depending on the muscle selected. They may be restricted to a narrow band across the muscle or they may be more widely distributed throughout the muscle tissue. Some investigators prefer to biopsy shorter muscles, maximizing the chance of finding the intramuscular nerves. The external intercostal muscle has been used for this reason. Many limb muscles have a single band of terminal motor innervation which corresponds to the so-called motor point. The motor point can be identified with the use of an electrical stimulator. After the administration of local anesthesia and incision of the skin, the muscle is stimulated using a metallic electrode before any tissue is removed. The nerve endings can be located at sites where a single fascicle, rather than the whole muscle, contracts after stimulation with a very weak current. Once the innervation zone is established electrically, the biopsy is removed.

Using a variety of techniques, different portions of the muscle innervation can be subsequently evaluated. Vital staining with methylene blue has been used to demonstrate the intramuscular nerve twigs, as well as the end-plates (65). This technique requires that the muscle be injected with a methylene blue solution before the muscle sample is actually taken. An undesirable complication of this technique is muscle pain, which many patients experience during the injection of the dye. To preserve the staining of the nerve endings, the biopsy must be oxygenated for one hour. This technique is obviously complicated and not recommended for most laboratories. A more simple, but less elegant technique for the demonstration of nerve twigs is the staining of muscle with silver methods such as the Bodian stain. The postjunctional portion of the end-plate can be stained histochemically for acetylcholinesterase activity (66). The reaction product is not restricted to the postjunctional membrane and, consequently, this is a relatively crude method of studying end-plates. More precise methods of studying end-plates involve the use of alpha-bungarotoxin and freeze fracture electron microscopy. Alpha-bungarotoxin is derived from cobra

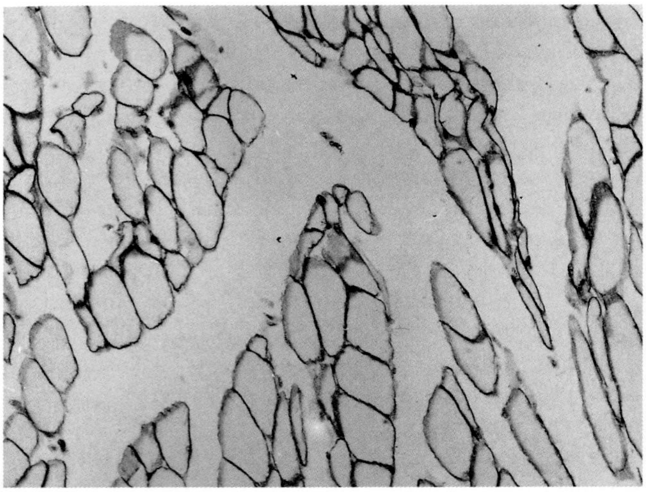

**FIG. 18.** Sarcolemmal regions are darkly stained (Immunostain for dystrophin).

venom and binds specifically with the actelycholine receptor. Immunoperoxidase techniques using alpha-bungarotoxin allow direct visualization of the postjunctional region of the motor end-plate, ultrastructurally (67). With the use of freeze fracture preparations, both the active zones of the presynaptic membrane and the acetylcholine receptors of the POS membrane can be studied in greater detail (68). In certain rare disorders of the neuromuscular junction, freeze fracture microscopy may be a useful ancillary diagnostic tool.

The nearly crystalline arrangement of filaments within muscle fibers renders them a suitable subject for x-ray diffraction studies. Diffractograms have provided considerable insight into the architecture and structure of the myofilaments (69). A major advantage of x-ray diffraction is its application to living muscle cells. Recently x-ray diffraction has been enhanced by the use of increasingly powerful x-ray sources and electronic signal detectors which have replaced photographic film. Reflection signals from a living muscle fiber can be adjusted to reveal equatorial reflections from the regular lateral spacing of the filaments or meridional reflections originating from the arrangement of subunits in the direction of the fiber axis, depending on the angle of the diffractogram and the camera light.

Finally, morphometric analysis of muscle tissue is indicated in the event that normal or abnormal findings such as variations in fiber diameters are minimal and subtle. In the past, morphometry has been performed manually, using an eyepiece micrometer, but this procedure is time consuming and tedious. More recently, it has been possible to conduct sophisticated morphometric analysis electronically, using a computer-assisted image analyzer (70). Automated image analysis can be adapted for quantitative measurements on photographs of microscopic sections, but systems also exist for totally automated analysis of images taken directly from microscopic slides or other types of tissue preparations.

## FUNCTION

Muscle has at least two major functions. In addition to the obvious role in locomotion, skeletal muscle is also an important participant in general protein metabolism. The reader will recall that muscles are a significant repository of protein for many systemic metabolic requirements. Protein metabolism depends on a number of factors in a healthy person. These include the rate of protein synthesis and breakdown. They are also determined by diet, hormonal influences, growth, and muscular activity. In general, protein synthesis and degradation are governed by the dietary intake of amino acids.

However, the aspect of muscle function which is most familiar relates to contraction, subsequent movement, and locomotion. It is this aspect of skeletal muscle function on which we will concentrate. When a muscle undergoes contraction, it usually exerts force on a moveable structure. Isotonic contraction refers to movement that changes the lengths of muscle fibers. If movement does not take place and fiber lengths do not shorten, the contraction is considered to be isometric. The sustained activity of the calf muscles, which do not change length while a person is standing erect, exemplifies isometric contraction. As a rule, a single muscle does not act alone functionally. The coordinated actions of several muscles are usually necessary in the performance of movement. The prime movers are those muscles directly responsible for the desired motion. Antagonists, muscles with opposite action, control the smoothness of the motion. Sometimes agonists and antagonists contract together to stabilize the joint.

An understanding of muscle contraction is predicated on the concept of the motor unit. In simple terms, the motor unit consists of the anterior horn cell which resides in the spinal cord, its motor axon, the intramuscular branches of the main axon (nerve twigs), and the muscle fibers innervated by the twigs. Each motor unit consists of an average of 50 to 100 muscle fibers. The interface between each muscle fiber and its terminal axon is the motor end-plate or neuromuscular junction.

There are at least seven critical steps in the process of muscle contraction, each of which will be briefly described (71):

1. The first step is initiated by the excitation and discharge of the motor neuron or anterior horn cell within the spinal cord. The neuronal discharge is associated with a nerve impulse or action potential that is propagated along the axon to its terminal. Nerve conduction is an active process so that the impulse travels along the nerve at a constant amplitude and velocity. The impulse is due to a change in ion concentration across the cell membrane which ultimately depends upon alterations in membrane ion channels. Commensurate with depolarization, the voltage-gated sodium channels open, permitting a massive influx of sodium ions.
2. It is useful to remember that the neuromuscular junction consists of presynaptic (PRS) and postsynaptic (POS) regions that are separated by a narrow, intercellular synaptic cleft. The process of neuromuscular transmission is heralded by a depolarization of the PRS axon terminal of the motor nerve that promotes an elevation of intracellular calcium. Calcium ions gain access to the axoplasm through calcium channels in the PRS membrane. In turn, the synaptic vesicles which contain acetylcholine (ACh) fuse with the axon membrane. This fusion is calcium dependent and leads to a release of ACh into the extracellular space.
3. ACh molecules then cross the synaptic cleft and bind to the nicotinic acetylcholine receptors (AChR) on the POS membrane of the muscle fiber. The binding of ACh to the AChR increases the sodium and potassium conductance of the muscle membrane. As a result, there is an influx of sodium ions which is accompanied by a de-

polarizing potential, representing the end-plate potential.

4. The motor end-plate potential is transmitted along the entire muscle fiber surface to initiate the contractile response. Since the transverse (T) tubules are an extension of the sarcolemma, depolarization spreads along the T tubules which ramify within the sarcoplasm. Depolarization of the transverse tubular membrane activates the sarcoplasmic reticulum (SR) by means of the so-called "dihydropyridine receptors." These are voltage-gated calcium channels in the transverse tubule membranes which trigger the release of calcium from the adjacent SR. Calcium is released from the SR through specific calcium channels known as ryanodine receptors (72).
5. Once calcium is released from the SR, it rapidly diffuses through the sarcoplasm. Calcium ions initiate contraction by binding to troponin C. In muscle at rest, troponin I is tightly bound to actin so that tropomyosin covers the sites where myosin can bind to actin. This troponin-tropomyosin complex inhibits the interaction between actin and myosin filaments. When calcium ion binds to troponin C, tropomyosin is displaced laterally, uncovering the binding sites for the myosin heads.
6. The molecular basis of muscle contraction involves the shortening of the contractile elements resulting from a sliding of the thin filaments across the thick filaments. The sliding of actin and myosin filaments occurs when the myosin heads bind to actin. X-ray crystallography has revealed that each myosin head has an actin-binding site and an ATP-binding site. The site that binds ATP is cleftlike, but when ATP is bound and hydrolyzed by ATPase, the conformation of the myosin head changes and the cleft appears to close. During this conformational change, the head, which was initially bent, appears to straighten out, producing a so-called power stroke that advances the myosin filaments along the actin molecules. Every power stroke shortens the muscle approximately 1%. During contraction, numerous power strokes occur each second and involve about 500 myosin heads on each thick filament.
7. Following contraction, the muscle relaxes as calcium ions are pumped back into the SR and calcium is released from troponin. This inhibits the interaction between actin and myosin.

Muscle is sometimes conceptualized as machinery that converts chemical energy into mechanical work. Muscle contraction requires large amounts of energy, which is derived from the intermediary metabolism of lipids and carbohydrates. The metabolism of these energy sources, which leads to the production of ATP, is beyond the scope of this chapter.

## GENDER, TRAINING, AND AGING

Some of the earliest studies addressing differences between males and females with regard to muscle fiber size and composition were conducted by Brooke and Kaiser (73). In a seminal study of the biceps muscle in six patients, they established certain principles that remain generally true concerning gender differences in skeletal muscle. Individual muscle fibers are larger in males than in females for several reasons. Explanations include the fact that males are generally bigger than females, being taller and heavier, with a larger muscle mass for body size. Males are also more active and frequently engage in more strenuous physical exertion. Androgens are also thought to play a role in the size of muscle fibers in males, because it is known that testosterone supplements produce muscle fiber hypertrophy. In males, type 2 fibers are usually larger than type 1 fibers, in contrast to females where type 1 fibers tend to be of greater diameter. An excellent summary of this subject was published by Bennington and Krupp (70) who showed that some of the differences between males and females is dependent on the muscles sampled. For example, studies of the biceps muscle essentially verify the findings of Brooke and Kaiser. However, examination of the vastus lateralis indicates no significant difference in diameter between type 1 and type 2 fibers in males. Another interesting conclusion from these studies addresses the question of fiber-type predominance in the two sexes. With regard to the biceps muscle, males have a much higher percentage of type 2 fibers, whereas females have almost equal numbers of each. On the other hand, in the vastus lateralis, both males and females have similar proportions of type 1 and type 2 fibers.

The effect of exercise and training on skeletal muscle has been examined by a host of investigations over the past 25 years. The results of many of these studies are conflicting, but certain general principles have emerged. It is clear that exercise and training of any type causes an increase in muscle fiber diameters. Activities that are basically anaerobic in nature promote hypertrophy of type 2 fibers, a common finding in sprinters. In long distance runners, in whom aerobic metabolism is more important, type 1 fibers tend to be larger. Most authorities agree that power training such as weight lifting results in remarkable hypertrophy of type 2 fibers and little, if any, enlargement of type 1 fibers. A more controversial topic is whether there is a change in fiber-type composition after long periods of training. It is well known that sprinters tend to have larger numbers of type 2 fibers than sedentary controls, and long distance runners tend to have more type 1 fibers than untrained counterparts. Many investigators tend to believe that these two groups of runners have genetically determined fiber-type composition and little, if any, conversion of fiber types takes place during training. However, some studies have shown that while conversion from type 1 to type 2 fibers probably does not occur, certain activities such as endurance running may be responsible for the conversion of type 2B to type 2A fibers over prolonged periods of time (74). Animal studies have shed minimal light on these questions, in part, because animal muscle responds differently to exercise and training than human muscle. In fact, animal experiments have more often clouded the issues

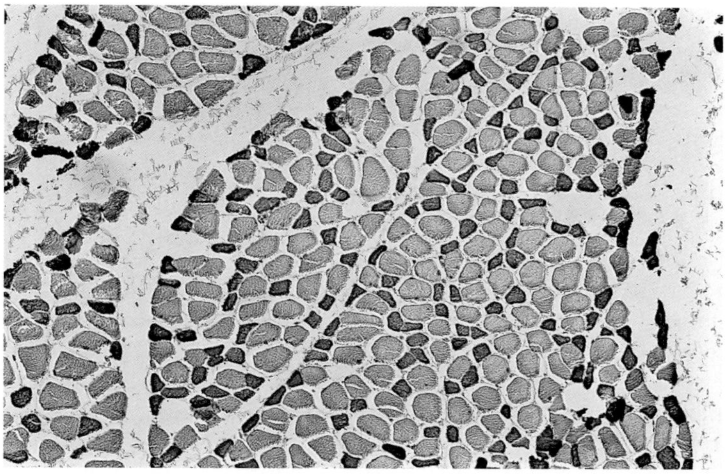

**FIG. 19.** Type 2 fiber atrophy (ATPase, pH 9.4).

of exercise and fiber composition instead of resolving the controversy.

During the process of aging, there is a functional and structural decline in skeletal muscle beginning in the sixth decade and accelerating after the age of 70 (75). By the age of 75, there is a 30 to 50% decline in muscle strength, the cause of which is complex. Because of the alterations in the makeup of their connective tissues, associated with decreased elasticity and flexibility, and because many older patients have joint disease of varying severity, the elderly become less active with a corresponding reduction in muscle volume and contractile strength. Some experts view this condition as a form of disuse. Their conclusions are supported by the fact that aging individuals, like young patients who do not use their muscles, for example, as a result of immobilization in a cast, have selective atrophy of type 2 fibers (Fig. 19). The effect of poor nutrition in the elderly has not been extensively studied, although it is well known that cachexia is also accompanied by atrophy of type 2 fibers.

A second problem in the elderly population is an insidious damage to the motor units, specifically to the anterior horn cells in the spinal cord. It has repeatedly been shown that with advancing age, there is a progressive loss of anterior horn cells. Due to degenerative spine disease, there is also injury to nerve roots with subsequent radiculopathy. The integrity of the muscle fiber is closely related to the maintenance of its nerve supply. Any sustained interruption of trophic influences from the motor neuron or nerve will culminate in atrophy of the denervated muscle fiber. In acutely denervated muscle, randomly distributed small fibers are

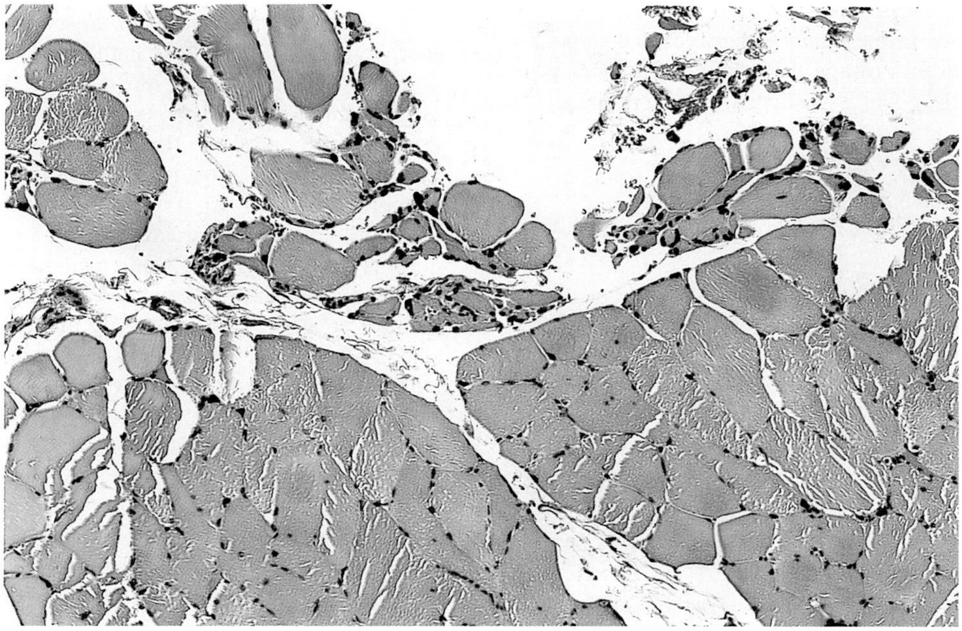

**FIG. 20.** Grouped atrophy (H&E).

seen. When sectioned transversely, atrophic fibers are characteristically angular or ensate. They appear flattened and bipolar with tapering ends. Most or all of the atrophic fibers are dark in alkaline ATPase reactions and are glycolytic in type. At this stage, selective atrophy of type 2 fibers is commonly the only pathologic abnormality, so that the proper diagnosis of denervation requires corroborative clinical information. With progressive denervation, the proportion of atrophic type 1 and type 2 fibers tends to equalize.

As long as atrophic fibers remain scattered and are not yet grouped together, from a diagnostic perspective, the pattern of atrophy is nonspecific. The esterase stain is very useful under these circumstances, since denervated fibers are extremely dark in esterase preparations, whereas atrophic fibers in other conditions are not. Atrophic fibers are also excessively dark in oxidative-enzyme reactions, but such staining applies to fiber atrophy of almost any cause. Small dark fibers are probably explained by the fact that mitochondria are relatively spared in the atrophic process and occupy a proportionately greater volume of sarcoplasm. The affinity of atrophic fibers for oxidative-enzyme stains means that the ATPase reaction is preferable for accurate fiber typing of small fibers, no matter what the pathogenesis of fiber atrophy is. Prima facie evidence of advanced denervation is a progression from random fiber atrophy to grouped atrophy, in which multiple collections of small, angular, or ensate fibers are present in the biopsy sample (Fig. 20). As a consequence of chronic denervation and of reinnervation, (76) the normal checkerboard-staining profile observed in histoenzymatic reactions is effaced. In an effort to reestablish the nerve supply to denervated muscle fibers, intact intramuscular nerves undergo collateral sprouting and new synapses are formed with atrophic fibers. As motor units enlarge, reinnervated fibers occupying a large area are converted to one histochemical type. The phenomenon of type grouping (Fig. 21) is explained by the fact that all muscle fibers within a single motor unit are of the same type—either type 1 or type 2—and the motor neuron, through the trophic influences of its axon and collaterals, governs the histochemical properties of its fibers. The plasticity of muscle fibers allows conversion from one histochemical type to the other when there is reinnervation by a motor neuron of the opposite type.

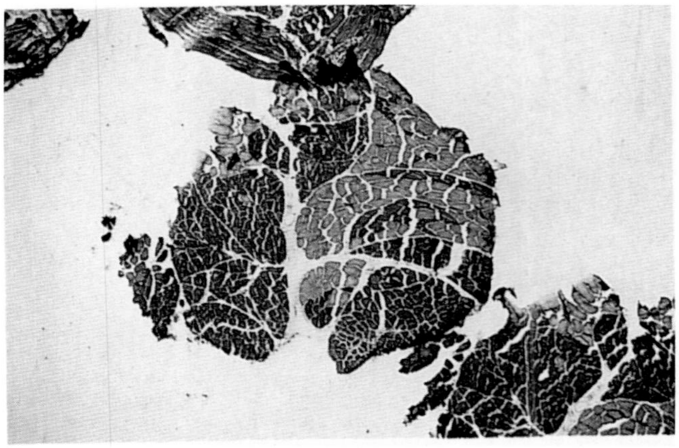

**FIG. 21.** Chronic denervation with reinnervation. Type grouping has altered the normal checkerboard staining profile (NADH-TR).

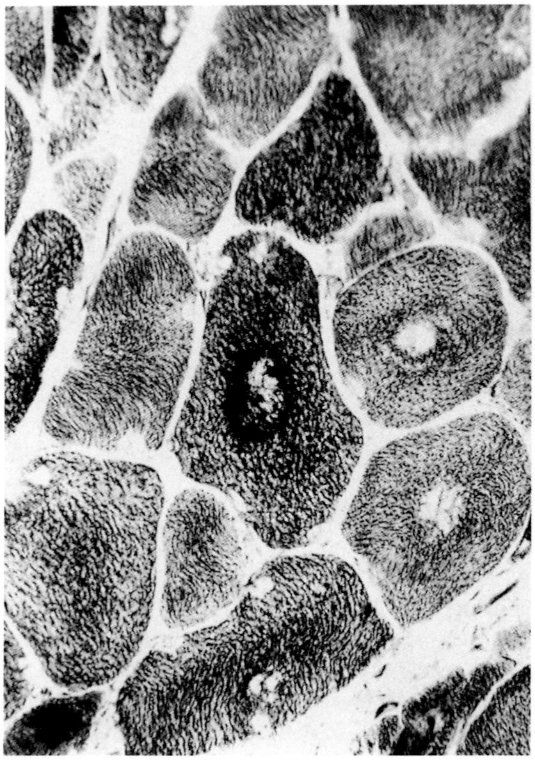

**FIG. 22.** Neurogenic atrophy. Target fiber at the center has an inner, unstained zone surrounded by a rim of increased enzyme activity (NADH-TR).

Along with type grouping, target fibers are pathognomic of denervation (77). Despite their unique specificity, regrettably, bona fide target fibers are present in less than 25% of cases of neurogenic atrophy. Although targets and cores are similar morphologically, they differ in three ways. While both tend to occur singly within a fiber, the target is larger in diameter. The target is limited in length, only extending across a few sarcomeres, in contrast to the core which may run the entire length of the fiber. Most important is the three-zone architecture of the target fiber (Fig. 22). The central zone, indistinguishable at the ultrastructural level from the unstructured core, is surrounded by an intermediate zone forming an intensely stained rim in oxidative-enzyme reactions. The intermediate zone, difficult to identify in most other stains, is absent from a core. By definition it is a zone of transition between the central zone of severe sarcoplasmic disruption and the other third zone that represents the normal portion of the muscle fiber. Targetoid fibers, which lack the intermediate zone of increased oxidative-enzyme activity, are morphologically identical to core fibers. The term "core" is conventionally used in cases of congenital central core disease and the term "targetoid" is applied to cores that are found in any other condition. In our experience, targetoid fibers are more commonly encountered in neurogenic atrophy than any other condition, and are more frequently seen than target fibers.

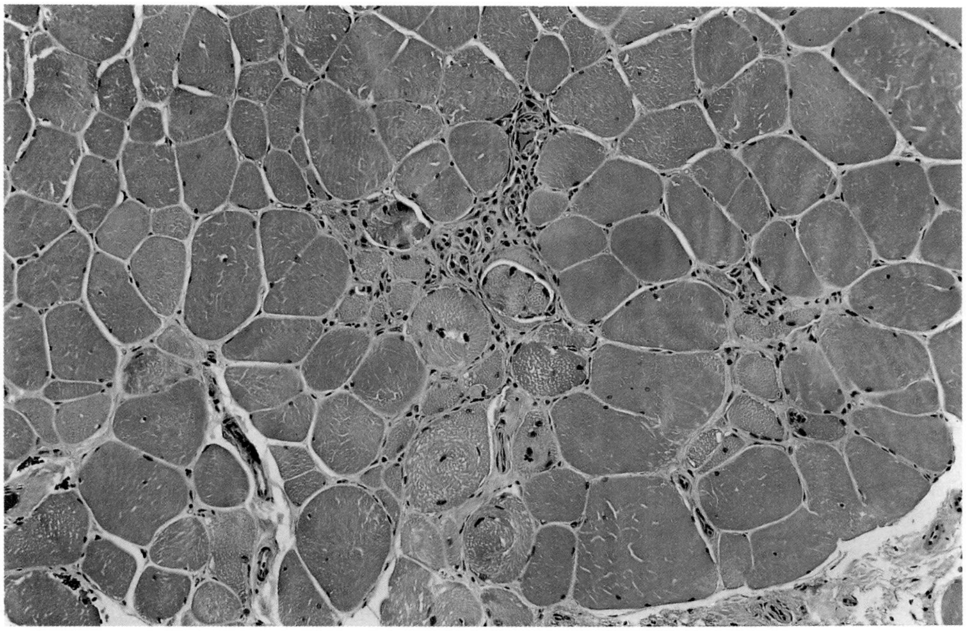

**FIG. 23.** Needle tract. Area of injury contains necrotic fibers and a small focus of lymphocytic inflammation (H&E).

## ARTIFACTS

The most common artifacts are related to unsuspected or inadvertent injury to the muscle specimen, irreverent handling at the time of removal, or to improper tissue sectioning and staining. When they are linear in configuration, needle tracts, such as those produced during electromyogram (EMG) studies, may easily be recognized. More often, needle tracts are cut tangentially so that the pathologist may be misled by a histologic picture of myopathy exemplified by fiber necrosis, regeneration, inflammation, and interstitial fibrosis (Fig. 23). This kind of artifact is generally traceable to poor communication between the physician requesting the biopsy and the individual performing the procedure who is unaware of the previous intramuscular injections.

Large numbers of neutrophils are occasionally observed within the intramuscular blood vessels. Typically, these cells are marginated and may have begun to penetrate the vascu-

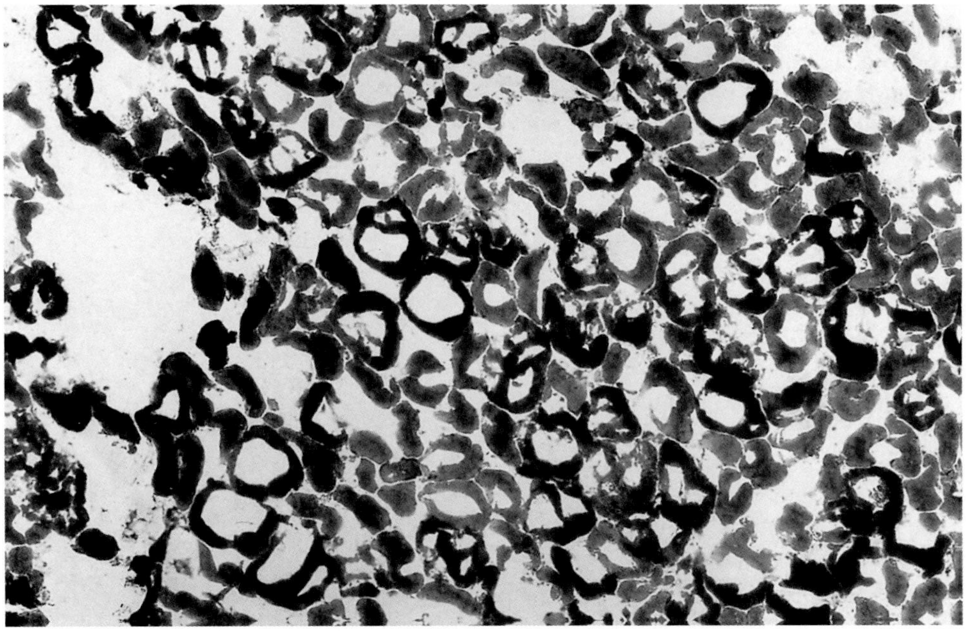

**FIG. 24.** Vacuolar artifact. Improper freezing has caused numerous clear holes to form within the fibers (NADH-TR).

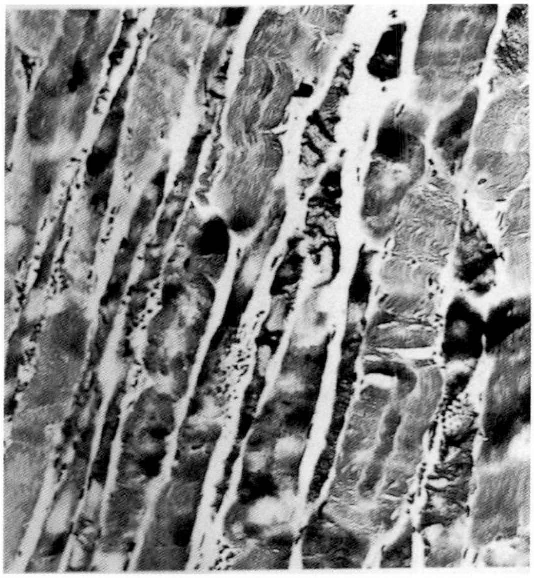

**FIG. 25.** Contraction artifact. Dark contraction bands and lucent zones of disruption are seen in longitudinally oriented fibers.

lar walls and enter the perimysium or endomysium. In the absence of other pathologic changes within the specimen, the presence of neutrophils usually means that the muscle has been crushed during the biopsy procedure or it has been infiltrated with an anesthetic agent.

Even with the best technical expertise available, muscle tissue is sufficiently fragile that most laboratories find vacuolization of muscle fibers produced during freezing is unavoidable in 10 to 20% of specimens. Vacuolization can be minimized by using proper techniques that permit rapid freezing, and by proper specimen storage to prevent thawing. Mild vacuolar artifacts may be tolerable, but large vacuoles that disrupt the sarcoplasm are especially troublesome (Fig. 24). Larger vacuoles may interfere with accurate biopsy interpretation by distorting the pathologic changes in the sample or by simulating the picture of vacuolar myopathy, such as glycogen or lipid storage disease.

Muscle that is unprotected by isometric clamping is vulnerable to contraction artifact. During uncontrolled contraction, a series of segmental contractions occur along the length of the muscle fiber as the contractile elements are pulled beyond the confines of their respective sarcomeres. This phenomenon is best observed in longitudinal sections where dark hypercontracted regions are punctuated by pale, ghostlike zones of myofibrillar disruption (Fig. 25). In transverse orientation, these disrupted segments are seen as irregular fissures in the sarcoplasm. Contraction artifact is particularly undesirable when electron microscopic studies are needed, even if the artifact is subtle and cannot be appreciated at the light microscopic level. The detection of ultrastructural abnormalities, which is dependent on the normal alignment of the myofibrils and myofilaments, is compromised by the distortion of sarcomeric structures.

Dark staining of the sarcoplasm in random fibers is often due to variations in section thickness. Fibers adjacent to the connective tissue of the perimysium are especially susceptible to this artifact. Inconsistencies of section thickness may be recognized when linear, bandlike regions of intense staining are visible within muscle fibers. Excessively pale histochemical reactions can result from the degradation of enzyme systems in the sarcoplasm. Artifacts are distinguished from legitimate abnormal staining if all histochemical reactions in the biopsy are pale. In our experience, this artifact is most often attributable to delayed freezing of the specimen because of a delay in transport. Laboratories that accept consultation specimens from institutions other than their own, should be aware of this problem to reduce the time required for transportation.

## DIFFERENTIAL DIAGNOSIS

Several findings in skeletal muscle biopsies are normal or are minor variations which may be mistaken for pathologic change. These include internal nuclei, ring fibers, hyaline fibers, excessive endomysial connective tissue, perivascular inflammation, and variations in fiber diameters.

One of the most common pathological abnormalities in muscle biopsies is nuclear internalization (Fig. 26). Quantitative analyses have demonstrated that the nuclei are periph-

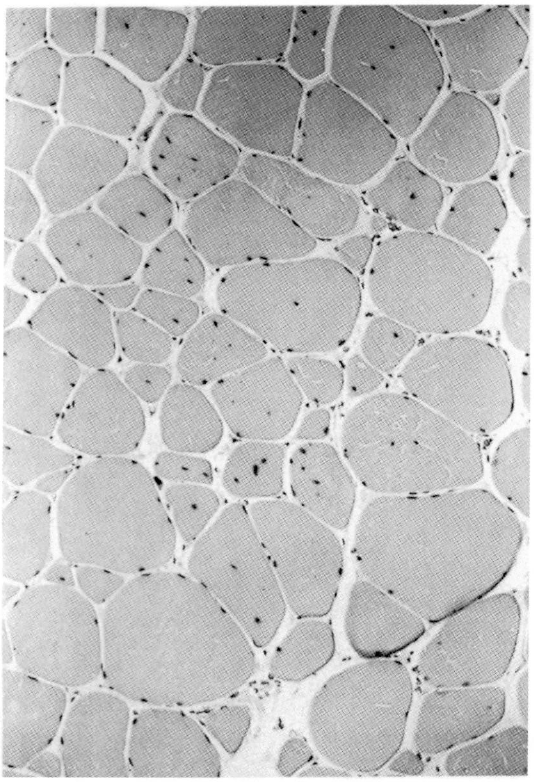

**FIG. 26.** Nuclear internalization. Many fibers contain internal pyknotic nuclei, a common nonspecific pathologic change.

erally located in 97 to 99% of normal muscle fibers, which means that up to 3% of fibers with internal nuclei is a normal finding. In many different conditions, an increase in internal nuclei is found, typically affecting 5 to 10% of fibers, particularly those that are mildly atrophic. Nuclear internalization has no specific diagnostic significance and appears to be a reaction to virtually any type of injury. The diagnosis of MyD should be strongly considered if the majority of fibers contain internal nuclei.

One must exercise caution in interpreting the significance of ring fibers in specimens disrupted by contraction artifact, because in this situation, ring fibers are not a genuine pathologic change. In properly processed, uncontracted muscle biopsies, ring fibers are a pathologic criterion of myotonic disorders. The ring is formed by a bundle of peripheral myofibrils, which are circumferentially oriented such that they encircle the internal portion of the sarcoplasm that is normal in structure and orientation. In cross sections of muscle, the ring is especially well visualized in PAS stains where the striations of the transversely oriented peripheral myofibrils are seen in contrast to the inner sarcoplasmic contents (Fig. 27). Rings are also seen to advantage in PTAH stains, resin sections, or under phase contrast microscopy. Under the electron microscope the pathologically oriented myofibrils are generally normal in structure except for hypercontraction of the sarcomeres (78).

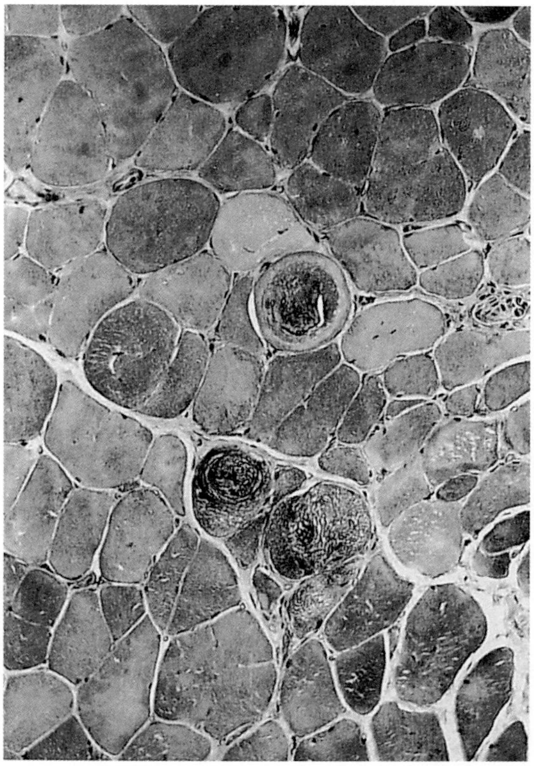

**FIG. 27.** Ring fibers. Bundles of myofibrils are circumferentially oriented, forming rings that encircle two transversely sectioned fibers (PAS).

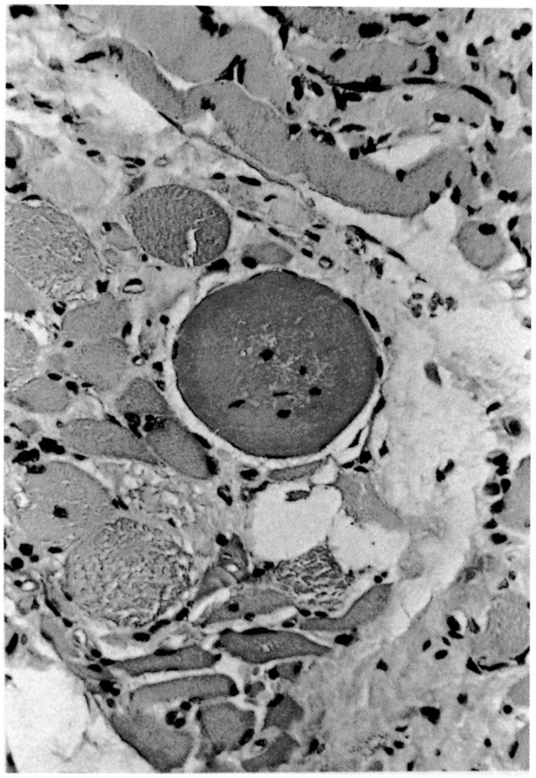

**FIG. 28.** Hyaline fiber. The fiber at the center is enlarged, rounded, and has darkly stained sarcoplasm containing several internal nuclei.

Along with ring fibers, hyaline fibers are evident in specimens damaged by contraction artifact. These fibers are abnormally increased in diameter and rounded in configuration. Their sarcoplasm in both paraffin and frozen sections is smudged or glassy and more deeply stained than in normal fibers (Fig. 28). The hyaline appearance is the legacy of hypercontraction, as shown in electron microscopic studies. In clamped specimens which are free of excessive contraction, true hyaline fibers are a common feature of Duchenne muscular dystrophy. The pathogenesis of true hyaline fiber formation, which is believed to precede subsequent fiber necrosis, (79) is apparently related to excessive irritability secondary to cell membrane instability. It is possible that sarcolemmal damage allows excessive contraction and also promotes cell necrosis. In serial sections of hyaline fibers, areas of necrosis may be found, indicating the importance of hyalinization as a sign of fiber destruction.

Excessive amounts of endomysial connective tissue usually represents reactive fibrosis accompanying neuromuscular disease. However, as pointed out previously, at the interface between muscle and tendons or fascia abundant connective tissue is normally present and should not be regarded as reactive fibrosis. Although endomysial connective tissue is not prominent in the biopsies of infants, as indicated previously, the perimysial connective tissue far exceeds the amount present in older children and adults (Fig. 29).

Interstitial and perivascular inflammatory cells almost always reflect clinical disease, most frequently immunologically mediated or idiopathic inflammatory myopathies such as polymyositis or dermatomyositis. However, in the biopsies of infants remember that small foci of hematopoiesis are normally present and do not represent true inflammatory infiltrates. Muscles subjected to trauma such as EMG needles may harbor foci of inflammation for months following the diagnostic study and are not clinically significant.

One of the most demanding challenges to the diagnostic pathologist is the muscle biopsy characterized by a variation in fiber diameters or by what appears to be atrophy or hypertrophy. The utility of enzyme histochemistry in these situations cannot be overstated. It is important to recall from previous discussions that: (a) a normal variation in fiber size occurs at the junctions of muscle fibers and either tendons or fascia; and (b) what at first seems to be atrophy may be normal, depending on the muscle examined and the patient's age and sex. Smaller muscles, and especially those devoted to finely coordinated activities, have much smaller diameters than large, bulky muscles. Muscle fibers are expected to be much smaller in infants and children than in mature adults. And, as previously noted, there is an increasing reduction in fiber diameters with advancing age. The significance of fiber hypertrophy should be evaluated in light of the patient's activity and level of regular exercise. In evaluating fiber size, it may be necessary to measure fiber diameters. Morphometric analysis of the muscle biopsy is imperative when the changes in fiber diameters are minimal and subtle. In order to obtain statistically significant morphometric data, the lesser diameter of each muscle fiber should be determined, based upon a minimum number of 200 fibers in the sample (80). The atrophic or hypertrophic process may be selective, affecting only one fiber type, or it may be nonselective (81). True selective atrophy of type 1 fibers is most commonly encountered in myotonic dystrophy. Type 2 fiber atrophy is a common finding in acute denervation, disuse, and myasthenia gravis. True hypertrophy of type 1 fibers is relatively specific for infantile spinal muscular atrophy. True type 2 fiber hypertrophy is generally restricted to congenital fiber-type disproportion.

The pattern of atrophy is important in distinguishing normal from abnormal. Randomly distributed small or large fibers may be normal, depending on other factors discussed earlier. Grouped atrophy, where five or more small angular fibers cluster together, is essentially diagnostic of chronic neurogenic disease. Panfascicular atrophy, in which the majority of fibers in each fascicle are atrophic, is virtually specific for infantile spinal muscle atrophy. Perifascicular atrophy is typical of dermatomyositis.

## SPECIMEN HANDLING

Muscle biopsies should be performed by physicians with expertise in biopsy technique and a sincere interest in obtaining the best possible specimen. The physician who has direct responsibility for the patient's care needs to be sure that the biopsy comes from an appropriate muscle, so that it is representative of the disease process. In some conditions, the disease process is widespread, such as in many metabolic diseases, and virtually any muscle is suitable for biopsy. However, in other disorders where, for example, symptoms are referable to the legs and spare the arms, a biopsy of the

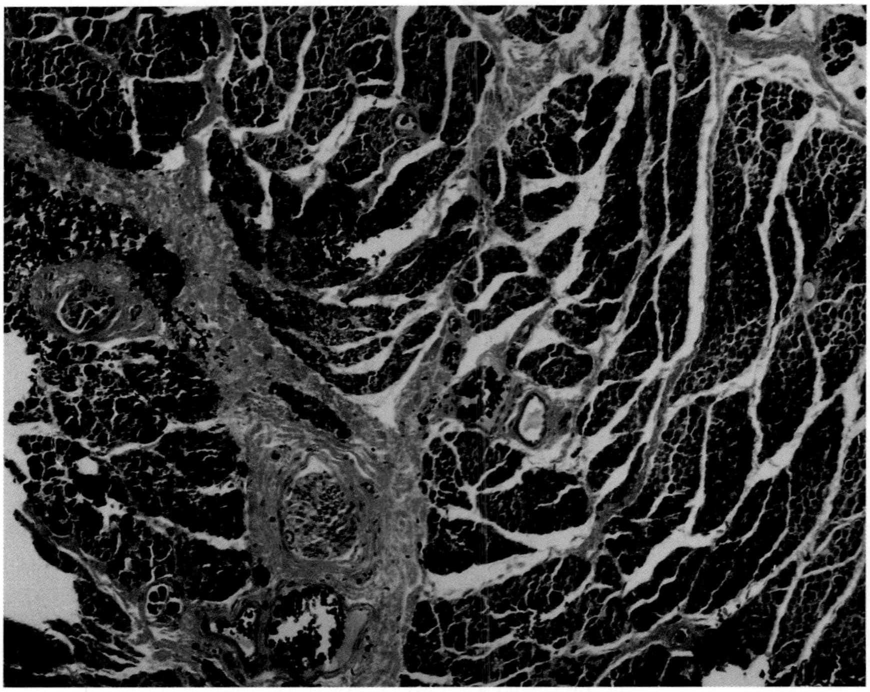

**FIG. 29.** Infant muscle. Relative increase in perimysial connective tissue is normal (Trichrome).

deltoid or biceps brachii muscle is unlikely to reflect the disease process accurately and may be normal or nondiagnostic. Moreover, whenever possible, the tissue sample should be obtained from a region in which the disease process remains active, rather than quiescent. In a muscle where the disease process has subsided, the biopsy is apt to be unremarkable. In severely involved muscle, particularly if there is marked weakness or wasting, the pathologic findings are likely to be those of end-stage disease which may defy conclusive pathologic interpretation. Muscles subjected to previous traumatic injury, such as needle tracts incurred during electromyography (EMG) or intramuscular injections of medications, and muscles altered by an unrelated disease process should not be biopsied. The pathologic picture in such muscles may simulate that associated with a variety of neuromuscular diseases and will confuse the pathologist.

The special handling of the muscle biopsy precludes submission of the specimen on weekends and holidays or late in the workday afternoon when laboratory personnel are not available to receive and process the tissue. If possible, a technician familiar with the biopsy technique should assist the physician performing the biopsy and collect the specimen properly. Two separate specimens from the same site are routinely required. The first specimen is maintained at isometric length by its insertion in a muscle clamp. This device is designed to minimize contraction artifact which inevitably results when an incision is made in the muscle and it is immersed in fixative. Because the muscle is introduced into the instrument lengthwise, the sample is conveniently oriented for further processing. The biopsy must extend entirely across the clamp, thereby ensuring an acceptable specimen size of at least 1 cm in length.

The biopsy should be of sufficient size to maximize the opportunity of observing the entire pathologic process. To attain this goal, some clinicians favor obtaining two biopsies routinely, one from the arm and one from the leg, for example. Thus, the major drawback to needle biopsy, which has certain advantages over open biopsy, is the limited size of the sample. Although there is some disagreement regarding the primary fixative for muscle biopsies, we have elected to use 10% formalin, buffered to a pH of 7.4 in a 0.1 M phosphate buffer. Strips of muscle 1 mm in width are dissected from the edges of the sample and postfixed in phosphate-buffered 2% glutaraldehyde for electron microscopic study. After fixation for a minimum of 24 hours in 10% phosphate-buffered formalin, the remainder of the sampled specimen is used for routine paraffin sections. A second unfixed specimen measuring $1 \times 0.5 \times 0.5$ cm is obtained for the preparation of frozen sections. Although the utilization of a muscle clamp is not mandatory, clamping the specimen will help in its orientation.

Several techniques are described for flash freezing, (82) but we prefer freezing the sample in liquid nitrogen after coating the surface of the specimen with talc. Whatever technique is employed, the condition on which the freezing technique is based is that it proceed with extreme rapidity, within 10 to 15 seconds. Freezing the tissue in a cryostat in a fashion similar to most specimens submitted for frozen section diagnosis from the operating room is contraindicated. The frozen sample should be oriented so that cross sections of muscle are cut. Serial frozen sections in our laboratory are stained with H&E, rapid Gomori trichrome (RTC), and three standard histochemical reactions-ATPase (pH 9.4 and 4.6) and NADH-TR. Other stains such as periodic acid-Schiff (PAS) for glycogen, phosphorylase, and fat stains are performed when indicated. Frozen tissue may also be used for biochemical analysis, for immunohistochemical preparations, and for immunofluorescence microscopy. Inasmuch as frozen tissue may be needed for future additional studies, muscle biopsies can be sealed in airtight plastic capsules or bags to prevent dessication and freezing artifact while stored in an ultra-low freezer at −70°C.

## REFERENCES


1. Jacob M, Christ B, Jacob HJ. On the migration of myogenic stem cells into the prospective wing region of chick embryos. *Anat Embryol (Berl)* 1978;153:179–193.
2. Larsen WJ. *Human embryology.* New York: Churchill Livingstone, 1983:281–307.
3. Okazaki K, Holtzer H. Myogenesis: fusion, myosin synthesis, and the mitotic cycle. *Proc Natl Acad Sci U S A* 1966;56:1484–1490.
4. Yaffe D. Developmental changes preceding cell fusion during muscle differentiation in vitro. *Exp Cell Res* 1971;66:33–48.
5. Wakshull E, Bayne EK, Chiquet M, Fambrough DM. Characterization of a plasma membrane glycoprotein common to myoblasts, skeletal muscle satellite cells, and glia. *Dev Biol* 1983; 100:464–477.
6. Keeter JS, Pappas GD, Model PG. Inter- and intramyotomal gap junctions in the axolotl embryo. *Dev Biol* 1975;45:21–33.
7. Chiquet M, Eppenberger HM, Turner DC. Muscle morphogenesis: Evidence for an organizing function of exogenesis fibronectin. *Dev Biol* 1981;88:220–235.
8. Kelly AM, Zacks SI. The histogenesis of rat intercostal muscle. *J Cell Biol* 1969;42:135–153.
9. Ishikawa H, Bischoff R, Holtzer H. Mitosis and intermediate-sized filaments in developing skeletal muscle. *J Cell Biol* 1968; 38:538–555.
10. Franklin GI, Yasin R, Hughes BP, Thompson EJ. Acetylcholine receptors in cultured human muscle cells. *J Neurol Sci* 1980;47:317–327.
11. Martin L, Joris C. Histoenzymological and semiquantitative study of the maturation of the human muscle fiber. In: Walton JN, Canal N, Scarlato G, eds. *Disease of muscle.* Amsterdam: Excerpta Medica, 1970:657.
12. Wohlfart G. Ueber das vorkommen verschiedener arten von muskelfarsern in der skelettmusculatur der menschen und einiger saugetiere. *Acta Psychiat Neurol* 1937;12 (Suppl):119.
13. Fenichel GM. A histochemical study of developing human skeletal muscle. *Neurology* 1966;16:741–745.
14. Goldspink G. Sarcomere length during post-natal growth of mammalian muscle fibers. *J Cell Sci* 1968;3:539–548.
15. Close RI. Dynamic properties of mammalian skeletal muscles. *Physiol Rev* 1972;52:129–197.
16. Goldspink G. Postembryonic growth and differentiation of striated muscle. In: Bourne GH, ed. *The structure and function of muscle, Vol. 1.* New York: Academic Press, 1972:179–236.
17. Stickland NC. Muscle development in the human fetus as exemplified by m. sartorius. *J Anat* 1981;132:557–579.
18. Adams RD, DeReuck J. Metrics of muscle. In: Kakulas BA, ed. *Basic research in myology.* Amsterdam: Excerpta Medica, 1973.
19. Kakulas BA, Adams RD. *Diseases of muscle.* New York: Harper and Row, 1985:8–9.
20. Hamburger V. History of the discovery of neuronal death in embryos. *J Neurobiol* 1992;23:1116–1123.
21. Sohal GS. Embryonic development of nerve and muscle. *Muscle Nerve* 1995;18:2–14.

22. Oppenheim RW, Prevette D, Haverkamp LJ, et al. Biological studies of a putative avian muscle-derived neurotrophic factor that prevents naturally occurring motorneuron death in vivo. *J Neurobiol*: 1993;24: 1065–1079.
23. Hughes RA, Sendtner M, Goldfarb M, et al. Evidence that fibroblast growth factor 5 is a major muscle-derived survival factor for cultured spinal motorneurons. *Neuron* 1993;10:369–377.
24. Houenou LJ, Turner PL, Li L, et al. A serine protease inhibitor, protease nexin I, rescues motorneurons from naturally occurring and axotomy-induced cell death. *Proc Natl Acad Sci U S A* 1995;92:895–899.
25. Sun D, Ziegler R, Milligan CE, et al. Apolipophorin III is dramatically up-regulated during the programmed death of insect skeletal muscle and neurons. *J Neurobiol*: 1995;26:119–129.
26. Haas AL, Baboshima O, Williams B, Schwartz LM. Coordinated induction of the ubiquitin conjugation pathway accompanies the developmentally programmed death of insect skeletal muscle. *J Biol Chem* 1995;270:9407–9412.
27. McClearn D, Medville R, Noden D. Muscle cell death during the development of head and neck muscles in the chick. *Dev Dyn* 1995; 202: 365–377.
28. Abood EA, Jones MM. Macrophages in developing mammalian skeletal muscle: evidence for muscle fiber death as a normal developmental event. *Acta Anat* 1991;140:201–212.
29. Fidzianska A, Goebel HH. Human ontogenesis. 3. Cell death in fetal muscle. *Acta Neuropathol (Berl)* 1991;81:572–577.
30. Tidball JG, Albrecht DE, Lokensgard BE, Spencer MJ. Apoptosis precedes necrosis of dystrophin-deficient muscle. *J Cell Sci* 1995; 108: 2197–2214.
31. Olive M, Blanco R, Rivera R, et al. Cell death induced by gamma irradiation of developing skeletal muscle. *J Anat* 1995;187:127–132.
32. McKenzie WC. *The action of muscles, including muscle rest and muscle re-education*. New York: Hoeber, 1921.
33. Feinstein B, Lindegard B, Nyman E, Wohlfart G. Morphological studies of motor units in normal human muscles. *Acta Anat* 1955; 23: 127–142.
34. Clemente CD, ed. *Gray's anatomy*. Philadelphia: Lea & Febiger, 1985: 434–436.
35. Blomfield LB. Intramuscular vascular pattern in man. *Proc Roy Soc Med* 1945;38:617–618.
36. Renkin EM, Hudlicka O, Sheehan RM. Influence of metabolic vasodilatation on blood-tissue diffusion in skeletal muscle. *Amer J Physiol* 1966;211:87–98.
37. Emslie-Smith AM, Engel AG. Microvascular changes in early and advanced dermatomyositis. A quantitative study. *Ann Neurol* 1990; 27: 343–356.
38. Schmalbruch H. Rote mupskelfasern. *Z Zellforsch Mikrosk Anat* 1971; 119:120–146.
39. Heuser JE, Reese TS, Landis DMD. Functional changes in frog neuromuscular junctions studied with freeze-fracture. *J Neurocytol* 1974; 3:109–131.
40. Ellisman MH, Rash JE, Staehelin LA, Porter KR. Studies of excitable membranes. II. A comparison of specializations at neuromuscular junctions and nonjunctional sarcolemmas of mammalian fast and slow twitch muscle fibers. *J Cell Biol* 1976;68:752–774.
41. Ross MJ, Klymkowsky MW, Agard DA, Stroud RM. Structural studies of a membrane-bound acetylcholine receptor from Torpedo californica. *J Mol Biol* 1977;116:635–659.
42. Carpenter S, Karpati G. *Pathology of skeletal muscle*. New York: Churchill Livingstone, 1984.
43. DeGirolami U, Smith TW. Pathology of skeletal muscle diseases. *Am J Pathol* 1982;107:235–276.
44. Dubowitz V, Brooke MH. Muscle biopsy. *A modern approach.* Philadelphia: WB Saunders, 1973.
45. Engel AG, Franzini-Armstrong C. *Myology, 2nd ed.* New York: McGraw-Hill, 1994.
46. Heffner RR, ed. *Muscle pathology*. New York: Churchill Livingstone, 1984.
47. Heffner RR. Muscle biopsy in the diagnosis of neuromuscular disease. *Semin Diagn Pathol* 1984;1:114–151.
48. Heffner RR. Muscle biopsy in neuromuscular disorders. In: Sternberg SS, ed. *Diagnostic surgical pathology, vol. 1*. New York: Raven Press, 1989:119–139.
49. Kakulas BA, Adams RD. *Diseases of muscle*. New York: Harper & Row, 1985.
50. Mastaglia FL, Walton JN, eds. *Skeletal muscle pathology*. New York: Churchill Livingstone, 1992.
51. Pearson CM, Mostofi FK, eds. *The striated muscle*. Baltimore: Williams & Wilkins, 1973.
52. Swash S, Schwartz MS. *Neuromuscular diseases*. New York: Springer-Verlag, 1981.
53. Schmalbruch H. *Skeletal muscle*. Berlin: Springer-Verlag, 1985:301.
54. Brooke MH, Engel WK. The histographic analysis of human muscle biopsies with regard to fiber types. 4. Children's biopsies. *Neurology* 1969;19:591–605.
55. Bowden DH, Goyer RA. The size of muscle fibers in infants and children. *Arch Pathol* 1960;69:188–189.
56. Vogler C, Bove KE. Morphology of skeletal muscle in children. *Arch Pathol Lab Med* 1985;109:238–242.
57. Kolliker A. *Mikrosckopische anatomie*. Leipzig; W. Engehmann, 1851.
58. Bakker GJ, Richmond FJR. The types of muscle spindles in cat neck muscles:a histochemical study of intrafusal fiber composition. *J Neurophysiol* 1981;45:973–986.
59. Swash M, Fox KP. Muscle spindle innervation in man. *J Anat* 1972; 112:61–80.
60. Campion DR. The muscle satellite cell:a review. *Internatl Rev Cytol* 1984;87:225.
61. Hoffman EP, Wang J. Duchenne-Becker muscular dystrophy and the nondystrophic myotonias. *Arch Neurol* 1993;50:1227–1237.
62. Johns DR. Mitochondrial DNA and disease. *New Engl J Med* 1995;333: 638–644.
63. Jay V, Becker LE. Fiber-type differentiation by myosin immunohistochemistry on paraffin-embedded skeletal muscle. *Arch Pathol Lab Med* 1994;118:917–918.
64. Ohlendieck K, Matsumura MD, Ionasescu VV, et al. Duchenne muscular dystrophy:deficiency of dystrophin-associated proteins in the sarcolemma. *Neurology* 1993;43:795–800.
65. Coers C, Woolf AL. *The innervation of muscle: a biopsy study*. Springfield, IL: Thomas, 1959.
66. Koelle GB, Friedenwald JS. A histochemical method for localizing cholinesterase activity. *Proc Soc Exper Biol Med* 1949;70:617–622.
67. Engel AG, Lindstrom JM, Lambert EH, Lennon VA. Ultrastructural localization of the acetylcholine receptor in myasthenia gravis and in its experimental autoimmune model. *Neurology* 1977;27:307–315.
68. Engel AG, Fukunaga H, Osame M. Stereometric estimation of the area of the freeze-fractured membrane. *Muscle Nerve* 1982;5:682.
69. Wray JS, Holmes KC. X-ray diffraction studies of muscle. *Annu Rev Physiol* 1981;43:553–565.
70. Bennington JL, Krupp M. Morphometric analysis of muscle. In:Heffner RR, ed. *Muscle pathology*. New York: Churchill Livingstone, 1984: 43–71.
71. Goodman SR. *Medical cell biology*. Philadelphia: JB Lippincott, 1994; 61–100.
72. MacLennan DH, Duff C, Zorzato F, et al. Ryanodine receptor gene is a candidate for predisposition to malignant hyperthermia. *Nature* 1990; 343:559–561.
73. Brooke MH, Kaiser KK. Muscle fiber types: how many and what kind? *Arch Neurol* 1970;23:369–379.
74. Gunby P. Runner's ability depends partly on muscle fiber type. *JAMA* 1979;242:1712–1713.
75. Lexell J, Henriksson-Larsen K, Winblad B, Sjostrom M. Distribution of different fiber types in human skeletal muscles: effects of aging studied in whole muscle cross sections. *Muscle Nerve* 1983;6:588–595.
76. Karpati G, Engel WK. "Type grouping" in skeletal muscles after experimental reinnervation. *Neurology* 1968;18:447–455.
77. Engel WK. Muscle target fibers, a newly recognized sign of denervation. *Nature* 1961;191:389–390.
78. Heffner RR. Electron microscopy of disorders of skeletal muscle. *Ann Clin Lab Sci* 1975;5:338–347.
79. Cullen MJ, Fulthrope JJ. Stages in fiber breakdown in Duchenne muscular dystrophy. *J Neurol Sci* 1975;24:179–200.
80. Dubowitz V, Brooke MH. *Muscle biopsy: a modern approach.* Philadelphia: WB Saunders, 1973.
81. Engel WK. Selective and nonselective susceptibility of muscle fiber types. A new approach to human neuromuscular diseases. *Arch Neurol* 1970;22:97–117.
82. Bossen EH. Collection and preparation of the muscle biopsy. In:Heffner RR, ed. *Muscle pathology*. New York: Churchill Livingstone, 1984:11–14.

# Serous Membranes

*Histology for Pathologists, second edition,*
Edited by Stephen S. Sternberg.
Lippincott-Raven Publishers, Philadelphia


# CHAPTER 10

# Serous Membranes

Darryl Carter, Lawrence True, and Christopher N. Otis



## ANATOMY

The mesothelium is the layer of cells that lines the serous membranes of the pleural, pericardial, and peritoneal spaces. Although mesothelial cells differentiate into a simple or cuboidal epithelium, they are of mesodermal origin. The serous membranes show functional differentiation according to their derivation from visceral or parietal mesoderm.

Because this is not a textbook of gross anatomy, the description of the areas covered by mesothelium must be somewhat truncated.

The pleura is a continuous membrane that covers the chest wall and the lungs. The visceral pleura coats the entire pulmonary surface including the major and minor fissures that divide the lung into lobes. The parietal pleura extends over the ribs, sternum, and supporting structures and is reflected over the mediastinal structures on either side. Posteriorly in the mediastinum, the two layers of parietal pleura are separated by a rather thin band of fibrovascular connective tissue. Superiorly, the cervical pleura is reflected into the retroclavicular area over the apex of the lung and is coated by a thickened layer of fibrous tissue and skeletal muscle; inferiorly, the diaphragmatic pleura represents its caudal extent. Anteriorly, the pleura is reflected over part of the pericardium. The posterior visceral pleura becomes continuous with the diaphragmatic pleura over the pulmonary ligament.

The pericardium is the sac surrounding the heart and great vessels, and it is lined by a continuous layer of mesothelium. The visceral side is termed epicardial and the parietal is the pericardial layer that rests on a dense fibrous tissue layer containing branches of the internal mammary and musculophrenic vessels and descending aorta as well as branches of the vagus, phrenic, and sympathetic nerves. The thoracic surface of the pericardium is coated with parietal pleura.

The peritoneum is a nearly continuous membrane lining the potential space between the intra-abdominal viscera and the abdominal wall. In the female, it is normally interrupted by the lumina of the fallopian tubes. Anatomically, it is more complex than either the pleura or pericardium. The parietal layer covers the abdominal wall, diaphragm, anterior surfaces of the retroperitoneal viscera, and the pelvis. The visceral peritoneum coats the intestine and the intra-abdominal viscera. The elongated structures in which the parietal and visceral layers come together are the mesentery, which contain blood vessels, lymphatics, lymph nodes, and nerves. The greater omentum is a double sheet with four layers of mesothelium between which there may be large quantities of adipose tissue. Blood vessels are numerous; lymphatics and lymph nodes are less prominent than in the mesentery. The peritoneal cavity is grossly divided into the greater sac over the intestines, the lesser sac that is retrogastric, the right and left retrocolic areas, and the pelvis.

There are several outpouchings of peritoneum which are often seen in pathology laboratories. Inguinal hernias are pouches of parietal peritoneum pushed through the abdominal musculature into the inguinal canal. The hernia sac is often invested with fibrous tissue and occasionally with skeletal muscle. The wide range of reactive processes in hernia sacs is not necessarily indicative of changes in the rest of the peritoneum. Umbilical or ventral hernias are also outpouchings of peritoneum, but the specimens received by pathologists after surgery for their repair are usually preperitoneal

D. Carter: Department of Pathology, Yale University School of Medicine, New Haven, CT 06510.
L. True: Department of Pathology, University of Washington, Seattle, WA 98195.
C. N. Otis: Department of Pathology, Bay State Medical Center, Springfield, MA 01199.

connective tissue pushed ahead of the parietal peritoneum rather than mesothelium itself.

The scrotum acquires a lining of parietal mesothelium, the processus vaginalis, into which the testes descend during the seventh month of gestation. A mesothelial layer forms the surface of the tunica vaginalis. Distention of this mesothelial sac on the tunica vaginalis results in a hydrocele—communicating with the peritoneal cavity when congenital but noncommunicating in hydrocele sacs formed subsequently. The sac of an inguinal hernia communicates with the peritoneal cavity and not with the mesothelium-lined space of the scrotum. Both hernia and hydrocele sacs are capable of a wide range of reactive changes.

## FUNCTIONAL ANATOMY

The functional anatomy of the pleura has been the subject of recent reviews by Sahn (1) and Pistolesi et al. (2). The pleura is a continuous membrane surrounding a space that normally contains approximately 10 ml of clear colorless fluid. The surface is lined by a single layer of mesothelial cells anchored to a basement membrane that lies on layers of collagen and elastic tissue. Vascular and lymphatic vessels are found in the subpleural layer. The lining mesothelial cells have rounded nuclei, which may contain a nucleolus and a relatively large amount of cytoplasm. The cell diameter is 16 to 40 $\mu$m. Although the visceral and parietal pleurae are opposing parts of the same continuous membrane, there are major differences between these two structures.

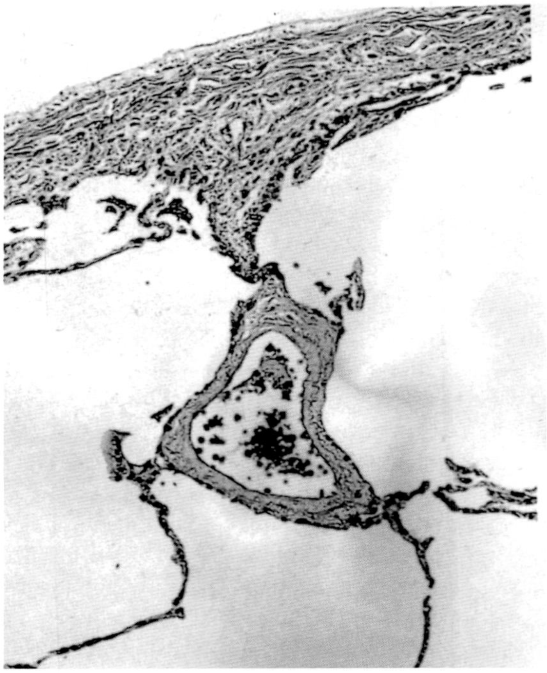

**FIG. 1.** Visceral pleura. The mesothelial cells on the surface are not apparent. The dense submesothelial layer from the posterior surface of the left lower lobe is composed of collagen and elastin. It extends into adjacent pulmonary interstitium and around pulmonary vessels.

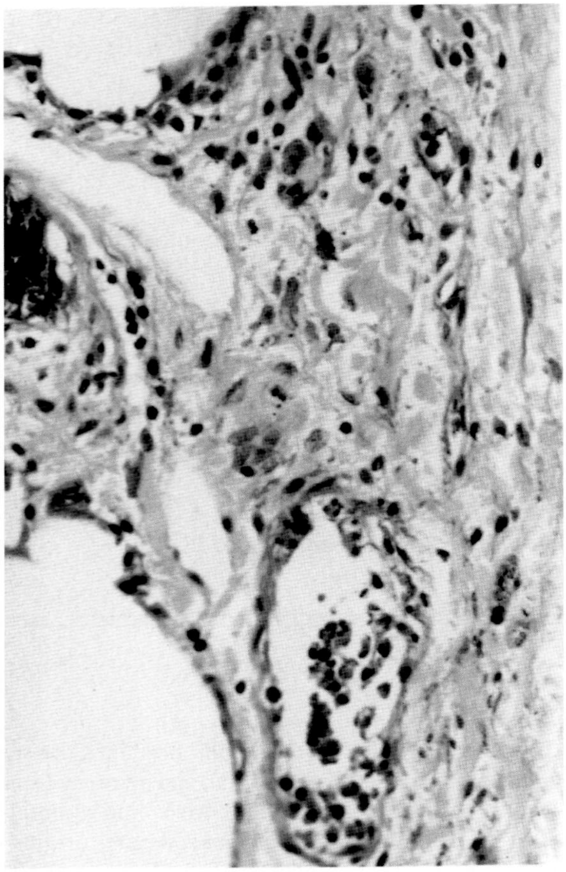

**FIG. 2.** Visceral pleura. Capillaries are prominent. The lymphatics are dilated but deeply placed and entirely invested by the submesothelial layer.

The visceral pleura in humans is thick relative to that seen in some other mammals (3) and is similar to that of horses, cattle, sheep, and pigs (4). The arterial blood supply of the visceral pleura is from the bronchial arteries, and the venous return passes first into the pulmonary veins and then into the left atrium except for certain hilar regions, which are drained by bronchial veins. The lymphatics that pass through the visceral pleura are the superficial layer of pulmonary lymphatics with extensive connections to the peribronchial, perivascular, and interlobular lymphatic spaces and lymphoid tissue (5). Blood and lymphatic vessels are invested by collagen and elastic fibers, which are divided into two layers: an external elastic lamina supporting the mesothelial cells and an internal layer investing the vessels and becoming continuous with the pulmonary interstitium (Figs. 1 and 2). Histologic identification of the layer of elastin has been considered clinically important because the relationship of a primary lung tumor to the visceral pleura helps define the stage of the tumor (6), but elastin may be interrupted in nonneoplastic conditions that scar the pleura. In sheep, and probably in humans, the thickness of the external layer increases in both craniocaudal and ventrodorsal directions (7). The visceral pleura is innervated by branches of the vagus nerves and sympathetic nerve trunks.

The parietal pleura is anatomically and, therefore, functionally different in its histology. Although the single layer of mesothelial cells that lie on the surface of the parietal pleura are cytologically similar to those that form the continuous membrane over the visceral pleura, they are separated from each other by stomata—discontinuities between the mesothelial cells—ranging in size from 2 to 12 um in diameter (8–12). The stomata communicate directly with lymphatic lacunae that are surrounded by bundles of collagen. The lymphatic vessels of the parietal pleura are not connected with the pulmonary lymphatics; they arise on the chest wall and drain into intercostal lymphatics and then into the mediastinum where they are particularly dense along the retrocardiac surface (13–16). Pulmonary fluid and particulate matter are collected in these lymphatics and passed into the mediastinum, where the mesothelium covers collections of macrophages that are designated Kampmeier foci (17,18). The arterial and venous blood supply to the parietal pleura is from the intercostal vessels. The thickness of the fibroelastic layer investing the parietal pleural lymphatics is relatively constant and considerably less than that of most of the visceral pleura, suggesting that it may serve as a membrane across which fluid may diffuse. The parietal pleura is innervated by branches of the intercostal nerves.

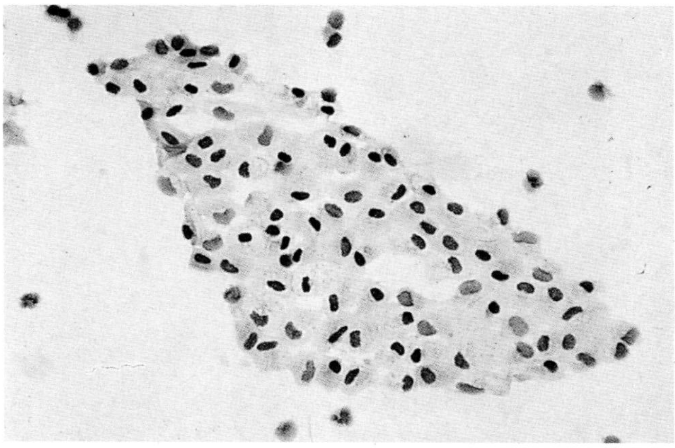

**FIG. 4.** In this peritoneal wash specimen, a sheet of normal mesothelial cells has been washed free.

The structure of the layers of the peritoneum is considered to be similar to that of the pleura (19,20).

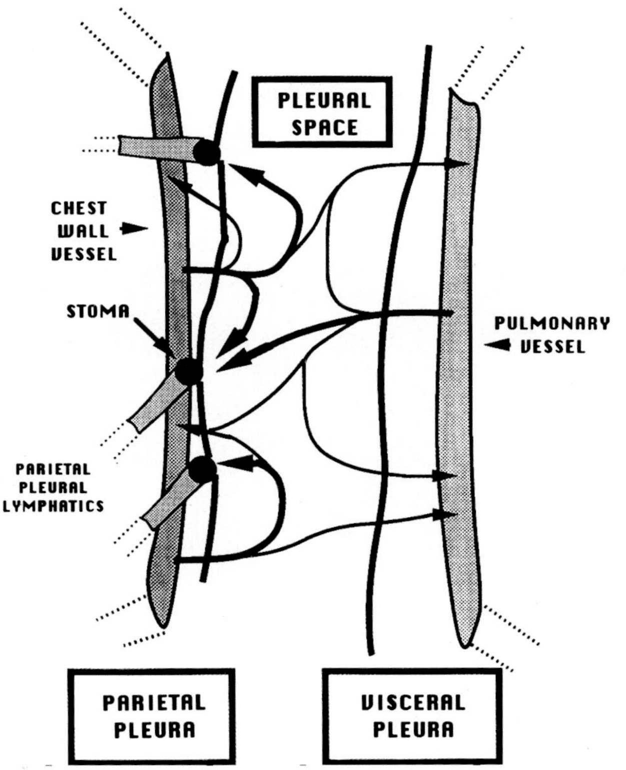


**FIG. 3.** Model of the dynamics of pleural fluid. A transudate of both visceral and parietal capillaries is partly reabsorbed by capillaries and partly diffuses into the pleural space. There it is resorbed, via stomata, into parietal pleural lymphatics.

## FUNCTIONS OF SEROUS MEMBRANES

Multiple functions are served by the serous membranes. The membranes are a selective barrier for fluid and cells. To maximize adherence of visceral and parietal pleurae, so that, for example, the lungs expand as the chest wall expands, a volume of fluid is required that is appropriate for adherence by capillary action, but minimal so that lung capacity is not affected. The elements of the serous membranes regulate this fluid interchange. Control appears to be at the capillary level, as fluid is freely diffusible through mesothelium and submesothelial stroma.

Another level of control results in the relatively low protein content (1.0 to 1.5 g/dl) of pleural fluid. The point of protein regulation is unknown, although speculation is that it is at the level of mesothelial microvilli (21).

In the thoracic cavity, the direction of flow appears to be via diffusion from capillaries of both visceral and parietal pleurae, with resorption primarily through parietal pleural capillaries. Turnover is estimated at 0.7 ml/hr (21) (Fig. 3).

The following structural elements of the serous membranes are responsible for control. Small molecules (less than 4 nm in diameter) diffuse through the intercellular spaces and junctions between mesothelial cells. Larger molecules, up to 50 nm in diameter, are transferred across the mesothelium by pinocytotic uptake and transcellular transport. Larger structures, such as cells in bloody effusions, are transported via the stomata and "crevices." An interesting finding is that mesothelial cells express the secretory component of IgA. This finding was a surprise as IgA transport was thought, by some, to be limited to surfaces that had direct contact with the environment (22).

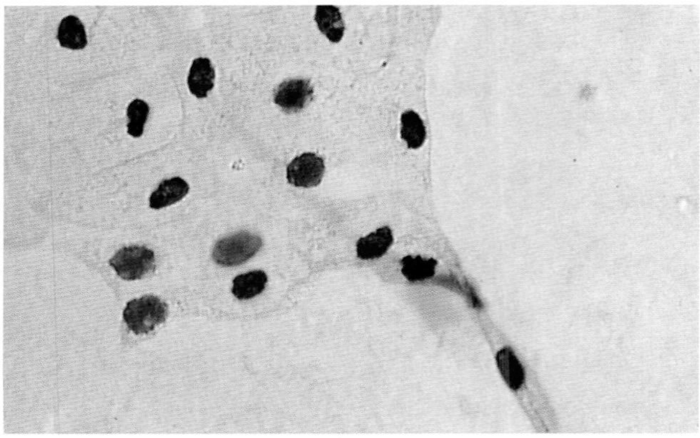

**FIG. 5.** At higher magnification of the sheet of relatively normal mesothelial cells, it is evident that the cells have an abundant and clear cytoplasm, which has crisply defined cell borders. The nuclei are small and centrally placed. The chromatin pattern is homogeneous.

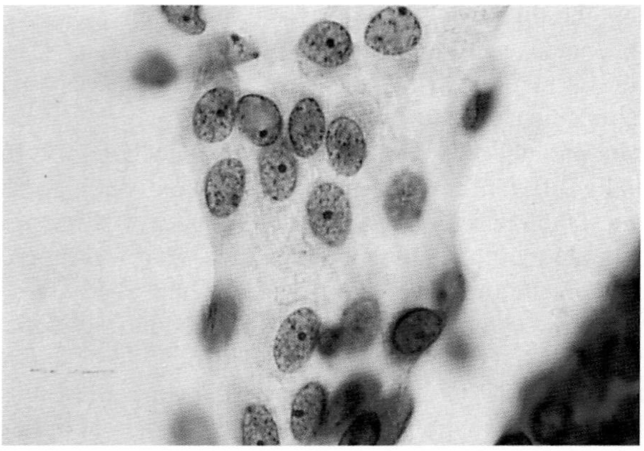

**FIG. 7.** These reactive mesothelial cells from the left side of Fig. 6 retain an abundant cytoplasm, but the nuclei are larger and the chromatin pattern is moving toward a more vesicular pattern. Nucleoli are present but are not prominent.

The submesothelial connective tissue distributes mechanical forces from the pleura uniformly throughout the lungs. Such a redistribution of forces is not required of the abdominal serosa. Both mesothelial cells and fibroblasts contribute to collagen synthesis.

Finally, a function of the glycoprotein-rich pleural fluid is as a lubricant to minimize friction between visceral and parietal pleurae. The site of synthesis and mechanisms of control of the carbohydrate-rich fractions of the pleural fluid are unknown.

## Mesothelial Cells

### *Morphology*

The normal mesothelium is rarely seen in histologic sections but may be evident in cytologic preparations of peritoneal washes taken during a laparotomy (Fig. 4). When visualized in such a case, mesothelial cells have abundant clear cytoplasm with crisply defined cell borders. The nuclei are

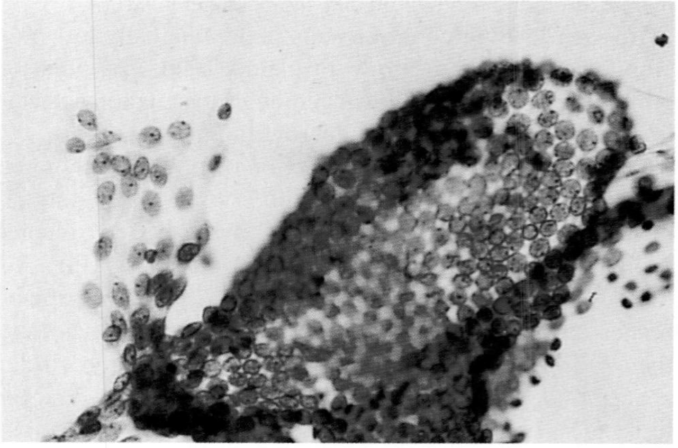

**FIG. 6.** This detached fragment of reactive mesothelium shows an intact mesothelial layer with cells in two phases of the reactive process. The small group of cells on the left are contrasted with those found in the larger group.

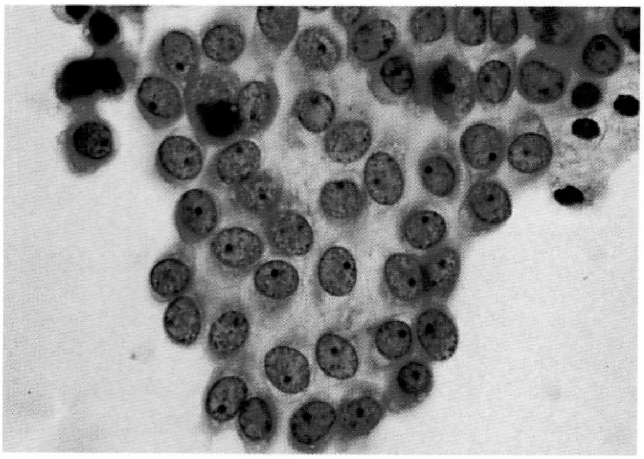

**FIG. 8.** These are the more reactive mesothelial cells from the right side of Fig. 6. The nuclei are larger, the chromatin pattern is more vesicular, and nucleoli are a more prominent feature. Less cytoplasm is present.

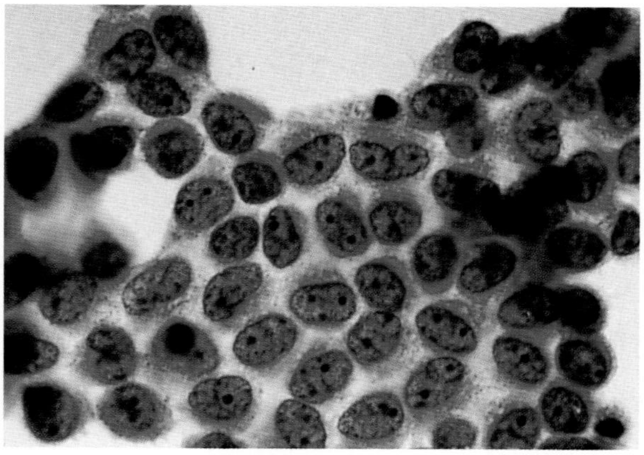

**FIG. 9.** In this more reactive sheet of mesothelial cells, the cytoplasm has grown smaller and the nuclei relatively larger. Irregularity of the chromatin pattern is more prominent.

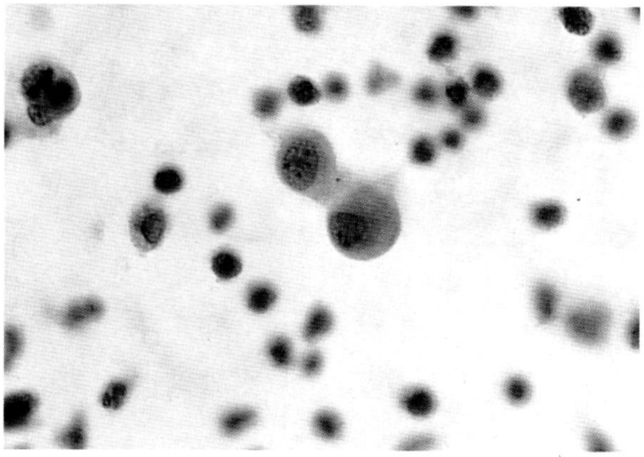

**FIG. 11.** Mesothelial reaction is frequently associated with inflammatory cells. These reactive mesothelial cells are joined in pairs. Each is several times the size of either polys or lymphocytes.

small and centrally placed with a homogeneous chromatin pattern usually without a nucleolus (Fig. 5).

In a variety of reactive processes, the mesothelial cells may undergo markedly proliferative and hyperplastic changes. A relatively abundant cytoplasm is maintained, but the cell borders are less sharply defined. The nuclei are larger, both absolutely and relatively, and the chromatin pattern is more hyperchromatic. Nucleoli are often present and may become prominent (Figs. 6–9).

As the hyperplastic changes in the reactive mesothelial cells progress, cell groups become smaller, with individual cells predominating. When clustered, reactive mesothelial cells present an irregular outside border. The nucleus, and especially the nucleolus, may enlarge dramatically but the nuclei are similar in size, shape, and pattern from cell to cell. Mitotic figures may be seen. The cytoplasm may become multivacuolated as the cells degenerate and imbibe fluid (Figs. 10–18).

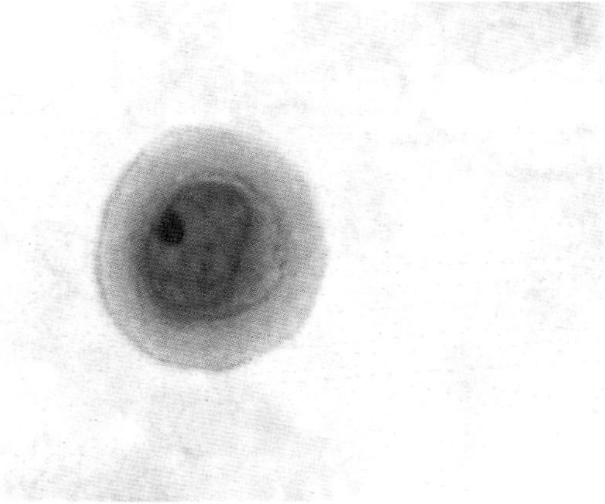

**FIG. 10.** This individual reactive mesothelial cell has a restricted amount of cytoplasm and a relatively large nucleus with a nucleolus. The cytoplasm is divided into an inner denser layer and an outer less dense layer. By electron microscopy the inner denser layer corresponds to the presence of intermediate filaments with the characteristics of keratin (see Fig. 25). The cell border is highly irregular, suggesting the presence of the numerous elongated microvilli, which are evident on electron microscopy (see Fig. 24).

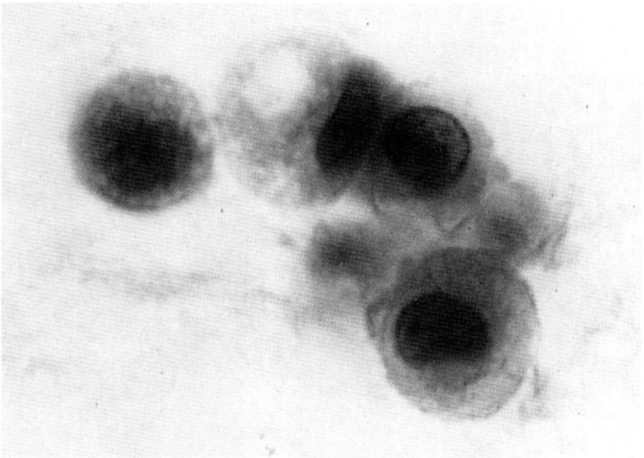

**FIG. 12.** These reactive mesothelial cells are loosely joined together. The uppermost cell has a vacuole in the cytoplasm, which may represent either a vesicle or an intracytoplasmic lumen.

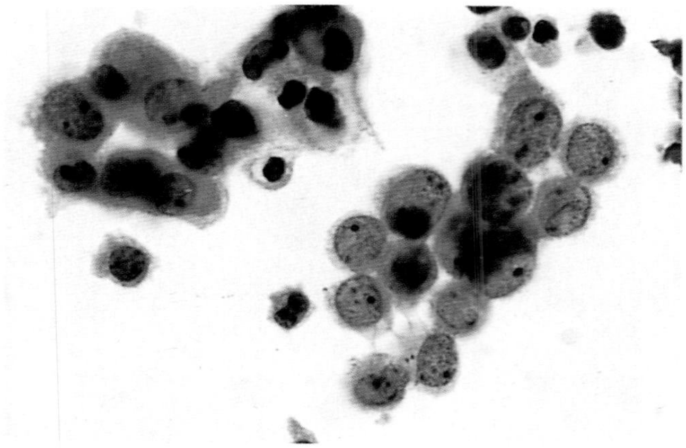

**FIG. 13.** When reactive mesothelial cells are in groups, an irregular or "knobby" outside border is formed.

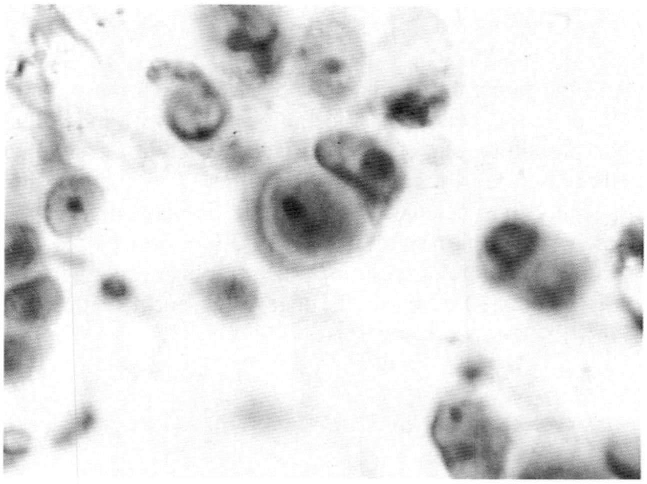

**FIG. 14.** Occasionally, very reactive mesothelial cells may show cellular interactions similar to that of a keratin pearl.

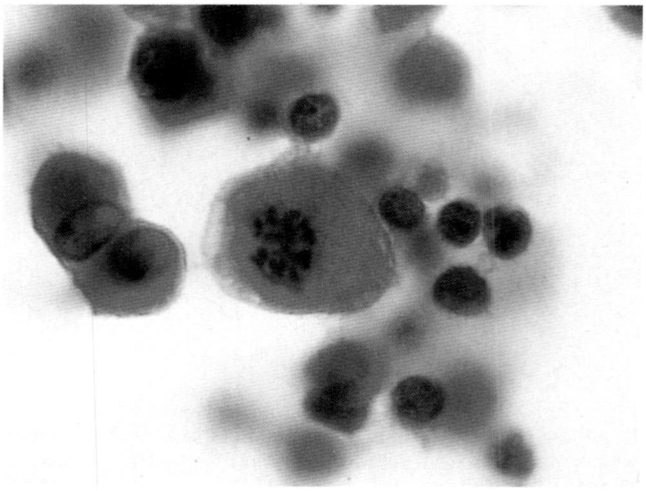

**FIG. 15.** Mitotic figures may be seen in the proliferating cells of reactive mesothelium.

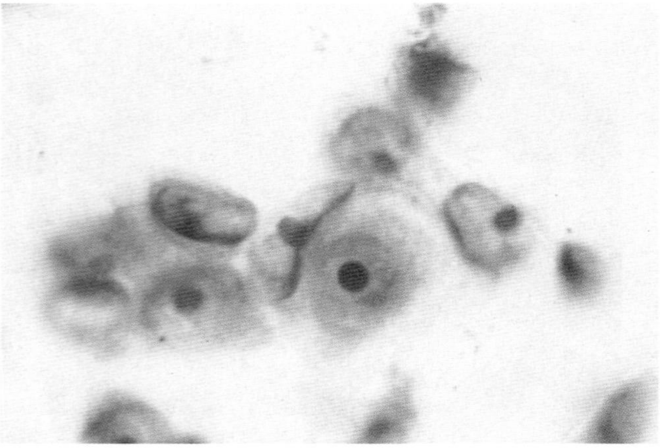

**FIG. 16.** Markedly reactive mesothelial cells may show large vesicular nuclei with a prominent nucleolus.

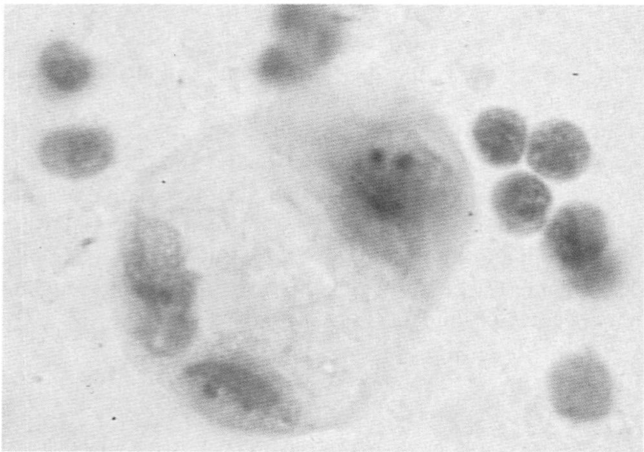

**FIG. 17.** Reactive mesothelial cells may degenerate and enlarge markedly. These three cells have both abundant multivacuolated cytoplasm and the large nuclei of the reactive mesothelial cells.

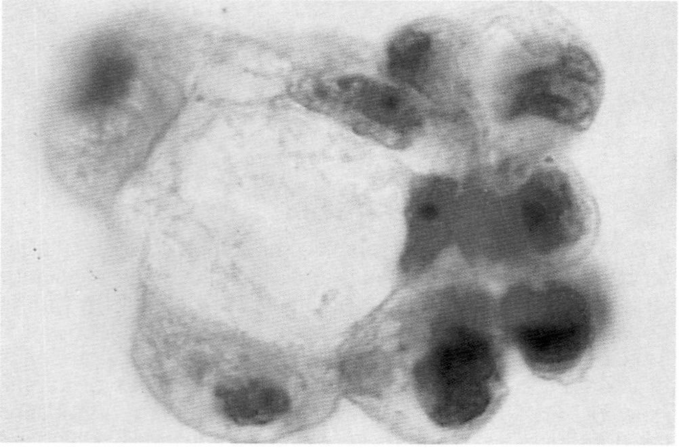

**FIG. 18.** When the markedly reactive mesothelial cells form irregular groups and are combined with degenerating forms, they may simulate a mucin-producing adenocarcinoma.

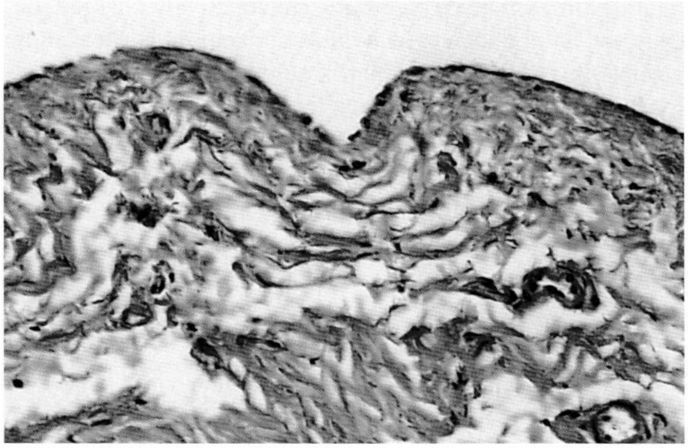

**FIG. 19.** Alcian blue stain of serosal membrane. Note staining of both mesothelium and of the matrix proteins, which contain abundant acid mucoproteins.

### *Histochemistry*

Histochemical stains have provided information about mucoprotein content of the mesothelium. Negativity for the periodic acid-Schiff (PAS) reaction is evidence that mesothelial cells lack significant quantities of neutral mucoproteins. In contrast, positivity for histochemical stains that detect negative groups, such as the positively charged dye alcian blue, is evidence of acid mucoproteins. That the intensity of staining reactions for acid mucosubstances is diminished by preincubating the tissue sections in hyaluronidase is evidence that at least some of the terminal hexose groups of the mucosubstances are either hyaluronic acid or chondroitin sulfate (Fig. 19). Furthermore, the fact that histochemical mucin is decreased, but not abolished, by incubating cells in neuraminidase prior to histochemical staining is evidence that some of the terminal carbohydrate groups are sialated (23). McDougall et al (24) have documented that neoplastic mesothelial cells may stain with mucicarmine.

The types of terminal carbohydrate groups of membrane proteins and lipids can also be characterized with lectins, which have specific and discrete ranges of sugar group affinities. Although little lectin histochemistry has been done with the mesothelium, concanavalin A mesothelial cell reactivity indicates the presence of terminal groups that are either alpha-mannose or alpha-glucose.

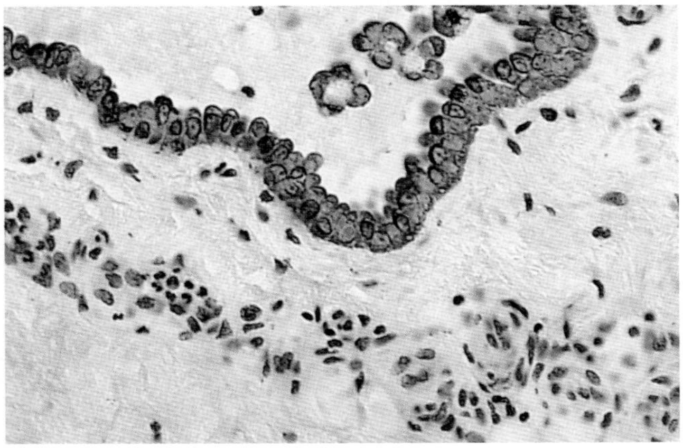

**FIG. 20.** Keratin expression by mesothelium and by detached mesothelial cells, defined by a mixture of monoclonal anti-keratin antibodies. Note that the pattern of staining is similar to the distribution of intermediate filaments, defined at the ultrastructural level.

### *Immunohistochemistry*

The mesothelial cell antigens that have been most studied include the membrane-associated glycoproteins, particularly carcinoembryonic antigen (CEA) and epithelial membrane antigen (EMA), and intermediate filaments. Virtually no significant expression of either CEA or EMA by mesothelial cells has been found. The expression of intermediate filaments, however, is quite interesting. Nonproliferating mesothelial cells express both vimentin and a variety of keratins (K7 of 55 kDa, K8 of 53 kDa, K18 of 44 kDa, and K19 of 40 kDa) that can be detected with monoclonal antibodies immunoreactive with the small, acidic, type I keratins (25). Mesothelium does not express keratin 20, using monoclonal antibodies (26). These keratins are distinct from those of epithelia, including the epidermis, glandular epithelia, and transitional epithelium (27). Of interest, ovarian epithelial tumors express a spectrum of keratins similar to the mesothelium. This phenomenon supports the putative mesothelial origin that some investigators have claimed for these tumors (27). The plasticity of the immunphenotype of mesothelial cells is demonstrable in abnormal states. Although mesothelium normally lacks sex steroid receptors, the reactive mesothelium adjacent to endometriosis expresses focal immunoreactivity for estrogen and progesterone receptors (28). Furthermore, reactive mesothelial cells can express the muscle cell cytoskeleton proteins desmin and muscle-specific actin (29).

There is experimental evidence that the pattern of intermediate filament expression by mesothelial cells is dependent on shape and cell-cell interaction. Induction of a spindle morphology inhibits keratin synthesis. In contrast, induction of an epithelioid morphology, for example, with retinoids, stimulates keratin synthesis and inhibits vimentin synthesis; the ability of cells to respond in this manner also depends on the presence of cell-cell interaction (30). The pattern of intermediate filament expression by intact mesothelium has not been analyzed in such detail (Figs. 20 and 21).

Mesothelial cells lack the determinant detected by Leu M1 (CD15) (31–34) but express that detected by HAM 56 (28) (Fig. 22). BER-EP4 was reported by Latza et al (35) and Sheibani et al. (36) to distinguish malignant epithelium (adenocarcinoma) from malignant mesothelioma, but Gaffey et al. (37), and Otis (38) reported BER-EP4 immunoreactivity in high proportions of both benign and malignant mesothe-

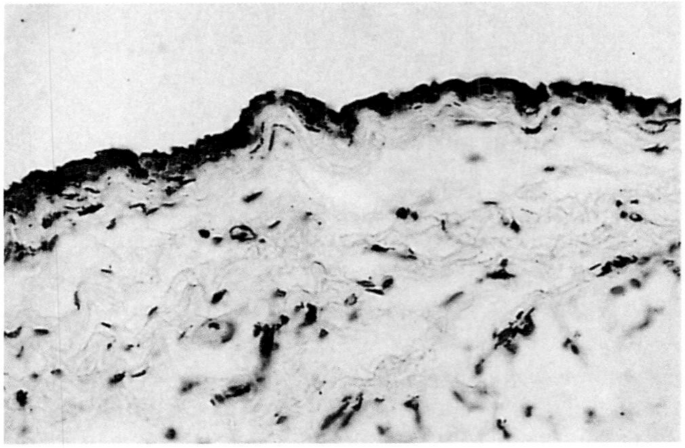

**FIG. 21.** Vimentin immunoreactivity of mesothelial cells and fibroblasts.

lial tumors as well as adenocarcinomas. CEA and CD15 remain the most useful pair of antibodies for demonstrating that epithelium is of epithelial (carcinomatous) rather than mesothelial origin. The identity of the determinants for these antibodies is not yet known.

### Ultrastructure

The most prominent feature is the presence of numerous long microvilli (Figs. 23 and 24). These microvilli measure up to 3 um in length and 0.1 um in diameter. There is heterogeneity in the nature of microvilli. They are more numerous in caudal portions of the pleura and in the visceral pleura.

The other organelles found in mesothelial cells are not specific for them. Junctions of all types are found—tight junctions that serve as a barrier to certain molecules, gap junctions for cell-cell transport, and desmosomes for cell-cell adherence. Intermediate filaments are somewhat prominent; although they do not aggregate into bundles, they are often arranged in a perinuclear, circumferential distribution (Figs. 25 and 26).

### Submesothelial Layer

Normally, the submesothelial layer contains few cells; most of these are fibroblasts. Much of the submesothelial layer is composed of collagen, elastin, and other extracellular proteins. During reactive processes, the submesothelial layer may become much more prominent as cells proliferate there.

#### *Histochemistry*

The main constituents of the submesothelial tissue are glycosylated proteins, including glycosaminoglycans. As the majority of carbohydrate groups are negatively charged, because of an abundance of hyaluronic acid and other acidic groups, this extracellular matrix stains in a manner characteristic of acidic mucoproteins; that is, it is alcian blue positive (Fig. 19). That staining intensity can be diminished by treating the section with hyaluronidase before histochemical staining is evidence that hyaluronic acid groups are responsible, in large part, for the intensity of staining (21).

#### *Immunohistochemistry*

The antigens of the submesothelial layer can be categorized into matrix constituents and antigens of the mesenchymal cells. The extracellular matrix materials are those typical of most connective tissue. Types I and III collagen and fibronectin are abundant. Elastin fibers are plentiful and basement membrane proteins, including type IV collagen and laminin, are found at the mesothelial cell-stromal interface.

Although proteoglycans are plentiful, they have not been immunohistochemically localized since antibodies to either the core proteins or the carbohydrate groups have not yet been generated and/or applied.

The pattern of intermediate filament expression by the submesothelial stromal cells varies with their state of "excitation." Quiescent cells contain only vimentin. In contrast, those stromal cells in regions of injury or inflammation also synthesize keratin, which is detectable with antibodies to type I keratins (30) (Fig. 27).

## RELATIONSHIP OF MESOTHELIAL AND SUBMESOTHELIAL CELLS

The submesothelial mesenchymal cell population serves as the anchoring substratum for the mesothelium. Both

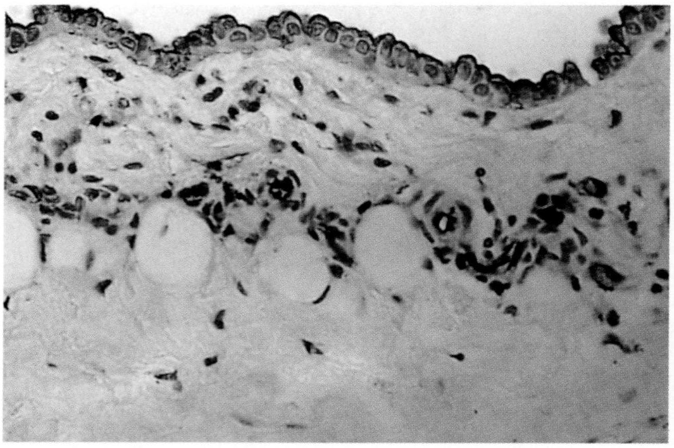

**FIG. 22.** HAM 56 staining of mesothelial cells. Note the apical localization of reaction product. Endothelial cells also stain.

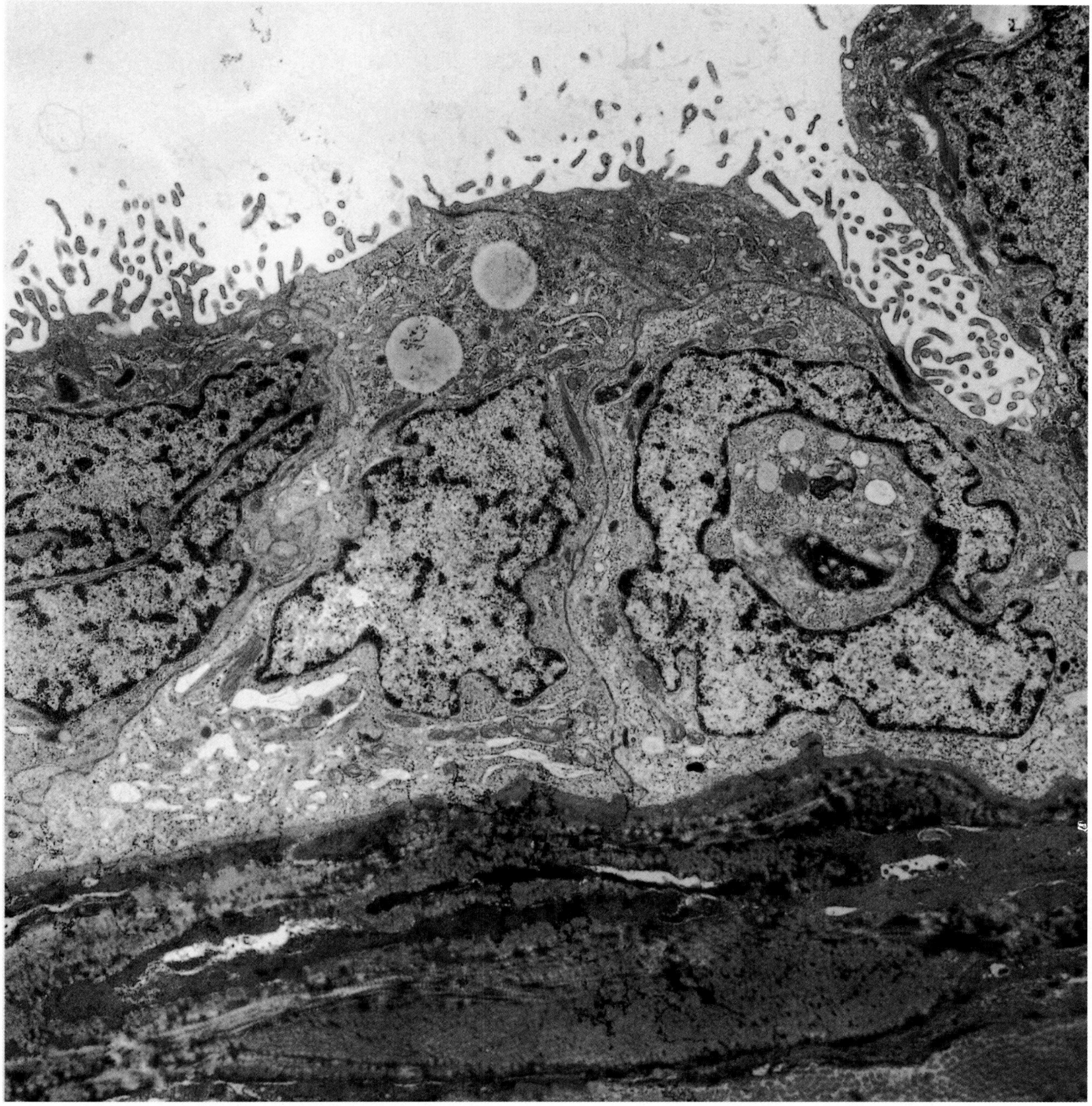

**FIG. 23.** Mesothelial cells, with prominent microvilli, cover the surface of the serosa. The subjacent stroma is composed of collagen and fibroblasts.

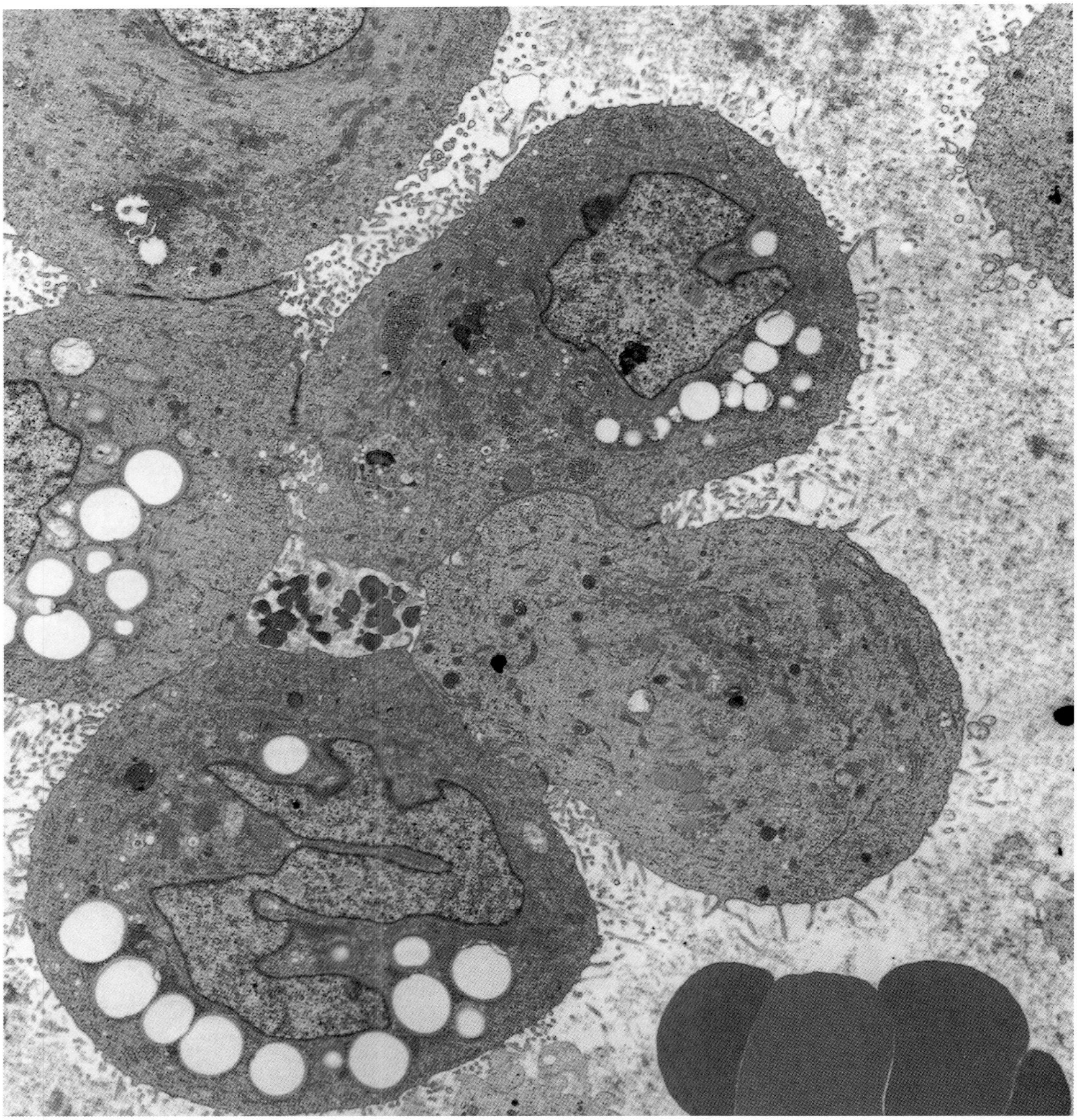

**FIG. 24.** A cluster of detached mesothelial cells within a pleural effusion. Cytoplasmic lipid droplets impart a vacuolated appearance to some cells. Note the long microvilli, which impart the "fuzzy" appearance to these cells at the light microscopic level.

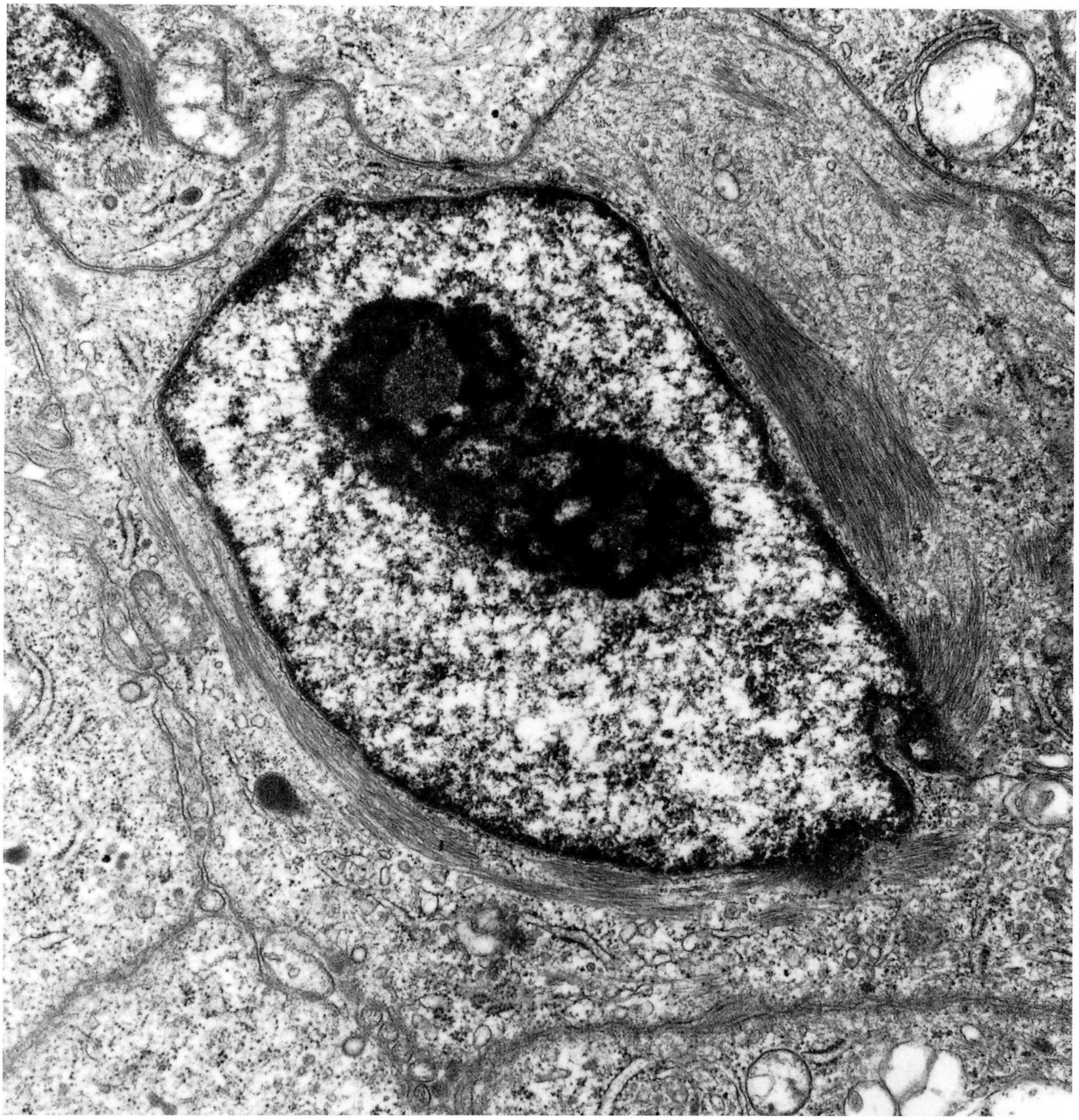

**FIG. 25.** Ultrastructure of a mesothelial cell. Intermediate filaments are arranged in a perinuclear distribution.

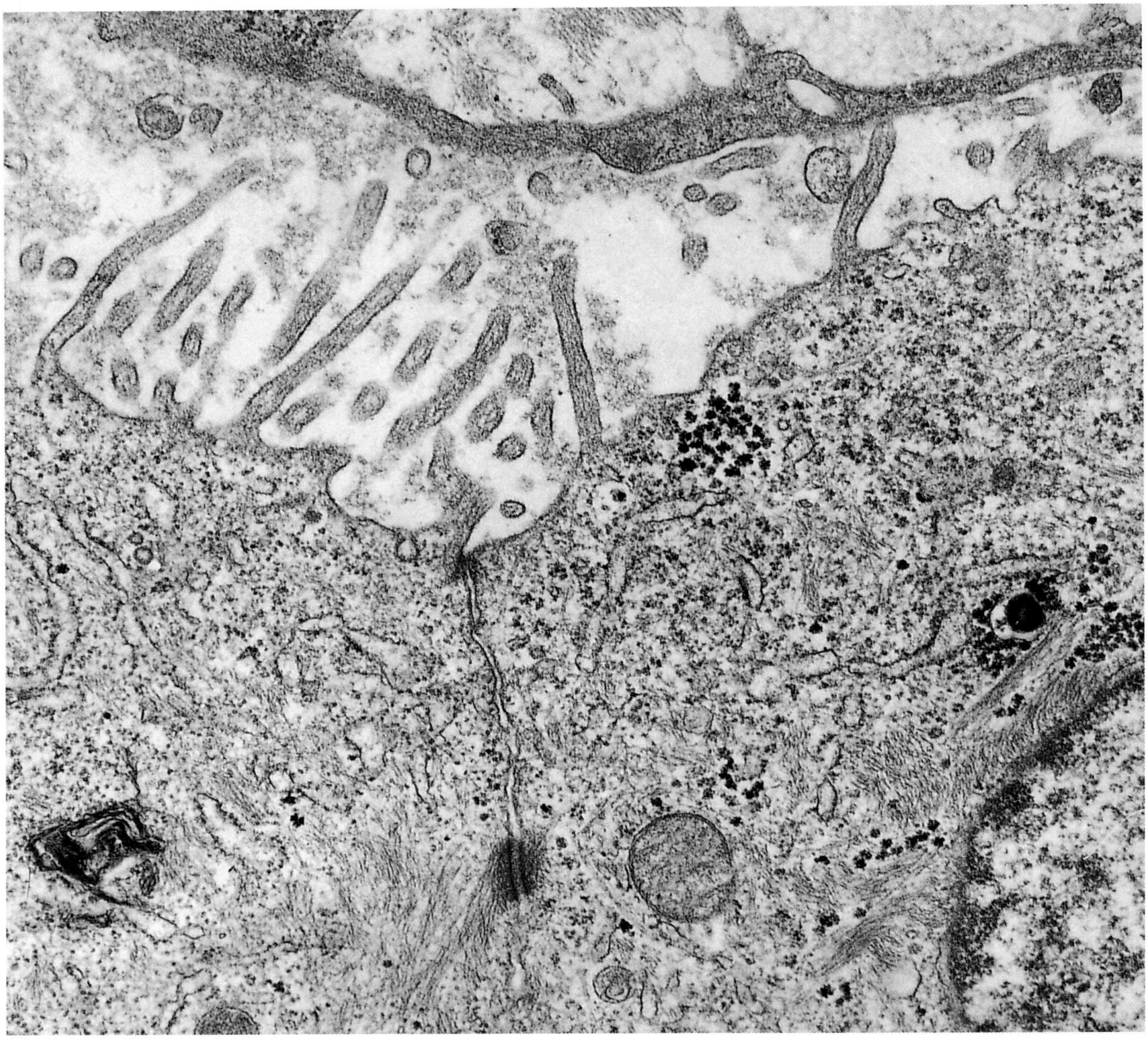

**FIG. 26.** High magnification of the luminal aspect of two mesothelial cells. Note the small tight junction, subjacent desmosome, and the cytoskeletal filaments within the microvilli.

mesothelial and submesothelial cells contribute to the extracellular proteins that comprise the matrix. Up to 3% of the total protein synthesized by mesothelial cells are collagens and laminin.

A controversial topic is whether submesothelial cells serve as a source of mesothelial cell renewal, either in normal development, which is the basis for regarding mesothelial cells as mesodermal in origin, or in conditions of rapid mesothelial cell turnover. Earlier ultrastructural and kinetics studies, using thymidine incorporation, suggested that the stromal cells contribute to the repopulation of denuded mesothelium (39,40). Consistent with this scheme is the observation that submesothelial cells, when stimulated to proliferate, synthesize keratin and assume a more epithelioid morphology. However, later studies have demonstrated that healing of injured serosa progresses by multiplication and migration of mesothelial cells at the edges of the wounded area (41).

The capacity for mesothelial and submesothelial cellular elements of serous membranes to proliferate, producing morphologic patterns mimicking neoplasia, is well known and frequently a source of diagnostic confusion (42,43). The

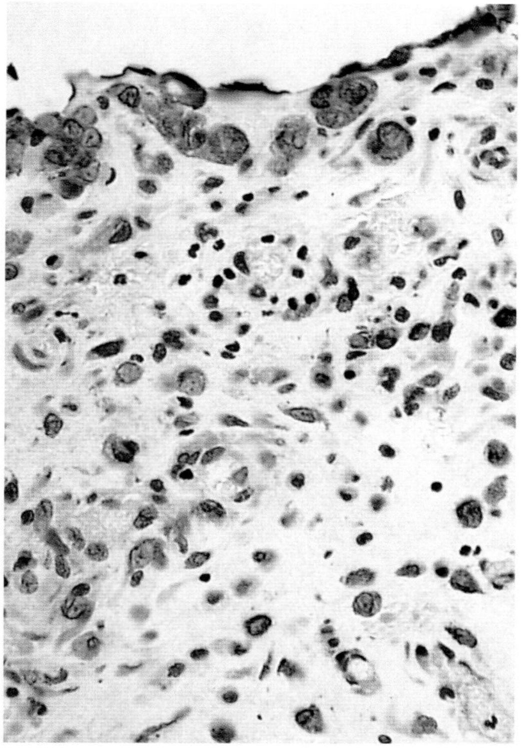

FIG. 27. Keratin immunoreactivity of proliferating submesothelial spindle cells.

process may be diffuse or localized (Fig. 28). The stimuli may be known in many instances (usually sustained trauma or irritation) or they may be unknown.

Mesothelial hyperplasia in herniorrhaphy specimens is well described (44). The hyperplasia may be nodular, may

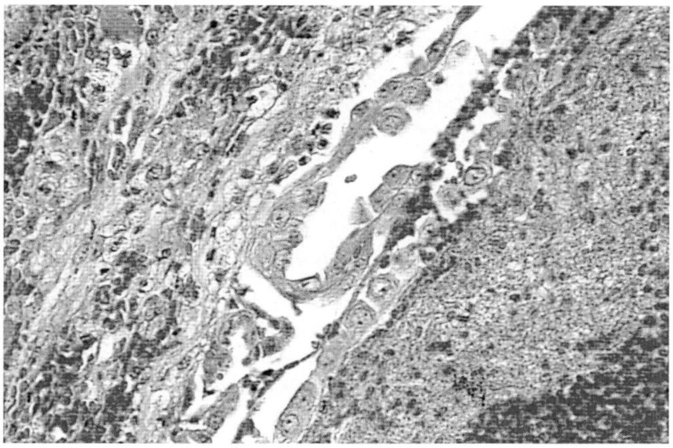

FIG. 28. In a variety of reactive processes, the mesothelial cells lining the surface of either the pleura or the peritoneum, undergo a markedly proliferative and hyperplastic change. This is a section through the pleura of a patient with severe active rheumatoid arthritis.

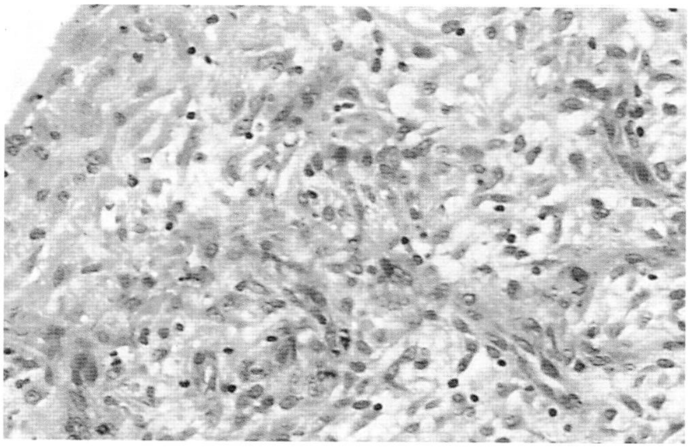

FIG. 29. This photomicrograph is from the mesothelium of a hernia sac of an 18-month-old boy. The reaction of the mesothelium is composed of a proliferation of epithelioid cells on the surface and of subjacent spindle-shaped cells that give the impression of proliferating fibroblasts.

demonstrate nuclear atypia and frequent mitotic figures, and may be accompanied by spindle cell elements (Figs. 29 and 30).

Reactive mesothelial cells in mediastinal lymph nodes have been reported by Brooks et al (45), although the mechanisms by which they enter lymphatics and survive in the sinuses of nodes are not known. This rare event may produce a difficult differential diagnosis. Clear demonstration of the mesothelial nature of these cells is necessary to exclude the much more commonly seen metastatic carcinoma. Having shown that the cells are mesothelial by electron microscopy or immunohistochemistry, it should be noted that Sussman and Rosai (46) showed that mesothelioma may present as a lymph node metastasis . Frequently, follow-up time is required to make the distinction between reactive benign mesothelial cells and metastatic malignant ones. See Figures 31 and 32.

An uncommon manifestation of mesothelial proliferation is the psammoma body. As a laminated calcific structure, it most likely arises through concentric calcification following cell death. The presence of psammoma bodies is usually nonspecific, since they may be observed in inflammatory processes accompanied by mesothelial hyperplasia, malignant mesothelial neoplasia, or epithelial neoplasia (Fig. 33). The significance of psammoma bodies depends on the setting in which they are observed.

Epithelial elements may be observed in glandular arrangements throughout the peritoneum, omentum, and within lymph nodes. Such glandular structures were recognized in the early 1900s and misinterpreted by some as metastatic carcinoma, a mistake that is unfortunately still committed today. These entities of endometriosis and endosalpingosis were expounded on by Sampson (47–49) earlier

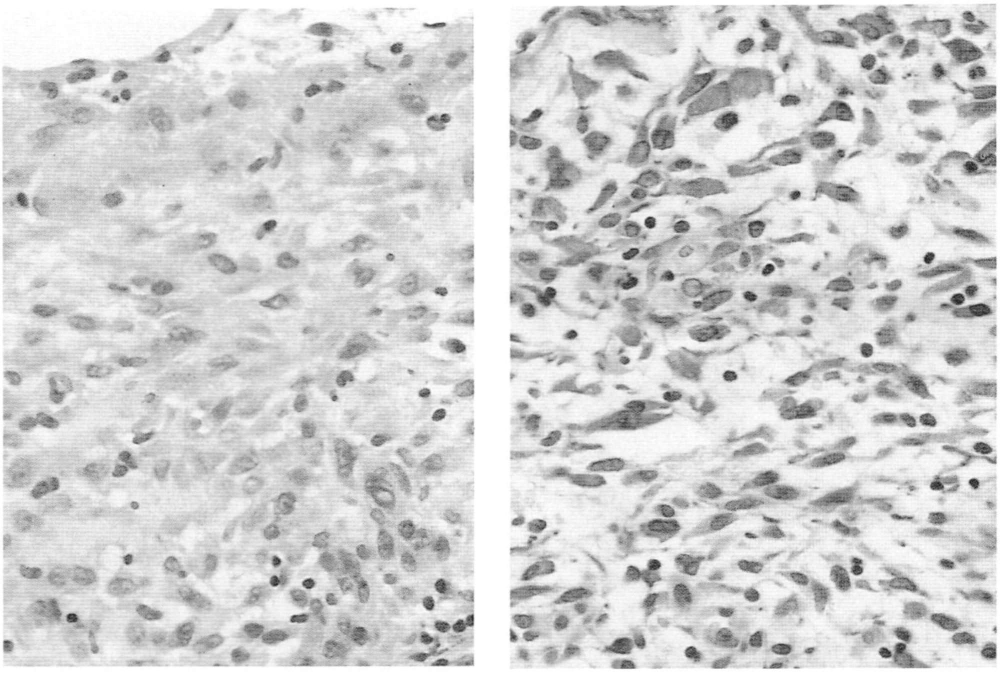

**FIG. 30.** The reactive peritoneum in the hernia sac shown in Fig. 29 is on the left. On the right is the immunohistochemical stain for keratin (AE1-AE3), which illustrates that both the surface lining mesothelial cells and the subjacent spindle-shaped cells are heavily decorated.

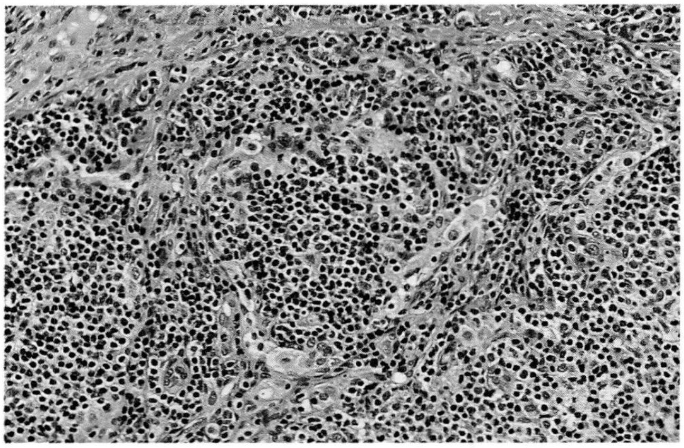

**FIG. 31.** Internal mammary lymph node found during coronary artery bypass surgery in a 61-year-old man with a monoclonal gammopathy and a lymphoproliferative disorder; but there is no evidence of a pleural lesion. Ascites was present but considered secondary to congestive heart failure and diminished after heart surgery. Note the large cells occurring singly and in small groups in the sinusoids.

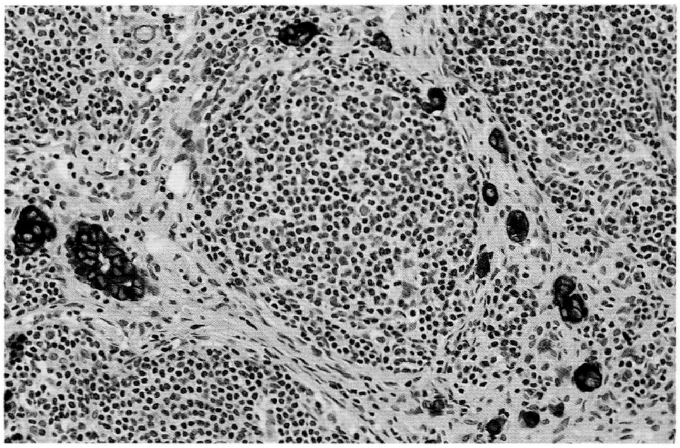

**FIG. 32.** A stain for Keratin (AE1-AE3) demonstrated the cells shown in Fig. 31. Stains for CEA, LeuM1, BER-EP4 and B72.3 were negative, consistent with mesothelial cell differentiation. Follow-up is brief and inconclusive.

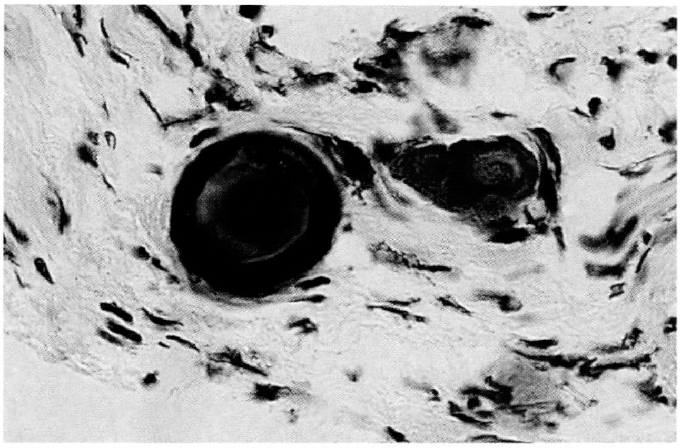

**FIG. 33.** Psammoma bodies in the left pelvic peritoneum of a 58-year-old woman.

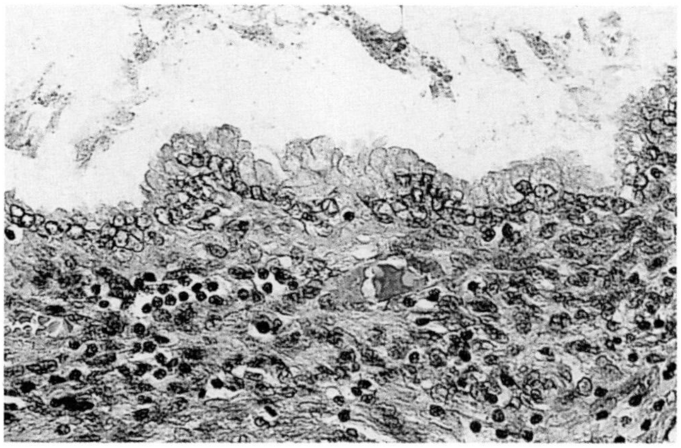

**FIG. 35.** Endosalpingosis involving the omentum contains cystic glands lined by mucinous epithelium with basally oriented nuclei and apical cytoplasm. Periglandular stroma contains chronic mononuclear inflammatory cells.

in this century, with reference to mechanisms of pathogenesis that are still debatable.

Endosalpingosis refers to glandular spaces lined by epithelium similar to fallopian tube epithelium, with three cell types (ciliated, secretory, and intercalated cells) (50) (Fig. 34). On occasion, psammoma bodies are present. Periglandular stroma containing chronic inflammatory cells is separated from epithelium by PAS-positive basement membrane. Endosalpingosis may be differentiated from endometriosis by the lack of endometrial stroma or evidence of stromal hemorrhage associated with endometriosis (47,50–53). This condition is seen exclusively in women and has been reported in 12.5% of omenta removed at surgery in females. A large proportion of these women have coexisting benign disease of the fallopian tube (50). The origin of the glandular inclusions is debated but is most likely either related to the influence of müllerian development on the peritoneal mesothelium (coelomic lining) or is a sequela of disease within the fallopian tube resulting in extratubal growth of displaced tubal epithelium (50,52). Although definitive evidence of neoplasia arising in endosalpingosis has not been documented (54), considerable difficulty may be encountered when differentiating extraovarian tumor implants removed in the setting of common epithelial ovarian tumors from endosalpingiosis with cellular atypia. Evaluation of the severity of epithelial atypia, mitotic activity, the presence of ciliated cells, and the presence of invasive characteristics may aid in establishing malignancy in this setting (50). Metaplasia in endosalpingosis may also be a source of diagnostic difficulty, particularly mucinous metaplasia, which may be mistaken for metastatic mucinous adenocarcinoma (Figs. 35 and 36).

Endometriosis may be defined by the presence of glands lined by endometrial-type epithelium surrounded by endometrial stroma, outside the uterine endometrial mucosa and myometrium (54). The condition occurs most frequently in women of childbearing age. It may occur in a variety of body sites ranging from the pelvic peritoneum to distant organs

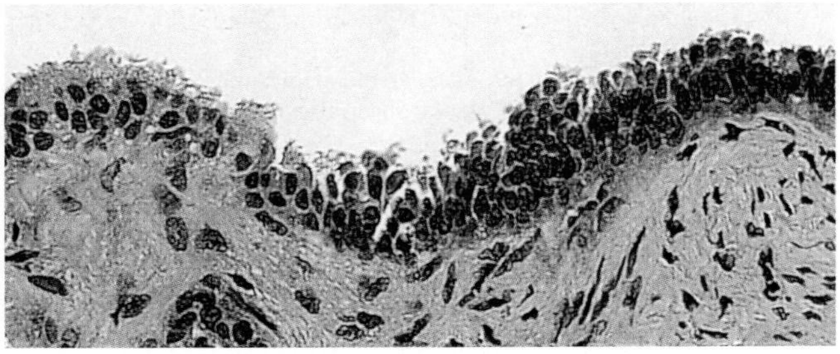

**FIG. 34.** Endosalpingosis involving the serosa of the uterus of a 56-year-old woman. Serous, intercalated, and occasional ciliated cells are present. Endometrial stroma is not present.

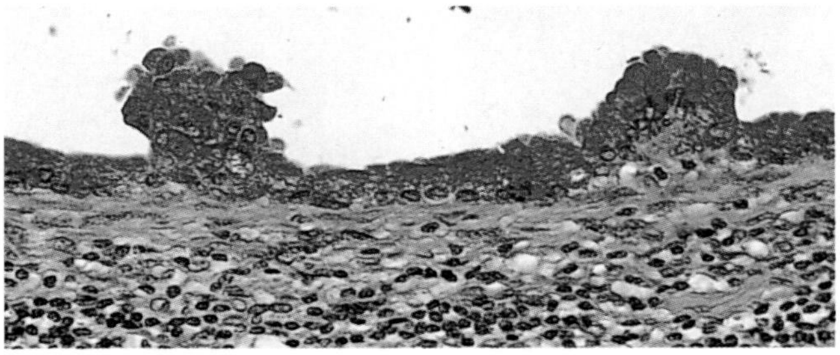

**FIG. 36.** Mucicarmine stain of mucinous change in endosalpingosis demonstrates intracytoplasmic mucin in apical cytoplasm.

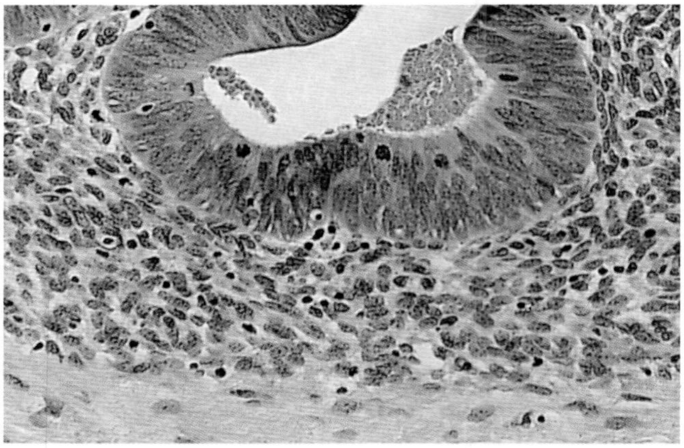

**FIG. 37.** Endometriosis involving the peritoneum with extension into the soft tissue of the anterior abdominal wall of a 23-year-old woman. Both endometrial glands and stroma are present.

such as lung, kidney, and skin. The most frequent site is the peritoneal lining of the pelvic organs (Fig. 37). Although the histogenesis of endometriosis remains unclear, two general theories have been proposed. The ectopic growth of endometrial elements may result from displacement of endometrial tissue, whether through local means such as entry of endometrium into the pelvis through the fallopian tubes or via vascular routes to distant organs (47,48). Another possibility includes metaplastic change of the pelvic peritoneum along müllerian lines of differentiation (55,56). Each mechanism may play a role in the histogenesis of endometriosis.

Endometriosis may appear as brown-maroon foci on the peritoneal surfaces and be accompanied by fibrosis or adhesions. Microscopically, endometrial stroma surrounding endometrial epithelium is present (47). Response to hormonal influences is often seen and may be synchronous with intrauterine endometrium. Metaplasia occurs in both epithelial elements and stromal elements, similar to metaplasias encountered in the endometrium of the uterus. The presence of hemosiderin-laden macrophages and fibrosis may be the only evidence that endometriosis had once been present. However, a definitive diagnosis of endometriosis may not be rendered unless both endometrial glands and stroma are seen.

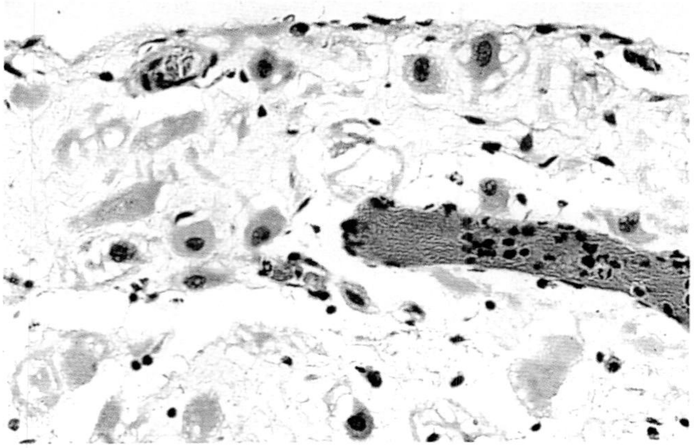

**FIG. 38.** Decidual change in the pelvis during pregnancy is seen in subserosal tissue. Loosely cohesive cells with abundant eosinophilic cytoplasm are present.

The metaplastic potential of a serosal surface is impressive. A common type of metaplasia, more frequently observed in pregnant than in nonpregnant women, is decidual change. Although usually encountered in the submesothelial layer of pelvic peritoneal surfaces, decidual change may be seen in distant sites including the serosal surfaces of the liver, spleen, diaphragm, and within lymph nodes. In these locations, decidual change may be mistaken for metastatic carcinoma or malignant mesothelioma (Fig. 38) (56).

## REFERENCES


1. Sahn SA. State of the art: The pleura. *Am Rev Respir Dis* 1988;138: 184–234.
2. Pistolesi M, Miniati M, Giuntini C. Pleural liquid and solute exchanges. *Am Rev Respir Dis* 1989;140:825–847.
3. Courtice FC, Simmonds WJ. Absorption of fluids from the pleura cavities of rabbits and cats. *J Physiol (*Lond) 1949;109:117–130.
4. Albertine KH, Wiener-Kronish JP, Roos PJ, Staub NC. Structure, blood supply and lymphatic vessels of the sheep s visceral pleura. *Am J Anat* 1982:165:227–294.
5. Grant T, Levin B. Lymphangiographic visualization of pleural and pulmonary lymphatics in a patient without a chylothorax. *Radiology* 1974;113:49–50.
6. Gallagher B, Urbanski SJ. The significance of pleural elastica invasion by lung carcinomas. *Hum Pathol* 1990;21:512–517.
7. Mariassy AT, Wheeldon EB. The pleura: a combined light microscopic scanning and transmission electron microscopic study in the sheep. I. Normal pleura. *Exp Lung Res* 1983;4:293–314.
8. Albertine KM, Wiener-Kronish JP, Staub NC. The structure of the parietal pleura and its relationship to pleural liquid dynamics in sheep. *Anat Rec* 1984;208:401–409.
9. Leak LV. Gross and ultrastructural morphologic features of the diaphragm. *Am Rev Respir Dis* 1979;119:S3–S21.
10. Wang NS. The preformed stomas connecting the pleural cavity and the lymphatics in the parietal pleura. *Am Rev Respir Dis* 1975;111:12–20.
11. Wang NS. Morphological data of pleura. Normal conditions. In: Chretien J, Hirsch A, eds. *Diseases of the pleura.* New York; Masson, 1983:10–24.
12. Wang NS. Anatomy and physiology of the pleura space. *Clin Chest Med* 1985;6:3–16.
13. Bernaudin JF, Fleury J. Anatomy of the blood and lymphatic circulation of the pleural serosa. In: Chretien J, Bignon J, Hirsch A, eds. *The pleura in health and disease.* New York; Marcel Dekker, 1985: 101–124.
14. Cooray GH. Defense mechanisms in the mediastinum with special reference to the mechanics of pleural absorption. *J Pathol Bacteriol* 1949; 6:551–567.
15. Courtice FC, Simmonds WJ. Physiological significance of lymph drainage of the serous cavities and lungs. *Physiol Rev* 1954;34: 419–448.
16. Staub NC, Wiener O, Kronish JP, Albertine KH. Transport through the pleura. Physiology of normal liquid and solute exchange in the pleura space. In: Chretien J, Bignon J, Hirsch A, eds. *The pleura in health and disease.* New York; Marcel Dekker, 1985:169–193.
17. Kampmeier OF. Concerning certain mesothelial thickenings and vascular plexuses of the mediastinal pleura associated with histiocyte and fat cell production. *Anat Rec* 1928;39:201–214.
18. Mixter RL. On macrophageal foci (Milky spots) in the pleura of different mammals, including man. *Am J Anat* 1941;69:159–186.
19. Nagel W. Kischinsky W. Study of the permeability of the isolated dog mesentery. *Eur J Clin Invest* 1970:1:149–154.

20. Tslibari E, Wissig SL. Lymphatic absorption from the peritoneal cavity: regulation of patency of mesothelioma stomata. *Microvasc Res* 1983;25:22039.
21. Chretien J, Bignon J, Hirsch A, eds. *The pleura in health and disease.* New York; Marcel Dekker, 1985:30.
22. Ernst CS, Brooks JJ. Immunoperoxidase localization of secretory component in reactive mesothelium and mesotheliomas. *J Histochem Cytochem* 1981;29:1102–1104.
23. Roth J. Ultrahistochemical demonstration of saccharide components of complex carbohydrates at the alveolar cell surface and at the mesothelial cell surface of the pleura visceralis of mice by means of concanavalin. *A Exp Pathol* 1973;8:S157–S167.
24. McDougall DB, et al. Mucin-positive epithelial mesothelioma. *Arch Pathol Lab Med* 1992;116:874–883.
25. Wu Y-J, Parker LM, Binder NE. The mesothelial keratins: a new family of cytoskeletal proteins identified in cultured mesothelial cells and nonkeratinizing epithelia. *Cell* 1982;31:693–703.
26. Moll R, Lowe A, Laufer J, Franke WW. Cytokeratin 20 in human carcinomas. A new histodiagnostic marker detected by monoclonal antibodies. *Am J Pathol* 1992;140:427–447.
27. Moll R, Franke W, Schiller DL, Geiger B, Krepler R. The catalog of human cytokeratins: Patterns of expression in normal epithelia, tumors and cultured cells. *Cell* 1982;31:11–24.
28. Nakayama K, Masuzawa H, Li S. Immunohistochemical anaylsis of the peritoneum adjacent to endometriotic lesions using antibodies for Ber-EP4 antigen, estrogen receptors, and progesterone receptors: implication of peritoneal metaplasia in the pathogenesis of endometriosis. *Int J Gynecol Pathol* 1994;13:348–358.
29. Pitt MA, Haboubi NY. Serosal reaction in chronic gastric ulcers: an immunohistochemical and ultrastructural study. *J Clin Pathol* 1995;48: 226–228.
30. Bolen JW, Hammer SP, McNutt MA. Reactive and neoplastic serosal tissue: A light-microscopic, ultrastructural and immunocytochemical study. *Am J Surg Path* 1986;10:34–47.
31. Otis CN, Carter D, Cole S, Battifora H. Immunohistochemical evaluation of pleural mesothelioma and pulmonary adenocardinoma. A bi-institutional study of 47 cases. *Am J Surg Path* 1987;11:445–456.
32. Sheibani K, Battifora H, Burke JS, Rappaport H. Leu-M1 antigen in human neoplasms: An immunohistologic study of 400 cases. *Am J Surg Pathol* 1986;10:227–236.
33. Sheibani K, Esteban JM, Bailey A, Battifora H, Weiss L. Immunopathologic and molecular studies as an aid to the diagnosis of malignant mesothelioma. *Hum Pathol* 1992;23:107–116.
34. Sheibani K. Immunopathology of malignant mesothelioma. *Hum Pathol* 1994;25:219–220.
35. Latza U, Niedobitck G, Schwarting R, Nekarda H, Stein H. Ber-EP4: new monoclonal antibody which distinguishes epithelia from mesothelia. *J Clin Pathol* 1990;43:213–219.
36. Sheibani K, Shin SS, Kezirian J, Weiss LM. Ber-EP4 antibody as a discriminant in the differential diagnosis of malignant mesothelioma versus adenocarcinoma. *Am J Surg Path* 1991;15:779–784.
37. Gaffey MJ, Mills SE, Swanson PE, Zarbo RJ, Shah AR, Wick MR. Immunoreactivity for Ber-EP4 in adenocardinomas, adenomatoid tumors, and malignant mesotheliomas. *Am J Surg Path* 1992;16:593–599.
38. Otis CN. Uterine adenomatoid tumors: Immunohistochemical characteristics with emphasis on Ber-EP4 immunoreactivity and distinction from adenocardinoma. *Int J Gynecol Pathol* 1996;15:146–51.
39. Raftery AT. Regeneration of parietal and visceral peritoneum in the immature animal: light and electron microscopic study. *Br J Surg* 1973; 60:969–975.
40. Raftery AT. Regeneration of parietal and visceral peritoneum: an electron microscopical study. *J Anat* 1984;115:375–392.
41. Whitaker D, Papdaimitrious JM. Mesothelial healing: morphological and kinetic investigations. *J Pathol* 1985;145:159–175.
42. Ackerman LV. Tumors of the retroperitoneum, mesentery, and peritoneum. In: *Atlas of tumor pathology, sec. VI, fasc. 23 and 24.* Washington, DC; Armed Forces Institute of Pathology, 1954.
43. McCaughey WTE, Kannerstein M, Chrug J. Tumors and pseudotumors of the serous membranes. In: *Atlas of tumor pathology, fasc. 20.* Washington, DC; Armed Forces Institute of Pathology, 1983.
44. Rosai J, Dehner LP. Nodular mesothelial hyperplasia in hernia sacs. A benign reactive condition simulating a neoplastic process. *Cancer* 1975;35:165.
45. Brooks JSJ, LiVolsi VA, Pietra GG. Mesothelial cell inclusions in mediastinal lymph nodes mimicking metastatic carcinoma. *Am J Clin Path* 1990;93:741–748.
46. Sussman J, Rosai J. Lymph node metastasis as the initial manifestation of malignant mesothelioma: report of six cases. *Am J Surg Path* 1990; 14:819–828.
47. Sampson JA. Heterotopic or misplaced endometrial tissue. *Am J Obstet Gynecol* 1925;10:649–664.
48. Sampson JA. Postsalpingectomy endometriosis (endosalpingosis). *Am J Obstet Gynecol* 1930;20:443–480.
49. Sampson JA. The pathogenesis of postsalpingectomy endometriosis in laparotomy scars. *Am J Obstet Gynecol* 1945;50:597–620.
50. Zinsser KR, Wheeler JE. Endosalpingosis in the omentum: a study of autopsy and surgical material. *Am J Surg Pathol* 1982;6:109–117.
51. Hsu YK, Parmley TH, Rosenshein NB, Bhagavan BS, Woodruff JD. Neoplastic and non-neoplastic mesothelial proliferations in pelvic lymph nodes. *Obstet Gynecol* 1980;55:83–88.
52. Karp LA, Czernobilsky G. Glandular inclusions in pelvic and abdominal para-aortic lymph nodes: A study of autopsy and surgical material in males and females. *Am J Clin Pathol* 1969;52:212–218.
53. Schnurr RC, Delgado G, Chun B. Benign glandular inclusions in para-aortic lymph nodes in women undergoing lymphadenectomies. *Am J Obstet Gynecol* 1978;130:813–816.
54. Clement PB. Endometriosis, lesions of the secondary müllerian system, and pelvic mesothelial proliferations. In: Blaustein's *Pathology of the female genital tract. 3rd ed.* New York; Springer-Verlag, 1987: 517–559.
55. Ferguson BR, Bennington JL, Haber SL. Histochemistry of mucosubstances and histology of mixed müllerian pelvic lymph node glandular inclusions: evidence for histogenesis by müllerian metaplasia on coelomic epithelium. *Obstet Gynecol* 1969;33:617–625.
56. Lauchlan SC. The secondary müllerian system. *Obstet Gynecol Surv* 1972;27:133–146.

# Central Nervous System

*Histology for Pathologists, second edition,*
Edited by Stephen S. Sternberg.
Lippincott-Raven Publishers, Philadelphia
© 1997.

# CHAPTER 11

# Central Nervous System

Gregory N. Fuller and Peter C. Burger



The central nervous system (CNS) is unparalleled among natural systems in terms of structural and functional complexity. As a consequence of its intricate regional architecture, heterogeneous cellular constituents, and an associated extensive and somewhat arcane lexicon, the nervous system is often viewed as a formidably Byzantine realm by many non-neuropathologists; and yet, a working familiarity with the normal morphology of this complex organ must precede competent evaluation of the many disease states that afflict it. To this end, this chapter will present the salient features of regional neuroanatomy followed by a description of the essentials of microscopic anatomy of the CNS, with special emphasis on those aspects that constitute potential diagnostic pitfalls, including normal anatomic variations, alterations associated with advancing age, reactive changes, and common artifacts.

G. N. Fuller: Department of Pathology, M. D. Anderson Cancer Center, Box 85, Houston, TX 77030.
P. C. Burger: Department of Pathology, The Johns Hopkins Medical Institutions, Baltimore, MD 21287.

## REGIONAL NEUROANATOMY

We have limited this discussion of regional neuroanatomy to those principles of structural organization that are of practical value to the diagnostician, emphasizing the rudiments of neuroembryology by which the basic organization of the nervous system is best understood. Further details about topographical neuroanatomy can be found in the list of suggested references provided at the end of the chapter.

### Organization of the Spinal Cord and Brain Stem

Embryologically, the nascent CNS begins as a hollow tube formed by the invagination of the neural plate ectoderm. This primitive cylinder is subdivided functionally into a dorsal sensory ("alar") plate and a ventral motor ("basal") plate. The two are separated by a lateral groove, termed the "sulcus limitans," along which develops the efferent autonomic system (Fig. 1). This primitive organizational pattern is retained, essentially unaltered, in the mature spinal cord. The central gray matter consists of: (a) dorsal horns that receive sensory input from the dorsal roots; (b) ventral horns that contain motor

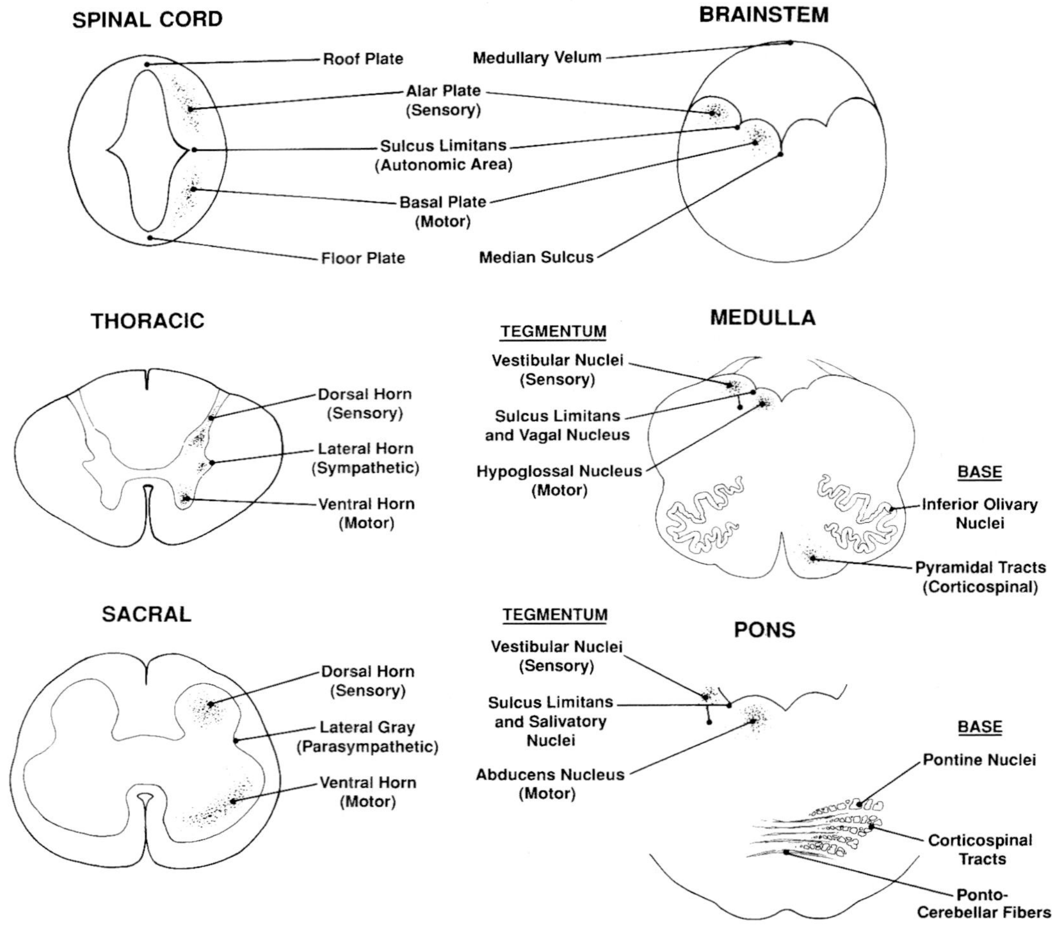


**FIG. 1.** Structural organization of the spinal cord and brain stem. (See text for discussion.)

neurons whose axons are conducted to the somatic periphery by the ventral roots; and (c) the lateral autonomic gray matter. Spinal autonomic neurons are confined to thoracic (sympathetic) and sacral (parasympathetic) levels, forming the intermediolateral cell columns. The axons of these "preganglionic" neurons exit the spinal cord through the ventral roots, ultimately to synapse on "postganglionic" neurons in the peripheral autonomic ganglia. The sympathetic intermediolateral cell column produces a third horn of gray matter in the thoracic cord, termed "the lateral horn" (Figs. 1 and 2). The parasympathetic intermediolateral cell column occupies a similar lateral position in the sacral cord (at the S-2, S-3, and S-4 levels), but does not form a distinct horn.

### *Spinal Cord*

The anatomy of the spinal cord varies according to the level (Fig. 2). Two enlargements of the ventral horns, one in the cervical region (Fig. 2A) and another in the lumbosacral region (Fig. 2C), provide motor innervation for the upper extremities and lower extremities, respectively. In contrast, the ventral horns of the thoracic cord provide innervation for the more limited axial musculature of the trunk and are, accordingly, much smaller (Fig. 2B). As mentioned earlier, the lateral horns of the gray matter (sympathetic neurons) are a unique feature of the thoracic cord. The thickness of the surrounding white matter fiber bundles (termed "funiculi") also varies with cord level, being greatest in the cervical cord, where the thickness reflects the summated accrual of ascending fiber tracts that have successively entered at lower levels, as well as the maximum content of descending tracts that are en route to lower levels, and thinnest in the lumbosacral cord. The terminus of the spinal cord, the filum terminale, is composed primarily of meningeal connective tissue in the human and is discussed separately with the pia-arachnoid (see Fig. 55).

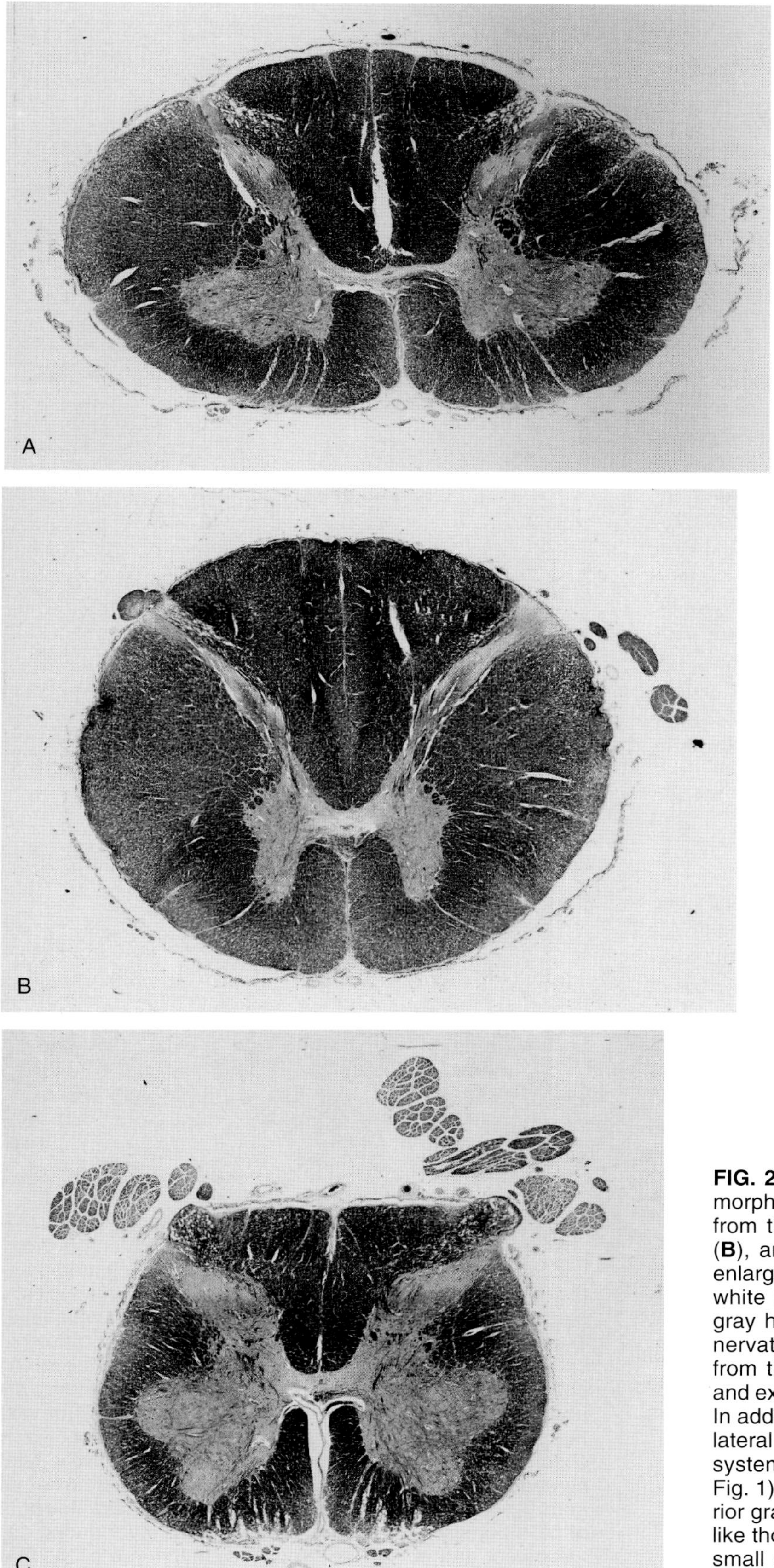


**FIG. 2.** Spinal cord: regional variation of spinal cord morphology is illustrated in these cross sections taken from the cervical enlargement (**A**), midthoracic cord (**B**), and lumbosacral enlargement (**C**). The cervical enlargement (**A**) is typified by an oval shape with large white matter funiculi and prominent, broad anterior gray horns which contain the motor neurons that innervate the upper extremities. In contrast, sections from thoracic cord (**B**) have a more rounded profile and exhibit small, slender, peglike anterior gray horns. In addition, lateral horns, which house the intermediolateral cell column neurons of the sympathetic nervous system, are unique to thoracic segments (see also Fig. 1). The lumbosacral cord (**C**) has very large anterior gray horns (motor supply to the lower extremities) like those of the cervical enlargement, but only a very small surrounding mantle of white matter (see also Fig. 1).

### *Brain Stem*

The brain stem is innately more complex than the spinal cord, but its basic organization is readily understood when viewed as a slightly modified version of the basic plan. Thus, the stem is also a neural tube, but one that has been stretched dorsally and splayed out laterally so that the ventrally located embryonic motor plate is now medial and the dorsal sensory plate is lateral (Fig. 1). Therefore, within the brain stem the cranial nerve motor nuclei are located medially, the sensory nuclei laterally, and the autonomic nuclei are intermediate in position.

The brain stem can be further subcategorized in cross section into tectum, tegmentum, and base. The tectum is the roof of the ventricular system, as exemplified by the superior and inferior colliculi (corpora quadrigemina) of the midbrain and the superior medullary vela of the pons and medulla. The tegmentum forms the floor of the cerebral aqueduct and fourth ventricle, and is divisible into the medial motor and lateral sensory areas discussed previously (Fig. 1). The "base" is located subjacent to the tegmentum and is the most ventral portion of the stem. It is composed principally of the so-called "long tracts," that is, the descending motor pathways and ascending sensory pathways that link the spinal cord with higher neural centers. The combination of long tract signs with dysfunction of specific cranial nerves allows for the precise anatomic localization of brain stem lesions by clinical examination.

### *Cerebellum*

Embryologically, the cerebellum arises as a dorsal outgrowth of the fetal brain stem and remains connected to it in the adult by the three pairs of cerebellar peduncles: the superior (brachium conjunctivum), middle (brachium pontis), and inferior (restiform body). They join with the midbrain, pons, and medulla, respectively. The cerebellum is composed of three structural and functional compartments: cortex, medulla, and deep nuclei. The cortex displays three distinct laminae: an outer hypocellular molecular layer, an intermediate single-cell thick Purkinje cell layer (described below), and a deep hypercellular granular cell layer (Fig. 3). Before 1 year of age, the cerebellar cortex is conspicuous for remnants of a fourth layer of small neurons, the fetal external granular cell layer, which is located immediately subjacent to pia (Fig. 3C). The external granular cells are gradually depleted during the first year of life as they descend the processes of Bergmann glia to reach their final position in the internal granular cell layer. Embedded within the white matter of the cerebellar medulla are four pairs of nuclei, from medial to lateral: fastigial, globose, emboliform, and dentate. The dentate is by far the largest, and is usually the only deep nucleus seen on routine sections. Its serpiginous profile is strikingly similar to that of the inferior olivary nucleus of the medulla oblongata (illustrated in Fig. 1) which is a major source of afferent fibers to the cerebellum.

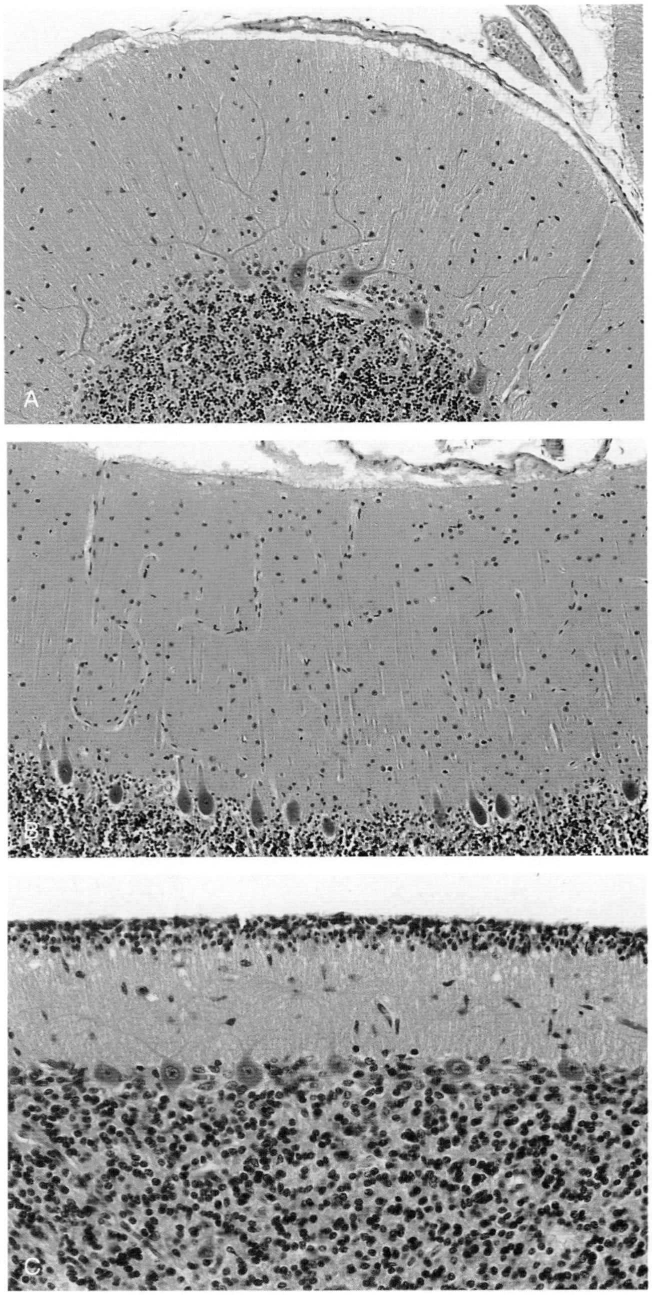


**FIG. 3.** Cerebellar cortex: the adult cerebellar cortex is composed of three layers: an outer hypocellular molecular layer, middle Purkinje cell layer, and inner densely populated granular cell layer. Whereas the Purkinje cells are prototypically neuronal in appearance, the small cells of the granular layer are hardly recognizable as neurons by traditional histologic criteria (see Fig. 7). A cross section of a cerebellar folium (**A**) shows the typical broadly branching Purkinje cell dendritic arbor. However, sections taken parallel to the folia (**B**) reveal the streamlined "on edge" appearance of the arbor, which should not be interpreted as pathological pruning. The fetal cerebellum (**C**) has an additional cortical lamina, the external granular layer, applied to the surface of the cortex. This pool of cells populates the internal granular cell layer during development and is, thereby, depleted by the end of the first year of postnatal life.

The Purkinje cell dendritic arbor extends into the molecular layer like a hand with outstretched fingers. Its broad, flat palm and radiating fingers are oriented perpendicular to the long axis of the cerebellar convolutions (folia). Thus, routine folia cross sections show the typical, elaborate dendritic branching pattern, whereas longitudinal sections present a dramatically different "on edge" view of the arbor (Fig. 3). This should not be mistaken for pathologic dendritic tree "pruning" seen in some disease states.

### *Diencephalon*

The diencephalon is interposed between the brain stem (midbrain, pons, and medulla) and the cerebrum. Four major divisions are recognized: epithalamus (pineal gland and habenula), thalamus, subthalamus, and hypothalamus. The medial and lateral geniculate nuclei of the thalamus are sometimes considered together as the metathalamus.

The strategic location of the thalamus is related to its major role in processing and relaying information passing between the cerebral cortex and brain stem and spinal cord. All sensory data (with the exception of olfaction) are processed by specific thalamic nuclei before distribution to the primary sensory cortices.

Of clinical significance to the pathologist, certain portions of the diencephalon immediately subjacent to the third ventricle, in particular, the large dorsomedial nuclei of the thalamus and the mamillary bodies of the hypothalamus, are often prominently involved in Wernicke's encephalopathy. The lesions at these sites are postulated to account for the memory disturbance that accompanies this disorder.

### *Cerebrum*

Supratentorially, the CNS becomes so much more complicated that it is difficult to describe in terms of any general pattern of orientation. It remains a hollow structure, but one that is no longer easy to consider as a tube of foldings and regional overgrowths. In light of this complexity, it is appropriate to review only those areas that are of particular diagnostic relevance.

### *Basal Ganglia*

The term *basal ganglia* refers to the deep gray matter masses of the telencephalon and encompasses the caudate nucleus, putamen, globus pallidus, and amygdala (Fig. 4). The term *ganglion* was formerly used interchangeably with *nucleus,* and *ganglion cell* was synonymous with *neuron* to earlier neuroanatomists. With the exception of the basal ganglia, the current definition of a ganglion is now generally restricted to mean a collection of neuronal cell bodies located outside the CNS, namely, the sensory and autonomic ganglia of the peripheral nervous system. Reference to CNS neurons as *ganglion cells* is still occasionally encountered, and this historical sense of the term is reflected in the names of such neoplastic entities as *ganglioglioma, ganglioneuroma,* and *ganglion cell tumor.*

The amygdala (archistriatum) is located in the mesial temporal lobe immediatly rostral to the hippocampus, and is functionally related to the limbic system. The remaining nuclei of the basal ganglia play an integral role in the modulation of motor function, and probably participate in other higher neural systems as well. The caudate nucleus, as the name implies, has a long tapering tail that intimately follows the curvature of the lateral ventricle. The caudate is morphologically and functionally closely related to the putamen. These two nuclei are appropriately referred to collectively as the neostriatum, or simply striatum. For descriptive pur-

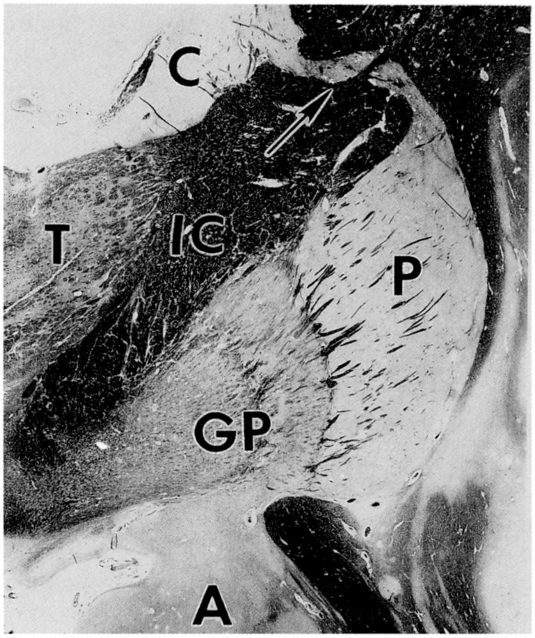


**FIG. 4.** Basal ganglia: the gray matter of the telencephalon is broadly divisible into two components—the superficial cortical gray matter mantle and the deep gray nuclei. The latter are known as the basal ganglia, and consist of the caudate nucleus (C), putamen (P), globus pallidus (GP), and amygdala (A). The lenticular nucleus is composed of the medially situated, diffusely myelinated globus pallidus and the laterally placed putamen, whose myelinated fibers are grouped into slender fascicles known as the pencil bundles of Wilson. The internal capsule (IC) separates the lenticular nucleus from the caudate and the thalamus (T). Gray matter bridges (*arrow*) occasionally span the capsule to connect the caudate and putamen, a reflection of the close functional relationship between these two nuclei. The lenticular nucleus receives its blood supply from several lenticulostriate arteries, which are direct branches of the middle cerebral artery, and is the most common site of intracerebral hypertensive hemorrhage and lacunar infarction. The large lenticulostriate artery coursing through the lateral putamen was known in former times as Charcot's artery, or, more colorfully, as the artery of internal hemorrhage. The lenticulostriate vessels are often surrounded by dilated perivascular spaces that should not be mistaken for lacunar infarcts.

poses, the putamen and the medially situated globus pallidus (paleostriatum or pallidum) are collectively referred to as the lentiform (lenticular) nucleus. The putamen and pallidum are separated from one another by the external medullary lamina of the pallidum, whereas the pallidum is itself divided into medial and lateral segments by the internal medullary lamina. The globus pallidus ("pale globe") is so named because of its pale appearance in the fresh state compared to the putamen. This contrast is attributable histologically to the dense meshwork of myelinated fibers in the pallidum. In contrast, myelinated axons in the putamen are grouped into slender fascicles ("pencil bundles of Wilson") that project medially to the pallidum and to the substantia nigra. The histologic appearance of the lentiform nucleus is distinctive and permits unambiguous identification of even very limited amounts of tissue from this site.

The basal ganglia are prominently involved in a variety of pathological processes, including kernicterus (literally, "nuclear jaundice") in the neonate and lacunar infarction in adults. Carbon monoxide poisoning classically produces selective necrosis of the inner segment of the pallidum. A frequent incidental finding of no diagnostic significance on routine sections of the lentiform nucleus is micronodular mineralization of small blood vessels, which is typically most prominent in the globus pallidus. Histologically, similar micronodular mineralization is also commonly seen in the hippocampus (see Fig. 5C).

### Hippocampal Formation

The hippocampal formation comprises the subiculum, Ammon's horn (hippocampus proper), and dentate gyrus (Fig. 5). In coronal sections of the medial temporal lobe, the subiculum forms the inferior base of the hippocampal formation, joining the parahippocampal gyrus with Ammon's horn. Ammon's horn, routinely abbreviated CA (for cornu Ammonis), is divided into four regions, CA1 through 4, based on cytological architecture and synaptic connectivity. (This nomenclature was introduced by Lorente de No in 1934.) CA1 arches superiorly, forming, along with CA2, the medial floor of the temporal horn of the lateral ventricle. The dorsally situated CA2 is usually recognizable by the greater compactness of the pyramidal cell layer, as compared to CA1. CA3 forms a descending medial arch that terminates in the hilus of the dentate gyrus. The final segment of Ammon's horn, CA4, lies within the hilus of the dentate gyrus and is often referred to as the end-plate. CA1, essentially equivalent to Sommer's sector, is the zone that is most sensitive to various insults, including seizures, ischemia, and Alzheimer's disease changes. In contrast, the adjacent CA2 segment is known as the dorsal resistant zone, in recognition of its relative sparing compared to the other three sectors. The exquisite sensitivity of CA1 to injury, with sparing of the adjacent CA2, is routinely observed as mesial sclerosis of the hippocampus, which is seen in many temporal lobes resected for intractable epilepsy. The classic histologic description of the pattern of neuronal loss in Ammon's horn was based on observations made on the brains of such epileptic patients by Wilhelm Sommer in 1880; E. Brotz coined the term *Sommer's sector* in 1920.

There are several notable features that are frequently encountered incidentally in the examination of routine hippocampal sections and can be mistakenly interpreted as evidence of disease. One is an asymptomatic micronodular mineralization comparable to that seen in the pallidum. In the hippocampal formation, it is most commonly seen just outside the apex of the dentate gyrus (Fig. 5B, C). A second common finding is a residual hippocampal fissure, which produces a rarefied lamina or cystic cleft that can be mistaken for a healed infarct (Fig. 5B, D). In addition, pyramidal neurons of Ammon's horn are often dark and shrunken in autopsy material and care must be taken not to overinterpret such changes as evidence of antemortem ischemia (see Figs. 16 and 17).

### Cerebral Cortex

From antiquity, neuroscientists have sought to divide the cortical mantle into discrete, functionally significant units. Early efforts yielded fanciful maps akin to those of phrenology and physiognomy. More recently, the application of light microscopy and special staining techniques for cell bodies (Nissl stains), dendritic arbors and unmyelinated axons (Golgi stains), and the myelin sheaths of myelinated axons (myelin stains such as the Weil, Weigert, and Luxol fast blue methods) have permitted a more scientific approach, although the details are beyond the scope of this chapter. In brief, the parcellation of the cortex is based on regional variation in the relative number, composition, and distribution of cortical neurons and their processes (cytoarchitectonics and myeloarchitechtonics). Various neuroanatomists have divided the cortex into a number of regions varying from 20 to more than 200, depending on the particular morphologic criteria and degree of subtlety employed. Currently, the most popular cortical map is that devised by Korbinian Brodmann in 1909. Brodmann's map and the classical nomenclature for the gross anatomy of the cerebral sulci and gyri are the two systems most commonly used at present for reference purposes in the neuroanatomical and clinical literature.

Within the context of even the simplest cortical map, it is generally not possible to assign a given histologic section of cortex to a precise anatomical locus without prior knowledge of the section's provenance. However, two cortical areas do exhibit distinctive features: primary motor cortex and primary visual cortex. The motor cortex, located on the precentral gyrus of the frontal lobe, is distinguished by the presence of the giant pyramidal cells of Betz. Pyramidal cells generally range from 10 to 50 $\mu$m in soma height from base to origin of the apical dendrite. By comparison, Betz cells may exceed 100$\mu$m in soma height. The primary visual cortex, located on the banks of the calcarine fissure of the medial oc-

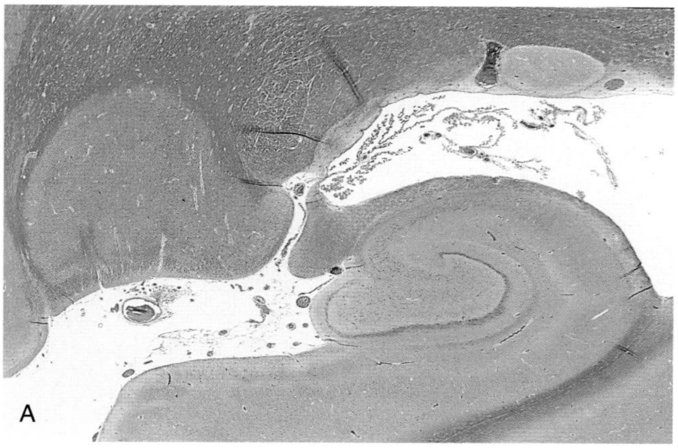

**FIG. 5.** Hippocampal formation: the hippocampal formation is composed of the subiculum, Ammon's horn (cornu Ammonis, abbreviated CA; divided into regions CA1-4), and the dentate gyrus (**A,B**). CA1 is equivalent to Sommer's sector and is the region of the hippocampus that is most sensitive to a variety of insults. In contrast, the adjacent CA2 region is known as the dorsal resistant zone. Two common incidental findings are also illustrated—micronodular mineralization (**B,C**), which is also seen in the globus pallidus, and a residual hippocampal fissure (**B,D**), which should not be misinterpreted as a healed infarct. CN, tail of the caudate nucleus; HF, residual hippocampal fissure; LGN, lateral geniculate nucleus (note the "Napoleon's hat" profile and distinctive lamination); MM, micronodular mineralization.

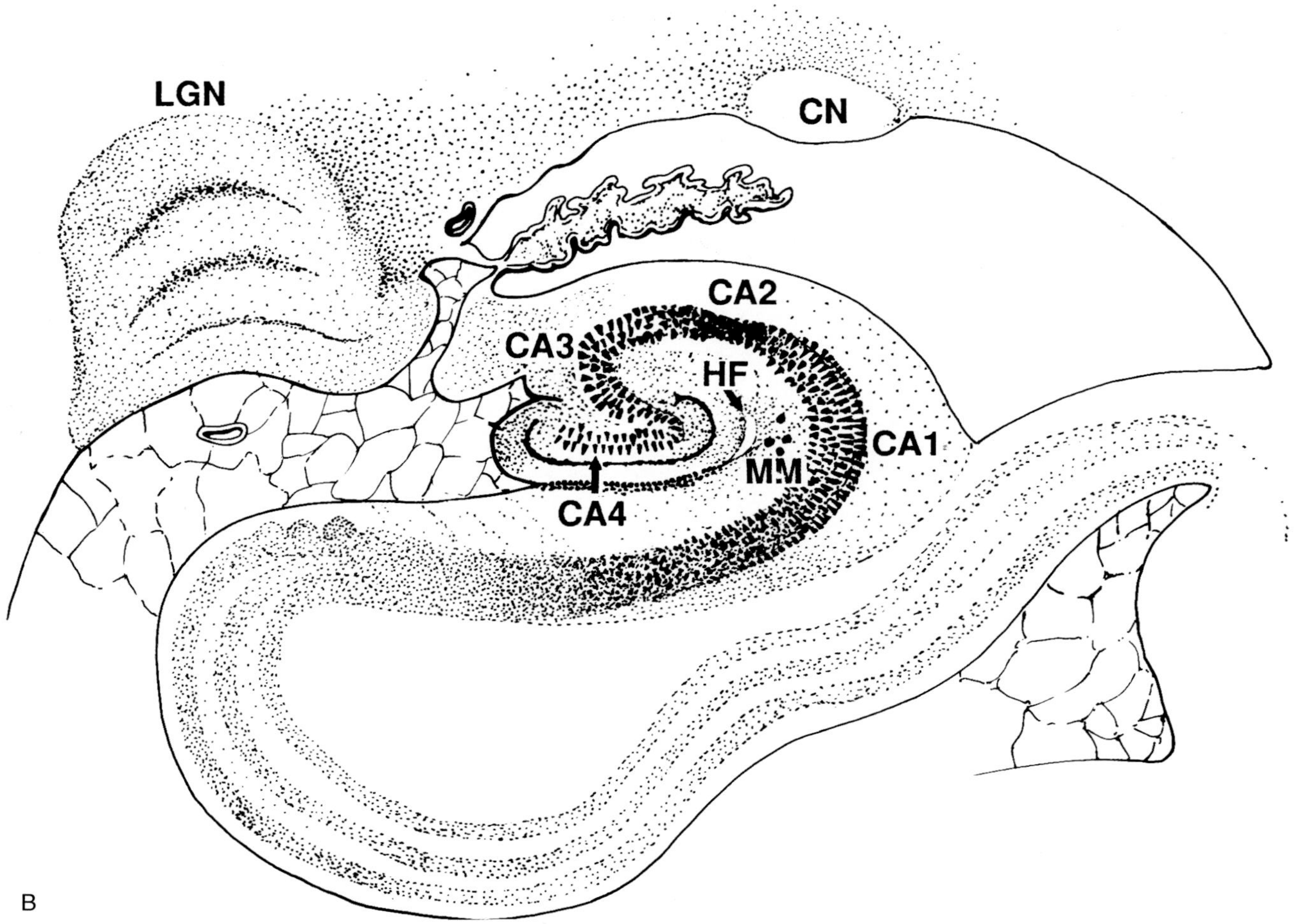


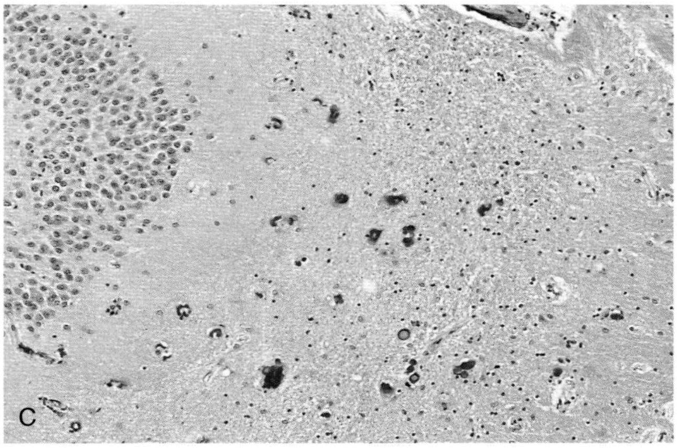

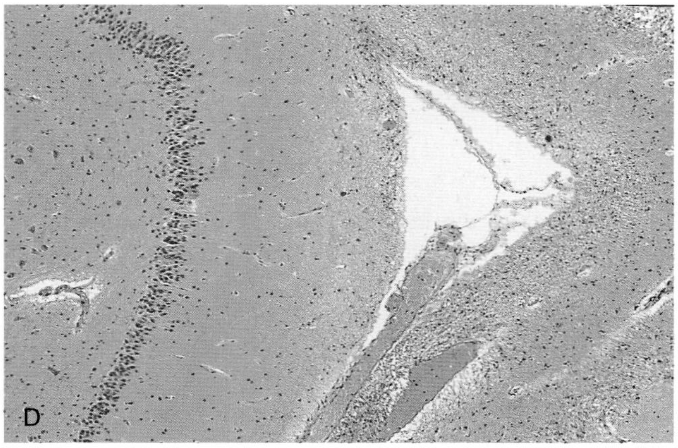

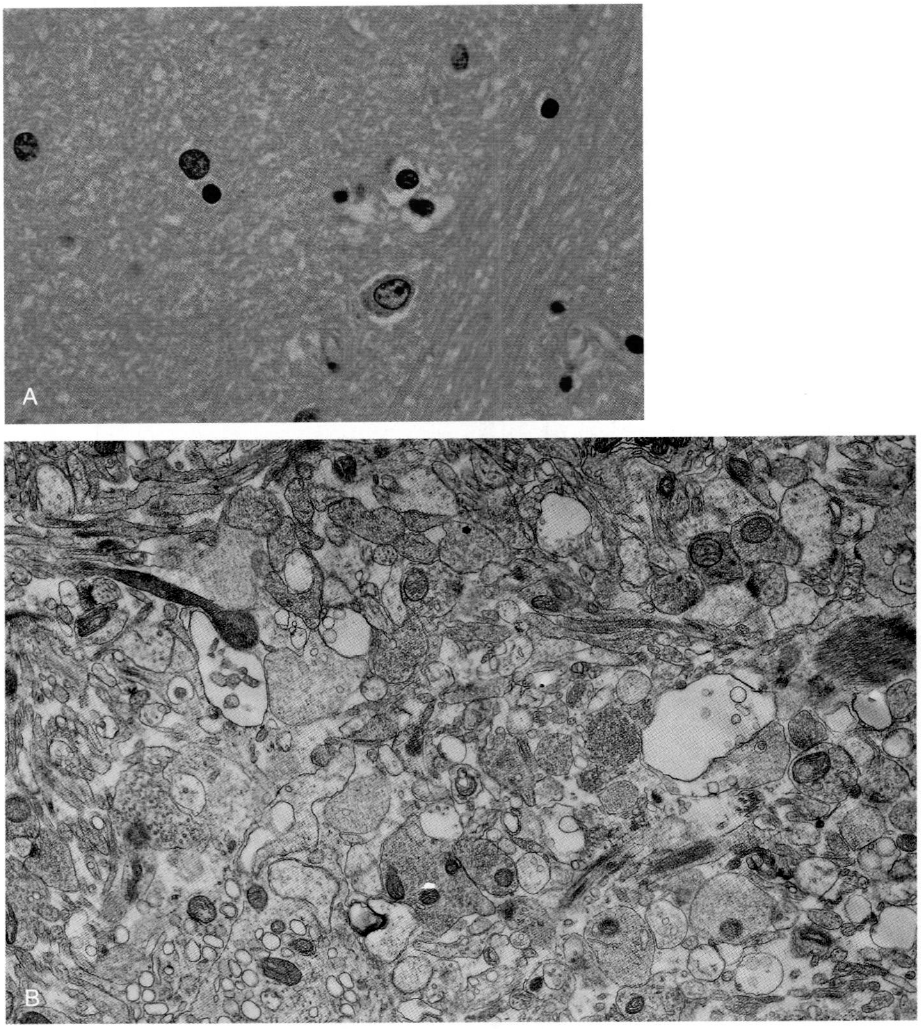

**FIG. 6.** Neuropil: neuropil is the term used for the fine "feltwork" background of gray matter that fills the expanses separating the cell bodies of neurons, astrocytes, and oligodendroglia (**A**). Ultrastructural examination reveals the neuropil to be composed of myriad intimately intermingling processes of the constituent cells (**B**).

cipital lobe, is remarkable for the presence of a prominent "external band of Baillarger," termed the "line (or stria) of Gennari." This myelinated stratum located in lamina IV is usually visible to the naked eye and permits exact delineation of the primary visual cortex (Brodmann area 17) from the adjacent visual association cortex (Brodmann area 18).

## CELLULAR CONSTITUENTS OF THE CENTRAL NERVOUS SYSTEM

### Neuropil

Before turning to the individual cellular constituents of nervous system tissue, mention should be made of the pervasive interwoven meshwork of neuronal and glial cell processes called *neuropil* (literally "nerve felt"). The individual component neurites that comprise the neuropil are not generally separable in routine hematoxylin-eosin (H&E)-stained sections. They appear as a finely textured eosinophilic background "feltwork" in which the perikarya of the parent cells are embedded (Fig. 6).

### Neurons

#### *Normal Microscopic Anatomy*

The prototypical neuron is exemplified by the large multipolar Betz cells of the motor cortex, the alpha motor neurons of the ventral horn of the spinal cord, and the Purkinje cells of the cerebellum. These neurons are characterized by large perikarya (cell bodies or somas) with abundant Nissl substance (rough endoplasmic reticulum), robust dendritic arborizations, and large nuclei with prominent single nucleoli (Fig. 7A). Such large multipolar forms, however, represent only one type of neuron; the diapason of neuronal morphologies is exceedingly broad. This is readily apparent by comparison of alpha motor neurons with granular cell neurons (Fig. 7A, C). These two neuronal populations typify the

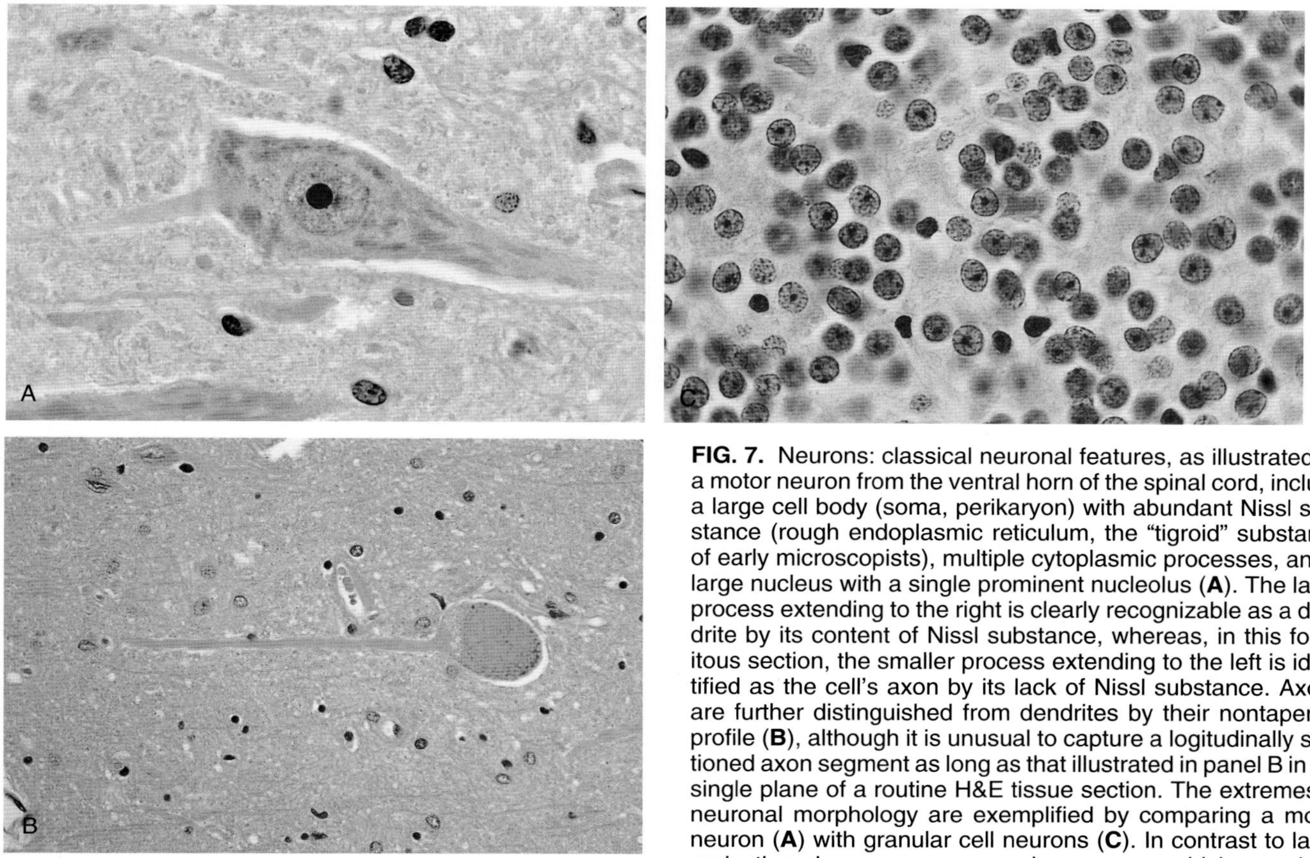


**FIG. 7.** Neurons: classical neuronal features, as illustrated by a motor neuron from the ventral horn of the spinal cord, include a large cell body (soma, perikaryon) with abundant Nissl substance (rough endoplasmic reticulum, the "tigroid" substance of early microscopists), multiple cytoplasmic processes, and a large nucleus with a single prominent nucleolus (**A**). The large process extending to the right is clearly recognizable as a dendrite by its content of Nissl substance, whereas, in this fortuitous section, the smaller process extending to the left is identified as the cell's axon by its lack of Nissl substance. Axons are further distinguished from dendrites by their nontapering profile (**B**), although it is unusual to capture a logitudinally sectioned axon segment as long as that illustrated in panel B in the single plane of a routine H&E tissue section. The extremes of neuronal morphology are exemplified by comparing a motor neuron (**A**) with granular cell neurons (**C**). In contrast to large projection class neurons, granular neurons, which are about the size of a motor neuron's nucleolus, lack recognizable Nissl substance (or even cytoplasm!) by routine light microscopy, although they do posses the characteristic single prominent central nucleolus.

classical dichotomous subdivision of CNS neurons into large extroverted projection neurons with long axons (Golgi type I neurons) and small introverts that function regionally with restricted connections (Golgi type II neurons). Between these two poles is a full spectrum of neuronal sizes and shapes, with an equally impressive variety of dendritic arbor configurations. The details of the latter are generally appreciable only with special stains for neuronal processes.

With respect to morphological variants, one unique population of CNS neurons merits brief mention. The mesencephalic nucleus of the trigeminal nerve, which is concerned chiefly with the mediation of jaw proprioception, is composed of true primary (first order) sensory neurons that possess only a single process emanating from the cell body (Fig. 8). This nucleus constitutes the only intraparenchymal example of this class of neurons; all other primary sensory neuronal perikarya are gathered outside the CNS in the spinal and cranial nerve ganglia.

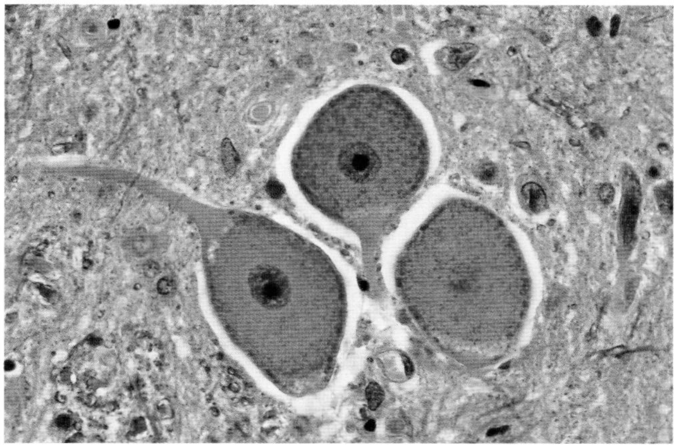

**FIG. 8.** Mesencephalic nucleus of the trigeminal nerve: the perfectly smooth contours of the somas are indicative of a complete absence of dendrites. A single process is seen emerging from two of the cell bodies. This extensive, but very sparsely populated nucleus, which may be seen in sections of the brain stem from the upper pons through the superior collicular level of the midbrain, is unique in comprising the only collection of primary somatic sensory neuronal cell bodies located intra-axially. The cell bodies of all other neurons of this class are found peripherally in ganglia of the spinal and cranial nerves.

### *Immunohistochemistry*

Antibodies have been raised against a wide variety of the many unique neuronal proteins that are being isolated

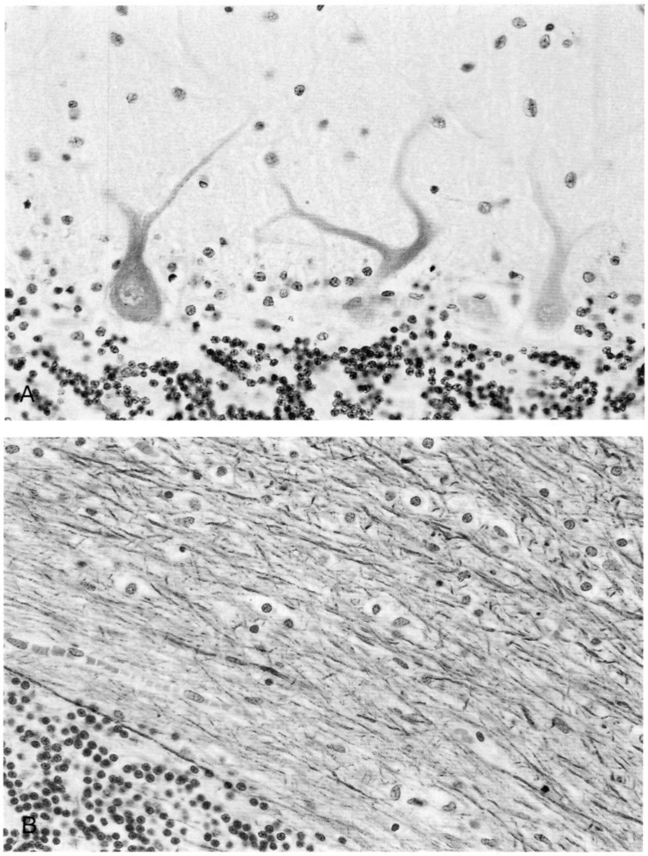


**FIG. 9.** Neurofilament proteins (NFPs): antibodies directed against neurofilament protein epitopes illuminate the cytoskeleton of neurons and their processes. As illustrated in the cerebellar cortex, specific antibodies directed against either nonphosphorylated (**A**) or phosphorylated (**B**) NFPs differentially identify cell bodies and dendrites or axons, respectively.

and characterized at an ever-increasing rate. A majority of these markers are confined to use for research purposes but several have found utility in the diagnostic laboratory. One of the earliest such markers, neuron specific enolase (NSE), has proven notoriously unreliable as a marker of neuronal differentiation. Its use for this purpose in evaluating neoplasms of the central nervous system is not recommended.

Antibodies directed against epitopes on the constituent proteins of neurofilaments, which are major cytoskeletal elements of the neuronal perikaryon and cytoplasmic processes, have been used extensively in both experimental and clinical studies (Fig. 9).

One of the most useful and widely employed neuronal markers is synaptophysin. Synaptophysin is an integral membrane protein of synaptic vesicles. In the normal nervous system, antisynaptophysin antibodies yield a diffuse, finely granular pattern throughout the gray matter neuropil (Fig. 10A). In addition, punctate granular decoration is seen along the cell bodies and proximal dendrites of several types of large, projection class neurons, including the Purkinje cells of the cerebellum, alpha motor neurons of the spinal cord, extraocular motor neurons of the brain stem, and Betz cells of the precentral gyrus (Fig. 10B).

### *Age-related Neuronal Inclusions*

A variety of inclusions, largely intracytoplasmic, appear with increasing frequency as we age. By far, the most common is lipofuschin (lipochrome or aging pigment), whose yellow-to-pale brown color is unaltered by most histologic procedures, including the H&E method (Fig. 11). Its autofluorescence and partial avidity for the acid-fast stain can be used to visualize differentially this "wear and tear" pigment,

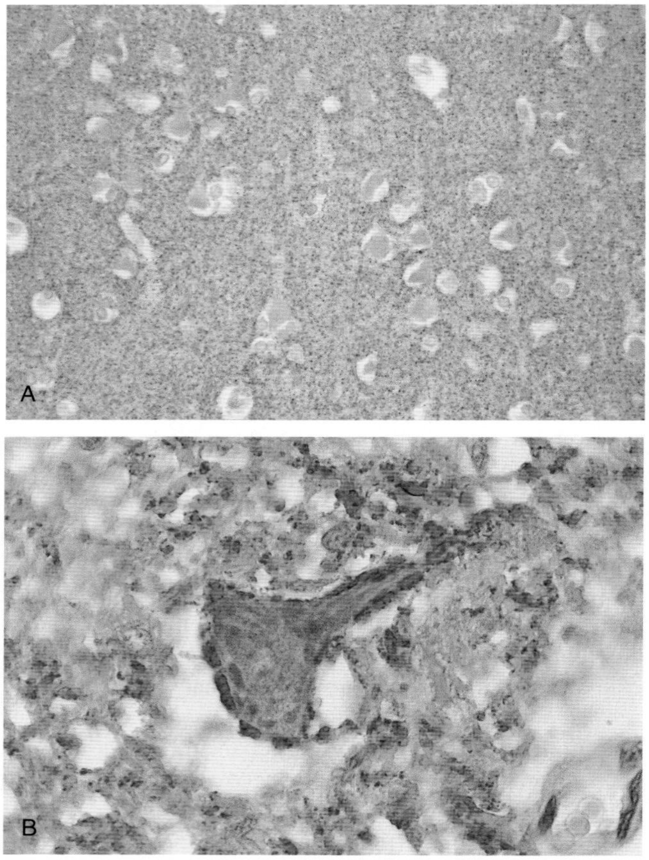


**FIG. 10.** Synaptophysin is one of the most useful and widely employed markers of neuronal differentiation. The neuropil of gray matter, which is rich in synaptic contacts, shows a diffuse, finely granular pattern (**A**). Several specific types of large projection class neurons show prominent punctate decoration of the cell body and proximal dendrites, as illustrated here by a motor neuron in the hypoglossal nucleus of the medulla (**B**). Other groups of large neurons exhibiting this pattern of synaptophysin immunopositivity include Purkinje cells of the cerebellum, motor neurons of the ventral horn of the spinal cord, and Betz cells of the precentral gyrus in the cerebral cortex.

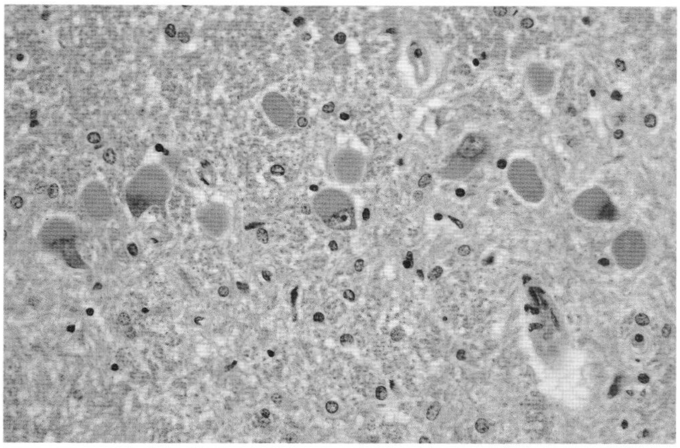

**FIG. 11.** Lipofuschin: extensive accrual of lipofuschin in aging neurons, as seen here in the lateral geniculate nucleus, can result in peripheral displacement of the nucleus and Nissl substance to such an extent as to mimic central chromatolysis. At higher power, however, the light brown color and finely granular texture distinguish lipochrome from the homogeneous eosinophilia of chromatolysis (see Fig. 18).

although little functional significance is generally assigned to lipochrome accumulation in normal aging. In larger neurons, lipofuschin may accumulate to such an extent that it displaces organelles, and creates an appearance similar to the cell swelling of central chromatolysis, described below (see Fig. 18). The lateral geniculate body provides an example of a densely populated nucleus whose constituent neuron's prominent accumulation of lipofuschin is often discernible macroscopically as a distinctly mahogany hue compared to adjacent cortex. Interestingly, lipofuscin accumulation is not simply a function of cell size because some classes of large neurons appear comparatively immune to significant accrual e.g., the cerebellar Purkinje cells.

Functionally more significant neuronal inclusions that may be seen in asymptomatic individuals are those associated with Alzheimer's disease. They are neurofibrillary tangles, neuritic plaques, granulovacuolar degeneration, and Hirano bodies. These illustrate the often ill-defined distinction between health and disease, because these changes can be seen in the elderly, albeit in limited numbers, in the absence of antemortem disturbances of mentation.

In some cases, neurofibrillary tangles may be found in asymptomatic individuals in occasional neurons of the subiculum or Ammon's horn. Although silver stains greatly aid visualization and quantitation, these structures may be identified on routinely stained H&E sections if the observer is familiar with their appearance. In pyramidal cells they appear as a slightly basophilic wisp of faintly fibrillar material that extends out into cell processes, most notably the apical dendrite, and they are often more prominent on one side of the nucleus (flame-shaped tangle; Fig. 12A). This morphology reflects the fact that tangles generally conform to the shape of the cell body. For example, in the pigmented neurons of the locus ceruleus, which are multipolar and lack the

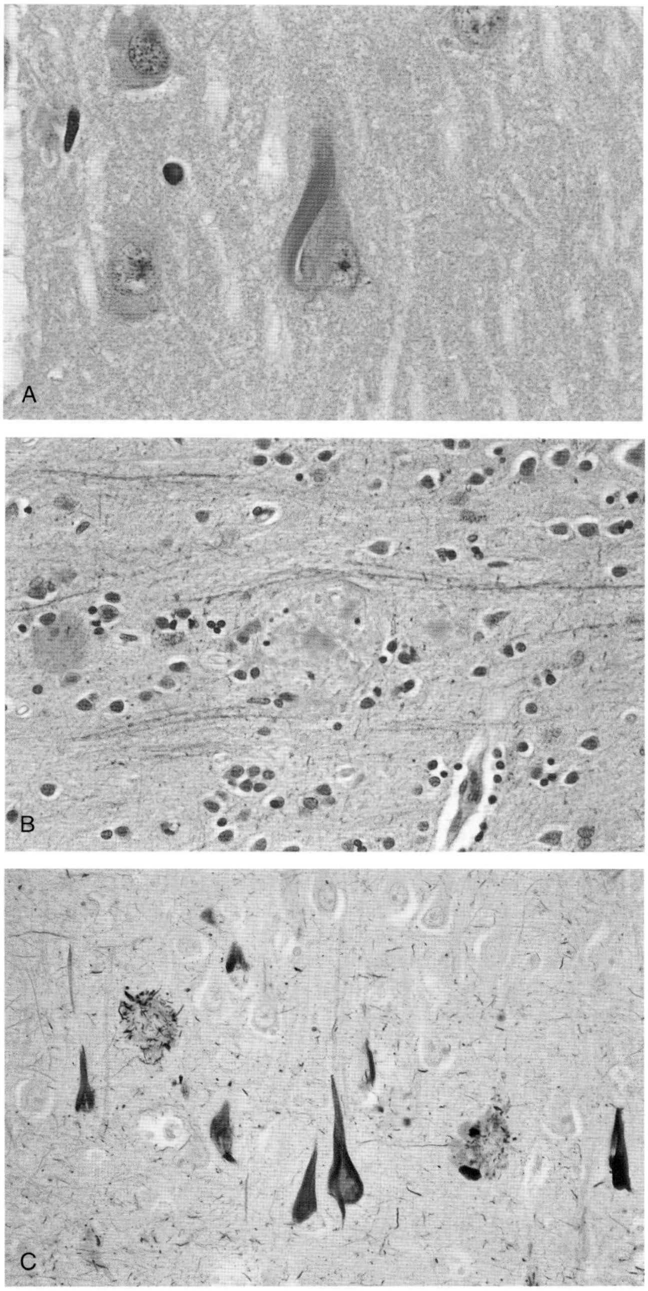


**FIG. 12.** Neurofibrillary tangles and neuritic plaques: neurofibrillary tangles (**A**) may be seen sporadically in the hippocampal formation of aging brains and have a fibrillary texture in H&E-stained sections. Mature senile (neuritic) plaques (**B**) deform the smooth texture of the neuropil and appear in H&E-stained sections as spherical, somewhat granular foci with a central eosinophilic core that is composed of amyloid. Note that adjacent myelinated axons are focally displaced as they pass by the plaque. In earlier stages, the plaques are less well defined and are not identifiable in H&E-stained sections. Although both neurofibrillary tangles and large mature neuritic plaques can be seen in H&E-stained sections, use of special techniques, such as silver stains (**C**), greatly facilitates visualization and quantitation.

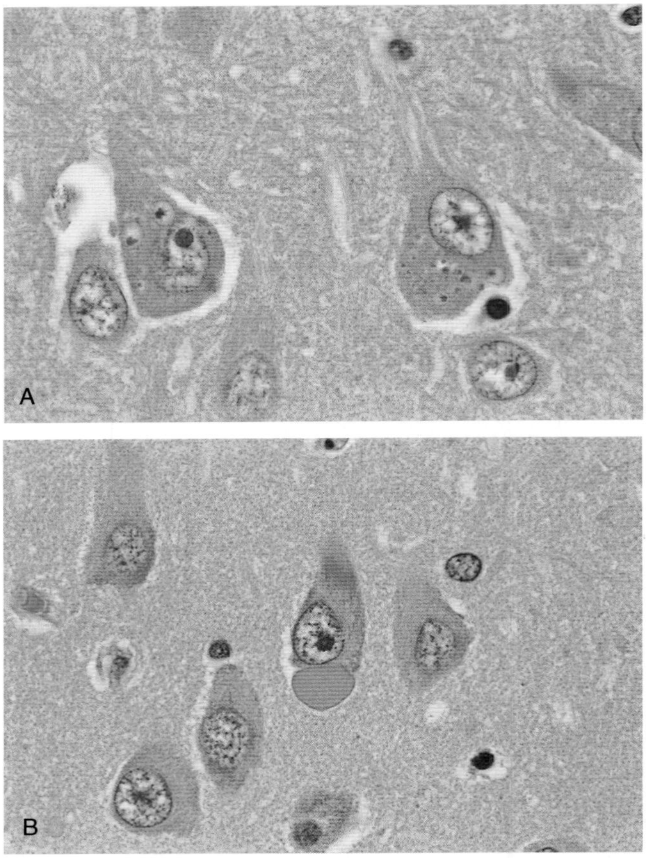

**FIG. 13.** Granulovacuolar degeneration (of Simchowitz) (**A**) and Hirano bodies (**B**): like neurofibrillary tangles, both of these intracytoplasmic inclusions can occasionally be seen in the hippocampal formation of normal older individuals. However, although these alterations are not pathognomonic for dementing illness, an appreciable number of affected cells should prompt a search for evidence of Alzheimer's disease in the form of a thorough examination for senile (neuritic) plaques and neurofibrillary tangles.

dominant apical dendrite of pyramidal neurons, tangles that are globular in shape are occasionally encountered as an incidental finding.

The senile plaque is also a manifestation of cell injury, but one that, like slight atherosclerosis, is not an unexpected finding in the brains of asymptomatic adults. In such individuals, the plaque is usually seen in its primitive form as a somewhat ill-defined, roughly circular region of abnormal argyrophilic neurites that is not visualized in the H&E-stained section. As the plaques mature they become visible in the latter preparation, particularly when a central core of eosinophilic amyloid appears (Fig. 12B). The latter can be more readily seen by Congo red or periodic acid-Schiff (PAS) staining. As noted earlier, both neurofibrillary tangles and neuritic plaques are more easily identified and quantitated with special techniques such as immunofluorescence or silver stains (Fig. 12C).

Two additional intraneuronal inclusions that are seen in Alzheimer's disease, but only rarely in nondemented individuals, are granulovacuolar degeneration (GVD) and Hirano bodies (Fig. 13). As the name implies, the inclusion of GVD consists of a dark, basophilic granule inside a small, clear vacuole. Clusters of these cytoplasmic inclusions may be present within a single neuron (Fig. 13A). Depending on the plane of section, Hirano bodies appear in H&E-stained sections as brightly eosinophilic oval, elliptical, or elongated rodlike refractile inclusions that are located either in very close apposition to a neuronal perikaryon (Fig. 13B), or within the neuropil. Ultrastructural examination supports a localization in neuronal cell bodies and processes, and immunohistochemical studies reveal the presence of actin and actin-associated proteins. Unlike neurofibrillary tangles and neuritic plaques, both GVD and Hirano bodies exhibit a very limited neuroanatomic distribution and are, in fact, virtually confined to the hippocampal formation. Encountering more than one or two cells with these alterations should raise the issue of Alzheimer's disease and prompt a search for other attendant histologic features.

A particularly striking cytoplasmic inclusion occasionally encountered in routine sections of the hypoglossal nuclei of the medulla (less often in the ventral horn motor nuclei of the spinal cord) is the hyaline (colloid) inclusion (Fig. 14). These inclusions, which consist of ectatic cisternae of endoplasmic reticulum, are rarely seen in the first few decades of life, but appear with increasing frequency thereafter. They are occasionally mistaken by the uninformed for viral inclusions.

Catecholaminergic neurons throughout the brain stem gradually accumulate neuromelanin as a by-product of neurotransmitter synthesis. The largest and most densely populated of these nuclei is the substantia nigra ("black substance"), which contains dopaminergic neurons. The locus ceruleus ("blue spot"), which is also seen by the unaided eye,

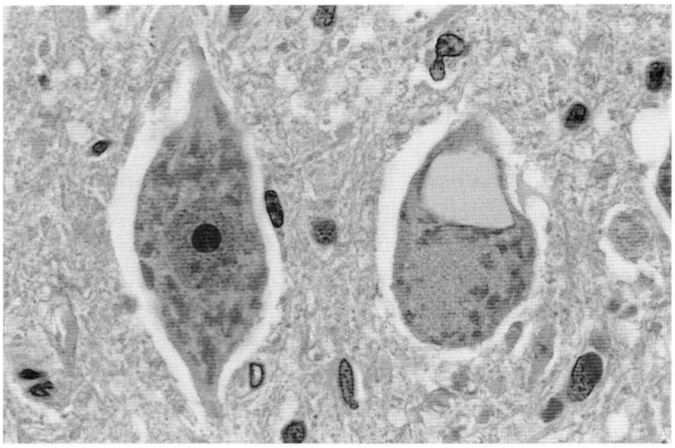

**FIG. 14.** Hyaline (colloid) inclusion: these eye-catching inclusions, as seen in the neuron on the right, may be observed sporadically throughout the neuraxis but are most commonly encountered in the large motor neurons of the hypoglossal nuclei in the medulla (as in this micrograph). Less frequently, they may be seen in the motor neurons of the ventral horn of the spinal cord. Electron microscopic examination reveals ectatic cisternae of endoplasmic reticulum.

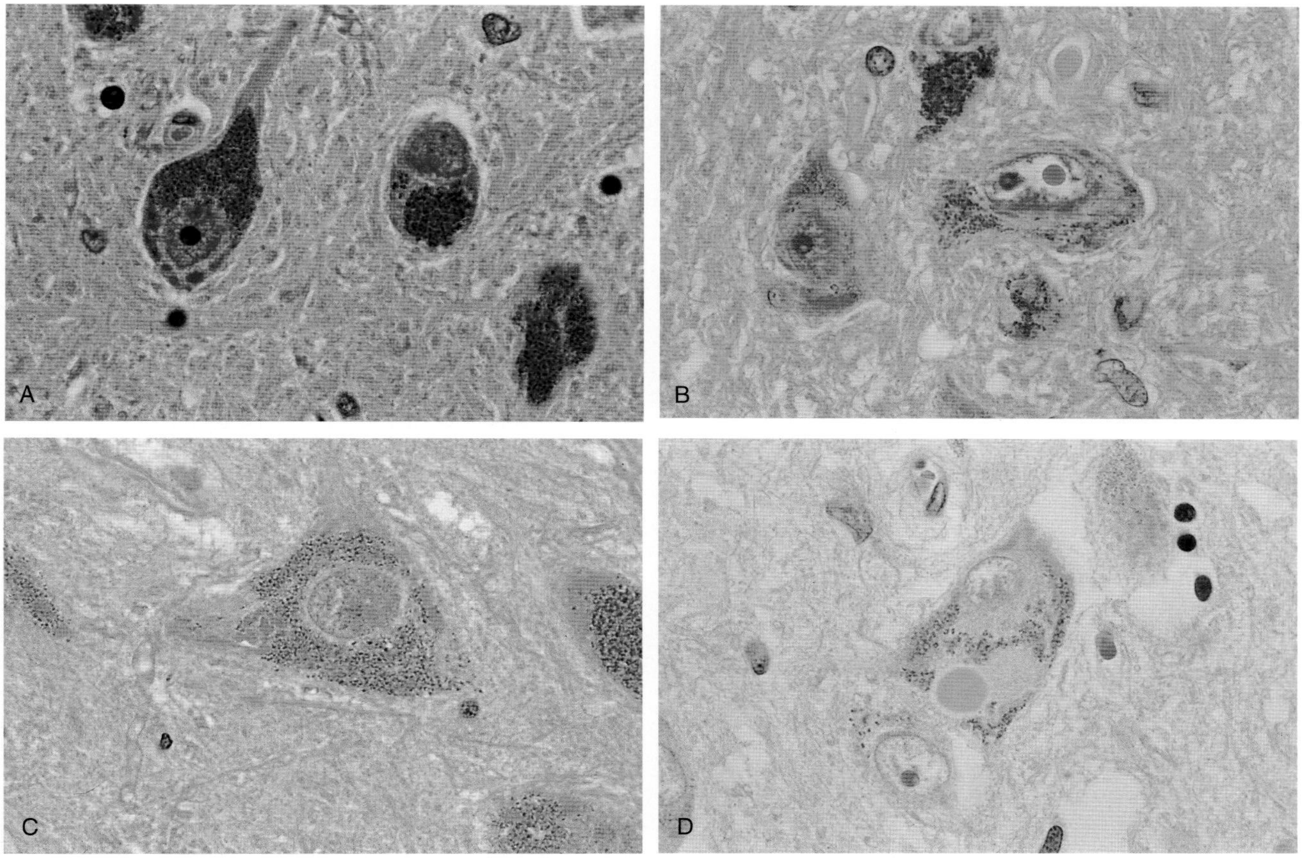


**FIG. 15.** Pigmented neurons of the brain stem: neuromelanin is a coarse, dark brown cytoplasmic pigment (**A**) that is formed as a by-product of catecholamine synthesis and is frequently encountered microscopically in scattered catecholaminergic neurons distributed widely throughout the brain stem. Two large populations are visible grossly: the substantia nigra ("black substance") of the midbrain and the locus ceruleus ("blue spot") of the pons. Marinesco bodies (**B**) are eosinophilic, spheroidal, paranucleolar bodies that are often observed in the nuclei of pigmented neurons, especially those of the substantia nigra. The number of Marinesco bodies increases with advancing age and can be quite striking in some individuals. They should not be mistaken for intranuclear viral inclusions. Clusters of minute intracytoplasmic eosinophilic granules (**C**), seen in this micrograph to the left of the nucleus, may occasionally catch the eye of an obsessive observer. They have no known pathologic significance and are much smaller than Lewy bodies (**D**), which are the characteristic intracytoplasmic inclusions of Parkinson's disease.

is a collection of noradrenergic neurons in the rostral pontine tegmentum. It is of practical importance that the Lewy bodies of Parkinson's disease can be found in both of these neuroanatomic locales. Of the smaller and more diffusely distributed pigmented neurons, those in the vicinity of the dorsal motor nucleus of the vagus nerve in the medulla oblongata are most commonly encountered during routine histologic examination. Microscopically, neuromelanin appears as coarse, dark brown granules (Fig. 15A), and should not be confused with melanocytic melanin. The latter is also present in the central nervous system, but is confined to leptomeningeal melanocytes as discussed below (see Fig. 56).

Several eosinophilic inclusions may be seen in pigmented brain stem neurons. The most striking of these are the commonly encountered Marinesco bodies (Fig. 15 B). These bright red, hyaline-appearing structures are located within the nucleus, often adjacent to and about the same size as a nucleolus (an alternative designation is "paranucleolar body"). Multiple Marinesco bodies may occur within a single nucleus and, in some cases, a large percentage of pigmented neurons exhibit these eye-catching inclusions. In such cases, they may raise concern about a viral infection to the unaccustomed observer, but are not pathologic and have yet to be correlated with any significant process except advancing age. Two types of eosinophilic inclusions may be encountered in the cytoplasm of pigmented neurons. Clusters of diminutive acidophilic granules are occasionally noted (Fig. 15C) but have no pathologic significance. Lewy bodies, in contrast, are much larger, notably displace the cytoplasmic neuromelanin from which they are separated by a small clear halo, and are associated with Parkinson's disease (Fig. 15D).

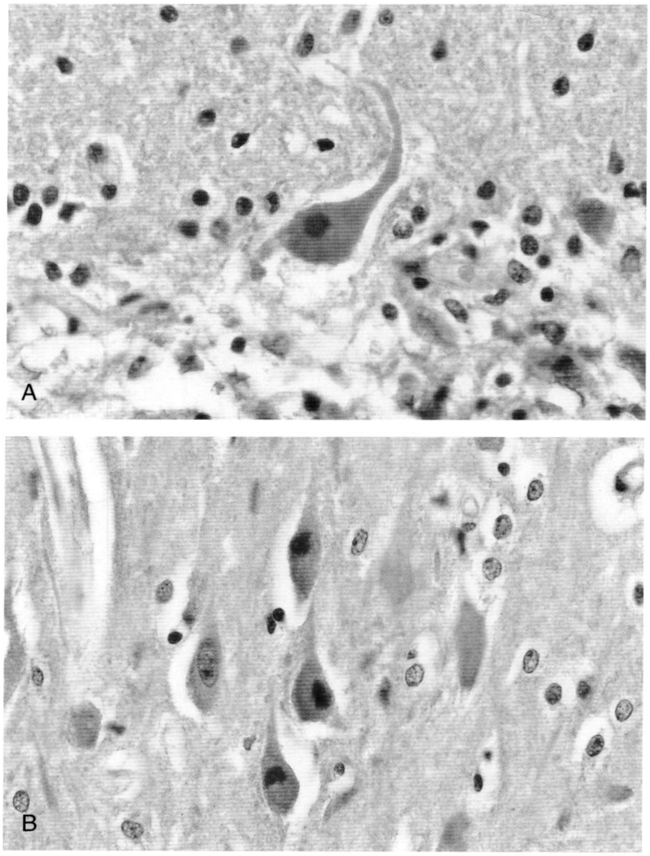


**FIG. 16.** Ischemic injury: the sine qua non of ischemic damage to the nervous system is the so-called red neuron. As illustrated here by a Purkinje cell of the cerebellum (**A**) and pyramidal neurons of the hippocampal CA1 region (**B**), the soma (cell body) is shrunken, the cytoplasm is intensely eosinophilic, and the nucleus is pyknotic with no discernible nucleolus. It is largely the pronounced eosinophilia that distinguishes this cellular alteration from autolytic neuronal condensation, in which the cytoplasm is dark and basophilic (see Fig. 17).

### *Autolysis and Basic Neuronal Reactions to Injury*

As captured in their normal state by perfusion fixation or rapid immersion fixation, neurons are generally rotund with lightly eosinophilic cytoplasm that is stippled with basophilic Nissl substance in the case of the larger neurons. The surrounding glia are inconspicuous and few clear vacuoles are seen. This perfection in fixation is rarely achieved in human material, however, and in virtually all autopsy and surgical specimens, autolysis alters this ideal appearance to a greater or lesser extent. Neurons are, thereby, rendered somewhat contracted and basophilic. Nuclei are also somewhat condensed. Simultaneously, the processes of glia that surround neurons and blood vessels imbibe water to produce clear vacuoles (see Fig. 29). The neuronal response to injury overlaps in some cases with these autolytic changes, and it may not be possible to distinguish agonal hypotensive injury

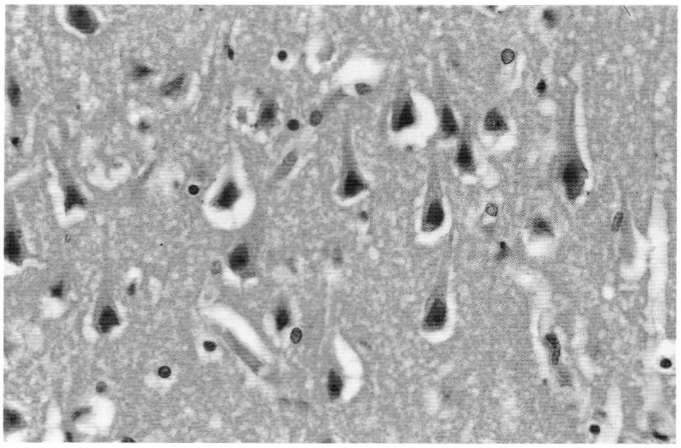

**FIG. 17.** Neuronal contraction as a tissue-handling artifact: in contrast to ischemic insult (Fig. 16), in "crush artifact" the cytoplasm is dark and basophilic rather than brightly eosinophilic.

from autolysis in autopsy specimens. In the former setting, the neuronal contraction is pronounced and the perineuronal and perivascular spaces are exceptionally prominent.

There are, however, three neuronal changes that provide unequivocal evidence of antemortem injury. One is the "red'" neuron, which is the sine qua non of ischemic damage. The second is central chromatolysis, and the third is ferruginization. The "red" neuron is characterized by a shrunken cell body and intense cytoplasmic eosinophilia with complete loss of Nissl basophilia (Fig. 16). The nucleus is dark and usually lacks a distinguishable nucleolus, but may be pale and demonstrate early karyolysis. At times, it has a somewhat fragmented look suggesting karyorrhexis,

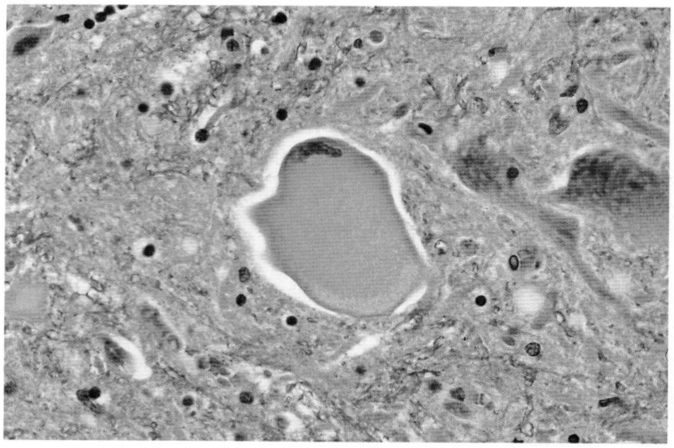

**FIG. 18.** Central chromatolysis: cytoplasmic hyalinization and swelling with peripheral displacement of the nucleus and lipofuschin can be a response to either intrinsic neuronal disease (such as in poliomyelitis or other viral infections) or to interruption of the axon in close proximity to the cell body. In the latter setting, the term axonal reaction is applied.

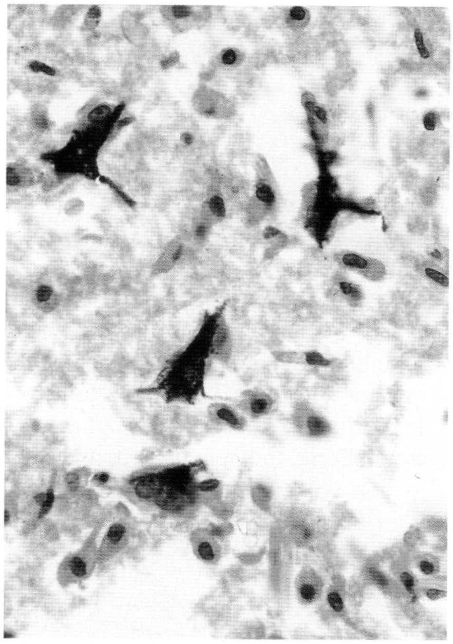

**FIG. 19.** Mineralized (ferruginized) neurons: these encrusted relics resembling petrified tree trunks are most commonly encountered around the margins of old infarcts.

although clearly defined karyorrhexis is rare. In surgical specimens, tissue-handling artifact ("crush" artifact) also results in dark, shrunken neuronal perikarya; however, as with autolytic autopsy specimens, these cells lack the distinctive cytoplasmic eosinophilia of ischemia (Fig. 17).

Central chromatolysis, the second unequivocally abnormal finding, consists of a loss of central basophilic staining of the cell body with peripheral margination of the Nissl substance (Fig. 18). It is seen in a number of pathologic states (the ballooned anterior horn cells of poliomyelitis being the classical example). There are numerous mimickers that lie in wait for the unwary. For example, some normal neuronal populations, such as the supraoptic and paraventricular nuclei of the hypothalamus and the dorsal nucleus of Clarke of the thoracic spinal cord, display Nissl substance that is preferentially distributed peripherally in the soma. Other neurons, such as those of the mesencephalic nucleus of the trigeminal nerve discussed previously (see Fig. 8), have large, exquisitely rounded somas and, hence, mimic that aspect of chromatolysis. The giant pyramidal cells of Betz in the motor cortex are so large in comparison to surrounding neurons, that at low magnification they may give an initial impression of chromatolytic swelling. Finally, as discussed earlier, one must be careful not to mistake the accumulation of various substances that displace the Nissl substance peripherally, such as lipofuschin, for central chromatolysis (see Fig. 11).

A striking finding sometimes encountered near old infarcts is the presence of ferruginized or fossilized neurons, in which both perikarya and axons are encrusted by blue-staining minerals (Fig. 19). This arresting phenomenon is not limited to the vicinal tissue of old infarcts, although this is the most common context, nor is it confined to the adult nervous

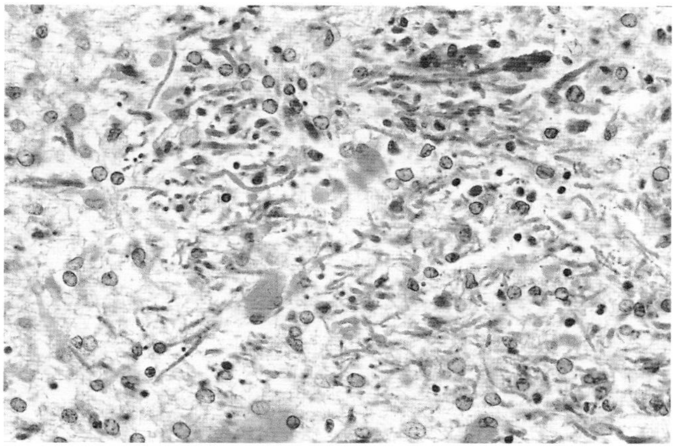

**FIG. 20.** Mineralized axons: clusters of mineralized axons have a superficial resemblance to fungal hyphae.

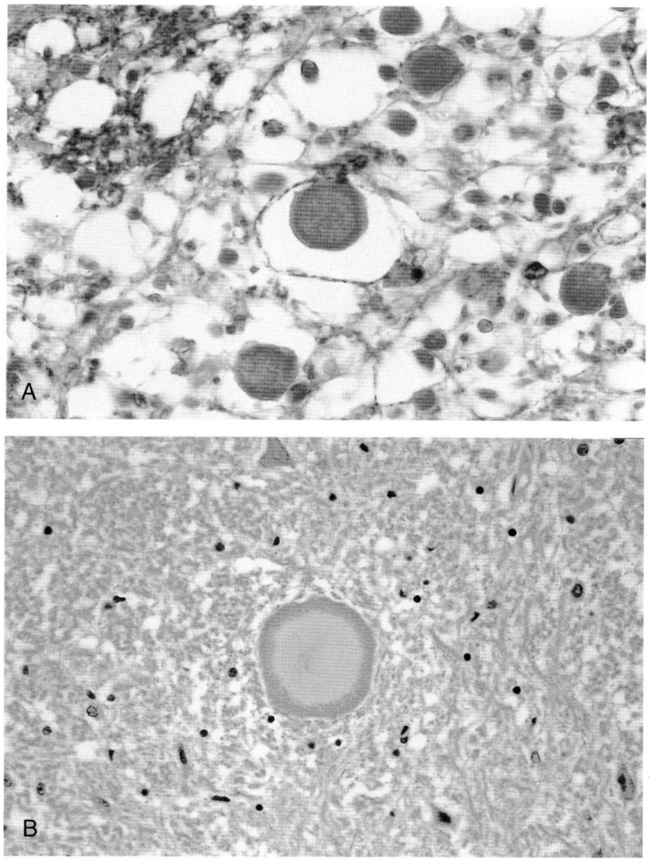


**FIG. 21.** Axonal spheroids: focal dilatations known as spheroids (**A**) are a common axonal reaction to injury that are seen in a wide array of pathologic conditions including radiation damage and posttraumatic diffuse axonal injury. Axonal spheroids are also frequently encountered incidentally in older individuals in the dorsal medulla oblongata (rostral fasciculus gracilis near nucleus gracilis) where, as in this example, they are often mineralized (**B**).

system, because prenatal insults may result in similar findings. Clusters of axons thus affected can be mistaken for fungal hyphae (Fig. 20).

A common reaction of axons to injury seen in a wide variety of pathologic states is the formation of localized dilatations known as axonal spheroids or axon "retraction balls" (Fig. 21A). Ultrastructural examination shows greatly distended axis cylinders filled with bundles of neurofilaments and cellular organelles. A regional variant of this process may be observed in the granular cell layer of the cerebellum where focal dilatations of Purkinje cell axons are termed *torpedoes.* These structures are seen in a number of cerebellar degenerative diseases as well as in normal aging. The most common site in the central nervous system where scattered axonal spheroids are routinely encountered as an incidental finding in aged individuals is in the rostral fasciculus gracilis of the medulla (Fig. 21B). Spheroids in this location are often mineralized.

## Astrocytes

### *Normal Microscopic Anatomy*

Like neurons, astrocytes are also heterogeneous. The cells of one class conform to the classic star shape, and occur as either the fibrillary or protoplasmic form. Fibrillary astrocytes populate the white matter, whereas the latter inhabit the gray matter. Other important subtypes of astrocytes include the "pilocytic" astrocytes of the periventricular region, cerebellum, and spinal cord, and the Bergmann astrocytes, which are distributed in a narrow lamina be-

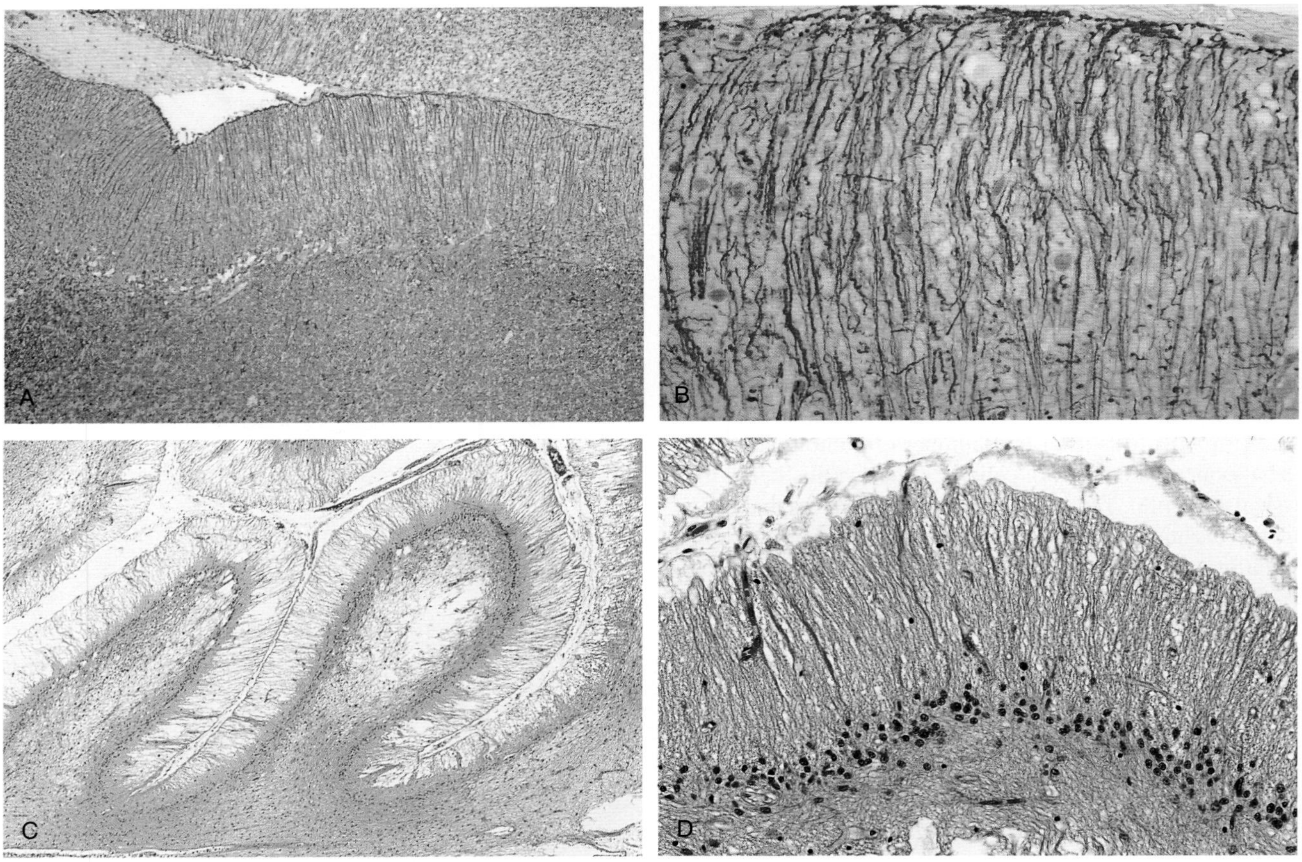


**FIG. 22.** Bergmann glia: these astrocytes illustrate the fact that specialization is not confined to neurons. Bergmann astrocytes have cell bodies distributed in a narrow lamina of the cerebellar cortex coextensive with that of the Purkinje cells. Each cell sends an elongated process through the molecular layer to the subpial surface. These processes are not usually well seen in healthy cerebellum with routine H&E staining (see Fig. 3A), but can be exquisitely visualized with immunohistochemistry for glial fibrillary acidic protein (GFAP; **A,B**). An equally striking unmasking of this elegant architecture is often seen without the use of specialized staining techniques in areas of cerebellar cortex adjacent to healed infarcts, in which the degree of ischemia was sufficient to kill the indigenous neuronal populations but spared the more resistant Bergmann glia (**C,D**). Like other astrocytes throughout the central nervous system, Bergmann glia respond to ischemic insult by proliferating, resulting in an increased thickness of the cell body lamina referred to as "Bergmann gliosis" (**D**).

tween the cell bodies of Purkinje neurons in the cerebellar cortex (Fig. 22).

In gray matter, nuclei of protoplasmic astrocytes cannot generally be distinguished from those of small neurons because the cytoplasm of both, blends imperceptibly into the surrounding neuropil and is not normally discernible as a discrete entity. In white matter, it is usually difficult in H&E-stained sections to distinguish fibrillary astrocytes from the much more numerous oligodendroglia. The nuclei of oligodendrocytes are smaller and more hyperchromatic, but usually these two cell types do not fall into two clearly defined groups. In sections stained for myelin, a very small amount of eosinophilic cytoplasm may occasionally, but not invariably, be seen surrounding normal astrocytic nuclei. This helps distinguish this cell from the oligodendrocyte whose cytoplasm, other than the myelin sheath, is not usually apparent by conventional light microscopy (see Fig. 32). Astrocytic cytoplasm becomes much more prominent when astrocytes respond to CNS injury, culminating in the abundant glassy cytoplasm of the gemistocyte (see Fig. 24).

To appreciate the distinctive morphology of the star cell, one must visualize its radiating processes. These threadlike extensions reach out to define a sphere of influence that is many times greater in extent than one would have suspected by looking at an H&E-stained section alone. Historically, this tinctorial feat was achieved through the technically capricious metallic impregnations, but now is accomplished with considerably greater ease and predictability by the immunohistochemical localization of glial fibrillary acidic protein (GFAP) (see Fig. 24). In the case of the fibrillary astrocyte, processes branch infrequently, whereas those of the protoplasmic astrocyte are more numerous and divide more frequently. They are often less well stained with GFAP than the fibrillary types. Neither type of resting astrocyte is as apparent immunohistochemically as are reactive astrocytes.

The polar forms of astrocytes include the pilocytic and Bergmann types. The pilocytic astrocyte is not conspicuous in its native state, but becomes so when responding as gliosis and forming Rosenthal fibers. The latter are hyaline, often corkscrew-shaped, eosinophilic structures that are wedged within one of the cell's bipolar processes (see Fig. 25). These structures are occasionally seen in normal brains in the hypothalamus or pineal gland, but become much more prominent in gliosis about such lesions as craniopharyngiomas, pineal cysts, cerebellar hemangioblastomas, and chronic lesions of the spinal cord.

The Bergmann astrocytes are confined to a one-to-two-cell thick lamina. Their polar processes extend to the pial surface of the cerebellum and are only faintly seen with difficulty in standard sections. Yet, they are well visualized with immunohistochemistry for GFAP and at the margins of old cerebellar infarcts (Fig. 22). The Bergmann glia provide an excellent illustration of astrocytic specialization. Their processes are a form of scaffold and serve as a reminder of the cooperative interplay between astrocytes and neurons during embryological development. At that time, the small

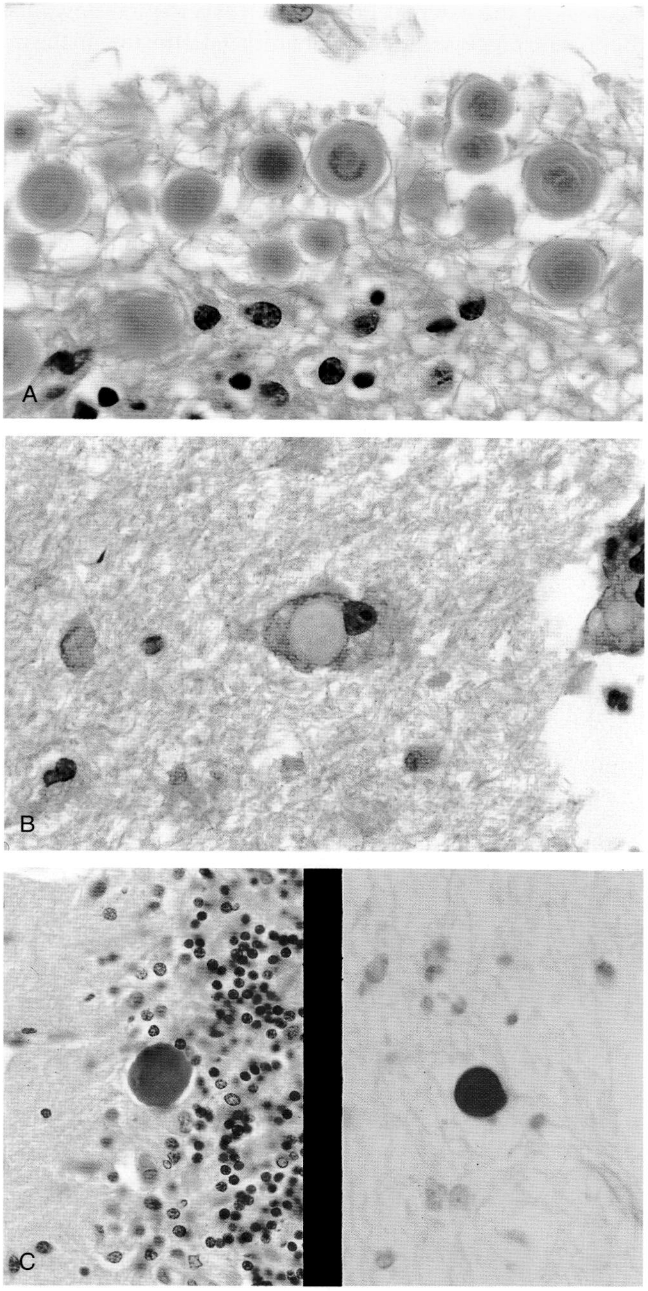


**FIG. 23.** Corpora amylacea: these basophilic, lamellated polyglucosan bodies accumulate in astrocytic processes with age (**A**). They are most numerous in the olfactory tracts (see Fig. 45), around blood vessels, and beneath the pia. In the latter location they are often artifactually dislodged during tissue sectioning and may appear to be freely disseminating within the subarachnoid space; they are also resistant to degradation and are sometimes observed within macrophages in resolving infarcts (**B**). In these instances they should not be mistaken for fungal yeast forms, with which they share an affinity for all of the routine stains used to detect fungal pathogens, including methenamine silver, alcian blue (**C**, left panel), and PAS (**C**, right panel).

neurons of the external granular cell layer spiral down the Bergmann processes to reach their final destination in the internal granular cell layer.

### *Age-related Inclusions in Astrocytes: Corpora Amylacea*

The ubiquitous corpora amylacea are, by far, the most salient astrocytic inclusions encountered in routine sections. These faintly laminated, slightly basophilic polyglucosan bodies accumulate with age and are observed in greatest numbers where astrocytic foot processes are most numerous, particularly around blood vessels and beneath the pia (Fig. 23). The olfactory tracts of adults are also typically rich in corpora amylacea (see Fig. 45).

The similarity between corpora amylacea and fungal yeast forms such as cryptococcus is a source of potential diagnostic error since both are strongly positive for methenamine silver, alcian blue, and periodic acid-Schiff (PAS) (Fig. 23).

In some individuals, corpora amylacea are strikingly numerous although no pathologic significance has yet been attributed to this abundance.

### *Astrocytic Reactions to Injury*

Although normally among the most morphologically demure of nervous system constituents (only naked nuclei are typically visible on routine H&E histology), astrocytes respond rapidly and dramatically to CNS injury. This response typically consists of two components: hypertrophy and hyperplasia. The initial hypertrophic response, an increase in cell size and cytoplasmic prominence, occurs rapidly following CNS insult. Conspicuous cytoplasm is generally indicative of reactive gliosis and constitutes prima facie evidence of CNS injury. Reactive astrocytes display a broad range of cytoplasmic quantity, from just barely perceptible to robustly embonpoint (Fig. 24). The latter cells are known

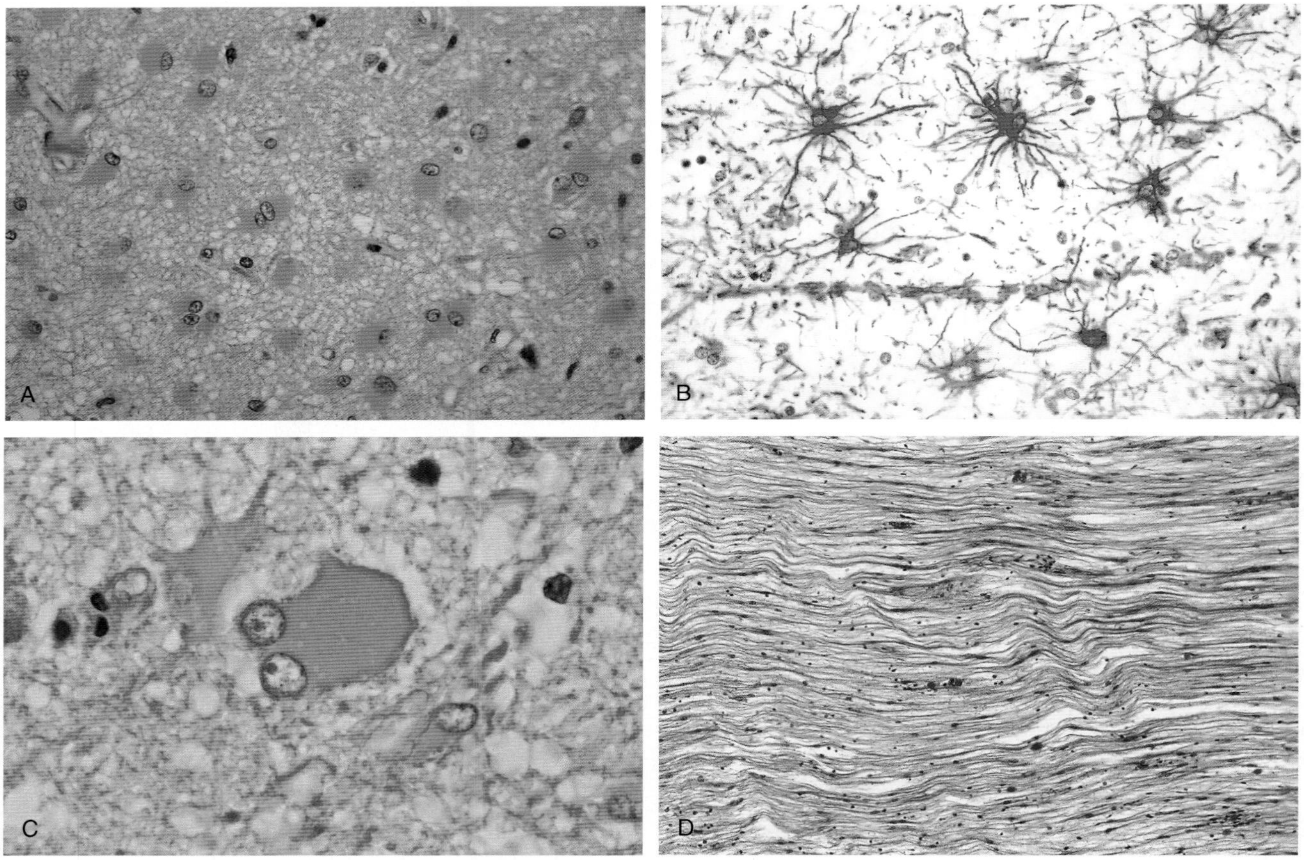


**FIG. 24.** Reactive astrocytosis: the plainly visible cytoplasm and processes of the astrocytes seen in panel **(A)** is proof of an insult to the nervous system. Under normal conditions, only bare nuclei are usually seen. The extensive, radiating cytoplasmic processes for which the astrocyte received its name are most readily appreciated when reactive astrocytes are immunostained for GFAP (**B**). Reactive astrocytes have been descriptively classified according to the amount and configuration of visible cytoplasm, and include the aptly named gemistocytic "laden" or "stuffed" cell (**C**), and pilocytic "hair cell" (**D**) types. Reactive gemistocytes are typical of the acute astrocytic reaction to CNS damage whereas dense fibrillary gliosis is commonly seen in longstanding lesions such as healed infarcts.

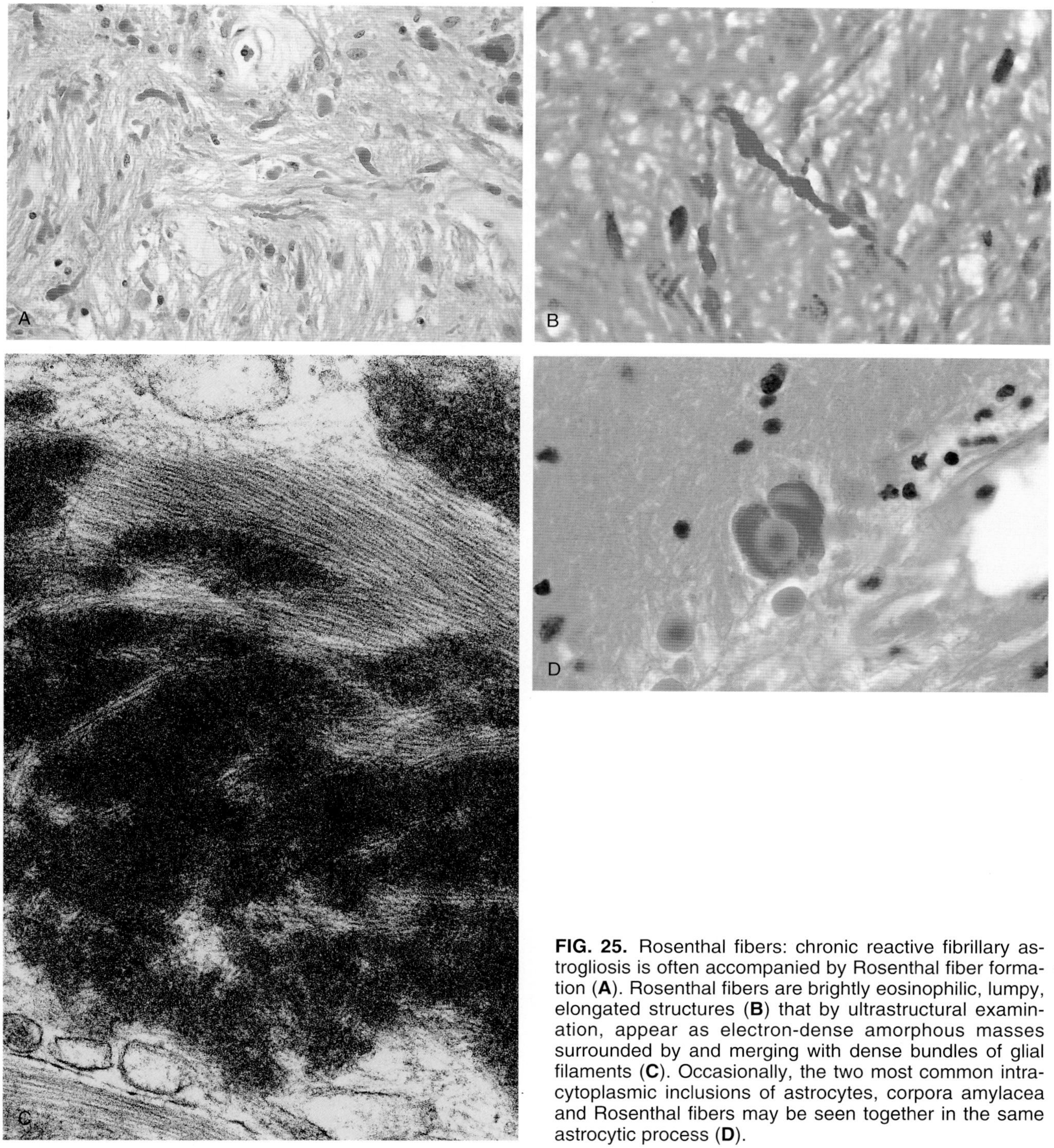


**FIG. 25.** Rosenthal fibers: chronic reactive fibrillary astrogliosis is often accompanied by Rosenthal fiber formation (**A**). Rosenthal fibers are brightly eosinophilic, lumpy, elongated structures (**B**) that by ultrastructural examination, appear as electron-dense amorphous masses surrounded by and merging with dense bundles of glial filaments (**C**). Occasionally, the two most common intracytoplasmic inclusions of astrocytes, corpora amylacea and Rosenthal fibers may be seen together in the same astrocytic process (**D**).

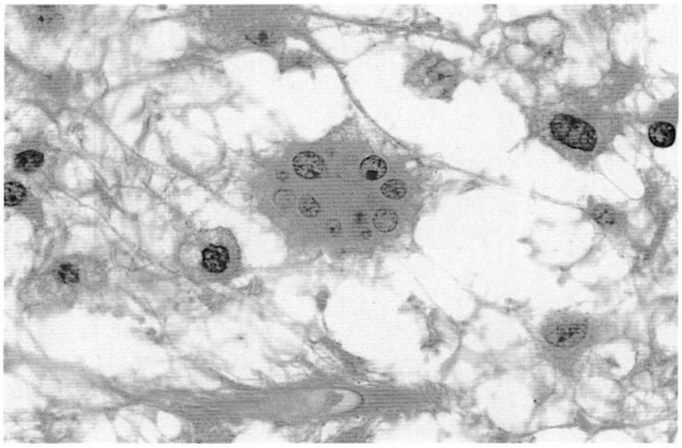

**FIG. 26.** Creutzfeldt astrocyte in demyelinating diseases: these distinctive reactive astrocytes exhibit multiple tiny nuclei "micronuclei." They may be seen in a variety of pathologic conditions, but are particularly characteristic of demyelinative lesions.

as *gemistocytes* (literally "stuffed cells"). Gliosis may, of course, also present as an increase in the number and density of astrocytic nuclei without attendant cytoplasmic prominence. This chronic type of gliosis is frequently subtle and often requires special stains for confirmation and quantitation.

The end result of acute reactive astrogliosis, such as that accompanying cerebral infarction, is frequently a dense fibrillary gliosis (Fig. 24D). The often-invoked analogy of the astrocyte as the "fibroblast of the CNS," i.e., a ubiquitously distributed cell with mitotic capability that responds with alacrity to a wide range of deleterious stimuli, is quite apt.

A distinctive cytoplasmic inclusion seen in fibrillary astrogliosis is the Rosenthal fiber (Fig. 25). These strikingly eosinophilic, elongated, anfractuous structures are observed in a wide variety of reactive states that share in common significant chronicity. Rosenthal fibers are also characteristic of several specific nosologic entities, including Alexander's disease and, perhaps most widely known, juvenile pilocytic astrocytoma. It should be stressed, however, that Rosenthal fibers may be strikingly abundant in the chronically compressed glial stroma surrounding a large number of nonneoplastic conditions (such as syringomyelia) and slowly expanding nonglial tumors (such as craniopharyngioma).

There are several specialized forms of reactive astrogliosis that deserve brief description. Reactive astrocytes with multiple small nuclei ("micronuclei"), termed "Creutzfeldt astrocytes," may be seen in a number of reactive states, but are especially typical of demyelinative processes (Fig. 26). A specific type of astrocytic reaction to injury is seen in a variety of hepatic diseases that produce hyperammonemia. The reaction consists of nuclear changes exclusively: swelling with contortion of the nuclear membrane, chromatin clearing, and development of one or two prominent nucleoli (Fig. 27). In sharp contrast to all of the other types of reactive astrocytes, these Alzheimer type II astrocytes fail to exhibit prominent (or even subtle!) cytoplasm by routine H&E microscopy. Alzheimer type II astrocytes may be seen throughout the neuraxis but are particularly prominent in certain locations, most notably the globus pallidus. Alzheimer type I astrocytes differ from type II astrocytes in displaying abundant eosinophilic cytoplasm (Fig. 27) and are only seen with frequency in Wilson's disease (hepatolenticular degeneration). As the eponyms imply, both types of reactive astrocytic morphologies were described by Alois Alzheimer

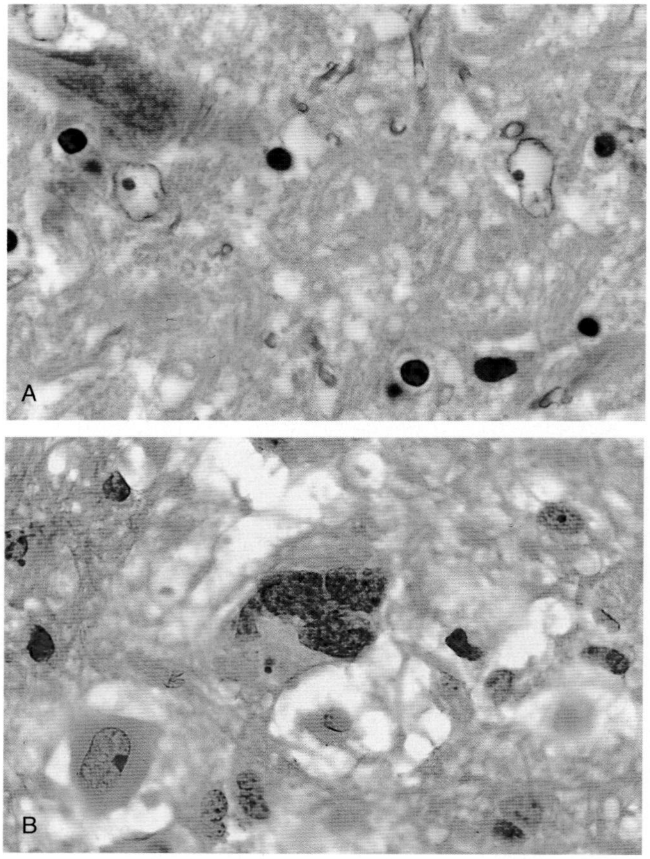


**FIG. 27.** Alzheimer astrocytes in hyperammonemia: two types of reactive astrocytic morphologies, termed Alzheimer type II and Alzheimer type I astrocytes, are associated with hyperammonemic conditions. They were described by Alois Alzheimer and bear his name but have nothing to do with the dementing disease that was also a subject of the famous neurologist's investigations. By far, the most frequently encountered are Alzheimer Type II astrocytes (**A**). Typical features include an enlarged pale nucleus with an irregular contour and one or more small nucleoli. In marked contrast to other types of reactive astrocytes, visible cytoplasm is lacking. Alzheimer type II astrocytes are commonly seen in a wide variety of diseases that result in increased blood ammonia. In contrast, Alzheimer type I astrocytes (**B**) have large, irregularly lobulated or multiple nuclei and clearly discernible eosinophilic cytoplasm. These cells are not seen in most hyperammonemic diseases, with the exception of hepatolenticular degeneration (Wilson's disease).

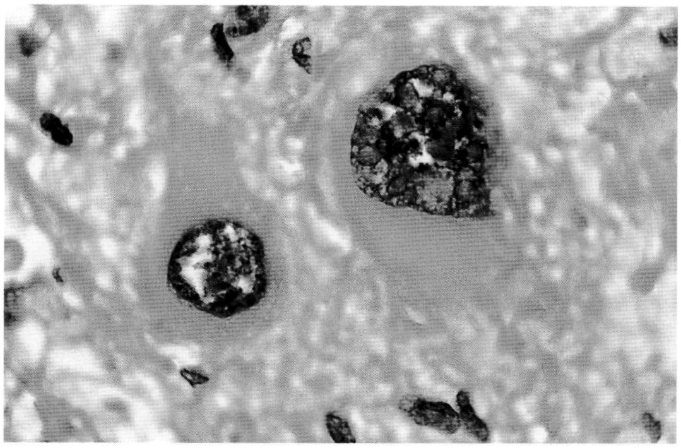

**FIG. 28.** Bizarre reactive astrocytes of progressive multifocal leukoencephalopathy (PML): atypical-appearing reactive astrocytes are sometimes the most striking finding in a PML biopsy and can be mistaken for neoplasia by the unprepared.

and have no relationship to the dementing disease of the same ilk.

Among astrocytic reactions to injury, none is more striking than that observed in some cases of progressive multifocal leukoencephalopathy (PML). Not infrequently, the most eye-catching aspect of a PML biopsy is an alarming nuclear hyperchromatism and pleomorphism exhibited by scattered astrocytes—a vignette that has on more than one occasion elicited a mental frisson from even the most experienced observer (Fig. 28).

Perivascular clearing is a routinely observed artifact of autolysis (Fig. 29). By electron microscopy, these clear spaces are revealed to be greatly dilated astrocytic perivascular foot processes. This phenomenon of water imbibition by astrocytes is seen both as an autolytic change in virtually all autopsy specimens and, when extreme, as a marker of antemortem hypoxic/ischemic injury.

## Oligodendroglia

The oligodendroglia ("few branch" glia) are small cells that are active in the formation and maintenance of myelin, and in the, as yet, poorly understood capacity of attending to neuronal cell bodies (satellitosis). In white matter, the oligodendrocytes' obligatory orientation to fiber pathways is occasionally made apparent by a fortuitous plane of section wherein the fascicular distribution of these cells is seen (Fig. 30). In gray matter, oligodendrocytes are encountered as two-to-three small, dark nuclei that are pressed against the cell membrane of larger neurons (Fig. 31). In surgical specimens obtained from infiltrating gliomas, these normal satellite oligodendroglia must be distinguished from infiltrating neoplastic cells that, like their nontransformed counterparts, are attracted to the immediate perineuronal region. Both astrocytomas and oligodendrogliomas may exhibit such satellitosis, but it is most prominent in the latter neoplasm. Gen-

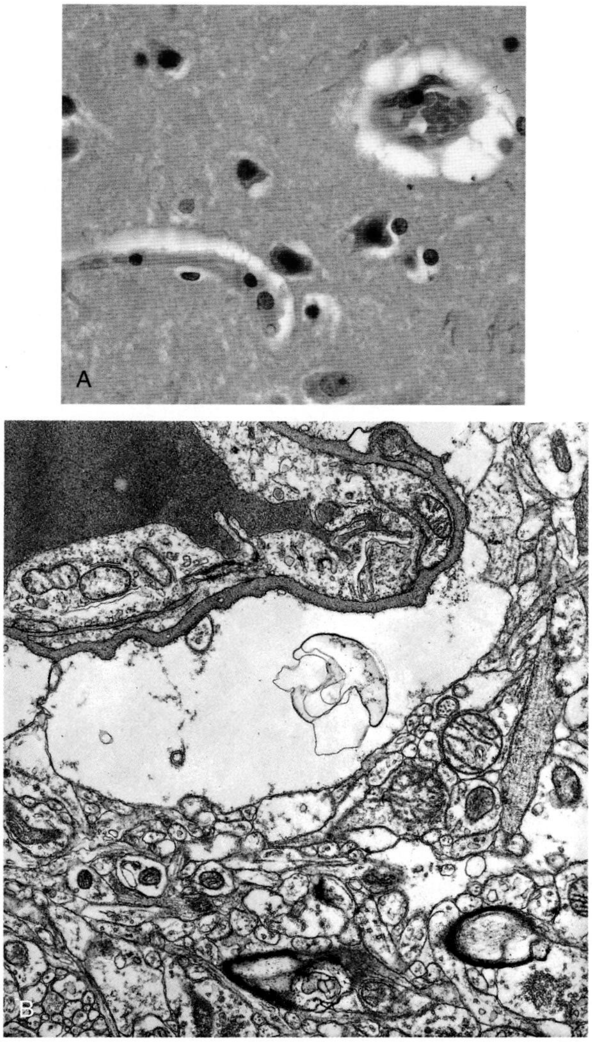


**FIG. 29.** Perivascular astrocytic foot process swelling in autolysis: this common artifact of routine tissue processing is observed by light microscopy as apparent perivascular clearing of the neuropil (**A**). As seen by electron microscopy, the clearing is due to dilated astrocyte foot processes (**B**).

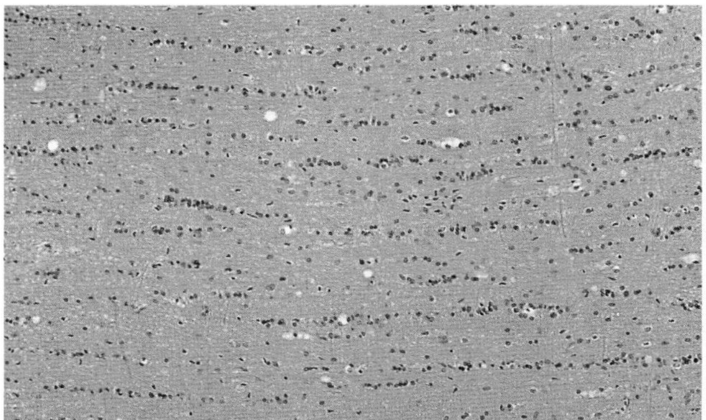

**FIG. 30.** Oligodendroglia: as seen here in a white matter tract (the corpus callosum) cut in longitudinal section, these glia may be identified, even at low power, as rows of nuclei queuing up between fascicles of myelinated axons.

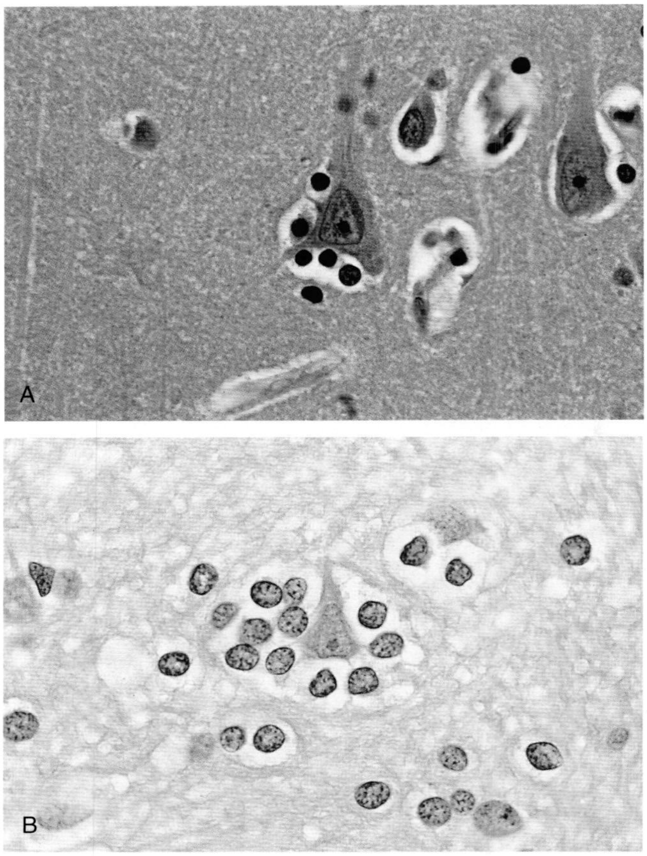

FIG. 31. Perineuronal satellitosis: normal perineuronal glia (**A**) consist primarily of oligodendroglial satellite cells, together with occasional astrocytes and microglia. This affinity of normal oligodendroglia for neuronal perikarya is often retained by their neoplastic counterparts, oligodendrogliomas, in the form of "neoplastic satellitosis" (**B**).

erally, the nuclei of the neoplastic satellites are larger, more pleomorphic, and more coarsely constructed than the normal orbiting cortical oligodendrocytes.

Identification of normal oligodendroglia in both gray and white matter is greatly facilitated by these cells' perinuclear halo (the so-called fried egg appearance), which results from swelling and vacuolation of the cytoplasm (Fig. 32A). This is analogous to the perivascular swelling and vacuolation of astrocytic foot processes. In oligodendroglial neoplasms (oligodendrogliomas), the perinuclear halo is a well-known, distinctive, and diagnostically useful feature (Fig. 32B). Oligodendroglia and their neoplastic counterparts exhibit strong immunopositivity for S-100 protein (Fig. 32C).

## Ependyma

This cuboidal-to-columnar epithelium provides a lining for the CNS ventricular system (Fig. 33), and specializes focally as a covering for the choroid plexus (see Fig. 47). The ciliated nature of the ependyma is readily appreciable in the child, but is generally less so thereafter. Tanycytes (literally "stretched cells") are specialized constituents of the ependyma whose elongated abluminal processes reach the subependymal vasculature. Thus, these cells provide a physical link between the ventricular, vascular, and intraparenchymal compartments of the CNS. Tanycytes are most

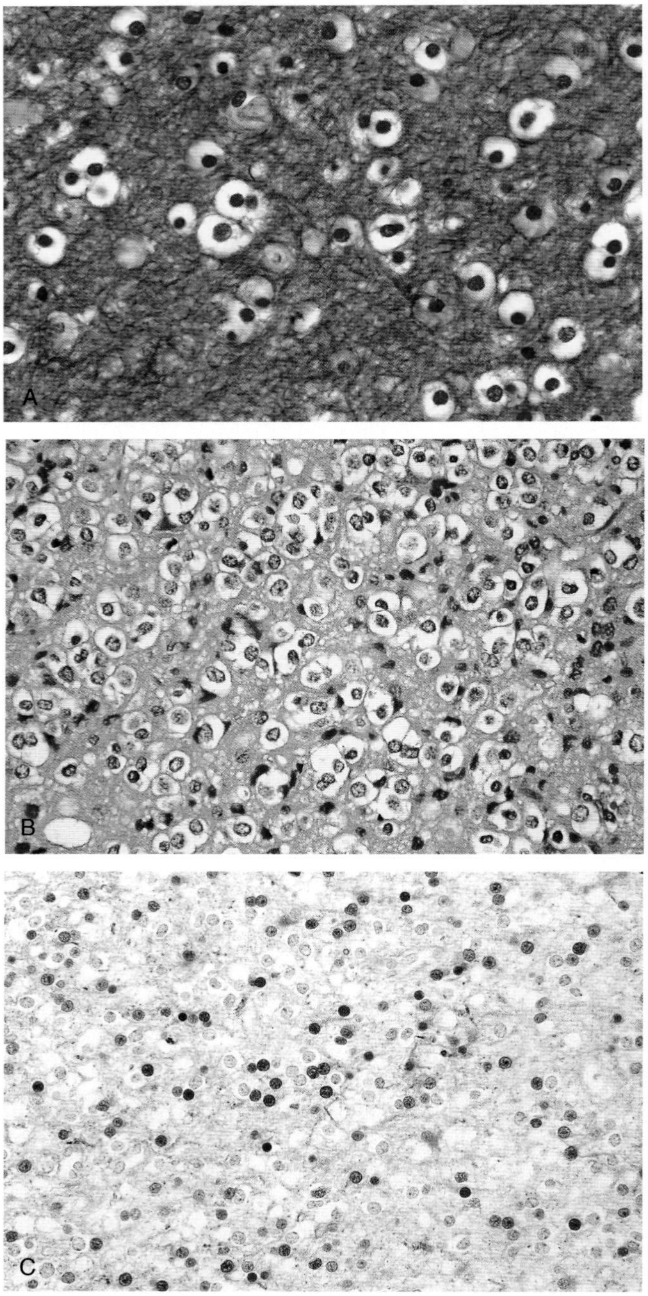

FIG. 32. Oligodendroglia: in many specimens, oligodendroglia exhibit characteristic perinuclear halos (**A**). This "fried egg" appearance is an artifact of hypoxia/ischemia and delayed fixation, and is a useful diagnostic feature that is also exhibited by oligodendrogliomas (**B**). Oligodendroglia, both normal and neoplastic, typically show strong nuclear immunopositivity for S-100 protein (**C**).

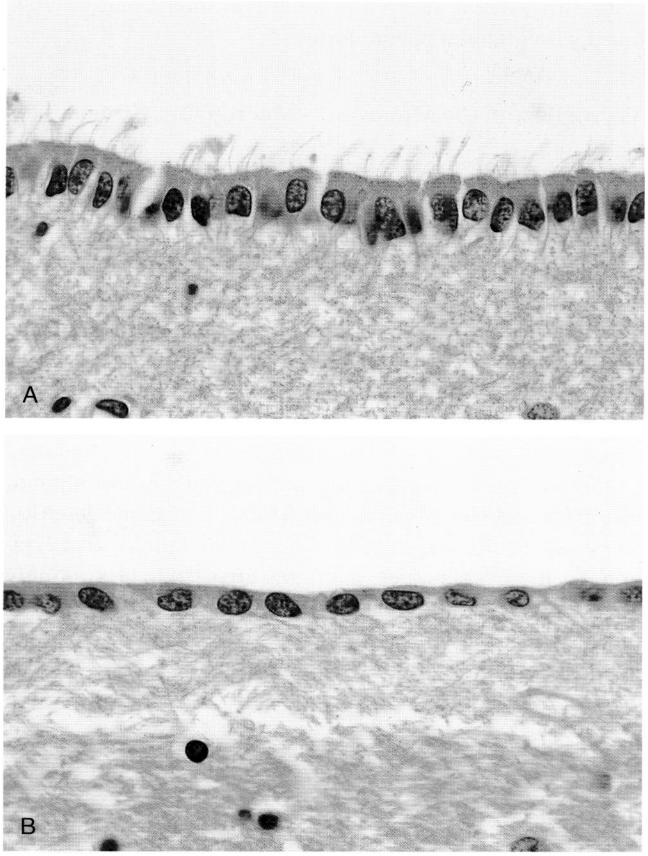


**FIG. 33.** Ependyma and the subependymal plate: the lining of the ventricular system varies from a robust ciliated-columnar epithelium (**A**) to nearly squamous flattened cuboidal (**B**). The relative abundance of cilia and the height of the ependyma vary with anatomic location and both decrease with age. The hypocellular fibrillary zone located immediately subjacent to the ependyma is known as the subependymal plate and contains scattered glia as single cells and in small clusters (see also Fig. 36B). Glia of the subependymal plate respond to ependymal injury with a proliferative response termed granular ependymitis (see Fig. 36A). Subependymomas originate from the glia of the ependyma and subependymal plate.

numerous in the modified ependyma covering many of the circumventricular organs (discussed below). Visualization of these cells is best effected through use of the Golgi stain.

The closely apposed ependymal surfaces of the tips of the lateral ventricle horns frequently fuse during development, resulting in cords of ependymal cell nests and rosettes. This is especially typical of the distal portions of the posterior horns in the occipital lobes (Fig. 34). The white matter in such areas appears pale and can simulate the rarefaction seen after ischemic insult. Detached ependymal rosettes may be encountered subjacent to the ventricular lining at any location throughout the neuraxis.

The ependyma-lined central canal of the spinal cord is patent in the child (Fig. 35) but generally becomes obliterated about the time of puberty, unless obstructive hydro-

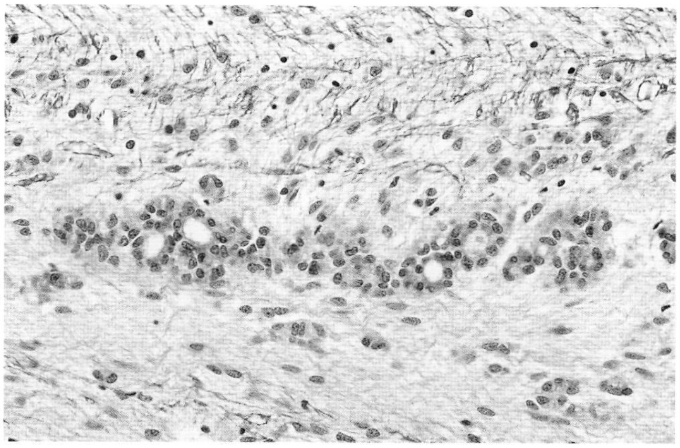

**FIG. 34.** Ependymal rosettes: clusters of ependymal rosettes may be found subjacent to the ependymal lining of the ventricular system throughout the neuraxis. They are particularly common in areas where opposed ventricular surfaces fuse during development, such as at the tips of the lateral ventricle horns, especially the occipital horns (as illustrated here), and at the lateral angles of the fourth ventricle. These normal rosette clusters are occasionally sampled in surgical specimens and should not be misinterpreted as evidence of disease.

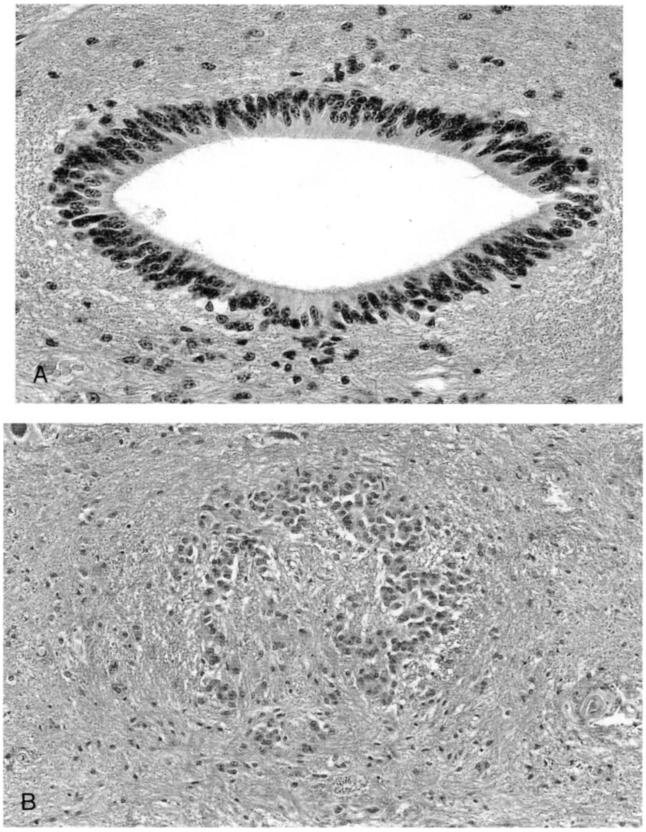


**FIG. 35.** Central canal of the spinal cord: in the child (**A**), the central canal is widely patent and exhibits the ciliated columnar ependymal lining expected in a young individual. In contrast, the central canal of adults is typically obliterated over much of its length, with only residual small nests and occasional rosettes of ependymal cells (**B**).

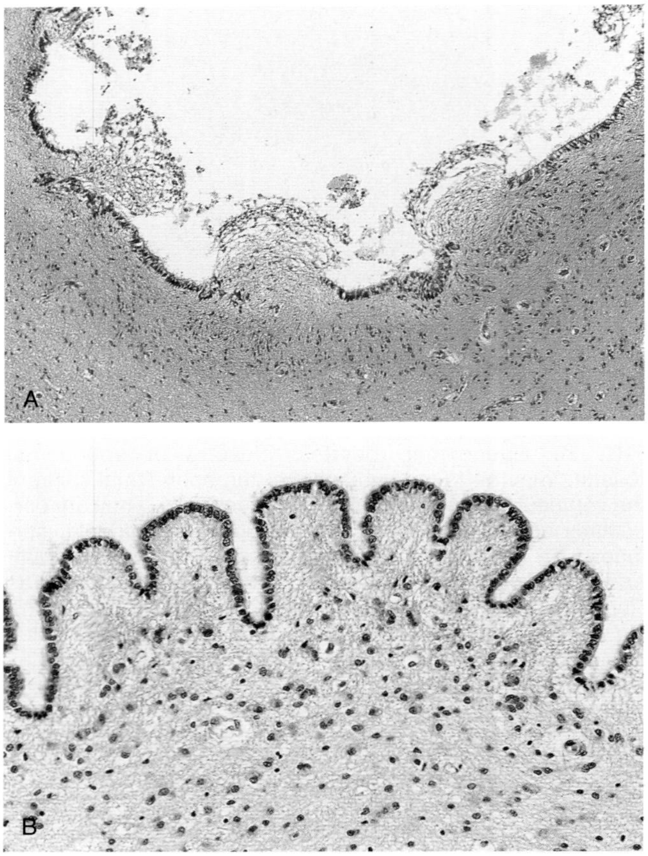

FIG. 36. Granular ependymitis: the combination of focal denudation of the ependyma, coupled with an exophytic fusiform proliferation of the subependymal glia constitutes granular ependymitis (**A**). Despite the implication of an inflammatory etiology inherent in the name, this common alteration can result from many diverse insults, ranging from hydrocephalus to viral infections. Normal undulations of the ependyma (**B**), termed *plicae,* should not be confused with granular ependymitis.

cephalus is present. In the latter case, the canal may remain patent and even become dilated (hydromyelia). In the normal adult, however, the spinal ependymal cells have completed their role as a generative epithelium and remain as scattered clumps and rosettes (Fig. 35). Occasional sections of adult spinal cord may exhibit a focally patent central canal.

The primary ependymal response to injury is loss. The resultant focal denudation of the ventricular wall is often accompanied by a proliferation of local cells, the subependymal glia. This nonspecific reaction, termed *granular ependymitis* (Fig. 36A), is the potential product of a broad range of disparate etiologies, from viral infection to hydrocephalus. It is seen frequently at autopsy as a very focal, limited response and has, in this setting, little diagnostic significance. The normal ependyma is commonly thrown into folds, termed *plicae,* in many parts of the ventricular system (Fig. 36B). These normal undulations should not be confused with granular ependymitis.

## Microglia and the Monocyte—Macrophage System

### *Normal Microscopic Anatomy*

The small, dark, elongated nuclei of microglia are ubiquitous in the normal brain. They are so small and inconspicuous in H&E-stained sections, however, that they are rarely noticed (Fig. 37A). They must be distinguished from the commonly encountered tangential or *en face* sections of endothelial cells, which possess similarly elongated, albeit somewhat larger and plumper, nuclei. Special staining techniques such as the classic silver carbonate method, the more predictable lectin histochemistry (Fig. 37B), and immunohistochemical markers such as Ham-56 uncloak the dendritic processes of microglia and permit unambiguous visualization. By these techniques, microglia are seen to be strikingly pervasive throughout the CNS parenchyma.

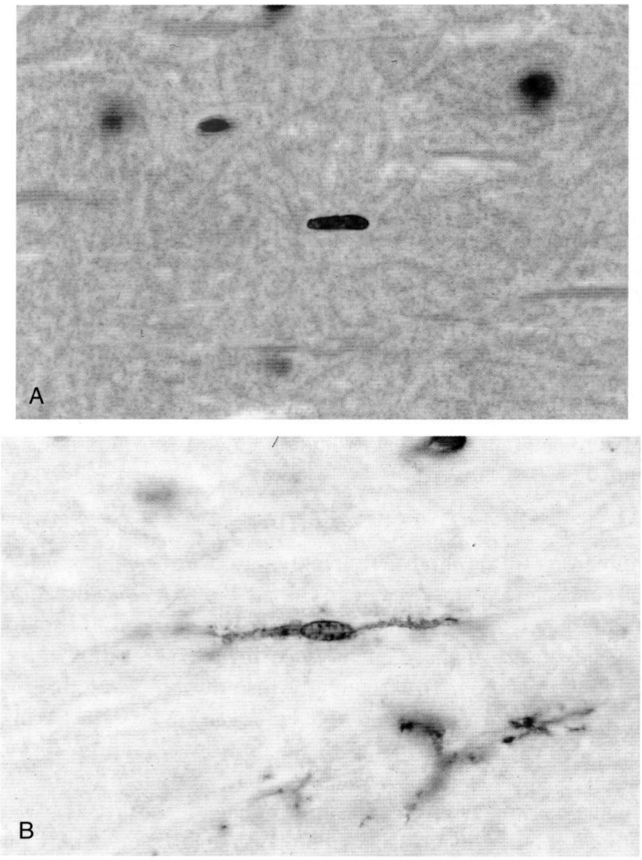

FIG. 37. Microglia: these normally inconspicuous residents of the CNS parenchyma are identifiable by their classical rod-shaped nuclei on routine H&E staining (**A**). Dendritic processes, often bipolar, are vividly demonstrated by lectin staining (**B**).

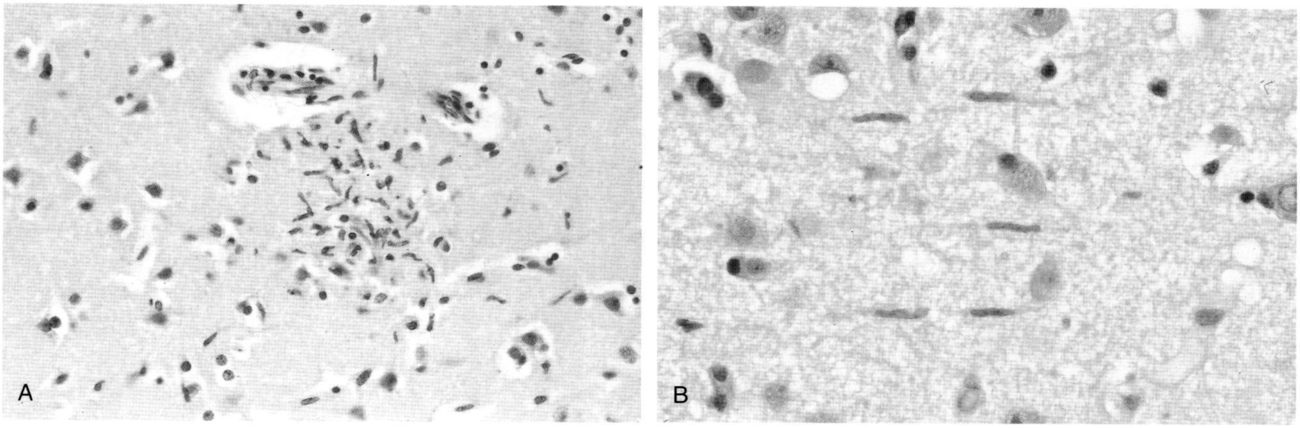


**FIG. 38.** Microglia: reactive microglia may take several forms. Microglial nodules (**A**) are focal hypercellular accumulations of microglia and astrocytes that commonly form as a response to viral and rickettsial infections. In diffuse microgliosis (**B**), seen in a variety of conditions including ischemia, the characteristic elongated rod-shaped nuclei are readily identified without the need for special stains.

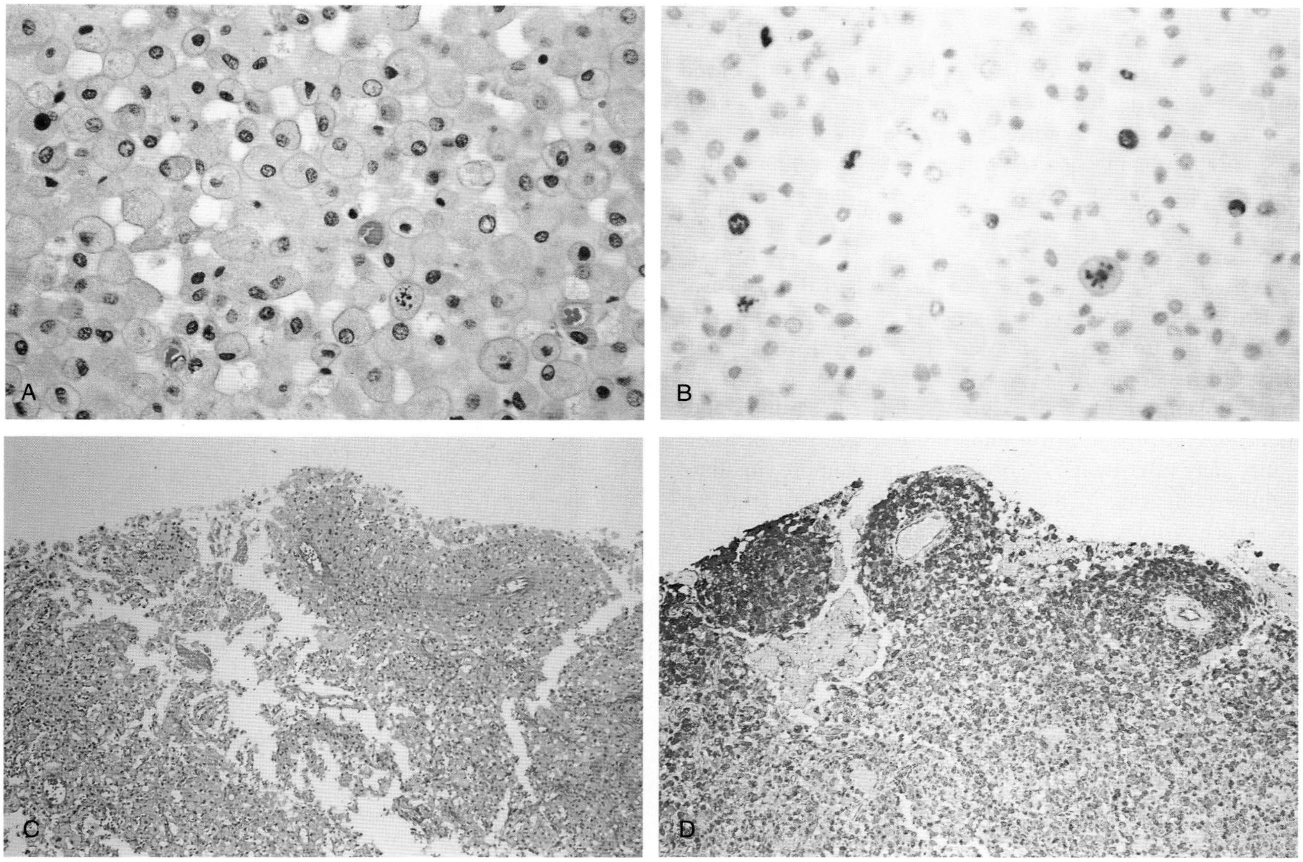


**FIG. 39.** Macrophages: discrete cell boundaries and vesicular cytoplasm serve to distinguish macrophages from other cellular constituents of the nervous system (**A**). Cognoscenti of the literature will be familiar with a number of colorful appellations given these cells in former times, including *Gitter cells (lattice cells)* and *compound granular corpuscles.* Macrophages are mitotically active cells and populations responding to CNS injury are readily labeled with proliferation markers such as the monoclonal antibody MIB-1 (**B**). Mitotic figures are, thus, to be expected in tissue samples from a wide range of nonneoplastic conditions that elicit a macrophage response, including infarcts and demyelinative diseases. In hypercellular biopsies (**C**), macrophages can be separated from other cellular constituents by a number of commercially available antibodies such as Ham-56 (**D**).

### Response to Injury

In contrast to the relative passivity and anonymity of microglia in healthy nervous tissue, their activity is by no means subtle when called to action by parenchymal injury. Two variants are seen: microglial nodules and diffuse microgliosis. Microglial nodules (also called microglial stars) are frequent concomitants of viral or rickettsial infection; and they are generally acknowledged to consist of both astrocytes and microglia (Fig. 38A). The microglia have an elongated shape and are known as rod cells. A form of glial nodule is also seen about degenerating neurons, as in amyotrophic lateral sclerosis. Diffuse microgliosis is equally distinctive. In this context, the rod-shaped nuclei of microglia are present in such numbers as to be easily discernible without the need for special stains (Fig. 38B). Cerebral intraparenchymal syphilis (general paresis) is the classic setting for this latter type of microglial response.

Destruction of nervous tissue, by whatever mechanism, generally elicits a macrophage response that serves to clear nonviable debris (Fig. 39A). Both the activation of autochthonous tissue microglia and the diapedesis of blood monocytes are sources for these scavengers. The weight of evidence suggests that the recruitment of blood monocytes plays a predominant role in large lesions such as infarcts, but that the supply of indigenous cells is sufficient for lesser insults.

Macrophages are proliferative cells (Fig. 39 A,B). Mitotic figures will, therefore, usually be present in disease processes that elicit a macrophage response, such as infarction and demyelination. They should not be interpreted as suggestive of a neoplastic process. Macrophages often contribute substantially to the cellularity of tissue samples and, depending on preservation and fixation conditions, their identity may not always be obvious. For example, in some specimens, clearing of the macrophage cytoplasm lends an appearance similar to that of oligodendroglial cells, to the extent that, together with the attendant hypercellularity, an infiltrating glioma might be suspected. In such instances a number of antibodies, such as KP-1 or Ham-56, can be used to identify the macrophage component (Fig. 39 C,D).

## SPECIALIZED ORGANS OF THE CENTRAL NERVOUS SYSTEM

### Pineal Gland

The pineal body (epiphysis or conarium) presents a singular histologic appearance among CNS tissues with a prominently lobulated architecture (Figs. 40 and 41). This glandular appearance might be mistaken for carcinoma by the unwary, and it can be difficult to distinguish the normal pineal gland from a well-differentiated pineocytoma in small surgical specimens.

Generally present in the pineal after puberty are corpora arenacea (acervuli cerebri or "brain sand"). These mineralized concretions accrue with age and confer the radiologic hyperdensity that, before the era of computerized tomography and magnetic resonance imaging, made the normal midline position of the pineal a useful radiologic landmark (Fig. 40).

The increase in corpora arenacea with senescence is accompanied by gradual gliosis and cystic change, with attendant effacement of the lush glandular appearance of the pineal seen in the earlier decades of life. The ubiquitous incidental pineal cysts typically have densely gliotic walls with

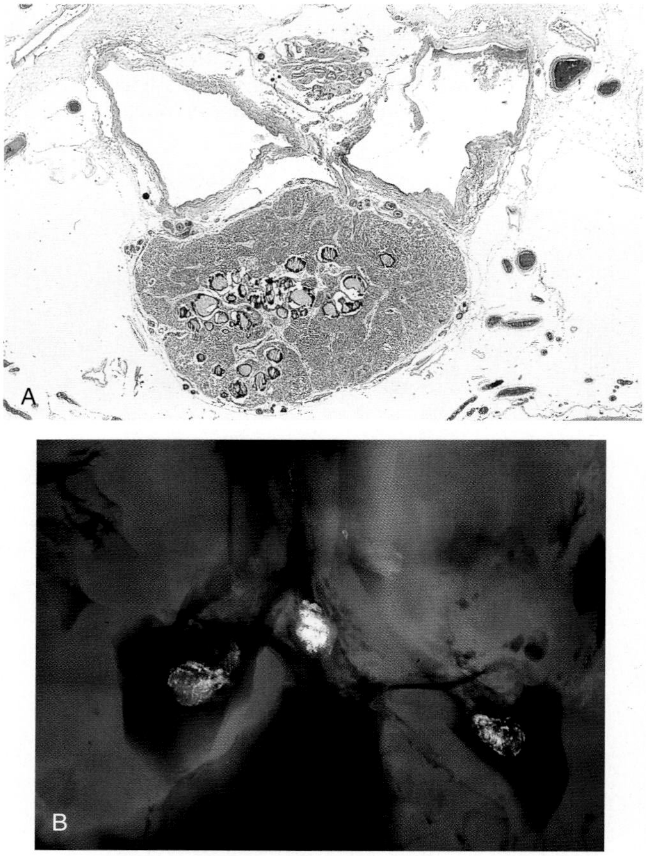


**FIG. 40.** Pineal gland (epiphysis): whole mount of a cross section of the pineal and its environs in situ (**A**) reveals the typical mineralized concretions variously referred to as corpora arenacea ("sand bodies"), acervuli cerebri ("little heaps"), or simply brain sand. Superior to the pineal are the paired internal cerebral veins, and between them is the suprapineal recess of the third ventricle which is lined with ependyma and often contains a tuft of choroid plexus. The loose connective tissue (redundant leptomeninges), in which all of these structures are located, is called the velum interpositum. The calcification of the pineal increases with age and was, thereby, quite useful as a radiographic midline marker prior to the advent of contemporary high resolution neuroimaging modalities (**B**). Also seen in this radiograph of a normal adult brain are prominently calcified tufts of choroid plexus (glomera choroidea; see Fig. 47) in the atria of both lateral ventricles.

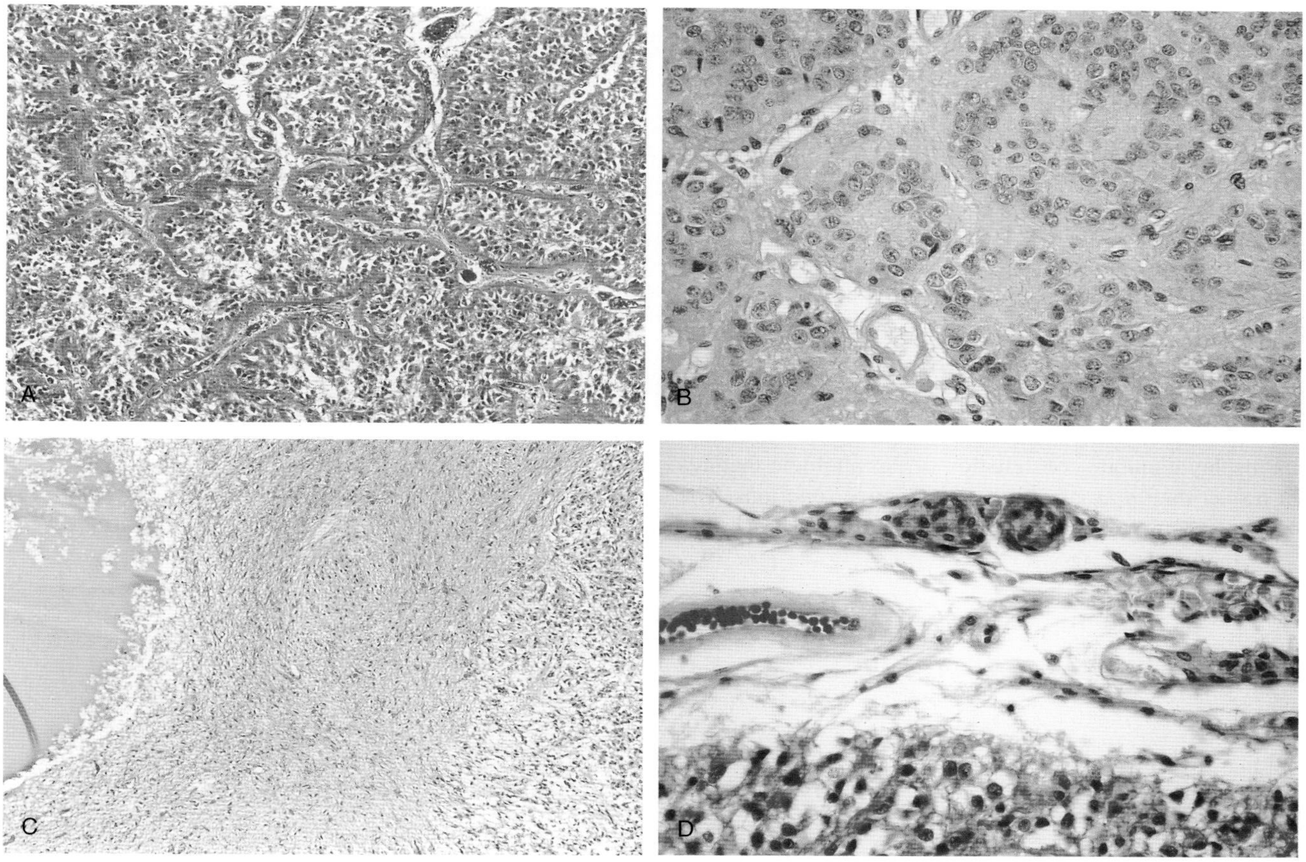


**FIG. 41.** Pineal histology: the pineal has a richly glandular architecture that is totally unlike any other region of the central nervous system. Salient features include a prominent lobular organization with connective tissue septa (**A**) and pineocytic rosettes (**B**). The latter impart a distinctly neuroendocrine character. Two additional histologic features of note are the ubiquitous incidental pineal cysts, whose walls (**C**) typically exhibit astrogliosis with scattered Rosenthal fibers, and arachnoid cell nests of the investing velum interpositum (**D**) that occasionally provide a source for meningiomas arising in this region.

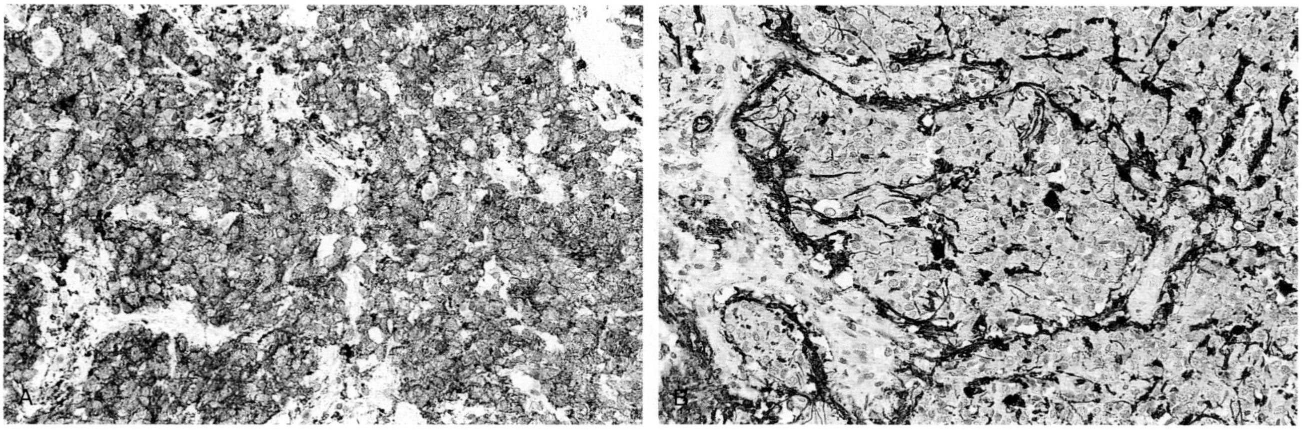


**FIG. 42.** Pineal immunohistochemistry: pineocytes (and their neoplastic progeny, the pineal parenchymal tumors) are strongly immunopositive for the neuronal marker synaptophysin (**A**). As expected, the indigenous population of pineal astrocytes are well visualized with antibodies directed against GFAP (**B**).

scattered Rosenthal fiber formation (Fig. 41C). The investing leptomeninges of the pineal contain arachnoid cell nests that occasionally give rise to meningiomas of the pineal region (Fig. 40).

Pineocytes express strong immunopositivity for the neuronal marker synaptophysin (Fig. 42A). This useful phenotypic marker is retained by most pineal parenchymal neoplasms. In addition to pineocytes, the pineal also contains an indigenous population of astrocytes whose distribution is revealed by immunostaining for GFAP (Fig. 42B).

### Median Eminence and Infundibulum

The median eminence and infundibulum of the hypothalamus display a unique constellation of morphologic features that reflect their specialized neuroendocrine functions. The background neuropil is highly fibrillar and exhibits two distinguishing structures: complex microvascular tangles, termed *gomitoli* ("coils"; Fig. 43A), which are composed of intricate capillary networks that invest terminal arterioles derived from the superior hypophyseal arteries, and spherical granular structures, termed *Herring bodies,* that constitute storage sites for oxytocin and vasopressin (Fig. 43B). The combination of a highly fibrillar pilocytic stroma, granular bodies, and microvascular tangles lends a superficial resemblance of this specialized tissue to that of juvenile pilocytic astrocytoma. The intrasellar continuation of the infundibulum, the posterior pituitary (neurohypophysis), is described in detail in Chapter 13.

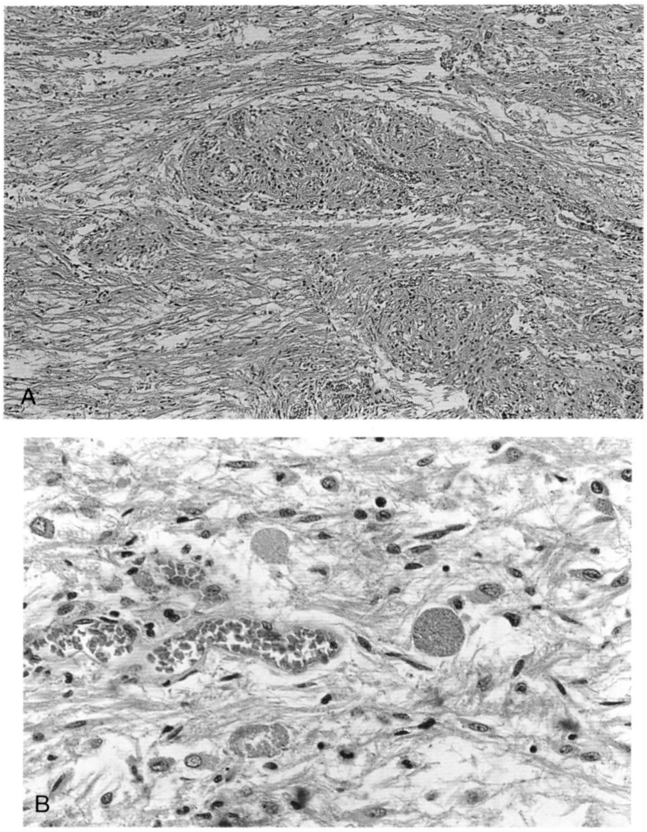


**FIG. 43.** Median eminence and infundibulum: this unique region of the CNS exhibits three distinguishing features: a highly spindled stroma, prominent capillary tangles of the hypothalamo-hypophyseal portal system called gomitoli (**A**), and spherical, eosinophilic axonal specializations for the storage of oxytocin and vasopressin called Herring bodies (**B**). The combination of spindled stroma, vascular tangles, and eosinophilic granular bodies lends a certain resemblance to juvenile pilocytic astrocytoma.

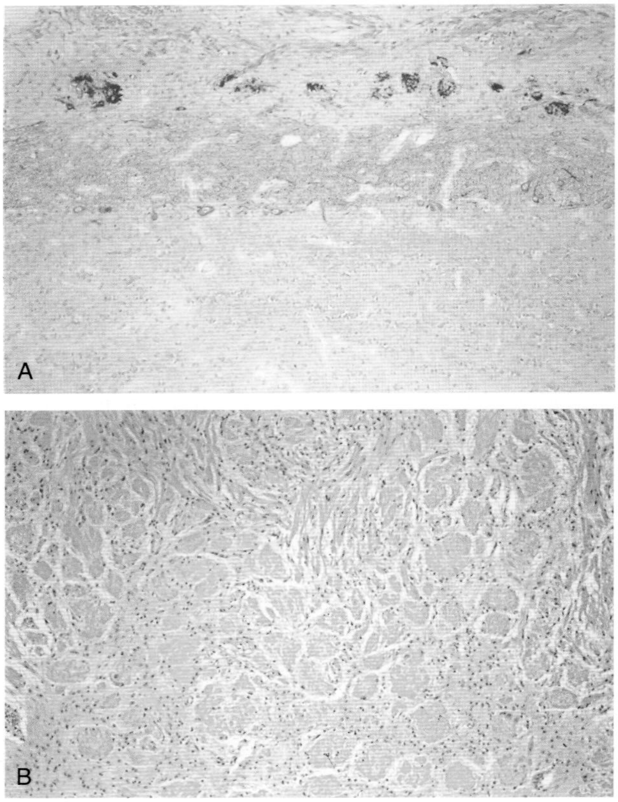


**FIG. 44.** Olfactory bulbs: the olfactory bulbs have a distinctive laminar organization consisting of a superficial spindled layer of entering olfactory nerve fascicles, glomerular layer, external plexiform layer, mitral cell layer, and granular cell layer. As illustrated in panel **A**, the glomeruli and mitral cells exhibit strong immunopositivity for synaptophysin, with diffuse neuropil positivity seen in the external plexiform and granular cell layers. The most distinctive and diagnostically useful architectural features of the olfactory bulbs are the glomeruli (seen at higher power with intermingling fascicles of olfactory nerve axons in panel **B**) and the dense lamina of granular neurons.

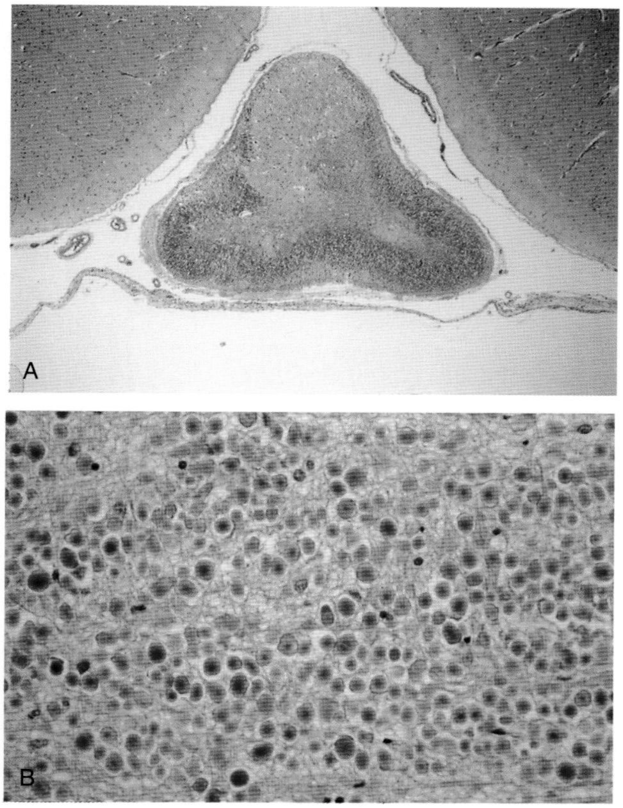


FIG. 45. Olfactory tracts: the olfactory tracts contain myelinated fiber bundles and are roughly triangular in cross section (**A**). A distinctive feature of the tracts frequently observed in adults is their remarkable content of corpora amylacea (**B**).

## Olfactory Bulbs and Tracts

The intracranial components of the olfactory apparatus (the olfactory bulbs and tracts) have a very distinctive histologic appearance. Familiarity with these structures is useful, not only for the neuropathologist, but also for the general surgical pathologist who may encounter them in resections performed as part of the surgical treatment for regionally invasive entities of the nasal and paranasal sinuses. In such situations, the surgical pathologist may be called upon to render an intraoperative frozen-section assessment of tissue resected superior to the cribriform plate. The ability to recognize the normal histologic features of olfactory bulb tissue is, thus, of more than pedantic importance.

The olfactory bulb has a laminar organization (Fig. 44). The outer layer is composed of spindled bundles of entering olfactory nerve fascicles intermixed with distinctive spherical, anuclear areas (termed "glomeruli") that constitute specialized zones of synaptic contact between olfactory nerve collaterals and the dendrites of intrinsic olfactory bulb neurons. Mitral cells are large neurons, so-named for a resemblance of the perikaryon shape to a bishop's mitre. Their cell bodies are located in a lamina deep to that of the glomeruli (Fig. 44). The deepest layer consists of a thick lamina of granular cell neurons that are comparable in size to those of the cerebellum and dentate gyrus.

The olfactory tracts (sometimes incorrectly referred to as olfactory nerves) extend posteriorly from the olfactory bulbs. They are triangular in cross section and, in adults, are notable for their profuse numbers of corpora amylacea (Fig. 45).

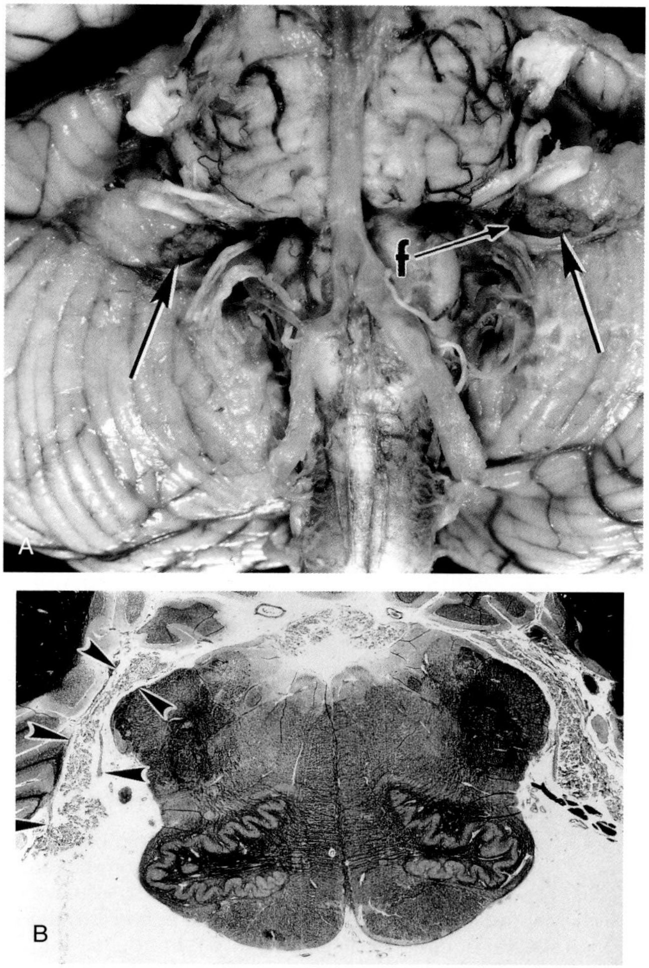


FIG. 46. Choroid plexus: **A:** Small tufts of choroid plexus are normally visible on the basal surface of the brain stem in the cerebellopontine angle (arrows), and indicate the location of the lateral foramina of Luschka (f) from which they protrude. The dusty discoloration of the inferior medulla is due to the presence of leptomeningeal melanocytes (see Fig. 56). **B:** The ependyma-lined sleeve of the lateral recess of the fourth ventricle (arrowheads), together with the protruding tuft of choroid plexus, is referred to in the older literature as the "flower basket of Bochdalek" or "cornucopia." Pieces of the ependymal cuff are often seen adherent to the lateral aspect of the medulla in autopsy brain stem sections and should be recognized as a normal finding.

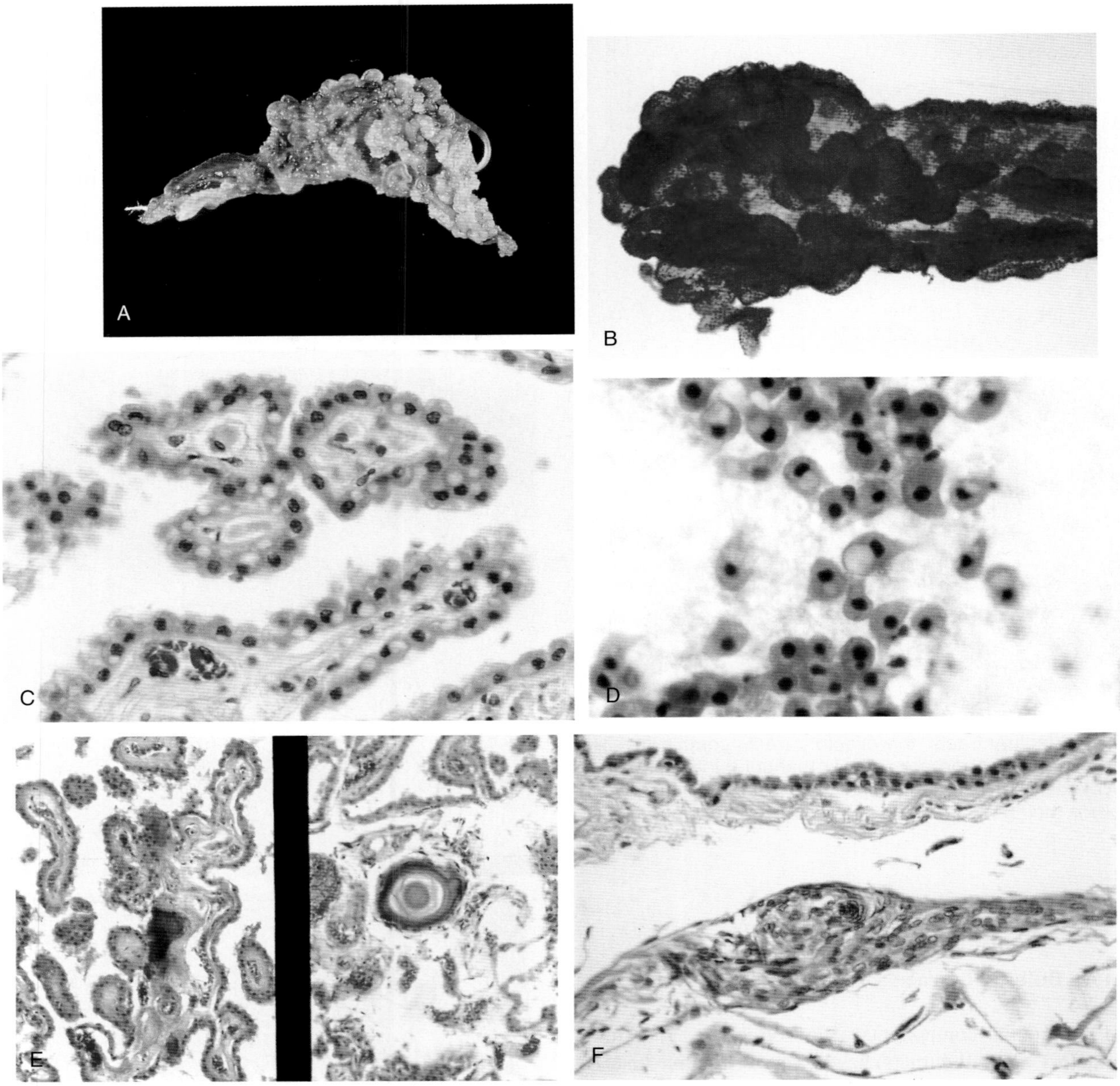


**FIG. 47.** Choroid plexus: the choroid plexus, as exemplified here by the glomus choroideum, is composed of a botryoid tangle of epithelium-covered blood vessels with a finely granular surface texture (**A**). This gross appearance is imparted by innumerable microscopic papillary tufts, as seen in squash preparations (**B**). The choroid plexus epithelium derives from modified ependyma and covers a highly vascular connective tissue core (**C**). In adults, many of the choroid epithelial cells bear a prominent paranuclear cytoplasmic vacuole (**C**). This feature can be particularly striking in touch (imprint) preparations (**D**), and should not be forgotten when interpreting biopsy specimens obtained from areas of the CNS that normally contain choroid plexus. Mineralization of the fibrovascular core occurs in two forms: nonspecific deposition of mineral salts onto the collagenous stroma (**E,** left-hand panel), and psammoma bodies (**E,** right-hand panel). Psammoma bodies originate in nests of meningothelial cells that are normal indigenous constituents of the plexus (**F**). Both forms of mineralization increase with age and impart radiodensity (see Fig. 40B). In addition to providing a nidus for psammoma body formation, the presence of meningothelial cells explains the occurrence of "intraventricular" meningiomas (which are actually choroid plexus meningiomas).

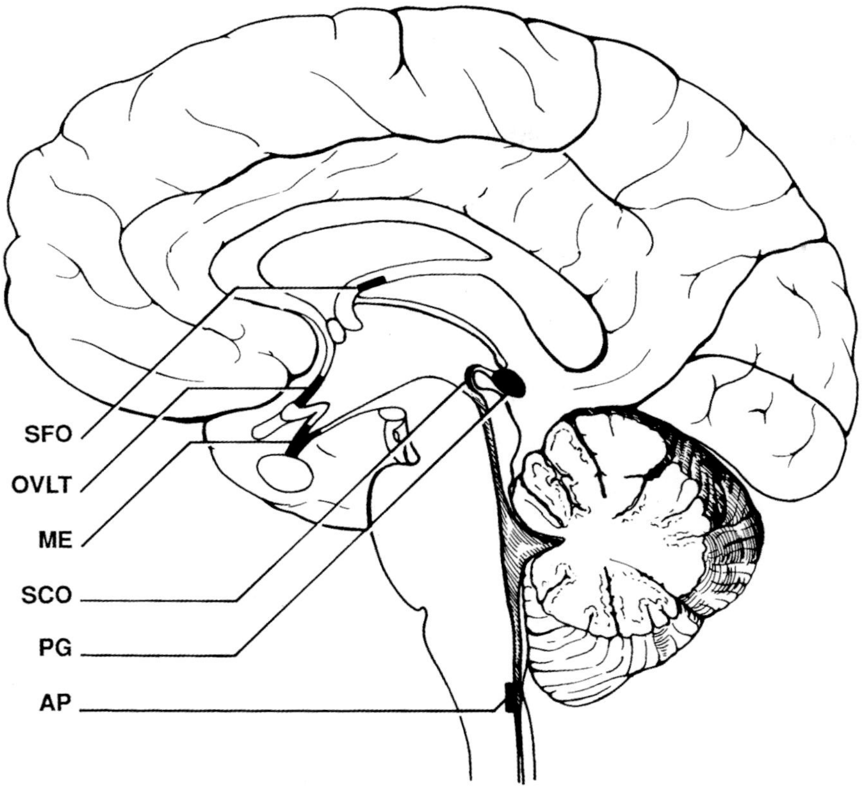


**FIG. 48.** Circumventricular organs: the circumventricular organs share a midline or paramidline position, proximity to the ventricular system, and lack of the usual blood-brain barrier. The subcommissural organ is present in the developing fetus but is vestigial in the adult. AP, area postrema; ME, median eminence and infundibulum; OVLT, organum vasculosum of the lamina terminalis; PG, pineal gland; SCO, subcommissural organ; SFO, subfornical organ.

### Choroid Plexus

The choroid plexus is a specialized organ of the CNS that is responsible for the production of cerebrospinal fluid. It is found in the body, atrium, and temporal horns of the lateral ventricles, in the interventricular foramina of Monro, in the roof of the third ventricle, and in the roof and lateral recesses of the fourth ventricle. The frontal and occipital horns of the lateral ventricles and the aqueduct of Sylvius are devoid of choroid plexus. The plexus is most obvious in the atria of the lateral ventricles (see Figs. 40B and 47), where prominent bilateral tufts (glomera choroidea) are formed. Cystic xanthomatous change is a common incidental finding in these botryoid structures. The plexus is also a normal resident in the subarachnoid space of the cerebellopontine angle (CPA) cisterns, which it reaches from the lateral recesses of the fourth ventricle by protruding through the foramina of Luschka (Fig. 46). The paired foramina of Luschka (lateral), which open laterally into the ventral basilar CPA cisterns, are to be distinguished from the single foramen of Magendie (median), which opens in the dorsal midline into the cisterna magna.

Microscopically, choroid plexus consists of invaginated fronds of vascular leptomeninges covered by an ependyma that is modified to become a highly secretory epithelium (Fig. 47). The cells are larger and more cobblestoned than those of the adjacent ependyma (Fig. 33). In addition to collagen and blood vessels, small nests of meningothelial (arachnoid) cells are common normal habitués of the choroid plexus; whorls of these cells frequently give rise to psammoma bodies (Fig. 47 E,F). Nonspecific deposition of mineral salts also occurs commonly throughout the connective tissue core with increasing age and accounts for most of the plexuses' radiodensity. An additional aging change of no specific pathological significance is cytoplasmic vacuolization of the ependyma-derived lining cells (Fig. 47 C,D).

### Circumventricular Organs

The circumventricular organs (CVOs) comprise a diverse group of specialized CNS centers with two shared morphologic features: a periventricular location and vasculature that lacks the typical properties of the blood-brain barrier. The five structures that represent the major human CVOs are the pineal gland (discussed previously), area postrema, subfornical organ (intercolumnar tubercle), organum vaculosum of the lamina terminalis (OVLT), and the median eminence and infundibulum of the hypothalamus (Fig. 48). The subcommissural organ, a prominent CVO of most vertebrates that is located on the ventral surface of the posterior commissure, regresses in the human near the end of gestation; vestigial

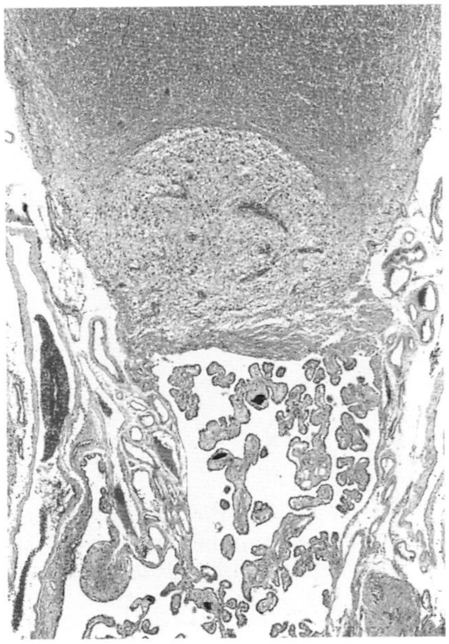

**FIG. 49.** Subfornical organ (intercolumnar tubercle): the microscopic appearance of all the circumventricular organs is remarkably similar. Typical features, as illustrated here by the subfornical organ, include a loose neuropil with prominent vascularity.

remnants may rarely be seen in a fortuitous section. Unfortunately, with the exception of the area postrema, these interesting structures are only rarely encountered in "routine" sections of the brain (Fig. 49).

## INTRADURAL ELEMENTS OF THE PERIPHERAL NERVOUS SYSTEM

The major intradural representatives of the peripheral nervous system are the cranial and spinal nerves and small autonomic fibers in the adventitia of blood vessels. In all of the cranial nerves except cranial nerve eight, the transition from central to peripheral nervous system occurs within 2 mm of the pial surface. In the eighth cranial nerve, the central nervous system extends out along the nerve for a centimeter or so to the level of the internal auditory meatus. At this point, the transition occurs between the medial central nervous system segment and the lateral peripheral segment that emerges from the apparatus for hearing and balance (Fig. 50). The myelin of the central nervous system is formed by oligodendrocytes, whereas that of the peripheral nervous system is formed by Schwann cells. Peripheral nerve is noted for its content of interstitial collagen and the elongated nuclei of Schwann cells.

Two additional intrathecal components of the peripheral nervous system may pique interest on fortuitous encounter. The first is the so-called microneuroma, which is usually found in the parenchyma of the spinal cord or, more rarely, the medulla (Fig. 51). These structures consist of a Gordian knot of unmyelinated axons that have been hypothesized to arise secondary to traumatic injury of peripheral nerve roots whose regenerating axons follow penetrating spinal or medullary arteries into the CNS parenchyma along the Virchow-Robin spaces. According to the hypothesis, the tapering perivascular spaces ultimately block further advance of the regenerating axons and, thereby, result in the observed neuroma.

An additional component of the peripheral nervous system that occasionally arouses interest is the unmyelinated terminal nerve (variously termed *nervus terminalis, cranial nerve zero,* and *cranial nerve T*), which courses in the subarachnoid space covering the gyri recti of the orbital surface of the frontal lobes. Although usually composed of multiple small anastomosing fascicles, it occurs as a single trunk in some specimens and can be quite striking. Rarely, intrafascicular ganglion cells may be observed.

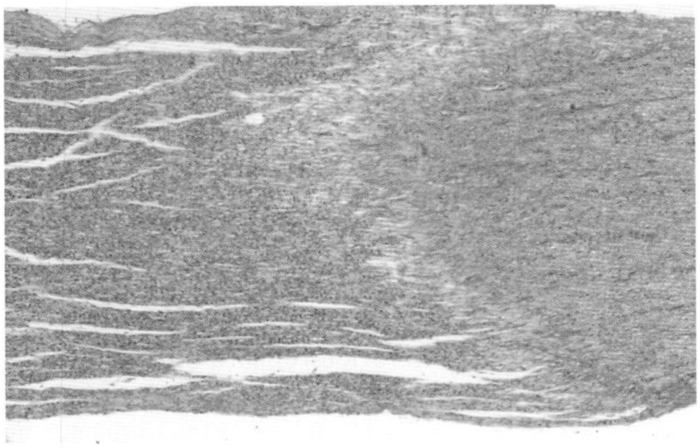

**FIG. 50.** Transition zone from central to peripheral nervous system myelin: for cranial nerve eight (vestibulo-cochlear) this transition occurs in the vicinity of the internal acoustic meatus.

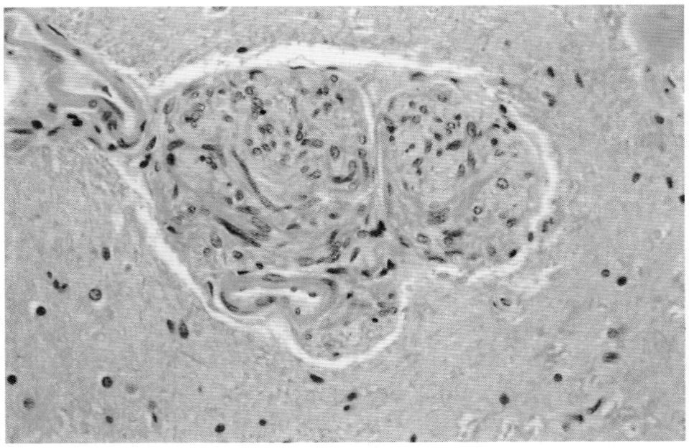

**FIG. 51.** Microneuroma: these tangled balls of unmyelinated axons are most often encountered in the spinal cord, less often in the medulla, as an incidental finding in an otherwise unremarkable specimen.

## MENINGES

### Dura Mater (Pachymenix)

The dura is composed of two tightly annealed layers of fibrous connective tissue. The outer layer functions as the periosteum of the cranium, whereas the inner meningeal layer is joined to the arachnoid membrane by weak intercellular junctions and focally forms the four dural reduplications that compartmentalize the cranial cavity: the falx cerebri, falx cerebelli, tentorium cerebelli, and diaphragma sellae. The two layers of the dura separate to accommodate the dural venous sinuses; the inner meningeal layer is pierced by draining veins and by arachnoid villi. The latter conduct CSF back into the venous circulation and are obvious over the superior parasagittal convexities of the cerebral hemispheres where they project into the superior sagittal sinus (Fig. 52). They are present in all other major venous sinuses, as well. They are often observed along the posterior margin of the cerebellar hemispheres in relation to the sinus confluens and the transverse venous sinuses. Small villi are also present intraspinally.

The epithelial properties of arachnoid granulations are reflected ultrastructurally in elongated, interdigitating cell processes bonded together with desmosomes and immunohistochemically, by positivity for epithelial membrane antigen (Fig. 52). These features are also characteristic of meningiomas.

With age, the deposition of collagen enlarges the arachnoid villi that are then referred to as pacchionian bodies (Fig. 52). Such large granulations frequently press through the overlying roof of the superior sagittal sinus and its lateral lacunae to produce small pits or depressions in the inner table of the calvarium. These are known as the *foveolae granulares* or *pacchionian foveolae.* Portions of the dura, particularly the falx cerebri and parasagittal dura associated with the superior sagittal sinus, often calcify nonspecifically with age. Cacification may also be seen in association with chronic renal failure. Focal ossification is sometimes encountered as an incidental finding.

### Pia-Arachnoid (Leptomeninges)

The arachnoid forms a continuous sheet immediately subjacent to the dura. Based on descriptive and experimental ultrastructural observations, it is now generally accepted that the dura and arachnoid exist in vivo as a physically continuous tissue, with sparse but unequivocal intercellular junctions linking these two historically discrete membranes. The

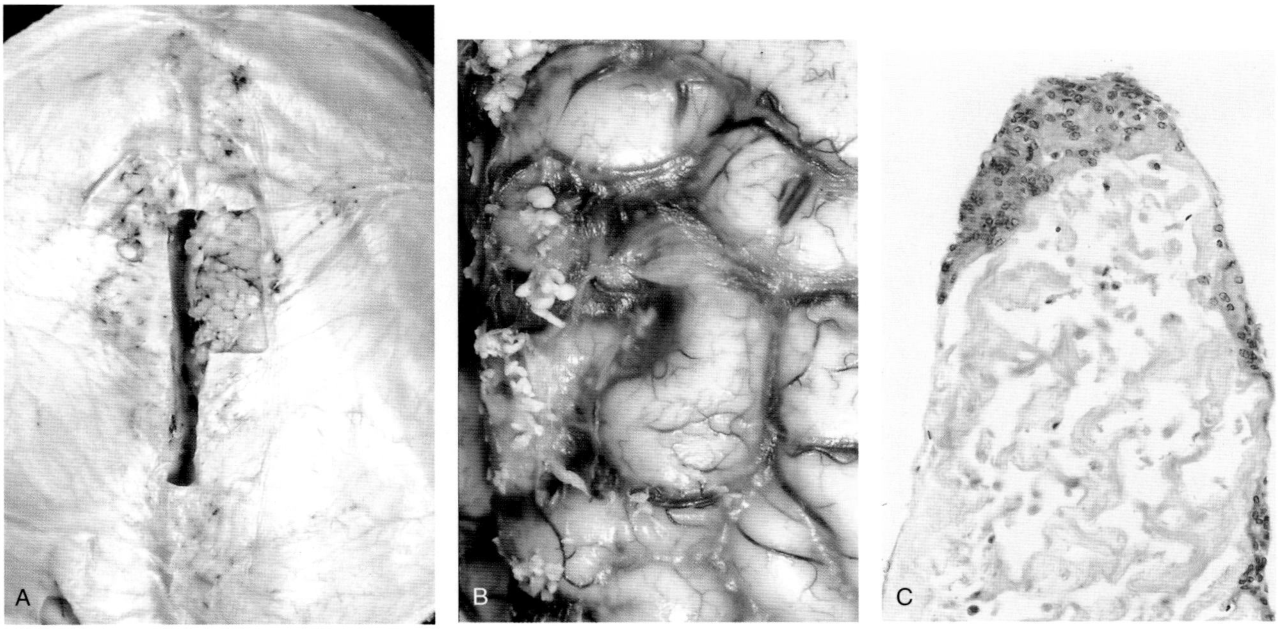


**FIG. 52.** Arachnoid granulations (villi): specialized structures of the arachnoid membrane serve to return cerebrospinal fluid from the subarachnoid space to the venous circulation and are accordingly found in relation to all major dural venous sinuses. The villi are most prominent in the superior sagittal (**A,B**) and transverse sinuses. With advancing age, they undergo collagenous hypertrophy, as seen in these micrographs, and may then be referred to as pacchionian bodies. The enlarged villi remodel the overlying bone of the inner table of the calvarium to produce small pits termed pacchionian foveolae, or foveolae granulares. Nests of meningothelial cells may be seen anywhere along the arachnoid membrane, but are especially prominent in the apical regions of arachnoid granulations where they are termed arachnoid cap cells (**C**), and in the arachnoid covering the orbitofrontal cortex. Normal meningothelial cells are innately inclined to form whorls and psammoma bodies, two features that are often retained by their neoplastic counterparts, meningiomas. *(figure continues)*

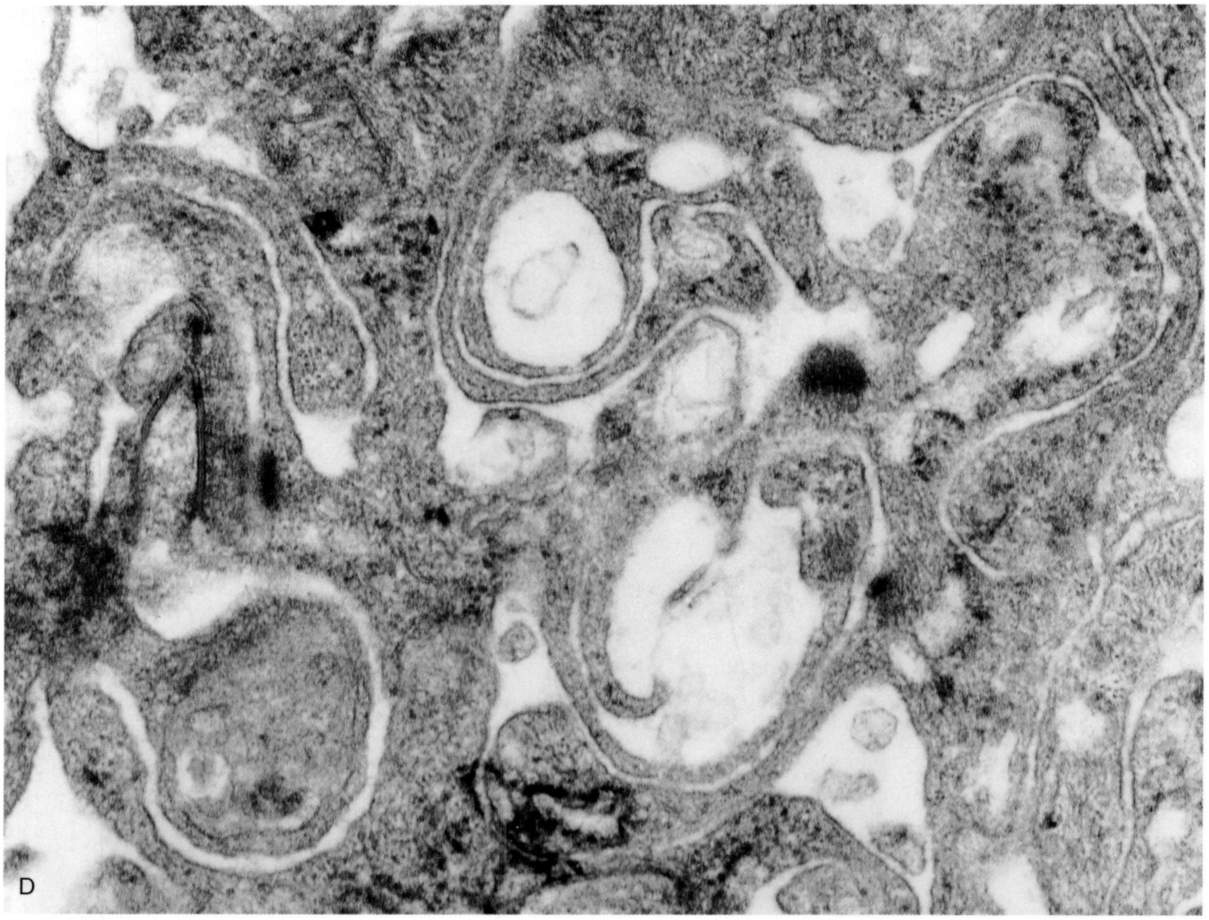


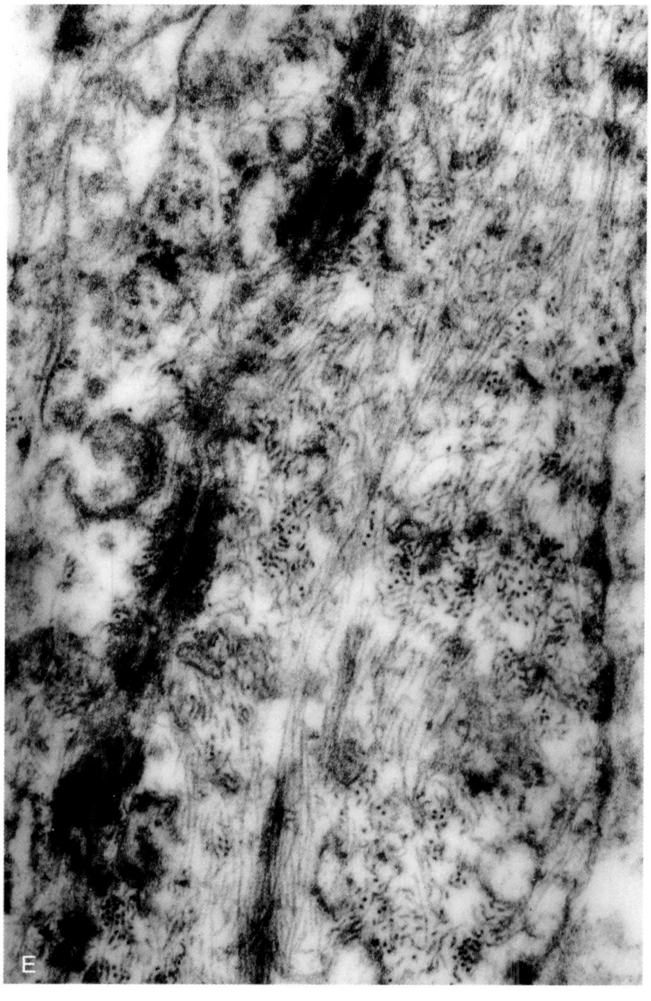


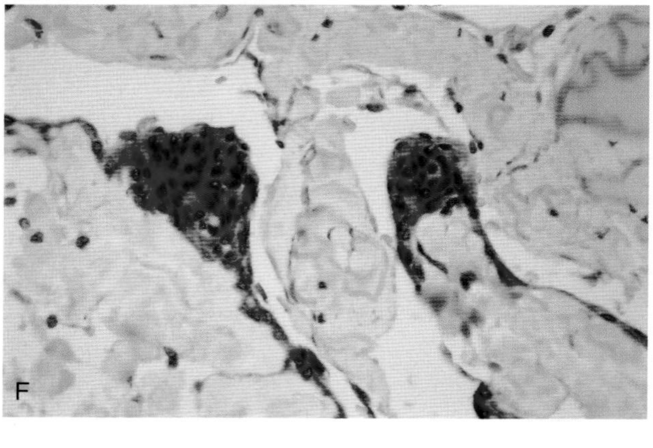


**FIG. 52.** *(continued)* The meningothelial cells of the arachnoid membrane, including the cap cells, serve an epithelial function. Accordingly, they possess elongated, intertwined cell processes (**D**) that are tightly spot welded together by numerous desmosomes (**E**) and exhibit strong immunopositivity for epithelial membrane antigen (EMA) (**F**). Like the tendency to form whorls and psammoma bodies, these epithelial phenotypic traits are retained by neoplastically transformed meningothelial cells and serve as useful diagnostic features of the vast majority of meningiomas which otherwise exhibit a very broad range of light microscopic morphologies.

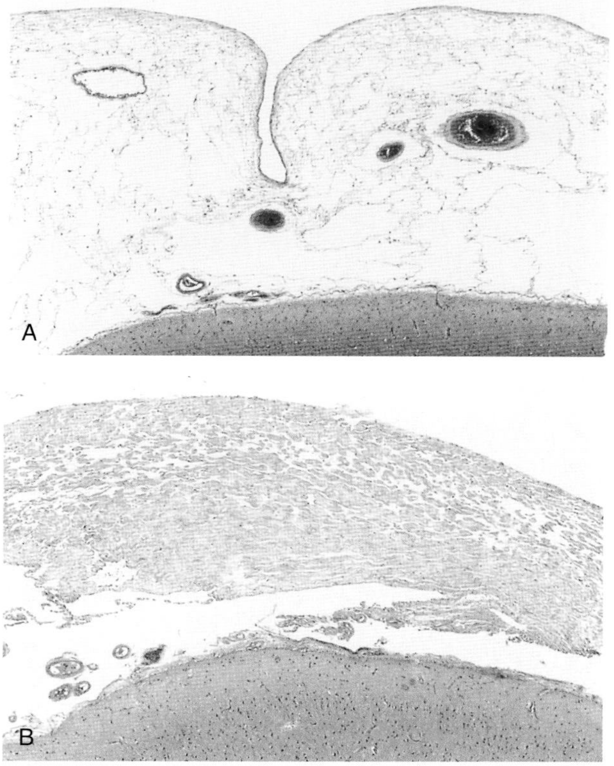


**FIG. 53.** Subarachnoid space: the subarachnoid space (**A**) is delimited by the arachnoid membrane externally and by the pia mater internally. Delicate arachnoid trabeculae course between these two membranes. In adults, gradual collagen deposition in the subarachnoid space (**B**) results in grossly appreciable "clouding" of the leptomeninges. This aging fibrosis appears grossly as diffuse opacification with focal plaques and small punctate nodules. It is characteristically most prominent along the dorsal cerebral convexities adjacent to the superior sagittal sinus.

storied subdural space has, thus, taken its rightful place in the pantheon of neuromythology, alongside brain lymphatics and the syncytial theory of the neural net. It has been proposed that the term *spatium subdurale* be eliminated from the standardized nomenclature of Nomina Anatomica. Nevertheless, there is no disputing the fact that the interface between dura and arachnoid constitutes the weak link or path of least resistance for pathologic processes that tend to disrupt the meninges. It seems unlikely that such venerable terms as *subdural hematoma* will soon be cashiered.

The pia mater and arachnoid are often considered as a single delicate covering of the brain and spinal cord (the pia-arachnoid or leptomeninges). The arachnoid is connected to the pia by delicate strands termed *arachnoid trabeculae* (Fig. 53A). In the young, the arachnoid is crystal clear, but with age it becomes gradually thickened. The extent of this change varies considerably. In some cases, it is severe enough to raise concern about a pathologic process – meningitis and meningeal carcinomatosis being the two usual suspects. This normal age-related arachnoid thickening is typically most pronounced over the dorsal parasagittal cerebral convexities. Microscopically, it results from the deposition of dense bundles of collagen (Fig. 53B), analogous to the collagenous hypertrophy of arachnoid villi that occurs prominently in the same vicinity.

Focal nests of arachnoid cells (also called meningothelial cells) may be seen throughout the arachnoid membrane, but are concentrated over the arachnoid villi (arachnoid cap cells) (Fig. 52C). These distinctive elements become more obvious and more clustered with advancing age and, in the adult, often form whorls with centrally placed psammoma bodies. At this point, the resemblance of these nests to those of the meningioma is inescapable. As mentioned previously, small nests of arachnoid cells are also present intraventricularly in the vascular connective tissue core of the choroid plexus (see Fig. 47F). Both normal and neoplastic meningothelial cells are immunoreactive for epithelial membrane antigen – an understandable property considering the epithelial phenotype of the desmosome-containing meningothelial cell (Fig. 52 D–F).

The dorsal leptomeninges of the thoracic and lumbosacral spinal cord occasionally contain white waferlike plaques (Fig. 54), a finding that is often termed *arachnoiditis ossificans.* In fact, in the majority (but not all) of cases these brittle lesions are roentgenographically and histologically devoid of bone or mineral. Rather, they most often consist of laminated, hyalinized fibrous tissue. True arachnoiditis ossificans generally occur in the context of prior symptomatic inflammation or trauma to the leptomeninges. Hyaline plaques, in contrast, are typically discovered as an incidental finding at autopsy in the absence of any relevant clinical history.

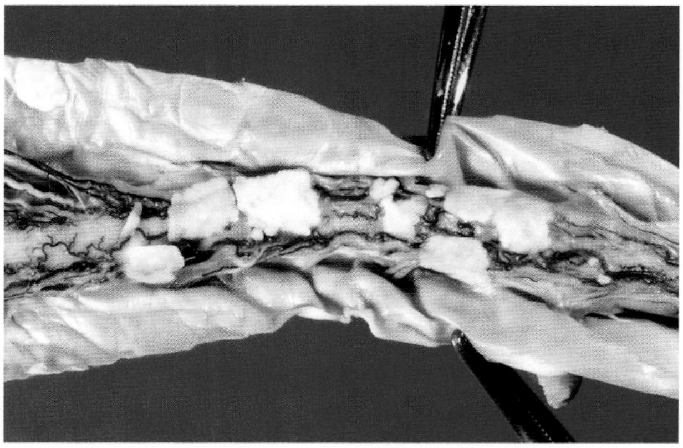

**FIG. 54.** Hyaline plaques of the spinal leptomeninges: these plaques are common incidental findings at autopsy and occur most frequently in the dorsal spinal arachnoid, although they may occasionally be seen in the cerebral leptomeninges as well.

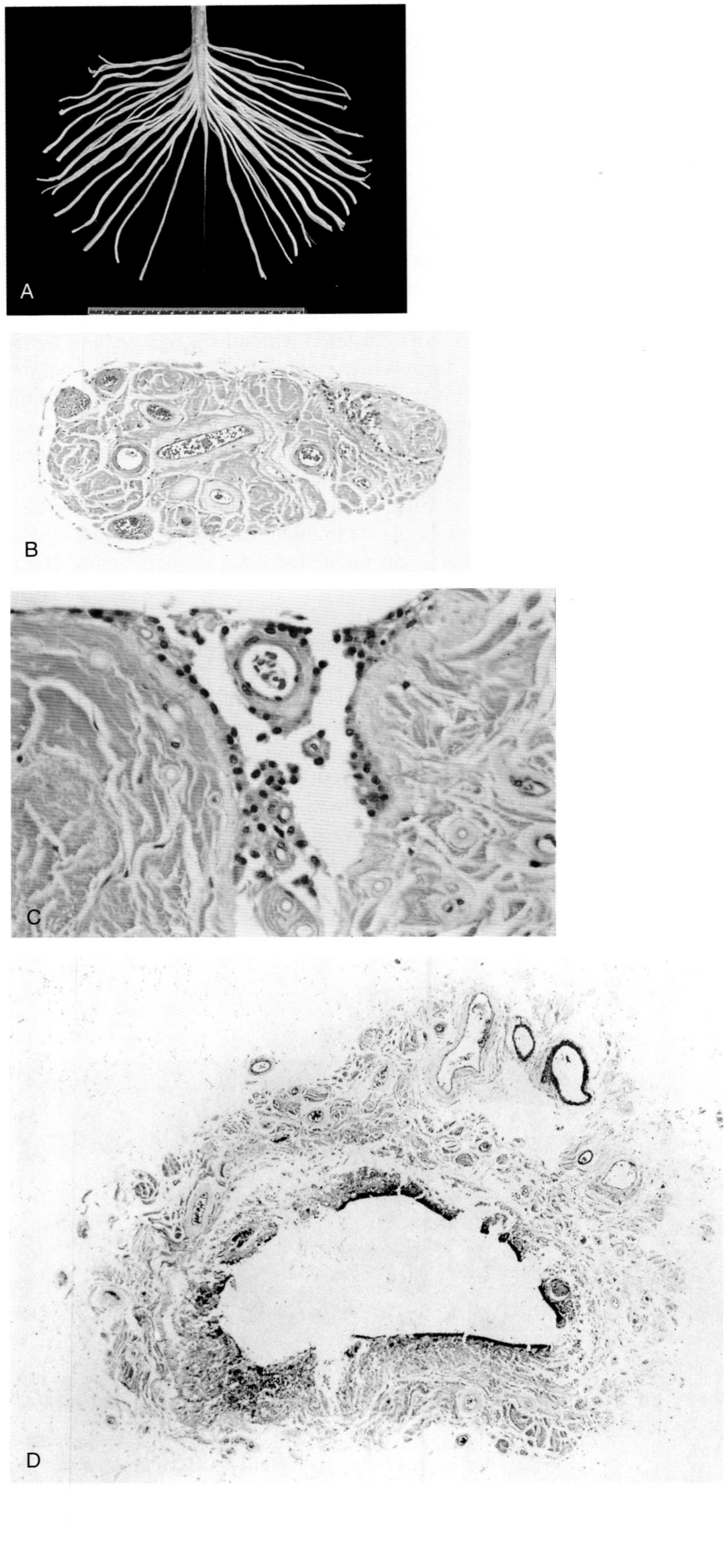


**FIG. 55.** Filum terminale: the filum terminale is the terminus of the spinal cord and extends downward from the conus medullaris surrounded by the nerve roots of the cauda equina (**A**). As seen in cross section (**B**), the filum is composed primarily of dense collagenous tissue and contains blood vessels, small peripheral nerve fascicles, and, of significant clinical importance, a small, often eccentrically located, ependymal remnant of the central canal (*upper right*). The latter structure, shown at higher magnification in **C**, is the origin of myxopapillary ependymoma. A remnant of the embryonic terminal ventricle of Krause (ventriculus terminalis), which consists of a focal dilatation of the central canal located in the region of the junction of the conus medullaris with the filum, may be encountered in sections from this vicinity (**D**).

Like the dura, the pia is traditionally divided into two layers: the epipia, which covers the surface of the CNS parenchyma and surrounds the vasculature, and the intima pia, which extends into the CNS parenchyma as the posterior median and intermediate septa of the spinal cord. Classically, three specialized structures of the epipia are recognized: the denticulate ligaments on either side of the spinal cord, the linea splendens adjacent to the anterior spinal artery, and the filum terminale. All three structures are composed primarily of dense bundles of collagen.

The filum terminale, which forms the terminus of the spinal cord, warrants additional brief description. As noted earlier, it is composed largely of leptomeningeal collagen but also contains small blood vessels, occasional small nerve fascicles, and may harbor focal collections of adiposites in a minority of normal individuals. Most importantly, however, is an ependymal remnant of the central canal (Fig. 55). This structure is the source of origin for a unique neoplasm of the conus medullaris and filum terminale: the myxopapillary ependymoma.

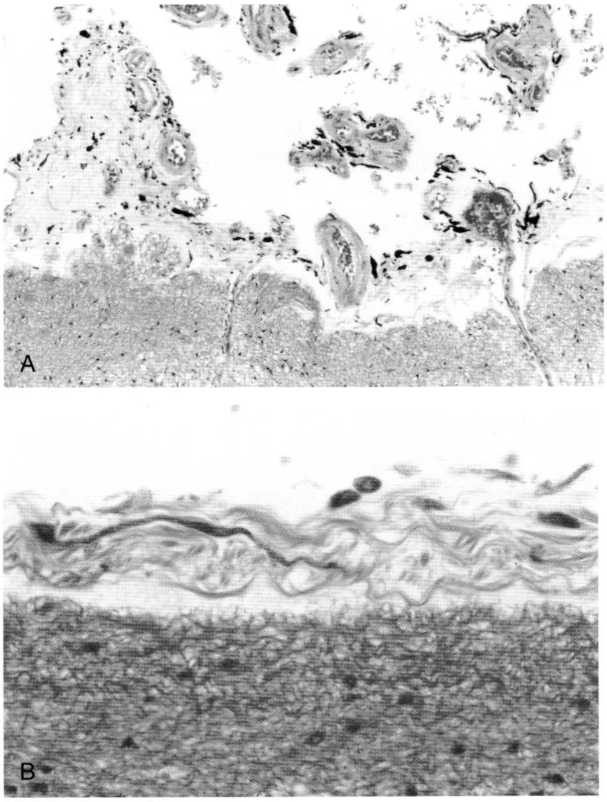


**FIG. 56.** Leptomeningeal melanocytes: true melanocytes (not to be confused with neuromelanin-containing catecholaminergic neurons) are normal constituents of the pia-arachnoid (**A**) and are often grossly appreciable as a dusky discoloration of the leptomeninges (see Fig. 46). On cross-section their rounded profiles might be confused with hemosiderin-laden macrophages but on longitudinal section their elongated, dendritic quality is evident (**B**).

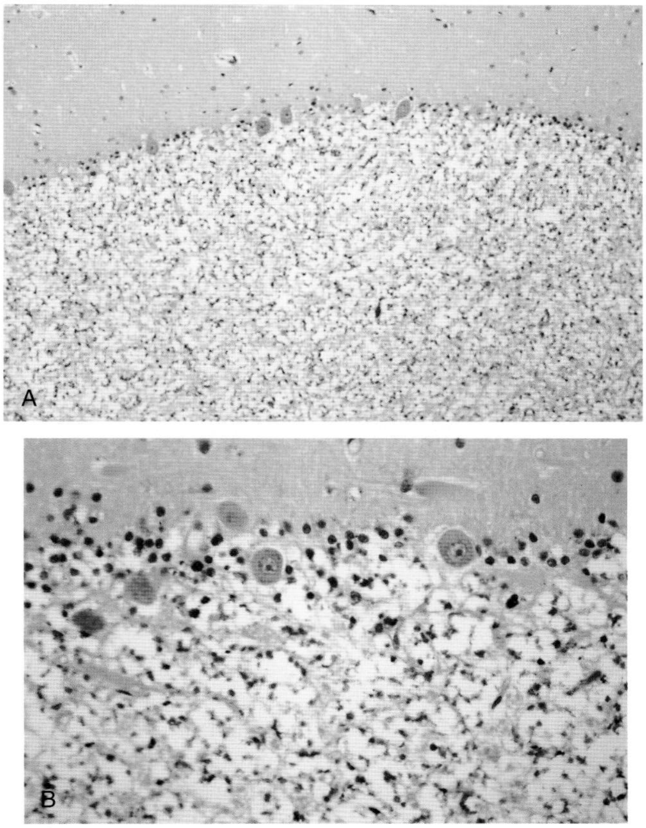


**FIG. 57.** Cerebellar conglutination (état glacé): conglutination appears as pallor of the granular cell layer (**A**) and at higher power, dissolution of granular neurons is seen (**B**). The Purkinje cells, however, are well preserved (note the clearly identifiable nucleoli), as are the Bergmann astrocytes, whose small cell bodies are located in the Purkinje cell layer (**B**). Conglutination is considered an autolytic phenomenon.

## Leptomeningeal Melanocytes

True melanocytes like those found in the skin are normal cellular constituents of the meninges. They are typically most concentrated in the leptomeninges of the ventral aspect of the upper cervical spinal cord and medulla oblongata (see Fig. 46A). In individuals with an abundant melanocytic presence, the distribution territory extends upward through the pontine cistern and mesencephalic interpeduncular fossa, lateral to the inferior cerebellar hemispheres and mesial aspects of the temporal lobes, and as far rostrally as the gyri recti of the orbitofrontal cortex. It is not unusual for melanocytes to follow the investing leptomeninges of the perivascular Virchow-Robin spaces around large penetrating arteries for short distances into the CNS parenchyma.

Intrinsic melanocytes of the leptomeninges may be involved in a spectrum of proliferative conditions ranging from benign melanocytoma to primary CNS melanoma, with all of these entities being exceptionally rare. In contrast, the normal presence of melanocytes in the leptomeninges must

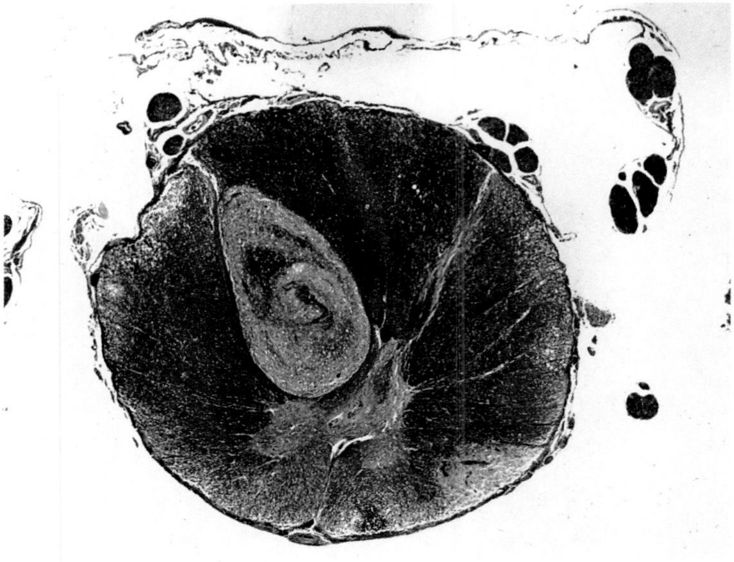

**FIG. 58.** "Toothpaste" ("squeeze") artifact: focal crushing of the spinal cord during removal at autopsy results in artifactual internal herniation of the central gray matter, producing an appearance on cross section that mimics malformation or heterotopia.

always be borne in mind when examining surgical biopsies from CNS sites known to harbor these distinctive elements; one must avoid misinterpreting them as evidence of a melanocytic neoplasm or as hemosiderin-laden macrophages. With regard to the latter, the long dendritic processes of the melanocytes are generally quite distinctive (Fig. 56).

## FETAL BRAIN

The two most distinctive histologic features of fetal brain compared to adult brain are active neurogenesis and paucity of myelin. The former is observed as a prominent, dense aggregation of neuroblasts and immature neurons in the periventricular and subpial zones. A similarly transient layer of migrating neurons in the fetal and infant cerebellum (the external granular layer) has been discussed. These generative laminae begin involuting during the latter part of gestation; remnants are present during the first year of postnatal life (see Fig. 3C).

## ARTIFACTS

A variety of macroscopic and microscopic artifacts may complicate evaluation of the central nervous system. Some are more typically seen at autopsy, whereas others are associated primarily with surgical specimens. The following entities are among the most frequently observed and warrant brief description because of the possibility that they may be misinterpreted as pathologic alterations.

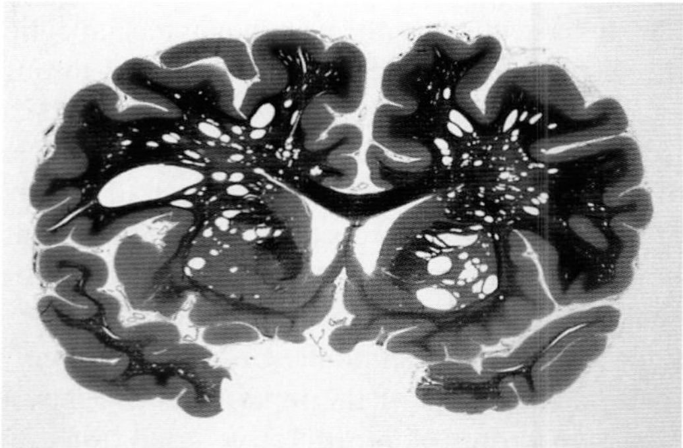

**FIG. 59.** "Swiss cheese brain": this striking macroscopic vacuolization of the brain results from postmortem proliferation of gas-forming bacteria.

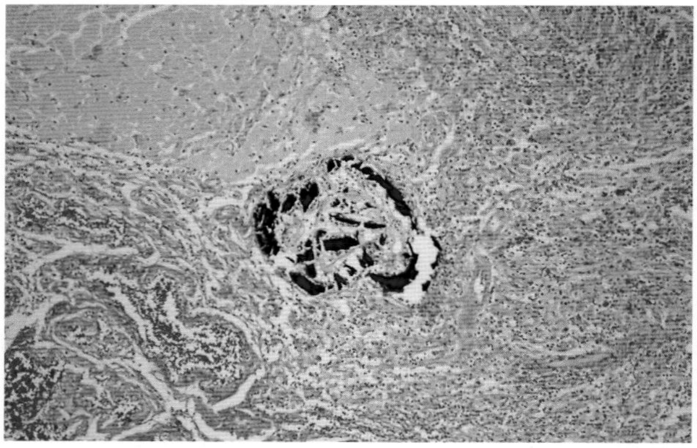

**FIG. 60.** "Bone dust": drilling of the calvarium during craniotomy often results in contamination of biopsy specimens with microscopic bits of bone, which may be artifactually admixed with tissue fragments and, thereby, mimic pathologic mineralization.

### Cerebellar Conglutination

Conglutination (also referred to as *état glacé*) is a very common change seen in the cerebellar cortex of autopsy specimens and is generally thought to reflect an autolytic process. On H&E-stained tissue sections, conglutination appears at low power as marked pallor of the granular cell layer (Fig. 57A). At higher resolution, disintegration of granular cell neurons is seen; however, there is preservation of Purkinje cell morphology (Fig. 57B).

### "Toothpaste" Artifact of the Spinal Cord

The most common artifact observed in the spinal cord is so-called toothpaste or squeeze artifact . Focal compression of the cord during removal at autopsy produces an artifactual internal herniation of the central gray matter, giving the general impression of a heterotopia or malformation (Fig. 58).

### "Swiss Cheese" Brain

A visually striking macroscopic artifact of the cerebral hemispheres is so-called Swiss cheese brain, seen when the ambient conditions and time interval between death and fixation allow for the growth of gas-forming bacteria (Fig. 59).

### "Bone Dust" Contamination

Obtaining tissue from the intracranial compartment necessitates drilling through cranial bone. Consequently, brain biopsy specimens often contain artifactually introduced microscopic bits of calvarium, referred to as bone dust. The adventitial nature of this material is usually apparent when found as scattered, free fragments. Frequently, however, intermixture of this microscopic scree with tissue fragments occurs during tissue handling and processing, such as to lend an appearance of intrinsic mineralization (Fig. 60). Awareness of the common inclusion of this material in brain biopsy samples mitigates the possibility of misinterpretation.

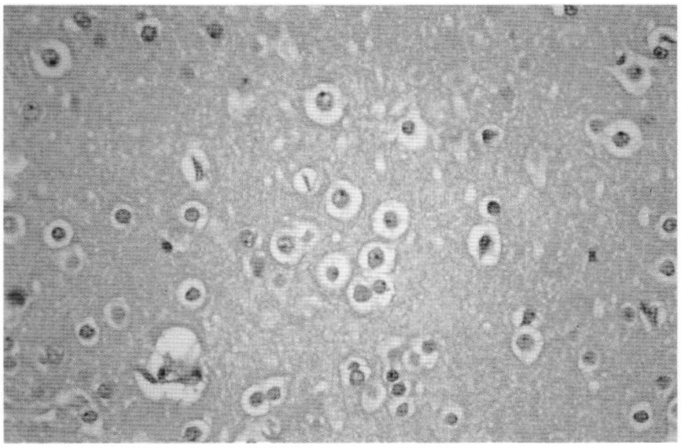

**FIG. 61.** Perineuronal halos: although much less commonly seen than the characteristic halo artifact associated with oligodendroglia, halos surrounding neuronal cell bodies are occasionally encountered in cortical biopsy specimens, and may be quite pronounced as in this example. Close inspection reveals prominent central nucleoli typical of neurons.

### Perineuronal Halos

Delayed fixation often produces prominent artifactual clear spaces around small blood vessels (Fig. 29) and oligodendroglial cells (Fig. 32). In the case of oligodendroglia, this is a useful artifact that is of value in the diagnosis of oligodendrogliomas. Less commonly, neurons in the cerebral cortex may also bear perikaryal "halos" (Fig. 61). The authors have, on more than one occasion, received a cortical biopsy consultation case in which this artifact was misconstrued as an infiltrating glioma (oligodendroglioma). Close scrutiny will usually reveal the prominent central nucleoli characteristic of neuronal nuclei.

## SUGGESTED REFERENCES

### Neuroanatomy Textbooks

Barr ML, Kiernan JA. *The human nervous system: an anatomical viewpoint.* 6th ed. Philadelphia; JB Lippincott, 1993.
Crosby EC, Humphrey T, Lauer EW. *Correlative anatomy of the nervous system.* New York; Macmillan, 1962.
Haines DE. *Fundamental neuroscience.* New York; Churchill Livingstone, 1996.
Heimer L. *The human brain and spinal cord.* 2nd ed. New York; Springer-Verlag, 1995.
Martin JH. *Neuroanatomy: text and atlas.* 2nd ed. Stamford; Appleton & Lange, 1996.
Nolte J. *The human brain: an introduction to its functional anatomy.* 3rd ed. St. Louis: CV Mosby, 1993.
Parent A. *Carpenter's human neuroanatomy.* 9th ed. Baltimore; Williams & Wilkins, 1996.
Paxinos G, ed. *The human nervous system.* San Diego; Academic Press, 1990.
Peele TL. *The neuroanatomic basis for clinical neurology.* 3rd ed. New York; McGraw-Hill, 1977.

### Neuroanatomical Terminology

Lockard I. *Desk reference for neuroscience.* 2nd ed. New York; Springer-Verlag, 1992.

### Neuroanatomical Approach to the Localization of CNS Lesions

Brazis PW, Masdeu JC, Biller J. *Localization in clinical neurology.* 3rd ed. Boston; Little, Brown, 1996.
Duus P. *Topical diagnosis in neurology.* 2nd English ed. Stuttgart; Georg Thieme Verlag, 1989. Lindenberg R, translator.
Haerer AF. *DeJong's the neurologic examination.* 5th ed. Philadelphia; JB Lippincott, 1992.
Mesulam M.M. *Principles of behavioral neurology.* Philadelphia; FA Davis, 1985.
Montgomery EB. *Principles of neurologic diagnosis.* Boston; Little, Brown, 1986.

Patten J. *Neurological differential diagnosis.* London; Springer-Verlag, 1977.

## Neuroanatomy Atlases

DeArmond SJ, Fusco MM, Dewey MM. *Structure of the human brain: a photographic atlas.* 3rd ed. New York; Oxford University Press, 1989.
Duvernoy HM. *The human hippocampus.* Berlin; Springer-Verlag, 1988.
England MA, Wakely J. *Color atlas of the brain and spinal cord.* St. Louis; CV Mosby, 1991.
Gluhbegovic N, Williams TH. *The human brain: a photographic guide.* Philadelphia; Harper and Row, 1980.
Haines DE. *Neuroanatomy: an atlas of structures, sections and systems.* 4th ed. Baltimore; Urban and Schwarzenberg, 1995.
Netter FH. *The CIBA collection of medical illustrations, vol 1, The nervous system.* West Caldwell; CIBA Pharmaceutical, 1991.
Nieuwenhuys R, Voogd J, Van Huijzen C. *The human central nervous system: a synopsis and atlas.* 3rd ed. Berlin; Springer-Verlag, 1988.
Nolte J, Angevine JB Jr. *The human brain in photographs and diagrams.* St. Louis; CV Mosby, 1995.

## Neurocytology

Andrews JM, Schumann GB. *Neurocytopathology.* Baltimore; Williams & Wilkins, 1992.
Bigner SH, Johnston WW. *Cytopathology of the central nervous system.* Hong Kong; ASCP Press, 1994.

## Neurohistology

Haymaker WE, Adams RD. *Histology and histopathology of the nervous system.* Springfield; Charles C Thomas, 1982.
Peters A, Jones EG, eds. *Cerebral cortex, vol 1, Cellular components of the cerebral cortex.* New York; Plenum Press. 1984.

## Ultrastructure of the Nervous System

Peters A, Palay SL, Webster H deF. *The fine structure of the nervous system: neurons and their supporting cells.* 3rd ed. Oxford; Oxford University Press, 1991.

## Neuropathology Textbooks

Adams JH, Graham DI. *An introduction to neuropathology.* Edinburgh; Churchill Livingstone, 1988.
Burger PC, Scheithauer BW. *Tumors of the central nervous system. Atlas of tumor pathology,* 3rd ser. Washington, DC: Armed Forces Institute of Pathology, 1994.
Burger PC, Scheithauer, BW, Vogel FS. *Surgical pathology of the nervous system and its coverings.* 3rd ed. New York; Churchill Livingstone, 1991.
Davis RL, Robertson DM. *Textbook of neuropathology.* 2nd ed. Baltimore; Williams & Wilkins, 1990.
Esiri MM, Oppenheimer DR. *Diagnostic neuropathology.* Oxford; Blackwell Scientific, 1989.
Graham DI, Lantos PL. *Greenfield's neuropathology.* 6th ed. Oxford; Oxford University Press, 1996.
Okazaki H. *Fundamentals of neuropathology: morphologic basis of neurologic disorders.* 2nd ed. New York; Igaku-Shoin, 1989.
Poirier J, Gray F, Escourolle R. *Manual of basic neuropathology.* 3rd English ed. Philadelphia; WB Saunders, 1990. Rubinstein LJ, translator.
Russell DS, Rubinstein LJ. *Pathology of tumours of the nervous system.* 5th ed. Baltimore: Williams & Wilkins, 1989. (6th edition in preparation, Bigner DD, Bruner JM, McLendon RL, eds.)
Weller RO, Symmers W Stc, eds. *Nervous system, muscle and eyes, vol 4, Systemic pathology.* 3rd ed. Edinburgh; Churchill Livingstone, 1990.

## Pediatric Neuropathology

Duckett S. *Pediatric neuropathology.* Baltimore; Williams & Wilkins, 1995.
Friede RL. *Developmental neuropathology.* 2nd ed. Berlin; Springer-Verlag, 1989.
Fuller GN. Central nervous system tumors. In: Parham DM, ed. *Pediatric neoplasia: morphology and biology.* Philadelphia; Lippincott-Raven, 1996.

## Neuropathology Atlases

Hirano A. *Color atlas of pathology of the nervous system.* 2nd ed. New York; Igaku-Shoin, 1988.
Kleihues P, Burger PC, Scheithauer BW. *Histologic typing of tumours of the central nervous system.* 2nd ed. Berlin; Springer-Verlag, 1993.
Mann DMA, Neary D, Testa H. *Color atlas and texts of adult dementias.* London; Mosby-Wolfe, 1994.
Okazaki H, Scheithauer BW. *Atlas of neuropathology.* New York; Gower Medical, 1988.
Schochet SS, Nelson J. *Atlas of clinical neuropathology.* East Norwalk; Appleton and Lange, 1989.
Weller RO. *Color atlas of neuropathology.* London; Oxford University Press, 1984.

## Comparative Neuroanatomy and Veterinary Neuropathology

Butler AB, Hodos W. *Comparative vertebrate neuroanatomy: evolution and adaptation.* New York; Wiley-Liss, 1996.
Cajal SR. *Histology of the nervous system of man and vertebrates.* Oxford; Oxford University Press, 1995. Swanson N and Swanson LW, translators.
Summers BA, Cummings JF, de Lahunta A. *Veterinary neuropathology.* St. Louis; CV Mosby, 1995.

# Peripheral Nervous System

*Histology for Pathologists, second edition,*
Edited by Stephen S. Sternberg.
Lippincott-Raven Publishers, Philadelphia


# CHAPTER 12

# Peripheral Nervous System

Carlos Ortiz-Hidalgo and Roy O. Weller



From a practical point of view, the pathology of peripheral nerves falls into two main categories: (a) peripheral neuropathies, which are diagnosed and treated by physicians and for which an elective nerve or muscle biopsy may be performed as a diagnostic procedure rather than as a therapeutic exercise; and (b) tumors and traumatic lesions, which are removed surgically mainly as a therapeutic measure to alleviate symptoms.

For the diagnosis of peripheral neuropathies, a detailed knowledge of the structure and ultrastructure of peripheral nerves and of clinicopathological correlations is essential. The diagnosis of tumors and traumatic lesions, conversely, relies more on identifying the cellular components within the lesion and their interrelationships. This chapter, therefore, concentrates first on how to identify different cellular components in normal peripheral nerves, and second, on how knowledge of the normal structure of peripheral nerves can be used to identify and assess pathologic lesions.

## DEVELOPMENT OF THE PERIPHERAL NERVOUS SYSTEM

The first anatomical evidence of nervous system differentiation is the neural plate, which develops as a thickened specialized area in the mid-dorsal ectoderm of the late gastrula stage of the developing embryo. This zone later becomes depressed along the axial midline to form a neural groove that folds inward to form the neural tube (1). Before fusion is completed, groups of cells become detached from the lateral folds of the neural plate to form the neural crests. Anteriorly, neural crests are located at the level of the presumptive diencephalon and extend backward along the whole neural tube (2).

The neural crests gives rise to a variety of cell types. In the peripheral nervous system, the neural crest is the source of neurons and satellite cells in the autonomic and sensory ganglia; ectodermal placodes may also give rise to ganglion cells in the cranial region. Schwann cells are also derived from the neural crest. Current evidence suggests that migrating neural crest cells are pluripotent, and their subsequent development is determined and progressively limited by environmental factors and by relations with other cell types (1).

Many of the events that occur during the later stages of development of peripheral nerves are recapitulated during the regeneration that follows nerve damage in postnatal life. Developing neuroblasts of the dorsal root ganglia (posterior sensory root ganglia) extend neurites both centrally into the neural tube and toward the periphery. Developing motor neurons in the anterior lateral parts of the neural tube extends their neurites toward the periphery. Schwann cells derived from the neural crest become associated with the developing peripheral nerves and, eventually, form myelin around many of the axons. The proximal portions of the anterior horn cell

C. Ortiz-Hidalgo: Department of Surgical Pathology, ABC Hospital, Mexico City 01120, Mexico.
R.O. Weller: Southampton University Hospital, Southampton, SO16 6YD England.

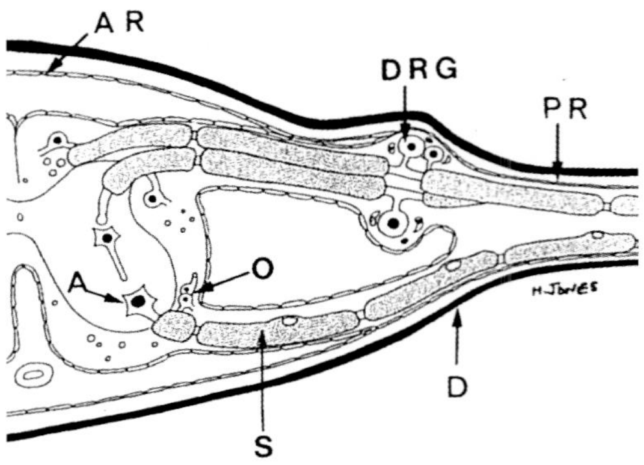


**FIG. 1.** Anatomy of spinal nerve roots. Motor axons arising from the anterior horn cell (A) are initially myelinated by oligodendrocytes (O) and then pass into the anterior root to be myelinated by Schwann cells (S). Sensory nerve axons pass into the dorsal root ganglion (DRG) and the central extension of the sensory neuron passes via the dorsal root into the spinal cord. Arachnoid (AR) appears to be continuous with the perineurium of the peripheral nerve (PR). Dura (D) extends from the spinal cord to coat the roots within the intervertebral foramen.

axons and the central axons of the sensory ganglion cells are myelinated within the neural tube by oligodendrocytes (Fig. 1).

## Growth of Axons

One of the major questions that has been raised is how neuronal processes grow over long distances and arrive at specific terminal regions. Genetic determinants, growth factors, and the extracellular matrix appear to play an important role in the appropriate guidance of neuronal processes (3,4). In 1909, Santiago Ramon y Cajal proposed the concept of neurotrophic substances to explain the directionality and specificity of axonal growth in the developing nervous system. But it was not until the 1960s that nerve growth factor (NGF) was discovered by Rita Levi-Montalcini and Stanley Cohen, as a target-derived neurotrophic factor that supports the survival and differentiation of sensory and autonomic ganglia in the peripheral nervous system (3). NGF is a protein composed of three subunits–alpha, beta, and gamma, but only the beta-NGF has nerve growth-promoting activity. Beta-NGF in humans is a 14,500 dalton polypeptide, gamma NGF is an arginyl esterase, whereas the function of the alpha subunit is not known (5,6). The tips of growing axons possess multiple surface receptors for soluble and bound molecules which provide information for the axons' growth course (7). NGF interacts with the NGF receptor on the surface of the axon, and promotes motility of the growing tip of the axon by interaction with the cytoskeleton of the cell. Mitochondria, neurotubules, neurofilaments, actin filaments, and some cisternae of smooth endoplasmic reticulum are incorporated into the axonal growth cone by axoplasmic flow. In addition to its growth promoting properties, NGF also promotes the early synthesis of neurotransmitters.

Schwann cells in the developing nerve produce NGF and possess NGF receptors on their surface membranes. However, expression of these receptors diminishes markedly as the peripheral nerve matures. As NGF binds to Schwann cell receptors and becomes concentrated on the surface of the primitive Schwann cell, it provides a chemotactic stimulus for growing axons (8).

The extracellular matrix also plays an important role in axonal growth and guidance. The tip of the growing axon has receptors for adhesion to extracellular substances such as collagen, fibronectin, laminin, and entactin; binding of extracellular components to these receptors promotes axonal elongation and stimulates cytoskeletal protein synthesis and, therefore, cell movement and axon growth. Some of these extracellular components are found within or near basement membranes surrounding Schwann cells (9,10).

## Schwann Cells and Myelination

Schwann cells move freely between and around developing peripheral nerve axons, forming primitive sheaths around the neurites and growing in parallel with them. Contact with axons stimulates Schwann cell division in vitro (11). In vivo Schwann cell multiplication virtually ceases in the normal adult animal, but mitotic activity is induced by peripheral nerve damage. It is thought that exposure of the axon to the Schwann cell following loss of myelin sheaths (demyelination) or during axonal regeneration following axonal degeneration (wallerian degeneration), promotes Schwann cell division, and that the relationship between Schwann cells and axons in the normal nerve induces some sort of contact inhibition in the Schwann cells. If axon regeneration does not occur following axon damage, Schwann cells gradually decrease in number, suggesting that Schwann cell growth and survival depend on contact with axons. Experimental evidence also suggests that continued axon regeneration depends on the presence of Schwann cells (12).

By the 9th week of gestation, fascicles of the human sural nerve are identifiable and contain large axon bundles surrounded by Schwann cell processes (13). Between weeks 10 and 15, Schwann cells extend several long flattened processes that wrap around large clusters of fine axons. At this stage, two to four Schwann cells are located within a common basement membrane and form Schwann "families" (14).

Myelination of peripheral nerves in humans commences between the 12th and 18th week of gestation (15). Initiation of myelination depends on the diameter of the axon and its association with Schwann cells. By the time that axons have increased in diameter to between 1.0 and 3.2 $\mu$m, they are in a one-to-one relationship with Schwann cells, and have either formed mesaxons or membrane spirals with compact sheaths of 3 to 15 layers (11). The reason why some nerves become myelinated and others do not is not clear. Schwann cells around myelinated fibers and around unmyelinated fibers are both able to produce myelin, but the factors that determine whether myelination occurs are unknown. Certain glycoproteins, such as myelin-associated glycoproteins, are believed to participate in establishing specific Schwann cell-axon interactions in the developing peripheral nervous system. Experimental studies have shown that axons may induce the formation of myelin if the unmyelinated sympathetic chain is grafted onto a myelinated nerve such as the saphenous nerve. Schwann cells that had not previously formed myelin will do so if they come into contact with large, regenerating axons that were previously myelinated (16). It appears also that Schwann cells may influence the caliber of axons since axonal diameter may be decreased markedly in some hereditary demyelinating neuropathies in which there is a genetic defect in Schwann cells and in myelination (11). Maintenance of an axon, therefore, appears to depend not only on influences from the neuron cell body, but also on interactions of the axon with the accompanying Schwann cells.

Some 70% of axons within a mixed sensory nerve, such as the sural nerve, are very small and will become segregated into groups of 8 to 15 axons lying in longitudinal grooves within one Schwann cell; these will form the unmyelinated fibers within the peripheral nerve. Thus, all axons in the peripheral nervous system are invaginated into the surfaces of Schwann cells, but myelin sheaths only form around the larger axons, which represent only a small proportion of peripheral nerve fibers.

## ANATOMY OF PERIPHERAL NERVES

An understanding of the anatomy of peripheral nerves is essential for the interpretation of clinical signs and symptoms, and for planning an autopsy to investigate a patient with a peripheral neuropathy (17).

Major nerves, such as the sciatic and median nerves, contain motor, sensory, and autonomic nerve fibers; they are, thus, compound nerve trunks. It was Sir Charles Bell, the Scottish physician who first demonstrated that motor function lay in the anterior roots; Francois Magendie, the French physiologist, showed that the sensory function lay in the posterior root. This (anterior–motor; posterior–sensory) is known as The Bell-Magendie law . Motor nerves are derived from anterior horn cells in the spinal cord or from defined nuclei in the brain stem. The initial segment of the axon lies within the central nervous system and is ensheathed by myelin formed by oligodendrocytes (Fig. 1). As the axons pass out of the brain stem or spinal cord they become myelinated by Schwann cells. Anterior spinal roots join the posterior roots as they pass through the intervertebral foramina to form peripheral nerve trunks. Cranial nerves leave the skull through a number of different foramina. Motor nerves end peripherally at muscle end-plates and many of the sensory nerves are associated with peripheral sensory endings.

The cell bodies of sensory nerves lie outside the central nervous system in the dorsal root ganglia or in cranial nerve ganglia (17). Each ganglion contains numerous, almost spherical, neurons (ganglion cells) with their surrounding satellite cells. Such satellite cells are derived from the neural crest and have an origin similar to that of Schwann cells (18). Satellite cells have been referred to in the past by a large variety of names such as amphicyte, capsular cells, perisomatic gliocyte, or perineuronal satellite Schwann cells.

Dorsal root ganglion cells were first described by the Swiss anatomist Albert von Kölliker in 1844. They are examples of pseudo-unipolar cells, which means that a single axon, or stem process, arises from each perikaryon but, at varying distances from the neuron, there is a T- or Y-shaped

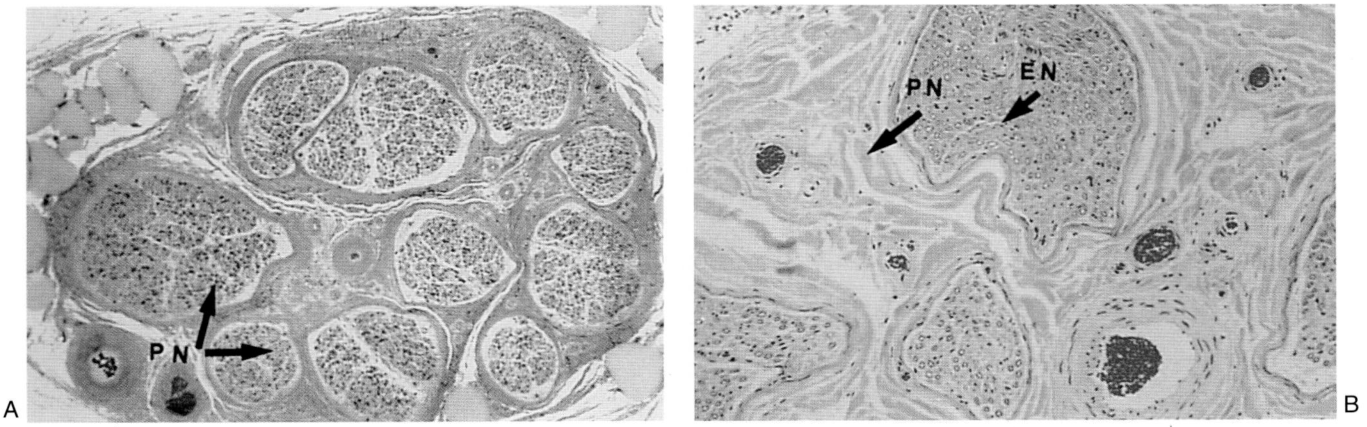


**FIG. 2.** Peripheral nerve sheaths and compartments. **A,** A low-power view of a transverse section of a normal sural nerve. The nerve fascicles with roughly circular outlines are surrounded by perineurium (PN) and embedded in the connective tissue of the epineurium. Epineurial blood vessels are also cut in cross section and there is adherent adipose tissue (*upper left*). The 1 $\mu$m resin sections are stained with toluidine blue (×**16**). **B,** The endoneurial compartment (EN) containing myelinated and nonmyelinated nerve fibers and their accompanying Schwann cells is surrounded by perineurium (PN). A large epineurial artery is seen in the lower right. Paraffin section stained with hematoxylin and eosin (×**45**).

bifurcation with the formation of central and peripheral axons. Thus, the initial segment of axon gives the impression that the cell is a unipolar neuron, but it actually has two axons (Fig. 1). The central axon passes into the spinal cord either to synapse in the posterior sensory horn of grey matter or to pass directly into the dorsal columns. Peripheral axons pass into the peripheral nerves.

Autonomic nerves are either parasympathetic or sympathetic. Preganglionic parasympathetic fibers pass out of the brain stem in the IIIrd, VIIth, IXth, and Xth cranial nerves and from the sacral cord in the second and third sacral nerves. Postganglionic neurons are situated near or within the structures being innervated. Sympathetic preganglionic fibers arise from neurons in the intermediolateral cell columns of grey matter in the thoracic spinal cord, and pass out in thoracic anterior roots. These preganglionic fibers are myelinated and reach the sympathetic trunk through the corresponding anterior spinal roots and synapse with the sympathetic ganglion cells in paravertebral or prevertebral locations. The autonomic nervous system innervates viscera, blood vessels, and smooth muscle of the eye and skin (17).

## HISTOLOGY, IMMUNOCYTOCHEMISTRY, AND ULTRASTRUCTURE OF PERIPHERAL NERVES

### Components of the Nerve Sheath

Macroscopic inspection of a normal peripheral nerve reveals glistening white bundles of fascicles bound together by connective tissue. Damaged peripheral nerves are often gray and shrunken due to the loss of myelin. Microscopically, transverse sections of a peripheral nerve (Fig. 2) show how endoneurial compartments containing axons and Schwann cells are surrounded by perineurium to form individual fascicles embedded in epineurial fibrous tissue.

#### *Epineurium*

The epineurium consists of moderately dense connective tissue binding nerve fascicles together. It merges with the adipose tissue that surrounds peripheral nerves (Fig. 2A), particularly in the subcutaneous tissue. In addition to fibroblasts, the epineurium contains mast cells. Although mostly composed of collagen, there are elastic fibers in the epineurium so that when a specimen of unfixed nerve is removed from the body there is some elastic recoil of the epineurium (19). The amount of epineurial tissue varies and is more abundant in nerves adjacent to joints. As nerve branches become smaller to consist of only one fascicle, epineurium is no longer present. In nerves that consist of several fascicles, one or more arteries, veins, and lymphatics run longitudinally in the epineurium parallel to the nerve fascicles (Fig. 2) (20). Inflammation and occlusion of such arteries is an important cause of nerve damage in vasculitic diseases (21).

#### *Perineurium*

Originally described by Friedrich G.H. Henle in the 19th century, the perineurium has, in the past, been known by a variety of different terms such as mesothelium, perilemma, neurothelium, perineurothelium, and, more recently, perineurial epithelium (22,23).

The perineurium consists of concentric layers of flattened cells separated by layers of collagen (Figs. 2–4). The number of cell layers varies from nerve to nerve and depends on the size of the nerve fascicle. In the sural nerve, for example, there are 8 to 12 layers of perineurial cells, but the number of layers decreases progressively so that a single layer of perineurial cells surrounds fine distal nerve branches. Perineurial cells eventually fuse to form the outer-core of the terminal sensory endings in pacinian corpuscles and muscle spindles (20,24,25). In motor nerves, the perineurial cells form an open funnel at the nerve ends at the motor end-plate.

With the use of electron microscopy, perineurial cells are seen as thin sheets of cytoplasm containing small amounts of

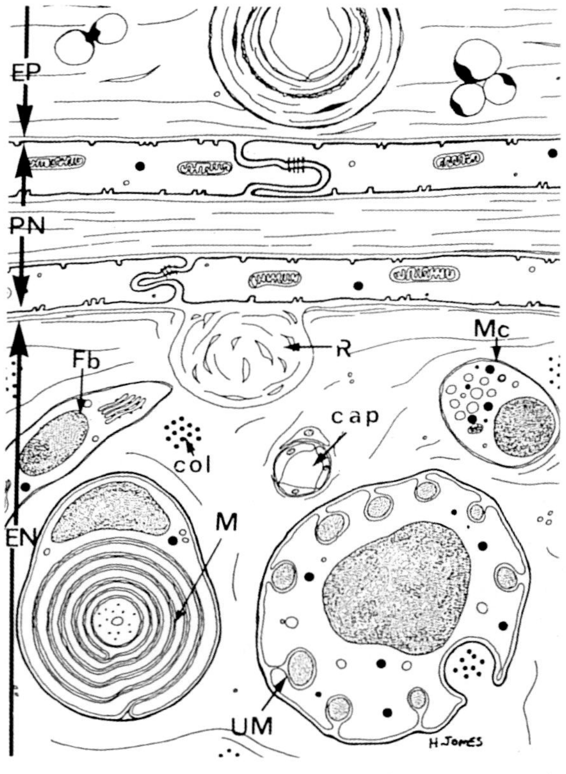


**FIG. 3.** Diagram to show the major elements of peripheral nerve compartments. The epineurium (EP) contains collagen, blood vessels, and some adherent adipose tissue. The flattened cells of the perineurium (PN) are joined by tight junctions and form-flattened layers separated by collagen fibers. Renaut bodies (R) project into the endoneurium (EN). Schwann cells forming lamellated myelin (M) (drawn uncompacted in this diagram) surround the larger axons. Multiple unmyelinated axons (UM) are invaginated into the surface of Schwann cells. Other elements include fibroblasts (Fb), mast cells (Mc), capillaries (cap), and collagen (col).

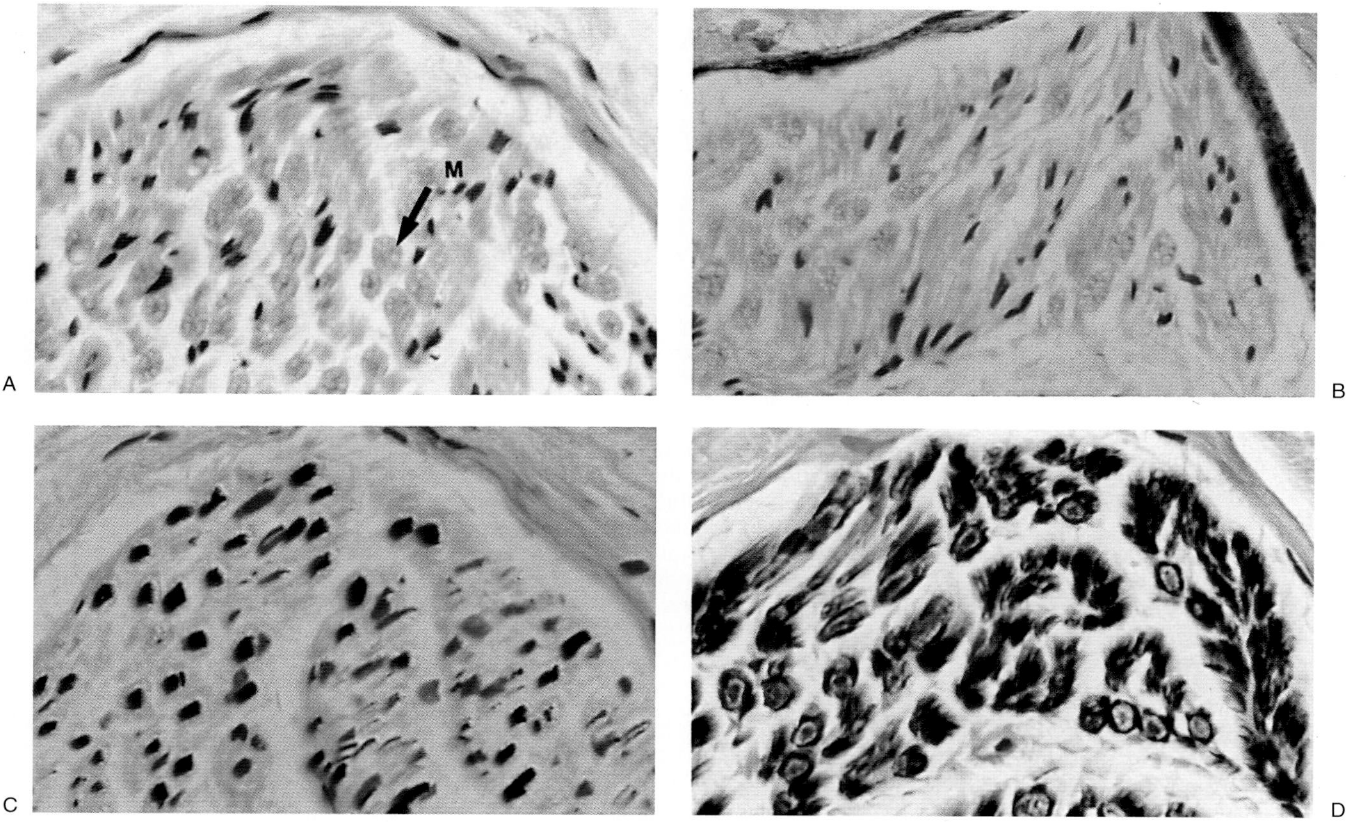


**FIG. 4.** Immunocytochemistry of a normal peripheral nerve. **A,** Part of single nerve fascicle, cut in transverse section. Perineurium (*top*) surrounds the endoneurium containing myelinated nerve fibers (M). The nuclei are mainly those of Schwann cells. Paraffin section stained with hematoxylin and eosin (×**160**). **B,** Similar field to (A) stained for epithelial membrane antigen. The perineurium (*top*) is densely stained. Immunoperoxidase technique (ABC) with anti-epithelial membrane antigen (EMA) antibody (×**160**). **C,** Part of a nerve fascicle stained for neurofilament protein. Large myelinated axons are well-stained but unmyelinated axons are difficult to detect. Immunoperoxidase technique (ABC) using an antibody against the 80 kDa neurofilament protein (×**160**). **D,** Part of a nerve fascicle stained for S-100 protein showing densely stained Schwann cells. Immunoperoxidase (ABC) using anti-S-100 protein antibody (×**160**).

endoplasmic reticulum, filaments, and numerous pinocytotic vesicles, which open on to the external and internal surfaces of the cell. Basement membrane is usually seen on both sides of each perineurial lamina (26,27). Tight junctions (zonulae occludentes) join adjacent cells within the same layer of perineurium. When tracer substances such as ferritin and horseradish peroxidase are injected into the blood, they do not enter peripheral nerves. Their entry is prevented by tight junctions in endoneurial capillaries, and in the inner layers of the perineurium (17). Thus, there is a blood-nerve barrier analogous to the blood-brain barrier. The blood-nerve barrier is present soon after birth and may prevent the entry of drugs and other substances into nerves, which may otherwise interfere or block nerve conduction (15,28). No such blood-nerve barrier exists in the dorsal root ganglia or in autonomic ganglia; these sites in the peripheral nervous system are vulnerable to certain toxins such as mercury (29).

Whereas the epineurial sheath of the nerve is continuous with the dura mater at the junction of spinal nerves and spinal nerve roots (Fig. 1), the perineurium blends with the pia-arachnoid. There are some morphological similarities between perineurium and arachnoid cells, although arachnoid cells are not usually coated by basement membrane. Immunocytochemically, perineurial cells and pia-arachnoid cells are positive for epithelial membrane antigen (EMA) (Fig. 4) and vimentin, and are negative for S-100 protein and Leu-7 (30,31). Epithelial membrane antigen is a collective term for a group of carbohydrate-rich, protein-poor, high-molecular-weight substances found originally on the surface of mammary epithelial cells (32), but present in the cells of virtually all epithelial tumors (33,34). EMA, however, is not restricted to epithelial structures and has been identified on plasma cells, on cells in certain lymphomas, and soft tissue tumors (22,32). Perineurial cells, arachnoid, and pia share

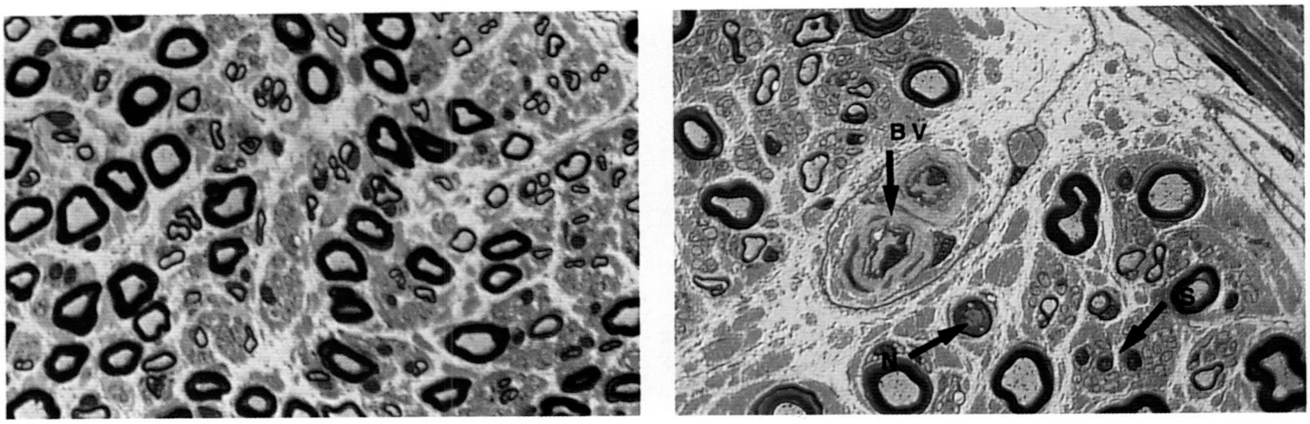


A B

**FIG. 5.** High-power histology of human sural nerve in transverse section. **A,** Large and small diameter myelinated fibers are seen. In the normal nerve, these fibers are separated from each other, but small numbers of clusters (see Fig. 14B) are seen in this illustration. The 1 $\mu$m resin section is stained with toluidine blue (×**160**). **B,** Part of a sural nerve fascicle cut in transverse section. Perineurium is at the top right. Both large and small myelinated fibers vary in cross-sectional outline (see Fig. 6). Splits within the sheath are Schmidt-Lanterman incisures. Endoneurial blood vessel (BV). Section through a fiber near the node of Ranvier (N). Unmyelinated axons are seen as unstained circles within Schwann cells (S). The 1 $\mu$m resin section (×**310**).

certain ultrastructural characteristics and EMA and vimentin in their cytoplasm. This suggests that these cells may have similar embryologic origins from the neural crest (2), although they do not contain S-100 protein, as do other neural crest derivatives such as Schwann cells and melanocytes. Recently it has been demonstrated by immunohistochemical studies that perineural cells constitute at least a part of some proliferative conditions such as traumatic neuroma, Morton's neuroma, neurofibroma, solitary circumscribed neuroma, neurothekeoma, pacinian neuroma, and mucosal neuroma associated with multiple endocrine neoplasia (see later) (35,36).

Some tumor cells break through the perineural sheath to grow along the perineural space; perineurial invasion has been correlated with decreased survival times in some cancers (37). The problem for the histopathologist, however, is that sometimes perineurial invasion cannot be unequivocally determined on hematoxylin-eosin (H&E)-stained sections. The recently described insulin-dependent glucose transporter protein 1 (GLUT-1) has been shown to be expressed in the perineurium and has been used to rapidly and accurately assess the presence of perineural invasion (38).

### *Endoneurium*

The endoneurium is the compartment that contains axons and their surrounding Schwann cells, collagen fibers, fibroblasts, capillaries, and a few mast cells (Figs. 3–5). In cross sections of peripheral nerves, some 90% of the nuclei belong to Schwann cells, 5% to fibroblasts, and 5% to other cells such as mast cells and capillary endothelial cells. Recently CD-34-positive bipolar cells with delicate dendritic processes have been identified within the endoneurium (Fig. 6). This CD-34 glycosylated transmembrane protein is encoded by a gene located on chromosome 1q and its amino acid structure has been sequenced (39). The CD-34-positive cells might represent precursor elements or play a supportive role for the Schwann cells (40). Other investigators have observed endoneural dendritic cells, distinct from Schwann cells and conventional fibroblasts, which may function as phagocytes under certain conditions (41). In this regard Bonnetti et al. have described within the human endoneurium, an intrinsic population of immunocompetent and potentially phagocytic cells (endoneural macrophages), that share several lineage-related and functional markers with macrophages, and may represent the

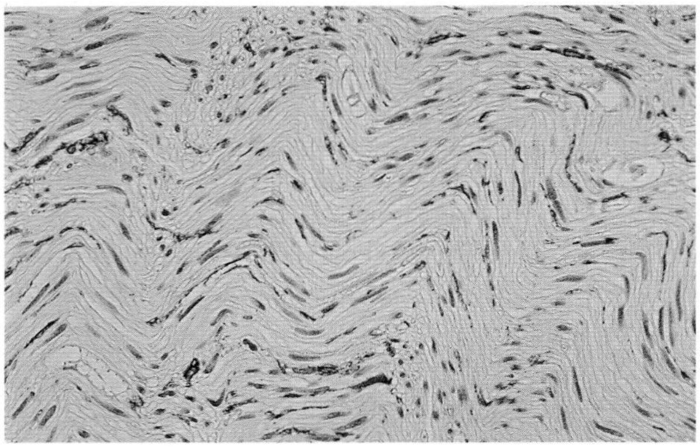

**FIG. 6.** Longitudinal section of a normal peripheral nerve showing CD-34 positive cells. These cells are clearly distinct from the Schwann cells that comprise the bulk of the nerve. Immunoperoxidase ABC using anti-CD-34 (×**160**)

peripheral counterpart of del-Rio-Hortega cells (microglia) of the CNS (42,43).

The nerve fibers may be myelinated or unmyelinated, but not all nerves have the same fiber composition. Most biopsies of peripheral nerves in humans are taken from the sural nerve at the ankle and it is the composition of this nerve that has been most closely studied (44). Fibroblasts are ultrastructurally identical to fibroblasts elsewhere in the body. Mast cells are a normal constituent of the endoneurium and are also seen in sensory ganglia and in the epineurial sheath of peripheral nerves. There is an increase in the number of mast cells in some pathological conditions such as axonal (wallerian) degeneration, and in some neoplastic entities such as von Recklinghausen's neurofibromatosis. A characteristically high number of mast cells is seen in neurofibromas, but they are only present in the Antoni B areas of schwannomas (24,45). Mast cells are thought to influence growth of neurofibromas, because some of their mediators may also act as growth factors. Likewise, mast cell stabilizers are claimed to reduce proliferation and itching of neurofibromas (46). Following nerve injury, there is breakdown of the blood-nerve barrier as endoneurial vessels become permeable to fluid and protein; this increase in permeability may be related to the release of biogenic amines from mast cells within the endoneurium. Proteases released from mast cells have a high myelinolytic activity and may play a role in the breakdown of myelin in certain demyelinating diseases (47).

Collagen within the endoneurial compartment is highly organized and forms two distinct sheaths around myelinated and unmyelinated nerve fibers and their Schwann cells (see Figs. 8 and 11). The outer endoneurial sheath (of Key and Retzius) is composed of longitudinally oriented large diameter collagen fibers; the inner endoneurial sheath (of Plenk and Laidlaw) is composed of fine collagen fibers oriented obliquely or circumferentially to the nerve fibers. The term "neurilemma" has been applied to the combined sheath formed by the basement membrane of the Schwann cell and the adjacent inner endoneurial sheath (24). The term "neurilemmoma" is, thus, inappropriate when used to describe tumors of Schwann cell origin (schwannomas). The longitudinal orientation of collagen fibers in the outer endoneurial sheath, together with the Schwann cell basement membrane tubes, may play an important role in guiding axons as they regenerate following peripheral nerve damage (20,24).

Renaut bodies (Fig. 3) are seen not infrequently in the endoneurium of human peripheral nerves. Described in the 19th century by the French physician Joseph Louis Renaut, they are cylindrical (circular in cross section), hyaline bodies attached to the inner aspect of the perineurium. Composed of randomly oriented collagen fibers, spidery fibroblasts and perineurial cells, Renaut bodies stain positively with alcian blue due to the presence of acid glycosaminoglycans. The rest of the endoneurium also contains alcian blue-positive mucoproteins (20). Renaut bodies express vimentin and EMA and produce extracellular matrix highly enriched in elastic fiber components (48). In longitudinal section, they may extend for some distance along the nerve and end in a blunt and abrupt fashion (48). These bodies are more prominent in horses and donkeys than in humans (2). Their precise function is not known but Renaut himself thought that they may act as protective cushions within the nerve. They increase in number in compressive neuropathies and in a number of other neuropathies, including hypothyroid neuropathy (22,48). In addition, they may be a reaction to trauma.

**Blood Supply of Peripheral Nerves**

Vasa nervorum supplying peripheral nerves are derived from a series of branches from associated regional arteries. Branches from those arteries enter the epineurium (Figs. 2 and 3) to form an intercommunicating or anastomosing plexus. From that plexus, vessels penetrate the perineurium obliquely and enter the endoneurium as capillaries often surrounded by pericytes (Fig. 5). Tight junctions between the endothelial cells of the endoneurial capillaries constitute the blood-nerve barrier (31).

Complete infarction of peripheral nerves is very uncommon, probably due to the rich anastomotic connections of epineurial arteries. However, inflammation and thrombotic occlusion of epineurial arteries is seen in vasculitides (49), and occlusion by emboli occurs in patients with atherosclerotic peripheral vascular disease; both these disorders result in ischemic damage to peripheral nerves with axonal degeneration and consequent peripheral neuropathy (29).

**Nerve Fibers**

Most peripheral nerves contain a mixture of myelin and unmyelinated nerve fibers. As the axons are oriented longitudinally along the nerve, quantitative estimates of the number of fibers in the nerve and their diameters are only adequately assessed in exact cross sections. Staining techniques that can be used to identify nerve fibers and other components within peripheral nerves are summarized in Table 1. Longitudinal sections of peripheral nerve are less valuable than transverse sections, but teased nerve fibers (see Fig. 18) are invaluable for detecting segmental demyelination and remyelination and for assessing past axonal degeneration and regeneration (50).

In a transverse section of a human sural nerve there are approximately 8000 myelinated fibers per $\mu$m2, whereas the unmyelinated axons are more numerous at 30,000 per mm2. Peripheral nerve fibers are classified as class A, class B, and class C fibers according to their size, function, and the speed at which they conduct nerve impulses (51). Class A fibers are myelinated and are further subdivided into six groups covering three size ranges. The largest are 10 to 20 $\mu$m diameter myelinated fibers which conduct at 50 to 100 m/sec; myelinated fibers 5 to 15 $\mu$m in diameter conduct at 20 to 90

**TABLE 12-1.** *Histologic techniques for peripheral nerves*

| Technique | Application |
|---|---|
| A. General | |
| 1. Hematoxylin and eosin | Detection of inflammation; myelin and axons, see Figs. 2B and 4A |
| 2. Hematoxylin van Giesen | Collagen, red; myelin, black |
| 3. Reticulin stains | Basement membrane around each Schwann cell in normal (e.g., Gordon-Sweet) nerve and in schwannomas |
| 4. Masson trichrome | Fibrinoid necrosis in vasculitides |
| 5. Alcian blue | Glycosaminoglycans, blue |
| 6. Toluidine blue | (a) Mast cells in paraffin sections, (b) general stain for 1 $\mu$m resin sections, (c) metachromatic stain for sulfatide lipid |
| B. Stains for myelin | |
| 1. Luxol-fast blue | Myelin, blue; can be combined with silver stains for axons |
| 2. Loyez | Myelin, black |
| 3. Osmium | Myelin, black |
| 4. Periodic acid-Schiff (PAS) | Myelin, bright pink (good for detecting small numbers of nerve fibers in muscle biopsies) |
| 5. Polarized light (frozen section) | Normal myelin, birefringent; degenerating myelin isotropic (nonbirefringent) |
| 6. Marchi | Degenerating myelin, black (due to presence of cholesterol esters); normal myelin, unstained |
| 7. Oil red O (frozen section) | Degenerating myelin, bright red; normal myelin, pink |
| C. Stains for axons (see also immunocytochemistry) | |
| 1. Palmgren or Bodian (silver stains) | Axons, black |
| D. 0.5 to 1 $\mu$m resin sections | |
| 1. Toluidine blue | Myelin, black; axons, unstained; Schwann cells and other cells, blue; collagen, blue; see Figs. 2A, 5, 12, 14, and 16A, B |
| 2. Toluidine blue and carbol fuchsin | Myelin, black; axons, unstained; cells and collagen, pink/blue (see Fig. 16C) |
| 3. Immunocytochemistry—can be performed on these sections | |
| E. Electron microscopy | See Figs. 7–10 and 17 |
| F. Teased fibers | |
| 1. Osmium stained | Myelin; nodes of Ranvier; demyelination and remyelination; see Fig. 16D |
| 2. Enzyme histochemistry | |
| a. Mitochondrial enzymes | Schwann cytoplasm; axoplasm |
| b. Acid phosphatase | Lysosomal activity associated with degenerating myelin |
| c. Polarized light | Myelin |
| 3. Lipid histochemistry | |
| a. Sudan black B | Myelin |
| b. Oil red O | Normal and degenerating myelin |
| G. Immunocytochemistry | |
| 1. S-100 Protein | Schwann cells (see Fig. 4D); schwannomas |
| 2. Leu-7 | Schwann cells; schwannomas |
| 3. Glial fibrillary acidic protein (GFAP) | Some Schwann cells—possibly unmyelinated |
| 4. Myelin basic protein | Myelin |
| 5. Neurofilament proteins | Axons, see Fig. 4C |
| 6. Epithelial membrane antigen | Perineurium, see Fig. 4B |
| 7. CD-34 | CD-34-positive endoneurial cell. See Fig. 6 |
| 8. LN-5 CD-68 | Endoneurial macrophages |

m/sec, and 1 to 7 $\mu$m diameter myelinated fibers conduct at 12 to 30 m/sec. Class B fibers are myelinated preganglionic autonomic fibers some 3$\mu$m in diameter and conducting at 3 to 15 m/sec. Unmyelinated fibers are small (0.2 to 1.5 $\mu$m in diameter), conduct impulses at 0.3 to 1.6 m/sec, and include postganglionic autonomic and afferent fibers, including pain fibers (51).

## Myelinated Axons

### *Ultrastructure*

Although myelinated nerve fibers can be demonstrated in paraffin sections (Fig. 4), they are best visualized by light microscopy in 0.5 to 1 $\mu$m thick toluidine blue-stained resin

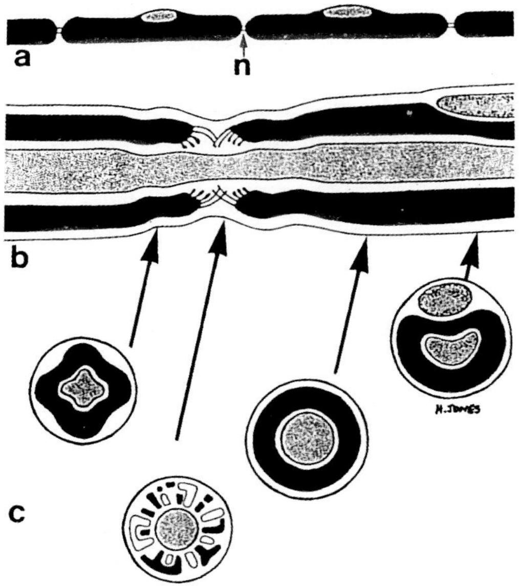


**FIG. 7.** Diagram to show the relationships between (A) teased fibers, (B) nerve fibers in longitudinal section, and (C) nerve fibers in transverse section. **a,** In teased fibers, nodes of Ranvier (n) are separated by internodal portions of the Schwann cell and myelin sheath. The Schwann cell nucleus is roughly in the center of the internode. **b,** Longitudinal section through the node of Ranvier shows how the myelin sheath terminates as a series of end-loops. The axon narrows as it passes through the node of Ranvier. **c,** Transverse sections of peripheral nerve as seen in electron micrographs and 1 μm resin sections are here related to the different portions of the internode and the node of Ranvier. From left to right, the paranodal region shows crenation of both axon and myelin sheath in larger fibers. At the node of Ranvier, the axon is small and coated by radially arranged Schwann cell processes and myelin end-loops. Throughout most of the internode the myelinated fiber is circular. In the region of the nucleus, the axon and the myelin sheath may be distorted on one side.

sections (Fig. 5). They exhibit a bimodal distribution of fiber diameter in the normal nerve with peaks at 5 and 13 μm and a range of 2 to 20 μm. Most axons above 3 μm in diameter are myelinated. Although along much of its length a myelinated nerve fiber has a circular outline in cross section, there is considerable variation in shape within the normal nerve, especially in the perinuclear regions and in the regions around the node of Ranvier (paranodal regions) (Fig. 7).

The axon itself is limited by a smooth plasma membrane (axolemma), which is separated from the encompassing Schwann cell by a 10 to 20 nm gap (periaxonal space of Klebs) (Fig. 8). The axonal cytoplasm (axoplasm) contains mitochondria, cisternae of smooth endoplasmic reticulum, occasional ribosomes and glycogen granules, peroxisomes, and vesicles containing neurotransmitters. The most prominent components of the axoplasm, however, are the filamentous and tubular structures. Microfilaments, 5 to 7 nm in diameter, are composed of chains of actin and comprise approximately 10% of the total axonal protein. They are virtually confined to the cortical zone of the axoplasm immediately beneath the axolemma (14). Neurofilaments (Figs. 8 and 10) are 8 to 10 nm intermediate filaments of indeterminant length. They constitute a major filamentous component in larger axons (52). They were described originally by Ramon y Cajal and Bielschowsky as argentophilic neurofibrillae. In the neuronal perikaryon, neurofilaments tend to appear in multiple whorled bundles with no clear orientation to elements of the cell. In the axons, however, neu-

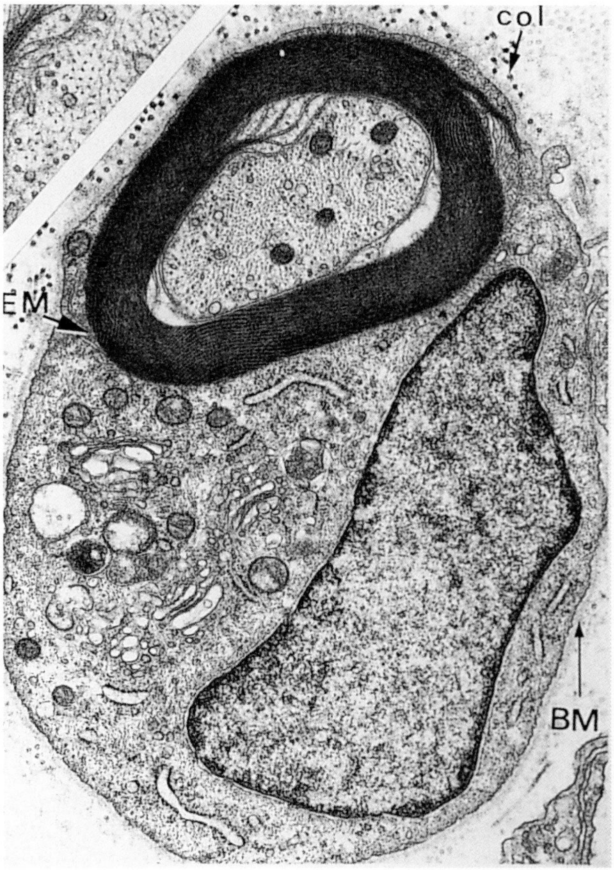


**FIG. 8.** Transverse section of a myelinated nerve fiber in the perinuclear region. The axon contains mitochondria, small vesicles, and numerous neurofilaments and neurotubules cut in cross section (*see inset, top left*). A distinct periaxonal space separates the axon from its encompassing Schwann cell. Myelin is compacted except at the external mesaxon (EM) and internally around the internal mesaxon near the axon itself. Part of a Schmidt-Lanterman incisure is seen on the inside of the myelin sheath. Abundant rough- and smooth-surfaced endoplasmic reticulum is seen in the perinuclear cytoplasm of the Schwann cell. A basement membrane (BM) surrounds the Schwann cell plasma membrane and endoneurial collagen fibers are seen cut in cross section (col). Electron micrograph (×**18,400**); inset (×**40,000**).

rofilaments appear in longitudinal, mostly parallel orientation (53). Small, armlike filaments are seen by electron microscopy. They project from the surface of the neurofilaments to form an irregular polygonal lattice. Neurofilaments are composed of protein triplets that are chemically and immunochemically distinct. Three major subunits are recognized and are classified according to their molecular weights of 68,000, 150,000, and 200,000 daltons. Within axons, neurofilaments are phosphorylated and are immunocytochemically distinct from the nonphosphorylated filaments within neuron cell bodies. Immunocytochemistry for neurofilament protein (Fig. 4) is often valuable for detecting large or medium-sized axons in normal nerves, and in traumatic lesions, in tumors involving peripheral nerves. It is also used occasionally, for detecting axonal processes in neuronal tumors.

The third "filamentous" component in the axoplasm is the microtubule (neurotubule). Microtubules are cylindrical (Figs. 8 and 10), unbranched, longitudinally oriented, 24 nm hollow tubules composed of globular subunits of tubulin 4 to 5 nm in diameter. Periodic radial projections of high-molecular-weight proteins, which are part of the microtubule-associated proteins (MAPs), arise from the surface of the neurotubules. These armlike projections bind neurofilaments and actin filaments, and together form neurotubule-neurofilament-actin filament lattices. The three-dimensional lattices form an ordered structure in the axoplasm, which appears to play an important role in axonal transport and contributes directly to the axon's shape (54). Microtubules also direct the transport of vesicular organelles between the cell body and the axon and thereby determine, in part, the composition of the axon (55).

### *Axoplasmic Flow*

In 1906, Scott proposed that neuron cell bodies secreted "growing substances" to maintain the function of the axon. He suggested that such substances pass down the axon cytoplasm to the axon terminals. This suggestion was endorsed by Ramon y Cajal when he observed how regeneration occurs from the proximal stump of a damaged axon as long as continuity with the cell body is maintained (14). More definitive evidence of axonal transport was provided later by experimental studies using autoradiography and other techniques. Not only can labeled substances such as tritiated leucine be traced by autoradiography as they are transported along axons from the cell body, but the transport of organelles within the axon can also be directly observed by the use of dark field microscopy or Nomarsky optics (55). The term *axoplasmic flow* was coined by Weiss to describe the movement of different materials along the axoplasm. Axoplasmic flow and transport occur in two directions: away from the cell body (anterograde) and toward the cell body (retrograde) (56).

Anterograde axoplasmic transport occurs at two velocities—fast and slow. Most organelles and large molecular-weight substances within the axon are conveyed by fast axoplasmic transport, up to 400 mm/day. If a ligature is placed around a nerve, transported material accumulates proximal to the ligature and, to some degree, distal to it, due to interference with anterograde and retrograde transport, which both occur at the same rate and by the same mechanisms. The filamentous lattice component of neurotubules-neurofilaments and actin filaments, is responsible for fast axoplasmic flow. These three elements probably act as rails, along which the various transported organelles and substances move. Fast axoplasmic transport is dependent on oxidative energy mechanisms and adenosine triphosphate (ATP); it also depends on calcium and magnesium ions and is blocked by calcium channel blocking agents. Some substances, such as trifluoperazine, which block calmodulin (calcium-activating protein) also block axoplasmic flow. Neurotubules, as an integral part of the axoplasmic transport mechanism, are depolymerized by cold and by colchicine; vincristine and vinblastine are known to bind tubulin and prevent the normal assembly of neurotubules. Such substances block fast axoplasmic flow (54).

Retrograde axoplasmic transport may convey information and organelles back to the cell body. In immature nerves, nerve growth factor is taken up by nerve terminals and retrogradely transported to the cell body where it may play a role in the maturation of neurons (57). It has been suggested that the transport of such growth factors may also influence the metabolism of mature neurons, and the absence of such signals from the distal part of the neuron when the axon is severed, may trigger chromatolysis (28). Retrograde transport is also a pathway by which certain toxins (tetanus neurotoxin) and some metals (lead, cadmium, and mercury) may bypass the blood-brain barrier and accumulate in neurons (58). Neurotropic viruses such as herpes, rabies, and poliomyelitis may be transported to the central nervous system via retrograde transport (59,60). In addition to toxic neuropathies, axonal transport has been shown to be defective in diabetes and peroneal muscular atrophy. It is also probably implicated in the pathogenesis of amyotrophic lateral sclerosis. Axoplasmic transport is reduced with age (61).

Slow axoplasmic transport at 1 to 3 mm/day concerns the distal movement of cytoskeletal elements such as neurofilaments, microtubules, and actin. It is a one-way process and neurofilaments are broken down by calcium-activated proteases at the distal end of the axon. Similarly, microtubules are depolymerized distally (62). Various toxins such as hexocarbons and their derivatives may interfere with slow axoplasmic transport so that neurofilaments accumulate and form large swellings within the axon (29). It is thought that neurofilaments within an axon may act primarily to maintain the bulk and the shape of large axons; neurofilaments are less numerous in small axons.

### *The Periaxonal Space of Klebs*

As the Schwann cell enwraps the axon, it leaves a space, 20 nm wide, between the Schwann cell membrane and the axolemma (Fig. 8); this is the periaxonal space of Klebs. This space is in continuity with the extracellular space at the node of Ranvier through a narrow helical channel at the site at which the terminal cytoplasmic processes of the Schwann cell approach the axolemma (14) (Figs. 7 and 10). The maintenance of the periaxonal space of Klebs appears to be mediated by an intrinsic 100,000 dalton myelin-associated glycoprotein (MAG) in the periaxonal membrane of the Schwann cell (63). This protein has a heavily glycosylated domain with sialic acid and sulfate residues on the external surface of the plasma membrane extending into the periaxonal space; in fact, about one half of the peptide of MAG is in the periaxonal space (64). Mutant mice that do not express MAG do not form a periaxonal space and the Schwann cell membrane fuses with the axolemma. Experimental studies with giant squid axons and mammalian nerve axons show that there is an increase in potassium concentration in the periaxonal space during repetitive conduction of nerve impulses. The full significance of the periaxonal space, however, is not clearly understood.

### *Schwann Cells*

In his book on the microscopic structure of animals and plants published in Berlin in 1839, Professor Theodore von Schwann identified a vague sheath of cells within nerve fibers; these cells have subsequently borne his name as Schwann cells. As described previously in the section on development of peripheral nerves, Schwann cells are derived from the neural crest and migrate with growing axons into the developing peripheral nerves. Schwann cells produce nerve growth factor both in development and during regeneration. As the nerves grow, Schwann cells divide axons into groups and eventually establish one-to-one relationships with the larger fibers, which they will ultimately myelinate (65,66). Immature proliferating Schwann cells have a relatively large volume of cytoplasm compared with mature Schwann cells. The Schwann cytoplasm is rich in mitochondria, polyribosomes, Golgi cisterns, and rough endoplasmic reticulum (Fig. 8). The cytoskeleton within the cells includes vimentin intermediate filaments and is particularly obvious during the active proliferative and migrating phases of development and regeneration.

Schwann cells in a normal adult peripheral nerve are associated with both myelinated fibers and unmyelinated fibers. In myelinated fibers the Schwann cytoplasm is divided into two compartments: around the nucleus and on the outside of the myelin sheath; and the thin rim of cytoplasm on the inside of the myelin sheath and around the internal mesaxon (Fig. 8). Using electron microscopy, Schwann cells within a nerve can be identified by their relationship with myelinated or unmyelinated fibers. Even in damaged peripheral nerves, however, Schwann cells can be identified most easily by the presence of an investing basement membrane (Fig. 8). Other cells within the endoneurium such as fibroblasts do not have a basement membrane, and although macrophages may invade the basement membrane tubes, they have a distinct ruffled border that distinguishes them from Schwann cells. Perineurial cells may be found in the endoneurial compartment, particularly in damaged nerves; they possess a basement membrane but can be distinguished from Schwann cells by the presence of tight junctions which are not a feature of Schwann cells (16). With increasing age, normal Schwann cells accumulate lipofuscin and lamellated structures in the paranuclear cytoplasm in the form of Pi granules of Reich. Such granules are composed of wide-spaced lamellated structures, and of amorphous osmiophilic material; they are rich in acid phosphatase and stain metachromatically with toluidine blue in frozen sections (67). Other inclusions, such as the corpuscles of Erzholz, are seen in Schwann cytoplasm; these bodies are spherical, 0.5 to 2.0 $\mu$m in diameter, and stain intensely with the Marchi method. Few Pi granules remain in Schwann cells following nerve damage in which there has been extensive Schwann cell mitosis and proliferation (67).

In addition to an investing basement membrane, composed of laminin, fibronectin, and entactin, Schwann cells also produce heparan sulfate, collagens type I, III, IV, and V, beta-1 and beta-4 integrin, and the protein BM-40 (68) . All these secreted products are incorporated into the basement membrane, except type I and type II collagen (69,70).

Schwann cells can be identified in paraffin sections by immunocytochemistry and by the presence of close investment by reticulin staining. There is a rich reticulin network investing each cell, not only in the normal peripheral nerve, but also in Schwann cell tumors. S-100 protein in the cytoplasm of Schwann cells can be identified by immunocytochemistry (Fig. 4); this acidic protein, which is 100% soluble in ammonium sulfate at neutral pH, has no known function but it is present in Schwann cells and not in fibroblasts or perineurial cells (Fig. 4) (71,72). Leu-7 is an antibody originally raised against cells of human T-lymphoblastoid lines which also recognizes a carbohydrate epitope on myelin-associated glycoprotein. Schwann cells are positively stained by immunocytochemistry using Leu-7 and perineurial cells are, again, negative (30). Occasionally, Schwann cells are labeled by anti-glial fibrillary acidic protein (GFAP) antibodies, but this may depend on the antibody used (73). GFAP immunoreativity in peripheral nerve sheaths (PNS) has been demonstrated in enteric ganglia, olfactory nerve cells, and in Schwann cells in the sciatic, splenic, and vagus nerves (74). A major intermediate filament in Schwann cells is vimentin.

### *Myelin*

Myelin sheaths appear as slightly basophilic rings in H&E-stained transverse paraffin sections of nerve (Fig. 4). They can be more prominently stained by Luxol fast blue or by hematoxylin stains such as Loyez (Table 1). In frozen sections, myelin is well depicted by Sudan-black staining and, in unstained frozen sections, can be identified due to its birefringence in polarized light: a technique that is particularly suitable for identifying myelin in enzyme histochemical preparations (49). Myelin is formed by the fusion of Schwann cell membranes and, by electron microscopy, it is seen as a regularly repeating lamellated structure with a 12 to 18 nm periodicity. On the outer and inner aspects of the sheath, external and internal mesaxons can be traced from the cell surface (Fig. 8). As the external aspects of the Schwann cell membranes fuse, they form an interrupted interperiod line in the myelin; the more densely stained period line is formed by fusion of the cytoplasmic aspects of the cell membrane. A narrow cleft can be resolved between the components of the interperiod line.

Biochemically, myelin is 75% lipid and 25% protein. The major lipids are cholesterol, sphingomyelin, and galactolipids, which are present in a rather higher proportion than they are in other cell membranes. It is the arrangement of the lipids that produces the liquid crystalline fluid birefringent myelin sheath and it is the esterification of the cholesterol in degenerating myelin that can be detected by Sudan dyes, by oil red O, and by the Marchi technique (Table 1). Ultrastructurally, as myelin degenerates and the cholesterol becomes esterified, the lamellated pattern of myelin is lost and replaced by the amorphous osmiophilic globules seen in electron micrographs. More than one-half the protein in myelin is a 28,000 to 30,000 dalton glycoprotein P0 (75); other proteins are P1 and P2. Although the lipid composition of myelin in the peripheral nervous system is very similar to that of the central nervous system, the protein components are markedly different. CNS myelin has no P0 protein but has a proteolipid that is soluble in organic solvents; it also has an 18,000 dalton basic protein that is probably homologous to the P1 protein of peripheral nerve. These biochemical differences may account for differences in the structure between peripheral and central nervous system myelin; for example, the spaces between the dense lines is less for CNS myelin (76). Biochemical differences in the proteins definitely account for the distinct antigenicities of peripheral and central nervous system myelin. Thus, injection of CNS myelin with Freund's adjuvant will produce allergic encephalomyelitis in experimental animals with destruction of myelin in the brain and spinal cord (77), whereas injection of peripheral nervous system myelin with Freund's adjuvant will produce allergic neuritis with demyelination in the peripheral nervous system.

Myelin sheaths are essential for the normal functioning of the peripheral nervous system. In those hereditary neuropathies in which myelination is defective, severe disability and retardation of development are seen (78). Acting as a biological electrical insulator, myelin allows discontinuous (saltatory) and very rapid conduction of a wave of depolarization along the fiber. It appears that myelination is an evolutionary adaptation that allows increased conduction velocities without excessive increases in axon diameter (79).

Myelination in the peripheral nervous system in humans occurs well in advance of that of the central nervous system (76). Although there is little myelin in human cerebral hemispheres at birth, myelin sheaths have already started to form around peripheral nerves at this time. Myelination is initiated by contact between Schwann cells and future myelinated axons. The Schwann cell rotates around the axon and may form 50 or more spirals, resulting in formation of the myelin sheath.

As the Schwann cell differentiates and produces a basement membrane, it acquires polarity via interaction of its cytoskeleton and some basement membrane components (mainly laminin and fibronectin) (70,80). The Schwann cell then begins to extend processes around individual axons. Once the lips of the Schwann cell starts to wrap around the axon, it generates traction to pull the whole cell around, and a spiral wrapping made up of many lamellae is formed (81). The importance of basement membrane formation as a prerequisite from the formation of myelin is emphasized by the lack of myelination when the basement membrane is deficient (80,82,83). Myelin-associated glycoprotein (MAG) also plays an important role in myelination (84). It is present in the membranes of Schwann cells around myelinated fibers but not in those cells associated with unmyelinated fibers. It

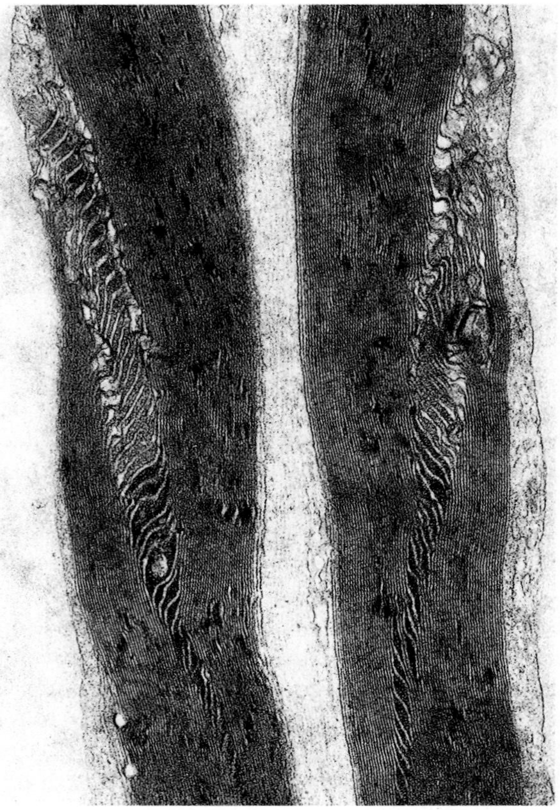

**FIG. 9.** Longitudinal section of peripheral nerve: a Schmidt-Lanterman incisure. Blebs of cytoplasm are seen running through the myelin sheath. Densities in the cytoplasm (*top left*) suggest some form of junction between the spiral turns of the incisure. The axon is cut tangentially. Electron micrograph (×**30,000**). (From ref. 19.)

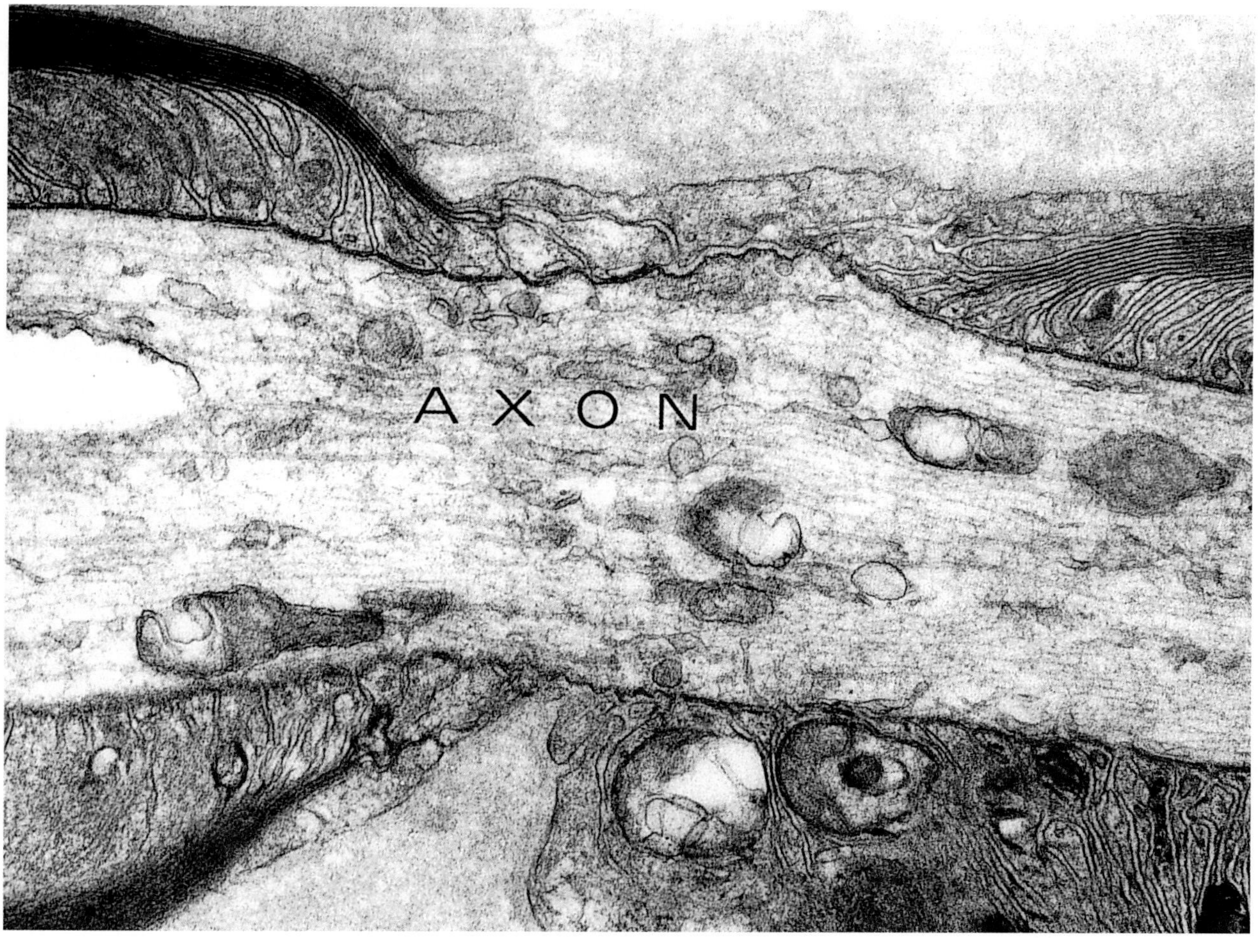


**FIG. 10.** Longitudinal section of a node of Ranvier showing how the myelin sheaths end as bulbs of cytoplasm (*top right and top left*). In the mid-nodal region, tongues of Schwann cytoplasm cover the axon. Within the axon, longitudinal profiles of microtubules, neurofilaments, mitochondria, and vesicles are seen. Electron micrograph (×**41,000**). (From ref. 19.)

is probable that MAG functions through its interaction with the Schwann cell cytoskeleton and this facilitates process lengthening and rotation during myelination (64). Recently a Schwann cell specific 47 Kd protein named periaxin has been described in the periaxonal region of Schwann cell plasma membrane that possibly interacts with myelin-associated glucoprotein during myelination (85). As myelination proceeds, cytoplasm is expressed from the spiral of Schwann cell processes and membranes compact to form the 12 to 18 nm lamellated structure of myelin.

The length of an embryonic Schwann cell is 30 to 60 $\mu$m and it becomes associated with that length of axon in the developing nerve. As the nerve lengthens, so does the Schwann cell; so that in an adult human sciatic nerve, the length of the Schwann cell or internodal distance (Fig. 7) in myelinated fibers reaches some 190 $\mu$m at 18 weeks gestation, and 475 $\mu$m at birth. In the adult nerve, normal Schwann cells may extend for up to 1 mm in length along myelinated fibers. Schwann cells associated with unmyelinated fibers lengthen to reach approximately 250 $\mu$m in the adult sural nerve. As emphasized later in the section on axonal degeneration and segmental demyelination, following damage to a peripheral nerve, Schwann cell lengths revert to their embryonic length and, thus, give short internodes in regenerating and remyelinating nerve fibers (see Figs. 14 and 16).

### *Schmidt-Lanterman Clefts or Incisures*

Once viewed as artifacts, the clefts or incisures described by H.D. Schmidt and A.J. Lanterman (Fig. 8) are now known to be fixed components of the myelin sheath (20). They consist of a continuous spiral of Schwann cytoplasm that runs from the outer (nuclear) to the inner (paraxonal) Schwann cell compartment in an oblique fashion at about 9° to the long axis of the sheath. The cleft splits the cytoplasmic membranes at the major dense line and forms a route for the passage of substances from the outer cytoplasmic layer through the myelin sheath to the inner cytoplasm. This function was suggested by Ranvier as early as 1897. Near the external surface of the cleft, stacks of desmosome-like structures are sometimes seen (Fig. 9), possibly maintaining the integrity of the spiral. Cytoplasm in the clefts contains membrane-bound dense bodies, lysosomes, an occasional mitochondrion, and a single microtubule (Fig. 8) that runs circumferentially around the fiber; this microtubule may be associated with transport and with stabilization of the cytoplasmic spiral (14).

The number of Schmidt-Lanterman clefts correlates with the diameter of the axon; the larger the fiber, the more clefts in the Schwann cell. The presence of these clefts throughout myelogenesis suggests that they are an important functional part of the sheath (20). It seems obvious that they are pathways of communication between the inner and outer Schwann cell cytoplasm, but their full significance remains to be elucidated.

### *Node of Ranvier*

With the introduction of techniques whereby individually separated or teased myelinated nerve fibers could be stained black with osmium tetroxide, a new view of nerve fibers was obtained. In his publication of 1876, Louis-Antoine Ranvier, Professor of Histology in Paris described and illustrated the constrictions or "étranglements annulaires," which are now known as the nodes of Ranvier (20). The functions of the node at that time were not known, but Ranvier did suggest that the constrictions may prevent displacement or flow of the semiliquid myelin along the nerve fibers (20). He also suggested that the gap in the myelin sheath at the node of Ranvier might allow diffusion of nutrients into the axon (14).

In teased fibers stained with osmium tetroxide or viewed in polarized light, the nodal gap is readily visible as is the bulbous swelling of the fiber on either side of the node of Ranvier (see Fig. 17). The distance between each node along a myelinated fiber (Fig. 7) is approximately proportional to the thickness of the myelin sheath. In a normal adult mammalian nerve, internodal segments between the nodes of Ranvier vary from 200 to 1500 $\mu$m in length; the Schwann cell nucleus is usually sited around the middle of the internode.

Histological study of 1 $\mu$m transverse resin sections of nerve and electron microscopic observations (Fig. 10) reveal a complex structure at the node of Ranvier and in the paranodal regions. As the axon approaches a node of Ranvier, it may become cruciform in cross section, especially in large fibers (Fig. 7). Deep furrows develop in the surrounding myelin sheath and those furrows are filled with cytoplasm, rich in mitochondria. As the axon passes through the node it is reduced to one third or one sixth of its internodal diameter. There may be a slight swelling at the midpoint of the node (Fig. 9). Amorphous, osmiophilic material rich in ankyrin (86,87) may be deposited under the axolemma (88). Ankyrin-binding proteins are also localized in the initial segment of the axon, the voltage-dependent sodium channel, the sodium/potassium ATPase, and the sodium/calcium exchanger (87). These specialized areas of axon membrane may reflect the site of high-ionic-current density during nerve impulse transmission. Numerous ionic channels are present in this region of the axolemma and they are responsible for the changes in ionic milieu that occur during the conduction of nerve impulses (89)

There is considerable specialization of the Schwann cell and the myelin sheath at the node of Ranvier. The myelin sheath terminates by forming dilated looplike structures, which are closely apposed to the axon surface (Fig. 10); occasionally, desmosome-like structures are formed between several terminal loops. The abundance of mitochondria in the paranodal cytoplasm is an indication of the high energy requirements of the node. Right in the center of the node, the myelin end-loops are replaced by multiple fingerlike processes (nodal villi) of Schwann cytoplasm 70 to 100 nm in diameter, which extend from the Schwann cell into the nodal gap and interdigitate with processes of adjacent Schwann cells. This interlacing pattern of cell processes around the axon at the node of Ranvier is more prominent and complex in larger fibers.

Basement membrane from the two adjacent Schwann cells is continuous over the nodal gap. Around the villous Schwann cell processes there is an electron-dense polyanionic-rich material that constitutes the extracellular matrix of the node. This gap substance creates a ringlike structure (ring of Nemiloff) and may provide an ionic pool necessary for nodal function. It has been demonstrated that the gap substance contains glycosaminoglycans with cation-binding substances (90).

The myelin sheath acts as a biological insulator for the internodal portion of the axons. Conduction of impulses along myelinated fibers proceeds in a discontinuous manner from node-to-node (saltatory conduction). Numerous sodium channels, with a suggested density of approximately 100,000 per $\mu$m2, are present on the axolemma at the node of Ranvier in contrast to the very low density of sodium channels (less than 25 per $\mu$m2) in the internodal axon membrane; the internodal membrane may be regarded as inexcitable (91). Potassium channels show a complementary distribution to that of the sodium channels; they are rarer than in the nodal membrane but are present in the paranodal and internodal axon membrane. They contribute to the stabilization of the axon by preventing repetitive firing responses to a single stimulus. Potassium channels also help to maintain the resting potential of the myelinated fiber (91).

In demyelinating diseases, when the myelin sheath is stripped from the axon, there is gross slowing or cessation of nerve conduction along the affected fibers. Spread of a continuous wave of depolarization along the axon membrane is prevented due to the absence of an adequate density of sodium channels in the internodal axon membrane. Furthermore, the exposure of the internodal axon cell membrane, rich in potassium channels, will also interfere with induction of the impulse (14,92).

### *Unmyelinated Axons*

Unmyelinated fibers can be detected as unstained structures by light microscopy in toluidine blue-stained 0.5 $\mu$m transverse resin sections of peripheral nerve (Fig. 5). However, at 1 to 3 $\mu$m diameter, they are almost at the limit of resolution and are only seen in good quality sections. Such fibers can be stained by silver techniques, such as Palmgren or Bodian, but are poorly visualized in immunocytochemical preparations using antineurofilament antibodies (Fig. 4), probably because unmyelinated fibers contain few neurofilaments and a high proportion of microtubules.

The structure of unmyelinated fibers and their quantitation are most adequately studied by transmission electron microscopy (Fig. 11). They are more numerous than myelinated fibers in mixed peripheral nerves by a factor of 3 or 4 to 1 (24,44); they were first recognized in 1838 by the Polish physician Robert Remak as "fibriae organicae"; the Schwann cells associated with unmyelinated axons are sometimes referred to as Remak cells (20). Schwann cells have the potential to differentiate into either myelinating or nonmyelinating ensheathing cell, depending on the signals received from the axon that they contact. Schwann cells must form basal lamine in order to myelinate axons. (20). Schwann cells around myelinated and unmyelinated axons may, thus, be regarded as originating from the same cell type, but developing morphologic, biochemical, and physiologic differences (93). The cytoplasm of Schwann cells associated with unmyelinated fibers contains a Golgi apparatus, rough endoplasmic reticulum, mitochondria, microtubules, and microfilaments and may exhibit centrioles near the nucleus. Pi granules, however, are not present although there are lysosomes containing acid phosphatase present in the cytoplasm (67). The nuclei of these cells are ellipsoid with one or more prominent nucleoli. A continuous basement membrane surrounds each cell (90). Schwann cells associated with unmyelinated fibers express different phenotypic characteristics from Schwann cells around myelinated axons. Although both types of Schwann cell contain immunocytochemically detectable vimentin intermediate filaments and S-100 protein, and almost the same basement membrane components, Schwann cells associated with unmyelinated axons are more likely to express GFAP (94). Such cells also lack myelin-associated glycoprotein (MAG), which is apparently necessary for segregation and myelination of axons.

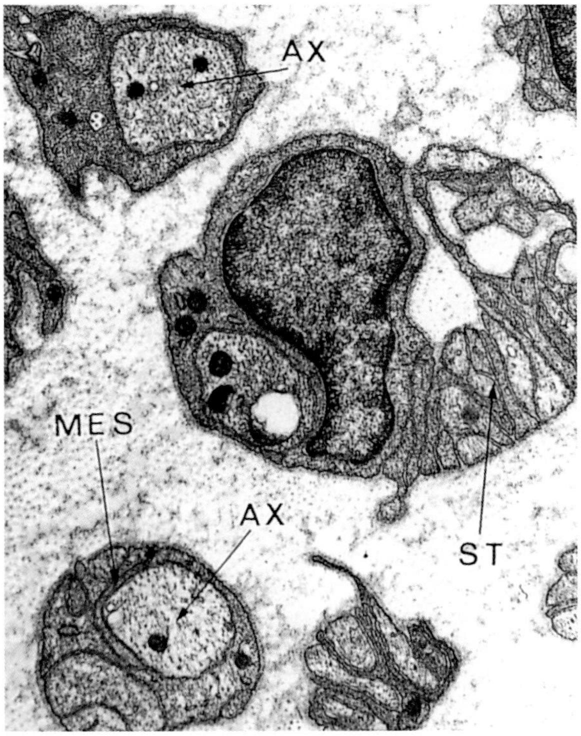


**FIG. 11.** Unmyelinated axons (1.3 $\mu$m in diameter) cut in transverse section. The axons (AX) are surrounded by Schwann cells, mesaxons (MES). Stacks of Schwann cell processes (ST) are commonly seen in adult nerves. Electron micrograph (×**13,000**).

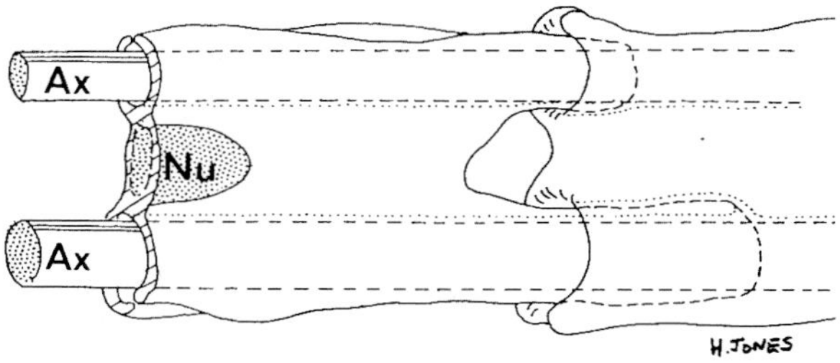


**FIG. 12.** A diagram to show the relationship between unmyelinated nerve fibers and their surrounding Schwann cells (Remak cells). As the unmyelinated axons (Ax) pass from one investing Schwann cell to the next, the Schwann cell processes interlock (*right center*). The nucleus (Nu) is shown to the left.

Electron microscopy of transverse sections of normal peripheral nerve show how numerous unmyelinated axons 0.2 to 3.5 $\mu$m in diameter are associated with a single Schwann cell. Short mesaxons extend from the surface of the cell (Fig. 11) and the Schwann cell is separated from the axon plasma membrane by a space 10 to 15 nm wide, which is analogous to the periaxonal space of Klebs seen around myelinated fibers. Although many axons may be gathered close to the cell body in the perinuclear region of the Schwann cell (20), as they move away from the nuclear region, single axons become more widely separated as they are enclosed by thin Schwann cell processes (Figs. 11 and 12). Each Schwann cell associated with unmyelinated axons in the sural nerve is between 200 and 500 $\mu$m in length. As axons pass from one Schwann cell to another, they are surrounded by flattened irregular, fingerlike processes that interlock and become telescoped into the adjacent Schwann cell (Fig. 12). The surface of the axon is, therefore, always in contact with the Schwann cell. In young children, only a thin layer of Schwann cytoplasm surrounds each axon away from the nuclear region but, in adult nerves, the picture is more complex with a number of Schwann cell processes stacked together and associated with each unmyelinated axon (Fig. 11).

Pockets of collagen bundles are frequently invaginated into the surface of Schwann cells associated with unmyelinated fibers (Figs. 3 and 11). They are more frequently seen in aging nerves and when there is loss of unmyelinated fibers. The collagen fibers are separated from the surface of the Schwann cell by a layer of basement membrane. The significance of this phenomenon is not fully known.

Endocrine cells have been identified within the perineurium in close contact with unmyelinated nerves in the lamina propria of the appendix (95). These cells were demonstrated in 1924 by Pierre Masson and later Auböck coined the term "endocrine cell nonmyelinated fiber complex," emphasizing the association between endocrine cells and unmyelinated fibers (96). These complexes are separated from the interstitial connective tissue by a common continuous basement membrane, leaving the cells in intimate contact with each other. It has been suggested that such endocrine cells could participate in the pathogenesis of the so-called neuromas of the appendix and appendiceal carcinoids (97,98). It is not known whether such endocrine cells exist in nerves other than those located in the wall of the appendix, but there are reports of extraepithelial carcinoid tumors in stomach, small intestine, and bronchus, which suggests that there may be endocrine cells related to nerves in these regions also (99).

Interesting immunological properties have been ascribed to Schwann cells. They express Ia determinants on their membranes and are able to present foreign antigens to specific synergic T cells. A role for Schwann cells has been suggested in myasthenia gravis (100). The cell of Schwann also expresses complement receptor CR1 (CD-35) and CD-59, a 19,00-25,000 mw glycoprotein, that binds to complement proteins C8 and C9 in the assembling cytolitic membrane attack complex. This may indicate that regulation of complement activation by these proteins is important in neural host defense mechanisms and may be implicated in the complement-mediated damage taking place in inflammatory demyelinating diseases such as multiple sclerosis and Guillian-Barré syndrome (101).

## CORRELATION OF NORMAL HISTOLOGY WITH THE PATHOLOGY OF PERIPHERAL NERVES

### Handling and Preparation of Peripheral Nerve Biopsy and Autopsy Specimens

The sural nerve is the nerve that is most commonly biopsied in the investigation of peripheral neuropathies. It is a sensory nerve so that in some motor neuropathies it may be totally normal, in which case, examination of small branches of motor nerves within a muscle biopsy (49) may be more fruitful. At autopsy, a wider range of motor and sensory

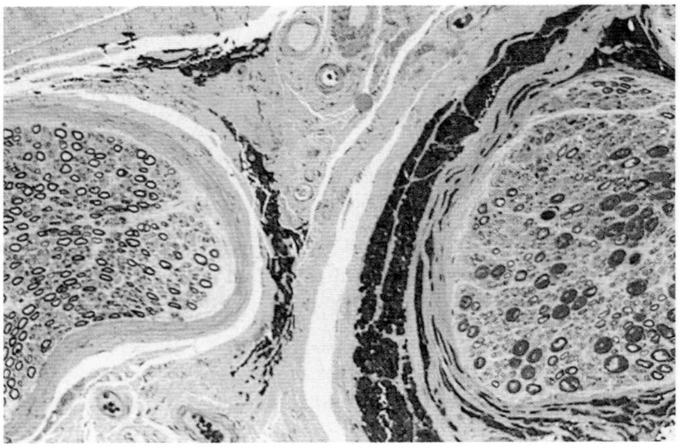

**FIG. 13.** Histologic artifact in a peripheral nerve. In this transverse resin section, the fascicle to the left of the picture is well preserved. However, there is extensive recent hemorrhage (*center*) that occurred during the biopsy procedure; the myelinated axons in the nerve fascicle are squeezed and distorted (*right*). The 1 μm resin section is stained with toluidine blue (×**40**).

nerves may be sampled depending on the clinical picture. Whether taken at biopsy or autopsy, peripheral nerves are very easily damaged. The myelin sheaths are semiliquid and may be crushed by indelicate handling (Fig. 13). The specimen should only be gripped at one end and then gently dissected free before laying it, (very gently stretched), on a piece of dry card, and placing it in fixative or in liquid nitrogen for snap freezing. Fresh, frozen nerve should be used for enzyme and lipid histochemical studies, whereas formalin-fixed nerve can be embedded in paraffin for the application of routine stains and immunocytochemistry (see Table 1). Although formalin-fixed material can be used for the preparation of 0.5 to 1 μm resin-embedded sections and for electron microscopy, ideally the tissue should be fixed in glutaraldehyde and postfixed in osmium for ultrastructural studies. Teased fibers can be prepared either from glutaraldehyde- or formalin-fixed material (20).

The method of preparation really depends on the information sought. Frozen sections are ideal for detecting abnormal lipids, such as sulfatide, in metachromatic leukodystrophy, and for detecting the cholesterol ester droplets of degenerating myelin by staining for Sudan red or oil red O. Increased lysosomal enzyme activity as in Krabbe's leukodystrophy or in human and experimental neuropathies in which axonal degeneration or segmental demyelination is suspected, can be detected in frozen sections stained histochemically for acid phosphatase (49). Brief formalin or glutaraldehyde fixation can be used in some cases for electron microscopic enzyme histochemistry (88,102). Frozen sections can also be used for immunofluorescence for the detection of immunoglobulin binding to myelin sheaths in paraproteinemias. Transverse frozen sections of nerve are ideal for these purposes although they are often more difficult to prepare than longitudinal sections.

There is a variety of methods of preparing and examining fixed specimens of peripheral nerve, and each method reveals different information (20). Ideally, exact transverse sections should be cut from the peripheral nerve; occasionally, longitudinal sections are also useful. Paraffin-embedded sections can be stained for a variety of histologic stains and for immunocytochemistry to reveal nerve components (Table 1). Blood vessels and inflammatory exudates are ideally studied in paraffin sections, but quantitation of nerve fibers, the detection of axon degeneration and regeneration, and the assessment of segmental demyelination and remyelination are more satisfactory in 0.5 to 1 $\mu$m toluidine blue-stained resin sections or by electron microscopy. The presence of amyloid in the endoneurium or giant axons in some hereditary neuropathies and in some toxic neuropathies, can be detected both in paraffin- and in resin-embedded sections. Teased preparations are most useful for detecting segmental demyelination and remyelination and for assessing whether axonal degeneration and regeneration have occurred within the nerve in the past (20).

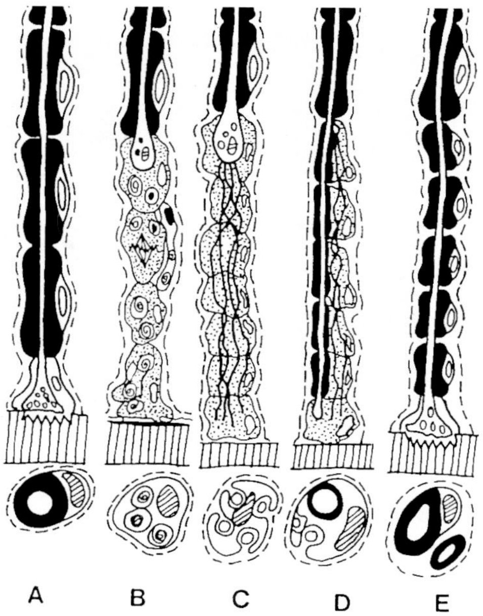


**FIG. 14.** Diagram summarizing the events occurring during axonal degeneration and regeneration. **A,** Normal nerve. **B,** Seven days after axonal damage; Schwann cells containing axon and myelin debris have divided to form bands of Büngner. **C,** Axon sprouts grow from the swollen end-bulb of the proximal axon. **D,** An axon becomes myelinated. **E,** Connection with the end-organ is reestablished; regenerated internodes are short. (From ref. 19.)

## Peripheral Neuropathies

The pathological diagnosis of a peripheral neuropathy usually requires close clinicopathologic correlation and knowledge of the electrophysiologic data such as nerve conduction speeds and electromyography. Moderate slowing of nerve conduction velocities usually indicates loss of large myelinated fibers, whereas excessive slowing of conduction velocity suggests that segmental demyelination has occurred. Although there are a number of specific histopathologic features that aid in the diagnosis of peripheral neuropathy [e.g., amyloid, the presence of lepra bacilli, abnormal lipids such as sulfatide within the nerve, giant axons and vasculitis (17,49)], for the most part, assessment of peripheral nerve pathology depends on detection and quantitation of general pathologic features.

### *General Pathology of Peripheral Nerves*

The pathologic reactions of peripheral nerves for most practical purposes are limited to axonal degeneration and regeneration, and segmental demyelination and remyelination. Hypertrophic changes with onion-bulb formation occur most commonly as a result of recurrent segmental demyelination and are most often seen in hereditary neuropathies.

### *Axonal Degeneration and Regeneration*

If a neuron in the anterior horn of the gray matter of the spinal cord or in a dorsal root ganglion dies, its axon degenerates and no regeneration occurs. Such neuronal destruction is seen in poliomyelitis, motor neuron disease, spinal muscular atrophy, and infarction of the spinal cord. Dorsal root ganglion cells may be lost in viral infections such as varicella zoster or in a variety of hereditary sensory neuropathies. If an axon in a peripheral nerve is injured, for example, by trauma, entrapment, or ischemia, the distal end of the axon degenerates and, subsequently, regeneration occurs from the proximal stump of the damaged axon (Fig. 14). The success of the regeneration depends on the distance of the site of damage from the nerve end-organ (either motor end-plate or sensory nerve ending) and the amount of scarring or other obstruction laid in the path of the regenerating axons.

Axonal degeneration was described by Augustus Vollney Waller in 1850 in London and the eponym "wallerian degeneration" is still used. Much of the fundamental work on nerve degeneration and regeneration, however, was performed by Ramon y Cajal (103). Twenty-four hours after nerve injury, most myelinated and nonmyelinated axons start to show degenerative changes. There is retraction of myelin from the nodes of Ranvier and dilatation of Schmidt-Lanterman incisures in the proximal, as well as the distal stump. By 48 hours, myelin and axon changes become more obvious as the axon disintegrates; myelin sheaths become disrupted and form globules (Fig. 15) in which axon fragments are enclosed. Disintegration of the myelin appears to start with dilatation of the Schmidt-Lanterman incisures during the first day or two after injury (20). Myelin debris is initially birefringent and has a lamellated ultrastructure, as does normal myelin. But, as proteins break down and lysosomal enzymes

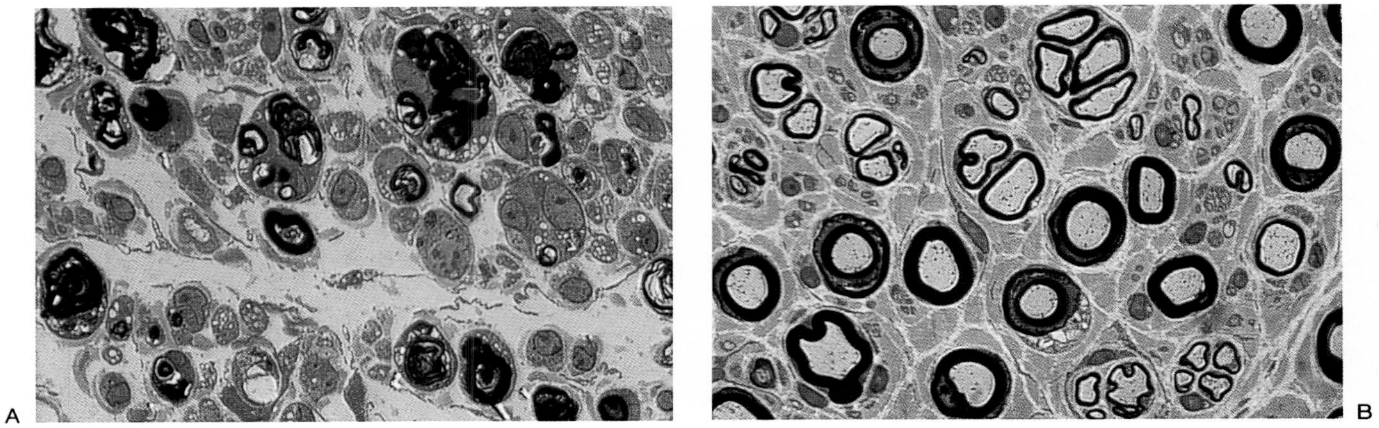


**FIG. 15.** Axonal degeneration and regeneration in transverse sections of peripheral nerve. **A,** Axonal degeneration 4 days after nerve section. Few axons are visible and myelin is forming globules in Schwann cells and macrophages. The 1 μm section is stained with toluidine blue (×**310**). **B,** Axonal regeneration in a human nerve biopsy. Normal myelinated fibers are interspersed with clusters of closely associated thinly myelinated regenerating fibers (*top and bottom right).* The 1 μm section is stained with toluidine blue (×**310**).

become active around the myelin debris (49,102), cholesterol within the myelin is esterified to cholesterol esters and lipid debris loses its birefringence in polarized light and its lamellated ultrastructure, to become amorphous globular lipid, which now stains strongly with Sudan dyes and oil red O. The Marchi technique also differentiates between normal myelin and degenerating myelin (49).

During the second week after nerve injury, much of the myelin debris is removed from the distal part of the nerve and regenerative features become more prominent. Axon fragments and myelin debris are broken down by both Schwann cells and macrophages (104,105) . Macrophages, in addition to their phagocytic function. may help to promote nerve repair through the elaboration of Schwann cell mitogens. They may also affect neurons and axonal growth directly through the release of neurotrophins (106–111).

Although Schwann cell mitoses are seen as early as 24 hours after nerve injury, the peak of proliferation is between 3 and 15 days after nerve damage (112). As Schwann cells proliferate, they form columns (bands of Büngner) surrounded by basement membrane (Fig. 14); often redundant, old, Schwann cell basement membrane is associated with these bands. Regenerating axons grow along the bands of Büngner and if regeneration fails, the bands shrink and Schwann cells may disappear and become replaced by fibrous tissue (113).

Several easily detectable histologic changes occur during axonal regeneration. The neuron cell bodies in the anterior horns of the spinal cord or in the dorsal root ganglia show changes of chromatolysis during the first 3 weeks after axonal injury (112). The nerve cell perikaryon swells by some 20%, and the nucleus becomes eccentric, as does the nucleolus. Nissl substance (a mixture of rough endoplasmic reticulum and polyribosomes) is dispersed so that the cytoplasm becomes pale when stained by H&E or by the Nissl stain (20,49). During this stage of chromatolysis, there is a marked increase in polyribosomal ribonucleic acid (RNA) and in peptides such as galanin and vaso-intestinal polipeptide (VIP), reflecting the metabolic events involved in axon regeneration (114,115).

Regenerative changes in axons are seen within the first few hours after nerve damage, but are most easily detected 5 to 20 days after injury. The proximal stump of the axon swells to create a balloonlike structure often 50 μm in diameter and 100 μm in length. The balloons are filled with organelles and fibrils, which can be detected by electron microscopy; they can be visualized by light microscopy using immunocytochemical stains for neurofilament protein, or by employing silver stains as used by Ramon y Cajal when he first described them. Myelin sheaths become stretched around the swollen axon balloons (103,116).

Starting around the fourth day after injury, multiple nerve sprouts or neurites extend from the axon balloon (growth cone) and grow distally at 1 to 2.5 mm/day. As the neurites enter the bands of Büngner, they become invaginated into the surface of the Schwann cell and, if growth continues, they become myelinated. Unmyelinated fibers regenerate in a similar way but they are smaller and no myelin sheaths form around them. Regenerating neurites can be detected in the classical way by silver staining; but in cross sections of peripheral nerve they are best demonstrated in 0.5 to 1 μm resin sections or by electron microscopy. Characteristically, regenerating axons form clusters encircled by a single basement membrane. In the light microscope, these clusters (Fig. 15) are recognized by the close association of small, thinly myelinated axons within the nerve; myelinated nerve fibers in a normal nerve are well separated from each other by endoneurial collagen (Fig. 5).

Axon growth and regeneration are stimulated by nerve growth factor synthesized by Schwann cells, fibroblasts, and macrophages and transported back along the axon by retrograde axoplasmic transport to stimulate nerve cell protein synthesis (57,107,117,118). Schwann cells also secrete an acidic 37,000 dalton protein that is released slowly after injury and may promote, and later maintain, axonal growth (119). In addition to growth factors, there appears to be topographical affinity between regenerating axons and certain pathways; for example, it appears that regenerating tibial nerve axons grow toward the distal tibial nerve rather than toward the distal peroneal nerves. Connective tissue elements may also play a role in guiding regenerating axons (9). Neurite-outgrowth-promoting factors on cell surfaces (cell adhesion molecules) or in the extracellular matrix promote extension of the axon by providing an appropriate "adhesiveness" in the substrate. (57) Both neurotrophic and neurite-outgrowth-promoting factors are essential for axonal growth after injury (57)

The success of regeneration, with axons reaching effective end-organs, may be influenced by several factors. If the injury is far proximal from the end-organ, few regenerating axons may make effective reconnections. But regeneration over short distances may be very effective in the peripheral nervous system. The presence of scar tissue or discontinuity of anatomical pathways may also inhibit regeneration. A number of grafting techniques are employed to overcome this problem (12,112). If regeneration to the distal stump of a nerve is blocked by scar tissue, axons may grow outside the original course of the nerve and even back alongside the proximal stump (terminals of Perroncito); thus, small bundles of regenerating neurites, often surrounded by perineurial cells, form amputation neuromas.

Microscopically, there are interlacing bundles containing axons surrounded by myelin sheaths and with fine perineurial coverings. Immunocytochemistry for neurofilament proteins (axons), EMA (perineurial cells), and S-100 (Schwann cells) may be very useful in establishing the structure and identity of the nerve bundles in an amputation neuroma. Immunohistochemical and radioimmunoassay data have shown a focal accumulation of sodium channels within the tips of injured axons that may be responsible, in part, for the ectopic axonal excitability, and the resulting abnormal sensory phenomena (pain and paresthesiae) which frequently complicate peripheral nerve injury (120). Macrophages migrate into the neuroma within the first two weeks after the injury. Later they are seen with numerous large cytoplasmic vacuoles filled with myelin fragments. This suggests that macrophages may also participate in the genesis of chronic pain after the neuroma has formed possibly by: (1) creating demyelinating axonal regions susceptible to external stimuli; (2) releasing substances which influence regeneration of axons; or (3) direct action on the denuded remodeling membranes (121).

Axon degeneration, often with regeneration, is a feature of numerous neuropathies including those associated with diabetes, amyloidosis, nerve root or peripheral nerve compression, trauma to peripheral nerve trunks, vascular disease, and metabolic diseases (20). Most toxic neuropathies (29) cause axonal degeneration at the extreme distal ends of sensory and motor nerves, in such a way that timely withdrawal of the toxin may allow effective regeneration to occur. Many peripheral neuropathies induced by the diseases itemized previously are slowly progressive, so that nerve biopsies in these conditions do not usually reveal the early stages of axonal degeneration and regeneration. More frequently, the histologic picture is characterized by loss of large myelinated axons and, to a lesser extent, by loss of small myelinated and unmyelinated axons. Regeneration may be recognized in transverse sections of peripheral nerve by the presence of clusters (Fig. 15). In teased fiber preparations, short internodes in the distal part of the nerve indicate that axonal degeneration and regeneration have occurred in the past (113).

### *Segmental Demyelination and Remyelination*

When demyelination occurs in peripheral nerves, it has a segmental distribution with each segment representing the internodal portion of an axon myelinated by one Schwann cell (Figs. 7 and 16). Such segments can be contiguous and thus demyelination may occur over long lengths of the nerve or in short sporadic segments (18). The axon remains intact except in severe demyelinating neuropathies in which secondary axonal degeneration occurs. Remyelination is often

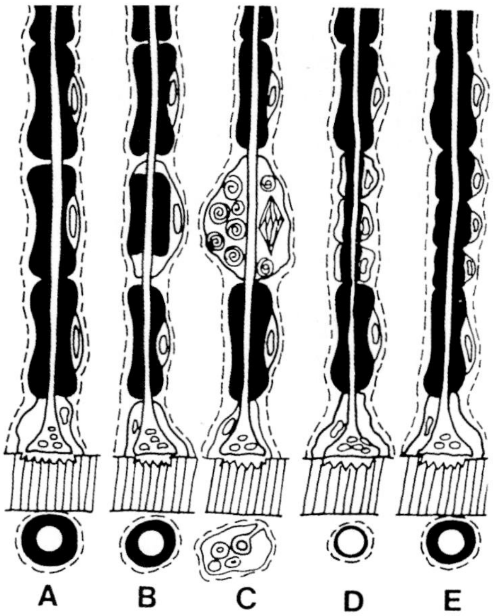


**FIG. 16.** Diagram to summarize the events occurring in primary segmental demyelination and remyelination. **A,** Normal nerve. **B,** Early segmental demyelination; retraction of paranodal myelin with widening of the nodal gap. **C,** Destruction of myelin sheath and Schwann cell mitosis. **D, E,** Remyelination; intercalated short segments. (From ref. 19.)

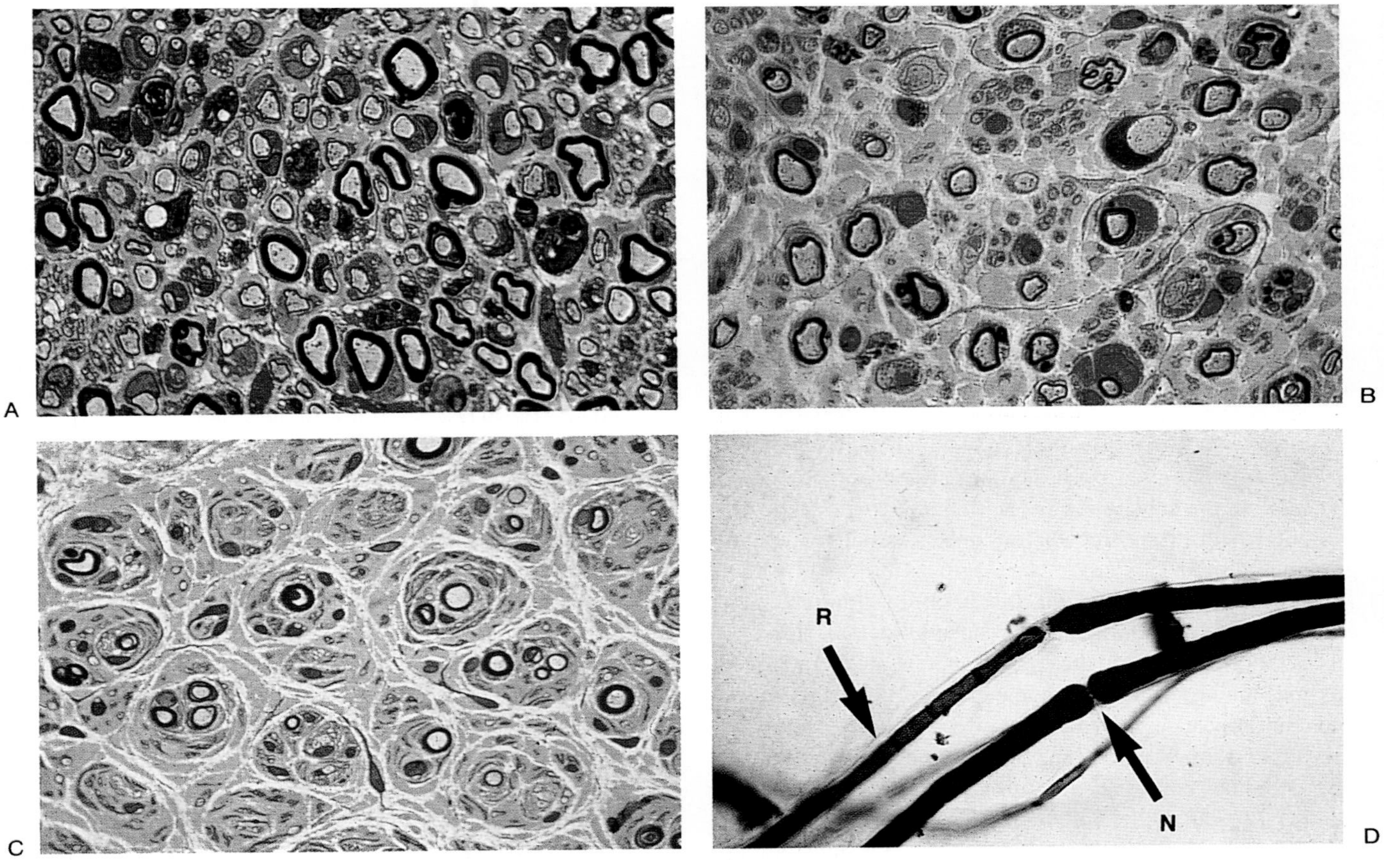


**FIG. 17.** Segmental demyelination and remyelination. **A,** Transverse section of peripheral nerve showing early remyelination in an experimental animal. There are normal, large myelinated fibers with axons 8 to 10 μm in diameter and axons 3 to 5 μm in diameter, which have thin myelin sheaths and are remyelinating. Myelin debris is seen in Schwann cells and macrophages. The 1 μm resin section is stained with toluidine blue (×**310**). **B,** Nerve biopsy from a child with metachromatic leukodystrophy (sulfatide lipidosis). Large axons with either thin myelin sheaths (remyelination) or with no myelin sheath at all (demyelinated) (*right of center*) are seen in the biopsy. Unmyelinated fibers (*center*) are unaffected. The 1 μm resin section is stained with toluidine blue (×**310**). (From ref. 35.) **C,** Hypertrophic neuropathy (Charcot-Marie-Tooth disease-HSMN type I). Demyelinated and remyelinated axons are seen at the centers of onion-bulb whorls formed by Schwann cell processes. There is abundant endoneurial collagen (*pink*). The 1 μm resin section is stained with toluidine blue and carbol fuchsin (×**240**). **D,** Teased fibers. Normal fiber (*lower*) with a normal node of Ranvier (N). The fiber above has a thin, remyelinating segment (R) on one side of the node and a normal segment on the other side. Osmium-stained teased fibers (×**200**). (From ref. 35.)

rapid and effective with restoration of nerve function. Demyelination may occur as a result of direct interference with Schwann cell metabolism, as in diphtheria; myelin sheaths are broken down through the lysosomal action of Schwann cells (88,89); although macrophages are later involved in the destruction of myelin debris (68). Another mechanism that is seen in the most common acute demyelinating neuropathy, Guillain-Barré syndrome, is an immunological attack on peripheral nerve myelin by lymphocytes and macrophages; segmental demyelination occurs and is followed by remyelination (Figs. 16 and 17). Functional recovery occurs following both types of demyelination, except in the most severe cases (122).

The first stages of segmental demyelination are seen at the node of Ranvier, where the nodal gap becomes widened; subsequently, the whole internode of myelin may be broken down (123). This results in severe slowing of conduction of nerve impulses across the demyelinated segment and the onset of symptoms for the patient. Preserved axons remain invaginated within Schwann cells as the myelin sheaths are broken down (Figs. 17 and 18). Schwann cells proliferate and within a few days, start to remyelinate the demyelinated axons by a similar mechanism to that seen during myelination in the fetus. Remyelination may be well advanced by 2 weeks after demyelination, as the thickness of myelin sheaths increases and conduction velocities return to normal.

Classically, segmental demyelination can be detected in teased nerve fibers, first by the presence of widening of the gap of the node of Ranvier and then by the presence of axons devoid of myelin sheaths. Intercalated thin myelin sheaths along the axon are seen as remyelination proceeds (Fig. 17). In electron micrographs or in resin-embedded light microscope sections, naked axons can be recognized in transverse section and remyelinating fibers detected by the presence of inappropriately thin myelin sheaths (Figs. 16–18). Segmental demyelination is a feature of mild vascular damage to peripheral nerves as in rheumatoid arthritis (124), diabetes (62), Guillain-Barré syndrome, occasional toxic neuropathies (125), and metabolic neuropathies such as metachromatic leukodystrophy (17,49) (Fig. 17). Throughout the range of neuropathies, however, segmental demyelination is less common than axonal degeneration.

### *Hypertrophic Neuropathy*

Recurrent segmental demyelination is a feature of a number of chronic hereditary neuropathies, particularly Charcot-Marie-Tooth disease, Déjérine-Sottas disease (hereditary motor and sensory neuropathy types I and III), and Refsum's disease (63,126,127). In such diseases, repeated segmental demyelination appears to be responsible for a florid proliferation of Schwann cells and the formation of onion-bulb whorls (128,129) (Figs. 17 and 18), giving a distinctive histologic picture of hypertrophic neuropathy to these peripheral neuropathies.

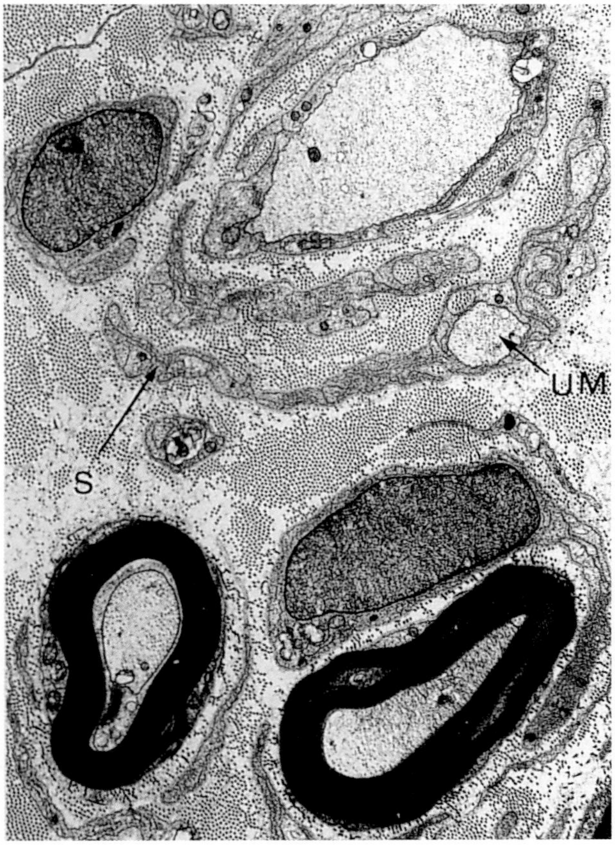


**FIG. 18.** Demyelination. A large diameter axon (*top*) is demyelinated and devoid of a myelin sheath. A small onion-bulb whorl has formed around this axon with the encirclement by Schwann cell processes (S), one of which contains an unmyelinated fiber (UM). Thickly myelinated fibers are seen at the bottom of the picture. Electron micrograph (× **6600**).

### Traumatic Lesions of Peripheral Nerve

An understanding of the structure and staining reactions of normal peripheral nerve is essential for unraveling the complexities of traumatic lesions of nerve. Identification of cell types, recognition of patterns of organization, and the detection of normal elements within a traumatic lesion allow a more confident diagnosis and description to be formulated.

Amputation neuromas may develop as painful swellings at the distal ends of amputated limbs or at sites of nerve damage without amputation. They consist of disoriented bundles of axons surrounded by Schwann cells and divided into compartments by perineurial cells. In H&E-stained paraffin sections, the tubular formation of the perineurial compartments can be recognized (49). By immunocytochemistry, axons can be stained with antibodies to neurofilament protein; the Schwann cells associated with them contain S-100 protein and the perineurial cells are EMA-positive but do not contain S-100 protein. Silver stains can also be used to identify the twisted and disoriented axons. The histologic picture reflects the processes seen in the normal regeneration of peripheral nerve, but in amputation neuromas, appropriate regeneration along the distal part of the nerve is prevented.

Morton's neuroma involves the plantar interdigital nerves and consists of small painful swellings on the nerves. Histologically, there is fibrosis and edema of the endoneurium and perineurium and the accumulation of mucosubstances similar to endoneurial glycosaminoglycans. The detection of axons and Schwann cells by immunocytochemistry is often a useful adjunct to the diagnosis of this lesion (130).

A pseudocyst or ganglion containing mucinous material, which stains with alcian blue, may form on a peripheral nerve, generally at a site of repeated trauma. Although the fibrous capsule of the cyst and its mucinous contents may dominate the picture, damaged nerve components can usually be detected adjacent to the cyst (129).

Compressive lesions of peripheral nerves have resulted in some debate regarding their origin. Because of the resemblance of whorls within these lesions to those seen in hypertrophic neuropathies, they have been labeled "localized hypertrophic neuropathy" (131). Such lesions usually occur at sites of compression over the fibula or on the posterior interosseous nerve (132); although, some lesions present with no obvious nerve compression. Although there is well-marked onion-bulb formation, ultrastructural studies have shown that the onion bulbs are formed not by Schwann cells as in hypertrophic neuropathies, but by perineurial cells (130,132). Immunocytochemistry has confirmed that the whorls are formed by EMA-positive perineurial cells (34) but the lesion has now, unfortunately, been interpreted as a tumor of perineurial cells – a perineuroma (26,27,34,133). From their considerable experience of peripheral nerve pathology, Johnson and Kline (134) have strongly emphasized that the designation of this lesion as neoplastic is probably erroneous. In reporting four cases, these authors (134) point out that no instance of progressive growth or recurrence of this lesion has been reported in the literature. "Localized hypertrophic neuropathy-perineuroma," therefore, appears to be a proliferative response to perineurial damage with the compartmentalization of the nerve well recorded at sites of nerve trauma or grafting (16,135).

### Tumors of the Peripheral Nervous System

A variety of cells and structures may be identified in tumors of the peripheral nervous system; they include perineural cells, Schwann cells, axons, and neurons. The diagnosis frequently depends on the histologic analysis of the tumor and, thus, the detection of cellular components forming the tumor and their relationship with normal nerve structures (130).

Perineuroma is true perineural neoplasm distinguishable from reactive localized hypertrophic neuropathy. It presents most often on the limbs or trunk of middle-aged adults with a female predominance. Histologically, perineuromas are well circumscribed lesions composed of spindle-shaped tumor cells that stain positively for EMA but fail to stain for S-100 protein, neurofilaments, and CD-34 (35). Perineuromas may be closely related to cutaneous meningioma because shared histologic features, and positive staining for vimentin and EMA in both conditions, suggest close similarities between these lesions (35).

Schwannomas (neurilemmomas) are tumors of peripheral nerves composed almost entirely of Schwann cells. They show the classical patterns of spindle cells in a compact (Antoni type A) or loose (Antoni type B) arrangement. Neoplastic schwann cells may exhibit different morphology (Fig.19). (136–139) Occasionally, the Schwann cells have an epithelioid appearance (epithelioid schwannomas), contain an abundant myxoid stroma (Neurothekoma) (135), or exhibit xanthomatous change with many foamy cells containing oil red O-positive neutral lipid (140). Schwannomas usually grow on the side of nerves and do not infiltrate nerve bundles

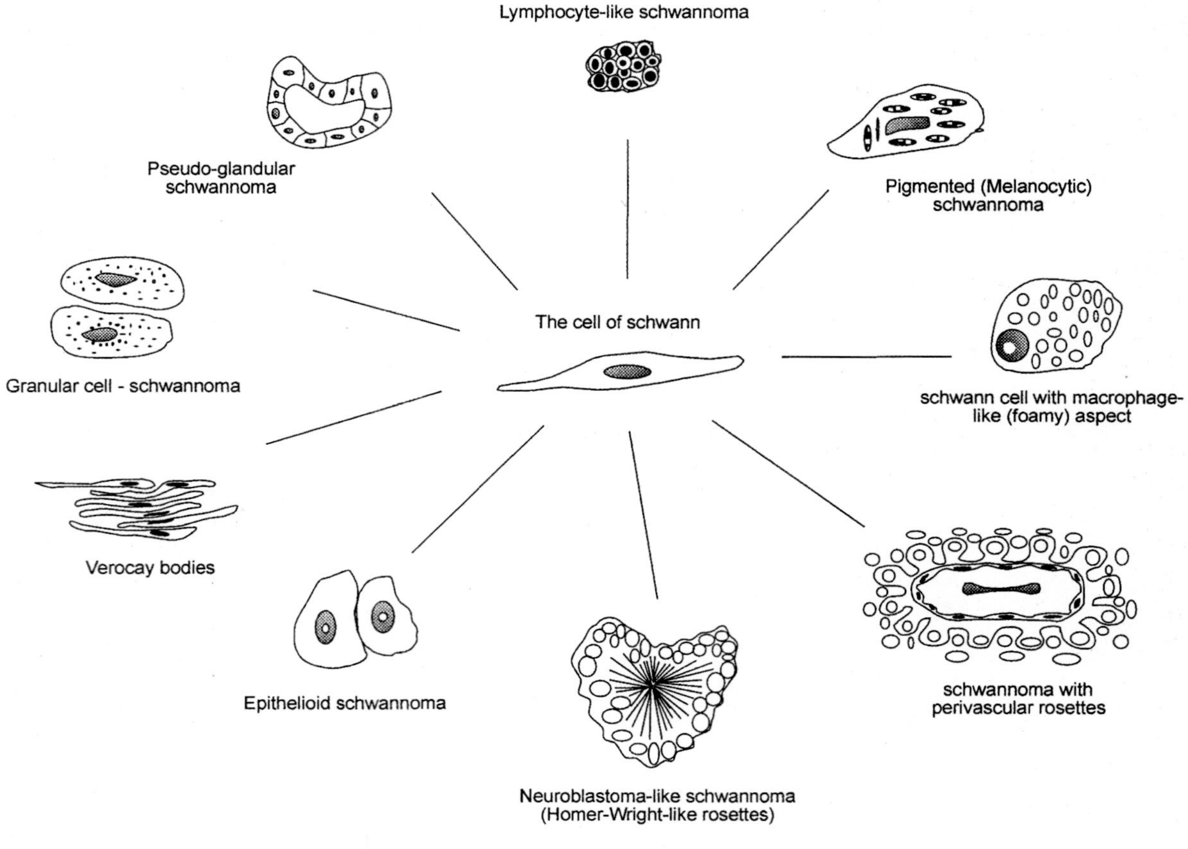


**FIG. 19.** Diagram to show the diferent morphology that the cell of Schwan may present in Schwannomas. [From refs. (136–140),146,147,150.]

(20). Thus, normal nerves may be seen within the fibrous capsule that is usually present around schwannomas. Histologically, the tumor cells have elongated nuclei and long eosinophilic processes often forming palisades first described by the Uruguayan pathologist Juan José Verocay and known today as Verocay bodies; they are, in effect, a series of palisades. The basement membrane investing each Schwann cell in the tumor is well demonstrated by electron microscopy, but can also be demonstrated in reticulin stains by light microscopy (20,141). Collagen bundles within schwannomas may have a distinctive long-spaced appearance (Luse bodies) (142). Immunocytochemistry shows the presence of S-100 protein and staining by Leu-7 in schwannoma cells, but they are negative for EMA (31). Some schwannomas associated with the spinal cord, and those deep in the body or close to major joints stain by immunocytochemistry for GFAP while the superficial, subcutaneous schwannomas are negative (143). Schwann cells associated with unmyelinated fibers are more likely to express GFAP. It has been proposed that the GFAP-positive schwannomas may arise from unmyelinated nerves (143,144). Melanin may be seen in schwannomas and by electron microscopy premelanosomes; melanosomes may be identified. Such structures emphasize the common origin of Schwann cells and melanocytes from the neural crest (145,146). Patients with melanocitic schwannomas may have evidence of Carney's syndrome (myxomas, spotty pigmentation, and endocrine overactivity producing Cushing's syndrome) (147).

Granular cell tumor (Abrikosoff tumor), also known as granular cell myoblastomas, is not a specific entity. Granular cytoplasmic change is the expression of a metabolic alteration occurring often, but not exclusively, in Schwann cells (148,149). The tumor cells have abundant granular cytoplasm and a small eccentric nucleus; they invade small nerve branches in the skin. Immunocytochemical studies have shown that the tumor cells, in some cases, contain S-100 protein and also, occasionally, express myelin (PO and P2) and myelin-associated proteins (136,150,151). Granular cells have also been described in nerves undergoing wallerian degeneration (149).

Neurofibromas are complex lesions frequently associated with neurofibromatosis. As distinct from schwannomas, neurofibromas are diffuse lesions in the skin or around peripheral nerves which invade the peripheral nerve endoneurium and enlarge nerve branches (49,130,141). They also diffusely invade surrounding tissues and may cause bone destruction. Histologically, neurofibromas contain a variety of cells that are associated with peripheral nerves; unlike schwannomas, they are not predominantly composed of Schwann cells. Mast cells (45) can be stained by toluidine blue or Giemsa techniques. By immunocytochemistry, S-100, and Leu-7-positive Schwann cells can be detected within the lesions, in addition to EMA-positive perineurial cells. Entrapped axons can be seen coursing through neurofibromas in immunocytochemical preparations for neurofilament protein or in silver-stained sections. Factor-XIIIa-positive fibroblasts-like cells are also found in neurofibromas which may play an important role in the formation of the large amount of extracelular matrix seen in these proliferations (152–154).

Neurofibromatosis, or von Recklinghausen's disease, presents as two major diseases, peripheral (type I) and central (type II) (155). Both type I and type II are inherited as autosomal-dominant traits but many cases are new mutations. Over 90% of cases of neurofibromatosis are type I (peripheral); a gene defect has been located on the long arm of chromosome 17 (NF1 gene) near the centromere and has been linked to the locus encoding for nerve growth factor (156–159). There is an increase in nerve growth factor in the serum of patients with this disorder (108,109). NF1 gene is a tumor-suppressor gene which spans over 350kb of genomic DNA and encodes a 2818 amino acid protein called neurofibromin. Neurofibromin has been shown to be associated with cytoplasmic microtubules and it is ubiquitously distributed in all tissues (160,161).

A wide variety of disorders occurs in type I neurofibromatosis, including elephantiasis nervosa in which there are redundant folds of skin associated with neurofibromata (20) and, more commonly, multiple cutaneous neurofibromata. Other tumors such as gliomas and pigmented hamartomas of the iris, (Lisch nodules), are also seen in patients with this disorder (162).

Central or type II neurofibromatosis is much less common than type I and is characterized by bilateral acoustic schwannomas; skin lesions are uncommon. A proportion of these patients have multiple tumors, including meningiomas, intramedullary spinal ependymomas, and glial microhamartomas of the cerebral cortex (163) A gene deletion on chromosome 22q12 (NF2 gene) has been identified in patients with this disorder and it is associated with abnormalities of glial growth factor and nerve growth factor activity (156). This NF2 gene spans 110kb and encodes a putative-membrane-organizing protein called merlin or schwannomin that is believed to act as a tumor-suppressor gene; the loss of its function is a fundamental event in the genesis of schwannomas.(163,164)

Neuronal tumors such as ganglioneuromas, occur in association with autonomic ganglia in the peripheral nervous system. Histologically, neurons can be identified within these tumors; axons and Schwann cells may be identified by immunocytochemistry. Electron microscopy reveals the presence of 100 nm dense-core vesicles resembling catecholamine granules in the neurons. In addition to well-differentiated ganglioneuromas, primitive neuroectodermal tumors such as neuroblastoma and ganglioneuroblastomas arise within the abdomen and thorax (165). Cell types within the more primitive tumors may be difficult to identify by immunocytochemistry. but electron microscopy usually reveals the presence of 100 nm dense-core catecholamine vesicles within the tumor cell cytoplasm (114).

Solitary circumscribed neuromas of the skin (palisaded encapsulated neuromas) are distinctive, small, benign cutaneous tumors usually on the face (166). The capsule is composed of EMA-positive perineurial cells. Partly enclosed within the capsule is a mass of S-100 protein-positive Schwann cells and many tiny neurofilament-positive axons in interlacing fascicles. Such lesions are not associated with von Recklinghausen's disease or multiple endocrine neoplasia type IIb.

Malignant peripheral nerve sheath tumors (MPNST) (167) (malignant schwannomas) show great histologic variation and many similarities to other soft tissue tumors (136). Immunocytochemistry has demonstrated EMA-positive and S-100 protein-positive cells in MPNST (168,169) as well as occasional tumors that are EMA-positive and S-100 protein-negative (170). This suggests that cells of MPNST may produce proteins characteristic of perineurial cells, or of both perineurium and Schwann cells. NSE, neurofilaments and myelin-basic protein have also been occasionally identified in MPNST (170). Unusual elements may be encountered sometimes in malignant nerve sheath tumors, such as cartilage, bone, squamous elements, and muscle. MPNST may also present with malignant glands (glandular malignant schwannoma) or rhabdomyosarcoma. In an attempt to explain the occurrence of malignant muscle differentiation (rhabdomyosarcoma) in malignant Schwannomas, Pierre Masson suggested that endoneurial cells might differentiate into muscle cells under the inductive influence of nerve cells, a situation which was thought to be operative in regenerating limbs in triton salamanders: hence the name "triton tumor" (Malignant schwannoma with rhabdomyoblastic differentiation) (171).

## ACKNOWLEDGMENTS

We thank the staff of the Neuropathology, Pathology, and Electron Microscope Laboratories of the Southampton General Hospital, Southampton England and the Immunohistochemistry section of the ABC Hospital in Mexico City for their generous and expert cooperation. Special thanks are due to Margaret Harris who typed the manuscript and to Dr. Hugh Jones who drew the diagrams.

## REFERENCES

1. Le Douarin NM, Smith J. Development of peripheral nervous system from the neural crest. *Annu Rev Cell Biol* 1988;4:375–404.
2. Maderson PFA. *Developmental and evolutionary aspects of the neural crest.* New York; Wiley-Interscience, 1987.
3. Cunningham TJ, Fisher C, Hawn F. Testing the trophic factor hypothesis in the visual system. In: Reider PJ, Bunge RP, Seil FJ, eds. *Current issues in neural regeneration research: neurology and neurobiology, vol 48.* New York; Alan R Liss, 1988;89–104.
4. Bhattacharyya A, Brackenbury R, Ratner N. Axons arrest the migration of Schwann cell precursors. *Development* 1994;120:1411–1420
5. Levi-Montalcini R, Calissano P. Nerve growth factor. In: Adelman G, ed. *Encyclopedia of neuroscience, vol II.* Boston; Birkhauser, 1987; 744–746.
6. Pérez-Polo JR. Neurotrophic factors In: Adelman G, ed. *Encyclopedia of neuroscience, vol II.* Boston; Birkhauser, 1987;827–828.
7. Sarpini E, Ross A, Rosen Brown MJ, Rostami A, Kropowski H, Lisak P. Expression of nerve growth factor during peripheral nerve development. *Dev Biol* 1988;125:301–310.
8. Johnson EM, Clark HB, Schweltzer JB, Taniuchi M. Expression of nerve growth factor receptors on Schwann cells after axonal injury. In: Reider PJ, Bunge RP, Seil FJ, eds. *Current issues in neural regeneration research: neurology and neurobiology, vol 48.* New York; Alan R Liss, 1988;179–188.
9. Carbonetto S, Douville P, Harvey W, Turner DC. Laminin, fibronectin, collagen and their receptors in nerve fiber growth. In: Reider PJ, Bunge RP, Seil FJ, eds. *Current issues in neural regeneration research: neurology and neurobiology, vol 48.* New York; Alan R Liss, 1988;147–158.
10. Leturneau P, Rogers S, Peach I, Palm S, McCarthy J, Furcht L. Cellular biology of neuronal interaction with fibronectin and laminin. In: Reider PJ, Bunge RP, Seil FJ eds. *Current issues in neural regeneration research: neurology and neurobiology, vol 48.* New York; Alan R Liss, 1988;137–146.
11. Webster HF, Favilla JT. Development of peripheral nerve. In: Dyck PJ, Thomas PK, Lambert EH, Bunge R, eds. *Peripheral neuropathy, 2nd ed., vol I.* Philadelphia; WB Saunders, 1984;329–359.
12. Nadim W, Anderson PN, Turmaine M. The role of Schwann cells and basal lamina tubes in the regeneration of axons through long lengths of freeze-killed nerve graft. *Neuropathol Appl Neurobiol* 1990;16: 419–429.
13. Shield LK, King RHM, Thomas PK. A morphologic study of human fetal sural nerve. *Acta Neuropathol (Berlin)* 1986;70:60–70.
14. Thomas PK, Ochoa J. Microscopic anatomy of peripheral nerve fibers. In: Dyck PJ, Thomas PK, Lambert EH, Bunge R, eds. *Peripheral neuropathy, 2nd ed., vol I.* Philadelphia; WB Saunders, 1984; 34–96.
15. Gamble HJ. Spinal and cranial nerve roots. In: Landon DN, ed. *The peripheral nerve.* London; Chapman and Hall, 1976;330–354.
16. Ahmed AH, Weller RO. The blood-nerve barrier and reconstitution of the perineurium following nerve grafting. *Neuropathol Appl Neurobiol* 1979;5:469–483.
17. Weller RO, Swash M, McLellan DL, Scholtz CL. *Clinical neuropathology.* Berlin; Springer-Verlag, 1983.
18. Liberman AR. Sensory ganglia. In: Landon DN, ed. *The peripheral nerve.* London; Chapman and Hall, 1976;188–278.
19. Ferreira JM, Caldini EM, Montes GS. Distribution of elastic fibers in peripheral nerves in mammals. *Acta Anat (Berlin)* 1987;130:168–173.
20. Weller RO, Cervos-Navarro J. *The pathology of peripheral nerves.* London; Butterworths, 1977.
21. Cavanagh JG Pathology of peripheral nerve diseases. In: Weller RO ed. *Systemic pathology Vol 4. Nervous system muscle and eyes. 3rd ed.* Edinburgh; Churchill Livingstone 1990;544–578.
22. Shantaveerappa TR, Bourne GH. The perineurial epithelium, nature and significance. *Nature* 1963;199:577–579.
23. Shantaveerappa TR, Bourne GH. Perineurial epithelium—a new concept of its role in the integrity of the peripheral nervous system. *Science* 1966;154:1464–1467.
24. Asbury AK, Johnson PC. *Pathology of peripheral nerve, vol 9. Major problems in pathology.* Philadelphia; WB Saunders, 1978.
25. Vega JA, Del Valle ME, Haro JJ, et al. The inner-core, outer-core and capsule cells of the human Pacinian corpuscles: an immunohistochemical study. *Eur J Morphol* 1994;32:11–18.
26. Lazarus SS, Trombetta LD. Ultrastructural identification of a benign perineural cell tumor. *Cancer* 1978;41:1823–1829.
27. Wendenheim KM, Campbell WG Jr. Perineural cell tumor immunocytochemical and ultrastructural characteristics. Relationship to other perineurial tumors with a review of the literature. *Virchows Arch [A]* 1986;408:375–383.
28. Low FN. The perineurium and connective tissue of peripheral nerve. In: Landon DN, ed. *The peripheral* nerve. London; Chapman and Hall, 1976;159–187.
29. Cavanagh JB. Toxic and deficiency disorders. In: Weller RO, ed. *Systemic pathology. 3rd ed., vol 4, Nervous system, muscle and eyes.* Edinburgh; Churchill Livingstone, 1990;244–308.
30. Perentes E, Rubinstein LJ. Recent applications of immunoperoxidase histochemistry in human neurooncology: an up-date. *Arch Pathol Lab Med* 1987;111:796–812.
31. Perentes E, Nakagawa Y, Ross G, Stanton C, Rubinstein LJ. Expression of epithelial membrane antigen in perineurial cells and their derivates: an immunohistochemical study with multiple markers. *Acta Neuropathol (Berlin)* 1987;75:160–165.
32. Pinkus GS, Kurtin PJ. Epithelial membrane antigen-a diagnostic discriminant in surgical pathology. *Hum Pathol* 1985;16:920–940.

33. Theaker JM, Gillet MB, Fleming KA, Gatter KC. Epithelial membrane antigen expression by meningiomas and perineurium of peripheral nerves. *Arch Pathol Lab Med* 1987;11:409.
34. Ariza A, Bilbao JM, Rosai J. Immunohistochemical detection of epithelial membrane antigen in normal perineurial cells and perineuromas. *Am J Surg Pathol* 1988;12:678–683.
35. Mentzel T, Dei Tos AP, Fletcher CDM. Perineuroma (storiform perineural fibroma): clinicopathological analysis of four cases. *Histopathology* 1994;25;261–267.
36. Erlandson RA. The enigmantic perineural cell and its participation in tumors and tumorlike conditions. *Ultrastruct Pathol* 1991;15: 335–351.
37. Shirouzu K, Isomoto H, Kakagawa T. Prognostic evaluation of perineural invasion in rectal cancer. *Am J Surg* 1993:165:233–237.
38. Fogt F, Capodieci P. Loda M. Assesment of perineural invasion by GLUT-1 immunohistochemistry. *Appl Immunohistochem* 1995; 3:194–197.
39. Van den Rijn M, Rouse RV. DC-34: a review. *Appl Immunohistochem* 1994;2:71–80.
40. Weiss SW, Nickoloff BJ. CD-34 is expressed by a distinctive cell population in peripheral nerve, nerve sheath tumors tumors and related lesions. *Am J Surg Pathol* 1993;17:1039–1045.
41. Stevens A, Schabet M, Schott K, Wiethölter H. Role of endoneural cells in experimental allergic neuritis and characterization of resident phagocytic cells. *Acta Neuropathol* 1989;77:412–419.
42. Bonetti B, Monaco S, Giannini C , Ferrari S, Zanusso G, Rizzuto N. Human peripheral nerve macrophages in normal and pathological conditions. *J Neurol Sci* 1993;118:158–168.
43. Griffin J, George R. The resident macrophages in peripheral nervous system. A renewed form of bone marrow: new variations of an old theme. *Lab Invest* 1993;3:257–260.
44. Weller RO. The pathology of peripheral nerves. *Wiss Z Friedrich-Schiller Univ* 1985;34:442–453.
45. Isaacson P. Mast cells in benign nerve sheath tumours. *J Pathol* 1975; 119:193–196.
46. Nurnberg M, Moll Y. Semiquantitative aspects of mast cells in normal skin and in neurofibromas of neurofibromatosis type 1 and 5. *Dermatology* 1994;188:296–299.
47. Johnson D, Seeldrayer PA, Weiner HL. The role of mast cells in demyelination. 1. Myelin proteins are degraded by mast cell proteases and myelin basic protein and P2 can stimulate mast cell degradation. *Brain Res* 1988;444:195–198.
48. Weis J, Alexianu ME. Heide G, Shroder JM. Renaut bodies contain elastic fiber component. *J Neuropathol* 1993;53:444–451.
49. Weller RO. *Colour atlas of* neuropathology. Oxford; Oxford University Press and Harvey Miller, 1984.
50. Lascelles RG, Thomas PK. Changes due to age in internodal length in the sural nerve of man. *J Neurol Neurosurg Psychiatry* 1966;22: 40–44.
51. Boyd IA, Davey MR. *Composition of peripheral nerves.* Edinburgh; Churchill Livingstone, 1968.
52. Xu Z, Dong DL, Cleveland DW. Neuronal intermediate filaments: new progress on an old subject. *Curr Opin Neurobiol* 1994; 4:655–661.
53. Hsieh S-T, Crawford TO, Griffith JW. Neurofilament distribution and organization in the myelinated axons of peripheral nervous system. *Brain Res* 1994;642:316–326.
54. Day-Allen R. The microtubule as an intracellular engine. *Sci Am* 1987;256:26–33.
55. Black MM. Microtubule transport and assembley cooperate to generate the microtubule array in growing axons. *Brain Res* 1994; 102: 61–77.
56. Brimijoin S, Capek P, Dyck PJ. Axonal transport of dopamine $\beta$-hydroxylase in human sural nerves in vitro. *Science* 1973;180:1295.
57. Lundborg G, Dahlin L, Danielsen N, Zhao Q. Trophism, tropism and specificity in nerve regeneration. *J Reconstr Microsurg* 1994;10: 345–354.
58. Arvidson B. A review of axonal transport of metals. *Toxicology* 1994; 88:1–14.
59. Price DL, Griffin JW, Hoffman PN. Axonal transport disorders. In: Adelman G, ed. *Encyclopedia of neuroscience, vol I.* Boston; Birkhauser, 1987;102.
60. Penfold ME, Armati P, Cunningham AL. Axonal transport of herpes simplex virions to epidermal cells; evidence for a specialized mode of virus transport and assembly. *Proc Natl Acad Sci* 1994;91:6529–6533.
61. Knox CA. Morphometric alterations of rat myelinated fibers with aging. *J Neuropathol Exp Neurol* 1989;42:119–139.
62. Thomas PK, Landon DP, King RHM. Disease of peripheral nerves. In: Adams JH, Corsellis JAN, Duchen LW, eds. *Greenfield's neuropathology, 4th ed.* London; Edward Arnold, 1984;779–806.
63. Li C, Tropak MB, Gerlai R, et al. Myelination in the absence of myelin-associated glycoprotein. *Nature* 1994;369:747–750.
64. Trapp B, Quartes R, Suzuki K. Immunocytochemical studies of quaking mice support a role for myelin associated glycoprotein in forming and maintaining the periaxonal space and periaxonal cytoplasmic collar of myelinating Schwann cells. *J Cell Biol* 1984;99:594–609.
65. Landon DL, Hall S. The myelinated fibre. In: Landon DN, ed. *The peripheral nerve.* London; Chapman and Hall, 1976;1–105.
66. Billings-Gagliardi S. Mode of locomotion of Schwann cells in vivo. *Am J Anat* 1977;150:73–79.
67. Weller RO, Herzog I. Schwann cell lysosomes in hypertrophic neuropathy and in normal human nerves. *Brain* 1970;93:347–356.
68. Jaakkola S, Savunen O, Halme T, Uitto J, Peltonen J. Basement membranes during development of human nerve: Schwann cells and perineurial cells display marked changes in their expression profiles for laminin subunits and beta 1 and beta 4 integrins. *J Neurocytol* 1993; 22:215–230.
69. Dziadek M, Edgar D, Paulsson M, Timpal R, Fleischajer R. Basement membrane proteins produced by Schwann cells and in neurofibromatosis. *Ann NY Acad Sci* 1986;486:248–259.
70. Bunge TM, Bunge RD. Linkage between Schwann cell extracellular matrix production and ensheathment function. *Ann NY Acad Sci* 1986; 486:241–247.
71. Fanó G, Biocca S, Fulle S, Mariggió M, Belia S, Calissano P. The S-100: A protein family in search of a function. *Prog Neurobiol* 1995; 46:71–82.
72. Vastapel MJ, Gatter KC, Wolf-Peeters C. New sites of human S-100 immunoreactivity detected with monoclonal antibodies. *Am J Clin Pathol* 1986;85:160–168.
73. Gould VE, Moll R, Moll I, Lee I, Schwechheimer K, Franke WW. The intermediate filament complement of the spectrum of nerve sheath neoplasms. *Lab Invest* 1986;55:463–474.
74. Kawahara E, Oda Y, Ooi A, Katsuda S, Nakanishi Y, Umeda S. Expression of glial fibrillary acidic protein (GFAP) in peripheral nerve sheath tumors. *Am J Surg Pathol* 1988;12:115–120.
75. Filbin MT, Tennekoon GI. Myelin PO-protein, more than just a structural protein?. *Bioessays* 1992;14:541–547.
76. Morell P. Myelin. In: Adelman G, ed. *Encyclopedia of neuroscience, vol II.* Boston; Birkhauser, 1987;727–732.
77. Raine CS. Multiple sclerosis and chronic relapsing EAE: comparative ultrastructural neuropathology. In: Halipike JF, Adams CWM, Tourtelotte WW, eds. *Multiple sclerosis.* London; Chapman and Hall, 1983;413–460.
78. Charnas L. Congenital absence of peripheral myelin: abnormal Schwann cell development causes lethal arthrogryposis multiplex congenita. *Neurology* 1988;9:625–638.
79. Aguayo AJ, Bray GM. Cell interaction studies in the peripheral nerve of experimental animals. In: Dyck PJ, Thomas PK, Lambert EH, Bunge R, eds. *Peripheral neuropathy, vol I.* Philadelphia; WB Saunders 1984;360–377.
80. Eldrige CF, Bunge MB, Bunge RP, Wood PM. Differentiation of axon-related Schwann cells in vitro. I. Ascorbic acid regulates basal lamina assembly and myelin formation. *J Cell Biol* 1987;105: 1023–1034.
81. Bunge RP, Bunge MB, Bates M. Movements of the Schwann cell nucleus implicate progression of the inner axon Schwann cell process during myelination. *J Cell Biol* 1989;109:274–284.
82. Eldrige CF, Bunge MB, Bunge RP. Differentiation of axon related Schwann cells in vitro. II. Control of myelin formation. *J Neurosci* 1989;9:625–638.
83. Bunge RP. Expanding roles of the Schwann cell:ensheathment, myelination, trophism and regeneration. *Curr Opin Neurobiol* 1993; 3:805–809.
84. Sternberg N, Quartes RH, Itoyama Y, Webster H. Myelin associated glycoprotein demonstrated immunohistochemically in myelin and myelin forming cells of developing rat. *Proc Natl Acad Sci U S A* 1979;76:1510–1514.
85. Guillespie CS, Sherman DL, Blair GE, Brophy PJ. Periaxin, a novel protein of myelinating Schwann cell with a possible role in axon ensheathment. *Neuron* 1994;12:497–508.

86. Balnes AJ. Ankyrin at the node of Ranvier. *TINS* 1990;13: 119–121.
87. Kordeli E, Lambert S, Bennett B. Ankyrin G. A new ankyrin gene with neural-specific isoforms localized at the axon initial segment and node of Ranvier. *J Biol Chem* 1995;270:2352–2359.
88. Weller RO. Diphtheritic neuropathy in the chicken; an electron microscope study. *J Pathol Bacteriol* 1965;89:591–598.
89. Scholz A, Reid G. Ion Channels in human axons. *J Neurophysiol* 1993;70:1274–1279.
90. Ochoa J. The unmyelinated fibre. In: Landon DN, ed. *The peripheral nerve.* London; Chapman and Hall, 1976;106–158.
91. Waxman SG, Ritchie JM. Organization of ion channels in myelinated nerve fiber. *Science* 1985;228:1502–1507.
92. Fernandez-Valle C, Fregien N, Wood PM, Bunge MB. Expression of the protein zero myelin gene in axon-related Schwann cells is linked to basal lamina formation. *Development* 1993:119:867–880.
93. Misky R, Jenssen K. The biology of non-myelin forming cells. *Ann NY Acad Sci* 1986;486:132–146.
94. Gray MH, Rosenberg AE, Dickersin GR, Bahn AK. Glial fibrillary acidic protein and keratin expression by benign and malignant nerve sheath tumors. *Hum Pathol* 1989;20:1089–1096.
95. Wilander E, Lundqvist M, Motin T. S-100 protein in carcinoid tumors of the appendix. *Acta Neuropathol (Berlin)* 1985;66:306–310.
96. Auböck L, Hofler H. Extraepithelial intraneural endocrine cells as starting points for gastrointestinal carcinoids. *Virchows Arch [A]* 1983;401:17–33.
97. Ortiz-Hidalgo C, Capurso-García M, Ortiz de la Peña J, Lasky-Marcovich D, Torres JE. Neuromas apendiculares (Obliteración fibrosa) de la punta apendicular. Estudio clinicopatológico e inmunohistoquímico de 10 casos. *Patología (México)* 1994;32:233–238.
98. Ortiz-Hidalgo C, de León-Bojorge B, Torres JE. Neuroma apendicular (obliteración fibrosa) asociado a microcarcinoide. *Patología (Mexico)* 1995;33;83–85.
99. Lunqvist M, Wilander E. Subepithelial neuro-endocrine cells and carcinoid tumours of the human small intestine. A comparative immunohistochemical study with regard to serotonin, neuron-specific enolase and S-100 protein reactivity. *J Pathol* 1986;148:141–147.
100. Zhana Y, Porter S, Wekerle H. Schwann cells in myasthenia gravis. *Am J Pathol* 1990;136:111–112.
101. Vedeler C, Ulvestad E, Borge L, et al. Expression of CD-59 in normal human nervous tissue. *Immunology* 1994;82:542–547.
102. Weller RO, Mellick RS. Acid phosphatase and lysozyme activity in diphtheritic neuropathy and wallerian degeneration. *Br J Exp Pathol* 1966;47:426–434.
103. [Anonymous] Neurotropism and nerve growth; the evolution of a concept [editorial]. *Acta Orthop Scand* 1987;58:91–92.
104. Scheidt P, Friede RL. Myelin phagocytosis in wallerian degeneration. Properties of millipore diffusion chambers and immunohistochemical identification of cell populations. *Acta Neuropathol (Berlin)* 1987;75: 77–84.
105. Reichert F, Saada A, Rotshenker S. Peripheral nerve injury induces Schwann cells to express two macrophage phenotypes: phagocytosis and galactose-specific lectine MAC-2. *J Neurosci* 1994;14: 3231–3245.
106. Ohara S, Takahashi H, Ikuta F. Specialized contacts of endoneurial fibroblasts with macrophages in wallerian degeneration. *J Anat* 1986; 148:77–85.
107. Perry VH, Brown MC, Gordon S. Macrophage response to central and peripheral nerve injury: a possible role of macrophages in regeneration. *J Exp Med* 1987;165:1218–1223.
108. Soube G, Taki T, Yasuda Mitsuma T. Gangliosides modulate Schwann cell proliferation and morphology. *Brain Res* 1988;474: 287–295.
109. Hall SM. Annotation: regeneration in the peripheral nervous system. *Neuropathol Appl Neurobiol* 1989;15:513–529.
110. Le Beau JM, La Corbiere M, Powell HC, Ellisman MH, Schubert D. Extracellular fluid conditioned during peripheral nerve regeneration stimulates Schwann cell adhesion, migration and proliferation. *Brain Res* 1988;459:93–104.
111. Khan S, Wigley C. Different efects of a marophage cytokine on proliferation in astrocytes and Schwann cells. *Neuro Report* 1994; 5:1381–1385.
112. Lundborg G. Nerve regeneration and repair. A review. *Acta Orthop Scand* 1987;58:145–169.
113. Blackemore WK. Myelination, demyelination and remyelination. In: Thomas Smith W, Cavanagh JB, eds. *Recent advances in neuropathology, vol 2.* Edinburgh; Churchill Livingstone, 1982;53–82.
114. Schreiber RC, Hyatt-Sachs H, Bennett TA, Zigmond RE. Galanin expression increases in adult rat sympathetic neurons after axotomy. *Neuroscience* 1994;60:17–27.
115. Mohney RP, Siegel RE, Zigmond RE. Galanin and vasoactive intestinal polypetide messenger RNAs increase following axotomy of adult sympathetic neurons. *J Neurobiol* 1994;25:108–118.
116. Janeka IP. Peripheral nerve regeneration: an experimental study. *Laryngoscope* 1987;97:942–950.
117. Nachemson AK, Hasson HA, Lundborg GL. Neurotropism in nerve regeneration. An immunohistochemical study. *Acta Physiol Scand* 1988;133:139–148.
118. Varon S, Conher JM. Nerve growth factor in CNS repair. *J Neurotrauma* 1994;11:473–486.
119. Skenne JH, Shooter EM. Denervated sheath cells secrete a new protein after injury. *Proc Natl Acad Sci U S A* 1983;80:4169–4173.
120. England JD, Gamboni F, Ferguson MA, Levinson SR. Sodium channels acumulate at the tip of injured axons. *Muscle Nerve* 1994;17: 593–598.
121. Frisen J, Risling M, Fried K. Distribution and axonal relations of macrophages in neuroma. *Neuroscience* 1993;55:1003–1013.
122. Bichem R, Mithen FA, L'Empereur KM, Wessels MM. Ultrastructural effects of Guillain-Barré serum in cultures containing only rat Schwann cells and dorsal root ganglion neurons. *Brain Res* 1987;421: 173–185.
123. Weller RO, Nester B. Early changes at the node of Ranvier in segmental demyelination: histochemical and electron microscopic observations. *Brain* 1972;95:665–674.
124. Weller RO, Bruckner FE, Chamberlain MA. Rheumatoid neuropathy: a histological and electrophysiological study. *J Neurol Neurosurg Psychiatry* 1970;33:592–604.
125. Weller RO, Mitchell J, Daves GD. Buckthorn (Karwinskia humboltiana) toxins. In: Spencer PS, Schaumburg HH, eds. *Experimental and clinical neurotoxicology.* Baltimore; Williams & Wilkins, 1980; 336–347.
126. Chance PF, Reilly M. Inherited neuropathies. *Curr Opin Neurol* 1994; 7:372–380.
127. Anthony DC, Hevner RF. Advances in genetics of hereditary peripheral neuropathies. *Adv Anat Pathol* 1995;5:283–298.
128. Weller RO. An electron microscopic study of hypertrophic neuropathy of Déjérine-Sottas. *J Neurol Neurosurg Psychiatry* 1967;30: 111–125.
129. Weller RO, Das Gupta TK. Experimental hypertrophic neuropathy: an electron microscope study. *J Neurol Neurosurg Psychiatry* 1966;31: 34–42.
130. Reed RJ, Harkin JC. *Tumors of the peripheral nervous system (supplement).* Washington DC: Armed Forces Institute of Pathology, 1983.
131. Weller RO. Localized hypertrophic neuropathy and hypertrophic polyneuropathy. *Lancet* 1974;2:529–593.
132. Lallemand RC, Weller RO. Intraneural neurofibromas involving the posterior intraosseous nerve. *J Neurol Neurosurg Psychiatry* 1973;36: 991–996.
133. Bilbao JM, Khoury NJS, Briggs SJ. Perineuromas (localized hypertrophic neuropathy). *Arch Pathol Lab Med* 1984;108:557–560.
134. Johnson PC, Kline DG. Localized hypertrophic neuropathy: a possible perineurial barrier defect. *Acta Neuropathol (Berlin)* 1989;77: 514–518.
135. Blumberg AK, Kay S, Adelaar S. Nerve sheath myxoma. *Cancer* 1989;63(6):1215–1218.
136. Enzinger FM, Weiss SW. *Soft tissue tumors.* St Louis; CV Mosby, 1995;821–889.
137. Goldblum JR, Beals TF, Weiss SW. Neuroblastoma-like neurilemoma. *Am J Surg Pathol* 1994;18:266–273.
138. Brooks JJ, Draffen RM. Benign glandular schwannoma. *Arch Pathol Lab Med* 1992;116:192–195.
139. Fisher C, Chapell ME, Weiss SW. Neuroblastoma-like epithelioid schwannoma. *Histopathology* 1995;26:193–194.
140. Escalona-Zapata J, Diez-Nav MD. The nature of macrophages (foam cells) in neurinomas. Tissue culture study. *Acta Neuropathol (Berlin)* 1978;44:71–75.
141. Weller RO. Tumours of the nervous system. In: Weller RO, ed. *Systemic pathology. 3rd ed., vol 4, nervous system, muscle and eye.* Edinburgh; Churchill Livingstone, 1990;427–503.

142. Dingemans KP, Teeling P. Long-spacing collagen and proteoglycans in pathologic tissue. *Ultrastruct Pathol* 1994;18:539–547.
143. Yen S-H, Fields KL. A protein related to glial filaments in Schwann cells. *Ann N Y Acad Sci* 1985;455:538–551.
144. Lodding P, Kindblom LG, Angeval L, Sterman G. Cellular schwannomas-a clinicopathological study of 29 cases. *Virchows Arch [A]* 1990;416:237–248.
145. Aso M. Expression of Schwann cell characteristics in pigmented nevus. Immunohistochemical study using monoclonal antibodies to Schwann cell associated antigen. *Cancer* 1988;62:938–943.
146. Kayano H, Katayama I. Melanocytic schwannoma arising in the sympathetic ganglion. *Hum Pathol* 1988;19:1355–1358.
147. Carney JA. Psammomatous melanocitic schwannoma: A distinctive heritable tumor with special association including cardiac myxoma and the Cushing syndrome. *Am J Surg Pathol* 1990;14:206–222.
148. Buley ID, Gatter KC, Kelly PMA, Haryet A, Millard PR. Granular cell tumour revisited. An immunohistological and ultrastructural study. *Histopathology* 1988;12:263–271.
149. Mentzel T, Wadden C, Fletcher CDM. Granular cell change in smooth muscle tumours of the skin and soft tissues. *Histopathology* 1994;24: 223–231.
150. Mittal KR, True L. Origin of granules in granular cell tumor. Intracellular myelin formation with autodigestion. *Arch Pathol Lab Med* 1988;112:302–303.
151. Clark HB, Minesky JJ, Agrawal D, Agrawal H. Myelin basic protein and P2 protein are not immunochemical markers for Schwann cell neoplasms. A comparative study using antisera to S-100 P2 and myelin basic proteins. *Am J Pathol* 1985;121:96–101.
152. Peltonen J, Pentinen R, Larjava H, Aho K. Collagen in neurofibromas and neurofibroma cell culture. *Ann NY Acad Sci* 1986;486:260–270.
153. Vitto J, Matsuoka Chu ML, Pihlajaniemi T, Prockop J. Connective tissue biochemistry of neurofibromas. *Ann NY Acad Sci* 1986;486: 271–286.
154. Takata M , Imai T, Hirone T. Factor-XIIIa-positive cells in normal peripheral nerves and cutaneous neurofibromas of type-1 neurofibromatosis. *Am J Dermatopathol* 1994;16;37–43.
155. Brill C. Neurofibromatosis. Clinical overview. *Clin Orthop* 1989;245: 10–15.
156. Fontain JM, Wallance MR, Bruce MA, et al. Physical mapping of a translocation breakpoint in neurofibromatosis. *Science* 1989;244: 1085–1087.
157. Barker D, Wright E, Nguyen L, et al. Gene for von Recklinghausen neurofibromatosis is in the pericentromeric region of chromosome 17. *Science* 1987;236:1100–1102.
158. Vinores SA. Nerve growth factor modification of ethylnitrosourea model for multiple schwannomas. *Ann NY Acad Sci* 1986;486: 124–131.
159. Sonnenfeld K, Bernard P, Rubinstein A, Sobue G. Nerve growth factor binding to the cells derived from neurofibromas. *Ann NY Acad Sci* 1986;486:107–113.
160. Gutman DH. New insights into the neurofibromatoses. *Curr Opin Neurol* 1994;7:166–171.
161. von Deimling A, Krone W, Menon AG. Neurofibromatosis type I: pathology, clinical features and molecular genetics. *Brain Pathol* 1995;5:153–162.
162. Huson SM. Recent development and diagnosis and management in neurofibromatosis. *Arch Dis Child* 1989;64:745–749.
163. Louis DN, Ramesh V, Gusella JF. Neuropathology and molecular genetics of neurofibromatosis 2 and related tumors. *Brain Pathol* 1995; 5:163–172.
164. Twist EC, Ruttledge MH, Rousseau M, et al. The neurofibromatosis type 2 gene is inactivated in schwannomas. *Hum Mol Genet* 1994; 3(1)147–151.
165. Lombart-Bosch A, Terrier-Lacombe MJ, Peydro-Olaya A, Contesso G. Peripheral neuroectodermal sarcoma (peripheral neuroepithelioma): a pathological study of ten cases with differential diagnosis regarding other round cell sarcoma. *Hum Pathol* 1989;20(6):273–280.
166. Dakin MC. Lepard B, Theaker JM. The palisaded, encapsulated neuroma (solitary circumscribed neuroma). *Histopathology* 1992;20: 405–410.
167. Erlandson RA, Woodruff JM. Peripheral nerve sheath tumors: an electron microscopic study of 43 cases. *Cancer* 1982;49:273–287.
168. Salisbury JR, Isaacson PG. Synovial sarcoma: an immunohistochemical study. *J Pathol* 1985;147:49–57.
169. Wick MR, Swanson PE, Schethauer BM, Manivel JC. Malignant peripheral nerve sheath tumor: an immunohistochemical study of 65 cases. *Am J Clin Pathol* 1987;87:425–433.
170. Hirose T, Sumitomo M, Kudo E, et al. Malignant peripheral nerve sheath tumor (MPNST) showing perineurial cell differentiation. *Am J Surg Pathol* 1989;13:613–620.
171. Ortiz-Hidalgo C. Pathology and mythology. *Am J Dermatopathol* 1992;14:572–575.

# Head and Neck

*Histology for Pathologists, second edition,*
Edited by Stephen S. Sternberg.
Lippincott-Raven Publishers, Philadelphia


# CHAPTER 13

# Normal Eye and Ocular Adnexa

Gordon K. Klintworth and Mark W. Scroggs



The eye and surrounding tissues are subject to a wide variety of primary ocular, as well as systemic disease processes. An understanding of ocular anatomy will enable the general surgical pathologist to appreciate morphologic abnormalities and will facilitate the diagnosis of many of the pathologic conditions affecting those structures. This chapter presents an overview of the normal histology of the eye and ocular adnexa. Several excellent texts are available for more detailed information on ocular anatomy and development (1–5).

The eye is roughly spherical in shape and external measurements are routinely obtained in three dimensions. In the adult, the anterio-posterior plane of the eye measures approximately 24 mm, whereas the vertical and the horizontal dimensions are both about 23 to 23.5 mm. Located midway between the anterior and posterior poles of the eye is the equator of the globe.

Several external landmarks allow the pathologist to orient the globe and to determine whether an eye is from the right or the left side (Fig. 1). By establishing the nasal (medial) and temporal (lateral) sides of the globe and the superior surface of the eye, the side of the eye can easily be deduced. The six extraocular muscles (four rectus and two oblique muscles) that arise in the posterior orbit and run forward to insert upon the sclera are important in this regard. The rectus muscles arise from a fibrous ring at the apex of the orbit, the annulus of Zinn, and are enveloped by a fascial membrane that creates a cone-shaped structure posterior to the globe. The levator palpebrae superioris also arises at the orbital apex and extends anteriorly to the eyelids. Of the extraocular muscles, only the inferior oblique has a muscular insertion upon the sclera; the other muscles have tendinous insertions. The extraocular muscle insertions are usually removed by the surgeon when the globe is excised (enucleated), but they are frequently present on eyes obtained postmortem. The superior and inferior oblique muscles are most useful in orientating the globe. The tendinous insertion of the superior oblique muscle behind the superior rectus muscle insertion indicates the top of the eye. The inferior oblique muscle inserts on the sclera temporally in the horizontal meridian, and its fibers run inferiorly toward the back of the orbit. The optic nerve is also useful in assessing orientation because it exits the globe slightly nasal to the posterior pole of the eye. Adjacent to the optic nerve, the prominent long posterior ciliary arteries course through the superficial sclera in opposite directions in a horizontal plane. Anteriorly, the dimensions of the cornea may be helpful in topographic orientation. In the adult, the cornea is elliptical in shape with its horizontal diameter being slightly greater than its vertical breadth. In young children this difference is less apparent.

The eye is traditionally described as having three tissue layers that surround the vitreous, the lens, and the spaces of the anterior and posterior chambers (Fig. 2). The outermost part of the eye is composed of the transparent cornea and the opaque sclera. The ocular middle layer is made up of the iris, ciliary body, and the choroid. The innermost retina is in direct contact with the vitreous body.

G. K. Klintworth and M. W. Scroggs: Departments of Pathology and Ophthalmology, Duke University Medical Center, Durham, NC 27710.

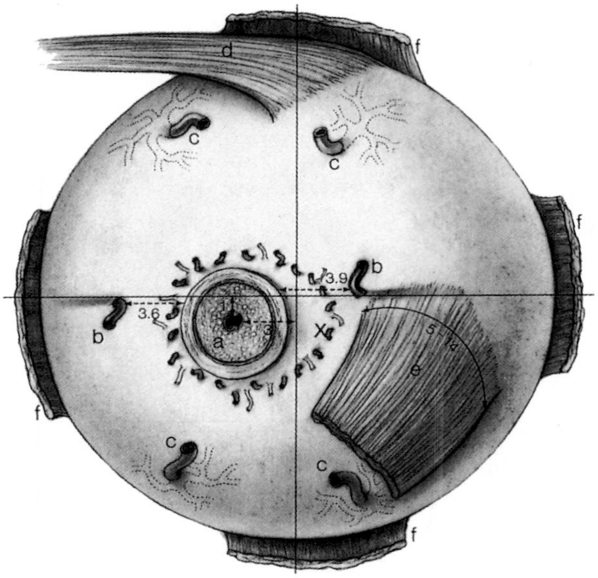


**FIG. 1.** This drawing depicts the right eye as seen from behind. Several external landmarks are useful in determining orientation of the globe. The optic nerve (a) is located approximately 1 mm inferior to and 3 mm nasal to the posterior pole of the eye. The long posterior ciliary arteries (b) are located in the horizontal plane and four vortex veins (c) exit the sclera posteriorly. The superior oblique muscle (d) inserts on the top of the globe, whereas the inferior oblique muscle (e) inserts temporally and its fibers run posteriorly and nasally. The rectus muscles (f) insert horizontally, inferiorly, and superiorly. The approximate location of the macula (x), the part of the retina responsible for the most distinct vision, is slightly temporal to the optic nerve. (Reproduced from ref. 2, with permission.)

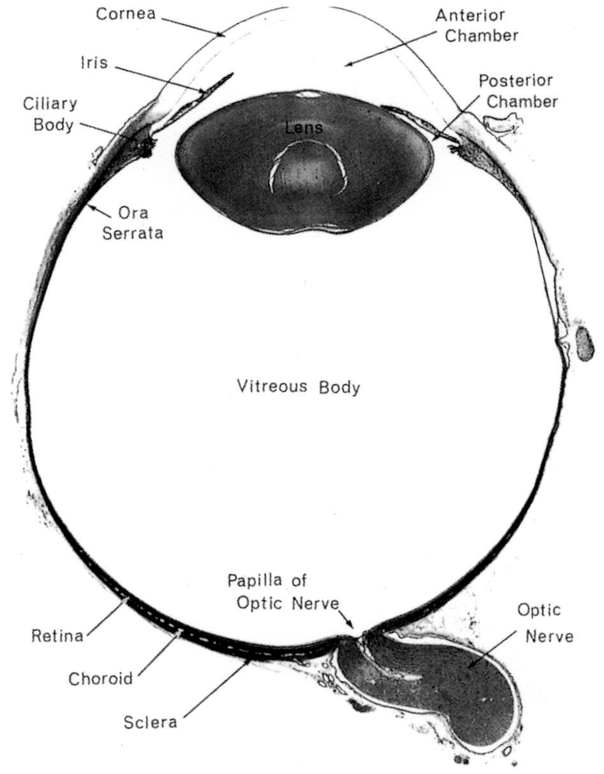


**FIG. 2.** This photomicrograph of a histologic section of an eye from a rhesus monkey illustrates the major tissue layers of the eye, the lens, the vitreous body, and the spaces of the anterior and posterior chambers. (Reproduced from ref. 5, with permission.)

## CORNEA

The transparent cornea occupies one sixth of the anterior surface of the globe and refracts the entering light. Although individual variation is common, the cornea measures approximately 11.7 mm in the horizontal plane and 10.6 mm in the vertical plane. Centrally, the cornea is about 0.5 mm thick, but peripherally it thickens to about 0.67 mm. Histologically, the cornea consists of six distinct layers: (a) the epithelium; (b) the basal lamina of the epithelium; (c) Bowman's layer; (d) the stroma; (e) Descemet's membrane; and (f) the endothelium (Fig. 3).

The corneal epithelium, which is composed of stratified nonkeratinized squamous cells, is about five cell layers thick centrally. The peripheral cornea is often twice as thick. The basilar epithelial cells are polygonal in shape and as they become displaced to the corneal surface during differentiation, a more flattened appearance is acquired. In the normal cornea, even the most superficial epithelial cells retain their nuclei. Mitotic figures are uncommon in the epithelium, but are observed in the basal cells occasionally. Some Langerhans' cells are present within the corneal epithelium, especially peripherally (6). Langerhans' cells are most readily identified by special histochemical and immunohistochemical methods, and are not normally recognizable in routinely stained tissue sections.

The corneal epithelium rests upon a basal lamina, which is difficult to see in hematoxylin and eosin (H&E)-stained tissue sections. Staining with the periodic acid-Schiff (PAS) reaction makes this layer apparent (Fig. 4). In certain pathologic conditions, the epithelial basal lamina assumes an intraepithelial location.

Bowman's layer is an acellular structure located just posterior to the epithelial basal lamina (Fig. 4). It is approximately 8 to 14 μm thick. As shown by transmission electron microscopy, Bowman's layer is not a true basement membrane, but is composed of randomly oriented delicate collagen fibers. The anterior face of Bowman's layer ends distinctly at its junction with the epithelial basal lamina. Posteriorly, Bowman's layer merges inconspicuously with the underlying corneal stroma. Unmyelinated sensory nerves reach the epithelium from the stroma after crossing Bowman's layer. However, nerve processes are difficult to detect in the cornea in standard tissue sections, even with the use of special histologic techniques.

The stroma accounts for approximately 90% of the cornea's thickness. It is composed of numerous layers of col-

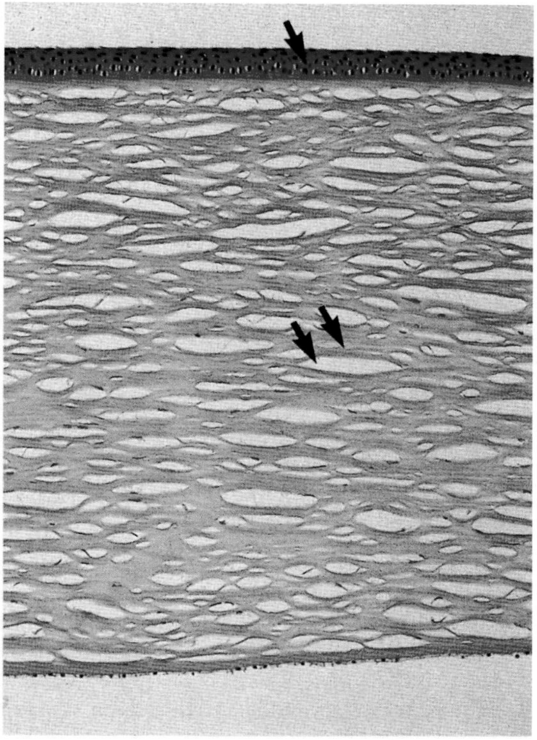

**FIG. 3.** The stratified squamous epithelium of the cornea (*arrow*) overlies the basal lamina and Bowman's layer. The clefts within the collagenous stroma (*double arrows*) represent artifacts of tissue processing. No blood vessels or lymphatics are normally present within the cornea. Descemet's membrane and the corneal endothelium are located just posterior to the stroma. (H&E × **33**.)

lagen fibers embedded in a proteoglycan-rich extracellular matrix. The stroma contains a tissue-specific keratan sulfate proteoglycan (lumican), as well as a galactosaminoglycan-rich proteoglycan (decorin). Transmission electron microscopy has disclosed that the corneal collagen fibers are regularly spaced and of a uniform diameter; this arrangement contributes to the transparency of the cornea. Surrounded by the stromal collagen lamellae are the corneal fibroblasts (keratocytes). Other cell types are seldom identified in tissue sections of the normal corneal stroma, but rarely an occasional mononuclear leukocyte or granulocyte may be present. The normal cornea lacks blood vessels and its nutrition is obtained from an arterial plexus at the junction of the cornea and sclera, and from direct contact with the aqueous of the anterior chamber. In tissue sections of routinely processed formalin-fixed corneas, clefts are almost invariably present between the collagen lamellae. Initially interpreted as lymphatic channels by early histologists, these clefts are artifacts of tissue processing. Lymphatic vessels are not present in the normal cornea.

Descemet's membrane, a true basal lamina elaborated by the underlying corneal endothelial cells, begins to form during fetal life. At birth, it is approximately 3 to 4 $\mu$m thick (Fig. 5). Basal laminar material is continuously added to the posterior part of Descemet's membrane throughout life so that by adulthood, this structure attains a thickness of approximately 10 to 12 $\mu$m. The fetal and postnatal regions of Descemet's membrane differ ultrastructurally. This difference is occasionally discernible by light microscopy.

The corneal endothelium (Fig. 5) is directly exposed to the aqueous in the anterior chamber. Although this cell layer does not line blood vessels or lymphatic spaces, the term "endothelium" is firmly entrenched in the literature. The endothelial cells of the cornea normally form a single flattened layer and, virtually, never regenerate by mitosis in human eyes. Under pathologic conditions (epithelial ingrowth and posterior polymorphous corneal dystrophy) cytokeratin-containing squamous cells replace the endothelium and form a layer that is more than one-cell thick.

After the second decade of life, age-related focal excresences (Hassall-Henle warts) commonly form on the periph-

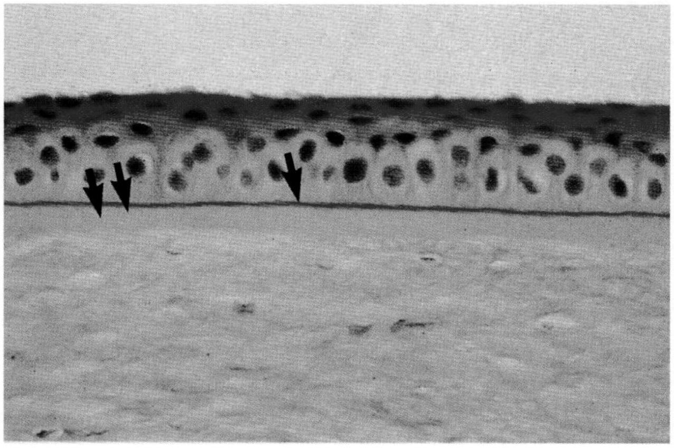

**FIG. 4.** The corneal epithelium rests upon a thin basal lamina (*arrow*), which is prominent in this section following periodic acid-Schiff staining. The acellular band directly underneath the basal lamina is Bowman's layer (*double arrows*). (Periodic acid-Schiff × **132**.)

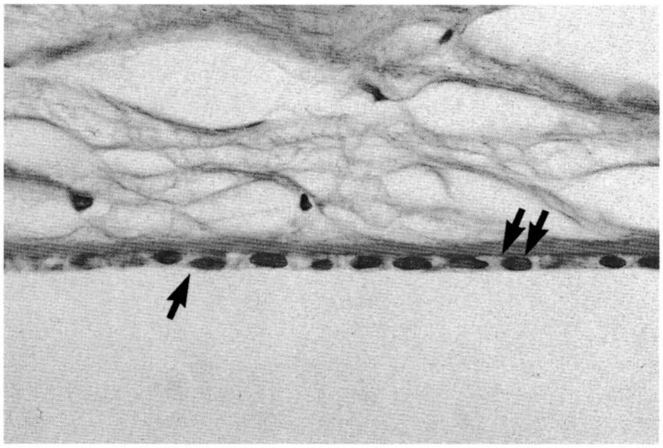

**FIG. 5.** A thin monolayer of corneal endothelial cells (*arrow*) is adjacent to Descemet's membrane (*double arrows*). These cells are in direct contact with the aqueous of the anterior chamber. (H&E × **132**.)

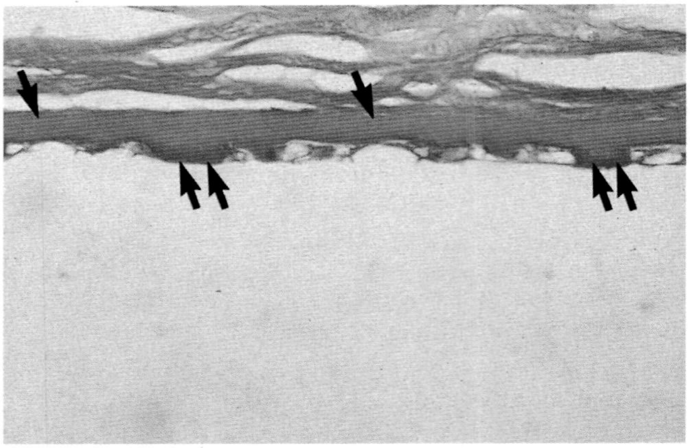

**FIG. 6.** Descemet's membrane *(single arrows)* is located immediately posterior to the corneal stroma. The excrescences on the peripheral portion of Descemet's membrane (Hassall-Henle warts) *(double arrows)* represent an aging change. Descemet's membrane also thickens with age. (H&E × **132**.)

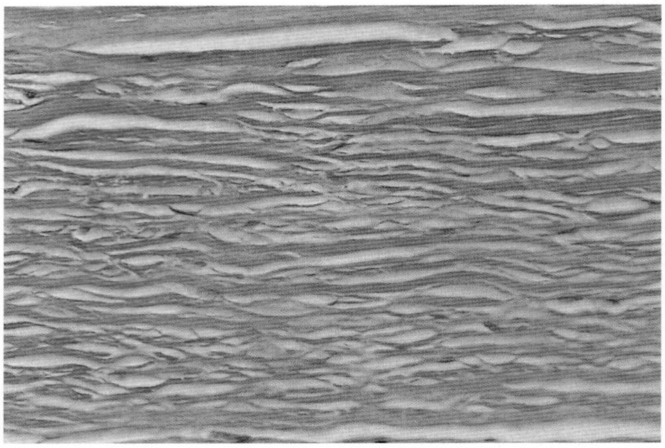

**FIG. 7.** The scleral stroma is predominantly composed of collagen fibers in haphazard array that vary in diameter. Scattered fibroblasts occur between the collagen bundles. (H&E × **100**.)

eral part of Descemet's membrane (Fig. 6). Virtually identical focal thickenings occur on the central part of Descemet's membrane (corneal guttata) under pathologic circumstances, and most notably in Fuchs' corneal dystrophy. The presence of excresences on Descemet's membrane in tissue sections of corneal buttons removed at penetrating keratoplasty (full-thickness corneal transplant) is always abnormal. Hassall-Henle warts are too peripheral in location to be present in a surgically excised corneal button.

## SCLERA

The sclera, which accounts for approximately five sixths of the surface area of the eye, begins at the periphery of the cornea and extends posteriorly to the optic nerve. The sclera's relatively rigid nature protects the eye from trauma and helps maintain intraocular pressure. Anteriorly, the sclera is visible underneath the transparent conjunctiva and is normally white in adults. The sclera varies in thickness, being about 0.8 mm thick near its junction with the cornea. At the insertions of the four rectus muscles approximately 5 to 8 mm posterior to the corneoscleral junction, the sclera is at its thinnest, measuring approximately 0.3 mm. From this point posteriorly, the sclera gradually thickens and attains its maximal width of about 1.0 mm adjacent to the optic nerve.

The sclera has three components: the episclera, the stroma, and the lamina fusca. The episclera, its most superficial part, is located between the fibrous structure that envelops the globe (Tenon's capsule), and the underlying scleral stroma with which it merges. The episclera is composed of loosely arranged collagen fibers and fibroblasts embedded in an extracellular matrix. Occasional melanocytes and mononuclear leukocytes are also present. Anteriorly, the episclera is richly vascularized.

The largest component of the sclera is its stroma, which consists of fibrous bands of collagen, occasional elastic fibers, and scattered fibroblasts (Fig. 7). The corneal and scleral stroma appear similar at the light microscopic level, but when viewed by transmission electron microscopy the individual collagen fibers within the sclera vary in diameter and are randomly arranged, in contrast to the orderly packed corneal collagen fibers of uniform diameter. This largely accounts for the opaque nature of the sclera.

Although the scleral stroma is relatively avascular, blood vessels, as well as accompanying nerves and scattered melanocytes, are present in perforating emissarial canals (Fig. 8). The anterior ciliary arteries perforate the sclera near the insertion of the rectus muscles. Venous channels draining the iris, ciliary body, and choroid (vortex veins) exit the

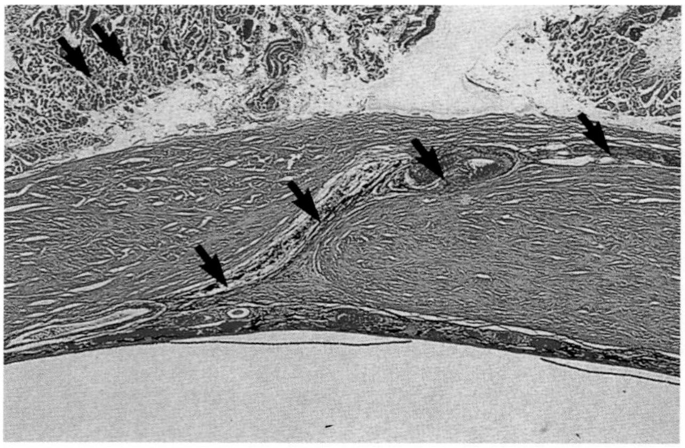

**FIG. 8.** This figure illustrates a blood vessel that penetrates the sclera and extends to the prominently vascularized choroid through an emissarial canal *(single arrows)*. Pigmented melanocytes are also present. The fibers of the inferior oblique muscle are present at site of insertion upon the outer sclera *(double arrows)*. (H&E × **50**.)

sclera several millimeters posterior to the equator of the eye. The posterior ciliary arteries pass through the sclera near the optic nerve. In some individuals, a nerve in an emissiarial canal near the corneoscleral junction may be prominent and attain a diameter of 1 to 2 mm. The nodular appearance of this so-called "nerve loop of Axenfeld" may mimic a neoplasm or conjunctival cyst clinically (7). To the unwary surgical pathologist, this totally normal nerve bundle may be mistaken for a neurofibroma (8).

The innermost layer of the sclera, the lamina fusca, contains loose collagen fibers, fibroblasts, and scattered melanocytes. It represents a region of transition between the sclera and the underlying choroid. The sclera is weakly attached to the choroid below by thin fibers of collagen.

With increasing age, several histologic changes occur in the sclera. Calcium may deposit diffusely between the individual collagen fibers throughout the entire scleral stroma. Localized abnormalities, known as senile scleral plaques, may occur just anterior to the insertion of the lateral or horizontal rectus muscles. These lesions are characterized by decreased stromal cellularity, abnormal collagen, and, in advanced cases, calcification (9).

## CORNEOSCLERAL LIMBUS

The corneoscleral junction, or limbus, is not a distinct anatomic site, but is a significant landmark clinically. Most surgical procedures on the anterior part of the eye are accomplished after access via an incision in the limbal area. For purposes of discussion, the trabecular meshwork and Schlemm's canal will be considered as part of the corneoscleral limbus.

The limbus is approximately 1.5 to 2.0 mm wide and separate layers of the cornea merge with components of the sclera or conjunctiva in this area (Fig. 9). The squamous epithelium of the cornea extends centrifugally beyond the limbus until it meets the epithelium of the bulbar conjunctiva. At the limbus, Bowman's layer of the cornea blends into the subepithelial tissues of the conjunctiva and the corneal and scleral stroma become continuous with each other. Descemet's membrane abruptly terminates in the limbal region and gives rise to the clinically significant landmark known as Schwalbe's ring. In about 15% of eyes, a prominent area of thickening is identified histologically at this site (Fig. 10) (2). Immediately adjacent to Schwalbe's ring is the most anterior aspect of the trabecular meshwork. Both the trabecular meshwork and Schlemm's canal constitute the apparatus responsible for the removal of aqueous from the eye (Fig. 11). Aqueous drainage occurs in the angle between the anterior surface of the iris and the sclera. Histologically, the meshwork appears as a collection of finely branching and delicately pigmented connective tissue bands. The cells, which line the trabecular meshwork, are continuous with the corneal endothelium. Posteriorly, the trabecular meshwork

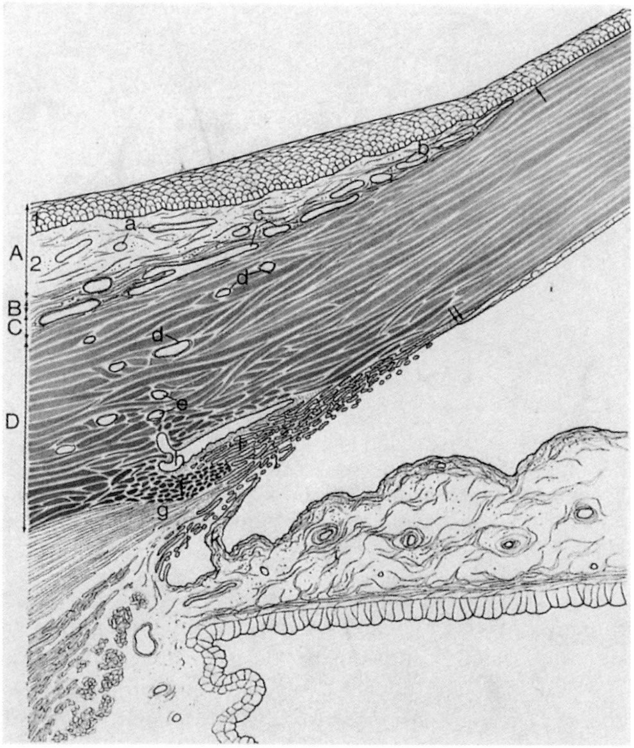


**FIG. 9.** The corneoscleral limbus represents the junction of the peripheral cornea with the anterior sclera, and is not a distinct anatomic site. Clinically the limbus is an important landmark. The conjunctiva of the limbus (**A**) is composed of epithelium (1) and stroma (2). The thin connective tissue layer of Tenon's capsule (**B**) overlies the episclera (**C**). The corneal and scleral stroma merge gradually in the area marked "**D**". Vessels of the conjunctival stroma (**a,b**), episclera (**c**) and limbal plexus (**d,e**) are illustrated. The projection of collagen fibers known as the scleral spur (**f**) merges with the smooth muscle fibers of the ciliary body (**g**). Schlemm's canal (**h**) and the trabecular meshwork (**i,j**) are responsible for removal of aqueous from the eye. Occasionally, processes from the iris (**k**) insert upon the trabecular meshwork. Bowman's layer (*arrow*) and Descemet's membrane (*double arrows*) both terminate in the area of the limbus. (Reproduced from ref. 2, with permission.)

extends to a roughly triangular-shaped projection of scleral connective tissue, known as the scleral spur.

Located slightly anterior and superficial to the trabecular meshwork is Schlemm's canal, an endothelial-lined venous channel that completely encircles the limbus. Because Schlemm's canal sometimes gives off smaller branches, two lumens are occasionally seen on histologic sections of the anterior chamber angle. Although the trabecular meshwork and Schlemm's canal appear to be in intimate contact in tissue sections, they are separated from each other by a thin layer of connective tissue and separate endothelial linings. Aqueous percolates among the delicate beams of the trabecular meshwork before becoming transported to Schlemm's canal. Ultrastructural examination of this region discloses

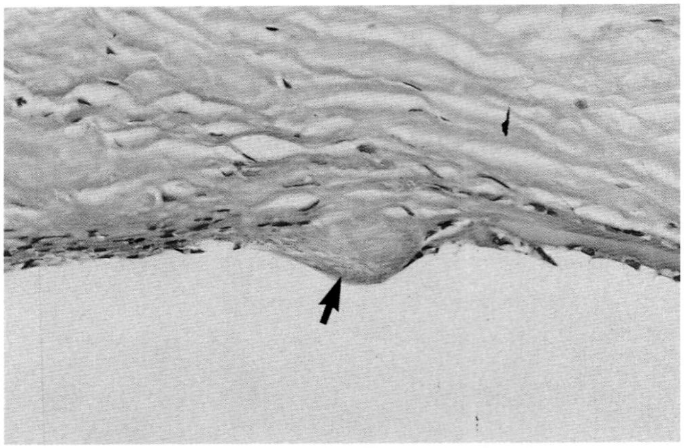

**FIG. 10.** Schwalbe's ring is a significant clinical landmark in the limbal area and represents the peripheral termination of Descemet's membrane. Prominent Schwalbe's rings (*arrow*) in this histologic section are identified in about 15% of eyes. (H&E × **80**.)

giant cytoplasmic vacuoles in the endothelial lining of Schlemm's canal, adjacent to the trabecular meshwork. These vacuoles are thought by some to contain fluid in the process of being transported from the trabecular meshwork into the lumen of Schlemm's canal (10). Once in Schlemm's canal, aqueous drains into the episcleral venous plexus by way of numerous small collector channels. Prolonged obstruction to the outflow of aqueous results in increased intraocular pressure and glaucoma.

## CONJUNCTIVA, CARUNCLE, AND PLICA SEMILUNARIS

The conjunctiva is a thin continuous mucous membrane lining the inner surface of the eyelids and much of the anterior surface of the eye. In addition to its protective function, the conjunctiva allows the eyelids to move smoothly over the globe. The conjunctival epithelium is composed of 2 to 5 layers of columnar cells and rests upon a basal lamina. Within the conjunctival epithelium are goblet cells that secrete mucoid material that becomes incorporated into the tear film (Fig. 12). Melanocytes are present in the basal epithelial layers and, like melanocytes in the skin, transfer melanosomes into adjacent epithelial cells. These pigmented epithelial cells are numerous in dark-skinned individuals (Fig. 13). The loose, fibrovascular subepithelial connective

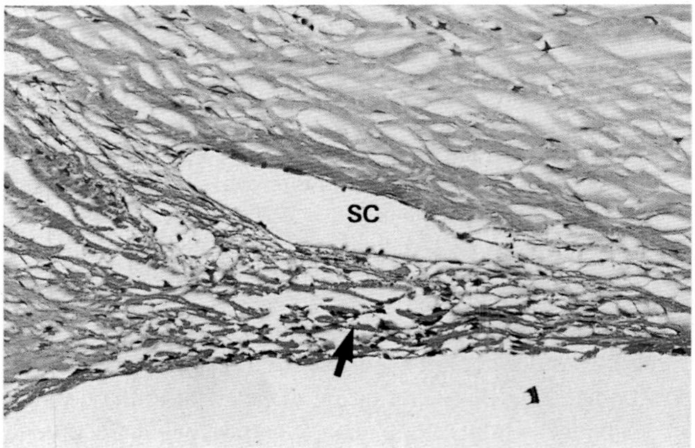


A

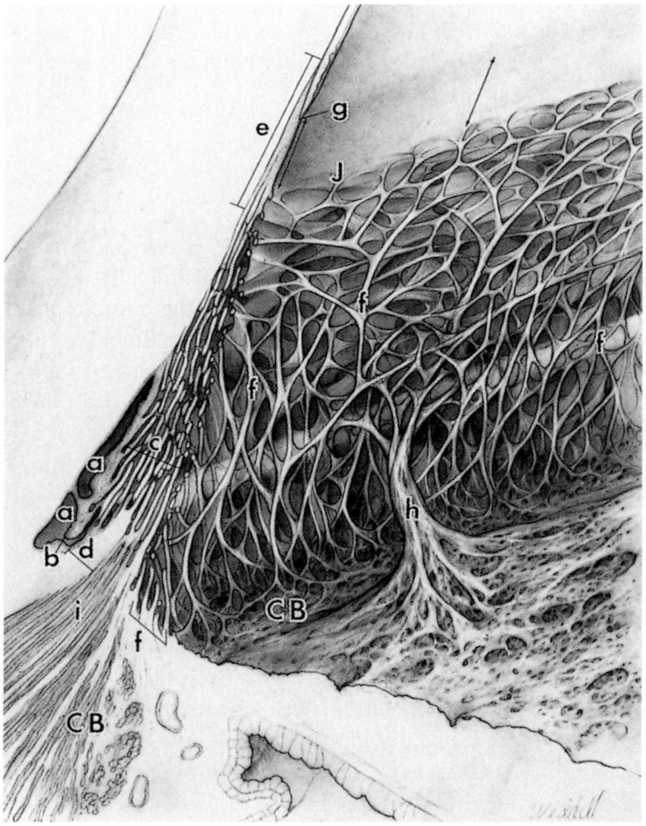


B

**FIG. 11. A,** Located in the angle of the anterior chamber is Schlemm's canal (SC) and the trabecular meshwork (*arrow*). Schlemm's canal is an endothelial channel which enables aqueous to drain from the eye. Aqueous reaches Schlemm's canal after percolating through the connective tissue strands of the trabecular meshwork. (H&E × **66**.) **B,** Structures within and near the angle of the anterior chamber are depicted in this drawing. In this illustration, Schlemm's canal (**a**) has two channels, one of which is in communication with a small collecting channel (**b**). The collecting channel is intimately associated with the limbal part of the trabecular meshwork (**c**). The scleral spur (**d**) is closely associated with the trabecular meshwork. Descemet's membrane terminates peripherally in the area denoted "**e**" and "**g**". Some components (**f**) of the trabecular meshwork arise at the ciliary body (CB). Isolated strands of meshwork merge with a nearby process (**h**) from the anterior surface of the iris. A muscle of the ciliary body (**i**) attaches to the trabecular meshwork as indicated by the *arrows.* The corneal endothelium merges with endothelial cells of the meshwork (**j**). (Reproduced from ref. 2 with permission.)

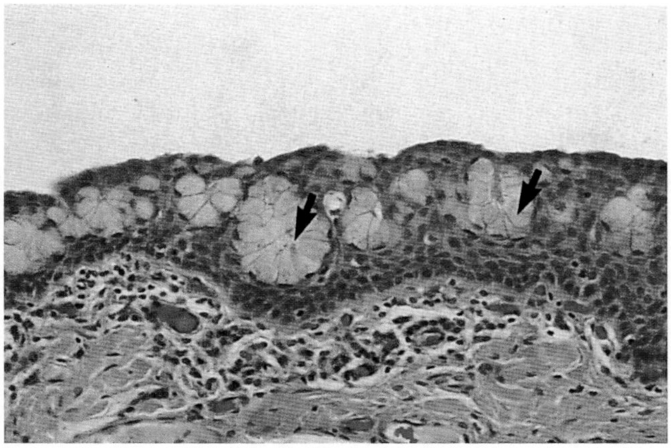

**FIG. 12.** Goblet cells (*arrows*) are prominent in this section of conjunctival epithelium. Scattered mononuclear cells are often present in apparently healthy individuals in the underlying conjunctival stroma. (H&E × **66**.)

tissue of the conjunctival stroma normally contains nerve cells, melanocytes, and accessory lacrimal glands. Lymphoid follicles with germinal centers reside in the conjunctiva (Fig. 14), particularly in areas where the conjunctiva lining the inner surface of the eyelid merges with the portion covering the eyeball (superior and inferior fornices); scattered lymphocytes are not unusual within the conjunctiva. Hence, their presence is not indicative of chronic conjunctivitis unless both plasma cells and significant numbers of lymphocytes are present. Three distinct areas of the conjunctiva are recognized (Fig. 15): the palpebral conjunctiva, the bulbar conjunctiva, and the conjunctiva lining the fornices.

The morphologic attributes of the conjunctiva vary in different parts of this tissue. Although goblet cells exist throughout the epithelium of the bulbar conjunctiva, they are more common in the inferior and nasal parts. Goblet cells are particularly abundant in the forniceal regions. The conjunctival stroma is thickest in the fornices and bulbar areas, and

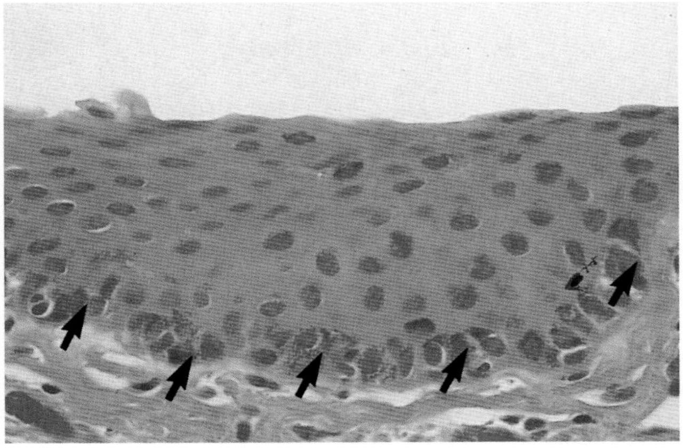

**FIG. 13.** In dark-skinned individuals, the basal layers of the conjunctival epithelium are pigmented (*arrows*). (H&E × **160**.)

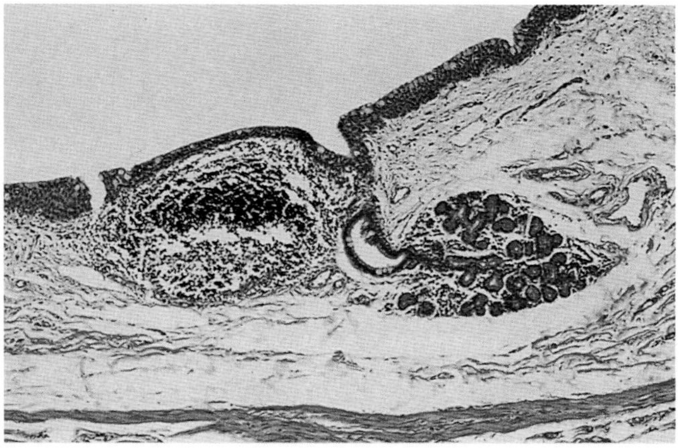

**FIG. 14.** A small lymphoid follicle and island of accessory lacrimal tissue are present in the stroma of the palpebral conjunctiva. (H&E × **25**.)

thinnest in the palpebral conjunctiva and at the corneoscleral limbus, where small conjunctival papillae, known as the palisades of Vogt, are evident. The palpebral conjunctiva is firmly attached to the inner surface of the eyelids, but the bulbar conjunctiva is loosely adherent to the underlying sclera by thin connective tissue strands.

The palpebral conjunctiva, which lines the posterior surface of the eyelids, extends from the fornices to the mucocutaneous junction at the eyelid margins, where the epithelium of the conjunctiva merges abruptly with the epidermis of the anterior surface of the eyelids. The palpebral conjunctiva contains several infoldings of epithelium (crypts of Henle). Islands of accessory lacrimal glands that are morphologically identical to the main tear-producing gland within the orbit, occur within the palpebral conjunctiva. The subconjunctival tissue of the upper fornix may contain over 40 such

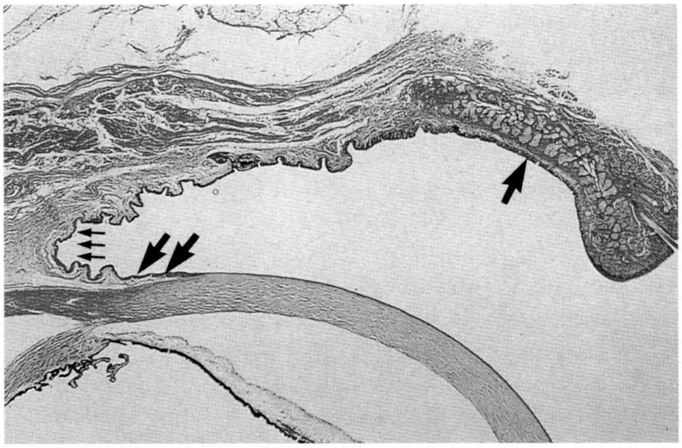

**FIG. 15.** The conjunctiva can be divided into three parts. The palpebral conjunctiva (*arrow*) lines the posterior surface of the eyelid. The bulbar conjunctiva (*double arrows*) extends from the limbus over the anterior sclera. The bulbar and palpebral conjunctiva converge upon the conjunctiva of the superior and inferior fornices (*triple arrows*). (H&E × **2.5**.)

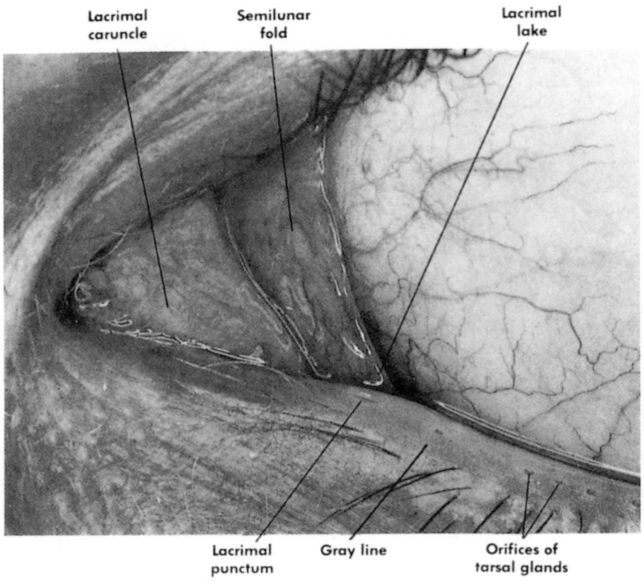


**FIG. 16.** The caruncle and semilunar fold are specialized portions of the conjunctiva and are located in the medial interpalpebral angle of the eye. Before tears enter the lacrimal drainage apparatus through the lacrimal punctum, they accumulate at the medial canthus (lacrimal lake). The demarcation between the conjunctival and cutaneous portions of the eyelid are discernible clinically at the so-called "gray line." The secretions of the meibomian glands (tarsal glands) reach the surface of the eyelids at small orifices. (Reproduced from Newell FW. *Ophthalmology; principles and concepts.* St Louis; CV Mosby, 1986, with permission.)

glands, but less than 10 accessory lacrimal glands are present in the lower fornix (glands of Krause). The upper eyelids have approximately 2 to 5 accessory lacrimal glands (glands of Wolfring) located at the superior aspect of the tarsus. The bulbar conjunctiva begins at the limbus, at which point the corneal epithelium gradually becomes replaced by conjunctival epithelium and continues over the sclera to the superior and inferior fornices There, the conjunctiva is thrown into small folds before becoming the palpebral conjunctiva.

Both the caruncle and plica semilunaris (semilunar fold), represent specialized segments of the conjunctiva (Fig. 16). The caruncle is the nodular mass of fleshy tissue located in the medial interpalpebral angle of the eye. Its surface is covered by a stratified nonkeratinized squamous epithelium. The subepithelial stroma of the caruncle contains hair follicles, smooth muscle, sebaceous glands, adipose connective tissue, and occasionally, accessory lacrimal glands, as well as sweat glands. The plica semilunaris, an arc-shaped fold of conjunctiva located immediately lateral to the caruncle, is thought to be a vestigial remnant of the nictitating membrane of lower species. The histologic features of the plica semilunaris are similar to those in other areas of the conjunctiva, except that the epithelium contains abundant goblet cells and, rarely, cartilage is present within the stroma.

## THE UVEAL TRACT

Located between the outer scleral covering and the inner retina is the uveal tract, which begins anteriorly as the iris, extends to the ciliary body, and then to the choroid posteriorly. The designated term *uvea* is derived from the Latin word *uva* (grape), because this portion of the eye resembles a grape macroscopically after the sclera and cornea are stripped from the globe.

### The Iris

The iris is a thin diaphragm of tissue with a central opening, the pupil, which functions to regulate the amount of light reaching the retina (Fig. 17). Muscles within the iris dilate or constrict the pupil in response to sympathetic or parasympathetic nerve impulses. The diameter of the iris is approximately 21 mm, whereas the diameter of the pupil ranges from 1 to 8 mm. The iris is thinnest at its point of attachment with the ciliary body peripherally, the iris root. Normally, the iris rests gently upon the crystalline lens and, therefore, bulges slightly forward. Structurally and developmentally, the iris consists of two main parts: the stroma and the posterior epithelial lining.

Numerous ridges and depressions may be identified in tissue sections of the anterior iris stroma. These correspond to the contraction folds and furrows seen on clinical examination. The anterior surface of the iris lacks a cellular lining. The stroma contains melanocytes, nerve cells, blood vessels, and smooth muscle in a loose connective tissue background. The color of the iris is due to the number of stromal melanocytes present. Lightly pigmented individuals with blue irises have relatively few stromal melanocytes. In contrast, darkly pigmented individuals with brown irises have numerous melanocytes within the iris stroma (Fig. 18). In

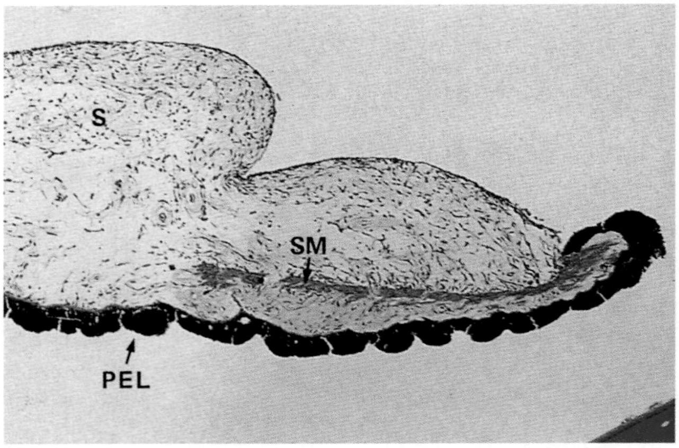


**FIG. 17.** The iris is composed of stroma (S) and a posterior epithelial lining (PEL). The sphincter muscle (SM) of the iris is evident within the stroma. The pigmented posterior epithelial lining normally extends around the lip of the pupil anteriorly for a short distance. (H&E × **25**.)

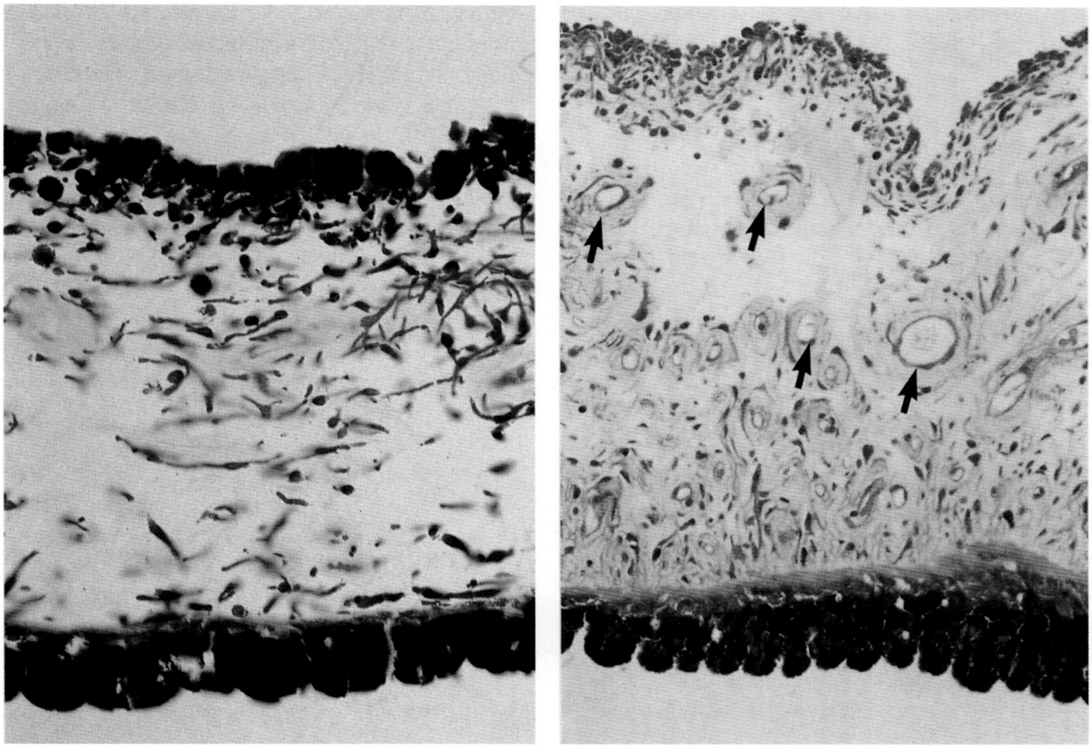

**FIG. 18.** The color of the iris is due to the number of stromal melanocytes which are more abundant in the stroma of an individual with a brown iris (*left*) than with a blue iris (*right*). The amount of pigment in the posterior epithelial lining is similar in irises of different color. Blood vessels in the iris stroma are normally surrounded by a thick collar of collagen fibers (*arrows*); this should not be confused as arteriolosclerosis. In contrast to the posterior surface of the iris, the anterior iris lacks a cellular lining. (Left: H&E × **66**; right: H&E × **66**.)

addition to melanocytes, melanosome-containing macrophages are also scattered within the iris stroma, particularly at the iris root. A thick collar of collagen fibers normally surrounds the blood vessels within the iris stroma. To the inexperienced observer, these normal vessels may appear to have arteriolosclerosis. In the pathologic process of iris neovascularization, thin-walled blood vessels, which lack such a collagenous coat, cover the anterior surface of the iris.

The sphincter muscle (sphincter pupillae), a bundle of circularly arranged smooth muscle innervated by parasympathetic nerves, acts to constrict the pupil. Located within the posterior stroma of the pupillary zone, the sphincter pupillae is nearly 1 mm wide. Radially oriented smooth muscle fibers with scattered cytoplasmic melanosomes are also located within the stroma of the iris (dilator pupillae). Innervated by sympathetic nerves, this muscle is active in pupil dilatation.

Posteriorly, the iris is lined by two separate, but closely apposed, epithelial layers derived from neuroectoderm. The cells of the anterior epithelial layer, which are in direct contact with the posterior aspect of the stroma, are continuous with smooth muscle fibers of the dilator pupillae; the sphincter pupillae are of similar developmental origin. The posterior iris pigment epithelial layer is in direct contact with the aqueous of the posterior chamber. The cytoplasm of both epithelial layers contains numerous melanosomes (approximately 1 micron in diameter), which are larger than those of the iris stroma (diameter of about 0.5 microns). The number of melanosomes in the iris epithelial layers does not vary significantly between lightly and darkly pigmented individuals. In persons with ocular and oculocutaneous albinism, the pigmented epithelia, as well as the stromal melanocytes, contain fewer melanin granules than in normal individuals. The pigmented epithelia of the iris normally extend around the lip of the pupil, anteriorly, for a short distance. In certain pathologic conditions, fibrovascular tissue on the anterior surface of the iris everts the pupillary margin and pulls the pigmented epithelia onto the anterior surface of the iris. This displaced pigmented epithelium may be apparent clinically and is known as ectropion uveae.

### The Ciliary Body

The middle segment of the uveal tract, the ciliary body, is located between the iris and the choroid. Situated interior to the anterior sclera, it is made up of two ring-shaped compo-

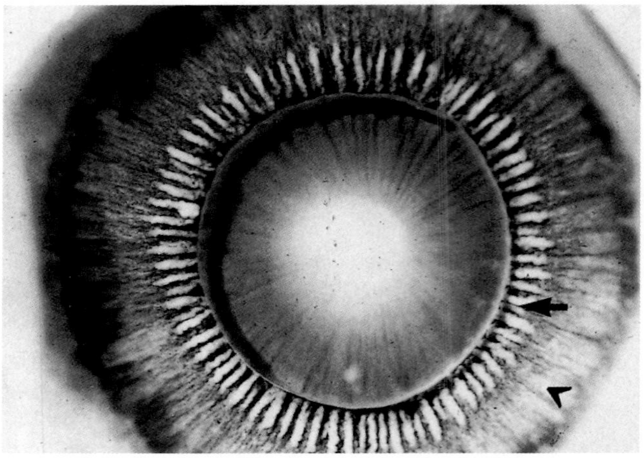

**FIG. 19.** The lens and ciliary body are viewed from behind in this photograph. The ciliary body has two components: the pars plicata and the pars plana. The pars plicata contains about 70 sagitally oriented folds or ciliary processes (*arrow*). The pars plicata gradually merges with the flat pars plana (*arrowhead*). (Reproduced from GK Klintworth and MB Landers III. *The eye: structure and function.* Baltimore; Williams & Wilkins, 1976, with permission.)

nents: the pars plicata and the pars plana (Fig. 19). The anteriormost aspect of the ciliary body, the pars plicata begins at the scleral spur and contains approximately 70 sagitally oriented folds (approximately 2 mm long and 0.8 mm high). Continuous with these folds the flat pars plana, which is approximately 4 mm wide, merges posteriorly with the serrated anterior border of the retina (ora serrata). Both portions of the ciliary body consist of epithelium, stroma, and smooth muscle.

The ciliary epithelium embraces two distinct layers, both of which share a similar development derivation from neural ectoderm (Fig. 20). The inner epithelial layer is virtually nonpigmented and is contiguous with the aqueous of the posterior chamber. At the ora serrata, the sensory retina converges into the nonpigmented ciliary epithelial monolayer, which extends anteriorly until it becomes the posterior epithelial layer of the iris. In contrast, the outer ciliary epithelial layer is pigmented and unites with the retinal pigment epithelium at the ora serrata. The pigmented epithelium of the ciliary body overlies a periodic acid-Schiff-positive basal lamina that is closely adherent to the adjacent stroma. The basal lamina of the pigmented epithelium can become conspicuously thickened in diabetes mellitus. Acellular fibers, known as zonules (Fig. 20), attach the crests of the nonpigmented ciliary epithelium in the pars plicata to the capsule of the crystalline lens.

The stroma of the ciliary body, composed of fibroblasts, blood vessels, nerve cells, and melanocytes, is most abundant in the ciliary processes of the pars plicata, and is least plentiful in the valleys between these processes and in the pars plana. During infancy, the stroma of the ciliary body is sparse (Fig. 21, *left*) but expands until adulthood. With advanced age, the ciliary body stroma becomes hyalinized (Fig. 21, *right*), and frequently calcifies.

The smooth muscle of the ciliary body (Fig. 22) forms three distinct bundles. The outermost muscle runs in a longitudinal or meridonal direction, whereas the middle layer contains radially oriented fibers, and the innermost muscle cells are aligned in a circular fashion. In routinely processed globes, histologic differentiation of these three muscular layers is difficult. Muscles of the ciliary body attach in large part to the scleral spur. The ciliary muscle assists in accommodation. As it contracts, the ciliary body extends forward, reducing pressure on the zonules, and enabling the lens to become less concave, thereby, increasing its refractive power.

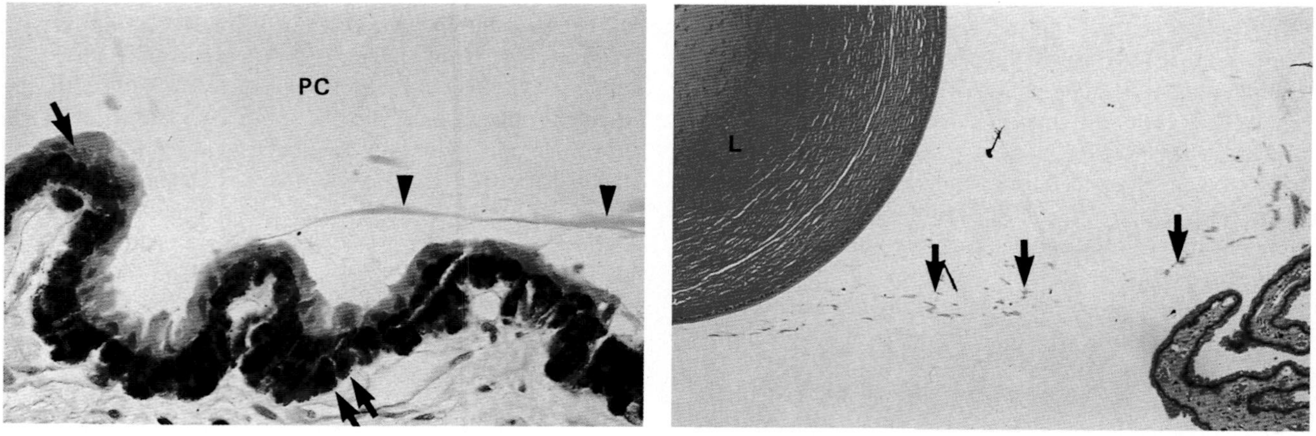


**FIG. 20.** ***Left:*** The epithelium of the ciliary body has two distinct layers. The inner nonpigmented layer (*arrow*) is in direct contact with the aqueous of the posterior chamber (PC). The outer pigmented epithelial layer (*double arrows*) is adjacent to the underlying stroma. Acellular eosinophilic fibers attach to the crests of the nonpigmented epithelium of the pars plicata (zonules) (*arrowheads*). Zonules do not originate in the valleys between the ciliary processes. (H&E × **132**)
***Right:*** Zonular fibers (*arrows*) span between the pars plicata of the ciliary body (CB) and the lens (L) and hold the lens in place. (H&E × **25.**)

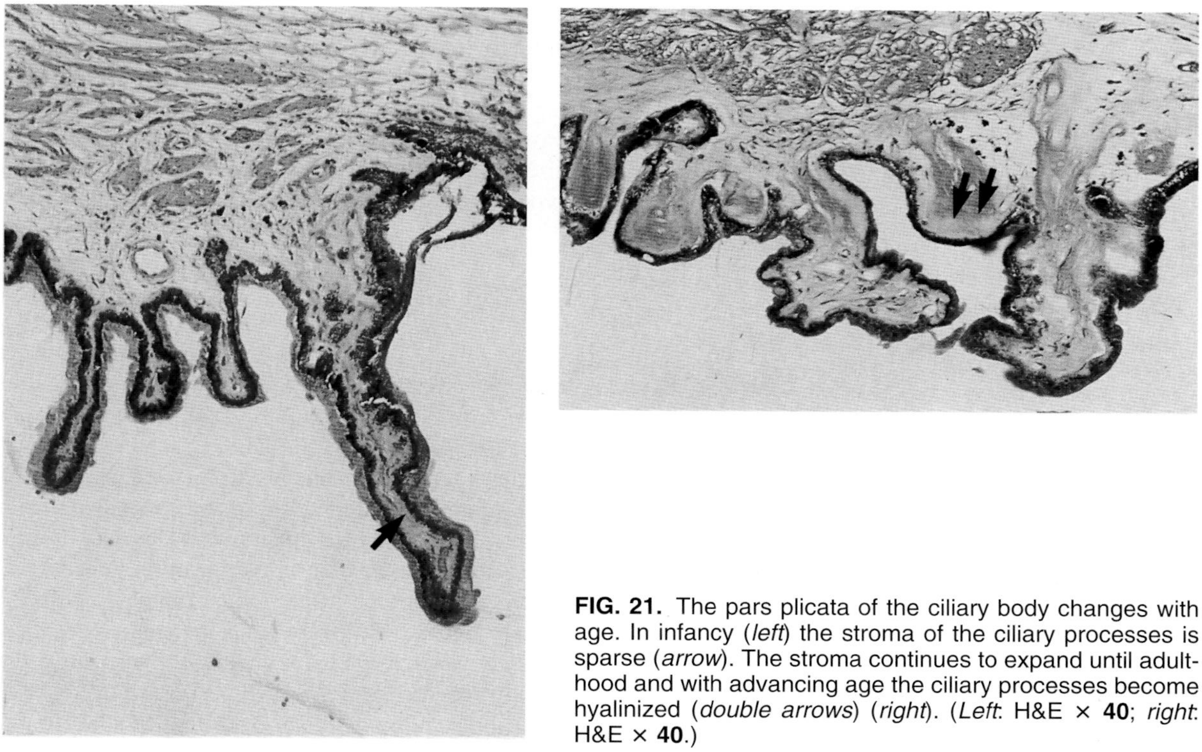

FIG. 21. The pars plicata of the ciliary body changes with age. In infancy (*left*) the stroma of the ciliary processes is sparse (*arrow*). The stroma continues to expand until adulthood and with advancing age the ciliary processes become hyalinized (*double arrows*) (*right*). (*Left*: H&E × **40**; *right*: H&E × **40**.)

### Choroid

The richly vascularized choroid (Fig. 23) extends from the ciliary body to the optic nerve. Its inner aspect is firmly adherent to the retinal pigment epithelium. The outer surface of the choroid is loosely attached to the overlying sclera. Bruch's membrane delineates the choroid from the overlying retinal pigment epithelium and is approximately 2 to 4 $\mu$m thick. Although Bruch's membrane appears as a thin acosinophilic layer in tissue sections, ultrastructural analysis has disclosed it to be composed of 5 distinct layers: the basal lamina of the overlying retinal pigment epithelium, a collagenous layer, an elastic fiber-rich component, another collagenous portion, and the basal lamina of the endothelial cells of the underlying capillary network (choriocapillaris). Located in the innermost choroidal stroma adjacent to Bruch's membrane, the choriocapillaris connects with arterial and venous channels from vessels in the outer choroidal stroma. Its function is to nourish the outer retinal layers. With age, Bruch's membrane thickens and commonly acquires focal excresences known as drusen (Fig. 24). Both drusen and Bruch's membrane may calcify.

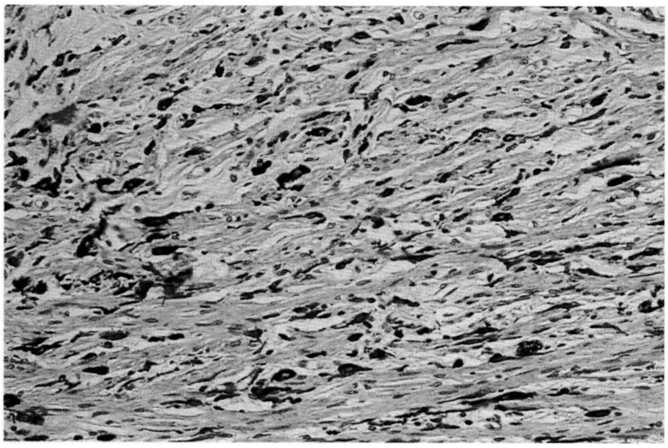

FIG. 22. Smooth muscle constitutes a large portion of the ciliary body. Pigmented melanocytes are often present in between the smooth muscle bundles. (H&E × **66**.)

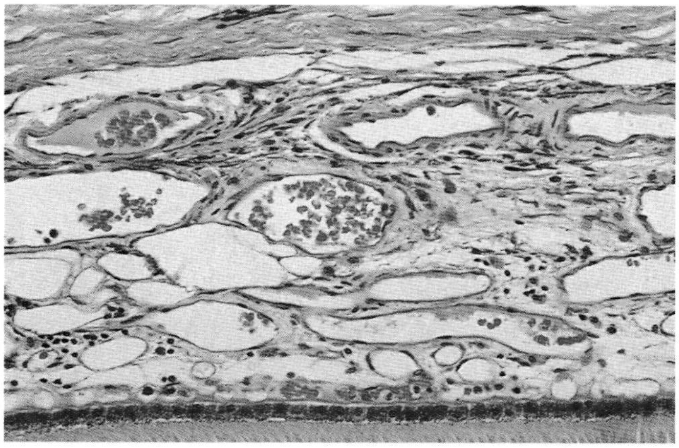

FIG. 23. This photomicrograph illustrates the well-vascularized choroid. At the top of the figure the choroid abuts the sclera. The single layer of retinal pigment epithelium is present at the bottom of the figure. (H&E × **66**.)

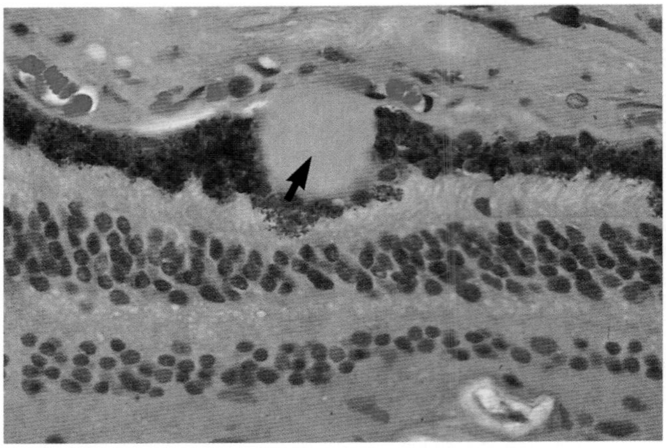

**FIG. 24.** An amorphous excresence (*arrow*) in Bruch's membrane appears to extend into the underlying retina. Such so-called "drusen" are common and, occasionally, calcify. (H&E × **160**.)

The choroidal stroma is thinnest anteriorly, near the ciliary body where it is approximately 0.1 mm thick. Posteriorly, at the optic nerve, the choroidal stroma thickens to nearly 0.22 mm. The tenuous connection between the choroidal stroma and the sclera is responsible for both the pathologic and artifactual separations often seen between these two layers in histologic sections. The stroma contains abundant pigmented melanocytes (Fig. 25), which are more numerous in heavily pigmented individuals than in persons with little pigment. Collagen fibers, some smooth muscle, neurons of the autonomic nervous system, and a prominent vascular system are also present. Large- and medium-sized arteries (branches of the posterior ciliary arteries) and veins (vortex veins) are situated in the outermost choroid.

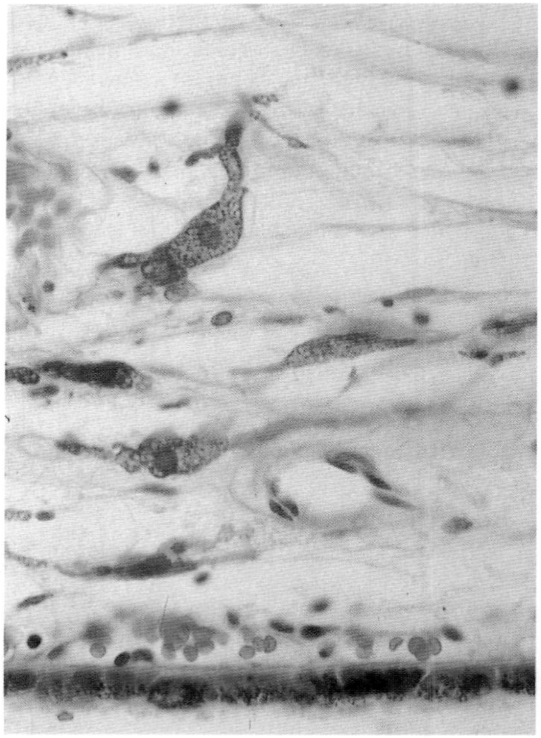

**FIG. 25.** Numerous pigmented melanocytes are located within the choroidal stroma. (H&E × **160**.)

## RETINA

The cellular components of the retina include the photoreceptors (rods and cones), a variety of different neurons (ganglion, bipolar, horizontal, and amacrine cells), and neuroglial cells (Müller cells and astrocytes). Many of these special types of cells can only be detected with the aid of specific staining techniques. These constituents of the retina are stratified into several distinct layers (Fig. 26). The rods and cones comprise the outermost part of the sensory retina and are closely apposed to the retinal pigment epithelium. The retina's anterior boundary has a serrated edge (ora serrata), at which point it is approximately 0.1 mm thick. Cysts develop in the peripheral retina (peripheral cystoid degeneration) in virtually everyone over age 20 (11) (Figs. 27 and 28). Here, the retina converges into a single layer of nonpigmented epithelium which continues anteriorly to where it merges with the nonpigmented epithelium of the ciliary body (Fig. 28). Posteriorly, the retina extends to the optic nerve where it is approximately 0.5 to 0.6 mm thick. The sensory retina is in direct contact with the vitreous and lies interior to the retinal pigment epithelium, which defines the outermost border of the retina.

The retinal pigment epithelium is a monolayer of cells. These epithelial cells contain numerous intracytoplasmic melanosomes; cellular processes envelop part of the overlying rods and cones as shown by transmission electron microscopy. The phagocytic function of the retinal pigment epithelium assists in the turnover of the photoreceptor elements. Undigested products of phagoliposomes culminate in the progressively increasing number of lipofuscin granules that accumulate within the retinal pigment epithelium, with time.

Some photoreceptors are cylindrical in appearance (rods), whereas others are conical shaped and somewhat longer and thicker (cones). Internal to the photoreceptors is the outer plexiform layer, formed from cell processes of the horizontal and bipolar cells and axonal extensions of the rods and cones. The inner nuclear layer embraces the nuclei of several cell types (the bipolar, Müller, horizontal, and amacrine cells). Constituents of the inner plexiform layer include bipolar and amacrine cell axons and dendrites of the ganglion cells. Near the vitreal aspect of the retina is the ganglion cell layer, composed predominantly of ganglion cell bodies. The axons of these large neurons make up the nerve fiber layer; these processes are usually unmyelinated, but as

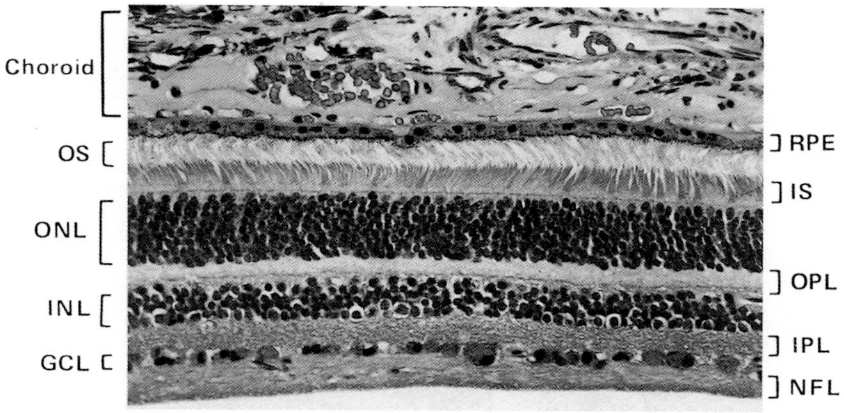


**FIG. 26.** The cellular components of the retina are organized in well-defined layers. The choroid is directly above the retinal pigment epithelium (RPE) in this figure. Specialized extensions of the photoreceptors known as the outer and inner segments (OS and IS) are located immediately adjacent to the RPE. Cell bodies of the photoreceptors are present in the outer nuclear layer (ONL); synapses between the bipolar cells, horizontal cells, and the photoreceptors occur in the outer plexiform layer (OPL); the inner nuclear layer (INL) embraces nuclei of the amacrine, bipolar, horizontal, and Müller cells; the inner plexiform (IPL) contains axons and dendrites of amacrine, bipolar, and ganglion cells; ganglion cell bodies are located in the ganglion cell layer (GCL); the nerve fiber layer (NFL) contains ganglion cell axons. (Reproduced from GK Klintworth and MB Landers III. *The eye: structure and function.* Baltimore; Williams & Wilkins, Baltimore, MD, 1976, with permission.)

an incidental developmental anomaly, bundles of some nerve fibers are occasionally myelinated. In older individuals, basophilic periodic acid-Schiff-positive intracellular rounded bodies (corpora amylacea), indistinguishable from similar structures in the brain, often accumulate in the nerve fiber layer of the retina near the optic disc. By light microscopy, two acellular zones can be distinguished within the retina: the external and internal limiting membranes. The so-called "external limiting membrane" is located between the photoreceptors and the outer nuclear layer. The membrane represents firm junctions between Müller cells and adjacent photoreceptors (zonula adherens). The basal lamina of the Müller cells accounts for the hyaline structure seen on light microscopy, and is known as the "internal limiting membrane."

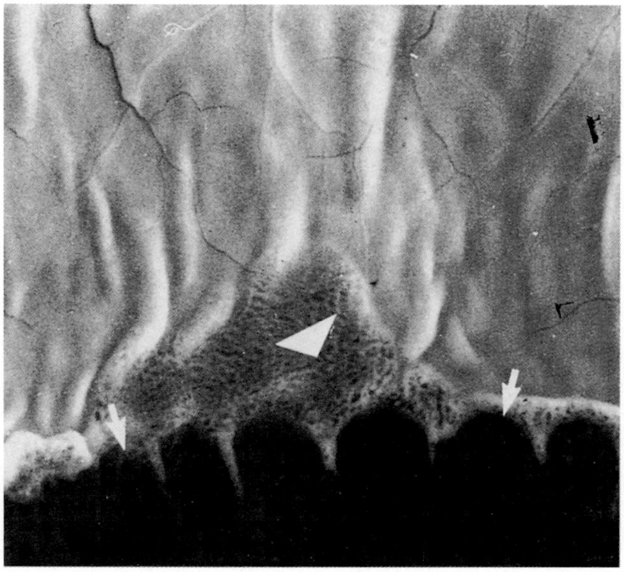

**FIG. 27.** The ora serrata marks the anterior boundary of the retina. An almost invariable finding in the retina of all human eyes after the age of 20 is peripheral cystoid degeneration. Macroscopically the peripheral retina immediately behind the ora serrata (*arrows*) has a focally vacuolated appearance (*arrowhead*). (Reproduced from GK Klintworth and MB Landers III. *The eye: structure and function.* Baltimore; Williams & Wilkins, 1976, with permission.)

Light passes through the entire sensory retina before it is converted by the photoreceptor cells into electric impulses. The impulses are eventually transmitted to the visual cortex in the occipital lobe of the brain through a complex series of intercellular connections.

The retina varies in structure in different sites (Fig. 29). A yellow specialized portion of the retina is located in the posterior pole of the eye (in an area slightly temporal to the optic disc). This is the macula lutea (yellow spot), where the bipolar and ganglion cells contain the pigment xanthophyll. In the macular region of the retina, the ganglion cells are several layers thick. The center of the macula contains a slightly depressed area (the fovea centralis) measuring almost 1.5 mm in diameter; it is responsible for most visual acuity. The walls of the fovea centralis are known as the clivus, and the precise center is designated the foveola. Blood vessels are absent in the foveola, which measures approximately 0.4 mm in diameter. The inner layers of the retina are displaced peripherally in the foveola so that only photoreceptors, the outer nuclear layer, and outer plexiform layer are present. Cones are located within the foveola, but rods are absent.

The microvasculature of the normal retina is composed of branches of the central retinal artery and tributaries of the central retinal vein. It contains arterioles, venules, and intervening capillaries (Fig. 30). In capillaries from normal individuals, endothelial cells and pericytes are present in a ratio of approximately 1 : 1. The retinal microvasculature is effected in hypertension, diabetes mellitus, and other conditions. Capillary microaneurysms and the loss of capillary pericytes are characteristics of diabetic retinopathy. These are best visualized in flat preparations of the retina after trypsin digestion of the retinal cells.

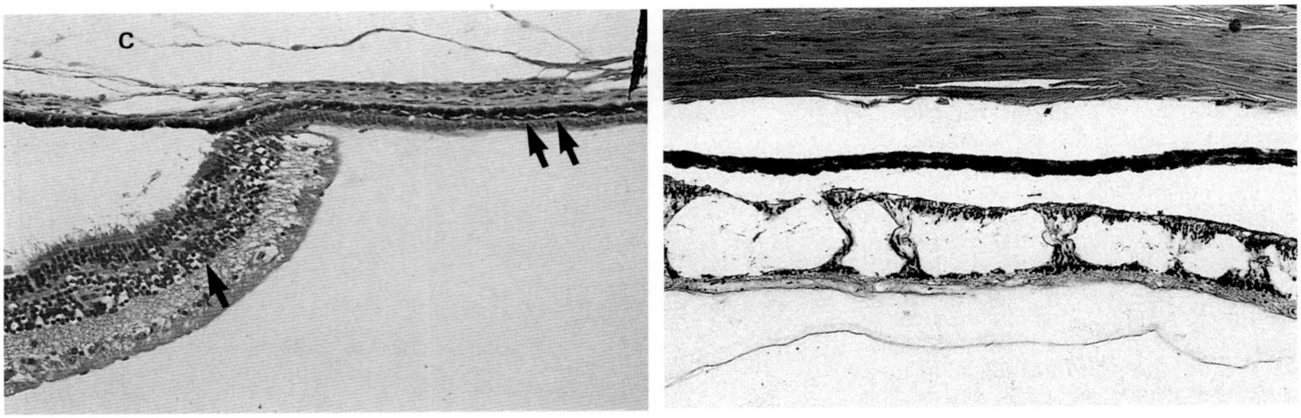


**FIG. 28.** ***Left:*** At the ora serrata, the multilayered retina (*arrow*) converges with the single layer of nonpigmented epithelium of the ciliary body (*double arrows*). The retina is loosely attached to the choroid (C) in the region of the ora serrata and is artifactually separated from it in this figure. (H&E × **50**) ***Right:*** Microscopically, peripheral cystoid degeneration is characterized by the presence of numerous cystlike spaces within the retina. (Reproduced with permission from GK Klintworth and MB Landers III. The eye: structure and function. Baltimore; Williams & Wilkins, 1976, with permission.)

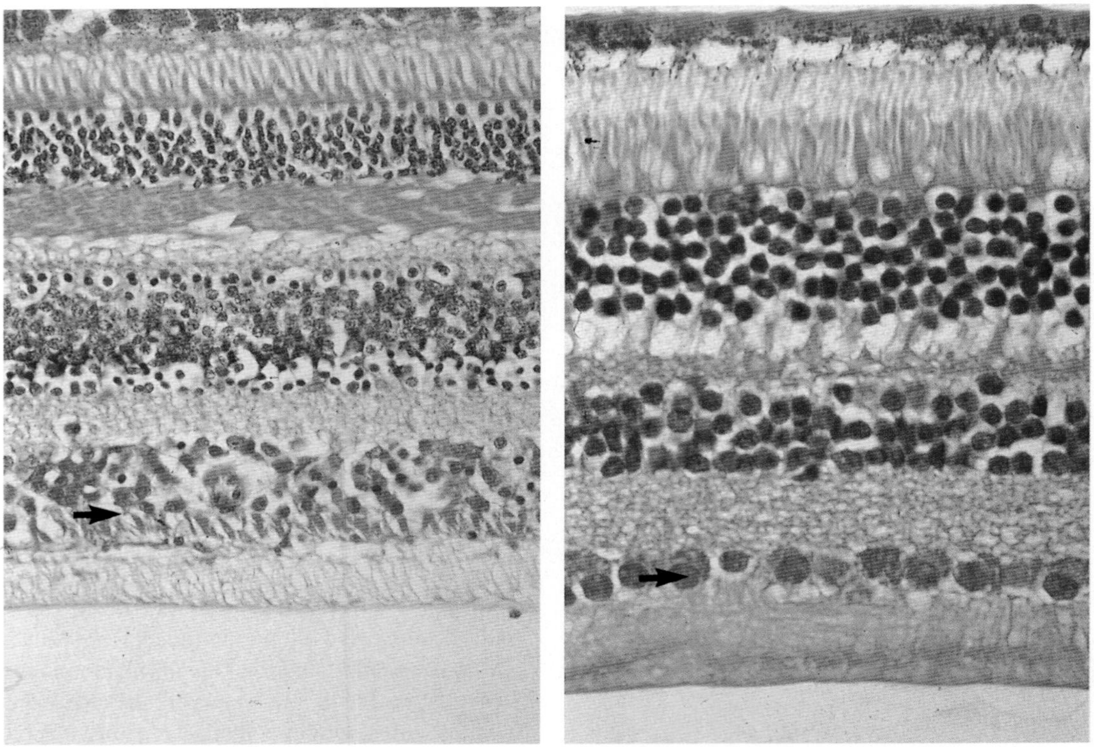

**FIG. 29.** The retina has regional histologic variations. In the macular region (*left*) the ganglion cells (*arrow*) are multilayered. In areas outside of the macula (*right*) ganglion cells (*arrow*) form a single layer. (*Left*: H&E × **80**; *right*: H&E ×**160**.)

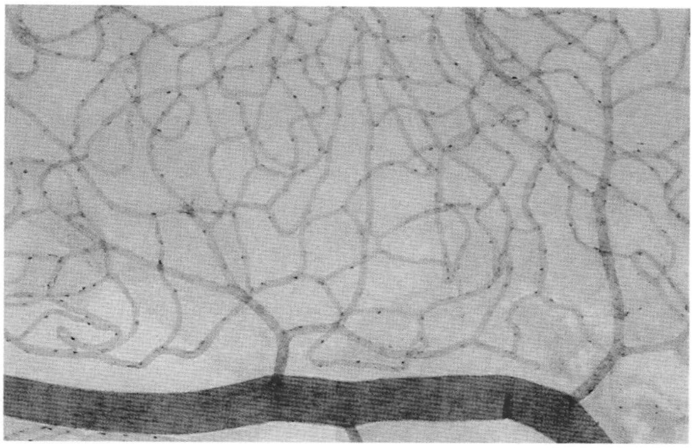

**FIG. 30.** This flat preparation of a normal retina following trypsin digestion discloses retinal capillaries adjacent to a retinal arteriole. (H&E × **25**.)

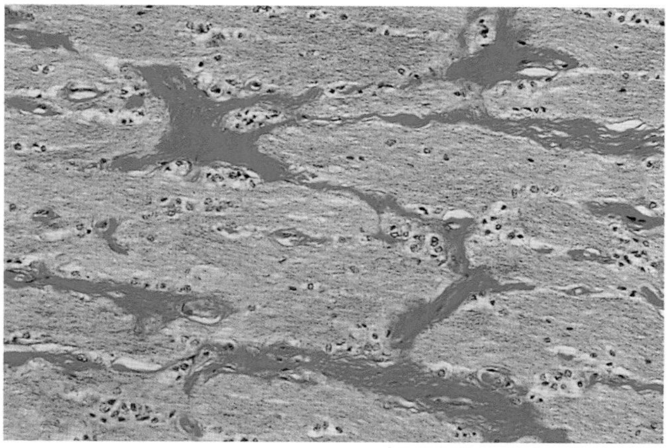

**FIG. 32.** Nerve fiber bundles within the optic nerve are surrounded by thin collagenous septae. (Masson trichrome × **50**.)

## THE OPTIC NERVE

More than one million axons from the retinal nerve fiber layer converge at the nerve head, the center of which accommodates the central retinal artery and vein within a slight depression lined by glial tissue (Fig. 31). The nerve head accounts for the physiologic blind spot in the normal visual field and represents the beginning of the optic nerve. From the nerve head, the axons extend for approximately 1 mm to a sievelike partition of connective tissue in the sclera, through which the nerve fibers pass on their way to the brain (the lamina cribrosa). Over one thousand nerve fiber bundles surrounded by astrocytes, oligodendroglia, and collagenous septae (Fig. 32) can be identified in cross sections of the optic nerve, which is a tract of the central nervous system. Like the brain, the optic nerve is surrounded by dura, arachnoid, and pia maters. Small focal meningothelial proliferations occasionally form within the leptomeninges surrounding the optic nerve. Some orbital meningiomas presumably arise from them. Laminated products of the meningothelial cells (psammoma bodies, corpora arencea) sometimes occur in the arachnoid mater (Fig. 33). After leaving the globe, each optic nerve continues posteriorly through the orbit to its respective optic foramen, and then to the optic chiasm, before terminating in the lateral geniculate bodies.

At the level of the lamina cribrosa, the axons within the optic nerve become myelinated by concentric membranous processes of the oligodendroglia. The rather abrupt transition between myelinated and nonmyelinated nerve fibers is eminently appreciated in tissue sections stained with Luxol fast blue or other dyes with an affinity for myelin (Fig. 34). As the axons acquire myelin coats, the diameter of the optic nerve doubles to nearly 3 mm. Located within the central core of the optic nerve, adjacent to the globe, are the central

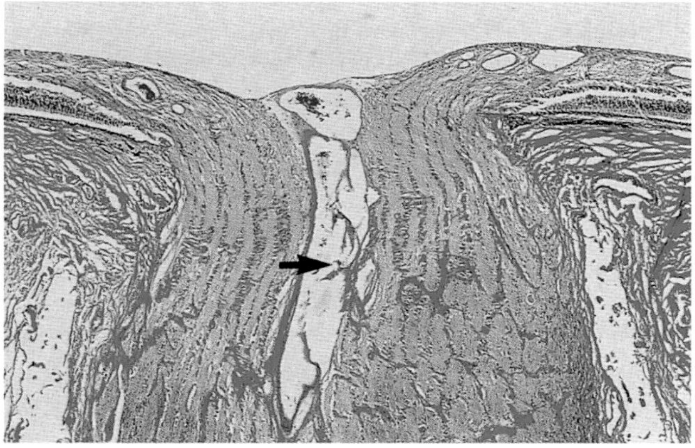

**FIG. 31.** The optic nerve penetrates the sclera near the posterior pole of the eye. This histologic section contains the central retinal artery (*arrow*) in the central part of the optic nerve. Both the central retinal artery and the central retinal vein traverse the optic nerve until they exit the nerve about 8 to 15 mm posterior to the eyeball. (Masson trichrome × **10**.)

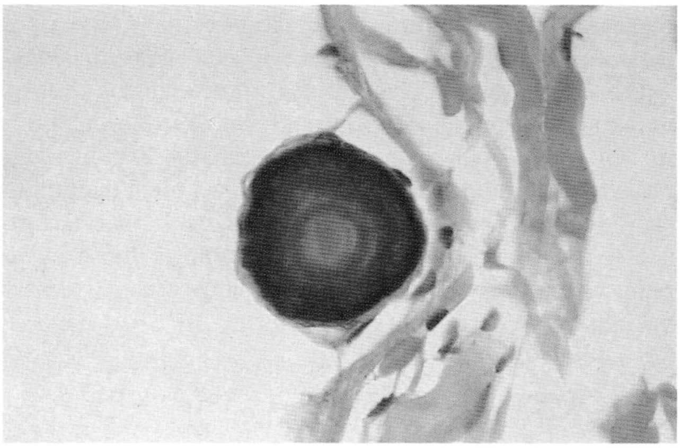

**FIG. 33.** Laminated psammoma bodies, such as this one, are often closely associated with the meningothelial cells of optic nerve. (H&E × **160**.)

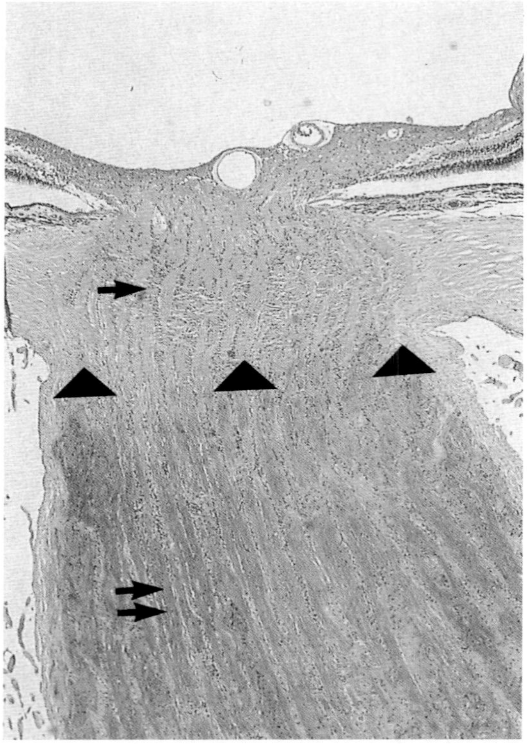

**FIG. 34.** The abrupt transition between nonmyelinated (*arrow*) and myelinated (*double arrows*) nerve fibers of the normal optic nerve at the level of the lamina cribosa (*arrowheads*) is dramatically illustrated in this tissue section stained with a dye that has an affinity for myelin. (Luxol fast blue × **10**.)

retinal artery and vein. Both of these vascular channels exit the nerve some 8 to 15 mm posterior to the lamina cribrosa; the channels are not evident within tissue sections of the optic nerve closer to the brain. The orbital portion of the optic nerve extends some 25 mm from the lamina cribrosa to the optic foramen at the apex of the orbit. If the optic nerve becomes compressed during enucleation of the globe, optic nerve tissue may extrude into the eye and become dislodged within vessels near the optic discs, between the sensory retina and the retinal pigment epithelium, and even within the vitreous. When such optic nerve tissue becomes displaced, like toothpaste from a compressed tube, the artifact should not be mistaken for ectopic intraocular nervous tissue. With age, corpora amylacea, similar to those in the retina and white matter of the brain, may become evident in the optic nerve.

## THE CRYSTALLINE LENS

The biconvex ocular lens (Fig. 35) is located directly behind the pupil and in front of the anterior face of the vitreous. In the adult, it measures approximately 10 mm in diameter and 4 to 5 mm in width. The lens is held in place by zonules that connect it to the pars plicata of the ciliary body. The lens is encircled by a collagen- and carbohydrate-rich capsule which serves as the site of attachment for the zonules. The capsule over the anterior surface of the lens thickens with time. At 2 to 3 years of age, the anterior capsule is almost 8 to 15 $\mu$m wide and increases to 14 to 21 $\mu$m by age 35. (Fig. 36). The posterior lens capsule becomes thinner with age. The maximum thickness of the posterior lens capsule ranges from 4 to 23 $\mu$m at age 35, and diminishes to 2 to 9 $\mu$m after age 70 (Fig. 37) (2). Directly interior to the anterior lens capsule is a single layer of cuboidal epithelium. These cells extend to about the level of the lens equator; they do not normally exist posterior to this point. Proliferating epithelial cells elongate at the lens equator and become displaced toward the center of the lens, known as the lens nucleus, where they are retained for life. This process continues throughout life and the long slender cells are designated lens fibers. In the peripheral part of the lens near the equator, the fibers retain their nuclei, but as the fibers become displaced toward the center of the lens their nuclei disintegrate so that the center of the lens lacks nuclei. In some cataractous lenses, such as the cataract of rubella, the fibers within the center of the lens retain their nuclei.

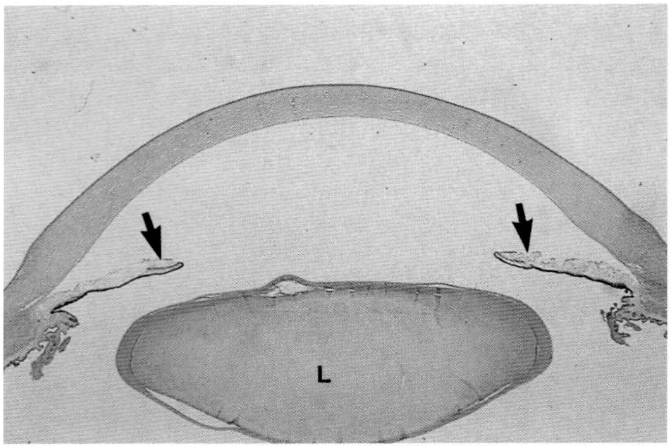


**FIG. 35.** The crystalline lens (L) is situated just posterior to the pupil and iris (*arrows*). (H&E × **2.5**.)

The normally transparent lens commonly opacifies with age. Discrete globules of degenerate lens fibers may form. They are frequently accompanied by the presence of an extension of epithelial cells, posterior to the equator. The high density of the lens fibers makes it difficult to obtain histologic sections of the lens that are free from artifact.

## INTRAOCULAR COMPARTMENTS

The eye accommodates two major fluid-containing intraocular compartments. One is filled with aqueous, the other with vitreous. The aqueous compartment is divided into an

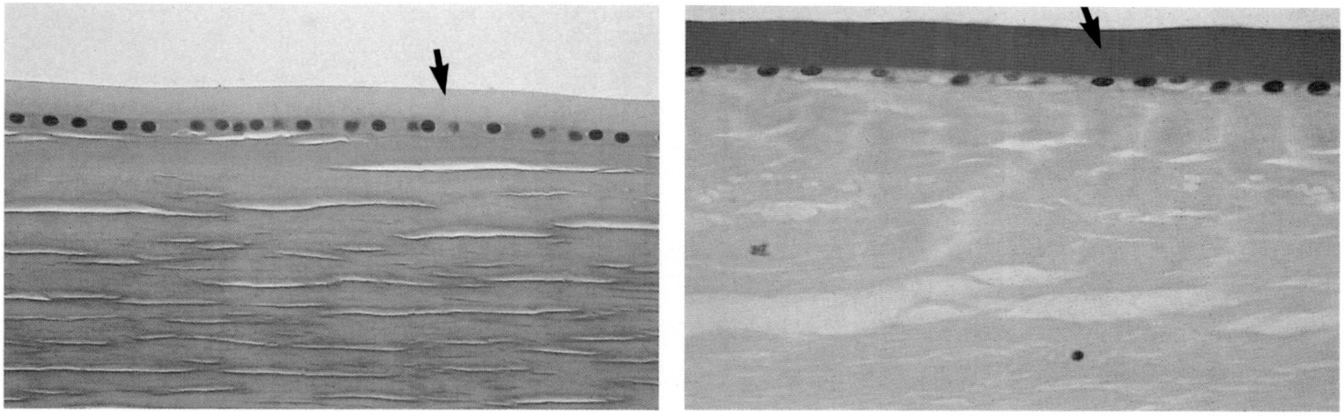

FIG. 36. The anterior lens capsule (*arrow*) appears as an eosinophilic acellular band overlying a single layer of epithelial cells in hematoxylin and eosin-stained preparations (*left*). The lens capsule is rich in carbohydrate and reacts intensely with the periodic acid-Schiff stain (*arrow*) (*right*). (*Left*: H&E × **132**; *right*: periodic acid-Schiff × **160**.)

anterior and posterior chamber (Fig. 38). The anterior chamber is delineated in front by the cornea, peripherally by the drainage angle of the eye, and posteriorly by the pupil and the iris. The small posterior chamber is situated between the pigmented epithelia of the iris, the ciliary body, the anterior face of the vitreous, and the lens. The aqueous, a watery solution, which does not normally stain with routine histologic techniques, is produced by the ciliary body and flows forward through the aperture of the pupil to the anterior chamber, where it leaves the eye through the trabecular meshwork and Schlemm's canal. The anterior chamber contains approximately 0.25 ml of aqueous; the posterior chamber has a volume of only approximately 0.06 ml. Normal human aqueous has a density slightly greater than water, and like plasma, it contains protein, ascorbic acid, electrolytes, and glucose. The major differences between aqueous and plasma are the relatively low-protein and high-ascorbic acid concentration of aqueous, relative to plasma.

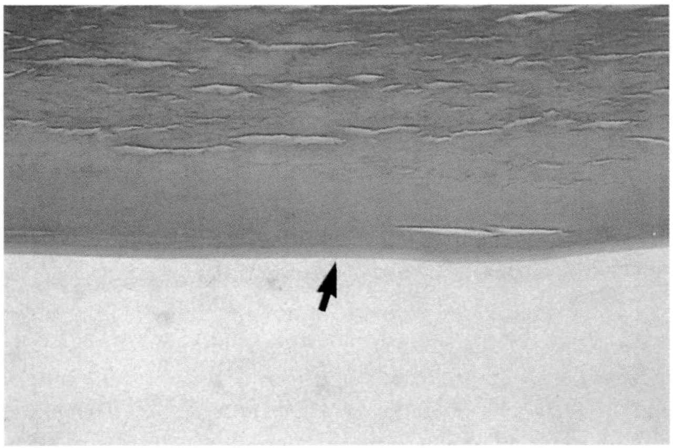

FIG. 37. Posteriorly, the lens capsule (*arrow*) is thinner than anteriorly, and epithelial cells are absent. (H&E × **132**.)

The vitreous extends from the sensory retina to the lens and contains a gel-like material composed of water, protein, hyaluronic acid, and a small population of cells, designated hyalocytes, which are rarely noted in standard tissue sections. These tissue macrophages are thought to synthesize collagen and hyaluronic acid. The gelatinous consistency of the vitreous is due to a framework of numerous, randomly oriented collagen fibrils. The concentration of glucose and ascorbic acid is much lower than in the aqueous, whereas the

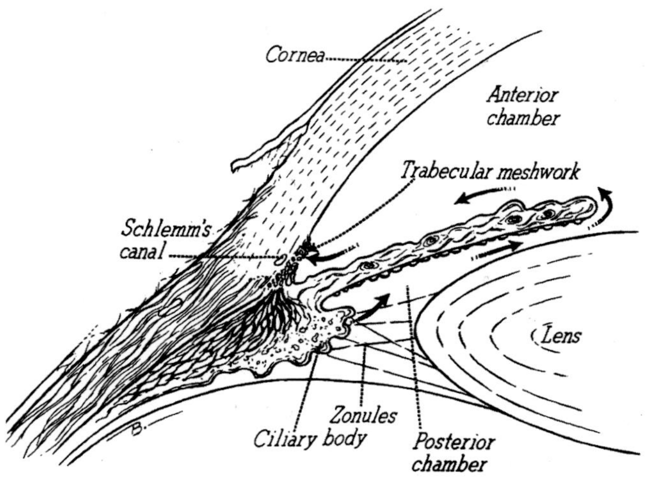


FIG. 38. The anterior chamber is defined by the cornea, anterior surface of the iris, and pupil. The boundaries of the much smaller posterior chamber include the posterior surface of the iris, the ciliary body, and the anterior face of the vitreous. Aqueous is produced by the ciliary body and circulates from the posterior chamber through the pupil into the anterior chamber. Aqueous drains from the eye by way of the trabecular meshwork and Schlemm's canal. (Reproduced with permission from GK Klintworth and MB Landers III. *The eye. structure and function*. Baltimore; Williams & Wilkins, 1976, with permission.)

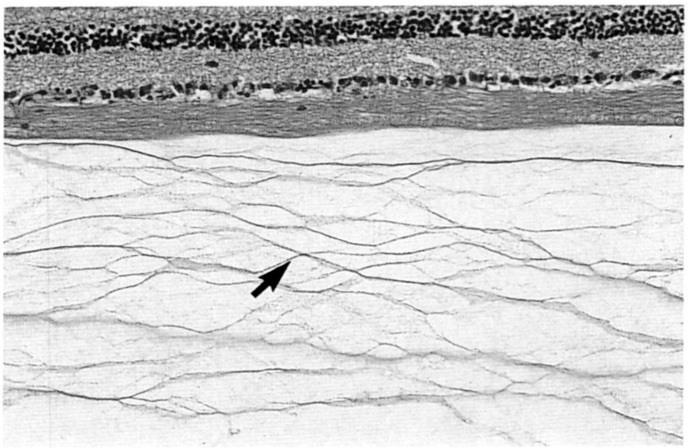

**FIG. 39.** The vitreous (*arrow*) appears as an amorphous material in standard tissue sections. (H&E × **50**.)

concentration of soluble protein is similar to that of the aqueous (12). The vitreous is attached securely to the retina at the ora serrata and near the optic disc. Occasionally, vitreous may be identified as an amorphous acellular material on H&E-stained sections (Fig. 39).

## THE EYELIDS

The eyelids (Fig. 40) can be divided into cutaneous and conjunctival portions. The cutaneous segment of the eyelid is composed of a stratified squamous epidermis overlying a loosely arranged dermis, beneath which is muscular tissue. The eyelids contain several types of skin appendages. Sebaceous glands deposit their secretions, together with decomposed whole cells via ducts, into hair follicles of the eyelashes (glands of Zeis), or into ducts that open into the lid margins (meibomian glands) (Fig. 41). Apocrine glands, whose secretions represent the pinched-off luminal aspect of the lining acinar cells, also open into the follicles of the eyelashes (glands of Moll) (Fig. 42). In addition, the dermis of the eyelid contains eccrine sweat glands, which discharge secretions directly onto the skin via a convoluted duct. The subcutaneous portion of the upper and lower eyelids contains concentrically arranged skeletal muscle fibers (orbicularis oculi), but very little adipose connective tissue. Striated muscle of the palpebral portion of the levator palpebrae superioris is also present in the upper eyelid; it terminates in a dense fibrocollagenous aponeurosis. Small bundles of smooth muscle fibers (Müller's muscle) are located within the upper and lower eyelids.

The junction between the cutaneous and conjunctival parts of the eyelid is demarcated clinically by a sulcus (the gray line), located between the ducts of the meibomian glands and the eyelashes. The conjunctival portion of the eyelid is made up of dense connective tissue containing the meibomian glands, (the tarsus), and the palpebral conjunctiva (Fig. 43). The tarsus, located immediately posterior to the muscles of the eyelid, accounts for most of the rigidity of the eyelids and is covered posteriorly by conjunctival epithelium and a thin subepithelial stroma. As described earlier, accessory lacrimal glands are present in the palpebral conjunctiva.

## THE ORBIT

The posterior and peripheral borders of the orbit are defined by bones of the skull, face, and nose. At the anterior orbital margin, the periosteum of the orbital bones gives rise to a dense connective tissue sheet, (the orbital septum) (Fig. 40), which extends forward to insert into the eyelids. Tissue posterior to this septum is considered to be within the orbit. In the human adult, the orbit measures approximately 40 mm in height, 45 mm in depth, and has a volume of almost 30 ml. Several bony canals allow for transmission of blood vessels and nerves into and out of the orbit, posteriorly. The contents of the orbit are organized in a complex three-dimensional arrangement (Fig. 44). Aside from the eye, the optic nerve and its meningeal coverings, Tenon's capsule, the extraocular muscles, the lacrimal gland, blood vessels, and a delicate framework of fibroadipose connective tissue constitute the major components of the orbit.

The only epithelial structure normally present in the orbit is the lacrimal gland (Fig. 45). Closely apposed to the globe and situated in the superolateral aspect of the orbit, this gland is traditionally divided into two parts: a larger orbital lobe and a smaller palpebral lobe. About a dozen ducts from the lacrimal gland open into the superior conjunctival fornices and transmit their secretions into the tear film. The lacrimal gland is not encapsulated and thin fibroconnective tissue septae divide the tissue into lobules composed of acini, lined by columnar-shaped cells. Some lobules, occasionally, extend posteriorly behind the globe. Most cells are serous in type and contain scattered intracytoplasmic fat droplets and granules. Mucinous cells similar to those of salivary glands are not usually present in the acini, but may be identified in the ducts. In addition to secretory cells, the lining of the larger peripheral ducts within the lacrimal gland contain myoepithelial cells external to the serous cells. Occasional lymphocytes and plasma cells are commonly present between the acini of the lacrimal gland.

The orbit contains the cranial nerves, which innervate the extrinsic muscles of the eye (abducent, oculomotor, and trochlear nerves), branches of the ophthalmic division of the trigeminal nerve, as well as parasympathetic and sympathetic nerves that innervate the cornea, conjunctiva, and the muscles of the ciliary body and iris. Neurons of the ciliary ganglion, which is located near the optic nerve close to the orbital apex and which measures approximately 2 mm in diameter, receive parasympathetic and sympathetic nerve fibers.

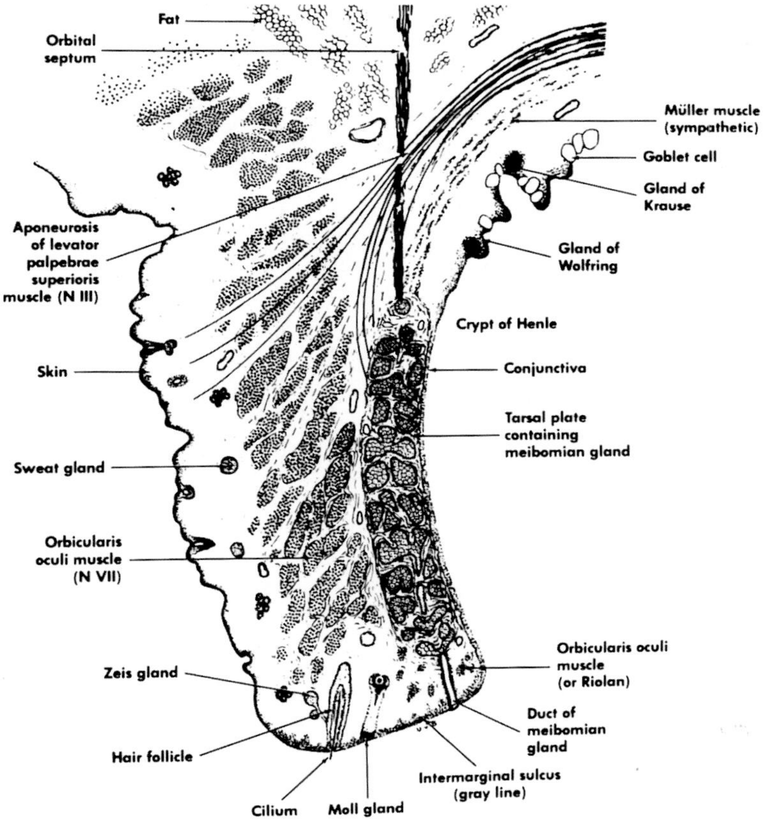


A

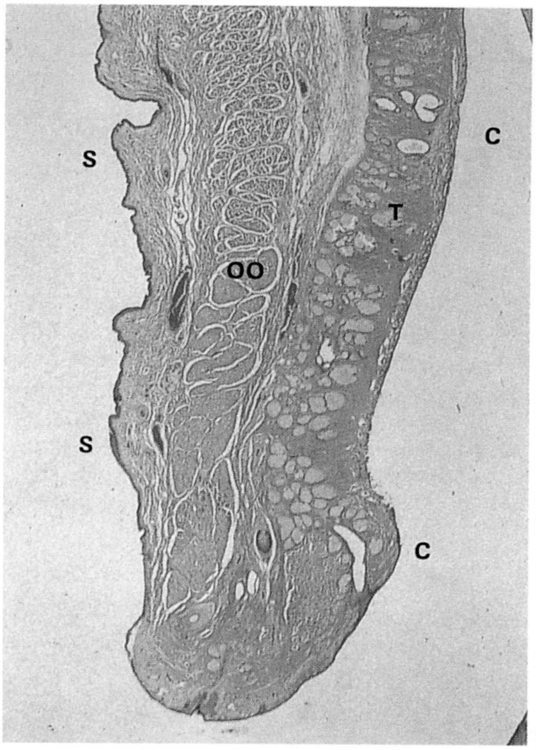


B

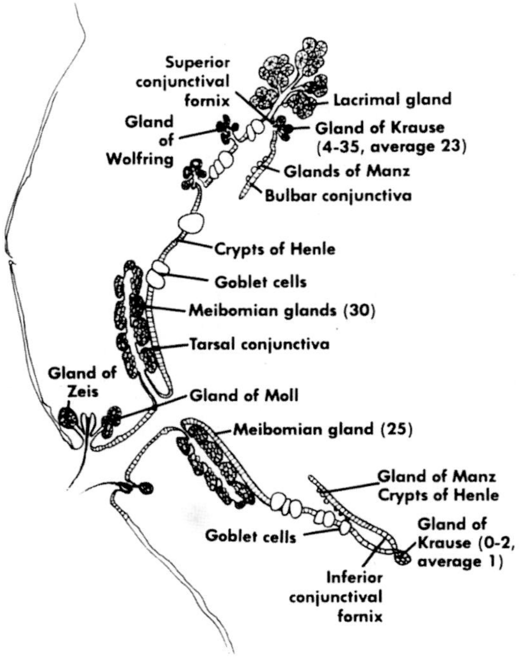


C

**FIG. 40. A:** Components of the eyelid as illustrated on this drawing include skin and cutaneous appendages, muscle, connective tissue, and conjunctiva. (Reproduced from FW Newell. *Ophthalmology: principles and concepts*. St. Louis; CV Mosby, 1986, with permission.) **B:** The skin surface (S), the orbicularis oculi muscle (OO), the tarsus (T) and the conjunctiva (C) are evident in this histologic section of an eyelid. (H&E × **3.3**)
**C**: Multiple foci of accessory lacrimal gland tissue (glands of Krause and Wolfring) are present in the eyelids. (Reproduced from FW Newell. *Ophthalmology: principles and concepts*. St. Louis; CV Mosby, 1986, with permission.)

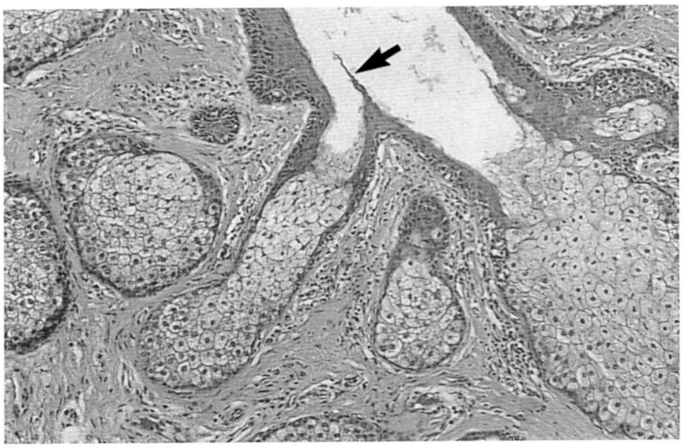

**FIG. 41.** Modified sebaceous glands, the meibomian glands, deposit secretions into ducts opening onto the eyelids. A valve is evident (*arrow*) in this duct of a meibomian gland. (H&E × **33**.)

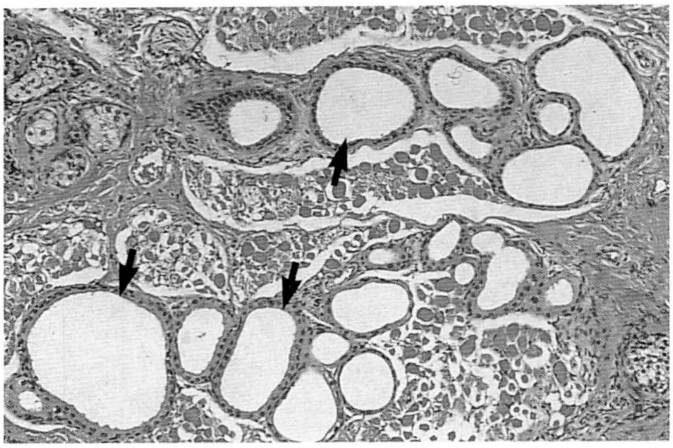

**FIG. 42.** Apocrine glands (glands of Moll) (*arrows*) occur in the eyelid and open into the follicles of the eyelashes. (H&E × **33**.)

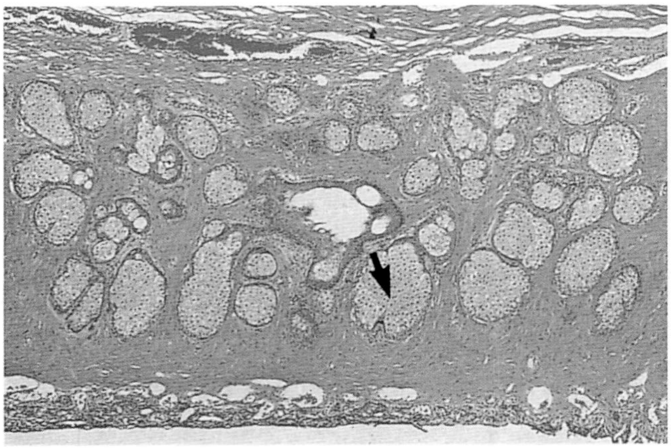

**FIG. 43.** The tarsus, composed of dense fibrous tissue, contains the meibomian glands (*arrow*). The palpebral conjunctiva is immediately beneath the tarsus at the bottom of this figure. (H&E × **13.2**.)

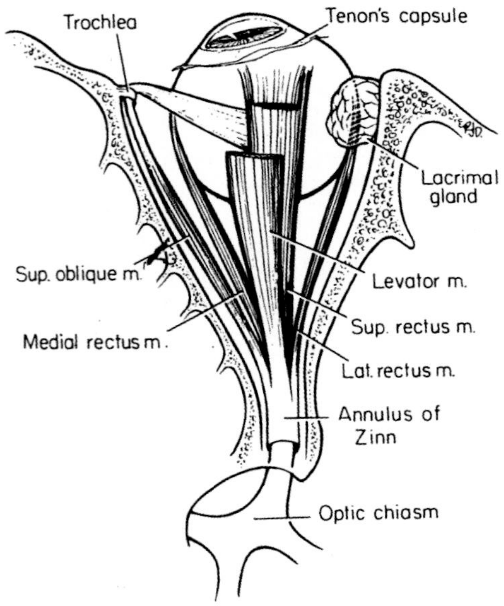


**FIG. 44.** The bony cavity of the orbit contains the eyeball and its fibrous covering (Tenon's capsule), the cartilagenous trochlea, the lacrimal gland, and the extraocular muscles. The trochlea and the lacrimal gland are located within the superonasal and superotemporal aspects of the orbit respectively. Some of the extraocular muscles originate from a ring of fibrous tissue in the posterior orbit known as the annulus of Zinn. (Reproduced from W Tasman and EA Jaeger, eds. Duane's clinical ophthalmology. vol. 2. Philadelphia; JB Lippincott, 1989, with permission.)

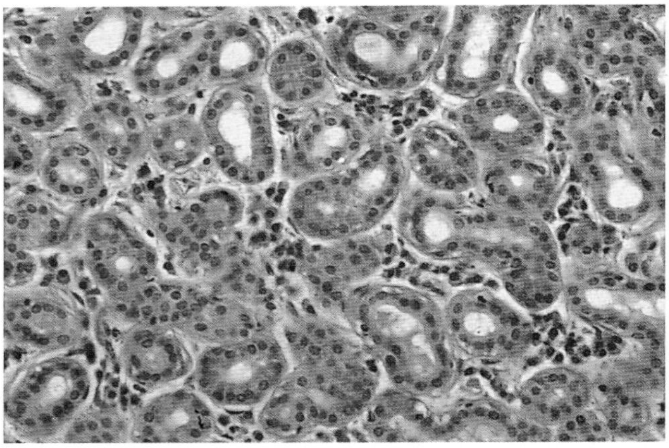

**FIG. 45.** Acini of the lacrimal gland are lined by columnar-shaped epithelial cells. Scattered lymphocytes and plasma cells are normally present in the gland. (H&E × **80**.)

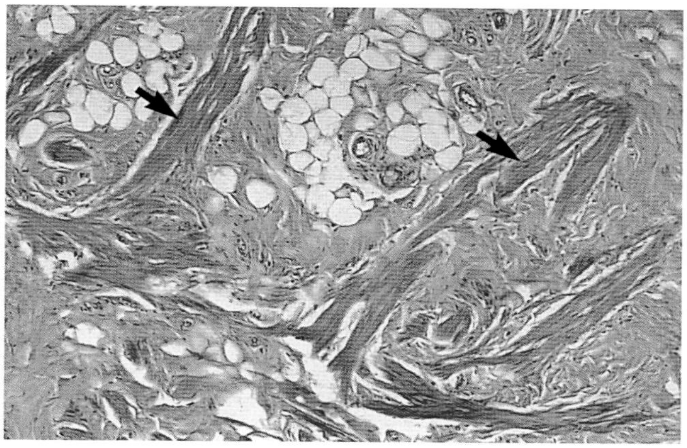

**FIG. 46.** Smooth muscle bundles (*arrows*) are present in the soft tissues of the orbit. (H&E × **10**.)

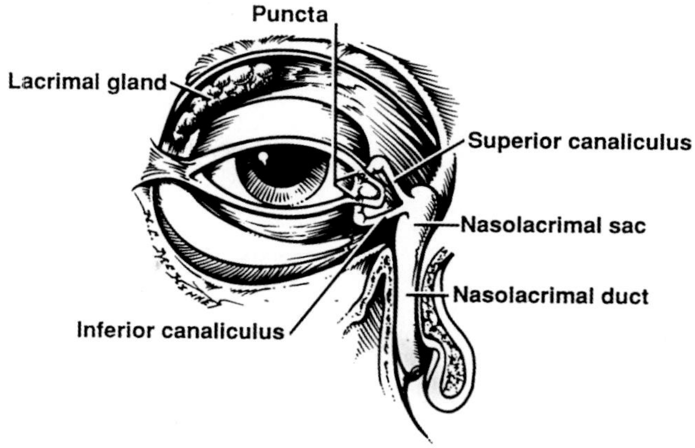


**FIG. 48.** The lacrimal gland and drainage apparatus are illustrated here. The lacrimal gland is located in the superotemporal aspect of the orbit and contributes secretions to the tear film. Tears enter the canaliculi through the puncta and drain through the nasolacrimal sac and duct, to eventually reach the inferior meatus within the nose.

Other constituents of the orbit include smooth muscle (Fig. 46) (13) and the arc-shaped structure, (trochlea), through which the tendon of the superior muscle passes before insertion upon the eyeball (Fig. 47). The trochlea is the only cartilaginous structure normally present in the orbit. It arises from the superior nasal aspect of the frontal bone.

Lymphatic channels do not exist in the orbit according to traditional teaching; but this point is disputed because lymphangiomas develop in the orbit on rare occasions (14). The orbit normally lacks lymphoid tissue, but contains scattered lymphocytes. These cells presumably give rise to the monoclonal and polyclonal lymphoid proliferations that frequently develop within the orbit, creating diagnostic and prognostic difficulty for the pathologist (15).

## LACRIMAL DRAINAGE APPARATUS

The lacrimal drainage apparatus (Fig. 48), composed of the puncta, canaliculi, lacrimal sac, and the nasolacrimal duct, collects the tears and drains them to the nose. Tear fluid drains toward the medial canthus and then passes through an opening in the medial aspect of each eyelid, known as the lacrimal punctum. The puncta drain into the lacrimal canaliculi, tubular structures approximately 0.5 mm in diameter. The canaliculi are, initially, oriented vertically, but within 2 mm of their origin, bend at right angles to become almost horizontal within the eyelids. The distal portions of the canaliculi exit the upper and lower eyelids. They merge to form the lacrimal sac, which is encased by bones located in the inferomedial wall of the orbit. A duct (the nasolacrimal duct) that is nearly 1 cm long drains the lacrimal sac into the inferior nasal meatus of the nose. The epithelium lining the lacrimal drainage apparatus, varies in different regions. In the canaliculi, it is a nonkeratinizing stratified squamous epithelium (Fig. 49), but in the lacrimal sac and duct, the epithelium is stratified columnar in type, and contains mucus-

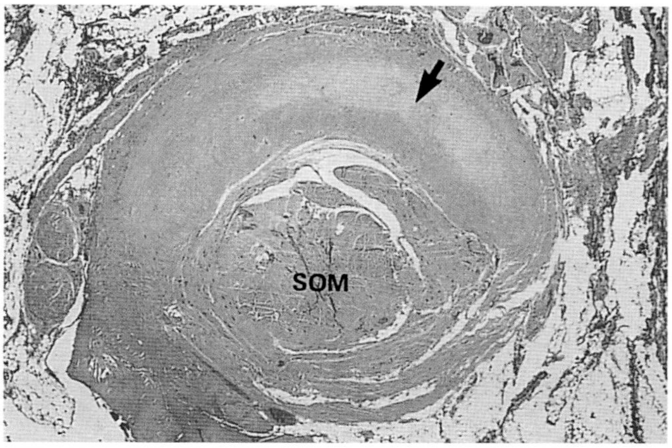


**FIG. 47.** The arc-shaped trochlea (*arrow*), the only cartilaginous structure of the normal orbit, envelops the skeletal muscle fibers of the superior oblique muscle (SOM). (H&E × **5**.)

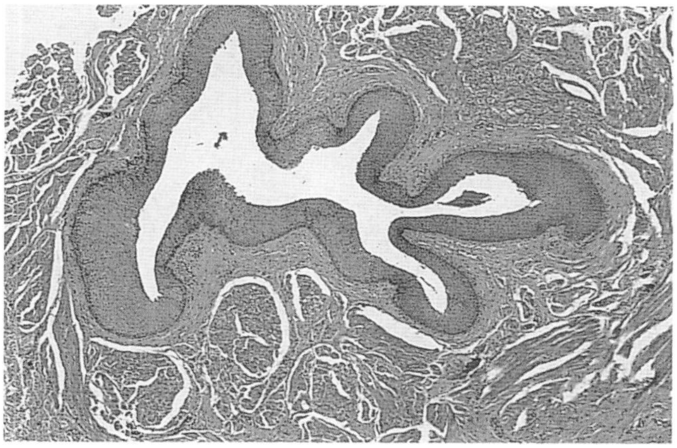

**FIG. 49.** The lacrimal canaliculi are lined by nonkeratinizing stratified squamous epithelium and are surrounded by fibrous tissue. (H&E × **13.2**.)

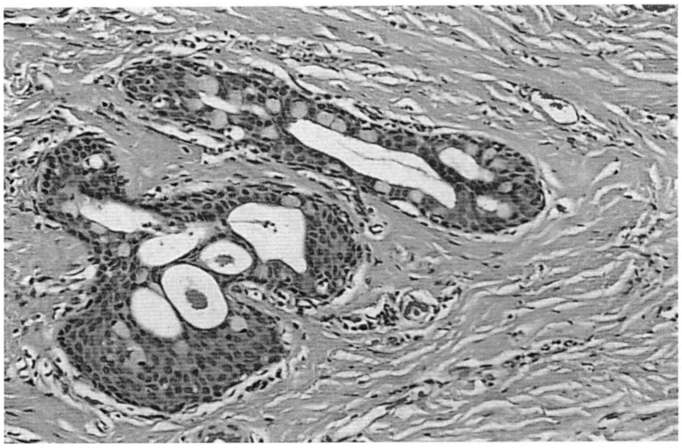

**FIG. 50.** The epithelium of the lacrimal sacs and ducts is stratified columnar and contains goblet cells. (H&E × **50**.)

secreting goblet cells surrounded by connective tissue (Fig. 50).

## REFERENCES


1. Last RJ. *Eugene Wolff's anatomy of the eye and orbit.* 6th ed. Philadelphia; WB Saunders, 1968.
2. Hogan MJ, Alvarado JA, Weddell JE. *Histology of the human eye.* Philadelphia; WB Saunders, 1971.
3. Fine BS, Yanoff M. *Ocular histology: A text and atlas. 2nd ed.* Hagerstown; Harper & Row, 1979.
4. Jakobiec FA, ed. *Ocular anatomy, embryology and teratology.* Philadelphia; Harper & Row, 1982.
5. Bloom W, Fawcett DW. *A textbook of histology. 11th ed.* Philadelphia; WB Saunders, 1986.
6. Gillette TE, Chandler JW, Greiner JV. Langerhans' cells of the ocular surface. *Ophthalmology* 1982;89:700–710.
7. Reese AB. Intrascleral nerve loops. *Arch Ophthalmol* 1931; 6:698–703.
8. Spencer WH. Sclera. In: Spencer WH, ed. *Ophthalmic pathology: an atlas and textbook. 4th ed.* Philadelphia; WB Saunders, 1996:337 (in press).
9. Cogan DG, Kuwabara T. Focal senile translucency of the sclera. *Arch Ophthalmol* 1959;62:604–610.
10. Tripathi RC. Aqueous outflow pathway in normal and glaucomatous eyes. *Br J Ophthalmol* 1972;56:157–174.
11. Straatsma BR, Foos RY. Typical and reticular degenerative retinoschisis. [XXVI Francis J. Proctor Memorial Lecture]. *Am J Ophthalmol* 1973;75:551–575.
12. Adler FH. *Physiology of the eye. 7th ed.* Saint Louis; CV Mosby, 1981: 261–262.
13. Koornneef L. New insights in the human orbital connective tissue. Result of a new anatomical approach. *Arch Ophthalmol* 1977; 95: 1269–1273.
14. Iliff WJ, Green WR. Orbital lymphangiomas. *Ophthalmology* 1979;86: 914–929.
15. Knowles DM, Jakobiec FA, McNally L, Burke JS. Lymphoid hyperplasia and malignant lymphoma occurring in the ocular adnexa (orbit, conjunctiva, and eyelids): a prospective multiparametric analysis of 108 cases during 1977 to 1987. *Hum Pathol* 1990; 21:959–973.

*Histology for Pathologists, second edition,*
Edited by Stephen S. Sternberg.
Lippincott-Raven Publishers, Philadelphia
© 1997.

# CHAPTER 14

# The Ear

Leslie Michaels



Pathologists have tended to bypass the ear as an organ of potential special interest because of its anatomical complexity and the difficulty in preparing and displaying its main parts postmortem for histological examination. Surgical specimens are small; they are usually taken from the external and middle ear. Those from the inner ear are few and related mainly to neoplasms of the internal auditory meatus and, occasionally, to fragments of the vestibular nerve removed during its ablation for severe Ménière's disease. The relative indifference of our specialty to the pathology of the ear is unfortunate. This organ presents as many problems of disease and disability, requiring the particular skills of the tissue pathologist for their interpretation, as does any other organ in the body.

## THE EAR AS A WHOLE

### Embryological Changes

The ear, in fact, is not a single organ, but two, subserving the separate functions of hearing and balance. Developmentally, these two functions are elaborated from a primordial invagination of ectoderm, the otocyst, which produces the epithelia of the membranous labyrinth of the inner ear. Superimposed upon, and developing slightly later, the first and part of the second branchial arch system provide structures that augment the hearing function. The endodermal component of the first branchial system, the branchial pouch, gives rise to the eustachian tube and middle ear epithelia and the corresponding ectodermal outgrowth, the first branchial groove, to the external ear epithelia (Fig. 1). The connective tissue part of the branchial system, the first and second branchial arches, produces the ossicles. The sensory epithelia lining the otocyst-derived cochlear and vestibular labyrinths link up with the eighth cranial nerve outflow from the central nervous system. The cartilaginous, bony and muscular conformations of the ear are developed from the mesenchyme surrounding these early epithelia.

#### *The External Ear*

The pinna develops from six knoblike protuberances arising from the first and second branchial arches, which fuse to form the various auricular components such as the helix, antihelix, and tragus. The external auditory meatus is derived

L. Michaels: Department of Histopathology, University College London Medical School, London WC1E 6JJ, United Kingdom.

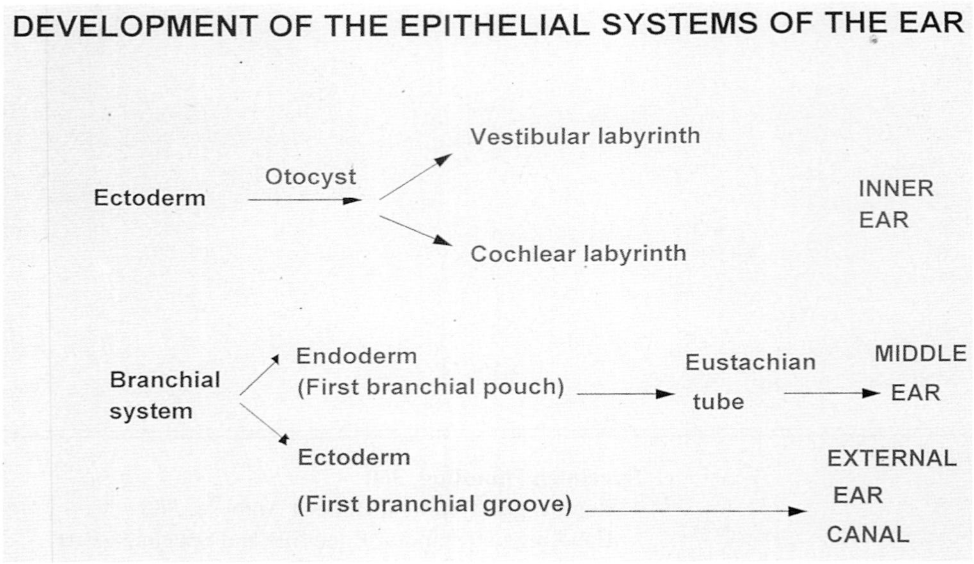


**FIG. 1.** Diagrammatic representation of the embryology of the epithelia of the inner, middle, and external ears.

from the first branchial groove, a depression of the ectoderm between the first (mandibular) arch and the second (hyoid) arch. The deep extremity of this groove meets the outer epithelium of the corresponding first pharyngeal pouch, separated from it by only a thin layer of connective tissue. The point of meeting produces the tympanic membrane. In the course of this development, a complex series of changes takes place, shown to be related to the function of auditory epithelial migration (1–3).

### *Auditory Epithelial Migration*

The stratified squamous epithelium of the tympanic membrane, like all epithelia of this type, matures continuously to produce keratin squames at its surface. In moist mucosal areas (such as the mouth and vagina), the squamous products of such epithelium are washed away. The surface of the deep ear canal and tympanic membrane is dry. Unless a mechanism would exist for the removal of keratin, this material would accumulate on the surface, resulting in defective sound transmission. There is a unique mechanism in this region by which keratin is removed: auditory epithelial migration. The whole epithelium with its keratin moves from the tympanic membrane onto the deep external canal; it then moves laterally, as far as the deep canal's junction with the

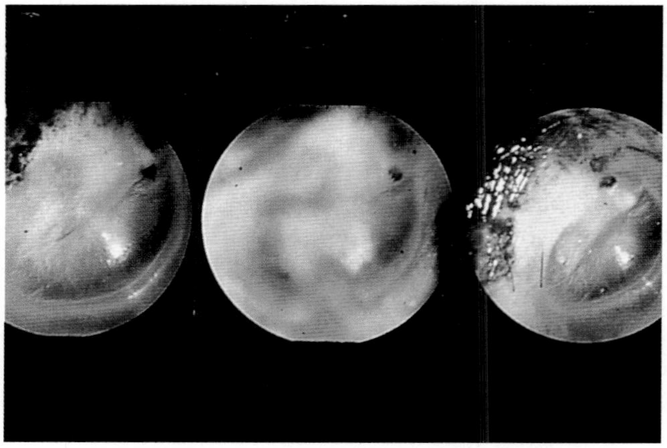

**FIG. 2.** Pathway of auditory epithelial migration as shown by movement of blue dye daubed on tympanic membrane. Dye is seen in the first photograph on the day at which it was daubed, just anterior and inferior to the lateral process of the malleus. In the next photograph, taken 9 days later, it has moved posteriorly and superiorly to lie over that structure. Thirteen days later, in the third photograph, it has crossed the pars flaccida region, moving in the same direction toward the external canal.

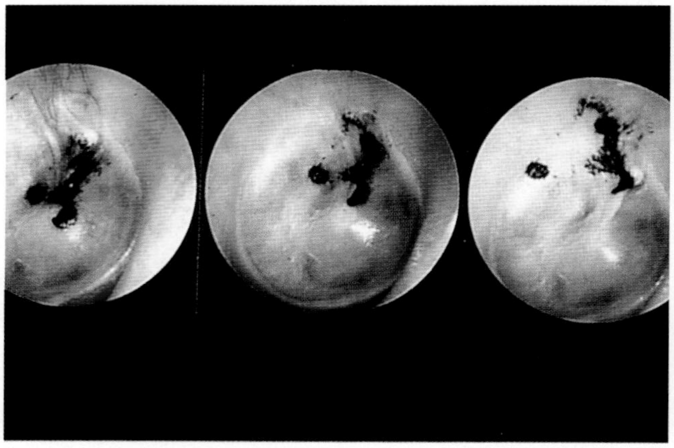

**FIG. 3.** In this daubed tympanic membrane, an irregular array of dye is seen on the handle of malleus region on the sixth day after its deposition, in the first photograph. By the 15th day, in the second photograph, a round dot that was just posterior to the handle of the malleus has separated and is commencing to travel backward, the main mass of dye moving discretely upward along the handle of the malleus. This process has advanced on the 27th day in the third photograph, the posterior dye having reached the back edge of the tympanic membrane and the large mass being now situated across the pars flaccida at an angle that has now changed to a posterosuperior one.

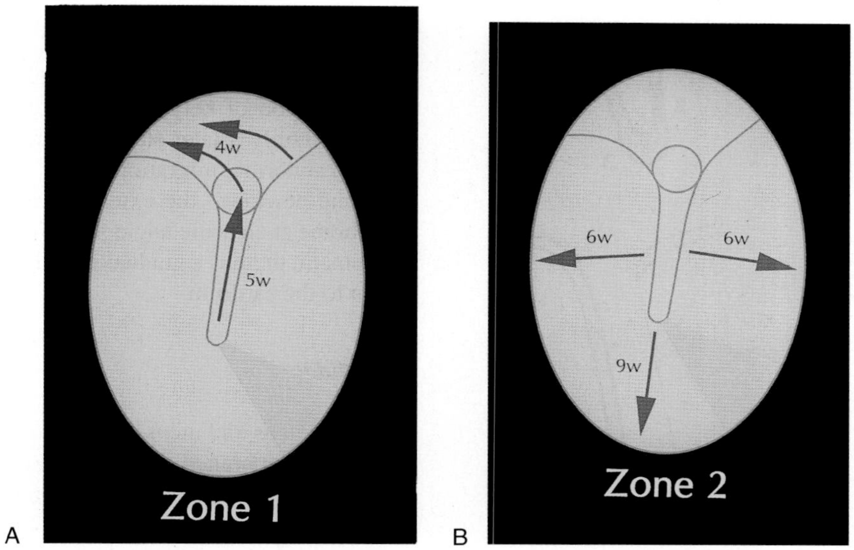


**FIG. 4.** Summary of pathways of migration on tympanic membrane as determined by serial photography of dye markings. The tympanic membrane and adjacent deep external canal epithelium are depicted as being viewed en face. Two discrete pathways are present: **A:** Passing upward along a tongue of epithelium over the handle of the malleus to join epithelium moving in a posterosuperior direction over the pars flaccida region (*zone 1*). **B:** A radial pathway moving centrifugally from the pars flaccida and handle of malleus regions to the periphery (*zone 2*). The times given for each region are the weeks required for dye to be completely cleared from that region.

cartilaginous canal, where it is desquamated. When serial photography of the tympanic membrane is carried out after dots of ink are daubed on its surface, two separate and discrete pathways of migration can be identified (4). The first is upward over the handle of the malleus and then posterosuperiorly across the pars flaccida, from which epithelium passes laterally over the deep canal. The second pathway is radially away from the handle of the malleus and pars flaccida—lower edge to the periphery of the eardrum, and then to the deep canal (Figs. 2–4).

These pathways have been related to the development of the epithelia of the tympanic membrane and deep external canal in the embryo and fetus. An understanding of this development explains the pathways of auditory epithelial migration as a persistence of developmental growth throughout life. It also clarifies the biology of this area and is likely to enhance knowledge on the pathogenesis of cholesteatoma.

From a primordial stage four zones of stratified squamous epithelium have been identified (Fig. 5) (1–3). These have developmental, morphological, and functional differences. Zone 1 is the fundus of the primary external canal. It will become the epithelial covering of the pars flaccida and the tongue of epithelium passing downward over the handle of the malleus. Zone 2 is the epithelium on the medial side of a prominent invagination, the meatal plate (MP). Zone 2 will become the thin epithelium covering the pars tensa. Zone 3, a thicker epithelium, is from the lateral side of the MP, and will produce the deep external canal epithelium. The fundal extension plate is an invagination from which, on its medial side, a large part of the pars flaccida-covering epithelium will develop (the adjacent deep external canal will be on its lateral side). Zone 4 is the side-wall of the primary external canal and from this will develop the superficial, adnexal-bearing, cartilaginous canal.

In the early development of the MP resides the origin of the fundamental processes of auditory epithelial migration. We have observed this development in daily sequence in the

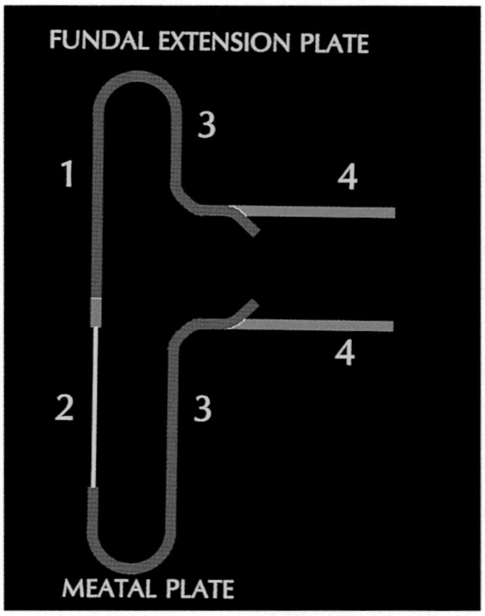


**FIG. 5.** Diagram of primary external canal (first branchial groove) in a 10- to 20-mm embryo showing the origin of the four component zones of epithelium (1, 2, 3 and 4) from the primordial ear canal and the meatal and the fundal extension plates. The inward projection of a bar of epithelium at the junction of zones 3 and 4 denotes loss of epithelium which has migrated from the eardrum.

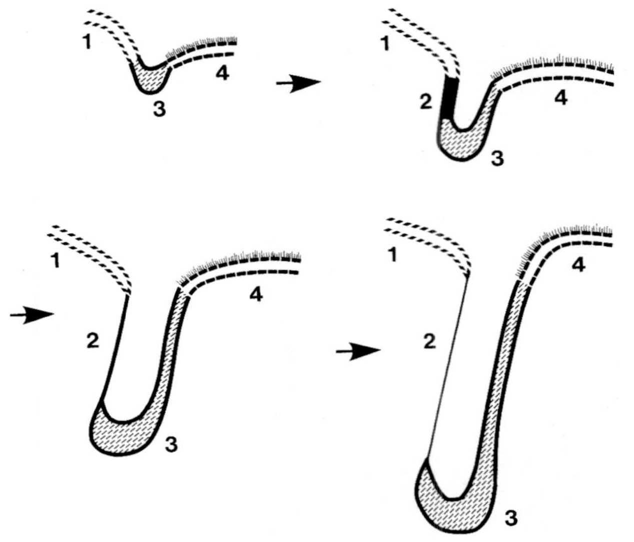


**FIG. 6.** (*Black and white*) Diagram of stages in development of meatal plate into pars tensa of tympanic membrane and adjacent deep external canal.

mouse embryo ear (Fig. 6) (2,3). Observations (though in fewer stages) in the human MP indicate, nevertheless, that it is similar to that of the mouse. Commencing as an ingrowth of cells with marked mitotic activity at the junction of zone 1 and zone 4, the MP becomes elongated towards the tubotympanic recess (early eustachian tube). As it does so, the marked thickening and mitotic activity of cells persists at its tip and, to a lesser extent, on the external side of the MP (zone 3), but there is a progressive attenuation of the internal layer of the MP, (zone 2) which becomes extremely thin and flattened.

Prominent rete ridges are formed in zone 3 in this area and are found there throughout life. Zone 3 extends for a short distance onto the zone 2 (medial) surface of the MP.

The mechanism of the unidirectional movement of auditory epithelial migration is unknown. The pars tensa-covering epithelium (zone 2) is very thin and may move over the basement membrane by an ameboid-flowing action, similar to the action of the epithelium (which it resembles) in wound healing. Mitotic activity favoring growth in the direction of the migration may be responsible for the flux of the thicker epithelia of zones 1 and 3.

The most frequently held concept in the pathogenesis of acquired cholesteatoma is that it is the result of the migration of stratified squamous epithelium from the outer surface of the tympanic membrane inward to the middle ear. However, there is no direct evidence linking cholesteatoma to auditory epithelial migration. Retraction pockets are considered to be frequent precursors of cholesteatoma. Deeply penetrating filaments of stratified squamous epithelium derived from the outer surface of the retracted eardrum have been observed in middle ears in which there are retraction pockets of the tympanic membrane (Fig. 7) (5,6).

Recognition of abnormalities of auditory epithelial migration is just beginning. A newly described condition, keratosis of the tympanic membrane and deep external canal, has been related to abnormal or absent migratory activity (7). The condition of keratosis obturans affecting the external canal, possibly a later stage of keratosis, has also been related to abnormal migration (8).

In the newborn, the external canal meets the tympanic membrane at an acute angle. In the course of subsequent development, there is a gradual straightening of the canal in relation to the eardrum.

### *The Middle Ear*

The malleus and incus are developed from connective tissue of the first branchial arch, Meckel's cartilage. The stapes is formed from the cartilaginous connective tissue of the second branchial arch or Reichert's cartilage. The vestibular wall of the footplate of the stapes is derived from tissue adjacent to the otocyst. The cavity and lining of the middle ear (tympanic cavity) arise from the expanding terminal end of the first pharyngeal pouch (the tubotympanic recess, later becoming the eustachian tube). Subsequently, the epitympanum and mastoid air cells become excavated and epithelialized. The fetal middle ear is filled with a loose connective tissue, known as primitive mesenchyme, which is interposed between the epithelium and the bone. Most of this tissue has disappeared by birth, although traces can still be identified up to 13 months of age.

The basis for the disappearance of primitive mesenchyme at approximately 9 months gestation has been obscure. A strong case has been put forward, based on image analysis of the volume of primitive mesenchyme and that of the middle ear cavity as a whole at different stages of development. The case is that primitive mesenchyme does not disappear, but

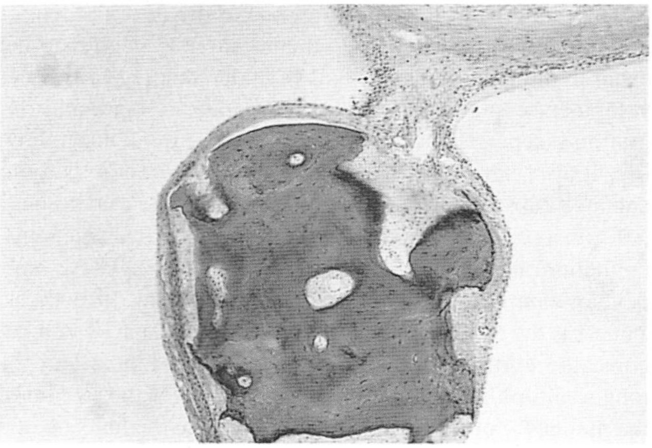

**FIG. 7.** Section of malleus from an adult ear with a retraction pocket of the tympanic membrane at autopsy. There is a thin layer of stratified squamous epithelium between the bone and middle ear epithelium. This was found on serial section to be an ingrowth of the stratified squamous epithelium from the outer epithelial covering of the retraction pocket.

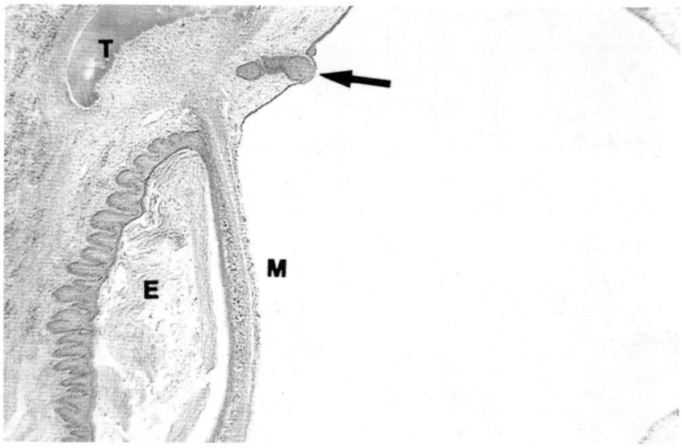


**FIG. 8.** Epidermoid formation (*arrow)* of plunging type at junction of middle ear with eustachian tube epithelium. Note its position in the epithelium, near the edge of the tympanic membrane and overhung by the anterior limb of the tympanic ring (T). It is always found in that position. E, external canal; M, tympanic membrane.

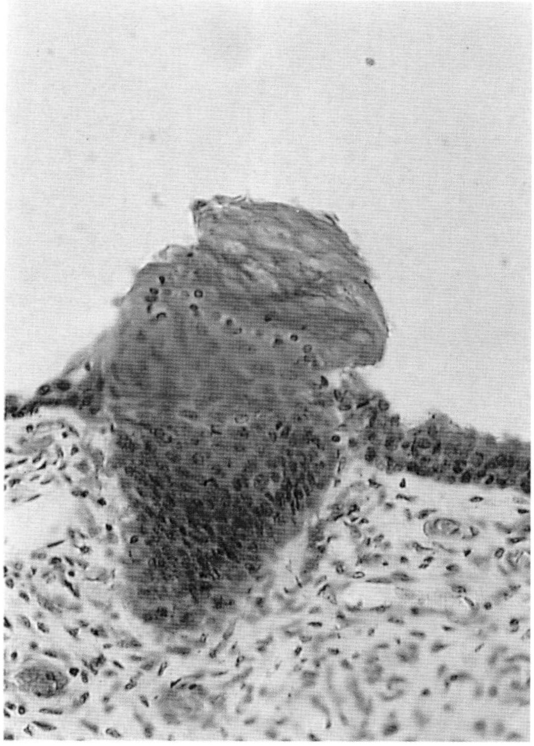

**FIG. 10.** Epidermoid formation with keratinous cap in epithelium at junction of eustachian tube (*columnar*) and middle ear (*cubical*).

simply fails to grow, so that it becomes relatively insignificant in the mature ear (9). The presence of a pathologically low volume of amniotic fluid surrounding the fetus (oligohydramnios) has been correlated with an increased amount of mesenchyme in the middle ear (10).

### *The Epidermoid Formation*

A stratified squamous cell rest, always in the same position, is frequently found in the middle ear of fetuses and young infants (11, 12). This epidermoid formation is prominent during early development when it may act as an organizer at the head of the upwardly migrating tubotympanic recess (13). It lies usually in the epithelium at the junction of the eustachian tube with the middle ear, in the region of the anterior superior quadrant of the tympanic membrane and approximately 0.3 mm anterior to it, adjacent to the bony annulus (Fig. 8). Recent studies have shown that this structure may sometimes be sited over the anterior-superior part of the eardrum, posterior to its anterior edge and even suspended into the tympanic cavity from the eardrum by a short stalk (Fig. 9). The epidermoid formation may appear as an elongated structure, sometimes with a superficial cap of keratin (Fig. 10). It may be spherical, often with central keratinization, sometimes featuring a space among the epidermoid cells (Fig. 11). It may be flat and superficial or even tubular

A

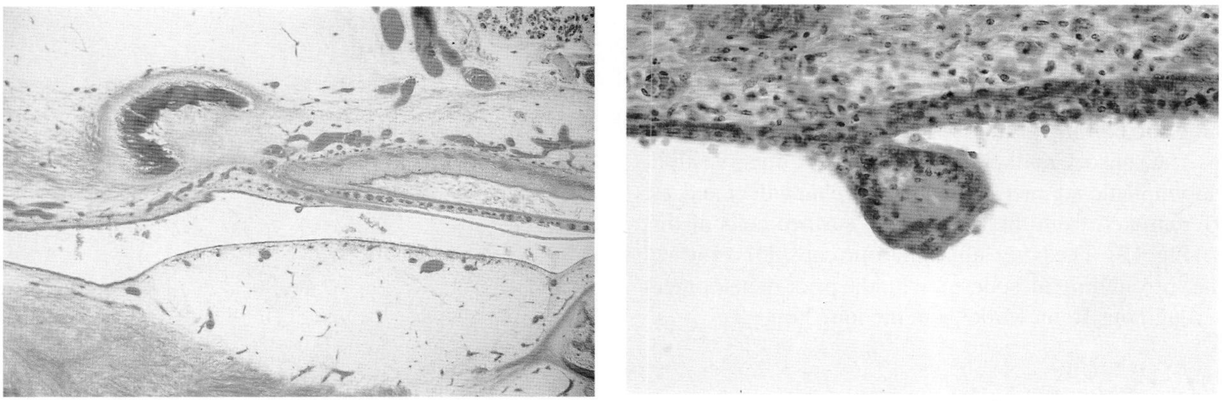

B

**FIG. 9. A:** Low power view of epidermoid formation (*arrow*) suspended into the tympanic cavity from the anterior part of the eardrum by a short stalk. P, primitive mesenchyme; **B:** Higher power of epidermoid formation from (**A**). Note central keratinization.

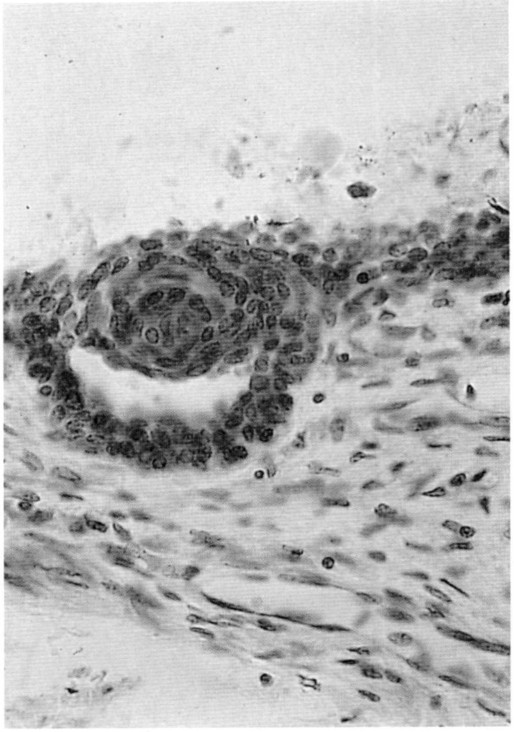

**FIG. 11.** Epidermoid formation with small vesicle giving it an organlike appearance.

with keratinization in the depths of the tube (Fig. 12). The epidermoid formation may be present as late as 6 months after birth; but is not seen in older children or adults.

It is almost certain that continued growth of the epidermoid formation beyond fetal life gives rise to the lesion of congenital cholesteatoma, which has been described recently with increasing frequency in young children. This is situated in the anterior-superior part of the tympanic cavity: in most cases, in the same position as the epidermoid formation (14, 15).

### *The Inner Ear*

The otocyst, after its initiation by invagination of ectoderm, becomes separated from the surface ectoderm and, by branching and coiling, gives rise to the whole endolymphatic system. The sensory epithelia of the cochlear duct, vestibular endolymphatic adjuncts, and endolymphatic duct and sac are differentiated from the inner lining surface cells of this otocyst (Fig. 13). The bony labyrinth (otic capsule) is formed from the surrounding mesoderm, with the prior development of a cartilaginous framework, as in the long bones.

### *Assessment of Maturity of Development*

In some fetal ears, a judgment is required to assess the possibility that there may be retarded development as a result of certain disease processes. This question arises, for instance, in fetuses delivered from mothers with rubella and those with trisomy or other genetic abnormalities. Table 1 lists the stages of the first appearance of some features that may be used in determining the developmental maturity in sections of fetal temporal bone. The table contains previously unpublished data derived from step sections of 61 ears from fetuses representing a broad spectrum of fetal life. Care was taken to use apparently normal fetal ears with no evidence of viral infection or chromosomal abnormality. Only such cases were utilized in which the crown–rump length was known, because this provides a more accurate determination of developmental stage than is given by the date of the last menstrual period. The third column, giving the fetal maturity in weeks, was obtained by reference to published figures relating the age in weeks to crown–rump length (16).

The vestibular structures, the saccule, utricle and semicircular canals, mature early in fetal life. The organ of Corti appears immature (Fig. 14) until a crown–rump length of 11.0 cm (15 weeks) is attained (Fig. 15). The otic capsule commences to ossify at 13.5 cm crown–rump length (18 weeks) (Fig. 15), and the ossicles at 15.5 cm (20 weeks). The stratified squamous epithelium of the deep external canal is fused solidly with that of the tympanic membrane early in fetal life (Fig. 16). Clearing of the deep external canal first begins at 16.5 cm crown–rump length (21 weeks), (Fig. 17) the subsequent development of the external canal showing widening and increase in the angle between the anterior tympanic membrane and deep canal epithelium. Before the 9.5 cm stage, primitive mesenchyme occupies all of the middle ear cleft, except for a small area of clearing continuous with eustachian tube lumen and extending posteriorly as far as the handle of the malleus (Fig. 16). This clearing, thereafter, expands a little posteriorly to the malleus, but it is not until the 25.5 cm crown–rump stage (29 weeks) that large areas of the middle ear cavity appear to be devoid of primitive mesenchyme.

Additional data for assessment of maturity is provided in Fig. 18 which plots the radius of the pars tensa of the tympanic membrane against the crown–rump length in the 61 fetuses. The radius measurement was obtained from the dis-

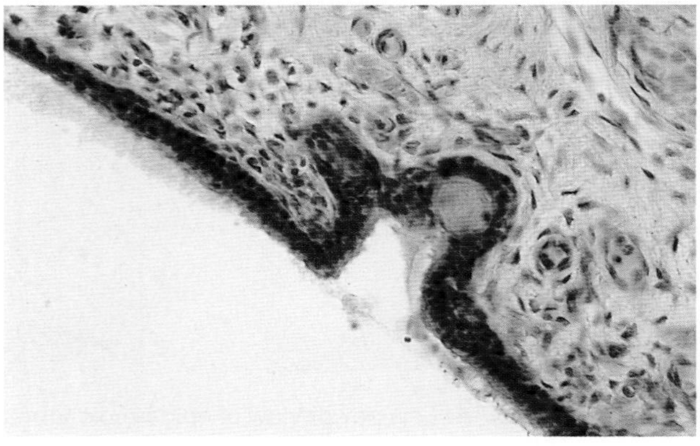

**FIG. 12.** Tubular epidermoid formation with keratinization at the bottom of the tube.

A
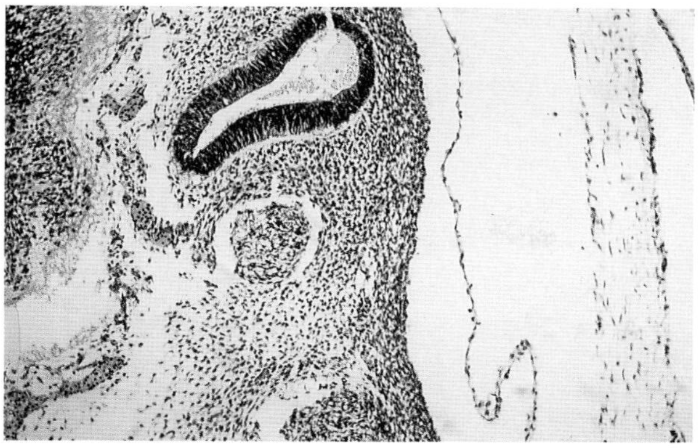

FIG. 13. **A:** Otocyst from 7-mm embryo. It lies just beneath the ectoderm at the side of the head region, from which it has originated and then becomes closed off. The branchial groove has not yet formed.
**B:** Diagram of the development of the labyrinthine system from the otocyst, based on literature sources.
Blue, cochlear development; Red, vestibular development; Green, endolymphatic duct and sac development; ED, endolymphatic duct; ES, endolymphatic sac; LSD, lateral semicircular duct; PSD, posterior semicircular duct; S, saccule; SSD, superior semicircular duct; U, utricle.

B
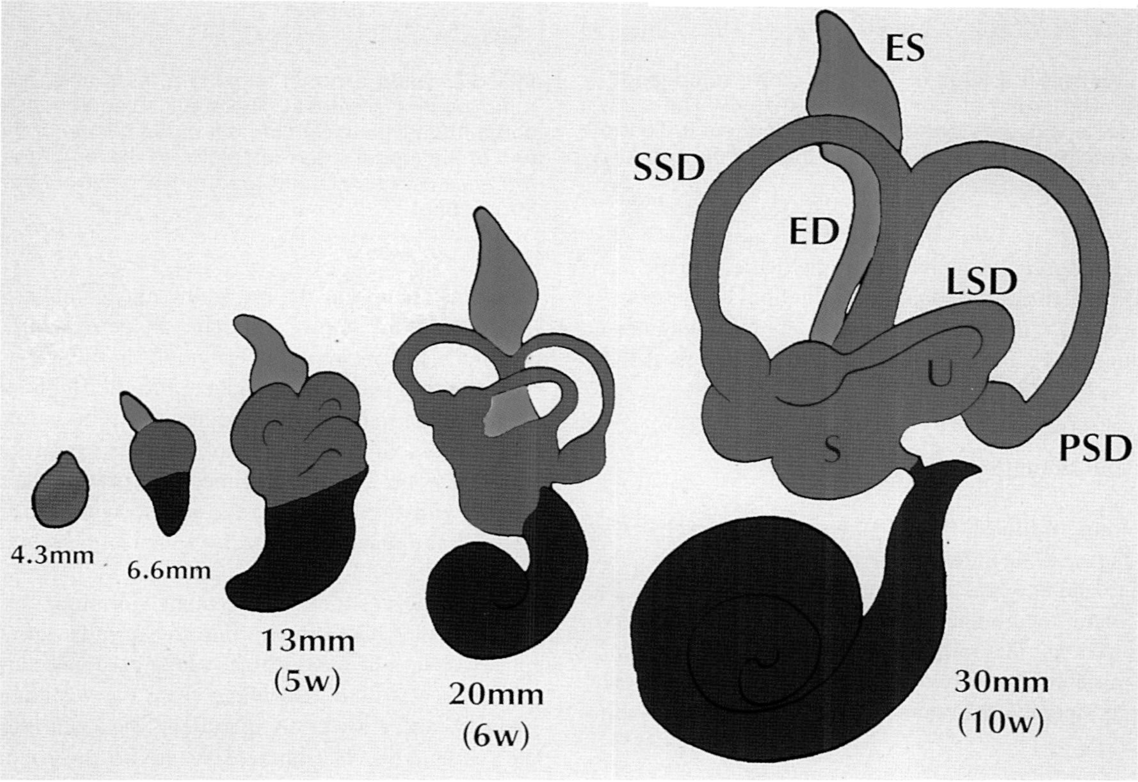


**TABLE 1.** *First appearance of some developmental features in the ear in relation to crown-rump length*

| Developmental feature | Crown-rump length (cm) | Approximate maturity (weeks) |
|---|---|---|
| Maturity of organ of Corti | 11.0 | 15 |
| Ossification of otic capsule | 13.5 | 18 |
| Ossification of ossicles | 15.5 | 20 |
| Cornification of stratified squamous epithelium in anterior part of deep external canal with clearing | 16.5 | 21 |
| Clearing of primitive mesenchyme from large areas of middle ear | 25.5 | 29 |

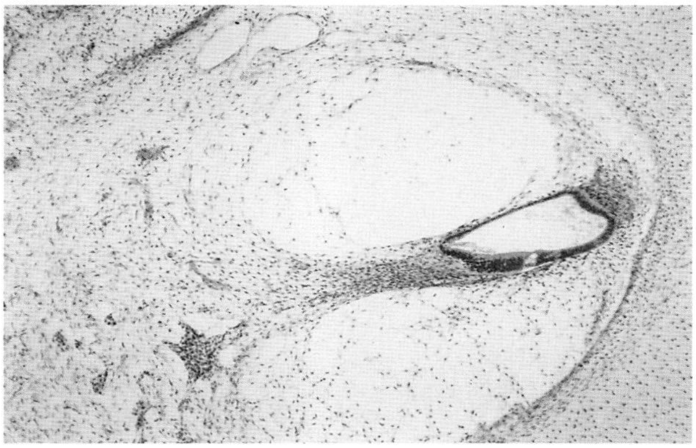

**FIG. 14.** Cochlear duct in one limb of basal cochlear coil in a fetus of 8.5 cm crown-rump length (13 weeks). Note that nerve fibers are in contact with the basilar membrane, but that the organ of Corti is not yet developed. The scala vestibuli has appeared from the mesenchyme, but the scala tympani has not yet formed. The otic capsule (*right*) is composed of cartilage.

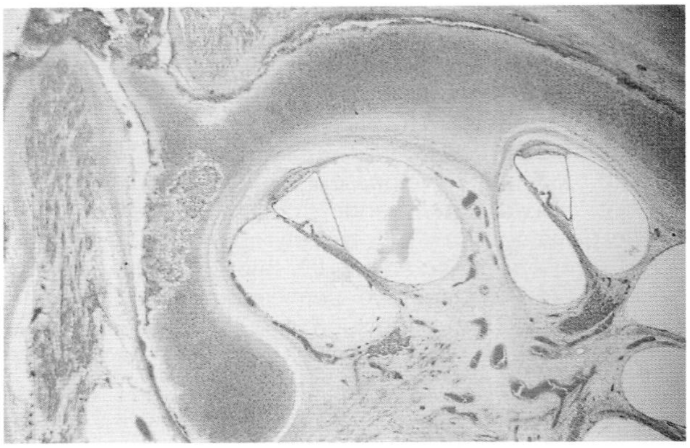

**FIG. 15.** Cochlea in a fetus of 14.0 cm crown-rump length (19 weeks). The organ of Corti appears mature. The cartilaginous otic capsule has started to ossify on the left. To the left of the cochlea is the facial nerve in the internal auditory meatus.

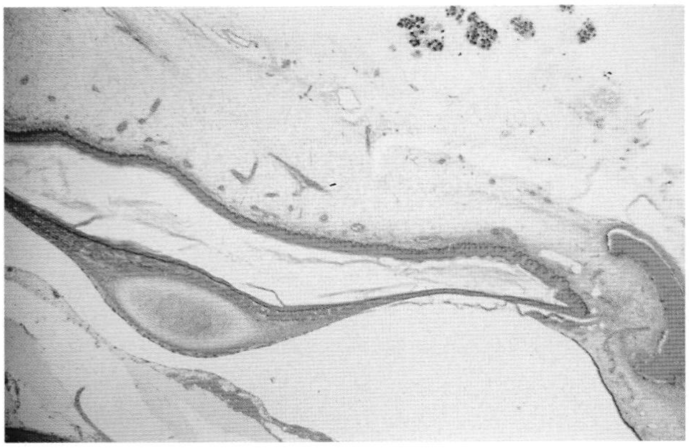

**FIG. 17.** Deep external canal in a fetus of 20.5 cm crown-rump length (25 weeks). The stratified squamous epithelium of the meatal plate (*to the right of the handle of the malleus*) and of the fundal extension plate (*to the left of the handle of the malleus*) has cleared to form the lumen of the deep external canal.

tance of the midpoint of the handle of the malleus to the anterior tip of the stratified squamous epithelium of the external surface of the tympanic membrane. The radius lengthens regularly until it is almost adult-sized in the 28-cm fetus (31 weeks).

### Anatomy and Functions

The anatomy of the ear (Fig. 19) may be assessed by reference to its functions in hearing and balance.

The pinna and external canal conduct sound waves in air to the tympanic membrane, which transmits them by very delicate vibrations. The middle ear enhances this sound energy transmission by conveying vibrations from the larger area of the tympanic membrane through the ossicular chain (malleus, incus and stapes), to the much smaller area of the footplate of the stapes, which lies in the oval window of the vestibule in contact with perilymph. In this way, vibrations representing sound are conducted to the fluids of the inner ear. The air space of the middle-ear cavity is magnified by the mastoid air cells which are complex expansions into the mastoid bone. There is a connection between the middle-ear space with the nasopharynx, and so with the external air through the eustachian tube, by which air pressure can be adjusted.

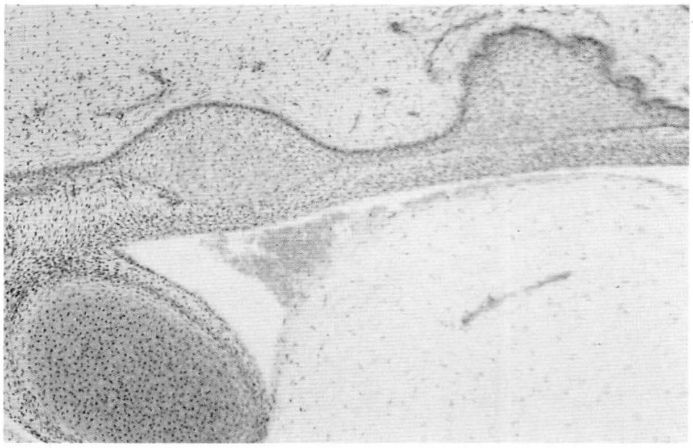

**FIG. 16.** Deep external canal in a fetus of 9.0 cm crown-rump length (14 weeks). The stratified squamous epithelium of the meatal plate, comprising that covering the deep part of the external canal and that of the pars tensa region of the tympanic membrane are fused as a band of epithelium across the upper part of the figure. The handle of the malleus is at the bottom left.

From the vestibular perilymph, vibrations derived from sound waves pass directly into the spirally coiled perilymphatic spaces of the cochlea, where an upper compartment, the scala vestibuli, ascending from the vestibule and oval window and a lower compartment, the scala tympani, may be recognized. The latter descends to the round window membrane, a connective tissue disc separating the perilymph compartment from the middle ear. Between the scalae vestibuli and tympani there is an endolymph-containing coiled middle compartment, the cochlear duct (scala media), which houses the sensory organ of sound reception, the organ of Corti. Waves of vibration are conveyed from the perilymph to the walls of the scala media, from which, through the endolymph, they affect the sensory cells of the organ of Corti.

The cochlear duct communicates with the vestibular endolymph-containing sacs through two fine canals so that the endolymphatic system of cochlea and vestibule is continuous, like the perilymphatic one. Gravitational acceleration of the head is detected in a sensory organ arranged within endolymph-containing sacs in the vestibule (the utricle and saccule), and angular acceleration is detected within tubes emanating in three dimensions from the utricle (lateral, posterior, and superior semicircular canals). The sensory cells are located as a thickened portion of epithelium, the macula, in the saccule and utricle, and as a raised prominence of ep-

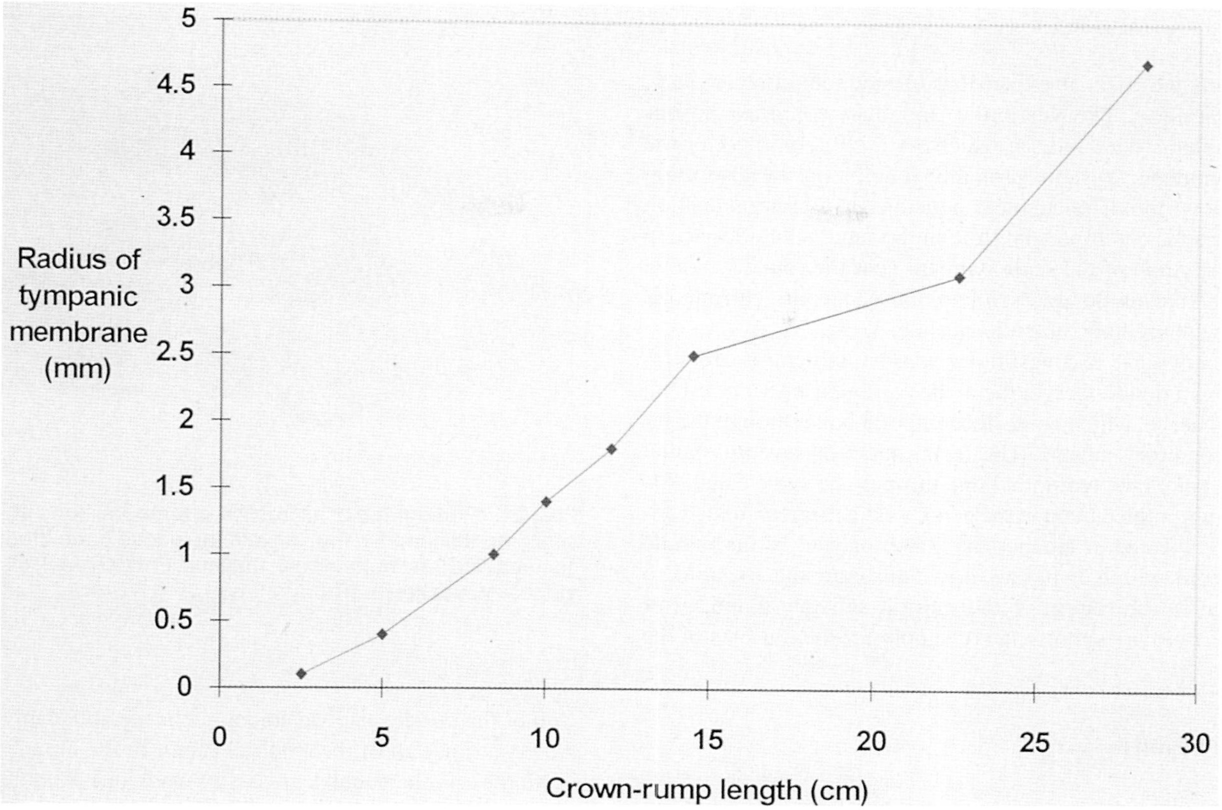


**FIG. 18.** Radius of the pars tensa portion of the tympanic membrane plotted against the crown-rump length in 61 fetuses.

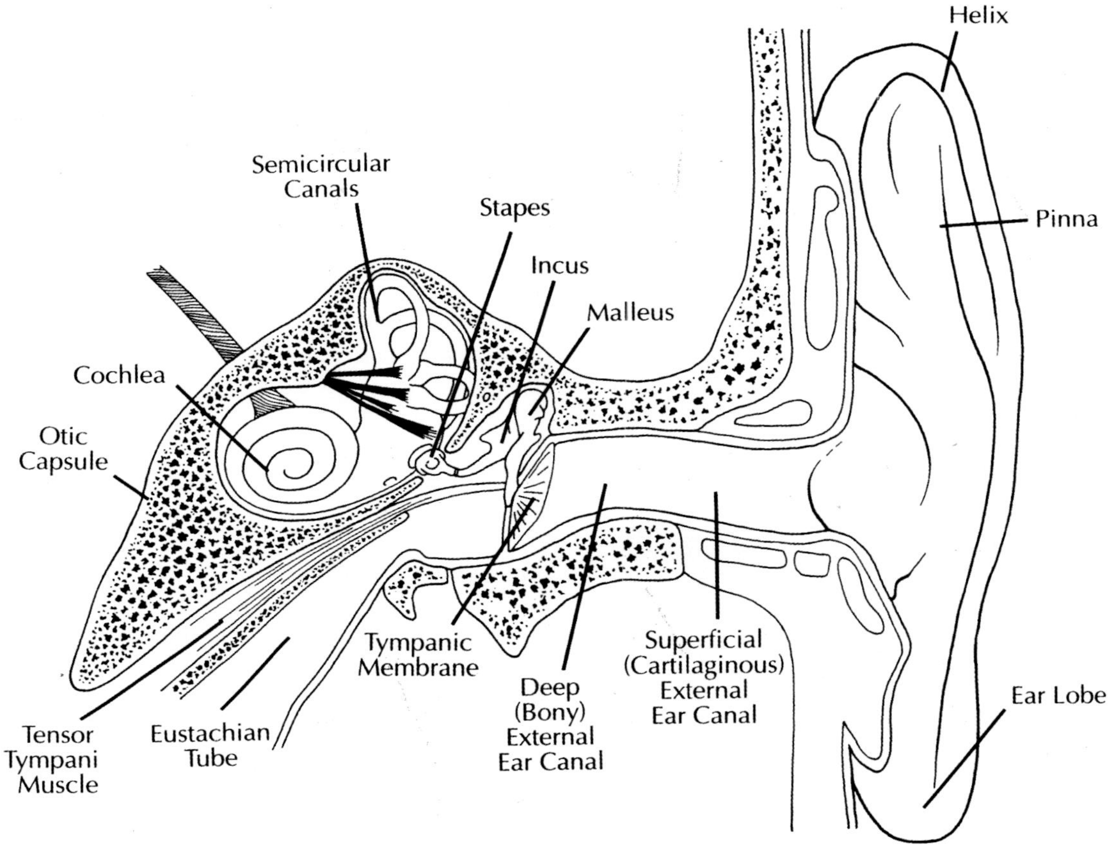


**FIG. 19.** (*Black and white*) Anatomic diagram of ear.

ithelium, the crista, in expansions of each semicircular canal, the ampullae. The vestibular aqueduct contains the endolymphatic duct and sac which are a blind offshoot of the endolymphatic system, probably functioning in absorption of endolymph. The cochlear aqueduct is a communication between the cerebrospinal fluid in the subarachnoid space to the perilymph of the scala tympani near the round window. Cochlea, vestibule, and semicircular canals are surrounded by very dense bone, the otic capsule.

The cochlear and vestibular sensory structures are supplied by a double nerve, the audiovestibular nerve or eighth cranial nerve, which enters the temporal bone through the internal auditory meatus. The facial nerve or seventh cranial nerve, enters the temporal bone through the same canal. After a right-angled bend in the genu, where the geniculate ganglion is located, it reaches the posterior wall of the middle ear, from which it passes down through the mastoid to emerge in the region of the parotid salivary gland, after which it provides motor nerve supply for the muscles of the face.

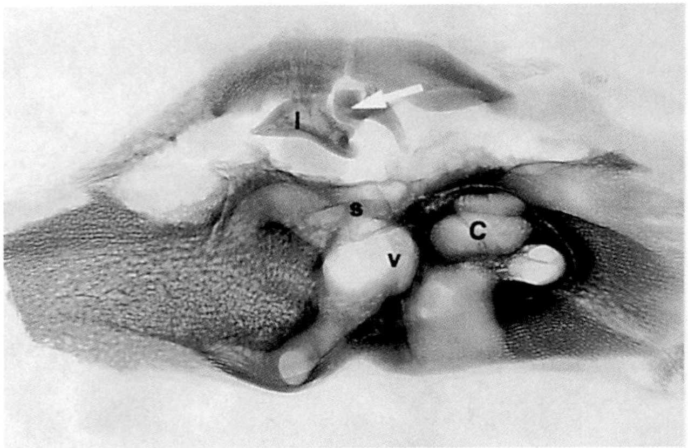


**FIG. 21.** Radiograph of microslice of temporal bone at a level similar to that seen in Fig. 3. Note the dense bone around the cochlea and vestibule. Arrow, malleus; C, cochlea; I, incus; S, stapes; V, vestibule. (From ref. 63.)

### Gross Features

Microslice preparation of the temporal bone (see following) yields a series of specimens in which the gross and radiographic features of external, middle, and inner ears and their neighboring tissues can be delineated (Figs. 20 and 21). The deeper osseous portion of the external auditory meatus terminating in the tympanic membrane, with its attached handle of the malleus, is identified. The ossicles themselves and the joints between the malleus and the incus, and between the incus and the stapes, can be seen. The eustachian tube is observed, opening onto the anterior wall of the middle ear and passing medially toward the nasopharynx. The tensor tympani muscle lies in a canal lateral to and above the eustachian tube. The facial nerve is present in the posterior wall of the middle ear. Mastoid air cells are abundant also in the posterior wall of the external canal. In the inner ear, the vestibule and the cochlea are easily made out. Although not notable in the two photographs, the three semicircular canals–superior, lateral, and posterior–are easily seen in slices at different levels.

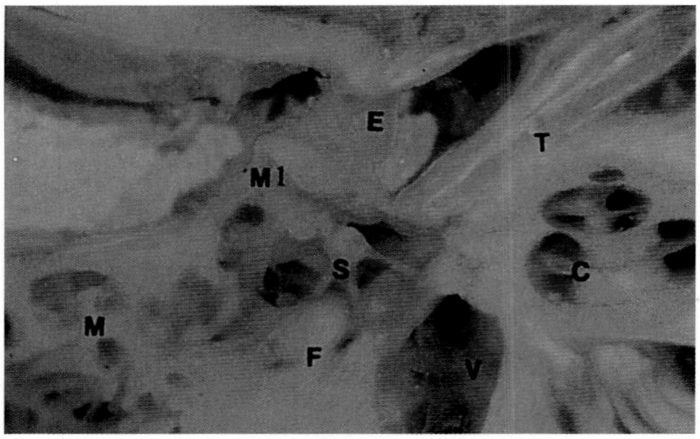


**FIG. 20.** Microslices through a normal temporal bone. C, cochlea; E, tympanic membrane; F, facial nerve; M, mastoid air cells; Ml, malleus; S, stapes; T, tensor tympani muscle; V, vestibule. (From ref. 63.)

### Apoptosis

The spent stratified squamous epithelium at the termination of auditory epithelial migration (see above) probably disappears as a result of apoptosis. Ballooned cells with peripheral, falciform, hyperchromatic nuclei, judged to be apoptotic cells on the basis of thier morphological similarity to some epidermal cells in lichen planus, are seen in large numbers in the stratified squamous epithelium of the deep external canal when developmental reconstruction of ear tissues is taking place, and in smaller numbers in the mature ear (16).

## EXTERNAL EAR

### Gross Features

#### *Diagonal Earlobe Crease*

A crease in the earlobe has been reliably associated with coronary heart disease (Frank's sign) (17), and so may be of interest to pathologists when performing an autopsy. Earlobes may be free or attached, the "soldered" form being an extreme version of the latter (18). Diagonal creases occur in all three forms of earlobes. The crease runs diagonally backward and downward across the lateral surface of the earlobe from the external meatus (Fig. 22). The crease may be classified as Grade 2 if it is superficial and runs across the whole

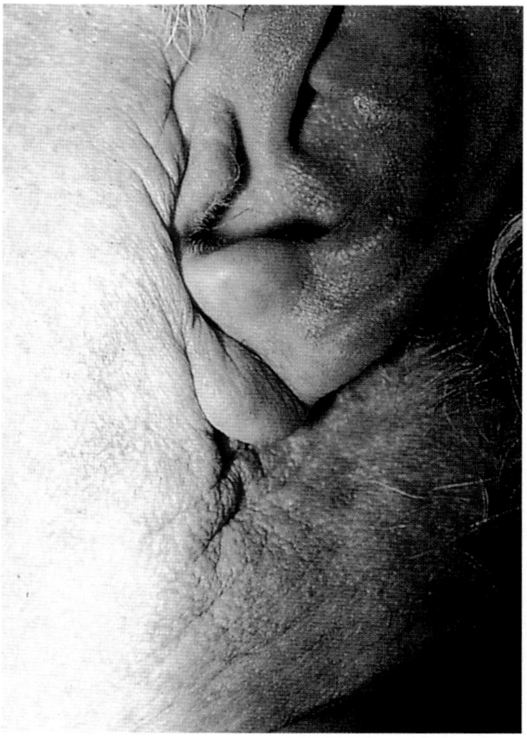

**FIG. 22.** Diagonal earlobe crease in a cadaver, a male aged 76, in whom autopsy revealed changes of severe ischemic heart disease.

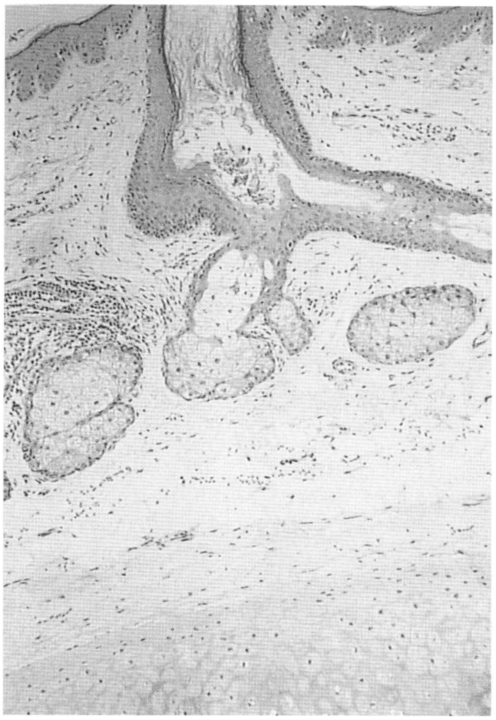

**FIG. 23.** Elastic cartilage, perichondrium, and skin of pinna showing hair follicle and sebaceous glands.

earlobe or, if it is deep but runs across more than 50%, but less than 100%, of the earlobe. Grade 1 is a less obvious-looking crease. It is Grade 3 if it is deep and runs across 100% of the earlobe as in Fig. 11. Bilateral Grades 2 and Grades 3 are associated with a significantly higher risk of death from atherosclerosis and myocardial infarction (19). Not only is there an increased cardiac mortality associated with diagonal creases (20), but also an increased cardiac morbidity (21).

## Light Microscopy

### *Pinna*

The pinna consists of elastic cartilage with a covering of skin containing appendages: hair with sebaceous glands, eccrine sweat glands, and a few ceruminous glands. There is hardly any subcutaneous connective tissue in the pinna except in the ear lobe, where the elastic cartilage is absent and is replaced by a pad of adipose tissue. The perichondrium is composed of loose vascular connective tissue, and is important as the tissue from which the avascular cartilage is nourished by diffusion from a network of capillary blood vessels derived from small arteries and arterioles running in a plane parallel to the surface of the cartilage (Fig. 23). Extensive collections of blood or pus following trauma or infection, respectively, may develop over the perichondrium and by compression of vessels there, lead to cartilage necrosis.

### *External Auditory Meatus*

The skin over the cartilaginous portion of the external auditory meatus shows hair follicles with sebaceous glands and apocrine (ceruminous) glands, but no eccrine glands. The ceruminous glands, of which there are between 1000 and 2000 in the average ear (22), closely resemble the apocrine glands of the axillary and pubic skin. They are found in the dermis at a deeper level than that of the sebaceous glands,

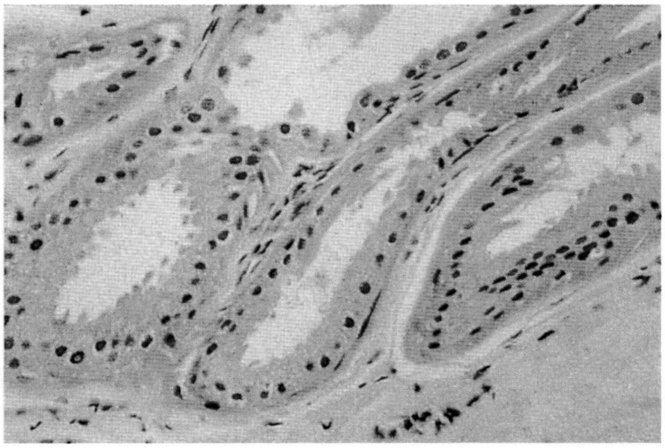

**FIG. 24.** Ceruminous glands of external auditory meatus. Note buds of cytoplasm projecting into the lumen. Brown pigment is present near the nuclei of many of the apocrine cells. An outer myoepithelial layer can be identified in the glands.

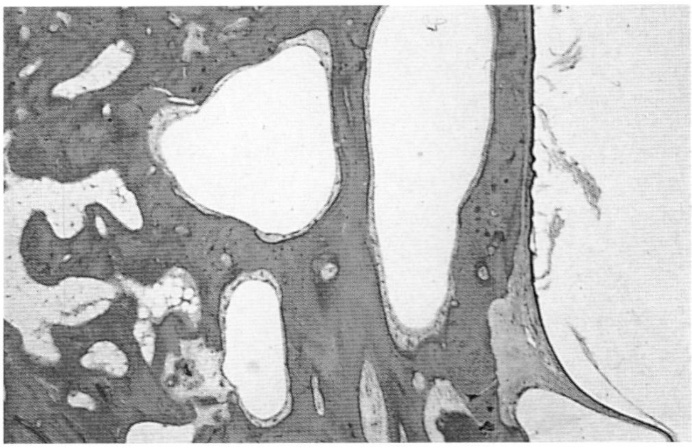

**FIG. 25.** Mastoid air cells (*center*), tympanic membrane (*lower right*), and squamous epithelium of the osseous portion of the external canal (*right*). Note the thin covering of skin over the external ear canal and the proximity of bone to it. (From ref. 63.)

just superficial to the perichondrium. In the ceruminous glands there are inner secretory cells displaying an apocrine-type secretion; that is, buds of cytoplasm that bulge from the surface of the cell into the lumen. There are also yellow-brown pigment granules near the nucleus that are acid-fast and show reddish fluorescence in ultraviolet light. Peripheral to the secretory cells are flattened myoepithelial cells (Fig. 24). The ducts of the ceruminous glands, which do not show apocrine or myoepithelial cells, terminate in a hair follicle or on the skin surface. The rare benign tumor of ceruminous glands, the ceruminal adenoma, usually displays both apocrine and myoepithelial cells.

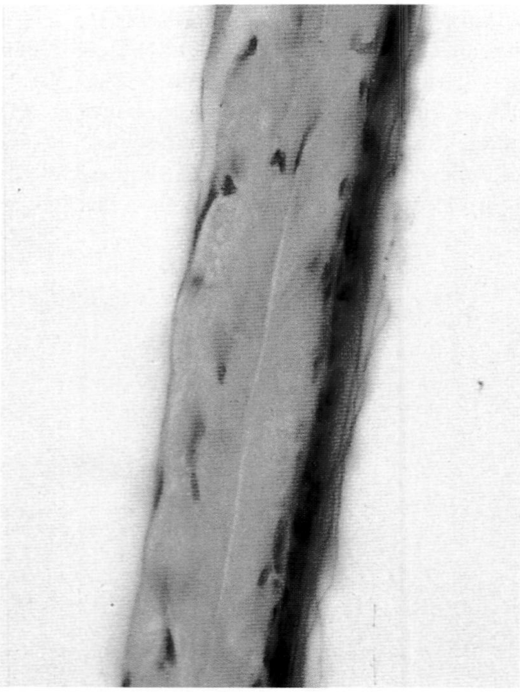

**FIG. 26.** Section of pars tensa of tympanic membrane. The following layers may be distinguished from right to left: stratified squamous epithelium, lamina propria, radial arrangement of collagenous fibers, circular arrangement of collagenous fibers (*i.e., at right angles to former layer*), lamina propria, and middle ear epithelium. (From ref. 63.)

In the deep bony portion of the external canal there are no adnexal structures, and the subcutaneous tissue and periosteum form a single thin layer. The distance between the epidermal surface and underlying bone is consequently small (Fig. 25). which explains the tendency for exostoses of the tympanic bone to develop in this region in cold water swimmers. The water dribbles into the deep canal and cools the bone surface, stimulating it to produce new bone.

#### *Tympanic Membrane*

The pars tensa consists of an external layer of stratified squamous epithelium, a central bilaminated zone (lateral radially arranged, and medial circularly arranged, collagenous fibers), and an internal mucosal layer (Fig. 26). It is a mark of previous inflammatory damage if this architecture is absent. Some elastic fibers are also present near the center and at the periphery of the membrane (23). The mucosal middle-ear surface is a single layer of cubical epithelium that rests on a thin lamina propria.

## MIDDLE EAR

### Light Microscopy

#### *Epithelium*

The epithelial covering of the middle ear is a single layer of flattened or cubical cells. In newborns, several layers of cubical epithelium may be seen in a few areas in response to inflammation (24), and true stratified squamous epithelium is found as the epidermoid formation in fetal life (see above) and in cholesteatoma. However, claims that stratified squamous epithelium is frequent in the middle ear as a result of squamous metaplasia (25) have not been confirmed.

Ciliated pseudostratified columnar epithelium can be seen in small patches among the cubical epithelial cells of the middle ear, but extensive "tracts" of ciliated cells that have been reported have not been substantiated (26). Inflammatory aural polyps, which grow from the medial surface of the middle ear, often show a partial covering of true ciliated epithelium (Fig. 27).

Periodic acid-Schiff positive (neutral mucopolysaccharide-containing) and alcian blue stained (acid mucopolysaccharide-containing) cells have been found in the middle ear, mostly adjacent to the eustachian tube in adults (27) and in children (28).

#### *Glandular Metaplasia*

The epithelium of most of the respiratory tract, including that of the cartilaginous portion of the eustachian tube, contains tubuloalveolar glands often with mucous and serous elements (see following). The middle ear, however, does not normally display these structures. Under pathological condi-

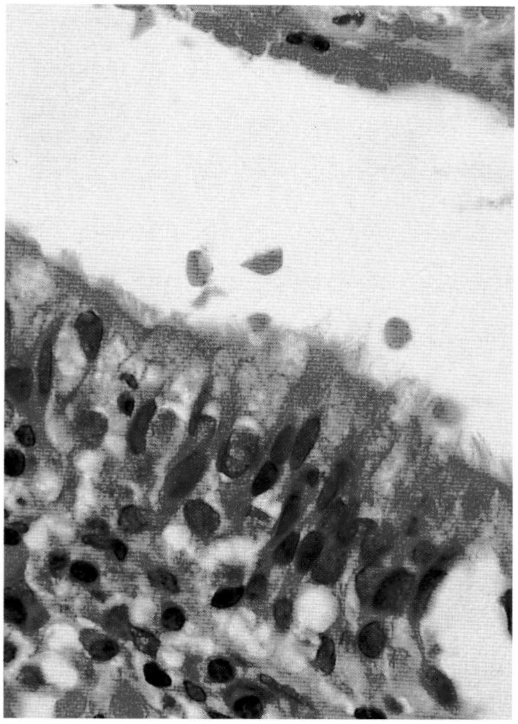

FIG. 27. Aural polyp derived from middle ear mucosa. The covering is of cells bearing cilia. (Oil immersion photograph.)

tions, however, the middle ear epithelium comes to resemble other parts of the respiratory tract by the formation of glands, but the middle ear glands consist only of a simple tubule of mucous-producing cells (Fig. 28). Glandular metaplasia of the middle ear has been described as the main lesion of chil-

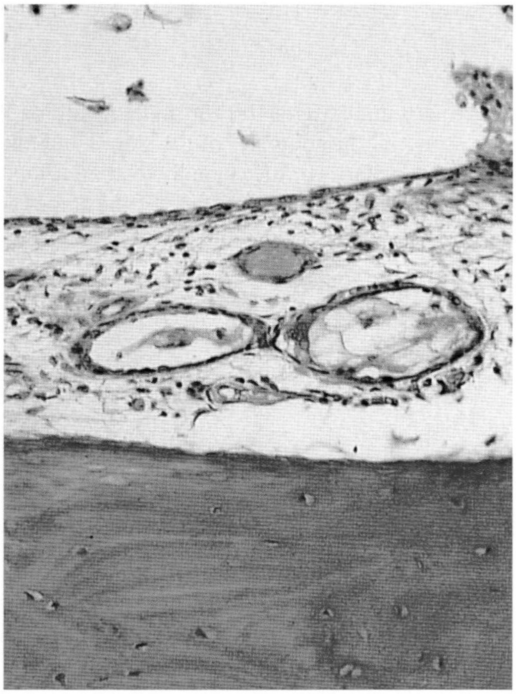

FIG. 28. Glands formed in mucosa of middle ear in association with an inflammatory process.

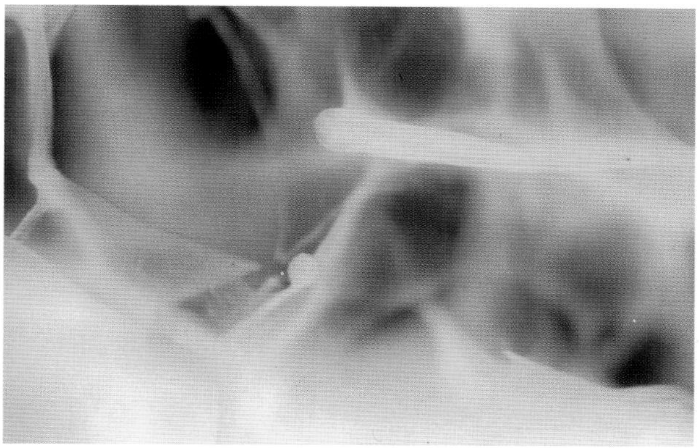

FIG. 29. Mastoid air cells in microsliced preparation showing numerous fibrous septa. Middle ear corpuscles are seen as spherical, elongated or pear-shaped swellings on some of the septa.

dren with secretory otitis media (29) and is also a prominent feature of the middle ear of patients with AIDS (30).

### *Mastoid Air Cells*

The mastoid air cells are a network of intercommunicating spaces that emanate from the tympanic cavity. Each air cell has a thin frame of lamellar bone, covered by a periosteum on which the middle ear epithelium rests (Fig. 25). In acute otitis media the mastoid air cells become filled with pus.

### *Middle Ear Corpuscles*

Middle ear corpuscles are smooth translucent, pear-shaped or oval-swelling usually found growing on fibrous septa, which appear in the mastoid air cells with advancing age (Fig. 29) (31). Microscopically, they are concentrically laminated masses of collagen, resembling corpora amylacea of the lung or prostate (Fig. 30). In frozen sections carried out on the middle ear, usually during operations for squa-

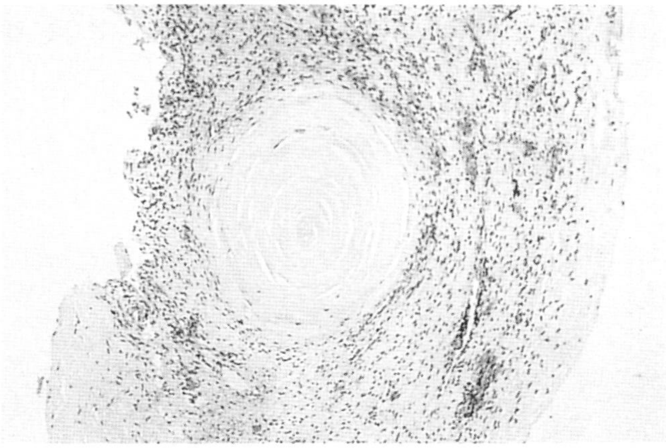

FIG. 30. Middle ear corpuscle composed of many layers of concentric lamellae. It is surrounded by inflammatory fibrous tissue. (From ref. 63.)

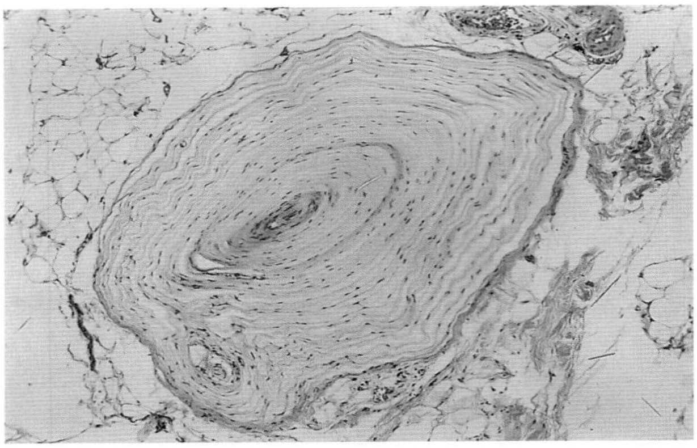

**FIG. 31.** Pacinian corpuscle from subcutaneous tissue near pinna. Note concentrically lamellated elongated cells, which are nucleated. The central condensation houses a nerve fiber.

mous cell carcinoma, they may be mistaken for pearls of keratinizing neoplasm. They have also been confused with pacinian corpuscles, but they lack the fine innervation and the nucleated concentric layers of the latter (Fig. 31).

### *Eustachian Tube*

The eustachian tube is covered by ciliated pseudostratified columnar (respiratory) epithelium, about one-fifth of which is composed of goblet cells; the proportion of the latter increases in middle ear infection (32). Beneath the epithelium are groups of lymphocytes, "Gerlach's tubal tonsil," (Fig. 32) probably the result of inflammation (33). Seromucinous glands are seen in the submucosa of the cartilaginous portion of the tube (Fig. 33) and, to a lesser extent, nearer the tympanic end of the tube. They are also increased in chronic otitis media (34,35). The cartilage at the nasopharyngeal end of the eustachian tube is a hyaline type. The mucosa of the osseous portion of the eustachian tube is separated from the carotid canal by a plate of bone, which is less than 1 mm in thickness (Figs. 34 and 35), and frequently shows dehiscence

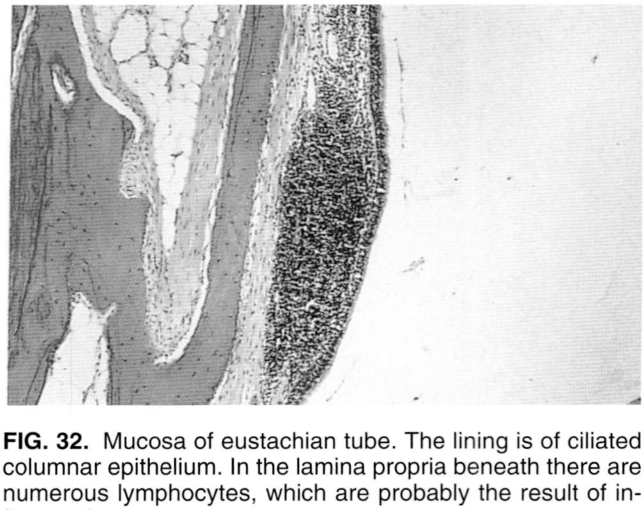

**FIG. 32.** Mucosa of eustachian tube. The lining is of ciliated columnar epithelium. In the lamina propria beneath there are numerous lymphocytes, which are probably the result of inflammation.

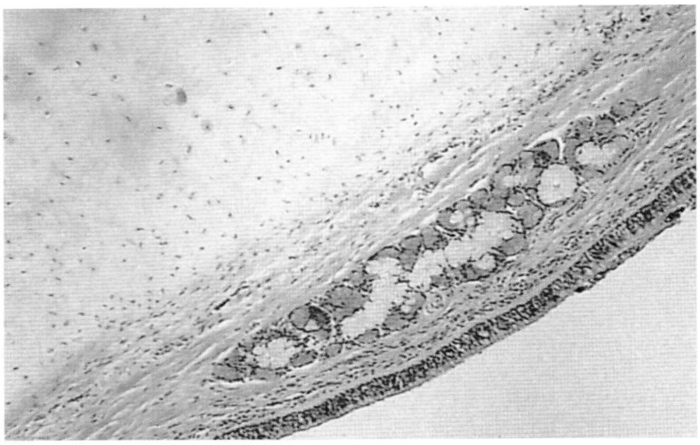

**FIG. 33.** Cartilaginous portion of eustachian tube with seromucinous glands.

(36). This can easily be penetrated by squamous carcinoma of the middle ear and eustachian tube to reach the carotid canal, where it tends to spread widely (37). The intactness or otherwise, of this thin plate of bone in the patient with squamous carcinoma of the middle ear, can be detected by imaging (38). Thin bone also separates the tube from the tensor tympani muscle superiorly and from air cells inferiorly and laterally.

### *Auditory Ossicles*

The auditory ossicles develop from cartilage with but a single center of ossification for each and no epiphyseal ossification. The persistence of cartilage in each of the ossicles and the bifurcation of the stapes to form the crura with the obturator foramen between them, distinguishes the auditory ossicles from other long bones (39) (Table 2).

### *Stapes*

Cartilage is retained as a thin horizontal lamina on the vestibular aspect of the footplate of the stapes and also covers the articular surfaces of the stapediovestibular joints (annulus fibrosus). The vestibular surface of the stapes is lined

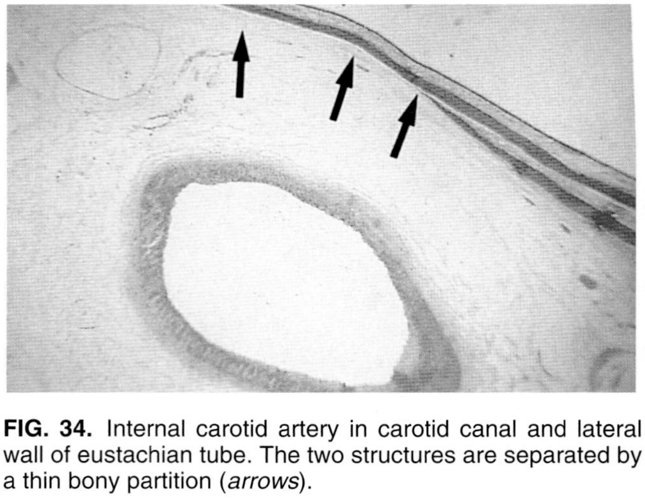

**FIG. 34.** Internal carotid artery in carotid canal and lateral wall of eustachian tube. The two structures are separated by a thin bony partition (*arrows*).

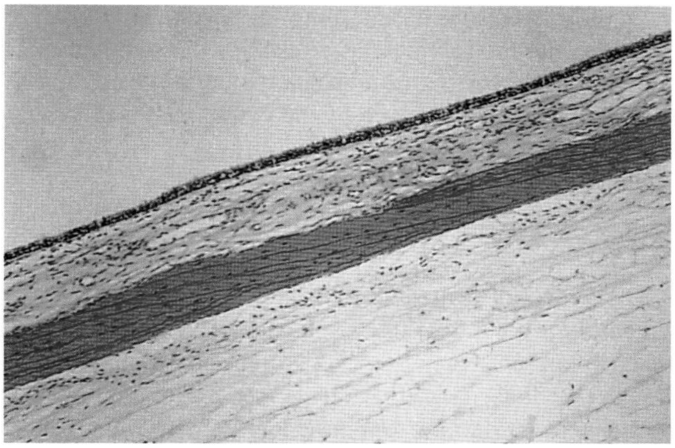

**FIG. 35.** Higher power view of bony portion of eustachian tube and thin partition of bone separating it from carotid canal.

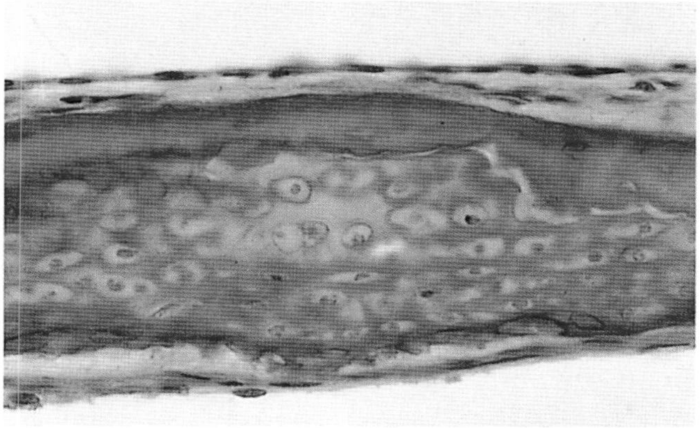

**FIG. 36.** Stapes footplate. Beneath the cubical epithelium of the middle ear above, there is a thin layer of bone. Below this the footplate consists of cartilage and there is a basal flattened layer of cells comprising the lining of the vestibule. (From ref. 63.)

by a single flattened layer of cells characteristic of the perilymphatic space. A thin layer of bone is exterior to the cartilage on the middle ear surface of the footplate. Occasionally, it contains areas of cartilage that extend from the vestibular to the tympanic surface (Fig. 36). The crura are formed of periosteal bone only (Fig. 37). Endochondral bone, which covered the inner part of the crura earlier in development, is completely eliminated during later development of the obturator foramen. The head of the stapes is composed of endochondral bone capped by a cartilaginous layer at the incudostapedial joint.

In a small proportion of temporal bone sections an artery, the persistent stapedial artery, is present. It arises from the internal carotid artery, passes into the middle ear, and then runs through the obturator foramen of the stapes, eventually entering the middle cranial fossa through the fallopian canal of the facial nerve.

### *Specimen After Stapedectomy*

Stapedectomy is performed to remove the fixation caused by otosclerosis. The fixed stapes is then replaced by a mobile prosthesis. The surgical pathology specimen of stapes is

**TABLE 2.** *Types of bone and persistence of cartilage in the parts of the auditory ossicles*

| | |
|---|---|
| *Stapes* | |
| Head: | Endochondral bone<br>Cartilaginous surface |
| Crura: | Periosteal bone only |
| Footplate: | Endochondral bone on tympanic surface<br>Cartilage on vestibular surface |
| Stapediovestibular joints: | Cartilage |
| *Incus* | |
| Body and long process: | Outer covering of periosteal bone<br>Inner core of endochondral bone<br>Islands of endochondral bone with cartilage occasionally retained |
| Articular process: | Articular cartilage |
| Short process: | Tip of cartilage |
| *Malleus* | |
| Head and upper handle: | Outer covering of periosteal bone<br>Inner core of endochondral bone |
| Articular process: | Articular cartilage |
| Lower part of handle: | Shell of cartilage (no periosteal bone). Perichondrium merges with central fibrous tissue of tympanic membrane<br>Inner core of endochondral bone |
| Anterior process: | Membrane bone |

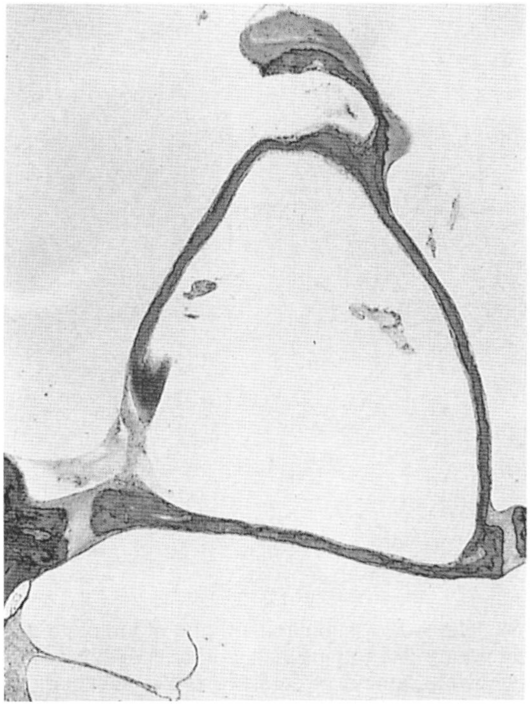

**FIG. 37.** Stapes showing two crura and footplate below. Note the stapediovestibular joints adjacent to the footplate on each side. (From ref. 63.)

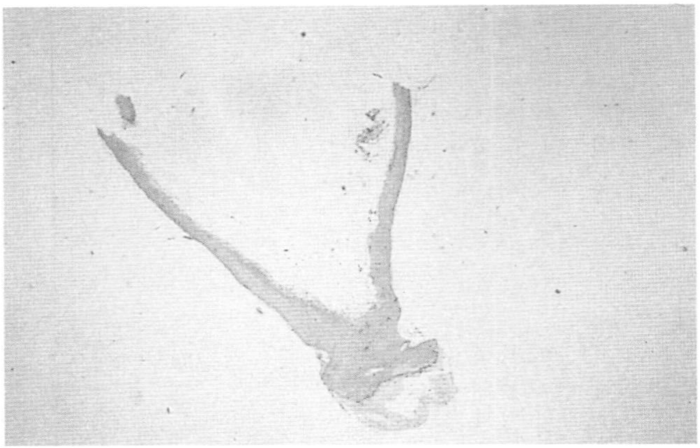

**FIG. 38.** Superstructure of stapes removed at partial stapedectomy. The footplate has not been removed. Such a specimen never shows changes of otosclerosis.

composed either of the superstructure (the head and crura) alone without the footplate (Fig. 38), or of the whole ossicle including the footplate. Otosclerosis is seen only in the footplate because the fixation causing deafness is often the result of extension of the otosclerotic process from the adjacent temporal bone across the annulus fibrosus (stapediovestibular joint) (Fig. 39). In many cases, not even the footplate will

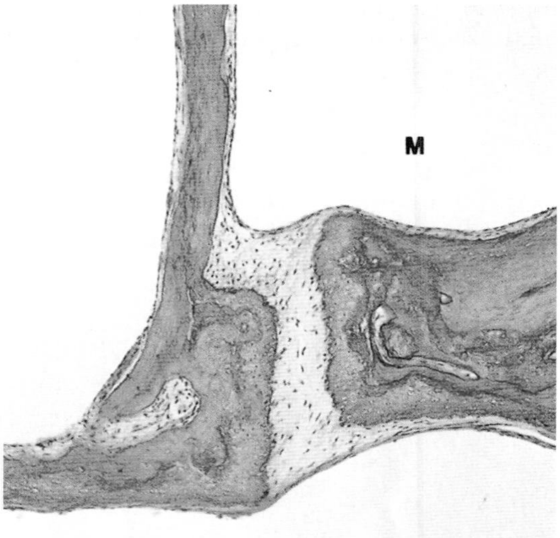


**FIG. 39.** Stapediovestibular joint, part of footplate of stapes, adjacent bony labyrinthine wall, and crus of stapes. The footplate shows a lamina of cartilage on its vestibular surface, which is continuous with the cartilage of the stapediovestibular joint. M, middle ear cavity; V, cavity of vestibule. (From ref. 63.)

show otosclerosis because fixation has been caused only by pressure onto the footplate as a result of the swelling of the otosclerotic process in the adjacent temporal bone. Thus, the specimen of stapes received by the pathologist is most often free from changes of otosclerosis.

### *Malleus and Incus*

The structure of malleus and incus is more like that of a typical long bone than that of the stapes. There is an outer covering of periosteal bone and an inner core of endochondral bone, both showing well-formed haversian systems. Both layers are subject to removal and replacement by new bone. Bone removal may give rise to pits on the surface of the ossicles, which should not necessarily be interpreted as the erosive effects of inflammation. The sites of fresh bony deposition are indicated by the presence of cement lines. Islands of endochondral bone with cartilage similar to the globuli ossei of the otic capsule (see following) are sometimes found in the incus and malleus.

Most of the malleus handle does not have a shell of periosteal bone; instead, there is a layer of retained cartilage. The handle merges with the middle collagenous layer of the tympanic membrane. Superiorly, the malleus handle is separated from the eardrum by a ligament covered by middle-ear epithelium. Lower down, the malleus handle is invested by the middle fibrous layer of the tympanic membrane (40). The inner core of the whole of the malleus handle is composed of endochondral bone like that of the rest of the malleus. The articular process of the malleus is covered by cartilage. The anterior process of the malleus is, unlike the rest of the malleus, formed in membrane early in fetal life, and merges with the malleus soon after its formation.

The short process of the incus shows a tip of unossified cartilage. Cartilage also covers the articular surfaces of the incus at its two joints.

### *Middle Ear Joints*

The incudomalleal and incudostapedial joints (Figs. 40 and 41) are diarthrodial. The space between the articular ends is occupied largely by fibrocartilage–the articular disc. The joint capsule is lined on its outer surface by middle-ear epithelium and on its inner surface by synovial membrane. The capsule is of fibrous tissue with a very high elastic fiber content.

The cartilaginous edge of the footplate of the stapes, the stapediovestibular joint, is bound to the cartilaginous rim of the vestibular window by a fibrous connection, the annular ligament (Fig. 39). A small cavity may be found in most adult annular ligaments (41). Elastic fibers are prominent near the surfaces of the ligaments (42).

In the bone just anterior to the joint, there is often seen a canal linking the middle ear with vestibule, the fissula ante fenestram. We have found that it develops as a slit filled with

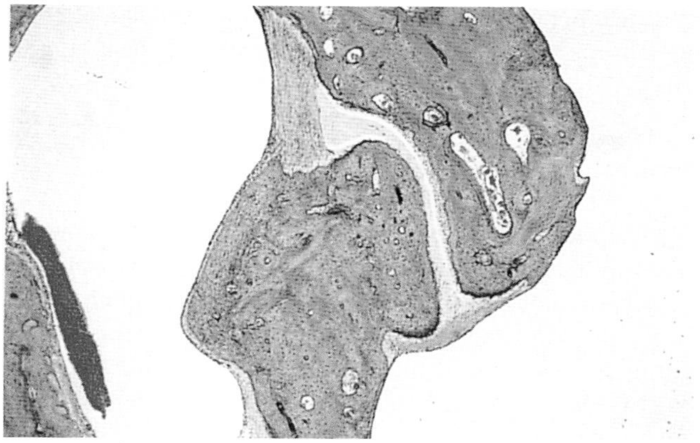

FIG. 40. Incudomalleal joint. Note the joint capsule at each end of the joint. The joint space is occupied by the fibrocartilage of the articular disc. (From ref. 63.)

fibrous tissue, often with associated cartilage. Its presence has been thought to be related to otosclerosis because both are seen in a similar position, but this is not yet confirmed.

### *Middle Ear Muscles*

The tensor tympani and stapedius muscles are composed of fibers with a penniform (i.e., feather-shaped) arrangement, showing a central tendon formed by elastic tissue with muscle fibers radiating from it (Fig. 42). The tensor tympani

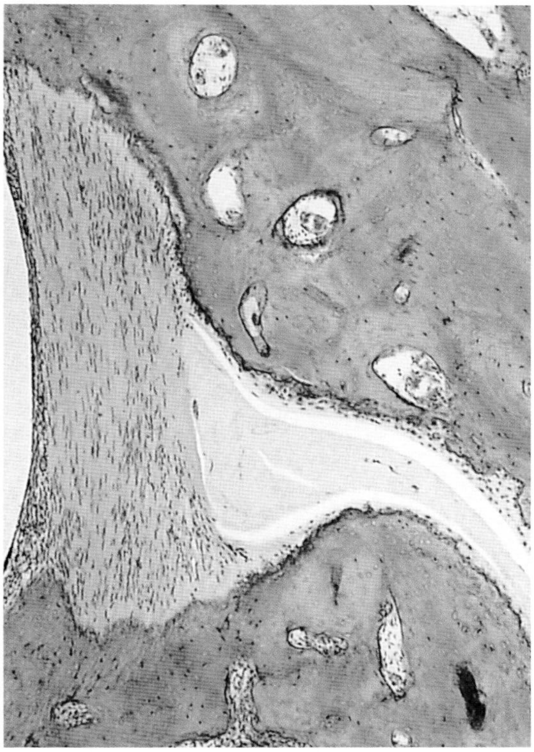

FIG. 41. Higher power of part of Fig. 40. Note one end of joint capsule and articular disc. (From ref. 63.)

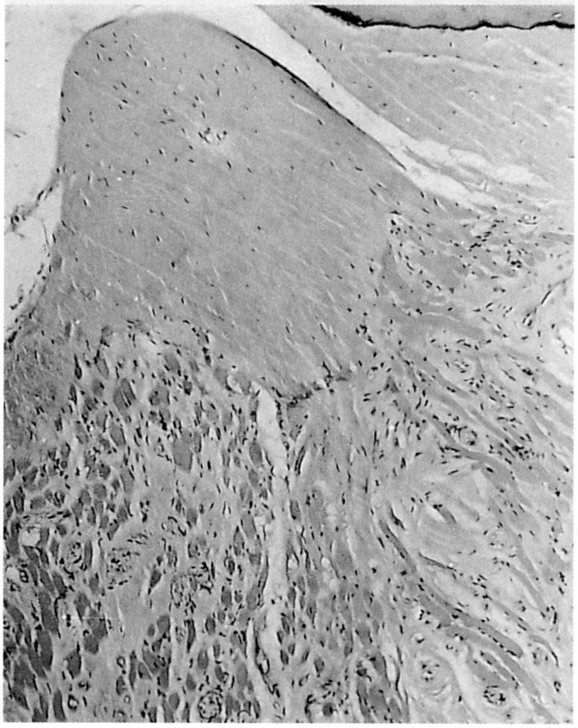

FIG. 42. Stapedius muscle and tendon. The skeletal muscle fibers and fibrous bands between them radiate to a tendon. (From ref. 64.)

often has a prominent content of adipose tissue, which may serve to insulate the nearby cochlea from the electric effects of its contraction.

### Aging Changes

Changes have been described in the incudomalleal and incudostapedial joints in the elderly, which are thought to cause a mild conductive deafness (43). The joint capsule and articular disc show hyalinization and later calcification. The articular cartilage frequently shows fraying, vacuolation, fibrillation, and even calcification. The joint becomes narrowed and eventually obliterated (44).

## INNER EAR

### Light Microscopy

#### *Otic Capsule*

The otic capsule surrounds and replicates the outline of the membranous labyrinth contained within it. Its extreme denseness is probably necessary to insulate and safeguard the extremely delicate vibrations of the fluids that it encloses, which subserve the functions of hearing and balance. Three layers may be recognized: an outer periosteal layer,

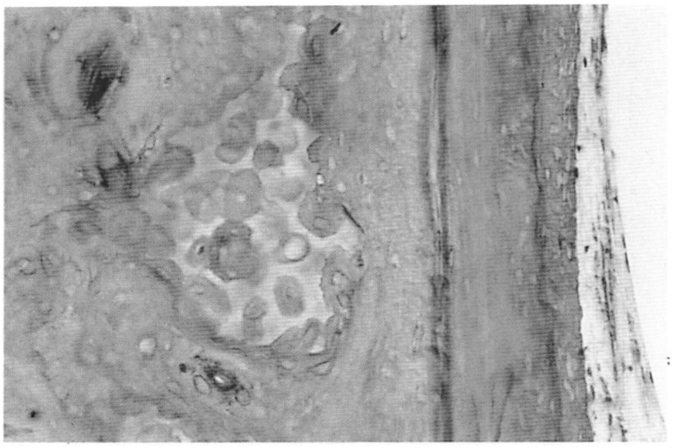

**FIG. 43.** Globuli ossei (*left*) and endosteum (*right*) of cochlea. (From ref. 63.)

which corresponds to the circumferential lamella of long bones; an inner layer, next to the membranous labyrinth, which is another periosteal layer, (although usually referred to as the "endosteal" layer of the otic capsule, suggesting, wrongly, correspondence to the osseous layer next to the bone marrow of long bones); and a middle layer, in which there is persistence of much of the calcified cartilaginous matrix, ("globuli interossei" or "globuli ossei" (Fig. 43) after the lacunae of the degenerated cartilage cells have been replaced by primitive bone. The bone of the adult otic capsule is neither lamellated nor woven bone, but somewhere inbetween. Thus, the otic capsule bone differs from any other adult bone by (a) lack of the normal developmental process of removal and replacement of calcified cartilaginous matrix, and (b) lack of removal and replacement of primitive bone. The interweaving of these persisting structures forms a unique tissue that is of extremely hard consistency.

### *Cochlea*

The modiolus is a axial core of spongy bone centrally placed in the cochlea. It is penetrated by blood vessels and the nerve bundles of the cochlear branch of the eighth nerve. At the origin of the three cochlear coils and forming nests within the modiolus lie the nerve cells of the spiral ganglion (Fig. 44) to which the axons derived from the sensory hair cells, carrying impulses of hearing, arrive and from which axons pass to the cochlear nucleus in the brain stem. The spiral ganglion cells are surrounded by Schwann cells.

The spaces of the cochlear coils are divided into two compartments, the scala vestibuli and the scala tympani, by a partially bony membrane, the spiral lamina which emanates from the modiolus in a spiral manner. Each scala contains perilymph. The scala vestibuli winds towards the apex of the cochlea at the helicotrema, where it becomes the scala tympani which coils back toward the round window (Figs. 44 and 45).

The inner zone of the spiral lamina is the osseous spiral lamina, composed of thin trabeculae of bone, the habenulae perforata. These surround nerve fibers composed of afferent fibers that run from the organ of Corti to the acoustic nerve and efferent fibers supplying the outer hair cells. The efferent fibers are derived from the olivocochlear system of Rasmussen, and follow the course of the cochlear branch of the eighth cranial nerve through the modiolus. The fibers then enter the osseous spiral lamina and basilar membrane, even-

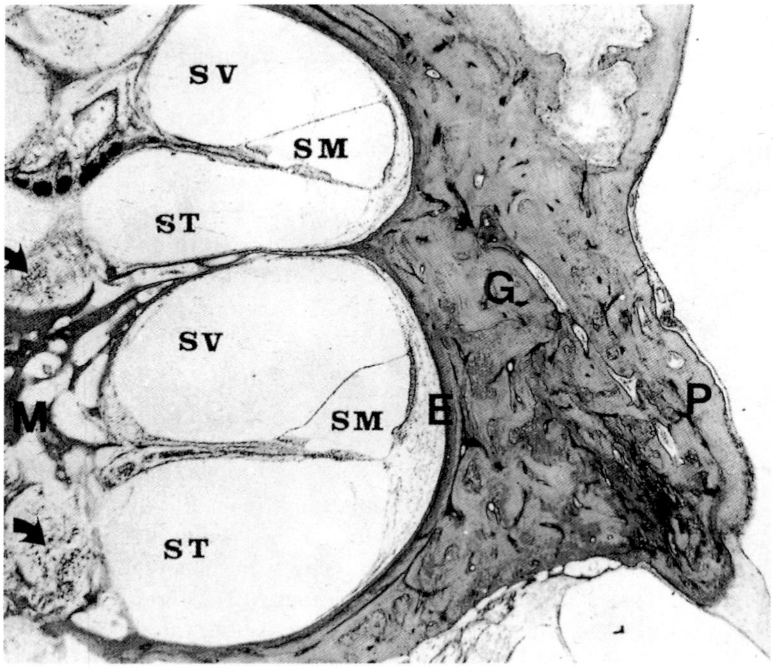


**FIG. 44.** Cochlea, bony cochlea, and modiolus. Arrows, spiral ganglion cells of basal and middle coils in modiolus; E, endosteal layer of bone; G, endochondral layer containing globuli interossei; M, modiolus; P, periosteal layer; SM, scala media; ST, scala tympani; SV, scala vestibuli. (From ref. 64.)

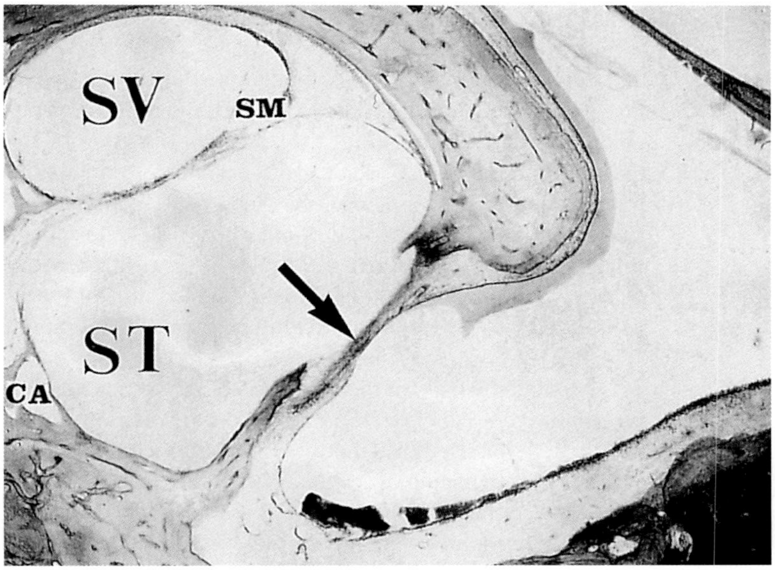


**FIG. 45.** Round window niche and membrane (*arrow*). The window separates the middle ear on the right from the scala tympani (ST). CA, cochlear aqueduct; SM, scala media; SV, scala vestibuli.

tually to supply the outer hair cells for arcane functions related to hearing. The outer zone of this lamina is known as the "basilar membrane." At the attachment of the latter to the cochlear wall, the periosteal connective tissue is thickened to form the spiral ligament. This appears in sections as a crescentic collagenous structure with a protruding peak on its concave surface to which the basilar membrane is anchored (unmarked in Fig. 44).

Sections of the scala tympani in the region of the basal coil and round window membrane usually show the cochlear aqueduct near its scala tympani opening (Fig. 45); this canal passes from the latter to the subarachnoid space near the jugular foramen. Thus, there is a connection between the labyrinth and the cerebrospinal fluid. The lumen of the aqueduct at its cochlear end is often filled by a meshwork of fibrous reticular tissue, but it still remains patent. Contaminated cerebrospinal fluid from the subarachnoid space in meningitis and red cells from subarachnoid hemorrhage can be conveyed to the perilymphatic space of the labyrinth along this channel (45).

The cochlear canal is further subdivided by a thin membrane, (Reissner's membrane), that extends from the osseous spiral lamina to the outer wall of the bony cochlea, so producing an additional scala, the scala media or cochlear duct. The cochlear duct is inserted between the other two (Figs. 44–46). Reissner's membrane consists of two thin layers of cells: an inner is ectodermal in origin and often contains epithelial-appearing clusters; an outer layer is mesodermal in origin and shows large, flat, and elongated cells. Reissner's membrane bulges upward into the scala vestibuli in conditions producing hydrops, notably Ménière's disease.

The outer vertical wall of the cochlear duct is the stria vascularis (Fig. 46). Under the light microscope lightly staining basal cells and darkly staining epithelial-like marginal cells can be recognized. The stria vascularis is frequently altered in ototoxic conditions such as those produced by the diuretic drugs frusemide and ethacrynic acid, and by the cytotoxic agent cisplatin.

The spiral prominence is a bulge of connective tissue covered by epithelial cells which lies at the outer end of the basilar membrane over the spiral ligament. The outer hair cells are present in rows which, in the mammalian organ of Corti,

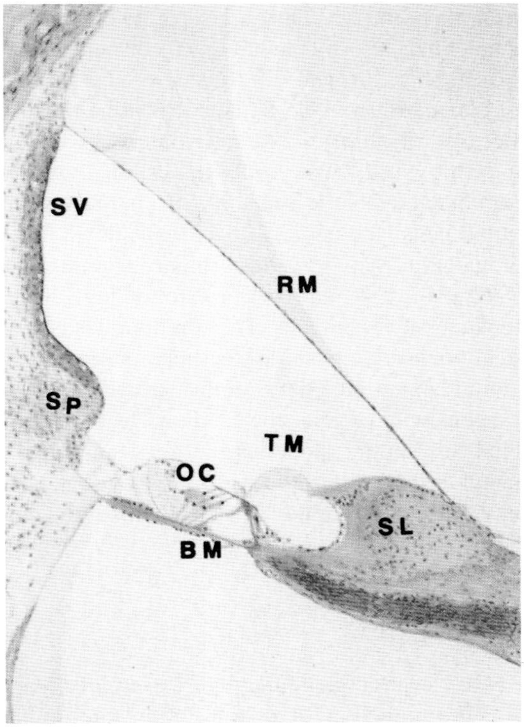


**FIG. 46.** Scala media of cat. BM, basilar membrane; OC, organ of Corti; RM, Reissner's membrane; SL, spiral limbus; SP, spiral prominence; SV, stria vascularis; TM, tectorial membrane. (From ref. 63.)

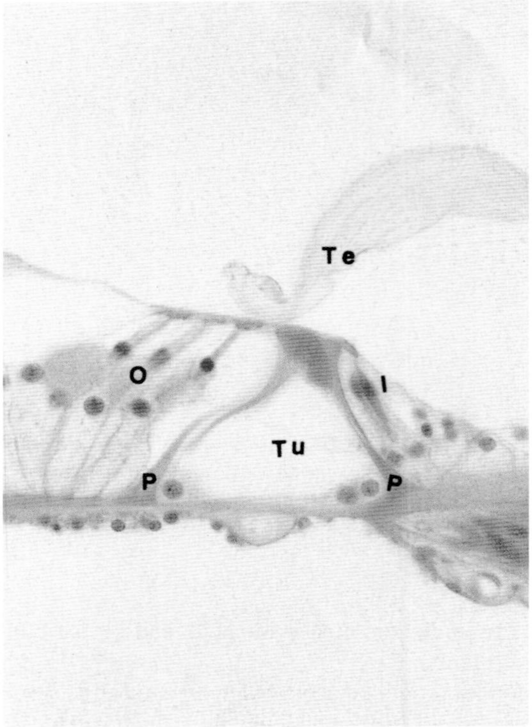


**FIG. 47.** Higher power of organ of Corti from Fig. 46. I, inner hair cells; O, outer hair cells; P, pillar cells (walls of tunnel); Te, tectorial membrane; Tu, tunnel of Corti. (From ref. 63.)

vary from three to five. They are separated from the single row of inner hair cells by the pillar cells that enclose the tunnel of Corti (Figs. 46 and 47). In many sectioned preparations of human organ of Corti, the cochlear hair cells are not seen because of autolysis; stereocilia are, moreover, observed with great difficulty only in sections. On the other hand, not only stereocilia and hair cells, but also supporting cells, pillar cells, and nerves can be well shown by the surface preparation method using ordinary staining and light microscopy (Figs. 48 and 49) (see following). Supporting cells separate outer hair cells. The spiral limbus is a bulge of periosteal connective tissue in the upper surface of the osseous spiral lamina. The fibers of this structure show a vertical arrangement to produce the "auditory teeth of Huschke." Epithelial cells on the upper margin of the spiral limbus, the interdental cells, secrete the tectorial membrane, a linear bundle of amorphous protein in which hairs of the outer hair cells lie.

### *Vestibular Structures*

The end of each semicircular duct is expanded to form the ampulla. The epithelium of the floor of the three ampullae is formed into a transverse ridge, the crista, and is their sensory epithelium. A viscous protein polysaccharide formation, known as the cupula, rests above each crista (Fig. 50). The remainder of the ampullary and semicircular duct lining is formed by flattened cells.

The two main membranous structures of the vestibule, the utricle and saccule (Fig. 51), are, in part, lined by a sensory epithelium, the macule (Fig. 52). The sensory cells of the maculae and the cristae are of two types when examined by tranmission electron microscopy. The type 1 cell is flask-shaped with a swollen basal portion. The type 2 cell is cylindrical. Type 1 cells are attached to the fibers of the sensory nerves by a wide chalicelike terminal. The terminal of type 2 cells is connected by buttonlike attachments of the nerve (Fig. 53).

Overlying the hairs of the sensory cells of the maculae are large numbers of crystalline bodies, known as otoliths, which are composed of a mixture of calcium carbonate and a protein, suspended in a jellylike polysaccharide.

In 1969, Schuknecht described in two cases of positional vertigo, a basophilic-staining homogeneous deposit on the cupula of the left posterior semicircular canal (46). He postulated that the calcific material derived from otoliths in a degenerated utricular macula will descend by gravity along the endolymph, and deposit on the crista of the posterior semicircular canal, the lowest point of the semicircular canal system. This ingenious theory, framed in the term "cupulolithiasis," is frequently used today as a synonym for the clinical condition of positional vertigo. Moreover, a surgical opera-

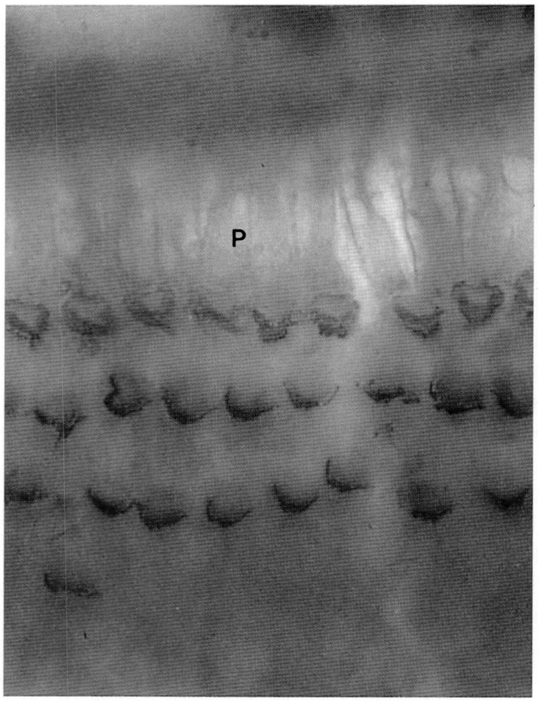


**FIG. 48.** Outer hair cells of basal coil of the normal cochlea in surface preparation. The stereocilia are short and arranged in a W formation in each hair cell. Osmic acid, alcian blue, and phloxine eosin (oil immersion). P, pillar cells. (From ref. 63.)

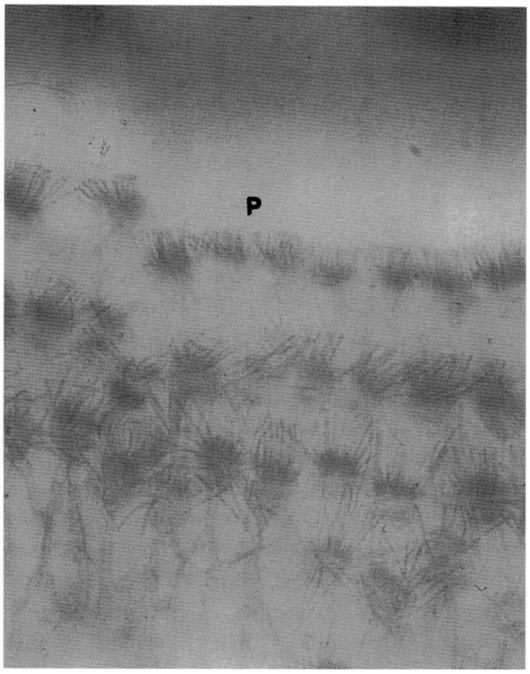


**FIG. 49.** Outer hair cells of middle coil of the normal cochlea in surface preparation. The stereocilia are long. Osmic acid, alcian blue, and phloxine eosin (oil immersion). P, pillar cells. (From ref. 63.)

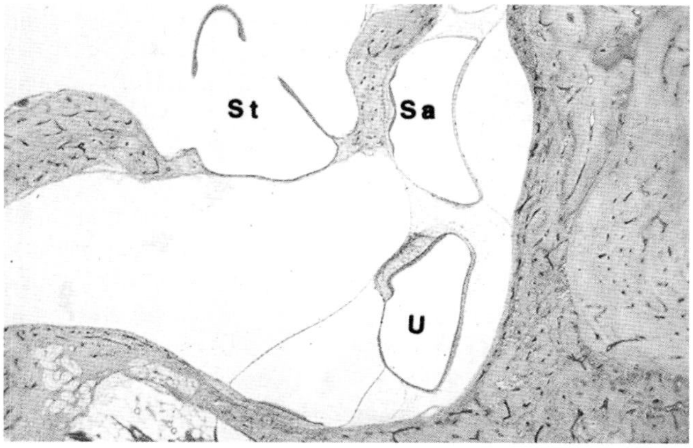


**FIG. 51.** Ventricle of cat showing utricle (U) and saccule (Sa). St, stapes. (From ref. 44.)

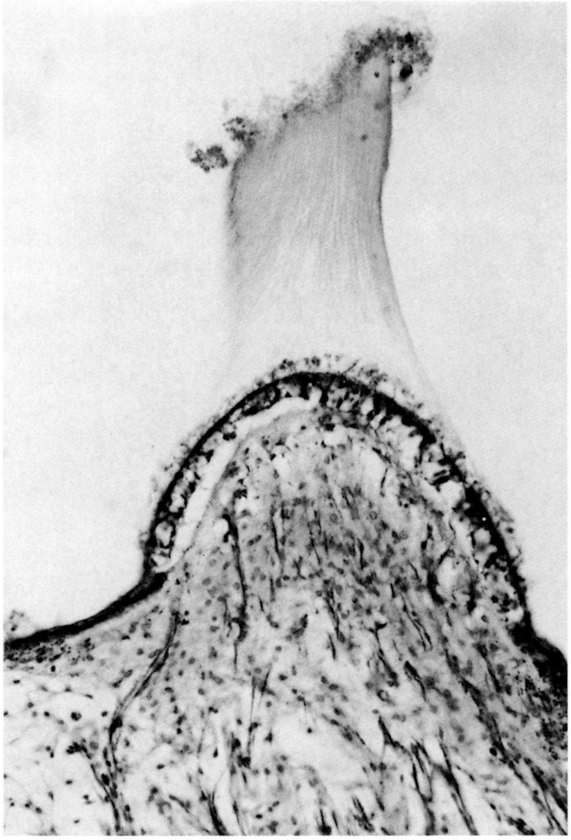

**FIG. 50.** Crista of ampulla of semicircular canal with cupula. (From ref. 64.)

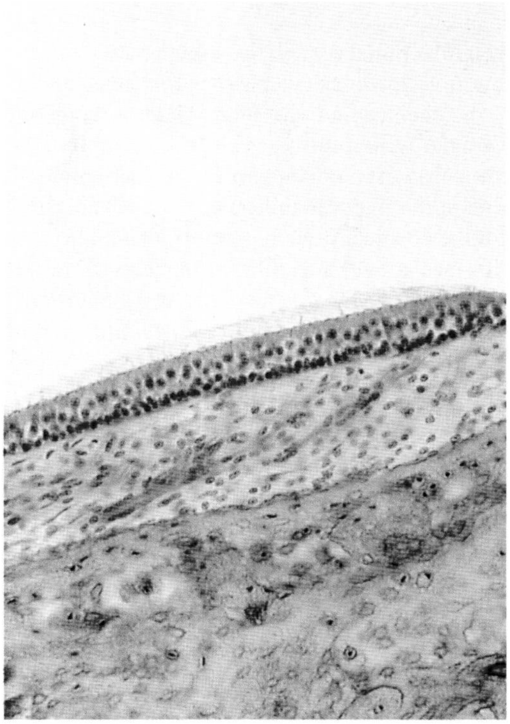

**FIG. 52.** Higher power of part of Fig. 51, showing macule of saccule. (From ref. 63.)

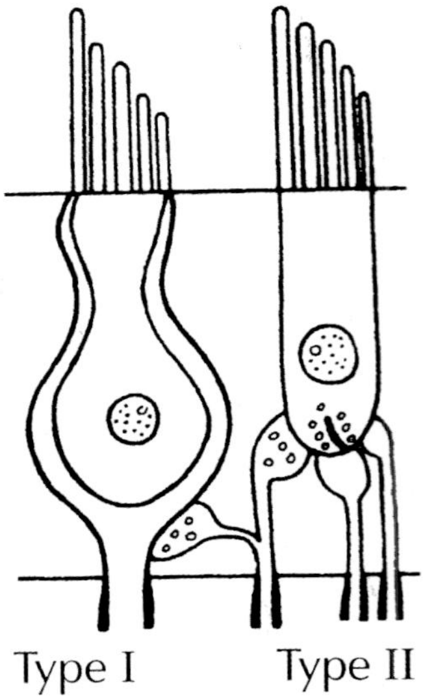


**FIG. 53.** Diagram of appearances of types 1 and 2 hair cells of maculae and cristae as seen by transmission electron microscopy.

tion to denervate the posterior semicircular canal in cases of positional vertigo has been devised and is claimed to be successful (47). No adequate confirmatory pathological studies have been reported on positional vertigo since Schuknecht's 1969 paper, however.

### *Cochleovestibular Nerve*

The eighth cranial (cochleovestibular) nerve lies in the internal auditory meatus in its passage to the peripheral end organs in the cochlea and vestibule. The afferent ganglion for the vestibular structures–the vestibular ganglion–is seen at the termination of the main part of the vestibular division of the nerve in the internal auditory meatus. The afferent ganglion for the cochlear division, the spiral ganglion, lies in the modiolus (see above). Near the entrance to the internal auditory meatus, where the cochlear and vestibular divisions are fused, the nerve changes from pale-staining proximally to dark-staining distally. This appearance is produced by the abrupt transition of the coverings of the nerve fibers from the pale-staining oligodendroglia to the darker Schwann cells (Fig. 54). It has been suggested that vestibular schwannomas (acoustic neuromas) are formed in the nerve at this junction, which could represent a region of Schwann cell instability.

### *Facial Nerve*

The facial nerve enters the temporal bone through the internal auditory meatus, where it lies above the eighth cranial nerve. It then passes Bill's bar, a pointed projection of bone that separates it from the superior division of the vestibular nerve. The facial nerve then enters the fallopian canal, making a right-angled bend at the genu. A bulge in the facial

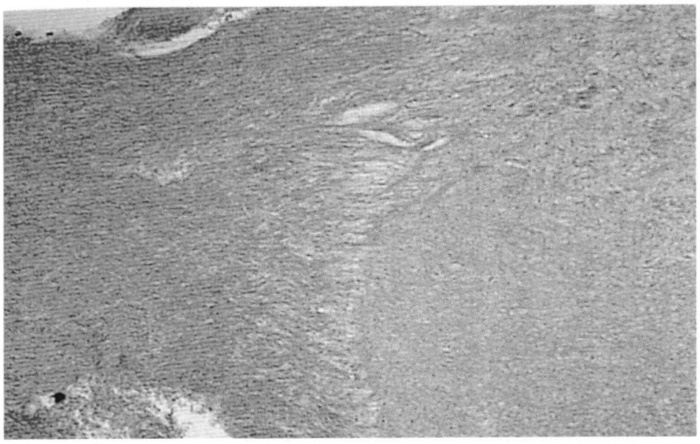

**FIG. 54.** Junction of glial region (*pale*) of cochleovestibular nerve in internal auditory meatus with Schwann sheath region (*dark*).

nerve below Bill's bar in the internal auditory meatus has mistakenly been regarded as a pathological feature of Bell's palsy (48). It is, in fact, a normal finding present in all temporal bones (Fig. 55). The facial nerve then lies in a bony canal in the posterior wall of the middle ear. It is surrounded here by a sheath of blood vessels. The bony covering separating the facial nerve from middle ear is often lacking. Such a "dehiscence" makes the nerve particularly vulnerable to damage by pathological change, especially inflammation, originating in the middle ear.

### *Paraganglia*

Small paraganglia with a structure similar to the carotid body have been described in the ear (49). More than 50% of these structures are situated in relation to the jugular bulb; a minority are found under the mucosa of the middle ear in the region of the medial promontory wall (Fig. 56). The tumors

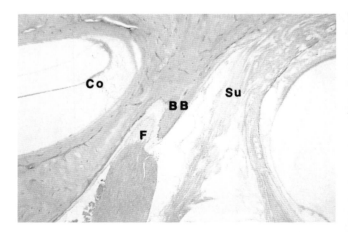

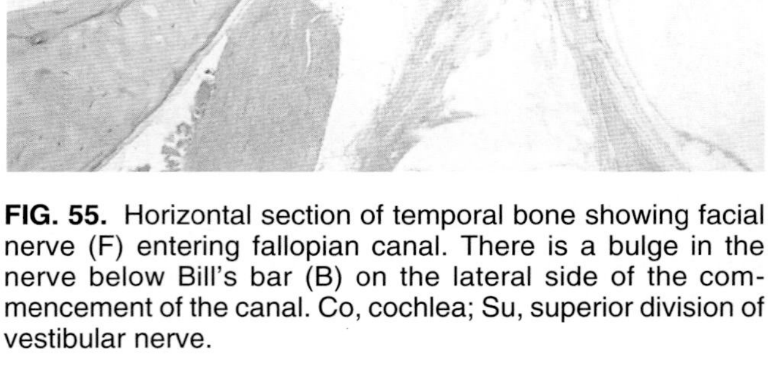


**FIG. 55.** Horizontal section of temporal bone showing facial nerve (F) entering fallopian canal. There is a bulge in the nerve below Bill's bar (B) on the lateral side of the commencement of the canal. Co, cochlea; Su, superior division of vestibular nerve.

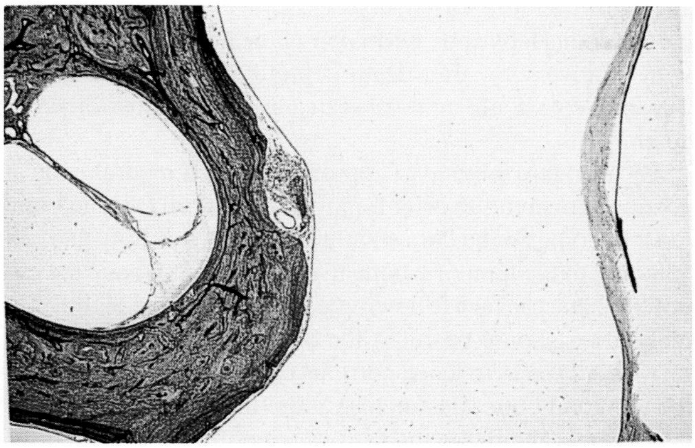

**FIG. 56.** Normal tympanic paraganglion under mucosa of medial side of middle ear over promontory. The tympanic membrane is on the right. Gomori's reticulin stain. (Courtesy of Dr. V. J. Hyams, Armed Forces Institute of Pathology, Washington, DC.)

arising from the paraganglia in these situations form the more frequent jugular paraganglioma (glomus jugulare) and the less frequent tympanic paraganglioma (glomus tympanicum), respectively.

### *Vestibular Aqueduct and Endolymphatic Duct and Sac*

The endolymphatic duct is linked by short canals to the utricle and saccule and passes posteriorly across the petrous bone to terminate in the blind endolymphatic sac, which projects into the dura in the posterior cranial fossa. In its course through the bone, the endolymphatic duct is housed within the vestibular aqueduct. The latter is identified easily in microsliced temporal bones and, particularly, in their radiographs. The lining epithelium of the endolymphatic duct is low cubical; (Fig. 57), the epithelium of the endolymphatic sac is taller and papillary (Fig. 58). An invasive tumor of this region, low-grade adenocarcinoma of probable endolymphatic sac origin, has been described, which has the character of a papillary-glandular neoplasm (50), presumed to be replicating the normal histology of the endolymphatic sac. About one-half of the patients with this condition have symptoms of Ménière's syndrome.

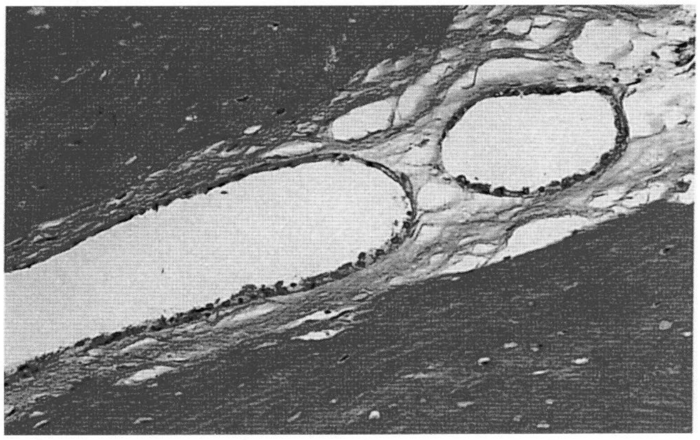

**FIG. 57.** Endolymphatic duct within the vestibular aqueduct. The duct is lined by low cubical epithelium.

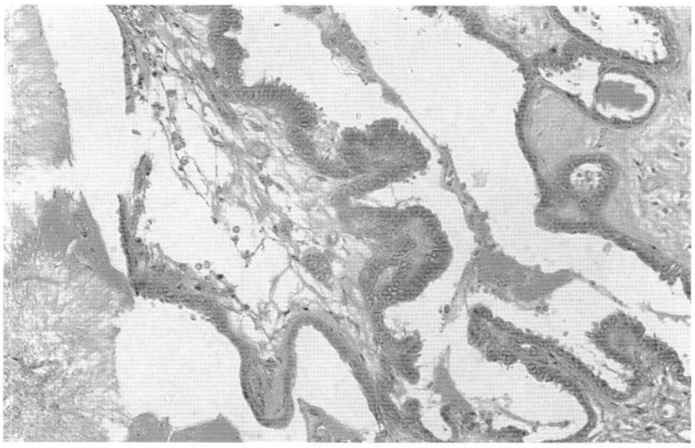

**FIG. 58.** Endolymphatic sac, which is lined by tall columnar epithelium arranged on papillae.

Obstruction of the duct by external fibrosis has been cited as a cause of hydrops, including Ménière's disease, but a variety of lesions causing such obstruction has been described, and not all cases have been associated with hydrops. Surgical drainage of the endolymphatic sac from the posterior cranial fossa is, nevertheless, sometimes carried out in the treatment of endolymphatic hydrops.

## Aging Changes

Presbycusis is a term in current use to denote the hearing loss in aged people that cannot be ascribed to any known cause other than old age. In recent years, degenerative changes at four different sites in the cochlea have been invoked as pathological bases for this hearing loss, namely, hair cells, spiral ganglion cells, stria vascularis, and basilar membrane (51). These options, together with two or more of these known sites combined or no known site at all, have provided no less than six possible bases for the pathogenesis of presbycusis. Electrophysiological and histopathological investigations in one human study have suggested, however, that it is damage to the outer hair cells alone that is responsible for the disorder. All subjects over 70 years of age in that study had high-tone deafness with specific changes in brain stem-evoked responses and electrocochleography, pointing to cochlear hair cell derangement (52, 53). Surface preparations of perfused cochleas stained for light microscopy by the method described previously showed atrophy of many outer hair cells in all coils of all cochleas from the elderly patients. Enumeration of hair cell losses showed that the inner hair cells had sustained little loss, the first row of outer hair cells had a greater loss, the second row loss was even greater, and in the third row, outer hair cells were very scanty or absent (Fig. 59). In addition, there was a complete loss of all

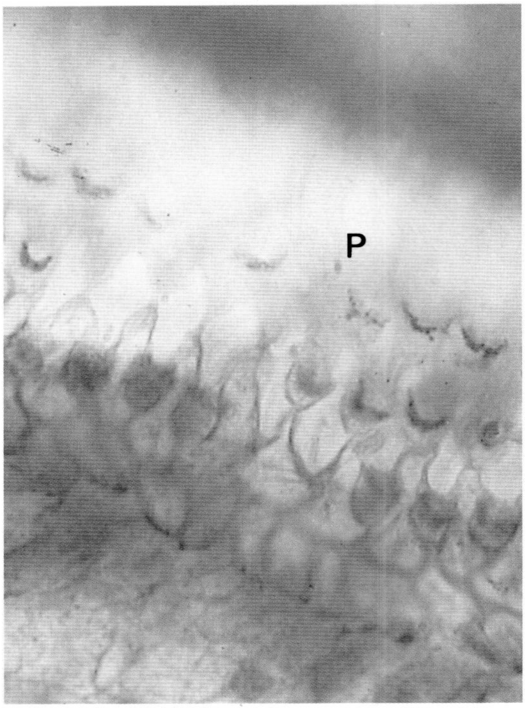


**FIG. 59.** Surface preparation of outer hair cells from basal coil of cochlea of elderly man. There are many gaps among the hair cells of the first two rows. P, pillar cells. Osmic acid, alcian blue, and phloxine eosin (oil immersion). (From ref. 63.)

hair cells of all rows, inner and outer, at the extreme lower end of the basal coil in every elderly cochlea. The other important change was the presence of enormously lengthened and thickened stereocilia, giant stereocilia, emanating from some surviving hair cells (Fig. 60). There is evidence that loss of outer hair cell stereocilia is an alteration that is slowly taking place throughout life, resulting eventually in presbycusis.

## SPECIMEN HANDLING

### Removal of Temporal Bone at Autopsy

Piecemeal removal of individual parts of the ear for postmortem examination is not satisfactory because the relationship of changes in adjacent structures is always important in ear disease and this is destroyed by such a means of examination. To examine the ear adequately the whole temporal bone should be removed as one block.

Autopsy and removal of the temporal bone should be carried out as soon after death as possible. Useful information may, however, still be obtained even 20 hours after death and longer. Autolysis of labyrinthine structures is prevented to some degree if 20% formalin is injected into the middle ear through the tympanic membrane soon after death (51). Such an injection will, of course, damage the tympanic membrane and some middle ear structures. For examination of the membranous labyrinth, perfusion of the perilymphatic space with fixative soon after death is preferable (see following). The cadaver should be refrigerated as soon as possible after death.

The standard method of approaching the temporal bone at postmortem involves prior removal of the skull cap and brain (54). In doing so the dura should be treated carefully and left adherent to the temporal bone in order not to damage the endolymphatic sac (see following). The seventh and eighth cranial nerves should be cut at the orifice of the internal auditory meatus so as to leave portions of the nerve trunks within the temporal bone specimen. A vibrating electric saw is satisfactory for removing the petrous temporal bone. A blade of triangular shape, measuring at least 5 cm (2 inches) from attachment to vibrating saw to edge is required. The more commonly employed circular blade is unsatisfactory for this purpose. Three vertical cuts and one horizontal cut are made with the saw (Figs. 61–63):

1. The first cut is set medial to the internal auditory meatus and extends vertically through the petrous temporal bone at right angles to the superior and posteromedial surfaces, to a depth of approximately 2.5 cm.
2. The second cut is made parallel with the first and at least 2.5 to 3 cm posterolateral to it, at the lateral end of the temporal bone. It also passes vertically to a depth of 2.5 cm. This cut leaves out most of the mastoid air cell system. A more extensive procedure by which these cells

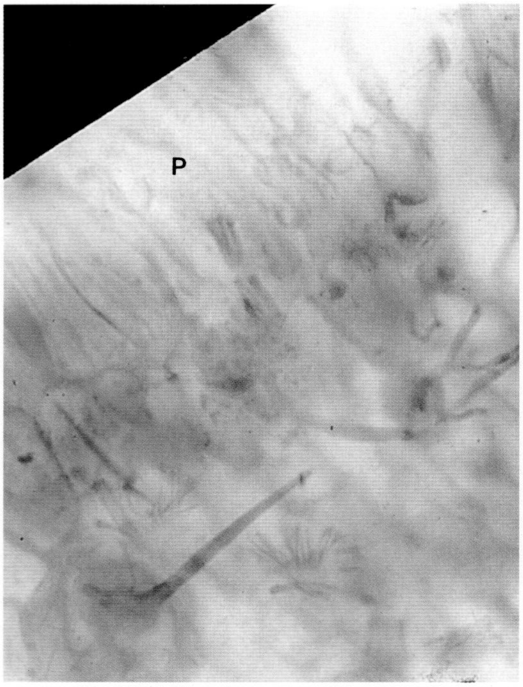


**FIG. 60.** Surface preparation of outer hair cells from middle coil of cochlea of elderly man. Note giant stereocilia. P, pillar cells. Osmic acid, alcian blue, and phloxine eosin (oil immersion). (From ref. 63.)

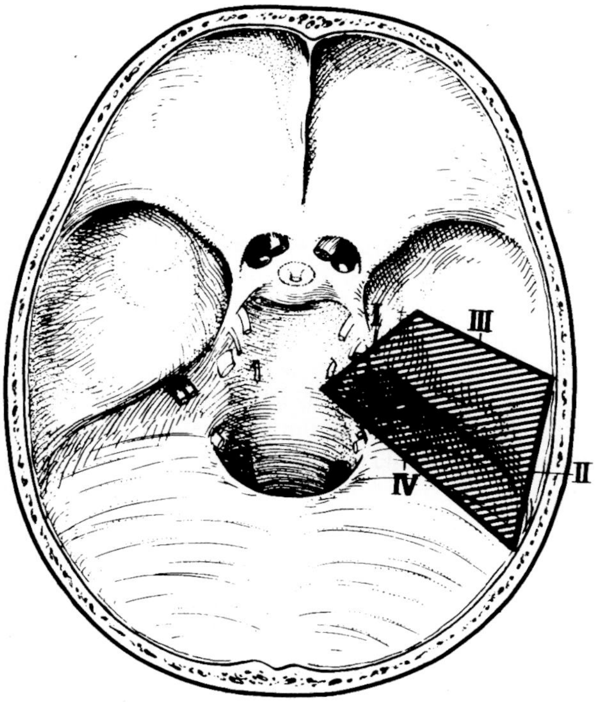


**FIG. 61.** Base of skull showing position of four saw cuts (roman numerals) that are required in removal of temporal bone. A more extensive procedure by which the mastoid process is removed is described in the text and shown in Fig. 59. (From ref. 58.)

may be removed involves extending cut 3 laterally to the lateral surface of the squamous temporal bone, anterior to the bony orifice of the external auditory meatus, after dissecting the pinna, scalp, and cartilaginous canal away from the latter. Cut 4 is also extended laterally posterior to the mastoid process and the two cuts are joined together below the bony ear canal. With care, this extended temporal bone resection does not result in an unsightly external disfigurement produced by skull base collapse as long as cut 1 on each side is placed just medial to the internal auditory meatus, and not further medially.

3. The third vertical cut is made connecting the forward ends of the two previous cuts, approximately parallel with the free (posterior) end of the petrous temporal bone at the anterior extent of the middle cranial fossa.
4. A horizontal cut is made beneath the petrous temporal bone at about 2.5 cm below the upper surface and parallel with it. The block can now be removed by gently "rocking" and cutting the ligamentous structures on its inferior surface. So removed it will include the deeper part of the external ear canal, the tympanic membrane, the middle ear, the labyrinthine structures, and the petrous portion of the seventh and eighth cranial nerves.

A method has been devised to remove and process the temporal bone so as to include the whole length of the eustachian tube (55).

### Handling of Temporal Bone Site and Specimen

After removing the specimen, plaster of Paris may be inserted in the space previously occupied by the temporal bone. To assist the subsequent embalming process, the internal carotid arteries may be clamped in the neck before removal of the temporal bones and then ligated after removal has been completed.

The specimen is then placed in fixative in a large screw-top plastic jar. For most purposes, the fixative may be buffered 4% formaldehyde solution. In some centers, another fixative is preferred, (e.g., Heidenhain Susa solution) (51), but this is unsatisfactory if modern immunochemical procedures are to be applied to sections.

### Surgical Specimens

The great majority of surgical biopsy specimens from the ear are small. Many contain some bone, and brief decalcifi-

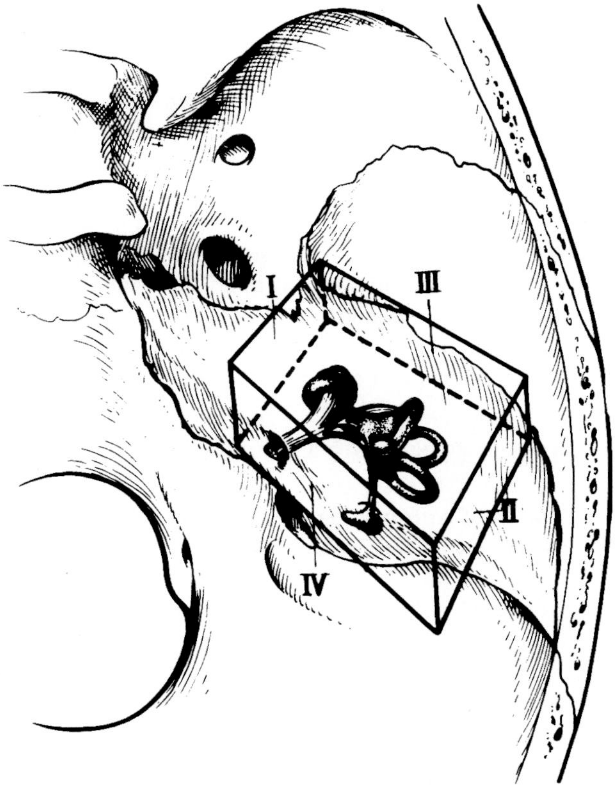


**FIG. 62.** Wedge of temporal bone that is removed from base of skull for histological examination. The outlines of the membranous labyrinth are drawn in. Roman numerals refer to the saw cuts required to remove the temporal bone. A more extensive procedure by which the mastoid process may be removed is described in the text and shown in Fig. 63. (From ref. 58.)

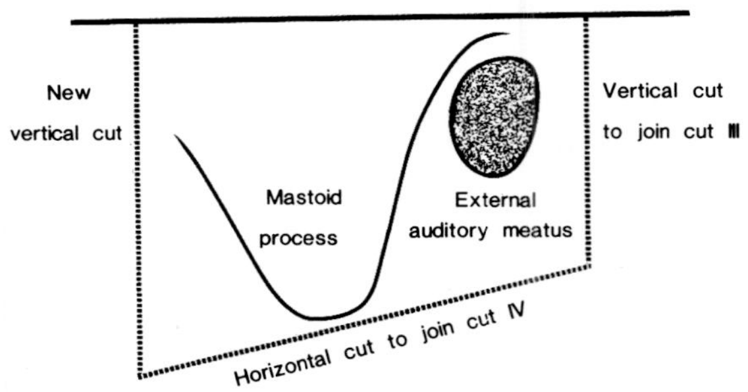


**FIG. 63.** Diagram of side view of skull in region of external auditory meatus to indicate the extended saw cuts, which may be carried out to remove mastoid process. (From ref. 64.)

cation is required. After decalcification, resection specimens of stapes superstructure or of the whole stapes should be oriented for embedding, so that the outline of the whole ossicle is revealed in the section; transverse sectioning is unsatisfactory. Care should be taken in orienting any skin or mucosal surface correctly in small biopsies during paraffin embedding so that sections will be cut at right angles to the epithelial surface. This can be carried out by observation with a hand lens or dissecting microscope at the time of embedding. Frozen sections from the ear region require no special handling procedures.

Occasionally, larger resection specimens are submitted, usually derived from the surgical treatment of squamous carcinoma of the external and/or middle ear. These include resection of the pinna and deep external canal and "petrosectomy." The last is far from being a resection of the whole petrous temporal bone, but consists usually of the external canal, tympanic membrane, and middle ear contents. The surviving normal anatomical structures should be identified in these specimens and resection margins should be carefully sampled for evidence of tumor extension.

## SPECIAL TECHNIQUES AND PROCEDURES

### Preparation of Autopsy Temporal Bones for Histological Examination and Molecular Techniques

The standard technique available for histological examination of the temporal as a whole bone has been to decalcify it and then embed it in celloidin; it is then cut into serial sections for histological staining. Hair cells, in particular, are not well displayed because their most characteristic feature, the stereocilia, are hardly visible in such sections. A more satisfactory method for examining the hair cells of the cochlea is by means of surface preparations of the basilar membrane. This has previously called for skilled drilling in exposing the inner ear (56). A method is available whereby slices of the undecalcified bone are first inspected, and chosen parts are then subjected to histological section. With suitably perfused material, surface preparations can, as an alternative, be obtained from the samples sliced by this method (see following).

### Technique of Serial Sectioning After Celloidin Embedding

Fixation is required for approximately 4 weeks. The bone should be roughly sawed to size before fixation. To decalcify the whole temporal bone, it is placed in 10% formic acid for a period of 4 to 8 weeks, with radiographs taken every week to check the progress of decalcification. On its completion, the final trimming of the specimen can be done by using a strong-bladed knife. It is important to keep the size of the bone to a minimum to allow adequate diffusion of impregnating substances during the processing of the bone; the trimmed block should measure not more than 4.0 cm long by 2.5 cm wide by 5.5 cm high. Dehydration of the whole specimen is carried out by placing it for 1 day in ascending grades of alcohol and alcohol-ether as follows: 30%, 50%, 95%, 100%, 100%, equal parts alcohol and ether.

Impregnation in a celloidin base dissolved in a mixture of equal parts of alcohol and ether is then required. For microtomy, a long heavy stellite-tipped knife is preferable. This should be sharpened to a final cutting edge bevel of about 28°. Sections are cut at 20 $\mu$m-thickness and it is necessary only to stain every tenth section, keeping the intermediate sections interleaved in vellum tissue, which may be stored indefinitely with the uncut blocks in 70% alcohol. Staining of sections may be carried out by the hematoxylin and eosin (H&E) method (preferably using Ehrlich's hematoxylin), as well as by a variety of other routine histological stains; immunohistochemical methods cannot normally be used in celloidin-embedded material, although a technique for this purpose has been described (60,61).

#### *Disadvantages of the Serial Sectioning Method*

Gross examination, an important prerequisite of the histological analysis of all other organs, cannot be carried by the serial sectioning method after celloidin.

Prolonged decalcification must precede embedding and marked alterations in the histological appearances of some of the tissues take place as a result of this. Some of the microscopic alterations ascribed to postmortem autolysis in serially sectioned temporal bones are likely to be the result of damage by acid. Decalcification by ethylenediamine tetracetate (EDTA) rather than acid, is less damaging and is carried out in some laboratories. Decalcification by EDTA is, however, very slow because it requires much more time than the use of acids.

The serial sectioning method after celloidin embedding makes special microscopic studies including histochemistry, immunohistochemistry, electron microscopy, and molecular biological investigations particularly difficult.

Processing of the whole temporal bone in toto is extremely slow, because not only decalcification, but also dehydration and embedding each require a long exposure. It takes at least 9 months from the autopsy to produce serial sections. This is discouraging in maintaining a sustained interest for research and teaching.

Serial sectioning of the embedded whole temporal bone is technically difficult and demands a high degree of skill on the part of the histologist in cutting sections through the whole of this structure, which is both tough and fragile.

Large numbers of serial sections are produced from a single temporal bone. Only a limited number are mounted and stained; the rest have to be stored in jars of alcohol. Sometimes the serial examination of a specific portion of the temporal bone is useful, but most of the sections are, as a rule, not required.

### *Slicing Method*

A method has been devised to obviate these disadvantages and to facilitate the examination of the temporal bone in the general histopathology laboratory (57). The temporal bone is removed at postmortem as described earlier. Fixation should take place for a minimum of 4 days. The bone is trimmed so that it is no larger than approximately 2.5 × 2.5 × 2.5 cm. It is then mounted with molten dental wax on a glass plate measuring 6.2 × 5 cm with a thickness of approximately 0.5 cm. The surface to be presented for slicing is arranged perpendicular to the glass plate. The glass plate, with the surface of the temporal bone that is to be cut to the front, is now mounted on the metal plinth attached with dental wax to the inner end of the lever of the slicing machine (Microslice 2 Precision Annular Saw)* (Fig. 64). This is a cutting machine with a circular steel blade that is bolted at 16 points to prevent lateral vibration. Cutting proceeds around a circular inner opening where the blade is tipped with diamond. The cutting edge is lubricated by a continuous jet of cold water. The speed of the rotatory motor may be adjusted by the left-hand knob on the front of the machine, a speed of about 200 r.p.m. usually being appropriate. The right-hand knob advances the lever with the specimen by the required length before each slice is made so that the thickness of the specimen can be regulated. Slices of 1-, 2-, or 3-mm thickness may be prepared. Slicing is carried out by gently lowering the weighted left-hand counterpoised end of the lever so that the specimen rotates up and is applied against the cutting edge. With this system, the specimen backs away from the blade when a particularly hard area is encountered, avoiding excessive mechanical and thermal stresses. The slices adhere together and are removed from the machine after the whole temporal bone has been treated. Each slice is radiographed with a laboratory x-ray machine (such as the Faxitron system made by Hewlett Packard).

*Available in Europe from Malvern Instruments Ltd., Spring Lane South, Malvern, Worcestershire WR14 1AT, UK. Telephone: **44 (0) 1684 892 456. Fax: **44 (0) 1684 892 456. E-mail: timh@vern.tcom.co.uk. World Wide Web: http://www.mmf.com/metal/home/malvern/

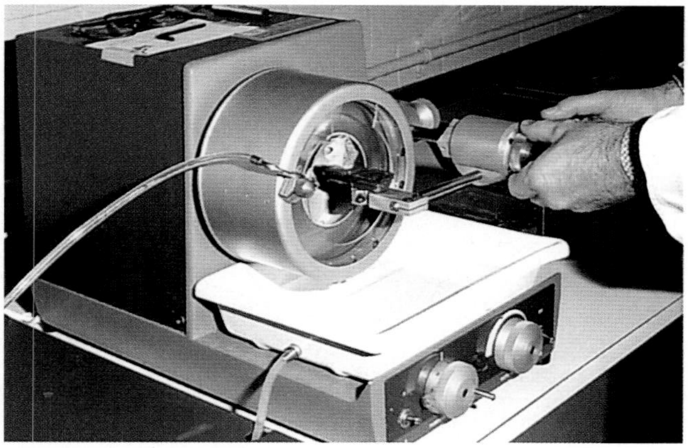

**FIG. 64.** Microslice 2 Precision Annular Saw used to prepare slices of undecalcified temporal bone. (From ref. 63.)

After careful examination of the slices with a hand lens or dissecting microscope, the whole series, a single slice, or selected areas may be subjected to celloidin or paraffin-embedding for light microscopy, special histological or histochemical methods, or even for electron microscopy (in the case of structures that have been sufficiently well-preserved).

### *Surface Preparation Method*

The surface preparation method has been applied mainly to the analysis of the hair cells of the organ of Corti and can be used in temporal bones in which the perilymphatic space has been perfused by fixative within 24 hours after death; the autolysis that takes place in the hair cells beyond that time, renders them unsuitable for this type of examination. Electron microscopy, particularly by the scanning method, is also frequently used to study specimens that have been perfused within 3 hours after death. This is often before permission for the autopsy has been granted and local legal restrictions have to be taken into account before this technique can be applied. A satisfactory method for perilymphatic perfusion has been described and has been well tested in a large number of cases (58). The procedure may be carried out directly on the cadaver in the autopsy room or in the histopathology laboratory on a temporal bone that has been removed by the method described previously. By using an ear speculum, the upper posterior part of the tympanic membrane may be folded forward. With a curette, any bony overhang is removed to expose the oval and round windows. The incudostapedial joint is divided and the stapes is luxated from the oval window. It can be left in the middle ear hanging from the stapedial muscle tendon, or removed for further study. The round window membrane is perforated with a small hook directed forward (toward the eustachian tube) (Fig. 65).

A glass pipette of tip diameter 0.5 to 1 mm, or a syringe

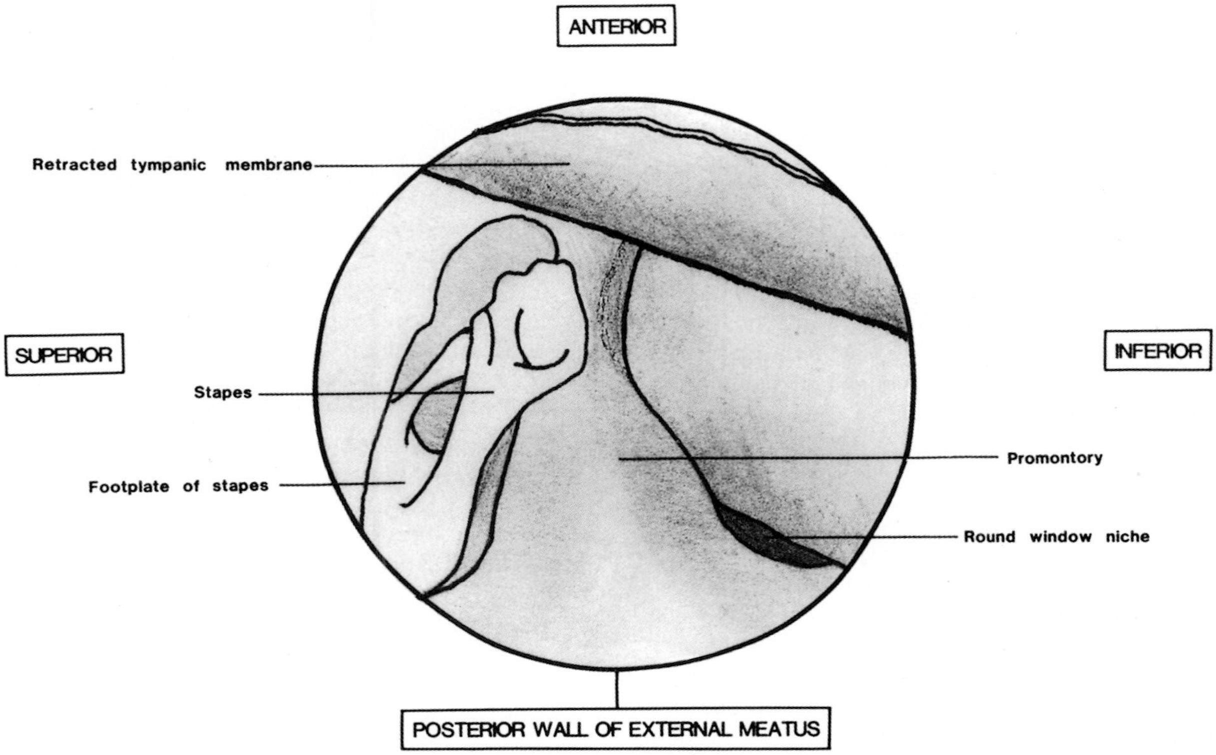


**FIG. 65.** Diagram of appearances of normal middle ear observed during perilymphatic perfusion. (From ref. 64.)

with an unsharpened needle of the same diameter, is filled by aspiration with 1 to 2 ml of fixative solution at room temperature. The tip is directed toward the oval window and the fixative injected. This causes a slight increase in pressure in the vestibule and some fixative will enter the scala vestibuli (see following) and perfuse the cochlea. The perilymphatic spaces are perfused in this way for 15 minutes, or at least 10 times. The fixative preferred if electron microscopy is to be carried out is the "reduced Karnovsky" solution (59). If surface preparation and staining by a light microscopic method is to be carried out, fixation by buffered formaldehyde solution is preferred.

### *Technique of Sampling the Membranous Labyrinth*

The method of drilling away the bony labyrinth to sample the membranous labyrinth is described by Johnsson and Hawkins (56). The method is difficult, requiring special training and a detailed knowledge of temporal bone anatomy. Because of its difficulty, damage to the membranous labyrinth is likely until the operator has acquired a high degree of skill in the procedure. Even then the drilling method requires hours of work on a single specimen. A further disadvantage is that in order to expose the membranous labyrinth in this way, it is necessary to destroy other parts of the middle and inner ear, which cannot, thereafter, be subjected to routine microscopic methods.

By contrast, the microsliced temporal bone prepared by the method previously described may be used to sample the membranous labyrinth without drilling, and with only slight damage to inner ear structures. By this method, the whole inner ear may be exposed within minutes. Moreover, there is no destruction of the rest of the ear. Thus, after portions of the inner ear have been selected and removed for the surface specimen technique, the rest of the temporal bone may be put through for routine histological study.

### *Staining the Surface Preparation*

The standard method for examination of the surface preparation, in both human and experimental investigations, has been to postfix the sample of the membranous labyrinth in osmic acid solution, and then to mount and view it microscopically by the phase contrast or Nomarski method. The following method of staining allows the microscopic examination of the specimen by ordinary light. After a short period of postfixation in dilute osmic acid solution, the sample is stained by an alcian blue solution followed by phloxine-eosin counterstain. Hairs (stereocilia), hair cells, supporting cells, pillar cells, and nerves are well-shown by this method using ordinary light microscopy (Figs. 48 and 49).

### *Molecular Techniques*

Although soft tissue specimens removed from the ear are fully amenable to modern methods of immunohistochemistry and molecular biology, a start has only just been made on the exploration of the bone-encapsulated tissues of the hearing and balance organ by these methods. There are large numbers of archival temporal bone sections available in many centers; if molecular methods could be adapted to their particular milieu, they might enhance understanding of pathologic processes in this region. The biggest hurdles to be overcome are the prolonged exposure to decalcifying agents and the widespread use of celloidin as an embedding medium.

The majority of archival temporal bone sections has been processed after prolonged acid decalcification. This may destroy antigens that are tested for by immunohistochemistry.

In one study in which temporal bones were embedded in paraffin wax after decalcification in 10% formic acid, sections showing cells with cytomegalovirus inclusions on H&E staining, did not display the virus antigen on immunohistochemistry (30). This failure was ascribed to the acid decalcification process. A technique for antigen retrieval in celloidin-embedded human temporal bone sections has recently been described, in which the sections are immersed in a saturated solution of sodium hydroxide in methanol before performing immunohistochemistry. Using this method on sections of temporal bone which had been decalcified in 5% trichloracetic acid, antigens of keratin, vimentin, neurofilament, glial fibrillary acidic protein and desmin intermediate filament proteins (60), and antigens of S-100 protein (61) were successfully demonstrated. The use of the sodium hydroxide method for antigen retrieval has not yet been confirmed by another group.

Studies have also been carried out in which the effects of celloidin embedding and decalcification on molecular biological methods have been examined. In temporal bones embedded in paraffin wax after decalcification in 10% formic acid, sections showing cells with cytomegalovirus inclusions on H&E staining displayed the virus DNA in fewer cells when the in situ hybridization method was used (30). The polymerase chain reaction (PCR) is an extremely sensitive method for augmenting small amounts of DNA and by its use, specific DNA fragments have been isolated in decalcified paraffin and celloidin sections. Using PCR for the detection of p53 gene DNA in temporal bone sections, we have found that after the use of a variety of decalcifying agents, sections of temporal bone celloidin-embedded sections yield ample amounts of the shorter fragments (gene exon 7: 38 base pairs); but longer fragments (gene exon 8 +6: 38 base pairs, and gene exon 7–9) were not amplified. EDTA-decalcified temporal bones also provide amplification of longer fragments (gene exon 8 +6: 320 base pairs), but not gene exon 7–9: 780 base pairs. Although there has been a reduced yield of p53 gene DNA from acid-decalcified specimens, herpes virus type 1 DNA has been successfully amplified from the geniculate ganglion of an acid-decalcified paraffin-embedded temporal bone of a patient with Bell's palsy (62).

Although the use of the PCR reaction, in particular, on archival sections of temporal bone is optimistic for future studies, it seems likely that prospectively planned investigations using optimally processed material from temporal bones may allow more significant results. The temporal bone material in inner ear investigations, for instance, would best be perfused with fixative into the perilymphatic space soon after death, and the bone would be subjected to microslicing. To avoid the necessity for decalcification, samples of the soft tissues of basilar membrane, stria vascularis, spiral ganglion, and eighth nerve, for instance, could be sampled by dissection from the microslices and embedded in paraffin wax. The techniques of immunohistochemistry, in situ hybridization, and PCR could then all be applied to the paraffin sections.

## REFERENCES


1. Michaels L, Soucek S. Development of the stratified squamous epithelium of the human tympanic membrane and external canal: the origin of auditory epithelial migration. *Am J Anat* 1989;184:334–344.
2. Michaels L, Soucek S. Stratified squamous epithelium in relation to the tympanic membrane: its development and kinetics. *Int J Pediatr Otorhinolaryngol* 1991;22:135–149.
3. Michaels L, Soucek S. Auditory epithelial migration: III. Development of the stratified squamous epithelium of the tympanic membrane and external canal in the mouse. *Am J Anat* 1991;191:280–292.
4. Michaels L, Soucek S. Auditory epithelial migration. II. The existence of two discrete pathways and their embryologic significance. *Am J Anat* 1990;189:189–200.
5. Michaels L. The biology of cholesteatoma. *Otolaryngol Clin North Am* 1989;22:869–881.
6. Wells M, Michaels L. Role of retraction pockets in cholesteatoma formation. *Clin Otolaryngol* 1983;8:39–45.
7. Soucek S, Michaels L. Keratosis of the tympanic membrane and deep external canal: a defect of auditory epithelial migration. *Eur Arch Otorhinolaryngol* 1993;250:140–142.
8. Corbridge RJ, Michaels L, Wright A. Epithelial migration in keratosis obturans. *Am J Otolaryngol*, in press
9. Piza JE, Northrop CC, Eavey RD. Neonatal mesenchyme temporal bone study: typical receding pattern vs increase in Potter's sequence. *Laryngoscope*, 1996; 106:856–864.
10. Eavey RD. Abnormalities of the neonatal ear: otoscopic observations, histologic observations, and a model for contamination of the middle ear by cellular contents of amniotic fluid. *Laryngoscope* 1993;103 (suppl 58):1–31.
11. Michaels L. An epidermoid formation in the developing middle ear; possible source of cholesteatoma. *J Otolaryngol* 1986;15:169–174.
12. Wang R-G, Hawke M, Kwok P. The epidermoid formation (Michaels' structure) in the developing middle ear. *J Otolaryngol* 1987;16: 327–330.
13. Michaels L. Evolution of the epidermoid formation and its role in the development of the middle ear and tympanic membrane during the first trimester. *J Otolaryngol* 1987;17:22–27.
14. Michaels L. Origin of congenital cholesteatoma from a normally occurring epidermoid rest in the developing middle ear. *Int J Pediatr Otolaryngol* 1988;15:51–65.
15. McGill TJ, Merchant S, Healy GB, Friedman EM. Congenital cholesteatoma of the middle ear in children: a clinical and histopathological report. *Laryngoscope* 1991;101:606–613.
16. Berry CL. Examination of the fetus and the neonatal autopsy. In: Berry CL, ed. *Paediatric pathology. Second edition.* London; Springer-Verlag, 1989;1–39.

16a. Lee TS, Liang J, Soucek S, Michaels L, Wright A. Auditory epithelial migration: loss of spent epithelial cells in the deep external canal by apoptosis. *Abstracts of the Midwinter Meeting of the Association for Research in Otolaryngology,* St. Petersburg Beach, Florida, 1997.

17. Frank ST. Aural sign of coronary heart disease. *N Engl J Med* 1973; 289:327–328.
18. Overfield T, Call EB. Earlobe type, race and age: effects on earlobe creasing. *J Am Geriatr Soc* 1983;31:479–481.
19. Patel V, Champ C, Andrews PS, Gostelow BE, Gunasekara NP, Davidson AR. Diagonal earlobe creases and atheromatous disease: a postmortem study. *J R Coll Physicians Lond* 1992;26;274–277.

20. Tranchesi B Jr , Barbosa V, de Albuquerque CP, et al. Diagonal earlobe crease as a marker of the presence and extent of coronary atherosclerosis. *Am J Cardiol* 1992;70:1417–1420.
21. Elliott WJ, Harrison T. Increased all-cause and cardiac morbidity and mortality associated with the diagonal earlobe crease: a prospective cohort study. *Am J Med* 1991;91:247–254.
22. Perry ET. *The human ear canal.* Springfield; Charles C Thomas, 1957.
23. Bloom W, Fawcett DW. *A textbook of histology. 9th ed.* Philadelphia; WB Saunders, 1968.
24. Michaels L. Histopathology of the middle ear in the newborn. In: Acute and secretory otitis media. *Proceedings of the International Conference on Acute and Secretory Otitis Media, Part 1.* Amsterdam; Kugler Publications, 1986.
25. Sade J. The biopathology of secretory otitis media. *Ann Otol Rhinol Laryngol Suppl* 1974;11:59–70.
26. Sade J. Middle ear mucosa. *Arch Otolaryngol Head Neck Surg* 1966; 84:137– 143.
27. Lim DJ, Shimada T, Yoder M. Distribution of mucus-secretory cells in the normal middle ear mucosa. *Arch Otolaryngol Head Neck Surg* 1973;98:2–9.
28. Akaan-Penttila E. Middle ear mucosa in newborn infants. A topographical and microanatomical study. *Acta Otolaryngol (Stockh)* 1982; 93:251–259.
29. Tos M. Pathogenesis and pathology of chronic secretory otitis media. *Ann Otol Rhinol Laryngol* 1980;89 (suppl 68):91–97.
30. Michaels L, Soucek S, Liang J. The ear in the acquired immunodeficiency syndrome: I. Temporal bone histopathologic study. *Amer J Otol* 1994;15:515–522.
31. Michaels L, Liang J. Structure and origin of middle ear corpuscles. *Clin Otolaryngol* 1993;18;257–262.
32. Bak-Pedersen K. Goblet cell population in the pathological middle ear and eustachian tube of children and adults. *Ann Otol Rhinol Laryngol* 1977;86:209–218.
33. Aschan G. The eustachian tube. Histologic findings under normal conditions and in otosalpingitis. *Acta Otolaryngol (Stockh)* 1954; **4:** 295–311.
34. Berger G. Eustachian tube submucosal glands in normal and pathological temporal bones. *J Laryngol Otol* 1993;107:1099–1105.
35. Matsune S, Sando I. Distributions of eustachian tube goblet cells and glands in children with and without otitis media. *Ann Otol Rhinol Laryngol* 1992;101:750–754.
36. Moreano EH, Paparella MM, Zelterman D, Goycoolea MV. Prevalence of carotid canal dehiscence in the human middle ear: a report of 1000 temporal bones. *Laryngoscope* 1994;104:612–618.
37. Michaels L, Wells M. Squamous cell carcinoma of the middle ear. *Clin Otolaryngol* 1980;5:235–248.
38. Phelps PD, Lloyd GAS. *Radiology of the ear.* Oxford; Blackwell Scientific, 1983.
39. Anson BJ, Donaldson JA. *Surgical anatomy of the temporal bone. 3rd ed.* Philadelphia; WB Saunders, 1981.
40. Graham MD, Reams C, Perkins R. Human tympanic membrane—malleus attachment. Preliminary study. *Ann Otol Rhinol Laryngol* 1978;87:426–431.
41. Bolz EA, Lim DL. Morphology of the stapediovestibular joint. *Acta Otolaryngol (Stockh)* 1972;73:10–17.
42. Davies DV. A note on the articulations of the auditory ossicles and related structures. *J Laryngol Otol* 1948;62:533–536.
43. Glorig A, Davis H. Age, noise and hearing loss. *Ann Otol Rhinol Laryngol* 1961;70:556–571.
44. Etholm B, Belal A. Senile changes in the middle ear joints. *Ann Otol Rhinol Laryngol* 1974;83:49–54.
45. Walsted A, Garbarsch C, Michaels L. Effect of craniotomy and cerebrospinal fluid loss on the inner ear. An experimental study. *Acta Otolaryngol (Stockh)* 1994;114:626–631.
46. Schuknecht HF. Cupolithiasis. *Arch Otolaryngol Head Neck Surg* 1969;90:765–78.
47. Gacek RR. Transection of the posterior ampullary nerve for relief of benign paroxysmal positional vertigo. *Ann Otol Rhinol Laryngol* 1974; 63:596–605.
48. Procter B, Corgill DA, Proud G. The pathology of Bell's palsy. *Trans Am Acad Ophthalmol Soc* 1976;82:70–80.
49. Guild SR. The glomus jugulare, a nonchromaffin paraganglion, in man. *Ann Otol Rhinol Laryngol* 1953;62:1045–1071.
50. Heffner DK. Low-grade adenocarcinoma of probable endolymphatic sac origin. A clinicopathologic study of 20 cases. *Cancer* 1989;64: 2292–2302.
51. Schuknecht HF. *Pathology of the ear. 2nd ed.* Philadelphia; Lea & Febiger, 1993.
52. Soucek S, Michaels L, Frohlich A. Pathological changes in the organ of Corti in presbyacusis as revealed by microslicing and staining. *Acta Otolaryngol Suppl (Stockh)* 1987:93–101.
53. Soucek S, Michaels L, Frohlich A. Evidence for hair cell degeneration as the primary lesion in hearing loss of the elderly. *J Otolaryngol* 1986; 15:175–183.
54. Baker RD. *Post mortem examination. Specific methods and procedures.* Philadelphia; WB Saunders, 1967.
55. Sando I, Doyle W, Takahara T, Kitajiri M, Coury WJ III. How to remove, process, and study the temporal bone with the entire eustachian tube and its accessory structures: a method for histopathological study. *Auris Nasus Larynx* 1985;12 (suppl 1):21–25.
56. Johnsson LG, Hawkins JE. A direct approach to cochlear anatomy and pathology in man. *Arch Otolaryngol Head Neck Surg* 1967;85: 599–613.
57. Michaels L, Wells M, Frohlich A. A new technique for the study of temporal bone pathology. *Clin Otolaryngol* 1983;8:77–85.
58. Iurato S, Bredberg G, Bock G. *Functional histopathology of the human audio-vestibular organ.* Eurodata hearing project. Commission of the European Communities, 1982.
59. Karnovsky MJ. A formaldehyde-glutaraldehyde fixative of high osmolality for use in electron microscopy. *J Cell Biol* 1965;27:137A–138A.
60. Shi S, Tandon AK, Haussmann RR, Kalra KL, Taylor CR. Immunohistochemical study of intermediate filament proteins on routinely processed, celloidin-embedded human temporal bone sections using a new technique for antigen retrieval. *Acta Otolaryngol (Stockh)* 1993;113: 48–54.
61. Shi S, Tandon AK, Coté C, Kalra KL. S-100 protein in human inner ear: use of a novel immunohistochemical technique on routinely processed, celloidin-embedded human temporal bone sections. *Laryngoscope* 1992;102:734–738.
62. Burgess RC, Michaels L, Bale JF, Smith RJ. Polymerase chain reaction amplification of herpes viral DNA from the geniculate ganglion of a patient with Bell's palsy. *Ann Otol Rhinol Laryngol* 1994;103:775–779.
63. Michaels L. *Atlas of ENT histopathology.* Lancaster:MTP Press, 1990.
64. Michaels L. *Ear, nose and throat histopathology.* London; Springer-Verlag, 1987.

*Histology for Pathologists, second edition,*
Edited by Stephen S. Sternberg.
Lippincott-Raven Publishers, Philadelphia


# CHAPTER 15

# Mouth, Nose, And Paranasal Sinuses

Karoly Balogh



## EMBRYOLOGY AND PRENATAL CHANGES

This chapter describes the development of a complex, highly specialized part of the head; for obvious reasons, our discussion is restricted to structures of importance to the surgical pathologist. Developmentally and functionally interrelated, the embryology of the organs covered are presented together. Only a broad and simplified outline of the intricate development is necessary here. For details, the reader is referred to other sources (1–4).

The oral region develops from an ectodermal depression, the stomodeum. The deep oral cavity is formed by the forward growth of structures about the margins of the stomodeum, giving rise to superficial parts of the face and jaws, as well as the walls of the oral cavity. The stomodeal prominence is surrounded by the right and left maxillary processes, the right and left mandibular processes, and rostrally by the unpaired frontal prominence. The ectoderm of the frontal prominence will form the lining of the nasal pits and ultimately the olfactory processes through the cribriform plate into the olfactory bulb. From the structures surrounding the stomodeum are cephalically derived the upper lip, maxilla, and nose; the caudal boundary of the oral cavity is formed by the paired mandibular processes, which during the second year of life fuse in the midline to form the mandible. Due to rapid proliferation of the mesenchyme beneath the surface, the paired maxillary processes likewise meet in the midline, crowding the nasal elevation and ultimately forming the maxilla and, by fusion in the midline, the palate. The nose is formed on either side of the frontonasal elevation by ectodermal invagination into the mesoderm to form two nasal pits, which gradually converge toward the midline and with the medial nasal elevations of either side gradually merge with each other. This way the mesenchyme under the ectoderm gives rise to the structures that develop into bone, cartilage, and skeletal muscle. At the end of the second month the formation of the bony structures begins; the maxilla is one of the first bones to calcify. Simultaneously the nasal pits become progressively deeper and extend downward toward the oral cavity. Later, elevations appear on the lateral walls of the right and left nasal cavity and will become the scroll-like nasal turbinates (conchae). The nasal cavities are communicating with chambers in the adjacent bones known as paranasal sinuses. Named for the bones in which they lie, they comprise the frontal, maxillary, and sphenoidal sinuses as well as the paired irregular group of bilateral small cavities, the ethmoid sinuses. The paranasal sinuses are first indicated at about the fourth month of fetal life, but most of their expansion occurs after birth and they attain full size many years later. The mucosa lining the nasal cavities invaginates into the surrounding bone, and the resulting chamber becomes the expanding sinus. The contours of the face change with the rapid growth of the nose and jaws (5). The nasolacrimal duct arises independently as an epithelial downgrowth from the conjunctival sac. The main part of the palate is derived from the maxilla; shelflike outgrowths arise from either side of the maxilla and grow toward the midline, where they later meet in a suture. While the palate has been taking shape from the roof of the mouth, the tongue has been forming in the floor. Simply put, the tongue can be considered a sac of mucous membrane that has become filled with a mass of growing muscle. The posterior part of the tongue

K. Balogh: Department of Pathology, Harvard Medical School, Boston, Massachusetts 02115.

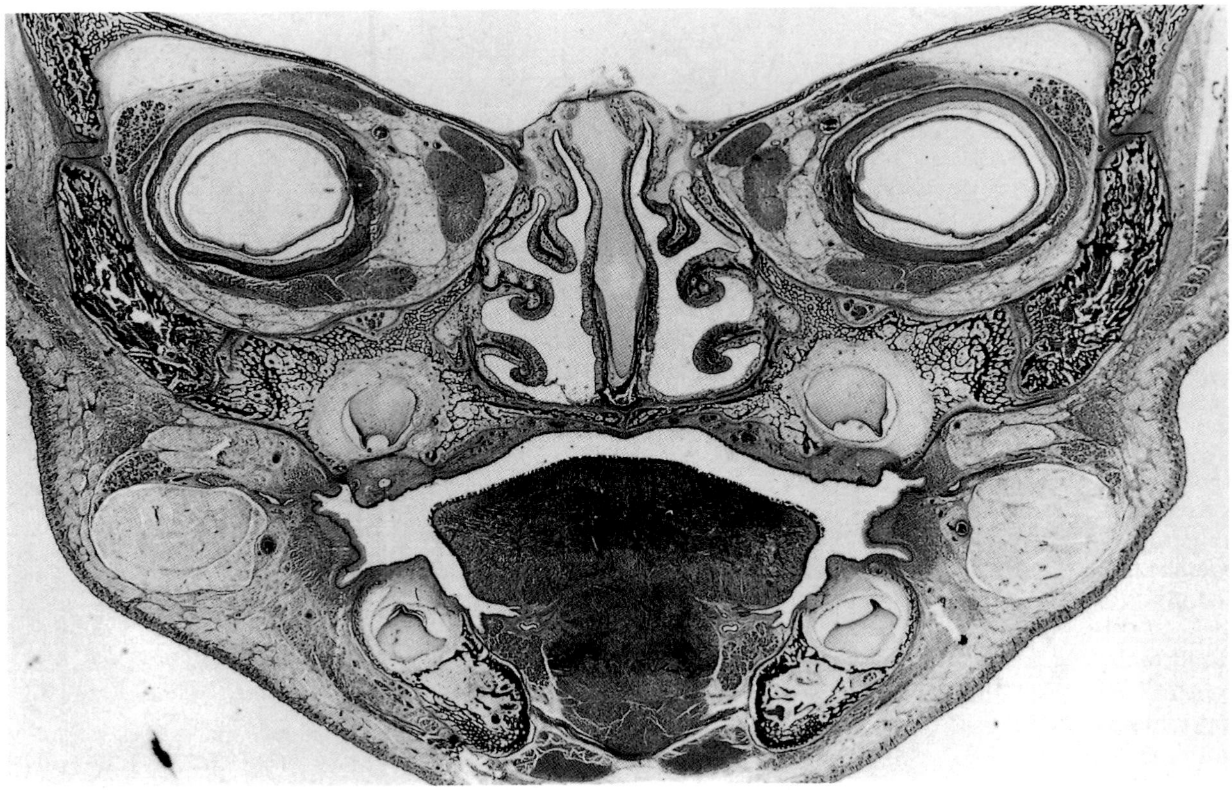

**FIG. 1.** Coronal section of head of a human fetus about 30 weeks of age (284 mm crown–rump length). The bell-shaped enamel organs are present in each quadrant. The tongue is relatively large. The paranasal sinuses are not yet discernible at this stage of fetal development. (Courtesy of Dr. Kenneth D. McClatchey, Ann Arbor, Michigan.)

(behind the sulcus terminalis) is derived from the midventral areas of branchial arches II, III, and IV.

The development of teeth is of considerable importance for the understanding of the pathogenesis of odontogenic tumors and cysts because most of them originate from some aberration in the normal development of the teeth. The teeth begin to develop inside the gums of the upper and lower jaw (Fig. 1). Initially, the oral epithelium shows definite thickening and grows into the subjacent mesenchyme around the entire arc of each jaw to form the dental lamina. From this horseshoe-shaped epithelial structure, buds arise to form the enamel organs at the site of each future tooth. Thus, the primordia for the deciduous teeth are formed. Shortly afterward, the primordia of the permanent teeth develop the same way. The developing enamel organ of each tooth takes the shape of a poorly formed goblet with the dental lamina as its stem. As the dental lamina disintegrates, the lining cells of the enamel organ differentiate to become columnar epithelial cells called ameloblasts, whereas the outer layer of the cells of the goblet-shaped enamel organ flattens into a layer of closely packed cells (outer enamel epithelium). Between the ameloblasts and the outer enamel epithelium is the loosely arranged epithelium of the stellate reticulum. Inside the goblet-shaped enamel organ, the mesenchymal cells proliferate to form a dense aggregation, the dental papilla. In the bell stage of the enamel organ the outer and inner enamel epithelium meet at their apical end; here the double row of epithelial cells proliferates to form Hertwig's sheath, which initiates the differentiation of the outermost cells of the papilla to become arranged in a row of single columnar cells to form the odontoblasts (Figs. 2 and 3). Nerves and blood vessels in the dental papilla appear to form the primitive dental pulp. The dental papilla grows toward the gum, crowding in on the enamel organ, which by then has lost its connection with the oral epithelium. The nonmineralized predentin is produced by the odontoblasts against the inner surface of the enamel organ. As the odontoblasts produce predentin, their cell bodies recede toward the center of the tooth, each odontoblast leaving behind a thin process (Tomes' fiber) that occupies a dentinal tubule. The organic matrix of the predentin eventually mineralizes to become dentin, which is arranged in the shape of tubules running from the pulp chamber toward the periphery. Meanwhile the enamel cap of the tooth is being formed by the ameloblasts (6). The formation of dentin and enamel begins at the tip of the crown and progresses toward the root of the tooth (7). As the developing root increases in length, the previously formed crown moves closer to the surface of the gum. Even when the crown of the tooth begins to erupt, the root is still incomplete and continues growing until the crown has completely emerged (8,9) (Figs. 4 and 5). The enamel is made by differentiated ameloblasts that produce long, thin enamel prisms, or rods; these rods become

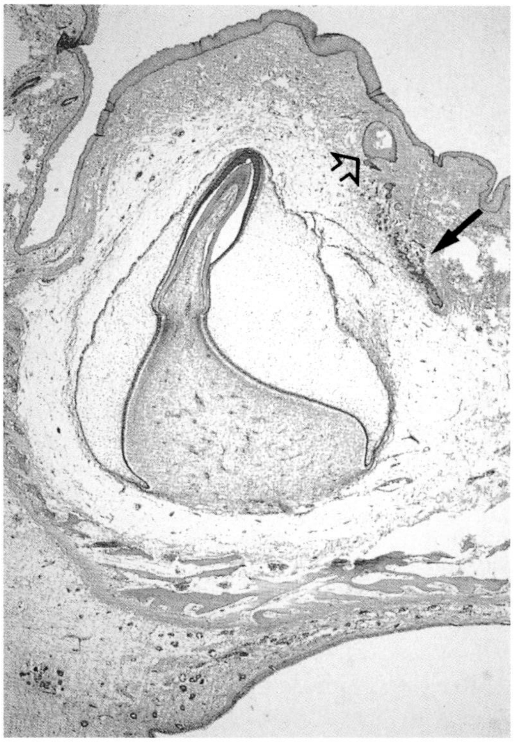

**FIG. 2.** Enamel organ of deciduous tooth. Formation of enamel and dentin has begun at the crown area of the tooth. *Arrow* points to remnants of dental lamina; *arrowhead* indicates a small epithelial cyst (rest of Serres). (Courtesy of Dr. Kenneth D. McClatchey, Ann Arbor, Michigan.)

calcified and are surrounded by a thin organic matrix. Enamel production is completed when the crown is mineralized and its final size attained (10). At this point in time the flattened ameloblasts and remainder of the cells of the enamel organ form a cuticle on the surface of the enamel; this membrane is then shed (11). After the root has attained its full length and definitive position in the jaw, a bonelike hard substance, cement, is deposited on it. Cement is produced by the mesenchymal cells adjacent to the root; these cells become differentiated into a cementoblast layer that resembles the osteogenic (cambial) layer of the periosteum (12,13). Fibers of the rest of the dental sac form the periodontal ligament, which firmly attaches the tooth in the bony alveolar socket (14).

The deciduous teeth, the first set of teeth, are temporary; the second set is permanent. The development of the permanent teeth is essentially the same as that of the deciduous teeth. The primordia of the permanent teeth appear early, budding off from the dental lamina close to the point from which the enamel organ of the corresponding deciduous teeth arose. The permanent tooth germs lie in a hollow of the alveolar sockets on the lingual side of the deciduous teeth. As the jaws approach their adult size, the latent primordia of the permanent teeth follow the same developmental process as did the deciduous teeth (15) (Fig. 6). When a developing permanent tooth increases in size, the root of the corresponding deciduous tooth is partly resorbed by osteoclastic

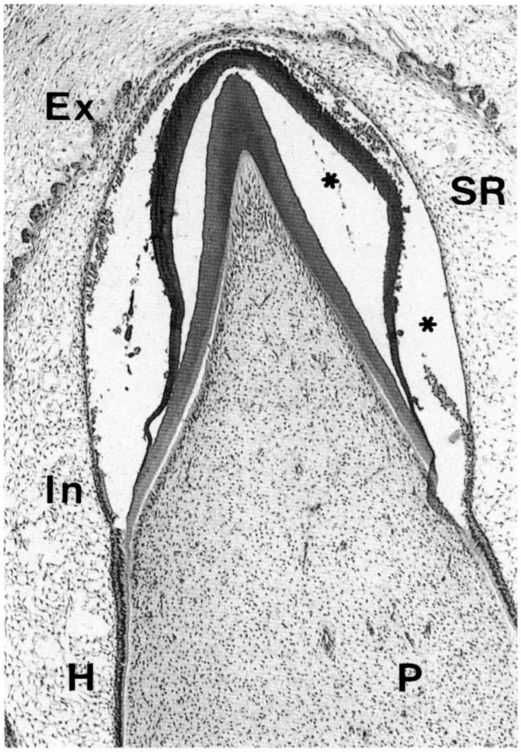


**FIG. 3.** Enamel organ. Amelogenesis and dentinogenesis progresses from crown to root. Early enamel and dentin appear as black bands, widest at the crown area and become thinner toward the root. Ex, external enamel epithelium; In, inner enamel epithelium; SR, stellate reticulum; H, root sheath of Hertwig; P, dental papilla; *, artifact (separation). (Courtesy of Dr. Kenneth P. McClatchey, Ann Arbor, Michigan.)

activity (Fig. 7). Thus, the anchorage of the deciduous tooth becomes weakened and the tooth is shed; consequently the underlying permanent tooth erupts.

Like the major salivary glands, the minor salivary glands also develop after a pattern of epithelial–mesenchymal inter-

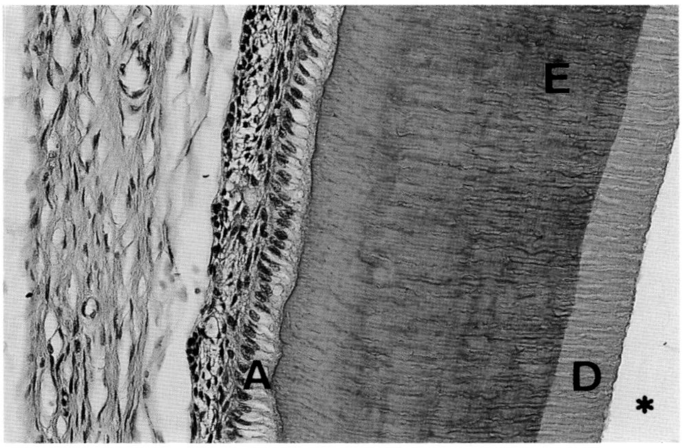


**FIG. 4.** Developing tooth, sagittal section. Ameloblasts (A) line the surface of the enamel matrix (E) which is partly mineralized. Dentin (D) is not mineralized (predentin) and has been separated by an artifact (*) from pulp (missing).

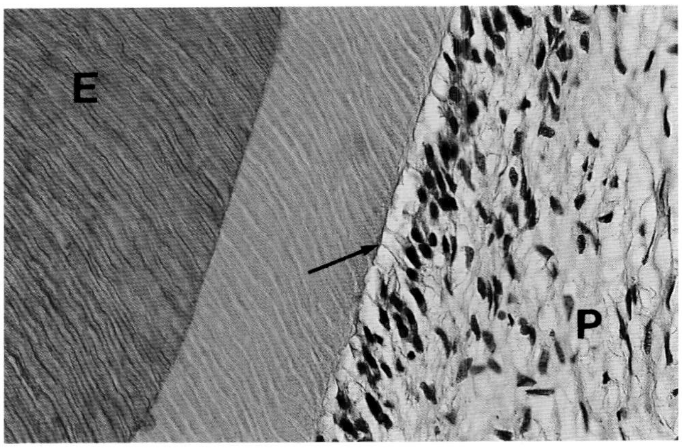


**FIG. 5.** Developing tooth. Layer of polarized odontoblasts with Tomes' fibers (*arrow*) extending into tubules of predentin. Fibroblasts of pulp (P) are loosely arranged. E, enamel matrix.

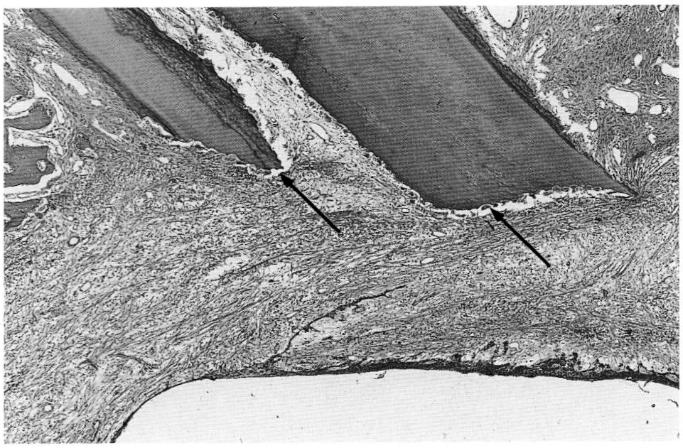

**FIG. 7.** Roots of deciduous molar tooth before shedding. Resorption of dentin is indicated by numerous Howship's lacunae and osteoclasts (*arrows*). The thin band (*bottom*) is the reduced internal enamel epithelium that covered the crown of the underlying permanent tooth; the enamel dissolved with decalcification.

actions between the outgrowth of an ectodermal bud from the lining of the stomodeum and the underlying mesenchyme. The proliferation, differentiation, and morphogenesis of the glands depend on intrinsic and extrinsic factors. The programmed pattern of cell-specific gene expression is established early in development; the extrinsic factors include cell–cell and cell–matrix interactions as well as growth factors (16).

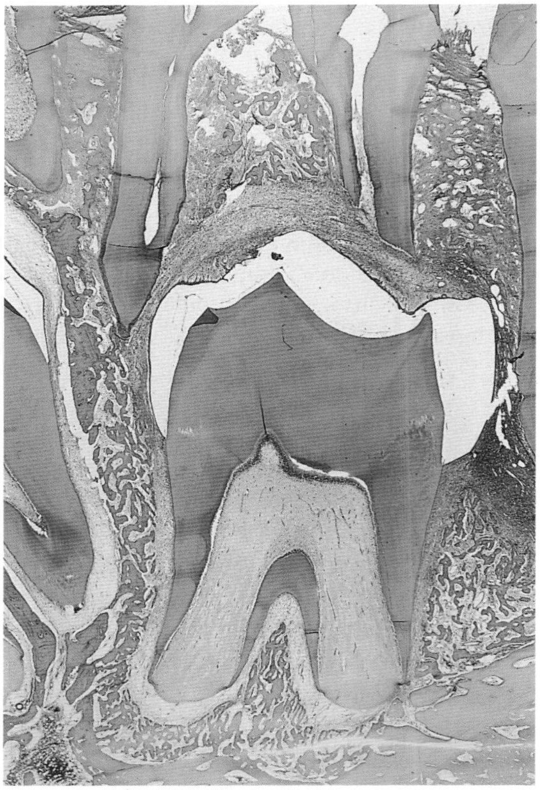

**FIG. 6.** Deciduous and unerupted permanent teeth in a 10-year-old child. Perpendicular section through the roots of two deciduous teeth with underlying permanent molar tooth. Empty space was left by enamel that was dissolved by decalcification. Note relationship between teeth and bone, respectively.

## GROSS ANATOMY

The anatomy of the structures discussed in this chapter makes their detailed description impractical and unnecessary. Therefore, we consider only those features that are important for the surgical pathologist.

### Jawbones

The mandible is a horseshoe-shaped bone; its horizontal part forms the body, which is continuous with the vertical parts of the two sides, the rami. The bone of the body has a thick cortex, and the compact shell contains plates of cancellous bone arranged along the trajectories. The upper part of the body is hollowed into sockets that on each side carry eight teeth. The ramus is a nearly vertical flattened oblong plate of bone; it is surmounted by two processes. The posterior articular process ends in the condyle, articulating with the articular disk of the temporomandibular joint. The anterior process (coronoid process) serves for the insertion of the temporal muscle.

The right and left maxilla jointly form the upper jaw; they participate in forming boundaries of four cavities: the roof of the mouth, the floor and lateral wall of the nose, the floor of the maxillary sinus, and the floor of the orbit. The alveolar processes of the maxillae together form the alveolar arch, holding eight teeth on each side.

### Nose and Paranasal Sinuses

The two orifices of the external nose, the nares, are separated from each other by a median septum that forms the medial wall of the two approximately symmetrical chambers, the right and left nasal fossae. The external nose as well as the nasal septum are partly cartilaginous and partly osseous. Externally the nose is covered by thin skin, which is rich in sebaceous glands. Inside the nares is the vestibule of the nose lined by skin that is continuous with the integument of the nose. The skin of the nasal vestibule contains coarse hairs and sebaceous glands and extends a small shallow recess toward the apex of the nose. In each nasal fossa is an olfactory region that occupies the superior part of the nasal cavity; the rest of the nasal fossa consists of the respiratory region. On the lateral wall of each nasal fossa are the superior, middle, and inferior conchae; these scroll-shaped structures hang over the corresponding funnel-shaped nasal passages or meatuses into which the various paranasal sinuses open. The mucous membrane lining the nasal cavity is continuous with the skin covering the vestibulum and nares. The nasal mucosa is also in continuity with the mucosa of the frontal, ethmoidal, sphenoidal, and maxillary sinuses through their corresponding openings. Posteriorly, the nasal mucosa is continuous with the mucosa of the nasopharynx through the posterior openings of the nasal cavities, the choanae. The nasal mucous membrane is most vascular and thickest over the conchae and is also relatively thick over the nasal septum, but it is thin on the floor of the nasal cavity, in the meatuses, and in the paranasal sinuses.

### Blood Vessels

The nasal cavity has an extraordinarily rich blood supply. The anterior and posterior ethmoidal branches of the ophthalmic artery supply the frontal sinuses, the ethmoidal sinuses, and the roof of the nasal cavity. The sphenopalatine branch of the maxillary artery supplies the mucosa of the conchae, the meatuses, and the nasal septum. The mucosa of the maxillary sinus is supplied by branches of the maxillary artery and the sphenoid sinus by the pharyngeal artery. The branches of all these vessels form a plexiform network in the mucous membrane and beneath it. The veins of the nasal mucosa are well developed, particularly in the inferior concha and in the posterior part of the nasal fossa forming a cavernous plexus. The veins of the lower jaw drain via the inferior central vein into the pterygoid plexus. From the upper jaw and facial structures they drain in two directions: the more anterior parts into the anterior facial vein, the more posterior parts into the pterygoid plexus. The pterygoid plexus drains the teeth, soft palate, fauces, and pharynx. These anatomic relationships are particularly important because infections and tumors of the face, mouth, nose, and paranasal sinuses can reach the cavernous sinus, i.e., enter the cranial cavity via the emissary vein of Vesalius, or by way of veins communicating with the inferior ophthalmic vein. Another, anterior route to the cavernous sinus occurs via the anterior facial and angular veins and then through the orbit by way of the superior ophthalmic vein. These veins drain the structures of the anterior face such as lips, cheek, external nose, eyelids, and forehead, as well as the mucosa of the frontal sinuses, ethmoidal cells, and upper lateral nasal wall. The cavernous sinus also receives veinous blood from the mucosa of the sphenoid sinus.

### Nerves

The regions discussed here have a rich and complex innervation, the description of which is beyond the scope of this chapter. However, many nerves of the head lie in close proximity to the mucosa and submucosa of the upper aerodigestive tract and are therefore prone to early invasion by carcinoma. Because of the functions of the nerves, their invasion by tumor often significantly influences the clinical course and prognosis.

### Lymphatics and Lymph Nodes

The face has an abundant lymphatic drainage. The afferent lymphatic vessels from the eyelids and conjunctiva run mainly to the parotid lymph nodes but partly also to the superficial facial (infraorbital, buccal, and mandibular) lymph nodes. These nodes also drain the skin and mucous membrane of the nose and cheek. Their efferent lymphatics run to the submandibular lymph nodes, which also drain the upper lip and the lateral parts of the lower lip. The lymphatics of the central part of the lower lip and of the anterior parts of the nasal cavities pass to the submental lymph nodes. Those from the posterior two thirds of the nasal cavities and the paranasal sinuses drain partly to the retropharyngeal and partly to the superior deep cervical lymph nodes. The lymphatics of the upper gum and anterior part of the hard palate end in the submandibular lymph nodes, and those of the posterior hard palate and soft palate terminate in the superior deep cervical lymph nodes. The soft palate also drains into the retropharyngeal and subparotid lymph nodes. The retropharyngeal lymph nodes that lie in the buccopharyngeal fascia can occasionally enlarge and present as pharyngeal masses; they should not be mistaken for pharyngeal lymphoid tissue or palatine tonsils. The lymphatics of the anterior floor of the mouth drain into the middle deep cervical or submental lymph nodes. Those of the posterolateral part of the floor of the mouth terminate in the submandibular and superior deep cervical lymph nodes. The lymphatics of the tongue end mainly in the deep cervical lymph nodes; the node at the bifurcation of the common carotid artery is considered to be the principal lymph node of the tongue. Of the numerous lymph nodes of the head, we mention here only those that relate to the regions covered in this chapter. These are the superficial facial lymph nodes, comprising the infraorbital, buccal, and mandibular groups. The deep facial lymph nodes are located deep to the ramus of the mandible near the maxillary artery. The lymphatics of the tongue drain into the lingual nodes. The superficial parotid nodes lie partially on the parotid gland. The deeper ones are situated partially in the parotid or on the lateral wall of the pharynx. The parotid lymph nodes drain the external ear canal and ear, frontotemporal region, eyelids, root of the nose, floor of the nasal cavity, and soft palate. The efferents of the parotid lymph nodes pass to the superior deep cervical nodes.

## MICROSCOPY

### Mouth

#### *Lips and Vermilion Border*

The entrance to the digestive tract is surrounded by two fleshy folds of skin, the lips. They are partly covered by skin that bears hairs, sweat glands, and sebaceous glands and is richly endowed with sensory nerves. The inner surface of the lips is covered by the oral mucosa and forms a part of the wall of the oral cavity. Between the external integument and the oral mucosa are the orbicularis oris muscle, the labial vessels, nerves, and fat tissue with numerous minor salivary glands. The latter are easily accessible for biopsies to diagnose Sjögren's syndrome. The junction between the skin and oral mucosa is known as the vermilion border, where the keratinized squamous epithelium of the skin changes to the mucous membrane of the oral cavity. The squamous epithelium of the vermilion border is thin, and the tall connective tissue papillae are close to the surface. The blood in the rich capillary network shows through the thin epithelium; these characteristics are the basis of the redness of the lips. The transition zone has no hairs. In adults ectopic sebaceous glands are commonly observed in the vermilion border, at the corners of the mouth, or in the buccal mucosa; these are termed Fordyce's spots (or Fox-Fordyce granules) and increase with age, so that 70% to 80% of elderly persons have them. These ectopic sebaceous glands are considered normal (Fig. 8) (17,18). Like the skin, the vermilion border is exposed to physical forces and chemical agents. For instance, actinic keratosis and solar elastosis can be seen on the vermilion border. The squamous epithelium of the transitional zone imperceptibly merges with the stratified squamous epithelium of the oral mucosa.

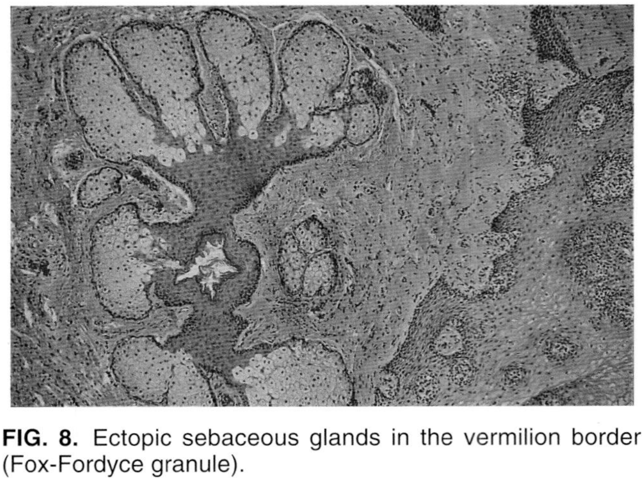

**FIG. 8.** Ectopic sebaceous glands in the vermilion border (Fox-Fordyce granule).

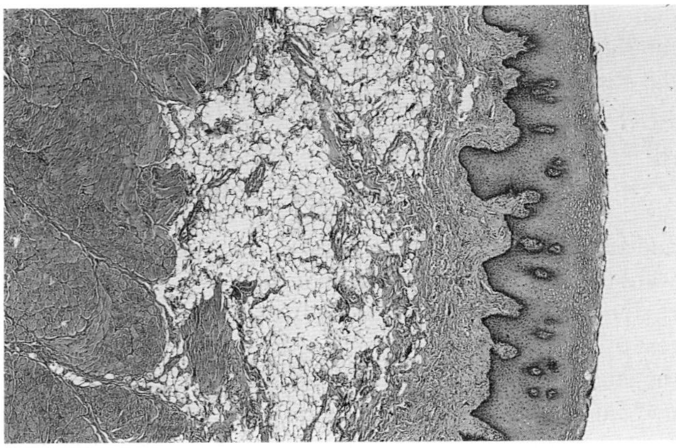

**FIG. 9.** Inner aspect of cheek, cross section. Right to left: buccal mucosa, lamina propria, adipose tissue, cross-striated muscle.

#### *Oral Mucosa and Submucosa*

The oral mucosa consists of an epithelial layer and an underlying layer of connective tissue, the lamina propria (Fig. 9). The mucosa of the oral cavity shows regional modifications that correspond to functional requirements. The stratified squamous epithelium of the oral mucosa has three functional types: the lining mucosa, masticatory mucosa, and specialized mucosa (19). Most of the oral mucosa is lined by nonkeratinized squamous epithelium of the lining mucosa. The palate, gingiva, and dorsum of the tongue are exposed to the forces of mastication and are covered by keratinized epithelium of the masticatory mucosa. Details of the specialized mucosa are described with the tongue. Throughout the oral cavity the epithelium is worn off by mastication and speaking; hence, epithelial cells are a normal constituent of the saliva and are frequently encountered by the pathologist in the sputum or as "contaminants" in bronchoscopic specimens. Squamous cells of the buccal mucosa also have been a convenient source for the microscopic demonstration of the sex chromosome (Barr body). (Fig. 10). The shed epithelial cells are replaced by the basal cells, which divide, then migrate to the surface and are worn off. The renewal of the oral mucosa takes about 12 days (20). As the name implies, the squamous epithelium of the mucosa is kept moist and glistening by mucus that is secreted by the numerous minor and paired major salivary glands. This thin film of mucus covers all intraoral structures, including the teeth, which are bathed by saliva, exerting an overall protective effect.

The interface of the epithelium and lamina propria is delineated by the basal lamina, or basement membrane. In hematoxylin and eosin (H&E)-stained sections it is sometimes hard to see the basal lamina, but special stains (e.g., reticulum) demonstrate it well (Fig. 11). The basal lamina is secreted by the epithelial cells and serves supportive and filtering functions. It also regulates differentiation, migration,

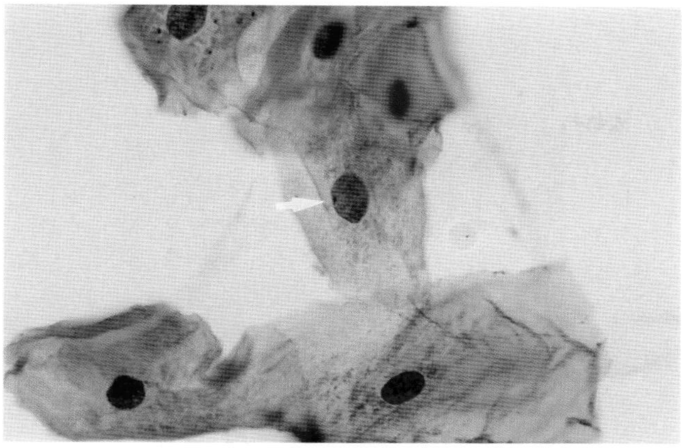

**FIG. 10.** Scraping of buccal mucosa. Intermediate squamous cell with sex chromatin body (Barr body) (*arrow*) lying against the inner nuclear membrane. Papanicolaou stain. (Courtesy of Dr. Imad Nasser, Boston, Massachusetts.)

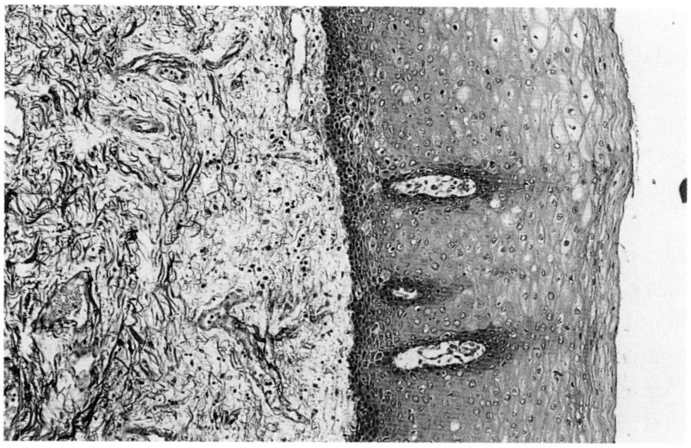

**FIG. 12.** Buccal mucosa showing maturation of squamous epithelium: row of small basal cells, larger cells of stratum spinosum, and parallel arranged flat surface cells. No keratinization is seen. Lamina propria shows delicate strands of connective tissue, blood vessels, and a few lymphocytes. Mallory's trichrome stain.

and polarity of the epithelial cells. The basal lamina is composed of type IV collagen and heparan sulfate, as well as by two glycoproteins, laminin and entactin, which interact with other components of the extracellular matrix. A single layer of basal cells rests on the basal lamina. The basal cells continuously divide, and the new cells push the overlying ones toward the surface. In this process of differentiation the small cuboidal basal cells become polyhedral and larger, forming the stratum spinosum. These cells contain abundant intracytoplasmic fibrils (tonofilaments) that attach to the desmosomes, connecting the squamous epithelial cells with each other. Toward the top layers the cells gradually become flat. The nonkeratinized squamous epithelium lacks the stratum granulosum and stratum corneum; the surface cells retain their nuclei, and the cytoplasm does not contain keratin filaments (Fig. 12) (21). In keratinizing epithelium the cells form a stratum granulosum, which is a prominent layer three to five cells thick. The cells of this layer have numerous intracytoplasmic granules, called keratohyaline granules, which stain with hematoxylin. As the process of keratinization advances, the nucleus and cytoplasmic organelles become disrupted and disappear; the cell becomes filled with an intracellular protein, keratin. Thus, the surface layer, the stratum corneum, is formed.

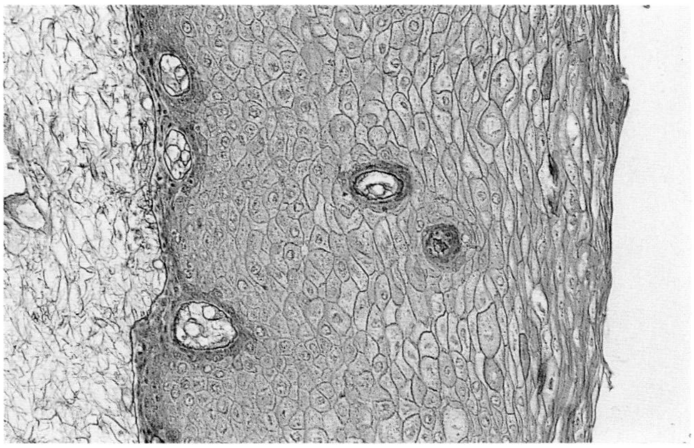

**FIG. 11.** Buccal mucosa. Reticulin stain delineates the plasma membrane of nonkeratinized squamous epithelial cells and the delicate basement membrane. Papillae of lamina propria contain blood vessels.

The oral mucosa from various sites exhibits striking differences in cytokeratin synthesis. The gingiva (masticatory mucosa) expresses a great complexity of cytokeratins, similar to that of the epidermis, containing proliferative keratinocytes. In contrast, the lining mucosa shows a paucity of cytokeratins, thus resembling some other stratified nonkeratinizing squamous epithelium, e.g., that of the esophagus. The differences in the distribution of cytoskeletal proteins can be well demonstrated immunohistochemically and reflect the relationship between morphology and function of these epithelia (22). From a practical point of view, however, immunohistochemical studies of cytokeratins in abnormal oral mucosa have not so far yielded consistent results that are diagnostically useful (23).

The lamina propria is a delicate layer of connective tissue under the squamous epithelium. It contains few elastic and collagenous fibers; the lamina propria is rich in blood vessels, lymphatics, and nerves. These all are arranged much like those are in the skin; the nerves belong to the sensory branches of the trigeminal nerve. The lamina propria also contains lymphocytes, which are often found migrating through the epithelium; consequently, lymphocytes are a normal constituent of the saliva (salivary corpuscles). Other sources of lymphocytes and polymorphonuclear leukocytes in the saliva are infections (e.g., periodontitis, tonsillitis).

The submucosa under the lining mucosa is composed of fairly loosely arranged connective tissue, which contains larger blood vessels, lymphatics, nerves, adipose tissue, and numerous minor salivary glands. Where the mucosa is in close proximity of the underlying bone, (e.g., the hard palate), there is no submucosa; the fibers of the lamina propria are directly and tightly attached to bone. In these areas the mucosa, lamina propria, and periosteum are joined together as one membrane and are generally referred to as a mucoperiosteum.

The number of lymphocytes in the lamina propria increases toward the posterior part of the oral cavity, where it merges with the submucosal lymphoid tissue known as Waldeyer's ring, a circular band of lymphoid tissue that guards the opening into the digestive and respiratory tract. The most anatomically distinctive portion of Waldeyer's ring are the palatine tonsils, the pharyngeal tonsil, and the lingual tonsil (see section on the tongue).

### *Palate and Uvula*

The roof of the oral cavity is formed by the palate, which consists anteriorly of the hard palate and posteriorly of the soft palate. The palate separates the oral and nasal cavities. Anteriorly and laterally it is bounded by the alveolar arches and gums; posteriorly it is continuous with the soft palate. The hard palate is covered by masticatory mucosa. The mucosal surface of the hard palate has a series of ridges (rugae) running across, but not crossing, the midline. The ridges are easily seen and palpated and can be felt with the tongue. Called palatal rugae, these prominent ridges are folds of squamous epithelium supported by a dense connective tissue of the lamina propria. The connective tissue fibers pass directly from the papillary layer of the lamina propria into the underlying bone. In the anterior lateral regions of the hard palate, the submucosa contains fat tissue, whereas more posteriorly its lateral regions contain minor salivary glands (palatine glands), which are pure mucous glands (Fig. 13). The soft palate is the mobile portion suspended from the posterior border of the palate like a curtain. Its oral surface is covered by lining mucosa, and its nasal surface, which is continuous with the floor of the nasal cavity, is mostly lined

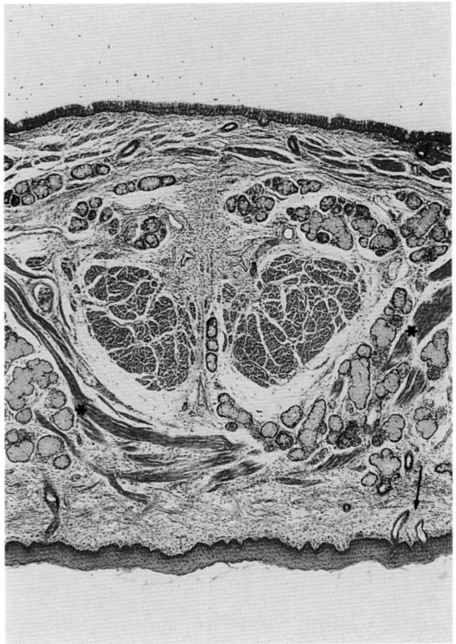

**FIG. 14.** Soft palate sectioned in the coronal plane. Nasal respiratory mucosa (*top*), oral squamous mucosa (*bottom*). Fascicles of pharyngopalatine muscle are right and left of the midline. Fibers of levator veli palatini muscle (*) are obliquely descending. Ducts of minor salivary glands are near the nasal and oral mucosa (*arrow*), respectively. (Courtesy of Dr. B. Csillik, Szeged, Hungary.)

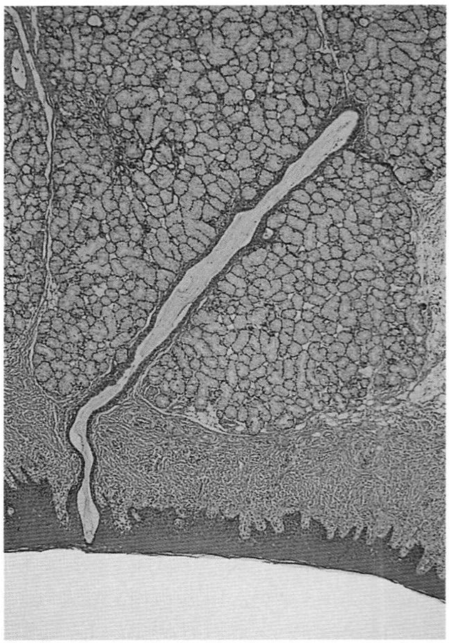

**FIG. 13.** Hard palate with pure mucous minor salivary glands and duct. Note dense connective tissue of lamina propria.

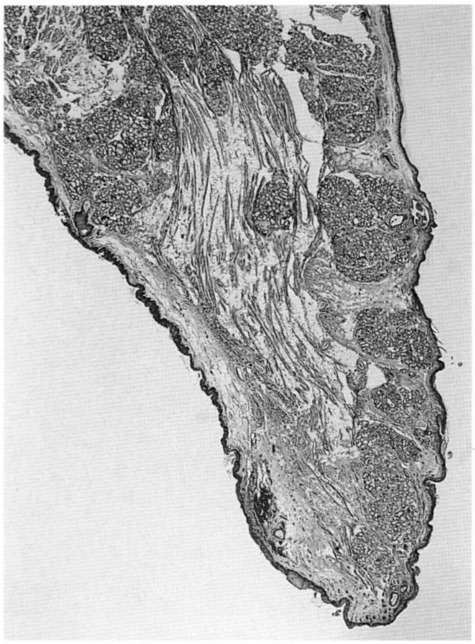

**FIG. 15.** Sagittal section of uvula with numerous mucous glands and bundles of cross-striated muscle. More glands are seen near the oral surface (*right*).

**TABLE 1.** *Minor Salivary Glands of Mouth, Nose and Paranasal Sinuses*

| Name | Location | Type of Acini |
|---|---|---|
| Labial (superior and inferior) | Lips | Mixed (predominantly mucous) |
| Buccal | Cheek | Mixed (predominantly mucous) |
| Glossopalatine | Anterior faucial pillar<br>Glossopalatine fold | Pure mucous |
| Palatine | Hard palate<br>Soft palate | Pure mucous |
| | Uvula | Mixed (predominantly mucous) |
| Sublingual | Floor of mouth | Mixed (predominantly mucous) |
| Lingual | Anterior tongue | Mixed (predominantly mucous) |
| Tongue | Circumvallate papillae | Pure serous |
| Lingual tonsil | Base of tongue | Pure mucous |
| Nasal and paranasal | Nose and sinuses | Mixed |

by ciliated respiratory epithelium. The soft palate contains fibers of striated muscle, blood vessels, and nerves (Fig. 14). Larger mucous glands underlie the oral epithelium, and smaller groups of mixed glands are present on the nasal surface under the respiratory epithelium. From the middle of the posterior border of the soft palate hangs a small, conical process of soft tissue, the uvula; it is microscopically similar to the soft palate and is not a lymphoid organ (Fig. 15).

### *Floor of the Mouth*

Here the mucous membrane is thin and loosely attached to the underlying structures. The rete ridges are short. The submucosa contains some adipose tissue and numerous minor salivary glands (sublingual mucous glands).

### *Minor Salivary Glands*

Numerous small glands are scattered throughout the submucosa of the oral cavity, nose and paranasal sinuses, as well as adjacent to the palatine and pharyngeal tonsils. These glands are not encapsulated and are named by their location; they can be classified as mucous, serous, and mixed seromucinous type (Table 1). The glands produce secretions similar to those of the major salivary glands and empty the secretion onto the mucosal surface through numerous small excretory ducts. The secretory activity of these glands appears to be continuous, although they can respond to specific local chemical or physical stimuli.

Structurally the minor salivary glands are compound tubular or tubuloacinar. Their secretory portions are the acini that are designated according to their secretion as mucous, serous, or mixed (both mucous and serous). The mucous and serous acini differ in shape and size; the mucous acini are more tubular. Within mixed, seromucinous acini, the mucous cells are nearest to the excretory duct; the serous cells are at the cul-de-sac of the acini and appear as crescents, called the demilunes of Gianuzzi (Figs. 16 and 17). The mucous cells are larger, and their flattened nuclei are at the bases of the cells. The mucous cells have a pale-appearing cytoplasm in H&E-stained sections (Fig. 13); their cytoplasm will stain with Alcian blue, periodic acid-Schiff (PAS) or mucicarmine (24,25). The serous cells are smaller, and their nuclei are rounded and situated near the bases of the cells. The serous cells have an eosinophilic cytoplasm that

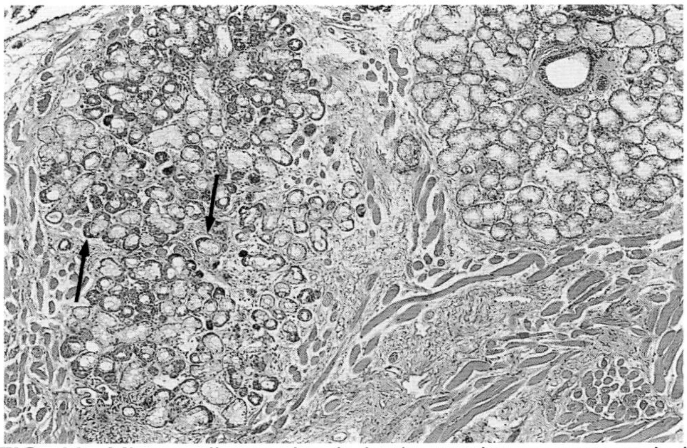

**FIG. 16.** Minor salivary glands in the uvula are surrounded by cross-striated muscle. The gland with the distinct duct is of the pure mucous type. The other gland is seromucinous, with the serous cells forming darker staining crescents (*arrows*).

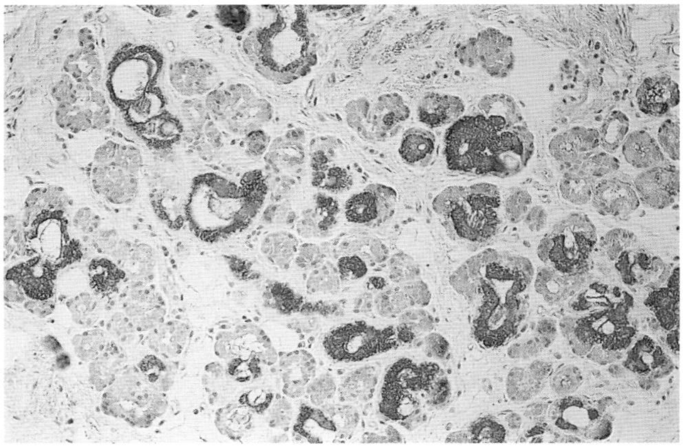

**FIG. 17.** Mixed minor salivary gland of the uvula. Acid mucopolysaccharides in mucous cells stain turquoise with Alcian blue (at pH 2.6).

contains zymogen granules. Contractile myoepithelial cells are wrapped around the acinus and squeeze the secretion from the acinar cells into the excretory ducts (26). The myoepithelial cells of the minor salivary glands are variably immunoreactive with antibodies to cytokeratin and muscle-specific actin, rarely to S-100 protein. Neoplastic myoepithelial cells, however, are more consistently reactive with these antibodies.

It is important to note that the minor salivary glands, wherever they occur in the mouth, nose, or paranasal sinuses, can become involved by the same pathologic processes as the major salivary glands. This is especially true for neoplasms, which arise from various cellular components of the minor salivary glands.

The surgical pathologist must be well aware of the fact that squamous metaplasia can occur in the excretory ducts and acini of minor salivary glands. For instance, epithelial regeneration after injury of various types may lead to squamous metaplasia that can mimic squamous cell carcinoma. A good example of this is seen in necrotizing sialometaplasia or in irradiated salivary glands. In the latter case, the dilemma is compounded by the possibility of a recurrence of known squamous cell carcinoma. Oncocytes are large, cuboidal, or columnar epithelial cells with a finely granular eosinophilic cytoplasm that have been identified in many exocrine or endocrine glands; because of their swollen appearance, Hamperl coined the term "oncocytes" ("swollen cells") (27). Up to 60% of their cytoplasm is occupied by mitochondria that can be visualized after long-term (48 hours) staining with phosphotungstic acid-hematoxylin or on fresh-frozen sections incubated for the histochemical demonstration of mitochondrial enzyme activity. Oncocytes are benign cells that occur with increasing frequency in older persons. Oncocytic cells are also found in minor salivary glands in varying numbers and distribution patterns; they develop by metaplasia of ductal and acinar epithelium to oncocytes (Fig. 18). The etiology and functional significance of oncocytic metaplasia is not clear. In the minor salivary glands, oncocytes can show nodular or diffuse oncocytosis, hyperplasia with or without cyst formation (cystadenoma), and very rarely an oncocytoma (28,29). Oncocytic carcinomas have been reported arising in the minor salivary glands of the palate and buccal mucosa (30).

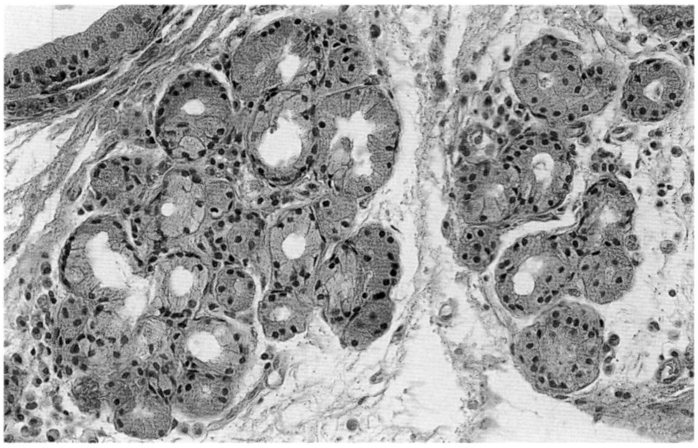

**FIG. 18.** Oncocytes in minor salivary gland appear as cuboidal swollen cells with a finely granular oxyphilic cytoplasm.

### *Cheeks*

The skin of the cheeks is part of the facial skin. The inner surface of the cheeks is covered by lining mucosa; the submucosa contains many minor salivary glands of the mixed type, embedded in loose connective tissue and some fat cells. The mucosa and submucosa are bound to the underlying buccal musculature by connective tissue fibers.

### *Juxtaoral Organ of Chievitz*

Deep in the wall of the cheeks sits an anatomically well-defined small structure, the juxtaoral organ of Chievitz, which is normally present in the buccotemporal space (31,32). In adults, it measures 0.7 to 1.7 cm in length and 0.1 to 0.2 cm in diameter. It is multilobulated, has a dense fibrous capsule, and consists of round or elongate nests of squamouslike epithelial cells embedded in fibrous stroma, which is rich in small nerves. These nests of epithelial cells appear in a cluster on histologic sections, but serial sectioning shows them to be small sprouts and folds in continuity with a mass of epithelium (32). Thus, cross sections through different portions of the juxtaoral organ can show considerable variation in number and shape of epithelial sprouts (Fig. 19). The larger nests of epithelium are composed of cells with a clear cytoplasm and round or oval nuclei; intercellular bridges can be seen toward the center of the cell nests. The cells in the smaller nests can show a whirl-like or concentric arrangement. Occasionally, a glandlike lumen or a follicle filled with colloidlike material are encountered. The seemingly esoteric and minute juxtaoral organ of Chievitz has considerable importance for the surgical pathologist because the presence of squamous epithelial nests intimately admixed with numerous small branches of the buccal nerve has been misinterpreted on frozen section biopsy as perineural invasion by squamous cell carcinoma (33). On the other hand, astute pathologists aware of this pitfall have, in a case of a mucoepidermoid carcinoma with lymphatic spread in the retromolar region, correctly recognized the epithelial nests of the juxtaoral organ (34). Such cases unequivocally demonstrate the importance of awareness of this small organ. It should be added that a case of nodular hyperplasia of the juxtaoral organ has been described (35), but so far no carcinoma originating from it has been reported. The function of the juxtaoral organ is unknown. Since Johan Henrik Chievitz, a Danish anatomist, in 1885 described this structure in a 10-week-old human embryo (36), it has been widely believed that the organ of Chievitz is a rudimentary structure, representing an abortive salivary gland anlage. More re-

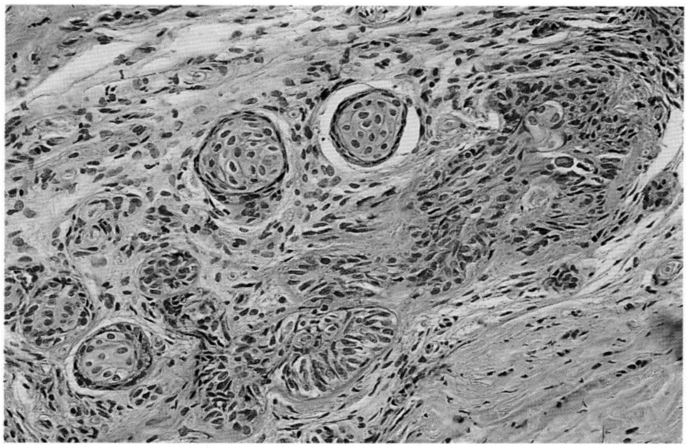

**FIG. 19.** Juxtaoral organ of Chievitz. Small nests of nonkeratinized squamous epithelial cells are delineated by basement membrane. The elongated cells outside the epithelial islands are fibroblasts and Schwann cells. Nerve is seen below and to the right. (Courtesy of Dr. T. Mikó, Szeged, Hungary.)

cently, based on electron microscopic and histochemical evidence, the possibility of a neurosecretory and receptor function of the organ has been raised. A thorough review of the relevant literature can be found in the small monograph by Zenker (32).

### *Tongue*

Situated in the floor of the mouth, the tongue is an organized mass of cross-striated muscle invested by mucous membrane. Its muscles are partly extrinsic (i.e., have their origins outside the tongue) and partly intrinsic, being contained entirely within it. The bundles of cross-striated muscle are embedded in connective tissue with some fat cells and are arranged three-dimensionally. The tongue is well supplied with blood vessels that form numerous anastomoses; its lymphatics drain mainly into the submandibular and deep cervical lymph nodes. The tongue is richly endowed with myelinated and nonmyelinated nerves containing motor, sensory, and vegetative nerve fibers, some with ganglion cells. The ventral surface of the tongue is covered by smooth lining mucosa that has short, blunt rete ridges (Fig. 20). Its submucosa merges with the connective tissue that intersects with the ventral muscle bundles of the tongue.

The upper (dorsal) surface of the tongue is divided into an anterior and posterior part by a V-shaped shallow groove, the sulcus terminalis. The anterior two thirds of the dorsum of the tongue is lined by specialized mucosa, which is bound by connective tissue fibers to the underlying skeletal muscle of the tongue. This specialized mucosa is modified keratinized squamous epithelium covered with small projections, papillae, which are visible to the naked eye. The pathologist has to be aware of these papillae so as not to mistake them for papillary epithelial hyperplasia, papillomas, or oral hairy leukoplakia. According to their shape, the papillae can be filiform, fungiform, foliate, or circumvallate. The great majority are filiform papillae, conical projections of the keratinized epithelium (Fig. 21). Among these are scattered the

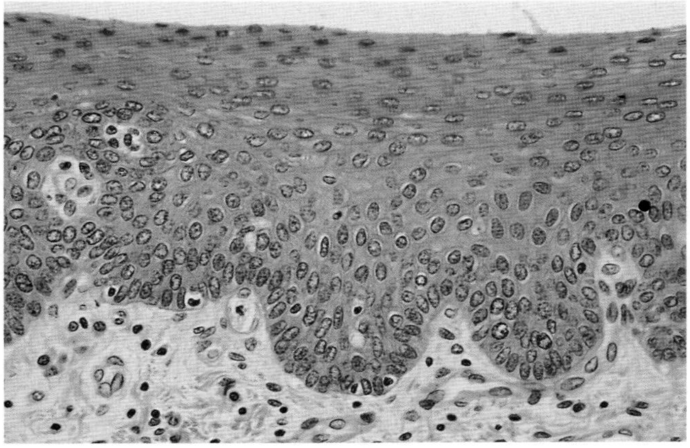

**FIG. 20.** Ventral surface of tongue. The stratified nonkeratinized squamous epithelium of the lining mucosa has a slightly wavy interface with the lamina propria. A few scattered lymphocytes are seen in the lamina propria and in the epithelium.

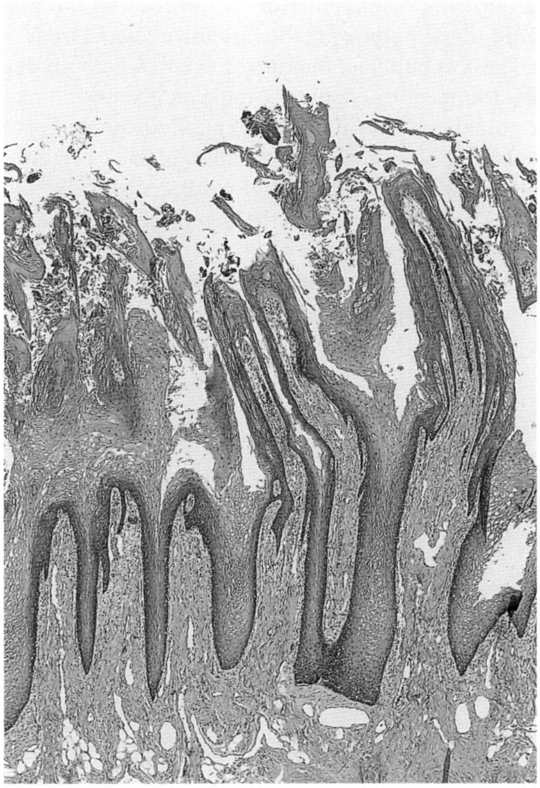

**FIG. 21.** Dorsal surface of tongue. Filiform papillae have a connective tissue core beset with secondary papillae with pointed ends. The superficial squamous cells are keratinized. Note the slender, pointed rete ridges.

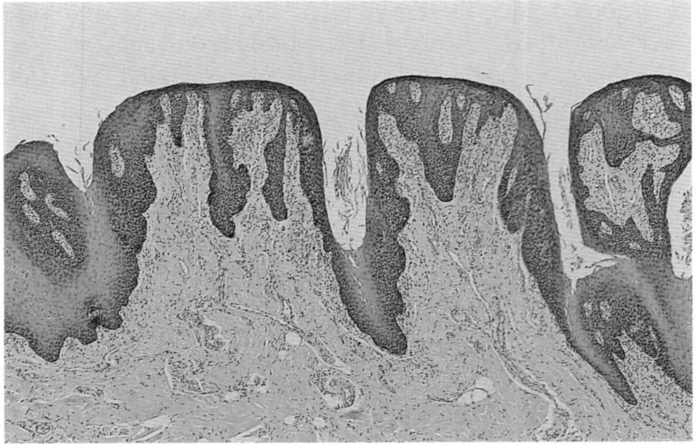

**FIG. 22.** Fungiform papillae. Slightly rounded, elevated structures with larger connective tissue core. Smaller connective tissue papillae project into the base of the surface epithelium.

fungiform papillae, which are rounded elevations above the surface of the tongue; their surface is not keratinized (Fig. 22). Clinically, fungiform papillae appear as small red nodules because the thin epithelium does not mask the underlying vascular connective tissue. Microscopically, fungiform papillae should not be misinterpreted as denture-induced fibrous hyperplasia or small traumatic fibromas. The foliate papillae are located posteriorly along the sides of the tongue. At the junction of the anterior two thirds and the posterior one third of the tongue are the circumvallate papillae. These are the largest papillae, measuring 0.1 to 0.2 cm in diameter and are arranged in a V shape immediately anterior to the sulcus terminalis. The circumvallate papillae number six to 12; a small, ring-shaped furrow surrounds each circumvallate papilla and separates it from a circular, palisadelike mucosal elevation (vallum), which is the outer border of the circumvallate papilla (Fig. 23).

Taste buds are present in large numbers on the side of the circumvallate papillae and in lesser numbers on the fungiform and foliate papillae, as well as elsewhere on the dorsum and lateral aspects of the tongue. Numerous small serous glands (von Ebner's glands) are located under the circumvallate papillae. The ducts of these glands empty their secretion into the small furrow around each papilla; this serous secretion flushes out the furrows, thus facilitating perception

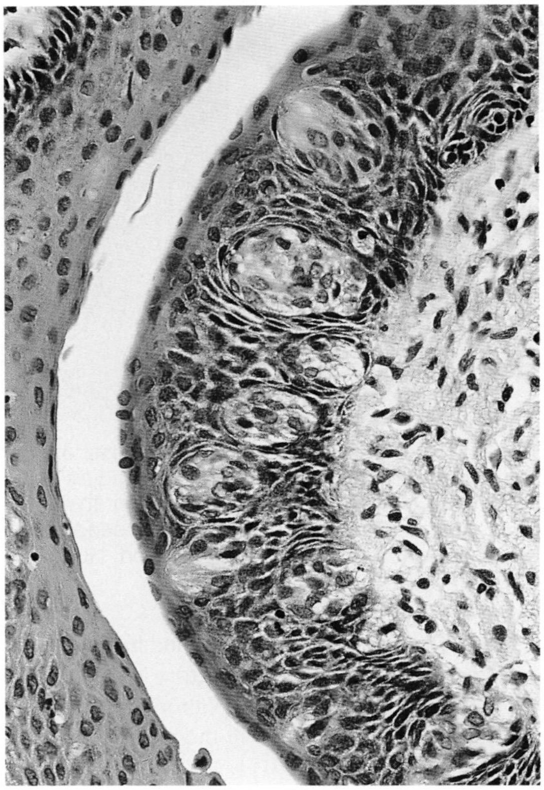

**FIG. 24.** Taste buds on the side of a circumvallate papilla. The cells of the intraepithelial taste buds are spindle shaped and oriented at a right angle to the surface. The cell nuclei are elongated and are situated mainly in the basal half of the buds. Nerve fibers ending on the sensory (gustatory) cells cannot be seen with H&E stain.

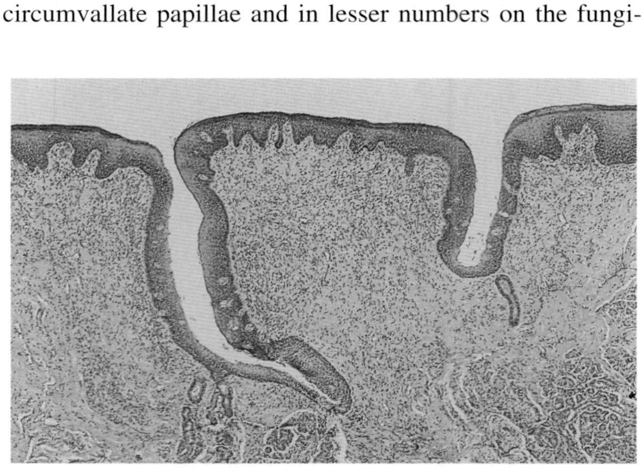

**FIG. 23.** Circumvallate papilla. Numerous taste buds are on the lateral walls of the papilla and on the epithelium facing the papilla within the furrow. Ducts of serous glands open into the furrow surrounding the circumvallate papilla.

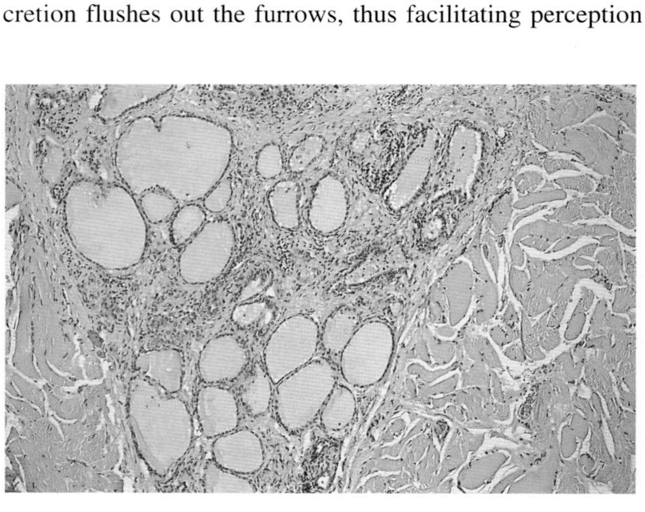

**FIG. 25.** Lingual thyroid. The glandular parenchyma is embedded in skeletal muscle. The thyroid tissue is not encapsulated, not to be mistaken for invasive growth.

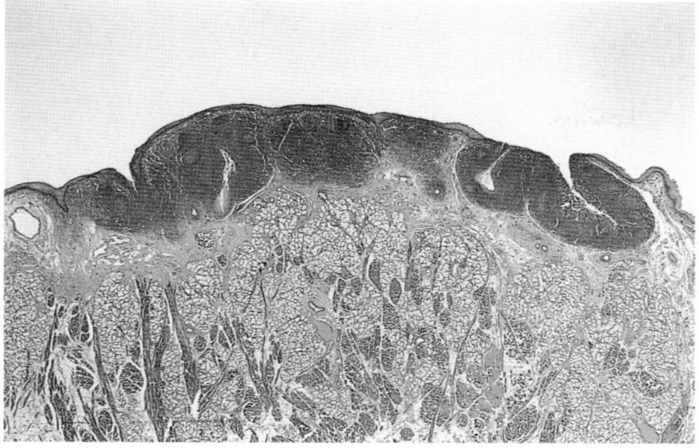

**FIG. 26.** Lingual tonsil. Low-power view of lymphoid tissue and underlying mucous glands that appear as pale areas among bundles of skeletal muscle.

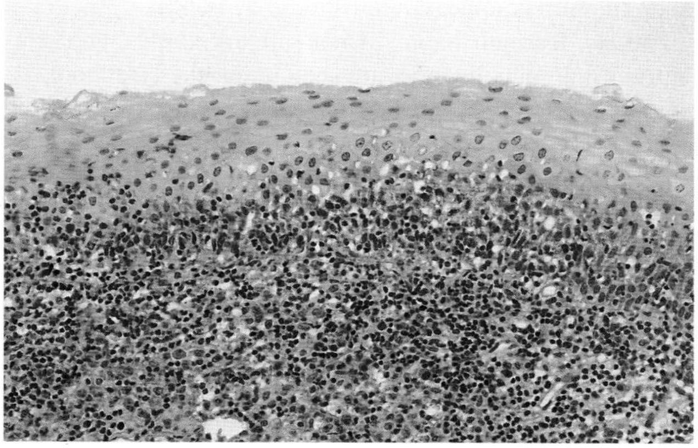

**FIG. 28.** Lingual tonsil. The mucosa (nonkeratinized stratified squamous epithelium) is infiltrated with numerous lymphocytes that obscure the basement membrane.

of new tastes (Fig. 23). The taste buds are barrel-shaped intramucosal sensory receptors that occupy the full thickness of the mucosa and communicate with the surface through a small opening, the gustatory pore (Fig. 24). The taste buds are composed of three types of cells: (a) gustatory or taste cells, (b) supporting, or sustentacular, cells, and (c) basal cells. The taste cells are crescent shaped, have lightly staining cytoplasm, and possess numerous fine microvilli that protrude through the taste pore as gustatory hairs. The basal end of the taste cells has intimate contact with many fine terminations of nerves that leave through the basement membrane and become myelinated outside the taste bud. The supporting cells are likewise crescentic, extending between the basement membrane and the surface; they form a shell for the taste bud and are also scattered between the gustatory cells. The supporting cells have a dark cytoplasm and possess microvilli that protrude through the taste pore. The basal cells are small and are situated between the bases of the other cells; they are giving rise to the other cells of the taste bud (37,38).

The apex of the V-shaped sulcus terminalis projects backward and is marked by a small pit, the foramen cecum, which is an embryologic remnant indicating the upper end of the thyroglossal duct. Correspondingly, ectopic thyroid tissue can occur at the base of the tongue (lingual thyroid) or anywhere along the tract of the thyroglossal duct caudally (Fig. 25). Ectopic thyroid tissue may undergo all the pathologic changes of the thyroid gland proper. Cysts of the thyroglossal duct are not uncommon and characteristically occur in the midline between the base of the tongue and the pyramidal lobe of the thyroid gland.

The lingual tonsil is situated on the dorsum of the tongue posteriorly, between the sulcus terminalis and the epiglottis. The lingual tonsil consists of lymphoid tissue with germinal centers and is covered by squamous epithelium. The lymphoid tissue is variable in amount, irregularly distributed, and is frequently well developed in adults. The overlying squamous epithelium forms several dozen nonbranching tubular infoldings (crypts) that are surrounded by lymphoid tissue (Figs. 26 and 27). Like in the palatine and pharyngeal tonsils, B- and T-lymphocytes migrate from the underlying lymphoid tissue into the epithelium of the crypts and to the surface of the lingual tonsils (Figs. 28 and 29). Sometimes

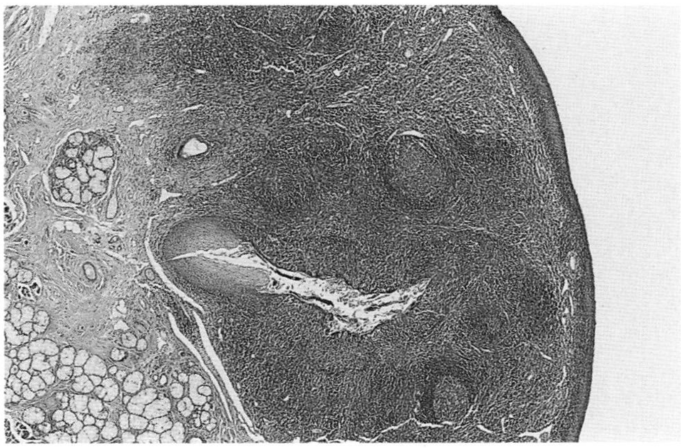

**FIG. 27.** Lingual tonsil. Lymphoid tissue with follicles under mucosa and around its infolding (crypt). Note mucous glands and ducts.

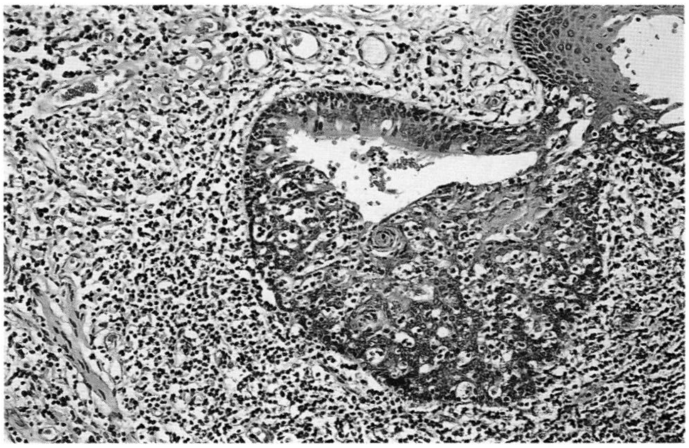

**FIG. 29.** Lingual tonsil. Squamous epithelium of crypt is disrupted by lymphocytes that have migrated into it.

the epithelium is so heavily infiltrated by lymphocytes that it is scarcely distinguishable. Minor salivary glands, predominantly of the mucous type, are seen under the lymphoid tissue and somewhat deeper in the muscle of the base of the tongue (Figs. 26 and 27).

### *Gingiva*

The gum is that portion of the oral mucosa that surrounds the neck of the teeth like a collar. Masticatory mucosa, i.e., parakeratinized or keratinized stratified squamous epithelium, covers the gum. There is no submucosal layer; the connective tissue of the lamina propria contains collagenous fibers that bind the epithelium tightly to the underlying alveolar periosteum and bone. The gingival epithelium interdigitates with the underlying connective tissue, forming long, interconnected rete ridges that are separated by connective tissue plates and papillae (Figs. 30 and 31). The short portion of gingiva apposed to the tooth (sulcular gingiva) differs from the rest of gingival epithelium in that it is thinner, lacks the characteristic rete ridges, and is not keratinizing (39,40).

The gingiva is highly vascular; its vessels originate in the periodontium and extend into the lamina propria, forming well-organized capillary loops. Occasionally random biopsies of gingiva have been performed to support the diagnosis of systemic diseases, e.g., amyloidosis or thrombotic thrombocytopenic purpura.

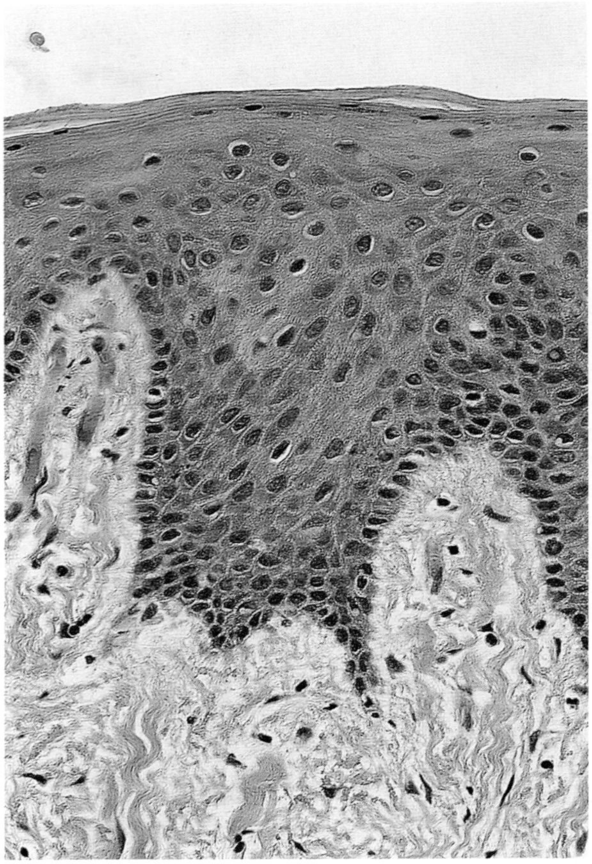

**FIG. 31.** Gum. Tall rete ridges and dense lamina propria with blood vessels in papillae.

### *Intraepithelial Nonkeratinocytes*

Four different nonepithelial cell types occur in the oral mucosa: melanocytes, Merkel cells, Langerhans cells, and lymphocytes.

Melanocytes occur normally in the oral mucosa; they are more common in people with darker complexions (41,42). Small areas of melanin pigmentation, mostly less than 10 mm in diameter, occur on the lips, gingiva, palate, and buccal mucosa and are called mucosal melanosis (melanotic macules) (43) (Fig. 32). The pigment is formed by melanocytes in the basal layer and is then transferred to the adjacent epithelial cells. Such changes can sometimes occur after inflammatory reactions, in Peutz-Jeghers syndrome or

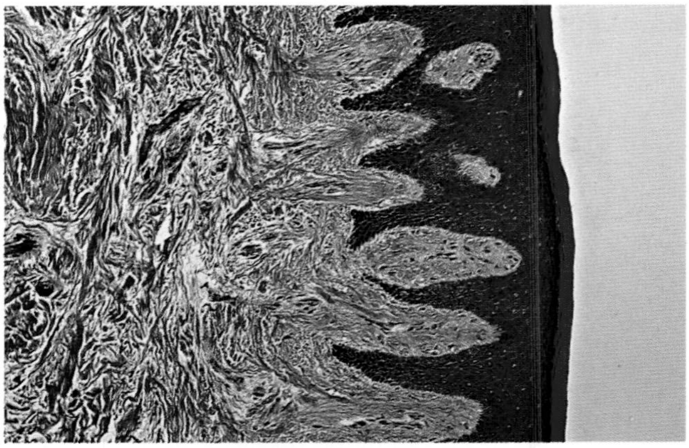

**FIG. 30.** Gum. The masticatory mucosa has tall rete ridges. A dense network of collagen fibers (blue) tightly anchors the epithelium to the underlying bone (not shown); the keratin layer (orange band) on surface of the epithelium imparts further strength to it. Mallory's trichrome stain.

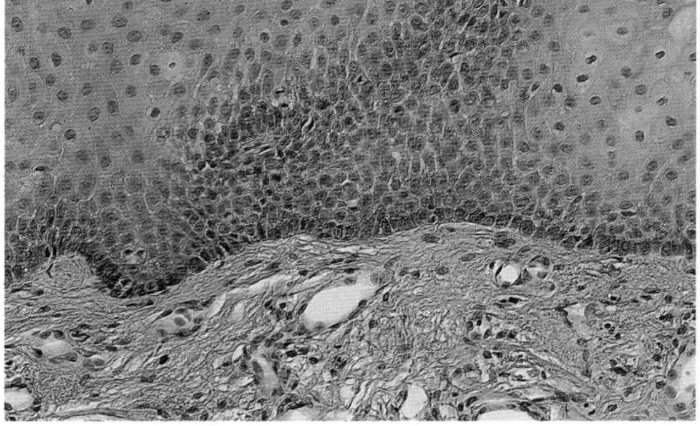

**FIG. 32.** Mucosal melanosis of the lip. Numerous melanocytes above the basal lamina appear as a brown ribbon.

in Addison's disease. Melanocytic hyperplasia (lentigo) and pigmented nevi also occur in the oral mucosa but less commonly than on the skin (44–47). Intramucosal nevi, similar to intradermal nevi, are the most common type histologically. Other types, such as compound nevi, junctional nevi, common blue nevi, and combined forms also can be observed on the vermilion border, cheeks, gum, palate, and tongue. Understandably, primary malignant melanomas can arise anywhere from the oral mucosa (48).

Merkel cells occur in the basal layer of the oral epithelium (49). On routine H&E-stained sections, their cytoplasm appears lighter than that of the surrounding basal cells. These neuroendocrine cells are morphologically and functionally identical to those in the skin. Their ultrastructure is characterized by many intracytoplasmic dense-core, membrane-bound granules, 80 to 100 $\mu$m in diameter (50,51) (Fig. 33).

Langerhans cells are microscopically similar to melanocytes and cannot be distinguished with certainty in routine H&E-stained sections. In the gingiva the Langerhans cells are structurally and functionally similar to those in the skin (52,53). Their cytoplasm appears clear, and the small nucleus stains heavily with hematoxylin. The dendritic processes among the cells of the stratum spinosum can be seen well with the immunohistochemical stain for S-100 protein (Fig. 34). Electron microscopy shows characteristic structures, the Birbeck granules, in their cytoplasm. Langerhans cells play an important role in the immune response; they are involved in the processing and presentation of antigens to subjacent lymphocytes. An increased number of Langerhans cells is seen in biopsy samples of the oral mucosa in oral lichen planus (53).

Numerous lymphocytes are present in the oral epithelium (see section on lingual tonsil).

### *Teeth and Supporting Structures*

The deciduous and permanent teeth have a similar microscopic appearance. The teeth are set in bony sockets on the alveolar processes of the maxillae and the mandible. The part of the tooth that lies within the socket is called the root. The alveolar processes are covered by the gum, and the crowns

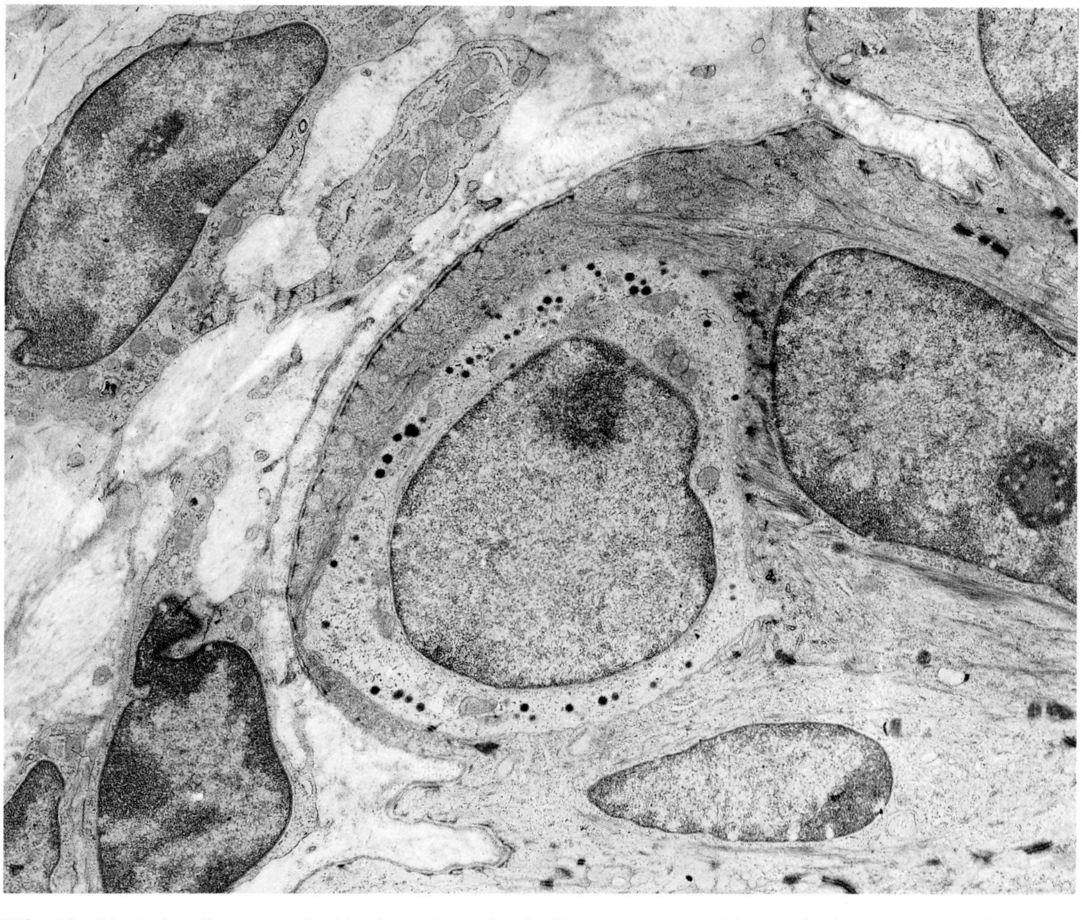

**FIG. 33.** Merkel cell surrounded by keratinocytes in the basal layer. Transmission electron micrograph shows the lighter staining cytoplasm with characteristic and subplasmalemmal, membrane-bound, dense core granules. The nucleus has no fibrous lamina, unlike melanocytes. The adjacent dermis contains fibroblasts. Original magnification ×11,500. (Courtesy of Dr. George Szabó, Boston, Massachusetts.)

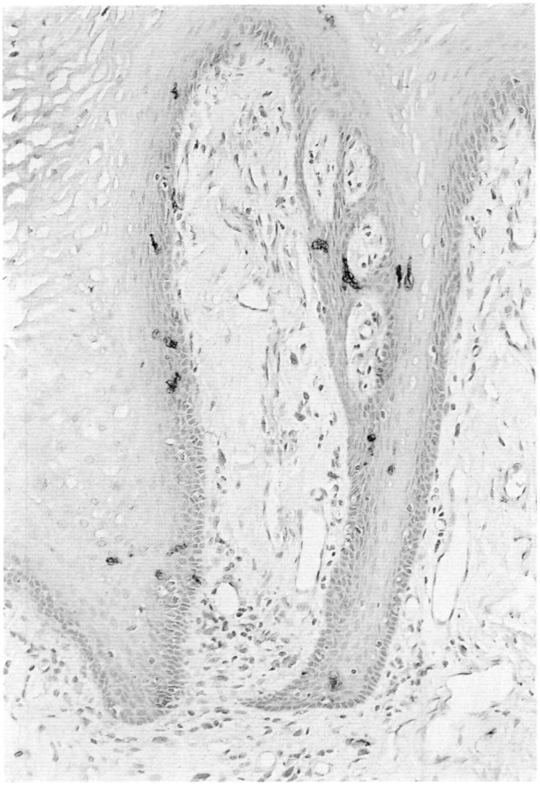

**FIG. 34.** Langerhans cells in mucosa of tongue. Dendritic cells in suprabasal epidermis demonstrate immunoreactivity for S-100 protein.

of the teeth project above the gums. The roots of the teeth are held securely in their sockets by bundles of collagen fibers called the periodontal ligament (periodontal membrane, periodontium) (14,40). In clinical parlance, however, periodontium includes the tissues investing and supporting the teeth, i.e., the cementum, periodontal membrane, alveolar bone, and gingiva (Figs. 35 and 36). The center of each tooth has a pulp chamber, or pulp cavity, which is filled with dental pulp containing loosely arranged fibroblasts, as well as nerves, blood vessels, and lymphatics (54) (Fig. 37). The pulp chamber narrows toward the root and becomes the root canal. The vessels and postganglionic sympathetic and sensory nerve fibers enter and leave the root canal through a small opening, the apical foramen. The pulp chamber of the growing tooth is lined by a single continuous layer of odontoblasts, tall columnar cells with oval nuclei. An elongated cell process, also known as Tomes' fiber, reaches from each odontoblast into the extracellular matrix secreted by them (Fig. 5). The matrix around the odontoblastic process eventually mineralizes, and the Tomes' fiber lies within a dentinal tubule (55,56). Besides the odontoblastic process, the tubules also contain 200 $\mu$m long unmyelinated nerve fibers, which account for the well-known sensitivity of dentin. The dentin is arranged in the shape of tubules running from the pulp chamber toward the periphery. The dentinal tubules and the meshwork of collagen between them are embedded in hydroxyapatite crystals; on a weight basis, 80% of dentin consists of inorganic calcium salts and 20% of organic material. Dentin makes up most of the wall of the tooth. In the mature tooth many odontoblasts become inactive but some continue producing predentin at a reduced rate throughout the life of the tooth. In response to injury, odontoblasts can upregulate their protein synthetic activity.

As the dental pulp ages, the number of fibroblasts decreases and concomitantly the number and size of collagen fibers increases. Pulp stones (denticles) are commonly observed in the dental pulp of aging individuals. True denticles contain dentinal tubules within a mineralized matrix and are surrounded by odontoblasts. False denticles are composed of a mineralized matrix arranged in concentric lamellae. Most denticles are asymptomatic.

Enamel covers the crown of the tooth. It is the hardest material found in the body and consists of 99.5% apatite crystals (57). Mature enamel is made up of long thin rods that dissolve during decalcification and are therefore not seen on conventional histologic sections. The dentin–enamel junction lies at the former interface between the inner enamel epithelium and dental mesenchyme. Coronal dentin is covered with enamel, and radicular dentin is covered with cementum. Thus, cementum covers the root of the tooth; it is similar in structure and composition to bone, but has fewer cells, called cementocytes, which occupy lacunae (12,13). Cementum is attached by the periodontal ligament to the surrounding bone (Fig. 36). In older persons, many cementocytes die, and only the surface layer appears viable. Another aging phenomenon are cementicles, which are small round calcified bodies on or in the cementum and in the periodontal ligament. Cementicles are of no clinical significance.

From the pathologist's point of view, it is noteworthy that examination of teeth involved in neoplastic growth shows in most cases tumor invading the periodontal ligament and the alveolar bone, destroying these structures. The roots of the teeth may remain intact or may undergo resorption; however, the dental pulp is rarely invaded by neoplasm.

### *Pathologic Correlates of the Rests of Serres and Rests of Malassez*

Developmental remnants of the dental lamina, called the rests of Serres, commonly occur under the gum as small nests of squamous epithelium (12,16) (Figs. 2 and 38). These epithelial islands may proliferate and may undergo cystic degeneration, which leads to the formation of gingival cysts. Similarly, epithelial remnants of Hertwig's root sheath, called the rests of Malassez, are universally present in the periodontal membrane and, exceptionally, even in the bone of the alveolar ridge. When dental caries causes a bacterial infection and necrosis of the pulp, the infection usually spreads toward the apical foramen, and a periapical granuloma may develop. As a result of the inflammatory stimulus, the nearby

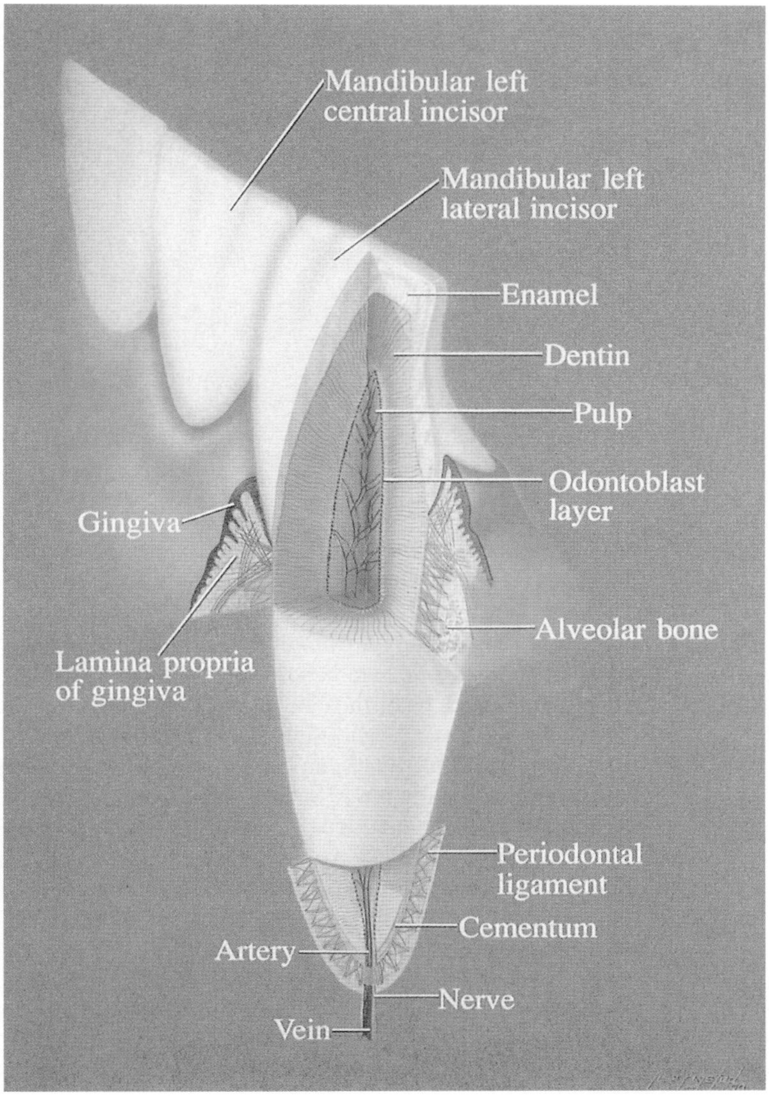


**FIG. 35.** Schematic drawing depicts the periodontium including the gingiva, alveolar bone, periodontal ligament, and cementum. (Courtesy of Dr. Kenneth D. McClatchey, Ann Arbor, Michigan.)

epithelium of the rests of Malassez begins to proliferate and forms an epithelial lining in these apical granulomas (Fig. 38). It is assumed that the rests of Serres and the rests of Malassez are potential sources of ameloblastomas and odontogenic cysts.

## Nose and Paranasal Sinuses

### *External Nose and Nasal Vestibule*

The external nose is covered by skin that contains many sebaceous glands. The nasal cavity extends from the nares anteriorly to the choanae posteriorly. Just behind the nares the nasal cavity widens and forms the vestibule. The skin of the external nose is continuous with the lining of the nasal vestibule, which has many hair follicles and sebaceous and sweat glands. The squamous epithelium of the vestibules merges with the respiratory mucosa, which covers the respiratory portion of the nasal cavity and all of the paranasal sinuses.

### *Nasal Mucosa*

The mucosa of the respiratory portion is continuous with that of the ostia and paranasal sinuses and consists of pseudostratified respiratory epithelium with the cells resting on a basal lamina. The mucosal lining contains three main cell types: basal cells, goblet cells, and ciliated cells (Fig. 39). Basal cells are the reserve cells that continuously replace the cells shed. The basal cells are confined to the vicinity of the basal lamina; they divide, and the newly formed daughter cells differentiate to become mucous or ciliated cells. The mucous cells stand on the basement membrane from which they arise with a slender stem, and the cytoplasm of their apical portion contains varying amounts of mucus. As the cells fill up with mucus, they resemble a goblet with a foot and a

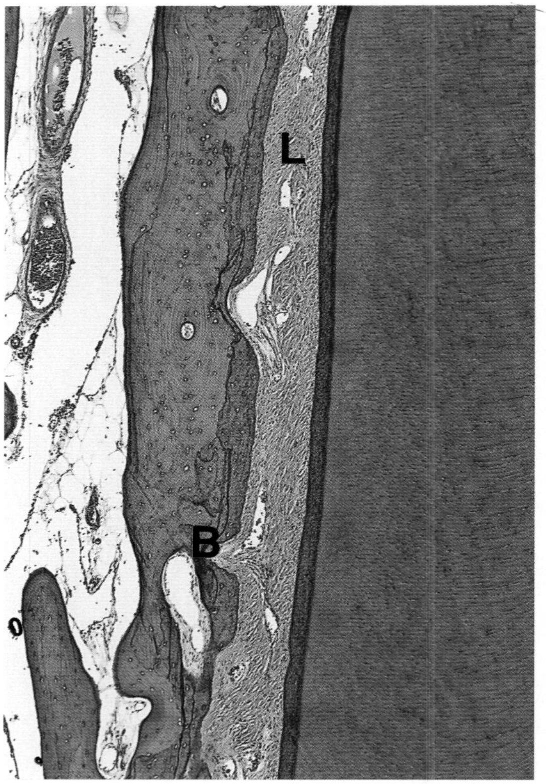


**FIG. 36.** Root of tooth and supporting structures, perpendicular section. Dentin is covered by a thin layer of cementum (appearing as a blue band). The periodontal ligament (L) holds the tooth in the bony socket of the alveolar process (B).

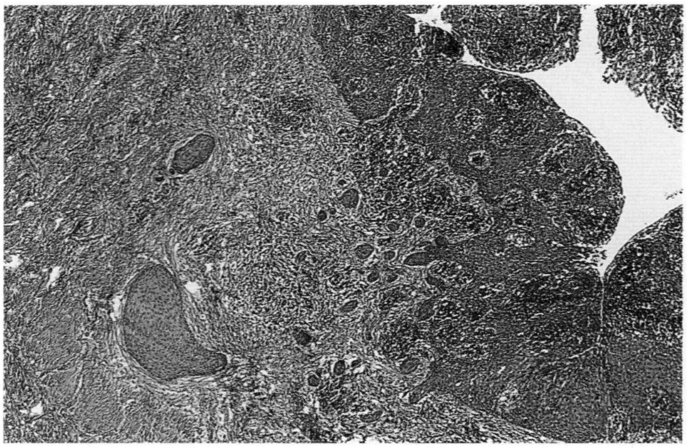

**FIG. 38.** Rests of Malassez in periodontium near the apical granuloma.

stem. The cells discharge their content to form the blanket of mucus covering the surface of the respiratory epithelium. Another source of the mucous coat are the seromucinous glands in the lamina propria. Normally the majority of the cells of the respiratory epithelium are made up of ciliated cells bearing small fingerlike cell processes, the cilia, which project from them into the lumen. Each cell has over 200 cilia, each about 5 $\mu$m long. Electron microscopically, the cilia are remarkably uniform. On cross section the ciliary shafts show a highly characteristic circular arrangement of nine pairs of microtubules (doublets), which are arranged symmetrically around two central microtubules (Fig. 40). Longitudinal sections of the cilia show that the ciliary shaft ends in a basal body (kinetosome), from which it is derived (58). The nasal mucosa is a convenient site for biopsy when ultrastructural abnormalities of cilia are suspected, e.g., in the immotile-cilia syndrome (59–61). The function of the ciliated cells in the nose is to constantly move the protective mucous blanket by the coordinated sweeping motion of the cilia toward the pharynx. The cilia beat 10 to 20 cycles/second; they have an effective whiplike stroke forward and a recovery stroke backward. The propulsive forward phase is much faster and more vigorous than the recovery phase (62). Ciliary activity is optimal at the normal nasal temperature of about 30°C. Cilia are hardy and persist under unfavorable conditions, e.g., under extreme cold and heat. They beat normally and forcefully in a pus-filled cavity. When injured or destroyed by an acute infection, they regenerate rapidly.

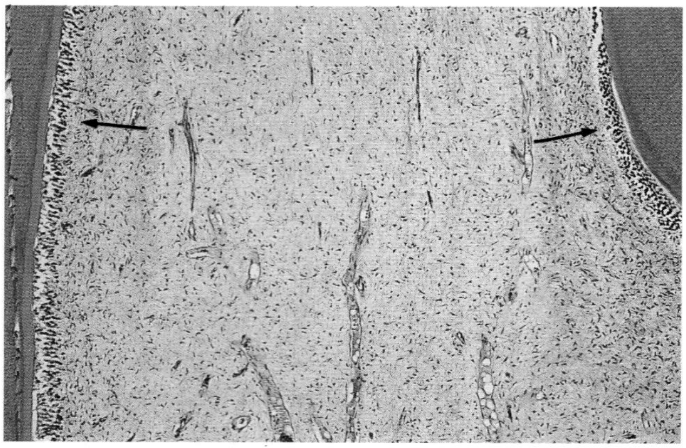

**FIG. 37.** Pulp of developing tooth. Odontoblasts (*arrows*) line dentin. The pulp consists mostly of loosely arranged fibroblasts. Note the delicate wall of blood vessels.

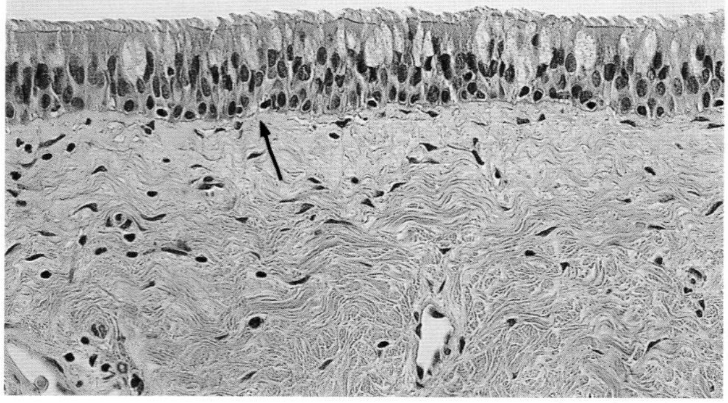

**FIG. 39.** Pseudostratified respiratory mucosa of the nose with predominantly ciliated cells. Goblet cells have clear cytoplasm. The basal cells (*arrow*) are lying on thin basal lamina.

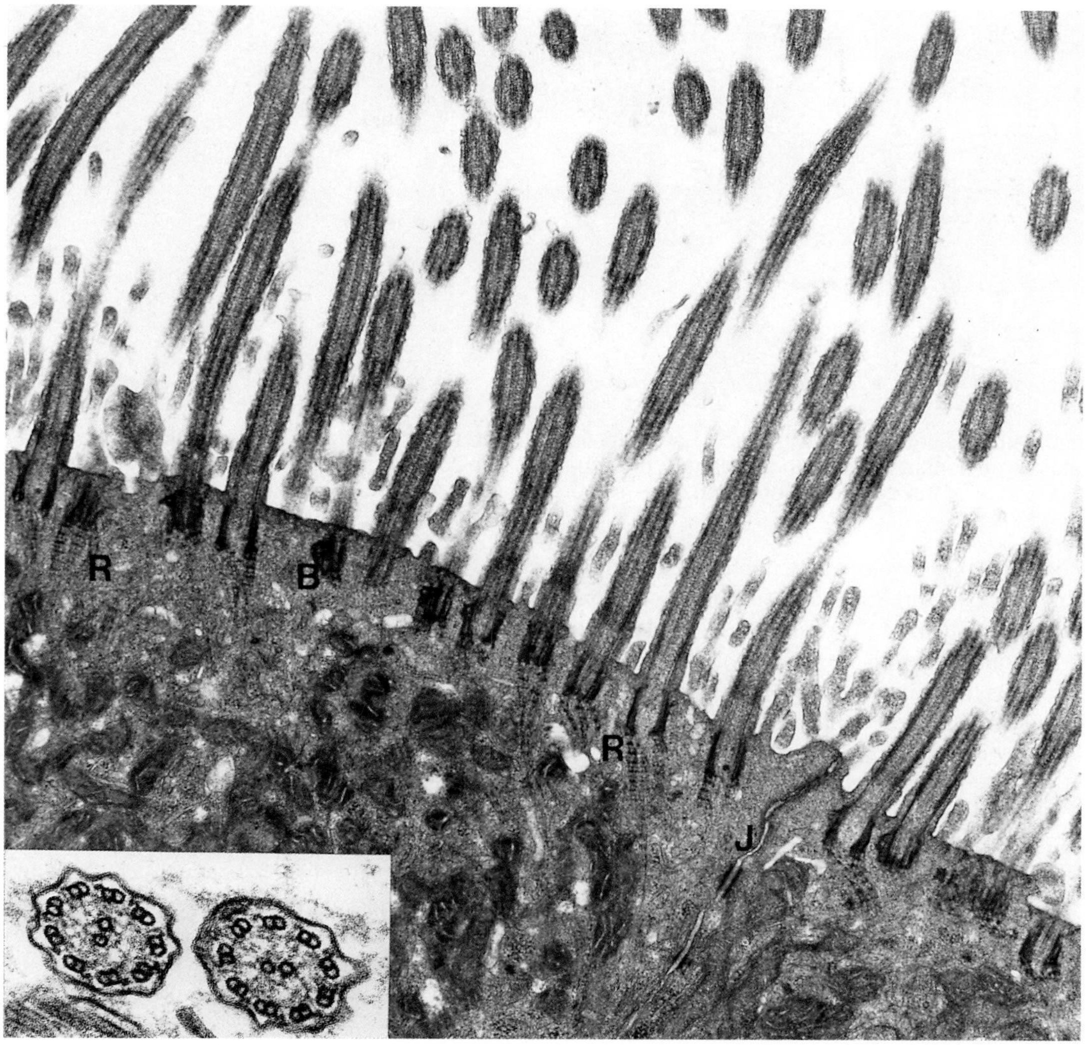


**FIG. 40.** Transmission electron micrograph of nasal mucosa. Vertical section shows ciliated epithelial cells extending to the surface. The shafts of the slender long cilia have peripheral and central microtubules that appear as darker linear structures extending from the kinetosome (basal body) (B). Cross-banded filamentous rootlets (R) are associated with kinetosomes. Note junctional complexes (J). Original magnification ×25,000. **Inset:** Cross section of the shaft of two cilia. Note the symmetrically arranged nine peripheral doublets and the central pair of single microtubules. Original magnification ×87,500. (Courtesy of Dr. Micheline Federman, Boston, Massachusetts.)

They do not, however, tolerate excessive drying but are dependent always upon a coating of moisture for their activity and preservation. The blanket of mucus covering the nasal mucosa and paranasal sinuses forms a conveyor of the bacteria and other foreign matter. The nasal mucociliary layer is the first line of defense against bacterial invasion. A secondary defense mechanism against bacteria is provided by the capillaries in the stroma of the mucous membrane: through the walls of these capillaries pass polymorphonuclear leukocytes, lymphocytes, and mononuclear cells to augment the local cellular defense mechanisms.

Melanocytes are also present in the normal mucosa of the upper airways. In the nasal cavity they can be seen in the respiratory epithelium and nasal glands. Melanocytes are commonly encountered in the lamina propria of the septum and turbinates, particularly in dark-skinned adults (63). Primary malignant melanomas are well known to arise in the nose and paranasal sinuses (64).

Beneath the mucous membrane is the lamina propria containing numerous small mucous and serous glands that discharge their secretion through their lobular ducts to the surface (Fig. 41). These glands are embedded in vascular fibroconnective tissue, which is attached to the perichondrium and periosteum of the cartilages and bones forming the nasal cavity (65–67).

The lateral nasal wall presents an irregular surface with convoluted structures, the nasal turbinates, hanging from it. The turbinates are somewhat curved structures that are sup-

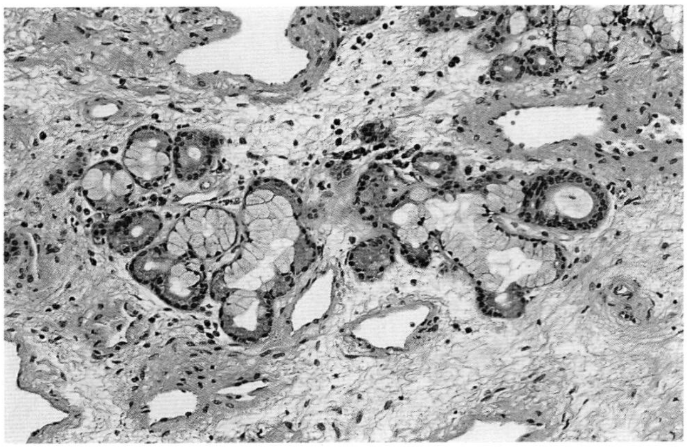

**FIG. 41.** Nasal seromucinous gland with duct. Serous cells with darker staining cytoplasm are at the periphery of tubuloacinar glands and form the demilunes of Gianuzzi.

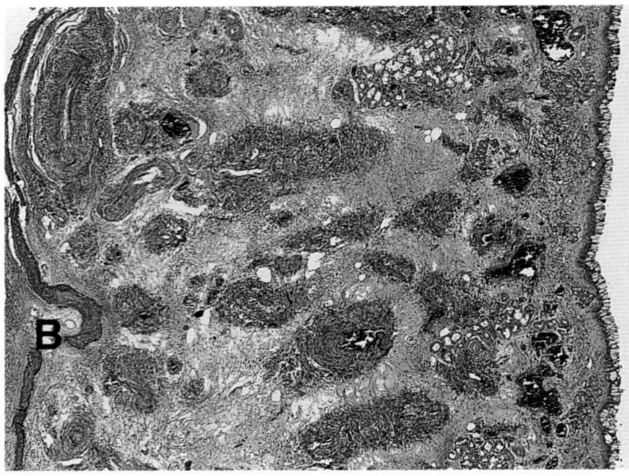

**FIG. 43.** Turbinate, coronal section. Mucosal blood vessels are surrounded by a thick sheath of connective tissue (blue). Note the large artery near the bone (B). Mallory's trichrome stain.

ported by an osseous axis enveloped by relatively thick mucosa (Figs. 1 and 42). The turbinates, or conchae, have a convex surface protruding toward the nasal cavity. Under their mucosa there is a tunica propria or stroma that attaches the mucosa to the underlying structures. The tunica propria is of variable thickness; it is thickest in the areas more exposed to inhaled and exhaled air, i.e., over the nasal septum and medial aspects of the inferior and middle turbinates, where the epithelium contains many goblet cells and the basement membrane is prominent (68). These areas have abundant blood vessels and clusters of mixed seromucinous glands (six to 10 glands per $mm^2$) (Fig. 43). The glands vary from the simple straight tubules lined with goblet cells to the tubuloalveolar type of glands. The chief ducts of the latter open on the mucosal surface by minute orifices. The glands tend to be at a level between the mucosa and the underlying bone. The turbinates are rich in venous sinuses, which are of variable size and shape, forming a dense network of large veins that resemble erectile tissue (Fig. 44). These blood vessels are of irregular shape, have muscular walls, and can rapidly dilate and constrict, thereby permitting fast adjustments of mucosal temperature and secretion to climatic changes. It is important for the surgical pathologist to know about the normal vascular anatomy of the turbinates in order to avoid mis-

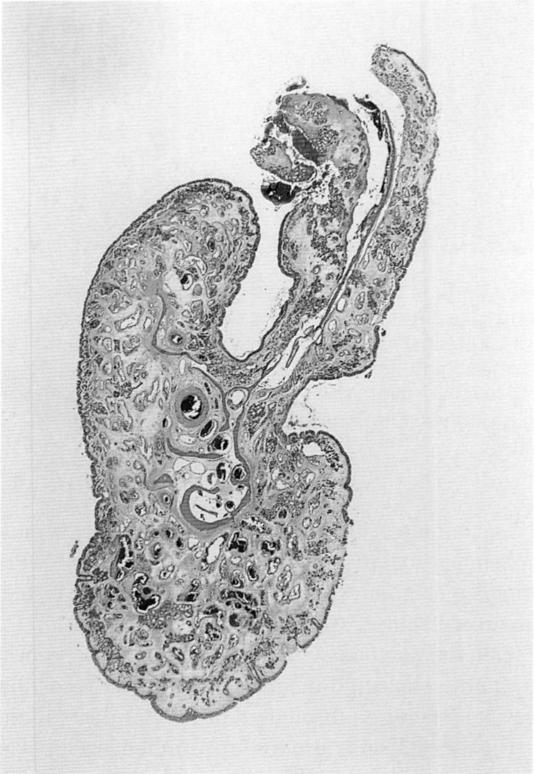

**FIG. 42.** Middle turbinate. Low-power view of coronal section. Bone in the axis of turbinate appears as a delicate, curled structure. The covering mucous membrane and tunica propria are rich in blood vessels and mucous glands, particularly on the convexity and inferior border of the turbinate, areas most exposed to the airstream in the nasal cavity.

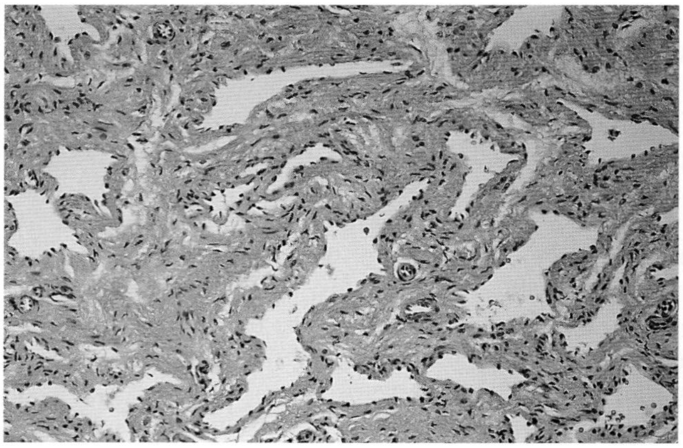

**FIG. 44.** Inferior turbinate. Numerous larger blood vessels of variable size and shape are closely packed and form a sponge-like vascular system resembling erectile tissue. The endothelial cells are evenly distributed. Capillaries are lacking.

taking them for a hemangioma, angiofibroma, or angioleiomyoma. The stroma of the nasal mucosa contains lymphatics, small nerves, and a sprinkling of round cells, mainly lymphocytes and plasma cells, but no lymphoid aggregates. A few mast cells and eosinophils are normally also present. The osseous portion of the turbinates consists of thin, interconnecting laminae of lamellar bone, forming a continuous shell that is interconnected with bone trabeculae. The interosseous spaces contain numerous large veins, arteries, and some nerves. In contrast to the submucosal veins, the intraosseous veins have a rather large, round or oval lumen on cross section and have proportionately thin walls. Occasional fat cells, but no hematopoietic marrow, are seen in turbinated bone.

Each nasal cavity is separated from the other by the nasal septum, constituting its medial wall. The septum consists of a large cartilaginous plate and four small osseous plates, all of which firmly unite with sutures (Fig. 45). The nasal mucosa covers these structures in close apposition; the periosteum and perichondrium attach so closely to the overlying submucosa as to constitute one membrane, called the mucoperiosteum. A common site of nosebleed is Little's area (or locus Kiesselbachii) on the anterior part of the cartilaginous nasal septum above the intermaxillary line; the submucosa of this area is particularly richly supplied with thin-walled dilated blood vessels (Fig. 46). Although rarely seen in surgical specimens, Little's area should not be mistaken for a pyogenic granuloma, which frequently occurs in this location. Pyogenic granulomas are raised nodules that have numerous capillary lumina and show considerable proliferation of endothelial cells.

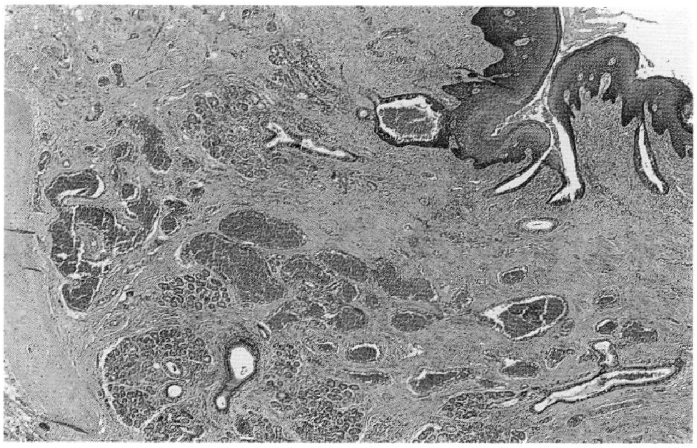

**FIG. 46.** Little's area. Teleangiectatic, thin-walled blood vessels are clustered under the epithelium in the anterior portion of the nasal septum. This area is above the level of mucous glands.

### *Vomeronasal Organ of Jacobson*

The vestigial remains of this paired embryonic structure are situated under the mucosa of the lower anterior side of the nasal septum covering an area of 0.2 to 0.6 cm. In adults it consists of a small tubular sac lined by columnar epithelium with microvilli, but has no sensory cells with cilia and lacks other well-differentiated olfactory structures (Fig. 47). The organ is best developed in the 20th week of embryonic life, after which regressive changes occur and it becomes rudimentary; in humans it has no known function and is of no pathologic significance (69). In many vertebrates Jacobson's vomeronasal organ is highly developed, particularly in animals of keen olfactory sensibility (70–72).

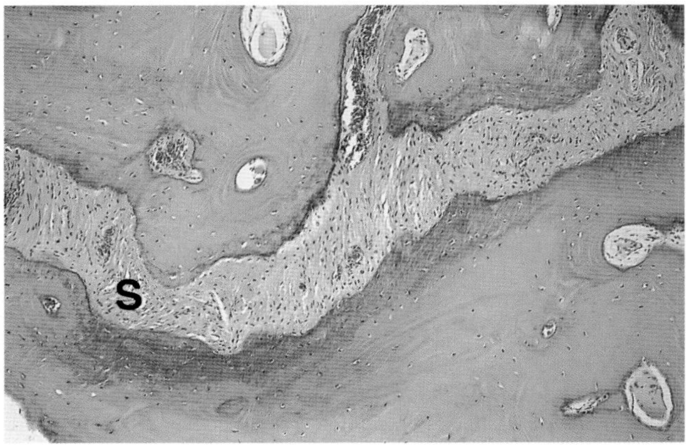


**FIG. 45.** Suture (S) in the nasal septum. Parallel edges of the vomer (*top*) and maxilla are connected by parallel, densely arranged collagen fibers that are anchored in the bones.

### *Olfactory Mucosa*

The roof of the nasal cavity and contiguous portions of the nasal septum and superior concha form the olfactory region (73). Here the ciliated columnar epithelium of the nasal mucosa is modified by liberally scattered cells of the organ of smell. The olfactory epithelium consists of three types of cells: (a) olfactory nerve cells, (b) supporting, or sustentacu-

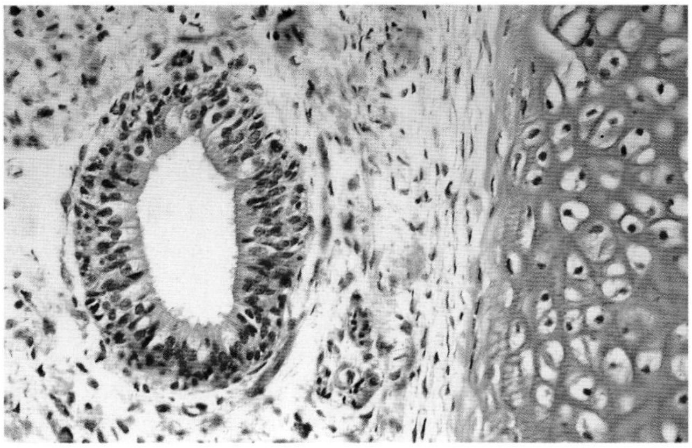

**FIG. 47.** Vomeronasal organ of Jacobson in a 22-week-old embryo (180 mm crown–rump length). Cross section of the tubular structure adjacent to vomeronasal cartilage. In humans the columnar epithelium has microvilli but no sensory epithelium.

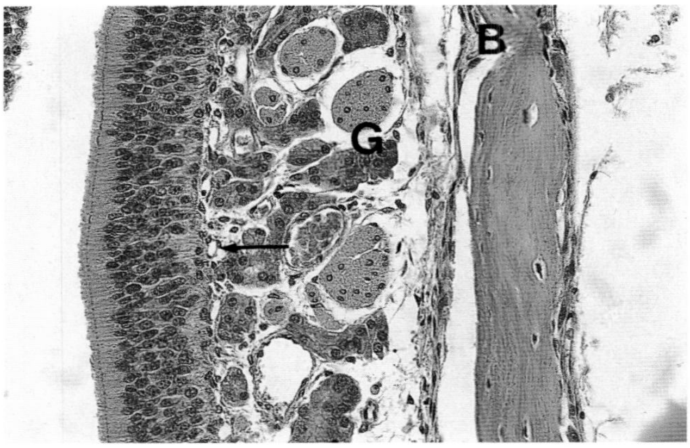


**FIG. 48.** Olfactory mucosa. The population of olfactory nerve cells and supporting cells forms a pseudostratified columnar epithelium with distinct microvilli. Basal cells lie on basal lamina (*arrow*). Bowman's glands (G) with excretory ducts and nerves are between the epithelium and bone of nasal septum (B).

lar, cells, and (c) basal cells that lie on the basal lamina (74,75) (Fig. 48). The olfactory nerve cells are spindle shaped and have a spherical nucleus. The dendrites of these bipolar cells extend to the surface of the pseudostratified olfactory epithelium and send out a tuft of fine processes known as olfactory cilia (hairs). The cilia are 2 $\mu$m long and lie along the surface of the mucosa embedded in mucus. The deep processes of these bipolar cells form axons that find their way through the basal lamina and join neighboring processes to become bundles of unmyelinated olfactory nerve fibers (75). These fibers collect to form myelinated nerves, which then pass through the cribriform plate of the ethmoid bone to end on the mitral cells in the olfactory bulb. The supporting cells are tall, cylindrical cells that in the elderly contain lipofuscin, giving the yellow hue of the olfactory mucous membrane. The free surface of these cells possesses many slender microvilli that protrude into the covering mucus. The basal cells are small and conical, lying with their base on the basement membrane. They are thought to give rise to new supporting cells. Under the mucosa is the lamina propria composed of loose connective tissue in which are found the olfactory glands of Bowman (76). The secretion of these tubuloalveolar glands is carried to the surface of the mucosa by narrow ducts.

### *Paranasal Sinuses*

These paired, air-filled cavities are located in the bones around the nasal cavity. The maxillary and frontal sinuses open into the middle meatus of the nose; the sphenoid sinus opens into the sphenoethmoidal recess above the superior concha. There are numerous ethmoid sinuses, forming small communicating cavities, also called ethmoid air cells (or ethmoid labyrinth). The ethmoid air cells have thin bony walls. According to their location, the ethmoid sinuses can be divided into three groups: the anterior and middle ethmoidal sinuses, which open into the middle meatus, and the posterior ethmoidal sinus, which opens into the superior meatus of the nose. There are many variations in size, shape, and location of all paranasal sinuses; one or more of them may even be underdeveloped or absent. The sinuses are lined with a mucous membrane that is continuous with the nasal mucosa; it is similar to that of the nasal cavity, but the epithelium and lamina propria are thinner and lack a rich vascular plexus. The mucus formed in the sinuses is moved by the action of the cilia through the apertures to the nasal cavities.

## REFERENCES


1. Larsen WJ. *Human embryology.* New York: Churchill-Livingstone; 1993.
2. Moore KL, Persaud TVN. *The developing human: clinically oriented embryology.* 5th ed. Philadelphia: WB Saunders; 1993.
3. Sadler TW. *Langman's medical embryology.* 7th ed. Baltimore: Williams & Wilkins; 1995.
4. Vander Zanden JW. *Human development.* 5th ed. New York: McGraw-Hill; 1993.
5. Sperber GH. *Craniofacial embryology.* 4th ed. London: Butterworth; 1989.
6. Listgarten MA. Phase-contrast and electron microscope study of the junction between reduced enamel epithelium and enamel in unerupted human teeth. *Arch Oral Biol* 1966;11:999–1016.
7. Schour I, Massler M. Studies in tooth development: the growth pattern of human teeth. *J Am Dent Assoc* 1940;27:1778–1793,1918–1931.
8. Gorski JP, Marks SC Jr. Current concepts of the biology of tooth eruption. *Crit Rev Oral Biol Med* 1992;3:185–206.
9. Marks SC Jr, Gorski JP, Cahill DR, Wise GG. Tooth eruption, a synthesis of experimental observations. In: Davidovich Z, ed. *The biological mechanisms of tooth eruption and root resorption.* Birmingham, AL: EBSCO Media; 1988:161–169.
10. Orban B, Sicher H, Weinmann JP. Amelogenesis (a critique and a new concept). *J Am Coll Dent* 1943;10:13–22.
11. Schroeder HE. Development and structure of the tissues of the tooth. In: *Oral structural biology.* New York, NY: Thieme Medical; 1986:4–184.
12. Bhaskar SN, ed. *Orban's oral histology and embryology.* 11th ed. St. Louis: CV Mosby; 1991.
13. Held AJ. Cementogenesis and the normal and pathologic structure of cementum. *Oral Surg Oral Med Oral Pathol* 1951;4:53–67.
14. Smukler H, Dreyer CJ. Principal fibres of the periodontium. *J Periodont Res* 1969;4:19–23.
15. Logan WHG, Kronfeld R. Development of the human jaws and surrounding structures from birth to the age of fifteen years. *J Am Dent Assoc* 1933;20:379–427.
16. Schroeder H. *Oral structural biology: embryology, structure and function of normal hard and soft tissues of the oral cavity and the temporomandibular joints.* New York: Thieme; 1991.
17. Miles EAW. Sebaceous glands in the lip and cheek mucosa of man. *Br Dent J* 1958;105:235–248.
18. Sewerin I. The sebaceous glands in the vermilion border of the lips and in the oral mucosa of man. *Acta Odontol Scand* 1975;33(suppl 68):13–226.
19. Meyer J, Squier CA, Gerson SJ, eds. *The structure and function of the oral mucosa.* New York: Pergamon Press; 1984.
20. Skougaard MR. Cell renewal with special reference to the gingival epithelium. *Adv Oral Biol* 1970;4:261–288.
21. Squier CA. Oral mucosa. In: Ten Cate AR, ed. *Oral histology, development, structure and function.* St. Louis, MO: CV Mosby; 1989: 341–382.
22. Ouhayoun J-P, Gosselin F, Forest N, Winter S, Franke WW. Cytokeratin patterns of human oral epithelia: differences in cytokeratin synthesis in gingival epithelium and the adjacent alveolar mucosa. *Differentiation* 1985;30:123–129.
23. Schulz J, Ermich T, Kasper M, Raabe G, Schumann D. Cytokeratin pattern of clinically intact and pathologically changed oral mucosa. *Int J Oral Maxillofac Surg* 1992;21:35–39.

24. Eversole LR. The histochemistry of mucosubstances in human minor salivary glands. *Arch Oral Biol* 1972;17:1225–1239.
25. Munger BL. Histochemical studies on seromucous- and mucous-secreting cells of human salivary glands. *Am J Anat* 1964;115:411–430.
26. Tandler B, Denning CR, Mandel ID, Kutscher AH. Ultrastructure of human labial salivary glands. III. Myoepithelium and ducts. *J Morphol* 1970;130:227–246.
27. Hamperl H. Über das Vorkommen von Onkocyten in verschiedenen Organen und ihren Geschwülsten: (Mundspeicheldrüsen, Bauchspeicheldrüse, Epithelkörperchen, Hypophyse, Schilddrüse, Eileiter). *Virchows Arch* 1936;298:327–375.
28. Chang A, Harawi SJ. Oncocytes, oncocytosis and oncocytic tumors. *Pathol Ann* 1992;27:263–304.
29. Balogh K, Roth SI. Histochemical and electron microscopic studies of eosinophilic granular cells (oncocytes) in tumors of the parotid gland. *Lab Invest* 1965;14:310–320.
30. Goode RK, Corio RL. Oncocytic adenocarcinoma of salivary glands. *Oral Surg Oral Med Oral Pathol* 1988;65:61–66.
31. Tschen JA, Fechner RE. The juxtaoral organ of Chievitz. *Am J Surg Pathol* 1979;3:147–150.
32. Zenker W. *Juxtaoral organ (Chievitz's organ). Morphology and clinical aspects.* Baltimore: Urban & Schwarzenberg; 1982.
33. Lutman GB. Epithelial nests in intraoral sensory nerve endings simulating perineural invasion in patients with oral carcinoma. *Am J Clin Pathol* 1974;61:275–284.
34. Mikó T, Molnár P. The juxtaoral organ—a pitfall for pathologists. *J Pathol* 1981;133:17–23.
35. Leibl W, Pflüger H, Kerjaschki D. A case of nodular hyperplasia of the juxtaoral organ in man. *Virchows Arch [A]* 1976;371:389–391.
36. Chievitz JH. Beiträge zur Entwicklungsgeschichte der Speicheldrüsen. *Arch Anat Physiol Abt* 1885;9:401–436.
37. Kruger L, Mantyh P. Gustatory and related chemosensory systems. In: Bjorklund A, Hökfelt T, Swanson LW, eds. *Handbook of chemical neuroanatomy.* Vol 7. Integrated Systems of the C.N.S. Part II. Amsterdam: Elsevier; 1989.
38. Oakley B. Neuronal–epithelial interactions in mammalian gustatory epithelium. In: *Regeneration of vertebrate sensory receptor cells.* Chichester, England: Wiley; 1991:277–287.
39. Ainamo J, Loe H. Anatomical characteristics of gingiva: clinical and microscopic study of the free and attached gingiva. *J Periodontol* 1966; 37:5–13.
40. Melcher AH, Bowen WH, eds. *The biology of the periodontium.* New York: New York Press; 1969.
41. Squier CA, Waterhouse JP. The ultrastructure of the melanocyte in human gingival epithelium. *Arch Oral Biol* 1967;12:119–129.
42. Schroeder HE. Melanin containing organelles in cells of the human gingiva. I. Epithelial melanocytes. *J Periodont Res* 1969;4:1–18.
43. Kaugars GE, Heise AP, Riley, WT, Abbey LM, Svisky JA. Oral melanotic macules: a review of 353 cases. *Oral Surg Oral Med Oral Pathol* 1993;76:59–61.
44. Buchner A, Merrell P, Hansen L, Leider A. Melanocytic hyperplasia of the oral mucosa. *Oral Surg Oral Med Oral Pathol* 1991;71:58–62.
45. Buchner A. Melanocytic nevi of oral mucosa: A clinico-pathologic study of 130 cases from northern California. *J Oral Pathol Med* 1990; 19:197–201.
46. Buchner A, Hansen L. Pigmented nevi of the oral mucosa: a clinicopathologic study of 36 new cases and review of 155 cases from the literature. Part I: A clinicopathologic study of 36 new cases. *Oral Surg Oral Med Oral Pathol* 1987;63:566–572.
47. Buchner A, Hansen L. Pigmented nevi of the oral mucosa: a clinicopathologic study of 36 new cases and review of 155 cases from the literature. Part II: Analysis of 191 cases. *Oral Surg Oral Med Oral Pathol* 1987;63:676–682.
48. Trodahl JN, Sprague WG. Benign and malignant melanocytic lesions of the oral mucosa. An analysis of 135 cases. *Cancer* 1970;25:812–823.
49. Hashimoto K. Fine structure of Merkel cell in human oral mucosa. *J Invest Dermatol* 1972;58:381–387.
50. Winkelmann RK, Breathnach AS. The Merkel cell. *J Invest Dermatol* 1973;60:2–15.
51. Gould VE, Moll R, Moll I, Lee I, Franke WW. Neuroendocrine (Merkel) cells of the skin: hyperplasias, dysplasias and neoplasms. *Lab Invest* 1985;52:334–353.
52. Waterhouse JP, Squier CA. The Langerhans cell in human gingival epithelium. *Arch Oral Biol* 1967;12:341–348.
53. Chou JM, Daniels TE. Langerhans cells expressing HLA-DQ, HLA-DR and $T_6$ antigens in normal oral mucosa and lichen planus. *J Oral Pathol* 1989;18:573–576.
54. Baume LJ. The biology of pulp and dentine. A historic terminologic-taxonomic histologic-biochemical, embryonic and clinical survey. *Monogr Oral Sci* 1980;8:1–220.
55. Holland GR. The odontoblast process: form and function. *J Dent Res* 1984;64:499–514.
56. Thomas HF. The dentin–predentin complex and its permeability: anatomical review. *J Dent Res* 1985;64:607–612.
57. Nylen UM, Termine JD, eds. Tooth enamel III. Its development, structure, and composition. *J Dent Res* 1979;58:675–1031.
58. Fawcett DW, Porter KR. A study of the fine structure of ciliated epithelium. *J Morphol* 1954;94:221–281.
59. Eliasson R. Mossberg B, Canner P, Afzelius BA. The immotile cilia syndrome. A congenital ciliary abnormality as an etiologic factor in chronic airway infections and male sterility. *N Engl J Med* 1977;297: 1–6.
60. Afzelius BA. The immotile-cilia syndrome and other ciliary disease. *Int Rev Exp Pathol* 1979;19:1–43.
61. Howell JT, Schochet SS, Goldman AS. Ultrastructural defects of respiratory tract cilia associated with chronic infections. *Arch Pathol Lab Med* 1980;104:52–55.
62. Sleigh MA, Blake JR, Liron N. The propulsion of mucus by cilia. *Am Rev Respir Dis* 1988;137:726–741.
63. Zak FG, Lawson W. The presence of melanocytes in the nasal cavity. *Ann Otol Rhinol Laryngol* 1974;83:515–519.
64. Cove H. Melanosis, melanocytic hyperplasia, and primary malignant melanoma of the nasal cavity. *Cancer* 1979;44:1424–1433.
65. Rhys-Evans PH. Anatomy of the nose and paranasal sinuses. In: Kerr AG, Groves J, Scott-Brown WG, eds. *Scott-Brown's otolaryngology.* 5th ed. Vol I. London: Butterworth; 1987:138–161.
66. Drake-Lee AB. Physiology of the nose and paranasal sinus. In: Kerr AG, Groves J, Scott-Brown WG, eds. *Scott-Brown's otolaryngology.* 5th ed. Vol I. London: Butterworth; 1987:162–182.
67. Ballenger JJ. The clinical anatomy and physiology of the nose and accessory sinuses. In: Ballenger JJ, ed. *Diseases of the nose, throat, ear, head and neck.* 14th ed. Malvern, PA: Lea & Febiger; 1991:3–22.
68. Trotter CM, Hall GH, Salter DM, Wilson JA. Histology of mucous membrane of human inferior nasal concha. *Clin Anat* 1990;3:307–316.
69. Zuckerkandl E. Das Jacobsonsche Organ. *Erg Anat Entwicklungsgesch* 1910;18:801–843.
70. Pearlman SJ. Jacobson's organ (Organon vomeronasale Jacobsoni): its anatomy, gross, microscopic and comparative, with some observations as well on its function. *Ann Otol Rhinol Laryngol* 1934;43:739–768.
71. Negus VE. The organ of Jacobson. *J Anat* 1956;90:515–518.
72. Seifert K. Licht- und elektronenmikroskopische Untersuchungen am Jacobsonschen Organ (Organon vomeronasale) der Katze. *Arch Klin Exp Ohr Nas Kehlk Heilk* 1971;200:223–251.
73. Naessen R. The identification and topographical localization of the olfactory epithelium in man and other mammals. *Acta Otolaryngol (Stockh)* 1970;70:51–57.
74. Schneider RA. The sense of smell in man—its physiologic basis. *N Engl J Med* 1967;277:299–303.
75. Palay SL. The general architecture of sensory neuroepithelia. In: *Regeneration of vertebrate sensory receptor cells.* Chichester, England: Wiley; 1991:3–24.
76. Seifert K. Licht- und elektronenmikroskopische Untersuchungen der Bowman-Drüsen in der Riechschleimhaut makrosmatischer Säuger. *Arch Klin Exp Ohr Nas Kehlk Heilk* 1971;200:252–274.

*Histology for Pathologists, second edition,*
Edited by Stephen S. Sternberg.
Lippincott-Raven Publishers, Philadelphia


# CHAPTER 16

# Larynx And Pharynx

Stacey E. Mills and Robert E. Fechner



## LARYNX

### Definition and Boundaries

The larynx is a complex organ with numerous connective tissue elements and a variety of epithelia. The superior border of the larynx is the tip of the epiglottis and the aryepigolottic folds. The inferior limit is the inferior rim of the cricoid cartilage. The anterior boundary is composed of the lingual surface of the epiglottis, the thyroid cartilage, the anterior arch of the cricoid cartilage, the thyrohyoid membrane, and the cricothyroid membrane. The posterior boundary is the cricoid cartilage and the arytenoid region. The piriform fossa is frequently, and erroneously, considered to be a part of the larynx. In reality, it is a pouch of the hypopharynx that passes on each side of the larynx. It is, thus, a conduit for food and water, not air.

Although not part of the larynx per se, the preepiglottic space is an important area for the spread of carcinoma. This more or less triangular space is filled with fat and loose connective tissue. It is bounded posteriorly by the epiglottis, anteriorly by the thyroid cartilage and thyrohyoid membrane, and superiorly by the hyoepiglottic ligament.

S. E. Mills and R. E. Fechner: University of Virginia, Health Sciences Center, Charlottesville, VA 22908

### Embryology

The supraglottic portion of the larynx is derived from the third and fourth branchial arches, and is, therefore, related to the development of the oral cavity and oropharynx. The glottis and subglottis arise from the sixth branchial arch, which also give rise to the trachea and lungs. Bocca et al. have demonstrated that the larynx virtually consists of two hemilarynges (superior and inferior), each of them with its own different derivation and its own largely independent lymphatic circulation (1). These authors also discuss the importance of this embryologic derivation with respect to the origin and spread of laryngeal carcinoma. Each of these hemilarynges may become invaded by cancer independent of one another. The extension of cancer is often limited within the boundaries of embryologic demarcation (1).

The first embryologic appearance of the respiratory apparatus occurs at approximately 21 days in the 3-mm embryo. At this time, an evagination, or groove, forms adjacent to the superior portion of the foregut, above the fourth branchial arch. The inferior portion of this evagination is the pulmonary anlage. The first portion of the larynx to develop is the epiglottis, but this does not appear as a definitively formed structure until approximately the 5th week of intrauterine development.

The outline of the larynx is recognizable in the 6-mm embryo. At this time, the respiratory groove described previ-

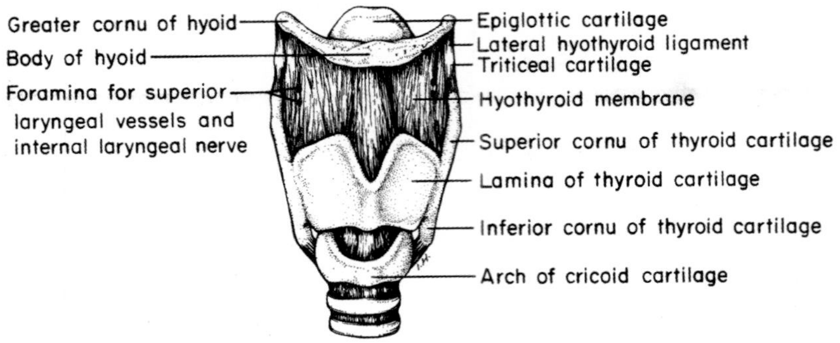


**FIG. 1.** Anterior view of an unopened larynx shows the lamina of thyroid cartilage, the arch of the cricoid cartilage, and the hyothyroid membrane as the major structures that define the anterior external surface of the larynx (From ref. 45.)

ously begins to close; this closure is completed with the formation of the arytenoid cartilages. By 60 to 70 days, at the stage of the 30 mm-embryo, the vocal cords begin to differentiate. The embryonic development of the larynx is complex, and it is not surprising that at least 30 different congenital malformations have been described (2).

### Gross and Functional Anatomy

The larynx is composed of an elastic cone, cartilages, intrinsic and extrinsic muscles, submucosa, and an overlying mucous membrane (Figs. 1–3). The elastic cone provides most of the structural strength to support the true vocal cords. The elastic tissue is thickened just under the mucosa of the free edge of the cord. This portion of the elastic cone is referred to as the vocal ligament. It is visible grossly as a white band beneath the mucous membrane (Fig. 3). The vocal ligament inserts on the thyroid cartilage anteriorly and the vocal process of the arytenoid cartilage posteriorly (Fig. 4).

The major cartilages of the larynx are the cricoid, thyroid, and the paired arytenoid cartilages (Fig. 5). These major structural cartilages are all of hyaline type. The epiglottis, in contrast, is composed of elastic cartilage containing numerous fenestrations. Calcification of the thyroid and cricoid cartilages begins during the second decade of life in males and somewhat later in females. In older individuals, the thyroid cartilage is frequently ossified, replete with fibrofatty and hematopoietic bone marrow elements. The ossification of the thyroid cartilage is important in regard to the spread of laryngeal carcinoma. This cartilage is involved by continuous or metastatic carcinoma only when ossified. Hyaline cartilage, perhaps because of its elaboration of angiogenesis inhibiting factors, is remarkably resistant to the spread of neoplasia.

The cricoid and thyroid cartilages articulate with one another, but their motion is limited by several dense ligaments that anchor the cartilages together. The arytenoid cartilages articulate with the cricoid cartilage. Both the cricothyroid and cricoarytenoid joints are diarthrodial and lined by flattened synovial cells. These tiny joints are susceptible to conditions such as gout and rheumatoid arthritis, that more commonly affect larger synovial-lined spaces.

Each arytenoid cartilage has a protrusion, the vocal process, that is the posterior point of insertion of the vocal ligament, and the thyroarytenoid muscle. The position of the arytenoid cartilage determines the tension of the vocal ligament. During adduction of the cords, the arytenoid cartilages move medially along the facets of the cricoid cartilage; they also pivot or rock (Fig. 4). The rocking motion causes the vocal processes to move downward and toward the midline to complete the adduction of the vocal cords.

The muscles of the larynx can be divided into two groups. The extrinsic muscles originate from neighboring structures outside the larynx and insert on the thyroid, cricoid, or hyoid cartilages. These muscles include the omohyoid, sternohyoid, sternothyroid, and thyrohyoid muscles; they act as a whole upon the larynx during swallowing.

The principle intrinsic muscles of the larynx are the cricothyroid, posterior cricoarytenoid, lateral cricoarytenoid,

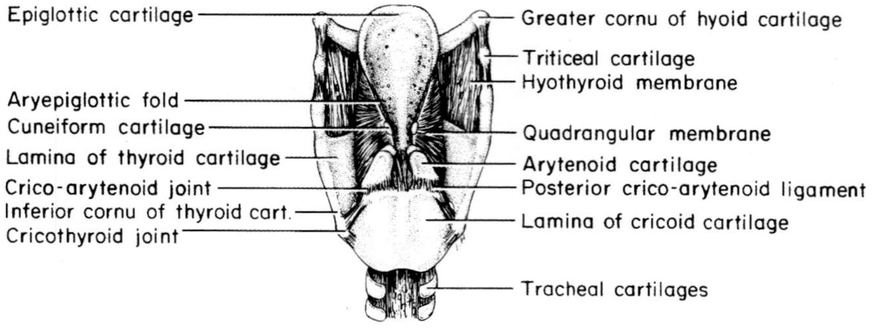


**FIG. 2.** Posterior view of an unopened larynx emphasizes the position of the arytenoid cartilages. Major support and posterior definition of the larynx are provided by the lamina of the cricoid cartilage. (From ref. 45.)

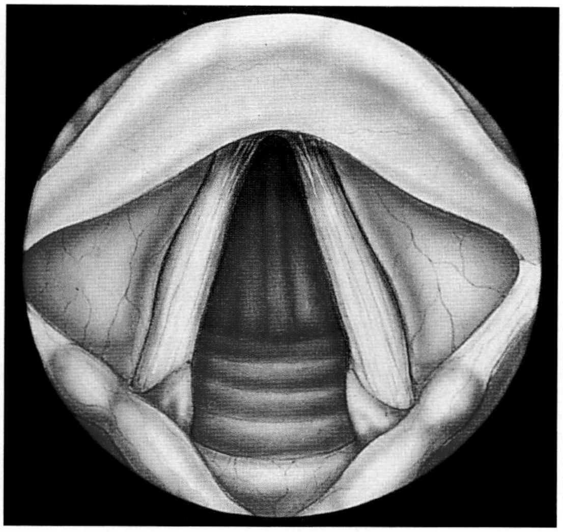

**FIG. 3.** Larynx as viewed endoscopically from above. The elastic cone is visible through the mucosa of the true cord as a gray-to-white zone. False cords are loose folds of mucosa without further distinguishing features.

and thyroarytenoid. There are also small strands of muscle that are in continuity with the thyroarytenoid muscle and insert along the length of the vocal ligaments. This is frequently referred to as the vocalis muscle. It should be remembered that the vocalis muscle is actually a component of the thyroarytenoid muscle, and some authors use these names interchangeably.

The lateral cricoarytenoid muscle adducts the vocal cord, and the posterior cricoarytenoid muscle abducts the cord. During phonation, the thyroarytenoid muscle slightly moves the thyroid cartilage. The degree of contraction of the thyroarytenoid muscle determines the length and tension of the vocal cord.

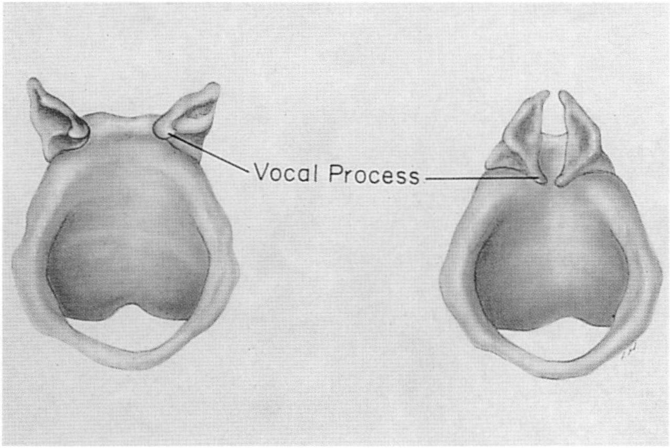


**FIG. 4.** The arytenoid cartilage articulates with the posterior lamina of the cricoid cartliagea. When the arytenoid cartilages are abducted, they are widely separated and the airway is open (*left*). When adducted, the arytenoid cartilages pivot, as well as move medially, thus bringing the vocal cords together (*right*). (From ref. 45.)

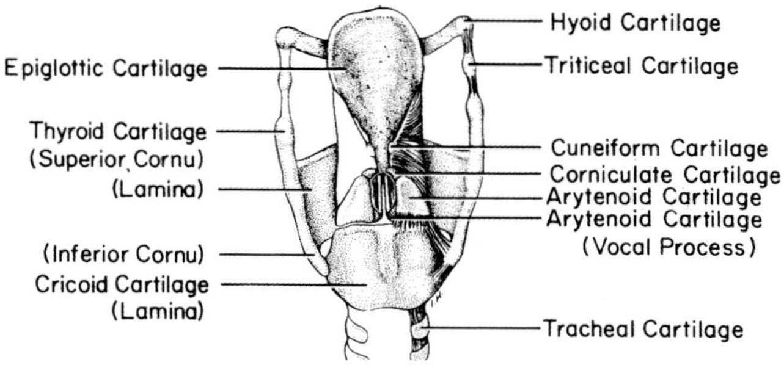


**FIG. 5.** The major cartilages of the larynx are better seen in this drawing that deletes the associated soft tissues. (From ref. 45.)

The larynx can be divided into three major compartments (supraglottic, glottic, subglottic) for purposes of discussing its submucosal and mucosal components. The supraglottic larynx extends from the tip of the epiglottis to the true cord (3). This portion of the larynx also includes the arytenoepiglottic (aryepiglottic) folds, false vocal cords, and ventricles. The arytenoepiglottic folds run posteriorly from the base of the epiglottis to the region of the arytenoid cartilages. The false vocal cords are soft, rounded protrusions of the mucous membrane that lie superior to the true cords. The ventricles form the lower boundary of the false cords and separate them from the inferiorly located true cords. The ventricles extend upward behind the false cords as elliptical pouches. The greatest extension of the ventricles is slightly forward, where they end as dilate, blind pouches called the saccules. Involvement of the ventricle is a frequent route of superior spread by glottic carcinoma, and this spread may be difficult to detect clinically.

The glottic compartment consists of the true vocal cords and the narrow band of mucous membrane called the anterior commissure, which bridges the vocal cords anteriorly (4,5). The subglottic compartment is the area between the lower border of the true vocal cords, where the squamous epithelium ends, and the first tracheal cartilage (6).

## Microscopic Anatomy

Studies of larynges from newborns have shown that, initially, the larynx is lined by ciliated epithelium, except for the true vocal cords (7) (Figs. 6 and 7). Squamous epithelium begins to appear on the false vocal cords by about 6 months of age, but does not necessarily completely replace the ciliated respiratory mucosa (8,9). The lingual or anterior surface of the epiglottis is invariably covered by stratified squamous epithelium. The posterior or laryngeal surface of the epiglottis is covered by stratified squamous epithelium in its upper portion, but this merges with respiratory-type epithelium inferiorly (10). About one-half of nonsmoking adults have patches of squamous epithelium intermixed with ciliated epithelium, both in the supraglottic and infraglottic regions. In smokers, the ciliated, respiratory epithelium of the larynx is, often, totally replaced by squamous epithelium.

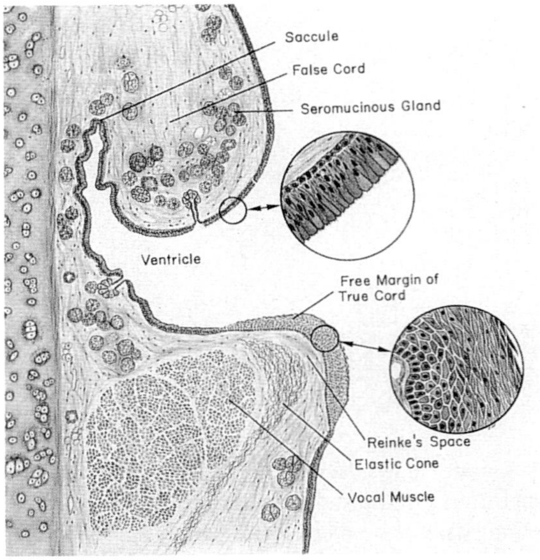


**FIG. 6.** Drawing of the normal microscopic anatomy of the larynx. Seromucinous glands are prominent in the false cord, and this cord is lined by ciliated columnar epithelium at birth. The vocalic muscle, elastic cone, and Reinke's space are also visualized in the true cord. (From ref. 45.)

The normal ciliated epithelium of the larynx has an innermost layer of small, round cells–the basal or reserve cell layer. This single cell layer of basal cells is overlaid by a second row of ciliated columnar cells. Variation in the position of the nuclei within the columnar cell layer imparts a psuedostratified appearance to the epithelium. The ciliated layer may vary considerably in thickness (Fig. 8). Mucus-secreting cells may be numerous or rare. When there is abundant mucin, the cells assume a goblet configuration and may be located either within the middle portion of the epithelium, or near the surface (Fig. 9). Other mucus-secreting cells are barely recognizable and have only a few faintly discernible vacuoles within otherwise eosinophilic columnar cells.

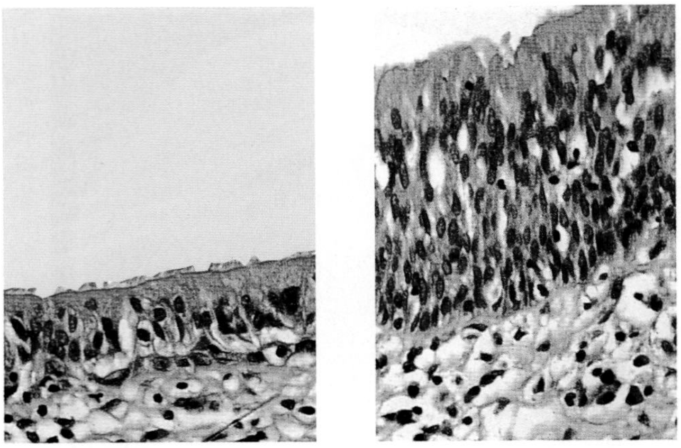

**FIG. 8.** The ciliated columnar epithelium of the larynx may be only a few cells in thickness (*left*), or it may form a considerably thicker layer (*right*). (From ref. 45.)

The squamous epithelium of the larynx has a basal layer of small cells with scant cytoplasm and ovoid nuclei that are typically oriented perpendicular to the surface. Mitotic figures are normally confined to this layer. Dendritic melanocytes may be present in the basal layer, especially in african-americans (11,12). The frequency with which this melanocytic change is observed, and whether it represents a congenital or acquired process, remain unclear. Rare laryngeal malignant melanomas presumably arise in such foci.

As the squamous cells in laryngeal mucosa mature and migrate toward the lumen, the nuclei enlarge, assume a more spherical shape, and have more vesicular chromatin. The eosinophilic cytoplasm becomes abundant and slight cell shrinkage during fixation produces numerous, thin strands of cytoplasm from adjacent cells that remain attached by desmosomes. Because of these thin cytoplasmic strands between cells, the term "prickle cell layer" (malpighian layer) has been applied to this zone. This is the broadest component of the squamous epithelium. The superficial layer is com-

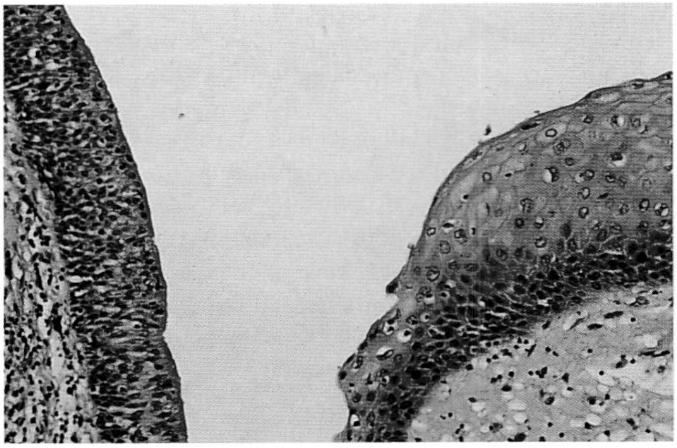

**FIG. 7.** Section through ventricle discloses squamous epithelium lining true cord (*right*) and ciliated columnar to intermediate epithelium lining false cord (*left*).

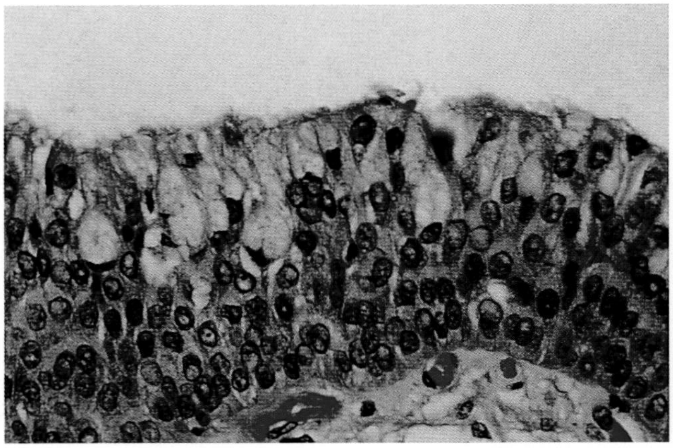

**FIG. 9.** Goblet cells and columnar mucinous cells may be present in variable numbers within the nonsquamous epithelium of the larynx.

posed of one to three flattened cells with small, condensed nuclei. The squamous epithelium of the larynx can vary from about five cells in total thickness to over twenty-five cells (Fig. 10). Normally, the larynx lacks a layer of parakeratotic surface cells. Continued exposure to irritants, such as cigarette smoke, may lead to foci of parakeratosis that may also be associated with orthokeratin formation.

The lamina propria of the true vocal cord is loose or dense connective tissue that lies between the vocal ligament and the squamous epithelium (Reinke's space) (Fig. 11). Reinke's space contains a few capillaries but lacks lymphatics, and only rarely has sparse seromucinous glands. As a result of this limited vascular access, carcinomas confined to the true vocal cords tend to remain localized, and are amenable to curative radiation or surgical therapy. The poor lymphatic drainage of Reinke's space also probably contributes to the development of vocal cord nodules and polyps when abnormal amounts of edema-like fluid collect in this region. The anterior commissure, unlike the true cords, contains more abundant capillaries, lymphatics, and seromucinous glands.

The junction between the ciliated columnar epithelium, inferior and superior to the squamous epithelium of the true vocal cords, may be abrupt, but usually there is a transitional zone that varies from several cells to a width of 1 to 2 mm. The transitional zone consists of columnar cells that are gradually replaced by small, basaloid or immature squamous cells (Fig. 12). In effect, this is a zone of immature squamous metaplasia in which the cells become progressively larger until they reach the size of the fully mature squamous epithelium that lines the true vocal cord.

The transitional zone often has a microscopically disorganized appearance when compared to the adjacent squamous and ciliated epithelium (Fig. 12). Furthermore, the epithelium in this zone may be thickened and consist predominantly of basaloid cells. The latter cells have uniform nuclei with mitotic figures confined to the basal-most cell layer.

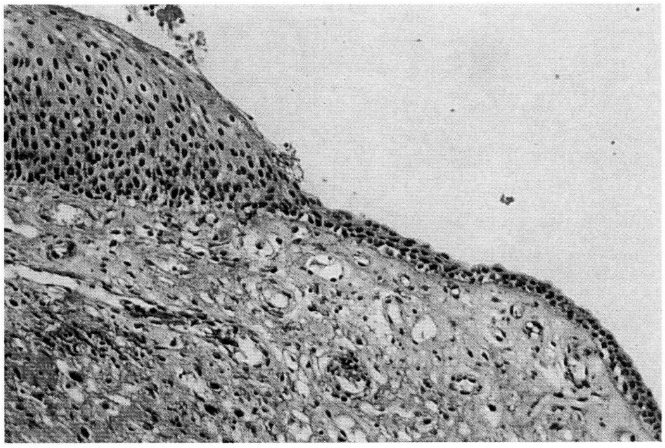

**FIG. 10.** The squamous epithelium of the larynx can vary from approximately 5 cells in total thickness to over 25 cells in thickness, even within the same larynx.

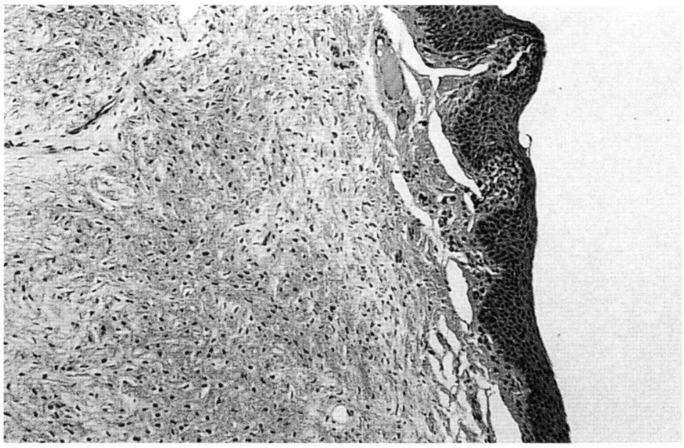

**FIG. 11.** The true vocal cord is lined by squamous epithelium. A narrow, sparsely vascular zone (Reinke's space) lies between the squamous epithelium and the underlying vocal ligament.

This normal pattern can easily be confused with dysplasia or so-called carincoma in situ, particularly in frozen sections or otherwise suboptimal preparations. Awareness of this transitional zone and attention to cytologic detail will avoid confusion.

Human Papillomavirus (HPV) subtypes have been implicated in the pathogenesis of a variety of squamous proliferations in the larynx and elsewhere in the head and neck. Using sensitive polymerase chain reaction (PCR) techniques, studies are beginning to document some HPV subtypes, such as type 11 in approximately 25% of light microscopically normal laryngeal specimens (13). Thus, the finding of this HPV subtype adjacent to a laryngeal carcinoma cannot be assumed to represent a causative assocation. HPV subtypes more commonly associated with malignancy (HPV 16,18) have not yet been demonstrated in light-microscopically normal laryngeal mucosa.

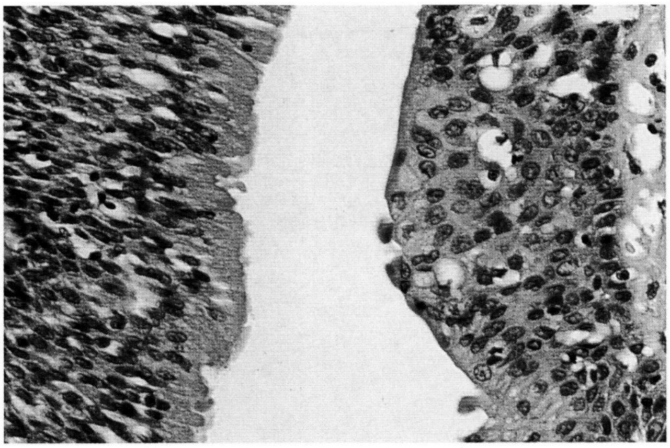

**FIG. 12.** Ciliated columnar epithelium lines the false cord at the left. A transitional zone is seen on the true cord at the right. This zone of immature squamous metaplasia has a disorganized appearance that should not be confused with dysplasia. (From ref. 45.)

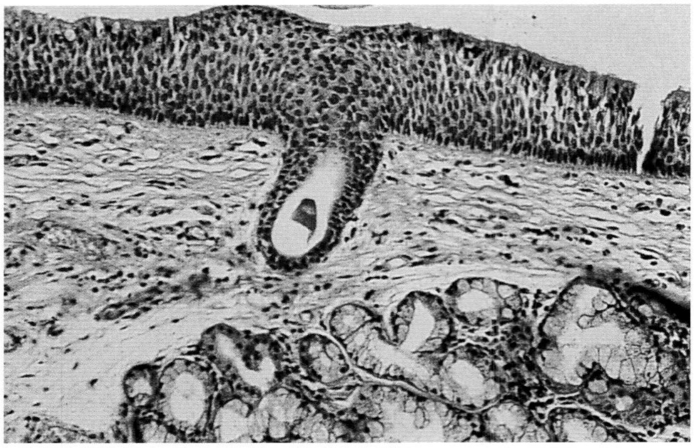

**FIG. 13.** Seromucinous glands in the false cord drain into a duct that enters the overlying ciliated columnar epithelium. (From ref. 45.)

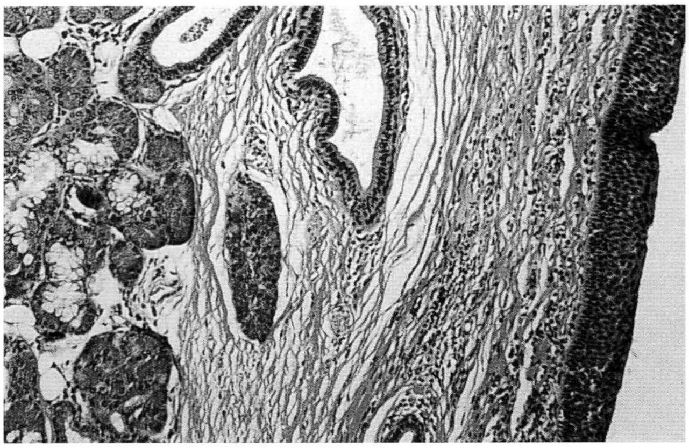

**FIG. 15.** Seromucinous glands and their ducts are most prominent in the false cord.

Seromucinous glands are present throughout most of the larynx and communicate with the surface epithelium by ducts that are lined either by squamous cells, columnar epithelium (Figs. 13 and 14), or a mixture of the two (14). The columnar epithelial component may or may not be ciliated. The glands are most abundant in the false cords (Fig. 15), and there is also an extensive group of seromucinous glands just below the anterior commissure. Just superior to the anterior commissure is a narrow zone, devoid of glands. In most cases, no glands are found beneath the squamous epithelium lining the free edge of the true vocal cords. Glands are present, however, beginning immediately at the squamocolumnar junction, both above and below the squamous epithelium of the true cords. Occasionally, there are glands in the stroma of the true vocal cord, and glands may be present in the underlying vocalis muscle (Fig. 16). The fenestration in the elastic cartilage of the epiglottis are filled with abundant seromucinous glands. These glands penetrate completely through the cartilage and afford a ready path for the spread of supraglottic carcinoma.

Laryngeal biopsies, particularly from the region of the false cords, will often contain seromucinous gland ducts lined by squamous epithelium and located deep beneath the surface mucosa. Because of tangential sectioning, these ducts may appear as seemingly isolated squamous nests. Distinction from infiltrating carcinoma should not be a problem in adequately prepared sections. However, changes of basal cell hyperplasia or dysplasia also can involve these ducts. Fortuitous sections of such ducts may then result in seemingly isolated nests of basaloid or overtly dysplastic epithelium that are much more likely to be mistaken for invasive carcinoma (Fig. 17).

Oncocytic metaplasia of ductal and acinar cells in the seromucinous glands of the larynx is a common, age-related change. Oncocytes are not seen in the seromucinous glands of individuals younger than 18 years of age, but oncocytes

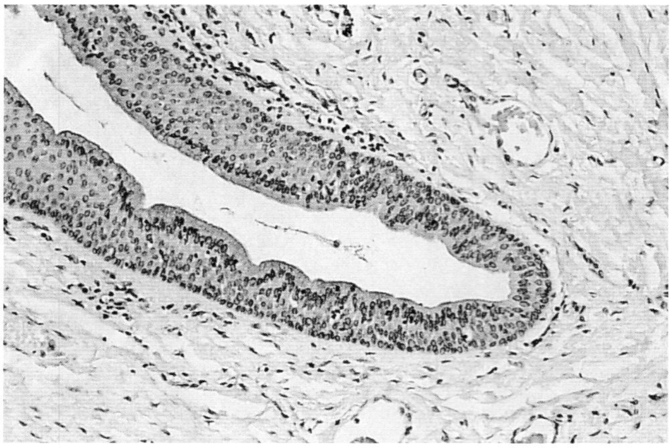

**FIG. 14.** Ducts from seromucionous glands may be lined by squamous cells, ciliated columnar epithelium, or a mixture of the two.

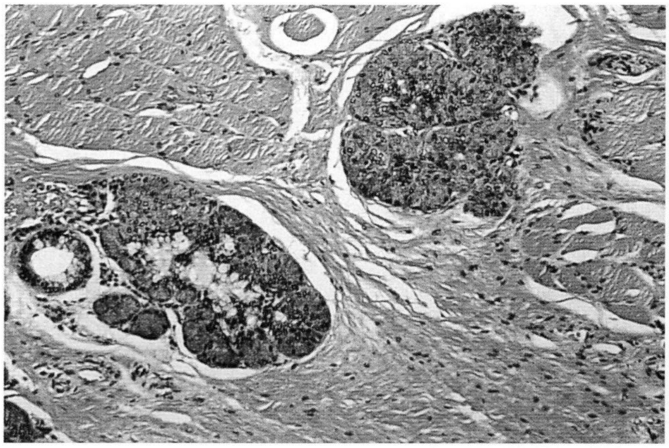

**FIG. 16.** Seromucinous glands are occasionally located deeply within the vocalic muscle.

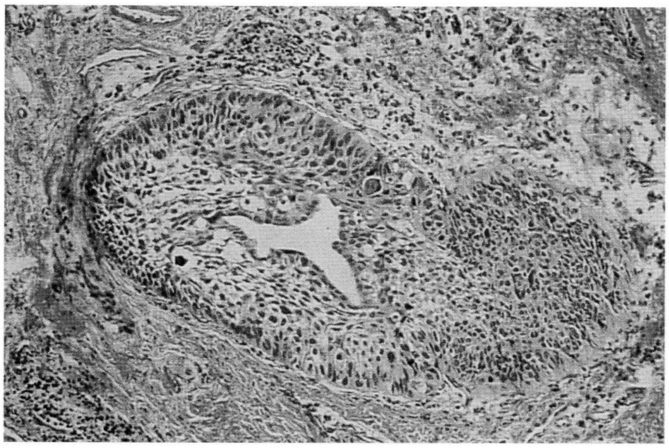

**FIG. 17.** When ducts are involved with cytologically atypical squamous epithelium resembling surface dysplastic changes, they should not be misinterpreted as invasive carcinoma. In this example, the inner columnar cell lining is retained.

are present in these glands in approximately 80% of people over the age of 50 (15,16). Uncomplicated oncocytic metaplasia is asymptomatic, but, occasionally, oncocytic metaplasia may become cystic (Fig. 18) and, if sufficiently large, produce symptoms.

The seromucinous glands of the larynx may also undergo infarction and associated squamous metaplasia. The resultant process, termed necrotizing sialometaplasia, is much more common in the oral cavity, and probably results from a traumatic or spontaneous ischemic event (17). The islands of metaplastic cells may be mitotically active and exhibit mild-to-moderate nuclear atypia. Confusion with mucoepidermoid or squamous cell carcinoma is common, particularly in frozen section specimens. At low power magnification, the preservation of the acinar pattern, in association with infarction, inflammation, and extravasation of mucin, will aid in the correct diagnosis.

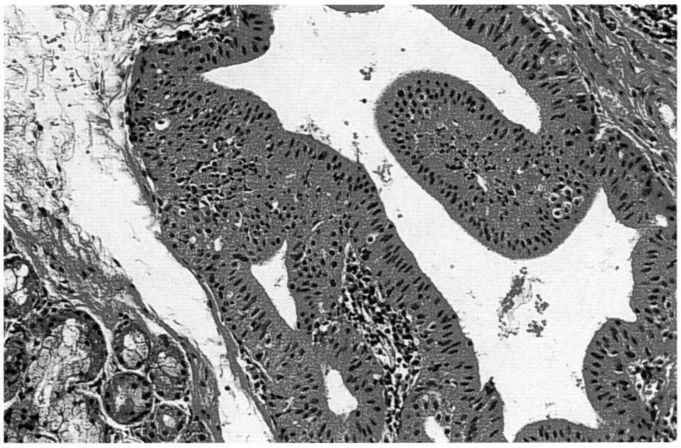

**FIG. 18.** Oncocytic transformation of Seromucinous epithelium can result in cystic structures.

If the external surface of the larynx is carefully sampled, it is not unusual to find microscopic islands of normal thyroid tissue within the fibrous capsule of the larynx and trachea, just external to the cricothyroid membrane (18). The thyroid follicles are small and appear normal, with well-formed colloid. Continuity with the main thyroid gland is not usually demonstrable (19). Less commonly, microscopic foci of thyroid tissue will be encountered internal to the cartilage of the larynx and trachea, usually at the junction of the cricoid cartilage and the first tracheal ring (18, 20). These isolated foci of extrathyroidal thyroid tissue probably lose their connection to the main portion of the thyroid gland during embryologic development (18). Awareness of this phenomenon and attention to the microscopic features will avoid confusion with invasive or metastatic thyroid carcinoma.

The normal larynx contains at least two pairs of paraganglia. The superior, supraglottic paraganglia are sharply localized to the upper, anterior third of the false cords, in close approximation to the margin of the thyroid cartilage and the internal branch of the superior laryngeal nerves (21,22). The paired inferior paraganglia are more variably situated, and may be found between the thyroid and cricoid cartilages or just below the cricoid cartilage (21,22). They are closely associated with the inferior laryngeal nerves. Aberrant or ectopic paraganglia have been described in various sites throughout the larynx. Laryngeal paraganglia are minute, neuroendocrine structures (0.1 to 0.4 mm) of unknown, physiologic activity. Their close association with neurovascular bundles suggests chemoreceptor function, but this has not been proved. Laryngeal paraganglia presumably give rise to the rare paragangliomas of the larynx.

The vocal process of the arytenoid cartilage is a normal structure that is occasionally encountered in biopsy specimens from the posterior portion of the true cord. It is a sharply circumscribed nodule of uniformly mature, elastic-type cartilage (Fig. 19). Its elastic nature, demonstrable with appropriate elastin stains, allows distinction from cartilagi-

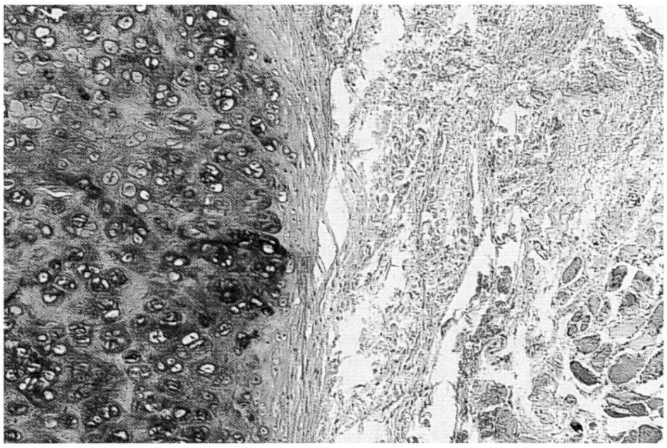

**FIG. 19.** The vocal process of the arytenoid cartilage is a sharply circumscribed nodule of elastic-type cartilage. (From ref. 45.)

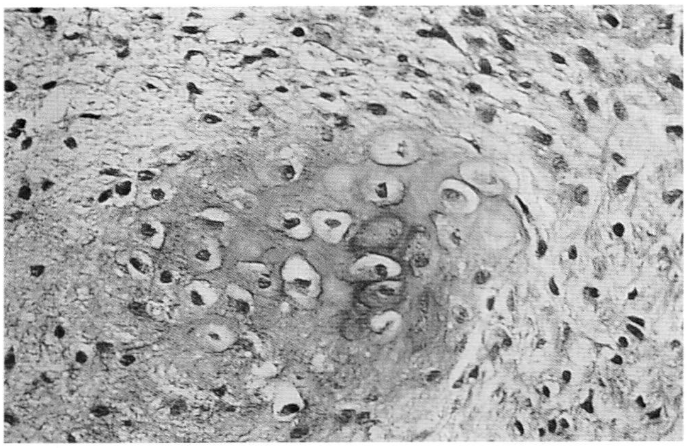

**FIG. 20.** Chondroid metaplasia of the larynx has ill-defined margins. (From ref. 45.)

nous neoplasms of the larynx, all of which are composed of hyaline-type cartilage. The sharp circumscription of the cartilaginous arytenoid process allows it to be differentiated from chondroid metaplasia of the vocal ligament described below. Chondroid metaplasia of the vocal cord is a common, usually asymptomatic, finding that typically affects the mid- and posterior portions of the vocal cord (23,24). The margins of the cartilage are blurred, and there is a peripheral zone of connective tissue that is rich in acid mucopolysaccharides (Fig. 20) (24). The metaplastic nodules contain dense aggregates of elastic fibers throughout the lesion. The multilobular pattern, typical of cartilaginous neoplasms, is absent. Chondroid metaplasia can occur in other soft tissues of the larynx, particularly in the region of the false cord. In one study, foci of chondroid metaplasia were found in 1 to 2% of larynges at autopsy (23).

### Neural, Vascular, and Lymphatic Components

The intrinsic laryngeal muscles are innervated by branches of the vagus nerve. The cricothyroid muscle is supplied by the superior laryngeal branch of the vagus, and the remainder of the intrinsic musculature has been conventionally viewed as being innervated by the recurrent laryngeal brance of the vagus nerve. The terminal portion of the recurrent laryngeal nerve is referred to as the "inferior laryngeal nerve" (25). More recently, it has been shown that branches of the superior and recurrent laryngeal nerves form anastomoses, most commonly within the interarytenoid muscle, but less consistently in the piriform sinus. Branches from the superior laryngeal nerve, referred to as the "communicating nerve," may pass through the cricothyroid muscle to partially innervate the vocalis muscle (26,27). It has been suggested that the ocmmunicating nerve may be the nerve of the elusive fifth branchial arch (27).

The lower portions of the larynx are supplied with blood from the inferior laryngeal artery, a small branch of the inferior thyroid artery that accompanies the inferior laryngeal nerve. The inferior laryngeal artery has anastomoses with the larger superior laryngeal artery, derived from the superior thyroid artery. The laryngeal arteries are accompanied by similarly named veins. The superior laryngeal vein joins the superior thyroid vein and drains into the internal jugular vein (25). The inferior laryngeal vein joins the inferior thyroid vein. Numerous anastomoses across the front of the trachea between the left and right inferior laryngeal veins may lead to contralateral venous return (25).

The lymphatics of the larynx tend to drain along with the vasculature. Therefore, supraglottic lymphatics drain superiorly, and subglottic lymphatics drain inferiorly (1,25). As discussed earlier, lymphatics are scarce in the glottis. Some of the laryngeal lymphatics end in very small lymph nodes on the thyrohyoid membrane, cricotracheal ligament, or superior trachea (25). These nodes, however, drain into the deep cervical nodes (25). Lymphatics in the supraglottic larynx are prominent and, typically, terminate in the anterior jugular chain (28). Subglottic lymphatics terminate in the midline pretracheal nodes or, less commonly, in the lower cervical lymph nodes (28).

## PHARYNX

### Definition and Boundaries

The pharynx has three functionally and structurally disperse subparts – the nasopharynx, oropharynx, and hypopharynx (Fig. 21). The nasopharynx is the portion of the pharynx that lies above the soft palate. It has anterior, posterior, and lateral walls. The anterior wall is perforated by the posterior nares (choanae). The posterior wall is an arch that includes the roof of the nasopharynx, as well as the posterior portion against the base of the skull. The posterior wall extends inferiorly and, at the level of the horizontal projection of the soft palate, continues inferiorly as the posterior wall of the oropharynx. The anterior and posterior walls are con-

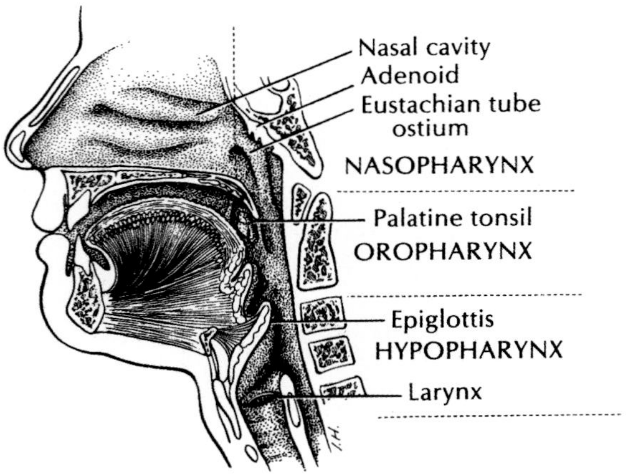


**FIG. 21.** This sagittal section delineates the boundaries of the nasopharynx, oropharynx, and hypopharynx.

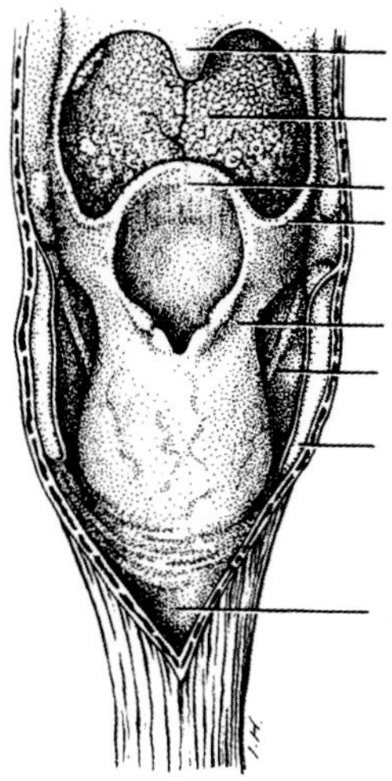


**FIG. 22.** The piriform sinuses are a conduit between the oropharynx and the opening of the esophagus. They surround the larynx laterally.

nected by the lateral walls into which the eustachian tubes empty.

The oropharynx lies between the soft palate and the tip of the epiglottis. By definition, its superior boundary is a horizontal projection of the soft palate. Anteriorly, it is bounded by the fauces or opening from the mouth and, below this, the posterior aspect of the dorsum of the tongue. The inferior margin of the anterior portion of the oropharynx is marked by the opening of the piriform recess at the level of the tip of the epiglottis. A horizontal projection posteriorly from this point, marks the posterior aspect of the inferior margin, which is continuous with the hypopharynx.

The hypopharynx is the portion of the pharynx below the tip of the epiglottis and extending downward to the beginning of the esophagus. The hypopharynx is wide superiorly, but rapidly narrows as it approaches the level of the cricoid cartilage and becomes continuous with the esophagus. The hypopharynx partially surrounds the larynx laterally, and is separated from it by the aryepiglottic folds. The latter extend from the upper posterior border of the larynx to the side of the epiglottis. The lateral extensions of the hypopharynx are called the "piriform recesses" or sinuses (25) (Fig. 22).

## Embryology

The embryologic pharynx is of endodermal derivation and, at its cephalic end, is in direct continuity with the ectoderm forming the stomodeum. Recent observations have suggested that the development of the roof of the pharynx is highly dependent on the closely adjacent notochord (29). The stomodeum and pharynx are separated by the buccopharyngeal membrane, which is lined on its external surface by ectoderm, and, internally, by endoderm. At the end of the 3rd week of embryologic development, the buccopharyngeal membrane ruptures, establishing contact between the stomodeum and the primitive pharyngeal portion of the foregut (29,30). Superiorly, the buccopharyngeal membrane corresponds to approximately the level of the nasal choanae. In the subsequent 5th through 7th weeks of gestation, the primitive nasal cavity forms and enlarges, with formation and later rupture of the bucconasal membrane, establishing the final connection between the nasal cavity and pharynx (29). In the 8th through the 10th gestational weeks, the secondary palate develops behind the primary palate, ending the formation of the basic pharyngeal structures. At this point, however, the pharynx is proportionally quite small and after the 10th week of gestation, remarkable growth in this region occurs with enlargement of the pharynx and downward movement of the palate and tongue (29).

Thus, the lining of the nasal cavity and paranasal sinuses is of ectodermal origin and constitutes the so-called Schneiderian membrane. The nasopharynx, oropharynx, and hypopharynx are, at least in large part, of endodermal origin. THe sharp demarcation between endoderm and ectoderm at the level of the nasal cavity, is of considerable practical importance. Certain neoplasms, such as angiofibromas and lymphoepitheliomas, are virtually confined to the endodermally derived nasopharynx. In contrast, schneiderian papillomas and intestinal-type adenocarcinomas arise from the ectodermally derived lining of the nasal cavity and paranasal sinuses; they do not occur in the nasopharynx.

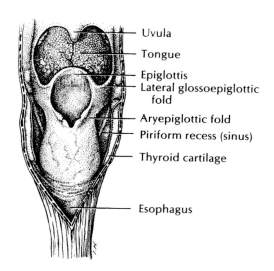

## Gross Anatomy

By nature of their boundaries and lack of resectability, the nasopharynx and oropharynx are practically never encountered as gross specimens. The roof of the nasopharynx is composed of mucosa overlying the basal portions of the sphenoid and occipital bones (25). The lateral and posterior walls of the nasopharynx are composed of the superior constrictor muscles and the pharyngobasilar fascia. The soft palate is the floor of the anterior portion of the nasopharynx: the only truly mobile portion of the nasopharynx (25). Although the opening between the nasopharynx and oropharynx is normally patent, the soft palate can be moved posteriorly and superiorly to completely separate the nasal and oral segments. This is important as a component of proper speech, and to keep food and water out of the nasal region during eating and drinking.

The most important gross features of the nasopharynx encountered by pathologists are the pharyngeal tonsil, Rosenmüller's fossa, and eustachian tube opening. The pharyngeal tonsil or adenoid is a prominent, convoluted mass in the roof of the nasopharynx in children. (It typically atrophies in adults.) The pharyngeal recess or Rosenmüller's fossa is a mucosal-lined depression in the posterolateral portion of the nasopharynx. Just anterior to the recess, located in the lateral wall, is the ostium of the eustachian tube. This opening is surrounded on its superior and posterior aspects by mucosa-covered cartilage, the tubal torus, from the eustachian tube wall (25).

The superior portion of the anterior oropharynx is bounded by the fauces or opening of the mouth into the oropharynx. The lateral walls of the fauces are composed, on each side, of the two tonsillar pillars, between which lies the palatine tonsil in the tonsillar fossa. The anterior tonsillar pillar is the palatoglossal arch. This structure curves downward and forward, from the soft palate to the tongue. The posterior tonsillar pillar or palatopharyngeal arch extends downward from the posterolateral border of the soft palate laterally along the pharyngeal wall. Each of the arches contains a similarly named muscle (25).

The palatine tonsil, more commonly referred to as simply the tonsil, varies tremendously in size, depending on its state of lymphoid reactivity. The surface of the tonsil is covered with epithelial-lined pits, the tonsillar crypts that pass into the underlying lymphoid tissue. Beneath the tonsil is the pharyngobasilar fascia, which sends branches of fibrous tissue into and around the tonsil, forming the so-called tonsillar capsule. Loose connective tissue between this capsule and the deeper superior constrictor muscle forms a plane of cleavage that facilitates surgical removal (25).

The parapharyngeal or lateral pharyngeal space is an important zone of loose connective tissue lying deep to the tonsil and lateral to the pharynx (Fig. 23). This space is roughly pyramidal, with the base of the skull forming the base of the pyramid superiorly (18, 25). Inferiorly, the apex is formed by the attachment of the cervical fascia to the hyoid bone. Medially, is the superior constrictor muscle of the pharynx and laterally, the pterygoid lamina, inner surface of the mandibular ramus, and the deep lobe of the parotid gland (18). Contained within the peripharyngeal space are the internal carotid artery, internal jugular vein, cranial nerves IX to XII, the cervical sympathetic chain, vagal and carotid bodies, and multiple lymph nodes (18). Mass-producing lesions involving any of these structures may cause medial displacement of the tonsil and lateral pharyngeal wall. Tonsilar abscesses or other sources of infection may also involve and rapidly spread throughout this space. Posteriorly, the parapharyngeal space is in direct continuity with loose connective tissue behind the pharynx and anterior to the prevertebral fascia of the vertebral column (25). This has been referred to as the retropharyngeal space (Fig. 23).

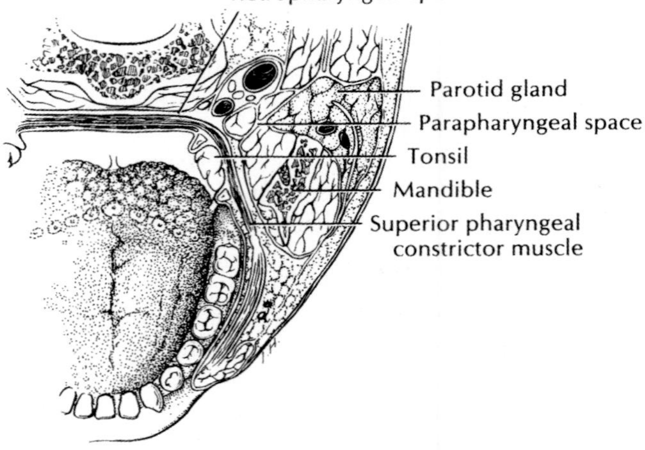


**FIG. 23.** The lateral pharyngeal space lies deep to the tonsil and contains several vital structures. It is in continuity, posteriorly, with the retropharyngeal space.

Inferior to the fauces, the oropharynx is bounded anteriorly by the posterior aspect of the immobile portion of the tongue. The base of the tongue contains abundant submucosal lymphoid tissue that constitutes the lingual tonsil. This structure, along with the palatine and pharyngeal tonsils, forms an oblique wreath of lymphoid tissue, encompassing the oropharynx and nasopharynx that is often referred to as Waldeyer's ring.

The most important structures in the hypopharynx are the piriform sinuses (Fig.22). These elongated, pear-shaped gutters extend laterally along both sides of the larynx, and posteriorly from the pharyngoepiglottic fold to the opening of the esophagus (28). Laterally, the piriform sinus lies against the thyroid cartlilage. Medially, it is separated from the laryngeal ventricle by a thin layer of muscles derived from the aryepiglottic fold and the opening of the esophagus (28). Just posterior and lateral to the piriform sinus, is the common carotid artery. Because of their close association, tumors arising in the hypopharynx often invade the larynx secondarily. These tumors should be distinguished from primary laryngeal neoplasms because of their poorer prognosis.

## Microscopic Anatomy

The nasopharyngeal mucosa in the adult has a surface area of about 50 $cm^2$. Most of it is lined by stratified squamous epithelium and about 40% is covered by respiratory-type, columnar epithelium (31). Squamous epithelium predominantly lines the lower portion of the anterior and posterior nasopharyngeal walls, as well as the anterior half of the lateral walls. Ciliated respiratory epithelium predominantly carpets the region of the posterior nares (choanae) and the roof of the posterior wall. The remainder of the nasopharynx, including the posterior lateral walls and the middle-third of the posterior wall, has alternating islands of squamous and respiratory epithelium.

The junction between squamous and respiratory epithelium may be sharp, or there may be zones of transitional or intermediate epithelium as previously described in the larynx. We prefer the term "intermediate epithelium," as opposed to "transitional epithelium," because these cells lack the ultrastructural features of urinary tract epithelium. Intermediate epithelium primarily forms a wavy ring at the junction of the nasopharynx and oropharynx. The intermediate cells may be basaloid with minimal cytoplasm, and they typically have a cuboidal or round configuration. As discussed under the larynx, biopsy specimens containing intermediate epithelium must not be overly interpreted as areas of dysplasia or carcinoma in situ. This is most likely to be a problem when this zone is encountered in a frozen section.

In addition to the pharyngeal tonsil, less-prominent collections of lymphoid follicles may be present submucosally throughout the nasopharynx (Fig. 24). These follicles are particularly abundant in the rim of the eustachian tube opening (Gerlach's tonsil), but they are also present under mucosa of the lateral and posterior walls of the nasopharynx, as well as on the nasopharyngeal surface of the soft palate (28). Thus, a submucosal follicular lymphoid infiltrate is normal in nasopharyngeal biopsies and should not be overinterpreted? as a pathologic inflammatory process.

Throughout the nasopharynx, there are numerous submucosal seromucinous glands that produce predominantly mucin. These glands are particularly numerous in the region of the eustachian tube opening. As with the laryngeal seromuncinous glands, oncocytic metaplasia in the glandular and ductal epithelium becomes increasingly frequent with advancing age (32,33).

The anterior portion of the pituitary gland forms from an intracranial invagination of epithelium in the form of Rathke's pouch. Microscopic remnants of Rathke's pouch epithelium are present in the roof of the nasopharynx in 95 to 100% of individuals (34–36). In most instances, this so-called pharyngeal pituitary is located in the midline, in the region of the vomerosphenoidal articulation. The nests of epithelial cells measure 0.2 mm to approximately 6 mm in greatest dimension. They are located deep in the mucosa or in the underlying periosteum (34). Most of the epithelial cells appear undifferentiated, but occasional basophilic and eosinophilic cells may be present. Although it is not entirely clear, the pharyngeal pituitary may not have any physiologic function. Most pituitary adenomas that involve the nasopharynx reach this location by invasion from the pituitary fossa. Occasionally, however, apparently ectopic pituitary adenomas present in the nasopharynx, and it is tempting to speculate that such lesions arise from the pharyngeal pituitary (37,38).

The pharyngeal bursa is a normal embryonic structure situated posterior to Rathke's pouch. Remnants of this bursa may be found in approximately 3% of normal adults (39,40). Cysts derived from this structure may be found in all ages, occasionally as an incidental finding, and occur in the regions of the adenoid (41). The cysts are separated from the adenoid by a fibrous membrane and will not be removed with routine adenoidectomy specimens (Fig. 25) (10). The median pharyngeal recess is a shallow depression formed normally in association with the pharyngeal tonsil. Unlike cysts derived from the pharyngeal bursa, those formed from the median pharyngeal recess are located within the adenoid and will be removed with it (10).

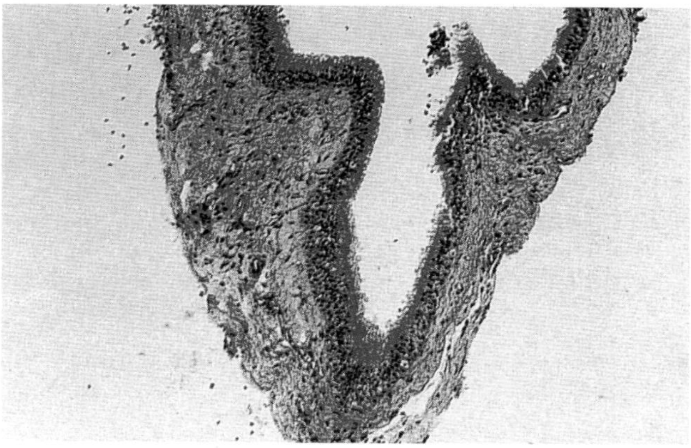

**FIG. 25.** Nasopharyngeal cysts are rimmed by fibrous tissue and lined by ciliated columnar epithelium.

The cranial end of the embryonic notochord is closely associated with the roof of the developing nasopharynx (42). Although most of the notochord degenerates during embryonic and fetal development, notochordal remnants have been demonstrated in the submucosa of the nasopharynx and other closely adjacent locations (10,43). Most chordomas involving the nasopharynx are down growths of cranio-occipital tumors, bur rare primary nasopharyngeal tumors presumably arise from these nasopharyngeal notochord remnants (42,43).

Both the oropharynx and hypopharynx are lined continuously by stratified squamous epithelium. This mucus is typically nonkeratinizing, although areas of parakeratin or orthokeratin may be seen secondary to chronic irritation. As in

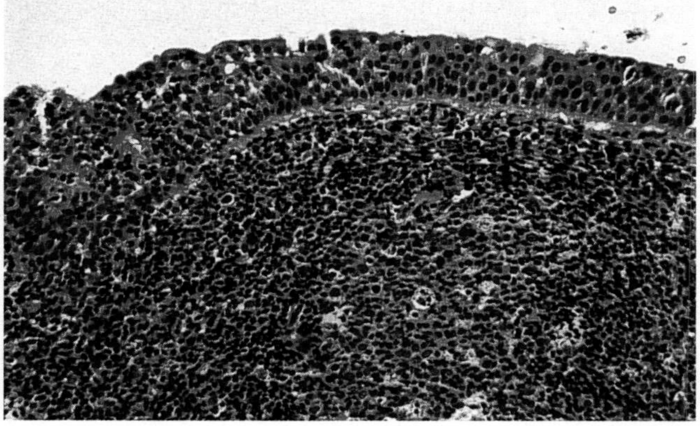

**FIG. 24.** Submucosal lymphoid aggregates are present normally throughout the nasopharynx and should not be overly interpreted as severe chronic inflammation.

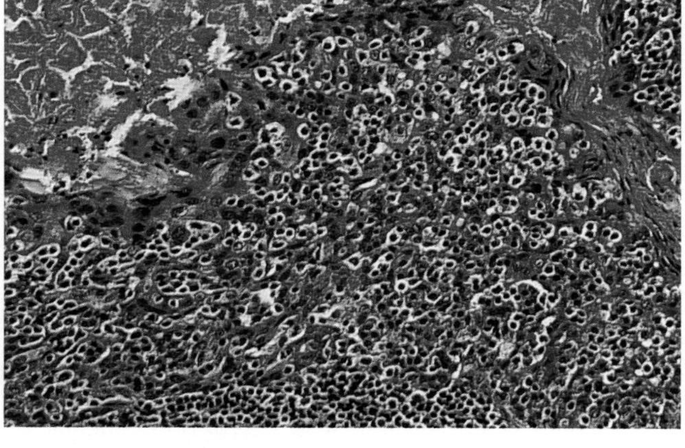

**FIG. 26.** The junction between lymphoid tissue and the squamous cells lining the tonsillar crypts is often blurred.

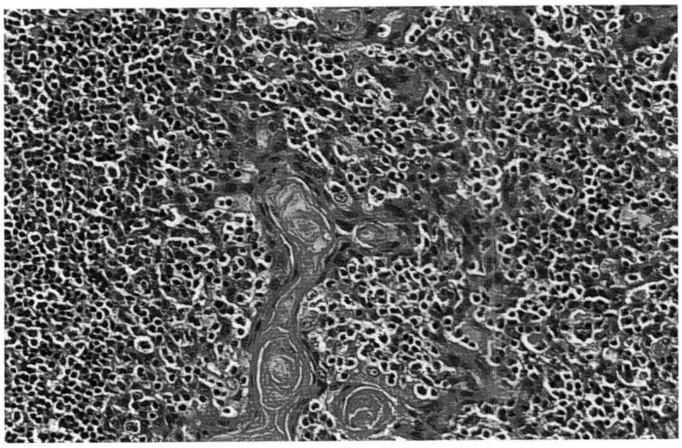

FIG. 27. Irregular nests of epithelium are frequently present deep within the tonsil. These are closely approximated to tonsillar crypts and are a normal finding not to be misinterpreted as carcinoma.

the nasopharynx, the submucosa of the oropharynx and hypopharynx contains scattered lymphoid aggregates, as well as prominent submucosal seromucinous glands.

The stratified squamous epithelium covering the tonsils extends into the tonsillar crypts for considerable distances. As these cords of epithelium merge with the underlying lymphoid tissue, the epithelial cells assume a more basaloid appearance and have uniform, but vesicular nuclei. The junction between the lymphoid cells and the islands of squamous cells is often blurred (Fig. 26). Apparently isolated, irregular nests of basaloid, focally keratinized squamous cells, often with vesicular nuclei, are common deep within the tonsil (Fig. 27), and such nests must not be confused with carcinoma.

Attention to the low-power architecture will confirm that these nests are closely approximated to tonsillar crypts and are a normal finding.

Occasionally, islands of metaplastic cartilage and bone are encountered within or immediately adjacent to the tonsils (18,44). This presumably represents a secondary, reactive change to prior inflammation. Eggston and Wolff described this change in about one-fifth of all resected tonsils (44). These authors noted that patients with this change had an average age of 24 years and, therefore, were older than most individuals undergoing tonsillectomy (44).

### Neural, Vascular, and Lymphatic Components

The nerves supplying the constrictor muscles of the phaynrx, the stylopharyngeus muscle, and the muscles of the soft palate are derived almost entirely from the pharyngeal plexus. The latter structure is formed by the union of the pharyngeal branches of the glossopharyngeal and vagus nerves. The inferior constrictor muscle may receive a portion of its innervation from the external laryngeal nerve, a separate branch of the vagus that primarily supplies the larynx (25).

The blood supply to the superior portion of the pharynx is from the ascending pharyngeal artery, which runs upward along the posterior lateral wall of the pharynx (25) (Fig. 28). The inferior portion of the pharynx is supplied by branches from the superior and inferior thyroid arteries. The veins draining the pharynx merge posteriorly to form the pharyngeal plexus, which in turn drains at irregular intervals into the pterygoid plexus and the superior and inferior thyroid veins (25).

The lymphatics from the roof and posterior wall of the nasopharynx join in the midline, and pass through the pharyngeal fascia. They then split to the right or left retropharyngeal lymph nodes. Some of the nasopharyngeal lymphatics terminate in the highest lymph nodes of the internal jugular and spinal chains (28). Most of the lymphatics from the soft palate converge at a group of lymph nodes located below the anterior belly of the digastric muscle, immediately in front of the jugular chain (28). Lymphatics from the tonsil pass through the lateral wall of the pharynx, and terminate in subdigastric nodes located anterior to the jugular chain (28). The hypopharynx is rich in lymphatics. These converge at an orifice in the thyrohyoid membrane, through which also passes the superior laryngeal artery. After exiting the thyrohyoid membrane, the lymphatics ramify into several trunks that terminate in lymph nodes of the internal jugular chain (28).

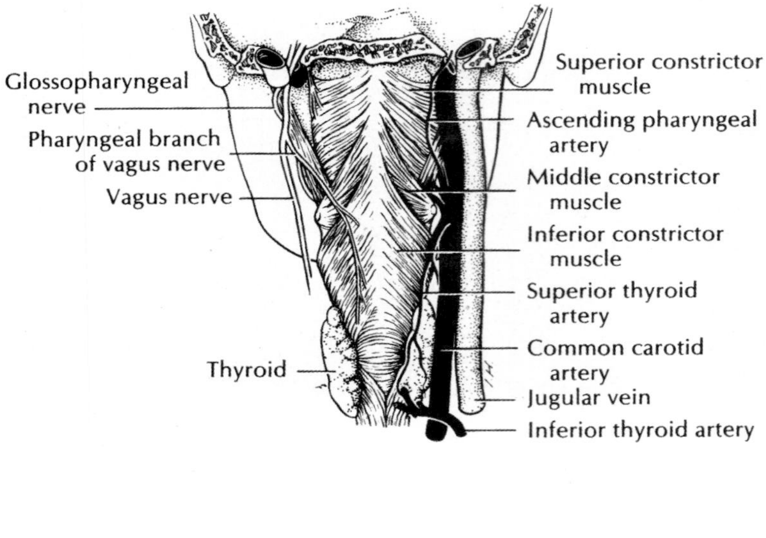


FIG. 28. Posterior view of the pharynx with emphasis on vascular and neural components.

## ACKNOWLEDGMENTS

The authors thank Linda Hamme for her expert artistic assistance, and Joshua Weikersheimer, director of the American Society of Clinical Pathologists Press, for obtaining and allowing the use of several illustrations from reference 45.

## REFERENCES

1. Bocca E, Pignataro O, Mosciaro O. Supraglottic surgery of the larynx. *Ann Otol Rhinol Laryngol* 1968;77:1005–1026.
2. Cotton A, Reilly JS. Congenital malformations of the larynx. In: Bluestone CD, Stool SE, eds. *Pediatric otolaryngology*. Philadelphia; WB Saunders, 1983;1215–1224.
3. Stell PM, Gudrun R, Watt J. Morphology of the human larynx. III. The supraglottis. *Clin Otolaryngol* 1981;6:389–393.
4. Stell PM, Gregory I, Watt J. Morphometry of the epithelial lining of the human larynx. I. The glottis. *Clin Otolaryngol* 1978;3:13–20.
5. Andrea M, Guerrier Y. The anterior commissure of the larynx. *Clin Otolaryngol* 1981;6:259–264.
6. Stell PM, Gregory I, Watt J. Morphology of the human larynx. II. The subglottis. *Clin Otolaryngol* 1980;5:389–395.
7. Hopp ES. The development of the epithelium of the larynx. *Laryngoscope* 1955;65:475–499.
8. Tucker JA, Vidic B, Tucker GF Jr, Stead J. Survey of the development of laryngeal epithelium. *Ann Otol Rhinol Laryngol* 1976;85(suppl 30):3–16.
9. Scott GBD. A quantitative study of microscopical changes in the epithelium and subepithelial tissue of the laryngeal folds, sinus, and saccule. *Clin Otolaryngol* 1976;1:257–264.
10. Hyams VJ, Batsakis JG, Michaels L. Tumors of the upper respiratory tract and ear. *Atlas of tumor pathology*, 2nd ser, fasc 25. Washington, DC; Armed Forces Institute of Pathology, 1988.
11. Busuttil A. Dendritic pigmented cells within human laryngeal mucosa. *Arch Otolaryngol Head Neck Surg* 1976;102:43–44.
12. Goldman JL, Lawson W, Zak FG, Roffman JD. The presence of melanocytes in the human larynx. *Laryngoscope* 1972;82:824–835.
13. Nunez DA, Astley SM, Lewis FA, Wells M. Human papilloma viruses: a study of their prevalence in the normal larynx. *J Laryngol Otol* 1994; 108:319–320.
14. Nassar VH, Bridger GP. Topography of the laryngeal mucous glands. *Arch Otolaryngol Head Neck Surg* 1971;94:490–498.
15. Lundgren J, Olofsson J, Hellquist H. Oncocytic lesions of the larynx. *Acta Otolaryngol (Stockh)* 1982;94:335–344.
16. Gallagher JC, Puzon BZ. Oncocytic lesions of the larynx. *Ann Otol Rhinol Laryngol* 1969;78:307–318.
17. Wenig BM. Necrotizing sialometaplasia of the larynx. A report of two cases and a review of the literature. *Am J Clin Pathol* 1995;103:609–13.
18. Michaels L. *Ear, nose, and throat histopathology*. New York; Springer-Verlag, 1987.
19. Richardson, GM, Assor D. Thyroid tissue within the larynx. Case report. *Laryngoscope* 1971;81:120–125.
20. Bone RC, Biller HF, Irwin TM. Intralaryngotracheal thyroid. *Ann Otol Rhinol Laryngol* 1972;81:424–428.
21. Lawson W, Zak FG. The glomus bodies (paraganglia) of the human larynx. *Laryngoscope* 1974;84:98–111.
22. Kleinsasser O. Das Glomas laryngicum inferior. Ein bisher unbekanntes, nichtchronaffines Paraganglion vom Bau der sog. Carotisdruse im menschlichen Kehlkopf. *Arch Ohr Nas Kehlkopfheilk* 1964;184: 214–224.
23. Hill MJ, Taylor CL, Scott GBD. Chondromatous metaplasia in the human larynx. *Histopathology* 1980;4:205–214.
24. Iyer PV, Rajagopalan PV. Cartilaginous metaplasia of the soft tissues of the larynx. Case report and literature review. *Arch Otolaryngol Head Neck Surg* 1981;107:573–575.
25. Hollingshead WH. *Textbook of anatomy*. 2nd ed. New York; Harper & Row, 1984.
26. Sanders I, WuB-L,Mu L, Li Y,Biller HF. The innervation of the human larynx. *Arch Otolaryngol Head Neck Surg* 1993;119:934–939.
27. Wu B-L, Sanders I, Mu L, Biller HF. The human communicating nerve. An extension of the external superior laryngeal nerve that innervates the vocal cord. *Arch Otolaryngol Head Neck Surg* 1994;120: 1321–1328.
28. del Regato JA, Spjut HJ, Cox JD. Ackerman and del Regato s cancer. *Diagnosis, treatment, and prognosis*. 6th ed. St. Louis: Mosby, 1985.
29. Sumida S, Masuda Y, Watanabe S, Nishizaki K, Slipka J. Development of the pharynx in normal and malformed fetuses. *Acta Otolaryngol (Stockh)* 1994;suppl 517:21–26.
30. Langman J. *Medical embryology*. 2nd ed. Baltimore: Williams & Wilkins, 1969.
31. Ali MY. Histology of the human nasopharyngeal mucosa. *J Anat* 1965; 99:657–672.
32. Morin GV, Shank EC, Burgess LPA, Heffner DK. Oncocytic metaplasia of the pharynx. *Otolaryngol Head Neck Surg* 1991;105:86–91.
33. Benke TT, Zitsch RP, Nashelsky MB. Bilateral oncocytic cysts of the nasopharynx. *Otolaryngol Head Neck Surg* 1995;112:321–324.
34. Melchionna RH, Moore RA. The pharyngeal pituitary gland. *Am J Pathol* 1938;14:763–772.
35. Boyd JD. Observations on the human pharyngeal hypophysis. *J Endocrinol* 1956;14:66–77.
36. McGrath P. Extrasellar adenohypophyseal tissue in the female. *Australas Radiol* 1970;14:241–247.
37. Langford L. Batsakis JG. Pituitary gland involvement of the sinonasal tract. *Ann Otol Rhinol Laryngol* 1995;104:167–169.
38. Kikuchi K, Kowada M, Sasaki J, Sageshima M. Large pituitary adenoma of the sphenoid sinus and nasopharynx: report of a case with ultrastructural evaluations. *Surg Neurol* 1994;42:330–334.
39. Hollender AR. The nasopharynx. A study of 140 autopsy specimens. *Laryngoscope* 1946;56:282–304.
40. Toomey JM. Cysts and tumors of the pharynx. In: Paparella MM, Shumrick DA, eds. *Otolaryngology*. Philadelphia; WB Saunders, 1980.
41. Nicolai P, Luzzago F, Maroldi R, Falchetti M, Antonelli AR. Nasopharygenal cysts. Report of seven cases with review of the literature. *Arch Otolaryngol Head Neck Surg* 1989;115:860–864.
42. Binkhorst CD, Schierbeek P, Petten GJW. Neoplasms of the notochord. Report of a case of basilar chordoma with nasal and bilateral orbital involvement. *Acta Otolaryngol (Stockh)* 1957;47:10–20.
43. Batsakis JG. *Tumors of the head and neck: clinical and pathological considerations*. 2nd ed. Baltimore; Williams & Wilkins, 1979.
44. Eggston AE, Wolff D. *Histopathology of the ear, nose and throat*. Baltimore; Williams & Wilkins, 1947.
45. Mills SE, Fechner RE. Pathology of the larynx. *Atlas of head and neck pathology series*. Chicago; American Society of Clinical Pathologists Press, 1985.

*Histology for Pathologists, second edition,*
Edited by Stephen S. Sternberg.
Lippincott-Raven Publishers, Philadelphia


# CHAPTER 17

# Major Salivary Glands

Fernando Martínez-Madrigal, Jacques Bosq, and Odile Casiraghi



The primary function of the salivary glands is to moisten the mucous membranes of the upper aerodigestive tract. In humans this function is fulfilled by the continuous exocrine secretion of numerous minor salivary glands. These glands are located in the submucosa throughout the oral cavity, pharynx, and upper airways. In developed species, most of the saliva is elaborated by three pairs of major glands or salivary glands named by their location: the parotid, the submaxillary or submandibular, and the sublingual glands. They are connected symmetrically to the oral cavity, where they empty their secretion only under specific stimuli. The saliva produced by these glands (750 to 1,000 ml per 24 hours) plays an important role in preparing food for digestion, as well as in controlling the bacterial flora of the mouth. The quality of the saliva produced by the major glands is variable and depends on both the stimuli and the predominant participating gland.

## EMBRYOLOGICAL AND POSTNATAL DEVELOPMENTAL CHANGES

### Parotid Gland

During embryologic life, the parotid is the first of the three major glands to appear and is seen by the 6th week. It derives from the ectoderm as an epithelial bud from the primitive oral epithelium, at the angle between the maxillary process and the mandibular arch (1). As the primordia grow, they ramify into a bush like system surrounded by mesenchymal tissue. This mesenchyma and, particularly, the basal lamina play an important role in the lobular organization of the gland (2–5), and in vascular and neural development. By the 7th week, the primitive gland moves in a dorsal and lateral direction and reaches the preauricular region. Development of the facial nerve divides the gland by approximately the 10th week into superficial and deep portions (6).

By the 3rd month, the gland has attained its general pat-

F. Martínez-Madrigal: Department of Pathology of the Hospital General "Dr. Miguel Silva," Hospital General de Zona N° 1, IMSS and the Medical Faculty of the Universidad Michoacana de San Nicolas de Hidalgo, Morelia, Michoacán, Mexico.

J. Bosq and O. Casiraghi: Department of Histopathology "A", Institut Gustave Roussy, 39 Rue Camille Desmoulins, 94805 Villejuif, Cedex, France.

tern of organization. The epithelial structures are arranged in lobules, limited by a capsule of loose connective tissue (Fig. 1A). The mesenchyma is then colonized by numerous lymphocytes that are later disposed in intraglandular and extraglandular lymph nodes. By the 6th month, the epithelial cordons are canalized and exhibit a double-cell ciliated cover. Cell differentiation begins in the excretory ducts with the progressive transformation of ciliated cells by columnar, squamous, and goblet cells (Fig. 1B) (7). Intralobular duct and acinar differentiation, including myoepithelial cell formation, begins about the 8th month (8). Recent studies have demonstrated myoepithelial cell differentation by the 19th- to 24th-week period. These cells, arranged in the basal portions of the acini and intercalated ducts, appear as clear cells with electron microscopy. Between 25 and 32 weeks the myoepithelial cells become flattened and show cytoplasma prolongations (9–11). Saliva production starts, at this time, as a mucinous liquid; but several studies in rodents suggest that full maturation is completed only after birth (12–15).

The definitive location of the parotid is behind the inferior maxillary branch, below and in front of the external ear. It is enclosed within a fibroadipose capsule in a depression whose anterior limit is the masseter muscle. Its superior limit is the zygomatic arch; the posterior limit is the tragus, and the inferior limit is the anterior border of the sternocleidomastoid muscle (16). The adult parotid is the largest of the three major salivary glands and weighs between 14 and 28 g. The gland is surrounded by a fine capsule and is divided into two portions by the facial nerve. The main portion, or superficial lobe, is flattened and quadrilateral; it is here that the majority of salivary tumors develop. This observation has permitted the development of conservative surgical treatment of many parotid tumors. The rest of the gland, called the deep lobe, is irregularly wedge-shaped in anatomical relationship with the parapharyngeal space (17). The surgical anatomic area where the parotid gland is located, is called the parotid region. In this region it is important to keep in mind the anatomical relations between the facial nerve, the gland and the subcutaneous planes. The facial nerve has four parts designated as retro-, inter-, intra-, and preglandular. The parotid gland is covered by a superficial musculoaponeurosis and the skin (18). Accessory parotid tissue is found in approximately 20% of cases. Nevertheless, in a recent study, the incidence was found to be 56% with no differences between right and left sides or between sexes (19). This accessory tissue may be found on the anterior surface of the gland, as well as along the parotid duct (20).

Like all the exocrine glands, the parotid is composed of numerous tubuloacinar units connected through the excretory ducts to a main duct (Stensens's duct) located in the an-

A

B

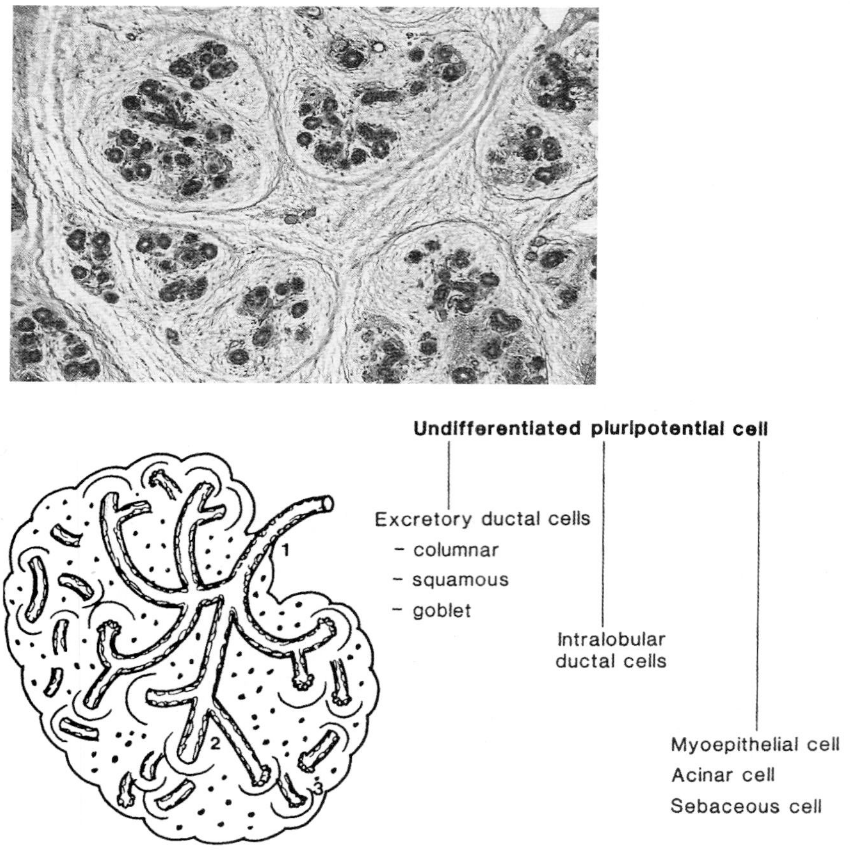


**FIG. 1.** Development and histogenesis of the epithelial constituents of the salivary gland. **A**, Fetal parotid gland at 4 months; a lobular architecture is present. **B**, Drawing of (A) showing excretory ducts, (1); interlobular ducts, (2); developing acini, (3); and the cellular lines of differentiation.

terior portion of the gland. The parotid duct follows a twisted course of 7 cm crossing the masseter muscle, the corpus adiposum of the cheek, and the buccinator muscle before opening into the oral vestibule. The secretion of the accessory parotid is emptied by an independent duct reaching the parotid duct in the masseter portion.

Blood supply is by arterial branches from the external carotid. The veins are tributaries of the external jugular, and the lymphatics join the superficial and deep cervical lymph nodes. Innervation is derived from the sympathetic and auriculotemporal nerves.

### Submaxillary Gland

In the submaxillary gland, the primordia appear at the end of the 6th week and, unlike the parotid, are probably of endodermal derivation (21,22). However, a recent study suggests that the sublingual process of the submandibular gland originates from a lateral ectodermal bud of the anlage of the submandibular gland (23). The epithelial bud appears in the groove between the lower jaw and tongue, at one side of the midplane. Extension of the glandular tissue in the mesenchyma goes backward beneath the lower jaw. Subsequent maturation and cell differentiation are similar to those of the parotid gland except for the lymphoid tissue, which is less obvious than in the parotid. In addition, there is no lymph node formation inside the gland.

The submaxillary gland is finely encapsulated; it lies inside the submandibular triangle, an osteofibrous cavity, from which it takes the form of a triangular prism. This gland weighs approximately 7 to 8 g and, like the other major salivary glands, is organized in lobules connected to a main excretory duct – the submaxillary duct (Wharton's duct) – which measures 5 cm in length and 2 to 3 mm in diameter. The duct originates near the surface; runs between the mylohyoideus, the hyoglossus, and genioglossus muscles; and finally opens through a narrow orifice in a small papilla called "caruncula sublingualis" on each side of the frenulum linguae. A submandibular gland having three ducts which opens separately into the oral cavity has also been reported (24). The blood supply is from branches of the facial and sublingual arteries. The secretomotor nerves are fibers from the cranial parasympathetic of the facial nerve; the vasomotor nerves are derived from the superior cervical ganglion. The lymph nodes are arranged in a row in the spaces between the mandible and the gland, and are disposed in anterior, medial, and posterior groups (16,17).

### Sublingual Gland

The sublingual glands are the last of the three major salivary glands to appear. Their primordia are located immediately lateral to the submaxillary glands for the greater sublingual glands, and in the linguogingival sulcus for the lesser sublingual glands. The epithelial buds grow downward from the groove between the lower jaw and the tongue. Parenchymal organization and differentiation are similar to those of the submaxillary gland and are also probably of endodermal derivation.

The principal sublingual gland weighs 3 g. It lies in the sublingual fossa of the mandible and is surrounded by loose connective tissue. Its secretion is drained through a main duct called "Bartholin's duct," which opens into the submandibular duct and various small ducts (Rivinus' ducts) opening separately into the mouth in the plica sublingualis or joining the submandibular duct (16,17).

Vascular supplies come from the sublingual and submental arteries; the veins are tributaries of the external jugular. Innervation is similar to that of the submaxillary gland.

## APOPTOSIS

In literature, the studies concerning apoptosis in salivary glands are not very frequent. Contrary to other glandular tissue, programmed cell death in the salivary glands has been sporadically studied in inferior species and developed species with experimental animals such as rats or monkeys, but less frequently in humans (25–29).

In normal salivary glands, apoptosis was uncommon when observed in acinar cells and epithelial duct cells and never observed in myoepithelial cells. In specific pathologic contexts, such as duct obstruction or irradiation of the salivary glands, programmed cell death was observed with many significant changes in the structure of the glands. Bcl-2 oncoprotein expression could also play a major role in the control of apoptosis in the salivary glands.

### Apoptosis and Salivary Gland Atrophy by Duct Obstruction

Duct obstruction due to calculi or strictures induces salivary gland atrophy. Histologically, the disappearance of acinar cells within the presence of groups of ductlike structures in a fibrous and inflammatory stroma was observed (28). The acinar cells had disappeared by apoptosis; this acinar cell death was observed a few hours after duct obstruction. In the first cell death, a few days after duct obstruction, the number of intraepithelial macrophages located in the acinar and duct epithelium of a normal salivary gland multiplied. These macrophages removed the dying cells and apoptosic cellular fragments by phagocytosis. Then they migrated to the interstitium. Simultaneous proliferation of duct epithelial cells by an increase in mitosis contributed to the groups of ductlike structures with some features of squamous metaplasia. Myoepithelial cells became more prominent at the periphery of residual ducts.

Similar morphologic modifications of salivary glands have also been observed in other pathologic conditions (e.g., ischiemia, Michulicz's disease, auto-immune sialadenitis) (30–32).

### Apoptosis and Radiation

Irradiation of the major salivary glands is unavoidable during radiotherapy for many head and neck cancers. In fact, radiotherapy induced dryness of the oral cavity, contributing to deterioration of oral mucosa and loss of teeth.

The death of salivary gland acinar cells by apoptosis was observed within 24 hours after irradiation. This mode of cell death occurs with relatively low doses of radiation. An acute inflammatory response located among the destroyed acini was observed.

In normal adult salivary glands, cell division is infrequent in the acini. Development and replenishment of acini destroyed by low doses of radiation comes from stem cells which are located in the terminal intralobular ducts. It is possible that radiation apoptosis of acinar cells could be a stimulus for replication of duct stem cells. However, the death of the ductal stem cells by high-dose radiation did not induce complete regeneration of the destroyed acini: the result being atrophy of salivary glands (29).

### Apoptosis and Bcl-2 Expression

The bcl-2 oncoprotein product is located in the inner mitochondrial, endoplasmic reticular, and nuclear membrane. Its main function is the inhibition of apoptosis blocking programmed cell death, producing extension of cell survival when it is overexpressed. This protein can also play a role in protecting some cells from c-myc-induced apoptosis (33). The inhibition of apoptosis by bcl-2 oncoprotein can be modulated by the interactions of TNF a and ionizing radiations (34).

Bcl-2 oncoprotein is expressed in several exocrine epithelial tissues such as salivary glands (27). In normal salivary gland, bcl-2 is detectable as fine, cytoplasmic granularity in some cells of ductal epithelium. Basal cells and a few luminal cells of the striated and excretory ducts expressed bcl-2. Very rarely, bcl-2-positive cells were detected in the intercalated ducts. Acinar cells and myoepithelial cells of both acini and ducts were negative (35).

This pattern of bcl-2 expression could confer the survival of stem cells (36). Bcl-2 function conferred longevity to progenitor cells in these tissues, but the role of bcl-2-positive luminal cells is unknown.

It was supposed that normal epithelial tissue would be renewed from stem cells (37). In the salivary glands, two reserve cell theories were proposed concerning the role and the meaning of the bcl-2 expression in the basal cells of ducts. The bcl-2 basal cells could be pluri or semipotential stem cells that generated a part or all cell types and could be responsible for differentiation of the functional units (37–39). Conversely, Dardick et al. have shown that all differentiated cells were capable of cell division, and that the mitotic rate of differentiated cells may even be higher than that of basal cells. All cells could have a reserve cell capacity, but the existence of stem cells is not necessarily excluded by this theory (40). At present, no direct evidence to support one of these two theories has been demonstrated.

## LIGHT MICROSCOPY

The salivary glands are compound exocrine tubuloacinar glands characterized by the aggregation of numerous secretory units. These units consist of acini where secretion is produced and a duct system that carries the secretion to the oral cavity and regulates the concentration of water and electrolytes. There are three types of salivary secretory units: the serous ones that contain amylase; the mucous ones where sialomucins are secreted; and mixed units made up of mucous and serous cells. According to the predominance of these types of secretory units, the salivary glands may be classified into three categories–serous, mucous, and mixed glands.

With the exception of some mucous units, the parotid gland is of the serous type (Fig. 2). The submaxillary and the sublingual glands are mixed with a predominance of serous units in the first category (Fig. 3) and a mucous predominance in the second (Fig. 4). In accessory parotid gland, mixed secretory units can be found (19).

The lobular architecture of the glands is well defined by the anastomosed connective tissue trabeculae carrying the vascular and neural branches, as well as the excretory ducts (41).

## SECRETORY UNITS

### Acini

Serous acini consist of pear-shaped groups of epithelial cells surrounded by a distinct basement membrane. The epithelial cells have a basal nucleus and dense cytoplasm packed with basophilic [periodic acid-Schiff (PAS-positive)] zymogen granules. They vary in number depending on the different phases of the secretory cycle (Fig. 2) (42). The primary enzyme present in the zymogen granules is amylase or ptyalin, which splits starch into smaller water-soluble carbohydrates. However, there are other proteins in these granules including agglutinin, proline-rich proteins, and histatins (43). Other enzymes such as nonspecific antibacterial lysozyme, lactoferrin, trypsin and chymotrypsin-like proteases, lisine endopeptidase, and histidine peptidase, also have been shown in the cytoplasm of acinar cells (44–46). The acini have a central lumen, rarely visible by light microscopy, through which the secretion drains into the intercalated ducts. The excretion seems to be promoted by the contraction of myoepithelial cells that lie between the outer surface of the acinus and the

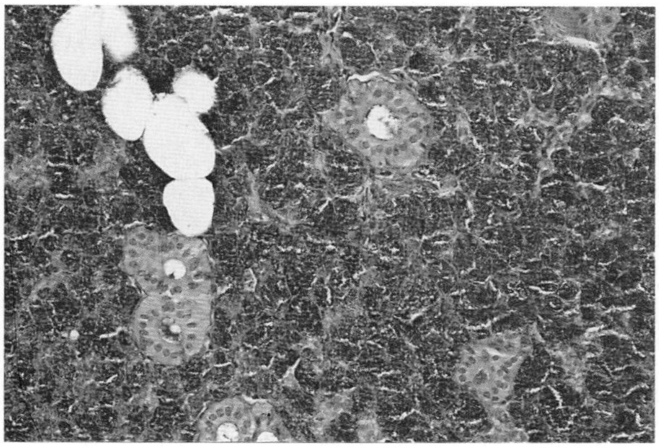

**FIG. 2.** Serous-type acini of a parotid gland, with dense secretory granules.

basement membrane (given the importance of myoepithelial cells in the pathology of salivary glands, a separate paragraph is devoted to their description).

Mucous acini are larger than the serous type and have an irregular pattern (Fig. 4). The secretory cells have abundant cytoplasm filled with clear mucous substance. They contain acid sialomucins (alcian blue and mucicarmine-positive) and neutral sialmucins (PAS-positive) in different concentrations (47). The characteristics of these sialmucins also differ between submandibular and sublingual glands (48).

Mixed acini (Fig. 3) are typically found in the submaxillary gland. These structures are characterized by the concentration of mucous cells near the intercalated duct and bordered by a crescent-shaped formation of serous cells. In mixed acini, the serous cells are more or less conspicuous, according to the amount of secretion accumulated in the mucous cells.

### Ducts

A peculiar duct system transports the saliva from the gland to the oral cavity, and modifies its water and electrolyte concentration. The first two segments, the intercalated and the striated ducts, are intralobular (Fig. 5). They are also known as secretory ducts because of their metabolic activity (49). The other segments are interlobular and are called excretory ducts (49).

The intercalated duct lies directly in contact with the acinus. It is lined with a single layer of cuboidal epithelium and an irregular layer of myoepithelial cells. The epithelial cells show a progressive transformation between the secretory and ductal cells and a strong cytoplasmic activity of lactoferrin and lysozyme (50). The lengths of the intercalated ducts are variable in the three major glands (Fig. 6). In the parotid gland, because they are relatively long, they are easy to recognize in the histologic sections (Fig. 5A). In contrast, they are short in the submaxillary gland and hardly visible in the sublingual gland (Fig. 4). Some authors have found undifferentiated cells on the basal side of the intercalated and striated ducts (51). These cells are positive for cytokeratins 13 and 16 on immunohistochemical staining (52,53). They are thought to be progenitor cells, but this remains a subject of controversy (38).

The striated ducts are obvious in routine sections, particularly in the submaxillary gland, where they are relatively longer (Figs. 3 and 6). The epithelial lining is simple columnar. On the basal side, it has characteristic parallel striations caused by the deep cell membrane invaginations and mitochondria (Fig. 5B). This structure represents a specialized surface on the epithelia involved in the transport of water and electrolytes. The numerous mitochondria are correlated with the strong eosinophilia of the duct. Various enzymes such as adenosinetriphosphatase (ATPase), succinyldehydrogenase, and carbonic anhydrase (54) are present in the cytoplasm of the striated ducts and provide them with a metabolic and energy system capable of concentrating some of the elements present in the saliva.

The striated ducts are connected with the interlobular ducts located in the septal connective tissue. These ducts are lined with a columnar pseudostratified epithelium with sparse goblet cells (Fig. 7). They become progressively

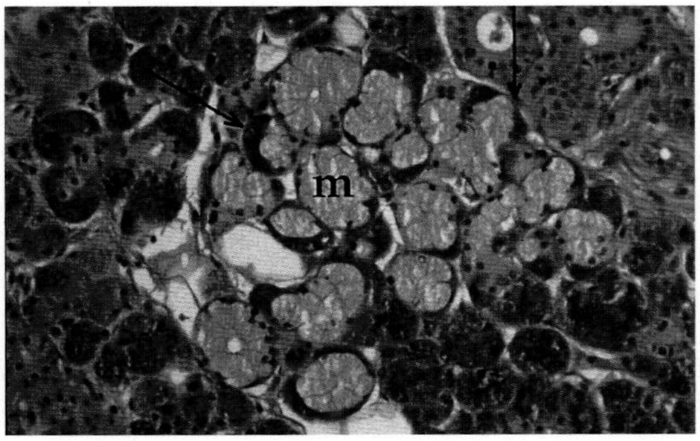


**FIG. 3.** Histologic section of a submaxillary gland. In mixed units (*arrows*) serous cells are grouped in a crescent-shaped formation on the periphery of the acini, whereas the mucous cells (m) are in direct contact with the duct system.

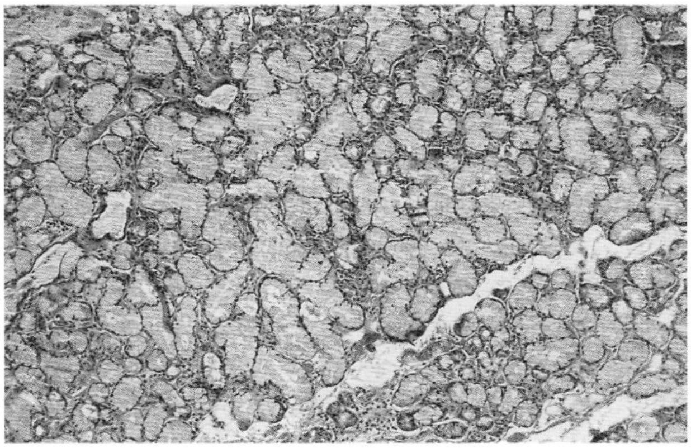

**FIG. 4.** Mucous-type acini of the sublingual gland, larger and more irregular than the serous and mixed types. Note an inconspicuous duct system.

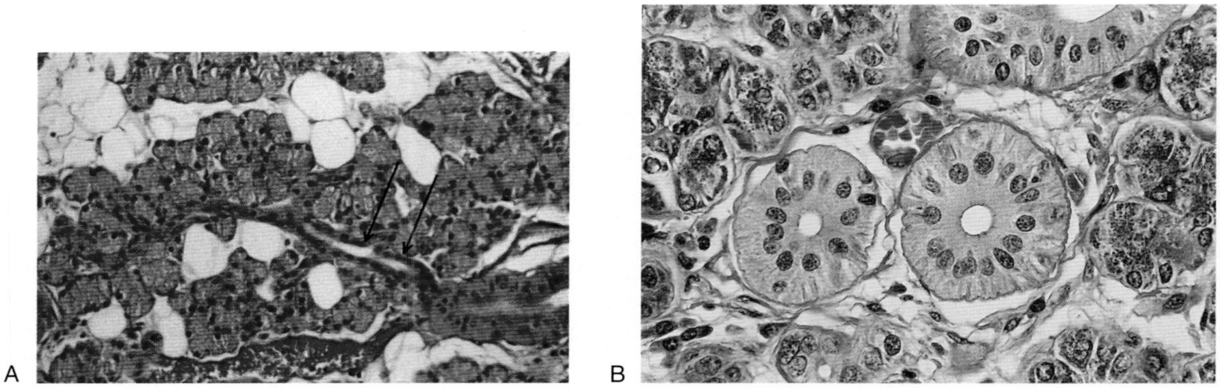


**FIG. 5.** Parotid intralobular ducts. The intercalated ducts (*arrows*)(sectioned longitudinally) lie in contact with the acinus (**A**). The striated ducts (**B**) (sectioned transversely) are lined with a columnar epithelium of basal-striated appearance.

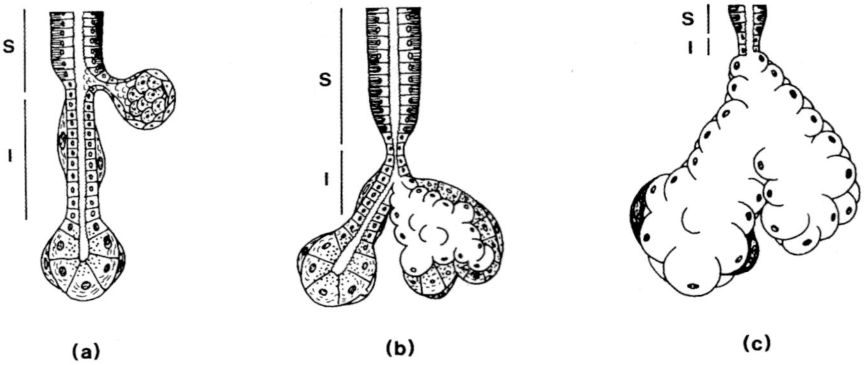


**FIG. 6.** The morphology of the major salivary glands is characterized by three types of secretory unit. In the parotid (**a**) the intercalated duct (I) is longer than in the submaxillary (**b**) and sublingual glands (**c**). In contrast, the striated duct (S) is longer in the submaxillary gland. Sebaceous glands are more frequent in the parotid gland; in the sublingual gland the intralobular ducts are inconspicuous.

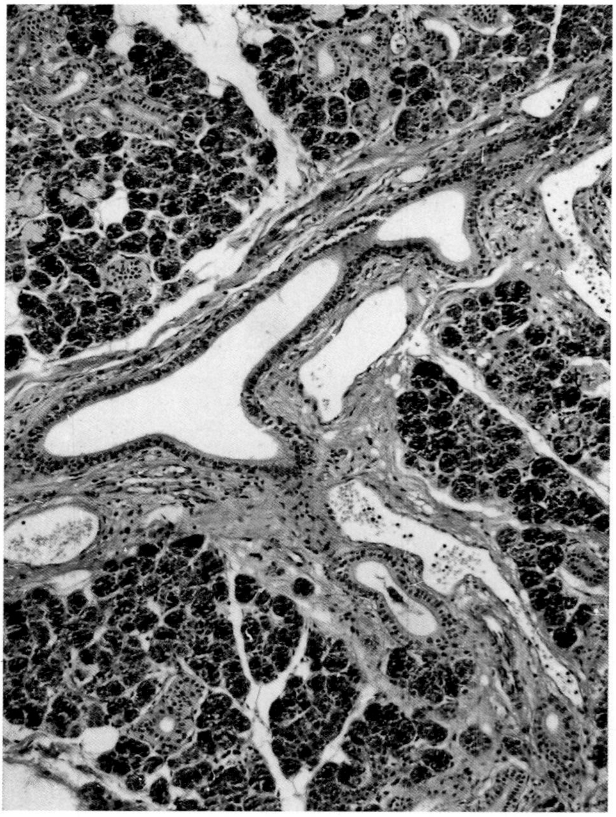

**FIG. 7.** Interlobular duct adjacent to vessels in the septal connective tissue.

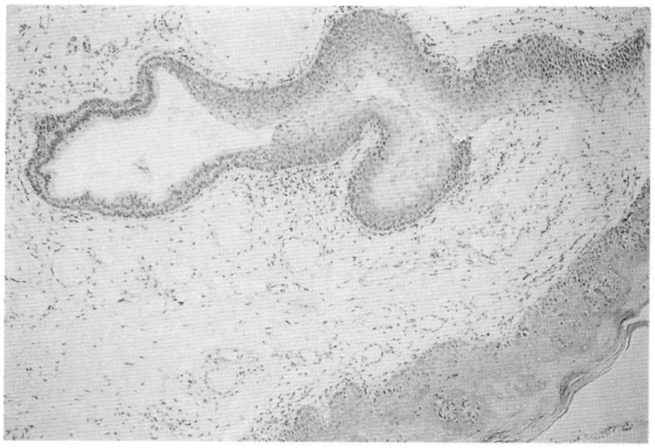

**FIG. 8.** Main excretory duct in the caruncula sublingualis. Near the oral surface, the duct is lined with a squamous stratified epithelium.

larger before joining the principal duct. The principal function of interlobular ducts is to transport saliva, but their role in regeneration is proposed by means of the hypothetical undifferentiated pluripotential cells. In theory, these cells may follow the same cellular lines as in embryonic development, (Fig. 1B), and are perhaps implicated in the metaplastic and neoplastic alterations of salivary glands (38,55) which are more frequent in these ducts.

The principal duct consists of a thick external fibrous coat of collagen, (similar to dermal collagen), and elastic fiber bundles. The epithelium is pseudostratified columnar and becomes squamous and stratified near the opening in the mucous membrane (Fig. 8).

## ULTRASTRUCTURE

At the electron microscopy level, the serous cells show all the characteristics of a specialized cell for secretion and export of proteins. The cytoplasm possesses abundant endoplasmic reticulum, Golgi vesicles, mitochondria, lipid droplets, and secretory granules (Fig. 9). The last are more common on the apical side of the cell. They consist of a membrane, which encloses the secretion, and a matrix of low-electron density and homogeneous aspect in immature granules and high-electron density in mature granules (56,57). The electron density of the granules differs according to the package of the different proteins within the same granule (43). All the cytoplasmic organelles increase during protein synthesis and decrease during discharge (54). The basal surface of the cell shows numerous folds of plasma and basal membranes. They cover the entire cell base and extend beyond the lateral margins in the manner of foot processes. Therefore, the basal surface of the cell is greatly expanded, facilitating diffusion of materials into the cell (57). Most of the cytoplasm in mucous cells is occupied by mucous vacuoles and Golgi apparatus. Only a small basal and lateral portion of the cytoplasm contains endoplasmic reticulum and mitochondria (56).

At the apical pole, the secretory cells are joined by an adhesive zone, whereas the basal side is adhered by desmosomes (54). Between the junctions, virtual spaces form the secretory capillaries, which are in continuation with the acinar lumen. Numerous microvilli protrude into the capillary lumen (Fig. 9).

The cytoplasm of myoepithelial cells may be separated into two portions (58): one, in contact with the basal lamina, is occupied by myofilaments and pinocytotic vesicles; the other portion is in contact with the secretory cell and contains mitochondria, endoplasmic reticulum, lysosome-like complexes, and Golgi vesicles. The visualization of myofilaments may vary in different myoepithelial cells; some of

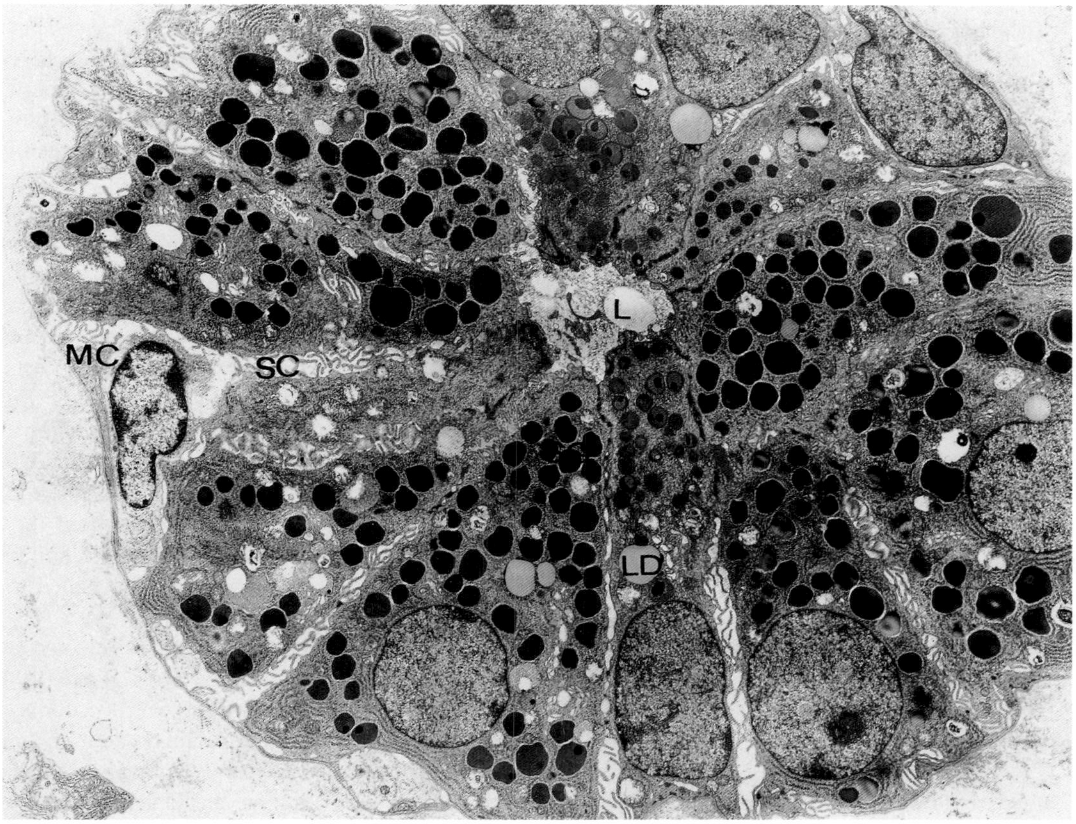


**FIG. 9.** Ultrastructure of a parotid acinus: lumen (L), secretory granules (SG), lipid droplets (LD), secretory capillaries (SC), and myoepithelial cell (MC) (×**6000**).

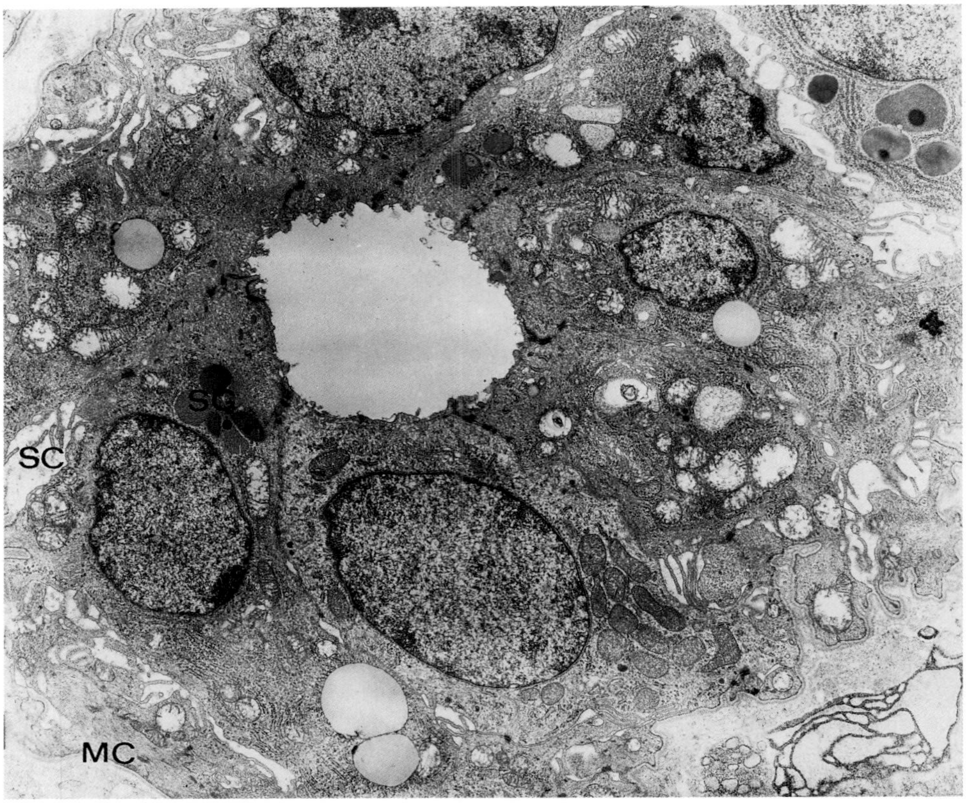


**FIG. 10.** Intercalated duct of parotid gland. Some secretory granules (SG) are present on the apical side as well as some secretory capillaries (SC). On the external surface myoepithelial cell prolongations are found (MC) (×**10,300**).

them have only focal aggregates of myofilaments, while others show a typical basal distribution resembling smooth muscle cells (59). The junction between myoepithelial and secretory cells is ensured by desmosomes.

Transition from acinus to intercalated duct is gradual. In the latter, epithelial cells have relatively large nuclei and few cytoplasmic organelles, consisting principally of mitochondria, some cisternae of endoplasmic reticulum, lipid droplets, and a few apical secretory granules (54,58) (Fig. 10). Scattered secretory capillaries may be found, as well. On the external surface, myoepithelial cell prolongations are usually present.

The striated ducts (Fig. 11) are composed of tall cylindrical cells with central nuclei. On the basal side, the cell membrane is extensively folded into fingerlike structures. The space between these folds is occupied by vertically oriented mitochondria. This cytoplasmic organization is specialized in the active transport of water and electrolytes from the vascular system to the lumen of the duct (60); the rest of the cytoplasm contains mitochondria and scattered endoplasmic reticulum.

## SEBACEOUS GLANDS

In 1931, Hamperl (61) described the presence of sebaceous glands histologically similar to those of the cutaneous adnexa. Other authors have indeed recognized such structures (62–65), which appear as isolated cells in the wall of either an intercalated or a striated duct (Fig. 12A) (70)). Larger cell accumulations form a sebaceous gland limited by a well-defined basal membrane (Fig. 12B,C). They vary in size, have a diverticular aspect, and are permanently linked to an interlobular duct. At the periphery of the gland, the cells are flattened with round or oval nuclei. The central cells have an abundant vacuolated cytoplasm rich in lipids, which may be stained, in frozen sections, with fat colorations (Sudan III and IV, oil red, osmic acid). The nuclei become irregular or pyknotic and finally disappear. When the gland reaches a certain size, the holocrine-type secretion is emptied into the ductal system and is mixed with the saliva (Fig. 12D).

The number of sebaceous glands in major salivary glands varies; they are common in the parotid gland, rare in the submaxillary gland, and probably absent in the sublingual gland. They are diffusely scattered throughout the parenchyma, where their numbers also vary greatly. Their presence or absence in the different lobules is not related to either age or sex (64).

In a review of 100 parotid glands selected at random from our material, we found sebaceous glands in 42% of cases. They were also found in 5% of 100 submaxillary glands. These findings are in agreement with other authors (64). Thus, we conclude that their incidence in the parotid gland is more frequent than imagined. The more sections that are examined, the more sebaceous glands are found; it is, therefore, merely a question of looking for them. If the entire parotid

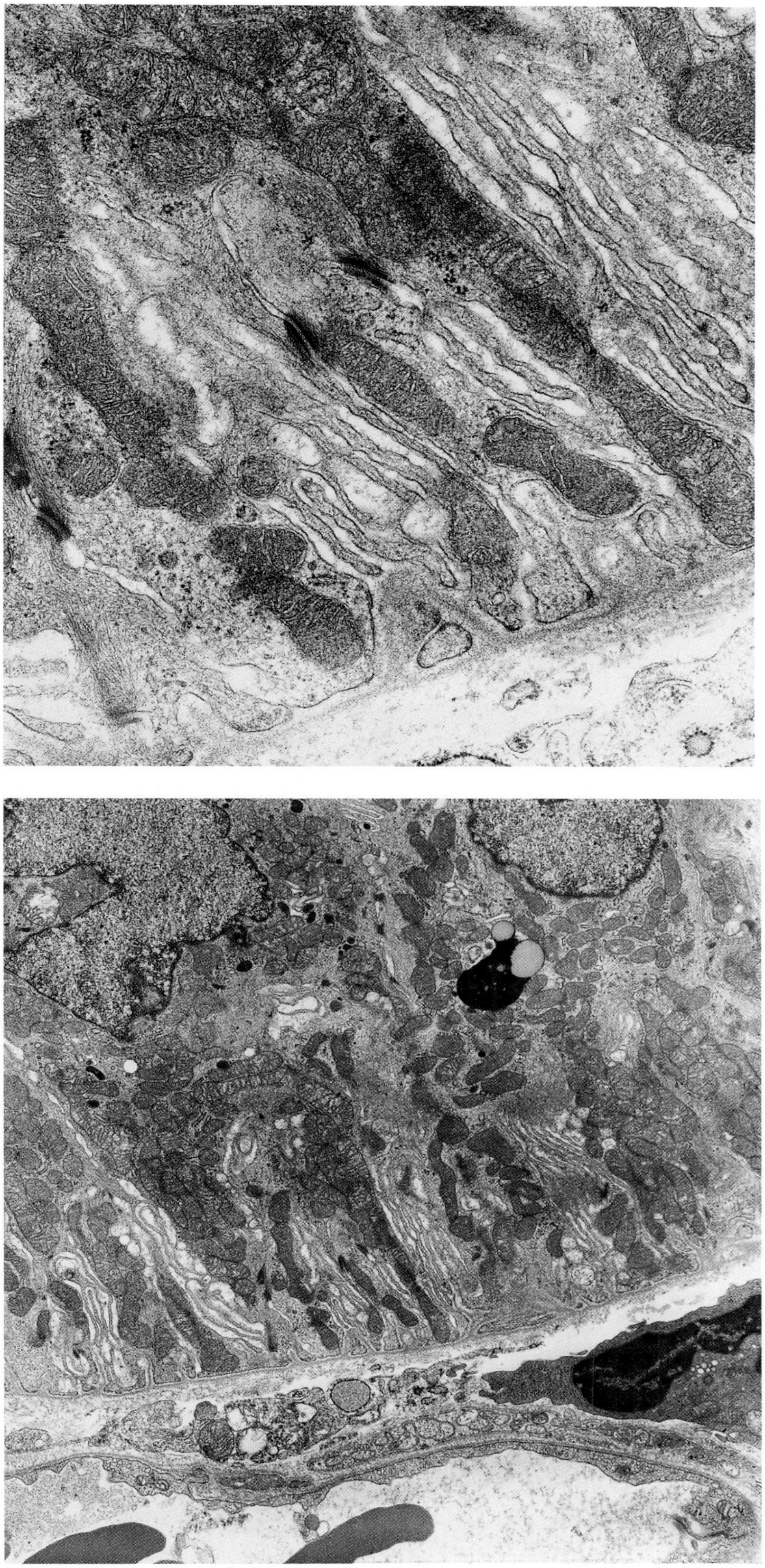

A

B

**FIG. 11.** **A**, Striated duct cells possess vertically oriented mitochondria and extensively folded plasma membrane. **B**, The basal side is in close relationship to the blood capillary (×**7920**).

gland were examined meticulously, it would be difficult not to find a sebaceous gland (66).

The presence of sebaceous glands in the salivary tissue has not been satisfactorily explained. A heterotopic phenomenon (62,63) similar to the occurrence of sebaceous glands in the oral mucosa (Fordyce's disease) seems unlikely. In the mouth, this condition may result from aberrant buds along the fetal line of closure (67); but in the parotid and submaxillary glands, there are no lines of closure. Metaplasia (61,68) beginning in the ducts does not explain the high frequency of sebaceous glands in parotid parenchyma. Therefore, it seems reasonable to consider the sebaceous glands as a normal holocrine differentiation. Their occurrence in the parotid gland appears to be related to a specific function that is not yet understood.

The belief that a potential for sebaceous differentiation exists in the salivary parenchyma is further supported by the fact that salivary tumors or tumorlike conditions with a sebaceous character or sebaceous gland participation, have been described. These rare lesions include sebaceous adenoma (69), sebaceous lymphadenoma (70–73), sebaceous carcinoma (74–76), and parotid cyst (77). They have also been noted in pleomorphic adenoma (66,78) and mucoepidermoid carcinoma (79).

## MYOEPITHELIAL CELLS

Myoepithelial cells, (basket cells), are derived from early modification and differentiation of primitive pluripotential salivary duct cells by the 10th week of gestation. It has also been suggested that the precursor of myoepithelial cells are the clear cells located in the terminal and striated ducts (58).

These cells lie between the epithelial cells and the basal lamina of acini, intercalated ducts, and probably also exist in the union of the striated and intercalated ducts (51,80). The cells are flat and have long cytoplasmic processes extending over the epithelial surface (Fig. 13) in a network that makes it difficult to discern them in routine histologic sections. Myoepithelial cells may assume, however, morphologic modification at different anatomic locations within the ductal acinar structure (51,59). These cells are best studied by electron microscopy.

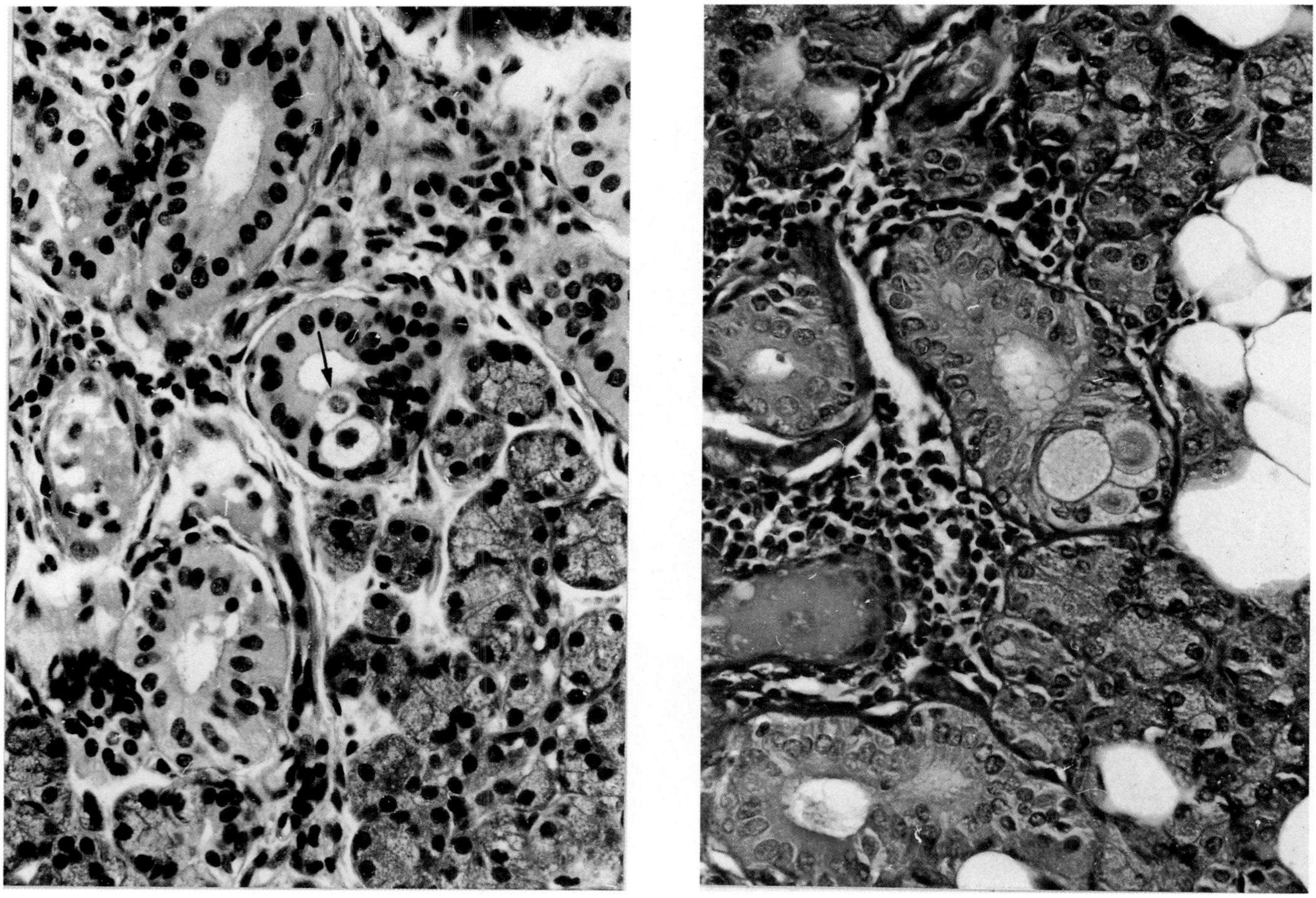

A B

**FIG. 12.** Sebaceous elements in a parotid gland. Isolated sebaceous cells can be seen in the duct wall (*arrows*). **A**, They proliferate to form a well-defined gland (**B, C**); secretion is present in the lumen of the duct (**D**) (*arrows*). Drawing (**E**) illustrates the above features.

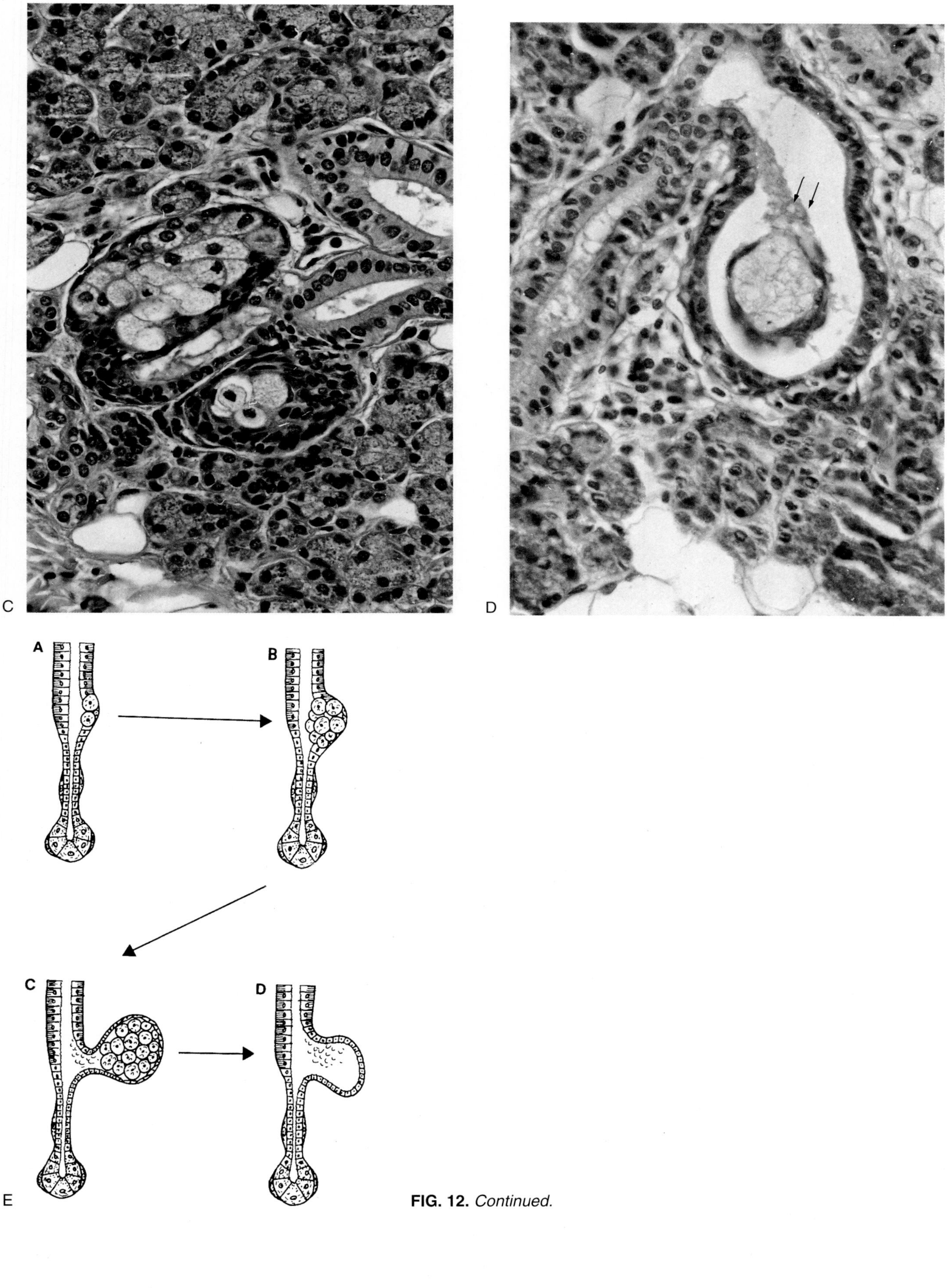


**FIG. 12.** *Continued.*

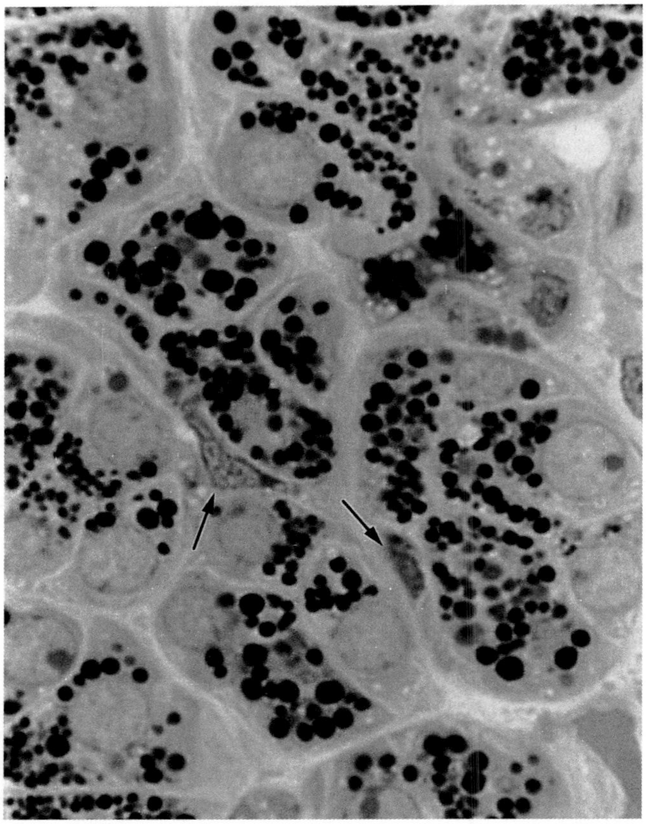

**FIG. 13.** Myoepithelial cells (*arrows*) on the acinic surface (semithin section, toluidine blue).

The most outstanding characteristic is the presence of cytoplasmic filaments on the basal side. Most of these consist of the myofilaments actin, tropomyosin, and myosin (58,81–83) which are arranged in a pattern similar to that of the smooth muscle. Tonofibril-like bundles of intermediate filaments are attached to the cellular junctions, particularly in desmosomes where the filaments are cytokeratin. Some forms of myoepithelial cells may also show scattered, rather than basal, cytoplasmic distribution of these filaments, which may reflect structural and functional differences (59). The presence of vimentin is not constant and the filament desmin is absent in normal myoepithelium (84). The cytoplasm shows a strong activity of ATPase and alkaline phosphatase (85,86).

It is generally accepted that myoepithelial cells are contractile. This function speeds up the outflow of the saliva by increasing the pressure on the excretory unit (87). It has been extensively studied in the mammary gland of the rat, where these cells are more frequently found. Oxytocin-induced contraction in the myoepithelial cells is similar to that of true muscle cells (88). The presence of myofilaments in the cytoplasm of these cells correlates strongly with this function. In addition, myoepithelial cells support the underlying parenchyma and participate in the elaboration of the basal lamina. This last function is important in some hyperplastic and neoplastic alterations, where the myoepithelial cells produce fibronectin laminin, and type III collagen (89–96). All these proteins are constituents of the basal lamina (97). In addition, myoepithelial cells are also involved in the production of tenascin, an extracellular matrix glycoprotein (98).

In spite of the endodermal or ectodermal origin, the myoepithelial cells share an epithelial and mesenchymal structure and function. Altered myoepithelial cells may manifest (in neoplastic proliferation) one or both characteristics. These cells are now considered the key factor in the morphology of many salivary neoplasms and in the morphologic variability of some tumors (Table 1).

The role of myoepithelial cells in the histogenesis of the pleomorphic adenoma has been extensively studied. This tumor, sometimes called "mixed tumor" on account of the epithelial and mesenchymal mixture of tissues, is the most frequent neoplasm of the major salivary glands (99,100). It is now accepted that myoepithelial cells play a crucial role in the neoplastic process, by expressing both epithelial and mesenchymal structures in the majority of pleomorphic adenomas (101–109). The participation of the contractile elements is also accepted in epithelial-myoepithelial carcinoma (clear cell carcinoma)–a malignant tumor that mimics the normal structure of the intercalated duct (110–115) and myoepithelioma, in which the myoepithelial cells are the only tumoral element showing different cellular forms (116–121). They also have been demonstrated in terminal duct adenocarcinoma (polymorphous low-grade adenocarcinoma) (122, 123), monomorphic adenoma which includes basaloid monomorphic adenoma (128), adenoid cystic carcinoma (89,93,105,129,130), and basaloid adenocarcinoma (131). Myoepithelial cell participation is also present in congenital tumors of salivary gland origin such as sialoblastoma (132) and the salivary gland anlage tumor (133). Although there are rare reports of myoepithelial cells in mucoepidermoid carcinoma (127,134), it is difficult to fully accept these statements because mucoepidermoid carcinoma arises from a ductal segment that lacks myoepithelial cells.

The principal morphologic types of altered myoepithelial cells are:

1. Stellate or myxoid cells, which are typically present in chondromyxoid areas of pleomorphic adenoma.
2. Spindle-shaped or myoid cells, which can be identified

**TABLE 1.** *Salivary gland tumors with myoepithelial cell participation*

| | |
|---|---|
| BENIGN TUMORS: | Myoepitheliomas |
| | Pleomorphic adenoma |
| | Basaloid adenomas |
| MALIGNANT TUMORS: | Epithelial-myoepithelial carcinoma |
| | Adenoid cystic carcinoma |
| | Teminal duct carcinoma |
| | Basaloid carcinoma |
| CONGENITAL TUMORS: | Sialoblastoma |
| | Salivary gland anlage tumor |

in pleomorphic adenoma and some types of myoepithelioma.

3. Hyalin or plasmocytoid cells (135), which can be seen in pleomorphic adenomas and can be present in myoepitheliomas. These cells show abundant cytoplasmic filaments that give a hyalin eosinophilic aspect.
4. Clear or epithelial cells, which are found in many salivary tumors on the external surface of ducts or ductlike structures. This is also characteristic in epithelial-myoepithelial carcinoma.

Bidirectional differentiation of the modified myoepithelium has been well documented. Myoepithelial cells with mesenchymal characteristics secrete mesenchymal mucins such as the acid glycosaminoglycans (hyaluronic acid, heparin sulfate, chondroitin-4-sulfate, and chondroitin-6-sulfate) (136,137), basement membrane constituents, elastin (103,104) and tenascin (98). In addition to contractile filaments (actin and myosin), vimentin becomes strongly positive, particularly in spindle-shaped form (138–140). S-100 protein, which is a common marker used for the myoepithelium, enhances its positivity in chondroid, myxoid, and stellate cells, particularly if they are associated with a myxoid stroma (104,141,142). Plasmocytoid myoepithelial cells are frequently negative for the muscular markers (143). However, these cells express several ultrastructural and immunomarkers characteristic of myoepithelial cells (121). On the other hand, epithelial differentiation may take the form of clear or squamous cells, which can contain both vimentin and keratin filaments in the same cell (104). Figure 14 illustrates the histologic and immunohistochemical patterns of modified myoepithelium. Myoepithelial cells are a central element in the histologic formation and organization of different salivary gland tumors. The cytomorphologic features and the variability of the extracellular products account for the morphologic heterogeneity of these lesions. The presence of these cells varies widely, from minimal as in monomorphic adenomas, to marked, as in myoepitheliomas (128). Malignant tumors containing myoepithelial cells usually tend to be less aggressive than tumors lacking these cells (144–149).

## LYMPHOID TISSUE

The immune system of salivary glands comprises two elements of the mucosa-associated immune system. One is the secretory component, a glycoprotein receptor for dimeric IgA and pentameric IgM that is produced by epithelial cells in the acini, intercalated ducts, and striated ducts (50,150,151). The other element is lymphoid tissue, which is either distributed diffusely, or organized in lymph nodes. Isolated lymphoid cells are present in the connective tissue near the acini and ducts. They are variable in number in the different glands (152) and yield principally IgA, (near 80% of the immunoglobulins in saliva), along with a lesser quantity of IgG and IgM (54). Small lymph nodes are usually present near the surface of the parotid gland, but not in the other salivary glands. Nevertheless, lymphoid cell aggregates are present in fetal submandibular and sublingual glands (153). These nodes usually contain salivary ducts and acini in the medullary region (Fig. 15A), a phenomenon probably due to the close relationship between developing gland and lymphoid tissue during embryonic life.

Lymph nodes are thought to participate in the histogenesis of Warthin's tumor. Although they have been pinpointed as the origin of the lymphoid tissue that characterizes this neoplasm, the theory is still under debate. Different mechanisms have been proposed, but the most widely accepted theory states that the lesion originates from the ducts inside

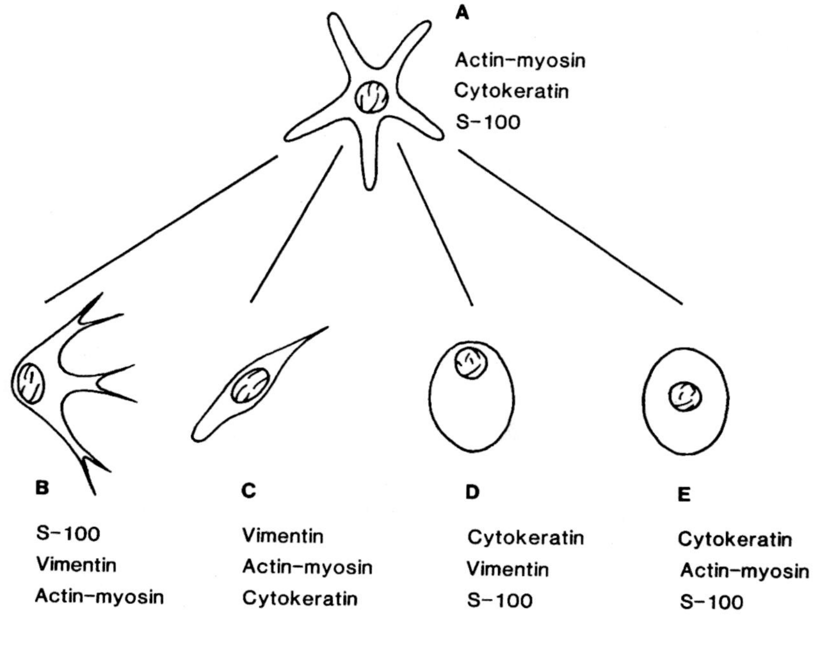


**FIG. 14.** Morphology and histologic markers of the normal (**A**) and modified myoepithelial cells (**B–E**). The most constant markers are present in order of frequency: chondromyxoid (B), spindle-shaped (C), hyalin or plasmocytoid (D), and epithelial (*clear*) (E).

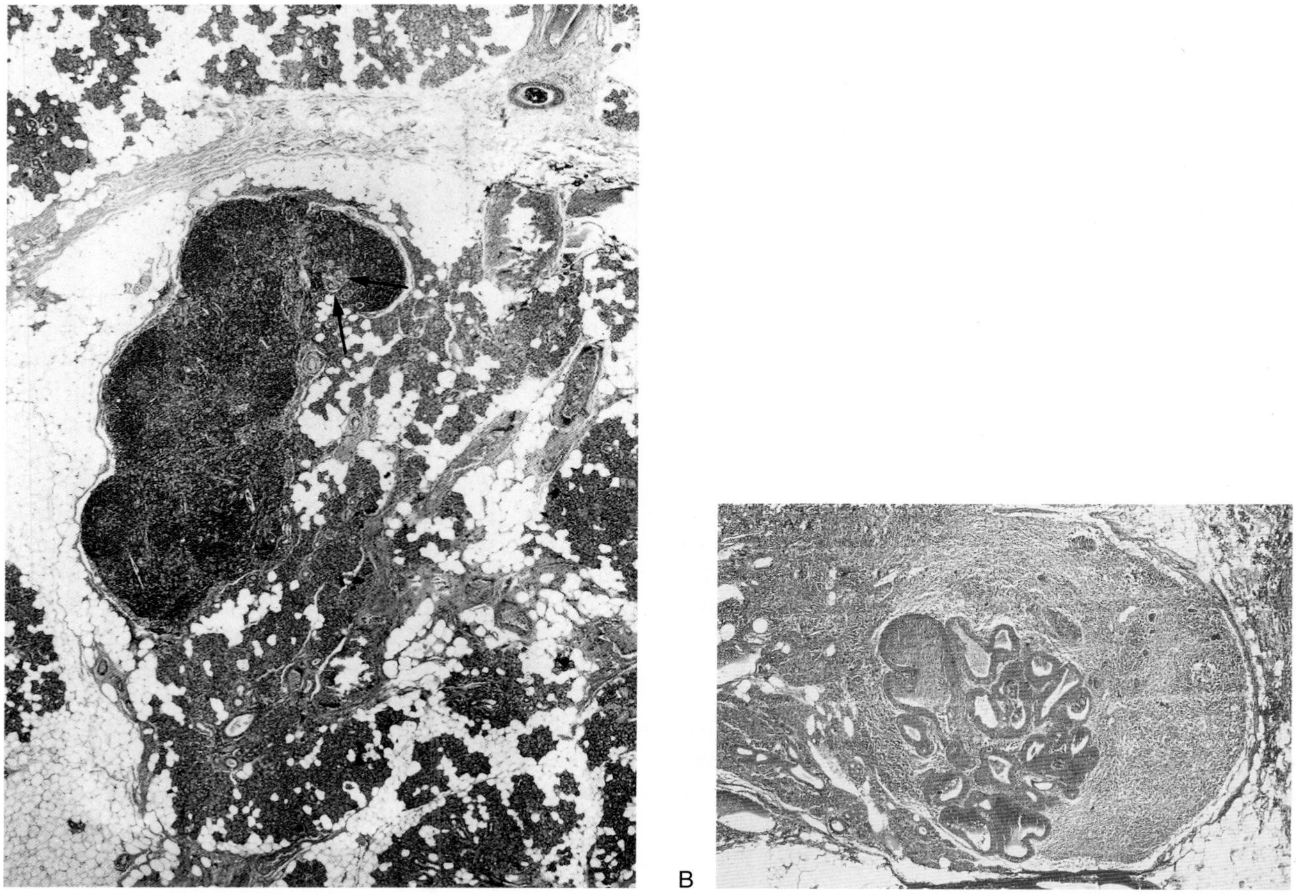

A B

**FIG. 15.** Lymph node of the parotid gland. **A**, Presence of glandular ducts in the medullary region (*arrows*). **B**, Duct dilatation and oncocytic transformation in another lymph node of the same patient.

lymph nodes within or adjacent to the parotid gland (72,78,154–156). According to this concept, the epithelial component of the tumor corresponds to altered ducts inside a lymph node and the lymphatic component is, in fact, a lymph node. The following arguments support this theory: salivary tissue is frequently present in intraparotid or periparotid lymph nodes (Fig. 15A); with the exception of a few cases, this tumor is exclusive to the parotid region; it is common to find early stages of oncocytic and papillary transformation in lymph nodes of the parotid region (Fig. 15B); and finally, tumors identical to the epithelial structure of Warthin's tumor occur outside the lymph nodes, but without lymphocytic components (154).

The diffuse lymphoid tissue may increase in chronic sialadenitis, particularly in immunologic reactions such as the benign lymphoepithelial lesion associated with Sjögren's syndrome. In these instances, lymphoid tissue may obscure the glandular parenchyma in a diffuse or nodular manner, and epimyoepithelial islands may be formed (91,154). The polyclonal character of the lymphoid cells and the presence of epimyoepithelial islands are useful criteria in the differential diagnosis of malignant lymphoma, which can occur in a preexisting benign lymphoepithelial lesion (157).

## THE HETEROTOPIC SALIVARY TISSUE AND ITS SIGNIFICANCE

The presence of salivary tissue outside the major salivary glands and the oral cavity, pharynx, and upper airways is considered heterotopia. This heterotopia may be classified as intranodal and extranodal in a number of locations in the head and neck.

Heterotopia is common in the lymph nodes near the parotid gland, but is much less frequent in the submaxillary region and in other upper cervical nodes (158,159). The glandular elements are either normal or atrophic; they consist mainly of ducts, but acini are also found. They are localized in the medullary region and comprise a variable proportion of lymphoid and salivary tissues. Although all types of secretory units are found, serous ones are predominant. The histologic architecture is similar to a normal gland. The lymph nodes exhibit a normal structure or some degree of lymphoreticular hyperplasia.

The incidence of heterotopic salivary tissue in the lymph nodes has been well documented (156,160). It is typically found in the parotid region of fetuses during various stages of development, usually in more than one lymph node. In adults, although the incidence is not constant, it is nonetheless frequent (161). In most of the reports, the histogenetic mechanisms of this phenomenon have been related to embryonic development. From this point of view, the salivary tissue is trapped during embryologic development. In the fetus, the parotid gland is closely related to lymphoid tissue from the beginning of the 2nd month. Moreover, Bairati (161) found that, at least in the first years of life, this salivary tissue is connected to the parotid gland. Although lymphatic dissemination has been proposed as a mechanism of salivary heterotopia in lymph nodes, in particular when they are located in the lower neck, this theory is only speculative (162).

Extralymphatic heterotopias are rare and often latent, but may be responsible for symptomatology. Depending on their site, they are classified as high or low heterotopia. High heterotopia is limited to the mandible, ear, palatine tonsil, mylohyoid muscle, pituitary gland, and cerebellopontine angle (159,163,164). All these sites, with the exception of the last, may be related to the embryonic migration of the salivary glands. The other group is known as a low heterotopia, which is localized in the base of the neck, particularly around the sternoclavicular joint and in the thyroid gland (Fig. 16) (162,165).

Most examples of high salivary heterotopia are explained in relation to lines of migration of the parotid and submaxillary glands. In the lower neck, an association with cysts and sinuses is frequent. This condition, along with the topographic presentation, has been related to the branchial apparatus (159,165) and, in particular, to a defective closure of the precervical His' sinus. The different abnormalities related to this defect (166) correspond embryologically to topographic distribution through the neck from the ear to the clavicle. When this defect occurs, the salivary tissue is the result of abnormal tissue differentiation (heteroplasia). Willis (167) has argued that this is the mechanism of heterotopia. This mechanism may also account for the salivary tissue in remnants of Rathke's pouch (164) and the thyroglossal duct.

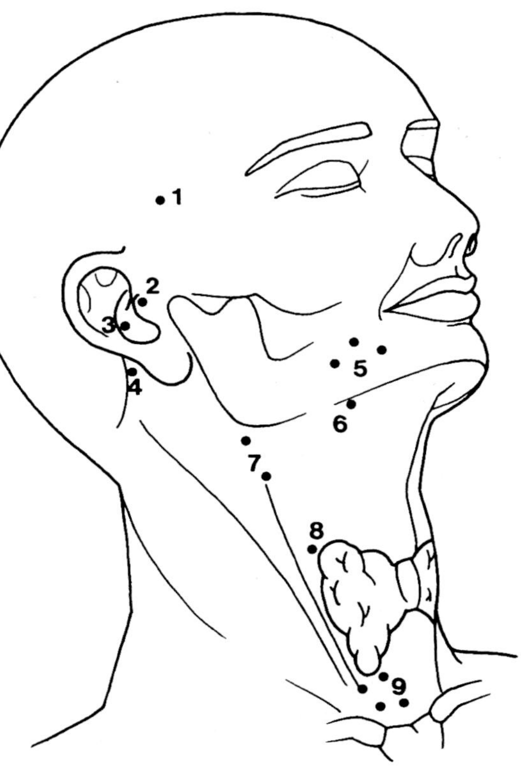


**FIG. 16.** Extranodal salivary heterotopias. Pituitary gland (1), middle ear (2), external auditory canal (3), cerebellopontine angle (4), mandible (5), oropharynx (6), cervical superior (7), thyroid capsule (8), and lower anterolateral neck (9).

Neoplastic transformation in heterotopic salivary tissue may pose a problem in differential diagnosis of metastasis in a cervical lymph node (158). Pleomorphic adenoma, mucoepidermoid carcinoma, and adenoid cystic carcinoma are the most frequent tumors arising in heterotopic salivary tissue. In fact, heterotopia is an explanation for many aberrant salivary tumors (162,168) and some cervical lymph node metastases which are thought to be metastases of an unknown primary (169).

## AGING CHANGES

### Oncocytes

The oncocyte is an altered swollen epithelial cell characterized by an abundant eosinophilic granular cytoplasm rich in altered mitochondria and enzymes (Fig. 17A) (170). This cell is frequently present in interlobular ducts and is less frequent in acinar cells. Oncocytes are more common in the parotid gland. They are rare before 50 years of age, increase in frequency with advancing years, and become constant after 70 years (61,171).

The nature and function of oncocytes are unknown. Their proliferative character is a common finding in organs with endocrine function or endocrine dependence (172). Numerous researchers are presently interested in the production of various peptides with endocrine function in the intralobular ducts of rodent salivary glands (173–175). On the other hand, a number of workers are investigating the presence of neuroendocrine peptides such as the substance P-like, beta-endorphin-like, (176,177) and a calcitonin-related peptide (178). In addition, neuroendocrine regulation of inflammation by the submandibular gland, has been explained by a immuno-neuroendocrine communication controlled by cervical sympathetic nerves (179).

The proliferation of oncocytes is called oncocytosis or oncocytic metaplasia when it is diffuse and generally without pathologic significance. In other cases, this proliferation presents a nodular pattern known as nodular hyperplasia (180). Histologically, it is easy to distinguish in the salivary parenchyma as one or several small foci of oncocytes that are well circumscribed, but not encapsulated. The cells may be arranged in solid cords or ductal structures (Fig. 17B). Oncocytes participate in various salivary gland tumors in ap-

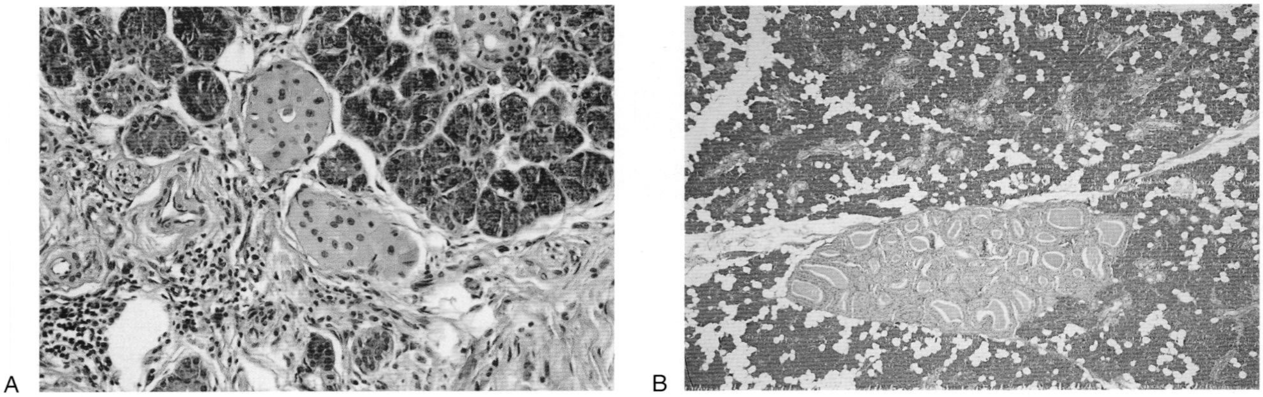

FIG. 17. **A**, Oncocytes in intralobular ducts of a normal submaxillary gland. Note the abundant and granulated cytoplasm. **B**, Nodular oncocytic hyperplasia.

proximately 10% of cases (181). The neoplastic proliferation called oncocytoma is rarely found in salivary glands (182).

### Fatty Infiltration

Normally, some adipose cells are present in the areolar connective tissue of the salivary glands. This fatty tissue increases in adults; in the elderly, it forms an important proportion of salivary gland tissue. Fatty infiltration may reach huge proportions, especially in alcoholics and the malnourished (183).

## REACTIVE CHANGES

### Metaplasia

Squamous metaplasia may be present in larger salivary ducts in chronic inflammatory processes, particularly when associated with calculi (Fig.18A) (184). (Remember that when the major salivary ducts open into the oral cavity, they are lined with a stratified squamous epithelium). Metaplastic squamous transformation is also present in intralobular ducts and acini in ischemia and radiation injury (185,186).

Mucous metaplasia is found on interlobular ducts, and less frequently on intralobular ducts in cases of obstructive and postradiotherapy forms of sialadenitis (187). An important proliferation of mucous goblet cells is accompanied by prominent ciliated cells mimicking the respiratory epithelium (Fig. 18B). Necrotizing sialometaplasia is a type of metaplasia peculiar to salivary tissue, but it is exceptional in major salivary glands (188). It consists of ischemic lobular infarction or necrosis of some acini, accompanied by extensive squamous metaplasia of salivary gland ducts and acini. Severe inflammation and granulation tissue are present. Necrosis of mucous acini is represented by small pools of mucin, that along with the squamous elements may be mistaken for mucoepidermoid carcinoma (189). The preservation of general lobular morphology and prominent granulation tissue are criteria in favor of benignity (146).

### Hyperplasia

Hyperplasia of mucous acini is an alteration exclusive to the minor salivary glands. In contrast, serous hyperplasia occurs in parotid and, rarely, in submaxillary glands; it is called sialadenosis (190). This hyperplasia is associated with a

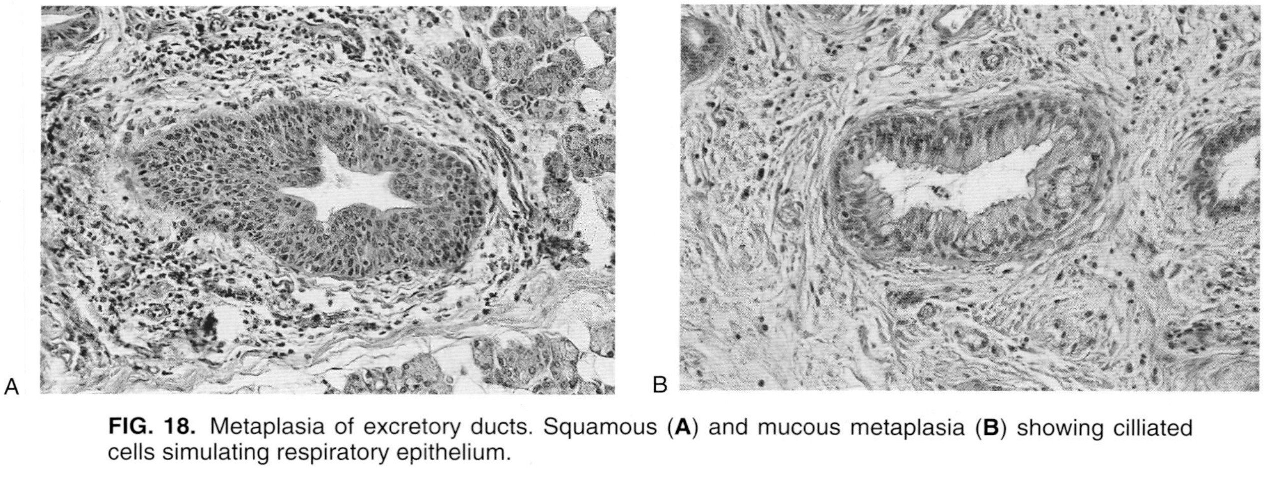

FIG. 18. Metaplasia of excretory ducts. Squamous (**A**) and mucous metaplasia (**B**) showing cilliated cells simulating respiratory epithelium.

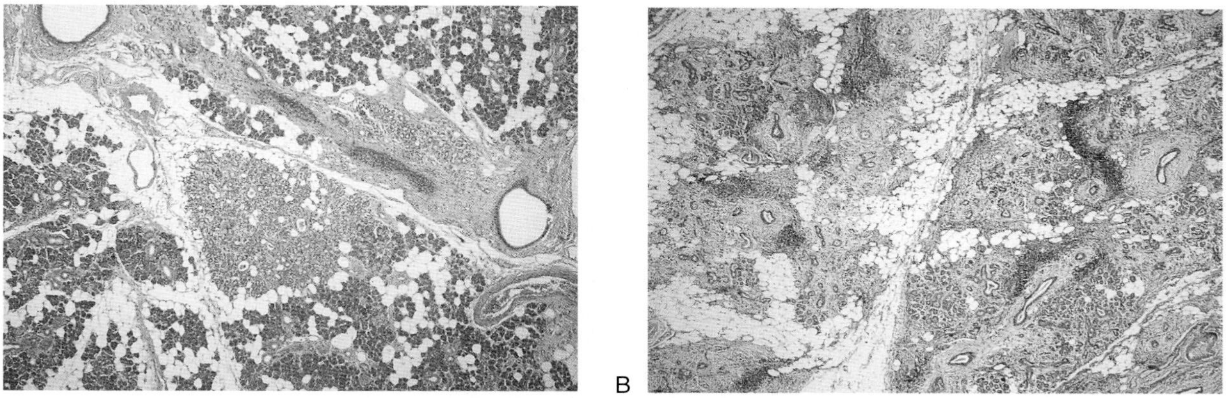

A B

**FIG. 19.** Atrophy of the salivary parenchyma. **A**, Focal atrophy in the vicinity of a parotid tumor; note the duct dilatation. **B**, Diffuse atrophy in chronic sialadenitis showing prominent periductal sclerosis.

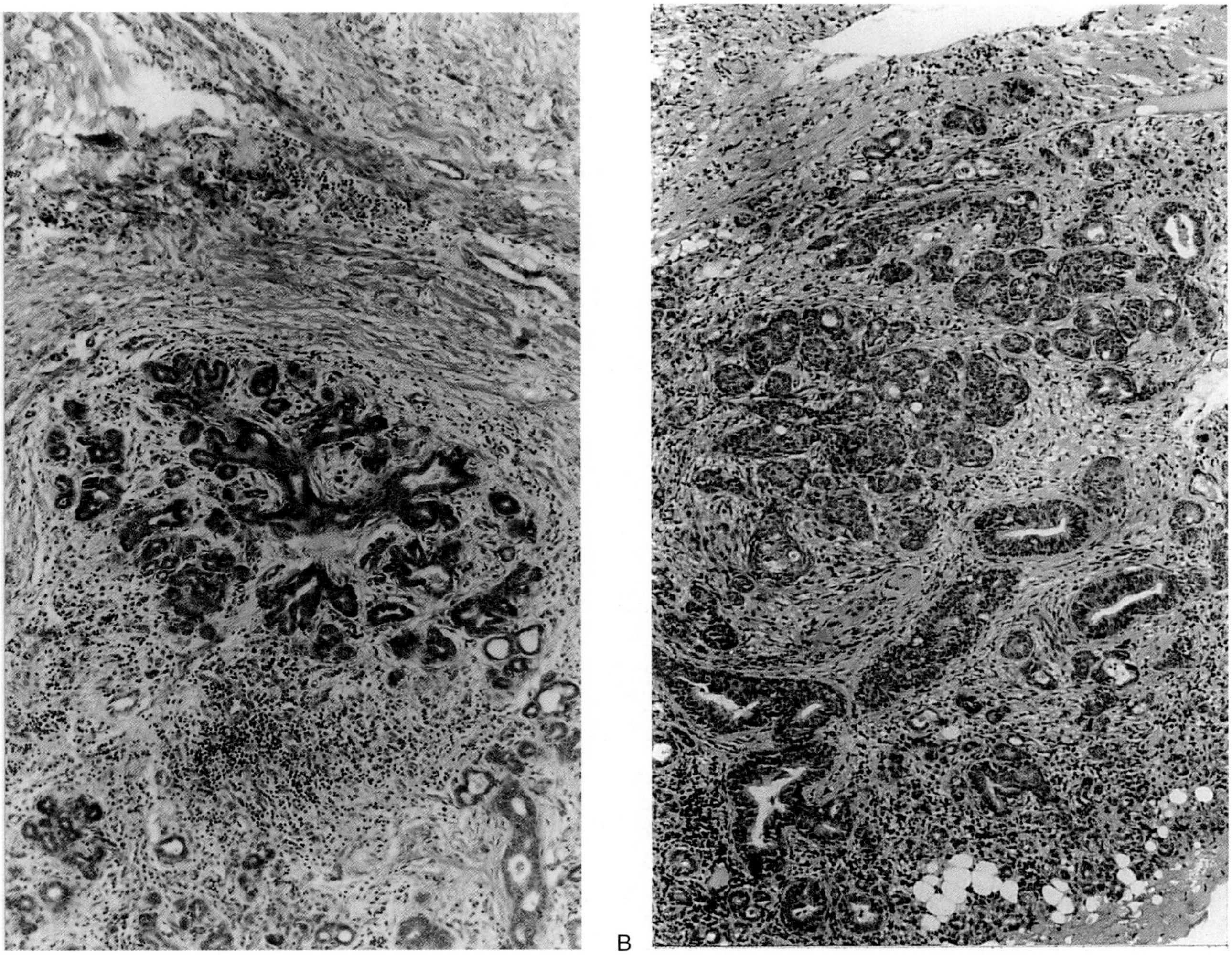

A B

**FIG. 20.** Regenerating salivary tissue of parotid gland. **A**, Formation of secretory units with an embryonic pattern. **B**, Atypical regenerating tissue; the lobular pattern is preserved.

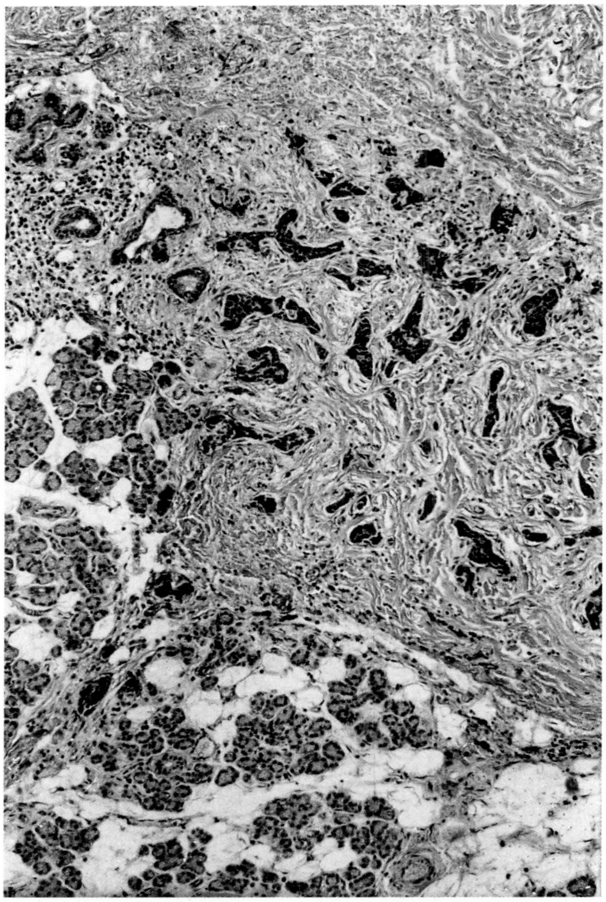

**FIG. 20.** *Continued.* **C**, Infiltrating residual adenoid cystic carcinoma in a parotid gland. Solid buds consist of undifferentiated cells without lobular arrangement.

number of metabolic, nutritional, and endocrine conditions or follows the ingestion of chemicals and drugs (22,191). In most cases, a bilateral swelling of the glands is caused by enlarged acini and an accumulation of secretory granules in the cytoplasm. In other cases, granulation is lost and the cytoplasm looks vacuolated (22). The myoepithelial cells may present nuclear pyknosis or cytoplasmic vacuolation.

### Atrophy

Atrophy of the salivary tissue is a common finding in surgical specimens of tumoral salivary glands that have one or more atrophied lobules. This atrophy is caused by partial or total obstruction of an excretory duct. Accordingly, secretory units distal to the obstructed duct are dilated, and the acinar lumina become visible. The secretory cells lose their granules and have a similar aspect to that of the intercalated duct. The atrophic lobule has an inflammatory component; the cells gradually disappear and the parenchyma is replaced by adipose tissue and collagen fibers (Fig. 19A). The extent of atrophy depends on the size of the affected duct. It is generally greater in lithiasic obstruction. The atrophy present in terminal stage chronic sialadenitis shows a diffuse pattern with prominent periductal sclerosis and dense inflammatory infiltration (Fig. 19B) (187). In the submaxillary gland, diffuse atrophy is frequent after radiotherapy and the gland has a firm consistency (Kuttner's tumor) that may be clinically mistaken for a submaxillary neoplasm. Atypical cells are often found in postradiotherapy atrophy. Dilated ducts lose cell polarity and exhibit hyperchromatic nuclei and prominent myoepithelium. In addition, interlobular ducts lose their continuity and the interstitium is densely infiltrated with plasma cells (186).

### Regeneration

The parenchyma of salivary glands have a capacity for regeneration. It is particularly notable in the salivary gland a few weeks after partial resection. In general, regenerating tissue follows an embryonic pattern, showing solid buds and branching columns of undifferentiated cells that eventually form excretory units (22)(Fig. 20A). In some cases, such regenerating tissue exhibits an atypical appearance. Proliferating, solid buds of undifferentiated cells may simulate basal cell adenoma (192) or other undifferentiated cell neoplasms (Fig. 20B). However, unlike neoplasms, the regenerating tissue preserves the lobular architecture characteristic of the normal salivary gland (Fig. 20B,C). In general, it is thought that salivary-regenerating tissue originates in the reserve cells of the duct system (22,39), but this theory has not been proved.

## CORRELATIVE NORMAL AND NEOPLASTIC HISTOLOGY

A characteristic of salivary glands is the ability to give rise to a large number of histologically distinct tumors (193). The histogenetic origin of these neoplasms is an interesting topic, but the numerous mechanisms that have been proposed remain hypothetical. The most attractive theories attempt to relate this phenomenon to embryonic development and, particularly, to the presence of ductal reserve cells (38,39,51,55,181,194). A conjectural role of these reserve cells is the regeneration of salivary parenchyma, as well as the development of metaplastic tissue in reactive conditions. Some researchers have demonstrated, by immunohistochemical methods, the presence of basal cells with an undifferentiated aspect in salivary ducts (52,53). However, this does not prove that they act as reserve cells. Conversely, experimental evidence exists of the proliferative capacity of differentiated acinar cells (195–197).

A correlation between the normal structure of the salivary gland and the histologic appearance of salivary tumors can help us to understand morphologic classifications. Nevertheless, we must realize that this histologic similarity does not necessarily imply that a particular tumor arises from the structure that it mimics (194).

The intercalated duct represents the most important seg-

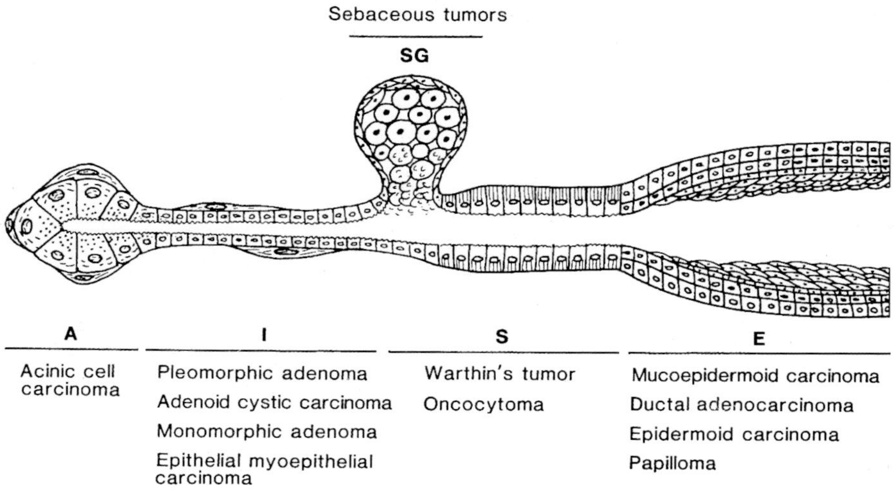


**FIG. 21.** Morphologic similarity of some salivary tumors and the different epithelial structures of the salivary gland: acinus (A), intercalated duct (I), striated duct (S), sebaceous gland (SG), and excretory ducts (E). Not necessarily related to histogenesis.

ment of the salivary gland in the morphologic organization of many salivary tumors (194). Many distinctive tumors have been related to it, including pleomorphic adenoma, adenoid cystic carcinoma, basal cell adenoma, epithelial-myoepithelial carcinoma, terminal duct carcinoma, basal cell carcinoma, and embryonic tumors (Fig. 21). These tumors show both epithelial and myoepithelial cell differentiation (89,93,101,104,105,110,123,124,126,128,131,139,140,194, 198), as does the normal intercalated duct. According to Batsakis (39), these tumors develop from "intercalated duct reserve cells" that follow the same direction as the embryonic terminal tubular cell. Statistically, approximately 80% of salivary tumors develop in the parotid gland where the intercalated ducts are relatively long (Fig. 6). In contrast, in the sublingual gland, which gives rise to less than 1% of salivary tumors (22,193), intercalated ducts are hardly visible.

A similar morphologic link exists between the acini, the most differentiated structure of the gland, and the acinic cell tumor, a well-differentiated neoplasm (199); between the mitochondria-rich cells of the striated duct, Warthin's tumor and oncocytomas (170–172); and between the sebaceous glands and sebaceous tumors (64,69,79). A morphologic analogy also may be found between the larger excretory ducts and mucoepidermoid carcinoma, salivary duct adenocarcinoma, epidermoid carcinoma, adenosquamous carcinoma, and papillary tumors (Fig.21) (144–149,200–202).

## IMMUNOHISTOCHEMISTRY

An important aspect of cytodifferentiation in normal and neoplastic salivary tissue is the expression of different intermediate filaments, enzymes, immunologic components, and other proteins. These proteins may be stained by immunohistochemical methods.

In normal salivary glands, the immunohistochemistry may be summarized as follows (Table 2): the expression of cytokeratin varies according to individual cell types of the secretory unit. Cytokeratins 6 and 12 are weakly positive in acinar cells, but strongly positive in ductal cells, especially in excretory ducts (Fig. 22) (52). Basal cells are stained with anticytokeratin 19 and 18 (52). Myoepithetial cells may co-

**TABLE 2.** *Histologic markers of salivary glands*

| | Structural markers (a) | | | | | | | | Functional markers (b) | | | | | |
|---|---|---|---|---|---|---|---|---|---|---|---|---|---|---|
| Structure | LMK | HMK | Vim. | A-M | CEA | EMA | S-100 | AFP | Amyl. | Lacto. | Lyso. | SC | ATPase | AP |
| Acinus | + + | + | − | − | + | − | − | − | + + | + | + | + | − | − |
| Intercalated duct | − | + + | − | − | + | + + | + + | + + | − | + + | + + | + | − | − |
| Striated duct | − | + + | − | − | − | − | − | + + | − | − | − | + | − | − |
| Excretory duct | − | + + | − | − | − | + + | − | − | − | − | − | + | − | − |
| Myoepithelial cell | + | − | ± | + + | − | − | + + | − | − | − | − | − | + + | + + |
| Basal cell | + + | − | − | − | − | − | − | − | − | − | − | − | − | − |

(a) LMK, low-molecular-weight keratin; HMK, high-molecular-weight keratin; Vim., vimentin; A-M, actin-myosin; CEA, carcinoembryonic antigen; EMA, epithelial membrane antigen; S-100, S-100 protein; AFP, alpha-foeto protein.

(b) Amyl., amylase; Lacto., lactoferrin; Lyso., lysozyme; SC, secretory component; AP, alkaline phosphatase.

+, weak positivity

+ +, strong positivity

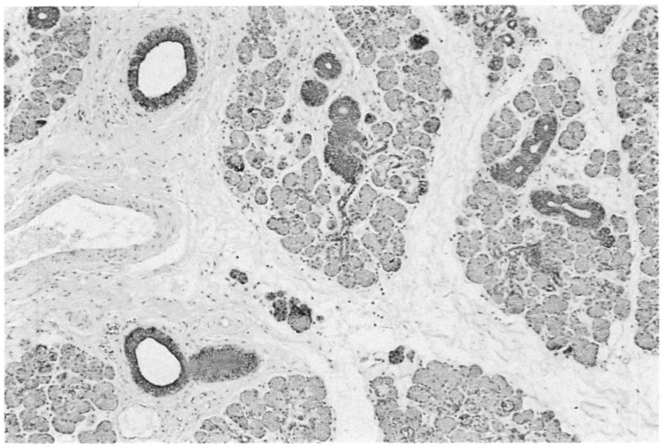

FIG. 22. Immunostaining for high-molecular-weight cytokeratin in a submaxillary gland. The acini are unstained but intercalated, striated, and excretory ducts show a progressive immunoreaction (peroxidase-antiperoxidase method).

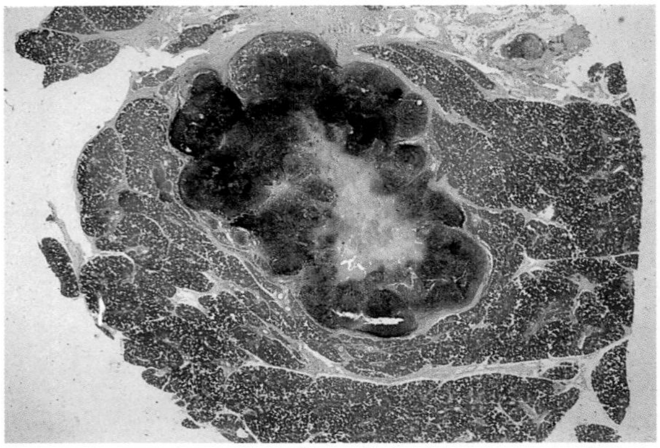

FIG. 24. Histologic section of a parotid gland showing a pleomorphic adenoma. The tumor is apparently well delimited; tumoral buds may be found separate from the principal tumor.

express cytokeratins 17 and 19 and vimentin (52,138,139); however, S-100 protein is the marker most often used for the myoepithelium (141). In addition, normal myoepithelial cells are sometimes stained with glial fibrillary protein (203). The secretory component is present in acinar cells, as well as intercalated and striated duct cells, except for the mucous units (50,204). Carcinoembryonic antigen (CEA) is present in acinar and intercalated duct cells; it is strongly positive in inflamed glands (205). Ductal epithelial cells of intercalated, striated, and interlobular ducts are strongly positive for epithelial membrane antigen (EMA)(207). Recently, the presence of alpha-fetoprotein in human submandibular gland has been documented (206). Used as functional markers, the following enzymes may be stained: amylase and lactoferrin in serous acinar cells (208), lysozyme in intercalated ducts (44,50), and alkaline phosphatase and ATPase in myoepithelial cells (85). When used as histologic markers, all these proteins have proved useful in surgical pathology.

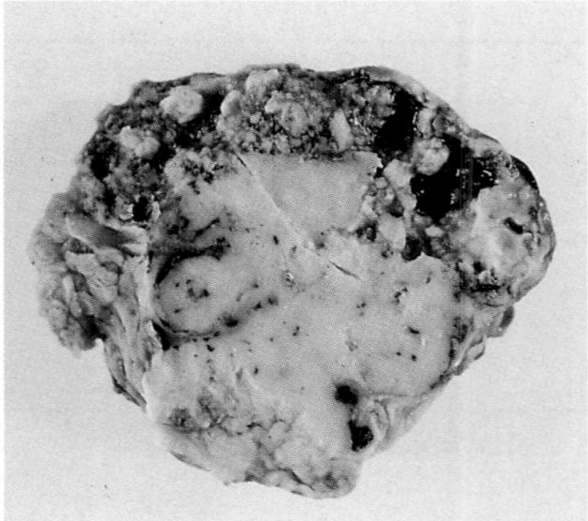

FIG. 23. Superficial parotidectomy for a pleomorphic adenoma. Note the tumor is well delimited within the normal gland.

## SPECIMEN HANDLING

The parotid gland is the most common location of major salivary gland tumors. Because most of them are benign and located on the superficial lobe, partial parotidectomy of the superficial lobe (lateral lobectomy) is the most common treatment. Superficial parotidectomy also suffices for small, well-differentiated, low-grade malignant neoplasms that have not compromised the facial nerve (209). The specimen should be sectioned horizontally and the relationship between the tumor and the gland should be stated (Fig. 23). The surgical limits should be described even in benign tumors (Fig. 24). Total parotidectomy with preservation of the facial nerve is usually indicated in recurrent or multiple benign tumors and large benign tumors of the isthmus and deep lobe.

Total parotidectomy including facial nerve resection (radical parotidectomy) is indicated in aggressive malignant tumors, malignant tumors situated in the deep lobe, or those that have compromised the facial nerve. All these specimens should be sectioned on their major axis to evaluate periparotid tissue infiltration (Fig. 25). Intraparotid and peri-

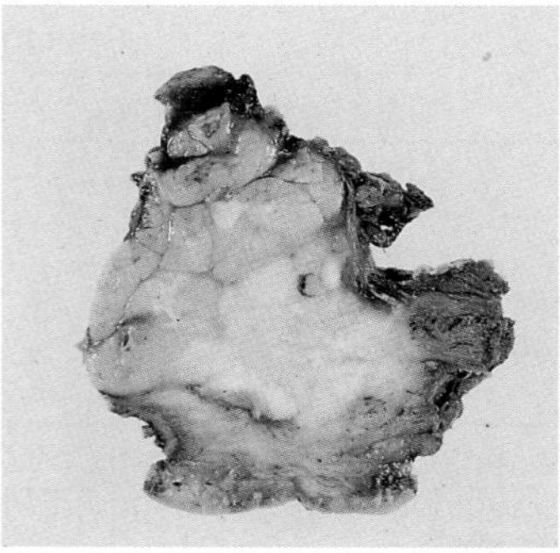

FIG. 25. Radical parotidectomy for a high-grade mucoepidermoid carcinoma. Note the infiltration of the periparotid tissues.

parotid lymph nodes should be identified, and when radical parotidectomy includes neck dissection, the lymph nodes should be separated according to the different anatomical regions.

Benign and malignant submandibular gland tumors are rare. Single gland resection is indicated for benign tumors, whereas malignant tumors are treated by a monobloc resection of the gland lesion along with associated muscles, nerves, and mucous membrane.

Sublingual tumors are rare and most (80%) are malignant. They are also treated by local monobloc resection, including the sublingual compartment and surrounding tissues (210).

## REFERENCES


1. Arey LB. *Developmental anatomy*. Philadelphia; WB Saunders, 1974.
2. Cohn RH. Banerjee SD, Bernfield MR. Basal lamina of embryonic salivary epithelia. Nature of glycosaminoglycan and organization of extracellular materials. *J Cell Biol* 1977;73:464–478.
3. Grobstein C. Epithelio-mesenchymal specificity in the morphogenesis of mouse submandibular rudiments in vitro. *J Exp Zool* 1953;124: 383–413.
4. Grobstein C. Mechanisms of organogenetic tissue interaction. Second Decennial Review Conference on cell tissue and organ culture. The Tissue Culture Association. *Natl Cancer Inst Monogr* 1967;26: 279–299.
5. Lawson KA. The role of mesenchyme in the morphogenesis and functional differentiation of rat salivary epithelium. *J Embryol Exp Morphol* 1972;27:497–513.
6. Gasser RF. The early development of the parotid gland around the facial nerve and its branches in man. *Anat Rec* 1970;167:63–78.
7. Azuma M, Sato. M. Morphogenesis of normal human salivary gland cells in vitro. *Histol Histopathol* 1994;9:781–790.
8. Donath K, Dietrich H, Seifert G. Enwicklung und ultrastrukturelle Cytodifferenzierung der Parotis des Menschen. *Virchows Arch A Pathol Anat Histopathol* 1978;378:297–314.
9. Lee SK, Hwang Jo, Chi JG, Yomada K, Mori M. Prenatal development of human submandibular gland observed by immunohistochemistry of smooth muscle actin and rhodamine-phalloidin fluorescence. *Pathol Res Pract* 1993;189:332–341.
10. Adi MM, Chisholm DM, Waterhouse JP. Stercological and immunohistochemical study of development of human fetal labial salivary glands and their S-100 protein reactivity. *J Oral Pathol Med* 1994;23: 36–40.
11. Lee SK, Kim EC, Chi JG, Mashimura K, Mori M. Immunohistochemical detection of S-100, S-100 alpha, S-100 beta proteins, glial fibrillary acidic protein, and neuron specific enolase in the prenatal and adult human salivary glands. *Pathol Res Pract* 1993;189: 1036–1043.
12. Line SE, Archer FL. The postnatal development of myoepithelial cell in the rat submandibular gland. *Virchows Arch B Cell Pathol Incl Mol Pathol* 1972;10:253–262.
13. Gresik EG. Postnatal developmental changes in submandibular glands of rat and mice. *J Histochem Cytochem* 1980;28:860–870.
14. Strum JM. Unusual peroxidase positive granules in the developing rat submaxillary gland. *J Cell Biol* 1971;51:575–579.
15. Yamashima S, Barka T. Localization of peroxidase activity in the developing submandibular gland of normal and isoproterenol treated rats. *J Histochem Cytoche*m 1972;20:855–872.
16. Testut L. *Traité d'Anatomie Humaine*. Paris; Octave Doin, 1901.
17. Mayo GCh. *Gray's anatomy*. Philadelphia; Lea & Febiger, 1973.
18. Gola R, Chossegros C, Carreu P. Anatomie chirurgicale de la région parotidienne. Concepts actuels. *Rev Stomatol Chir Mayillofac* 1994; 95:395–410.
19. Toh H, Kodama J, Fujuda J, Rittman B, Mackenzie I. Incidence and histology of human accessory parotid glands. *Anat Rec* 1993;236: 586–590.
20. Frommer J. The human accessory parotid gland: its incidence, nature and significance. *Oral Surg Oral Med Oral Pathol* 1977;43:671–676.
21. Hamilton WJ, Boyd DJ, Mossman HW. *Human Embryology, Prenatal Development of Form and Function*. London; Williams & Wilkins, 1972.
22. Evans RW, Cruickshank AH. *Epithelial Tumors of the Salivary Glands*. Philadelphia; WB Saunders, 1970.
23. Merida-Velasco JA, Sanchez-Montesinos I, Espin-Ferra J, García-García ID, García-Gomez S, Roldan-Shilling V. Development of the human submandibular salivary gland. *J Dent Res* 1993;73: 1227–1232.
24. Gaur V, Choundry R, Anand C, Chaundry S. Submandibular gland with multiple ducts. *Surg Radiol Anat* 1994;16:439–440.
25. Bowen ID, Morgan SM, Mullarkey K. Cell death in the salivary glands of metamorphosing calliphora vomitoria. *Cell Biol Int* 1993; 17:13–33.
26. Tomei LD, Cope FO. *Apoptosis: the molecular basis of cell death*. Plainview; Cold Spring Harbor Lab Press, 1991.
27. Lu Q, Poulsom R, Wong L, Hanby AM. Bcl-2 expression in adult and embryonic non-haematopoietic tissues. *J Pathol* 1993;169:431–437.
28. Walker NI, Gobé GC. Cell death and cell proliferation during atrophy of the rat parotid gland induced by duct obstruction. *J Pathol* 1987; 153:333–344.
29. Stephens LC, Schultheiss TE, Price RE, Ang KK, Peters LJ. Radiation apoptosis of serous acinar cells of salivary and lacrimal glands. *Cancer* 1991;67:1539–1543.
30. Hand AR, Ho B. Liquid-diet-induced alterations of rat parotid acinar cells studied by electron microscopy and enzyme cytochemistry. *Arch Oral Biol* 1981;26:369–380.
31. Sharawy M, White SC. Morphometric and fine structural study of experimental autoallergic sialadenitis of rat submandibular glands. *Virchows Arch B Cell Pathol Incl Mol Pathol* 1978;28:255–273.
32. Chaudhry AP, Cutler LS, Yamane GM, Satchidanand S, Labay G, Sunderraj M. Light and ultrastructural features of lymphoepithelial lesions of the salivary glands in Mickulicz's disease. *J Pathol* 1986;146: 239–250.
33. Fanidi A, Harrington EA, Evan GI. Cooperative interaction between c-myc and bcl-2 proto-oncogenes. *Nature* 1992;359:554–556.
34. Chen M, Quintans J, Fuks Z, Thompson C, Kufe DW, Weichselbaum RR. Suppression of Bcl-2 messenger RNA production may mediate apoptosis after ionizing radiation, tumor necrosis a and ceramide. *Cancer Res* 1995;55:991–994.
35. Pammer J, Horvat R, Weninger W, Ulrich W. Expression of bcl-2 in salivary glands and salivary adenomas. *Pathol Res Pract* 1995;191: 35–41.
36. Hockenbery DM, Zutter M, Hickey W, Nahm M, Korsmeyer SJ. Bcl-2 proteinis topographically restricted in tissues characterized by apoptotic cell death. *Proc Natl Acad Sci U S A* 1991;88:6961–6965.
37. Sell S, Pierce GB. Biology of disease. *Lab Invest* 1994;70:6–22.
38. Eversole LR,. Histogenetic classification of salivary tumors. *Arch Pathol Lab Med* 1971;92:433–443.
39. Batsakis JG. Salivary gland neoplasia: an outcome of modified morphogenesis and cytodifferentiation. *Oral Surg Oral Med Oral Pathol* 1980;49:229–232.
40. Dardick I, Byard RW, Carnegie JA. A review of the proliferative capacity of major salivary glands and the relationship to current concepts of neoplasia in salivary glands. *Oral Surg Oral Med Oral Pathol* 1990;69:53–67.
41. Bloom W, Fawcett DW. *A textbook of histology*. 10th ed. Philadelphia; WB Saunders, 1986.
42. Donath K. *Sialadenose der Parotis. Ultrastruktirelle, Klinische und Experimentelle Befunde zur Sekretiospathologie*. Sttutgart; Fischer, 1976.
43. Takano K, Malaumd D, Bennick A, Oppenheim F, Hand AR. Localization of salivary proteins in granules of human parotid and submandibular acinar cells. *Crit Rev Oral Biol Med* 1993;4:399–405.
44. Caselitz J, Jaup T, Seifert G. Lactoferrin and lysozyme in carcinomas of the parotid gland. A comparative immunocytochemical study with the occurrence in normal and inflamed tissue. *Virchows Arch A Pathol Anat Histopathol* 1981;394:61–73.
45. Reitamo S, Kontinnen YT, Sgerber-Kontinnen M. Distribution of lactoferrin in human salivary glands. *Histochemistry* 1980;66: 285–291.

46. Xu L, Lal K, Santarpia RP, Pollock JJ. Salivary proteolysis of histidine-rich polypeptides and antifungal activity of peptide degradation products. *Arch Oral Biol* 1993;38:277–283.
47. Quinatrelli G. Histochemical identification of salivary mucins. *Ann N Y Acad Sci* 1963;106:339–363.
48. Reddy MS, Bobek LA, Harasztty GG, Biesbrock AR, Levine MJ. Structural features of the low-molecular-mass human salivary mucin. *Biochem J* 1992;287:639–643.
49. Greep RO, Weiss L. *Histology*. New York; McGraw-Hill, 1973.
50. Korsrud FR, Brandtzaeg P. Characterization of epithelial elements in human major salivary glands by functional markers. Localization of amylase, lactoferrin, lysozyme, secretory component and secretory immunoglobulins by paired immnunofluorescence staining. *J Histochem Cytochem* 1982;30:657–666.
51. Riva A, Serra GP, Proto E, Faa G, Puxeddu R, Riva FT. The myoepithelial and basal cells of ducts of human major salivary glands: a SEM study. *Arch Histol Cytol* 1992;55 (suppl):115–124.
52. Born A. Schwechheimer K, Maier H, Offo NF. Cytokeratin expression in normal salivary glands and in cystadenolymphomas demonstrated by monoclonal antibodies against selective cytokeratin polypeptides. *Virchows Arch A Pathol Anat Histopathol* 1987;411: 583–589.
53. Burns BF, Dardick I, Dorks WR. Intermediate filament expression in normal salivary glands and in pleomorphic adenomas. *Virchows Arch A Pathol Anat Histopathol* 1988;413:103–112.
54. Seifert GA, Miehlke A, Hanubrich J, Chilla R. *Diseases of the Salivary Glands: pathology, diagnosis, treatment, facial nerve surgery*. Sttutgart; Georg Thiem, 1986.
55. Regezi JA, Batsakis JG. Histogenesis of salivary gland neoplasms. *Otolaryngol Clin North Am* 1977;10:297–307.
56. Scott BL, Pease DC. Electron microscopy of the salivary and lacrimal glands of the rat. *Am J Anat* 1954;104:115–161.
57. Tandler B. Ultrastructure of the human submaxillary gland. I. Architecture and histological relationship of the secretory cells. *Am J Anat* 1962;111:287–307.
58. Tandler B, Denning CR, Mandel ID, Kutscher AH. Ultrastructure of human labial salivary glands. III. Myoepithelium and ducts. *Morphol* 1970;130:227–246.
59. Norberg L. Dardick I, Leung R, Burford-Mason AP, Rippstein P. Immunogold localization of actin and cytokeratin filaments in myoepithelium of human parotid salivary gland. *Ultrastruct Pathol* 1992;16: 555–568.
60. Sjöstrand FS. Rhodin J. The ultrastructure of the proximal convoluted tubules of the mouse kidney as revealed by high resolution electron microscopy. *Exp Cell Res* 1953;4:426–465.
61. Hamperl H. Beitraäge zur normalen und pathologischen Histologic menschlicher Speicheldrüsen. *Z Mikrosk Anat Forsch* 1931;27:1–55.
62. Harts PH. Development of sebaceous glands from intralobular ducts of the parotid gland. *Arch Pathol* 1946;41:651–654.
63. Marshall L Jr. Intraparotid sebaceous glands. *Ann Surg* 1949;129: 152–155.
64. Meza-Chavez L. Sebaceous glands in normal and neoplastic parotid glands. *Am J Pathol* 1949;25:627–645.
65. Micheau C. Les glandes dites sébacées de la parotide et de la sousmaxillaire. *Ann Anat Pathol* 1969;14:119–126.
66. Patey D., Thackray AC. The treatment of parotid tumors in the light of a pathological study of parotidectomy material. *Br J Surg* 1958;45: 477–487.
67. Margolies A,. Weidman F. Statistical and histologic studies of Fordyce's disease. *Arch Dermatol Syph* 1921;3:723–742.
68. Brocheriou C. Les tumeurs des glandes salivaires. In: Nezelof C, ed. *Nouvelles acquisitions en pathologie*. Paris; Hermann, 1983;223–268.
69. Albores-Saavedra J, Morris AW. Sebaceous adenoma of the submaxillary salivary gland. Report of a case. *Arch Otolaryngol* 1963;77: 500–503.
70. Assor D. Sebaceous lymphadenoma of the parotid gland: a case report. *Am J Clin Pathol* 1970;53:100–103.
71. Cheek R, Pitcock JA. Sebaceous lesions of the parotid. Report of two cases. *Arch Pathol* 1966;86:147–150.
72. Seifert G, Bull HG, Donath K. Histologic subclassification of the cystadenolymphoma of the parotid gland. Analysis of 275 cases. *Virchows Arch A Pathol Anat Histopathol* 1980;388:13–38.
73. Wasan SM. Sebaceous lymphadenomas of the parotid gland. *Cancer* 1971;28:1019–1022.
74. Kleinsasser O, Hübner G, Klein HJ. Talgzellcarcinom der Parotis. *Arch Klin Exp Ohr Nas Ukehlkopfheilk* 1970;197:59–71.
75. Silver H, Goldstein MA. Sebaceous cell carcinoma of the parotid region. A review of the literature and a case report. *Cancer* 1966;19: 1173–1179.
76. Martínez-Madrigal F, Casiraghi O, Khattech, Nasr-Khattech, Richard JM, Micheau C. Hypopharyngeal sebaceous carcinoma: a case report. *Hum Pathol* 1991;22:929–931.
77. Ginepp DR, Sporck T. Benign lymphoepithelial parotid cyst with sebaceous differentiation. Cystic sebaceous lymphadenoma. *Am J Clin Pathol* 1980;74:683–687.
78. Peel RL, Gnepp DR. Diseases of the salivary gland. In: Barnes L, ed. *Surgical pathology of the head and neck*. New York; Marcel Dekker, 1985.
79. Rawson AJ. Horn RC. Sebaceous glands and sebaceous gland containing tumors of the parotid salivary gland. *Surgery* 1950;27:93–101.
80. Cutter LS, Chandhry A, Innes DJ. Ultrastructure of the parotid duct. Cytochemical studies of the striated duct and papillary cystadenoma lymphomatosum of the human parotid gland. *Arch Pathol Lab Med* 1977;101:420–424.
81. Archer FL, Kao VCY. Immunohistochemical identification of actomyosin in myoepithelium of human tissues. *Lab Invest* 1968;18: 669–674.
82. Drenckhan DU, Gröschel-Stewart U, Unsicker K. Immunofluorescence microscopic demonstration of myosin and actin in salivary glands and exocrine pancreas of the rat. *Cell Tissue Res* 1977;183: 273–279.
83. Tandler B. Ultrastructure of the human submaxillary gland. III. Myoepithelium. *Z Zell Forsch Mikrosk Anat* 1965;68:852–863.
84. Franke WW, Schmid E, Frendenstein C, Appelhans B, Osborn M, Weber K, Keenan TW. Intermediate sized filaments of the prekeratin type in myoepithelial cells. *J Cell Biol* 1980;84:633–654.
85. Hamperl H. The myoepithelia (myoepithelial cells). *Curr Top Pathol* 1970;53:161–220.
86. Shear M. The structure and function of myoepithelial cells in salivary glands. *Arch Oral Biol* 1966;11:769–780.
87. Garrett JR, Emmelin N. Activities of salivary myoepithelial cells: a review. *Med Biol Eng Comput* 1979;57:1–28.
88. Schroeder BT, Chakraborty J, Soloff MS. Binding of (3 H) oxytocin to the cells isolated from the mammary gland of the lactating rat. *J Cell Biol* 1977;74:428–440.
89. Azumi N, Battifora H. The cellular composition of adenoid cystic carcinoma. An immunohistochemical study. *Cancer* 1987;670: 1589–1598.
90. D'Ardenne AJ, Kirkpatrick P, Wells CA, Davies DJ. Laminin and fibronectin in adenoid cystic carcinoma. *J Clin Pathol* 1986;39: 138–144.
91. Donath K, Seifert G. Ultrastrucktur and Pathogenese der myoepithelialen Sialadenitis. Über das Vorkommen von Myoepithelzellen bei der benignen lymphoepithelialen Läsion. *Virchows Arch A Pathol Anat Histopathol* 1972;356:315–329.
92. Kallioinen M. Immunoelectron microscope demonstration of the basement membrane components laminin and type IV collagen in the dermal cylindroma. *J Pathol* 1985;147:97–102.
93. Orenstein JM, Dardick I, Van Nostrand AWP. Ultrastructural similarities of adenoid cystic carcinoma and pleomorphic adenoma. *Histopathology* 1985;9:623–638.
94. Seifert G, Donath K. Classification of the pathology of diseases of the salivary glands. Review of 2,600 cases in the salivary gland register. *Beitr Pathol Biol* 1976;159:1–32.
95. Skalowa A, Leivo I. Extracellular collagenous spherule in salivary gland tumors. *Arch Pathol Lab Med* 1992,116:649–653.
96. Skalova A. Leivo I. Basement membrane proteins in salivary gland tumors. Distribution of type IV collagen and laminin. *Virchows Arch A Pathol Anat Histopathol* 1992;420:425–431.
97. Laurie GW, Leblond CP, Martin GR. Localization of type IV collagen, laminin, heparan sulfate proteoglycan and fibronectin to the basal lamina of basement membranes. *J Cell Biol* 1982;95:340–344.
98. Sunardhi-Widyaputra S, Van-Damme B. Immunohistochemical expression of tenascin in normal human salivary glands and in pleomorphic adenomas. *Pathol Res Pract* 1993;189:138–143.
99. Eneroth CM. Salivary gland tumors in the parotid gland, submandibulary gland and the palate region. *Cancer* 1971;27:1415–1418.
100. Thackray AC, Sabin LH. Histological typing of salivary gland tumors.

In: *International histological classification of tumors,* No. 7. Geneva; World Health Organization, 1972.
101. Dardick I, Van Nostrand AWP, Asrt DJ. Rippstein P, Edwards V. Pleomorphic adenoma. I. Ultrastructural organization of "epithelial regions." *Hum Pathol* 1983;14:780–797.
102. Dardick I, Van Nostrand AWP, Phillips MJ. Histogenesis of salivary gland pleomorphic adenoma (mixed tumor) with an evaluation of the role of the myoepithelial cell. *Hum Pathol* 1982;13:62–75.
103. David R, Buchner A. Elastosis in benign and malignant salivary gland tumors. A histochemical and ultrastructural study. *Cancer* 1980;45: 2301–2310.
104. Erlandson RA, Cardon-Cardo C, Higgins PJ. Histogenesis of benign pleomorphic adenoma (mixed tumor) of the major salivary glands. An ultrastructural and immunohistochemical study. *Am J Surg Pathol* 1984;8:803–820.
105. Hubner G, Klein HJ, Kleinsasser O, Shiefer HG. Role of myoepithelial cells in the development of salivary gland tumors. *Cancer* 1971; 27:1255–1261.
106. Seifert G, Langrock I, Donath K. Pathomorphologische Subklassifikation der pleomorphen Speicheldrüsenadenome. Analyse von 310 pleomorphen Parotisadenomen. *HNO* 1976;24:415–426.
107. Shirasuma K, Sato M, Migazaki T. A myoepithelial cell line established from a human pleomorphic adenoma arising in a minor salivary gland. *Cancer* 1980;45:297–305.
108. Yanagawa T, Hayashi Y, Nagamine S, Yoshida H, Yura Y, Sato M. Generation of cells with phenotypes of both intercalated duct-type and myoepithelial cells in human parotid gland adenocarcinoma cell grown in athymic nude mice. *Virchows Arch B Cell Pathol Incl Mol Pathol* 1986;51:187–195.
109. Gallo O, Bani D, Toccafondi G, Almerigogna F, Storchi OF. Characterization of a novel cell line from pleomorphic adenoma of the parotid gland with myoepithelial phenotype and producing interlenkin-6 as an autocrine growth factor. *Cancer* 1992;70:559–568.
110. Corio RL, Sciubba JJ, Brannou RB, Batsakis J. Epithelial-myoepithelial carcinoma of intercalated duct origin. A clinicopathological and ultrastructural assessment of sixteen cases. *Oral Surg Oral Med Oral Pathol* 1982;53:280–287.
111. Donath K, Seifert G. Zur Diagnose und Ultrastruktur des tubulären Speichelgangcarcinomas. Epithelial-myoepitheliales Schaltstück carcinom. *Virchows Arch A Pathol Anat Histopathol* 1972;356:16–31.
112. Luna MA, Ordonez NG, Mackay B, Batsakis JG, Gillamandegui O. Salivary epithelial-myoepithelial carcinomas of intercalated ducts: a clinical, electron microscopic and imunohistochemical study. *Oral Surg Oral Med Oral Pathol* 1985;59:482–490.
113. Batsakis JG, El Naggar AK, Luna MA. Epithelial-myoepithelial carcinoma of salivary glands. *Ann Otol Rhinol Laryngal* 1992;101: 540–542.
114. Nistal M, García-Viera M, Martínez-García C, Paniagua R. Epithelial-myoepithelial tumor of the bronchus. *Am J Surg Pathol* 1994;18: 421–425.
115. Palmer RM. Epithelial-myoepithelial carcinoma: an immunocytochemical study. *Oral Surg Oral Med Oral Pathol* 1985;59:511–515.
116. Crissman JD, Wirman JA, Harris A. Malignant myoepithelioma of the parotid gland. *Cancer* 1977;40:3042–3049.
117. Leifer C, Miller AS, Putang PB, Harwick RD. Myoepithelioma of the parotid gland. *Arch Pathol Lab Med* 1974;98:312–319.
118. Luna MA, Mackay B, Gomez-Araujo J. Myoepithelioma of the palate. *Cancer* 1973;32:1429–1435.
119. Sciubba JJ, Brannon RB. Myoepithelioma of the salivary glands: report of 23 cases. *Cancer* 1982;49:562–572.
120. Dardick I, Canell S, Bovin M, Hoppe D, Parks WR, Stinson I, et al. Salivary gland myoepithelioma variants, histological, ultrastructural and immunological features. *Virchows Arch A Pathol Anat Histolpathol* 1989;416:25–42.
121. Martínez-Madrigal F, Santiago-Payan H, Meneses-García A, Domínguez-Malagón H, Rojas ME. Plasmocytoid myoepithelioma of the laryngeal region: a case report. *Hum Pathol* 1995;26:802–804.
122. Frierson HR, Mills SE, Gerland TA. Terminal duct carcinoma of minor salivary glands. A non-papillary subtype of polymorphous low-grade adenocarcinoma. *Am J Clin Pathol* 1985;84:8–14.
123. Gnepp D, Chen CH, Warren C. Polimorphous low-grade adenocarcinoma of minor salivary gland. An immunohistochemical and clinicopathologic study. *Am J Surg Pathol* 1984;8:367–374.
124. Dardick I, Kahn HJ, Van Nostrand AWP, Baumal R. Salivary gland monomorphic adenoma. Ultrastructural, immunoperoxidase and histogenetic aspects. *Am J Pathol* 1984;115:334–348.
125. Dardick I, Van Nostrand AWP. Myoepithelial cells in salivary gland tumors-revised. *Head Neck Surg* 1985;7:395–408.
126. Hoa W, Kech PC, Swerdlow MA. Ultrastructure of the basal cell adenoma of parotid. *Cancer* 1976;37:1322–1333.
127. Kahn HJ, Baumal R, Morks A, Dardick I, Van Nostrand AWP. Myoepithelial cells in salivary gland tumors: an immunohistochemical study. *Arch Pathol Lab Med* 1985;109:190–195.
128. Batsakis JG, Luna MA, El Naggar AK. Basaloid monomorphic adenomas. *Ann Otol Rhinol Laryngol* 1991;100:68-69.
129. Chaudry AP, Leifer C, Cutles LS, Satchidanand S, Labay GR, Yamane GM. Histogenesis of adenoid cystic carcinoma of the salivary glands. Light and electron microscopic study. *Cancer* 1986;58:72–82.
130. Chen JC, Gnepp DR, Bedrossianm CW. Adenoid cystic carcinoma of the salivary glands: an immunohistochemical analysis. *Oral Surg Oral Med Oral Pathol* 1988;65:316–326.
131. Williams SB, Ellis GL, Auclair PL. Immunohistochemical analysis of basal cell adenocarcinoma. *Oral Surg Oral Med Oral Pathol* 1993;75: 64–69.
132. Hsueh C, Gonzalez-Crussi F. Sialoblastoma: a case report and review of the literature on congenital tumors of salivary glands origin. *Pediatr Pathol* 1992;12:205–214.
133. Dehner LP, Valbuena L, Perez-Atayde A, Reddick RL, Askin FB, Rossi J. Salivary gland anlage tumor ("congenital pleomorphic adenoma"). A clinicopathologic, immunohistochemical and structural study of nine cases. *Am J Surg Pathol* 1994;18:25–36.
134. Dardick I, Daya D, Hardie J, Van Nostrand AWP. Mucoepidermoid carcinoma: ultrastructural and histogenetic aspects. *J Oral Pathol Med* 1984;13:342–358.
135. Lomax-Smith JD, Azzopardi JG. The hyaline cell: a distinctive feature of "mixed salivary tumors." *Histopathology* 1987;2:77–92.
136. Quintarelli G, Robinson L. The glycosaminoglycans of salivary gland tumors. *Am J Pathol* 1967;51:19–37.
137. Takeuchi J, Sobue M, Yoshida M, Esaki T, Katoh Y. Pleomorphic adenoma of the salivary gland. With special reference to histochemical and electron microscopic studies and biochemical analysis of glycosaminoglycans in vivo and in vitro. *Cancer* 1975;36:1771–1789.
138. Caselitz J, Osborn M, Seifert G, Weber K. Intermediate-sized filament proteins (prekeratin, vimentin, desmin,) in the normal parotid gland and parotid gland tumors. Immunofluorescence study. *Virchows Arch A Pathol Anat Histopathol* 1981;393:273–286.
139. Caselitz J, Osborn M, Wustrow J, Seifert G, Weber K. The expression of different intermediate-sized filaments in human salivary gland and other tumors. *Pathol Res Pract* 1982;175:266–278.
140. Morinaga S, Nakajma T, Shimosato Y. Normal and neoplastic myoepithelial cells in salivary glands. An immunohistochemical study. *Hum Pathol* 1987;18:1218–1226.
141. Hara K, Ito M, Takeuchi MJ, Iijima S, Endo T, Hidaka H. Distribution of S-100 protein in normal salivary glands and salivary gland tumors. *Virchows Arch A Pathol Anat Histopathol* 1983;401:237–249.
142. Markaki S, Beuropenlen V, Milas Ch. S-100 protein and neuron specific enolase (NSE), immunoreactivity in pleomorphic adenomas of the salivary glands and its relationship to the composition of their extracellular matrix. *Arch Anat Cytol Pathol* 1987;35:211–216.
143. Franquemont DW, Mills SE. Plasmocytoid monomorphic adenoma of salivary glands. Absence of myogenous differentiation and comparison to spindle cell myoepithelioma. *Am J Surg Pathol* 1993;17: 146–153.
144. Mills SE, Garland TA, Allen MS Jr. Low grade papillary adenocarcinoma of palatal salivary gland origin. *Am J Surg Pathol* 1984; 8:367–374.
145. Garland TA, Innes DJ, Fechner RE. Salivary duct carcinoma: an analysis of four cases with review of the literature. *Am J Clin Pathol* 1984; 81:436–441.
146. Chen KTK, Hafez GR. Infiltrating salivary duct carcinoma. A clinicopathologic study of five cases. *Arch Otolaryngal* 1981;107:37–39.
147. Allen MS Jr, Fitz-Hugh GS, Marsh WL Jr. Low-grade papillary adenocarcinoma of the palate. *Cancer* 1974;33:153–158.
148. Batsakis JG, McClatchery KD, Johns M, Regezi JA. Primary squamous cell carcinoma of the parotid gland. *Arch Otolaryngol Head Neck Surg* 1976;102:355–357.
149. Martínez-Madrigal F, Baden E, Casiraghi O, Micheau C. Oral and pharyngeal adenosquamous carcinoma. A report of four cases with

immunohistochemical studies. *Eur. Arch. Oto-Rhinol-Laryngol* 1991; 248:25-258.
150. Brandtzaeg P. Mucosal and glandular distribution of immunoglobulin components. Immunohistochemistry with a cold ethanol fixation technique. *Immunology* 1974;26:1101–1114.
151. Brandtzaeg P. Mucosal and glandular distribution of immunoglobulin components: differential localization of free and bound sc in secretory epithelial cells. *J Immunol* 1974;112:1553–1559.
152. Korsrud FR, Brandtzaeg P. Quantitative immunohistochemistry of immunoglobulin and J-chain-producing cells in human parotid and submandibular salivary glands. *Immunology* 1980;39:129–140.
153. Lee SK, Lim CY, Chi JG, Hashimura K, Yamada K, Kunikata M. Mori M. Immunohistochemical study of lymphoid tissue in human fetal salivary gland. *J Oral Pathol Med* 1993;22:23–29.
154. Bernier JL. Bhaskar SN. Lymphoepithelial lesions of salivary glands. *Cancer* 1958;11:1156–1179.
155. Hsu SM, Hsu PL, Nayak RN. Warthin's tumor: an immunohistochemical study of its lymphoid stroma. *Hum Pathol* 1981;12: 251–257.
156. Thompson AS; Bryant HC. Histogenesis of papillary cystadenoma lymphomatosum (Warthin's tumor) of the parotid gland. *Am J Pathol* 1950;26:807–829.
157. Azzopardi JG, Evans DJ. Malignant lymphoma of parotid gland associated with Mikulicz's disease (benign lymphoepithellial lesion). *J Clin Pathol* 1971;24:744–752.
158. Browun RB, Gaillard RA, Turner JA. The significance of aberrant or heterotopic parotid gland tissue in lymph nodes. *Ann Surg* 1953;138: 850–856.
159. Micheau C. Les ectopies salivaires. *Arch Anat Cytol Pathol* 1969;17: 179–186.
160. Neisse R. Über den Einschluss von Parotisläppen in Lymphknoten. *Anat Hefte* (Wisbaden) 1898;10(1):289–306.
161. Bairati A. Constate concrescenza fra noduli linfatici ed adenomeri delle ghiandole salivari nellúomo durante lo sviluppo e nell adulto. *Arch Biol* (Paris) 1932;43:415–450.
162. Youngs LA. Scofield HH. Heterotopic salivary gland tissue in the lower neck. *Arch Pathol Lab Med* 1967;83:550–556.
163. Curry B, Yaylor Ch W, Fisher AWF. Salivary gland heterotopia. A unique cerebellopontine angle tumor. *Arch Pathol Lab Med* 1982;106: 35–38.
164. Schochef JR, McCormick WF, Hapni NS. Salivary gland rests in the human pituitary: light and electron microscopic study. *Arch Pathol Lab Med* 1974;98:193–200.
165. Jernstrom P, Prieto C. Accessory parotid gland tissue at base of neck. *Arch Pathol Lab Med* 1962;73:53–60.
166. Willis RA. *The borderline of embryology and pathology.* London; Butterworth, 1962.
167. Willis RA. Some unusual developmental heterotopias. *BMJ* 1968; 3:267–272.
168. Dhawan IK, Bhargava S, Nayak NC. Gupta RK. Central salivary gland tumors of jaws. *Cancer* 1970;26:211–217.
169. Singer MI, Appelbaum EL, Ley KD, Heterotopic salivary tissue in the neck. *Laryngoscope* 1979;89:1772–1778.
170. Micheau C, Riou G. Oncocytes et oncocytomes. Histoenzymologie, ultrastructure et description de l' ADN mitochondrial. *Arch Anat Cytol Pathol* 1975;23:123–132.
171. Meza-Chavez L. Oxyphilic granular cell adenoma of the parotid gland (oncocytoma). Report of five cases and study of oxyphilic granular cells (oncocytes) in normal parotid gland. *Am J Pathol* 1949;25: 523–548.
172. Hamperl H. Oncocyten und Oncocytome. *Virchows Arch A Pathol Anat Histopathol* 1962;335:452–483.
173. Barka T. Biologically active polypeptides in submandibular glands. *J Histochem Cytochem* 1980;28:836–859.
174. Bing J, Paulsen K, Hackenthal E, Rix E, Taugner R. Renin in the submaxillary gland. A review. *J Histochem Cytochem* 1980;28:874–880.
175. Murphy RA, Watson AY, Metz J, Forssmann WG. The mouse submandibular gland: an exocrine organ for growth factors. *J Histochem Cytochem* 1980;28:890–902.
176. Whitley BD, Ferguson JW, Harris AJ, Kardos TB. Immunohistochemical localization of substance P in human parotid gland. *Int J Oral Maxillofac Surg* 1992;21:54–58.
177. Pikula DL, Harris EF, Desiderio DM, Fridland GH, Lovelace JL. Methionine enkephalin-like, substance P-like, and beta-endorphin-like immunoreactivity in human parotid saliva. *Arch Oral Biol* 1992,37: 705–709.
178. Salo A, Ylikoski J, Uusitalo H. Distribution of calcitonin gene-related peptide immunoreactive nerve fibers in the human submandibular gland. *Neurosci Lett* 1993,19:137–140.
179. Mathison R, Davison JS, Befus AD. Neuroendocrine regulation of inflammation and tissue repair by submandibular gland factors. *Immunol Today* 1994;15:527–532.
180. Blanck C, Eneroth CM, Jakibsson PA. Oncocytoma of the parotid gland: neoplasm or nodular hyperplasia. *Cancer* 1970;25:919–925.
181. Batsakis JG. *Tumors of the head and neck.* Baltimore; Williams & Wilkins, 1974.
182. Gray SR, Cornog JL, Seo IS. Oncocytic neoplasms of salivary glands. A report of fifteen cases including two malignant oncocytomas. *Cancer* 1976;38:1306–1317.
183. Hemenway WG, Allen GW. Chronic enlargement of the parotid gland. Hypertrophy and fatty infiltration. *Laryngoscope* 1959;69: 1508–1523.
184. Isacsson G, Lundquist PG. Salivary calculi as an aetiological factor in chronic sialadenitis of the submandibular gland. *Clin Otolaryngol* 1982;7:231–236.
185. Dradick I, Jeans MTD, Sinnot NM, Wittkuhn JF, Kahn HJ, Baumal R. Salivary gland components involved in the formation of squamous metaplasia. *Am J Pathol* 1985;119:33–43.
186. Fajardo LF, Berthrong M. Radiation injury in surgical pathology. Part III. Salivary glands, pancreas and skin. *Am J Surg Pathol* 1981; 5:279–296.
187. Seifert G, Donath K. Zur Pathoegenese des Küttner-Tumors der Submandibularis. *HNO* 1977;25:81–92.
188. Beer GM, Neuwirth A. Nekrotisierende Sialometaplasie (Speicheldrüseninfarkt) der Glandula submandibularis. *Laryngol Rhinol Otol* (Stuttg) 1983;62:468–470.
189. Abrams AM, Melrose RT, Howell FV. Necrotizing sialometaplasia. A disease simulating malignancy. *Cancer* 1973;32:130–135.
190. Seifert G, Donath K. Die Sialadenose der Parotis. *Dtsch Med Wochenschr* 1975;100:1545–1548.
191. Mandel L, Baurmash H. Parotid enlargment due to alcoholism. *J Am Dent Assoc* 1971;82:369–373.
192. Daley TD, Dardick I. An unusual parotid tumor with histogenetic implications for salivary gland neoplasms. *Oral Surg Oral Med Oral Pathol* 1983;55:374–381.
193. Thackray AC, Lucas RB. Tumors of the Major Salivary Glands. In: *Atlas of tumor pathology*, ser II, fasc 10. Washington DC; Armed Forces Institute of Pathology, 1974.
194. Dardick I, Van Nostrand AWP. Morphogenesis of salivary gland tumors. A prerequisite to improving classification. *Pathol Annu* 1987; 22:1–53.
195. Barka T. Induced cell proliferation: the effect of isoproteresol. *Exp Cell Res* 1965;37:662–679.
196. Dardick I, Dardick AM, Aackay AJ, Pastolero GC, Guillane PJ. Pathobiology of salivary glands IV. Histogenetic concepts and cycling cells in human parotid and submandibular glands cultured in floating collagen gels. *Oral Surg Oral Med Oral Pathol* 1993;76:307–318.
197. Dardick I, Burford-Mason A.P. Current status of the histogenetic and morphogenetic concepts of salivary gland tumorigenesis. *Crit Rev Oral Biol Med* 1993;4:639–677.
198. Dardick I, Van Nostrand AWP, Asrt DJ. Rippstein P, Edwards V. Pleomorphic adenoma. II. Ultrastructural organization of "stromal" regions. *Hum Pathol* 1983;14:798–809.
199. Micheau C, Lacour J. Epithelioma acineux de la parotide. *Ann Anat Pathol* 1971;16:173–188.
200. Luna MA, Batsakis JG, Ordonez NG, Mackay B, Tortoledo ME. Salivary gland adenocarcinomas: a clinicopathologic analysis of three distinctive types. *Semin Diagn Pathol* 1987;4:117–135.
201. Micheau C, Lacour J. Genin J. Brugère J. Tumeurs mucoépidermoïdes de la parotide et de la cavité buccale. *Ann Anat Pathol* 1972;17:59–71.
202. White DK, Miller AS, McDaniel RK, Rothman BN. Inverted ductal papilloma: a distinctive lesion of minor salivary gland. *Cancer* 1982; 49:519–524.
203. Zarbo RJ, Haffield JS, Trojanowski JQ, et al. Immunoreactive glial fibrillary acidic protein in normal and neoplastic salivary glands: a combined immunohistochemical and immunoblot study. *Surg Pathol* 1988;I:55–63.

204. Fantasia JE, Cally ET. Localization of free secretory component in pleomorphic adenomas of minor salivary gland origin. *Cancer* 1984; 53:1786–1789.
205. Caselitz J, Jaup T, Seifert G. Immunohistochemical detection of carcioembryonic antigen (CEA) in parotid gland carcinomas. *Virchows Arch A Pathol Anat Histopathol* 1981;394:49–60.
206. Tsuji. T, Nagai N. Production of alpha-fetoprotein by human submandibular gland. *Int J Dev Biol* 1993;37:497–498.
207. Gusterson BA, Lucas RB, Ormerod MG. Distribution of epithelial membrane antigen in benign and malignant lesions of the salivary glands. *Virchows Arch A Pathol Anat Histopathol* 1982;397:227–233.
208. Caselitz J, Seifert G, Grenner G, Schmidtberger R. Amylase as an additional marker of salivary gland neoplasms. An immunoperoxidase study. *Pathol Res Pract* 1983;176:276–283.
209. Cenley J, Baker DC. *Cancer of the salivary glands in cancer of the head and neck.* New York; Churchill Livingstone, 1981.
210. Rankow RM, Mignogna F. Cancer of the sublingual gland. *Am J Surg Pathol* 1969;118:790–795.

# Lungs

*Histology for Pathologists, second edition,*
Edited by Stephen S. Sternberg.
Lippincott-Raven Publishers, Philadelphia


# CHAPTER 18

# Lungs

Thomas V. Colby and Samuel A. Yousem



## NORMAL STRUCTURE AND HISTOLOGY

The following review is based on several standard references on the topic (1–12).

### General

The lungs are paired intrathoracic organs that are divided into lobes (three on the right—right upper lobe, right middle lobe, right lower lobe; two on the left—left upper lobe, left lower lobe), and the lobes are further divided into bronchopulmonary segments (Table 1). The segmental anatomy of the lung is important for radiologists, bronchoscopists, and pathologists in defining the location of lesions. The lobes are divided by fissures and have their own pleural investments. The segments are not separated by fissures and do not normally have separate pleural investments, although they are recognizable on the basis of their supplying bronchi (segmental bronchi).

The primordial lungs arise as ventral buds of the primitive foregut extending into the primitive thoracic mesenchyme. Bronchial cartilages, smooth muscle, and other connective tissues are derived from the mesenchyme that surrounds these dichomatously branching buds. The phases of airway and lung parenchymal development are summarized in Table 2.

### Airways

The airways serve as conduits for air traveling to and from alveoli, for evacuation of material along the mucociliary escalator, and for immunologic, protective, air-moisturizing, and warming functions.

The airways arise by dichotomous branching of the bronchial buds. In a normal individual, there are approximately 20 generations extending from the trachea to the respiratory bronchioles. Airways are tubular structures with muscle in their walls and an inner epithelial lining. In histologic sections from normal lungs, the diameter of an airway is approximately the same size as its accompanying artery (and vice versa) (13). Disparities in size (of either airway or artery) suggest a pathologic condition. Airways are defined as follows:

**Bronchi** are cartilaginous airways, more than 1 mm in diameter. They are conducting airways with cartilage in their walls that prevent their collapse.

**Bronchioles** are airways less than 1 mm in diameter that lack cartilage (Fig. 1).

T.V. Colby: Department of Laboratory Medicine and Pathology, Mayo Clinic, Rochester, Minnesota 55905.

S.A. Yousem: Department of Pathology, Presbyterian University Hospital, Pittsburgh, Pennsylvania 15213.

**TABLE 1.** *Bronchopulmonary segments*[a]

| | |
|---|---|
| Right upper lobe | Left upper lobe |
| 1. Apical | 1,2. Apical posterior |
| 2. Posterior | 3. Anterior |
| 3. Anterior | Lingula |
| Right middle lobe | 4. Superior |
| 4. Lateral | 5. Inferior |
| 5. Medial | Left lower lobe |
| Right lower lobe | 6. Superior |
| 6. Superior | 7. Anterior-medial basal |
| 7. Medial basal | 8. Lateral basal |
| 8. Anterior basal | 9. Posterior basal |
| 9. Lateral basal | |
| 10. Posterior basal | |

[a] Modified from reference 12.

These nonrespiratory bronchioles include terminal bronchioles which represent the bronchioles just proximal to respiratory bronchioles.

Respiratory bronchioles are airways that have alveoli budding from their walls.

Cell types lining the airways include basal cells, Kulchitsky's cells, ciliated cells, serous cells, Clara cells, goblet cells, intermediate cells, and brush cells. Ultrastructural abnormalities in the ciliated cells of the respiratory tract are known to be associated with pathologic conditions (e.g., immotile cilia syndrome). (For a review of the normal structure of the cilia, the reader is referred to reference 12.) Goblet cells and ciliated cells decrease in number as the terminal bronchioles are approached; there is a concomitant increase in Clara cells, and the mucosa becomes less columnar and more cuboidal in appearance. Clara cells have secretory functions (e.g., surfactant-like material) and also act as progenitor cells after bronchiolar injury. Clara cell differentiation in tumors of the lung may be appreciated by the presence of apical periodic acid-Schiff (PAS)-positive, diastase-resistant granules, as well as by their electron microscopic apical-dense granules. Kulchitsky's cells contain dense core granules and are part of the diffuse neuroendocrine system. Aggregates of neuroepithelial cells are called "neuroepithelial bodies." They tend to occur at airway bifurcations. The cell types in the airways and parenchyma are summarized in Table 3 and illustrated in Figures 2, 3, and 4.

Submucosal salivary-type glands containing both serous and mucous cells are found in the larger bronchi. In older individuals, oncocytic metaplasia can be seen in these glands (Fig. 5). Within the walls of the large airways, ganglia, nerves, and bronchial arteries are found.

Lambert's canals are direct communications between bronchioles and adjacent alveolar parenchyma that are rarely visible in histologic sections. They are thought to be involved in collateral ventilation of adjacent parenchyma, as well as the origin of metaplastic bronchiolar epithelium lining peribronchiolar alveoli following bronchiolar injury (Fig. 6).

## Lobule and Acinus

The lung lobule is grossly visible and represents the smallest anatomic subunit of the lung that is bounded by connective tissue (interlobular) septa (Fig. 7). Lobules are approximately 2 cm in diameter and are visible to the naked eye on both the pleural surface of the lung and on cut surfaces of the parenchyma. Lobules are accentuated in fibrotic conditions in which the septa contract (e.g., honeycombing). Pulmonary lobules are identifiable with high-resolution computerized tomography (CT) scanning of the lung. The term "lobule" as used here has also been referred to as the secondary lobule of Miller (12). The use of the term *secondary lobule* is discouraged because it implies that there is a primary lobule, and the latter term is not in current usage.

The functional unit of the lung is the acinus where gas transfer takes place (Fig. 8). The precise definition of the acinus has varied. For the purpose of this review, the acinus includes the lung tissue supplied by a single terminal bronchiole (10,12). According to this definition of the acinus, each pulmonary lobule comprises some 3 to 10 acini. The acinus has also been defined as a respiratory bronchiole and its supplied alveolar ducts and sacs; using this definition, each lobule comprises some 20 to 30 acini.

Squamous (type 1 pneumocytes) and cuboidal (type 2 or granular pneumocytes) epithelial cells line the alveoli (Table 3). Gas exchange takes place across the cytoplasm of type 1 cells. Type 2 cells are the progenitor cells for type 1 cells, produce surfactant, and proliferate after injury to restore alveolar epithelial integrity. Type 2 cell hyperplasia represents a nonspecific marker of alveolar injury and repair. Macrophages are a common finding, lining the surfaces of the alveoli and percolating into the interstitium; a number of

**TABLE 2.** *Phases of lung development*

| Phase | Gestation | Major Events |
|---|---|---|
| Embryonic | 26 days to 6 weeks | Development of major airways |
| Pseudoglandular | 6 to 16 weeks | Development of airways to terminal bronchioles |
| Canalicular | 16 to 28 weeks | Development of the acinus and its vascularization |
| Saccular | 28 to 36 weeks | Subdivision of saccules by secondary crests |
| Alveolar | 36 weeks to term (and up to 4 years of age) | Acquisition of alveoli |

**TABLE 3.** *Major cell types of the lower respiratory tract*[a]

| Cell Type | Features | Function(s) | Location | Comments |
|---|---|---|---|---|
| Ciliated | Columnar, cuboidal, ciliated bronchial lining cells; each cell has approximately 250 cilia at the apical surface and each cilium is approximately 6 μm long | Proximal transport of mucus stream (mucociliary escalator) | Bronchi and bronchioles | Decreased number and morphologic abnormalities seen with chronic irritation |
| Goblet | Columnar mucus-secreting cells; contain mucus glycoprotein which discharges apically | Contribute to airway mucus | Bronchi, more numberous proximally; small numbers in bronchioles | Increased number in chronic airway irritation |
| Basal | Short cells with relatively little cytoplasm oriented along the basement membrane; do not reach the luminal surface of the epithelium | Precursor cell of ciliated and goblet cells | Bronchi; rare in bronchioles | — |
| Neuroendocrine (Kulchitsky or K cells) | Basal-oriented cells with numerous dense core (neurosecretory) granules; single or in groups (neuroepithelial bodies), the latter near sites of airway bifurcation | Specific functions not known in detail; considered part of the diffuse neuroendocrine system | Bronchi; rare in bronchioles | — |
| Neuroendocrine bodies | Clusters of 4–10 neuroendocrine cells adjacent to the subepithelial basement membrane | Unknown; some suggest chemoreceptor, tactile receptor, basoconstrictive functions | Bronchi, bronchioles, and alveoli | — |
| Oncocytic | Eosinophilic mitochrondral-rich cells in submucosa gland rich cells in submucosal gland ducts | Ion secretory functions | Submucosal glands | Increasing number with aging |
| Squamous | Stratified squamous epithelium as an abnormal reaction replacement; normal pseudostratified respiratory epithelium | Protective, reparative | Bronchi, bronchioles, and occasionally alveoli | Metaplastic response to irritation or repair |
| Clara | Columnar nonciliated bronchiolar cells; protuberant apical cytoplasm with large ovoid electron-dense granules, comprise the majority of nonciliated bronchiolar cells | Secretory functions contributing to the mucus pool and maintaining extracellular lining fluid; progenitor for other bronchiolar cells; role in surfactant production | Predominantly in bronchioles | — |
| Type 1 alveolar pneumocyte | Large, flat, squamous alveolar lining cells; cover some 93% of alveolar surface area; incapable of division | Provide a thin air/blood interface for gas transfer | Alveoli | — |
| Type 2 alveolar pneumocyte | Columnar alveolar lining cells; microvillous surface; synthesize and secrete surfactant (lamellar ultrastructural inclusions); capable of division | Maintain alveolar stability; stem cell alveoli acting as progenitor for type 1 pneumocytes | Alveoli | Increased in reparative states and as a response to chronic injury |
| Minor salivary tissue<br>Serous cells<br>Mucus cells<br>Ductal cells | Submucosal minor salivary glands identical to other sites with serous and mucinous acinar cells which secrete into the ducts which empty at the mucosal surface | Secretion and contribution to airway mucus stream | Bronchial submucosa | — |
| Other cells | Endothelial cells and pericytes<br>Interstitial fibrocytes, fibroblasts, and myofibroblasts<br>Macrophages<br>Lymphoid cells<br>Mast cells<br>Mesothelial pleural lining<br>Cartilage and bone<br>Smooth muscle<br>Peripheral nerves<br>Myoepithelial cells | | | |

[a] Modified from reference 41.

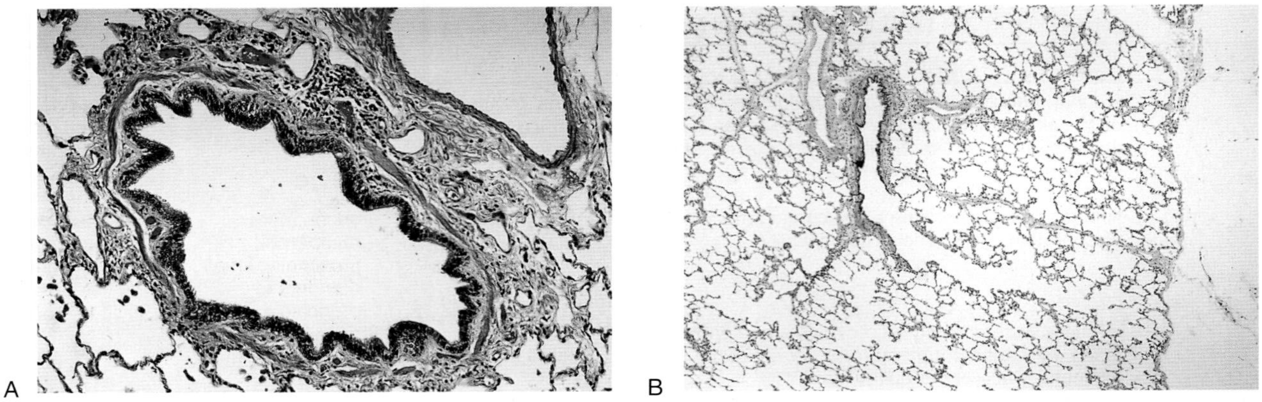


**FIG. 1.** Normal bronchioles. The bronchiole depicted in (**A**) has a luminal diameter approximately the same as that as of its accompanying pulmonary artery (the latter is not completely shown). The mucosa is low columnar, and there is no thickening of the submucosa. There is a circumferential layer of smooth muscle and an adventitial layer. The small amount of lymphoid tissue present in the wall of the bronchiole is probably abnormal but is a relatively common finding that often has no apparent clinical significance. The terminal bronchiole depicted in (**B**) (*left upper center*) is continuous with a respiratory bronchiole (*center left*) which leads into alveolar ducts and, ultimately, alveoli.

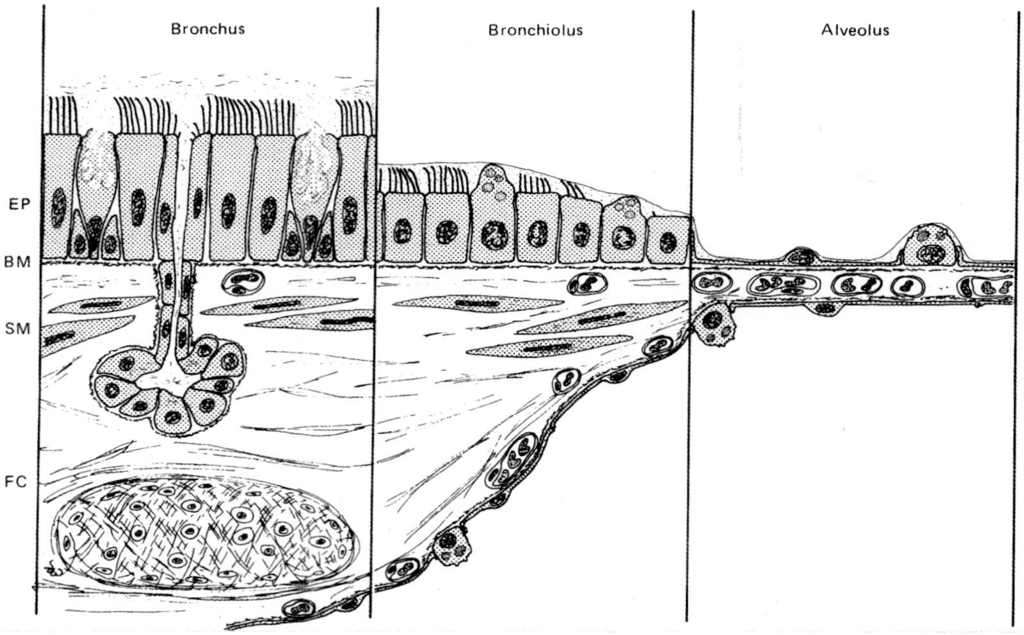


**FIG. 2.** Respiratory tract epithelia. There is a progression of pseudostratified columnar epithelium in the large airways to a more cuboidal epithelium in the small airways, to large squamous-type epithelial cells (type 1 pneumocytes) in the alveoli. The epithelium in the large airways is designed for maintaining and moving the mucus stream, whereas the squamous pneumocytes in the airspaces facilitate gas transfer. (Fig. 2 is reproduced from Weibel ER, Taylor CR. Design and Structure of the Human Lung. In: Fishman AP, ed. *Pulmonary diseases and disorders,* Vol 1. 2nd ed. New York; McGraw-Hill, 1988;p. 14, with permission.)

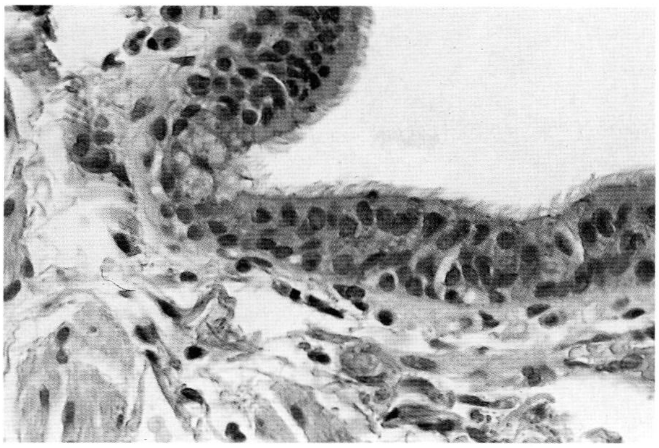

A

**FIG. 3.** Bronchial epithelium. Normal bronchial epithelium is pseudostratified and columnar with numerous ciliated cells and scattered basophilic and flocculent-appearing goblet cells (**A**). An ultrastructural schematic (**B**) of bronchial epithelium shows the various cell types present. (Fig. 3B reproduced from Sorokin SP. The respiratory system. In: Weiss L, ed. *Cell and tissue biology: a textbook of histology. 6th ed.*. Baltimore; Williams & Wilkins, 1988; p. 769, with permission.)

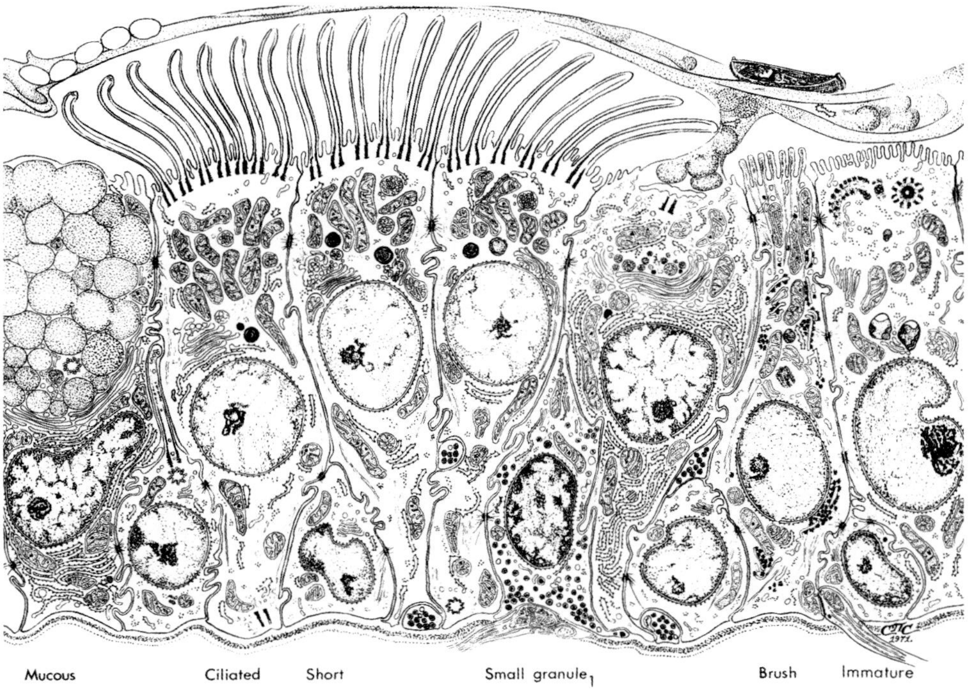


B

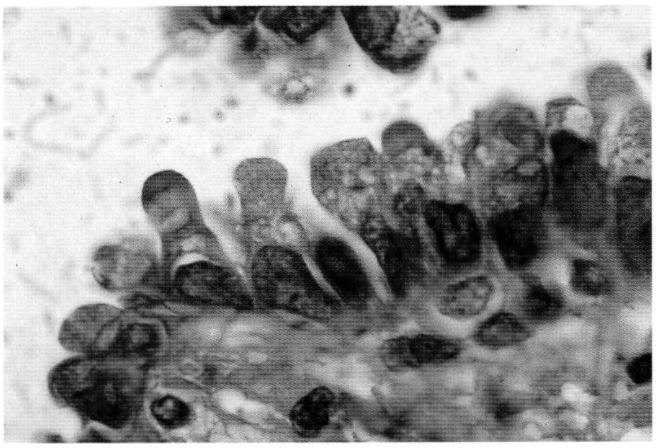

**FIG. 4.** Clara cells. Although Clara cells can sometimes be identified in bronchioles, they are seen to best advantage in neoplasms such as in this nonmucinous bronchioloalveolar carcinoma. The apical snouting and increased cytoplasmic density are well seen.

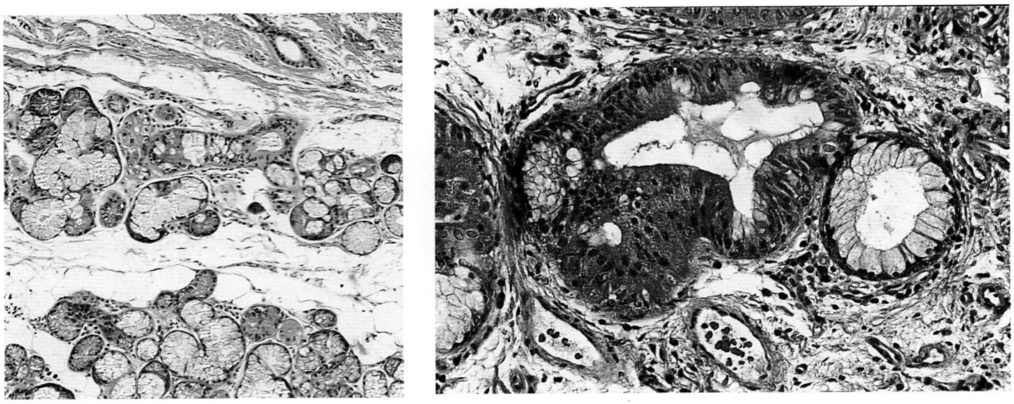

A B

**FIG. 5.** Bronchial submucous glands. The bronchial submucosal glands are normally located in the submucosa above the bronchial cartilage and contain mixed seromucous glands with a duct leading to the bronchial mucosal surface (**A**). Oncocytic metaplasia involving bronchial submucosal gland ducts is relatively common (**B**).

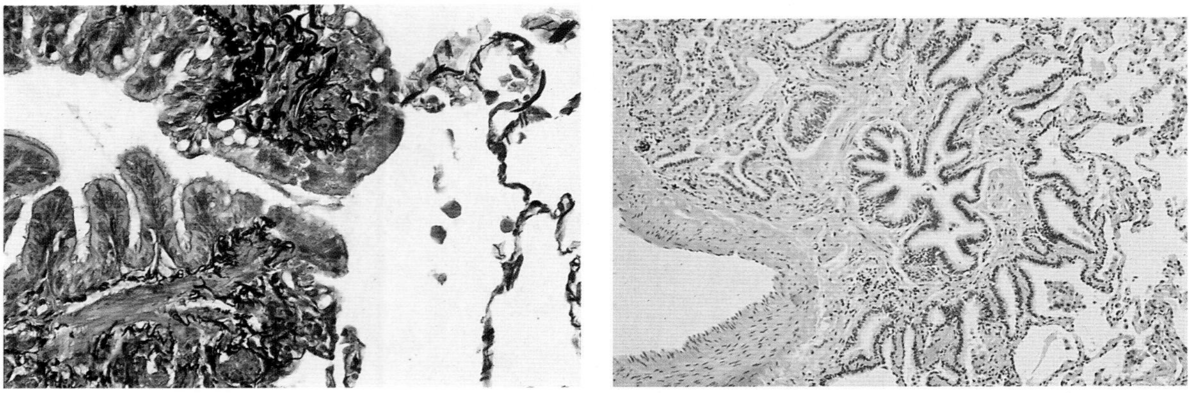

A B

**FIG. 6.** Lambert's canals. These canals (communications between nonrespiratory bronchioles and adjacent alveoli) are only rarely seen in histologic sections (**A**). It is these canals that are thought to be the origin of the bronchiolar metaplasia (lambertosis) which is seen as a repair phenomenon involving peribronchiolar alveoli after bronchiolar injury (**B**).

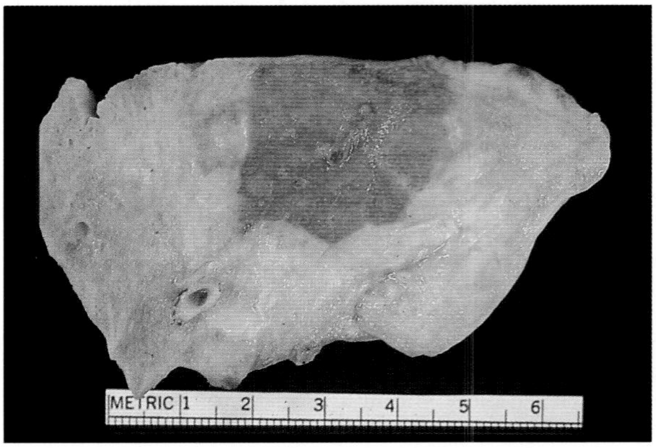


**FIG. 7.** Pulmonary lobule. This cut section of normal lung tissue (from an explanted lung that could not be used for transplantation) shows focal hemorrhage highlighting a pulmonary lobule. The hemorrhage stops abruptly at the interlobular septa and, centrally, a bronchovascular bundle can be appreciated. This lobule is approximately 2 cm in diameter.

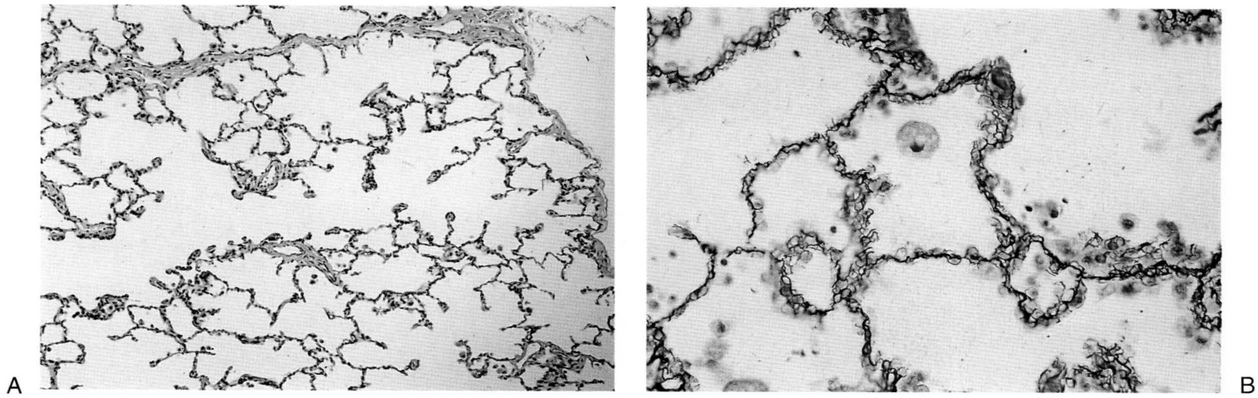

**FIG. 8.** Distal lung parenchyma. The acinus is the functional unit of the lung where gas transfer takes place. An alveolar duct extends from the left to right and communicates directly with alveolar spaces (**A**). A small interlobular septum is present at the top of the figure and the pleura is present at the right. (From the case as illustrated in Fig. 1B.) Reticulin stain (**B**) highlights the vasculature of the alveolar septum, showing pulmonary capillaries winding around the axis of the alveolar wall to maximize gas transfer surface area. A foamy alveolar macrophage is present (*upper center*), a normal finding in lung parenchyma.

subpopulations of pulmonary macrophages are definable, based on their anatomic locations and their role in most defense clearance functions (14).

The epithelial and capillary basement membranes in the alveolar septum are irregularly fused. Gas transfer takes place across the alveolar-capillary membrane, which includes the attenuated cytoplasm of the type 1 cell, the endothelial cell cytoplasm and their fused basement membranes. Pores of Kohn represent direct communications between adjacent alveoli via a "pore" in the alveolar wall. They are thought to be involved in collateral ventilation. Pores of Kohn are rarely visible with the light microscope.

An interstitial space is present in some regions of the alveolar wall and perivascular areas, and it contains collagen, elastic fibers, mesenchymal cells, and a few inflammatory cells. This space is normally inconspicuous in adults. In children (up to approximately age 4) apparent interstitial widening and increased cellularity are a normal histologic finding.

Given the concentration of nuclei of the various cell types comprising the alveolar wall, it may be difficult to decide what degree of cellularity is pathologic. Although one may attempt to count nuclei in a single alveolar wall, it is more practical to look for inflammatory cell infiltrates in the perivenular regions and to compare various foci in the biopsy, since interstitial infiltrates are rarely perfectly uniform.

## Vasculature

The pulmonary vasculature includes bronchial (systemic) arteries and veins, pulmonary arteries and veins, and the alveolar microvasculature. Large (elastic) pulmonary arteries in infants are similar to the aorta in structure, although the elastic fiber lamellae become more irregular, fragmented, and less compact in adulthood. The muscular pulmonary arteries and arterioles have an internal and external elastic membrane; pulmonary veins have only a single (outer) elastica (Fig. 9) and a smudgy hyalinized collagenous cuff. Small parenchymal pulmonary veins merge into larger veins in the interlobular septa.

It may be difficult to separate small pulmonary arterioles from venules, especially since a single elastic lamina forms as arterioles get smaller. In pathologic states the veins may develop muscular hypertrophy and increased mural thickening (arterialization). The location of the vessel, particularly whether it is in a septum or accompanied by an airway, is extremely helpful (and sometimes the only way) to separate pulmonary veins from pulmonary arteries. In mild or early pulmonary hypertension, the pulmonary arteries may appear normal; in general, pressure measurements taken at catheterization are more reliable than histologic subtleties in determining the pressure and degree of pulmonary hypertension.

## Lymphatics and Lymphoid Tissue

The lung is invested with a rich supply of lymphatics and lymphoid tissue. Lymphatic channels are found along bronchovascular structures and pulmonary veins, and in the septa and pleura. Lymphatics do not extend into alveolar walls. The lymphatics are inconspicuous except in pathologic states such as pulmonary edema or lymphangitic carcinoma. Lymphoreticular infiltrates and some pneumoconioses have a distribution along the lymphatic routes, but the lymphatic vessels themselves may not be prominent.

Lymphoid tissue may be seen as small collections of lymphocytes along the lymphatic routes, especially branch points of the bronchovascular bundles; lymphoid tissue is generally absent or inconspicuous except in pathologic states. Lymphoid tissue along the airways is part of the diffuse mucosa-associated lymphoid tissue (MALT), and in the

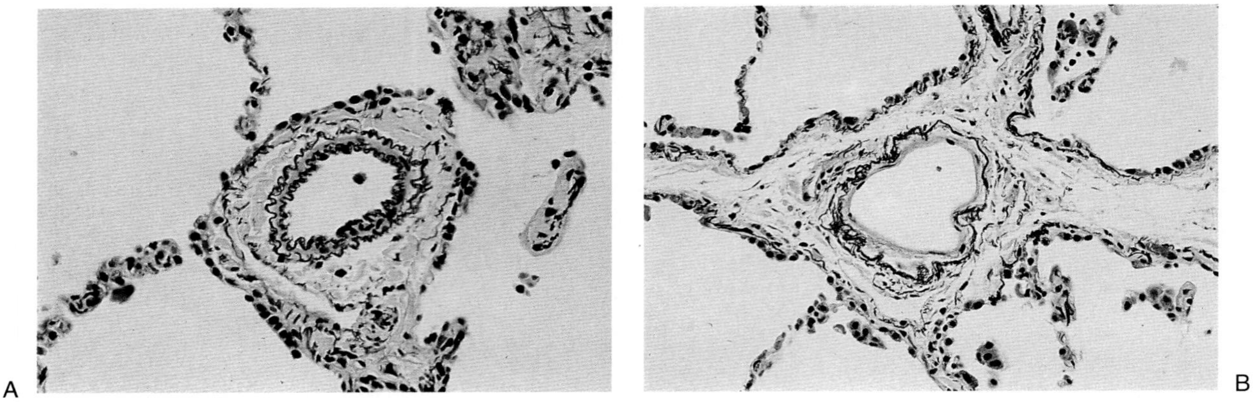


**FIG. 9.** Pulmonary vasculature. Normal pulmonary arteries contain two elastic lamina (A), whereas veins have a single elastic lamina (**B**). The location of a vessel within a septum (B) is also very helpful in identifying it as a vein.

lung is labeled bronchus-associated lymphoid tissue (BALT). Submucosal lymphoid tissue in the intermediate and small airways is associated with flattening and attenuation of the overlying respiratory mucosa ("lymphoepithelium"). At these sites, lymphocyte emperipolesis is common and is thought to reflect active antigen processing by the BALT. BALT displays the same reactions observed in lymphoid tissue at other sites, for example, reactive hyperplasia and immunoblastic proliferation which can be confused with lymphoreticular malignancies. BALT also shares features of MALT as seen at other sites. In normal adult lungs, BALT is rarely present, and its presence correlates with some form of chronic antigenic stimulation (15–17). According to Tschernig et al., BALT is not present at birth, but is found normally with increasing age, probably due to exposure to environmental antigens (17). After the individual has been exposed to most of the common antigens, the BALT regresses and dendritic cells in the airways assume the role of antigen uptake and presentation. Its reappearance in adults follows chronic antigen stimuli such as chronic infection.

As currently defined, BALT refers only to lymphoid tissue along the airways (18) and not to the lymphoid tissue that may be seen in the pleura and septa as part of diffuse lymphoid hyperplasia in the lung. To any casual observer of lung pathology, hyperplasia of BALT is frequently accompanied by lymphoid hyperplasia at these other sites, and whether lymphoid tissue at these other sites is separate and distinct from BALT, or part of the BALT system, remains to be clarified.

Intrapulmonary peribronchial lymph nodes are a normal finding, but peripheral intraparenchymal lymph nodes are unusual. Although in smokers and others with high dust exposure, they are increasingly recognized (and biopsied) with current imaging techniques (19). Intrapulmonary lymph nodes are usually septal or subpleural in location. Anthracosis in the nodes is common.

### Pleura

The visceral pleura contains connective tissue, an elastic lamina, and an outer mesothelial layer. Elastic tissue stains are useful in assessing whether a given pathologic process is confined within or transgresses the visceral pleura (20). When the pleura is fibrotic and in foci of pleural adhesions, vessels may be thick and sclerotic or pseudoangiomatous in appearance. Fatty metaplasia is often striking in foci of pleural and subpleural scarring. Because of its separate vascular supply, the pleura often remains viable over pulmonary infarcts. Submesothelial fibroblasts may undergo mesothelial metaplasia (and become cytokeratin-positive) in inflammatory lesions of the pleura.

## PATTERN RECOGNITION BASED ON NORMAL ANATOMIC LANDMARKS

It is useful to define pathologic conditions in the lung in terms of the normal anatomic landmarks (Fig. 10). This can usually be done with diffuse diseases and often with localized processes. Such an exercise in diffuse lung disease is extremely useful in correlation with gross findings, as well as with high-resolution CT scanning. The following patterns can be recognized:

Angiocentric (e.g., vasculitis, emboli)
Broncho/bronchiolocentric (e.g., viral bronchiolitis)
Pleural/subpleural
Lymphatic (e.g., lymphoreticular lesions)
Peripheral acinar, which may be deceptive because peripheral acinar regions are found in subpleural, paraseptal, and peribronchial regions (e.g., usual interstitial pneumonia)
Septal (e.g., chronic passive congestion)
Airspace (e.g., bacterial pneumonia)
Diffuse interstitial (e.g., drug reaction)
Random (e.g., miliary infection)

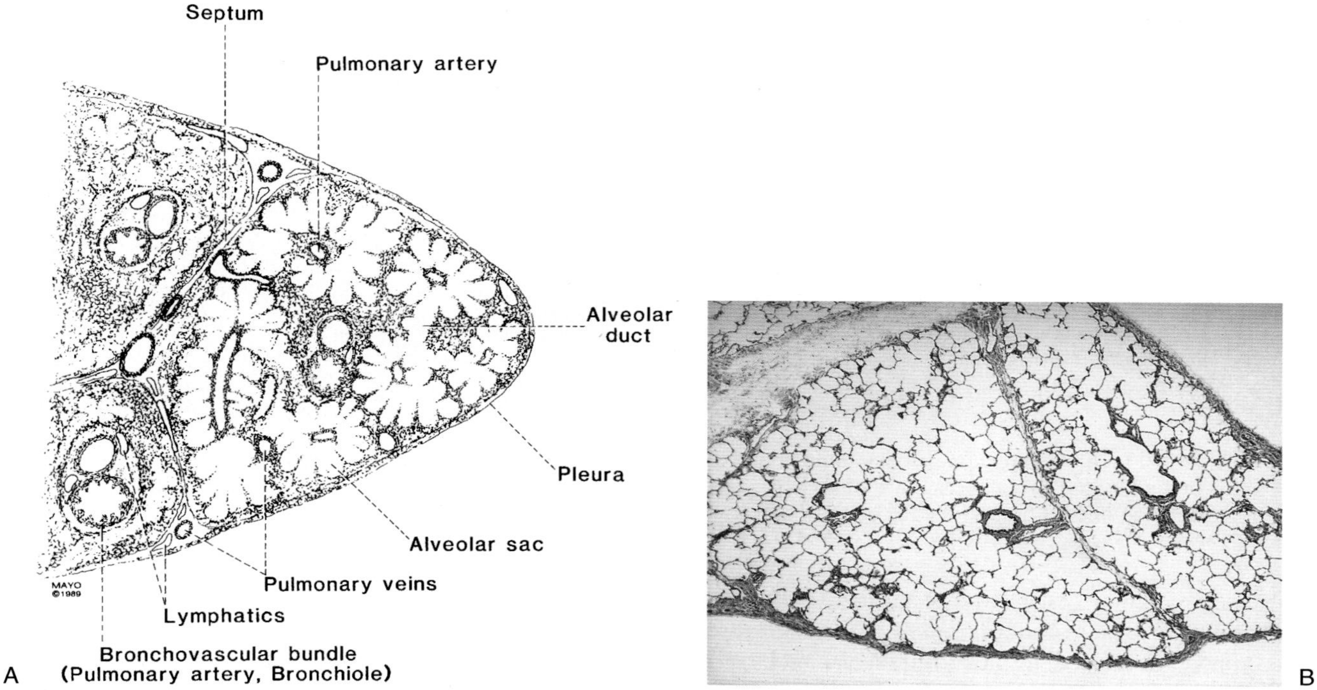


**FIG. 10.** Wedge lung biopsy. The stylized diagram (**A**) is used to depict anatomic landmarks. Structures depicted in (A) can be appreciated in an actual wedge biopsy specimen (**B**).

## SITE-SPECIFIC CHANGES COMMONLY SEEN IN SURGICAL PATHOLOGY MATERIAL

Site-specific changes that may be primary lesions or incidental findings in surgical material are shown in Table 4.

Biopsies from lobar tips, particularly from the lingula or right middle lobe, may show nonspecific and incidental inflammatory changes (21). These sites are frequently biopsied because of their accessibility. They may show nonspecific interstitial fibrosis, epithelial metaplasia, and even focal honeycombing, all of which may not be representative of an underlying process, but are, instead, due to old pneumonias that have left residual scars in these poorly drained and vascularized regions of the lung. Biopsy specimens from these sites should be discouraged in chronic interstitial lung disease, but if they are to be taken, the pathologist should insist that they be at least 3 cm in greatest dimension in order to help avoid sampling error. The possibility of middle lobe syndrome (22,23) and its lingular counterpart should be considered for persistent infiltrates in these sites.

**TABLE 4.** *Site-specific changes*

1. Inflammatory changes at lobar tips, especially lingula and right middle lobe
2. Apical caps: pleural and subpleural fibrosis in the apex
3. Upper lobe centriacinar emphysema
4. Visceral pleural/subpleural fibrosis ("subpleural blebs")

Apical caps (Fig. 11) were once thought to be the result of healed tuberculosis, but they are quite nonspecific, common in patients who have never had tuberculosis, and are now thought to be an ischemic alteration related to their apical position (24,25). Apical caps are regions of fibrosis in the pleura and immediate subpleural parenchyma that are rich in thickened elastic fibers; the background structure of collapsed alveolar walls and interposed eosinophilic collagen can often be discerned in the tissue; elastic tissue stains enhance their recognition. Ossification and nests and tubules lined by metaplastic atypical pneumocytes may be present. The changes are sufficiently distinctive that apical caps can often be recognized histologically, even when one does not know the site of origin; although, any ancient lung scar may sometimes show a similar elastotic appearance. Apical caps in older individuals may be biopsied to exclude a carcinoma or a visceral pleural tumor.

Centriacinar (centrilobular) emphysema is a pathologic abnormality that is more severe in the upper lobes; it is found predominantly in cigarette smokers and is a common finding in lobes resected for bronchogenic carcinoma. Emphysematous changes are frequently accompanied by some degree of fibrosis, particularly where bullous change is present. The fibrosis tends to appear as strands of dense, hypocellular collagenous septa traversing the emphysematous spaces, often with distinctive terminal collagenous knots. Anthracosis is also a common finding in smokers and urban dwellers. Patchy nonspecific pleural and subpleural fibrosis (Fig. 12)

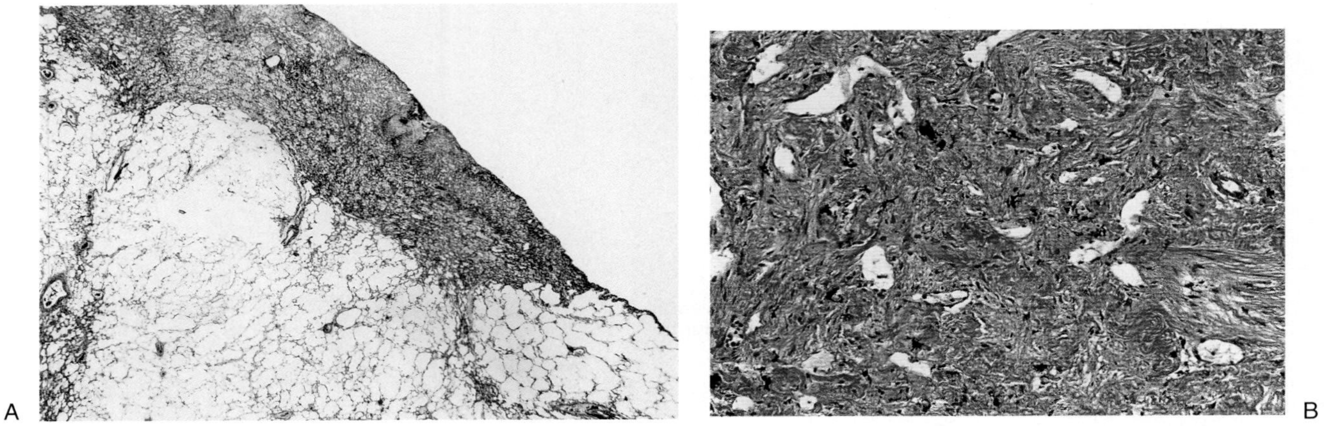

FIG. 11. **A**, Apical caps are biconvex zones of fibrosis with patchy, chronic inflammation in the apices of the lungs. **B**, Apical caps are often rich in elastic tissue fibers and anthracotic pigment, and the ghost outlines of background alveoli occasionally can be discerned.

is extremely common, especially as an incidental microscopic finding in lobar resections from smokers with a carcinoma. Abnormal airspaces formed by irregular fibrous septa are accompanied by smooth muscle hyperplasia, mucostasis, bronchiolar metaplasia, and occasional granulomas.

Subpleural blebs (Fig. 12) are often the only pathologic change found in patients who have had recurrent pneumothoraces (26). By convention blebs are less than 1.0 cm in diameter and are usually derived from air dissection into the visceral pleura; bullae are 1.0 cm or greater in diameter (27). Their rupture introduces air into the pleural space, inciting a mesothelial proliferation with numerous macrophages and giant cells, and eosinophils called eosinophilic pleuritis. This reaction may accompany any condition that is associated with pneumothorax (28). Collections of interstitial air, with or without giant cell reaction, may be an accompanying finding. Focal subpleural scarring can usually be distinguished from chronic fibrosing interstitial pneumonias by its restriction to the subpleural region, lack of fibroblastic proliferation, and the relative abrupt transition to normal alveolar walls. Clinical history and radiographic findings may also be supportive.

When an interstitial lung disease such as eosinophilic granuloma or lymphangioleiomyomatosis has resulted in pneumothorax, both the primary process and the secondary eosinophilic pleuritis may be recognizable on the biopsy.

Adhesions between the pleura and chest wall are composed of fibrovascular tissue with pockets of bland mesothelial cells, and are identical to their intraperitoneal counterparts. Dense, hyalinized fibrotic pleural plaques (29–31) are the consequence of a variety of prior inflammatory events. Their presence bilaterally often is an incidental finding, and

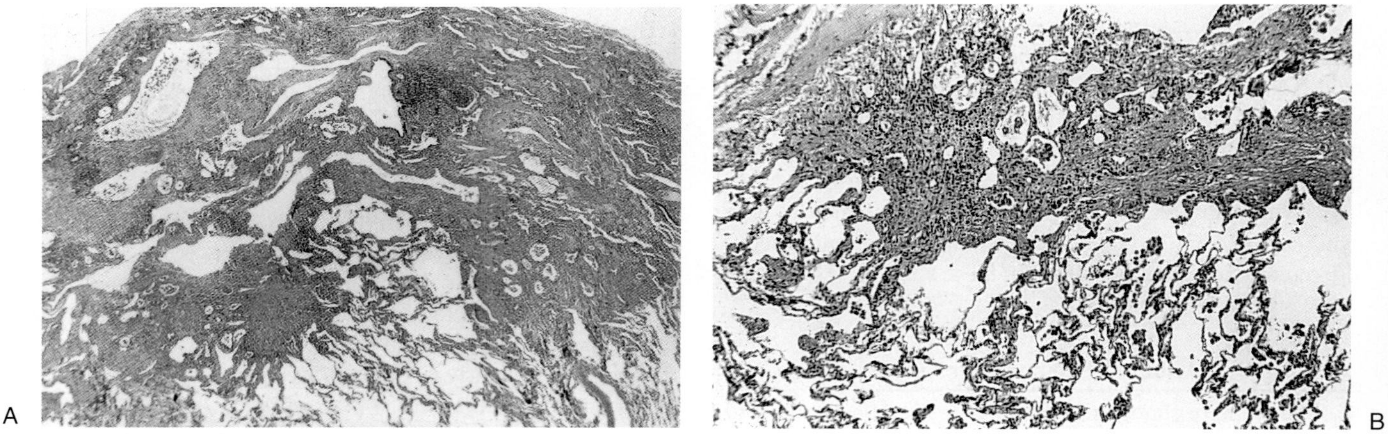

FIG. 12. Subpleural blebs and focal subpleural fibrosis. **A**, An open lung biopsy from a patient with a normal chest radiograph and history of pneumothorax shows zones of pleural and subpleural scarring with bleb formation. **B**, The subpleural fibrosis shows sharp demarcation from chest and normal lung. The presence of normal underlying lung and a negative chest radiograph in an asymptomatic patient exclude the possibility of diffuse lung disease.

if there is no obvious inflammatory cause, prior asbestos exposure is likely.

## ARTIFACTS SEEN IN LUNG BIOPSY AND RESECTION MATERIAL

Artifacts related to lung biopsy of prior procedures are shown in Table 5.

Knowledge of the clinical course of events prior to lung biopsy usually allows the pathologist to avoid misinterpreting changes of prior instrumentation. Previous bronchial biopsies may cause airway inflammation, ulceration, and a granulation tissue reaction. Strips of epithelium may be dislodged by mechanical trauma and embedded in inspissated mucus, but they are not associated with submucosal inflammation. Residual basal cells may be all that is left adhering to the basement membrane. Bronchoalveolar lavage can produce vacuolation of alveolar pneumocytes and macrophages. Previous needle biopsies may induce necrosis and hemorrhage, followed by organization and reactive epithelial atypia (Fig. 13). Patients who have been on positive-pressure ventilation (Fig. 14) may have disproportionate bronchiolar and alveolar duct distension, especially when high inspiratory pressures are used in the adult respiratory distress syndrome (ARDS). Some associated acute inflammatory exudate in the lumen is common, often with relative absence of associated inflammation in the airway wall.

Compression of lung tissue, particularly in transbronchial biopsies, may produce rounded spaces in alveoli that resemble fat vacuoles and can easily be mistaken for exogenous lipoid pneumonia (Fig. 15). This artifactual change can be recognized because there are no macrophages with small intracytoplasmic lipid vacuoles (all the vacuoles are extracellular), and there is usually little fibrosis which is a constant feature of chronic exogenous lipoid pneumonia.

Compression of airways produces crinkling and telescoping of the epithelium, similar to that seen in endometrial biopsies; sometimes entire strips of mucosa are displaced into the alveolar spaces. Compression-induced nuclear smearing artifact can be produced in any cellular tumor and even in normal bronchial mucosa. It may suggest small cell carcinoma. Lymphomas and carcinoid tumors may be extremely difficult to distinguish from small cell carcinoma when this phenomenon is present. Recognition of these diagnostic pitfalls, examining multiple levels, and enlisting the aid of concomitant cytology specimens and immunohistochemistry, allows resolution of most cases. In rare instances, rebiopsy may be necessary.

Atelectasis may be misinterpreted as interstitial pneumonia or interstitial fibrosis because the apposition of alveolar walls produces apparent scarring and hypercellularity (Fig. 16). With experience this change can be recognized on routine hematoxylin and eosin (H&E) sections; connective tissue stains show an absence of scarring and a normal background of supporting fibrous tissue along vessels and in septa. In atelectatic lung, the vessels and septa may appear to have more collagen than normal and to be thickened because they are contracted and shortened. Careful assessment of the nuclei in atelectatic lung shows that most are endothelial or epithelial in origin, rather than inflammatory, because they lack the typical chromatin of lymphocytes or plasma cells. Leukocyte common antigen stain and stains for other lymphoid markers may be useful in this setting. It is also unusual in open biopsies (and larger specimens) for the entire specimen to be uniformly atelectatic, and, therefore, a low-power

**TABLE 5.** *Artifacts seen in lung biopsies and resections*

1. Changes related to prior instrumentation including bronchoscopy, bronchoalveolar lavage, needle aspiration, and ventilatory assistance
2. Compression/atelectasis; pseudolipoid change
3. Hemorrhage/inflammatory changes
4. Septal edema, lymphatic dilatation
5. Material from surgical gloves, for example, talc and starch
6. Inflation-induced alveolar distension resembling emphysema and patchy atelectasis in underinflated zones

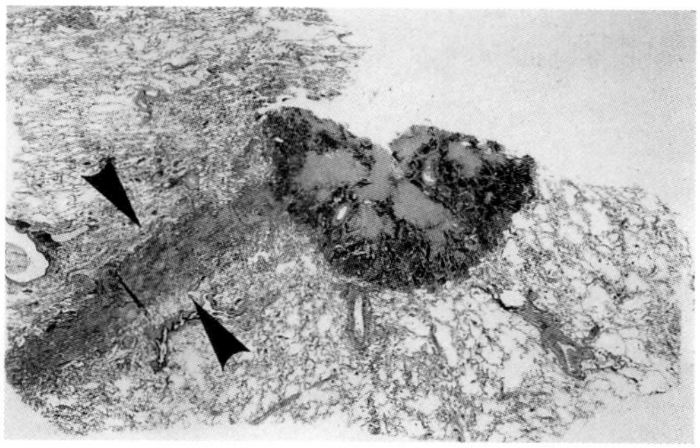

**FIG. 13.** Needle tract to a small peripheral adenocarcinoma. The biopsy had been performed a week earlier, and the needle tract shows evidence of hemorrhage, necrosis, organization, and epithelial regeneration.

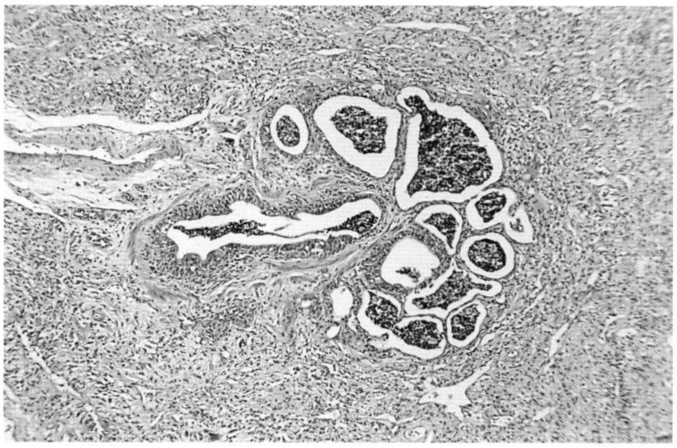

**FIG. 14.** The changes of positive-pressure respirator therapy in this patient with diffuse alveolar damage (clinically ARDS) are distension of the bronchioles, flattening of their epithelium, and an acute inflammatory exudate in the lumen with minimal change in the surrounding airway walls.

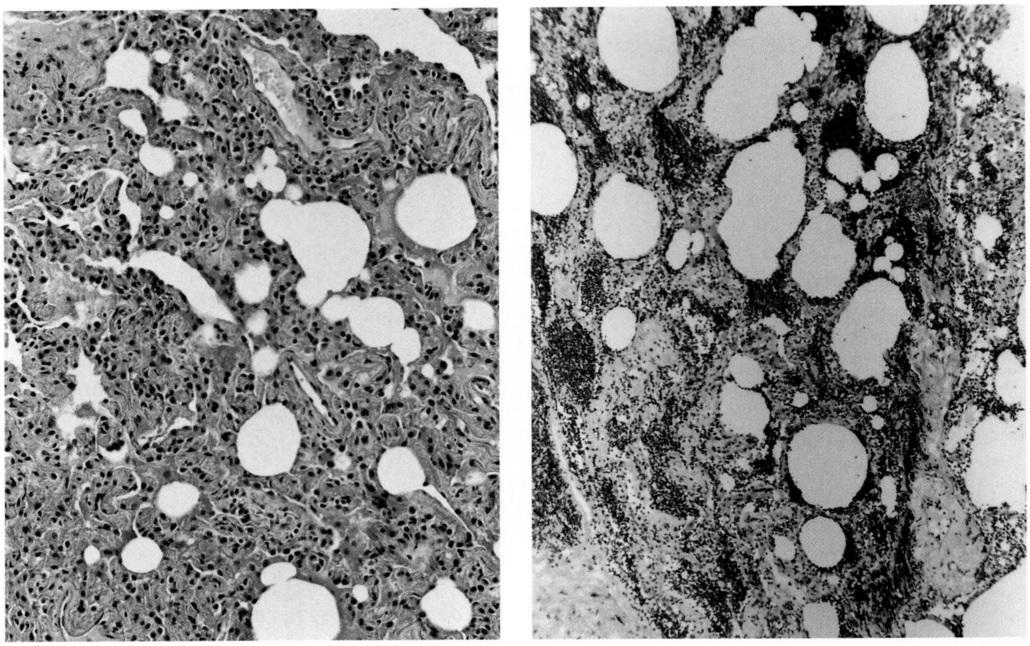

A B

FIG. 15. Pseudolipoid change in surgically induced pulmonary hemorrhage. **A**, Compression of a lung biopsy has produced round spaces resembling lipoid pneumonia. **B**, In other regions of the same biopsy, hemorrhage was also found, also with spaces suggesting lipoid pneumonia.

survey of the entire pattern generally helps one appreciate atelectasis merging with more normal lung. In fact, when significant fibrosis is present (usually associated with foci of honeycombing), atelectasis is rarely a problem because the more rigid fibrotic lung tissue tends to retain its configuration.

Fresh intra-alveolar hemorrhage due to the trauma of surgery is extremely common in biopsy material and should not be overinterpreted as pathologic (Fig. 15). One can approach this problem from three points of view: the statistical, the histologic, and the clinical. Statistically, the vast majority of cases of fresh alveolar hemorrhage are traumatic since

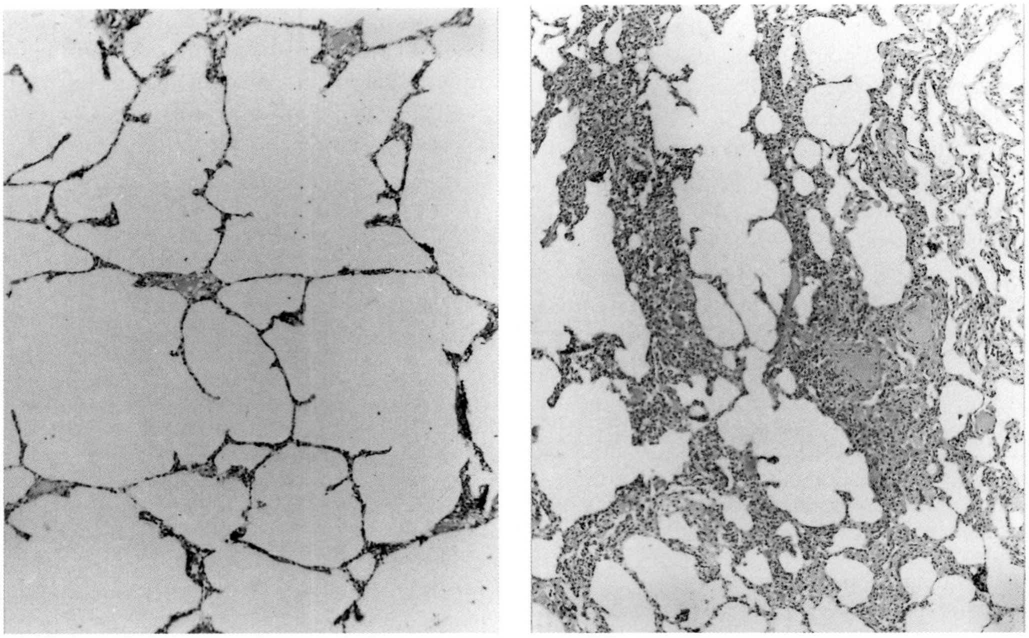

A B

FIG. 16. Atelectasis. In well-inflated regions (**A**) much of the lung architecture is normal, whereas in the compressed regions (**B**) the apposed alveolar walls create an impression of fibrosis and interstitial infiltrate. In fact, only a minimal inflammatory infiltrate and increase in alveolar macrophages were present.

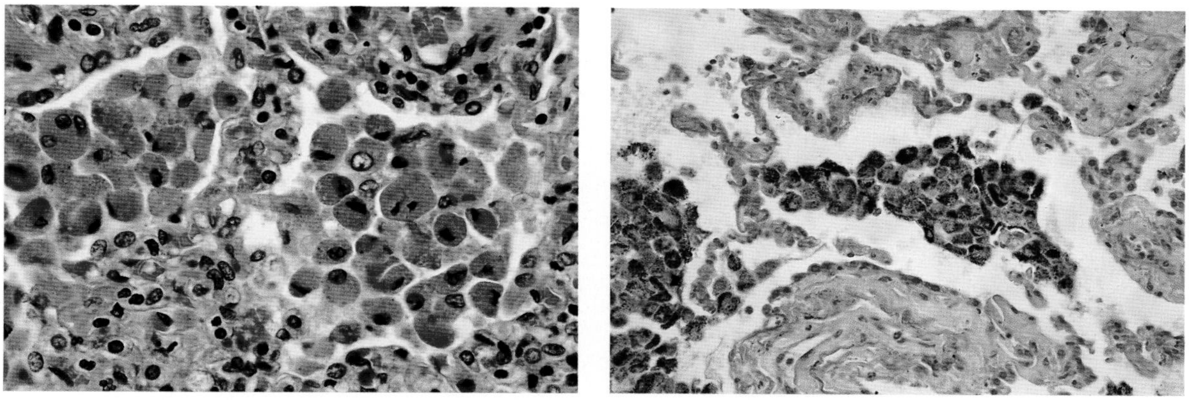

A B

**FIG. 17.** Tan-brown macrophages (**A**) associated with cigarette smoking often stain positively with iron stains (**B**). The staining is finely granular and less intense than in alveolar hemorrhage syndromes.

pathologic alveolar hemorrhage is relatively uncommon; thus, in any given case, acute hemorrhage is unlikely to be significant. When pathologic hemorrhage is present, there are usually (but not always) an associated fibrinous exudate of hyaline membranes, distention of alveoli with blood, and evidence of prior hemorrhage manifested by hemosiderin-filled macrophages in the interstitium or airspaces; this last finding is not a reliable histologic criterion in patients with venous obstruction or chronic passive congestion. The most common cause of macrophages staining positively with iron stains is smoking (Fig. 17). The hemosiderin in smokers macrophages is finely granular and gray-blue, in contrast to the coarse, dark blue staining in chronic hemorrhage. Nevertheless, it is surprising how many Prussian blue-positive cells can be seen in smokers. Finally, the clinician can usually confirm whether an alveolar hemorrhage syndrome or alveolar hemorrhage due to some other cause, (e.g., cardiac), is in the realm of possibility in any given patient.

Prolonged surgery prior to resection, and even multiple transbronchial biopsies, can lead to margination of neutrophils in capillaries (especially those in the pleura) that also mimic capillaritis. Clamping of the biopsy specimen prior to removal can result in lymphatic obstruction, dilatation, and septal edema.

Careful inflation of a lung biopsy specimen (32) may be helpful diagnostically, and is aesthetically pleasing since the lung architecture is more easily appreciated (and particularly amenable to photography). A heavy hand can create overdistension of alveoli and an emphysematous appearance. If this occurs, clinical correlation may be required to assess whether emphysema is actually a clinical consideration. Patchy atelectatic (uninflated) portions of lung tissue are common in biopsies that have been nonuniformly inflated. In general, it is also worthwhile to cut sections perpendicular to the pleural surface; sections taken parallel to the pleura may give an artificial honeycomb appearance. A problem that may be encountered in inflated biopsies is that cells and fluid may be "washed out" of the airspaces. This is especially true of smoker's (respiratory) bronchiolitis which may be quite subtle in inflated specimens.

Video-assisted thoracoscopic lung biopsies (thoracoscopic biopsies) have largely replaced traditional open lung biopsy as a diagnostic procedure for obtaining lung tissue for histologic evaluation. Although there are minor disadvantages in comparison to traditional open lung biopsy, diagnostic accuracy does not appear to be compromised (33). Allowing for the fact that bimanual palpation is not as feasible with thoracoscopic biopsies, and that the tissue is forcibly pulled through a small hole in the chest wall, sampling error and specimen artifacts are only a minor problem. The specimen size approaches that achieved with traditional open lung biopsy, and the minor degrees of hemorrhage, atelectasis/overinflation, and neutrophil margination represent artifactual changes that do not compromise diagnostic accuracy (33).

## INCIDENTAL FINDINGS IN LUNG BIOPSY AND RESECTION TISSUE

There are a number of incidental findings in lung tissue that may be overinterpreted as pathologic lesions (Table 6).

Findings related to smoking and emphysema are extremely common, especially in lungs resected for bronchogenic carcinoma. They may be divided into three broad groups: large airway changes, small airway lesions, and abnormalities of the alveolar parenchyma.

In the large airways, one often sees goblet cell hyperplasia, squamous metaplasia (with or without dysplasia), basement membrane thickening, hypertrophy and hyperplasia of bronchial glands with dilated ducts and mucostasis, and, often, a mild submucosal chronic inflammatory infiltrate (27).

The changes in the small airways may be quite dramatic and may mimic or even produce an interstitial lung disease (34,35). Smoking-induced respiratory bronchiolitis (Fig. 18) includes goblet cell metaplasia, an inflammatory infiltrate in the airway walls, metaplasia of type 2 cells in the surrounding alveoli, mild peribronchiolar fibrosis, and accumulations of macrophages in adjacent airspace and the bronchiolar lumen. The pigmented macrophages (smokers macrophages)

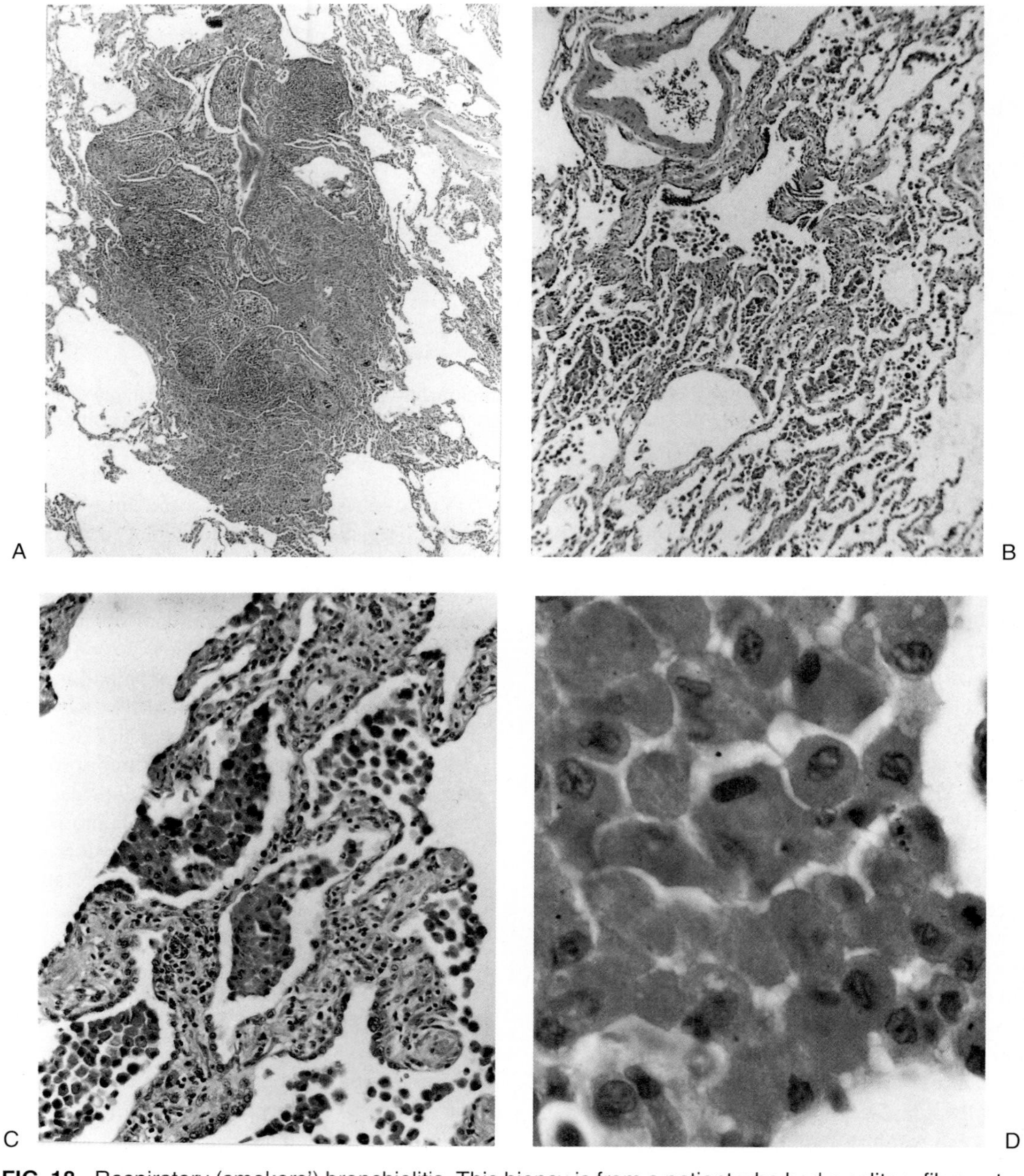

**FIG. 18.** Respiratory (smokers') bronchiolitis. This biopsy is from a patient who had a solitary fibrous tumor resected, but was asymptomatic and had an otherwise normal chest radiograph. In some zones (**A**) there is dense peribronchiolar hypercellularity and lymphoid hyperplasia, whereas in others (**B**) there is only mild inflammatory interstitial thickening, and the histology is reminiscent of desquamative interstitial pneumonia. There is an accumulation of intra-alveolar macrophages containing granular intracytoplasmic flecks of debris. **C**, High-power scans of macrophages in part (**D**).

**TABLE 6.** *Incidental findings in lung tissue*

1. Effects of smoking: emphysema, chronic bronchitis, respiratory (smoker's) bronchiolitis, intraparenchymal lymph nodes
2. Changes of asthma
3. Ossification and marrow formation in bronchial cartilages, bronchial submucosal fatty infiltration, and elastotic change
4. Parenchymal nodules
   a. Carcinoid tumorlets
   b. Minute (meningothelial-like nodules) pulmonary chemodectomas
   c. Bronchioloalveolar cell adenomas
   d. Healed granulomatous disease, infarcts, and so on
   e. Hamartomas
   f. Focal incidental scars
   g. Occasional (anthraco-) silicotic nodules (in the absence of clinical pneumoconiosis)
   h. Metaplastic bone
   i. Intrapulmonary lung nodes
   j. Small carcinomas (rarely) and other tumors
5. Intracellular/intra-alveolar/interstitial structures
   a. Macrophages
   b. Corpora amylacea
   c. Blue bodies
   d. Schaumann's bodies
   e. Asteroid bodies
   f. Calcium oxalate crystals
   g. Mallory's hyaline-like material in type 2 cells
   h. Ferruginous bodies
   i. Anthracotic pigment/birefringent material (including silica and silicates)
   j. Metaplastic bone
6. Epithelioid and/or cholesterol granulomas, giant cells, lipogranulomas
7. Intravascular/vascular
   a. Megakaryocytes
   b. Thrombi (mimic emboli)
   c. Bone marrow emboli
   d. Calcification and iron encrustation of the elastic tissue
   e. Senile amyloid
   f. Foreign material
8. Hilar/peribronchial nodes
   a. Sinus and paracortical histiocytosis (may simulate granulomas)
   b. Occasional silicotic or anthracosilicotic nodules
   c. Anthracosis/birefringent material
   d. Hamazaki-Wesenberg bodies
9. Pleural adhesions; hyaline pleural plaques

contain phagocytosed debris from inhaled cigarette smoke and have prominent secondary lysosomes in their cytoplasm. This results in a dirty granular-tan or brown appearance to the cytoplasm. They contain PAS-positive (lysosomes) and finely granular Prussian blue-positive (hemosiderin) material, as well as tiny, irregular flecks of brown-black material.

The changes in the most distal pulmonary parenchyma represent centriacinar emphysema with permanent airspace enlargement and loss of alveolar walls (27). Histologic quantification of emphysema on biopsy material is difficult and not advised, given the relatively small size of the specimens, although one can often determine as to whether it is present. Bullous emphysema is more common in the upper lobes and is usually associated with fibrosis in the septa of the bullae and adjacent alveolar walls. The fibrosis is relatively acellular, noninflammatory, and poorly vascularized. Metaplasia and ulceration of the epithelium and interstitial dissection of air occur in bullae and may induce a giant cell response analogous to that seen in persistent interstitial emphysema in infants.

Asthmatics are predisposed to a number of lung conditions that may lead to lung biopsy, although the asthmatic changes themselves may not be the dominant lesion. These changes include goblet cell metaplasia in the airway epithelium, thickening of the basement membrane, smooth muscle hypertrophy and hyperplasia, lymphoid hyperplasia, and a variable infiltrate of eosinophils, lymphocytes, and a few neutrophils, and fibrous tissue in the wall (27). Mucostasis (including Curschmann's spirals) may be an accompanying feature, but when mucostasis is extensive and is associated with sloughing of epithelial fragments into the airways (Creola bodies), one should suspect that the asthma itself is the main lesion; such an appearance is typical of status asthmaticus. In patients with quiescent asthma or past history of asthma, the airways may be entirely normal or show only minor inflammatory or fibrotic changes.

Metaplastic bone, including bone marrow and calcification, is an aging change that is occasionally seen in bronchial cartilages (36). Metaplastic bone may also be seen in regions of scarring (dystrophic ossification), particularly in apical caps. Small bony nodules may also be seen with no apparent associated pathologic changes. In some older individuals with chronic bronchitis, the bronchial submucosa may have a gray elastotic appearance, particularly in bronchoscopic biopsies.

Carcinoid tumorlets (37–39) and minute pulmonary chemodectomas (40) are nodular proliferations that are quite common. They may be mistaken for each other, other lesions, or even metastases. Carcinoid tumorlets (Fig. 19) represent well-circumscribed proliferations of neuroendocrine cells that usually occur in the walls of and around small airways, particularly in scarred or bronchiectatic airways and in a small number of patients with airflow destruction. They lack mitotic figures and necrosis, although there is a superficial resemblance to small cell carcinoma. Tumorlets are actually more reminiscent of spindle cell carcinoid tumors. Tumorlets are often multiple; some may become large enough to be recognized radiographically and to be removed to exclude carcinoma. Exactly where one draws the line between a carcinoid tumorlet and a carcinoid tumor, particularly in cases with multiple lesions, is quite arbitrary, although a cutoff point of 1 cm diameter or larger for carcinoid tumor is reasonable (41).

Minute pulmonary meningothelial-like nodules (minute pulmonary chemodectomas) (Fig. 20) were originally thought to represent an intrapulmonary proliferation of perivenular chemoreceptor cells (40,42). However, the accumulated evidence suggests that the cellular constituents are

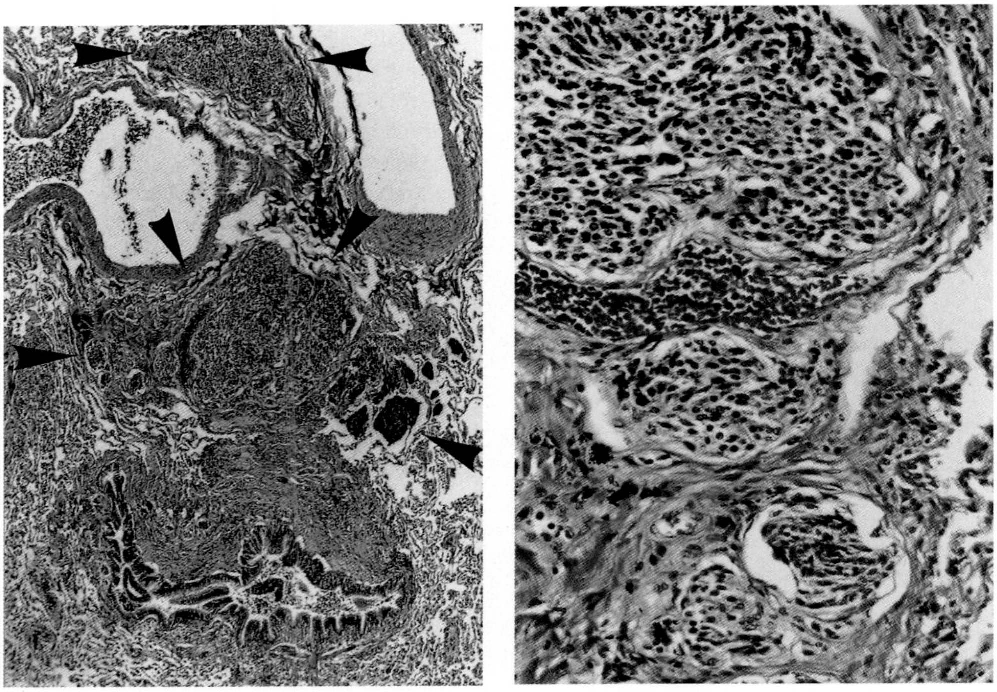

A B

**FIG. 19.** Carcinoid tumorlet. **A**, A nodular proliferation of fusiform hyperchromatic cells is seen between a bronchial and its adjacent pulmonary artery (*arrowheads*). **B**, Some cell clusters extend into alveolar spaces. Cytologically, the lesion resembles a spindle cell carcinoid tumor.

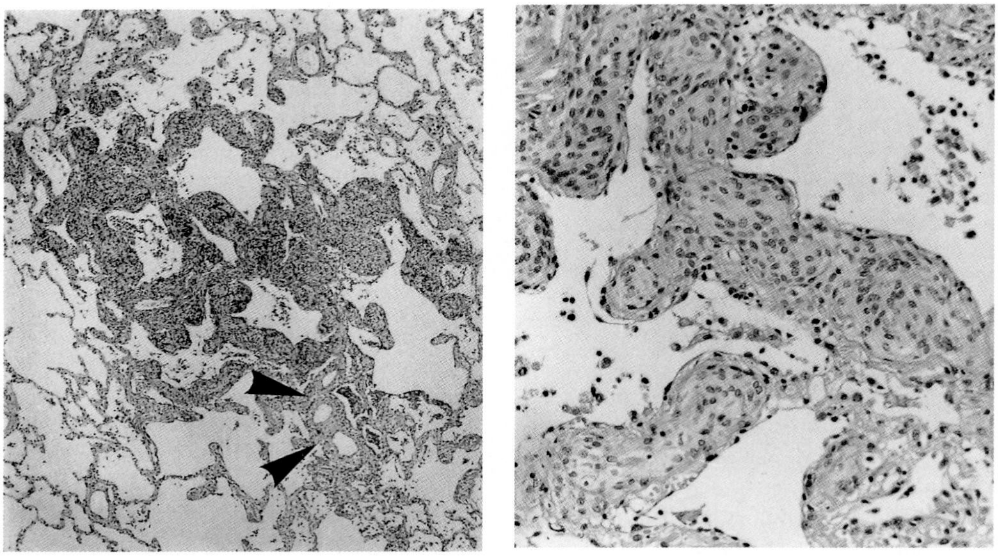

A B

**FIG. 20.** Pulmonary meningothelial-like nodule. There are perivenular (*arrowheads*) nodular accumulations (**A**) of interstitial cells resembling (**B**) arachnoidal lining cells of the meninges.

more closely related to meningothelial cells. Minute pulmonary meningothelial-like nodules are composed of interstitial clusters of fusiform cells with pale eosinophilic cytoplasm, forming small stellate nodules (occasionally, grossly appreciable) near small veins. Their location and characteristic bland cytology resembling meningothelial cells, are very distinctive.

Bronchioloalveolar cell adenomas (atypical adenomatous hyperplasia) represent small nodular lesions in the lung parenchyma (Fig. 21) that were first recognized in resection specimens for carcinoma (43). Miller found these lesions in 23 of 247 consecutive resection specimens for carcinoma (43). They are most easily recognized in cases that are inflated with Bouin's fixative. Bronchoalveolar adenomas are seen as incidental nodules 1 to 7 mm in diameter and located in the centrilobular zones of the lung parenchyma unrelated to the carcinoma. Histologically, bronchoalveolar cell adenomas are composed of a localized proliferation of cytologically benign or mildly atypical type 2 cells growing in a lipidic fashion on alveolar walls. The alveolar walls may show slight thickening and inflammatory change. Miller concluded that bronchoalveolar cell adenomas may represent a premalignant phase of glandular neoplasia in the lung. In general, we advocate a conservative approach to these lesions, since there are many causes of type 2 proliferation, many of them reactive.

Focal scars (see following), healed granulomatous disease, and organized infarcts are among other incidental nodular lesions occasionally encountered in the lung. Early infarcts have a wedge shape with hemorrhagic necrosis, and the overlying pleura is viable with a fibrinous pleuritis. They often also have a rim of granulation tissue. Older infarcts are often round and have a rim of fibrous tissue; they can be mistaken for healed granulomas. Necrotic tumor nodules sometimes mimic infarcts. Squamous metaplasia is common in the airspaces adjacent to recent and organizing infarcts, and around bronchioles in organizing diffuse alveolar damage may be sufficiently exuberant to be mistaken for a neoplastic process. A single anthracosilicotic nodule is an occasional finding that may be accepted as incidental and insignificant if there is no clinical or radiological evidence of pneumoconiosis. When silicotic nodules are multiple, the occupational history and the possibility of pneumoconiosis should be explored.

Although extensive parenchymal scarring is clearly a pathologic process, focal scars (Fig. 22) are a common incidental finding in biopsy material. There are a number of nonspecific histologic changes that accompany pulmonary scarring, regardless of cause. These include vascular intimal thickening, sometimes to the point of luminal occlusion (endarteritis obliterans); smooth muscle and myofibroblastic hyperplasia in the interstitium; metaplasia and hyperplasia of type 2 cells or bronchiolar-type epithelium; accumulations of intra-alveolar macrophages, mucostasis, carcinoid tumorlets (particularly along scarred small airways); dystrophic calcification or ossification; microscopic pericicatricial emphysema; and metaplastic adipose tissue in the pleural and peribronchial regions. The proliferation of type 2 cells associated with scars may be confused with bronchioloalveolar carcinoma. Bronchioloalveolar carcinoma generally has uniform dense cellularity with abrupt transition to normal alveolar walls, significant cytologic atypia, and lack of ciliated cells.

In rare instances, mature bone is observed in normal alveoli; it may represent the residue of an organized airspace exudate from chronic passive congestion of mitral stenosis or an ancient organized pneumonia (44). Extensive dystrophic ossification occasionally accompanies lesions with diffuse pulmonary fibrosis (Fig. 23) (45).

A large number of intra-alveolar and intracellular structures are seen in the lung. Small numbers of intra-alveolar macrophages are a normal finding, and an increase in their numbers is nonspecific and a common reaction in smokers. Desquamative interstitial pneumonia-like reactions are seen in many pathologic conditions, especially those with fibrosis and architectural disorganization (46). When hemosiderin is

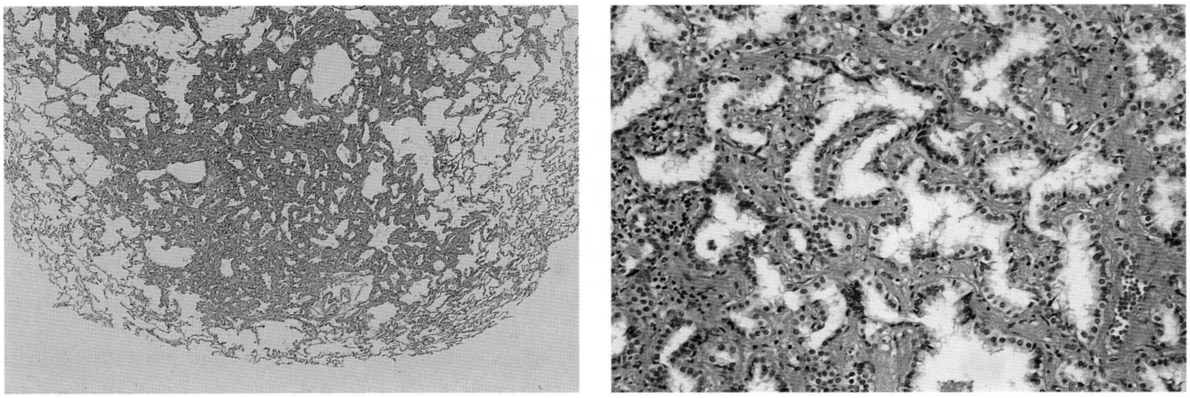

A B

**FIG. 21.** Bronchioloalveolar cell adenoma. This relatively large bronchioloalveolar cell adenoma shows a nodular zone in the lung parenchyma with mild alveolar septal thickening (**A**). The lining cells are cytologically bland and show features of type 2 cells (**B**).

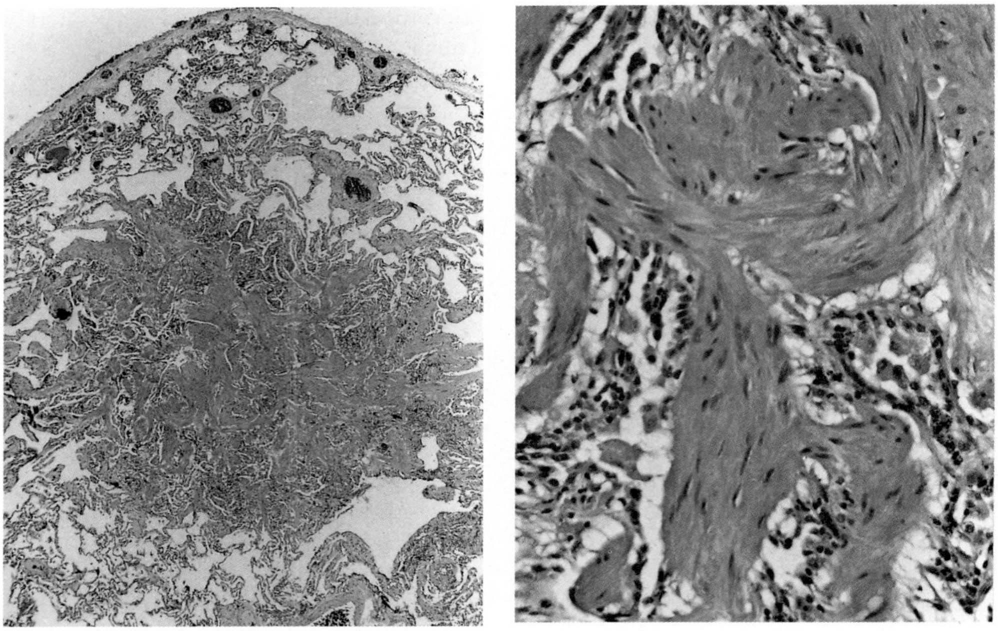

A B

**FIG. 22.** An incidental pulmonary scar (**A**) associated with prominent smooth muscle metaplasia (**B**) from a lobectomy for carcinoma.

present, causes for alveolar hemorrhage (both primary and secondary) should be excluded.

Corpora amylacea (47,48) are eosinophilic, rounded, slightly lamellated proteinaceous bodies (Fig. 24) that stain positively with PAS stains and faintly with Congo red stain; they are more common in the lungs of older individuals. Sometimes there is a blue-gray, calcified, or polarizable crystalline particulate body in the center and a macrophage or giant cell response around them. The exact nature and cause of corpora are unclear, but they are of no clinical significance.

Blue bodies (Fig. 25) are intra-alveolar, lamellated, basophilic, calcified structures found in airspaces associated with alveolar macrophages and giant cells (48). They are a nonspecific finding in a number of diffuse lung diseases related to accumulation of macrophages, and are of no diagnostic significance. They are thought to be related to macrophage catabolism; they are composed primarily of calcium carbonate.

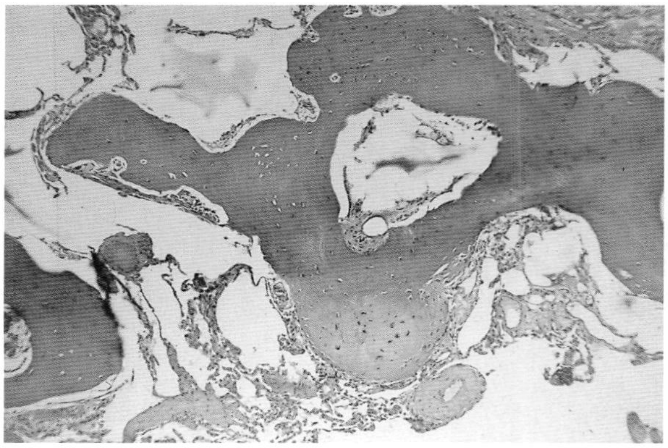

**FIG. 23.** An incidental focus of pulmonary ossification from a patient with usual interstitial pneumonia.

Schaumann's bodies (Fig. 26) are similar lamellated, calcified bodies seen in giant cells and associated with granulomas (48–50). They are also of no diagnostic significance and may be found in granulomas from diverse causes. Schaumann's bodies are endogenously derived and may be mistaken for exogenous material since they may be partially birefringent, due to concomitant presents of oxalate crystals (see following).

Asteroid bodies (Fig. 27) represent a starlike array of crystallized protein and are seen in the giant cells of many granulomatous conditions; other than being aesthetically pleasing, they are nonspecific.

Calcium oxalate crystals are lucent, birefringent, platelike crystals, often in giant cells, that may be mistaken for exogenous material (48,49) (Fig. 28). Accumulation of oxalate crystals around aspergillomas and in patients with forms of invasive aspergillosis is also common.

Material resembling Mallory's hyaline (Fig. 29) may be found in the reactive type 2 cells of a number of interstitial diseases. It is distinctive, but nonspecific.

Ferruginous bodies, the majority of which are asbestos bodies, are indicative of significant inhalational exposure to the ferruginated material, but their presence does not necessarily correspond to clinically significant lung disease. Recent studies with electron-probe analysis have helped eluci-

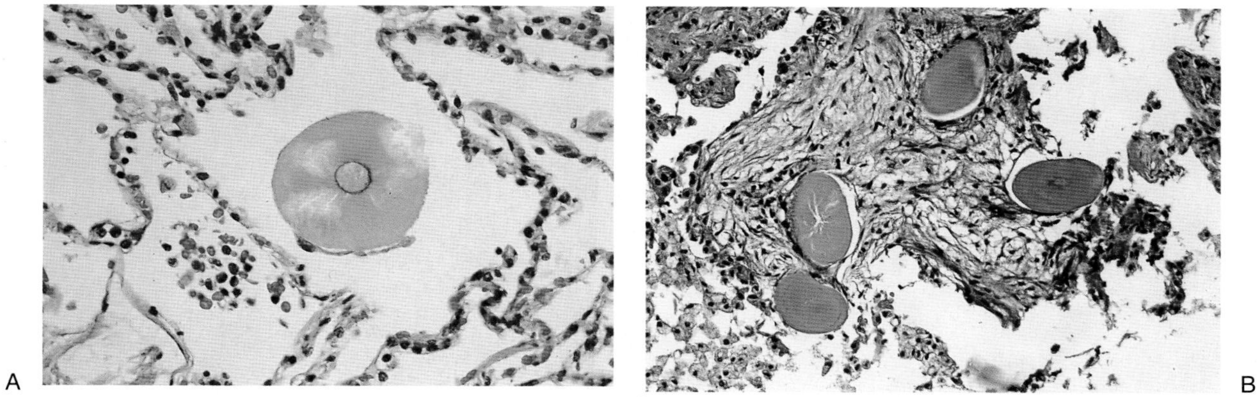

FIG. 24. Pulmonary corpora amylacea. These may show a central bluish nidus (**A**) and a giant cell or macrophage reaction around them. Others may have radiating proteinaceous arrays and show cracking in histologic sections. In (**B**), multiple corpora amylacea are an incidental finding associated with an organizing pneumonia.

date the variety of materials that may become iron encrusted, of which asbestos fibers comprise only a portion (51).

In virtually any urban adult, one may find short, needle-like, birefringent material (usually silica or silicates) in association with anthracotic pigment (Fig. 30). Silicates are more brightly birefringent than silica. The amount of birefringent material may be quite impressive in individuals (particularly smokers) who have no significant occupational exposure. This material should be distinguished from formalin pigment, as well as from surgical glove talc or starch, which is limited to the handled surfaces and often has a Maltese-cross configuration with polarization. The diagnosis of silicosis (and silicatosis) is not based solely on the presence of birefringent material; it requires clinicopathologic correlations: appropriate chest radiograph findings, and parenchymal silicotic nodules or masses of histiocytes (within which early fibrotic nodules may be seen to form) along lymphatic routes. Precise characterization of any material identified requires special techniques such as electron-probe analysis.

An occasional nonnecrotizing epithelioid granuloma may be found in the lungs of patients who have no evidence of granulomatous disease; they are analogous to the occasional granuloma seen at many sites in the body. Likewise, cholesterol granulomas or single giant cells containing cholesterol clefts may also be an occasional incidental finding (Fig. 31). In some instances, the presence of cholesterol granulomas has been linked to prior alveolar hemorrhage, mucostasis, or pulmonary hypertension (52), but usually no significance can be ascribed to them. Lipogranulomas are an occasional nonspecific finding, said to be more common in diabetics (53).

An interesting finding is the presence of scattered megakaryocytes in alveolar walls (Fig. 32), predominantly within alveolar capillaries. Large numbers can be seen, particularly during sepsis. They are of no diagnostic signifi-

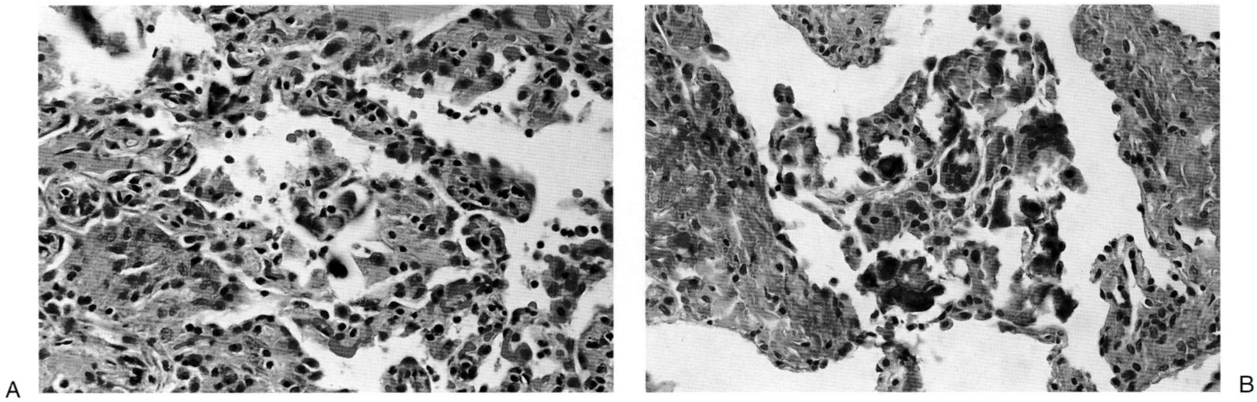

FIG. 25. **A, B:** Blue bodies are gray or blue intra-alveolar, calcified, lamellated structures often associated with clusters of macrophages, including giant cells.

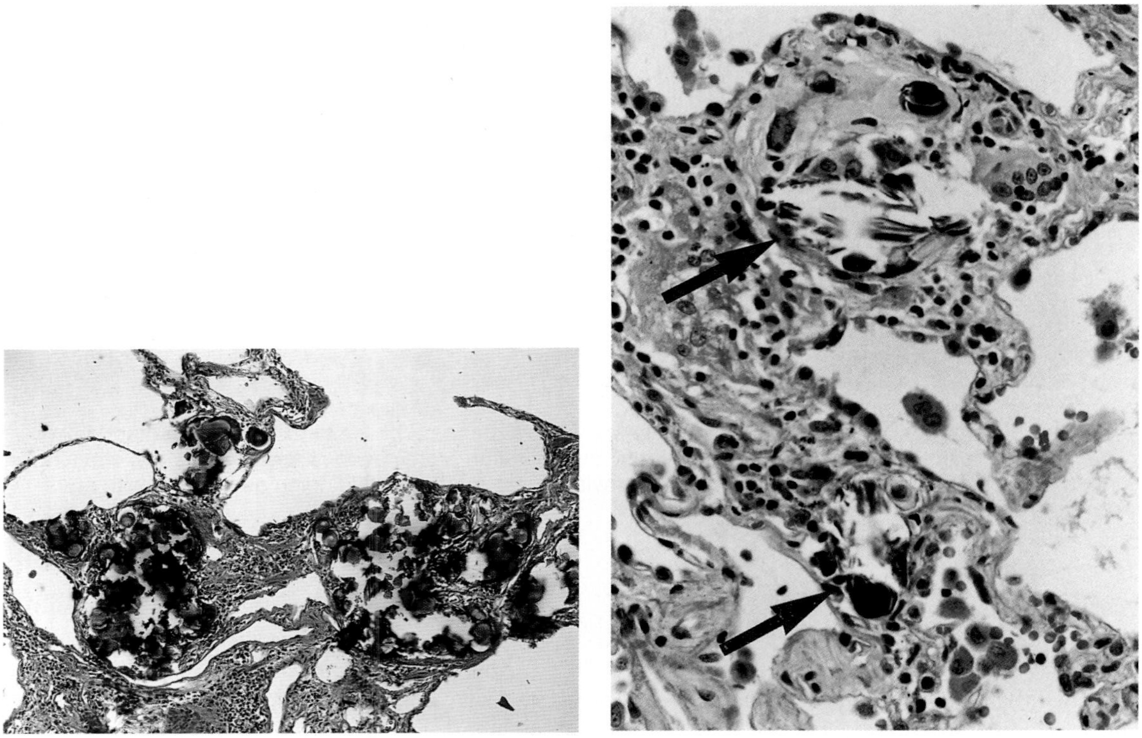

A B

**FIG. 26. A, B:** Schaumann's bodies are quite similar to blue bodies and are calcified, lamellated, often cracked bodies, seen interstitially and in giant cells associated with granulomatous diseases. After the granulomas disappear, Schaumann's bodies may be left behind.

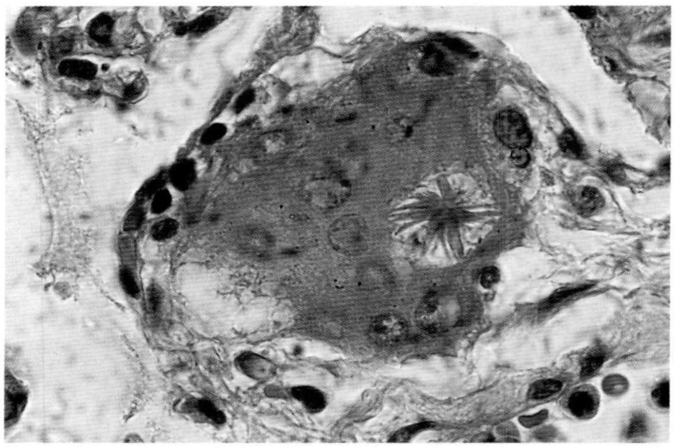

**FIG. 27.** An asteroid body in a giant cell from a case of asbestosis.

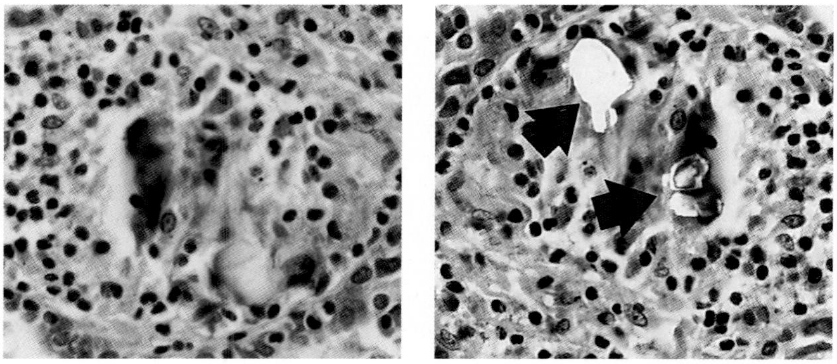

A B

**FIG. 28.** Calcium oxylate crystals (**A**) may be difficult to appreciate on routine microscopy, but the lucent platelike crystals (**B**) are brightly birefringent (*arrows*).

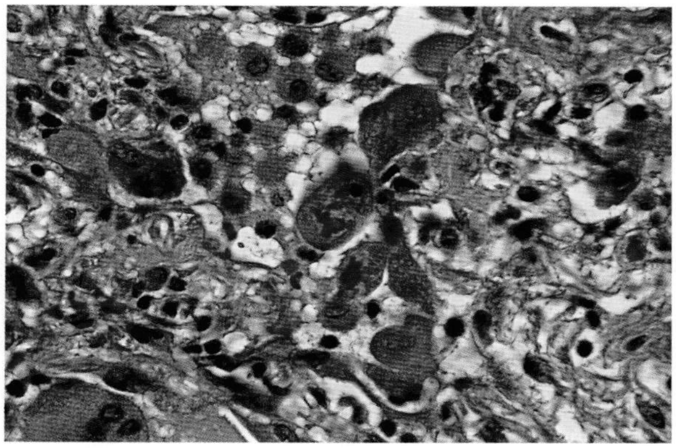

**FIG. 29.** Material resembling Mallory's hyaline may be seen in reactive type 2 cells in a number of conditions.

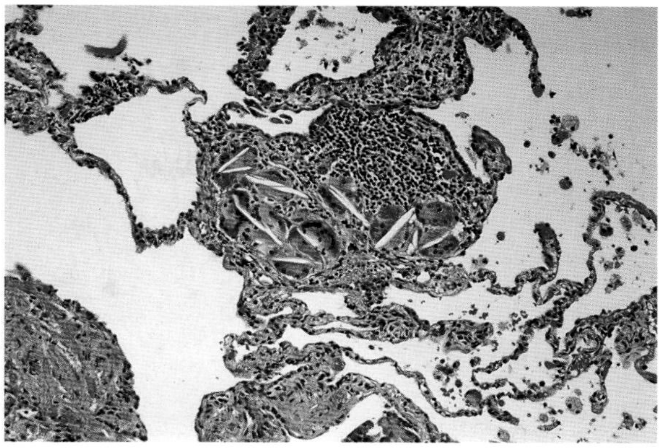

**FIG. 31.** Granulomas and clusters of giant cells containing cholesterol clefts are a frequent nonspecific finding in interstitial lung disease.

cance but should not be overinterpreted as malignant or virally infected cells. Along with the bone marrow and spleen, the lung acts as a major reservoir for megakaryocytes.

Bone marrow emboli, common in autopsy material, are also seen in biopsy specimens (Fig. 33). Rarely correlated with any clinically significant process, they may be a consequence of bony trauma or excision of ribs. In some cases, however, such as thoracoscopic biopsies, bony trauma cannot be implicated and the marrow emboli are an unexplained incidental finding.

Recent intravascular thrombi (probably formed in situ) are a relatively common accompanying finding in any severe acute inflammatory lung disease (Fig. 34), and they should not be considered evidence of pulmonary emboli without corroborating clinical information.

In patients with chronic hemorrhagic, chronic pulmonary congestion, or metabolic abnormalities, calcification and iron encrustation of the pulmonary elastic tissue may occur and even elicit a giant cell reaction (Fig. 35). This phenomenon has been inappropriately labeled endogenous pneumoconiosis (54).

Intravascular foreign material is usually birefringent and may have a giant cell reaction. While it usually occurs in intravenous drug abuse (IV talcosis), occasional fragments of foreign material are seen in patients without a history of drug abuse, perhaps related to intravenous lines during hospitalization or surgery.

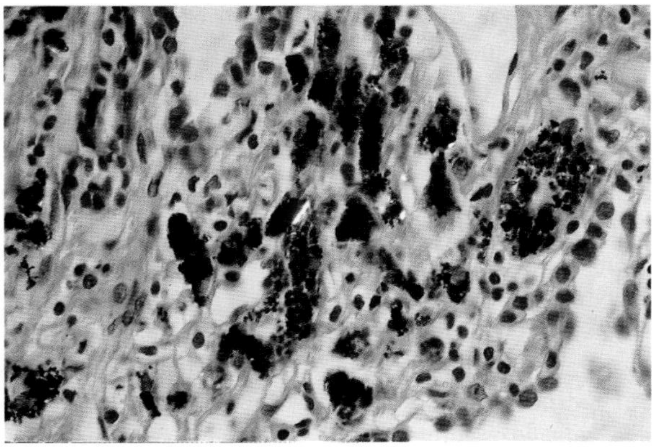

**FIG. 30.** Birefringent silica and silicate particles are a common nonspecific finding in and around the anthracotic pigment that is so commonly seen in urban adults and smokers.

A

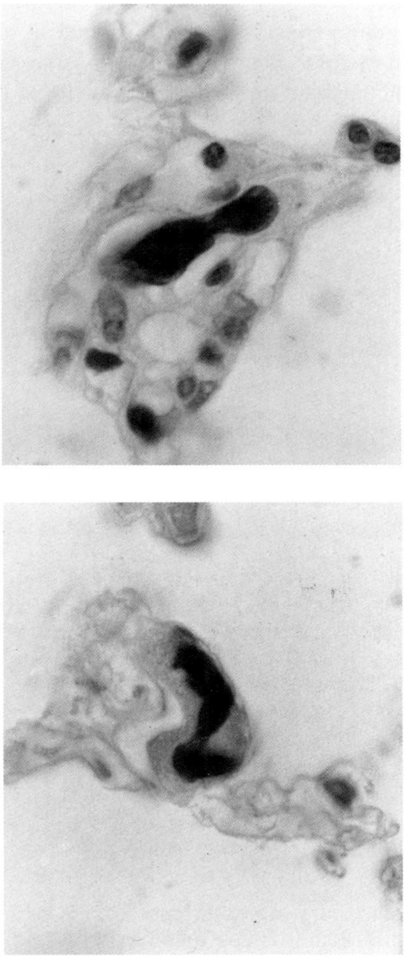

B

**FIG. 32. A, B:** Megakaryocytes, usually in alveolar capillaries, are a common nonspecific finding in lung biopsies.

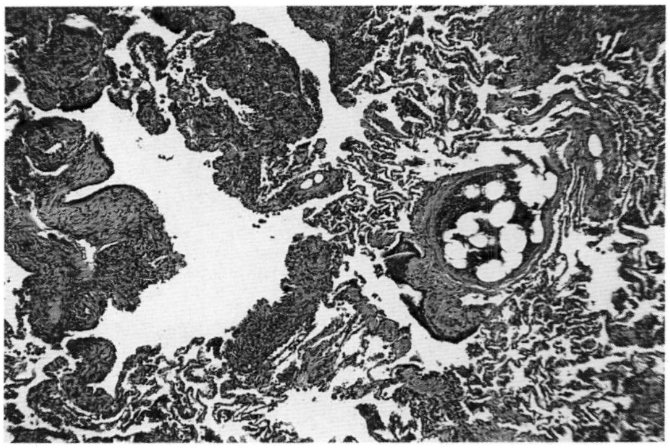

**FIG. 33.** An incidental bone marrow embolus (*right center*) identified in a pulmonary artery in a biopsy from a patient with lymphangioleiomyomatosis (*left*).

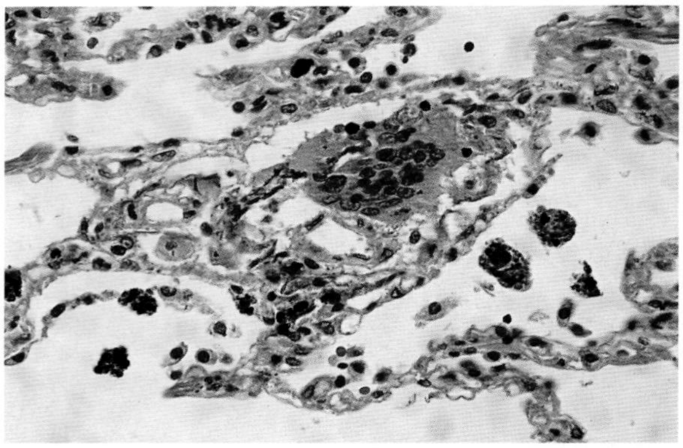

A

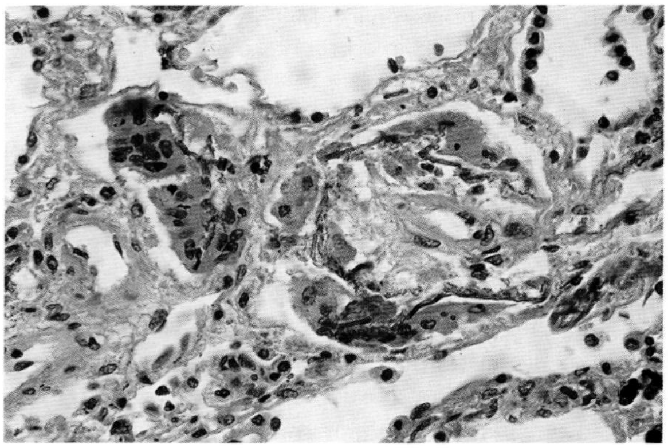

B

**FIG. 35. A, B:** Severe chronic passive congestion with concomitant chronic microhemorrhages may result in encrustation of interstitial and vascular elastic fibers by hemosiderin. A giant cell reaction is a frequent accompanying finding.

Hilar and peribronchial lymph nodes are rarely carefully examined beyond the evaluation for metastatic carcinoma. Nevertheless, they frequently exhibit a number of characteristic changes. Clusters of dust-filled macrophages in the sinuses and paracortical areas may resemble small granulomas (Fig. 36). Silicotic or anthracosilicotic nodules, old healed infectious granulomas, and sinus histiocytosis are also common. When sarcoidosis is a consideration, one may have difficulty distinguishing the normal histiocytosis of hilar nodes from the granulomas of sarcoidosis. Generally, this problem can be approached by maintaining a high threshold for granulomas, requiring well-formed, rounded granulomatous masses (particularly with accumulations of intergranulomatous fibrinoid or hyalinized material), giant cells, and careful clinicopathologic correlation.

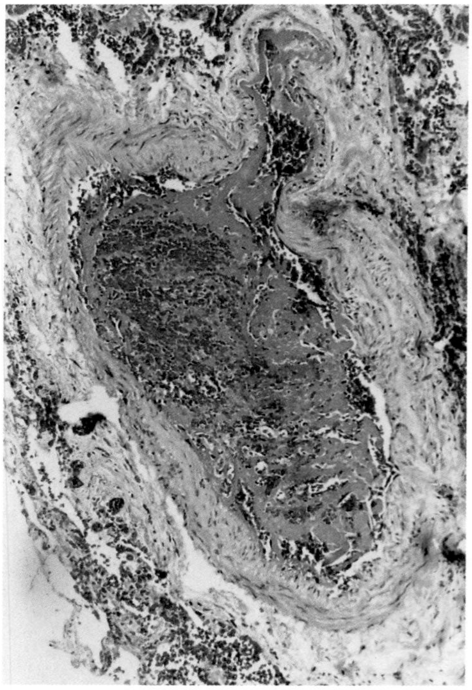

**FIG. 34.** Pulmonary artery thrombi are of common nonspecific finding in acute diffuse inflammatory lung disease, regardless of cause. They are rarely of clinical significance, although their presence should be noted.

Although multiple intraparenchymal silicotic nodules should make one suspect the possibility of silicosis, anthracosilicotic nodules in hilar nodes are quite common in the absence of silicosis. The nodules are composed of concentric whorled and layered hyalinized collagen, and are usually surrounded by a nonpalisaded rim of dust-filled macrophages that contain birefringent material when examined with polarized light. Central degenerative changes may be evident. Silicotic nodules should be distinguished from old/healed granulomatous disease.

Hamazaki-Wesenberg bodies (55) are small (average 5 microns in length), oral yellow-brown intracellular or extracellular structures associated with sinus histiocytes in lymph nodes, especially lung hilar nodes. The cause of these bodies is unknown, but they resemble lipofuscin. Positive staining with methenamine silver and PAS stains may lead to their

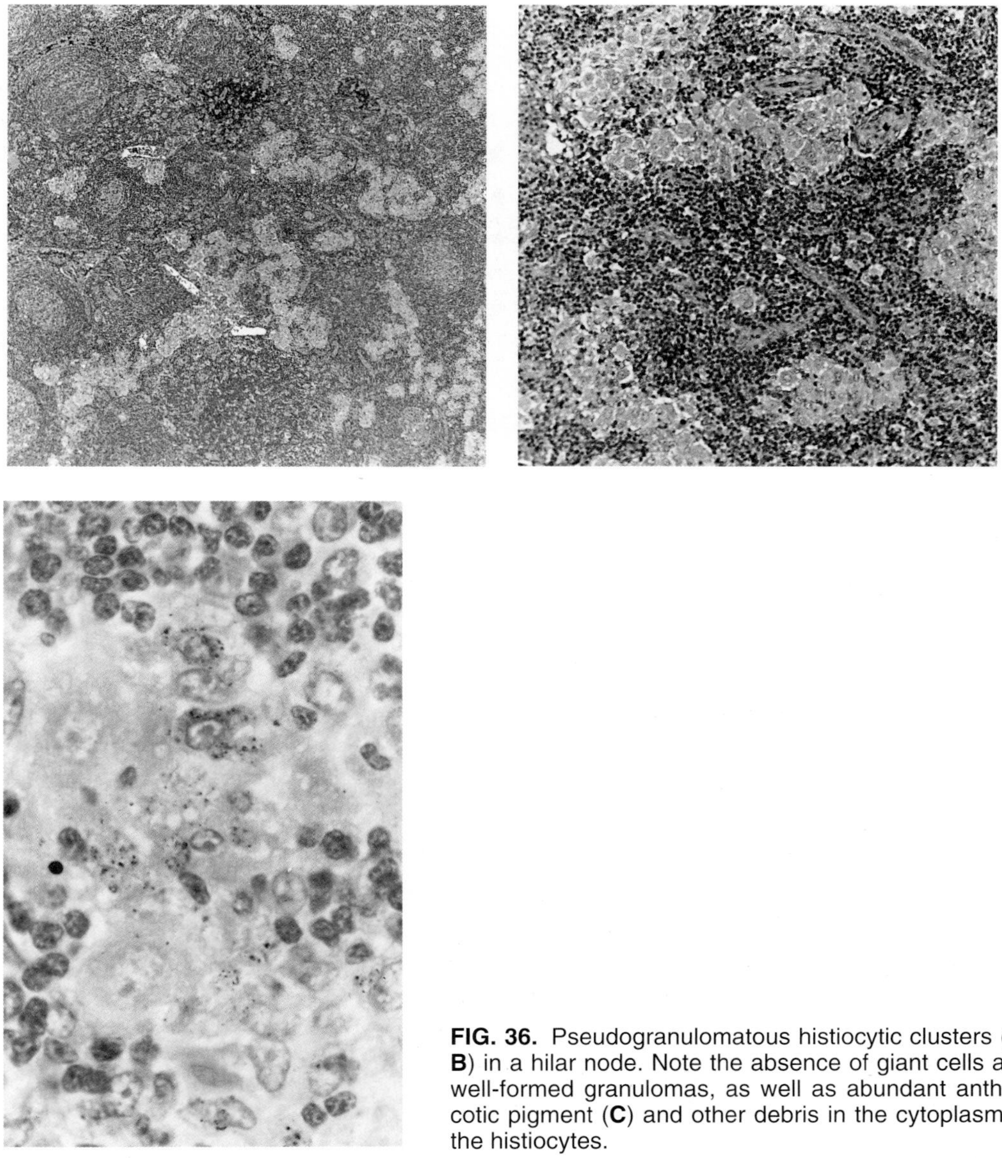

FIG. 36. Pseudogranulomatous histiocytic clusters (**A**, **B**) in a hilar node. Note the absence of giant cells and well-formed granulomas, as well as abundant anthracotic pigment (**C**) and other debris in the cytoplasm of the histiocytes.

confusion with yeast forms, but their H&E appearance, lack of associated necrosis or inflammation, and positive staining with Fontana-Masson stain should facilitate their recognition and distinction from fungi.

## EFFECTS OF AGING

Some of the effects of aging on the lung are shown in Table 7. Calcification and ossification of cartilages in the large airways may be seen. Intimal thickening is an age-related change in pulmonary arteries and veins (Fig. 37) and apical pulmonary arteries are effected more often (2). Intimal thickening of veins is often hyaline and sclerotic in character and should be distinguished from the more cellular intimal and muscular proliferation seen in pulmonary veno-occlusive disease and chronic passive congestion. Mural hyalinization of small arterioles is also an aging change (as well as being common in emphysematous lungs). Some degree of alveolar enlargement accompanies aging (56), so-called senile emphysema.

Senile amyloid is usually an incidental finding, is perivascular, and increases in incidence with age (57).

**TABLE 7.** *Effects of aging seen in lung biopsies*

1. Tracheobronchial cartilage ossification, submucosal fatty metaplasia, oncocytic metaplasia and/or hyperplasia in bronchial glands, and elastotic appearance of the submucosa
2. Pulmonary arterial and venous intimal thickening and hyalization of arterioles
3. Alveolar enlargement (rarely appreciated in biopsy material)
4. Medial calcification in bronchial arteries
5. Senile vascular amyloidosis
6. Anthracosis (urban dwellers)

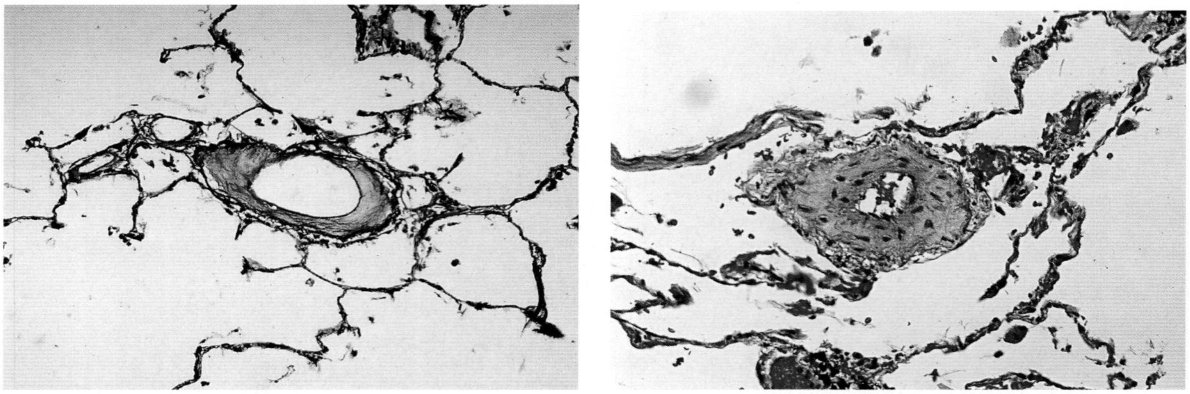

A B

**FIG. 37.** Intimal thickening of pulmonary veins (**A**, elastic tissue stain) and hyaline thickening of arteries (**B**) are common nonspecific aging changes.

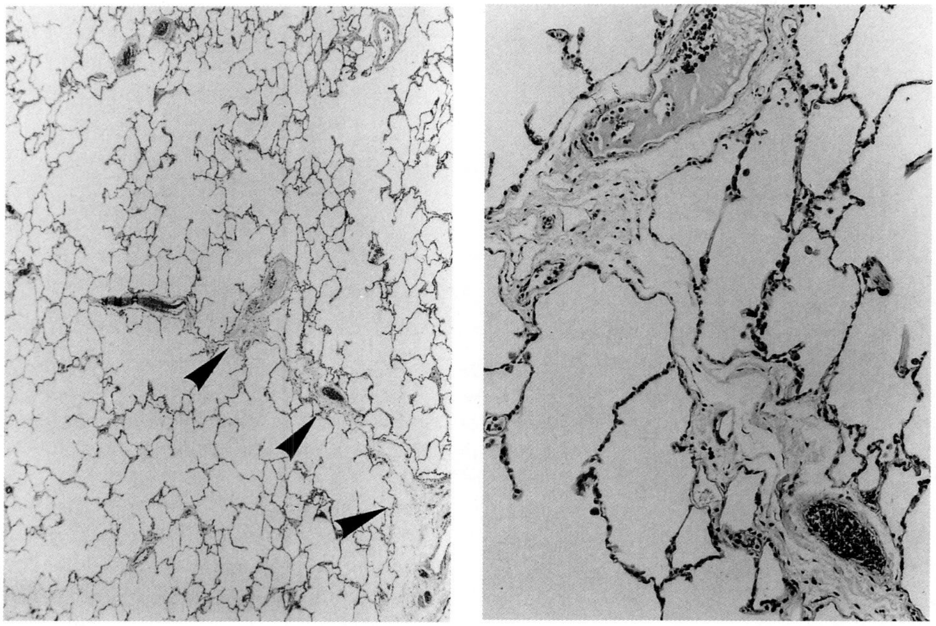

A B

**FIG. 38. A, B:** An apparently normal biopsy from a patient with systemic lupus erythematosus and acute pulmonary infiltrates. Clinical follow-up confirmed the diagnosis of acute pulmonary edema; review of the biopsy revealed septal thickening and lymphatic dilatation.

**TABLE 8.** *Situations in which a lung biopsy may appear normal*

1. Sampling error
2. Pulmonary vascular disease
3. Small airway (bronchiolar) disease
4. Pulmonary edema and early diffuse alveolar damage
5. Emboli, including fat emboli
6. A very subtle interstitial infiltrate
7. Cardiac disease with secondary pulmonary abnormalities

## THE BIOPSY THAT LOOKS NORMAL AT FIRST GLANCE

When a lung biopsy for presumed diffuse lung disease initially appears normal, a number of possibilities should be considered (Table 8), especially pulmonary edema (Fig. 38).

Although one can argue that interstitial infiltrates that are so subtle as to be overlooked are probably not clinically significant, their recognition is necessary. This situation can arise, for example, with biopsy material from the less severely effected portions of lung in patients with interstitial pneumonias, in cases in which the inflammatory infiltrate has been suppressed by steroids or immunosuppressive therapy, and in pathologic entities characterized by patchy inflammation. The presence of inflammatory cells in the perivenular regions and alveolar wall with reactive type 2 cells is usually indicative of an interstitial pneumonia.

## REFERENCES


1. Nagaishi C. *Functional anatomy and histology of the lung.* Baltimore; University Park Press, 1972.
2. Wagenvoort CA, Wagenvoort N. *Pathology of pulmonary hypertension.* New York; John Wiley, 1977.
3. Kuhn C. Ultrastructure and cellular function in the distal lung. In: Thurlbeck WM, Abell MR, eds. *The lung.* Baltimore; Williams & Wilkins, 1978.
4. Fishman AP. *Pulmonary disease and disorders.* New York; McGraw-Hill, 1980.
5. Scadding JG, Cumming G. *Scientific foundations of respiratory medicine.* Philadelphia; WB Saunders, 1981.
6. Gail DB, Lenfant CJM. Cells of the lung: biology and clinical implications. *Am Rev Respir Dis* 1983;127:366–387.
7. Bienenstock J, Befus AD. Gut-and-bronchus-associated lymphoid tissue. *Am J Anat* 1984;170:437–445.
8. Langston C, Kida K, Reed M, Thurlbeck WM. Human lung growth in late gestation and in the neonate. *Am Rev Respir Dis* 1984;129: 607–613.
9. Murray JF. *The normal lung. 2nd ed.* Philadelphia; WB Saunders, 1986.
10. Corrin B. The lungs. In: St. Claire Symmers W, ed. *Systemic Pathology. 3rd ed.* New York; Churchill Livingstone, 1990.
11. Dail DH, Hammar SP. *Pulmonary pathology. 2nd ed.* New York; Springer-Verlag, 1994.
12. Thurlbeck WM, Churg AM. *Pathology of the lung. 2nd ed.* Thieme, New York, 1995.
13. Yaegashi H, Takahashi T. The airway dimension in ordinary human lung. *Arch Pathol Lab Med* 1994;118:969–974.
14. Lehnert BE. Pulmonary and thoracic macrophage subpopulations and clearance of particles from the lung. *Environ Health Perspect* 1992;97: 17–46.
15. Gould SJ, Isaacson PG. Bronchus-associated lymphoid tissue (BALT) in human fetal and infant lung. *J Pathol* 1993;169:229–234.
16. Richmond J, Pritchard GE, Ashcroft T, Avery A, Corris PA, Walters EH. Bronchus associated lymphoid tissue (BALT) in human lung: its distribution in smokers and non-smokers. *Thorax* 1993;48:1130–1134.
17. Tschernig T, Kleemann WJ, Pabst R. Bronchus-associated lymphoid tissue (BALT) in the lungs of children who had died from sudden infant death syndrome and other causes. *Thorax* 1995;50:658–660.
18. Bienenstock J. Bronchus-associated lymphoid tissue. *Int Arch Allergy Immunol* 1985;76:62–69.
19. Kradin RL, Spirn PW, Mark EJ. Intrapulmonary lymph nodes. *Chest* 1985;87:662–667.
20. Gallagher B, Urbanski SJ. The significance of pleural elastica invasion by lung carcinomas. *Hum Pathol* 1990;21:512–517.
21. Newman SL, Michel RP, Wang NS. Lingular biopsy: is it representative? *Am Rev Respir Dis* 1985;132:1084–1086.
22. Albo RJ, Grimes OF. The right middle lobe syndrome: a clinical study. *Dis Chest* 1966;50:509–518.
23. Kwon KY, Myers JL, Swensen SJ, Colby TV. Middle lobe syndrome: a clinicopathological study of 21 patients. *Hum Pathol* 1995;26: 302–307.
24. Renner RR, Markarian B, Pernice NJ, Heitzman ER. The apical cap. *Radiology* 1974;110:569–582.
25. McLoud TC, Isler RJ, Noveline RA, Putman CE, Simeone J, Stark P. The apical cap. *AJR* 1981;137:299–306.
26. Lichter I, Gwynne JF. Spontaneous pneumothorax in young adults: a clinical and pathologic study. *Thorax* 1971;26:409–417.
27. Thurlbeck WM. *Chronic airflow obstruction in lung disease.* Philadelphia; WB Saunders, 1976.
28. Askin FB, McCann BG, Kuhn C. Reactive eosinophilic pleuritis. *Arch Pathol Lab Med* 1977;101:187–191.
29. Churg A. Asbestos fibers and pleural plaques in a general autopsy population. *Am J Pathol* 1982;109:88–96.
30. Meurman L. Asbestos bodies and pleural plaques in a Finnish autopsy series. *Acta Pathol Microbiol Immunol Scand [Suppl]* 1966;181:7–107.
31. Roberts GH. The pathology of parietal pleural plaques. *J Clin Pathol* 1971;24:348–353.
32. Churg AC. An inflation procedure for open-lung biopsies. *Am J Surg Pathol* 1983;7:69–71.
33. Kadokura M, Colby TV, Myers JL, Allen MS, Deschamps C, Trastek, Pairolero PC. Pathologic comparison of video-assisted thoracic surgical lung biopsy with traditional open lung biopsy. *J Thorac Cardiovasc Surg* 1995;109:494–498.
34. Neiwohner DE, Kleinerman J, Rice DB. Pathologic changes in the peripheral airways of young cigarette smokers. *N Engl J Med* 1974;291: 755–758.
35. Myers JL, Veal CF, Shin MS, Katzenstein ALA. Respiratory bronchiolitis causing interstitial lung disease. *Am Rev Respir Dis* 1987;135: 880–884.
36. Ashley DJB. Bony metaplasia in trachea and bronchi. *J Pathol* 1970; 102:186–188.
37. Churg A, Warnock ML. Pulmonary tumorlets. *Cancer* 1976;37: 1469–1477.
38. Gould VE, Linnoila I, Memoli VA, Warren WH. Neuroendocrine components of the bronchopulmonary tract: hyperplasias, dysplasias, and neoplasms. *Lab Invest* 1983;49:519–537.
39. Ranchod M. The histogenesis and development of pulmonary tumorlets. *Cancer* 1977;39:1135–1145.
40. Kuhn C, Askin FB. The fine structure of so-called minute pulmonary chemodectomas. *Hum Pathol* 1975;6:681–691.
41. Colby TV, Koss MN, Travis WD. Tumors of the lower respiratory tract. In: *Atlas of Tumor Pathology, 3rd. ed.* Fascicle 13, AFIP, Washington DC, 1995.
42. Gaffey MJ, Mills SE, Askin FB. Minute pulmonary meningothelial-like nodules. A clinicopathologic study of so-called minute pulmonary chemodectoma. *Am J Surg Pathol* 1988;12:167–175.
43. Miller RR. Bronchioloalveolar cell adenomas. *Am J Surg Pathol* 1990; 14:904–912.
44. Elkeles A, Glynn LE. Disseminated parenchymatous ossification in the lungs in association with mitral stenosis. *J Pathol* 1946;58:517–522.
45. Green JD, Harle TS, Greenberg SD, Weg JG, Nevin H, Jenkins DE. Disseminated pulmonary ossification. *Am Rev Respir Dis* 1970;101: 293–298.
46. Bedrossian CWM, Kuhn C, Luma MA, et al. Desquamative interstitial pneumonia-like reactions accompanying pulmonary lesions. *Chest* 1977;101:166–169.
47. Hollander DH, Hutchins GM. Central spherules in pulmonary corpora amylacea. *Arch Pathol Lab Med* 1978;102:629–630.

48. Koss MN, Johnson FB, Hochholzer L. Pulmonary blue bodies. *Hum Pathol* 1981;12:258–266.
49. Visscher D, Churg A, Katzenstein ALA. Significance of crystalline inclusions in lung granulomas. *Mod Pathol* 1988;1:415.
50. Schaumann J. On the nature of certain peculiar corpuscles present in the tissue of lymphogranulomatosis benign. *Acta Med Scand* 1941;61: 239–253.
51. Churg A, Warnock ML. Asbestos and other ferruginous bodies. *Am J Pathol* 1981;102:447–456.
52. Glancy DL, Frazier PD, Roberts WC. Pulmonary parenchymal cholesterol-ester granulomas in patients with pulmonary hypertension. *Am J Med* 1968;45:198–210.
53. Reinila A. Perivascular xanthogranulomatosis in the lungs of diabetic patients. *Arch Pathol Lab Med* 1976;100:542–543.
54. Walford RL, Kaplan L. Pulmonary fibrosis and giant cell reaction with altered elastic tissue: "endogenous pneumoconiosis." *Arch Pathol* 1957;65:79–90.
55. Ro JY, Luna MA, MacKay B, Ramos O. Yellow-brown (Hamazaki-Wesenberg) bodies mimicking fungal yeast. *Arch Pathol Lab Med* 1987;111:555–559.
56. Gillooly M, Lamb D. Airspace size in lungs of lifelong non-smokers: effect of age and sex. *Thorax* 1993;38:39–43.
57. Kunze WP. Senile pulmonary amyloidosis. *Pathol Res Pract* 1978;164: 413–422.

# Alimentary Canal

*Histology for Pathologists, second edition,*
Edited by Stephen S. Sternberg.
Lippincott-Raven Publishers, Philadelphia


# CHAPTER 19

# Esophagus

Franco G. DeNardi and Robert H. Riddell



## EMBRYOLOGY

In the early stages of development, the notochord induces the formation of the foregut from endoderm (1). At about 21 days' gestation, septa arise from the lateral walls of the foregut, fuse, and divide the foregut into the esophagus and trachea. This process of septation begins at the carina and extends cephalad, being completed by 5 to 6 weeks' gestation (Fig. 1).

The esophagus is initially lined by a thin layer of stratified columnar epithelium, which proliferates to almost occlude the lumen (2). At 6 to 7 weeks the lumen is reformed as a result of epithelial vacuolization (2) (Fig. 2). As early as 8 weeks' gestation and beginning in the middle third of the esophagus, ciliated cells appear and extend cephalad and caudally to almost cover the entire stratified columnar epithelium (2–4). At approximately 10 weeks a single layer of columnar cells populates the proximal and distal ends of the esophagus (2). At approximately 4 months' gestation the esophageal cardiac-type glands form as a result of the downward growth of these columnar cells into the lamina propria, with subsequent proliferation and differentiation (2,3).

At approximately 5 months' gestation stratified squamous epithelium initially appears in the middle third of the esophagus and extends cephalad and caudally, replacing the ciliated epithelium (3,4). The upper esophagus is the last area to be replaced by squamous epithelium, and if this process of squamous replacement is not completed at birth there may be persistence of ciliated cells in the upper esophagus (2,4) (Fig. 3). These residual cells are short lived, being replaced by squamous epithelium within 2 to 3 days postpartum (4,5). The single layer of columnar cells is also replaced by squamous epithelium, although some cells may persist at birth, usually located over the esophageal cardiac glands. The submucosal glands develop after the appearance of the squamous epithelium and are likely derived from this squamous epithelial layer (4,5).

At about 6 weeks' gestation the circular muscle layer develops, followed by the development of the longitudinal layer at approximately 9 weeks' gestation. Initially, the muscularis propria consists entirely of smooth muscle, after which striated muscle gradually develops in the upper esophagus so that by 5 months the normal ratio and arrangement of both muscle types are established (4).

F. G. DeNardi: Department of Anatomical Pathology, Henderson General Hospital, and McMaster University, Hamilton, Ontario L8N 3Z5, Canada.
R. H. Riddell: Department of Anatomical Pathology, McMaster University Medical Centre, McMaster University, Hamilton, Ontario L8N 3Z5, Canada.

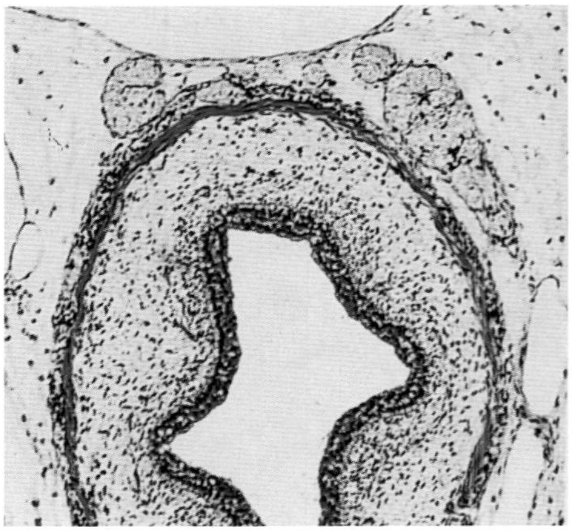

FIG. 1. Fetal esophagus (late first trimester). Transverse section overview of the esophagus demonstrating inner mucosal layer, middle submucosal layer, and thin outer muscle layer. Note the vagus nerves lying over the esophagus.

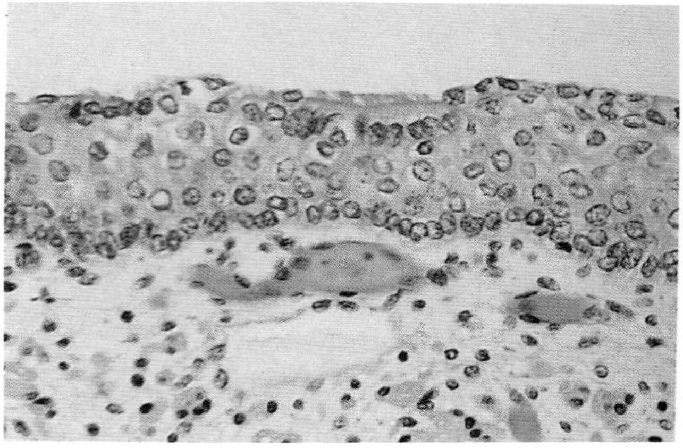

FIG. 3. Fetal esophagus (third trimester). The epithelial layer at this stage consists of stratified squamous epithelium with occasional ciliated cells on the surface. Note the individual smooth muscle cells of developing muscularis mucosae.

Developmental defects of the esophagus can be attributed to errors in this morphogenetic sequence. The notochord can induce the formation of the neural tube, gastrointestinal tract, and other organ systems. It has been shown experimentally that a split notochord can result in the duplication of any region of the gastrointestinal tract (1), which may include duplications of the esophagus ranging from the more common cysts to esophagus segments of variable length (1,6,7). As a consequence of this ability to induce development of more than one organ system, any patient presenting with duplications, segmental or cystic, should undergo radiologic evaluation that specifically explores for axial skeletal defects. Abnormalities during the phase of foregut septation is one proposed mechanism for the formation of tracheoesophageal fistulas with or without atresia or mediastinal cysts of bronchogenic or esophageal origin (8,9). It has been suggested that esophageal duplications also may occur as a result of segments of fused vacuoles formed during the vacuolization phase persisting and differentiating toward esophageal structures (1).

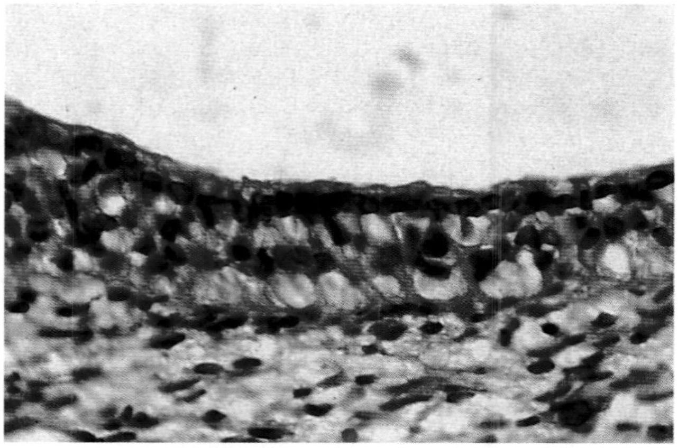

FIG. 2. Fetal esophagus (late first trimester). The epithelial layer is composed of stratified columnar epithelium. Note the lack of muscularis mucosae.

## TOPOGRAPHY AND RELATIONS

The esophagus begins in the neck at the cricoid cartilage, passes through the thorax within the posterior mediastinum, and extends for several centimeters past the diaphragm to its junction with the stomach. The overall length varies with trunk length, but in the adult the average length is approximately 23 to 25 cm. In practice, endoscopic distances are measured from the incisor teeth, and in the average male the junction of the esophagus and stomach is generally considered to be approximately 40 cm from the incisors. This length may vary from 38 to 43 cm. Although convenient and commonly used in practice, the use of this distance is a crude and unreliable measurement for locating the gastroesophageal junction. It has been found that in children the esophageal length correlates with height (10).

For the purpose of classification, staging, and reporting of esophageal malignancy, the International Union Against Cancer suggests division into four segments, with distances measured from the incisors (11) (Fig. 4). The cervical esophagus extends from the cricoid cartilage (15 cm) to the level of the thoracic inlet (18 cm). The upper thoracic segment extends from the thoracic inlet to the tracheal bifurcation (24 cm). The midthoracic segment extends to the level of the eighth cervical vertebra (approximately 32 cm), and the lower thoracic segment extends to the junction with the stomach (40 cm).

Along its course the normal esophagus has several points of constriction (Fig. 5). These occur at the cricoid origin of the esophagus, along the left side of the esophagus at the aortic arch, at the crossing of the left main bronchus and left atrium, and where the esophagus passes through the dia-

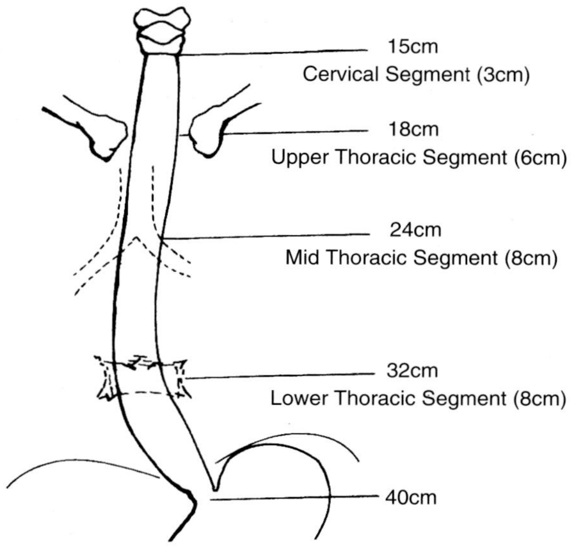


**FIG. 4.** Segments of the esophagus.

phragm. These constrictions may become clinically significant if food or pills become lodged at these sites of luminal narrowing, with the possibility of contact mucosal injury. The most common sites for lodgement are at the level of the aortic arch and left atrium, where, especially in patients with left atrial enlargement, compression may become significant (12).

Knowledge of the relationships of the esophagus with other anatomic structures is important because these relationships may be directly affected by esophageal diseases such as carcinoma or diverticula. Disease of adjacent structures may cause local compression of the esophagus, resulting in dysphagia or lodgement of food or pills. The cervical esophagus is posterior to the trachea and bounded on both sides by the recurrent laryngeal nerve and the carotid sheath and its structures. The thyroid gland overlaps the esophagus in its cervical segment. In the thoracic segment, the esophagus continues posterior to the trachea to the level of bifurcation, a site for the formation of the rare midesophageal diverticula secondary to traction from inflamed mediastinal lymph nodes (13,14). The esophagus courses posterior to the left atrium. The azygous veins ascend on either side of the thoracic segment.

Initially, the right and left vagus nerves run lateral to the esophagus, giving branches that form plexi on the posterior and anterior esophageal surfaces. At variable sites in the lower thoracic segment, the left and right nerves course onto the anterior and posterior surfaces of the esophagus, respectively, divide to form the anterior and posterior plexuses, and then reunite to form the anterior and posterior vagal trunks that course down to the stomach. An awareness that variations of this pattern exist is most important for the surgeon performing vagotomies. In the abdomen, the liver forms an impression on the anterior aspect of the esophagus. On the right side the junction with the stomach is smooth, whereas on the left the junction forms a sharp angle known as the incisura or angle of His.

The esophagus enters the abdomen by passing through the esophageal hiatus, which is formed by muscles of the di-

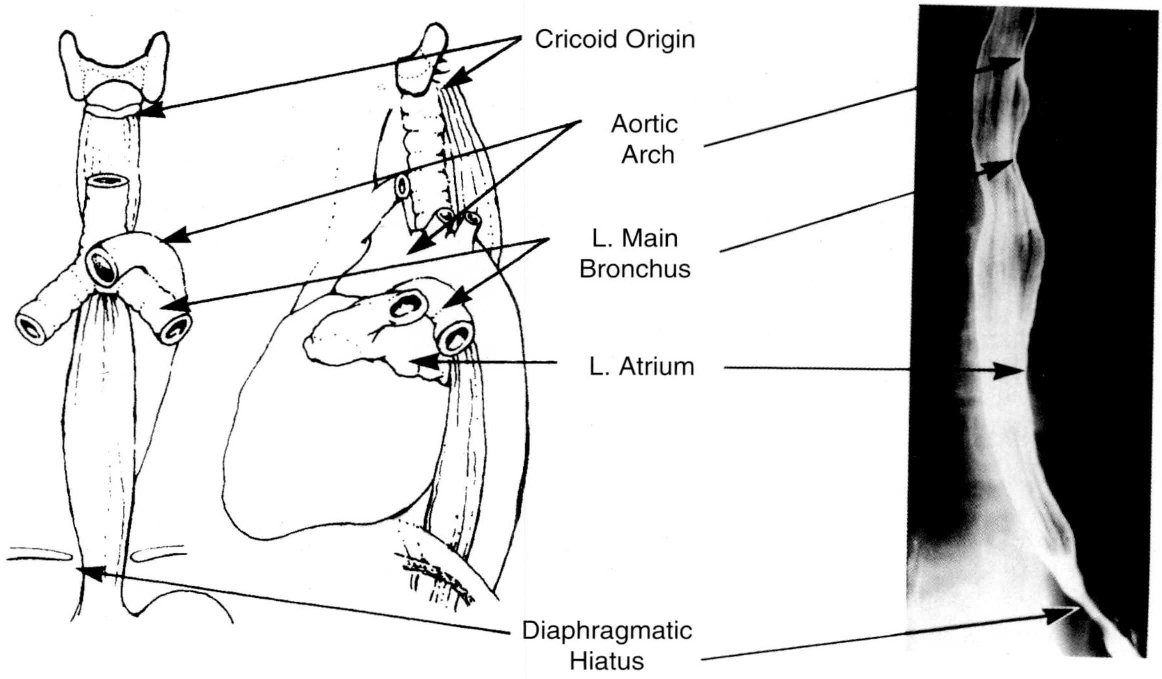


**FIG. 5.** Relationship of the esophagus with normal esophageal constrictions. Barium swallow of the normal esophagus demonstrates narrowing of the lumen at the sites of constriction.

aphragm and contains the phrenoesophageal ligament. In most cases the muscle sling encircling the esophagus is formed entirely from the right diaphragmatic crus (15), although variations of this pattern do occur. The phrenoesophageal ligament arises from the fascia of the abdominal diaphragm and divides into an ascending and descending leaf. The former passes up through the hiatus to insert approximately 2 to 3 cm above the hiatus, whereas the descending leaf has a variable insertion at or below the gastroesophageal junction or even into the gastric fundus (16). Proposed functions of the phrenoesophageal ligament include (a) assisting in maintaining the pressure differential between the thorax and abdomen, (b) providing fixation mechanisms with maintenance of the gastroesophageal junction within the abdomen during episodes of increased intraabdominal pressure, and (c) contributing to the competence of the lower esophageal sphincter (LES), thus representing a possible mechanism for the absence of reflux in some patients with hiatal hernias (16,17).

## MACROSCOPIC/ENDOSCOPIC FEATURES

In the empty state, the esophagus has an irregular outline as a result of the mucosa and submucosa being thrown into longitudinal folds. During endoscopy, insufflation causes distension so that these folds may not be appreciated and the mucosa is seen to be a uniform white–pink.

### Glycogenic Acanthosis

Glycogenic acanthosis can be seen in 25% of the population with the combined use of endoscopy and barium studies (18). Macroscopically, glycogenic acanthosis interrupts the uniformity of the mucosa and presents as white nodules or small plaques on the mucosal folds primarily in the distal third of the esophagus (19,20). These lesions vary in size and may be up to 1 cm in diameter and if extensive may coalesce to larger plaques. Microscopically, glycogenic acanthosis consists of hyperplasia of the cells of the prickle layer containing abundant glycogen. Glycogenic acanthosis may resemble, and thus may be confused macroscopically with, monilial plaques or leukoplakia. Glycogenic acanthosis should be considered a variant of normal with as yet no defined relationship to infection or malignancy.

### Heterotopias

Heterotopias are defined as normal tissue occurring in sites not expected for that tissue. In the literature, structures accepted as esophageal heterotopias are inconsistently defined. Esophageal cardiac-type glands and ciliated epithelium have been considered as heterotopias (5,21,22) or as embryologic remnants (4) by some investigators. The categorization of melanocytes and argyrophilic cells presents a similar problem because these cells have not been regularly found in the esophagus. Gastric body–type mucosa and sebaceous glands have been accepted as heterotopias without controversy.

Gastric body–type mucosa has been described occurring in the upper third of the esophagus, usually within 3.0 cm of the upper esophageal sphincter (4,5,23), hence the designation "inlet patch" (23) (Fig. 6). These heterotopias have been found in approximately 2% to 4% of esophagi (5,23) and can be found at all ages (5). Macroscopically they have a deep pink, velvety appearance, and the junction with squamous epithelium is similar in appearance to the mucosal gastroesophageal junction (23). Associated small peptic erosions or ulcers occasionally are identified nearby.

Microscopically the heterotopic mucosa contains a variable number of parietal and chief cells with a variable chronic inflammatory cell infiltrate (4,5,23) (Fig. 7). Acid production and symptoms have been attributed to heterotopias of larger size (23). These heterotopias along with the esophageal cardiac-type glands have been implicated as possible origins for the rare occurrence of adenocarcinoma of the upper esophagus (24). Theories for the origin of these heterotopias include a metaplastic change in preexisting cardiac-type glands (4) or cell arrest where cells destined to become body mucosa remain in the esophagus rather than descend to the site of the future stomach (23).

Sebaceous glands are occasionally found in the esophagus (Fig. 8) (25), and symptoms have been attributed to the presence of such glands (4). Thyroid tissue also has been described as heterotopic tissue in the esophagus (4). Pancreatic metaplasia is probably the most common form of metaplasia in the cardia, usually close to the Z line, although it also may be found in Barrett's esophagus (Fig. 9).

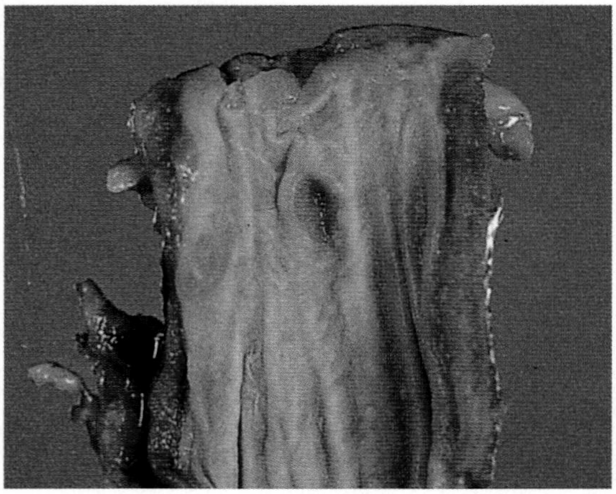

**FIG. 6.** Proximal esophagus. Gastric body heterotopia situated slightly distal from the esophageal origin.

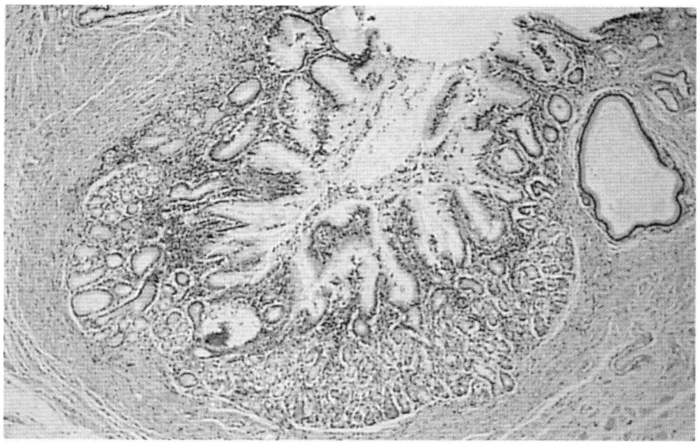
A

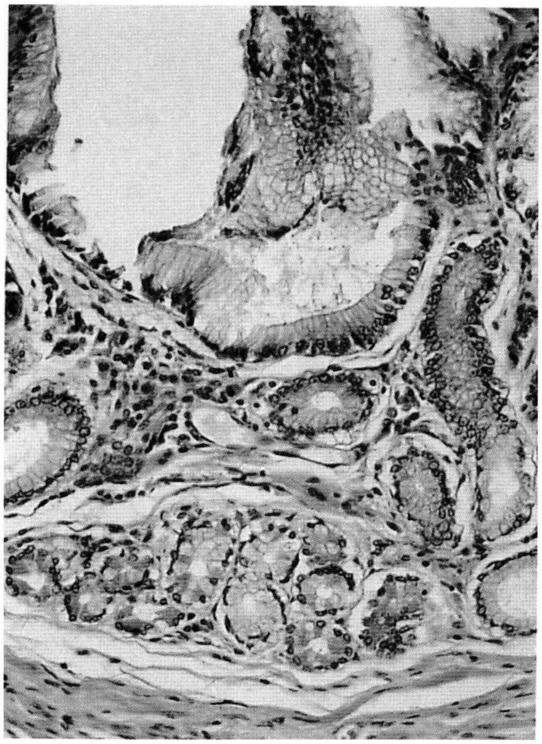
B

**FIG. 7.** Proximal esophagus. Gastric body heterotopia composed of cardiac-type mucosa with scattered chief cells and a mild chronic inflammatory cell infiltrate.

### Esophageal Musculature

The muscular coat of the esophagus consists of an outer longitudinal and inner circular layer. The esophageal entrance is bounded superiorly by the cricopharyngeal and inferior pharyngeal constrictor muscles, both of which contribute muscle fibers to the esophageal musculature (17). Horizontal fibers from both these muscles form the upper esophageal sphincter, which manometrically is a localized zone of increased pressure measuring 2 to 4.5 cm in length (15). Together these muscle groups act in tandem to control the act of swallowing, but when this ability is lost, disorders classified as "oropharyngeal dysphagia" may arise (4).

The longitudinal layer originates as two bands from its origin at the cricoid cartilage. The muscles sweep dorsally where they incompletely interdigitate, leaving a bare V-shaped area (area of Laimer) exposing the underlying circular layer. This area represents an area of potential weakness where a posterior pulsion diverticulum (Zenker's) may form (4,17). The circular layer is slightly thinner than the longitudinal layer, a pattern that is reversed from the remainder of the gastrointestinal tract (17).

At the gastroesophageal junction the esophageal longitudinal layer is continuous with the outer longitudinal layer of the stomach. The circular layer continues over the stomach, dividing in the region of the cardia to form the middle circular and inner oblique muscle layers of the stomach. The fibers of the inner oblique layer pass in a slinglike manner at the incisura and cross at right angles with the more horizontally oriented fibers of the middle layer, forming a muscular ring (collare Helvetti) to which a possible sphincter function has been ascribed (17).

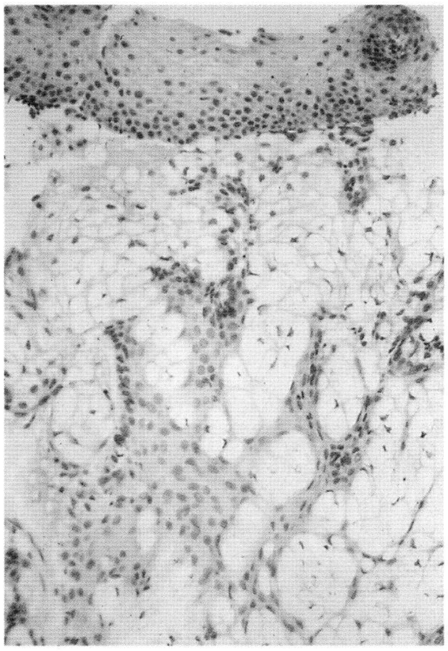

**FIG. 8.** Sebaceous glands that in this case formed a nodule that was examined via biopsy.

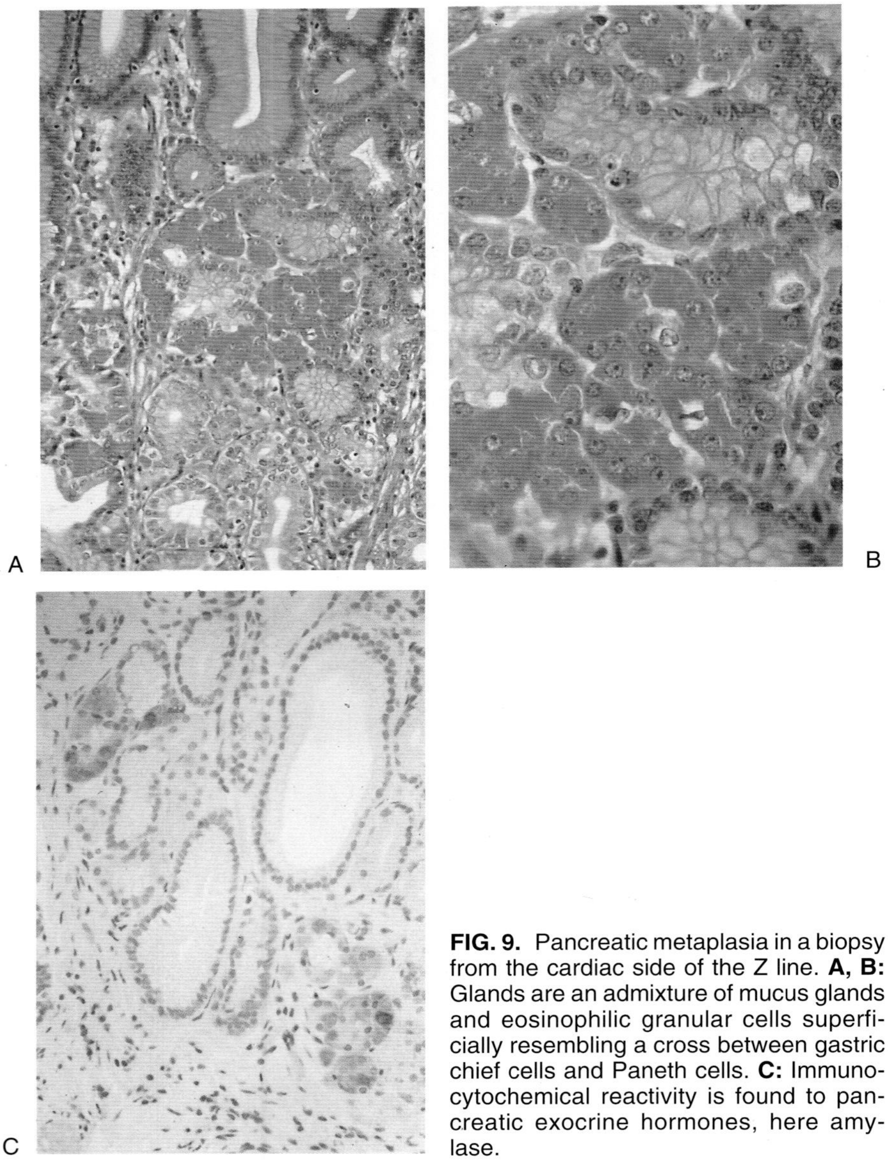


**FIG. 9.** Pancreatic metaplasia in a biopsy from the cardiac side of the Z line. **A, B:** Glands are an admixture of mucus glands and eosinophilic granular cells superficially resembling a cross between gastric chief cells and Paneth cells. **C:** Immunocytochemical reactivity is found to pancreatic exocrine hormones, here amylase.

### Lower Esophageal Sphincter

The LES is best defined manometrically, where it presents as a 2- to 4-cm zone of pressure that is higher than intragastric or intraesophageal pressure. The distalmost end of the LES defines the gastroesophageal junction (26). At rest, the sphincter maintains an average pressure of 20 mm Hg (range 10–26) (15). The function of the LES is to keep the lumen closed during rest, thus preventing reflux, and to relax during swallowing, thereby allowing food to pass through. Physiologically, a competent sphincter exists, yet until recently attempts to identify a corresponding anatomic structure have been unsuccessful. Various changes in the musculature of the distal esophagus, thought to represent such a sphincter, have been described (15,17,27,28).

### Gastroesophageal Junction

The gastroesophageal junction can be defined physiologically, anatomically, or microscopically and can be considered as being either muscular or mucosal in nature. The muscular gastroesophageal junction is most accurately defined physiologically by manometric studies in which the distalmost segment of the LES defines the junction (26). Unfortunately, in disease states such as severe gastroesophageal reflux disease (GERD) or Barrett's esophagus, the pressure may be so low as to not allow for localization by these means.

Anatomic landmarks that can be used to define the gastroesophageal junction include the peritoneal reflection from the stomach onto the diaphragm or the incisura (angle of His)

A 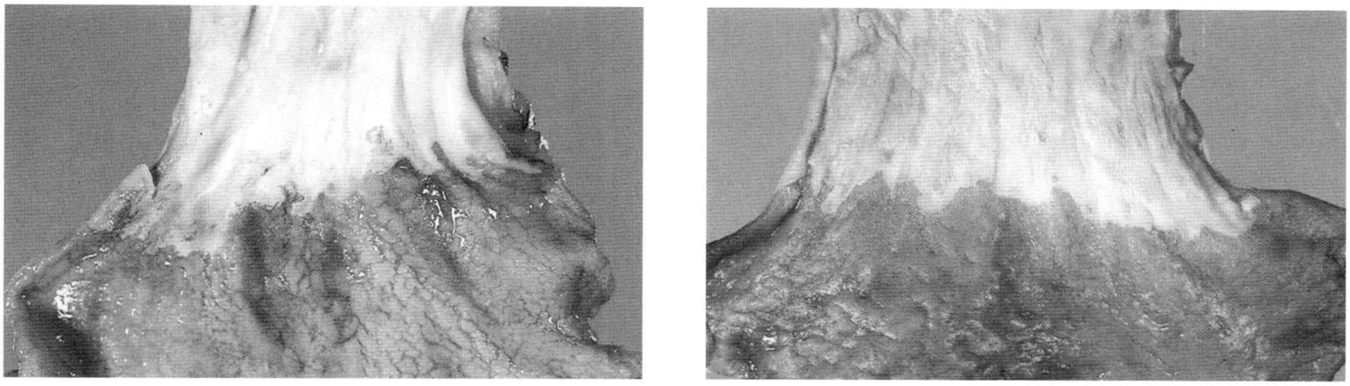 B

**FIG. 10.** Gastroesophageal region. Formalin-fixed specimen demonstrates the variation of the normal squamocolumnar junction (Z-line).

(29); however, their use is limited to the resected surgical specimen. Endoscopically, the upper margin of the diaphragmatic indentation has been used as a guide to define the gastroesophageal junction; however, in the presence of a hiatal hernia this demonstrates variable movement (18). The proximal margin of the gastric folds has been shown to closely approximate the muscular gastroesophageal junction (16) and thus may provide a fixed and reproducible anatomic landmark for the muscular gastroesophageal junction (30).

The mucosal squamocolumnar junction is seen macroscopically as a serrated line of contrast known as the Z line or ora serrata (Fig. 10). The Z line consists of small projections of red gastric epithelium, up to 5 mm long and 3 mm wide, extending upward into the squamous epithelium. Although extension of this gastric mucosa may be circumferentially symmetric, it often is asymmetric (26). The mucosal gastroesophageal junction may be straight rather than serrated, this occurring most often in the presence of a lower mucosal ring (31).

The mucosal gastroesophageal junction does not correspond to the muscular gastroesophageal junction as defined above. The mucosal junction normally lies within the LES, found usually within 2 cm of the muscular junction as defined by the proximal edge of the gastric folds (30); thus, the distal 2 cm of the esophagus may be lined by columnar epithelium that is identical to that found in the gastric cardia. The length of these extensions may be unusually exaggerated, sometimes extending 3 cm into the esophagus and thus endoscopically resembling early Barrett's esophagus. Pancreatic metaplasia occasionally is identified in biopsy specimens from the columnar side of the Z line (Fig. 9) and also may be associated with Barrett's esophagus (32).

### Lower Esophageal Rings

Two thin, annular structures known as the lower mucosal ring (Schatzki's, type B) (Fig. 11) and lower muscular ring (type A) may be identified in 10% and 5% of normal esophagi, respectively (31). The lower muscular ring is situated slightly more proximal than the Schatzki ring, with both being confined to the LES. These rings are usually asymptomatic but may be associated with intermittent dysphagia, sometimes becoming progressive or associated with attacks of sudden dysphagia (15). The lower mucosal ring is thought to mark the mucosal gastroesophageal junction, and the presence of such a ring is said to indicate the existence of a sliding hiatal hernia; however, these views are not universally accepted (27,31,33,34).

Histologically, the upper surface of the lower mucosal ring is lined by stratified squamous epithelium, whereas the undersurface is lined by columnar-type epithelium with the junction of both usually, but not invariably, being found at the apex of the ring. The core of the ring consists of connective tissue plus fibers of the muscularis mucosae without

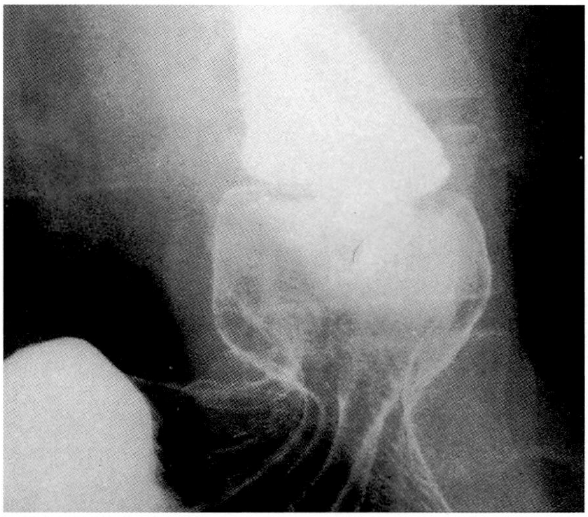

**FIG. 11.** Lower esophageal mucosal ring (Schatzki's ring). The mucosal ring is outlined by the column of barium.

contribution from the muscularis propria. Some have equated the lower muscular ring with the inferior esophageal sphincter (27,31). Microscopically, this ring is composed of a thickened circular smooth muscle with overlying squamous mucosa.

## HISTOLOGY

The four layers that characterize the gastrointestinal tract—mucosa, submucosa, muscularis propria, and serosa—form the wall of the esophagus.

### Mucosa

The mucosa consists of a nonkeratinizing, stratified squamous epithelium, lamina propria, and muscularis mucosae (Fig. 12).

#### *Epithelium*

The squamous epithelium can be divided into the basal, prickle, and functional cell layers. In addition, argyrophilic positive endocrine cells, melanocytes, and various inflammatory cells can be found in the epithelium of the normal esophagus. The basal layer occupies approximately 10% to 15% of the epithelium, being one to three cells thick; however, in the distal 3 cm approximately 60% of normal individuals (without objective or subjective evidence of gastroesophageal reflux) may show basal cell hyperplasia of greater than 15% (35). The upper extent of the basal zone has been arbitrarily defined as the level where the nuclei are separated by a distance equal to their diameter (36,37). Periodic acid-Schiff (PAS) stain may be used to demonstrate the upper extent of the glycogen-poor basal cells (Fig. 13). Above the basal cell layer, the prickle and functional cell layers consist of glycogen-rich cells that become progressively flatter toward the surface. Glandular mucosa of the distal esophagus is typical cardiac mucosa with variable numbers of specialized gastric cells and cardiac glands as described in the following chapter.

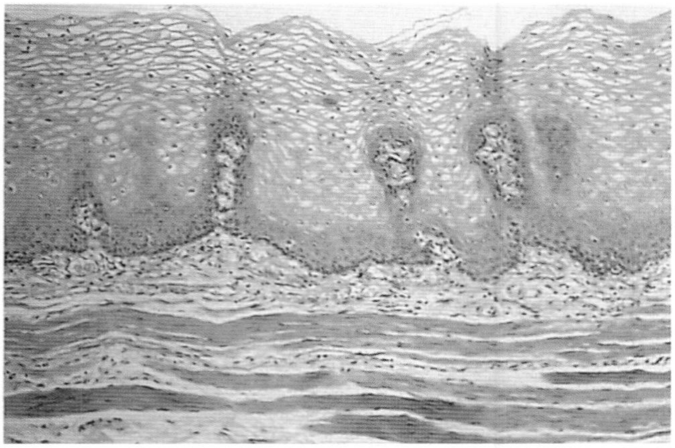

**FIG. 12.** Midesophagus. The esophageal mucosa consists of a surface epithelial layer, middle lamina propria, and lower muscularis mucosae, which consist of longitudinally oriented smooth muscle bundles.

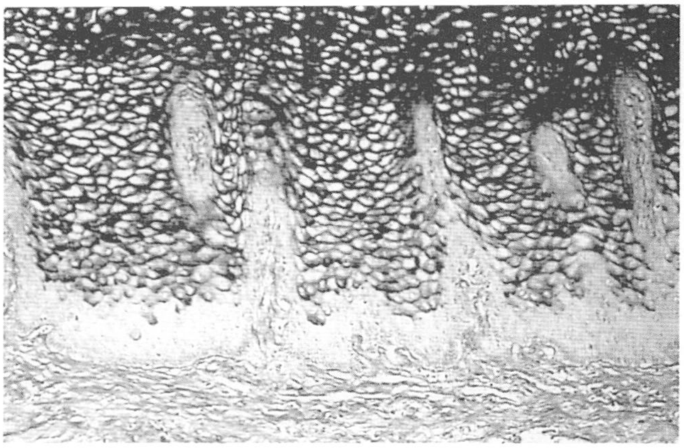

**FIG. 13.** Midesophagus. The basal cell layer of the esophageal epithelium shows lack of glycogen, allowing for ready distinction from the overlying glycogen-rich cells (PASD).

Argyrophilic-positive endocrine cells and melanocytes have been found scattered among the basal cells in approximately 25% (38) and 4% to 8% (38,39) of normal individuals, respectively. The presence of melanocytes, referred to as melanosis (38,40), accounts for the occurrence of primary melanoma of the esophagus (40), whereas the presence of argyrophilic positive cells accounts for the rare occurrence of small cell carcinoma (38).

Occasional lymphocytes are a normal finding in the epithelium and usually are located in a suprabasal location (37,41–43). As they interdigitate between the epithelial cells, their nuclei become convoluted and may be confused with the nuclei of neutrophils. The term "squiggle cell" is used to describe this appearance (Fig. 14). As in the rest of the gastrointestinal tract, intraepithelial lymphocytes are CD3/CD8 positive, indicating suppressor/cytotoxic function. Langerhans cells, which are CD6 and la positive, also are located in a suprabasal location (41) (Fig. 15). Langerhans cells function as antigen-presenting cells, similar to Langerhans cells of the skin (41).

The cytology of the esophagus is represented by stratified squamous epithelium, gastric-type epithelium representing the distal 1 to 2 cm, and contaminants from the oropharynx, respiratory tract, and foreign material such as food particles. The squamous epithelium in cytologic material consists predominantly of superficial and intermediate squamous cells, with the deeper parabasal cells or squamous "pearls" occasionally observed. The gastric-type epithelium from the lower 1 to 2 cm of the esophagus is brushed as cohesive

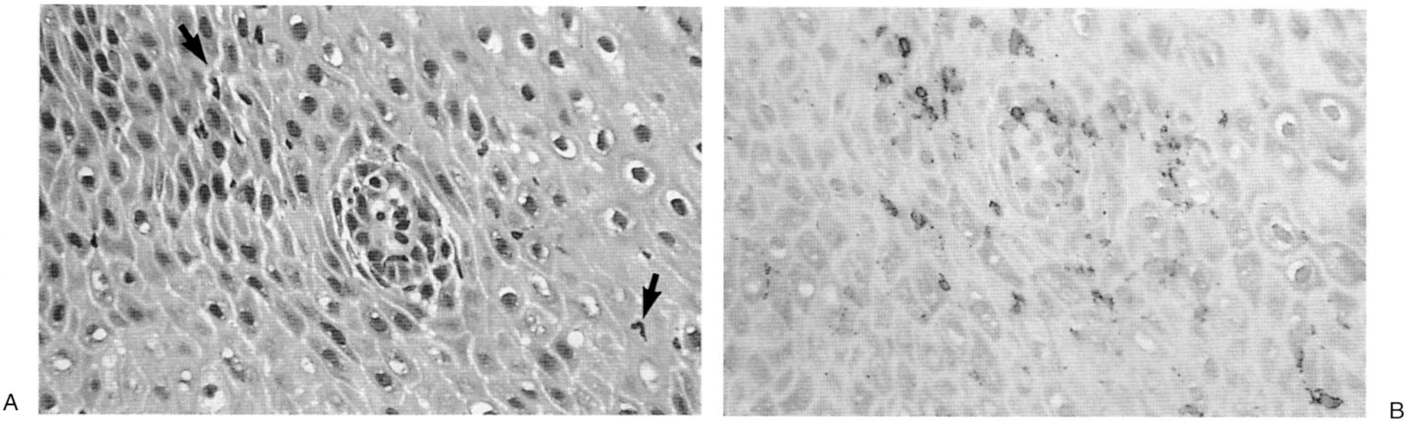

FIG. 14. A: Numerous lymphocytes within the esophageal epithelium, some of which have a "squiggle" appearance (*arrows*). B: These intraepithelial lymphocytes are of T-cell origin, as demonstrated using the T-cell marker UCHL-I.

fragments of uniform cells displaying a honeycomb arrangement. The peripheral cells of the cluster are flattened. The nuclei are regular and paracentrally situated and contain a few granules of chromatin and occasionally a small nucleolus.

The electron microscopic appearance of the epithelial layer demonstrates similarities to nonkeratinizing squamous epithelium elsewhere (Fig. 16). The cuboidal basal cells are attached to the basement membrane by hemidesmosomes. Progressing superficially, the epithelial cells become more flattened and the nuclei more pyknotic (41). Cell processes and desmosomes are most extensive in the prickle cell layer, becoming fewer and more simplified superficially (44). Membrane-bound, acid phosphatase–containing structures measuring 200 to 300 nm in diameter are identified within the epithelial cells and are postulated to have a lysosomal function, possibly involved in the digestion of cell junctions necessary for epithelial sloughing (20,44).

Cell kinetics of the human esophagus have not been studied extensively. The basal cells are responsible for epithelial regeneration, and although data on human esophageal mucosal renewal are not available, epithelial turnover in the esophagus is slower than in the small bowel (45). In the mouse, basal cell proliferation has been shown to have a circadian rhythm (46), and the epithelial turnover time in the

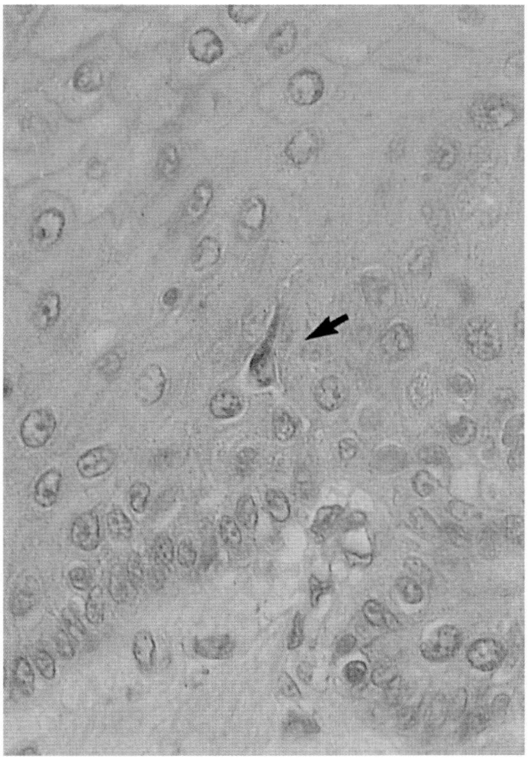

**FIG. 15.** Langerhans cell (*arrow*) in a suprabasal position demonstrated using S-100.

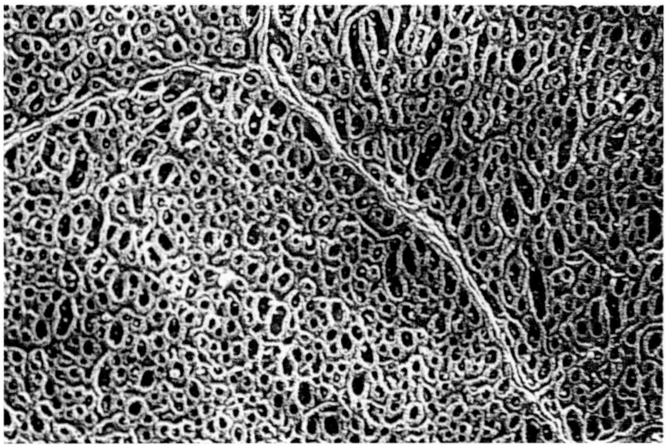

**FIG. 16.** Scanning electron micrograph of the surface esophageal mucosa in which intercellular junctions are readily appreciated.

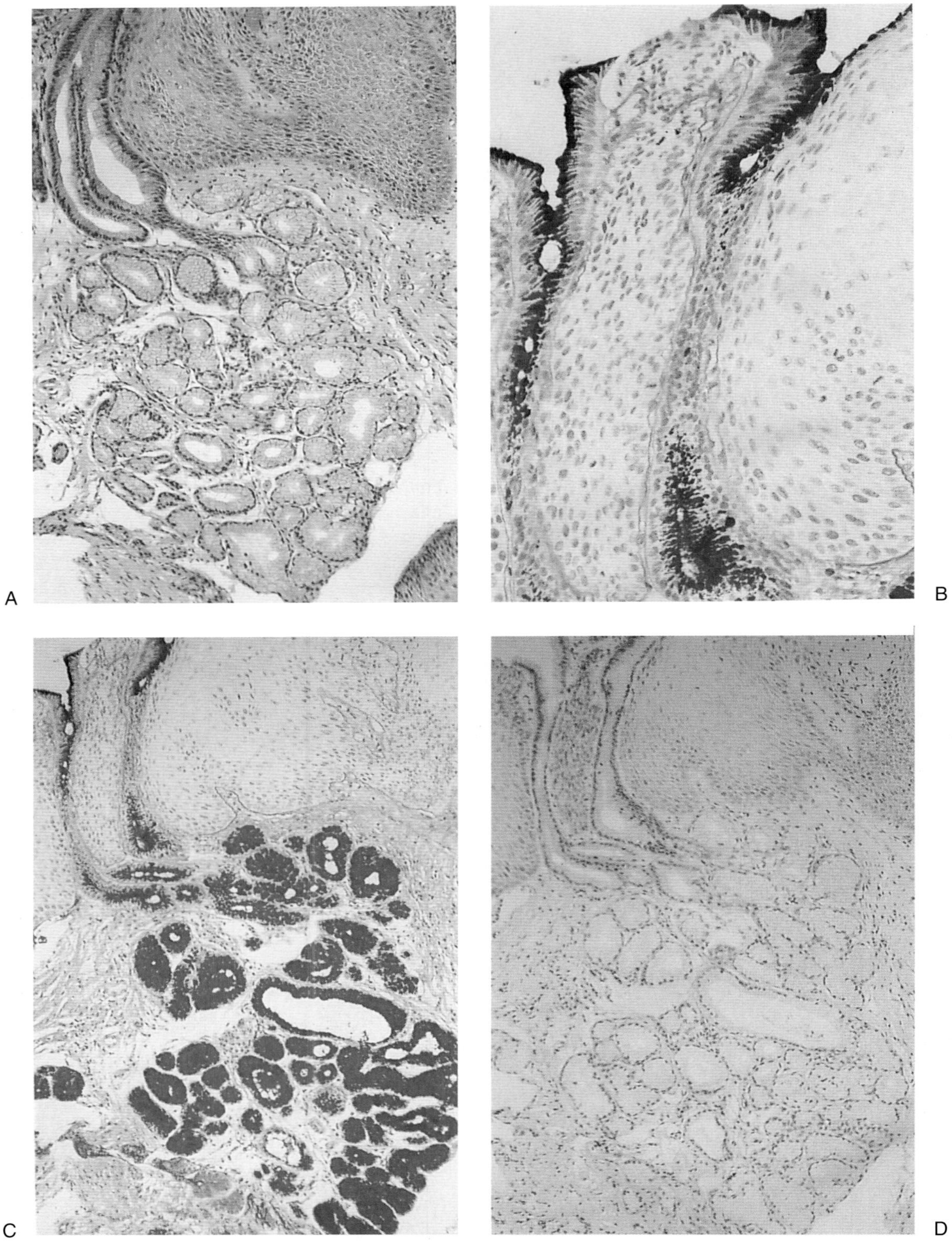

**FIG. 17.** Midesophagus. **A:** Esophageal cardiac-type glands are located within the lamina propria. The ducts are lined by gastric foveolar–like cells. **B:** The duct-lining cells may extend over the stratified squamous epithelium for variable distances (PASD). **C, D:** The glands stained PASD positive and alcian blue at pH = 2.5 negative, characteristic of neutral mucins.

normal rat esophagus is approximately 7 days (47). In patients with GERD, there is an increased proliferative activity of the basal cells, resulting in basal cell hyperplasia (48).

### *Lamina Propria*

The lamina propria is the nonepithelial portion of the mucosa above the muscularis mucosae consisting of areolar connective tissue and containing vascular structures, scattered inflammatory cells, and mucus-secreting glands. In adults, the presence of scattered inflammatory cells, including lymphocytes and plasma cells, is considered a normal finding and does not correlate with acid reflux (36,42). Lymphocytes identified in the lamina propria are both CD4 and CD8 positive, with the T4 population predominating (41). IgA-producing B cells (plasma cells) predominate, with a smaller population of immunoglobulin (Ig)G- and IgM-producing B cells (plasma cells) (41).

Fingerlike extensions of lamina propria, termed papillae, extend into the epithelium, with the maximum depth of extension allowable in the normal esophagus varying from 50% (42) to 75% (49). In the distal 3 cm of the esophagus, up to 60% of individuals without objective evidence of reflux demonstrate papillary lengths that may exceed these values (35).

Esophageal cardiac-type glands are diffusely scattered in the lamina propria through all levels of the esophagus, predominating in the distal and proximal regions (4,21). They have been variably considered as heterotopias (5,21,22), normal constituents, or embryologic remnants and are not always identified in the esophagus, having been found in 6% to 16% of esophagi in various studies (4,5,21). Histologically, these glands are located within the lamina propria, resemble the cardiac glands of the stomach, and are composed of cells secreting neutral mucins (50) (Fig. 17). The glands open directly into the lumen through ducts lined by gastric foveolarlike cells that may extend over the squamous epithelial surface. Although there is uncertainty as to the cell of origin for Barrett's esophagus, the cells lining the gland duct may be considered as a possible source (26).

### *Muscularis Mucosae*

The muscularis mucosae are composed of smooth muscle bundles oriented longitudinally (26), rather than having both a circular and longitudinal arrangement as in the stomach. The muscularis mucosae begin at the cricoid cartilage of the pharynx and become thicker distally. At the gastroesophageal junction the esophageal muscularis mucosae are thicker than those of the stomach and may be so thick as to be mistaken for muscularis propria on biopsy (Fig. 18). This thicker appearance along with the longitudinal arrangement is used sometimes to indicate an esophageal origin for the biopsy, and the differences between the muscularis mucosae

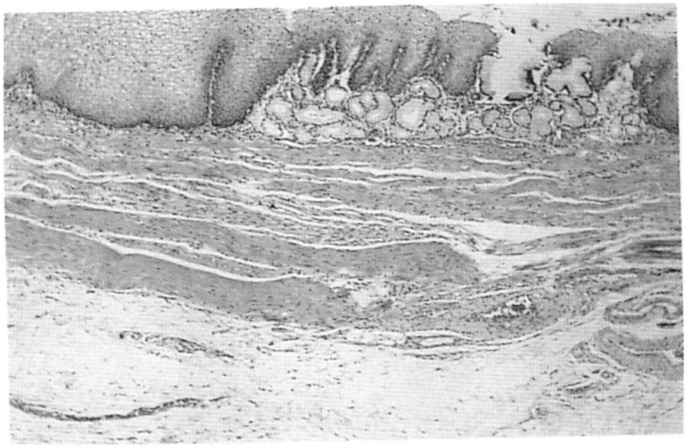

**FIG. 18.** Distal esophagus. The mucosal layer at the gastroesophageal junction is characterized by muscularis mucosae that are thicker than the muscularis mucosae of the more proximal esophagus (compare with Fig. 10). Note the esophageal cardiac-type gland situated above the muscularis mucosae.

of the stomach and esophagus can be used to identify the muscular gastroesophageal junction.

### Submucosa

The submucosa consists of loose connective tissue containing vessels, nerve fibers including Meissner's plexus, lymphatics, and submucosal glands (Fig. 19). The submucosal glands are considered to be a continuation of the minor salivary glands of the oropharynx (4) and are scattered throughout the entire esophagus but are more concentrated in the upper and lower regions (4). The glands consist of muci-

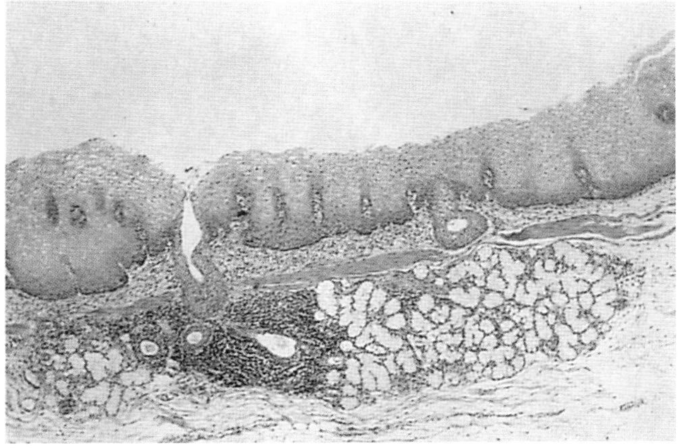

**FIG. 19.** Midesophagus. Submucosal glands of the esophagus are located within the submucosa just beneath the muscularis mucosae. Periductal and periglandular chronic inflammation can be a normal finding. Note that in contrast to the columnar-lined glands of the lamina propria, the ducts of the submucosal glands are lined by squamous epithelium.

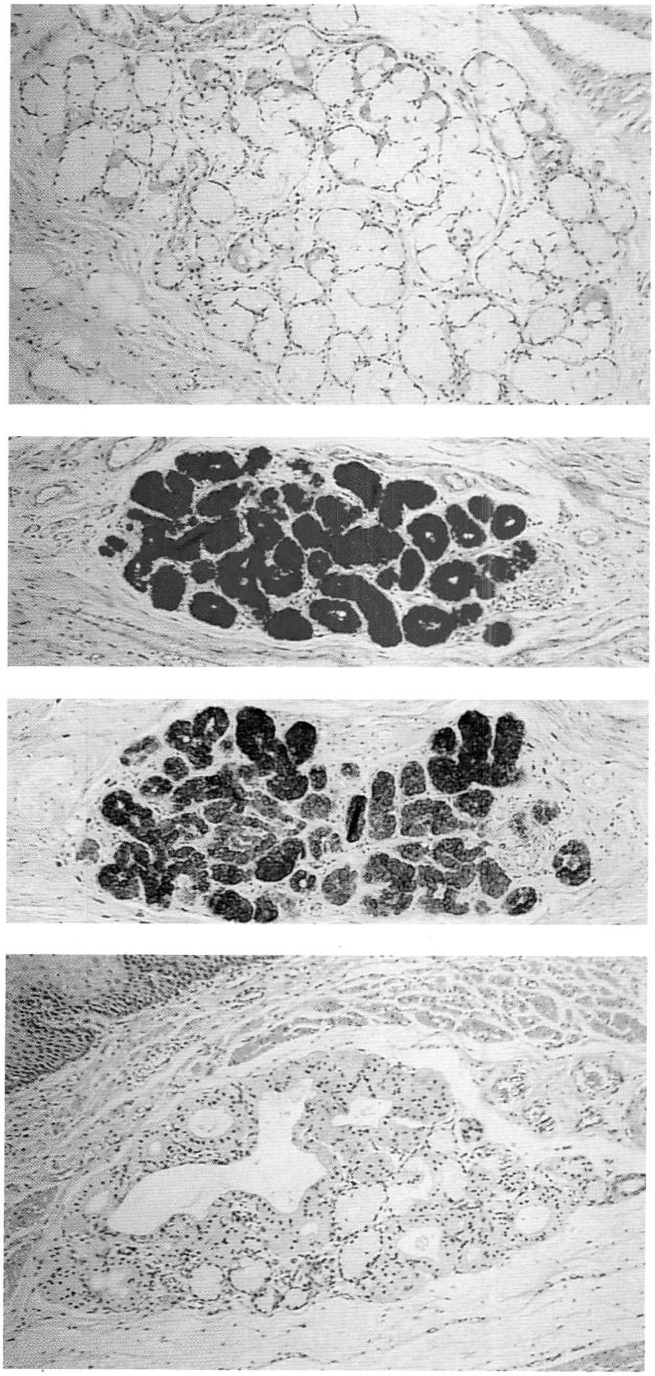

A B C D

**FIG. 20.** Midesophagus. **A:** The submucosal glands are composed predominantly of mucus-secreting cells with a variable serous component. **B,C:** The submucosal glands stained PASD and alcian blue pH at = 2.5 positive, characteristic of acid mucins. **D:** Submucosal glands may demonstrate oncocytic metaplasia.

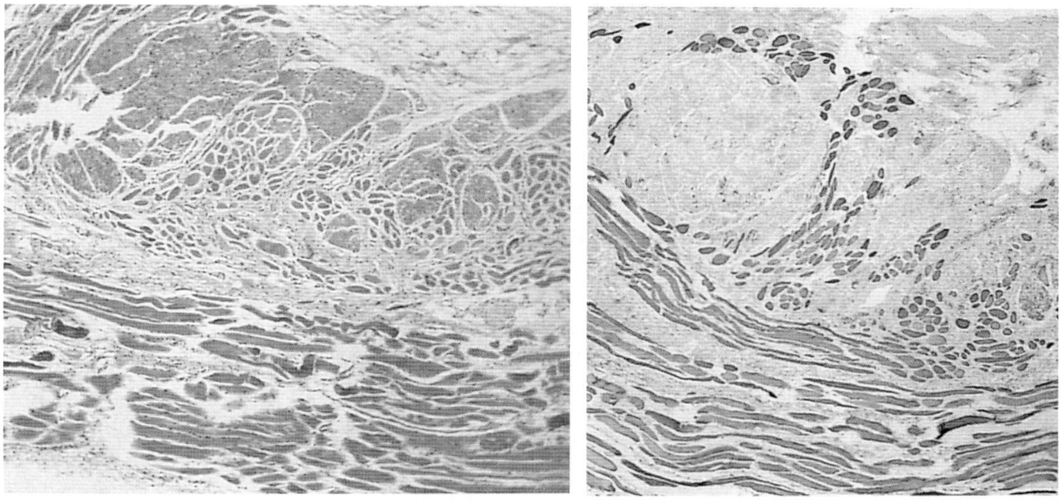

A B

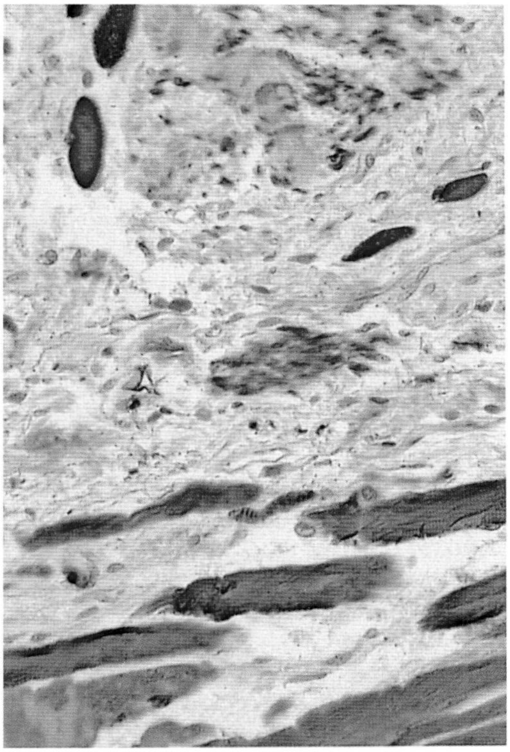

C

**FIG. 21.** Proximal esophagus. **A:** The muscularis propria demonstrates a mixture of smooth and striated muscle bundles. **B:** This mix of smooth (weakly stained) and striated (strongly stained) muscle is demonstrated using a myoglobin antibody. **C:** Detail photomicrographs of myoglobin-stained section demonstrates cross-striations and peripherally located nuclei typical of striated muscle.

nous cells with or without a minor serous component and produce acid mucins (Fig. 20). The glands are drained by ducts, initially lined by a single layer of cuboidal epithelium, becoming stratified squamous in type, which penetrate the muscularis mucosae and epithelium to open into the esophageal lumen. Microscopic periductal aggregates of chronic inflammatory cells and duct dilatation are not uncommon findings in the normal esophagus (51). The presence of submucosal glands is indicative of an esophageal origin because these glands are not present in the stomach; unfortunately, submucosal glands are almost never present in biopsy specimens. Esophageal intramucosal pseudodiverticulosis arises from postinflammatory obstruction of the ducts with subsequent duct dilatation (51,52)

### Muscularis Propria

It is generally stated that as much as the upper quarter to upper third of the proximal muscularis propria is composed of striated muscle (17); however, recently is was shown that only a short length (approximately 5%) of the proximal muscularis propria is composed of striated muscle (53). Immediately distal to this, smooth and striated muscle intermix, with smooth muscle predominating, whereas slightly more than 50% of the distal muscularis propria is composed solely of smooth muscle (53) (Fig. 21). Despite the presence of these two different muscle types, they can function as a unit. Auerbach's plexus is found between the two muscle layers. Disease processes may preferentially involve only one of the muscular layers, as in scleroderma, in which atrophy predominantly involves the circular layer (4), or in achalasia, in which the circular layer may become hypertrophied (4).

### Serosa

Only short segments of the thoracic and intra-abdominal esophagus are lined by serosa derived from the pleura and peritoneum, respectively (4). The majority of the esophagus is surrounded by fascia, which condenses around the esophagus, forming a sheathlike structure. In the upper mediastinum, the esophagus is given support as this fascial tissue extends out to surround and form a similar sheathlike arrangement around adjacent structures (17).

## ARTERIAL SUPPLY

The cervical portion of the esophagus is supplied by branches of the inferior thyroid artery with contribution from various intercostal arteries. Branches of the bronchial arteries, intercostal arteries, and aorta supply the thoracic segment, whereas the abdominal segment is supplied by branches of the left gastric and inferior phrenic artery (4,17,54). Branches from these arteries run within the muscular layer, giving rise to branches that course within the submucosa. Anastomoses are extensive, explaining the rarity of esophageal infarction (4).

## VENOUS DRAINAGE

The venous return from the upper two thirds of the esophagus drains into the inferior thyroid vein and azygous system, eventually reaching the superior vena cava. The lower esophageal segment drains into the systemic system through branches of the azygous vein and left inferior phrenic vein. The lower esophageal segment also drains into the portal system from branches of the left gastric vein and through the short gastric veins that empty into the splenic vein (4,17,54).

The anatomy of the lower esophageal system has been shown to consist of four layers (55). Radially arranged intraepithelial channels drain into the superficial venous plexus, which is found in the upper submucosa. This superficial venous plexus communicates with the deep intrinsic veins consisting of three to five main trunks located in the lower submucosa. Perforating veins connect this layer with the adventitial layer of veins located on the esophageal surface. The venous system appears to be mainly distributed within the esophageal mucosal folds (56).

The portal and caval systems communicate through the esophageal and gastric submucosal veins, and with increased blood flow, as occurs in portal hypertension, all the venous channels of the normal esophagus dilate and are referred to as varices. In portal hypertension, varices are complicated by ulceration and rupture with hemorrhage. It has been suggested that a major variceal hemorrhage occurs as a result of rupture of a varix of the deep intrinsic veins, whereas minor variceal hemorrhages occur as a result of rupture of a varix in the superficial venous plexus or even from the intraepithelial channels (55).

## LYMPHATIC DRAINAGE

A rich network of lymphatics in the lamina propria and submucosa connect with lymphatics in the muscular and adventitial layers. Lymphatics in the muscular layer are predominantly oriented in a longitudinal direction (4). In view of this longitudinal arrangement, extensive intramucosal and submucosal spread beyond a grossly visible tumor is not uncommon. This becomes an important consideration when assessing resection margins at frozen section.

In general, the cervical esophagus drains into the internal jugular and upper tracheal lymph node groups. The thoracic esophagus drains into the superior, middle, and lower mediastinal lymph node groups, whereas the abdominal segment drains into superior gastric, celiac axis, common hepatic artery, and splenic artery lymph nodes (57). Despite this drainage pattern, in practice the extensive communication of lymphatics results in a varied and unpredictable metastatic pattern (57).

## INNERVATION

The esophagus receives both parasympathetic and sympathetic nerve supply containing afferent and efferent fibers that innervate glands, blood vessels, and muscles of the esophagus. The vagus nerve carries both parasympathetic and some sympathetic fibers. Sympathetic fibers originating in cervical and paravertebral chains run with vascular structures, ending at the esophagus.

As in the rest of the gastrointestinal tract, the esophagus has an intrinsic innervation system. This consists of ganglion cells in the submucosa (Meissner's plexus) and between the circular and longitudinal muscle layers (Auerbach's plexus). These plexuses are less well developed in the esophagus when compared with the remainder of the gastrointestinal tract, and the density of neurons increases as one proceeds toward the stomach (17). The submucosal plexus is less well developed than the myenteric nerve plexus.

The plexuses of the esophagus receive input from postganglionic sympathetic and preganglionic and postganglionic parasympathetic fibers as well as from other intrinsic ganglion cells (15). Three cell types are described in the plexuses (53). Type I neurons are multipolar, confined to Auerbach's plexus, and their axons establish synapses with type 2 cells. Type II neurons are more numerous, are multipolar, and are found in both Auerbach's and Meissner's plexuses. These cells supply the muscularis propria and muscularis mucosae and stimulate secretory activity. Interstitial cells of Cajal are found associated with the terminal networks of sympathetic nerves.

Regulatory peptides identified within nerve fibers and around smooth muscle bundles include vasoactive intestinal peptide (VIP), substance P, enkephalin, and neuropeptide Y (NPY) (58,59). Nerve fibers containing VIP and NPY are the most abundant types present in the esophagus, and the pattern of innervation by these peptide-containing neurons differs from that in the stomach and small intestine (60).

## DIAGNOSTIC CONSIDERATIONS

Commonly received biopsy specimens from the esophagus are for the diagnosis of reflux esophagitis or Barrett's esophagus. The problems of interpretation present in these cases involve the mucosal changes occurring primarily within the confines of the LES.

### Barrett's Esophagus

There is not a single reliable definition of Barrett's esophagus. Both macroscopic and microscopic definitions exist, each proposed in an effort to address diagnostic problems encountered in this disease. It has been recommended that for a macroscopic diagnosis, columnar-lined mucosa of any type should be seen extending at least 3 cm into the tubular esophagus (61), but this is unsatisfactory and misses patients with short-segment Barrett's esophagus (less than 3 cm of specialized epithelium including most tongues). The microscopic definition is dependent on the presence of intestinalized glandular epithelium (62,63), which works well except in children, in whom it is rarely found in the first decade of life. A false-negative rate of 15% has been observed in patients with previously diagnosed Barrrett's esophagus. However, the importance of using this criterion is that virtually all lower esophageal adenocarcinomas occur in intestinalized mucosa, so that in its persistent absence there is almost certainly no increased risk of cancer.

The macroscopic definition of 3 cm allows for the presence of the gastric-type mucosa normally found within the distal 1 to 2 cm of the esophagus and thus avoids its misinterpretation as Barrett's esophagus (61). Among patients with short segments of the distal esophagus suspicious for Barrett's esophagus (less than 3 cm), the endoscopic identification of the LES may be imprecise and the stomach may be inadvertently examined via biopsy, resulting in a false-positive diagnosis. In such cases, manometrically guided biopsies can be used to identify the gastroesophageal junction.

Macroscopically, Barrett's esophagus demonstrates a red velvety mucosa corresponding to the columnar epithelium, with an apparent focal or diffuse cephalad migration of the Z line relative to the previous normal mucosal gastroesophageal junction (Fig. 22). Barrett's mucosa merges imperceptibly with the gastric mucosa distally. The junction with the esophageal squamous epithelium may appear as a symmetric or asymmetric Z line (as at the normal gastroesophageal junction) or as islands of columnar mucosa alternating with the squamous epithelium ("island pattern"). Foci of squamous epithelium occasionally are identified within Barrett's mucosa. Inflamed squamous mucosa may be indistinguishable from Barrett's mucosa endoscopically, and therefore also the squamo-Barrett junction, when both are present.

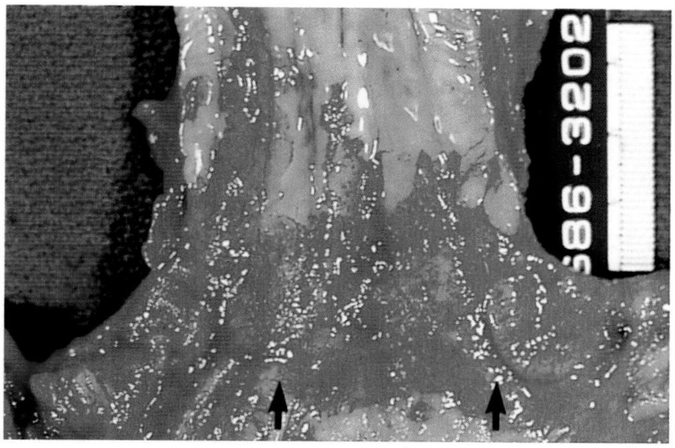


**FIG. 22.** Gastroesophageal region. Barrett's esophagus demonstrating proximal extension of columnar-lined mucosa well into the tubular esophagus. This columnar-lined mucosa extends more than 2 cm from the proximal gastric folds (*arrows*).

The diagnosis of Barrett's esophagus should always be confirmed histologically. If potential Barrett's mucosa is identified endoscopically, it should be examined via biopsy, as outlined below, to confirm the presence of specialized epithelium, as well as to exclude dysplasia or carcinoma, both of which may be inapparent endoscopically. Histologic confirmation is also important in cases of short-segment Barrett's esophagus, in which the short tongues of mucosa present may endoscopically resemble hiatal hernias (which are lined by gastric mucosa), inflammatory changes at the gastroesophageal junction, or an exaggerated and asymmetric yet normal mucosal gastroesophageal junction (62–64). Histologic confirmation is also necessary in cases of suspected childhood Barrett's esophagus, where Barrett's mucosa may be indistinguishable from the normal squamous epithelium (61,62,65).

Microscopically, Barrett's esophagus can be defined as the replacement of the esophageal squamous epithelium by metaplastic specialized (intestinalized) columnar epithelium. In adults, specialized epithelium is by far the most frequent epithelial type identified, so much so that the presence of this epithelium is increasingly being used as the sole criterion for the diagnosis of Barrett's esophagus (62,63,66). Other epithelial types are of much less value diagnostically

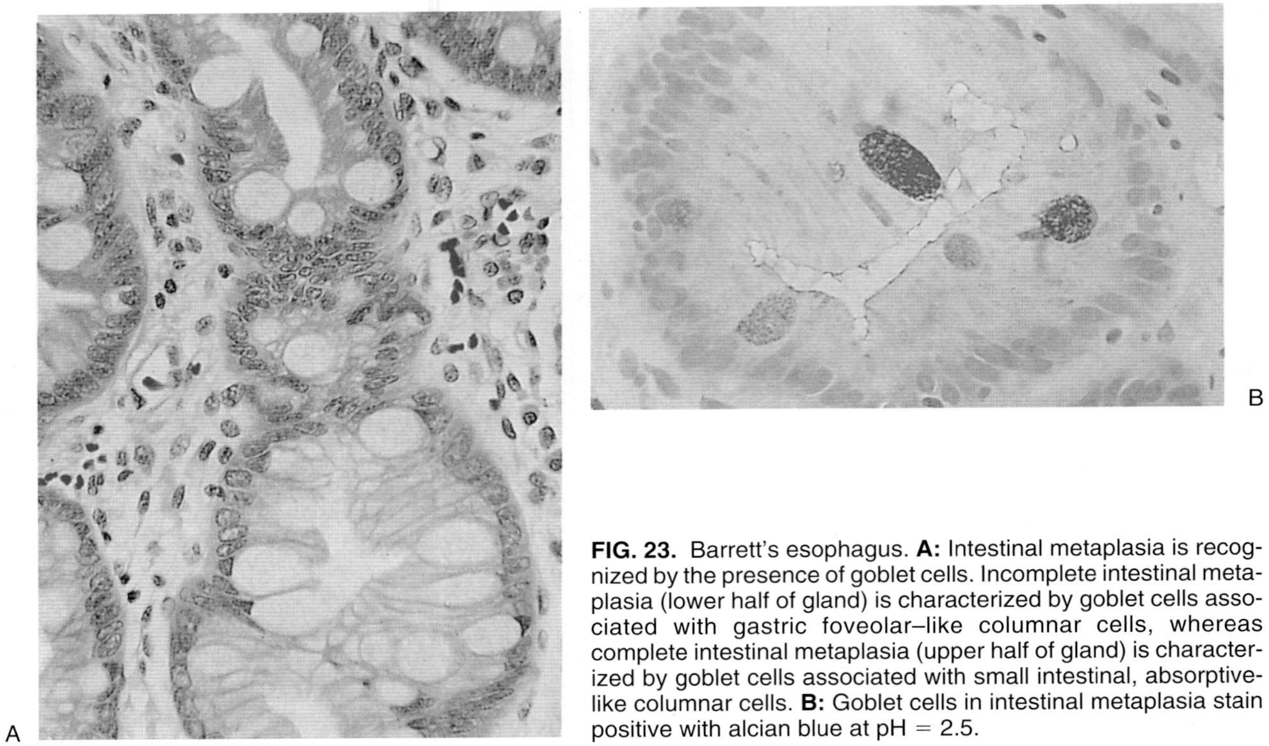

**FIG. 23.** Barrett's esophagus. **A:** Intestinal metaplasia is recognized by the presence of goblet cells. Incomplete intestinal metaplasia (lower half of gland) is characterized by goblet cells associated with gastric foveolar–like columnar cells, whereas complete intestinal metaplasia (upper half of gland) is characterized by goblet cells associated with small intestinal, absorptive-like columnar cells. **B:** Goblet cells in intestinal metaplasia stain positive with alcian blue at pH = 2.5.

and include fundic, junctional, and regenerative epithelium. Superimposed dysplasia, primarily of intestinalized epithelium, also may be present.

Specialized-type epithelium is characterized by the presence of goblet and columnar cells. The goblet cells contain acid mucins, predominantly sialomucins, thus staining positive with alcian blue at pH 2.5. The columnar epithelial cells may resemble either small intestinal absorptive cells (complete intestinal metaplasia) or gastric foveolar cells (incomplete intestinal metaplasia); however, these metaplastic cells demonstrate abnormal features that distinguish them from their normal counterparts (Fig. 23). In the case of complete intestinal metaplasia, the small intestinal-like columnar cells may demonstrate a brush border, but it is not well developed and lacks the uniform enzymatic activity normally found in the brush border of the small intestine (67). Ultrastructurally, these metaplastic cells have been shown to contain mucin granules, which are not present in the absorptive cells of the small intestine (62,63,67). The gastric foveolar-like columnar cells frequently contain alcian blue–positive acid mucin, in contrast to those that normally populate the stomach, which contain alcian blue–negative neutral mucins (67).

Other types of gastric mucosa may be present in Barrett's esophagus, but cannot easily be distinguished from mucosa arising from the normal gastric mucosa; their definitive presence in Barrett's esophagus can be accepted only in resections or other circumstances under which specialized mucosa has been identified above the gastroesophageal junction. In the adult, fundic-type mucosa is uncommon and if present resembles the transitional epithelium seen at the junction of the gastric body with the antrum or cardia, with only a scattering of parietal and chief cells. Fundic-type mucosa without intestinalization and resembling normal gastric fundus mucosa can be seen in childhood Barrett's esophagus; otherwise, it is rare and if present one must consider the possibility that the invariably present hiatal hernia has been examined via biopsy. The lack of intestinalized mucosa is a feature usually confined to children; it is likely that specialization occurs later in early adult life. Similarly, junctional-type mucosa that histologically is indistinguishable from normal gastric cardiac mucosa may be present, so much so that if seen as the only mucosal type in a case of suspected short-segment Barrett's esophagus, a normal exaggerated Z line cannot be excluded.

The diagnosis of Barrett's esophagus is best established by taking biopsy samples from various levels of the gastroesophageal region (68), beginning in the stomach just distal to the upper end of the gastric folds, ideally along the lesser curve, and then every 1 to 2 cm, up into the tongues of mucosa or the most irregular portion of the squamocolumnar junction until squamous epithelium is reached. Obvious islands of columnar-lined epithelium also should be examined via biopsy. This series of biopsy samples yields tissue that initially originates in a site that is clearly of gastric origin (thereby excluding gastric intestinal metaplasia as a cause of proximal intestinalized epithelium)—continues through mucosa in which intestinalized epithelium is present, thereby confirming the diagnosis of Barrett's esophagus and finishes in squamous mucosa. Intestinal metaplasia may be focal and thus may be missed on biopsy. In such cases, if the diagnosis of Barrett's esophagus is suspected, follow-up with repeat biopsy is necessary.

## Intestinal Metaplasia Limited to the Cardiac Region

In an unselected successive group of patients undergoing endoscopy in whom two large particle biopsy samples were taken from the cardia, intestinal metaplasia (IM) was found in 6% of patients with no endoscopic evidence of Barrett's esophagus (69) (the investigators report a rate of 18%, but tongues up to 3 cm in length were not considered diagnostic of Barrett's esophagus; the 6% value is derived from those patients without endoscopic abnormality). Other recent reports in abstract form have confirmed a high prevalence of intestinal metaplasia in short-segment Barrett's esophagus (variously defined as less than 2- or less than 3-cm tongues or circumferential extension) (70,71). One of these studies conducted on primarily Hispanic patients found a prevalence of 17% but with a female predominance and dysplasia in 3% (70), unlike carcinoma in this region which (currently) has a male predominance. The second study involved the analysis of eight radial biopsy samples taken from 80 patients immediately below the Z line. Short-segment Barrett's esophagus was diagnosed in 10 of 27 patients in whom it was suspected, but goblet cells were found in a further six patients (7.5% of the total) in whom it was not suspected (71). It is currently unclear if these changes are GERD related or whether isolated carditis is necessary for intestinal metaplasia to occur at the cardia. Their potential significance, particularly with reference to cancer risk, while unknown, cannot be completely ignored. Furthermore, the likelihood of detecting intestinal metaplasia at the cardia may be increased if biopsy samples are taken of the Z line through the retroflexed scope as viewed from beneath. This increased the prevalence of IM from 18% to 25% (72); however, it is unclear whether taking the same number of additional biopsy samples in the conventional manner would not have yielded the same result.

This raises several issues. First, there is no generally accepted definition of short-segment Barrett's esophagus; neither is it clear whether a generally accepted definition is possible. The notion that a predefined length of intestinalized epithelium is required for the diagnosis, a notion dating back to the days of blind suction biopsies (73), which is now obsolete. Second, do these changes represent intestinal metaplasia in preexisting (native) cardiac mucosa or ultra–short-segment Barrett's esophagus, that is metaplasia in what was formerly squamous mucosa, and what is the effect on our current definitions of Barrett's esophagus? Clearly, Barrett's esophagus has to begin somewhere, but this distinction is currently impossible because differences between metaplasia in native cardiac mucosa and metaplasia in what was formerly squamous mucosa have yet to be demonstrated. The third and critical issue regarding the type of epithelium in which intestinal metaplasia is occurring is in part the pathogenesis issue but also its implication. Does intestinal metaplasia in what is believed to be the native cardiac side of the Z line have the same malignant potential as recognized Barrett's mucosa? If it does not, then it becomes critical to attempt to separate the two, but if it does, then the exercise is futile because both diseases are premalignant and the issue becomes the extent of the risk and whether this justifies surveillance. Assuming that the risk of malignancy is similar in both, then the detection of intestinal metaplasia anywhere in the lower esophagus immediately puts the patient at increased risk of developing dysplasia and carcinoma, with the need to make a decision regarding potential surveillance. Because the risk of cancer appears to be intimately associated with intestinal metaplasia, perhaps Barrett's esophagus should be redefined simply as intestinal metaplasia of the lower esophagus.

## Gastroesophageal Reflux Disease

The problems encountered in GERD are related to squamous epithelial changes in the distal 3 cm of the esophagus and to the significance of intraepithelial inflammatory cells. Reflux-associated squamous hyperplasia (RASH) consists of basal cell hyperplasia of greater than 15% and extension of the papillae into the upper third of the epithelium (74,75) (Fig. 24). Practically, in well-oriented biopsy samples, the esophageal mucosa can be divided into thirds; the papillae should not be seen extending into the upper third and the basal cell layer should not extend more than halfway into the lower third. This is operatively a simple and rapid technique for assessing the degree of RASH. However, similar changes have been described in the distal 3 cm of the esophagus in approximately 60% of patients without objective or subjective evidence of acid reflux (34); thus, if present in biopsy samples originating from this zone, such hyperplastic changes must be considered normal. Changes of RASH are much more likely to be indicative of reflux if the biopsy sam-

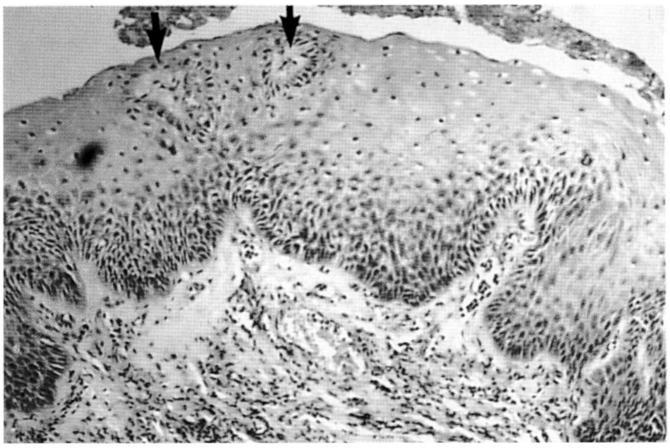

**FIG. 24.** Reflux esophagitis. Basal cell hyperplasia and lengthening of the papillae are present. The papillae have extended almost to the surface of the mucosa.

ples are taken above the distal 3 cm of the esophagus (35,36). It should be remembered that squamous hyperplasia is a nonspecific reaction to any form of esophageal injury and needs to be interpreted in light of the clinical context.

Intraepithelial eosinophils (IEEs) and intraepithelial neutrophils (IENs) are generally not considered to be normal constituents of the epithelium throughout its entire length, although recent studies have demonstrated rare IEEs in the distal 3 cm of approximately one third of patients considered normal (76). The presence of IEEs has been considered a sensitive indicator of reflux esophagitis (36,37,42,49,77), although this sensitivity is in question, and not infrequently it is the only pathologic change (35,36,41,48,77) (Fig. 25). IEEs are not absolutely specific, having been described in esophagitis due to alkaline reflux, allergic disorders, and infections (49). In children, however, it has been suggested that, although not an absolute criterion, eosinophils within the lamina propria may be a significant finding in GERD (37).

The presence of IENs is reasonably specific for esophagitis, correlating with the presence of erosion or ulceration, and is less sensitive for mild GERD (36,75,78). When present, IENs are invariably accompanied by the other histologic features of esophagitis. The use of IEEs and IENs as histologic criteria of GERD has the advantage that localization and orientation of the biopsy is not important.

Vascular changes such as dilated capillaries and extravasated red blood cells in the lamina propria should not be considered as criteria for GERD (36,42,74). Increased vascularization in the lamina propria, thought of as indicative of RASH (79) is not at present considered a diagnostic criterion although it may account for red streaks seen endoscopically. The presence of inflammatory cells within the lamina propria has no diagnostic relevance (36,42). There may be an increase in the number of intraepithelial lymphocytes in GERD (41), but this is not a documented criterion.

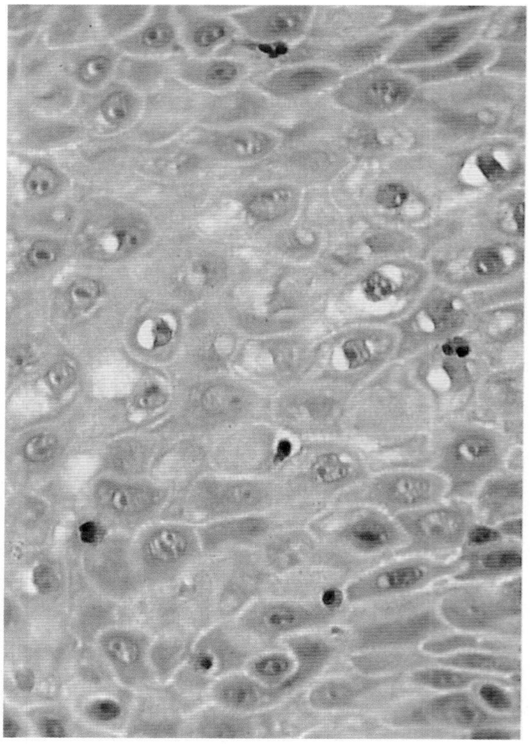

**FIG. 25.** Reflux esophagitis. Intraepithelial eosinophils are present between the epithelial cells.

In the assessment of biopsy tissues for RASH, well-oriented biopsy specimens of full epithelial thickness are necessary. Quite often biopsy samples are taken with small pinch forceps, resulting in a specimen that is small, superficial, and difficult to orient. If endoscopy is being performed to obtain a tissue diagnosis, an appropriate endoscope with large-particle grasp forceps should be used. Changes of GERD may have a patchy distribution; thus, multiple biopsies are recommended. It is important to avoid the use of picric acid containing dyes and fixatives such as Bouin's solution because this interferes with the staining of the eosinophil granules, thus preventing their recognition (42,49).

### *Inflammatory Changes on the Cardiac Side of the Z Line*

Because of the increasing use of biopsy samples immediately on the squamous side of the Z line to detect inflammatory cells, some biopsy samples inevitably contained cardiac mucosa immediately distal to the Z line. Some of these specimens contained an excess of chronic and sometimes acute inflammatory changes, which were not only unaccompanied by inflammatory changes elsewhere in the stomach, as might be expected with *Helicobacter pylori gastritis,* but inflammation appeared to be completely limited to the gastric cardia and therefore was appropriately termed gastric carditis. However, preliminary findings suggest that this may be a more sensitive marker for GERD than inflammatory changes in the squamous mucosa, as judged by correlation with 24 hour pH studies (73).

### Adenocarcinomas of the Gastroesophageal Region

Adenocarcinomas arising in the gastroesophageal region may have their origin from the gastric cardia, from Barrett's mucosa, or theoretically from the gastric cardiac-type mucosa present in the distal 2 cm of the esophagus. Gastric cardiac adenocarcinomas can be defined macroscopically as those occurring at or below the gastroesophageal junction, with the bulk of the tumor found in the gastric cardia and not involving the body or distal stomach (80). The presence of premalignant changes in the adjacent cardiac epithelium, such as a villous adenoma or dysplasia, would be confirmatory. Adenocarcinoma arising from Barrett's esophagus are predominantly located in the esophagus and are usually associated with demonstrable Barrett's mucosa histologically. Those arising from the gastric epithelium of the distal 2 cm of the esophagus can be classified with those of the gastric cardia unless associated with Barrett's mucosa. Occasionally, an adenocarcinoma may involve both the lower esophagus and gastric cardia equally, with obliteration of the landmarks of the gastroesophageal junction and any premalignant mucosa. In these cases, identification of the site of origin may be impossible; however, from a practical viewpoint, this distinction may not be important because their clinical behaviors are similar (30).

### ACKNOWLEDGMENTS

We thank J. Butera for her secretarial assistance and Dr. G. W. Stevenson for radiographic material.

## REFERENCES

1. Vaage S, Knutrud O. Congenital duplications of the alimentary tract with special regard to their embryogenesis. A follow-up study in 16 surgically corrected cases. *Prog Pediatr Surg* 1974;7:103–123.
2. Johns BAE. Developmental changes in the oesophageal epithelium in man. *J Anal* 1952;86:431–442.
3. Berardi RS, Devaiah KA. Barrett's esophagus. *Surg Gyncol Obstet* 1983;156:521–538.
4. Enterline H, Thompson J. *Pathology of the esophagus.* New York: Springer-Verlag, 1984.
5. Rector LE, Connerley ML. Aberrant mucosa in the esophagus in infants and in children. *Arch Pathol* 1941;31:285–294.
6. Le Roux BT. Intrathoracic duplication of the foregut. *Thorax* 1962;17: 357–362.
7. Tarnay TJ, Chang CH, Nugent RG, Warden HE. Esophageal duplication (foregut cyst) with spinal malformation. *J Thorac Cardiovasc Surg* 1970;59:293–298.
8. Abell MR. Mediastinal cysts. Arch Pathol 1957;61:360–379.
9. Rosenthal AH. Congenital atresia of the esophagus with tracheoesophageal fistula. Report of eight cases. *Arch Pathol* 1931;12:756–772.
10. Strobel CT, Byrne WJ, Ament ME, Euler AR. Correlation of esophageal lengths in children with height: application to the Tuttle test without prior esophageal manometry. *J Pediatr* 1979;94:81–84.
11. International Union Against Cancer (UICC). TNM. In: Hermanek P, Sobin LH, eds. *Classification of malignant tumours. 4th ed.* Berlin: Springer-Verlag, 1987.
12. Kikendall JW, Friedman AC, Oyewole MA, Fleischer D, Johnson LF. Pill-induced esophageal injury. Case reports and review of the medical literature. *Dig Dis Sci* 1983;28:174–182.
13. Jenkins DW, Fisk DE, Byrd RB. Mediastinal histoplasmosis with esophageal abscess. Two case reports. *Gastroenterology* 1976;70: 109–111.
14. Scully RE, Galdabini JJ, McNeely BU. Weekly clinicopathological exercises. *N Engl J Med* 1977;296:384–389.
15. Sleisenger MH, Fordtran JS. *Gastrointestinal disease. Pathophysiology, diagnosis and management. 4th ed.* Philadelphia: WB Saunders, 1989.
16. Bombeck CT, Dillard DH, Nyhus LM. Muscular anatomy of the junction and the role of phrenoesophageal ligament. Autopsy study of sphincter mechanism. *Ann Surg* 1966;164:643–654.
17. Netter FH. Upper digestive tract. In: *Digestive system. Part I of CIBA collection of medical illustrations. Vol 3.* Summit, NJ: CIBA-Geigy, 1957.
18. Blackstone MO. *Endoscopic interpretation. Normal and pathologic appearances of the gastrointestinal tract.* New York: Raven Press, 1984.
19. Bender MD, Allison J, Cuartas F, Montgomery C. Glycogenic acanthosis of the esophagus: a form of benign epithelial hyperplasia. *Gastroenterology* 1973;65:373–380.
20. Geboes K, Desmet V. Histology of the esophagus. *Front Gastrointest Res* 1978;3:1–17.
21. De La Pava S, Pickren JW, Adler RH. Ectopic gastric mucosa of the esophagus. A study on histogenesis. *NY State J Med* 1964;64: 1831–1835.
22. Variend S, Howat AJ. Upper oesophageal gastric heterotopia: a prospective necropsy study in children. *J Clin Pathol* 1988;41: 742–745.
23. Jabbari M, Goresky CA, Lough J, Yaffe C, Daly D, Cote C. The inlet patch: heterotopic gastric mucosa in the upper esophagus. *Gastroenterology* 1985;89:352–356.
24. Christensen WN, Sternberg SS. Adenocarcinoma of the upper esophagus arising in ectopic gastric mucosa. Two case reports and review of the literature. *Am J Surg Pathol* 1987;11:397–402.
25. Merino MJ, Brand M, LiVolsi VA, McCallum RW. Sebaceous glands in the esophagus diagnosed in a clinical setting. *Arch Pathol Lab Med* 1982;106:47–48.
26. Goyal RK. Columnar cell–lined (Barrett's) esophagus: a historical perspective. In: Spechler SJ, Goyal RK, eds. *Barrett's esophagus. Pathophysiology, diagnosis and management.* New York: Elsevier, 1985:1–18.
27. Goyal RK. The lower esophageal sphincter. *Viewpoints Dig Dis* 1976; 8:1–4.
28. Liebermann-Meffert D, Allgower M, Schmid P, Blum A. Muscular equivalent of the lower esophageal sphincter. *Gastroenterology* 1979; 76:31–38.
29. Haggitt RC, Dean PJ. Adenocarcinoma in Barrett's epithelium. In: Spechler SJ, Goyal RK, eds. *Barrett's esophagus. Pathophysiology, diagnosis and management.* New York: Elsevier, 1985:153–166.
30. McClave SA, Boyce HW Jr, Gottfried MR. Early diagnosis of columnar-lined esophagus: a new endoscopic diagnostic criterion. *Gastrointest Endosc* 1987;33:413–416.
31. Goyal RK, Bauer JL, Spiro HM. The nature and location of lower esophageal ring. *N Engl J Med* 1971;284:1175–1180.
32. Krishnamurthy S, Dayal Y. Pancreatic metaplasia in Barrett's esophagus. *Am J Surg Pathol* 1995;19:1172–1180.
33. Kramer P. Location of the squamocolumnar mucosa junction. *Gastroenterology* 1977;73:194–195.
34. Hendrix TR. Schatzki ring, epithelial junction and hiatal hernia—an unresolved controversy. *Gastroenterology* 1980;79:584–585.
35. Weinstein WM, Bogoch ER, Bowes KL. The normal human esophageal mucosa: a histological reappraisal. *Gastroenterology* 1975;68: 40–44.
36. Groben PA, Siegal GP, Shub MD, Ulshen MH, Askin FB. Gastroesophageal reflux and esophagitis in infants and children. *Perspect Pediatr Pathol* 1987;11:124–151.
37. Cooper HS, Dayal Y, Gourley WK, et al. Proceedings of the 1988 subspecialty conference on gastrointestinal biopsy pathology at the US-CAP. Diagnostic nonproblems in gastrointestinal biopsy pathology. *Mod Pathol* 1989;2:244–259.
38. De La Pava S, Nigogosyan G, Pickren JW, Cabrera A. Melanosis of the esophagus. *Cancer* 1963;16:48–50.
39. Tateishi R, Taniguchi H, Wada A, Horai T, Taniguchi K. Argyrophil cells and melanocytes in esophageal mucosa. *Arch Pathol* 1974;98: 87–89.
40. DiCostanzo DP, Urmacher C. Primary malignant melanoma of the esophagus. *Am J Surg Pathol* 1987;11:46–52.
41. Seefeld U, Krejs GJ, Siebenmann RE, Blum AL. Esophageal histology in gastroesophageal reflux. Morphometric findings in suction biopsies. *Am J Dig Dis* 1977;22:956–964.
42. Goldman H, Antonioli DA. Mucosal biopsy of the esophagus, stomach and proximal duodenum. *Hum Pathol* 1982;13:423–448.
43. Geboes K, de Wolf-Peeters C, Rutgeerts P, Janssens J, Vantrappen G, Desmet V. Lymphocytes and Langerhans cells in the human esophageal epithelium. *Virchows Arch [A]* 1983;401:45–55.
44. Hopwood D, Logan KR, Bouchier IAD. The electron microscopy of normal human oesophageal epithelium. *Virchows Arch [C]* 1978;26: 345–358.
45. Bell B, Almy TP, Lipkin M. Cell proliferation kinetics in the gastrointestinal tract of man. II. Cell renewal in esophagus, stomach and jejunum of a patient with treated pernicious anemia. *J Natl Cancer Inst* 1967;38:615–628.
46. Burns ER, Sehezing LE, Fawcett DF, Gibbs WM, Galatzan RE. Circadian influence on the frequency of labelled mitoses in the stratified squamous epitheliurn of the mouse esophagus and tongue. *Anat Rec* 1976;184:265–273.
47. Eastwood GL. Gastrointestinal epithelial renewal. *Gastroenterology* 1977;72:962–975.
48. Livstone EM, Sheahan DG, Behar J. Studies of esophageal epithelial cell proliferation in patients with reflux esophagitis. *Gastroenterology* 1977;73:1315–1319.
49. Brown LF, Goldman H, Antonioli DA. Intraepithelial eosinophils in

endoscopic biopsies of adults with reflux esophagitis. *Am J Surg Pathol* 1984;8:899–905.
50. Fenoglio-Preiser CM, Lantz PE, Listrom MB, Davis M, Rilke FO. *Gastrointestinal pathology. An atlas and text.* New York: Raven Press, 1989.
51. Muhletaler CA, Lams PM, Johnson AC. Occurrence of oesophageal intramural pseudodiverticulosis in patients with preexisting benign oesophageal stricture. *Br J Radiol* 1980;53:299–303.
52. Medeiros U, Doos WG, Balogh K. Esophageal intramural pseudodiverticulosis: a report of two cases with analysis of similar, less extensive changes in "normal" autopsy esophagi. *Hum Pathol* 1988;19: 928–931.
53. Meyer GW, Austin RM, Brady CE III, Castell DO. Muscle anatomy of the human esophagus. *J Clin Gastroenterol* 1986;8:131–134.
54. Shackelford RT. *Surgery of the alimentary tract. Vol 1.* Philadelphia: WB Saunders, 1978.
55. Kitano S, Treblanche J, Kahn D, Bornman PC. The venous anatomy of the lower esophagus in portal hypertension: practical implications. *Br J Surg* 1986;73:525–531.
56. Vianna A, Hayes PC, Moscoso G, Driver M, Portmann B, Westaby D, Williams R. Normal venous circulation of the gastroesophageal junction. A route to understanding varices. *Gastroenterology* 1987;93: 876–889.
57. Akiyama H, Tsurumaru M, Kawamura T, Ono Y. Principles of surgical treatment for carcinoma of the esophagus. Analysis of lymph node involvement. *Ann Surg* 1981;194:438–445.
58. Aggestrup S, Uddman R, Sundler F, et al. Lack of vasoactive intestinal polypeptide nerves in esophageal achalasia. *Gastroenterology* 1983;84: 924–927.
59. Aggestrup S, Uddman R, Jensen SL, et al. Regulatory peptides in lower esophageal sphincter of pig and man. *Dig Dis Sci* 1986;31:1370–1375.
60. Wattchow DA, Furness JB, Costa M, O'Brien PE, Peacock M. Distribution of neuropeptides in the human esophagus. *Gastroenterology* 1987;93:1363–1371.
61. Spechler SJ, Goyal RK. Barrett's esophagus. *N Engl J Med* 1986;315: 362–371.
62. Reid BJ, Weinstein WF. Barrett's esophagus and adenocarcinoma. *Annu Rev Med* 1987;38:477–492.
63. Reid BJ, Haggit RC, Rubin CE. Barrett's esophagus and esophageal adenocarcinoma. In: Hill L, Kozarek R, McCallum R, Mercer CD, eds. *The esophagus: Medical and surgical management.* Philadelphia: WB Saunders, 1988:157–166.
64. Bozymski EM. Barrett's esophagus: endoscopic characteristics. In: Spechler SJ, Goyal RK, eds. *Barrett's esophagus. Pathophysiology, diagnosis and management.* New York: Elsevier, 1985:113–120.
65. Hassall E, Weinstein WM, Ament ME. Barrett's esophagus in childhood. *Gastroenterology* 1985;89:1331–1337.
66. Gottfried MR, McClave SA, Boyce HW. Incomplete intestinal metaplasia in the diagnosis of columnar lined esophagus (Barrett's esophagus). *Am J Clin Pathol* 1989;92:741–746.
67. Trier JS. Morphology of the columnar-cell lined (Barrett's) esophagus. In: Spechler SJ, Goyal RK, eds. *Barrett's esophagus. Pathophysiology, diagnosis and management.* New York: Elsevier, 1985:19–28.
68. Mangla JC. Barrett's esophagus; an old entity revisited. *J Clin Gastroenterol* 1981;3:347–356.
69. Spechler SJ, Zeroogian JM, Antonioli DA, Wang HH, Goyal RK. Prevalence of metaplasia at the gastro-oesophageal junction. *Lancet* 1994;344:1533–1536.
70. Abo SR, Stevens PD, Abedi M, et al. Prevalence of short segment Barrett's epithelium in patients with gastroesophageal reflux disease [Abstract]. *Gastroenterology* 1995;108:43.
71. Cameron AJ, Kamath PS, Carpenter HC. Barrett's esophagus. The prevalence of short and long segments in reflux patients [Abstract]. *Gastroenterology* 1995;108:65.
72. Clark GWB, Ireland AP, Chandrasoma P, DeMeester TR, Peters JH, Bremner CG. Inflammation and metaplasia in the transitional mucosa of the epithelium of the gastroesophageal junction: a new marker for gastroesophageal reflux disease [Abstract]. *Gastroenterology* 1994; 106:63.
73. Paull A, Trier JS, Dalton MD, Camp RC, Loeb P, Goyal RK. The histologic spectrum of Barrett's esophagus. *N Engl J Med* 1976;295: 476–480.
74. Ismail-Beigi F, Horton PF, Pope CE II. Histological consequences of gastroesophageal reflux in man. *Gastroenterology* 1970;58:163–174.
75. Behar J, Sheahan DC. Histologic abnormalities in reflux esophagitis. *Arch Pathol* 1975;99:387–391.
76. Tummala V, Barwick KW, Sontag SJ, Vlahcevic RZ, McCallum RW. The significance of intraepithelial eosinophils in the histologic diagnosis of gastroesophageal reflux. *Am J Clin Pathol* 1987;87:43–48.
77. Winter HS, Madara JL, Stafford RJ, Grand RJ, Quinlan J, Goldman H. Intraepithelial eosinophils: a new diagnostic criterion for reflux esophagitis. *Gastroenterology* 1982;83:818–823.
78. Collins BJ, Elliott H, Sloan JM, McFarland RJ, Love AHJ. Oesophageal histology in reflux oesophagitis. *J Clin Pathol* 1985;38: 1265–1272.
79. Kobayashi S, Kasugai T. Endoscopic and biopsy criteria for the diagnosis of esophagitis with a fiberoptic esophagoscope. *Am J Dig Dis* 1974;19:345–352.
80. Kalish RJ, Clancy PE, Orringer MB, Appelman HD. Clinical, epidemiologic, and morphologic comparison between adenocarcinomas arising in Barrett's esophageal mucosa and in the gastric cardia. *Gastroenterology* 1984;86:461–467.

*Histology for Pathologists, second edition,*
Edited by Stephen S. Sternberg.
Lippincott-Raven Publishers, Philadelphia
© 1997.

# CHAPTER 20

# Stomach

David A. Owen



## EMBRYOLOGY AND POSTNATAL DEVELOPMENT

The stomach develops as a fusiform dilatation of the foregut caudal to the esophagus. This occurs first when the embryo is 7 mm in length. Initially, it is attached to the back of the abdomen by the dorsal mesogastrium and to the septum transversum (diaphragm) by the ventral mesogastrium. As the stomach enlarges, the dorsal mesogastrium becomes the greater omentum and the ventral mesogastrium becomes the lesser omentum.

The stomach is derived from endoderm, and early glandular differentiation of the mucosal lining occurs first at the 80-mm stage of fetal development. Enzyme and acid production first occur at the fourth month of fetal life and are well established by the time of birth. The newborn stomach is fully developed and similar to that of the adult.

## GROSS MORPHOLOGIC FEATURES

The stomach is a flattened J-shaped organ located in the left upper quadrant of the abdomen. At its upper end, it joins the esophagus several centimeters below the level of the diaphragm. At its distal end, it merges with the duodenum, just to the right of the midline. The stomach is extremely distensible and its size varies, depending on the volume of food present.

For the purposes of gross description, the stomach can be divided into four regions: cardia, fundus, corpus (or body), and antrum (1,2) (Fig. 1). The superomedial margin is termed the lesser curvature and the inferolateral margin is termed the greater curvature. The cardia is found just distal to the lower end of the esophagus. It is a small and ill-defined area, extending 1 to 3 cm from the gastroesophageal junction. The fundus is that portion of the stomach that lies above the gastroesophageal junction, just below the left hemidiaphragm. The antrum comprises the distal third of the stomach, proximal to the pyloric sphincter (pylorus), with the remainder of the stomach referred to as the corpus. The junction between the antrum and corpus is ill defined. By external examination, it comprises the portion of stomach distal to the incisura, a notch on the lesser curvature (1). Internally, the gastric mucosa is usually thrown into coarse folds called rugae. These are prominent when the stomach is empty, but flattened out when the organ is distended. The rugae are most prominent in the corpus and fundus because this is where the major dilatation to accommodate food occurs. The antrum may be distinguished because its mucosa is flatter and more firmly anchored to the underlying submucosa (Fig. 2).

D. A. Owen: Department of Pathology, University of British Columbia, and Division of Anatomical Pathology, Vancouver Hospital and Health Sciences Centre, Vancouver, British Columbia, V5Z 1M9, Canada.

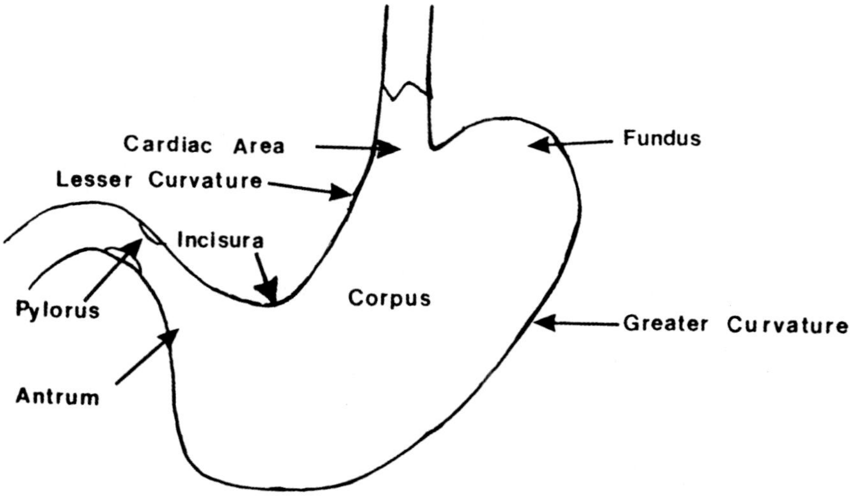


**FIG. 1.** Gross anatomical zones of the stomach.

The wall of the stomach has four layers: mucosa, submucosa, muscularis propria, and submucosa. Apart from the mucosa, these layers are structurally similar to the bowel wall elsewhere in the gastrointestinal tract. When viewed close up, the surface of the mucosa is dissected up by thin shallow grooves termed areae gastricae (3). These are structurally fixed and do not flatten out when the stomach is distended. They are best seen when the mucosa is viewed en face with a hand lens. Areae gastricae are best demonstrated radiologically via double-contrast barium examination, but also can be recognized on histologic sections, particularly from gastrectomy specimens where they appear as shallow depressions on an otherwise monotonously smooth surface (Fig. 3).

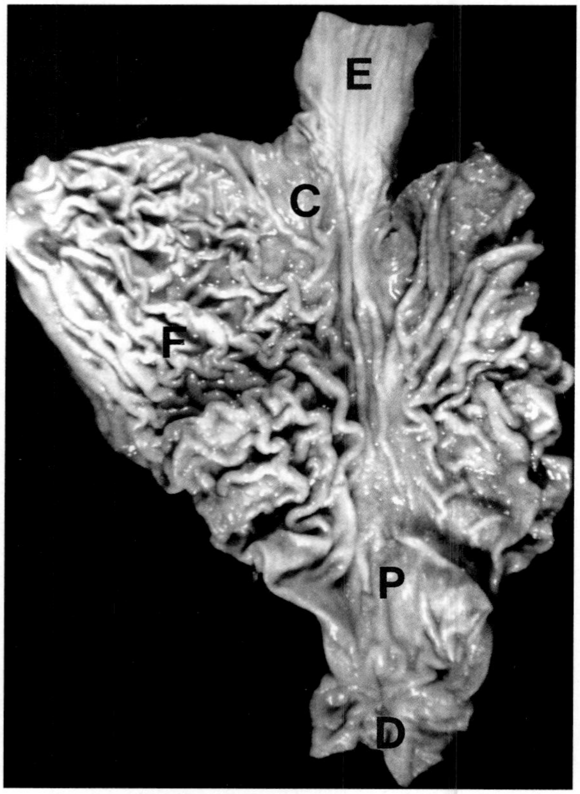


**FIG. 2.** Mucosal zones of the stomach. The cardiac mucosa (C) is present distal to the lower end of the esophagus (E). The pyloric mucosa (P) occupies a triangular zone proximal to the duodenum (D). Elsewhere, the fundic mucosa (F) shows prominent rugal folds.

### Blood Supply

Five arteries supply blood to the stomach. The left gastric artery arises directly from the celiac axis and supplies the cardiac region. The right gastric artery, which supplies the lesser curve, and the right gastroepiploic artery, which supplies the greater curve, arise from the hepatic artery. The left gastroepiploic and the short gastric arteries arise from the splenic artery and also supply the greater curvature. All these vessels anastomose freely, both on the serosal surface of the

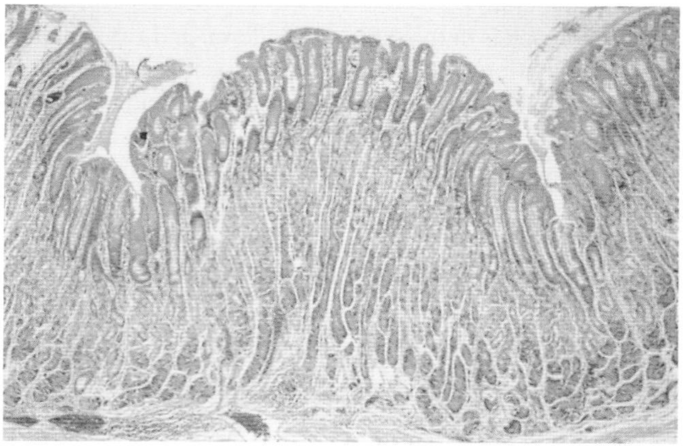

**FIG. 3.** Low-power view of the gastric fundal mucosa. The grooves in the mucosa are fixed anatomical features called areae gastricae.

stomach and in the muscularis propria, with extensive true plexus formation present within the submucosa. This richness of blood supply explains why it is so unusual to see gastric infarcts. The mucosal arteries are derived from this submucosal plexus but are end-arteries and supply an area of mucosa that is largely independent of the adjacent mucosal arteries (4).

### Nerve Supply

The sympathetic nerve supply to the stomach is derived from the celiac plexus via nerves that follow the gastric and gastroepiploic arteries. Branches also are received from the left and right phrenic nerves. The parasympathetic supply is the vagus nerve via the main anterior and posterior trunks that lie adjacent to the esophagogastric junction. Shortly after entering the abdomen, the anterior vagus nerve gives off a hepatic branch and the posterior vagus nerve gives off a celiac branch. Therefore, truncal vagotomy above these branches results in denervation of not only the stomach but the entire intestinal tract. Sectioning below these nerves results only in gastric denervation. A highly selective vagotomy (gastric fundal denervation) is achieved by sectioning lateral branches because the two main gastric nerves pass along the lesser curvature, with preservation of the terminal portion of the vagi that supply the antrum. No true nerve plexuses occur on either serosal surface of the stomach, but they are concentrated in Meissner's plexus in the submucosa and Auerbach's plexus between the circular and longitudinal fibers of the muscularis propria.

### Lymphatics

Recent studies (5,6) have disproved the former view that lymphatic channels are present at all levels of the lamina propria. By using careful ultrastructural techniques, lymphatics have been demonstrated to be limited to the portion of the lamina propria immediately superficial to the muscularis mucosae. From there, efferents penetrate the muscle and communicate with larger lymphatic channels running in the submucosa. This arrangement implies that an early gastric cancer may have lymphatic metastases, even though the primary tumor is all superficial to the muscularis mucosae.

The lymphatic trunks of the stomach generally follow the main arteries and veins. Four areas of drainage can be identified, each with its own group of nodes. The largest area comprises the lower end of the esophagus and most of the lesser curvature, which drains along the left gastric artery to the left gastric nodes. From the immediate region of the pylorus, on the lesser curvature, drainage is to the right gastric and hepatic nodes. The proximal portion of the greater curvature drains to pancreaticosplenic nodes in the hilum of the spleen, and the distal portion of the greater curvature drains to the right gastroepiploic nodes in the greater omentum and to pyloric nodes at the head of the pancreas. Efferents from all four groups ultimately pass to celiac nodes around the main celiac axis.

## GENERAL HISTOLOGIC FEATURES

Histologically, the mucosa has a similar pattern throughout the stomach. It consists of a superficial layer containing pits (foveolae), which represent invaginations of the surface epithelium and a deep glandular layer consisting of coiled glands that empty into the base of the pits (Fig. 4). The glandular layer differs in structure and function in different zones of the stomach that correspond roughly, but not precisely, to the gross anatomic regions (Fig. 1). Extending distally from the gastroesophageal junction for approximately 1 to 2 cm is the cardiac mucosa, where the glands are mucus secreting.

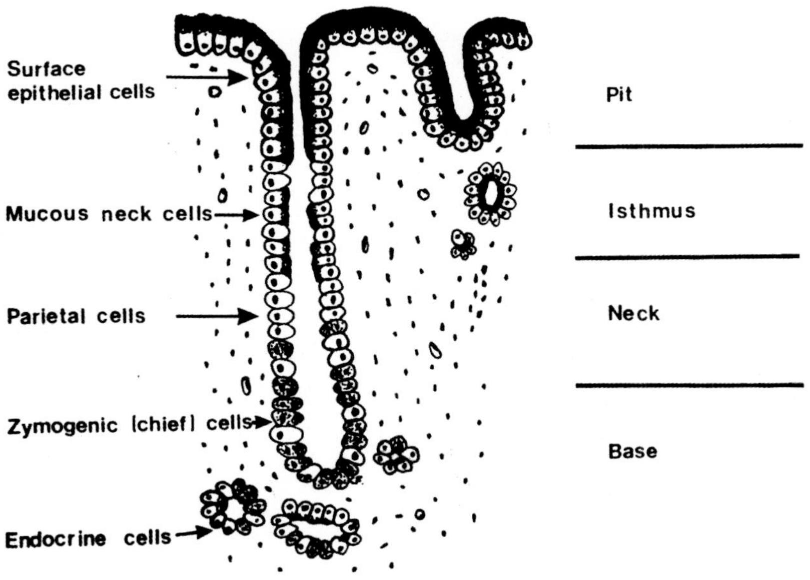


**FIG. 4.** Diagrammatic representation of gastric fundal mucosa. Chief cells are seen mainly in the basal portion of the glands and parietal cells mainly in the isthmic portion. The neck portion contains chief cells, parietal cells, and mucus neck cells. A small number of endocrine cells are present in the basal zone.

Extending proximally from the pylorus is the pyloric mucosa (sometimes called the antral mucosa), where the glands are also mucus secreting. This zone is triangular, extending much further (5–7 cm) proximally along the lesser curvature than it does along the greater curvature (3–4 cm). The pyloric mucosal zone is not identical to the antral region, although some investigators use these terms interchangeably. Also, contrary to what is implied in some accounts, the incisura has no fixed relationship to the proximal margin of the pyloric mucosal zone. Elsewhere within the stomach (corpus and fundus), the mucosa is exclusively fundic in type, where the glands are specialized to secrete acid and pepsin. Histologic transition between all zones is gradual rather than abrupt, with intervening junctional mucosae (1–2 cm in width) having a mixed histologic appearance.

A broad mucosal transition zone is also present at the pylorus, where gastric and duodenal mucosae merge. However, at the lower end of the esophagus, there is a change from nonkeratinizing squamous epithelium to columnar epithelium, which is abrupt, both grossly and microscopically. The position of this squamocolumnar junction is variable and does not coincide with the strict anatomic esophagogastric junction, that is, the point where the tubular esophagus becomes the saccular stomach. The mucosal junction commonly is located 0.5 to 2.5 cm proximal to the anatomic junction and often is serrated, rather than being a regular circumferential line (Z line) (2). The lower portion of esophagus, below the Z line, is therefore covered by cardiac-type gastric mucosa.

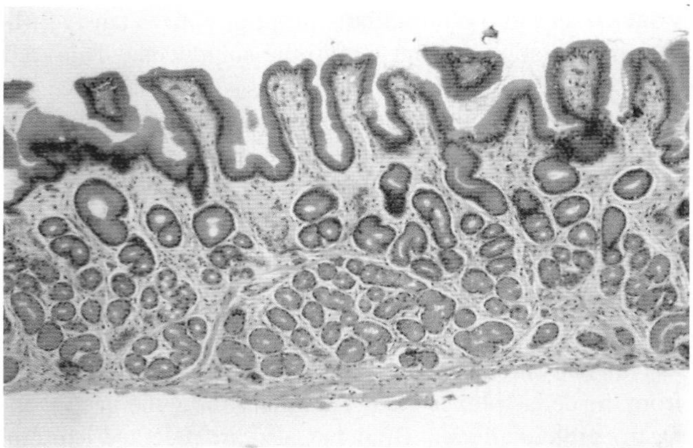

**FIG. 6.** Gastric pyloric mucosa. Note that the glands are loosely packed and occupy about half the mucosal thickness. The surface epithelium appears slightly villous.

### Surface Epithelium

Histologically, the gastric mucosa is covered by a tall, columnar, mucus-secreting epithelium (Fig. 5). There are intervening pits (or foveolae) that are lined by a similar epithelium. These surface cells are similar throughout all the mucosal zones of the stomach. Emptying into the base of the pits are convoluted gastric glands that, as mentioned, are of different types in the different mucosal zones. The bases of the glands abut the superficial surface of the muscularis mucosae. Between both the pits and the glands is the lamina propria. In the cardiac and pyloric mucosal zones, the pits are wider than in other areas, sometimes giving the mucosa a slightly villous appearance (Fig. 6).

The cells of the surface epithelium and pits are tall and columnar with basally situated nuclei and superficial cytoplasm that is almost entirely filled with mucus (Fig. 7). The nuclei have an even distribution of chromatin, with a single inconspicuous nucleoli. On hematoxylin and eosin (H&E)-stained sections, the appearance of the mucus varies, depending on the staining routine and type of eosin used. For example, with alcoholic eosin, the mucus appears as a single vacuole that is clear or lightly eosinophilic. With aqueous eosin, the mucus is more heavily eosinophilic and is seen to

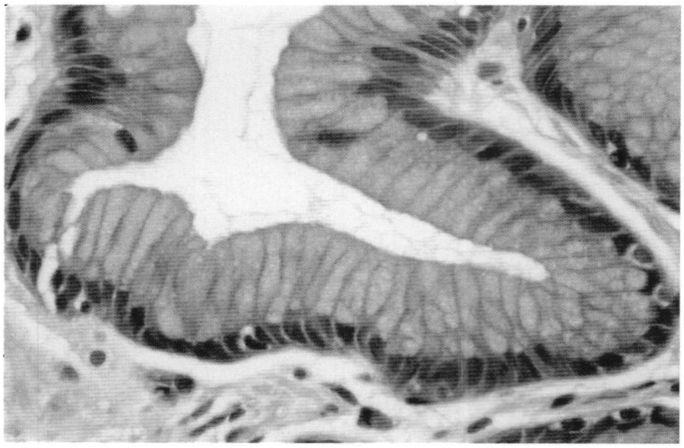

**FIG. 5.** Gastric surface epithelium with each cell having a mucous globule in the superficial cytoplasm. Intraepithelial lymphocytes are present. These are surrounded by a clear halo (formalin fixation artifact).

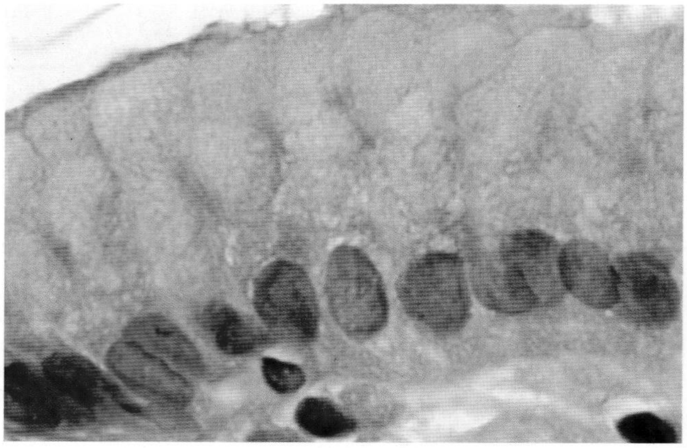

**FIG. 7.** Gastric surface epithelium showing cytoplasmic mucus present in multiple small vacuoles.

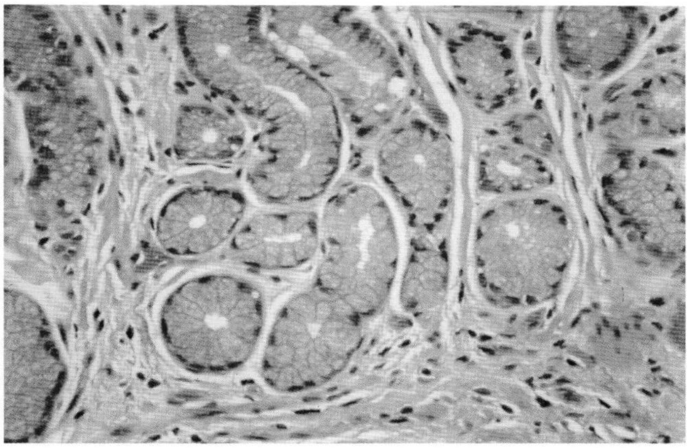

**FIG. 8.** Pyloric glands, containing cells with a bubbly, foamy appearance.

be present in numerous, small, closely aggregated vacuoles. Histochemically, the mucus is all neutral, periodic acid-Schiff (PAS)-positive, but alcian blue negative at pH 2.5 and lower (7).

## Cardiac and Pyloric Mucosa

In the cardiac and pyloric zone, the pits occupy approximately one half of the mucosal thickness (Fig. 6). The cardiopyloric glands are exclusively mucus secreting and are loosely packed with abundant intervening lamina propria (Fig. 8). Occasional cystic glands, lined by mucus-secreting epithelium, are a characteristic feature of the cardiac mucosa but usually are not found in the pyloric mucosa. The cells of the mucus glands have ill-defined borders and a bubbly cytoplasm that is different from the pit and surface epithelium. They resemble Brunner's glands of the duodenum. Parietal cells are not infrequently found either singly or in small groups, particularly in the pyloric mucosa and especially at the junctional zone, where it meets the fundic mucosa (1). However, it is uncommon for chief cells to be present outside of the fundic mucosa and junctional area. The pyloric glands secrete neutral mucin only. The cardiac glands secrete predominantly neutral mucin with small amounts of sialomucin (7).

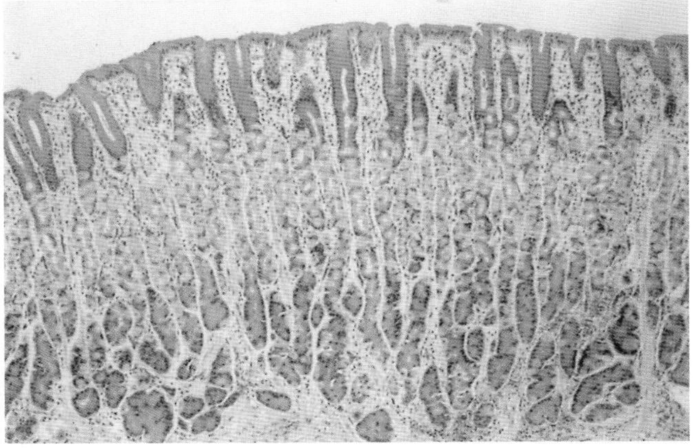

**FIG. 9.** Gastric fundic mucosa. Note the short pits and the tightly packed glands. Bluish chief cells predominate at the base and pinkish parietal cells predominate in the upper part of the glands.

## Fundic Gland Mucosa

The fundic (or oxyntic) gland mucosa has pits that occupy less than one quarter of the mucosal thickness. In contrast with the cardiac and pyloric mucosa, the glands are tightly packed and are straight, rather than coiled (Fig. 9). For descriptive purposes, they can be divided into three portions: base, neck, and isthmus. The basal portion consists mainly of chief cells (pepsinogen secreting). These are cuboidal and have a basally situated nucleus, which typically contains one or more small nucleoli and cytoplasm that usually stains pale blue-gray with some variation, depending on the type of hematoxylin used (Fig. 10). The isthmic portion of the glands contains predominantly parietal cells (acid and intrinsic factor secreting). These are roughly triangular, with their base along the basement membrane. The nuclei are centrally placed with evenly distributed chromatin, and the cytoplasm stains a deep pink on a well-differentiated H&E section (Fig. 10). The neck portion of the fundic glands contains a mixture of chief and parietal cells, together with a third type, the mucus neck cells (Fig. 11). These are difficult to recognize on an H&E stain, but are easily identified using a PAS stain, where they are seen to resemble the mucus-secreting cells of the cardiac and pyloric glands. These cells produce neutral and acidic mucin, especially sialomucin, which stains positively with alcian blue at pH 2.5 (8). Mucous neck cells are also found in lesser numbers in the isthmic portion of the glands, and occasional parietal cells can be encountered in the basal portion of the glands. Mucous neck cells are also present in the pyloric mucosa.

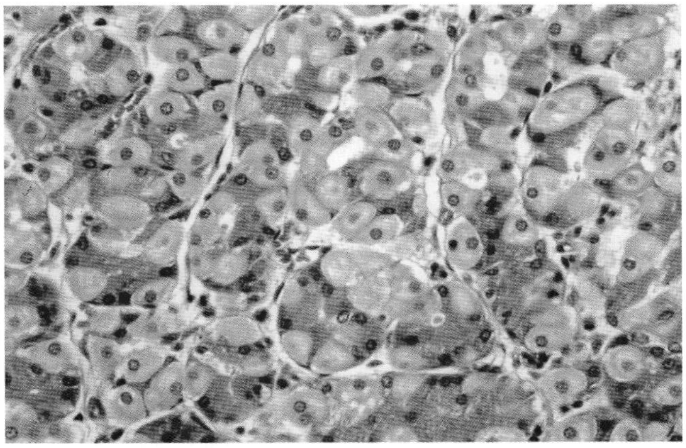

**FIG. 10.** Fundic glands, showing parietal cell cytoplasm staining light pink and chief cell cytoplasm staining purplish.

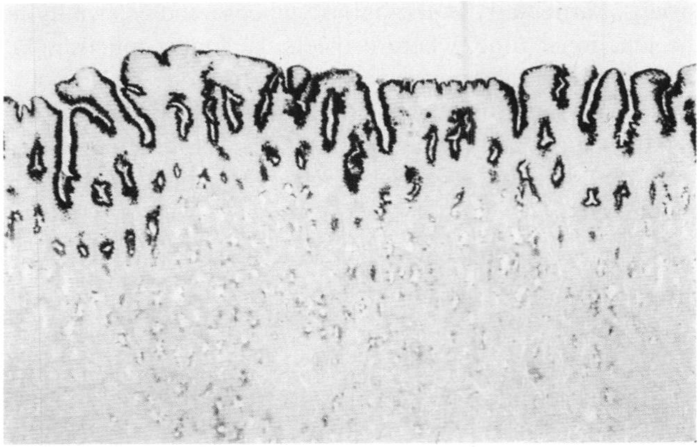

**FIG. 11.** Fundic mucosa with a PAS stain. The surface and pit lining epithelium is intensely positive. Paler staining mucus neck cells are present within the glands.

Studies indicate that the mucous neck cells located in glands from all areas of the stomach have as their major function proliferation and mucosal regeneration. These undifferentiated cells act as stem cells and may migrate upward to renew pit and surface epithelium or downward to renew chief, parietal, or neuroendocrine cells (9). It has been estimated that, in humans, the gastric surface epithelium is normally replaced every 4 to 8 days. The parietal and chief cells turn over much more slowly, likely every 1 to 3 years.

### Endocrine Cells

The stomach contains a wide variety of hormone-producing cells. In the antrum, about 50% of the whole endocrine cell population are G cells (gastrin producing), 30% are enterochromaffin (EC) cells (serotonin producing), and 15% are D cells (somatostatin producing). In the fundic mucosa, however, a major portion of the endocrine cells are enterochromaffin-like (ECL). These are histamine secreting. Small numbers of X cells (secretion product unknown) and EC cells are also present. In the fundic mucosa, the cells secreting these hormones are mostly located in the glands, particularly toward the base. In the pyloric mucosa, they are most common in the neck region just below the pits. Within these neuroendocrine cells, the hormones are present as cytoplasmic granules located between the nucleus and basement membrane, but because the granules are generally inconspicuous on H&E sections, special techniques are required for their demonstration (Fig. 12). The location of endocrine granules within the epithelial cells is functionally significant. Unlike other secretory products of the mucosa, endocrine cells discharge their granules into the mucosal lamina propria rather than into the gastric lumen. From here, the hormones enter the blood to exert an endocrine effect or influence other locally situated cells (paracrine effect).

The EC cells and some of the ECL cells have argentaffin granules, which can be stained by Fontana, Masson, or the diazo technique. The other cells are argyrophilic, but not argentaffinic. Traditionally, the Grimelius technique (10) was commonly used for their demonstration. Although sensitive, silver stains are not specific in distinguishing cell types, and reliance has to be placed on immunologic techniques for showing specific hormones. An excellent method for demonstrating endocrine cells of all types is an immunostain using antichromogranin (11). This seems to be more sensitive than the silver methods and is less prone to background staining. In addition to the presence of hormones in epithelial cells, some hormones also are found in neurons and nerve endings present in the stomach wall and mucosa. It is generally believed that vasoactive intestinal peptide is predominant in neural tissue and that catecholamines, bombesin, substance P, enkephalins, and possibly gastrin are also found at these sites. Quantitation of antral G cells may be important, especially in disease states, and various methods are available for this (12,13). Hyperplasia is generally linear. Overgrowth of ECL cells in the fundic mucosa occurs secondary to pernicious anemia. This has been divided into five patterns: pseudohyperplasia, hyperplasia, dysplasia, microinfiltration, and neoplasia (14).

### Lamina Propria

The epithelial cells of the surface, pits, and glands all rest on a basement membrane, which is similar to that seen elsewhere in the intestinal tract. Within the mucosa is a well-developed lamina propria that provides structural support, consisting of a fine meshwork of reticulin with occasional collagen and elastic fibers that are condensed underneath the basement membrane (Fig. 13). The lamina propria is more abundant in the superficial portion of the mucosa between the pits, especially in the pyloric mucosa. It contains numerous cell types, including fibroblasts, histiocytes, plasma cells, and lymphocytes. It is also normal to find occasional

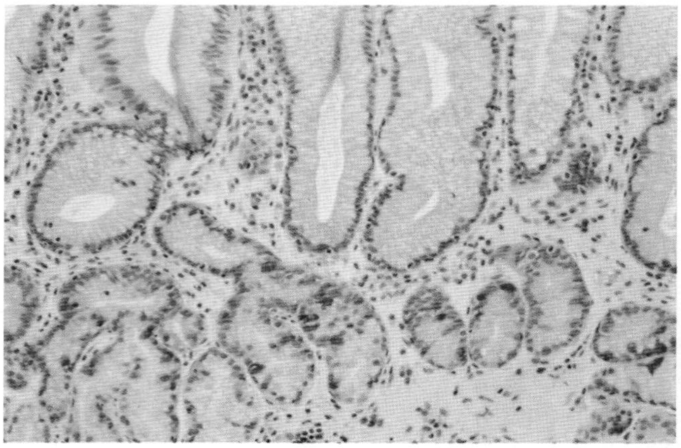

**FIG. 12.** Endocrine cells in gastric antral glands. The granules are located between the nucleus and the basement membrane (immunostain for chromogranin).

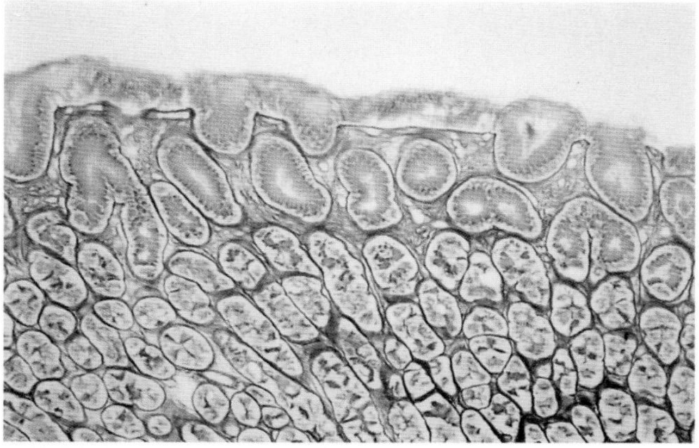

**FIG. 13.** Normal gastric fundic mucosa (reticulin).

polymorphs and mast cells. As mentioned, the lamina propria also contains capillaries, arterioles, and nonmyelinated nerve fibers. A few fibers of smooth muscle extend upward from the muscularis mucosa into the lamina propria, occasionally reaching the superficial portion of the mucosa, especially in the antrum.

The lymphoid tissue of the stomach has not been studied as extensively as that of the small bowel. The isolated lymphocytes and plasma cells in the lamina propria are predominantly of the B-cell type and IgA secreting. Intraepithelial lymphocytes are present in the stomach but are much less frequent than in the small bowel. They are commonly surrounded by a clear halo, which represents a formalin fixation artifact. These lymphocytes, as well as small numbers of lamina propria lymphocytes, are of T-cell origin.

Recently it was shown that small numbers of primary lymphoid follicles (aggregates of small lymphocytes) can be found in the normal stomach (15). However, secondary lymphoid follicles (follicles with germinal centers) are found only in gastritis, usually secondary to infection with *Helicobacter pylori.* The causative organism may not always be demonstrated via biopsy, especially in individuals recently treated with antibiotics, although there will be serologic evidence of infection.

### Submucosa

The submucosa is located between the muscularis mucosae and the muscularis propria and also forms the cores of the gastric rugae. It consists of loose connective tissue, in which many elastic fibers are found. The autonomic nerve plexus of Meissner is found in the submucosa, as are plexuses of veins, arteries, and lymphatics.

### Muscular Components

In classical anatomy texts (16,17), the main muscle mass of the stomach is referred to as the muscularis externa. In North America, however, the alternative name, muscularis propria, is widely used and preferred. This is because the term "muscularis externa" is ambiguous and it is sometimes not clear whether it refers to the whole of the muscle mass or only its external layer.

Three layers of fibers can be recognized in the muscularis propria: outer longitudinal, inner circular, and innermost oblique. The external fibers are continuous with the longitudinal muscle of the esophagus. The inner circular layer is aggregated into a definite sphincter mass at the pylorus, where it is sharply separated from the circular fibers of the duodenum by a connective tissue septum. The oblique muscular fibers are an incomplete layer present interior to the circular fibers and are most obvious in the cardiac area. Evidence for the presence of a circular sphincter at the cardia is controversial (18). Histologic examination is not conclusive, and although radiologic techniques show arrest of swallowed food at this level, this may be due to external compression from the adjacent crura of the diaphragm.

The muscularis mucosae consist of two layers, the inner circular and outer longitudinal, together with some elastic fibers. Thin bundles of smooth muscle also penetrate into the lamina propria, where they terminate in the basement membrane of the epithelium. This is most obvious in the antral area.

## ULTRASTRUCTURE

The surface and pit lining epithelial cells are ultrastructurally similar. They are characterized by multiple, rounded, electron-dense mucous vacuoles in the superficial cytoplasm and stubby microvilli projecting from the luminal surface. The basal cytoplasm contains moderate amounts of rough endoplasmic reticulum and some mitochondria. Adjacent epithelial cells are joined by tight junctions (zona occludens) at their luminal aspect and by adherence junctions along the rest of the cell interfaces. These tight junctions are considered to play an important role in maintaining mucosal integrity and the gastric mucosal barrier.

Parietal cells are unique ultrastructurally (Fig. 14) (19). In the unstimulated state, the cytoplasm contains an apical crescent-shaped canaliculus lined by stubby microvilli (Fig. 14). Between the microvilli are elongated membrane invaginations termed microtubules. Upon stimulation, the microtubules disappear to be replaced by a dense meshwork of intracellular canaliculi (20). The canalicular system is considered essential for the formation of hydrochloric acid. This is achieved by active transport of hydrogen ions across the canalicular membrane. Because this process has high energy requirements, the remainder of the parietal cell cytoplasm is occupied by mitochondria.

The chief cells are similar to protein-secreting exocrine cells elsewhere in the body. They have rough-surfaced vesicles in the superficial cytoplasm and abundant rough endoplasmic reticulum in the remainder of the cell.

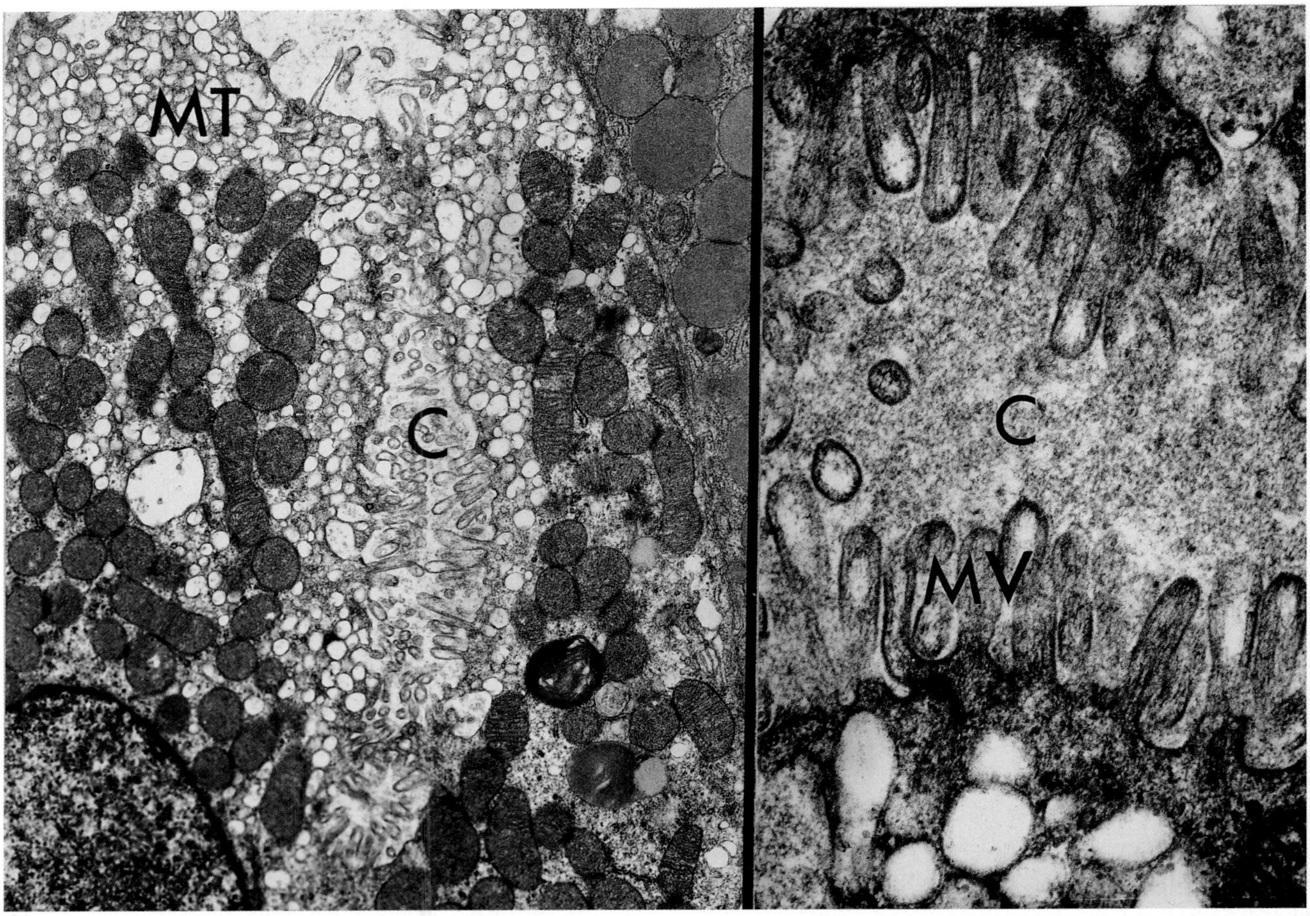


**FIG. 14.** Ultrastructural appearances of the parietal cell canaliculus (C). Note the fingerlike microvilli (MV) and the microtubular invaginations (MT). (Original magnifications: *left,* ×**9000**; *right,* ×**41,000**.)

## GASTRIC FUNCTION

The function of the stomach is to act as a reservoir and mixer of food and to initiate the digestive process. Gastric secretion of acid, pepsin, and electrolytes is partly under nervous control by the vagus and partly under the control of gastrin, a hormone produced by neuroendocrine G cells of the antrum. It is not yet clear if gastrin and acetylcholine produced by the vagal nerve endings act directly on acid-secreting cells or whether they act by stimulating the release of histamine from mast cells within the lamina propria. Gastrin release from the G cells may occur either as a result of distention of the antrum or by direct stimulation from ingested food, particularly amino acids and peptides. Hydrochloric acid is produced by the active transport of hydrogen ions across the cell membrane. This is an energy-consuming process, requiring adenosine triphosphate. Such high concentrations of hydrochloric acid are achieved that most ingested microorganisms are killed and the contents of the stomach are normally sterile.

Gastric mucus is secreted in two forms: a soluble fraction produced by the gastric glands and an insoluble form produced by the surface and pit lining cells. Biochemically, the mucus is a complex glycoprotein consisting of a protein core with branched carbohydrate side chains. Histochemically, gastric mucin is almost entirely neutral, although the mucous neck cells may secrete small amounts of sulfomucin and sialomucin (7). The physiologic role of gastric mucin is somewhat controversial. Clearly, the soluble mucin plays a role in lubrication, but it has been suggested that the insoluble fraction acts as a surface layer, forming a mucosal barrier and thus preventing back diffusion of acid and gastric autodigestion. However, the current view (21) is that although the mucus may have some protective action, the actual mucosal barrier is formed by the continuous layer of luminal mucosal cells and the tight junctions between adjacent cells.

The gastric parietal cells are also the source of intrinsic factor. Production is stimulated by histamine, gastrin, and acetylcholine but is inhibited by $H_2$ receptor antagonists. The exact control mechanism has yet to be elucidated, but it is unlikely that it is different from the regulation of acid and pepsin secretion.

## SPECIAL TECHNIQUES AND PROCEDURES

Relatively few special techniques are applicable to routine diagnosis. Mucin stains are the most widely used and the best is the combined PAS/alcian blue. This stains neutral mucin magenta, acid mucin light blue, and combinations purple. The combined stain is preferred over a straight PAS because the mucus in some carcinomas is PAS-negative. A mucicarmine stain is not recommended because it does not permit identification of the mucin type and is also negative with some varieties of mucin. Sialomucin and sulphomucin may be distinguished by a combined high iron diamine and alcian blue stain, which stains sulphomucin black and sialomucin light blue. At the present time, however, this distinction does not have diagnostic utility.

Endocrine cells of all types are best detected using an immunostain for chromogranin. Antral G cells can be distinguished if a specific antiserum to gastrin is available. ECL cells cannot be specifically detected immunohistochemically. The silver stains of Grimelius and Sevier-Mungier appear to be less reliable than a chromogranin technique.

Usually there is no difficulty in distinguishing chief and

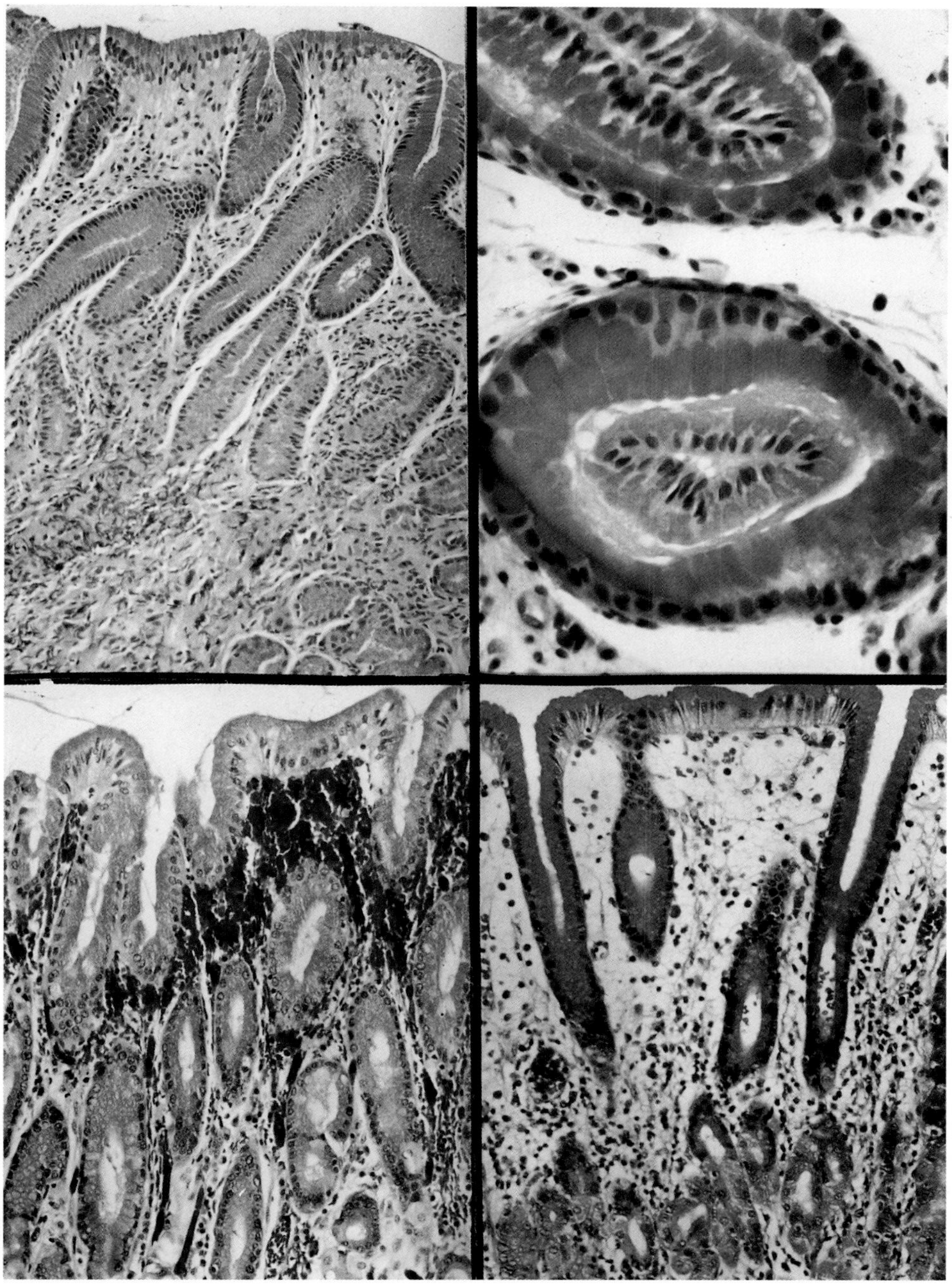

**FIG. 15.** Biopsy artifacts: crushing, producing an apparent lamina propria infiltrate (*top left*); crushing, resulting in displacement (telescoping) of cells into pit lumen (*top right*); biopsy-induced hemorrhage (*bottom left*); and stretching, producing an appearance of superficial edema (*bottom right*).

parietal cells on a good H&E stain (Fig. 10). If necessary, special stains, such as a Maxwell stain (22), can aid this distinction. Parietal cells can be recognized and quantified by use of a human milk fat globulin antibody (23).

## AGE CHANGES

Many older adults have a reduced gastric acid output (24,25). Histologically, this is characterized by a reduction in the area of fundic mucosa with expansion of the zone of pyloric mucosa. This results in proximal displacement of the pylorofundic junction, a change termed pyloric metaplasia (26). However, recently it was recognized (27) that hypochlorhydria of the elderly is not the result of a simple age change but is secondary to chronic gastritis. Older individuals without gastritis may have normal, or even elevated, acid secretion. This can be accompanied by elevated serum pepsinogen and gastrin levels (28).

## ARTIFACTS

A variety of artifacts may occur in gastric biopsy specimens (Fig. 15). Most of these artifacts relate to rough handling of the specimen, either at the time the biopsy sample is taken or when it is removed from the forceps. Crushing is common and can result in compression of the lamina propria, leading to a false impression of an inflammatory infiltrate. Crush artifact also produces telescoping of the pit lining cells. Stretching of the mucosa results in separation of the pits and glands, leading to the impression of edema. Hemorrhage into the lamina propria is also common in gastric biopsy samples and has to be distinguished from hemorrhagic gastritis. This can be difficult in small biopsy samples, but usually the endoscopic appearances of hemorrhagic gastritis are characteristic.

Gastrointestinal mucosa at all sites may contain intraepithelial lymphocytes. In formalin-fixed tissue, these are frequently surrounded by a clear halo. This represents a shrinkage artifact.

## DIFFERENTIAL DIAGNOSIS

One of the problems for pathologists examining gastric biopsy samples is determining whether the specimen is normal or shows minor degrees of gastritis. It is therefore appropriate to review briefly certain aspects of the classification, diagnosis, and epidemiology of gastritis. Specific types of gastritis, for example, acute hemorrhagic gastritis (29) or granulomatous gastritis, are usually so distinct that confusion with a normal stomach is unlikely. On the other hand, *H. pylori* gastritis may be patchy or may be associated with atrophy. In the early stage of *H. pylori* gastritis (chronic superficial gastritis), an infiltrate of inflammatory cells may be observed in the superficial portion of the mucosa, particularly in the lamina propria between the gastric pits (Fig. 16). Later, the inflammation spreads deeply to involve the whole thickness of the mucosa and is accompanied by atrophy of gastric glands (chronic atrophic gastritis). Ultimately, the inflammation may burn itself out and all glands are destroyed, leaving only a thinned mucosa containing pitlike structures (gastric atrophy) (29).

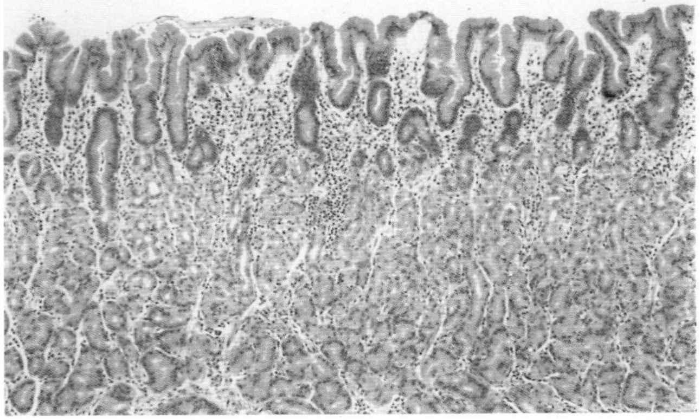

**FIG. 16.** Mild chronic superficial gastritis with chronic inflammatory cells present in the superficial lamina propria in excess of normal. This is a borderline biopsy sample and illustrates the least number of cells acceptable for a diagnosis of gastritis.

As described, the superficial gastric lamina propria normally contains some chronic inflammatory cells. It is often a matter of judgment whether these are normal or increased in number because there is no simple satisfactory method of objective measurement. In actual practice, it may be even more difficult to evaluate these cells because the gastric biopsy samples obtained by endoscopists are frequently distorted by crushing or stretching. In assessing possible minor degrees of inflammation, therefore, study should also be made of the superficial and pit lining epithelium, where a number of useful diagnostic features may be identified, depending on the degree of activity of the inflammation. The

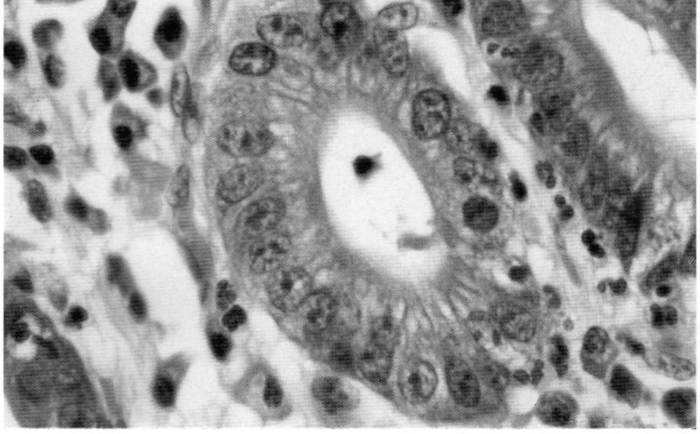

**FIG. 17.** Gastritis showing cytoplasmic mucin loss with enlarged nuclei containing prominent nucleoli.

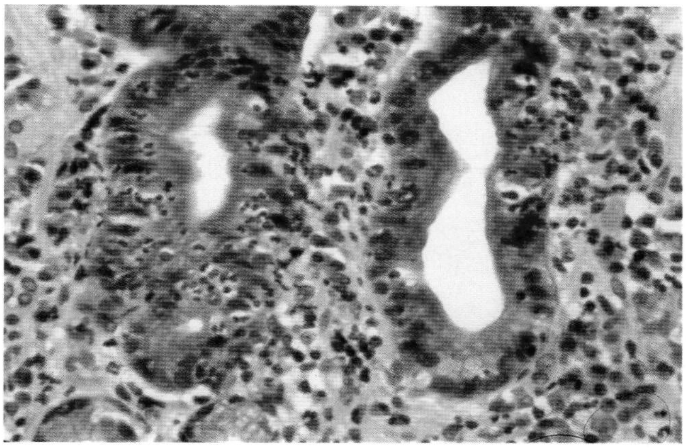

**FIG. 18.** Gastric pits infiltrated by neutrophils in a case of *Helicobacter pylori* gastritis.

earliest changes seen are a reduction in the mucin content of the cytoplasm, an increase in nuclear size, and the presence of one or more prominent nucleoli (Fig. 17). At the base of the pits, there may be increased numbers of mitoses, reflecting a more rapid cell turnover. These findings are features of epithelial damage and regeneration and are common to all forms of gastritis. In severe active inflammation, the epithelium and the lamina propria are infiltrated by acute inflammatory cells (Fig. 18) and organisms may be seen on the mucosal surface (Fig. 19). Optimum recognition of organisms is enhanced by using special stains.

Where low-grade gastritis has been present for some time, there may be atrophy of the mucosal glands, which can be accompanied by an increase in inflammatory cells. On an H&E section, this is seen as a separation of the glands with increased intervening lamina propria. However, minor degrees of atrophy may be difficult to distinguish, particularly if there is biopsy artifact. In these instances, a reticulin stain can be useful in confirming atrophy by demonstrating coarse condensation of fibers in the lamina propria (Fig. 20).

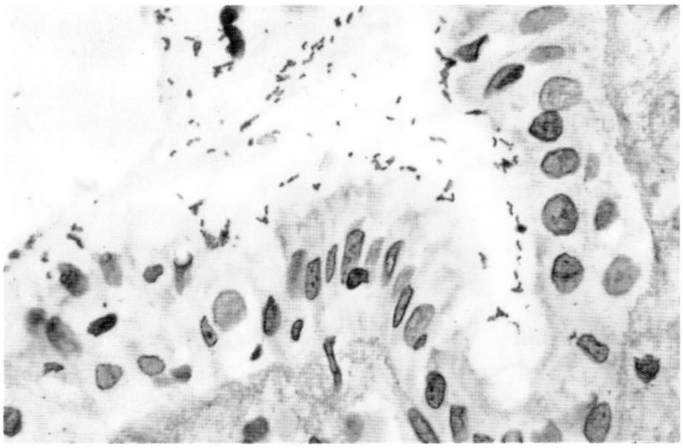

**FIG. 19.** *Helicobacter pylori* organisms present in the mucus layer on the gastric mucosal surface. These are always considered abnormal.

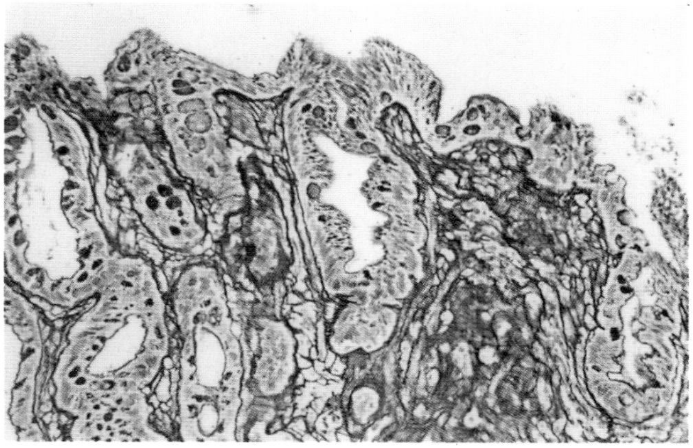

**FIG. 20.** Coarse condensation of mucosal fibers in atrophic gastritis (reticulin).

Information collected in a systematic fashion on the prevalence of *H. pylori* gastritis, suggests that in both Europe (30) and North America (31) it is uncommon in children and young adults, but thereafter steadily increases in frequency with age. Beyond the age of 60 years, it affects 40% to 60% of the general population (32). However, in developing countries, up to 50% of children and 70% to 90% of adults (31) are affected.

## Metaplasia

There are two major types of metaplasia that are seen in the stomach: intestinal metaplasia (IM) and pyloric metaplasia. Both are thought to be the result of chronic gastritis, and consequently both are more frequently encountered in elderly individuals; neither type is considered symptomatic.

In pyloric metaplasia, there is a replacement of the specialized acid and enzyme-secreting cells of the fundic glands by mucus-secreting glands of the type present in normal pyloric mucosa. This change occurs in the zone of fundic mucosa adjacent to the histologic fundopyloric junction, and what were typical fundic glands now come to resemble typical pyloric glands. Therefore, in persons with extensive pyloric metaplasia, the fundic gland area of the stomach contracts, the pyloric gland area expands, and the junctional zone is moved proximally toward the cardia (26).

In IM, there is a change in the cells of the surface and pit epithelium so that they morphologically and histochemically come to resemble the cells of either the small or large bowel. IM may be complete (type I) or incomplete (type II) (33,34). In complete small bowel IM, the gastric mucosa changes to normal small bowel epithelium, characterized by fully developed goblet cells and enterocytes with a brush border (Fig. 21). In advanced cases, the contour of the mucosa changes with the development of villi and crypts. Paneth cells may be present in the base of the crypts. In incomplete metaplasia, recognizable absorptive cells are not seen. The epithelium consists of a mixture of intestinal-type goblet

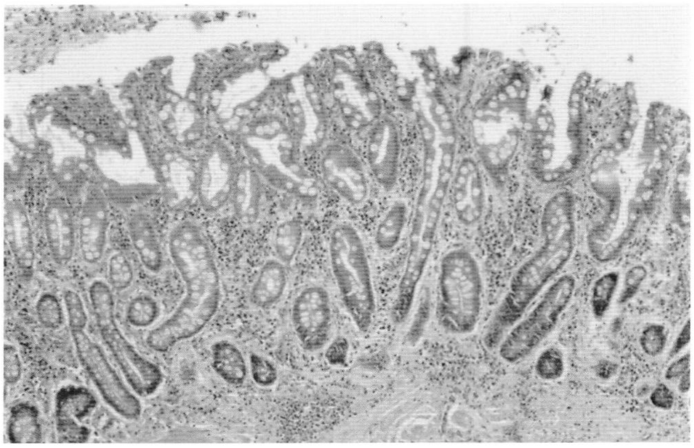

**FIG. 21.** Complete intestinal metaplasia.

cells and columnar mucus-secreting cells, morphologically resembling those of the normal gastric epithelium.

Histochemical changes detected in the mucus production of the various types of IM are interesting and complex (7,33). In the normal stomach, mucus secreted by the columnar cells is neutral in type, recognized histochemically as PAS-positive and alcian blue-negative. In complete IM, the enterocyte cytoplasm, apart from the brush border, is mucin-negative, but the goblet cells secrete either sialomucin, an acid mucin that is PAS-positive, alcian blue-positive at pH 2.5, but alcian blue-negative at pH 0.5, or sulfomucin, a strongly acidic mucin that is weakly PAS-positive and alcian blue-positive at pH 2.5 and at pH 0.5 (Fig. 22). In incomplete small bowel metaplasia, sialomucin is present in the columnar cells, and in incomplete large bowel metaplasia (also called type III) (34), the columnar cells contain sulfomucin (Fig. 23). Sulfomucin may be recognized separately from sialomucin because it is also positive with high iron diamine (34). The details of these methods are well described in standard textbooks of histochemistry (35).

Minor degrees of gastric IM are relatively common in persons both in North America and elsewhere. The variants described above rarely exist as a pure entity, and mixtures of the various types within the same gastric pit frequently are encountered. IM should never be considered normal and almost always reflects some degree of gastric damage, usually from chronic gastritis.

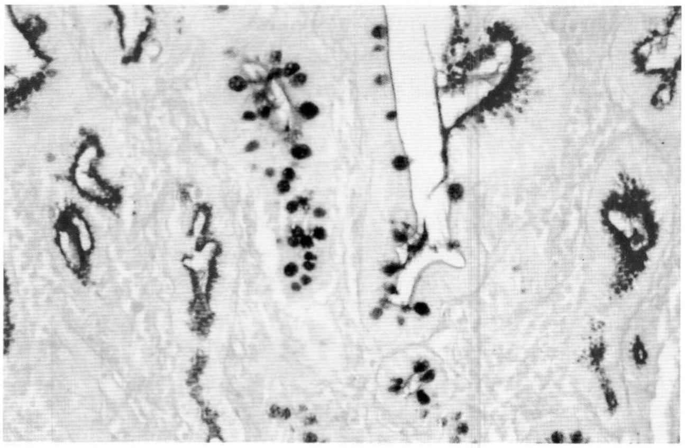

**FIG. 22.** Complete IM. (PAS/alcian blue).

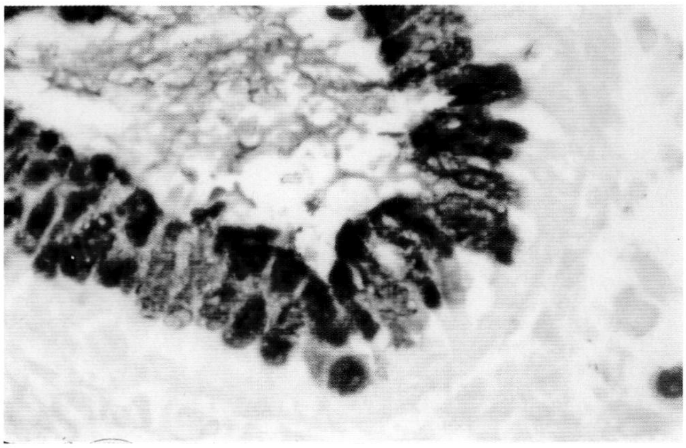

**FIG. 23.** Incomplete large bowel metaplasia. The pit contains columnar cells with cytoplasmic sulphomucin (high iron diamine and alcian blue).

Less commonly encountered forms of metaplasia include subnuclear vacuolation (36), ciliated metaplasia (37), and pancreatic acinar metaplasia (38). These changes all involve the pyloric mucus glands. Subnuclear vacuolation is not strictly a metaplastic change because it does not simulate the appearance of any other type of normal cells and probably represents a degenerative change secondary to gastritis or duodenal reflux. The vacuoles are clear on H&E sections and indent the nucleus. Ultrastructurally, they consist of a membrane-lined space derived either from endoplasmic reticulum or Golgi and probably contain nonglycoconjugated mucus core protein (39). Ciliated cells are found at the base of antral glands where there is superficial IM (37). The cause and significance of this change is not known. Pancreatic acinar metaplasia (38) may be present in up to 1.2% of gastric biopsy samples or 13% of gastrectomy specimens. The cells, which are indistinguishable from normal acinar cells, also produce lipase and trypsinogen. Seventy-five percent of cases are positive for amylase. Cells are present in nests and variably sized lobules, scattered among the antral glands. The majority of patients with acinar metaplasia also have intestinal or pyloric metaplasia.

## SPECIMEN HANDLING

Gastric mucosa is delicate and should be handled with care. Tissue should be gently removed from the biopsy forceps and oriented before being placed flat on a supportive mesh, such as filter paper or gelfoam. A variety of fixatives are suitable, depending on personal preferences, although routine formalin is suitable for most purposes. Sections are cut in ribbons, usually at two or three levels.

For the best results, it is suggested that gastrectomy specimens be opened and pinned out on a cork board or wax platform before being immersed in formalin and fixed overnight. If sections are taken directly from a fresh specimen, they almost invariably curl up, resulting in irregular orientation of the final slide.

## REFERENCES


1. Lewin KJ, Riddell RH, Weinstein WM. Normal structure of the stomach. In: *Gastrointestinal pathology and its clinical implications.* New York: Igaku Shoin, 1992:496–505.
2. Antionioli DA, Madara JL. Functional anatomy of the gastrointestinal tract. In: Ming SC, Goldman H, eds. *Pathology of the gastrointestinal tract.* Philadelphia: WB Saunders, 1992:14–36.
3. Mackintosh CE, Kreel L. Anatomy and radiology of the areae gastricae. *Gut* 1977;18:855–864.
4. Piasecki C. Blood supply to the human gastro-duodenal mucosa. *J Anat* 1974;118:295–335.
5. Lehnert T, Erlandson RA, Decosse JJ. Lymph and blood capillaries in the human gastric mucosa. *Gastroenterology* 1985;89:939–950.
6. Listrom MB, Fenoglio-Preiser CM. Lymphatic distribution of the stomach in normal, inflammatory, hyperplastic and neoplastic tissue. *Gastroenterology* 1987;93:506–514.
7. Felipe I. Mucins in the human gastrointestinal epithelium: a review. *Invest Cell Pathol* 1979;2:195–216.
8. Goldman H, Ming SC. Mucins in normal and neoplastic gastrointestinal epithelium. *Arch Pathol* 1968;85:580–586.
9. Matsuyama M, Suzuki H. Differentiation of immature mucous cells into parietal, argyrophil and chief cells in stomach grafts. *Science* 1970; 169:385–387.
10. Grimelius L. A silver stain for $\alpha_2$ cells in human pancreatic islets. *Acta Soc Med Upsalla* 1968;73:243–270.
11. Rindi G, Buffa R, Sessa F, et al. Chromogranin A, B and C immunoreactivities of mammalian endocrine cells: distribution, distinction from costored hormones/prohormones and relationship with the argyrophil component of secretory granules. *Histochemistry* 1986;85:19–28.
12. McIntyre RLE, Piris J. Quantification of human gastric G cell density in endoscopic biopsy specimens. Effect of shape on specimen. *J Clin Pathol* 1980;33:513–516.
13. Stave R, Brandtzaeg P. Immunohistochemical investigation of gastrin producing (G) cells. The distribution of G cells in resected human stomachs. *Scand J Gastroenterol* 1975;11:705–711.
14. Solcia E, Frocca R, Villani L, et al. Hyperplastic, dysplastic and neoplastic enterochromaffin-like cell proliferations of the gastric mucosa. *Am J Surg Pathol* 1995;19(suppl1):S1–S7.
15. Genta RM, Hamner HW, Graham DY. Gastric lymphoid follicles in *Helicobacter pylori* infection: frequency, distribution and response to triple therapy. *Hum Pathol* 1993;24:577–583.
16. Ham AW, Cormack DH. *Histology.* Philadelphia: JB Lippincott; 1979: 669–677.
17. Leeson CR, Leeson TS, Paparo AA. *Textbook of histology.* Philadelphia: WB Saunders, 1985:334–343.
18. Bowden RE, El Ramli HA. The anatomy of the esophageal hiatus. *Br J Surg* 1967;54:983–989.
19. Rubin W, Ross LL, Sleisenger MH, Jeffries GH. The normal human gastric epithelia. A fine structural study. *Lab Invest* 1968;19:598–626.
20. Forte JG, Forte TM, Black JA, Okamoto C, Wolosin JM. Correlation of parietal cell structure and function. *J Clin Gastroenterol* 1983; 5(suppl1):17–27.
21. Piper DW. Mucus, chemistry and characteristics. In: Sircus W, Smith AN, eds. *Scientific foundations of gastroenterology.* Philadelphia: WB Saunders, 1980:333–343.
22. Maxwell A. Alcian dyes applied to the gastric mucosa. *Stain Technol* 1963;38:286–287.
23. Walker MM, Smolka A, Waller JM, et al. Identification of parietal cells in gastric body mucosa with HMFG-2 monoclonal antibody. *J Clin Pathol* 1995;48:832–834.
24. Baron JH. Studies of basal and peak acid output with an augmented histamine test. *Gut* 1963;4:136–144.
25. Vakil BJ, Mulekar AM. Studies with the maximal histamine test. *Gut* 1965;7:364–371.
26. Kimura K. Chronological transition of the fundic pyloric border determined by stepwise biopsy of the lesser and greater curvatures of the stomach. *Gastroenterology* 1972;63:584–592.
27. Kekki M, Samloff IM, Ihamaki T, et al. Age and sex-related behaviour of gastric acid secretion at the population level. *Scand J Gastroenterol* 1982;17:737–743.
28. Goldschmiedt M, Barnett CC, Schwarz BE, et al. Effect of age on gastric acid secretion and serum gastrin concentrations in healthy men and women. *Gastroenterology* 1991;101:977–990.
29. Owen DA. Stomach. In: Sternberg SS, ed. *Diagnostic surgical pathology. 2nd ed.* New York: Raven Press; 1994:1279–1310.
30. Siurala M, Isokoski M, Varis K, Kekki M. Prevalence of gastritis in a rural population. *Scand J Gastroenterol* 1968;3:211–223.
31. Drumm B, Sherman P, Cutz E, Karmali M. Association of *Campylobacter pylori* on the gastric mucosa with antral gastritis in children. *N Engl J Med* 1987;316:1557–1561.
32. Megraud F, Brassens-Rabbe MP, Denis F, et al. Seroepidemiology of *Campylobacter pylori* infection in various populations. *J Clin Microbiol* 1989;27:1870–1873.
33. Jass JR, Filipe MI. The mucin profiles of normal gastric mucosa, intestinal metaplasia and its variants and gastric carcinoma. *Histochem J* 1981;13:931–939.
34. Filipe MI, Potet F, Bogomoletz WV, et al. Incomplete sulphomucin-secreting intestinal metaplasia for gastric cancer. Preliminary data from a prospective study from three centres. *Gut* 1985;26:1319–1326.
35. Filipe MI, Lake BD. *Histochemistry in pathology.* Edinburgh: Churchill Livingstone, 1983:310–313.
36. Rubio CA, Slezak P. Foveolar cell vacuolization in operated stomachs. *Am J Surg Pathol* 1988;12:773–776.
37. Rubio CA, Hayashi T, Stemmerman G. Ciliated gastric cells: a study of their phenotypic characteristics. *Mod Pathol* 1990;3:720–723.
38. Doglioni C, Laurino L, Dei Tos AP, et al. Pancreatic (acinar) metaplasia of the gastric mucosa. Histology, ultrastructure, immunocytochemistry and clinicopathologic correlations of 101 cases. *Am J Surg Pathol* 1993;17:1134–1143.
39. Thompson IW, Day DW, Wright NA. Subnuclear vacuolated mucous cells: a novel abnormality of simple mucin-secreting cells of non-specialized gastric mucosa and Brunner's glands. *Histopathology* 1987;11: 1067–1081.

*Histology for Pathologists, second edition,*
Edited by Stephen S. Sternberg.
Lippincott-Raven Publishers, Philadelphia


# CHAPTER 21

# Small Intestine

Glenn H. Segal and Robert E. Petras



## GROSS ANATOMY AND SURGICAL PERSPECTIVE

The small intestine, located within the abdominal cavity, is a multiply coiled tubular organ that extends from the gastric pylorus to the junction of the cecum and ascending colon. Its average length in the human adult is 6 to 7 m (1). Three subdivisions—the duodenum, jejunum, and ileum—are defined and characterized by various anatomic relationships. The duodenum is the most proximal portion of the small intestine; it measures about 12 inches (20 to 25 cm) in length and extends from the pylorus to the duodenojejunal flexure. The duodenum, excluding the most proximal several centimeters, is a fixed, retroperitoneal structure that forms a C or U shape around the head of the pancreas (2). Four subdivisions of the duodenum have been described: (a) the first portion, also known as the duodenal cap or bulb, is the most proximal and superior segment; (b) the descending or second portion into which the common bile duct and major and minor pancreatic ducts empty into their respective papillae; (c) the horizontal or third portion; and (d) the ascending or fourth portion, which veers forward at the level of the second lumbar vertebra, just left of midline, to become continuous with the remainder of the small bowel (1,2).

The origin of the jejunum is marked by a strip of fibromuscular tissue, the so-called ligament of Treitz, which anchors the terminal duodenum and duodenojejunal flexure to the posterior abdominal wall (3). Distal to the ligament of Treitz, the remainder of the small bowel is arbitrarily subdivided into the jejunum, the proximal two fifths, and the ileum, which is the distal three fifths terminating at the ileocecal junction within the right iliac fossa (1).

Although a discrete point demarcating jejunum from ileum does not exist, several relatively distinctive features become gradually more apparent from proximal to distal; these features help surgeons isolate specific segments of the small bowel. For example, the proximal jejunum has a thicker wall and is about twice the diameter of distal ileum. In addition, jejunal segments have more prominent permanent circular folds (plicae circulares) that can be palpated externally at surgery (1,4). The quantity of mesenteric adipose tissue is greater in the ileum, thus imparting a dense opaque appearance that contrasts with the less fatty translucent mesentery of the jejunum (4). Finally, most of the jejunum lies within the upper abdominal cavity, whereas most of the ileum lies within the lower abdominal cavity and pelvis.

The arterial vascular supply of the small bowel originates from two major aortic axes: the celiac and superior mesenteric trunks (5). The duodenum is supplied by branches and

G. H. Segal: Division of Anatomic Pathology, University of Utah Health Sciences Center, Salt Lake City, Utah 84132.
R. E. Petras: Department of Pathology, Cleveland Clinic Foundation, Cleveland, Ohio 44195.

interanastomosing arcades of both trunks, and its blood supply is intimately associated with that of the pancreatic head (1). The jejunum and ileum receive their blood from more distal branches of the superior mesenteric artery (5). The lymphatic and venous drainage systems follow the arterial supply and flow into regional lymphatics and lymph nodes or the portal venous system, respectively.

Sympathetic neural input to the small bowel is carried by the celiac and superior mesenteric plexuses, whereas the parasympathetic supply is derived from distal branches of the vagus nerve; these both closely follow the arterial paths into the bowel wall.

## PHYSIOLOGY

The small intestine has several functional roles, the most important of which is the processing and absorption of ingested nutrients. Pancreatic enzymes act on the larger ingested carbohydrates and proteins to produce more appropriately sized molecules for further digestion. The brush border created by the numerous apical microvilli on absorptive epithelial cells offers an array of peptidases and carbohydrases, which act as key enzymes in additional nutrient breakdown and processing (6). The resulting smaller molecules are subsequently absorbed across the epithelial layer, and most pass into the portal venous system for eventual systemic distribution.

Fat digestion differs somewhat in that pancreatic lipase and bile act intraluminally to create free fatty acids and monoglycerides that direct diffusion through the lipid-soluble plasma membrane of enterocytes, without surface processing or active transport (7). Most undergo intracytoplasmic resynthesis with directed packaging into chylomicrons and are released into regional lymphatic vessels. Water and electrolytes, vitamins, minerals, and various drugs also are absorbed at points along the mucosa of the small bowel. Therefore, the structural integrity of this viscus is critical to the maintenance of nutritional status as well as in appropriate drug handling.

The small intestine also functions to propel and segmentally mix both newly accepted gastric contents and the residual material left after initial digestive efforts. Although a number of factors influence gut motility, the most basic contractile activity is initiated at the level of the individual smooth muscle cells within the wall (8). Important functional differences exist based on whether an individual is feeding or fasting. With feeding, a distended bowel segment initiates peristalsis, a forward propulsive motion that is mediated through the enteric nervous system; the intrinsic neurons of the myenteric plexus of Auerbach are most important in this regard (8,9). In contrast, during fasting or between meals, a slow yet continually recurring set of contractions attempts to clear the enteric lumen of any residual debris. The hormone motilin is believed to be important in the generation of these migratory motor complexes (9). Other endocrine influences, as well as the autonomic and central nervous systems, play a modulatory role in these intrinsic activities.

Advances in the burgeoning field of endocrine gut physiology and immunohistology have disclosed a variety of hormones within individual cells lining the small intestinal mucosa (10). Although the precise physiologic role of most of these cells and their secretory products remains to be determined, some are thought to exert a modulatory effect on gut motility or to influence the function of nearby epithelial cells (9,11).

The gut in general and the small bowel in particular have a crucial function in mucosal immunity. The mucosa/gut-associated lymphoid tissues, which are discussed in detail later in this chapter, are important in the local defense against mucosally encountered microorganisms and generate the initial immunologic responses to these various agents (12). Additionally, these tissues are the breeding ground for various reactive and neoplastic pathologic conditions.

## HISTOLOGY

Although regional histologic differences exist within the small intestine, the general microscopic structure is similar throughout its length. The wall of the small bowel can be divided into four basic layers; mucosa, submucosa, muscularis externa or propria, and serosa.

### Mucosa

#### *Mucosal Architecture and Design*

Because the principal function of the small intestine is absorption of ingested nutrients, the mucosa, which is the layer in contact with luminal contents, is specifically designed for this purpose. Several architectural adaptations augment the otherwise limited surface area of the small intestine (13). One of these, the grossly evident permanent circular folds (plicae circulares), course perpendicular to the longitudinal axis of the bowel (13,14) (Fig. 1). These mucosa-covered folds contain submucosal cores and traverse nearly the entire circumference of the bowel lumen before overlapping with adjacent permanent folds. In addition to enhancing surface area, they act as partial barriers that attenuate the forward flow of intraluminal contents, thus increasing the time of contact with absorptive surfaces.

The mucosa is composed of an epithelial component, a lamina propria, and a muscularis mucosae. The surface epithelium and lamina propria form intraluminal projections called villi. These microscopic fingerlike and leaflike projections cover the entire luminal surface of the small bowel and are the most important morphologic modification responsible for enhancing surface area (13,15,16) (Figs. 2 and 3). Each villous surface is covered by a single layer of epithelium consisting of various cell types. Beneath this ep-

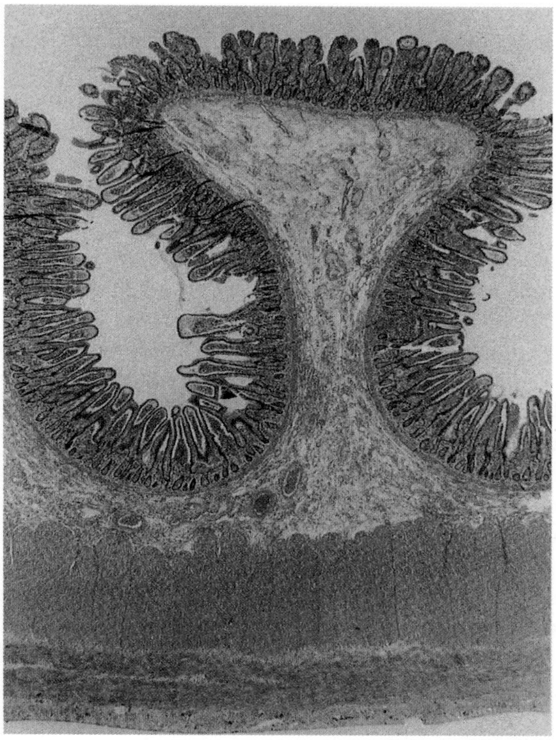

**FIG. 1.** A single plica, or permanent circular fold, with its submucosal core and mucosal surface. The absorptive surface area is further augmented by intraluminal mucosal projections (villi).

ithelial layer lies a core of lamina propria that contains a centrally located, blind-ended lymphatic channel (lacteal), an arteriovenous capillary network, and an abundant migratory cell population (17–19) (Fig. 4). In the intervening regions, and beneath the villi, lie the crypts of Lieberkühn. These tubular intestinal glands open between the villi and extend down to the muscularis mucosae (Fig. 3). The crypts are depressions of the surface epithelium, whereas the villi are extensions above it. However, these mucosal compartments are contiguous in that the lamina propria forming the villous cores also surrounds the crypts. The ratio of villous length to crypt length in normal small bowel varies from about 3:1 to 5:1 (13) (Fig. 3). The crypts and surrounding lamina propria lie upon the muscularis mucosae, a thin fibromuscular layer that separates the mucosa from the underlying submucosa.

### *Mucosal Components and Their Composition*

#### *Epithelium*

The mucosal epithelium is divided into the villous and crypt compartments. Although similar in appearance, the cell types differ somewhat and their basic functions are distinct. Common to both, however, is a basic polarity of cellular organization, with nuclei aligned side by side typically in a basal location within each cell.

*Villous Epithelium.* The absorptive cell is the major villous epithelial cell type encountered. It is tall, columnar, with

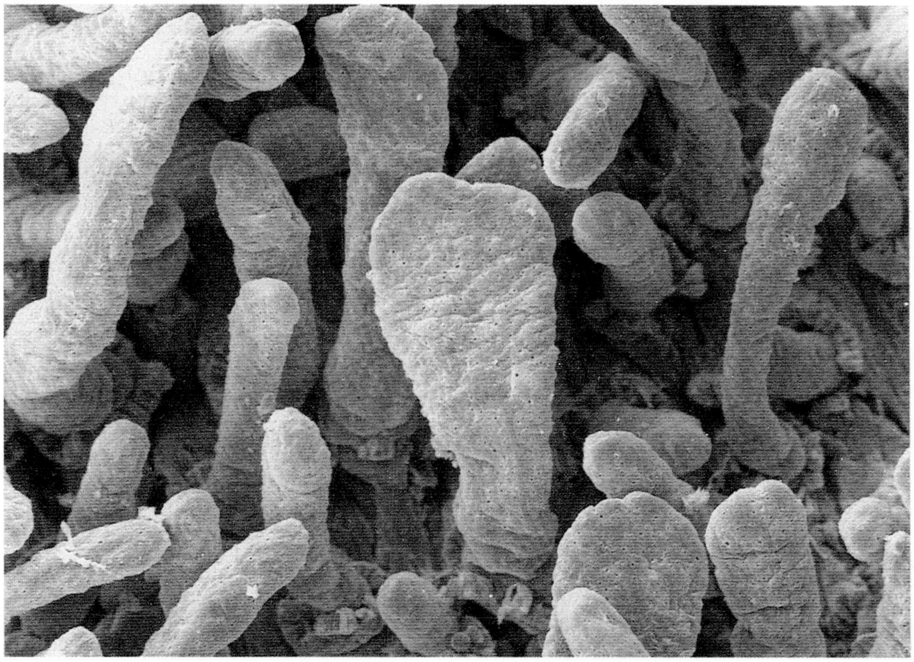

**FIG. 2.** Scanning electron micrograph of small intestinal mucosa discloses the fingerlike and leaflike appearance of villi. Fingerlike villi predominate in the more distal segments of small bowel (jejunum and ileum), whereas leaflike villi are more common in the duodenum. Mixed populations, as in this micrograph, are considered normal.

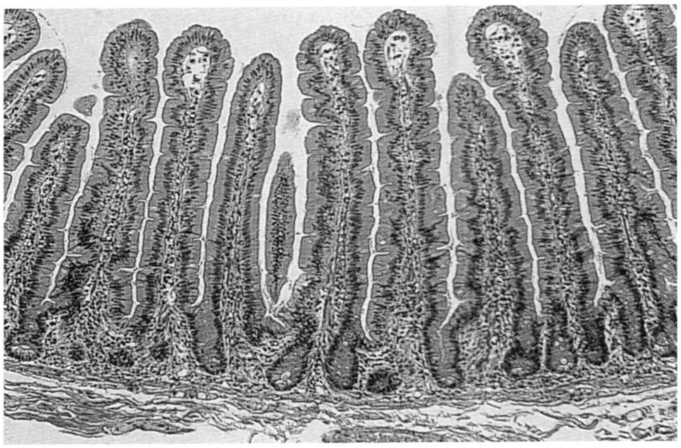

**FIG. 3.** Normal jejunal villi. These villi are long and slender mucosal projections with a core of lamina propria covered by a luminal epithelial layer. A single row of intestinal glands (crypts) is found at the base of the mucosa. These crypts lie between adjacent villi and are surrounded by the same lamina propria that forms the villous cores.

a basally situated round-to-oval nucleus and an eosinophilic cytoplasm (Fig. 5). The apical surface contains a brush border that appears densely eosinophilic, stains positive with periodic acid-Schiff (PAS), and is composed of microvilli and the glycocalyx, or fuzzy coat (Figs. 5 and 6). Microvilli, which are best seen on ultrastructural examination, are evenly spaced surface projections that also augment the mucosal surface area of the small intestine (20) (Fig. 7). Multiple filamentous structures emanating from and contiguous with their surface comprise the glycocalyx (17). The microvillous membrane–glycocalyx complex houses important enzymes—peptidases and disaccharidases—that function in terminal digestive processes. This layer probably also acts as a barrier to microorganisms and other foreign matter (21). Components forming the glycocalyx are continually synthesized within the absorptive cell and transported to the surface to replace the preexisting coat in a dynamic fashion (17,21,22). Although its functional capacities are uncertain, absence of the glycocalyx of the small bowel mucosa was the sole detectable histologic abnormality found in one recent study in some children with allergic enteropathy (i.e., cow's milk allergy) (21).

Interspersed among the absorptive cells are goblet cells, which have a characteristic apical mucin droplet and an attenuated, basally situated, bland nucleus (Fig. 5). They contain both neutral and acid mucin and function as secretory cells, sustaining a moist viscid environment within the lumen (20). In a combined alcian blue–PAS stain, the droplets appear blue–purple (Fig. 8). The acid mucins of the small intestine are primarily sialomucins, in contrast to the colonic goblet cell, which contains predominantly acid sulfomucins (23,24). The number of goblet cells increases with distal progression along the small bowel (20).

Scattered endocrine cells are present within the villous epithelium, but they are more abundant within the crypts. In-

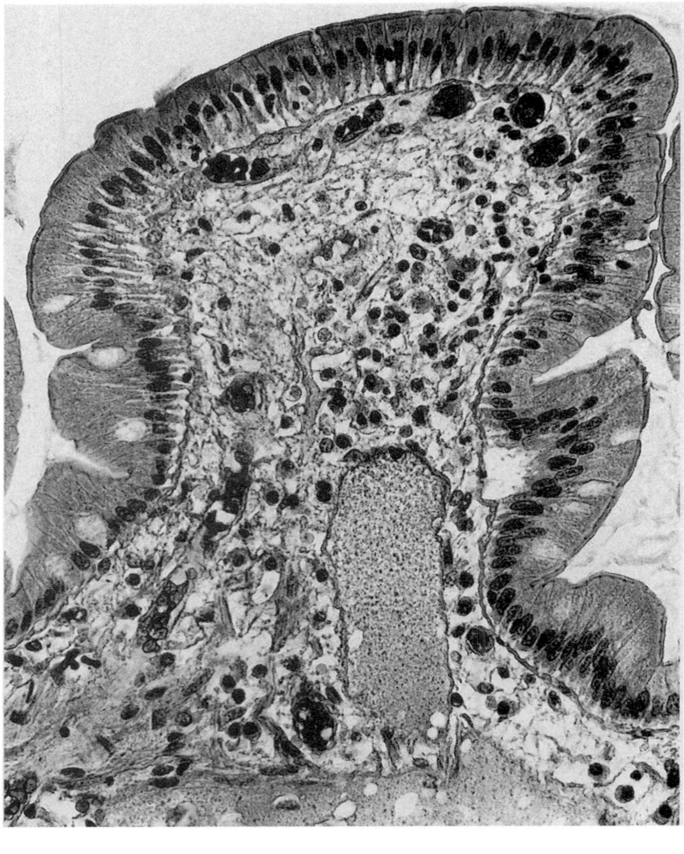

**FIG. 4.** This duodenal villous surface is covered by a single layer of tall columnar epithelial cells. The underlying lamina proprial core contains lymphoid and plasma cells and a connective tissue framework including a lymphatic vessel (lacteal) and a subepithelial capillary network.

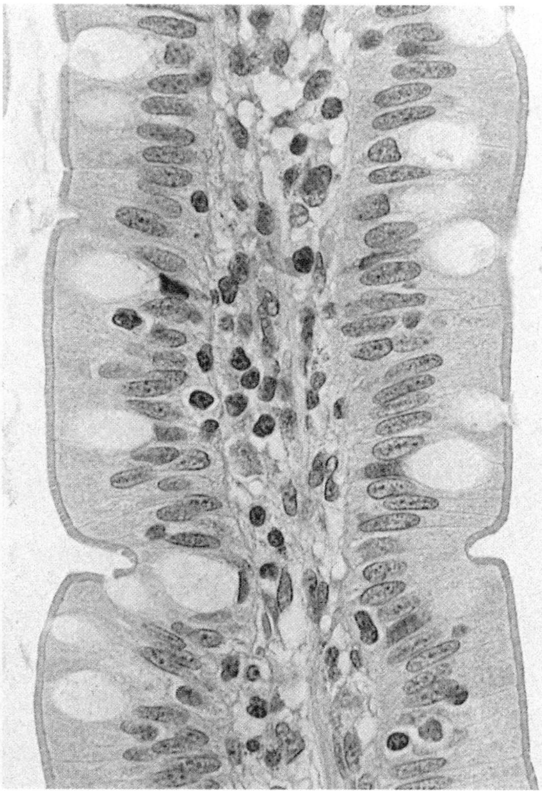

**FIG. 5.** High magnification view of a jejunal villus disclosing the general features of villous morphology. Both columnar absorptive cells and goblet cells (with apical clear vacuole) cover the villous surfaces; each cell type has a basally situated oval-to-round nucleus. Microvilli (brush border) are seen extending from the columnar absorptive cell surface. Note the intraepithelial lymphocytes scattered among and between the epithelial cells.

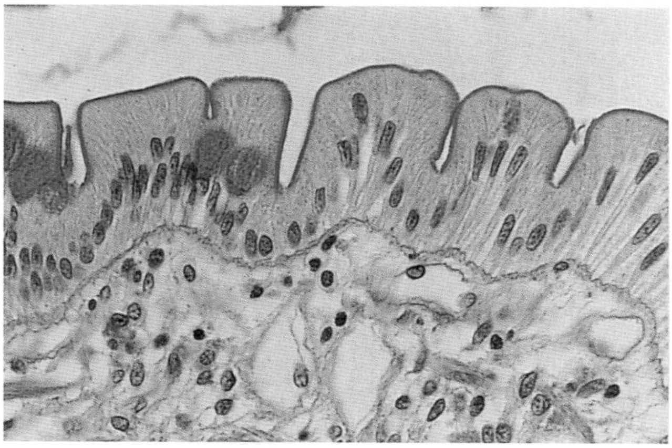

**FIG. 6.** Periodic acid–Schiff (PAS) stain highlights the microvillous membrane–glycocalyx complex along the apical surface of the absorptive cells. The thin subepithelial basement membrane that separates the lamina propria from the epithelial compartment also stains with PAS but to a lesser degree. The neutral subgroup of mucins contained within the goblet cells are PAS positive as well.

traepithelial lymphocytes are scattered among and lie between individual epithelial cells, usually just above the basement membrane; normally there is about one lymphocyte for every five epithelial cells (25,26) (Fig. 5). Intraepithelial lymphocytes mark as T cells (Fig. 9), and most are of the T-suppressor/cytotoxic (CD8-positive) variety (27–29). An increase in the number of intraepithelial lymphocytes is characteristic of several disorders, including gluten-sensitive enteropathy (celiac sprue), tropical sprue, and giardiasis (30,31).

*Crypt Epithelium.* The crypt epithelium primarily functions in epithelial cell renewal (20), and as a consequence of this regenerative function, mitoses are seen frequently within the crypts (normal range one to 12 mitoses/crypt) (32). Goblet cells and columnar cells, some of which are undifferentiated or stem cells, are conspicuous. The four major epithelial cell types of the mucosa (absorptive, goblet, endocrine, and Paneth cells) arise from this stem cell (33). Differentiation and maturation occur in about 5 to 6 days as the cells migrate from the crypt depths to the villous tips, where they are subsequently sloughed into the lumen (20,33); however, the Paneth cell remains within the crypt base (34). It is thought that apoptosis probably functions as a regulator of cell migration toward the villous surface; however, it is not certain whether this form of programmed cell death is responsible for epithelial cell sloughing from the villous tip (35). Morphologically, cells undergoing apoptosis show nuclear condensation and cell shrinkage with subsequent detachment from adjacent epithelium. In addition, the cell disintegrates into so-called apoptotic bodies and is phagocytosed by local histiocytes (35).

Endocrine cells are relatively abundant in the crypts, occurring as single cells or in discontinuous groupings along the intestinal tract (10). They are of two morphologic types. The "open" type have a pyramidal shape that tapers toward the glandular lumen with which they communicate, whereas "closed" cells are spindle shaped and have no luminal connection (10). The former are the most frequent type found in the small bowel. Some endocrine cells disclose eosinophilic basal (infranuclear) granules on hematoxylin and eosin staining so that they are easily identified on routine preparations (Fig. 10); however, not all enteroendocrine cells have such a quality, and their identification remains elusive unless special methods are used. Silver (argyrophilic, argentaffinic) preparations or immunocytochemical techniques are useful for visualization in these cases. The disadvantage of silver stains is that no information can be gleaned with respect to endocrine cell type or hormonal composition, and some cells do not reduce silver preparations (10). Immunocytochemistry is, therefore, the best method for definitive evaluation. Antibody preparations to chromogranin and neuron-specific enolase have been shown to be useful nonspecific markers for endocrine cells (36) (Fig. 11). Precise identification of endocrine chemical content requires specific monoclonal or polyclonal antibody preparations. Although most often used in experimental settings, specific hormonal content im-

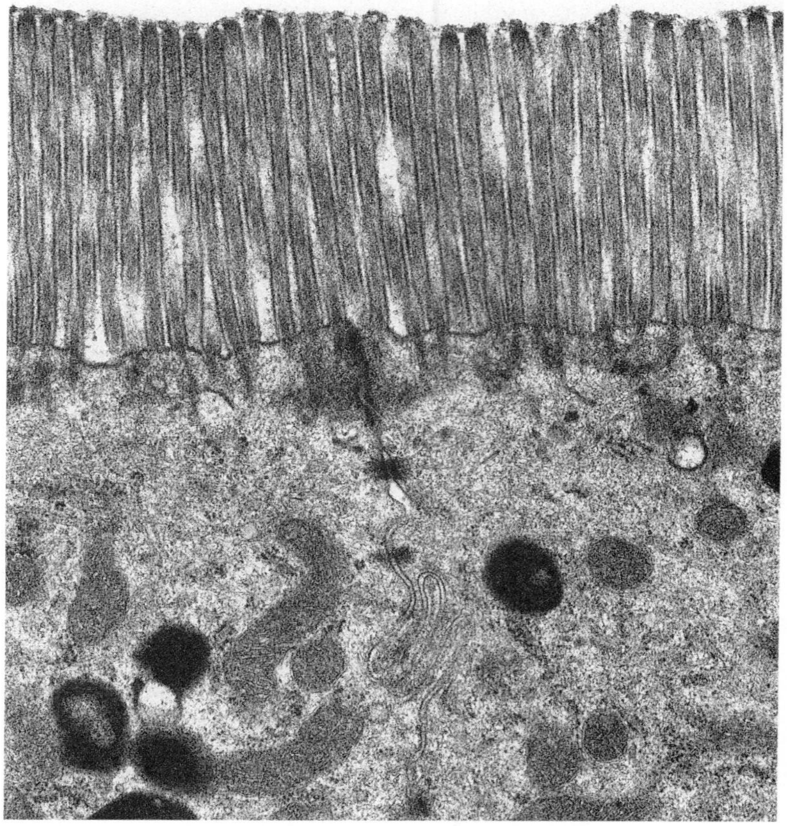

**FIG. 7.** Transmission electron micrograph of microvilli emanating from the absorptive columnar cell surfaces. The glycocalyx component is the filamentous layer overlying the microvilli, but most of this has been artifactually removed during processing.

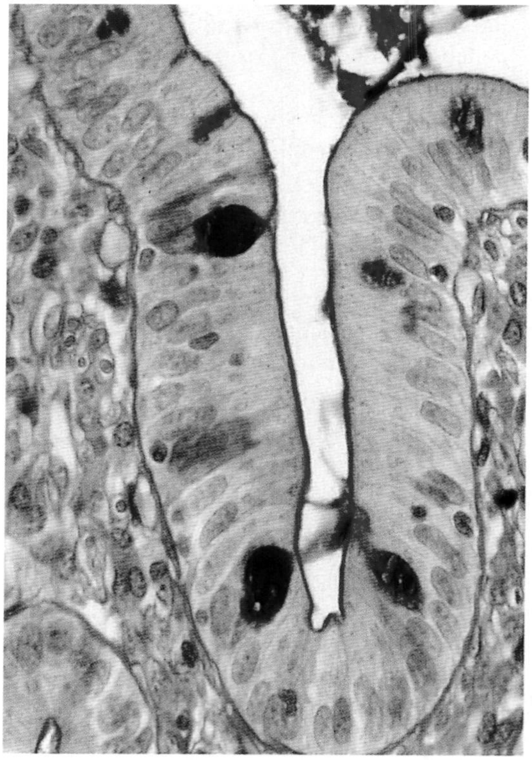

**FIG. 8.** Alcian blue–PAS combination stain showing characteristic blue–purple apical mucin droplet of intestinal goblet cells. The heterogeneous composition (neutral and acid mucins) allows for both stains to be incorporated into the droplet, imparting this distinctive color.

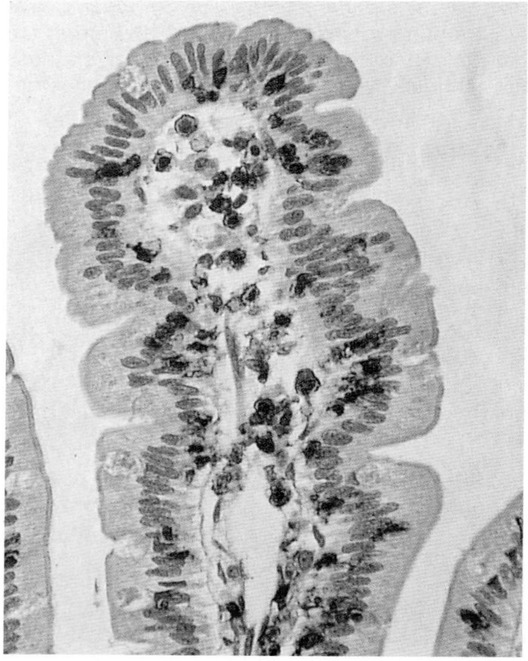

**FIG. 9.** Small intestinal mucosa immunostained for UCHL1 (CD45 RO), a pan–T-lymphocyte marker. The positive red–brown reaction highlights both the intraepithelial and lamina proprial T cells. Although CD8-positive T-suppressor/cytotoxic lymphocytes predominate within the epithelium, lamina proprial T cells usually mark for CD4, the T-helper/inducer subset.

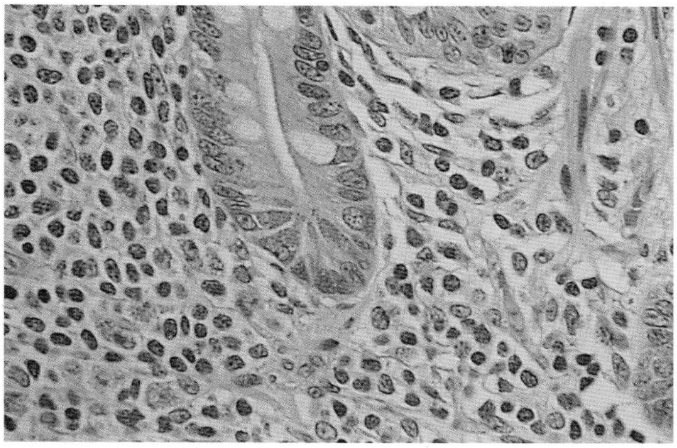

**FIG. 10.** A single crypt surrounded by normal cellular lamina propria with abundant migratory cells. Both absorptive columnar and goblet cells are seen lining the crypt. In addition, an endocrine cell (infranuclear eosinophilic granules) and several Paneth's cells (supranuclear granules) are clearly evident.

munostaining also may have diagnostic value in studying neuroendocrine tumors (37). Electron microscopy also can be used to identify cytoplasmic neurosecretory granules.

At least 16 distinct types of endocrine cell have been described along the gut (38) with a characteristic regional distribution and composition. Individual cells containing cholecystokinin, secretin, gastric inhibitory polypeptide, and motilin populate more proximal segments of the small bowel, whereas enteroglucagon-, substance P–, and neurotensin-storing cells are seen in greater frequency in the ileum (38,39). Serotonin- and somatostatin-containing cells are not as regionalized and are found throughout the gastrointestinal tract (38). Some of these endocrine cells are known to play key roles in daily gastrointestinal activity. For example, secretin and cholecystokinin are released in response to various foodstuffs and modulate pancreatic secretion and gallbladder function, respectively (39). Most other gut endocrine cells are still of uncertain or unknown physiologic significance (11,39).

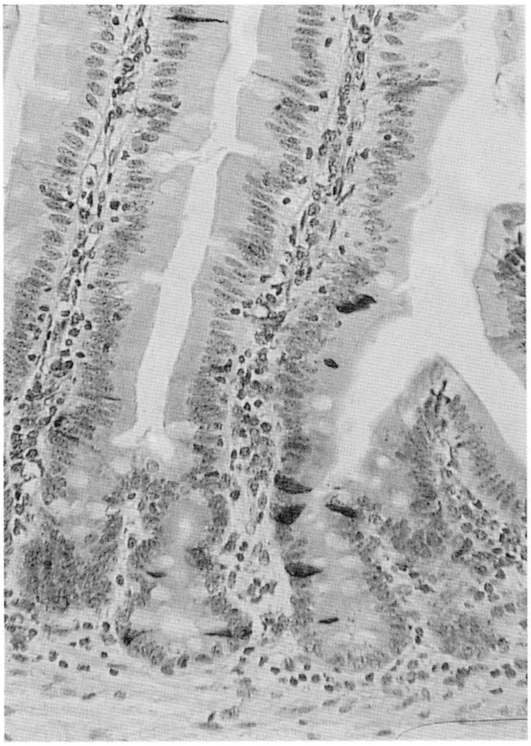

**FIG. 11.** Immunostain for chromogranin shows numerous endocrine cells within the crypts and several scattered along the villous surface.

The Paneth's cells, normally found only in the crypt, comprise most of the base of individual crypts throughout the entire small intestine (40). They also are encountered to a lesser degree in the appendix and ascending colon (41). Paneth's cells have a pyramidal shape with their apices pointing toward the lumen. Their cytoplasm contains characteristic supranuclear, intensely eosinophilic granules that are easily visualized in hematoxylin and eosin–stained sections (Fig. 10). Interestingly, fixatives containing picric acid (e.g., Hollande's, Bouin's) mask the eosinophilic staining of these granules, often disclosing only unstained cytoplasmic vacuoles (40) (Fig. 12). Their round nuclei often contain a prominent nucleolus (20,29). The exact function of Paneth's cells is still uncertain, but they are known to contain lysozyme and immunoglobulin, and they are capable of phagocytic activity. These features suggest that they play a role in regulating the intestinal microbial flora (41,42).

The crypt epithelium also contains intraepithelial lymphocytes that are predominantly T-suppressor/cytotoxic (CD8-positive) cells (43). Other inflammatory cell types such as the neutrophil or the plasma cell are not normally present within either the crypt or villous epithelial compartments; their presence would indicate a pathologic state (31,44).

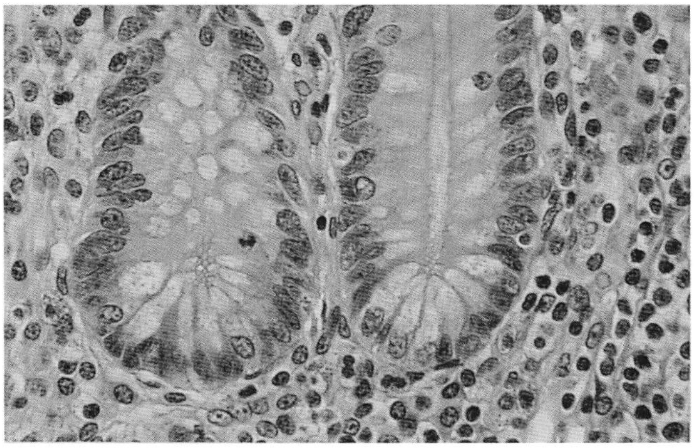

**FIG. 12.** Although Hollande's and other picric acid-containing fixatives are superior preservers of cytomorphologic detail, the characteristic supranuclear eosinophilic granules of Paneth's cells are not as easily visualized when compared with the appearance in 4% formaldehyde solution (see Fig. 10). Clear vacuoles replace the distinct eosinophilic granules within the Paneth's cells (along the crypt bases). Note that the single endocrine cell in this crypt maintains its infranuclear granular staining quality.

*Immunostaining Patterns of the Epithelium.* Carcinoembryonic antigen (CEA) is present on the apical surfaces of cells covering the villi and lining the crypts, and it has been shown to localize to the glycocalyx surface component (45). Additionally, the mucin droplets of goblet cells contain an abundance of CEA and consequently mark intensely with polyclonal anti-CEA. However, no intracytoplasmic immunostaining for CEA is evident in the normal small bowel (45).

Human leukocyte antigen (HLA)-DR–like antigens have been shown to be present in a scattered, focal distribution on the apices of small intestinal columnar-shaped cells (46). Immunostaining with anti–HLA-DR discloses a diminishing intensity of reactivity from the villous surfaces to the crypt bases. Immune-related cells such as lymphocytes (mostly B cells) and macrophages along with the walls of capillaries in the lamina propria also show immunoreactivity for HLA-DR (46).

### *Lamina Propria*

The lamina propria, the intermediate layer of the mucosa, functions both structurally and immunologically. It rests upon the muscularis mucosae, surrounds the crypts, and extends upward as the cores of the intestinal villi. The crypt epithelium and villous epithelium rest upon the lamina propria and are separated from it by a distinct basement membrane recognized as a slender eosinophilic, PAS-positive band at their interface (Figs. 4–6). This subepithelial basement membrane is a continuous structure composed of an ultrastructurally apparent basal lamina and a deeper network of collagenous/reticular fibers and ground substance (17). Interweaving collagen bundles and other connective tissue fibers, fibroblasts, mature fibrocytes, and smooth muscle cells comprise the framework of the lamina propria (44), whereas blood capillaries, lymphatics, and nerves course through this layer on their various routes to and from all portions of the bowel wall.

The most conspicuous feature of the lamina propria is its abundant immunocompetent and migratory cell component (Figs. 10 and 12). Five types of immunocompetent or inflammatory cells are normally encountered in the lamina propria: plasma cells, lymphocytes, eosinophils, histiocytes, and mast cells. Neutrophils are not usually encountered in the lamina propria, or for that matter anywhere in the small bowel wall, with the exception of those confined to vascular lumina.

Plasma cells are the most abundant cellular lamina proprial constituent; most contain cytoplasmic immunoglobulin (Ig)A but some contain IgM (Fig. 13). In contrast to extraintestinal sites (e.g., peripheral lymph nodes) (30,47), IgG-secreting plasma cells are scant. Lymphocytes, both B and T cells, are also common. T-lymphocytes with the helper/inducer immunophenotype (CD4 positive) are the predominant subset of T cells within the lamina propria (27,47,48)

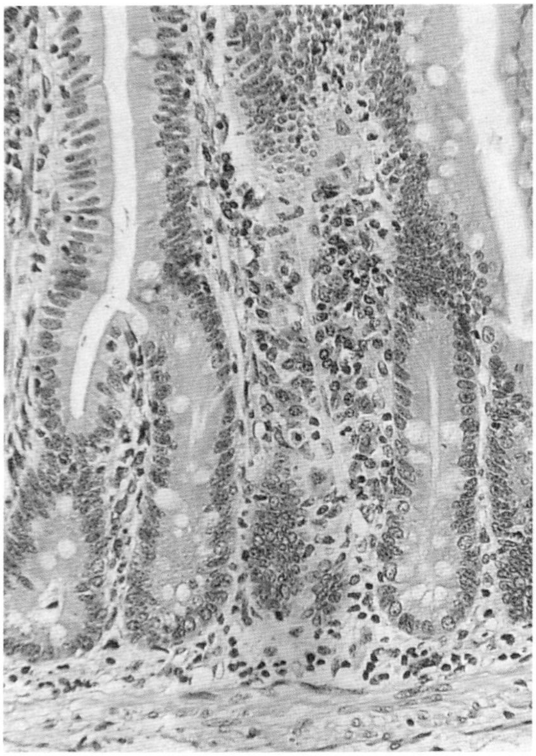

**FIG. 13.** Numerous IgA-containing plasma cells (red–brown cytoplasmic staining) within the lamina propria of normal small intestine, immunostained for alpha heavy chain. Note that in contrast to T cells (see Fig. 9), the plasma cells localize to the lamina propria and are not normally found in the epithelium.

(Fig. 9). Lymphocytes are found throughout the lamina propria but often form more dense infiltrates just above the muscularis mucosae (44). Moreover, lymphoid aggregates and nodules, many with germinal centers, are scattered along the small bowel and are found in increasing concentration distally. These lymphoid aggregates are based in the lamina propria, but they often extend to some degree into the underlying submucosa.

Histiocytes or macrophages are also seen in the lamina propria but in fewer numbers than lymphocytes or plasma cells. Most are located along the superiormost aspect of the lamina propria near the tips of the villi (28). They function in T-cell regulation as antigen presenters and phagocytes (30). Exaggerated expression of this latter function can be seen pathologically in disseminated *Mycobacterium avium-intracellulare* complex infection and in Whipple's disease, where the lamina propria becomes filled with macrophages engorged with microorganisms (30,49–51).

The only granulocytes normally found in the lamina propria are eosinophils and mast cells. Eosinophilic leukocytes usually are conspicuous, but their role in the normal bowel is uncertain (52). The numbers of eosinophils in the lamina propria increase under various conditions, including those comprising the eosinophilic gastroenteropathies (53–57).

Mast cells are relatively abundant in the small intestinal lamina propria, as compared with other body sites (30), but in absolute numbers appear to decrease with distal progression along the small bowel (58). Their function in the gastrointestinal tract in normal and disease states is unknown. Increased numbers of mast cells can be found in inflammatory bowel disease and in the specimens of some individuals with eosinophilic gastroenteropathy (56,59). According to some investigators, a specimen disclosing more than eight mast cells per high magnification field should suggest the diagnosis of systemic mast cell disease (60). Mast cells can be seen on hematoxylin and eosin–stained sections, but they are more easily visualized with special techniques such as toluidine blue, sulfated alcian blue, or Giemsa stains. Rarely, subepithelial (lamina proprial) endocrine cells may be found in the small bowel; however, these are much more prominent in the vermiform appendix (61). Occasionally, in apparently healthy individuals and in certain disease states (e.g., Crohn's disease), ganglion cells are found in the lamina propria of the small bowel. These could potentially be confused with cytomegalovirus infection–induced cellular changes.

#### *Muscularis Mucosae*

The muscularis mucosae, which is the outermost layer or limit of the mucosa, is a slender band of tissue composed of elastic fibers and smooth muscle arranged in an outer longitudinal and inner circular layer (Fig. 14). However, these layers are usually not well delineated on routine light microscopy. Tufts of smooth muscle radiate from the muscularis mucosae into the lamina propria and extend into the villi. The muscularis mucosae provides an important structural foundation for the mucosa, and its absence in some biopsy specimens can cause a loss of villous orientation, an artifact that may interfere with optimal evaluation (52).

### Submucosa

Between the muscularis mucosae and muscularis externa is the submucosa, a loose, paucicellular layer composed of a regular, honeycomb-like arrangement (at the ultrastructural level) of collagenous and elastic fibers and related fibroblasts. The submucosa also may contain scattered, rather inconspicuous migratory cells (e.g., histiocytes, lymphoid and plasma cells, and mast cells) and adipose tissue (62). Its histologic appearance and principal role in maintaining the structural integrity of the small bowel are similar throughout the gastrointestinal tract (62). The submucosa is a major focus of vascular routing and related distribution of regional blood and lymphatic flow. Relatively large caliber arterioles, venules, and lymphatic vessels form extensive individual plexuses and networks within this layer (5,19) (Fig. 15). From this "vascular center," numerous penetrating capillary vessels supply and drain most of the mucosa and muscularis externa (5,19). Lymphatic vessels may be distinguished from blood vessels by the thinner wall of the former and the lack of luminal erythrocytes. However, certain immunohistologic patterns and electron microscopic characteristics are more helpful for definitive identification (18,63,64). Specifically, the endothelial cells of blood capillaries immunostain for PAL-E and Factor VIII–related antigen, whereas lymphatic capillary endothelia typically lack these antigenic sites and remain unstained with such antibody preparations (63,64). In addition, blood capillaries as seen by ultrastruc-

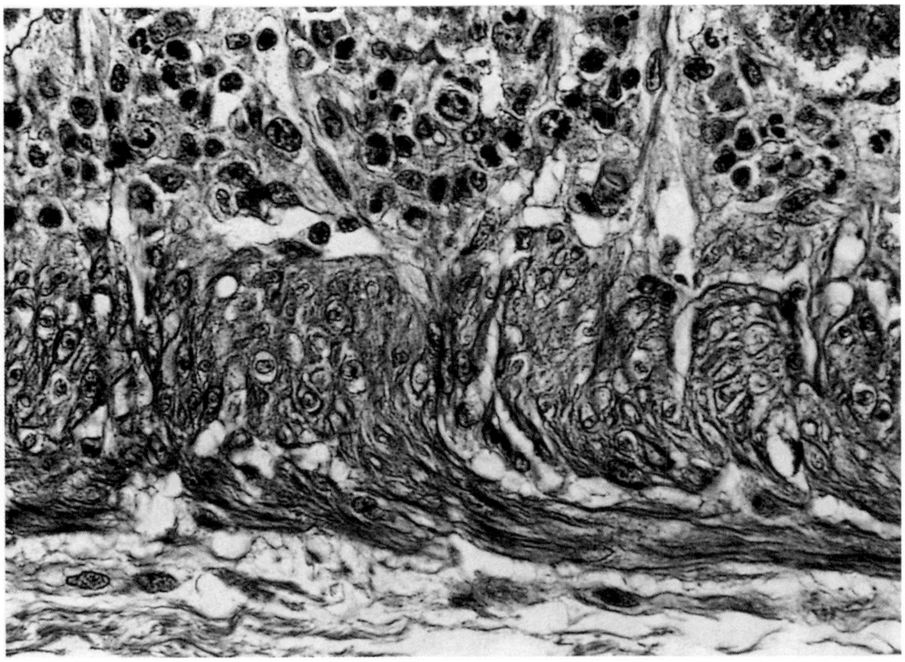

**FIG. 14.** High-magnification photomicrograph disclosing inner circular and outer longitudinal smooth muscle bands of the muscularis mucosae; this layering is often inconspicuous on hematoxylin and eosin preparations, where the muscularis mucosae appears as a thin eosinophilic strip between the lamina propria and underlying submucosa (Masson's trichrome).

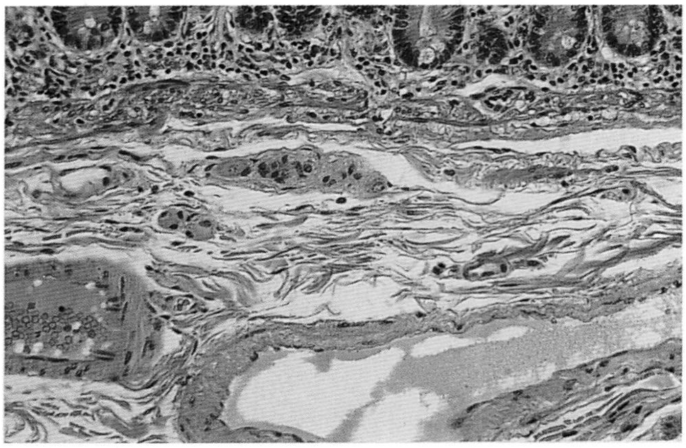

FIG. 15. Normal submucosa separated from overlying mucosa by the eosinophilic staining muscularis mucosae. The submucosa is paucicellular, disclosing fibrocollagenous tissue and a prominent vascular component. Note the ganglion cells of Meissner's plexus just beneath the muscularis mucosae.

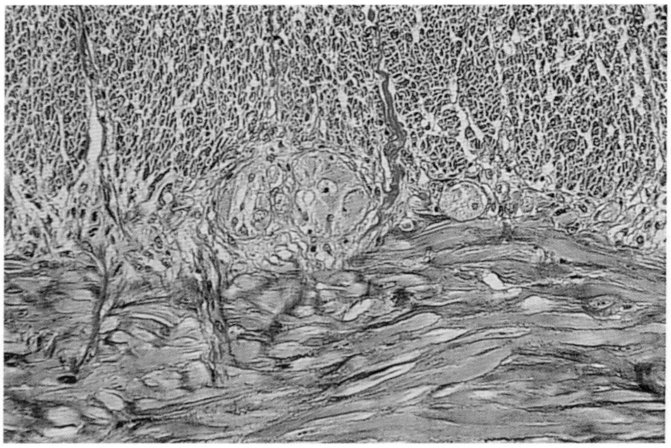

FIG. 16. Masson's trichrome stain clearly delineates the inner circular (*above*) from the outer longitudinal (*below*) smooth muscle bands of the muscularis externa. The prominent muscular component (red) is partitioned into bundles of varying size by delicate collagenous fibers (blue). Note ganglia of the myenteric (Auerbach's) plexus characteristically located between the two muscle bands. Fibrous tissue is minimal within the muscularis externa and is also not normally part of the plexus.

tural analysis have a continuous basal lamina, endothelial fenestrations, and ensheathing pericytes. However, lymphatic capillaries have a discontinuous basal lamina and lack both fenestrations and surrounding pericytes (17,18). Although small lymphatic vessels are a conspicuous submucosal component, prominent, dilated lymphatic structures in this layer, as well as in the mucosa, can be seen in pathologic states such as intestinal lymphangiectasia or Crohn's disease (31,65).

Neural structures are also prominent in the submucosa. The submucosal plexus of Meissner forms one of the two major integrative centers of the enteric nervous system. It consists of a network of ganglia that interconnect through neural processes (66). The ganglia contain compact aggregates of neurons (ganglion cells) routinely identified on hematoxylin and eosin preparations by their characteristic large oval shape, abundant pink cytoplasm, vesicular nucleus, and single prominent, often eosinophilic nucleolus (Fig. 15). Abundant S-100–positive Schwann cells, glial-like cells, and neural processes are also present in Meissner's plexus. The entire plexus, including the ganglia, contains no connective tissue elements or vascular structures in the normal state (66–69). The plexus is also normally devoid of inflammatory cells; therefore, if these are seen, an injury pattern specific to the neural plexus such as an inflammatory neuropathy should be considered, as long as primary inflammatory bowel disease can be excluded (68). Neural interconnections exist between Meissner's plexus and the myenteric plexus of Auerbach (discussed later), as well as with extrinsic (autonomic) neural processes.

### Muscularis Externa

The muscularis externa (or propria) is the thick outer smooth muscle layer that surrounds the submucosa. It is covered externally by subserosal connective tissue and in most places by a serosa. Its two distinct muscular layers, oriented perpendicular to each other, are arranged as an outer longitudinally running muscle fiber layer and an inner circular muscle band (Fig. 16). Blood vessels, lymphatics, and nerves course through the muscularis externa and slender collagenous septa surround groups of smooth muscle cells creating characteristic bundles and packets of muscle (Fig. 16). However, fibrous tissue in this layer is minimal in the normal small bowel (68). Therefore, even slight fibrous alterations or collagen deposition may be significant. Moreover, the fact

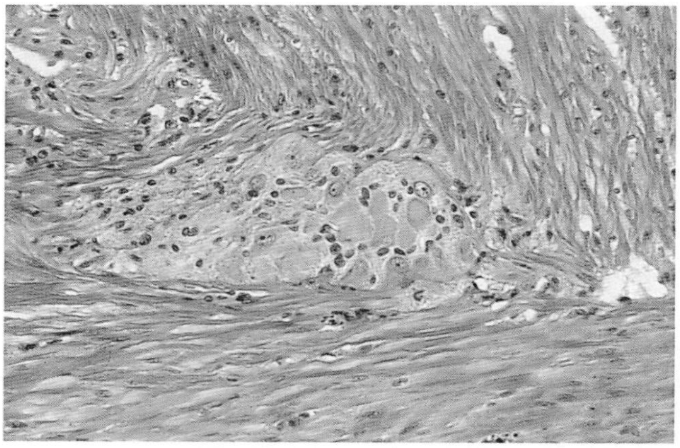

FIG. 17. A single ganglion of the myenteric plexus of Auerbach located at the interface of the inner (*above*) and outer (*below*) smooth muscle layers of the muscularis externa. Ganglion cells (neuronal cell bodies) are evident and characterized by a polygonal shape, abundant pink cytoplasm, and an eccentric nucleus; spindled neural projections and Schwann cells are also intermixed.

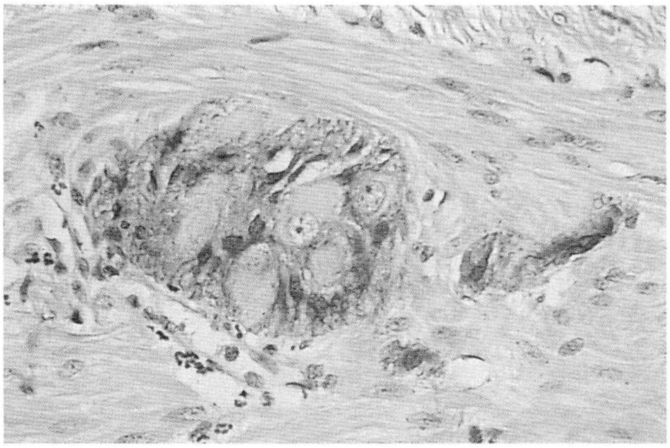

**FIG. 18.** This S-100 immunostain highlights the otherwise inconspicuous spindled Schwann cell component of the ganglion. It also marks the Schwann cells accompanying the neural projections that interconnect these ganglia to one another within the plexus system. Note that the ganglion cells show no such immunoreactivity.

that only a few disease entities are associated with fibrosis of the muscularis propria, including ischemia, irradiation, familial visceral myopathy, scleroderma, and mycobacterial infection, aids in narrowing a broad differential diagnosis (31).

The myenteric plexus of Auerbach, the other major neural plexus of the enteric nervous system, lies between the outer longitudinal and inner circular muscle layers (Figs. 16–18). Auerbach's plexus is similar in composition to the submucosal plexus, although it typically has larger ganglia, a greater number of neurons, and a more compact plexus network (67,68). As a consequence of these features, it is best to evaluate the myenteric plexus for specific disease processes involving the enteric nervous system, such as the various visceral neuropathies. Because routine processing allows only a small portion of the plexus to be visualized and because many of these conditions cause no detectable changes on routine hematoxylin and eosin-stained sections, special preparations of thicker, larger, and silver-stained sections cut en face are currently necessary to diagnose many of these disorders (68). Finally, although of lesser importance, a deep muscular, subserous plexus and several mucosal plexuses are also present within the small bowel (67).

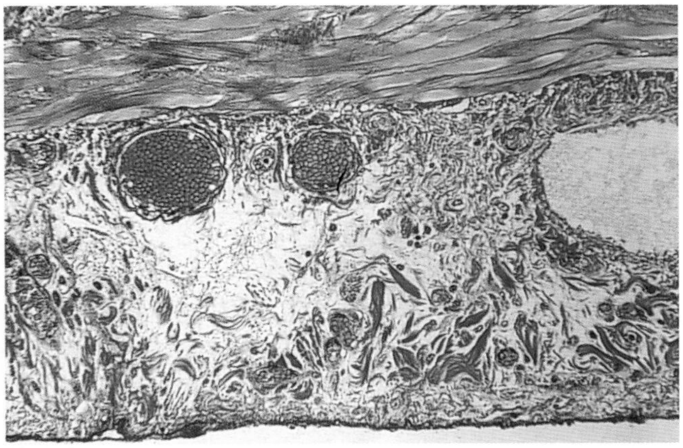

**FIG. 19.** The subserosal region contains a delicate fibrocollagenous network, blood vessels, lymphatics, and nerves. The serosa consists of a thin fibrous layer (*blue and bottom*) covered by a single layer of mesothelial cells; however, the mesothelium is often denuded in surgical specimens. A portion of the outer layer of the muscularis externa is also present in this field (*top*). (Masson's trichrome.)

### Serosa and Subserosal Region

The serosa is the covering that envelops most of the external surface of the small bowel. Its outermost layer consists of a single row of cuboidal mesothelial cells, under which lies a thin band of loose connective tissue. A subserosal zone of connective tissue lying between this mesothelial covering and the muscularis externa also contains ramifying branches of blood vessels, lymphatics, and nerves (Fig. 19).

## DISTINCTIVE REGIONAL CHARACTERISTICS OF THE SMALL BOWEL

### Duodenum

The duodenum exhibits several distinctive histologic features, many related to its proximal location in direct continuity with the pylorus. The gastroduodenal junction, although well delineated grossly, is poorly demarcated histologically (70) (Figs. 20 and 21). A gradual transition in epithelial types occurs, with three distinct subtypes in the duodenum (71): (a) an antral type mucosal epithelium that is identical to the

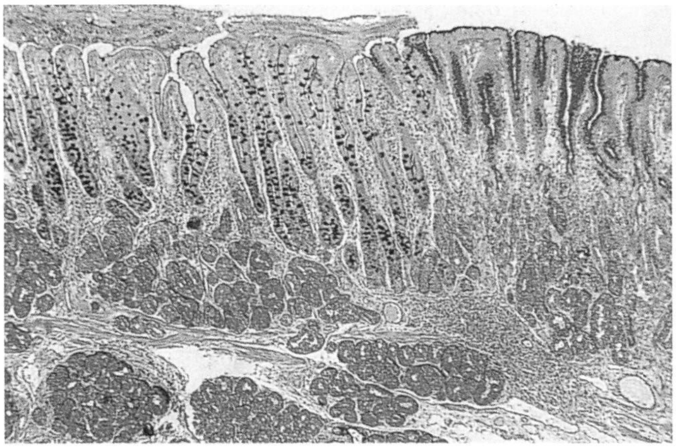

**FIG. 20.** Gastroduodenal junction. Note the transition from PAS-positive (red) gastric foveolar epithelium and underlying pyloric glands (*right*) to a villous mucosal architecture of the duodenum (*left*) lined predominantly by alcian blue–PAS-positive (blue–purple) goblet cells and absorptive cells. Note that both pyloric (*right*) and Brunner's (*left*) glands are composed predominantly of cells containing only neutral, PAS-positive mucin. Brunner's glands, however, are predominantly submucosal in location, while pyloric glands are an intramucosal structure. (Alcian blue–PAS.)

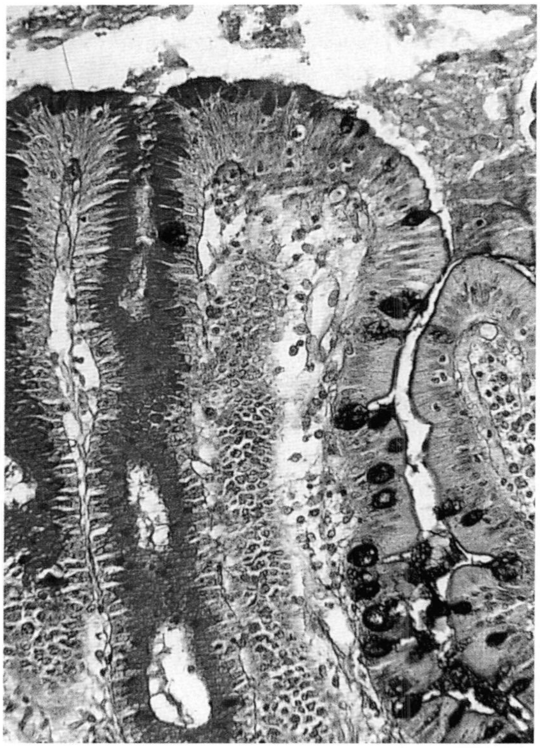

**FIG. 21.** Several villi within the confines of the gastroduodenal junction disclosing both "usual small intestinal type" epithelium and antral type, PAS-positive, foveolar epithelium. This transitional type epithelium is a characteristic "hybrid" found in this region. At more distal small intestinal sites, this transitional type epithelium is termed gastric metaplasia. (Alcian blue–PAS.)

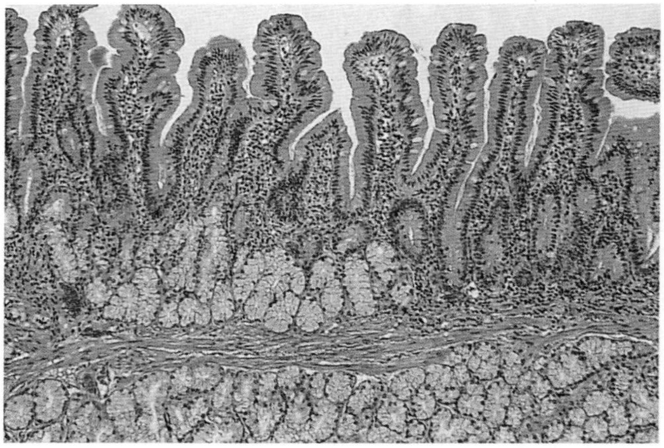

**FIG. 22.** Short, slightly broader villi predominate in the duodenum. The underlying submucosal Brunner's glands are a distinctive feature of this portion of small bowel. Note that a fair portion of Brunner's glands normally occurs above the muscularis mucosae.

pyloric mucosa; (b) a "usual small intestinal type" (jejunal type) characterized by villi covered by absorptive cells and interspersed goblet cells; and (c) a transitional type (Fig. 21), in which the same villus is covered by epithelium having features of both antral type and usual small intestinal type epithelia. In the region of the gastroduodenal junction, irregular undulating slips of antral type mucosa extend about 1 to 2 mm into the anatomic duodenum, which then abuts a 2- to 3-mm segment of transitional type epithelium (71). Distal to this, only the usual small intestinal type mucosa is found (71). The transitional type epithelium occurring in more distal aspects of the duodenum and in the rest of the small intestine is termed gastric metaplasia (31).

Although the duodenal mucosa may demonstrate long villi with a villous-to-crypt length ratio on the order of 3:1 to 5:1, more commonly, particularly in the first portion (the duodenal cap or bulb), the villi are shorter and broader with occasional branching extensions (72) (Fig. 22). They often have a leaflike shape with few fingerlike forms when viewed under a scanning electron or dissecting microscope (20,72,73) (Fig. 23). Also, the number of mononuclear cells within the lamina propria is increased in the duodenum when compared with the rest of the small intestine (72,73). This varied constellation of findings is considered normal and is probably a consequence of the effect of acidic gastric contents on this most proximal intestinal site (40,73).

The submucosa of the gastrointestinal tract lacks glands except at two sites: the esophagus and the duodenum. The submucosal glands of Brunner are the type localized to the duodenum. Indeed, these glands are typically used by the pathologist to identify histologically a segment of small intestine as duodenum. These glands, which begin just distal to the gastroduodenal junction, are most concentrated in this region and gradually decrease in quantity along the duodenum (74). Beyond the entrance of the ampulla of Vater, only scattered groups can be found. In rare instances, Brunner's glands extend beyond the duodenojejunal flexure for a short distance (75–77).

Brunner's glands are lobular collections of tubuloalveolar glands predominantly located within the submucosa; however, they often extend through the muscularis mucosae into the deep portions of mucosa beneath the crypts of Lieberkühn (Figs. 22 and 24). On average, about one third of the gland population resides within the mucosa (75). Brunner's glands are lined by cuboidal-to-columnar cells with pale, uniform cytoplasm and an oval, basally situated nucleus. Their cytoplasm contains neutral mucins that are PAS positive and diastase resistant (Fig. 20). Occasionally, mucous cells with apically concentrated mucin and perinuclear vacuolization or clearing are seen. Although opinions vary, these changes are thought to represent the secretory phase of the gland (i.e., recently fed state) (78,79). The glands empty by way of ducts lined by a similar epithelium, which are often seen passing through slips of muscularis mucosae (Fig. 24). These ducts drain into the crypts at varying levels (77). Brunner's glands and their ducts can be distinguished from surrounding crypts by the absence of goblet cells and by their diffuse cytoplasmic PAS positivity (77).

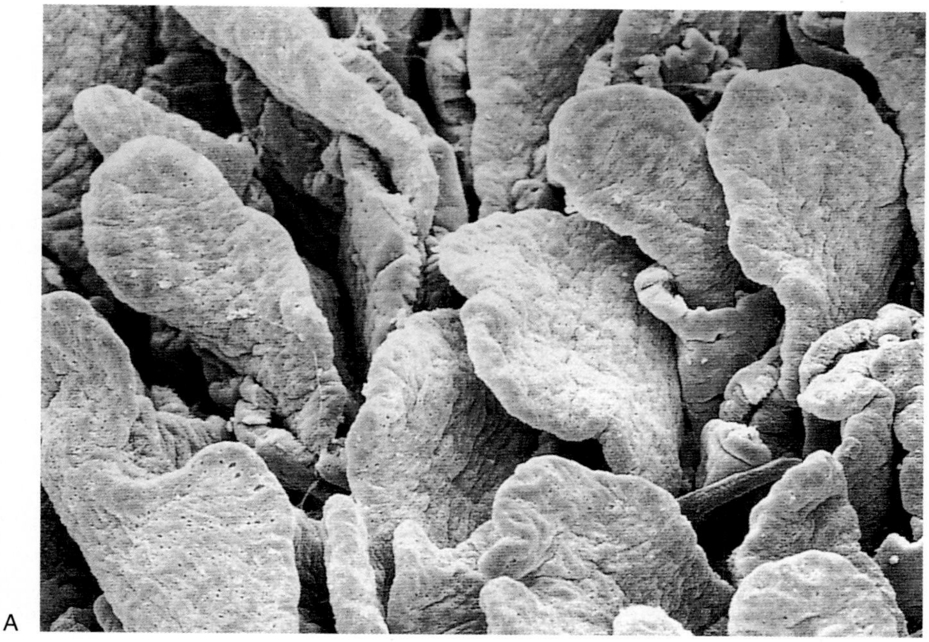

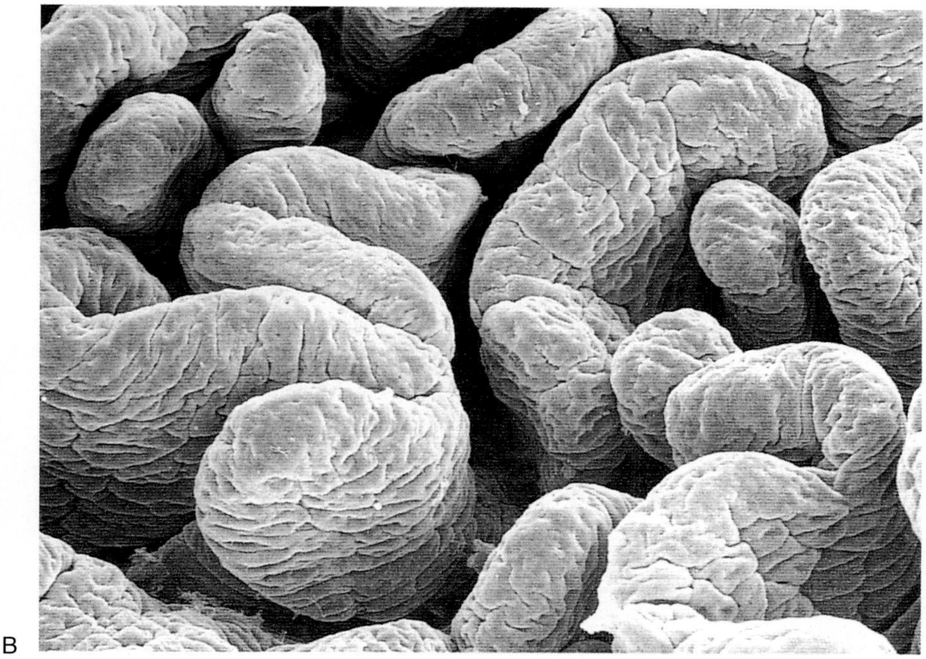

**FIG. 23.** Two views of duodenal mucosa using scanning electron microscopy: leaflike (**A**) and ridged-shaped (**B**) villi predominate in these normal duodenal specimens.

Although most of the lining epithelial cells of the Brunner's glands are of the mucous type, scattered endocrine cells are present as well. Many can be detected on routine hematoxylin and eosin–stained sections because of their basal eosinophilic granulated cytoplasm (80). By using immunohistologic methods, some have been shown to contain somatostatin, gastrin, and peptide YY (81). However, the ducts that drain Brunner's glands are devoid of endocrine cells (81).

Peptidergic neural fibers, predominantly those with immunoreactivity for vasoactive intestinal peptide and substance P, course within and between individual Brunner's glands. These neuroendocrine substances are probably important in local regulation of acinar secretion, although this function has been verified only for vasoactive intestinal peptide (81). The function of Brunner's glands has not been fully elucidated, but their mucus is felt to be of prime importance for protection of the duodenal mucosa from the potentially damaging effects of the delivered acidic gastric contents (76).

Hyperplasia of Brunner's glands exists in three forms: (a) diffuse glandular proliferation, imparting a coarse nodularity

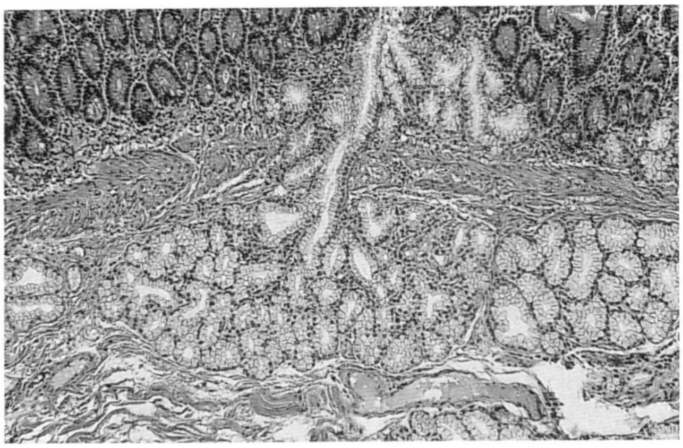

**FIG. 24.** Submucosal Brunner's gland lobule with draining duct extending through muscularis mucosae. Note the stark contrast between the crypt epithelium and that of the Brunner's glands and their ducts.

to most of the duodenum; (b) isolated discrete nodules in the proximal duodenum; and (c) a solitary nodule, often designated as an "adenoma" of Brunner's glands (75,82,83). All three types are typically composed of an increased quantity of normal-appearing Brunner's glands, accompanied by variable proportions of smooth muscle (Fig. 25). The distinction between adenoma and hyperplasia is arbitrary, and no substantial evidence exists to suggest that any of these proliferations are truly neoplastic (82). Moreover, carcinoma arising from a population of Brunner's glands has yet to be convincingly documented (31). Nodules or polypoid structures composed of collections of these submucosal glands in the duodenum are probably best termed Brunner's gland nodules (31).

Pseudomelanosis duodeni, or brown–black pigment, located primarily within lamina proprial macrophages, rarely may be observed in the proximal duodenum (84) (Fig. 26). Iron and sulfur are the prime constituents of these apparently acquired deposits; however, their accumulation is of uncertain etiology and significance (84).

### Jejunum

The jejunum is the least distinctive segment of the small bowel, and as such its histologic features are most similar to those described for the small bowel in general. However, a characteristic feature is the prominent development of the plicae circulares, or permanent circular folds, also termed valves of Kerckring and valvulae conniventes (Fig. 1). These folds are tallest and most numerous (i.e., closely spaced) in this portion of the small bowel (20). Histologically, the jejunal villi are tall with a villous-to-crypt ratio on the order of 3:1 to 5:1. The vast majority of jejunal villi are slender and fingerlike (Figs. 2 and 3), in contrast to the slightly shorter villi of the ileum and to the leaflike, occasionally branched and blunted villi of the proximal duodenum (20,40). These morphologic transitions are gradual, particularly in the mobile small intestine, where the separation between jejunum and ileum is arbitrarily defined.

### Ileum

The ileum has a number of distinctive features, including its unique junction with the large intestine. The ileum protrudes approximately 2 to 3 cm into the large intestine at the junction of the cecum and ascending colon. This nipplelike extension of the terminal ileum is encircled by large bowel mucosa and has been likened to the relationship of the uterine cervix with the vagina (85). A muscular sphincter at this site, along with external ligamentous support, is responsible for modifying its function in order to prevent reflux and to allow forward passage of ileal contents (85,86). Histologically, the mucosal transition demonstrates a gradual loss of villi occurring at variable lengths along the short intracecal

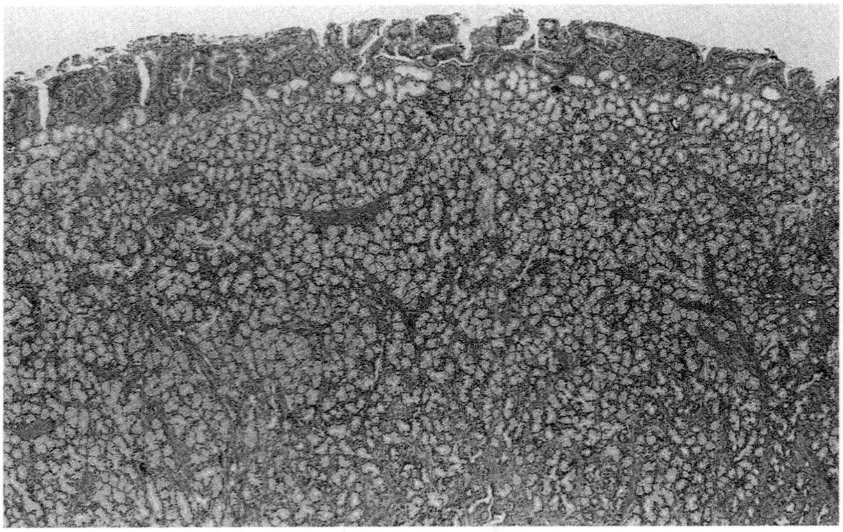

**FIG. 25.** A relatively minute field of a Brunner's gland nodule (nearly 10 cm in greatest dimension) disclosing abundant normal-appearing submucosal glands of Brunner intermixed with smooth muscle, underlying an unremarkable duodenal mucosal villous surface.

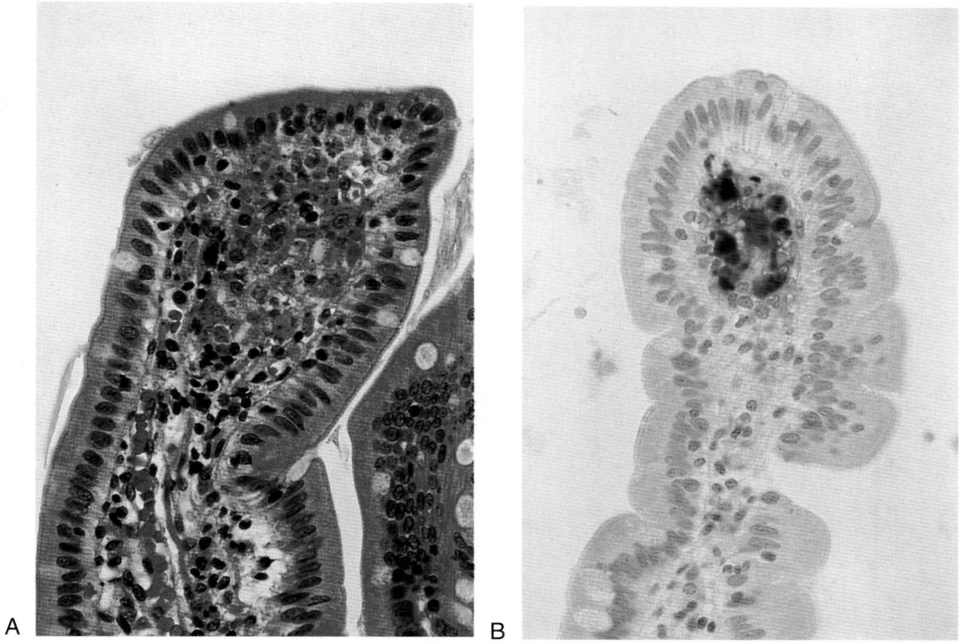

**FIG. 26.** **A:** Macrophages containing granular brown pigment within the lamina propria of the duodenum characteristic of pseudomelanosis duodeni. **B:** Prussian blue stain disclosing the prominent iron content of the pigment.

ileal segment; the ileal mucosa blends rather imperceptively with the mucosa of the large bowel (Fig. 27). The ileocecal region normally can contain abundant fat within its submucosa, diffusely distributed and proportional to adipose content in the rest of the abdominal cavity (87) (Fig. 27). In fact, on rare occasion, a distinct mass of fat is evident. This benign entity, so-called lipohyperplasia of the ileocecal region, reportedly can cause variable symptoms, including abdominal pain and lower gastrointestinal bleeding (87).

The distinctive mucosal characteristics of the ileum when compared with both jejunum and duodenum include shorter and fewer plicae circulares and an increased proportion of goblet cells within the epithelium (Fig. 28). The villi are typically shorter than at more proximal sites and have a predominantly fingerlike shape (20). These features become gradually more apparent along the length of the small intestine and are most evident in the distal ileum. With distal progression, lymphoid nodules that can be found anywhere in the small intestine gradually increase in quantity (20). In addition, specialized clusters of lymphoid aggregates, or Peyer's patches, are most prominent in the ileum.

Peyer's patches are located along the antimesenteric bor-

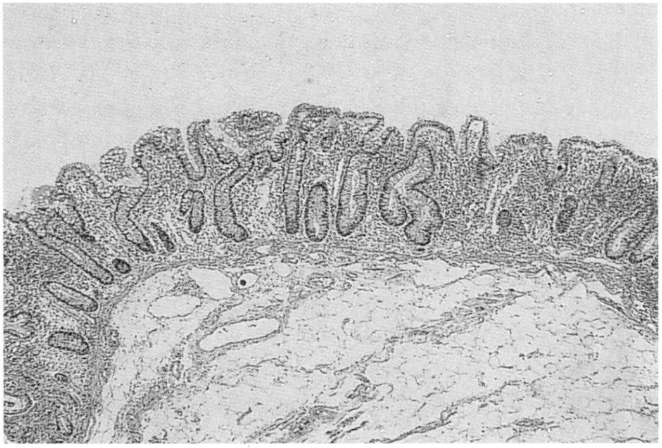

**FIG. 27.** Transition from villous mucosal surface of ileum (*left*) to flat mucosa of large intestine (*right*) at the ileocecal junction. Note the prominent submucosal adipose tissue characteristic of this region.

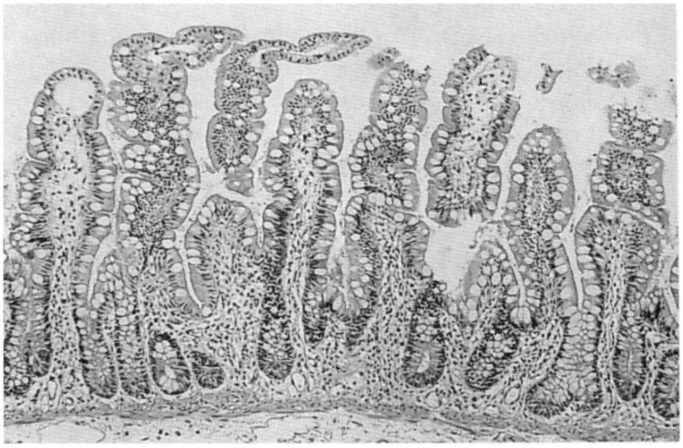

**FIG. 28.** Characteristic ileal mucosa with slender relatively short villi (compare with jejunal villi in Fig. 3) lined by abundant goblet cells with a lesser number of absorptive columnar cells.

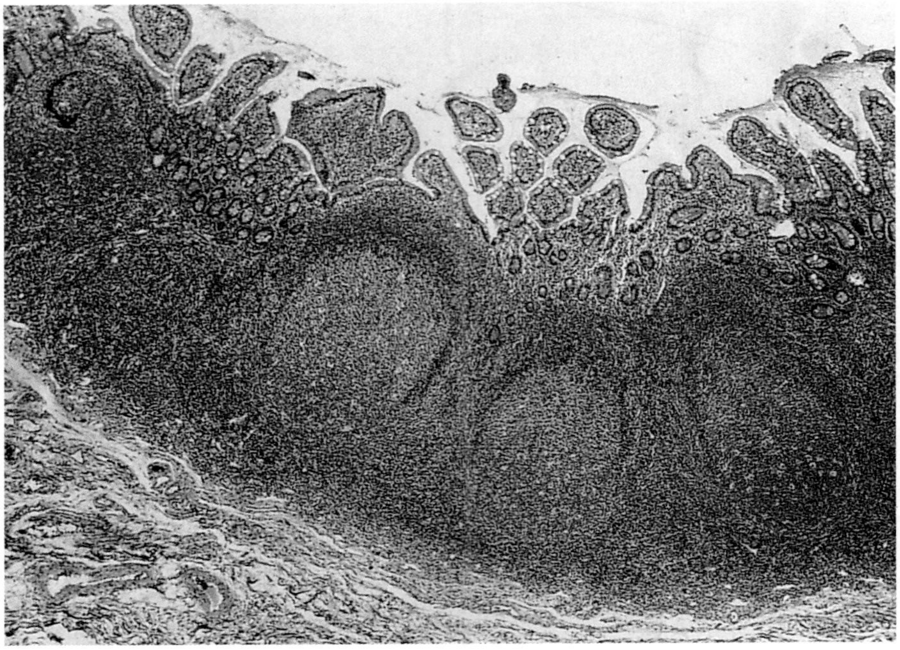

**FIG. 29.** Confluent lamina proprial lymphoid aggregates of a Peyer's patch. This organized lymphoid tissue typically extends into the underlying submucosa. The four components of the Peyer's patch are seen and include lymphoid nodules with germinal centers, an overlying flattened follicle-associated epithelium, and an intervening pale-staining dome region. The abundant lymphoid population between the follicles is the T-cell–rich interfollicular zone.

der of the small bowel. They consist of varying numbers of lymphoid follicles, ranging from five to over 900, and have been shown to be present during fetal life (88). Until puberty they increase in size and number and subsequently regress steadily thereafter; nonetheless, Peyer's patches are invariably present even into extreme old age (88). In children, these patches can be grossly visualized near the ileocecal junction (89); although on the whole, they cannot be seen with the naked eye (90). Moreover, hyperplastic Peyer's patches (or focal lymphoid hyperplasia) may be found in the terminal ileum during childhood and have been linked to more than one third of the cases of idiopathic intussusception occurring in the ileocecal region in this age group (91–93).

Peyer's patches are basically specialized groups of lymphoid follicles that occupy the mucosa and a variable portion of the submucosa. Structurally, four distinct compartments exist: follicle, dome, follicle-associated epithelium, and interfollicular regions (30,94) (Fig. 29). Most lymphoid follicles within a Peyer's patch contain a germinal center that is populated by numerous surface IgA-positive B cells, with occasional CD4-positive T cells and macrophages (30,90) (Figs. 29 and 30). However, the surrounding mantle zone contains a population of small B-lymphocytes (predominantly surface IgD and IgM positive). The dome is the area between the follicle and the overlying surface epithelium; this region contains a heterogeneous population of cells, including B-lymphocytes of all immunoglobulin isotypes (except IgD), macrophages, and plasma cells (90). The specialized or follicle-associated epithelium overlying lymphoid aggregates is distinct from surrounding villous epithelial surfaces. It characteristically has fewer goblet cells and contains membranous cells, or M cells, interspersed among the usual columnar absorptive cells (30,95) (Fig. 30). The M cell is a specialized columnar epithelial cell that transports luminal antigens to adjacent extracellular spaces, thus allowing access to immunocompetent cells. These cells play a key role in mucosally based immunity, antigen tolerance, and probably in certain immunopathologic disease states (95). Morphologically, M cells have an attenuated brush border with diminished alkaline phosphatase staining intensity (94,96), a thin strip of apical cytoplasm, and a basally situated round nucleus. The dependent portion of the M cell's cytoplasm is often deformed by several lymphocytes (95). However, definitive M-cell characterization rests upon the identification of specific ultrastructural features (94,95). The follicle-associated epithelium also has a distinctive migratory cell composition because the intraepithelial lymphocyte population is more abundant and has a greater proportion of CD4-positive (T-helper/inducer) cells than does the usual villous epithelium (approximately 40% versus 6%) (94). Last, the fourth component of the Peyer's patch is called the interfollicular region. As in the lymph node, it is predominantly a T-cell zone with CD4-positive T-lymphocytes outnumbering CD8-positive lymphocytes by a seven-to-one margin (90).

Plasma cells are a scant component of Peyer's patches, in contrast to the surrounding lamina propria, but they may frequently be found in the dome compartment. Peyer's patches are believed to be important in the generation of the mucosal immune response, in part by supplying the lamina propria with immunocompetent surface IgA-positive B cells that become functional secretory plasma cells (30,89,90,95).

Irregularly distributed, granular brown–black pigment can commonly be found in the deep portions of Peyer's patches in adults (97) (Fig. 31). Although its origin is controversial, atmospheric or dietary sources are most probable (97,98).

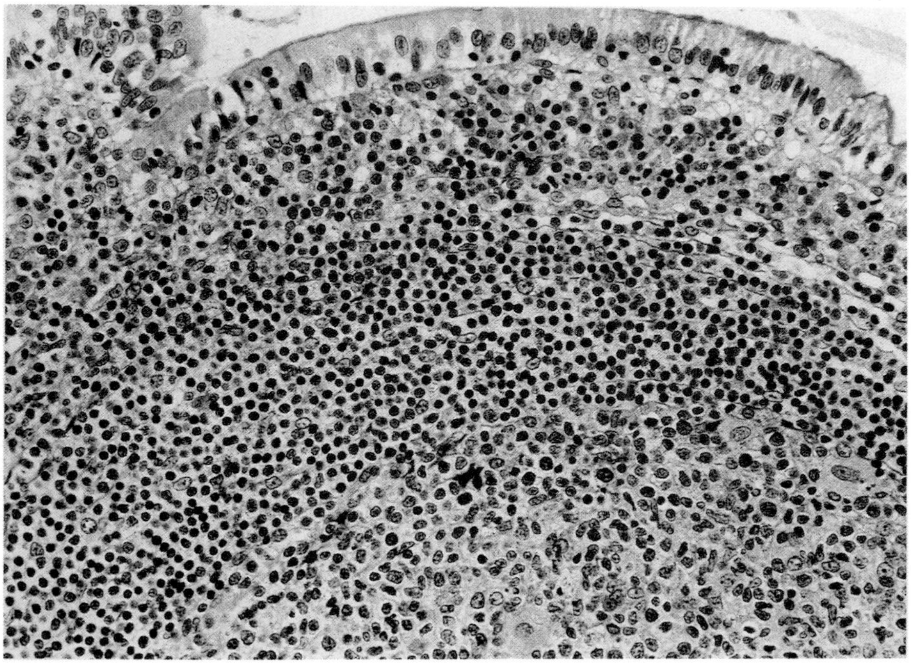

**FIG. 30.** High magnification of surface epithelium above a lymphoid nodule within a Peyer's patch. The polymorphous germinal center (*below*) is surrounded by monotonous, small round lymphocytes that comprise the nodule's mantle zone. Above this lies the dome region with lymphocytes, plasma cells, and macrophages. The follicle-associated epithelium characteristically has few, if any, goblet cells; ultrastructurally, most of these cells would be identified as M cells.

Accumulating principally within macrophages, this pigment has been shown by x-ray spectroscopy to contain a distinct mineral composition that includes silicates, aluminum, and titanium (97,98). The pigment is inert and has no known clinicopathologic significance.

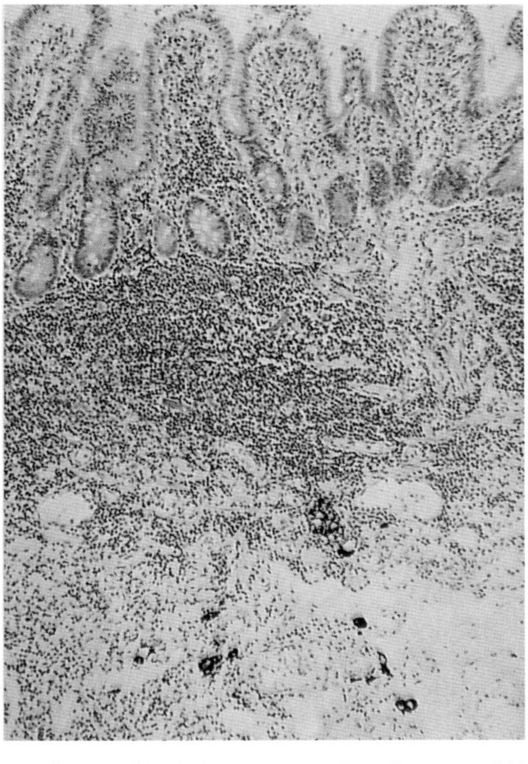

**FIG. 31.** Dense black–brown granular pigment within the depths of a Peyer's patch of ileum. The pigment is typically confined to macrophages.

A final distinctive feature often seen in the ileum is Meckel's diverticulum; it is the most common intestinal congenital anomaly and is found in 1% to 2% of the general population (31). Meckel's diverticulum is an antimesenteric outpouching of the terminal ileum usually located approximately 20 cm from the ileocecal junction. It represents the persistence of the omphalomesenteric duct. Although Meckel's diverticulum is usually an incidental finding, it can cause lower gastrointestinal bleeding or small bowel obstruction (99,100). Histologically, small intestinal mucosa alone lines the diverticulum in about 50% to 70% of cases. Ectopic gastric or pancreatic tissues are found in the remainder, typically encountered at the distalmost aspect (100).

## SPECIAL CONSIDERATIONS

### Geographic, Age-Related, and Dietary Factors

Because geographic and local environmental factors can affect small bowel morphology, historical data about the residence or recent travel of an individual are essential to evaluate histologic material accurately. Specimens from individuals residing in, or visiting at length, certain underdeveloped" tropical locations such as Africa, southern India, and Thailand show a distinctly different villous appearance from those of individuals who live in temperate climate zones (44,101–104). The morphologic alterations seen in individuals from "underdeveloped" tropical areas include leaflike villi predominating over fingerlike forms in jejunal segments examined via biopsy and an increased number of lamina proprial mononuclear cells (105). This difference in the villous population is reflected histologically as stubby villi with a pyramidal shape (i.e., a broader base than apex) and occasional branched and fused villous tips (44,101,102). Interesting, although the villi are shorter, the villous-to-crypt length ratio usually remains constant in both geographic settings (44,102). Such alterations should probably be considered a normal variant because these individuals are typically asymptomatic and otherwise healthy (101). The cause of these morphologic changes is uncertain, but environmental factors, particularly regional enteric flora, presumably play a role (101). Similar mucosal changes, as mentioned previously, are seen in normal individuals in temperate environments, but only in proximal portions of the duodenum. Therefore, these particular mucosal alterations must be analyzed in the context of both the patient's residence and the site within the small intestine in order to prevent misinterpretation as a pathologic change, such as tropical sprue.

Aging also modifies small bowel mucosal architecture. Although the literature on humans is limited, it has been shown that specimens from elderly individuals generally have shorter and broader villi than those from younger individuals (106). Moreover, lower animal and human fetuses have been documented as having fingerlike villi exclusively, suggesting that exposure to the environment or aging itself modifies villous architecture (106,107). However, the functional significance of these changes is uncertain (106).

Diet alters villous architecture in laboratory animals. A diet high in fiber results in broad and fused villi, whereas a fiber-free diet seems to prevent the formation of leaflike forms (17). If this finding is valid in humans, it may be one factor related to the presence of stubby, leaflike villi seen in patients in underdeveloped countries where high-fiber diets are common.

### Metaplastic and Heterotopic Tissues

Gastric type mucosa is not an unusual finding in the small intestine. A distinction can be made between metaplasia, an acquired alteration, and heterotopia, thought to be congenital in origin. Gastric metaplasia characteristically consists solely of antral type, PAS-positive, foveolar columnar cells lying along the surface epithelium (Fig. 21). This change is focal and often in direct continuity with usual columnar absorptive epithelium on the same villus (73). Gastric metaplasia may be encountered in more than 60% of healthy asymptomatic individuals in the duodenal bulb, where it can be regarded as within normal limits (73). More distally, however, it is less commonly seen in the asymptomatic person but rather is frequently associated with duodenitis or mucosal ulceration (73,108). Scattered chief and parietal cells without any organized arrangement are also associated with this type of metaplasia or with reparative processes (108).

In contrast, gastric heterotopia is usually a grossly evident mucosal polyp that contains all cellular elements encountered in the normal gastric fundic mucosa. Characteristically, mucous foveolar epithelium overlies an organized arrangement of glands lined by chief and parietal cells; this is typically well demarcated from the surrounding usual intestinal villous epithelium. Gastric heterotopia is also fairly common, being reported in up to 2% of the population (109); it may be found anywhere along the gastrointestinal tract (108). Gastric heterotopia is a well-defined entity in the proximal duodenum and usually presents as a mucosal nodule on the anterior wall. Although they are usually of no clinical significance, larger ones may cause obstructive symptoms (109). In contrast, gastric heterotopia distal to the ligament of Treitz is usually symptomatic and often causes intussusception (110). This relationship to clinical symptoms may derive from patient selection bias because asymptomatic gastric heterotopias at a distal site would not be routinely detectable.

Heterotopic pancreas tissue also can be found anywhere along the small intestine but most commonly is found in the duodenum and jejunum (111,112). It can form submucosal, intramural, or serosal nodules and is composed of various admixtures of pancreatic acini, ducts, and islets of Langerhans' (111,113) (Fig. 32). Isolated ductal structures admixed with smooth muscle may be the predominant or exclusive component, and in these instances the alternative term adenomyoma has been used (31,112). Nodules of pancreatic tissue within the small intestine are usually asymptomatic, al-

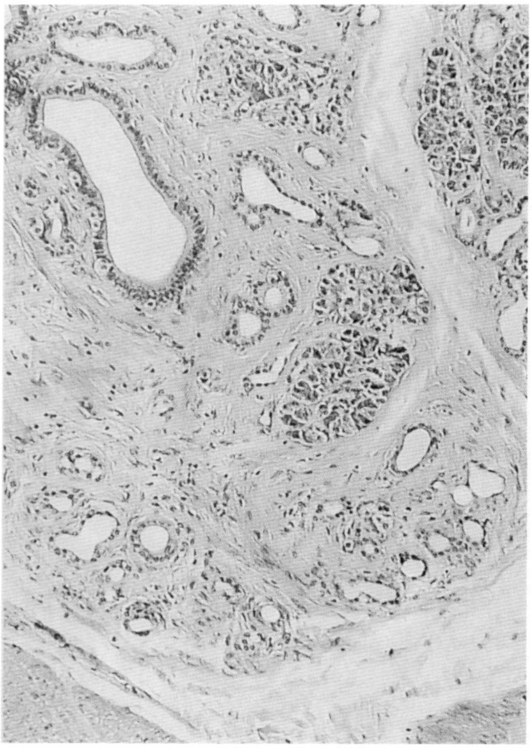

**FIG. 32.** Heterotopic pancreas in the duodenum characterized in this instance by variably sized ducts, acini, and abundant smooth muscle.

though larger lesions (greater than 1.5 cm) with prominent mucosal involvement may become clinically significant (112,113). A single case of a combined submucosal pancreatic heterotopia with overlying gastric type mucosa in the duodenal bulb recently was reported (114).

### Lymphoid Proliferations

Lymphoid tissue is a prominent feature of the small bowel. The gut-associated lymphoid system in this region, as in the entire gastrointestinal tract, is compartmentalized into lymphocytes of the epithelium, lamina propria, isolated lymphoid aggregates, and Peyer's patches (115). The normal appearance and immunologic composition of these distinct lymphoid populations have been detailed earlier in the chapter. All these compartments participate at some level in mucosal immune response, but they also provide the milieu for various hyperplastic and neoplastic immunoproliferations, as well as for certain immunodeficiency states. Some of these disorders have histologic features that deviate only slightly from a normal appearance and from one another. Additionally, some are believed to be preneoplastic.

Lymphoid hyperplasias are divided into two broad categories: focal and diffuse forms (116). Focal lymphoid hyperplasia is a localized, well-circumscribed proliferation of benign lymphoid tissue characterized by a polymorphic infiltrate of lymphocytes within which numerous benign follicles with reactive germinal centers are dispersed. These proliferations often involve only the mucosa and submucosa, but they may extend through the entire wall (116). Focal lymphoid hyperplasia is predominantly found in the terminal ileum of children or adolescents who present either with ileocecal intussusception or with a clinical syndrome mimicking appendicitis (91,93,116).

Diffuse or nodular lymphoid hyperplasia is a distinct entity in which multiple nodules composed of aggregates of benign lymphoid follicles disfigure the mucosa and submucosa along extensive lengths of the small intestine, with or without colonic involvement (116–118). It is usually asymptomatic and incidentally encountered (116). However, a distinct clinicopathologic variant exists that is characterized clinically by associated, combined variable immunodeficiency and giardiasis-related diarrhea, and histologically by a greatly diminished or absent plasma cell population in the nearby lamina propria (116). Nodular lymphoid hyperplasia with or without combined variable immunodeficiency has been associated with an increased risk for the development of various malignancies (e.g., malignant lymphoma, carcinoma) (116–119).

Differentiation of these benign lymphoid lesions from malignant lymphoma can be problematic. However, recognizing the diagnostic morphologic features of malignant lymphoma, such as the usual cytologic monotony of the lymphoid population, the lack of a reactive follicular architecture, and the presence of mucosal ulceration, should resolve most dilemmas (116,120–122). Additionally, because the majority of small bowel malignant lymphomas are of B-cell lineage (122), demonstration of light-chain restriction by immunohistologic techniques or flow cytometric analysis or detection of heavy- or light-chain immunoglobulin gene rearrangements (e.g., monoclonality) by molecular diagnostic methods can aid in certain cases (123–125); T-cell receptor gene rearrangement analysis may be necessary in a minority of cases.

### Morphologic Changes Associated with Ileal Diversion and Continence-Restoring Procedures

With the increasing number of diversion and continence-restoring procedures being performed after total colectomy, it has become common to see biopsy and revision specimens after such operations. As a consequence, familiarity with the altered yet "normal" morphology within these ileal creations must be appreciated in order to evaluate them optimally. The expected mucosal changes include villous shortening and crypt lengthening (approximate 1:1 to 2:1 ratio), increased numbers of goblet cells and lymphoid follicles, and a denser mononuclear cell infiltrate within the lamina propria (31,126,127). These alterations are similar after either colectomy with conventional ileostomy or after ileoanal anastomosis with ileal reservoir formation (e.g., pouch) (127–129). However, ileostomy stomas in particular show additional changes of mucosal prolapse exemplified by fibromuscular obliteration of the lamina propria and superficial erosions and microhemorrhages (31). Additionally, goblet cell mucin alterations have been seen in nearly 50% of pouches examined with conversion to predominantly sulfomucins (i.e., colonic epithelial mucin) (129). However, another group of investigators saw no change in goblet cell mucin from the typical small bowel acid sialomucins in ileal segments after either ileoanal anastomosis with pouch formation or conventional ileostomy (127). Nonetheless, all these changes should be interpreted as "normal" because more definitive and specific criteria need to be met to establish persistent, recurrent, or novel disease in these specimens.

## MUCOSAL BIOPSY SPECIMEN EVALUATION IN SUSPECTED MALABSORPTION

### Specimen Procurement and Processing

The usefulness of small bowel mucosal biopsy is unquestioned (130), particularly in the evaluation of malabsorptive states. In the past, up to four biopsy samples were usually obtained from the area of the ligament of Treitz via a suction biopsy device attached to a long tube (131). In recent years, the standard upper endoscope has been used, and comparable specimens have been procured (74,132). Because this technique is performed under direct visualization, many more biopsy specimens can be obtained. Regardless of the biopsy technique used, the most critical part of the procedure is proper orientation of the specimen. Ideally, specimens are immediately mounted mucosa side up on a solid substance such as filter paper or plastic mesh and then placed into Hollande's or other fixative. After processing, the histotechnologist embeds the tissue perpendicular to the mounting material. Alternatively, biopsy specimens may be placed unmounted into fixative immediately. The tissue can then be properly oriented after processing at the time of embedding. Because the specimen will naturally curl, some tangential sectioning can be expected. Proper specimen evaluation requires examination of optimally oriented intestinal villi obtained from the central region of the biopsy specimen. Although serial sectioning is advocated by some investigators (105), step sectioning (usually seven levels) is a reasonable alternative.

Our standard small bowel biopsy procedure consists of obtaining four to six endoscopic biopsy specimens. One is used to make a touch preparation that is then fixed in alcohol and stained via the Giemsa technique. The other tissue samples are placed in Hollande's fixative and routinely processed. Seven step-section slides are obtained: five are stained with hematoxylin and eosin, one with PAS, and one with trichrome stain. The PAS stain is a useful screen for Whipple's disease and *Mycobacterium avium-intracellulare* complex infection, whereas the trichrome stain confirms collagen deposition seen in ischemia or collagenous sprue. In addition, the iron hematoxylin counterstain used in the trichrome technique makes it easier to identify.

## Specimen Interpretation and Common Artifacts

With appropriate specimen procurement, the mucosa with muscularis mucosae and a small portion of upper submucosa should be available for histologic examination. These specimens should be evaluated in a systematic fashion, including assessment of (a) villous architecture, (b) surface and crypt epithelia, (c) lamina propria constituents, and (d) submucosal structures (52). A well-oriented specimen is essential for optimal evaluation. However, it must be remembered that villi vary in length and shape, particularly in the proximal duodenum, and that villous apices bend and twist in various planes to create unusual forms; these variations should not be misinterpreted as a villous abnormality (40,52). Generally, if four normal villi in a row are observed, the villous architecture of the entire specimen is probably normal (52,105). This does not mean that specimens with fewer than four well-aligned normal villi should be considered inadequate because even one normal intestinal villus in a proximal small bowel biopsy specimen rules out celiac sprue (31). Conversely, identification of four normal villi in a row does not necessarily exclude focal lesions, although it almost always does (105). The pathologist must be wary of certain common artifacts that may lead to erroneous interpretations. Careful attention to certain features (described later) within the various mucosal compartments will aid in their recognition.

### *Tangential Sectioning*

Inappropriate orientation of the specimen, occurring at any point during processing, will lead to various tangential cuts or sections. The mucosa must be sectioned perpendicular to its long axis, or a distorted pattern disclosing apparently short and broad villi and an expanded lamina proprial compartment will be observed. However, several features aid in recognizing an oblique cut: (a) numerous elliptically shaped glands, (b) a multilayered arrangement of the crypts (Fig. 33), or (c) a multilayered surface epithelium (52) (Fig. 34). If any of these features are present, the villous architecture must be interpreted with caution.

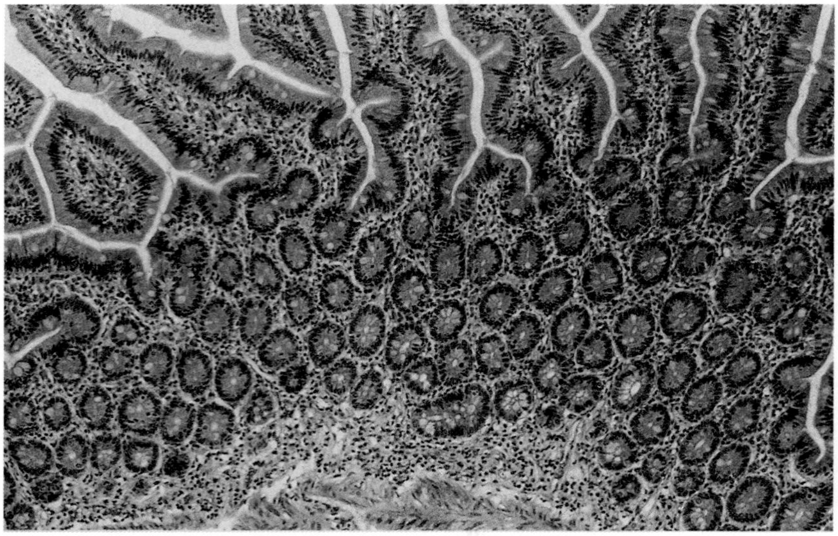

**FIG. 33.** Multilayering of crypts indicates a tangential or oblique section of small intestine. The villous architecture overlying the crypts is normal, albeit unusual in appearance; this is also a product of malorientation of the biopsy specimen.

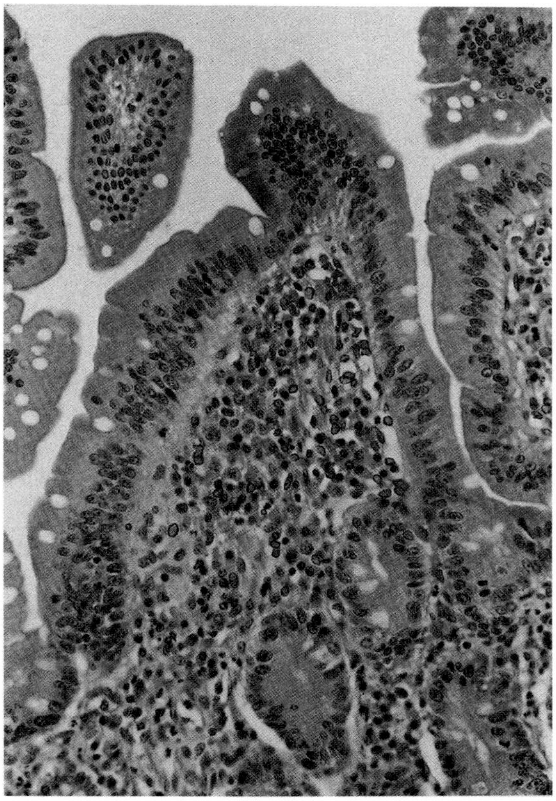

**FIG. 34.** Another clue in identifying a tangential cut is multilayering, or "stratification," of the surface epithelium (left portion of central villus). The normal surface layer is one cell thick. This broad and short villous appearance is a consequence of malorientation and should be interpreted accordingly.

### *Brunner's Gland–Related Artifact*

Brunner's glands have an inconsistent effect on villous architecture (31). Occasionally, normal length villi can be encountered overlying the Brunner's glands (Fig. 35), but more commonly the villi appear distorted, short, broad, and stubby (31,40) (Fig. 22). To minimize the potential effects of this artifact on interpretation, biopsy specimens of the small bowel for evaluation of malabsorptive states are routinely obtained as distally as possible in the duodenum or from the proximal jejunum (i.e., near the ligament of Treitz) (74,132). Occasionally, however, more proximal small bowel biopsies are necessary for evaluation of duodenitis or ulcer disease. In these instances, such villous characteristics must not be misinterpreted.

### *Lymphoid Aggregate–Related Artifact*

Mucosal lymphoid aggregates, or nodules, are scattered along the small bowel and often distort the villous architecture. Villi are usually absent over lymphoid aggregates, and nearby villous forms may be distorted, short, and stubby (52)

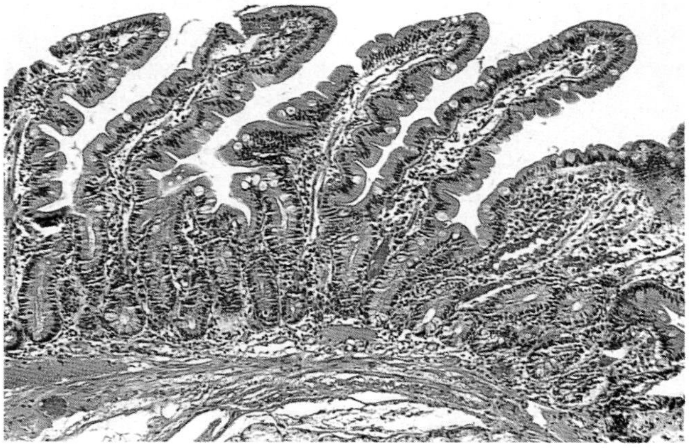

**FIG. 35.** Occasionally, long slender villi, similar to those seen in the jejunum, are found overlying Brunner's glands. However, villi associated with Brunner's glands are more commonly shorter and broader (see Fig. 22).

(Fig. 29). Therefore, when a lymphoid aggregate is seen below an isolated flat portion of the surface epithelium, it should not be misinterpreted as a severe villous abnormality.

### *Absence of Muscularis Mucosae*

As mentioned earlier, the muscularis mucosae is an important structural component of the mucosa. In its absence, for instance, in a very superficial mucosal biopsy specimen, the tissues tend to spread laterally, resulting in villi becoming more widely spaced and appearing short and broad (52,133) (Fig. 36).

### *Biopsy-Trauma–Related Artifacts*

As a direct result of the traumatic pinch or suction biopsy procedures, certain alterations of normal mucosa can be

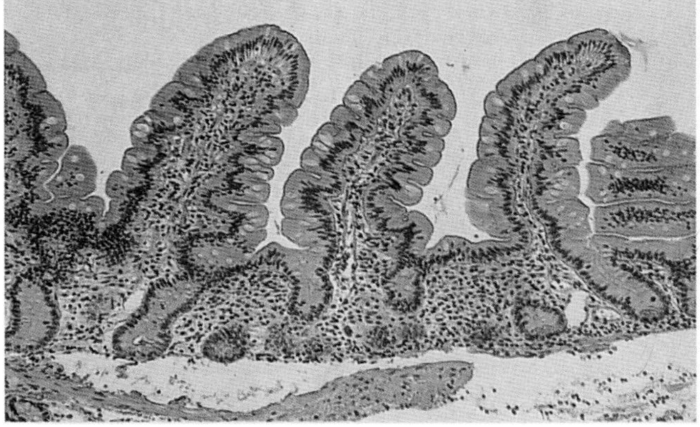

**FIG. 36.** Absence of muscularis mucosae in a small bowel biopsy specimen, resulting in shorter- and broader-appearing villi that are widely spaced.

seen. Separation of the villous surface epithelium from the underlying lamina propria or focally denuded epithelium are not unusual (52,133). The lack of acute erosive changes (e.g., neutrophilic infiltrate, cellular necrosis) or chronic evidence of ulceration (e.g., granulation tissue, regenerative epithelium) allow this alteration to be recognized as biopsy related. Additionally, focal hemorrhage and scattered polymorphonuclear leukocytes may be observed in the lamina propria as a consequence of the biopsy procedure. Crush or compression artifact can occur at the site of closure of the endoscopic forceps, resulting in a condensation of the lymphoplasmacytic component that can be misinterpreted as increased chronic inflammation (134). Additionally, the connective tissue may be altered in such a way that it appears more tightly packed, mimicking fibrosis or excessive collagen deposition (134).

### *Fixative-Related Artifacts*

Certain fixatives other than formalin (4% formaldehyde solution) can cause interpretive problems. Although Hollande's fixative better preserves cytologic and nuclear detail, several artifacts may interfere with evaluation. The brightly eosinophilic granules of Paneth's cells and sometimes eosinophilic leukocytes seen readily in formalin-fixed tissue are not as well preserved by Hollande's fixative. Additionally, suboptimal clearing of Hollande's fixative from the specimens before paraffin embedding can result in residual minute, round, basophilic structures that resemble yeast forms or parasites (e.g., cryptosporidium, *Giardia lamblia*) (134)

## ACKNOWLEDGMENTS

We thank James T. McMahon, Ph.D., for the scanning electron micrographs.

## REFERENCES

1. Williams PL, Warwick R, Dyson M, Bannister LH, eds. *Gray's anatomy. 37th ed.* New York: Churchill Livingstone; 1989.
2. Thorek P. *Anatomy in surgery. 3rd ed.* New York: Springer-Verlag; 1985.
3. Costacurta L. Anatomical and functional aspects of the human suspensory muscle of the duodenum. *Acta Anat* 1972;82:34–46.
4. Trier JS, Winter HS. Anatomy, embryology, and developmental abnormalities of the small intestine and colon. In: Sleisenger MH, Fordtran JS, eds. *Gastrointestinal disease. 4th ed.* Philadelphia: WB Saunders; 1989;991–1021.
5. Parks DA, Jacobson ED. Physiology of the splanchnic circulation. *Arch Intern Med* 1985;145:1270–1281.
6. Alpers DH. Digestion and absorption of carbohydrates and proteins. In: Johnson LR, ed. *Physiology of the gastrointestinal tract. 2nd ed.* New York: Raven Press; 1987;1469–1487.
7. Davenport HW. *Physiology of the digestive tract. 5th ed.* Chicago: Year Book Medical 1982.
8. Quigley EMM. Small intestinal motor activity-its role in gut homeostasis and disease. *Q J Med* 1987;246:799–810.
9. Fiorenza V, Yee YS, Zfass AM. Small intestinal motility: normal and abnormal function. *Am J Gastroenterol* 1987;82:1111–1114.
10. Lewin KJ. The endocrine cells of the gastrointestinal tract: the normal endocrine cells and their hyperplasias. In: Sommers SC, Rosen PP, Fechner RE, eds. Part 1. *Pathology annual.* Norwalk, CT: Appleton-Century-Crofts; 1986;1–27.
11. Solcia E, Capella C, Buffa R, Usellini L, Fiocca R, Sessa F. Endocrine cells of the digestive system. In: Johnson LR, ed. *Physiology of the gastrointestinal tract. 2nd ed.* New York: Raven Press; 1987:111–130.
12. Elson CO, Kagnoff MF, Fiocchi C, Befus AD, Targan S. Intestinal immunity and inflammation: recent progress. *Gastroenterology* 1986; 91:746–768.
13. Rubin W. The epithelial "membrane" of the small intestine. *Am J Clin Nutr* 1971;24:45–64.
14. Wilson JP. Surface area of the small intestine in man. *Gut* 1967; 8:618–621.
15. Holmes R, Hourihane DO, Booth CC. The mucosa of the small intestine. *Postgrad Med J* 1961;37:717–724.
16. Toner PG, Carr KE. The use of scanning electron microscopy in the study of the intestinal villi. *J Pathol* 1969;97:611–617.
17. Madara JL, Trier JS. Functional morphology of the mucosa of the small intestine. In: Johnson LR, ed. *Physiology of the gastrointestinal tract. 2nd ed.* New York: Raven Press; 1987:1209–1249.
18. Dobbins WO. The intestinal mucosal lymphatic in man. A light and electron microscopic study. *Gastroenterology* 1966;51:994–1003.
19. Golab B, Szkudlarek R. Lymphatic vessels of the duodenum—deep network. *Folia Morphol (Warsz)* 1980;39:263–270.
20. Neutra MR, Padykula HK. The gastrointestinal tract. In: Weiss L, ed. *Modern concepts of gastrointestinal histology.* New York: Elsevier; 1984:658–706.
21. Poley JR. Loss of the glycocalyx of enterocytes in small intestine: a feature detected by scanning electron microscopy in children with gastrointestinal intolerance to dietary protein. *J Pediatr Gastroenterol Nutr* 1988;7:386–394.
22. Trier JS. The surface coat of gastrointestinal epithelial cells. *Gastroenterology* 1969;56:618–622.
23. Dawson IMP. Atlas of gastrointestinal pathology as seen on biopsy. In: Gresham GA, ed. *Current histopathology. Vol. 6.* Philadelphia: JB Lippincott; 1983.
24. Filipe MI. Mucins in the human gastrointestinal tract: a review. *Invest Cell Pathol* 1978;2:195–216.
25. Dobbins WO. Human intestinal intraepithelial lymphocytes. *Gut* 1986;27:972–985.
26. Ferguson A, Murray D. Quantitation of intraepithelial lymphocytes in human jejunum. *Gut* 1971;12:988–994.
27. Selby WS, Janossy G, Bofill M, Jewell DP. Lymphocyte subpopulations in the human small intestine: the findings in normal mucosa and in the mucosa of patients with adult coeliac disease. *Clin Exp Immunol* 1983;52:219–228.
28. Cerf-Bensussan N, Schneeberger EE, Bhan AK. Immunohistologic and immunoelectron microscopic characterization of the mucosal lymphocytes of human small intestine by the use of monoclonal antibodies. *J Immunol* 1983;130:2615–2622.
29. Greenwood JH, Austin LL, Dobbins WO. In vitro characterization of human intestinal intraepithelial lymphocytes. *Gastroenterology* 1983; 85:1023–1035.
30. Kagnoff MF. Immunology and disease of the gastrointestinal tract. In: Sleisenger MH, Fordtran JS, eds. *Gastrointestinal disease.* Philadelphia: WB Saunders; 1989:114–144.
31. Petras RE. Non-neoplastic intestinal disease. In: Sternberg SS, ed. *Diagnostic surgical pathology. Vol. 2.* New York: Raven Press; 1989: 967–1014.
32. Ferguson A, Sutherland A, MacDonald TT, Allan F. Technique for microdissection and measurement in biopsies of human small intestine. *J Clin Pathol* 1977;30:1068–1073.
33. Lipkin M. Proliferation and differentiation of normal and diseased gastrointestinal cells. In: Johnson LR, ed. *Physiology of the gastrointestinal tract. 2nd ed.* New York: Raven Press; 1987:255–284.
34. Williamson RCN. Intestinal adaptation: structural, functional, and cytokinetic changes. *N Engl J Med* 1978;298:1393–1402.
35. Watson AJM. Necrosis and apoptosis in the gastrointestinal tract. *Gut* 1995;37:165–167.
36. Facer P, Bishop AE, Lloyd RV, Wilson BS, Hennessy RJ, Polak JM. Chomogranin: a newly recognized marker for endocrine cells of the human gastrointestinal tract. *Gastroenterology* 1985;89:1366–1373.
37. Albrecht S, Gardiner GW, Kovacs K, Ilse G, Kaiser U. Duodenal so-

matostatinoma with psammoma bodies. *Arch Pathol Lab Med* 1989; 113:517–520.
38. Sjolund K, Sanden G, Hakanson R, Sundler F. Endocrine cells in human intestine. *Gastroenterology* 1983;85:1120–1130.
39. Walsh JH. Gastrointestinal peptide hormones. In: Sleisenger MH, Fordtran JS, eds. *Gastrointestinal disease. 4th ed.* Philadelphia: WB Saunders; 1989:78–107.
40. Goldman H, Antonioli DA. Mucosal biopsy of the esophagus, stomach, and proximal duodenum. *Hum Pathol* 1982;13:423–448.
41. Sandow MJ, Whitehead R. The Paneth cell. *Gut* 1979;20:420–431.
42. Geller SA, Thung SN. Morphologic unity of Paneth cells. *Arch Pathol Lab Med* 1983;107:476–479.
43. Jenkins D, Goodall A, Scott BB. T-lymphocyte populations in normal and coeliac small intestinal mucosa defined by monoclonal antibodies. *Gut* 1986;27:1330–1337.
44. Lee FD, Toner PG. *Biopsy pathology of the small intestine.* Philadelphia: JB Lippincott; 1980.
45. Isaacson P, Judd MA. Carcinoembryonic antigen (CEA) in the normal human small intestine: A light and electron microscopic study. *Gut* 1977;18:786–791.
46. Scott H, Solheim BG, Brandtzaeg P, Thorsby E. HLA-DR–like antigens in the epithelium of the human small intestine. *Scand J Immunol* 1980;12:77–82.
47. Chiba M, Ohta H, Nagasaki A, Arakawa H, Masamune O. Lymphoid cell subsets in normal human small intestine. *Gastroenterol Jpn* 1986; 21:336–343.
48. Brandtzaeg P, Halstensen TS, Kett K, et al. Immunobiology and immunopathology of human gut mucosa: Humoral immunity and intraepithelial lymphocytes. *Gastroenterology* 1989;97:1562–1584.
49. Comer GM, Brandt LJ, Abiss CJ. Whipple's disease: a review. *Gastroenterology* 1983;78:107–114.
50. Strom RL, Gruninger RP. AIDS with *Mycobacterium avium-intracellulare* lesions resembling those of Whipple's disease. *N Engl J Med* 1983;309:1323–1324.
51. Roth RI, Owen RL, Keren DF, Volberding PA. Intestinal infection with *Mycobacterium avium* in acquired immune deficiency syndrome (AIDS). Histological and clinical comparison with Whipple's disease. *Dig Dis Sci* 1985;30:497–503.
52. Perera DR, Weinstein WM, Rubin CE. Small intestinal biopsy. *Hum Pathol* 1975;6:157–217.
53. Klein NC, Hargroove RL, Sleisenger MH, Jeffries GH. Eosinophilic gastroenteritis. *Medicine* 1970;49:299–319.
54. Johnstone JM, Morson BC. Eosinophilic gastroenteritis. *Histopathology* 1978;2:335–348.
55. Goldman H, Proujansky R. Allergic proctitis and gastroenteritis in children. *Am J Surg Pathol* 1986;10:75–86.
56. DeSchryver-Kecskemeti K, Clouse RE. A previously unrecognized subgroup of "eosinophilic gastroenteritis." Association with connective tissue diseases. *Am J Surg Pathol* 1984;8:171–180.
57. McNabb PC, Fleming CR, Higgins JA, Davis GL. Transmural eosinophilic gastroenteritis with ascites. *Mayo Clin Proc* 1979;54: 119–122.
58. Heatley RV. The gastrointestinal mast cell. *Scand J Gastroenterol* 1983;18:449–453.
59. Befus D, Goodacre R, Dyck N, Bienenstock J. Mast cell heterogeneity in man. Histologic studies of the intestine. *Int Arch Allergy Appl Immunol* 1985;76:232–236.
60. Scott BB, Hardy GJ, Losowsky MS. Involvement of the small intestine in systemic mast cell disease. *Gut* 1975;16:918–924.
61. Lundgvist M, Wilander E. Subepithelial neuroendocrine cells and carcinoid tumors of the human small intestine and appendix. A comparative immunohistochemical study with regard to serotonin, neuron specific enolase and S-100 protein reactivity. *J Pathol* 1986;148: 141–147.
62. Lord MG, Valies P, Broughton AC. A morphologic study of the submucosa of the large intestine. *Surg Gynecol Obstet* 1977;145:55–60.
63. Lee AKC, DeLellis RA, Silverman ML, Wolfe HJ. Lymphatic and blood vessel invasion in breast carcinoma: A useful prognostic indicator? *Hum Pathol* 1986;17:984–987.
64. Schlingemann RO, Dingjan GM, Emeis JJ, Blok J, Warnaar SO, Ruiter DJ. Monoclonal antibody PAL-E specific for endothelium. *Lab Invest* 1985;52:71–76.
65. Vardy PA, Lebenthal E, Schwachman H. Intestinal lymphangiectasia: a reappraisal. *Pediatrics* 1975;55:842–851.
66. Gershon MD, Erde SM. The nervous system of the gut. *Gastroenterology* 1981;80:1571–1594.
67. Goyal RK, Crist JR. Neurology of the gut. In: Sleisenger MH, Fordtran JS, eds. *Gastrointestinal disease.* Philadelphia: WB Saunders; 1989:21–52.
68. Krishnamurthy S, Schuffler MD. Pathology of neuromuscular disorders of the small intestine and colon. *Gastroenterology* 1987;93: 610–639.
69. Ferri G-L, Probert L, Cocchia D, Michetti F, Marangus PJ, Polak JM. Evidence for the presence of S-100 protein in the glial component of the human enteric nervous system. *Nature* 1982;297:409–410.
70. Lawson HH. The duodenal mucosa in health and disease: A clinical and experimental study. *Surg Annu* 1989;21:157–180.
71. Lawson HH. Definition of the gastroduodenal junction in healthy subjects. *J Clin Pathol* 1988;41:393–396.
72. Korn ER, Foroozan P. Endoscopic biopsies of normal duodenal mucosa. *Gastrointest Endosc* 1974;21:51–54.
73. Kreuning J, Bosman FT, Kuiper G, van der Wal AM, Lindeman J. Gastric and duodenal mucosa in "healthy" individuals: An endoscopic and histopathologic study of 50 volunteers. *J Clin Pathol* 1978;31: 69–77.
74. Dandalides WM, Carey WD, Petras RE, Achkar E. Endoscopic small bowel mucosal biopsy: A controlled trial evaluating forceps size and biopsy location in the diagnosis of normal and abnormal mucosal architecture. *Gastrointest Endosc* 1989;35:197–200.
75. Robertson HE. The pathology of Brunner's glands. *Arch Pathol* 1941; 31:112–130.
76. Lang IM, Tansy MF. Brunner's glands. In: Young JA, ed. *Gastrointestinal physiology. IV. International review of physiology. Vol. 28.* Baltimore, MD: University Park Press; 1983:85–102.
77. Treasure T. The ducts of Brunner's glands. *J Anat* 1978;127:299–304.
78. Leeson TS, Leeson RC. The fine structure of Brunner's glands. *J Anat* 1968;103:263–276.
79. Thompson CW, Day DW, Wright NA. Subnuclear vacuolated mucus cells: a novel abnormality of simple mucin-secreting cells of non-specialized gastric mucosa and Brunner's glands. *Histopathology* 1987; 1:1067–1081.
80. Kamiya R. Basal-granulated cells in human Brunner's glands. *Arch Histol Jpn* 1983;46:87–101.
81. Bosshard A, Chery-Croze S, Cuber JC, Dechelette MA, Berger F, Chayvialle JA. Immunocytochemical study of peptidergic structures in Brunner's glands. *Gastroenterology* 1989;97:1382–1388.
82. Silverman L, Waugh JM, Huizenga KA, Harrison EH. Large adenomatous polyp of Brunner's glands. *Am J Clin Pathol* 1961;36: 438–443.
83. Franzin G, Musola R, Ghidini O, Manfrini C, Fratton A. Nodular hyperplasia of Brunner's glands. *Gastrointest Endosc* 1985;31:374–378.
84. Rex DK, Jersild RA. Further characterization of the pigment in pseudomelanosis duodeni in three patients. *Gastroenterology* 1988;95: 177–182.
85. Rosenberg JC, Didio LJA. Anatomic and clinical aspects of the junction of the ileum with the large intestine. *Dis Colon Rectum* 1970;13: 220–224.
86. Kumar D, Phillips SF. The contribution of external ligamentous attachments to function of the ileocecal junction. *Dis Colon Rectum* 1987;30:410–416.
87. Axelsson C, Anderson JA. Lipohyperplasia of the ileocecal region. *Acta Chir Scand* 1974;140:649–654.
88. Cornes JS. Number, size, and distribution of Peyer's patches in the human small intestine. Part I. The development of Peyer's patches. Part II. The effect of age on Peyer's patches. *Gut* 1965;6:225–233.
89. MacDonald TT, Spencer J, Viney JL, Williams CB, Walker-Smith JA. Selective biopsy of human Peyer's patches during ileal endoscopy. *Gastroenterology* 1987;93:1356–1362.
90. Spencer J, Finn T, Isaacson PG. Human Peyer's patches: an immunohistochemical study. *Gut* 1986;27:405–410.
91. Pang LC. Intussusception revisited: clinicopathologic analysis of 261 cases with emphasis on pathogenesis. *South Med J* 1989;82:215–228.
92. Schenken JR, Kruger RL, Schultz L. Papillary lymphoid hyperplasia of the terminal ileum: an unusual cause of intussusception and gastrointestinal bleeding in childhood. *J Pediatr Surg* 1975;10:259–265.
93. Fieber SS, Schaefer HJ. Lymphoid hyperplasia of the terminal ileum—a clinical entity? *Gastroenterology* 1966;50:83–98.
94. Bjerke K, Brandtzaeg P, Fausa O. T cell distribution is different in fol-

licle-associated epithelium of human Peyer's patches and villous epithelium. *Clin Exp Immunol* 1988;74:270–275.
95. Wolf JL, Bye WA. The membranous epithelial (M) cell and the mucosal immune system. *Annu Rev Med* 1984;35:95–112.
96. Owen RL, Jones AL. Epithelial cell specialization within human Peyer's patches: an ultrastructural study of intestinal lymphoid follicles. *Gastroenterology* 1974;66:189–203.
97. Shepherd NA, Crocker PR, Smith AP, Levison DA. Exogenous pigment in Peyer's patches. *Hum Pathol* 1987;18:50–54.
98. Urbanski SJ, Arsenault AL, Green FHY, Haber G. Pigment resembling atmospheric dust in Peyer's patches. *Mod Pathol* 1989; 2:222–226.
99. Mackey WC, Dineen P. A fifty-year experience with Meckel's diverticulum. *Surg Gynecol Obstet* 1983;156:56–64.
100. Artigas V, Calabuig R, Badia F, Rius X, Allende L, Jover J. Meckel's diverticulum: value of ectopic tissue. *Am J Surg* 1986;151:631–634.
101. Bennett MK, Sachdev GK, Jewell DR, Anand BS. Jejunal mucosal morphology in healthy northern Indian subjects. *J Clin Pathol* 1985; 38:368–371.
102. Cook GC, Kajubi SK, Lee FD. Jejunal morphology of the African in Uganda. *J Pathol* 1969;98:157–169.
103. Lindenbaum J, Gerson CD, Kent TH. Recovery of small-intestinal structure and function after residence in the tropics. Studies in Peace Corps volunteers. *Ann Intern Med* 1971;74:218–222.
104. Gerson CD, Kent TH, Saha J, Siddiqi N, Lindenbaum J. Recovery of small intestinal structure and function after residence in the tropics. II. Studies in Indians and Pakistanis living in New York City. *Ann Intern Med* 1971;75:41–48.
105. Dobbins WO III. Small bowel biopsy in malabsorptive states. In: Norris HT, ed. *Pathology of the colon, small intestine, and anus.* New York: Churchill Livingstone; 1983:121–165.
106. Webster SGP, Leeming JT. The appearance of the small bowel mucosa in old age. *Age Ageing* 1975;4:168–174.
107. Chacko CJG, Paulson KA, Mathan VI, Baker SJ. The villus architecture of the small intestine in the tropics: A necropsy study. *J Pathol* 1969;98:146–151.
108. Wolff M. Heterotopic gastric epithelium in the rectum: a report of 31 new cases with a review of the 87 cases of gastric heterotopia in the alimentary canal. *Am J Clin Pathol* 1971;55:604–616.
109. Lessels AM, Martin DF. Heterotopic gastric mucosa in the duodenum. *J Clin Pathol* 1982;35:591–595.
110. Tsubone M, Kozuka S, Taki T, Hoshimo M, Yasui A, Hachisuka K. Heterotopic gastric mucosa in the small intestine. *Acta Pathol Jpn* 1984;34:1425–1431.
111. Lai ECS, Tompkins RK. Heterotopic pancreas. A review of a 26-year experience. *Am J Surg* 1986;151:697–700.
112. Dolan RV, ReMine WH, Dockerty MB. The fate of heterotopic pancreatic tissue. A study of 212 cases. *Arch Surg* 1974;109:782–785.
113. Armstrong CP, King PM, Dixon JM, McCleod IB. The clinical significance of heterotopic pancreas in the gastrointestinal tract. *Br J Surg* 1981;68:384–387.
114. Tanemura H, Uno S, Suzuki M, et al. Heterotopic gastric mucosa accompanied by aberrant pancreas in the duodenum. *Am J Gastroenterol* 1987;82:685–688.
115. Tomasi TB. Mechanisms of immune regulation at mucosal surfaces. *Rev Infect Dis* 1983;5:784–792.
116. Ranchod M, Lewin KJ, Dorfman RF. Lymphoid hyperplasia of the gastrointestinal tract: a study of 26 cases and review of the literature. *Am J Surg Pathol* 1978;2:383–400.
117. Rambaud JC, DeSaint-Louvert P, Marti R, et al. Diffuse follicular lymphoid hyperplasia of the small intestine without primary immunoglobulin deficiency. *Am J Med* 1982;73:125–132.
118. Matuchunsky C, Touchard G, Lemaire M, et al. Malignant lymphoma of the small bowel associated with diffuse nodular lymphoid hyperplasia. *N Engl J Med* 1985;313:166–171.
119. Hermans PE, Diaz-Buxo JA, Stobo JD. Idiopathic late-onset immunoglobulin deficiency: clinical observations in 50 patients. *Am J Med* 1976;61:221–237.
120. Lewin KJ, Kahn LB, Novis BH. Primary intestinal lymphoma of "Western" and "Mediterranean" type, alpha chain disease and massive plasma cell infiltration: A comparative study of 37 cases. *Cancer* 1976;38:2511–2528.
121. Lewin KJ, Ranchod M, Dorfman RF. Lymphoma of the gastrointestinal tract: A study of 117 cases presenting with gastrointestinal disease. *Cancer* 1978;42:693–707.
122. Grody WW, Weiss LM, Warnke RA, Magidson JG, Hu E, Lewin KJ. Gastrointestinal lymphomas: immunohistochemical studies on the cell of origin. *Am J Surg Pathol* 1985;9:328–337.
123. Tubbs RR, Sheibani K. Immunohistology of lymphoproliferative disorders. *Semin Diagn Pathol* 1984;1:272–284.
124. Little JV, Foucar K, Horvath A, Crago S. Flow cytometric analysis of lymphoma and lymphoma-like disorders. *Semin Diagn Pathol* 1989; 6:37–54.
125. Grody WW, Gatt RA, Naeim F. Diagnostic molecular pathology. *Mod Pathol* 1989;2:553–568.
126. Goldman H, Antonioli DA. Mucosal biopsy of the rectum, colon, and distal ileum. *Hum Pathol* 1982;13:981–1012.
127. Bechi P, Romagnoli P, Cortesini C. Ileal mucosal morphology after total colectomy in man. *Histopathology* 1981;5:667–678.
128. Philipson B, Brandberg A, Jagenburg R, Kock NG, Lager I, Ahren C. Mucosal morphology, bacteriology, and absorption in intra-abdominal ileostomy reservoir. *Scand J Gastroenterol* 1975;10:145–153.
129. Shepherd NA, Jass JR, Duval I, Moskowitz RI, Nicholls RJ, Morson BC. Restorative proctocolectomy with ileal reservoir: pathological and histochemical study of mucosal biopsy specimens. *J Clin Pathol* 1987;40:601–607.
130. Trier JS. Diagnostic value of peroral biopsy of the proximal small intestine. *N Engl J Med* 1971;285:1470–1473.
131. Brandborg LL, Rubin GE, Quinton WE. A multipurpose instrument for suction biopsy of the esophagus, stomach, small bowel, and colon. *Gastroenterology* 1959;37:1–16.
132. Achkar E, Carey WD, Petras R, Sivak MV, Revta R. Comparison of suction capsule and endoscopic biopsy of small bowel mucosa. *Gastrointest Endosc* 1986;32:278–281.
133. Whitehead R. Mucosal biopsy of the gastrointestinal tract. *Modern problems in pathology. Vol. 3. 3rd ed.* Philadelphia: WB Saunders; 1985.
134. Haggitt RC. Handling of gastrointestinal biopsies in the surgical pathology laboratory. *Lab Med* 1982;13:272–278.

*Histology for Pathologists, second edition,*
Edited by Stephen S. Sternberg.
Lippincott-Raven Publishers, Philadelphia


# CHAPTER 22

# Colon

Douglas S. Levine and Rodger C. Haggitt



## EMBRYOLOGY

The colon, which consists of epithelial, glandular, neural, vascular, muscular, and fibrous tissues, develops from the endoderm, ectoderm, and splanchnic mesoderm (1,2). The cecum, appendix, ascending colon, and proximal portion of the transverse colon are derived from the midgut, and the distal transverse colon, descending colon, sigmoid colon, and rectum are derived from the hindgut. During development, the midgut elongates, projects or "herniates" into the umbilical cord, rotates, and ultimately returns to a fixed position within the abdominal cavity. The hindgut lengthens, the cloaca differentiates into the urogenital sinus and rectum, and the membrane covering the cloaca ruptures to form the anal canal.

Several congenital abnormalities result from failure of normal rotation and fixation of the midgut (1,2), examples of which include omphalocele, gastroschisis, and congenital umbilical hernia (failure of return to or of fixation in the abdominal cavity); and nonrotation, mixed rotation, reverse rotation, volvulus, subhepatic cecum, and mobile cecum (rotational abnormalities). Examples of other abnormalities that result from failures of programmed cell death or proper growth of tissue elements include stenoses and atresias, Meckel's diverticulum, duplications, aganglionic megacolon (Hirschsprung's disease), and imperforate anus.

D. S. Levine: Department of Medicine, Division of Gastroenterology, University of Washington, Seattle, Washington 98195.
R. C. Haggitt: Departments of Pathology and Medicine, Division of Gastroenterology, University of Washington, Seattle, Washington 98195.

## APOPTOSIS

Programmed cell death is recognized as a normal aspect of growth control during embryogenesis and in tissues in which there is continuous cellular turnover (3,4). The epithelial cells of the colon are remarkable for short life spans lasting only several days, during which time they move from crypts to surface (2). Therefore, apoptosis of colonocytes is a normal phenomenon that can be recognized during microscopic examination of the surface epithelium (5). Apoptotic bodies are only rarely encountered within the normal crypt. Although cellular necrosis is characteristic of many diseases of the colon, apoptosis may be increased in some diseases, such as acute graft-versus-host disease, or in response to physical or chemical agents (6,7). Neoplasia in the colonic epithelium is associated with an attenuation of apoptosis, which may be brought about by abrogation of the normal loss of intercellular contact between colonocytes (8) or somatic genetic aberrations that characterize the neoplastic process (9,10).

## GROSS ANATOMY

### Surgical Perspective

The colon comprises the terminal 1 to 1.5 m of the gastrointestinal tract and lies completely within the abdominal cavity or is invested in peritoneum, except for its most distal part, the rectum (11) (Fig. 1). Beginning at the ileocecal valve, the anatomic terminology for various regions of the colon corresponds to their configurations and locations: the cecum (that part of the proximal colon lying below the ileocecal valve) and the appendix lie in the right lower abdominal quadrant; the ascending or right colon extends cephalad to the hepatic flexure; the transverse colon connects the hepatic to the splenic flexure; the descending or left colon proceeds caudad to the left lower quadrant; the S-shaped sigmoid colon extends with variable redundancy from the descending colon to the peritoneal reflection; and the rectum forms the distal 8 to 15 cm of extraperitoneal colon that lies within the pelvis and ends at the anal canal. Anatomic relationships between portions of the colon and other intraabdominal organs may vary (12) because of developmental variation among individuals.

Peritoneal folds (mesocolon) and fascial attachments anchor the colon to the posterior abdominal wall (11). Serosa and subserosal tissues encase the colon, but through them the external, longitudinal muscle layers of the muscularis propria are visible and reveal three distinct bands (taeniae coli) on the right side that become confluent on the left. Contractions and relative lengths of the external longitudinal muscle layer and the inner, circular muscle layer of the muscularis propria may account for the bulges (haustrations) along the viscus (11,13). Distension of the colon, as occurs during air-contrast barium enema examination and colonoscopic evaluation, can produce changes in normal colonic structure (14).

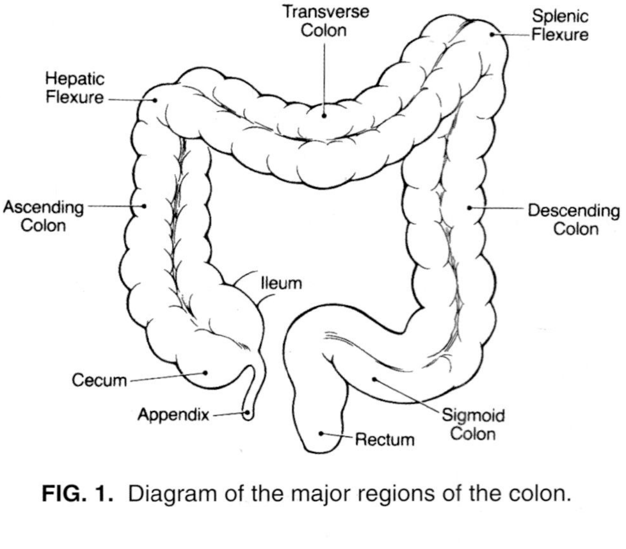


**FIG. 1.** Diagram of the major regions of the colon.

A rich vasculature supplies the colon in a fanlike distribution within the mesentery (15,16) and is derived primarily from branches of the superior mesenteric artery (from cecum to splenic flexure) and the inferior mesenteric artery (splenic flexure distally). Some of the rectum is supplied by the middle and inferior rectal arteries, which are branches of the internal iliac arteries. Venous blood leaves the colon predominantly via portal tributaries, but systemic veins drain portions of the rectum via the hemorrhoidal plexus. Lymphatic drainage occurs via channels that generally parallel the blood vessels. The colon is innervated by parasympathetic branches of the vagus and nervi erigentes and by sympathetic nerves from the superior mesenteric, inferior mesenteric, and pelvic ganglia.

### Endoscopic View

Although the colonoscopist's luminal view is limited to the mucosa, reasonably accurate anatomic localization within the colon can be obtained by regional landmarks, transillumination of the abdominal wall, and the use of fluoroscopy (17–23). The cecum is reliably identified when the ileocecal valve and the appendiceal orifice are seen. Sometimes, the mucosa is molded by the intersecting taeniae coli to a configuration that is unique to the cecum. The hepatic flexure is frequently identified by noticing the bluish mucosal coloration that results from the venous circulation of the juxtaposed liver. The transverse colon often appears to the endoscopist as a triangular lumen that results from the configuration of the taeniae coli. The splenic flexure is identified by an acute bend and slitlike opening at the junction of the transverse colon and the descending colon. Decreased luminal diameter, thickened mucosal folds, and numerous diverticular orifices (24), when present, all suggest localization in the descending or sigmoid colon; however, endoscopic landmarks in this vicinity are not reliable and compensation for this is achieved by calibration marks on the colonoscope and by fluoroscopic guidance.

## LIGHT MICROSCOPY

### Normal Mucosal Architecture

The colonic mucosa is composed of a single-cell layer of columnar epithelium covering the luminal surface and lining the crypts, along with the lamina propria and a thin, underlying muscle layer, the muscularis mucosae (25–30) (Fig. 2). As suggested before, mucosal folds and ridges can be created by contractions of the deeper muscularis propria. Surface deformations of a lesser degree also can be created by contractions of the muscularis mucosae.

An en face view of an area of colonic surface shows the openings of numerous crypts (Fig. 3). Sections cut perpendicular to the surface show a characteristic "row of test tubes" appearance created by crypts in parallel alignment (Fig. 2). Some variation in space between the crypts and slight alterations in the configuration of crypts can be present in the mucosal samples from healthy individuals, particularly in biopsy samples that do not include muscularis mucosae, but branching of crypts rarely occurs normally. This crypt architecture is normally maintained throughout the colon, except in the presence of mucosal lymphoid collections, in zones of transition to small intestinal mucosa (ileocecal valve), or to squamous epithelium (anorectum) (31), and in normally occurring grooves in the surface of the mucosa. Sections from these innominate grooves show cloverleaflike crypt structures in which all crypts connect to a single common lumen (32) (Fig. 4).

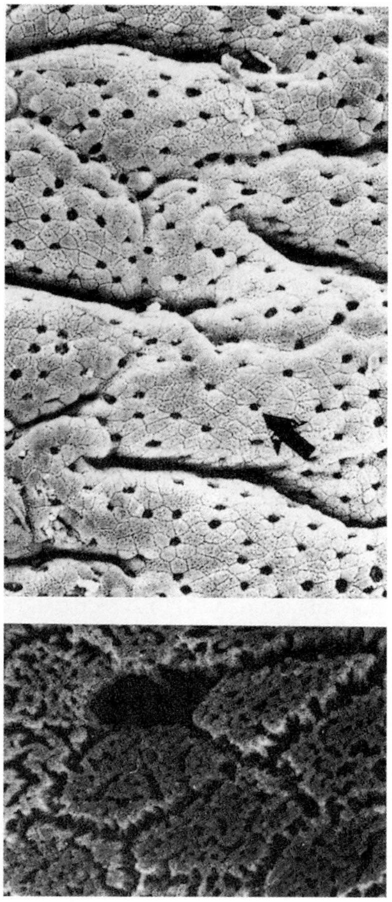
A
B

**FIG. 3.** Scanning electron micrographs of normal colonic surface epithelium. These en face views demonstrate circular and longitudinal openings corresponding to the mouths of the crypts and innominate grooves, respectively (compare with Figs. 2 and 4). (Original magnifications: **A**, ×**450**; *arrow* indicates area enlarged in **B**, ×**2400**). [Reprinted with permission (152).]

## Surface Epithelium

The colonic surface epithelium is a simple columnar or cuboidal epithelium that serves as a protective barrier between the host and the luminal environment. It is composed of absorptive and goblet cells (33–35). Both cell types are polarized and rest on a subepithelial basement membrane complex. Absorptive cells (Fig. 5) are responsible for colonic ion and water transport. Luminally directed apical striate borders are visible by light microscopy and correspond to the microvilli and glycocalyx seen by transmission electron microscopy (36). The cytoplasm of mature surface absorptive cells is eosinophilic and does not contain mucin. Absorptive nuclei are oval, basally oriented, and uniform in size with their long axes parallel to the long axes of the cells; they often contain nucleoli. Specialized absorptive and antigen-processing M cells, which are characteristically present in the small intestine, serve as conduits for the transport of luminal antigens to the underlying lymphoid tissue, but cannot be discriminated by light microscopy (37–39).

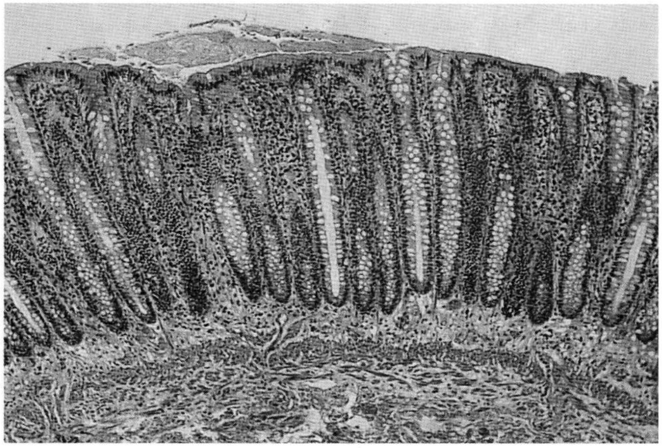

**FIG. 2.** Normal colonic mucosa. The histologic section of this endoscopic mucosal biopsy specimen is oriented so the simple columnar surface epithelium facing the lumen is at the top of the figure and the cut surface of the specimen is at the bottom. The mucosal crypts are lined up in parallel, and their mouths are open to the lumen. The lamina propria consists of the stromal elements investing the crypts and extending from the surface epithelium to the smooth muscle cells of the muscularis mucosae at the bottom.

Goblet cells (named for their wine goblet shape) (Fig. 5) synthesize, store, and secrete mucous granules by exocytosis (40). Luminally directed apical microvilli of small and irregular size are visible by electron microscopy, except in cells that are actively extruding mucous granules. Goblet cells seem to contain vacant cytoplasm by light microscopy after routine hematoxylin and eosin (H&E) staining, but granules become obvious with mucin stains (35,41–44). Mucin gly-

A 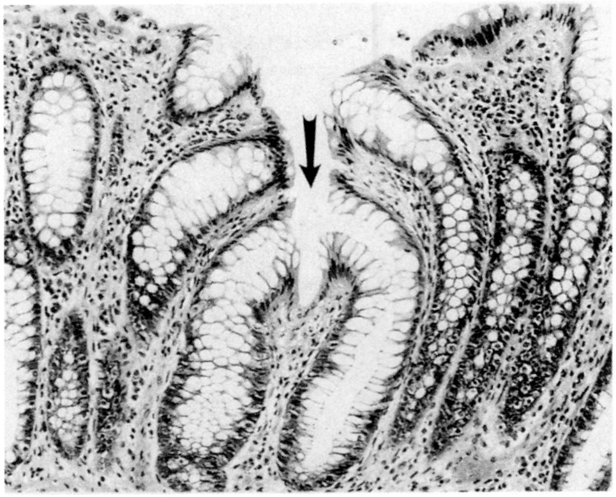 B 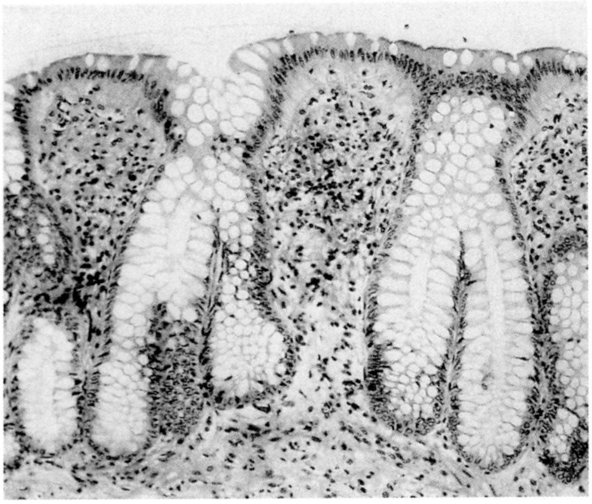

**FIG. 4. A:** Innominate grooves of colonic mucosa. Cross section of longitudinally oriented innominate grooves (see Fig. 3) shows a cloverleaf-like structure that should not be misinterpreted as pathologic distortion of the normal crypt architecture. Multiple crypts open into the lumen of the groove (*arrow*), which communicates with the colonic lumen. **B:** Quiescent chronic idiopathic ulcerative colitis. This histologic section demonstrates pathologic distortion of crypt architecture characterized by true branching of multiple crypts, which often is seen in idiopathic inflammatory bowel disease and which can be differentiated from the normal innominate grooves illustrated in (A) by noting that the branches open into the lumen through a single common orifice rather than independently.

coprotein structure in goblet cells is regionally variable throughout the colon, as suggested by variations in mucin histochemical-staining patterns (42,43) and differences in lectin binding (45). Goblet cell nuclei are basally oriented, often more densely stained than the nuclei of absorptive cells by hematoxylin (rendering nucleoli inapparent), and indented or otherwise deformed by their mucous granule-filled cytoplasm.

Lymphocytes and occasional eosinophils may normally be present between surface epithelial cells, as may occasional apoptotic vacuoles containing cellular debris and nuclear dust (Figs. 5 and 6). Care must be taken not to confuse apoptotic cells with neutrophils, which are not normally found in colonic epithelium.

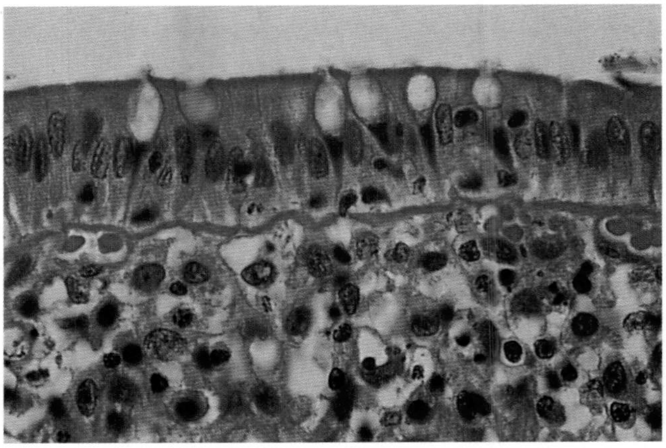

**FIG. 5.** Normal colonic surface epithelium. Absorptive cells and goblet cells are anchored to the underlying basement membrane complex. Intraepithelial lymphocytes are present between the surface epithelial cells. Note the nuclear dust in the lamina propria.

A thin basement membrane complex (Fig. 5) composed of collagen (46) and other proteins (47) that anchor epithelial cells supports the colonic epithelium. The components of the basement membrane cannot be resolved by light microscopy. This structure is permeable to absorbed or secreted ions, water, and protein and also must allow egress of the lamina propria lymphocytes into the epithelial cell layer. Fenestrations of the basement membrane, through which lamina propria cells may pass, are demonstrable by ultrastructural techniques (48). Connective tissue stains clearly show the normal subepithelial basement membrane to be only a few microns thick on sectioned profile (46,49–52).

### Crypt Epithelium

The simple columnar epithelium lining the colonic crypts (Fig. 7) comprises a more heterogeneous population of cells than does the surface epithelium. In addition to mature absorptive cells and goblet cells, immature and undifferentiated precursor cells as well as specialized endocrine and Paneth's cells are found in the crypts. Absorptive cells and goblet cells in the crypts have structures similar to those in the surface epithelium, but the less mature, less differentiated cells deeper in the crypts are more cuboidal than their mature surface, columnar counterparts. The least differentiated cells of the crypt contain little or no mucus.

Endocrine cells (Fig. 7) usually display a polarity opposite

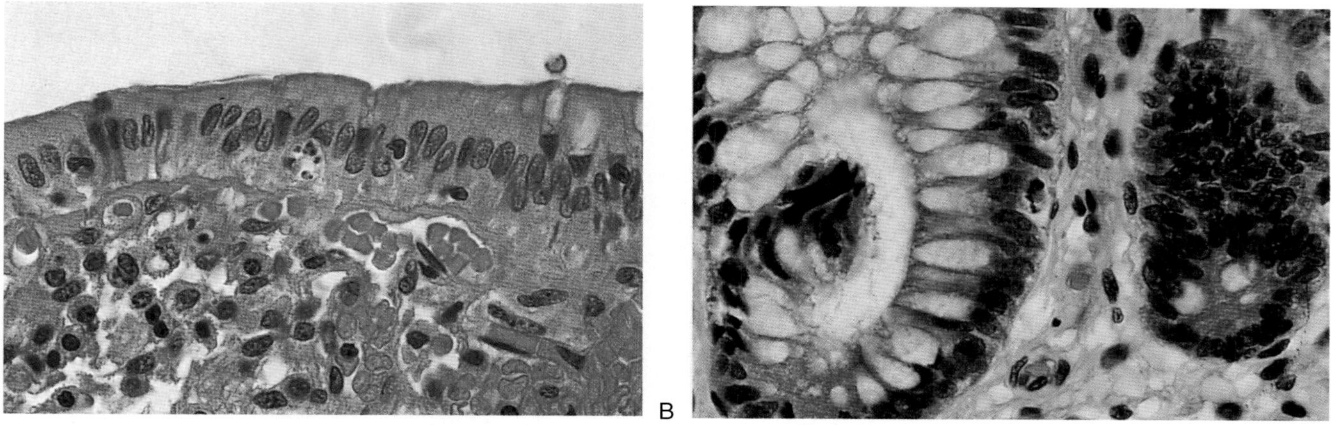

A B

**FIG. 6.** Apoptotic vacuoles (center of field) in colonic surface (**A**) and basal crypt (**B**) epithelium.

to that of the more numerous absorptive and goblet cells: the majority of the granule-containing cytoplasm is oriented abluminally below the nucleus. Although it is not well recognized, these cells are readily visible in good quality H&E-stained sections. The eosinophilic granules that identify the endocrine cells are smaller in size than Paneth's cell granules and are located between the nucleus and the base of the cell rather than on the luminal side of the nucleus, as in Paneth's cells. The endocrine cells in the colon can readily be identified by silver staining techniques: most of them are argyrophilic (precipitate metallic silver from a solution of silver salts only after addition of an external reducing agent), whereas a few are argentaffin (precipitate metallic silver from a solution of silver salts without an external reducing agent) (53). Various hormones within the cytoplasmic secretory granules are visible in these cells by light and transmission electron microscopy using peptide-specific antibodies in various immunohistochemical protocols (53–65). So much information exists on these cells, the peptides they contain, and their putative function that a discussion of them would require a separate full-length chapter. The interested reader is referred to the references cited above for additional information.

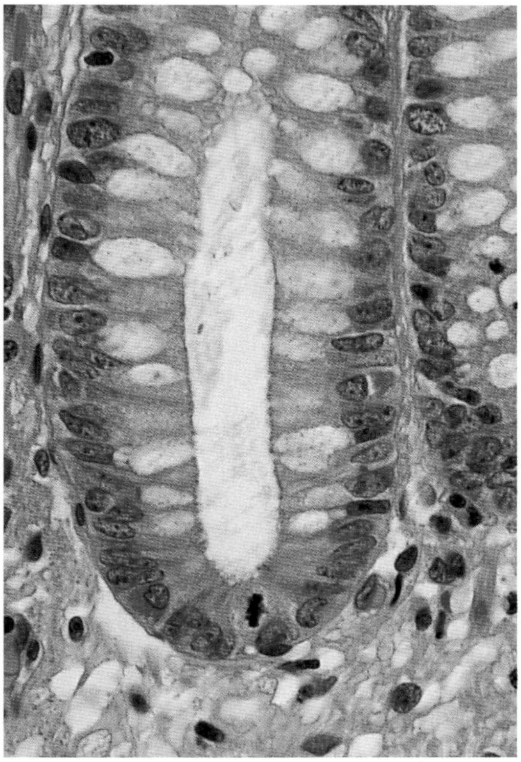

**FIG. 7.** Normal colonic basal crypt epithelium. Among the absorptive cells and goblet cells are a mitotic figure and endocrine cells with basally oriented secretory granules.

Paneth's cells are secretory cells whose precise function is not established with certainty. They are pyramid shaped and retain a base-to-lumen polarity like absorptive and goblet cells. Their most notable feature is their eosinophilic secretory granules, which are the largest seen in all gastrointestinal epithelia (66–68). These granules contain lysozyme, epidermal growth factor, and arginine-rich basic protein as well as glycoprotein. Paneth's cells are normally found only in the cecum and proximal right colon; their presence in other regions of the colon indicates metaplasia, usually as a result of chronic inflammation (69).

An important function of the colonic crypts is to renew the surface epithelium, the cells of which have finite lifetimes and are exfoliating constantly into the lumen or are being lost through the process of programmed cell death known as apoptosis (70–72). The proliferative zone at the base of the crypts is defined by mitotic figures within epithelial precursor cells that retain the ability to divide (Fig. 7). This zone can be located more precisely by incubation of colonic mucosal biopsy samples with tritiated thymidine or other thymidine analogues, such as bromodeoxyuridine (73), which are incorporated by cells synthesizing DNA as a prelude to cell division. Tissue sections of these biopsy samples are processed for autoradiography or immunohistochemistry, and proliferating cells that are labeled by uptake of radioactive thymidine or by immunolabeling are mostly confined to the basal 50% of the crypt but occasionally may be seen closer to the surface. The luminal 25% of the crypt represents the maturational zone. Most of the epithelial cells within this latter zone have lost the ability to divide, but they continue to differentiate and become more functionally mature until they eventually exfoliate from the surface.

## Lamina Propria

The lamina propria forms the investing stroma of the colonic mucosa and extends from the subepithelial basement membrane complex to the muscularis mucosae. It contains a wide variety of cells arranged among loosely organized strands of collagen, occasional slips of smooth muscle, and nerve twiglets (Fig. 8) (74–76). Most of the cells of the lamina propria are responsible for local, immunologically mediated host defense against noxious agents delivered in the luminal contents (77).

Plasma cells (B cells) (Fig. 9) in various numbers are the predominant normal round cell of the lamina propria. They are easily recognized by their characteristic cartwheel-shaped chromatin pattern in the nucleus and eccentric cytoplasmic clear areas corresponding to protein-synthesizing organelles. The chief protein products of colonic mucosal plasma cells are of the immunoglobulin (Ig)A variety, although IgM, IgG, and IgE also are synthesized (78–83). IgA and IgM become available for translocation across the intestinal epithelium into the colonic lumen (84,85). Plasma cells in normal rectal mucosa tend to be concentrated in the more superficial regions of the lamina propria (86).

T-lymphocytes are normally present not only within the lamina propria (Fig. 9), but also in the colonic epithelium and in the submucosa (87–89). The nuclei of lymphocytes are densely and homogeneously stained by hematoxylin, and usually only a thin rim of perinuclear cytoplasm is visible. The majority of these T cells are helper/suppressor cells that participate in complex immunological processes, with a small percentage being of the killer cell or natural killer cell variety (90,91). Intraepithelial lymphocytes may have a host defense function and can easily be distinguished from the nuclei of absorptive cells and goblet cells (Figs. 5 and 10).

Lymphocytes within the lamina propria proper are both diffusely distributed and organized into lymphoid follicles (Fig. 10) (92,93). The latter may be confined wholly within

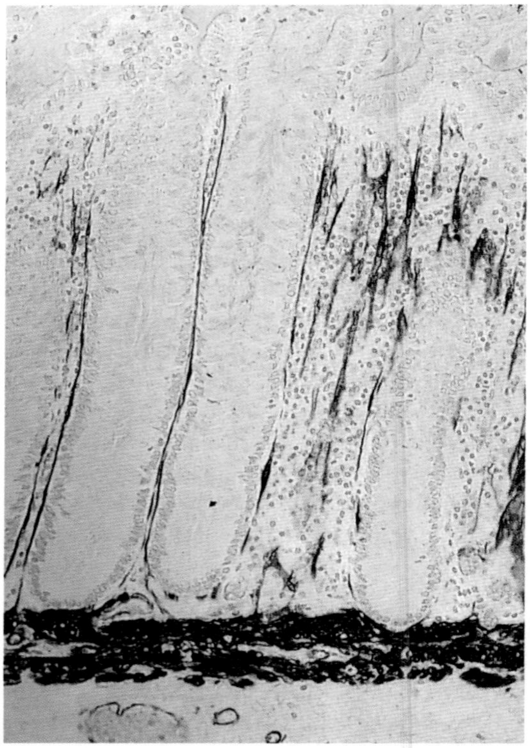

**FIG. 8.** Normal colonic mucosa after labeling with monoclonal antibody HHF-35 to muscle actins. Note the strands of smooth muscle in the lamina propria between crypts as well as the positive reaction of the cells of the pericryptal fibroblast sheath. The muscularis mucosae and vessels in the submucosa are also labeled by this antibody (*bottom*).

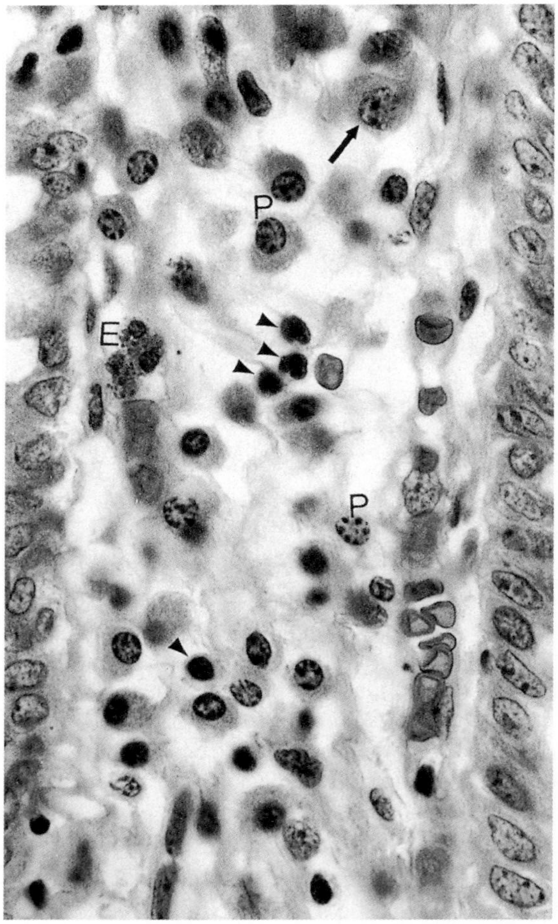


**FIG. 9.** Colonic lamina propria cells. The common cellular constituents of this stromal tissue that are illustrated are plasma cells (P), lymphocytes (*arrowheads*), macrophages (*arrow*), and occasional eosinophils (E).

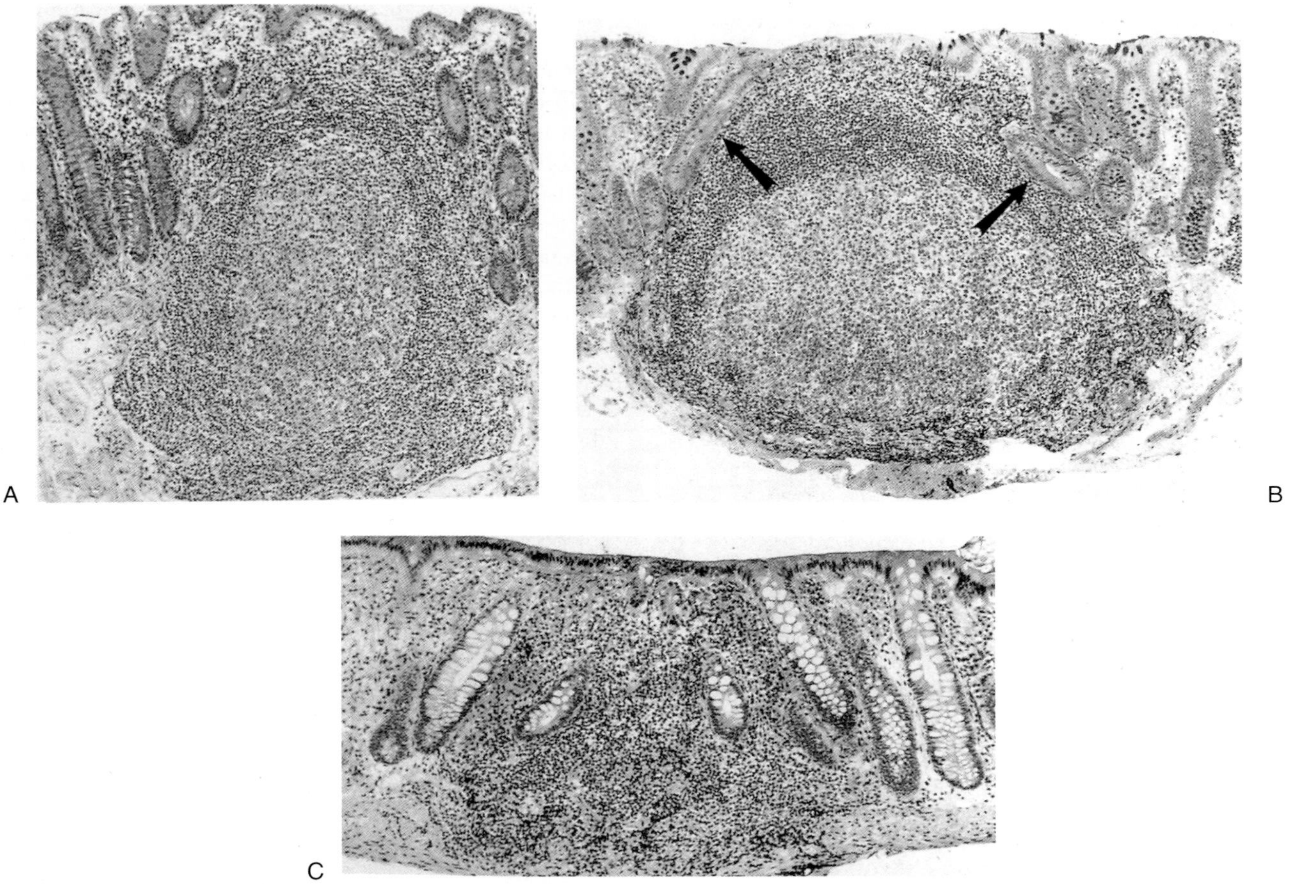


**FIG. 10.** Colonic lymphoid follicles. **A:** Lymphoid follicle with a prominent germinal center extends from the mucosa through the muscularis mucosae to the submucosa (hematoxylin and eosin, alcian blue at pH 2.5, and saffron). **B:** Lymphoid follicle with a prominent germinal center also produces splaying of adjacent crypts. Goblet cells are absent in crypt epithelium (*arrows*) immediately adjacent to the lymphoid follicle and increased numbers of intraepithelial lymphocytes are present within the surface epithelium superficial to the lymphoid nodule (hematoxylin and eosin, alcian blue at pH 2.5, and saffron). **C:** A less organized lymphoid collection in this section splays adjacent crypts.

the lamina propria or within the submucosa, or they may extend across the muscularis mucosae and occupy both. When this occurs, there is often a discontinuity in the muscularis mucosae through which crypts may extend to produce "lymphoglandular complexes" (37,94,95) (Fig. 11) that must not be mistaken for a pathologic process. The surface epithelium overlying lymphoid follicles differs from the adjacent surface in that the cells may be cuboidal and heavily infiltrated by lymphocytes.

Myeloid cells that normally reside in the lamina propria include eosinophils and mast cells (96,97) (Fig. 9). In the normal colon, the number of eosinophils is highly variable, but they are relatively rare compared with plasma cells and lymphocytes and are randomly distributed throughout the lamina propria. Mast cells, or tissue-based basophils, are less numerous than eosinophils, and their density appears to be increased in the ileocecal region compared with other sites of the colon (98). Occasional eosinophils and mast cells may permeate the surface epithelium in normal colonic mucosa. However, neutrophils should not be present normally in either the surface or crypt epithelium. A rare neutrophil loose within the lamina propria in otherwise normal colonic mucosa is probably within normal limits. Neutrophils may be found normally within the lumina of capillaries in the lamina propria and within areas of hemorrhage secondary to the trauma of biopsy.

Fibroblasts (Figs. 8 and 12) are located in two different sites: randomly distributed throughout the lamina propria or in the pericryptal fibroblast sheath surrounding the crypts and at the most superficial portion of the lamina propria, tightly apposed to the subepithelial basement membrane complex (99). Fibroblasts are typically fusiform and produce collagen, thereby contributing to the subepithelial basement membrane. Abundant rough endoplasmic reticulum for collagen biosynthesis can be demonstrated in fibroblasts by transmission electron microscopy. Immunohistochemical localization of muscle-specific actins using monoclonal antibody HHF-35 discloses that the pericryptal "fibroblasts"

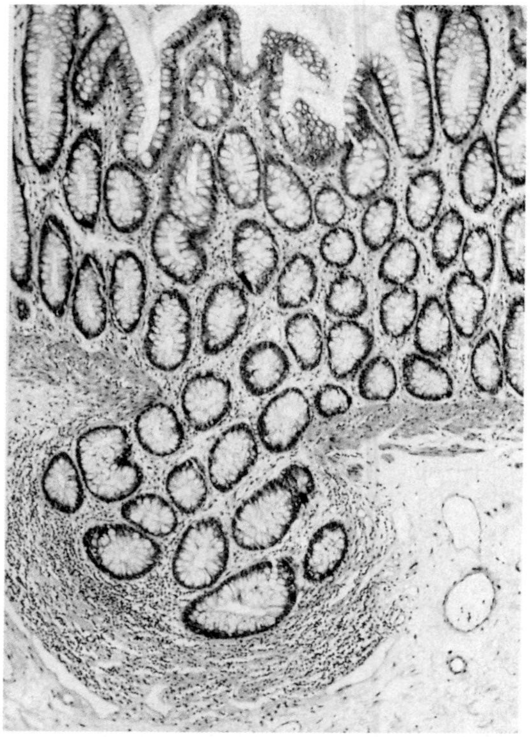

**FIG. 11.** Lymphoglandular complex. In this tangential section crypt epithelium is present within a lymphoid follicle that extends from the mucosa through the muscularis mucosae into the submucosa.

contain muscle actins and might more appropriately be designated pericryptal myofibroblasts or smooth muscle cells (Fig. 8).

Macrophages are common inhabitants of the lamina propria (Fig. 9) (100,101) and probably represent tissue-based monocytes. Macrophages are important for processing and presentation of antigenic materials to other immunocytes. This is accomplished in part by this cell's ability to subject these materials to phagocytosis, the results of which are readily apparent on transmission electron microscopy as numerous cytoplasmic endocytic vesicles and lysosomal structures. Light microscopic evaluation of colonic mucosa may not permit easy identification of macrophages unless stainable pigment is present. Intracellular brown pigment may represent deposits from ingested anthracene-type laxatives (melanosis coli) (102,103) or hemosiderin deposits from prior mucosal hemorrhage. Muciphages, or macrophages containing mucin extruded by goblet cells abluminally through the subepithelial basement membrane complex into the lamina propria, are often present in biopsy samples from healthy individuals (Fig. 13) (104,105). The foamy cytoplasm of these cells contains mucin that stains most intensely with periodic acid-Schiff (PAS)-diastase but is most specifically demonstrated by alcian blue or other histochemical stains for mucus. All varieties of macrophages are present in normal colonic mucosa, but the presence of sufficient numbers of these cells to fill the lamina propria is pathologic and may represent infection with *Mycobacterium avium-intracellulare* or various metabolic storage disorders.

In biopsies from healthy individuals, one occasionally sees nuclear dust and cellular debris in the lamina propria immediately beneath the basement membrane of the surface epithelial cells or within the cytoplasm of macrophages in the upper part of the lamina propria (Fig. 5). The dust and debris probably originate from apoptotic cells in the overlying surface epithelium; because these cells are broken down, particulate debris from them may be extruded through the basement membrane complex into the lamina propria. In addition, macrophages may migrate through the gaps in the basement membrane complex, phagocytize apoptotic debris, then migrate back into the superficial lamina propria.

Neuroendocrine cells are present in the lamina propria outside the basement membranes of the crypts in normal colon, as well as in small intestine and appendix (106–108). These cells may be identified with specific antibody markers and probably are the cells of origin of neuroendocrine tumors, such as carcinoids.

Vascular structures within the lamina propria are limited to capillaries, easily identified by their thin walls of endothelium and containing erythrocytes, round cells, and neutrophils within their lumina. The lymphatic vessels of the

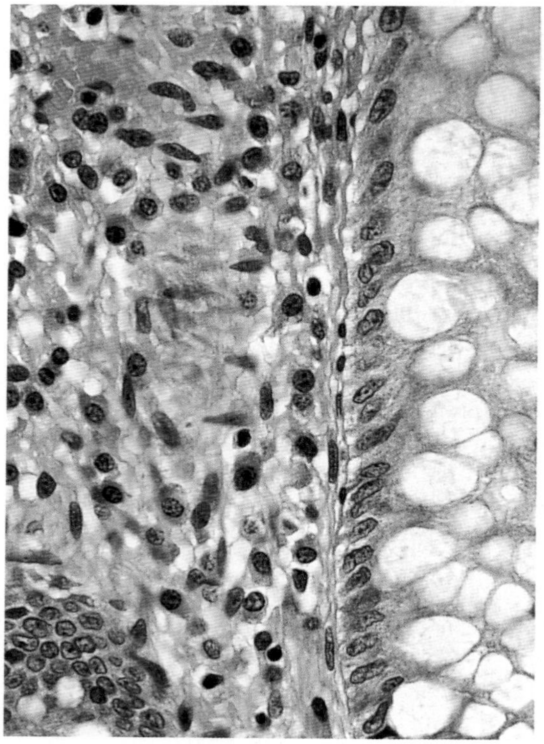

**FIG. 12.** Colonic pericryptal fibroblasts are parallel to the basement membrane complex. A tangential section of an adjacent crypt (*left center*) that is not centered in the plane of section shows many pericryptal fibroblasts that have a superficial resemblance to a granuloma.

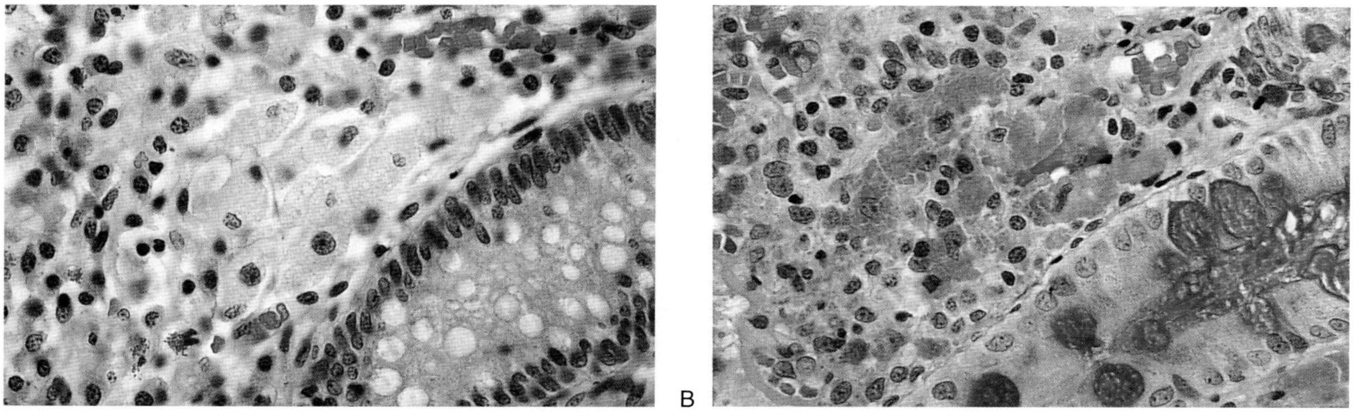

**FIG. 13.** Colonic muciphages are macrophages containing mucin that are easily demonstrated with mucin stains: **A:** Hematoxylin and eosin stain. **B:** Hematoxylin and eosin stain with alcian blue at pH 2.5.

colonic mucosa are limited to the region immediately above the muscularis mucosae and are not found extending above this region in the upper part of the lamina propria (Fig. 14) (109). Although lymphatic vessels generally appear to have thinner walls than capillaries and contain no red cells, differentiation of these vascular structures may require immunohistochemical techniques or electron microscopy (110–112).

A thin layer of muscle, the muscularis mucosae (Figs. 2, 8, and 15), separates the mucosa (epithelium and lamina propria) from the deeper submucosa. Some smooth muscle cells from this layer may normally extend upward into the lamina propria (Fig. 8) (113,114) and may become more numerous whenever there is traction on the mucosa as, for example, when there is mucosal prolapse (115). The thickness of the muscularis mucosae is variable, and it often forms the deep margin in shallow endoscopic biopsy samples. Contractions of this muscle layer deform the mucosa and may affect the normal physiologic (absorptive, secretory, and proliferative) processes of the epithelium. The muscularis mucosae is normally traversed by lymphoglandular complexes, vascular channels, and neural twiglets.

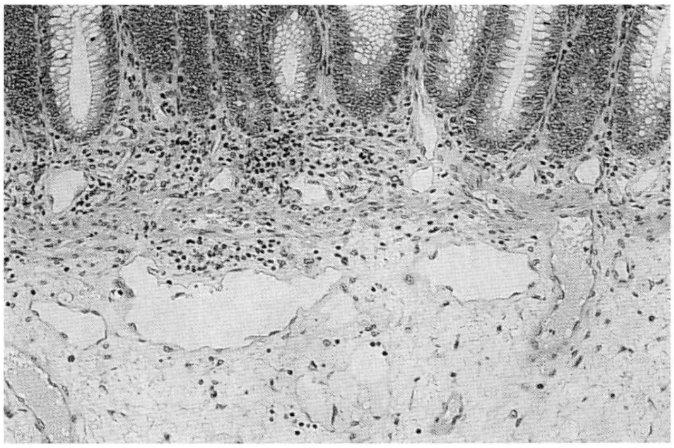

**FIG. 14.** Colonic lymphatics are present in the mucosa between the bases of crypts and the muscularis mucosae and within the submucosa. For comparison note capillary containing lysed erythrocytes and polymorphonuclear leukocytes in submucosa at lower right-hand portion of illustration.

### Submucosa

Many of the same cellular constituents of the lamina propria also reside within the submucosal stroma (lymphocytes, plasma cells, fibroblasts, macrophages) (116), so their de-

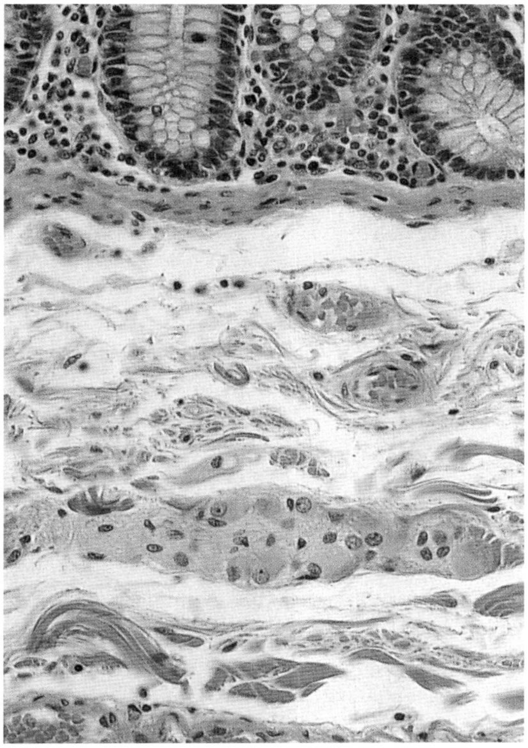

**FIG. 15.** Colonic submucosal plexus of Meissner. Neural tissue of the plexus is present amid the stromal elements of the submucosa deep to the muscularis mucosae. Ganglion cells, nerve axons, and Schwann cell nuclei are visible within the plexus.

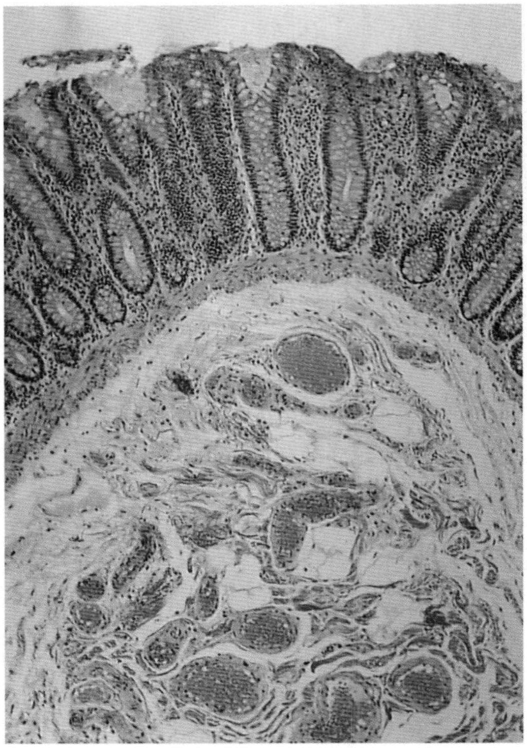

**FIG. 16.** Colonic submucosal vasculature. Most of the blood vessels in this section contain erythrocytes.

scriptions are not repeated in this section. Certain structures in the submucosa, such as fat cells, are not normally present in the lamina propria.

Two neural plexuses occupy the submucosal region (117–119). The first plexus lies immediately beneath the muscularis mucosae and is known as the submucosal plexus of Meissner (Fig. 15). The neural tissue of Meissner's plexus is composed of neurons and glial cells interspersed among the stromal elements. The second plexus lies along the inner aspect of the muscularis propria and is known as Henle's or the deep submucosal plexus; it is probably analogous to the myenteric plexus of Auerbach. Cell bodies of neurons, or ganglion cells, have a characteristic appearance in tissue sections: round or oval nuclei that contain a prominent nucleolus are surrounded by ample basophilic cytoplasm stippled by Nissl substance. Ganglion cells are not normally found in the lamina propria. When several ganglion cells are grouped together, their appearance can be confused with giant cells, epithelioid cells, and granulomas. Nerve axons of the plexus have a fibrillar appearance and traverse in and out of the plane of section. Nucleated cells associated with nerve axons are Schwann cells. The normal appearance of neural tissues in the submucosal and myenteric plexuses is best discerned by silver staining techniques that more easily differentiate artifactual from pathologic changes (117). Investigations of the three-dimensional organization of the enteric nervous system, its anatomic relationships to other colonic wall structures, and its functions have been described using ultrastructural, immunohistochemical, and retrograde axonal labeling techniques (120–133). A report of these is beyond the scope of this chapter, and the reader is referred to the references cited above.

Vascular structures in the submucosa include arterioles, venules, and lymphatics (Figs. 14 and 16). These submucosal vessels not infrequently appear large and tortuous in otherwise normal colons, especially when the colon is contracted, as is usually the case after fixation, and should not be mistaken for a vascular anomaly. Venules or capillaries that lack erythrocytes may be differentiated from lymphatic channels by immunohistochemistry (110–112) or electron microscopic evaluation of the endothelial cells. Blood vessels and lymphatics are normally free of surrounding inflammatory cells but may contain marginating polymorphonuclear leukocytes.

### Muscularis Externa, Subserosal Zone, and Serosa

The external smooth muscle layers of the colon, the muscularis propria, include a circular inner layer and a longitudinal outer layer (117,134) (Fig. 17). Structural variations of the muscularis propria have been identified and perhaps reflect different motility and storage functions of different colonic regions (135,136). The neural tissue of Auerbach's plexus lies between these two muscle layers and has histologic features like those of Meissner's plexus. The muscularis is perforated by blood and lymphatic vessels and encased in a subserosal zone of variable thickness that is in turn covered by the serosal lining of mesothelial cells. The term "serosa" is frequently used incorrectly; strictly speaking, it applies only to the mesothelium and the immediately adjacent fibroelastic tissue. The layer of connective tissue between the serosa and muscularis propria constitutes the subserosal tissue.

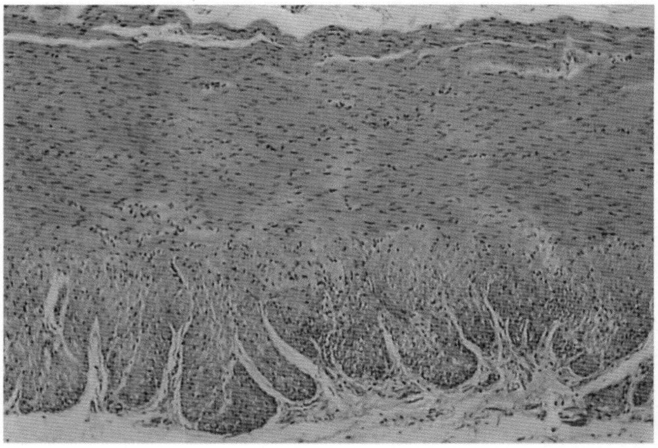

**FIG. 17.** Colonic muscularis propria includes the circular inner layer subjacent to the submucosa and the longitudinal external layer superficial to the subserosal zone.

## FUNCTION

The colon serves primarily as a depot for desiccation and storage of feces (137–141). Water and electrolyte absorption by the mucosa convert a daily liter of ileal output into a compact, formed stool weighing less than 200 g when a standard Western diet is consumed. Mass movements of colonic content from right to left are neurally and hormonally regulated (142–144). The voluntary nervous system controls defecatory stimuli and functions.

Short-chain fatty acids, flatus, and water are produced as metabolic products of undigested carbohydrate and dietary fiber by carbohydrate-consuming bacterial flora of the colon. A rumenlike function of the colon is attributable to these bacteria because metabolic breakdown products of complex carbohydrates, such as short-chain fatty acids, can be absorbed and used by colonic mucosal epithelial cells and can serve as a significant source of dietary calories (145,146).

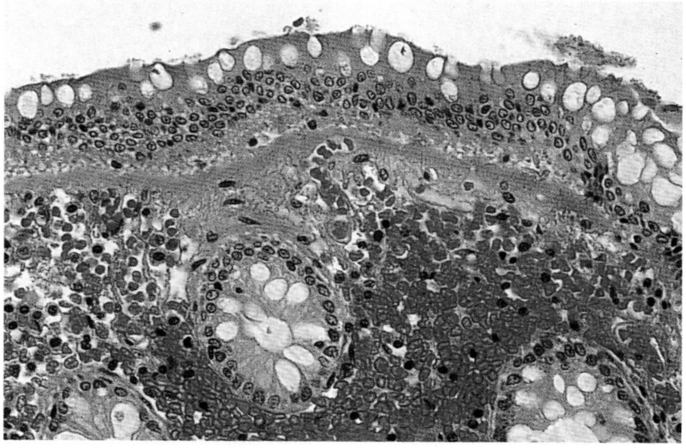

**FIG. 18.** Tangential sectioning artifact in normal colonic mucosa creates the false impression that the subepithelial basement membrane complex is thickened. Tangential sectioning is indicated by the cross section of epithelial crypts producing acinus-like structures and the pseudostratification of surface epithelial nuclei.

## SPECIAL TECHNIQUES AND PROCEDURES

Enhanced visualization of the colonic mucosa in vivo is possible during colonoscopy with magnification endoscopy and after application of structure-specific dyes (chromoendoscopy). These and other physical methods, such as laser-induced fluorescence microscopy and video-enhanced microscopy (40,147,148) can be applied to excised colon.

H&E staining of fixed and processed colonic tissue usually suffices for most routine clinical diagnostic practice. However, a variety of special techniques, some of which are mentioned above, are used to facilitate histopathologic diagnosis, and others are being developed as part of research investigations of the normal structure of the colon and its various disease states (149). Computerization and digitization of histologic data are becoming routine for the acquisition of quantitative research information. Special histochemical, immunohistochemical, and in situ hybridization staining of colonic tissue provides enhancement of specific structures and molecules for investigational study. Nonhistologic, degradative analyses are performed for subcellular and molecular analyses.

## ARTIFACTS AND VARIATIONS IN NORMAL COLONIC HISTOLOGY

### Incorrect Tissue Orientation and Tangential Sectioning

The colonic tissue obtained by endoscopic biopsy or by surgical resection is interpreted most accurately if tissue sections are taken perpendicular to the plane of the surface epithelium. Improper orientation of tissue with resultant tangential sectioning produces appearances in normal mucosa that may be interpreted as pathologic changes. The presence of cross sections of acinus-like structures rather than normal parallel crypts indicates tangential sectioning. With tangential sectioning, the thickness of the subepithelial basement membrane complex may be exaggerated and lead to an improper diagnosis of collagenous colitis (Fig. 18; compare with Fig. 5). Tangential sections made through the most basal portions of the colonic crypts show cross sections of crypt epithelium with diminished cytoplasmic mucus and undifferentiated nuclear characteristics. These features can be incorrectly interpreted as those of a tubular adenoma.

### Laxatives and Enema Preparations Before Colonic Biopsy

Mucosal endoscopic biopsy samples are best obtained from an unprepared colon or after administration of gentle isotonic saline enemas or oral, nonabsorbable lavage solutions because these electrolyte solutions do not produce histologic changes in the mucosa. Other commonly used preparations (sodium phosphate enemas, bisacodyl enemas and suppositories, dioctyl sodium sulfosuccinate, soapsuds enemas) can produce abnormalities in the mucosa (150–156) (Fig. 19) that may be mistaken for or may preclude the diagnosis of subtle inflammatory disease. Surface epithelial cells may be detached from the mucosal surface, leaving the false diagnostic impression of epithelial erosions; the intact basement membrane devoid of overlying epithelium and the absence of polymorphonuclear leukocytes rule out the possibility of erosions. The surface epithelial cells may be flattened or cuboidal and atypical, falsely suggesting regeneration of the epithelium after a pathologic insult (other than the insult of an irritating enema). Diminution or depletion of goblet cell mucus, which is a nonspecific finding in colonic inflammation, may occur. Mild acute inflammation with neutrophilic infiltration of the surface and crypt epithelium and within the lamina propria may be observed (Fig. 19).

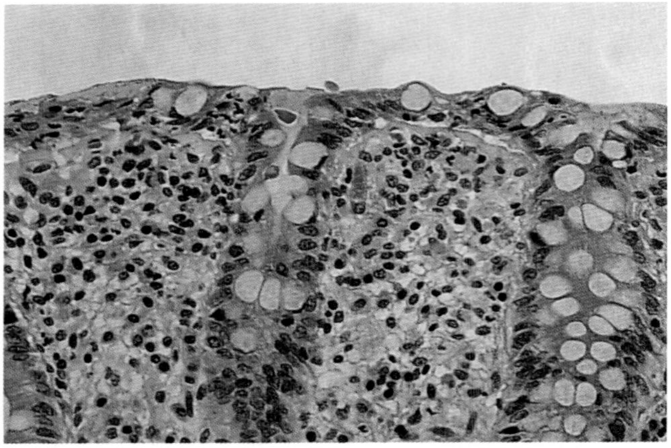

**FIG. 19.** Bisacodyl-induced artifact in normal colonic mucosa. Mucosal biopsy samples were obtained 2 hr after bisacodyl was given. A high-power view shows increased numbers of inflammatory cells in the superficial portion of the lamina propria and surface epithelial abnormalities. The loss of columnar shape of the surface epithelium and neutrophilic infiltration of the superficial lamina propria and surface epithelium can be mistaken for colitis.

Edema and hemorrhage within the lamina propria, which may be caused by the trauma of the biopsy procedure, can be exaggerated after administration of laxatives and enemas.

### Tissue Trauma

Traumatic artifacts in normal colonic mucosa can be produced by faulty endoscopic technique, by improper handling of biopsy specimens before fixation, and during tissue processing. Endoscopic trauma to the mucosa can produce edema, petechiae, friability, tears, and bleeding (18,20–22,157). Because biopsy samples from this traumatized mucosa commonly show edema and hemorrhage in the lamina propria, such abnormalities should not be considered pathologic unless they are accompanied by other evidence of significant injury such as neutrophilic infiltration of the epithelium (Fig. 20) (157). White plaques in colonic mucosa may result from endoscopic air insufflation or accidental lavage with hydrogen peroxide (inappropriately placed in the water pumping system of the endoscope). Biopsy of these plaques shows vacuolated areas within the lamina propria that may resemble adipocytes but are actually gas-filled pockets (158) (Fig. 21). This entity, which has been referred to as pseudolipomatosis, lacks inflammation and is thereby differentiated from pneumatosis cystoides intestinalis (159).

Endoscopic biopsy samples are best obtained with a large, double-cup forceps with a central spike to impale the mucosa when approaching it tangentially (Fig. 22) or forceps of similar size with a cutting-edge cup design. These forceps are designed to grasp the mucosa when they are closed. The biopsy is then removed from the mucosa by avulsion. This biopsy technique produces tissue damage, including edema and hemorrhage in the lamina propria (Fig. 20). The ends of the biopsy often show crush artifact where the forceps jaws have closed on the tissue (Fig. 23). Crush artifacts and perforations may be seen in a small, central region of the biopsy because of the central spike. Such artifactually crushed tissue may have atypical nuclei that are hyperchromatic to the point of being opacified, angulated, and irregularly shaped. These distorted nuclei can be mistaken for dysplasia or carcinoma if the observer is not aware of the potential problem. These and other artifacts may result from the use of rigid, "long-jawed" types of cutting biopsy forceps, which are used with rigid proctosigmoidoscopes (160).

Colonic polyps are often removed endoscopically by

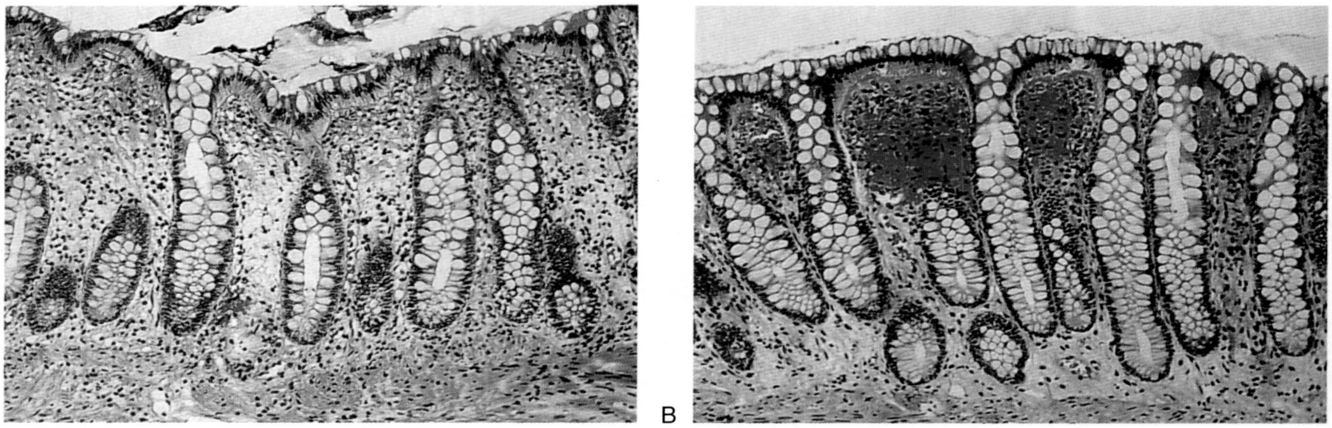

A B

**FIG. 20.** Traumatic artifacts in normal colonic mucosa. **A:** Increased cell-free space within the lamina propria creates the appearance of edema and separates adjacent crypts. **B:** Mucosal hemorrhages without associated histologic abnormalities should not be interpreted to be part of a disease process because they are frequently seen in biopsy samples from normal mucosa.

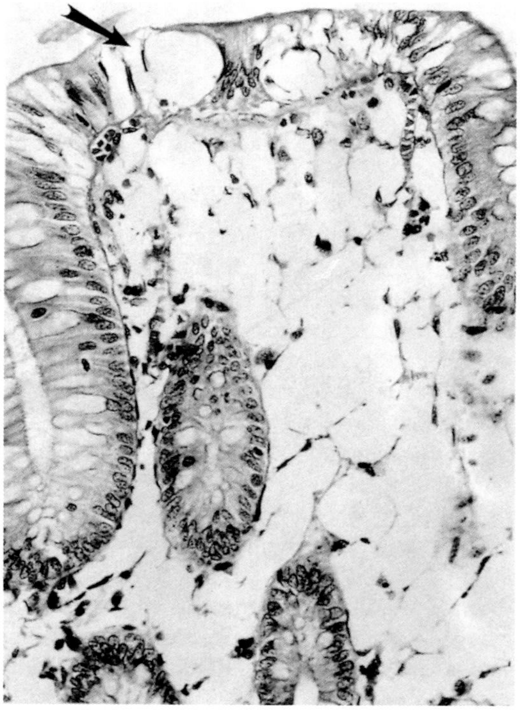

**FIG. 21.** Colonic pseudolipomatosis. Vacuolated areas are present within the lamina propria as well as within the surface epithelium (*arrow*).

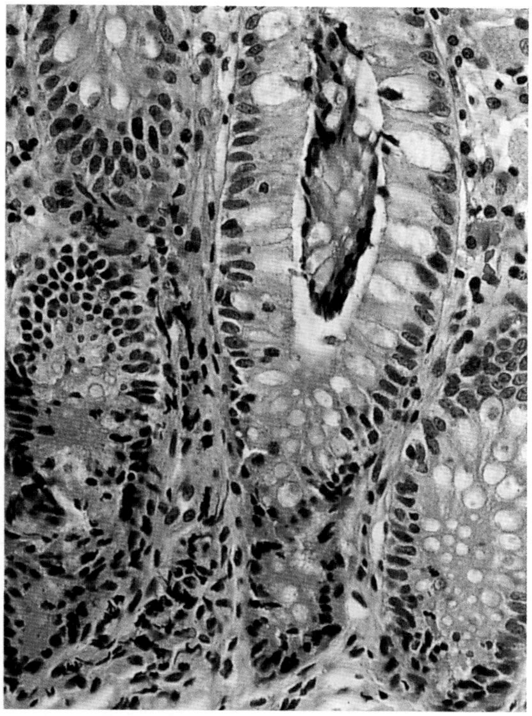

**FIG. 23.** Biopsy crush artifact in normal colonic mucosa. Distortion and crowding of epithelial cells are apparent in the bases of adjacent crypts. Stripped epithelial cells and debris have been traumatically relocated to the lumen of one of these crypts.

tightening a wire snare around the stalk of the polyp, applying electrocautery current through the wire to coagulate the tissue, and cutting through the stalk (18–23). Histologic examination of polyps resected in this manner often shows artifacts secondary to electrodesiccation and compression by the wire snare (Fig. 24). Crush artifacts similar to those pro-

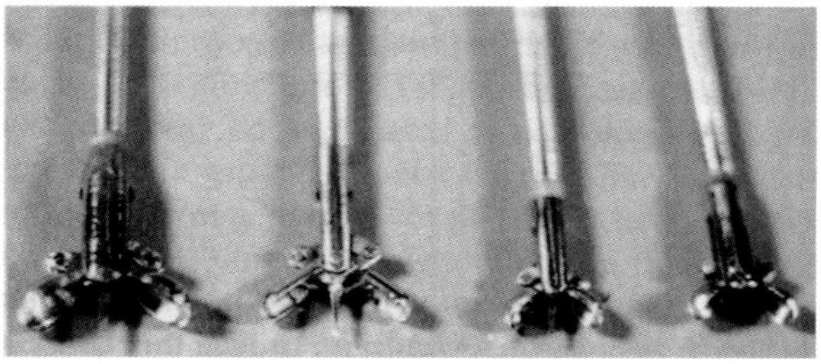

**FIG. 22.** Endoscopic biopsy forceps. All four instruments are double-cup forceps of varying sizes, and three have a central spike for impaling the mucosa before closure of the forceps. We favor the use of the largest ("jumbo" size) pinch biopsy forceps at the left to permit safe acquisition of the most tissue and to facilitate orientation of biopsy samples. Use of this large forceps is not associated with an increased risk of perforation or hemorrhage, and at least twice as much tissue is obtained as with the smaller forceps.

duced using biopsy forceps may be seen. Electrocautery also produces nuclear pyknosis, elongation, and "streaming" in the direction of the current, sometimes making it difficult or impossible to differentiate between normal and neoplastic epithelium.

Traumatic damage to surface epithelium can occur during the orientation of biopsy specimens before fixation. Surface epithelium may be cuboidal, flattened, or stripped off. Other crush artifacts may result during tissue processing if polyfoam pads are placed with the tissue in embedding cassettes (161).

## Edema

Apparent edema in colonic mucosal biopsy samples, as indicated by a wider than normal separation of the cellular components of the lamina propria or a horizontal, relatively empty-appearing band between the crypt bases and the muscularis mucosae (Fig. 20), is nonspecific because it can be seen in biopsy samples from healthy individuals who have had neither laxatives nor preparatory enemas. Edema can be produced by many different disease states, may merely reflect the secretory or absorptive state of normal mucosa, and,

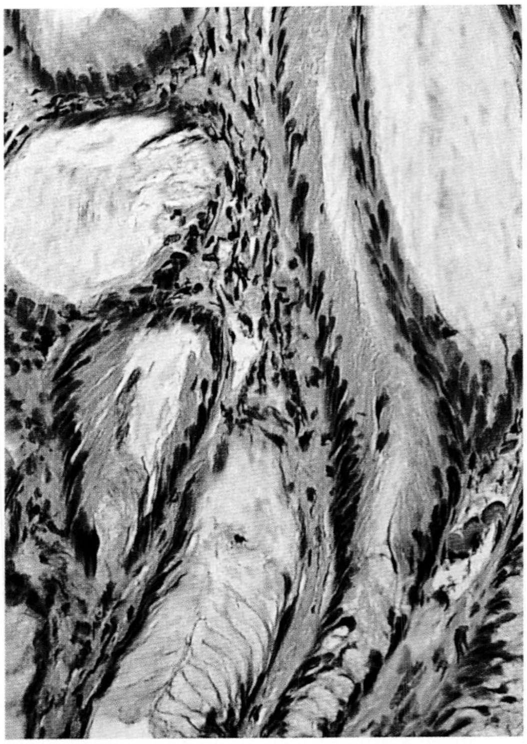

FIG. 24. Electrodesiccation and compression artifact in the bases of adjacent crypts in normal colonic mucosa produced by an endoscopic electrocautery snare. Affected nuclei are pyknotic and elongated. Colonic crypts distorted by this artifact may be difficult or impossible to differentiate from the tubules of an adenoma.

as indicated previously, may be an artifact of the biopsy procedure. The degree of edema can vary considerably within the same biopsy and among different biopsies.

### Mononuclear Cell Density

Normal colonic mucosa has a complement of "inflammatory" cells located within the epithelium and the lamina propria. These plasma cells, lymphocytes, and occasional eosinophils do not represent chronic inflammation (162). A common error is to diagnose "mild chronic nonspecific colitis" after biopsy of a normal colon because of the normal population of mononuclear cells. As a general rule, the diagnosis of colitis should not be made unless there is evidence of injury to the colonic epithelium. For example, inflammation is present if there are sufficient mononuclear cells within the lamina propria to splay, separate, or otherwise distort colonic crypts provided they do not represent a normal lymphoid aggregate. Other evidence of epithelial injury is less subtle and includes neutrophilic or lymphocytic infiltration of the crypt epithelium, epithelial erosions, granulomas, multinucleated giant cells, and distorted crypt architecture (163,164).

### Architectural Changes Associated with Lymphoid Aggregates

One to two mucosal lymphoid follicles and/or lymphoglandular complexes may be present in the normal colorectal biopsy sample. Tangential sections through the periphery of lymphoid follicles should not be mistaken for increased mononuclear density due to inflammation. Serial sections of the isolated lymphoid aggregate usually show its compact nature or demonstrate a germinal center, either of which establishes its true nature (Fig. 10). Multiple, small, basally located lymphoid aggregates are pathologic and may be due to Crohn's disease or ulcerative colitis (163).

Lymphoid aggregates in normal mucosa may distort the architecture of the crypts immediately adjacent to them (Fig. 10). Absence of goblet cells in crypts adjacent to lymphoid aggregates also can occur normally. Such features should not be misdiagnosed as idiopathic inflammatory bowel disease.

## SPECIMEN HANDLING

### Value of Diagnosing Normal Colonic Histology

There are occasions in the practice of pathology when normal colonic or rectal biopsy results have diagnostic value. For example, because ulcerative colitis, by definition, involves the rectal mucosa, normal rectal biopsy results in a patient who has not been treated with steroid enemas exclude that diagnosis. If the differential diagnosis had previously been narrowed to ulcerative colitis or Crohn's disease, normal rectal biopsy results become diagnostic of Crohn's disease. In patients with ulcerative colitis who have been treated with steroid enemas, the rectal mucosa often appears normal endoscopically, but biopsies show distortion of the crypt architecture, indicating healed colitis. Rarely, the biopsy sample from such a patient may show only subtle abnormalities and can be misinterpreted as normal. Biopsy samples containing normal mucosa may also document "skip" lesions or focal inflammation in Crohn's disease. Often, normal colonic biopsy results are of great value to the clinician in excluding organic disease and suggesting that the patient suffers from irritable bowel syndrome.

Biopsy samples of "polyps" that show only normal colonic mucosa after step sectioning of the entire biopsy specimen suggest that the endoscopist missed a target lesion, took a biopsy sample of a normal fold of mucosa that had a polypoid configuration, or obtained a biopsy sample of mucosa overlying a lymphoid follicle or submucosal nodule. Identification of the normal colonic mucosal margin in endoscopic polypectomy specimens assures that the electrocautery snare was appropriately placed on the polyp stalk or adjacent colonic mucosa.

## Biopsy Techniques

Cutting biopsy forceps, which are sometimes used through the rigid proctosigmoidoscope, are capable of taking large and deep samples, thereby increasing the risk of complications (bleeding, perforation) from the biopsy procedure. Smaller pinch forceps that are passed through the instrument channels of flexible video or fiberoptic colonoscopes and sigmoidoscopes are used more frequently because they take a safer, relatively superficial sample that is limited to the mucosa and superficial submucosa, which is usually adequate for histologic diagnostic purposes. We recommend "jumbo" pinch biopsy forceps with a central spike or cutting-edge cup design that have at least a 9-mm open span rather than the "standard" size pinch forceps with smaller open spans (Fig. 22). The larger forceps increase the amount of mucosa available for diagnosis and facilitate orientation of the biopsy sample. Endoscopic biopsy techniques, such as the "turn-and-suction" method, also safely augment biopsy sample size (165).

Ideally, biopsy samples should be oriented submucosal side down on a support material before fixation (166,167). Our practice is to lift the sample gently from the biopsy forceps with a wooden spatula fashioned from a broken applicator stick. The sample is gently rolled epithelial side down on the gloved index finger, and the curled edges are flattened with the shaft (not the point) of a dissecting needle. A small square of monofilament mesh screening material is placed on the cut side of the sample and is gently squeezed against the index finger by apposition of the thumb. With the aid of the side of the dissecting needle, the tip of the index finger is rolled off the luminal surface of the mounted sample, which

**TABLE 1.** *Formula for Hollande's solution*

| | |
|---|---|
| Formalin (40% formaldehyde) | 100 ml |
| Glacial acetic acid | 15 ml |
| Picric acid | 40 g |
| Cupric acetate | 25 g |
| Water | 1000 ml |

Dissolve cupric acetate in water without heat; add picric acid slowly with stirring. When dissolved, filter then add formalin and acetic acid. Hollande's solution has a shelf life of at least 1 year.

Alternative:

| | |
|---|---|
| Saturated picric acid | 1000 ml |
| Cupric acetate | 24 g |
| Formalin (40% formaldehyde) | 100 ml |
| Glacial acetic acid | 15 ml |

Add in order given.

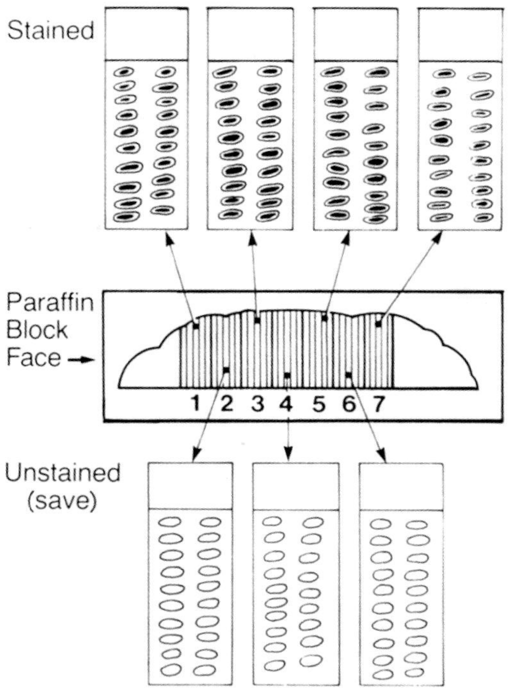


**FIG. 25.** Diagram of how colonic mucosal biopsy samples are step-serial sectioned. A single biopsy sample oriented with its surface epithelium up and its cut surface down within a paraffin block is depicted in the center. Sectioning perpendicular to the plane of the illustration proceeds from left to right through the seven numbered regions. Ribbons of serial sections from regions 1, 3, 5, and 7 were stained and evaluated, whereas the serial sections from regions 2, 4, and 6 were saved and not stained.

is then placed in fixative. Other support materials that can be used are millipore filter paper, cucumber slices, and gelfoam.

## Fixation, Processing, Sectioning, and Staining Procedures

We recommend the use of Hollande's (Table 1), Bouin's, or B-5 fixatives rather than formalin for routine histology. The definition of features in gastrointestinal mucosa fixed in Hollande's, Bouin's, or B-5 is superior to those achieved with formalin: shrinkage is minimized and nuclear detail becomes more clear. Hollande's has the advantage of not lysing eosinophil granules and of not laking red cells as does Bouin's.

Colonic biopsy samples are step-serial sectioned (Fig. 25) to permit adequate sampling of the entire biopsy specimen and to allow better evaluation of architecture in the well-oriented, more central core of the biopsy sample. Examination of adjacent serial sections increases diagnostic accuracy by making it possible to identify small granulomas, to differentiate between lymphoglandular complexes and increased

**TABLE 2.** *Method for H&E alcian blue saffron stain*

*Rationale:* Alcian blue and saffron used in combination with routine hematoxylin and eosin (H&E) stain have the added benefits of demonstrating acidic mucins (alcian blue) and staining collagen yellow (saffron). When used as a routine stain on GI material, it results in earlier diagnosis because it eliminates the need to do separate special stains for mucin and collagen.

*Precautions:* Care must be taken not to overstain in saffron. If sections are overstained, decolorize slides in ammonia water, wash well, and restain starting with eosin.

*Results:* Nuclei: blue; cytoplasm: pink to red; mucin: aqua blue; collagen: yellow; smooth muscle: salmon pink; other elements: shades of pink and blue.

*Fixation:* Hollande's, Bouin's, B-5

*Technique:* Paraffin sections, 4$\mu$m.

*Solutions:* Routine H&E

**3% Acetic acid**

| | |
|---|---|
| Glacial acetic acid | 30.0 ml |
| Distilled water | 970.0 ml |

**1% Alcian Blue**

| | |
|---|---|
| Alcian blue 8 GN | 10.0 ml |
| 3% Acetic acid | 1000.0 ml |

Mix until dissolved and add a crystal of thymol as a preservative.

Alcian blue usually has a normal shelf life of about 3 mo, but one must be aware of the more rapid deterioration of solutions when large numbers of slides are stained. Change accordingly.

**Alcoholic Saffron**

| | |
|---|---|
| Saffron | 1.5 g |
| Absolute alcohol | 100.0 ml |

Mix filter and add:

| | |
|---|---|
| Acetic acid | 1.0 ml |

Keeps well but for consistent staining change once a week.

**0.5% Lithium Carbonate**

| | |
|---|---|
| Lithium carbonate | 5.0 g |
| Distilled water | 1,000.0 ml |

Mix well

The remaining solutions are the routine solutions used in the H&E procedure.

*Procedure*

| | | |
|---|---|---|
| 1. | Deparaffinize | |
| 2. | 3% Acetic acid | 3 min |
| 3. | Alcian blue | 10 min |
| 4. | Water | wash |
| 5. | Check microscopically and dip several times in 3% acetic acid to remove background staining when necessary | |
| 6. | Water | wash |
| 7. | Lithium carbonate | 1 min |
| 8. | Water | wash |
| 9. | Hematoxylin | 6 min |
| 10. | Water | wash |
| 11. | Acid alcohol | dip as needed |
| 12. | Water | wash |
| 13. | Ammonia water | dip to blue |
| 14. | Water | wash |
| 15. | Check microscopically for nuclear detail | |
| 16. | Eosin | 2 min |
| 17. | Water | wash |
| 18. | 95% Alcohol | several dips |
| 19. | Absolute alcohol | 1 min |
| 20. | Absolute alcohol | 1 min |
| 21. | Saffron | 30 s |
| 22. | Absolute alcohol | 10 dips |
| 23. | Absolute alcohol | 10 dips |
| 24. | Xylene | 10 dips |
| 25. | Xylene | 2 dips |
| 26. | Xylene | 2 min |
| 27. | Coverslip | |

Metanil yellow (C.I. 13065) can be substituted for saffron for purposes of economy. Staining time in saffron is variable: five dips seem to work well with freshly made batches. The solution should be topped up with absolute alcohol to compensate for evaporation.

mononuclear cell density, and to detect less obvious abnormalities of crypt architecture.

We routinely perform a multipurpose screening stain consisting of H&E with special stains added to demonstrate mucin (Alcian blue at pH 2.5) and collagen (saffron). Our staining protocols are listed in Table 2.

## REFERENCES


1. Moore KL. *The developing human.* Philadelphia: WB Saunders, 1973.
2. Cohn SM, Birnbaum EH. Colon: Anatomy and structural anomalies. In: Yamada T, ed. *Textbook of gastroenterology. 2nd ed.* Philadelphia: JB Lippincott, 1995:1735–1747.
3. Bowen ID, Locksin RA, eds. *Cell death in biology and pathology.* London: Chapman & Hall, 1981.
4. Tomei LD, Cope FO, eds. *Apoptosis: the molecular basis of cell death.* Plainview, NY: Cold Spring Harbor Laboratory Press, 1991.
5. Hall PA, Coates PJ, Ansari B, Hopwood D. Regulation of cell number in the mammalian gastrointestinal tract: the importance of apoptosis. *J Cell Sci* 1994;107:3569–3577.
6. Potten CS. The significance of spontaneous and induced apoptosis in the gastrointestinal tract of mice. *Cancer Metastasis Rev* 1992;11: 179–195.
7. Lee FD. Importance of apoptosis in the histopathology of drug-related lesions in the large intestine. *J Clin Pathol* 1993;46:118–122.
8. Bates RC, Buret A, van Helden DF, Horton MA, Burns GF. Apoptosis induced by inhibition of intercellular contact. *J Cell Biol* 1994;125: 403–415.
9. Merritt AJ, Potten CS, Watson AJ, et al. Differential expression of bcl-2 in intestinal epithelia. Correlation with attentuation of apoptosis in colonic crypts and the incidence of colonic neoplasia. *J Cell Sci* 1995; 108:2261–2271.
10. Payne CM, Bernstein H, Bernstein C, Garewal H. Role of apoptosis in biology and pathology: resistance to apoptosis in colon carcinogenesis. *Ultrastruct Pathol* 1995;19:221–248.
11. Warwick R, Williams PL. *Gray's anatomy. 35th British ed.* Philadelphia: WB Saunders, 1973.
12. Jaques PF, Warshauer DM, Keefe B, Mauro MA, McCall JM. Variations in liver-colon anatomic relationship: relevance to interventional radiology. *J Vasc Interv Radiol* 1994;5:637–641.
13. Meyers MA, Volberg F, Katzen B, Abbott G. Haustral anatomy and pathology: a new look. I. Roentgen identification of normal patterns and relationships. *Radiology* 1973;108:497–504.
14. Rubesin SE, Furth EE, Rose D, Levine MS, Laufer I. The effects of distention of the colon during air-contrast barium enema on colonic morphology: anatomic correlation. *Am J Roentgenol* 1995;164: 1387–1389.
15. Parks DA, Jacobson ED. Physiology of the splanchnic circulation. *Arch Intern Med* 1985;145:1278–1281.
16. Parks DA, Jacobson ED. Mesenteric circulation. In: Johnson LR, ed. *Physiology of the gastrointestinal tract. 2nd ed.* New York: Raven Press, 1987:1649–1670.

17. Abramson DJ. The valves of Houston in adults. *Am J Surg* 1978;136: 334–336.
18. Blackstone MO. *Endoscopic interpretation: normal and pathologic appearances of the gastrointestinal tract.* New York: Raven Press, 1984.
19. Cotton PB, Williams CB. *Practical gastrointestinal endoscopy. 2nd ed.* Oxford: Blackwell Scientific, 1982.
20. Hunt RH, Waye JD. *Colonoscopy techniques: clinical practice and color atlas.* London: Chapman & Hall, 1981.
21. Nagasako K. *Differential diagnosis of colorectal diseases.* Tokyo: Igaku-Shoin, 1982.
22. Shinya H. *Colonoscopy: diagnosis and treatment of colonic diseases.* Tokyo: Igaku-Shoin, 1982.
23. Silverstein FE, Tytgat GNJ. *Atlas of gastrointestinal endoscopy. 2nd ed.* New York: Gower, 1991.
24. Whiteway J, Morson BC. Pathology of the ageing—diverticular disease. *Clin Gastroenterol* 1985;14:829–846.
25. Donnellan WL. The structure of the colonic mucosa: the epithelium and subepithelial reticulohistiocytic complex. *Gastroenterology* 1965; 49:496–514.
26. Flick AL, Voegtlin KF, Rubin CE. Clinical experience with suction biopsy of the rectal mucosa. *Gastroenterology* 1962;42:691–705.
27. Goldman H, Antonioli DA. Mucosal biopsy of the rectum, colon, and distal ileum. *Hum Pathol* 1982;13:981–1012.
28. Hamilton SR. Structure of the colon. *Scand J Gastroenterol* 1984; 19(suppl 93):13–23.
29. Lumb G. Normal human rectal mucosa and its mechanism of repair. *Am J Dig Dis* 1960;5:836–840.
30. Neutra MR, Padykula HA. The gastrointestinal tract. In: Weiss L, ed. *Modern concepts of gastrointestinal histology.* New York: Elsevier, 1984:696–702.
31. Flick AL, Voegtlin KF, Rubin CE. Clinical experience with suction biopsy of the rectum. *Gastroenterology* 1962;42:691–705.
32. Williams I. Innominate grooves in the surface of mucosa. *Radiology* 1965;84:877–880.
33. Fenoglio CM, Richart RM, Kaye GI. Comparative electron microscopic features of normal, hyperplastic and adenomatous human colonic epithelium. II. Variations in surface architecture found by scanning electron microscopy. *Gastroenterology* 1975;69:100–109.
34. Kaye GI, Fenoglio CM, Pascal RR, Lane N. Comparative electron microscopic features of normal, hyperplastic, and adenomatous human colonic epithelium. Variations in cellular structure relative to the process of epithelial differentiation. *Gastroenterology* 1973;64:926–945.
35. Shamsuddin AM, Phelps PC, Trump BF. Human large intestinal epithelium: light microscopy, histochemistry, and ultrastructure. *Hum Pathol* 1982;13:790–803.
36. Rifaat MK, Iseri OA, Gottlieb LS. Ultrastructural study of the "extraneous coat" of human colonic mucosa. *Gastroenterology* 1965;48: 593–601.
37. O'Leary AD, Sweeney EC. Lymphoglandular complexes of the colon: structure and distribution. *Histopathology* 1986;10:267–283.
38. Pappo J, Owen RL. The lymphoid system and immunologic defense of the digestive tract. In: Motta PM, Fujita H, eds. *Ultrastructure of the digestive tract.* Boston: Martinus Nijhoff, 1988:181–199.
39. Fujimura Y, Hosobe M, Kihara T. Ultrastructural study of M cells from colonic lymphoid nodules obtained by colonoscopic biopsy. *Dig Dis Sci* 1992;37:1089–1098.
40. Terakawa S, Suzuki Y. Exocytosis in colonic goblet cells visualized by video-enhanced microscopy. *Biochem Biophys Res Commun* 1991; 176:466–472.
41. Culling CFA, Reid PE, Dunn WL, Freeman HJ. The relevance of the histochemistry of colonic mucins based upon their PAS reactivity. *Histochem J* 1981;13:889–903.
42. Filipe MI. Mucins in the human gastrointestinal epithelium: a review. *Invest Cell Pathol* 1979;2:195–216.
43. Sipponen P. Histochemical reactions of gastrointestinal mucosubstances with high iron diamine after prior oxidation and methylation of tissue sections. *Histochemistry* 1979;64:297–305.
44. Ueda T, Fujimori O, Yamada K. A new histochemical method for detection of sialic acids using a physical development procedure. *J Histochem Cytochem* 1995;43:1045–1051.
45. Jacobs LR, Huber PW. Regional distribution and alterations of lectin binding to colorectal mucin in mucosal biopsies from controls and subjects with inflammatory bowel disease. *J Clin Invest* 1985;75: 112–118.
46. Gledhill A, Cole FM. Significance of basement membrane thickening in the human colon. *Gut* 1984;25:1085–1088.
47. Scott DL, Morris CJ, Blake AE, Low-Beer TS, Walton KW. Distribution of fibronectin in the rectal mucosa. *J Clin Pathol* 1981;34: 749–758.
48. Mestres P, Diener M, Mai H, Rummel W. The epithelial basal lamina of the isolated colonic mucosa: scanning and transmission electron microscopy. *Acta Anat Basel* 1991;141:74–81.
49. Bogomoletz WV. Collagenous colitis: a clinicopathological review. *Surv Dig Dis* 1983;1:19–25.
50. Hwang WS, Kelly JK, Shaffer EA, Hershfield NB. Collagenous colitis: a disease of pericryptal fibroblast sheath? *J Pathol* 1986;149: 33–40.
51. Levine DS, Surawicz CM, Ajer TN, Dean PJ, Rubin CE. Diffuse excess mucosal collagen in rectal biopsies facilitates the differential diagnosis of solitary rectal ulcer syndrome from other inflammatory bowel diseases. *Dig Dis Sci* 1988;33:1345–1352.
52. Teglbjaerg PS, Thaysen EH, Jensen HH. Development of collagenous colitis in sequential biopsy specimens. *Gastroenterology* 1984;87: 703–709.
53. Smith DM Jr, Haggitt RC. A comparative study of generic stains for carcinoid secretory granules. *Am J Surg Pathol* 1983;7:61–68.
54. Bottcher G, Alumets J, Hakanson R, Sundler F. Coexistence of glicentin and peptide YY in colorectal L-cells in cat and man. An electron microscopic study. *Regul Pept* 1986;13:283–291.
55. Buffa R, Capella C, Fontana P, Usellini L, Solcia E. Types of endocrine cells in the human colon and rectum. *Cell Tissue Res* 1978; 192:227–240.
56. Facer P, Bishop AE, Lloyd RV, Wison BS, Hennessey RJ, Polak JM. Chromogranin: a newly recognized marker for endocrine cells of the human gastrointestinal tract. *Gastroenterology* 1985;89:1366–1373.
57. Inokuchi H, Kawai K, Takeuchi Y, Sano Y. Identification of EC cells in the human intestine: a comparative study between immunohistochemical and silver impregnation techniques. *Histochemistry* 1983; 79:9–16.
58. Lechago J. The endocrine cells of the digestive and respiratory systems and their pathology. In: Bloodworth JMB, ed. *Endocrine pathology. 2nd ed.* Baltimore: Williams & Wilkins, 1982:513–555.
59. Lehy T, Cristina ML. Ontogeny and distribution of certain endocrine cells in the human fetal large intestine: histochemical and immunocytochemical studies. *Cell Tissue Res* 1979;203:415–426.
60. Lewin KJ. The endocrine cells of the gastrointestinal tract. The normal endocrine cells and their hyperplasias. *Pathol Annu* 1986;21:1–27.
61. Lukinius AIC, Ericsson JLE, Lundqvist MK, Wilander EMO. Ultrastructural localization of serotonin and polypeptide YY (PYY) in endocrine cells of the human rectum. *J Histochem Cytochem* 1986;34: 719–726.
62. Sjolund K, Sanden G, Hakanson R, Sundler F. Endocrine cells in human intestine: an immunocytochemical study. *Gastroenterology* 1983;85:1120–1130.
63. Smith DM Jr, Haggitt RC. The prevalence and prognostic significance of argyrophil cells in colorectal carcinomas. *Am J Surg Pathol* 1984; 8:123–128.
64. Sokolski KN, Lechago J. Human colonic substance P-producing cells are a separate population from the serotonin-producing enterochromaffin cells. *J Histochem Cytochem* 1984;32:1066–1074.
65. Wilander E, Portela-Gomes G, Grimelius L, Westermark P. Argentaffin and argyrophil reactions of human gastrointestinal carcinoids. *Gastroenterology* 1977;73:733–736.
66. Geller SA, Thung SN. Morphologic unity of Paneth cells. *Arch Pathol Lab Med* 1983;107:476–479.
67. Lewin K. The Paneth cell in disease. *Gut* 1969;10:804–811.
68. Sandow MJ, Whitehead R. Progress report: the Paneth cell. *Gut* 1979; 20:420–431.
69. Symonds DA. Paneth cell metaplasia in diseases of the colon and rectum. *Arch Pathol* 1974;97:343–347.
70. Bristol JB, Williamson RCN. Large bowel growth. *Scand J Gastroenterol* 1984;19(suppl 93):25–34.
71. Eastwood GL. Gastrointestinal epithelial renewal. *Gastroenterology* 1977;72:962–975.
72. Lipkin M. Proliferation and differentiation of normal and diseased gastrointestinal cells. In: Johnson LR, ed. *Physiology of the gastrointestinal tract. 2nd ed.* New York: Raven Press, 1987:255–284.
73. Darmon E, Pincu-Hornstein A, Rozen P. A rapid and simple in vitro method for evaluating human colorectal epithelial proliferation. *Arch Pathol Lab Med* 1990;114:855–857.
74. Eidelman S, Lagunoff D. The morphology of the normal human rectal biopsy. *Hum Pathol* 1972;3:389–401.

75. Kolodej P, Yakimets WW. Topography of the human colonic lamina propria. *J Electron Microsc* (Tokyo) 1981;30:334–335.
76. Malchiodi AF, Ciaralli F, Giuliani A. Increased osmiophilia of glycosaminoglycan-like structures after fixation with cetylpyridinium chloride in human colonic mucosa. *J Submicrosc Cytol Pathol* 1991; 23:415–418.
77. Elson CO, Kagnoff MF, Fiocchi C, Befus AD, Targan S. Intestinal immunity and inflammation: recent progress. *Gastroenterology* 1986; 91:746–768.
78. Bjerke K, Brandtzaeg P, Rognum TO. Distribution of immunoglobulin producing cells is different in normal human appendix and colon mucosa. *Gut* 1986;27:667–674.
79. Crabbe PA, Heremans JF. The distribution of immunoglobulin-containing cells along the human gastrointestinal tract. *Gastroenterology* 1966;51:305–316.
80. Gelzayd EA, Kraft SC, Fitch FW. Immunoglobulin A: localization in rectal mucosal epithelial cells. *Science* 1967;157:930–931.
81. Gelzayd EA, Kraft SC, Kirsner JB. Distribution of immunoglobulins in human rectal mucosa. I. Normal control subjects. *Gastroenterology* 1968;54:334–340.
82. Regadera J, Paniagua R, Nistal M, Santamaria L. Quantitative distribution of Ig-containing cells in the mucosa of the human large intestine. *Cell Mol Biol* 1983;29:387–395.
83. Scott BB, Goodall A, Stephenson P, Jenkins D. Rectal mucosa plasma cells in inflammatory bowel disease. *Gut* 1983;24:519–524.
84. Brown WR, Isobe Y, Nakane PK. Studies on translocation of immunoglobulins across intestinal epithelium. II. Immunoelectron-microscopic localization of immunoglobulins and secretory component in human intestinal mucosa. *Gastroenterology* 1976;71:985–995.
85. Brown WR, Isobe Y, Nakane PK, Pacini B. Studies on translocation of immunoglobulins across intestinal epithelium. IV. Evidence for binding of IgA and IgM to secretory component in intestinal epithelium. *Gastroenterology* 1977;73:1333–1339.
86. Leonard RCF, MacLennan ICM. Distribution of plasma cells in normal rectal mucosa. *J Clin Pathol* 1982;35:820–823.
87. Bartnik W, ReMine SG, Chiba M, Thayer WR, Shorter RG. Isolation and characterization of colonic intraepithelial and lamina propria lymphocytes. *Gastroenterology* 1980;78:976–985.
88. Bull DM, Bookman MA. Isolation and functional characterization of human intestinal mucosal lymphoid cells. *J Clin Invest* 1977;59: 966–974.
89. Greenwood JH, Austin LL, Dobbins WO III. In vitro characterization of human intestinal intraepithelial lymphocytes. *Gastroenterology* 1983;85:1023–1035.
90. Chiba M, Shorter RG, Thayer WR, Bartnik W, ReMine S. K-cell activity in lamina proprial lymphocytes from the human colon. *Dig Dis Sci* 1979;24:817–822.
91. Hogan PG, Hapel AJ, Doe WF. Lymphokine-activated and natural killer cell activity in human intestinal mucosa. *J Immunol* 1985;135: 1731–1738.
92. Burbige EJ, Sobky RZF. Endoscopic appearance of colonic lymphoid nodules: a normal variant. *Gastroenterology* 1977;72:524–526.
93. Watanabe H, Margulis AR, Harter L. The occurrence of lymphoid nodules in the colon of adults. *J Clin Gastroenterol* 1983;5:535–539.
94. Kealy WF. Colonic lymphoid-glandular complex (microbursa): nature and morphology. *J Clin Pathol* 1976;29:241–244.
95. Kealy WF. Lymphoid tissue and lymphoid-glandular complexes of the colon: relation to diverticulosis. *J Clin Pathol* 1976;29:245–249.
96. Heatley RV. The gastrointestinal mast cell. *Scand J Gastroenterol* 1983;18:449–453.
97. Sanderson IR, Slavin G, Walker-Smith JA. Density of mucosal mast cells in the lamina propria of the colon and terminal ileum of children. *J Clin Pathol* 1985;38:771–773.
98. Bacci S, Faussone-Pellegrini S, Mayer B, Romagnoli P. Distribution of mast cells in human ileocecal region. *Dig Dis Sci* 1995;40:357–365.
99. Kaye GI, Pascal RR, Lane N. The colonic pericryptal fibroblast sheath. Replication, migration, and cytodifferentiation of a mesenchymal cell system in adult tissue. III. Replication and differentiation in human hyperplastic and adenomatous polyps. *Gastroenterology* 1971; 60:515–536.
100. Sawicki W, Kucharczyk K, Szymanska K, Kujawa M. Lamina propria macrophages of intestine of the guinea pig: possible role in phagocytosis of migrating cells. *Gastroenterology* 1977;73:1340–1344.
101. Yunis E, Sherman FE. Macrophages of the rectal lamina propria in children. *Am J Clin Pathol* 1970;53:580–591.
102. Steer HW, Colin-Jones DG. Melanosis coli: studies of the toxic effects of irritant purgatives. *J Pathol* 1975;115:199–205.
103. Walker NI, Bennett RE, Axelsen RA. Melanosis coli: a consequence of anthraquinone-induced apoptosis of colonic epithelial cells. *Am J Pathol* 1988;131:465–476.
104. Azzopardi JG, Evans DJ. Mucoprotein-containing histiocytes (muciphages) in the rectum. *J Clin Pathol* 1966;19:368–374.
105. Lou TY, Teplitz C, Thayer WR. Ultrastructural morphogenesis of colonic PAS-positive macrophages ("colonic histiocytosis"). *Hum Pathol* 1971;2:421–439.
106. Aubock L, Hofler H. Extraepithelial intraneural endocrine cells as starting-points for gastrointestinal carcinoids. *Virchows Arch* [A] 1983;401:17–33.
107. Lundqvist M, Wilander E. Subepithelial neuroendocrine cells and carcinoid tumors of the human small intestine and appendix. A comparative immunohistochemical study with regard to serotonin, neuron-specific enolase and S-100 protein reactivity. *J Pathol* 1986;148: 141–147.
108. Miettinen M, Lehto V-P, Dahl D, Virtanen I. Varying expression of cytokeratin and neurofilaments in neuroendocrine tumors of human gastrointestinal tract. *Lab Invest* 1985;52:429–436.
109. Fenoglio CM, Kaye GI, Lane N. Distribution of human colonic lymphatics in normal, hyperplastic, and adenomatous tissue: its relationship to metastasis from small carcinomas in pedunculated adenomas, with two case reports. *Gastroenterology* 1973;64:51–66.
110. Lee AKC, DeLellis RA, Silverman ML, Wolfe HJ. Lymphatic and blood vessel invasion in breast carcinoma: a useful prognostic indicator? *Hum Pathol* 1986;17:984–987.
111. Martin SA, Perez-Reyes N, Mendelsohn G. Angioinvasion in breast carcinoma: an immunohistochemical study of factor VIII-related antigen. *Cancer* 1987;59:1918–1922.
112. Saigo PE, Rosen PP. The application of immunohistochemical stains to identify endothelial-lined channels in mammary carcinoma. *Cancer* 1987;59:51–54.
113. Fulcheri E, Cantino D, Bussolati G. Presence of intra-mucosal smooth muscle cells in normal human and rat colon. *Basic Appl Histochem* 1985;29:337–344.
114. Fulcheri E, Baracchini P, Lapertosa G, Bussolati G. Distribution and significance of the smooth muscle component in polyps of the large intestine. *Hum Pathol* 1988;19:922–927.
115. Levine DS. "Solitary" rectal ulcer syndrome: are "solitary" rectal ulcer syndrome and "localized" colitis cystica profunda analogous syndromes caused by rectal prolapse? *Gastroenterology* 1987;92: 243–253.
116. Lord MG, Valies P, Broughton AC. A morphologic study of the submucosa of the large intestine. *Surg Gynecol Obstet* 1977;145:55–60.
117. Krishnamurthy S, Schuffler MD. Pathology of neuromuscular disorders of the small intestine and colon. *Gastroenterology* 1987;93: 610–639.
118. Meier-Ruge W. Hirschsprung's disease: its etiology, pathogenesis and differential diagnosis. *Curr Top Pathol* 1974;59:131–179.
119. Weinberg AG. Hirschsprung's disease—a pathologist's view. *Perspect Pediatr Pathol* 1975;2:207–239.
120. Faussone-Pellegrini MS, Pantalone D, Cortesini C. Smooth muscle cells, interstitial cells of Cajal and myenteric plexus interrelationships in the human colon. *Acta Anat Basel* 1990;139:31–44.
121. Rumessen JJ, Peters S, Thuneberg L. Light- and electron microscopical studies of interstitial cells of Cajal and muscle cells at the submucosal border of human colon. *Lab Invest* 1993;68:481–495.
122. Rumessen JJ. Identification of interstitial cells of Cajal. Significance for studies of human small intestine and colon. *Dan Med Bull* 1994; 41:275–293.
123. Timmermans JP, Barbiers M, Scheuermann DW, et al. Nitric oxide synthase immunoreactivity in the enteric nervous system of the developing human digestive tract. *Cell Tissue Res* 1994;275: 235–245.
124. O'Kelly TJ, Davies JR, Brading AF, Mortensen NJ. Distribution of nitric oxide synthase containing neurons in the rectal myenteric plexus and anal canal. Morphologic evidence that nitric oxide mediates the rectoanal inhibitory reflex. *Dis Colon Rectum* 1994;37:350–357.
125. Faussone-Pellegrini MS, Bacci S, Pantalone D, Cortesini C, Mayer B. Nitric oxide synthase immunoreactivity in the human ileocecal region. *Neurosci Lett* 1994;170:261–265.
126. Matini P, Manneschi LI, Mayer B, Faussone-Pellegrini MS. Nitric oxide producing neurons in the human colon: an immunohistochemical and histoenzymatical study. *Neurosci Lett* 1995;193:17–20.
127. Faussone-Pellegrini MS, Bacci S, Pantalone D, Cortesini C. Distribu-

tion of VIP-immunoreactive nerve cells and fibers in the human ileocecal region. *Neurosci Lett* 1993;157:135–139.
128. Trudrung P, Furness JB, Pompolo S, Messenger JP. Locations and chemistries of sympathetic nerve cells that project to the gastrointestinal tract and spleen. *Arch Histol Cytol* 1994;57:139–150.
129. Krammer HJ, Karahan ST, Sigge W, Kuhnel W. Immunohistochemistry of markers of the enteric nervous system in whole-mount preparations of the human colon. *Eur J Pediatr Surg* 1994;4:274–278.
130. Messenger JP, Furness JB, Trudrung P. Locations of postganglionic nerve cells whose axons enter nerves originating from prevertebral ganglia. *Arch Histol Cytol* 1994;57:405–413.
131. Ibba-Manneschi L, Martini M, Zecchi-Orlandini S, Faussone-Pellegrini MS. Structural organization of enteric nervous system in human colon. *Histol Histopathology* 1995;10:17–25.
132. Wattchow DA, Brookes SJ, Costa M. The morphology and projections of retrogradely labeled myenteric neurons in the human intestine. *Gastroenterology* 1995;109:866–875.
133. Park HJ, Kamm MA, Abbasi AM, Talbot IC. Immunohistochemical study of the colonic muscle and innervation in idiopathic chronic constipation. *Dis Colon Rectum* 1995;38:509–513.
134. Fraser ID, Condon RE, Schulte WJ, DeCosse J, Cowles VE. Longitudinal muscle of muscularis externa in human and nonhuman primate colon. *Arch Surg* 1981;116:61–63.
135. Stoss F. Investigations of the muscular architecture of the rectosigmoid junction in humans. *Dis Colon Rectum* 1990;33:378–383.
136. Faussone-Pellegrini MS, Cortesini C, Pantalone D. Neuromuscular structures specific to the submucosal border of the human colonic circular muscle layer. *Can J Physiol Pharmacol* 1990;68:1437–1446.
137. Binder HJ, Sandle GI. Electrolyte absorption and secretion in the mammalian colon. In: Johnson LR, ed. *Physiology of the gastrointestinal tract. 2nd ed.* New York: Raven Press, 1987:1389–1418.
138. Bustos-Fernandez L, ed. *Colon structure and function.* New York: Plenum Medical, 1983.
139. Carey WD. Colon physiology: A review. *Cleve Clin Q* 1977;44: 73–81.
140. Gebbers J-O, Laissue JA, Otto HF. Modern aspects of the functional morphology of the colon. *Coloproctology* 1981;3:211–226.
141. Phillips SF. Functions of the large bowel: an overview. *Scand J Gastroenterol* 1984;19(suppl 93):1–12.
142. Christensen J. The response of the colon to eating. *Am J Clin Nutr* 1985;42:1025–1032.
143. Christensen J. Motility of the colon. In: Johnson LR, ed. *Physiology of the gastrointestinal tract. 2nd ed.* New York: Raven Press, 1987: 665–694.
144. Huizinga JD, Daniel EE. Control of human colonic motor function. *Dig Dis Sci* 1986;31:865–877.
145. Cummings JH. Fermentation in the human large intestine: evidence and implications for health. *Lancet* 1983;1:1206–1209.
146. Roediger WEW. Role of anaerobic bacteria in the metabolic welfare of the colonic mucosa in man. *Gut* 1980;21:793–798.
147. Schomacker KT, Frisoli JK, Compton CC, et al. Ultraviolet laser-induced fluorescence of colonic tissue: basic biology and diagnostic potential. *Lasers Surg Med* 1992;12:63–78.
148. Romer TJ, Fitzmaurice M, Cothren RM, et al. Laser-induced fluorescence microscopy of normal colon and dysplasia in colonic adenomas: implications for spectroscopic diagnosis. *Am J Gastroenterol* 1995; 90:81–87.
149. Rubin CE, Haggitt RC, Levine DS. Endoscopic mucosal biopsy. In: Yamada T, ed. *Textbook of gastroenterology.* New York: JB Lippincott, 1991:2479–2523.
150. Leriche M, Devroede G, Sanchez G, Rossano J. Changes in the rectal mucosa induced by hypertonic enemas. *Dis Colon Rectum* 1978;21: 227–236.
151. Lutzger LG, Factor SM. Effect of some water-soluble contrast media on the colonic mucosa. *Radiology* 1976;118:545–548.
152. Meisel JL, Bergman D, Graney D, Saunders DR, Rubin CE. Human rectal mucosa: proctoscopic and morphological changes caused by laxatives. *Gastroenterology* 1977;72:1274–1279.
153. Pike BF, Phillippi PJ, Lawson EH. Soap colitis. *N Engl J Med* 1971; 285:217–218.
154. Pockros PJ, Foroozan P. Golytely lavage versus a standard colonoscopy preparation: effect on normal colonic mucosal histology. *Gastroenterology* 1985;88:545–548.
155. Saunders DR, Sillery J, Rachmilewitz D. Effect of dioctyl sodium sulfosuccinate on structure and function of rodent and human intestine. *Gastroenterology* 1975;69:380–386.
156. Saunders DR, Sillery J, Rachmilewitz D, Rubin CE, Tytgat GN. Effect of bisacodyl on the structure and function of rodent and human intestine. *Gastroenterology* 1977;72:849–856.
157. Levine DS. Proctitis following colonoscopy. *Gastrointest Endosc* 1988;34:269–272.
158. Snover DC, Sandstad J, Hutton S. Mucosal pseudolipomatosis of the colon. *Am J Clin Pathol* 1985;84:575–580.
159. Pieterse AS, Leong AS-Y, Rowland R. The mucosal changes and pathogenesis of pneumatosis cystoides intestinalis. *Hum Pathol* 1985; 16:683–688.
160. Dankwa EK, Davies JD. Smooth muscle pseudotumors: a potentially confusing artifact of rectal biopsy. *J Clin Pathol* 1988;41: 737–741.
161. Carson FL. Polyfoam pads—a source of artifact. *J Histotechnol* 1981; 4:33–34.
162. Binder V. Cell density in lamina propria of the colon: a quantitative method applied to normal subjects and ulcerative colitis patients. *Scand J Gastroenterol* 1970;5:485–490.
163. Surawicz CM, Belic L. Rectal biopsy helps to distinguish acute self-limited colitis from idiopathic inflammatory bowel disease. *Gastroenterology* 1984;86:104–113.
164. Surawicz CM. Rectal biopsy diagnosis of inflammatory bowel disease. *Surv Dig Dis* 1984;2:164–172.
165. Levine DS, Reid BJ. Endoscopic biopsy technique for acquiring larger mucosal samples. *Gastrointest Endosc* 1991;37:332–337.
166. Allen TV, Achord JL. The pickle of proper bowel biopsy orientation. *Gastroenterology* 1977;72:774–775.
167. Haggitt RC. Handling of gastrointestinal biopsies in the surgical pathology laboratory. *Lab Med* 1982;13:272–278.

*Histology for Pathologists, second edition,*
Edited by Stephen S. Sternberg.
Lippincott-Raven Publishers, Philadelphia
© 1997.

# CHAPTER 23

# Vermiform Appendix

Glenn H. Segal and Robert E. Petras



## GROSS ANATOMY/SURGICAL PERSPECTIVE

The vermiform (wormlike) appendix is a slender tubular extension of the posteromedial aspect of the cecum originating below, and within 1 to 3 cm of, the ileocecal junction. Although the appendix has a relatively constant relationship with the cecum at the appendiceal base, the remainder of its length can be found in a variable number of positions, including retrocecal, subcecal, pelvic, and juxtaileal (1–3). A retrocecal position occurs most commonly, being present in nearly 70% of the population (3,4). Unusual locations including a vermiform appendix buried within the cecal wall have been documented (5). Although the appendix itself lacks taeniae, the base of the vermiform appendix lies at the convergence of the three cecal/ascending colon taeniae. These aid in locating the appendix when it is not readily apparent; the prominent anterior taenia is most easily traced for this purpose (1,6).

Vermiform appendices can vary remarkably in length but average 7 to 10 cm (2,4). The peritoneum covers almost all its external surface. The mesoappendix (mesentery of the appendix), a fold of peritoneum contiguous with the mesentery of the terminal ileum, extends along its length, terminating just proximal to the tip (1).

G. H. Segal: Division of Anatomic Pathology, University of Utah Health Sciences Center, Salt Lake City, Utah 84132.

R. E. Petras: Department of Pathology, Cleveland Clinic Foundation, Cleveland, Ohio 44195.

The appendiceal vascular supply courses within the mesoappendix, and with distal progression, these vessels gradually rest nearer to the appendiceal muscular wall. In the proximity of the tip where there is no mesoappendix, blood vessels lie essentially "unprotected" on its external surface (1). The appendicular artery, a derivative of the inferior branch of the ileocolic artery of the superior mesenteric trunk, provides the majority of blood to the appendix (4,7). However, a variable supply with accessory arterial contributions is not unusual (8). Branches of the ileocolic vein drain the appendiceal venous network into the superior mesenteric vein, and eventually into the portal circulation, whereas lymphatic vessels drain into regional (e.g., ileocolic) lymph nodes (6). Innervation is derived from branches of the vagus nerve (parasympathetic) and superior mesenteric plexus (sympathetic). Venous, lymphatic, and neural components closely follow the arterial vasculature (6).

Grossly, the external surface of the vermiform appendix appears smooth, pink–tan or gray, and glistening. The appendiceal diameter typically measures 5 to 8 mm. The wall is tan–white and the mucosal lining is light yellow, often disclosing a nodular appearance imparted by the characteristic and prominent lymphoid component (9). Because of these lymphoid aggregates, the central lumen on cross section is often irregular (stellate), rather than round. The normal luminal diameter measures 1 to 3 mm; however, in one study a luminal diameter of 1.2 cm or more was arbitrarily defined as dilatation (10). Focal occlusions of the appendiceal lumen are not uncommon (9).

## DEVELOPMENT OF THE VERMIFORM APPENDIX AND CONGENITAL ANOMALIES

The vermiform appendix originates from the primordial structure termed the cecal diverticulum (5,11). First apparent during the sixth week of fetal life, this blind-ended sac progressively develops. Its most proximal portion, in continuity with the remainder of the large bowel, enlarges and expands, forming the cecum proper, whereas its distal aspect or apex simply elongates, remains narrow, and becomes the vermiform appendix (11). Continued growth through infancy and childhood leads to differing cecoappendiceal relationships over this period. For example, the "infantile" cecoappendiceal junction lacks a conspicuous transition; the appendix arises from the inferior aspect of the cecum in this age group. In contrast, an abrupt, easily recognizable junction on the posteromedial cecum is observed in the adult (2).

Abnormal embryologic development can result in agenesis, hypoplasia, and various duplications or even triplication of the appendix (5,9,12–14). Duplication of the appendix can mimic cecal duplication. In general, appendiceal duplication is recognized by the presence of complete and separate inner circular and outer longitudinal muscle bands and the presence of a prominent lymphoid component (12).

Duplications have been well described and categorized and can be associated with other complex and life-threatening congenital anomalies. The classification of appendiceal duplications includes (a) type A, an appendix with a common base, single cecum, and bifurcated distal portion; (b) type B, two separate appendices with distinct bases arising from a single cecum; and (c) type C, two cecal structures, each with its own single appendix (12,13). The type C anomaly is always associated with other organ duplications and often necessitates extensive operative correction in infancy; a type B variant is also associated with other systemic anomalies (12). However, the majority of type B and all type A duplications are found incidentally or during operation for suspected appendicitis in older children and adults.

## FUNCTION

The exact role of the appendix is uncertain. However, rather than simply representing a vestigial, functionless structure, the abundant quantity of organized lymphoid tissue suggests involvement in mucosal immunity (15). It has been suggested that B-lymphocytes derived from the appendix migrate and populate distant sites of the gastrointestinal tract lamina propria and evolve in these widespread foci into functional immunoglobulin (Ig)A-secreting plasma cells (15,16). In this role, the appendix can both attenuate potentially harmful immunoglobulin responses and enhance regional mucosal immunity (16).

## NORMAL HISTOLOGY OF THE APPENDIX

The histologic composition of the appendix is similar to that of the large bowel. The four layers, from its luminal to external surface, include the mucosa, submucosa, muscularis externa (or propria), and serosa. The distinctive features of the appendix are emphasized.

### Mucosal Architecture and Design

A single layer of surface epithelium covers the luminal aspect of the appendiceal mucosa. This overlies the lamina propria within which crypts, or intestinal glands, contiguous with the surface epithelial cells are irregularly dispersed (Fig. 1). The lamina propria is a cellular layer with an abundant migratory cell component and prominent, often confluent, lymphoid aggregates. In contrast to the scattered lymphoid nodules within the large bowel proper, the appendix, particularly in young individuals, contains abundant and organized lymphoid structures spread around its entire luminal circumference. These lymphoid nodules often distort the luminal contour (9,17). The outermost component and limit of the mucosa is the muscularis mucosae. This slender fibromuscular band is poorly developed in the appendix and often focally deficient.

#### *Surface Epithelium*

Several different cell types comprise the surface epithelium. A prominent cell that can be identified at the light microscopic level is tall, columnar with eosinophilic cytoplasm, and has a round, basally located nucleus (Fig. 2). These cells represent several distinct cell types that can be differentiated at the ultrastructural level, including "senescent" mucous cells, so-called absorptive cells, and membranous or M cells (18–21). Goblet cells with distinctive apical mucin droplets surrounded by eosinophilic cytoplasm and undermined by an attenuated basal nucleus intermix with the

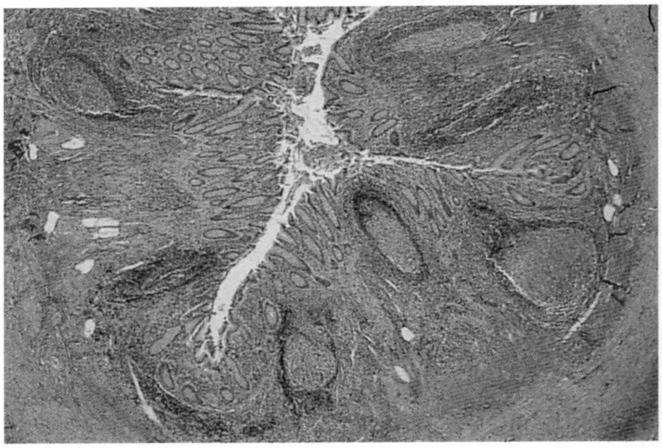

**FIG. 1.** Low-magnification view of a cross section of the vermiform appendix. The irregular (stellate) lumen is lined by a single layer of surface epithelium. The remainder of the mucosa (crypts, surrounding lamina propria, and the rather inconspicuous muscularis mucosae) surround this surface epithelial layer. Note the characteristic lymphoid nodules within the lamina propria that also extend into the submucosa.

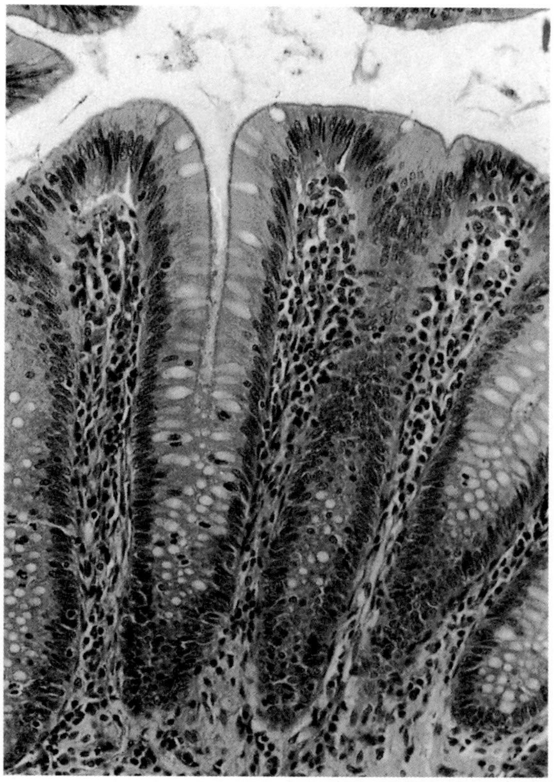

**FIG. 2.** The surface epithelium is composed of a single layer of predominantly columnar cells with rare interspersed goblet cells. The crypts are lined by a similar cellular composition but contain more goblet cells.

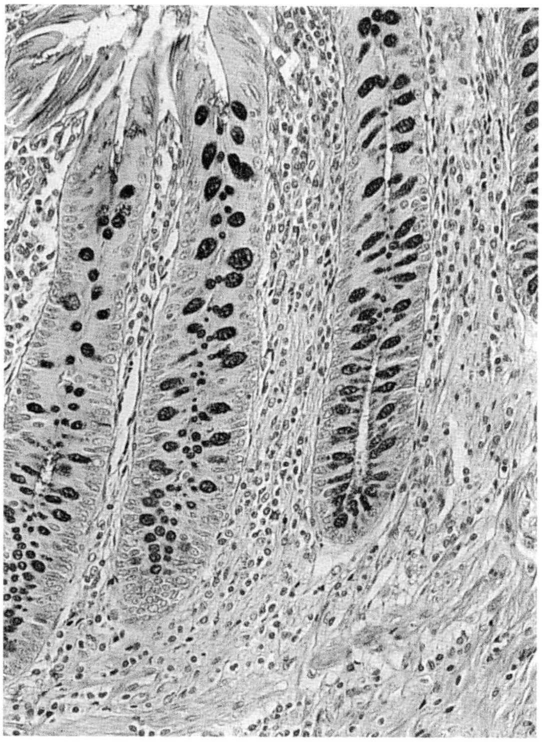

**FIG. 3.** Because goblet cells contain both neutral and acid mucopolysaccharides, their apical mucin droplets stain blue–purple with the mixed alcian blue–PAS preparation.

columnar cells (Fig. 2). The goblet cell apical mucin droplet contains both periodic acid-Schiff (PAS)-positive neutral mucin and alcian blue–positive acid sulfomucin. This combination results in the formation of a blue–purple color in a mixed alcian blue–PAS stain (19,22) (Fig. 3). Overlying lymphoid aggregates, as in other portions of the small and large bowel, is a specialized or follicle-associated epithelium that is distinct from the surrounding surface epithelium. It characteristically has fewer goblet cells, and many of the columnar cells are of the M-cell type (22) (Fig. 4). The M cell, a specialized epithelial cell, assists in luminal transport of antigens into the epithelium for appropriate immunologic processing (23,24). M cells are columnar in shape with an attenuated brush border; several lymphocytes are often seen deforming their dependent cytoplasm. Definitive characterization rests on ultrastructural examination, which shows apical cytoplasmic vesicles and shortened microvilli or microfolds (21,23). Because circumferentially distributed orga-

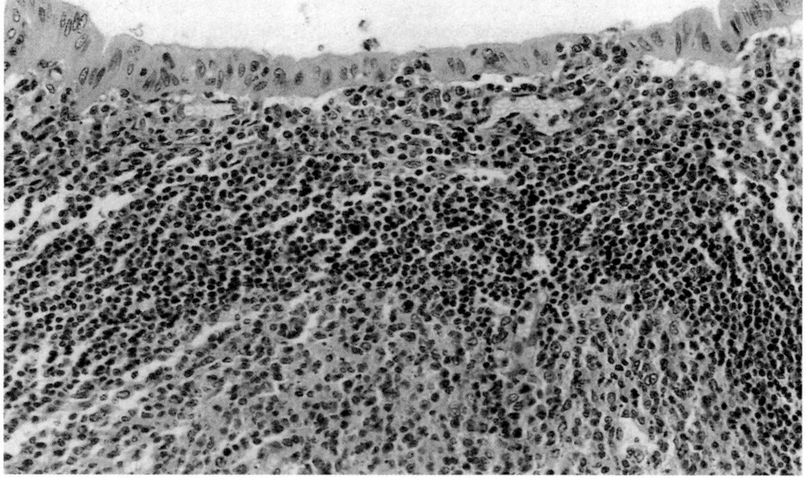

**FIG. 4.** Surface epithelium overlying a lymphoid aggregate composed solely of tall columnar cells without intermixed goblet cells. Ultrastructurally, most of these would be classified as membranous or M cells. Note the increased numbers of intraepithelial lymphocytes between the individual columnar cells. Directly beneath the epithelium is the dome region of the lymphoid nodule. The apical portion of the germinal center with surrounding mantle zone is present near the bottom of the micrograph.

nized lymphoid aggregates and lymphoid tissue are prominent in the normal appendix, the specialized follicle-associated epithelium often lines the majority of the appendiceal lumen. Thus, functionally, the surface epithelium is probably primarily involved in antigen processing as well as in forming a barrier to luminal contents. The luminal surface is also the site where senescent cells are sloughed into the lumen (19,20). Scattered endocrine cells can be seen within the surface epithelium but are more abundant in the underlying crypts. Migratory T- and B-lymphocytes can be found anywhere within the surface epithelium (25,26) but are more abundant in the follicle-associated epithelium (Fig. 4).

### *Crypt Epithelium*

In contrast to the colon, where crypts line up evenly like test tubes in a rack, appendiceal crypts are more irregular in shape, length, and distribution (27). In areas with abundant lymphoid tissue or lymphoid aggregates, crypts are typically absent (28) (Fig. 5).

Several different cell types line the crypts. The goblet and columnar cell variants discussed above are the most abundant (Figs. 2 and 6). Undifferentiated stem cells are scattered about but are inconspicuous. These are typically located at the crypt base, rest on the basement membrane, and do not extend to the crypt lumen; they are best identified by ultrastructural means (19). Isolated or clustered endocrine cells are seen along the crypt epithelium. Their appearance varies from a flask-shaped cell with a narrow strip of apical cytoplasm contiguous with the surface to a spindle-shaped cell with no luminal connection (29,30). Although some endocrine cells can be recognized on hematoxylin and eosin–stained sections by their eosinophilic, infranuclear granules (31) (Fig. 6), definitive identification rests on immunohistologic analysis for chromogranin (or other pan-reactive neuroendocrine marker) (Fig. 7) or ultrastructural analysis, which discloses neurosecretory granules within their cytoplasm. More specific immunohistologic methods show that endocrine cells within the appendiceal epithelium contain a variety of amine and polypeptide substances, including serotonin, substance P, somatostatin, and enteroglucagon (32). Paneth's cells also can be found in the crypt bases within the normal appendix in nearly 96% of specimens (33–35). This cell has a basally situated, round nucleus with a conspicuous nucleolus and abundant eosinophilic supranuclear granules (Fig. 8); their function remains unknown, but they probably play a role in microbial regulation (33).

Intraepithelial lymphocytes occur within the crypt epithe-

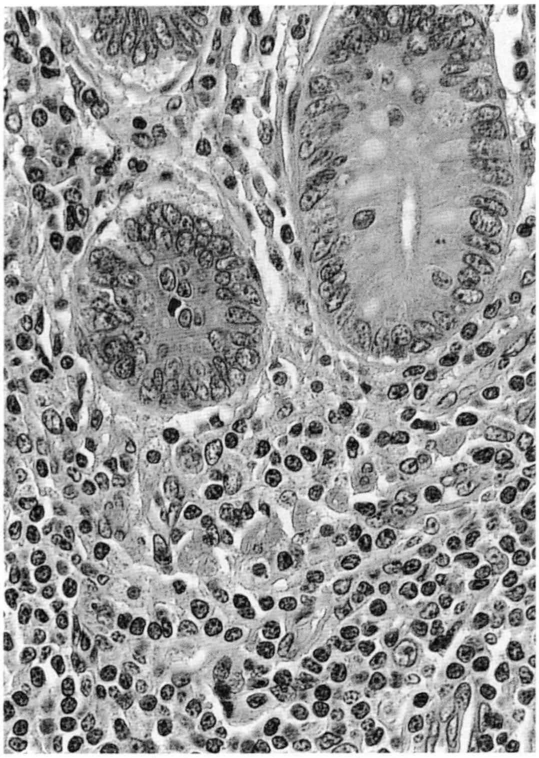

**FIG. 6.** Crypts lying within a normocellular lamina propria. The round or ovoid crypts are lined predominantly by eosinophilic columnar cells and goblet cells. A single endocrine cell (infranuclear eosinophilic granules) is present at the base of each crypt. The lamina propria contains plasma cells, lymphocytes, and scattered eosinophils. Note the polygonal cells with abundant eosinophilic cytoplasm within the lamina propria. These are the subepithelial (laminal proprial) endocrine cells that are often found near the crypt bases.

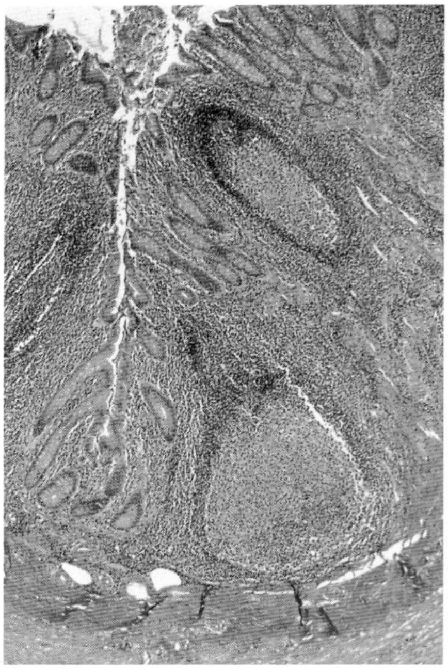

**FIG. 5.** Lymphoid aggregates are often a prominent component within the appendiceal mucosa. Note the absence of crypts in the region of the lymphoid nodules and the distortion of surrounding crypts. This is a normal finding in the appendix and is similar to the alteration associated with isolated lymphoid aggregates in the colon.

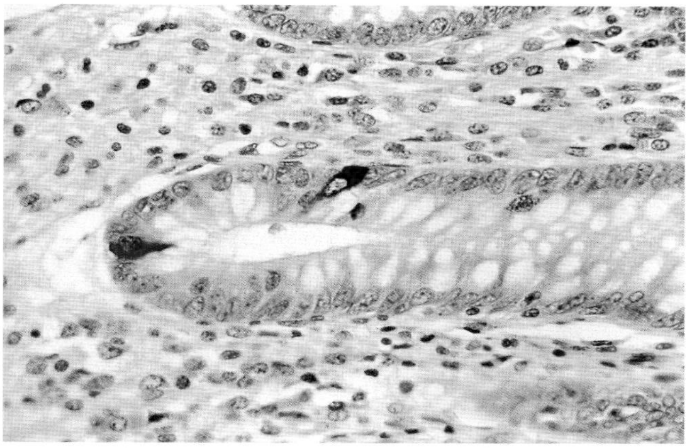

**FIG. 7.** Scattered endocrine cells within the epithelium of an appendiceal crypt highlighted with antichromogranin. Intense red–brown cytoplasmic staining is evident in these endocrine cells.

lium (36,37), but neutrophils and plasma cells are not normal constituents of either epithelial compartment. Rarely, gastric, ileal, or esophageal squamous type mucosa can be seen interrupting the normal appendiceal lining; some recognize these as true heterotopias (38–40).

The crypt functions in cell production and renewal because all cells of both epithelial compartments originate from the crypt's stem cells. Most of these cells travel to the surface epithelium, where they are subsequently sloughed intraluminally; the exception (Paneth's cell) remains in the crypt base (36,37). It is believed that apoptosis within the crypt probably functions to regulate cell migration toward the surface; however, it is uncertain whether this type of cell death is responsible for epithelial cell loss into the lumen (41).

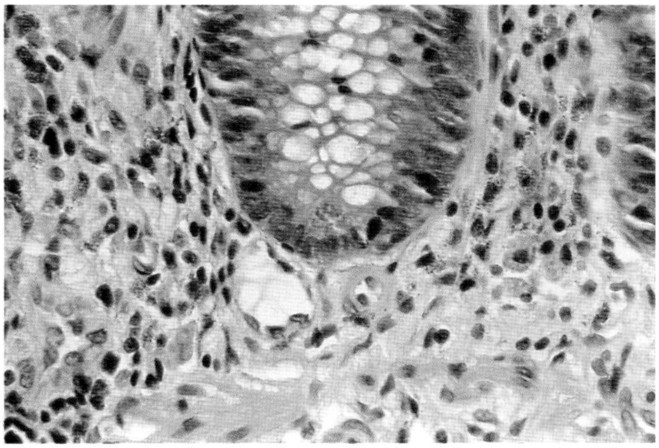

**FIG. 8.** Appendiceal crypt disclosing Paneth's cell (at its base) with characteristic supranuclear eosinophilic granules. The surrounding lamina propria has a conspicuous, albeit normal, quantity of eosinophils. Also, note the golden brown, granular pigment within the macrophages characteristic of melanosis "coli."

### *Subepithelial Basement Membrane*

A slender zone separates the epithelial compartments from the lamina propria and is composed of collagen and other matrix components (42). The subepithelial basement membrane stabilizes the epithelial layers. A PAS stain can be used to highlight this layer, which measures only microns in thickness (20,42) (Fig. 3).

### *Lamina Propria*

The lamina propria, the central layer of the mucosa, surrounds the crypts and forms a connective tissue framework around them. Its structural components are collagen and elastic fibers and associated fibroblasts intermingled with blood capillaries, lymphatics, and nerve fibers (18–20). As in the large bowel, its migratory cell component consists primarily of plasma cells and T-lymphocytes along with scattered macrophages, eosinophils, B-lymphocytes, and mast cells (18,26,43) (Figs. 6 and 8). However, depending on an individual's age, a varying number of organized lymphoid nodules distort the lamina proprial architecture. These lymphoid aggregates can extend beneath the muscularis mu-

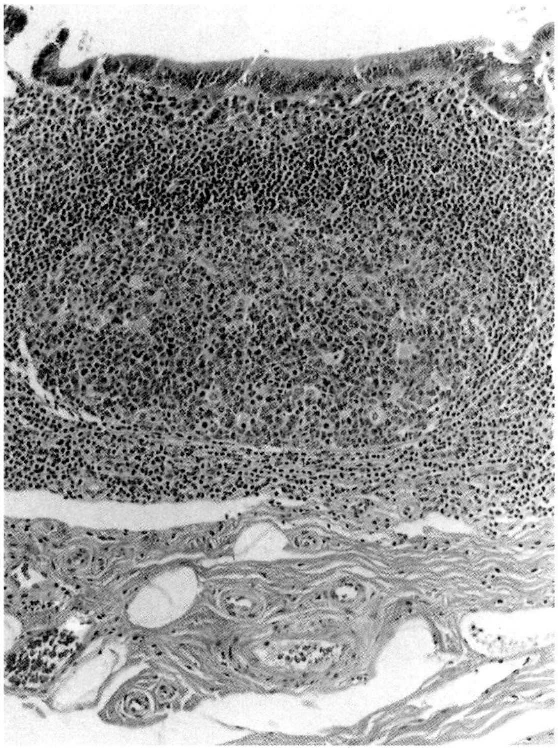

**FIG. 9.** Characteristic lymphoid nodule within lamina propria of appendix. A germinal center forms the "core" of the follicle and is surrounded, at least in part, by a mantle zone of small round lymphocytes. Between the overlying epithelium and the mantle is the dome, which contains a mixed cellular population of lymphocytes, plasma cells, and macrophages. A portion of the parafollicular area (T-cell zone) is seen at the right. Lymphatic and blood vessels are seen beneath the lymphoid nodule in the underlying superficial submucosa.

cosae into the underlying submucosa (Figs. 1 and 5), are often confluent, and appear similar in composition and function to the Peyer's patches of the small bowel (21). As in Peyer's patches (see Chapter 21), this lymphoid network of the appendix is compartmentalized into (a) follicle, (b) dome, (c) interfollicular (or parafollicular) region, and (d) follicle-associated epithelium (44–46) (Fig. 9). The follicle has, in most cases, a germinal center containing a polymorphic cellular population of small and large B-lymphocytes in various stages of maturation, occasional CD4-positive T-helper cells, and tingible body macrophages; these reactive centers invariably contain mitoses (15,45–47) (Fig. 10). Immediately surrounding the germinal center is the mantle zone, a darkly staining cuff of small, round B-lymphocytes. Overlying the lymphoid aggregate and beneath the epithelium is the dome region (mixed cell zone) composed of a heterogeneous population of cells including B- and T-lymphocytes, macrophages, and occasional plasma cells (21,46). Both the lymphoid aggregate and the dome region are supported by a structural framework provided by dendritic reticulum cells and their processes (16,47). A prominent collagenous network and closely associated lymphatic vessels surround and define the lymphoid nodule (16). This collagenous/fibrous border is contiguous with the connective tissue framework of the interfollicular zones and adjacent lamina propria (16). The zone surrounding a single lymphoid nodule (parafollicular region) and the area between confluent lymphoid aggregates (the interfollicular region) consist predominantly of T cells (46) (Fig. 11). Moreover, the ratio of T-helper/inducer (CD4-positive) to T-suppressor/cytotoxic (CD8-positive) lymphocytes is normally about 8:1 in these T cell–rich areas (46). Finally, the overlying epithelium as detailed previously is specialized and distinct from the usual surface epithelium.

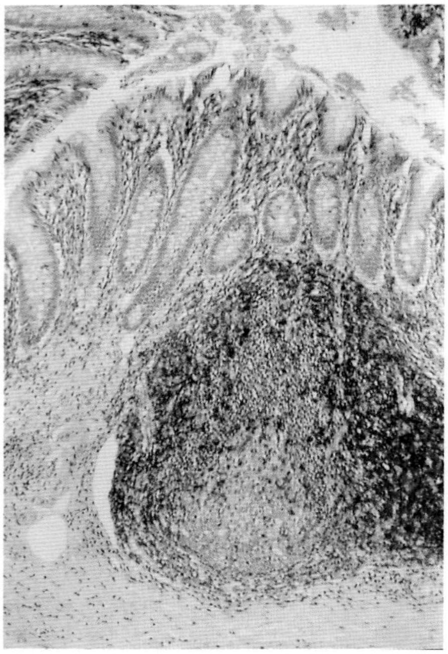

**FIG. 11.** Leu 22 (CD43), a pan–T-cell immunomarker, disclosing the characteristic T-lymphocyte distribution within the appendiceal mucosa. The lamina propria and interfollicular regions (between lymphoid follicles) are normally populated by numerous T-lymphocytes. There is a sprinkling of T cells within the germinal center; these are predominantly T-helper/inducer (CD4-positive) lymphocytes.

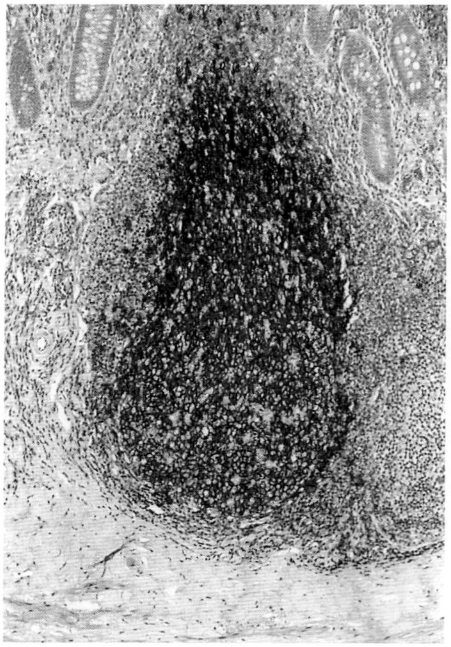

**FIG. 10.** The germinal center and mantle zone contain predominantly B-lymphocytes. L26, a pan–B-cell immunomarker, discloses this characteristic immunophenotype. Scattered macrophages and occasional T cells (see Fig. 11) are also normally found within the germinal center. Only scattered B cells are present within the interfollicular zone and adjacent lamina propria.

The immunophenotypic cellular composition of the appendiceal mucosa is different from the colon. Although the quantity of lymphoid and plasma cells containing IgA and IgM is similar in both, IgG-containing cells are more abundant in the appendix (15,46) (Fig. 12). In fact, nearly 50% of the those along the follicle borders, including the dome region, are IgG immunoreactive, whereas IgA-containing cells are more abundant in distant lamina proprial sites (15).

Lymphoid tissue, although a characteristic feature of the appendix, varies in quantity with age. The newborn's appendix contains scant or no lymphoid tissue. With increasing age the lymphoid nodules accumulate, peaking in the first decade (17,48). Lymphoid aggregates then steadily diminish in quantity throughout the remainder of life. However, appendices excised incidentally from middle-aged adults can still occasionally show a prominent organized lymphoid component (10). In contrast, lymphoid nodules and associated lymphocytes can be scant in the central obliterative

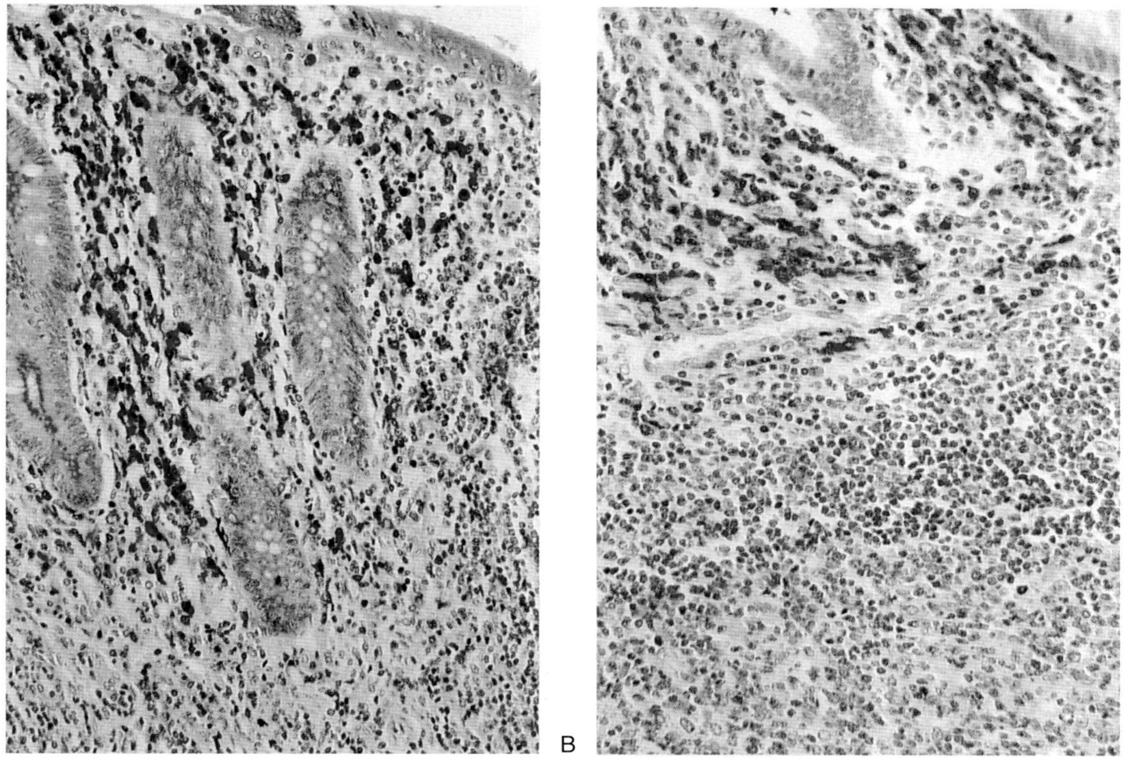

A B

**FIG. 12.** **A:** Immunohistologic preparation showing abundant IgA-containing plasma cells within lamina propria; the epithelial staining is a consequence of the secretory nature of the IgA molecule. **B:** Abundant IgG-bearing cells are characteristically located within the dome region and along the margins of lymphoid nodules in the appendix.

form of appendiceal neuroma (fibrous obliteration of the appendiceal lumen) and occasionally in appendices removed from normal patients at any age (10). Thus, a great range of normal variation exists in the appendix with respect to its lymphoid content.

Histiocytes with intracellular golden-brown pigment (lipofuschin), not infrequently observed in the colonic mucosa, can also be found in the appendiceal lamina propria; this alteration results from anthracene-containing laxative abuse and has been termed melanosis coli when seen in the colon proper (9,49) (Fig. 8). Interestingly, this pigmentation is a result of apoptosis induced by anthraquinones (41).

The lamina propria of the appendix contains a well-developed mucosal nervous plexus that is different from the more prominent submucosal and myenteric plexuses. Although all contain neurons (ganglion cells), Schwann cells, and neural processes (axons and neuropil), only the mucosal plexus contains endocrine (neurosecretory) cells. As a consequence, this network has been termed the mucosal neuroendocrine complex (50). These complexes located just beneath the crypts are composed of collections of endocrine cells, seen on hematoxylin and eosin–stained preparations as polygonal cells with pale granular cytoplasm (Fig. 6), often intimately associated with spindled Schwann cells, neural processes, and occasional neurons. These collections, or neuroendocrine ganglia, are interconnected by neural fibers that can be highlighted immunohistologically with antibody preparations to neuron-specific enolase and, in a subset, to substance P (32); anti–S-100 also can outline this network as it marks the accompanying Schwann cells. The mucosal plexus also communicates with other neural networks of the enteric nervous system (50–53). The subepithelial endocrine cells are not always conspicuous but can be highlighted using general neuroendocrine immunomarkers such as anti-chromogranin (Fig. 13) and anti–neuron-specific enolase or by using electron microscopy (54,55). Most of these cells have been shown to contain serotonin by specific immunohistologic analysis (51,55). The mucosal neuroendocrine complex is believed to modulate neural communication, through serotonin mediators, between the epithelium and the deeper submucosal and intermuscular plexuses (55). Interestingly, because most appendiceal carcinoids are biphasic, consisting of an admixture of endocrine cells and S-100–positive Schwann cells (similar to the architecture of the mucosal neuroendocrine complex), the majority of these appendiceal neoplasms are believed to be derived from these lamina proprial endocrine cells rather than from the epithelium-based ones (51).

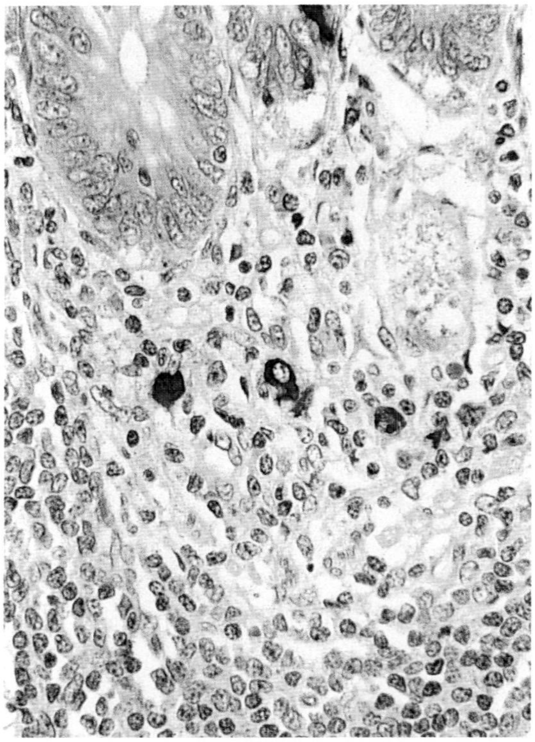

**FIG. 13.** Anti-chromogranin highlights the subepithelial (lamina proprial) endocrine cells beneath the crypts. These are more prominent and abundant in the appendix than in any other portion of gastrointestinal tract. Note also the epithelial-based endocrine cell in the overlying crypt.

### *Muscularis Mucosae*

The muscularis mucosae is a thin band of fibromuscular tissue separating the lamina propria and mucosal epithelium from the underlying submucosa. It characteristically forms a continuous layer in the large bowel (18), but in the appendix the muscularis mucosae is attenuated, poorly developed, and often focally absent, particularly in the region of penetrating lymphoid aggregates (28,56) (Fig. 14). In these areas the muscularis mucosae may exist solely as isolated smooth muscle cells in the underlying submucosa (56).

### Submucosa

The submucosa separates the mucosa from the muscularis externa. Its loose architectural framework contains a meshwork of collagenous and elastic fibers and associated fibroblasts (Fig. 15). The submucosa can also contain inconspicuous migratory cells such as macrophages, lymphoid and plasma cells, and mast cells along with adipose tissue (17,57) (Fig. 14). The morphologic appearance of the appendiceal submucosa and its primary role in maintaining structure are similar throughout the gastrointestinal tract (57). Arterioles, venules, blood capillaries, and lymphatic vessels are a prominent component of the submucosa (7,18) (Fig. 15). Lymphatic vessels (or sinuses) are most prominent just beneath the bases of lymphoid aggregates (16). Neural structures, particularly Meissner's plexus, are also conspicuous (Fig. 16). This plexus consists of ganglia, collections of neurons (ganglion cells) with associated neuronal processes, and Schwann cells that interconnect, creating a neural network throughout the submucosal layer (58,59). The ganglion cell is large and oval with abundant eosinophilic cytoplasm; its vesicular nucleus is often eccentrically placed and contains a prominent nucleolus. The surrounding spindle and wavy Schwann cell component of the ganglia is less conspicuous on hematoxylin and eosin–stained preparations but can be highlighted with anti–S-100 (Fig. 16).

### Muscularis Externa, Subserosal Region, and the Serosa

The thick smooth muscle layer lying between the submucosa and serosal portions of the appendix is the muscularis externa or propria. It is separated into an inner circular layer

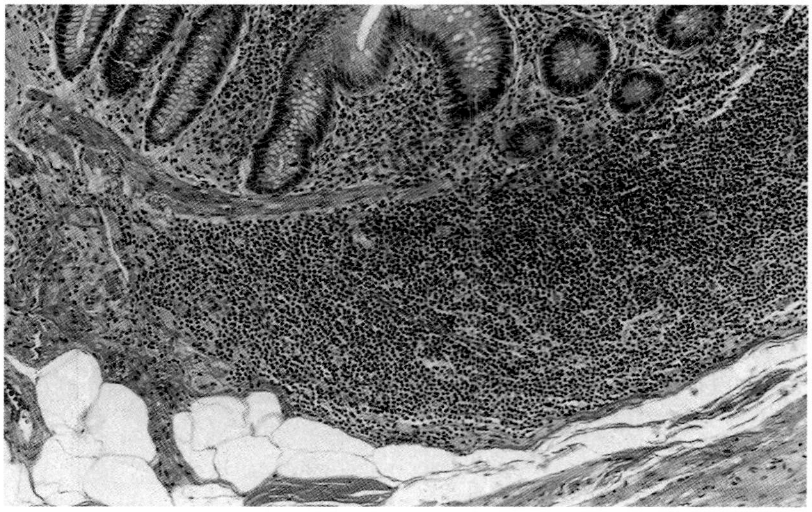

**FIG. 14.** Characteristic focal deficiency of muscularis mucosae in region of lymphoid nodule. There is adipose tissue within the submucosa; this is a normal finding.

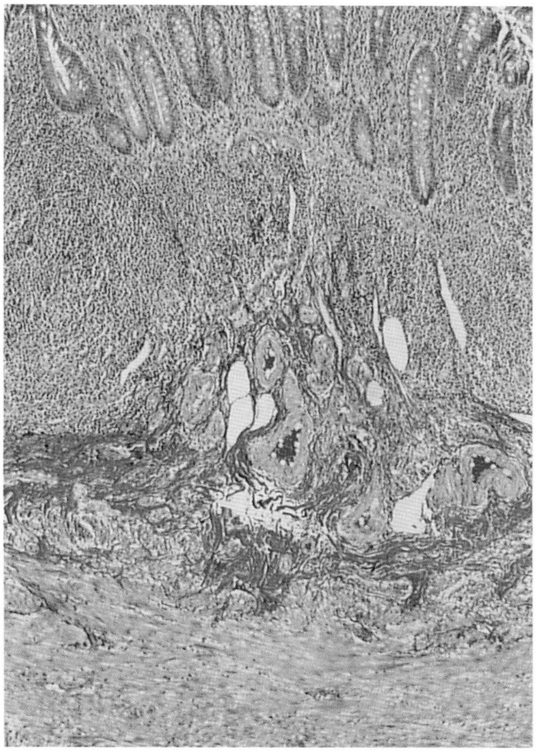

**FIG. 15.** Normal appendiceal submucosa outlined in blue, highlighting its prominent collagenous framework. Numerous vascular spaces are also present within this layer. The mucosa (crypts) is above and the inner circular layer of the muscularis externa is below (Masson's trichrome.)

and an outer longitudinal band (28). The individual smooth muscle cells are oval with blunted ends and form bundles of varying size. Occasionally, granular degeneration (eosinophilic cytoplasmic granularity) of individual or groups of smooth muscle cells is seen, particularly within the inner circular layer (56,60). Between the two muscle bands lies the myenteric (Auerbach's) plexus, which is similar morphologically and functionally to the previously described submucosal plexus of Meissner (59) (Fig. 17). Additionally, blood and lymphatic vessels and nerve fibers course through this muscular layer (16). Just external to the outer longitudinal smooth muscle layer is the subserosal region, consisting of loose connective tissue and ramifying blood vessels, lymphatics, and nerves. The exteriormost surface, or serosa, is lined by a single layer of cuboidal mesothelial cells that overlies a slender band of fibrous tissue. Only the attachment of the fibrofatty mesoappendix lacks a serosa (1).

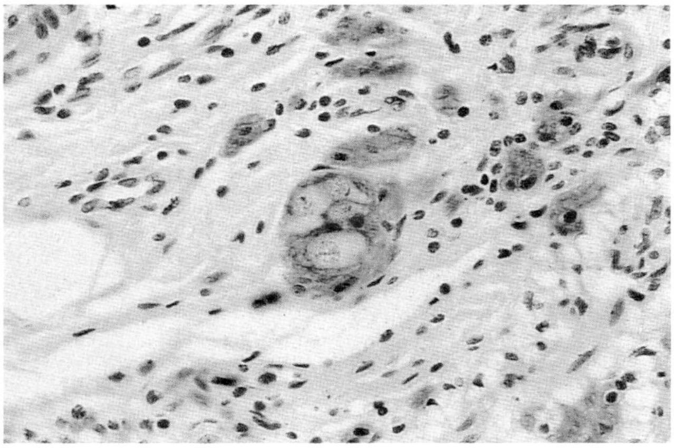

**FIG. 16.** Submucosal neural network outlined with anti–S-100. A single ganglion of Meissner's plexus is at the center; the ganglion cells (neurons) have abundant pale cytoplasm, a large eccentric nucleus, and show no immunoreactivity. The Schwann cells of the ganglion and those ensheathing the neuronal processes of the remainder of the plexus are highlighted.

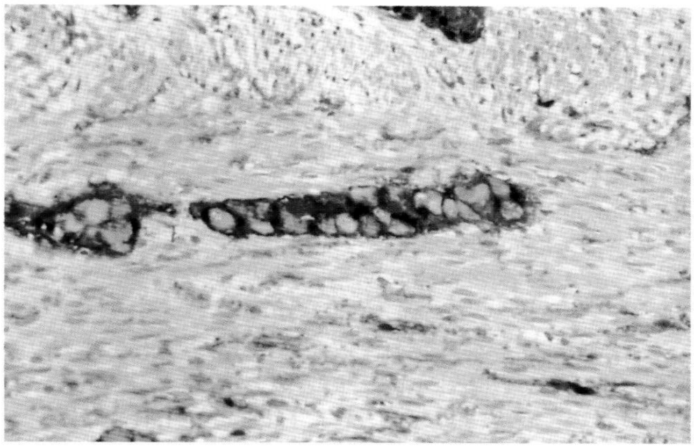

**FIG. 17.** Anti–S-100 highlighting Schwann cells of the neural network of the muscularis externa and a ganglion of the myenteric (Auerbach's) plexus.

## SPECIAL CONSIDERATIONS

### Normal Variation of Mucosal Inflammation Versus Acute Appendicitis

Acute appendicitis is usually characterized by an abundant neutrophilic and eosinophilic infiltrate within the mucosa, submucosa, and often muscularis externa with at least focal mucosal ulceration; frequently suppurative inflammation extends into and through the appendiceal wall (9,10). However, the changes seen in early appendicitis can be quite minimal, and criteria considered sufficient to diagnose early acute appendicitis have varied (9,10,61–66). We agree that "reactive" lymphoid follicles are not a reliable sign of acute appendicitis (9). Focal collections of neutrophils within the lumen and lamina propria have been considered nondiagnostic by some investigators because many "incidental" appendectomy specimens contain these changes (9,10,61, 64–66). However, we believe that if care is taken to recognize marginating neutrophils and early mucosal migration of these acute inflammatory cells (i.e., a result of the operative procedure alone), then other collections of neutrophils within the mucosa or intraluminal pus reflect stasis, infection, and changes of early appendicitis (62–64). Whether acute appendicitis becomes chronic or whether it can be recognized in a chronic state has long been debated (63). Fibrous obliteration of the appendiceal lumen is probably not a sequelae of acute appendicitis (53). However, prominent fibrosis, a marked chronic inflammatory cell infiltrate within the wall, and granulation tissue are abnormal and suggest an organizing appendicitis (9). Occasional specimens exhibit infiltration of the appendiceal wall by eosinophilic leukocytes with no other apparent abnormality (10). This change could reflect appendicitis elsewhere in the specimen that was not sampled; however, it remains possible that an infiltrate composed predominantly of eosinophils could represent appendicitis in a resolving phase or be a manifestation of "eosinophilic gastroenteritis" (62,67,68).

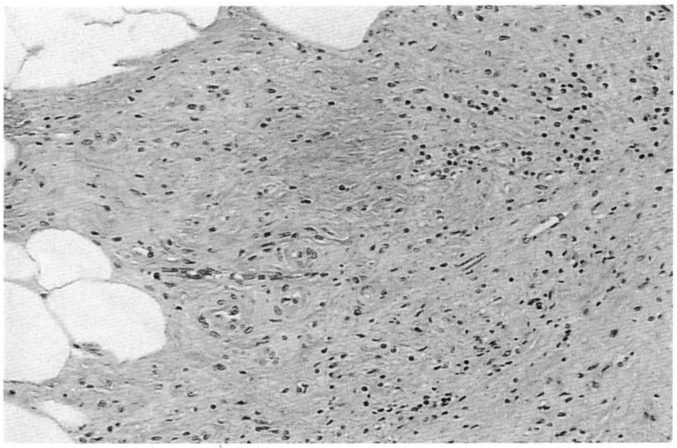

**FIG. 19.** High magnification of Fig. 18 showing spindled cell proliferation in an eosinophilic, fibromyxoid background.

### Obliteration of the Appendiceal Lumen (Appendiceal Neuromas)

Obliteration of the appendiceal lumen with absence of the lining mucosa and underlying crypts frequently occurs and has a prevalence in surgical specimens of nearly 30% (9,53). This process usually affects the distal aspect or just the tip, but occasionally the entire lumen is obliterated. This process is often termed fibrous obliteration; however, more recent studies have shown that in some cases the occlusive proliferation appears to be predominantly neurogenic (32,53,69). Other diagnostic terms have been proposed, including neurogenic appendicopathy and appendiceal neuroma. The typical appendiceal neuroma, or the central obliterative form, is composed of a collection of spindle cells in a loose myxoid background with varying amounts of collagen, fat, and chronic inflammatory cells (Figs. 18 and 19). This typically occludes the lumen and blends imperceptibly with the surrounding submucosa (53). The involved segment usually lacks a mucosa, and lymphoid follicles are typically not seen

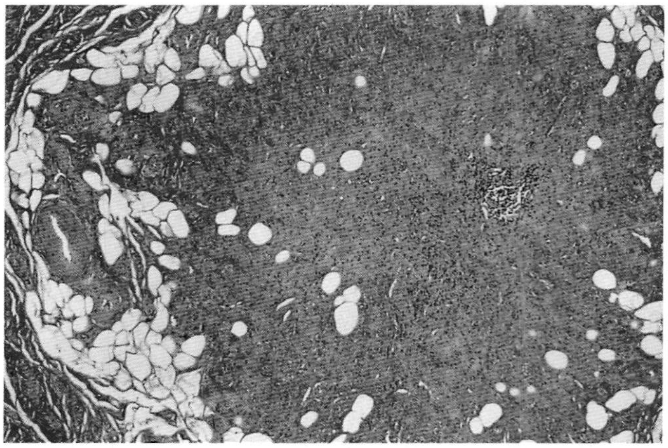

**FIG. 18.** Obliteration of appendiceal lumen. The occlusive proliferation is composed of spindled cells within a collagenous and myxoid background, along with scattered adipocytes. A focus of chronic inflammatory cells is also present.

(20). Immunostaining for neuron-specific enolase and S-100 highlights the spindle cells and identifies their neuronal (axons) and perineuronal (Schwann cell) nature, respectively (32,53) (Fig. 20). Moreover, endocrine cells visualized with anti–neuron-specific enolase and anti-chromogranin (Fig. 21) occur in many of the cases, usually intermingled with the other elements; serotonin and somatostatin have been identified in some of these endocrine cells by immunohistologic methods (32,53). Ultrastructural analysis discloses neuronal processes, Schwann cells, and cells with neurosecretory granules (endocrine cells) corroborating the immunostaining results (53).

Another variant of this entity, the intramucosal appendiceal neuroma, primarily affects the mucosa, causing no luminal obliteration. Although morphologically similar to the central obliterative form, this intramucosal variant deceptively expands the lamina propria, separates the crypts, and replaces the usual prominent migratory cell population (53) (Fig. 22). S-100 immunostaining can be helpful in visualizing these more subtle changes.

Both of these entities are believed to be proliferative rather than involutional, progressing through consecutive

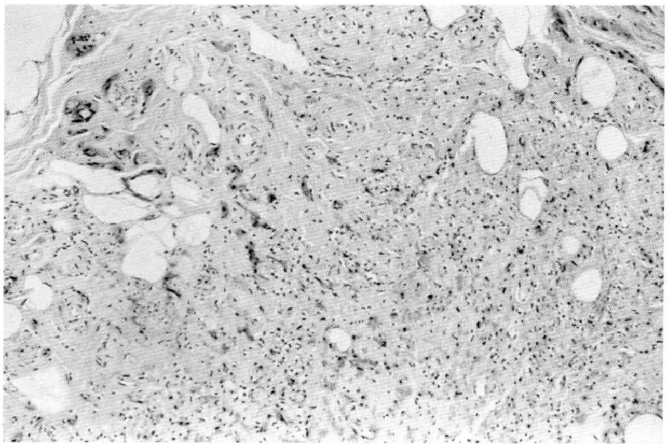

**FIG. 20.** Prominent neurogenic (Schwann cell) component highlighted by anti–S-100 within the obliterated lumen.

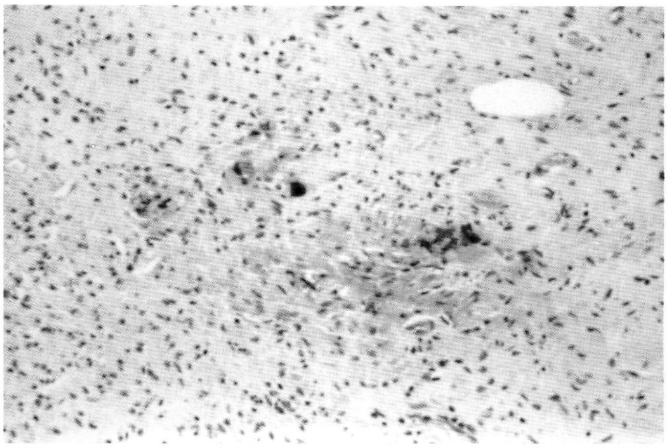

**FIG. 21.** Scattered endocrine (neurosecretory) cells are evident within the obliterative luminal proliferation as highlighted by antichromogranin; specific immunomarkers show some of these to contain serotonin or somatostatin.

stages of growth, regression, and finally an end-stage with fibrosis (53,70). Overlapping features are therefore expected with varied admixtures of neurogenic components, collagen, and fat. It is hypothesized that associated endocrine cell hyperplasia often found in adjacent uninvolved appendiceal segments may be responsible for painful stimuli mimicking typical acute appendicitis (53). However, appendiceal neuromas are often found in specimens removed at incidental appendectomy.

### Mucocele of the Appendix

The term *mucocele* has been used to describe a dilated appendiceal lumen filled with mucin (71). *Mucocele,* however, should not be used as a specific diagnostic term because the condition is almost always caused by a neoplastic proliferation, either a mucinous cystadenoma or mucinous cystadenocarcinoma (63,71,72). Characteristic architectural and cytologic features should permit identification of these entities.

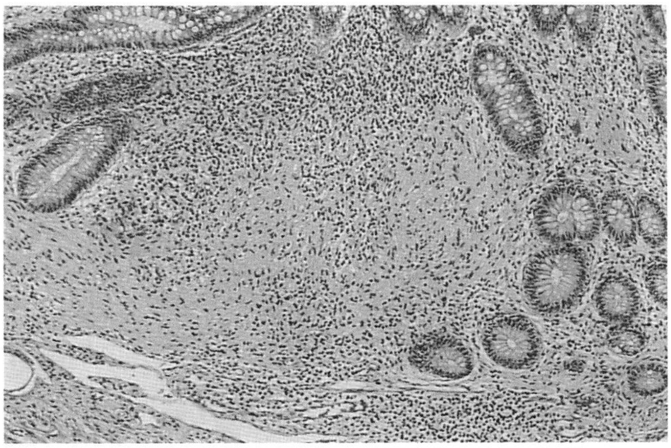

**FIG. 22.** Intramucosal variant of appendiceal neuroma. The characteristic subtle spindle cell (schwannian) proliferation expands the lamina propria and separates the crypts. A diminished number of migratory cells is evident in this area.

### Dissection and Processing Techniques

Gross dissection and processing of the appendix are generally straightforward. Routine description of size, appearance, and any unusual lesions should be recorded. Luminal patency should be assessed (i.e., obliteration or dilatation) along with the focality and regional distribution of any changes. The tip should be closely inspected for carcinoid tumors because these commonly occur in the distal portion of the appendix (9,73). When grossly evident, they often appear as bulbous, tan–yellow expansions or nodules. However, a routine section of the tip is standard at most institutions and will identify small, grossly unidentifiable tumors (9). The common recommendation of a longitudinal section of the distal several centimeters is often difficult to orient, and we prefer a cross section of the tip. In the usual specimen, 1-cm serial cross-sectioning is performed along the entire length of the appendix. Two cross sections, one from the middle and one of the proximal line of resection, should be submitted for embedding. Because neoplastic proliferations of the appendix (e.g., mucinous cystadenoma/cystadenocarcinoma, carcinoid tumor, and its variants) are not infrequently discovered incidentally during microscopic evaluation of the specimen, we routinely sample the margin of resection. Otherwise, it could be difficult to reconstruct the gross specimen in an attempt to assess the adequacy of excision. The choice of a fixative is not crucial. However, we prefer the superior nuclear detail afforded by Hollande's solution over routine 4% formaldehyde solution. Modifications of dissection and processing may be necessary in certain situations.

## REFERENCES


1. Williams PL, Warwick R, Dyson M, Bannister LH, eds. *Gray's anatomy. 37th ed.* New York: Churchill Livingstone; 1989.
2. Buschard K, Kjaeldgaard A. Investigation and analysis of the position, fixation, length, and embryology of the vermiform appendix. *Acta Chir Scand* 1973;139:293–298.
3. Wakeley CPG. The position of the vermiform appendix as ascertained by an analysis of 10,000 cases. *J Anat* 1933;67:277–283.
4. Thorek P. *Anatomy in surgery. 3rd ed.* New York: Springer-Verlag; 1985.
5. Abramson DJ. Vermiform appendix located within the cecal wall. Anomalies and bizarre locations. *Dis Colon Rectum* 1983;26:386–389.
6. Hollinshead WH, Rosse C. *Textbook of anatomy. 4th ed.* New York: Harper & Row; 1985.
7. Parks DA, Jacobson ED. Physiology of the splanchnic circulation. *Arch Intern Med* 1985;145:1270–1281.
8. Solanke TF. The blood supply of the vermiform appendix in Nigerians. *J Anat* 1968;102:353–361.
9. Gray GF Jr, Wackym PA. Surgical pathology of the vermiform appendix. In: Sommers SC, Rosen PP, Fechner RE, eds. *Pathology annual. Part 2.* Norwalk, CT: Appleton-Century-Croft; 1986:111–144.
10. Butler C. Surgical pathology of acute appendicitis. *Hum Pathol* 1981; 12:871–878.
11. Moore KL. *Clinically oriented embryology. 3rd ed.* Philadelphia: WB Saunders; 1982.
12. Bluett MK, Halter SA, Salhany KE, O'Leary JD. Duplication of the ap-

pendix mimicking adenocarcinoma of the colon. *Arch Surg* 1987;122: 817-820.
13. Wallbridge PH. Double appendix. *Br J Surg* 1963;50:346–347.
14. Tinckler LF. Triple appendix vermiformis—a unique case. *Br J Surg* 1968;55:79–81.
15. Bjerke K, Brandtzaeg P, Rognum TO. Distribution of immunoglobulin producing cells is different in normal human appendix and colon mucosa. *Gut* 1986;27:667–674.
16. Bockman DE. Functional histology of appendix. *Arch Histol Jpn* 1983; 46:271–292.
17. Hwang JMS, Krumbhaar EB. The amount of lymphoid tissue of the human appendix and its weight at different age period. *Am J Med Sci* 1940;199:75–83.
18. Hamilton SR. Structure of the colon. *Scand J Gastroenterol* 1984; 19(suppl 93):13–23.
19. Shamsuddin AM, Phelps PC, Trump BF. Human large intestinal epithelium: light microscopy, histochemistry and ultrastructure. *Hum Pathol* 1982;13:790–803.
20. Levine DS, Haggitt RC. Normal histology of the colon. *Am J Surg Pathol* 1989;13:966–984.
21. Bockman DE, Cooper MD. Early lymphoepithelial relationships in human appendix: a combined light and electron microscopic study. *Gastroenterology* 1975;68:1160–1168.
22. Filipe MI. Mucins in the human gastrointestinal epithelium: a review. *Invest Cell Pathol* 1979;2:195–216.
23. Owen RL, Jones AL. Epithelial cell specialization within human Peyer's patches: an ultrastructural study of intestinal lymphoid follicles. *Gastroenterology* 1974;66:189–203.
24. Wolf JL, Bye WA. The membranous epithelial (M) cell and the mucosal immune system. *Annu Rev Med* 1984;35:95–112.
25. Dobbins WO. Human intestinal intraepithelial lymphocytes. *Gut* 1986; 27:972–985.
26. Bartnik W, ReMine SG, Chiba M, Thayer WR, Shorter RG. Isolation and characterization of colonic intraepithelial and lamina proprial lymphocytes. *Gastroenterology* 1980;78:976–985.
27. Fawcett DW. *Bloom and Fawcett: A textbook of histology. 11th ed.* Philadelphia: WB Saunders; 1986.
28. Neutra MR, Padykula HA. The gastrointestinal tract. In: Weiss L, ed. *Modern concepts of gastrointestinal histology.* New York: Elsevier; 1984:658–706.
29. Lewin KJ. The endocrine cells of the gastrointestinal tract: the normal endocrine cells and their hyperplasias, part 1. In: Sommers SC, Rosen PP, Fechner RE, eds. *Pathology annual.* Norwalk, CT: Appleton-Century-Croft; 1986:1–27.
30. Sjolund K, Sanden G, Hakanson R, Sundler F. Endocrine cells in human intestine. *Gastroenterology* 1983;85:1120–1130.
31. Millikin PD. Eosinophilic argentaffin cells in the human appendix. *Arch Pathol Lab Med* 1974;98:393–395.
32. Hofler H, Kasper M, Heitz PU. The neuroendocrine system of normal human appendix, ileum, and colon and in neurogenic appendicopathy. *Virchows Arch [A]* 1983;399:127–140.
33. Sandow MJ, Whitehead R. The Paneth cell. *Gut* 1979;20:420–431.
34. Geller SA, Thung SN. Morphologic unity of Paneth cells. *Arch Pathol Lab Med* 1983;107:476–479.
35. Vestfrid MA, Zabala Suarez JE. Paneth's cells in the human appendix: a statistical study. *Acta Anat* 1977;97:347–350.
36. Eastwood GL. Gastrointestinal epithelial renewal. *Gastroenterology* 1977;72:962–975.
37. Lipkin M. Proliferation and differentiation of normal and diseased gastrointestinal cells. In: Johnson LR, ed. *Physiology of the gastrointestinal tract. 2nd ed.* New York: Raven Press; 1987:255–284.
38. Aubrey DA. Gastric heterotopia in the vermiform appendix. *Arch Surg* 1970;101:628–629.
39. Ashley DJB. Aberrant mucosa in the vermiform appendix. *Br J Surg* 1957;45:372–373.
40. Droga BW, Levine S, Barber JJ. Heterotopic gastric and oesophageal tissue in the vermiform appendix. *Am J Clin Pathol* 1963;40:190–193.
41. Watson AJM. Necrosis and apoptosis in the gastrointestinal tract. *Gut* 1995;37:165–167.
42. Gledhill A, Cole FM. Significance of basement membrane thickening in the human colon. *Gut* 1984;25:1085–1088.
43. Heatley RV. The gastrointestinal mast cell. *Scand J Gastroenterol* 1983;18:449–453.
44. Tomasi TB. Mechanisms of immune regulation at mucosal surfaces. *Rev Infect Dis* 1983;5:5784–5792.
45. Kagnoff MF. Immunology and disease of the gastrointestinal tract. In: Sleisenger MH, Fordtran JS, eds. *Gastrointestinal disease.* Philadelphia: WB Saunders; 1989:114–144.
46. Spencer J, Finn T, Isaacson PG. Gut associated lymphoid tissue: a morphological and immunocytochemical study of the human appendix. *Gut* 1985;26:672–679.
47. van der Valk P, Meijor CJLM. The histology of reactive lymph nodes. *Am J Surg Pathol* 1987;11:866–882.
48. Berry RJA. The vermiform appendix of man and the structural changes therein coincident with age. *J Anat Physiol* 1905;40:247–256.
49. Walker NI, Bennett RE, Axelson RA. Melanosis coli: a consequence of anthraquinone-induced apoptosis of colonic epithelial cells. *Am J Pathol* 1988;131:465–476.
50. Papadaki L, Rode J, Dhillon AP, Dische FE. Fine structure of a neuroendocrine complex in the mucosa of the appendix. *Gastroenterology* 1983;84:490–497.
51. Lundgvist M, Wilander E. Subepithelial neuroendocrine cells and carcinoid tumors of the human small intestine and appendix. A comparative immunohistochemical study with regard to serotonin, neuron-specific enolase and S-100 protein reactivity. *J Pathol* 1986;148: 141–147.
52. Millikin P. Extraepithelial enterochromaffin cells and Schwann cells in the human appendix. *Arch Pathol Lab Med* 1983;107:189–194.
53. Stanley MW, Cherwitz D, Hagen K, Snover DC. Neuromas of the appendix. A light-microscopic, immunohistochemical and electron-microscopic study of 20 cases. *Am J Surg Pathol* 1986;10:801–815.
54. Facer P, Bishop AE, Lloyd RV, Wilson BS, Hennessy RJ, Polak JM. Chromogranin: a newly recognized marker of endocrine cells in the human gastrointestinal tract. *Gastroenterology* 1985;89:1366–1373.
55. Rode J, Dhillon AP, Papadaki L. Serotonin-immunoreactive cells in the lamina propria plexus of the appendix. *Hum Pathol* 1983;14:464–469.
56. Sobel HJ, Marquet E, Schwarz R. Granular degeneration of appendiceal smooth muscle. *Arch Pathol* 1971;92:427–432.
57. Lord MG, Valies P, Broughton AC. A morphologic study of the submucosa of the large intestine. *Surg Gynecol Obstet* 1977;145:55–60.
58. Gershon MD, Erde SM. The nervous system of the gut. *Gastroenterology* 1981;80:1571–1594.
59. Krishnamurthy S, Schuffler MD. Pathology of neuromuscular disorders of the small intestine and colon. *Gastroenterology* 1987;93:610–639.
60. Hausman R. Granular cells in musculature of the appendix. *Arch Pathol* 1963;75:360–372.
61. Pieper R, Kager L, Nasman P. Clinical significance of mucosal inflammation of the vermiform appendix. *Ann Surg* 1983;197:368–374.
62. Petras RE. Non-neoplastic intestinal diseases. In: Sternberg SS, ed. *Diagnostic surgical pathology.* New York: Raven Press; 1989:967–1014.
63. Morson BC, Dawson IMP, Day DW, Jass JR, Price AB, Williams GT. *Morson and Dawson's gastrointestinal pathology. 3rd ed.* Oxford: Blackwell Scientific; 1990.
64. Schenken JR, Anderson TR, Coleman FC. Acute focal appendicitis. *Am J Clin Pathol* 1959;26:352–359.
65. Campbell JS, Fournier P, Da Silva T. When is the appendix normal? A study of acute inflammations of the appendix apparent only upon histologic examination. *Can Med Assoc J* 1961;85:1155–1157.
66. Touloukian RJ, Trainer TD. Significance of focal inflammation of the appendix. *Surgery* 1964;56:942–944.
67. Johnstone JM, Morson BC. Eosinophilic gastroenteritis. *Histopathology* 1978;2:335–348.
68. Klein NC, Hargroove RL, Sleisenger MH, Jeffries GH. Eosinophilic gastroenteritis. *Medicine* 1970;48:299–319.
69. Aubock L, Ratzenhofer M. "Extraepithelial enterochromaffin cell–nerve-fibre complexes" in the normal human appendix and in neurogenic appendicopathy. *J Pathol* 1982;136:217–226.
70. Olsen BS, Holck S. Neurogenous hyperplasia leading to appendiceal obliteration: an immunohistochemical study of 237 cases. *Histopathology* 1987;11:843–849.
71. Qizilbash AH. Mucoceles of the appendix: their relationship to hyperplastic polyps, mucinous cystadenomas and cystadenocarcinomas. *Arch Pathol* 1975;99:548–555.
72. Higa E, Rosai J, Pizzimbono CA, Wise L. Mucosal hyperplasia, mucinous cystadenoma, and mucinous cystadenocarcinoma of the appendix: a reevaluation of appendiceal "mucocele." *Cancer* 1973;32: 1525–1541.
73. Glasser CM, Bhagavan BS. Carcinoid tumors of the appendix. *Arch Pathol Lab Med* 1980;104:272–275.

*Histology for Pathologists, second edition,*
Edited by Stephen S. Sternberg.
Lippincott-Raven Publishers, Philadelphia


# CHAPTER 24

# Anal Canal

Claus Fenger



The anal canal has a complex anatomy and histology and in the past few decades much new information has been collected with regard to its structure and function. Because the spectrum of diseases found in this area has widened considerably, a detailed knowledge of the normal variants is important in diagnostic histopathology.

Unfortunately much confusion exists about definitions and nomenclature; therefore, this chapter includes a historical review and a discussion of the terms used for the different structures (1).

## HISTORICAL REVIEW

Anal diseases and their treatment are mentioned as far back as the Egyptian papyri (2). Nevertheless, there are few early descriptions of anal anatomy. Of note is Galenos (130–200 A.D.), who compared the anus to a laced-up purse (3). The first observations on the anal canal mucosa were published by Franciscus Glisson (1597–1677) (4), who noted the anal valves. In 1717 Morgagni (5) mentioned the anal columns and included the now famous drawing in the *Adversaria* (Fig. 1); in addition, it shows pronounced papillae. In 1727 Heister (6) described the smooth zone between the anal valves and the perianal skin, and in 1732 Winslöw (7) described the semilunar lacunae between the valves and the bases of the anal columns.

The first exact microscopic description of the different epithelial zones in the anal canal was given by Robin and Cadiat in 1874 (8). The perianal apocrine glands were found by Gay in 1871 (9), and in 1878 Chiari introduced the theory of the anal sinus infection in the pathogenesis of anal fistulas (10). Hermann and Desfosses' microscopic description of anal glands followed shortly afterward (11).

In 1877 Hilton (12) introduced the term "white line" for the junction between the skin and the mucous membrane, corresponding to the linear interval between the internal and external sphincter muscle. In 1896 Stroud (13) introduced the term "pecten" for the smooth area between the anal valves and Hilton's white line. However, later investigators recommended that use of the term "Hilton's white line"

C. Fenger: Department of Pathology, Odense University Hospital, DK-5000 C Odense, Denmark.

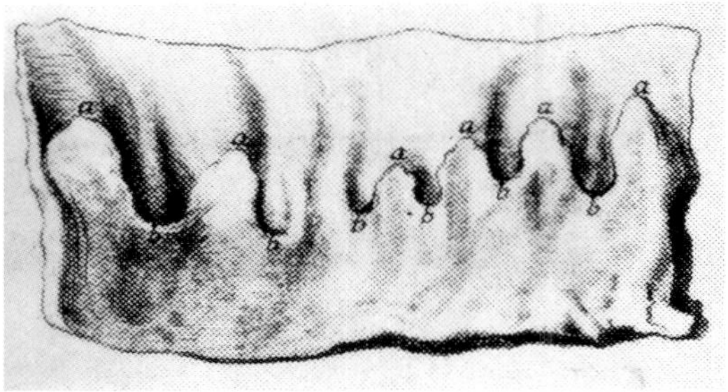

**FIG. 1.** The anal canal as seen by Morgagni (5).

should be discontinued because no anatomic feature identified it (14,15). Detailed macroscopic and stereomicroscopic investigations of surgical specimens of the anal canal have not shown any such structure (16,17).

The term "anal canal" was proposed by Symington in 1888 (18) for what had earlier been described as the third or perineal part of the rectum, that is, the part extending from the level of the pelvic floor backward and downward to the anal opening. This definition corresponds to the "surgical" anal canal, whereas the term "anatomic" anal canal has been used for the area between the line of anal valves and sinuses [dentate line (DL)] and the anal verge alone (19) (Fig. 2). The anal verge can be defined as the point (line) where the walls of the anal canal come in contact in their normal resting state (20).

As to embryology, Tourneux in 1888 (21) and Retterer in 1890 (22) wrote that the cloacal membrane was divided into anal and urogenital membranes by a descending septum, thus giving basis for the often quoted but never illustrated delusion that the DL is the site of a former anal membrane.

## EMBRYOLOGY

Earlier (23) as well as recent investigations (24) on human embryos have shown that in the sixth week [(10 to 14-mm crown-rump (CR) length] the hindgut and the urogenital sinus open into a common cloaca. The inferior boundary of this is the cloacal membrane, which at this time is rather thick (Fig. 3). By regression of the dorsal part of the cloacal membrane after the rapidly growing ventral part of the genital tubercle, the anorectum finds its place at the tail groove. Thinning and rupture of the cloacal membrane, which occur at about the 7th week (16 to 22-mm CR length), expose the orifices of the anorectal and urogenital systems simultaneously, and a special anal membrane does not exist (23,24).

The cloacal membrane is situated caudally to the anal crypts and columns as well as to the anlage of the internal sphincter, the epithelial lining coming from the dorsal cloaca (24–27). After the rupture, squamous epithelium begins to extend cranially to reach the anal sinuses at about 180-mm CR length (26). At this time the characteristic epithelium of the anal transitional zone is already present (Fig. 4). The anal cushions are also present in fetal life (28).

Anorectal anomalies occur once in every 3,000 to 5,000 births. Many of these may be due to a lack of regression of the dorsal part of the cloacal membrane (24). The anomalies can be classified according to their relation to the puborectalis part of the levator muscle in high (supralevator), intermediate, low (translevator), and a miscellaneous group (29). In the high anomalies (anorectal agenesis) the anal canal is absent and the rectum ends above the levator muscle and is often connected with a fistulous tract to the bladder, urethra, or vagina. The intermediate anomalies are rare and include anal agenesis, anorectal stenoses, and the rare anorectal membrane, situated above the site of the cloacal membrane. It is considered that some of these high and intermediate anomalies are part of the intestinal atresias and stenoses rather than of anorectal malformations (24). The low anomalies comprise the ectopic (perineal, vestibular, or vulvar) anus, anal stenosis, and covered anus. In the last case a track usually runs forward to open somewhere in the midline. Occasionally, the cover of the track becomes stretched, giving the impression of being a membrane (30).

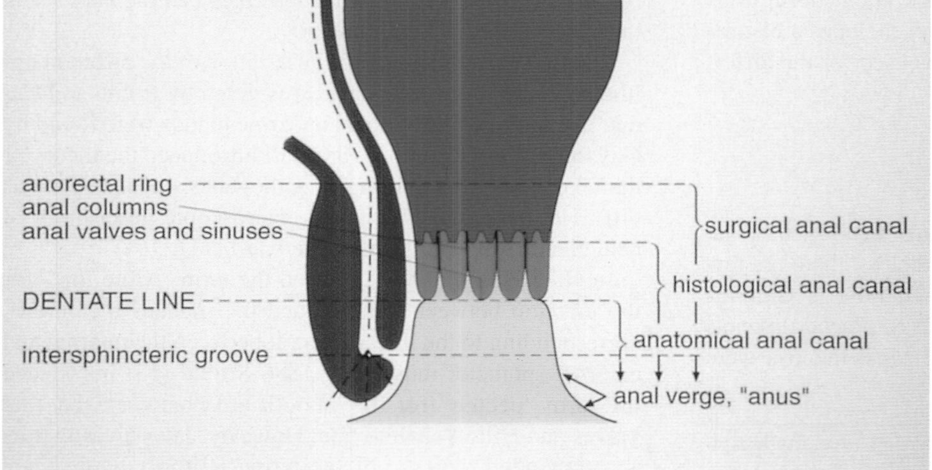


**FIG. 2.** Schematic drawing of the anal canal showing the macroscopic landmarks. The "surgical" and "anatomical" anal canals have their lower border at the rather ill-defined anal verge or anus. This point has sometimes been called the anal margin, whereas other authors have used this term for the same area as the anatomic anal canal. Hilton's "white line" was meant to be located at the intersphincteric groove; Stroud's "pecten" was the area between the DL and Hilton's line. The "histologic" anal canal begins at the irregular upper border of the ATZ (compare to Figs. 9–13).

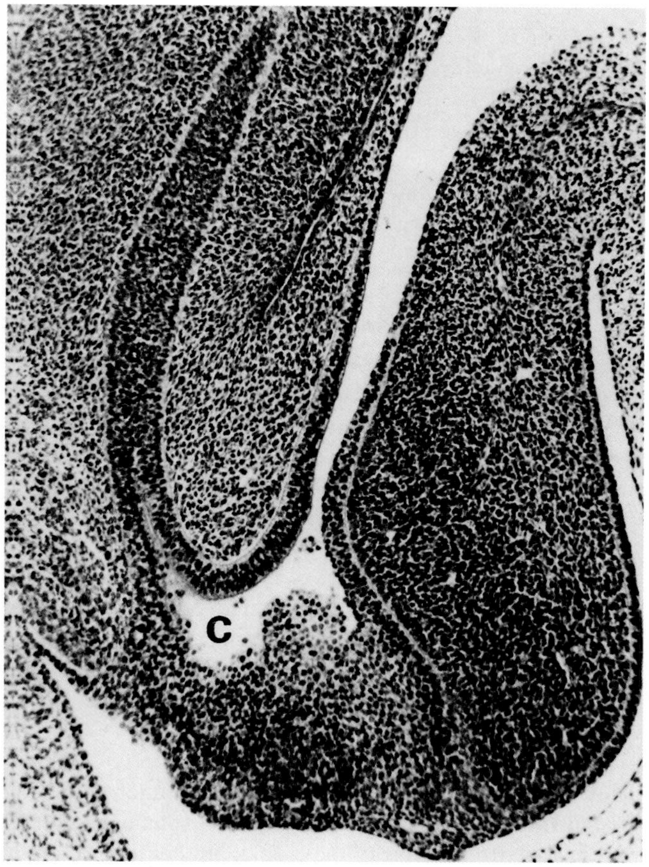


**FIG. 3.** Midsagittal section through a 13-mm (~6 week) human embryo showing the position of the cloaca (C) located between the urorectal "septum" (*up*), postanal swelling (*left*), and cloacal membrane (*down*). (H&E, original magnification ×**120**.) [Reprinted with permission (24).]

## APOPTOSIS

Apoptosis, a distinct mode of cell death that is responsible for deletion of cells in normal tissues, also occurs in various pathologic situations in the gastrointestinal tract. There is no reason to doubt that it also can be found in the anal canal, but so far no reports on its significance in this area have been published.

## NOMENCLATURE OF THE ANAL CANAL

It would seem natural to start with a definition of the anal canal, but because there are several definitions and new ones are still introduced (31), a description of the anatomical landmarks and epithelial zones may be the best introduction to this never-ending discussion.

### Official Terms

Official terms (32) for the structures seen on the anal canal surface include columnae anales, sinus anales, valvulae anales, and linea anorectalis. However, the latter term is not generally accepted, and many synonyms have been used. Official names for the epithelial zones in the anal canal mucosa do not exist, but numerous terms have been introduced during the last century.

When discussing anal nomenclature, one must always bear in mind that the terms "anal columns," "valves," and "sinuses" and the line composed by the latter two structures are macroscopic landmarks. However, the different zones in the anal canal are microscopic structures, although they can be visualized by using macroscopic staining (33), and they do not correspond exactly to the macroscopic landmarks (16). The most important macroscopic landmark is the line composed of the anal valves and sinuses and the bases of the anal columns (Figs. 5 and 6).

A list of names introduced for this line is given in Table 1 (1). Among these, the term "dentate line," also widely used in textbooks and by the World Health Organization (31,34,35), is the one that most prefer. Anal valves and papillae are not present as often as reported in anatomy textbooks, and crypts and sinuses may be found over a larger area than compatible with the definition of a line. Anorectal and anocutaneous refer to special definitions of the anal canal. When no valves, columns, or papillae are present, the line should be defined by the lowest sinuses visible.

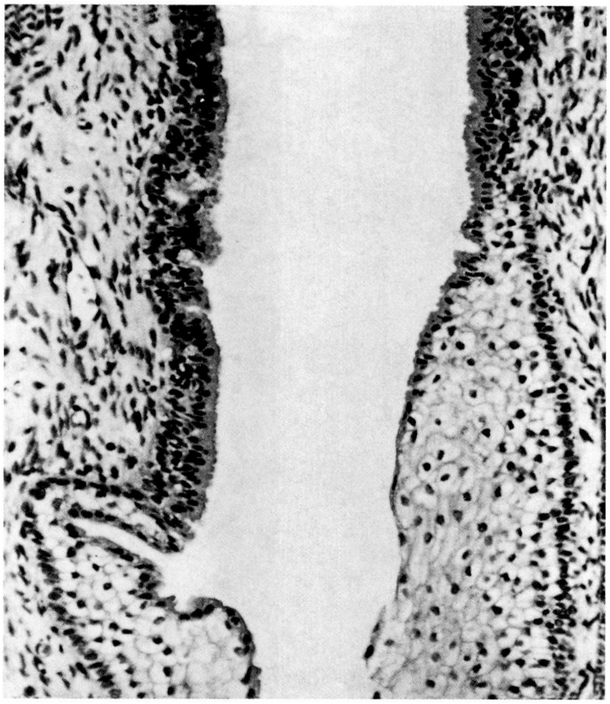

**FIG. 4.** Longitudinal section through the middle of an anal canal in a 13-week-old fetus. Squamous epithelium is seen in the lower part; anal transitional zone with the characteristic epithelium is seen in the upper part.

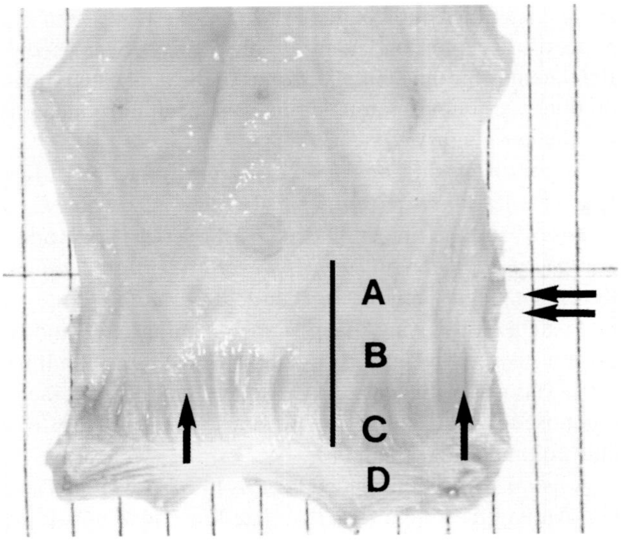


FIG. 5. Autopsy specimen of the lower rectum and anal canal from an infant. The DL is composed of the bases of the well-defined anal columns. Only a narrow rim of perianal skin is at the bottom. The *black vertical line* indicates the extent of the anal canal, the *single arrows* the DL, and the *double arrows* the upper border of the ATZ. A to D are explained in Fig. 7 (formalin).

### Epithelial Zones

Whatever definition of the anal canal is used, the sequence of epithelial zones in this area (i.e., rectum to perianal skin) is described as follows (Fig. 7):

1. The zone covered with uninterrupted mucosa of colorectal type.
2. The zone with epithelial variants [anal transitional zone (ATZ)].
3. The zone covered with uninterrupted squamous epithelium.
4. The perianal skin with keratinized squamous epithelium and skin appendages.

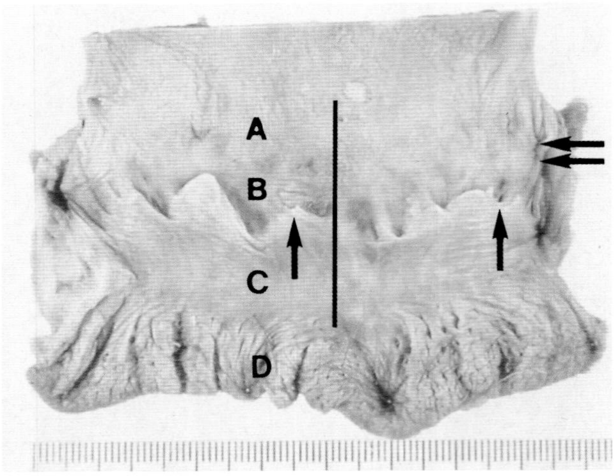


FIG. 6. Surgical specimen of the lower rectum and anal canal from an adult. Here the DL is composed of anal sinuses, valves, and pronounced papillae, whereas the anal columns are nearly invisible. At the bottom, there is a broad rim of wrinkled perianal skin with hairs. Symbols as in Figs. 5 and 7 (formalin).

These zones have been given many different names over the past century (Table 2) based on macroscopic, histologic, and embryologic considerations. Among the terms applied to the zone with epithelial variants, situated between the colorectal-type mucosa above and the squamous epithelium below, the term "anal transition or transitional zone" is now widely accepted (33). The term "zona columnaris" refers to a macroscopic observation; the names "membranous," "cloacogenic," and "junctional" zones all indicate the site of the cloacal membrane in early fetal life and the meeting point of endoderm and ectoderm, a theory that was rejected decades ago. The terms "intermediate" or "middle" zone could be used, but neither gives any information about the character of the epithelial lining. "Hemorrhoidal zone" is misleading because hemorrhoids are not confined to this area.

The definition of the anal transitional zone is as follows. The ATZ is the zone interposed between uninterrupted colorectal mucosa above and uninterrupted squamous epithelium below, irrespective of the type of epithelium present in the zone itself (33).

From this it follows that names related to the histologic appearance also would be appropriate for the other zones. One can therefore use the term "colorectal zone" for the mucosa above the ATZ and "squamous zone" for the area below, which gradually merges into the perianal skin (Fig. 7).

These zones are not always clearly visible to the clinician, and biopsy specimens should therefore be forwarded to the pathologist with an explanation of their location in relation to the DL. Biopsy samples from the lower part of the anal canal can be guided using a colposcope (Fig. 8) (36,37).

**TABLE 1.** *List of terms introduced for the line corresponding to the anal valves, papillae, and sinuses and the bases of the anal columns*[a]

| | | |
|---|---|---|
| Cruveilhier | 1843 | Ligne sinueuse |
| Robin and Cadiat | 1874 | Ligne anale cutanée |
| Symington | 1912 | Mucocutaneous junction |
| | | Pectinate line |
| Abel | 1932 | Dentate line |
| Goligher et al. | 1955 | Valvular line |
| Parks | 1956 | Crypt line |
| Morgan and Thompson | 1956 | Anorectal line |
| Walls | 1958 | Papillary line |
| Grobler | 1977 | Hilton's line |

[a] For references, see ref. 37.

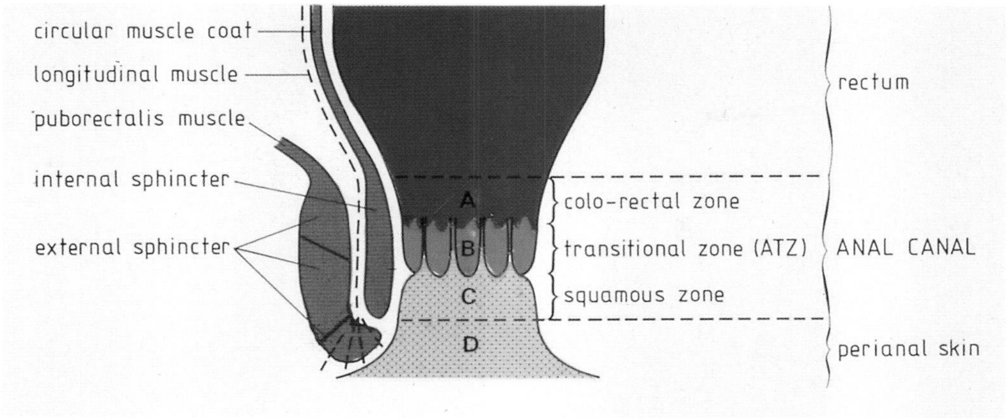


**FIG. 7.** Schematic drawing of the anal canal showing the different zones and the proposed nomenclature. Colorectal zone (of anal canal) above (**A**). The extent of the anal transitional zone (**B**) is highly variable. The squamous zone (**C**) gradually merges into the perianal skin (**D**).

**TABLE 2.** *List of terms for the various zones in the anal canal and perianal skin*[a]

| Reference | | A | B | C | D |
|---|---|---|---|---|---|
| Robin and Cadiat | 1874 | | Zone muqueuse | Zone cutanée lisse | |
| Duret | 1879 | Zone muqueuse | Zone moyenne<br>Zone fibroide | | |
| Hermann | 1880 | | Muqueuse anale | | |
| Hermann and Desfosses | 1880 | | Region cloacale | | |
| Stroud | 1896 | | | Pecten | |
| Waldeyer | 1899 | | Zona columnaries | Zona intermedia | Zona cutanea |
| Szent-Gyórgyi | 1913 | Zona intestinalis | | | |
| Tucker and Helwig | 1935 | | Intermediate zone | | |
| Tucker and Helwig | 1938 | Upper zone | Middle zone | Cutaneous zone | Cutaneous zone |
| Parks | 1956 | | Zone of stratified columnar epithelium | | |
| Grinvalsky and Helwig | 1956 | | Membraneous zone | | |
| Walls | 1958 | | Junctional zone | | |
| Duthie and Gairns | 1960 | | Transitional zone | | |
| Spanner | 1970 | | | Zona haemorrhoidalis | |
| Hollinshead | 1974 | | Zona haemorrhoidalis | | |
| Ferner and Staubesand | 1975 | | | Zona alba | |
| Williams and Warwick | 1980 | | | Transitional zone | |
| Singh | 1981 | | Zone III | Zone II | Zone I |
| Haas, Fox, and Haas | 1984 | | | Anoderm | |

[a] For detailed references, see ref. 37.

A, zone covered with uninterrupted mucosa of colorectal type; B, zone with epithelial variants; C, zone covered with uninterrupted squamous epithelium; D, perianal skin with keratinized squamous epithelium

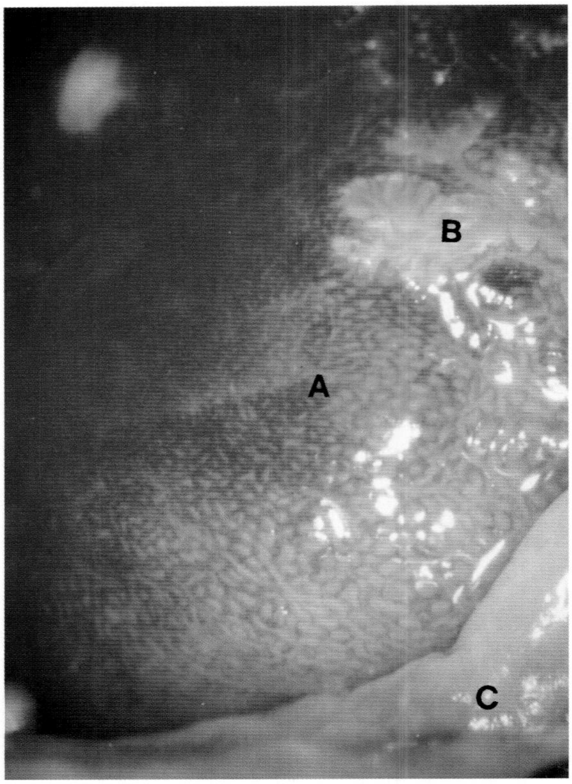


**FIG. 8.** Colposcopy of the anal canal at the level of the DL. Symbols as in Fig. 7. Compare the irregular outlines of the ATZ with Fig. 15.

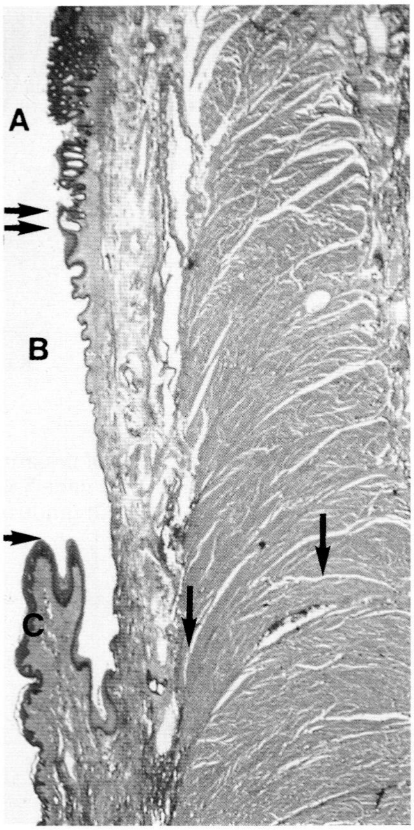


**FIG. 9.** Longitudinal section of the anal canal showing the ATZ and parts of the neighboring zones. At the upper border of the ATZ, a little island of squamous epithelium can be seen. The ATZ extends down into an anal sinus. The vertical arrows indicate anal glands in the submucosa and internal sphincter. Symbols as in Figs. 6 and 8.

## Extent of the Zones

The colorectal zone, ATZ, and the area covered by squamous epithelium can easily be distinguished on longitudinal histologic sections (Fig. 9). However, this method gives only limited information regarding the extent of the zones because the outlines are highly irregular. A better impression is provided by staining the whole anal canal with alcian dye. This method results in dark staining of the abundant mucus in the colorectal zone and an absence of staining in the squamous zone. The interposed ATZ is turquoise, due to sparse mucin production in the surface epithelium and scattered crypts (16). Subsequent serial sectioning of the whole specimen and comparison with the macroscopic picture gives a reliable measurement of the extent of the zones in the whole circumference of the anal canal (33).

By using this method on a consecutive series of 113 anal canals, four main variants could be visualized. In most cases (88%), the ATZ started at the DL and extended on average 9 mm cranially (range 3–20 mm) (Fig. 10). In a few cases (7%) the ATZ started below the DL (Fig. 11) or above the DL (4%) (Fig. 12). In one case the ATZ was totally absent (Fig. 13). In addition, the method clearly demonstrated the highly irregular outlines of the ATZ, especially at the upper border, as visualized by stereomicroscopy (Fig. 14) (17).

The squamous zone normally extends downward from the DL, but squamous epithelium is often found covering parts of the anal columns (17). The lower border of the squamous zone is difficult to determine because the squamous zone gradually merges into the perianal skin. If the transition is

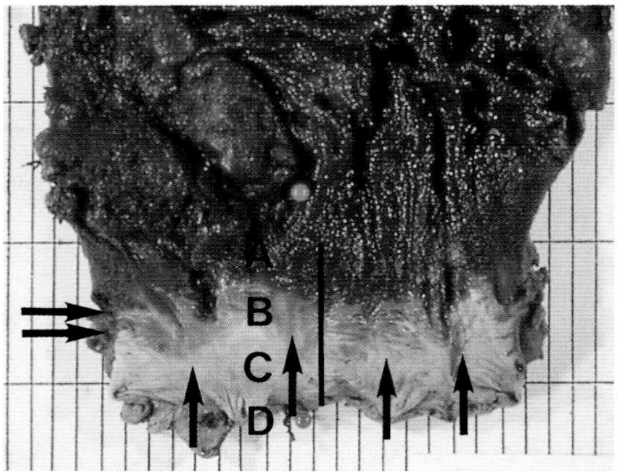


**FIG. 10.** Surgical specimen of adult anal canal: normal location of ATZ (stained with alcian green for 15 min). Symbols as in Figs. 6 and 8.

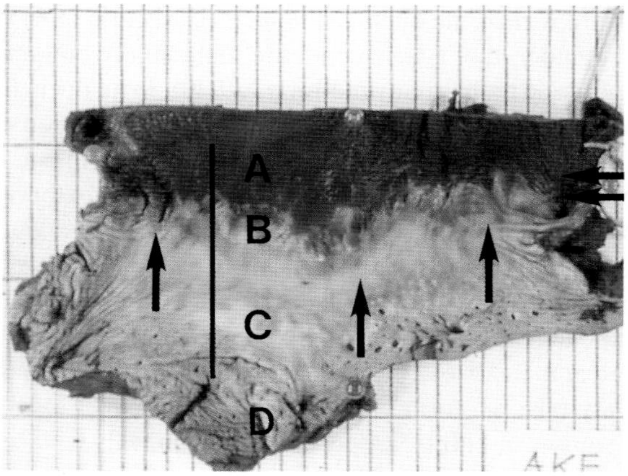


**FIG. 11.** Surgical specimen of adult anal canal: low location of ATZ (stained with alcian green for 15 min). Symbols as in Figs. 6 and 7.

defined by the occurrence of skin appendages, the lower border of the squamous zone is located outside the anal canal. This is particularly the case when hemorrhoids or prolapse is present. From this it follows that the histologic transition to perianal skin does not necessarily correspond to the definitions of the lower border of the anal canal.

### Definitions of the Anal Canal

Various definitions of the anal canal have been suggested through the ages. Some are based on macroscopic landmarks (Fig. 2), others on the extent of the epithelial zones (Figs. 2 and 7). Of the two based on macroscopy, the anatomic anal canal, which extends from the DL down to the anal verge, has been abandoned by most investigators as the definition leaves the ATZ and the characteristic tumors in this area outside the anal canal. The question is, therefore, to choose between the definitions of the "surgical anal canal" and "histologic anal canal," and there are advantages and drawbacks to both.

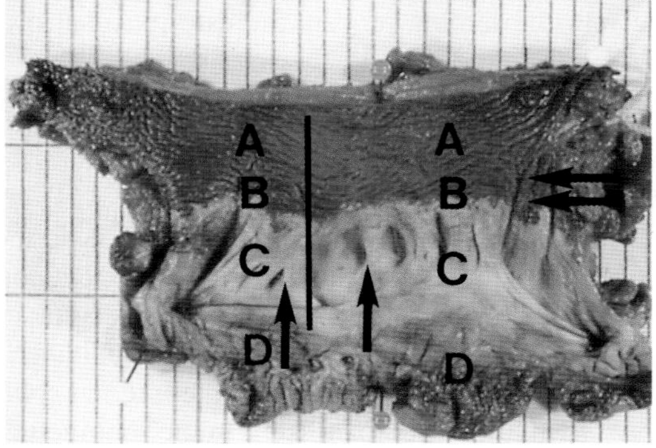


**FIG. 12.** Surgical specimen of adult anal canal: high location of ATZ, which here is very narrow (stained with alcian green for 15 min). Symbols as in Figs. 6 and 7.

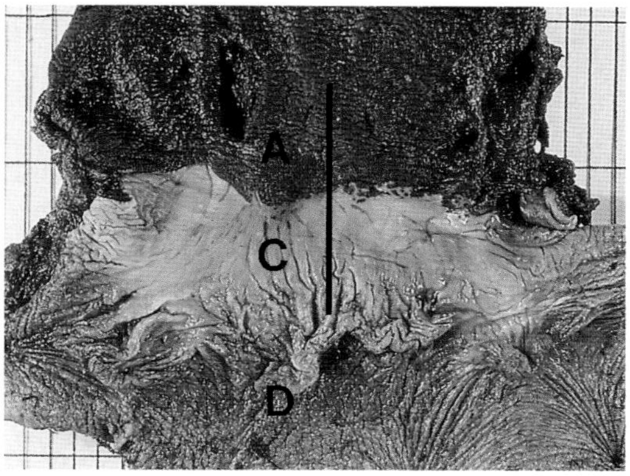


**FIG. 13.** Surgical specimen of adult anal canal: no ATZ (stained with alcian green for 15 min). Symbols as in Figs. 6 and 7.

The histologic anal canal is defined by the extent of the special mucosa in this area, i.e., the ATZ and the squamous epithelium down to the perianal skin. Using this definition, microscopic identification of the canal is reasonably easy and all the special tumors in this area have their origin in the canal, whereas rectal tumors are excluded. The drawback is that the extent of the anal canal cannot be estimated by the clinicians and that colorectal neoplasias can have their origin inside the histologic anal canal because it also harbors colorectal-type epithelium scattered in the ATZ.

The surgical anal canal can be identified easily by the clinician and described in the surgical report, thus making communication between surgeon and pathologist easier. The surgical anal canal is also regarded as a functional unit. However, with regard to the mucosal lining, the surgical anal

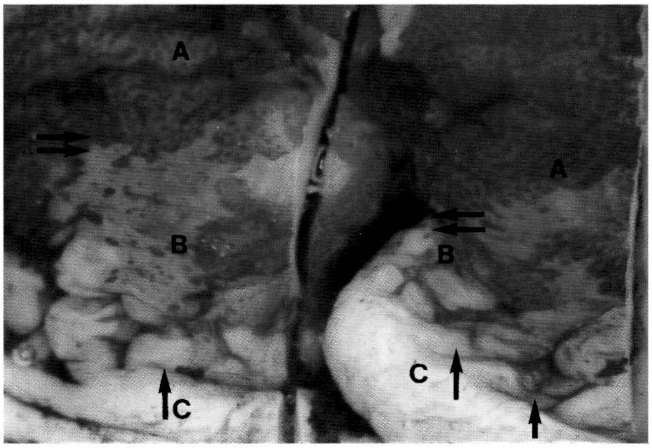


**FIG. 14.** Close-up of the anal canal mucosa at the level of the DL. The highly irregular outlines of the ATZ (**B**) contrasts to the heavily stained colorectal-type mucosa above (**A**) and the unstained squamous zone below (**C**). The vertical line is for later histologic control of the macroscopic staining (alcian blue 15 min).

canal most often includes a ring of more or less normal appearing colorectal mucosa at its upper border.

The lack of agreement between macroscopic and microscopic definitions is well known from other areas, i.e., the cervical transformation zone and the esophagogastric junction, and must be accepted. The essential point is that when the clinician describes the location of a process or a biopsy, the position in relation to the DL is the important message. The pathologist will then report what epithelial types are present in the material and, considering the above-mentioned variations, decide whether it is normal. In the following text the anal canal is described using the definition of the surgical anal canal.

## ANATOMY

### Mucosal Surface

Following the definition of the surgical anal canal (18), the structure extends from the level of the pelvic floor (pelvic visceral aperture, anorectal ring) to the anal opening (anal verge) (Fig. 2) and in a living person has an average length of 4.2 cm (38). Histologically, the anal canal extends from the upper to the lower border of the internal anal sphincter (34) and has, on formalin-fixed specimens, an average length of 3 cm (16). This slight difference in definitions and measurements must be accepted because the curved appearance of the anal verge cannot be evaluated histologically and because loss of tonus and the fixation procedures may influence the appearance of the specimens.

The anal lumen often forms a more or less triradiate slit when seen at anoscopy. The stem of the Y so formed approaches the midline posteriorly and the arms embrace a pad of tissue anteriorly. Thus, three folds are seen (Fig. 15); these folds are named the anal cushions (39). According to some investigators, the Y is asymmetric and usually embraces a pad of tissue to the right anteriorly (39,40). In an opened surgical specimen, these cushions are often inconspicuous.

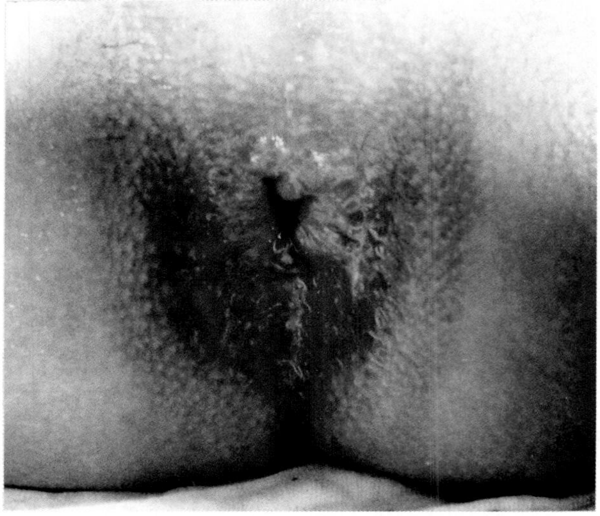

**FIG. 15.** The anus seen from below in a woman with labor pains. Note the Y shape created by the anal cushions.

The surface relief of the anal canal varies with age. The characteristic relief described in all anatomy textbooks is most distinct in children (Fig. 5). Here the mucosa shows six to ten vertical mucosal folds (the anal columns) that extend from a little below the middle of the anal canal and gradually disappear near the upper end. The anal columns are connected at their bases by small semilunar valves, which occasionally take the form of small papillae. Small pockets, the anal sinuses or crypts, are found behind the valves.

In adults (Figs. 6, 10–13) the mucosa often shows less pronounced valves and columns and may exhibit a smooth surface with or without scattered anal sinuses and papillae (16).

The three epithelial zones are faintly visible to the naked eye on unstained, formalin-fixed specimens (Fig. 6). The upper third shows the same relief as the mucosa of the rectum above. The area immediately above the anal valves and sinuses usually appears more smooth and gray–blue. This is the ATZ. Distal to the sinuses, the squamous epithelium appears as a smooth gray–brown area (Stroud's pecten). At the lower border of the anal canal, the dull, wrinkled perianal skin with hair follicles is obvious.

### Musculature

The exact arrangement of the anal musculature is still a subject of debate, and new information recently was added using anal endosonography, magnetic resonance imaging, and manometry. For a comprehensive review, see the article by Rasmussen (41). The muscles here are described from the inside out (Fig. 7).

#### *Muscularis Mucosae*

The well-defined muscularis mucosae of the rectum continue in the colorectal zone of the anal canal (Fig. 16) and can be found in the upper part of the ATZ (Fig. 17). Fibers extending into the lamina propria indicate mucosal prolapse syndrome.

#### *Musculus Submucosae Ani*

The musculus submucosae ani, originally described by Treitz (42), also have been called musculus sustentator tunicae mucosae, musculus mucosus ani, and musculus canalis ani (43). They consist of fibers from the intersphincteric longitudinal muscle, which pass through the internal sphincter, and from the internal sphincter itself. In the submucosa, they form a network around the vascular plexus (Fig. 17) and are sometimes connected to the muscularis mucosae upward. Caudally, they rejoin the muscles from which they came.

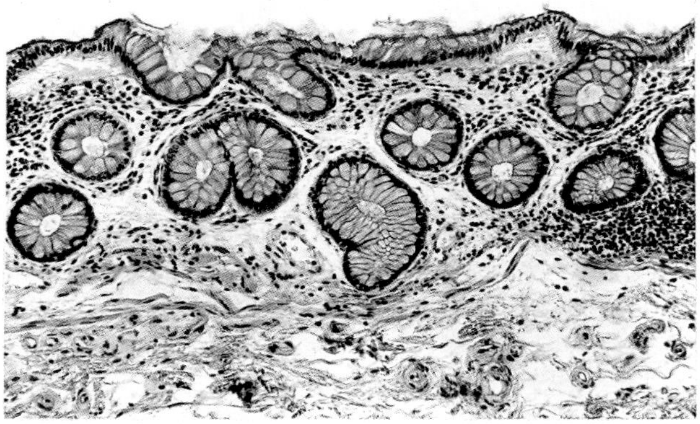

**FIG. 16.** Colorectal zone of the anal canal: short, slightly irregular crypts. Muscularis mucosae still present (H&E).

Some fibers fan out in the perianal skin, where they may join fibers from the corrugator cutis ani muscle (39,43).

### *Internal Anal Sphincter*

The internal anal sphincter is a continuation of the circular muscle coat of the rectum but is considerably thicker. In histologic sections it measures 5 to 8 mm in thickness and ends 5 to 19 mm (average 11.4) below the DL (16). Using anal endosonography, the thickness is only 1 to 4 mm and its lower border is found 8 to 12 mm below the DL (41). The muscle receives symphathetic (motor) fibers and parasympathetic (inhibitory) fibers from the inferior hypogastric plexus. In contrast to the adjacent rectum, the internal sphincter contains no enkephalin-immunoreactive fibers, few substance P–reactive fibers, but moderate numbers of fibers reactive for neuropeptide Y and vasoactive intestinal peptide (44). Collagen fiber deposition increases with age (45) and is higher in patients with neurogenic fecal incontinence (46).

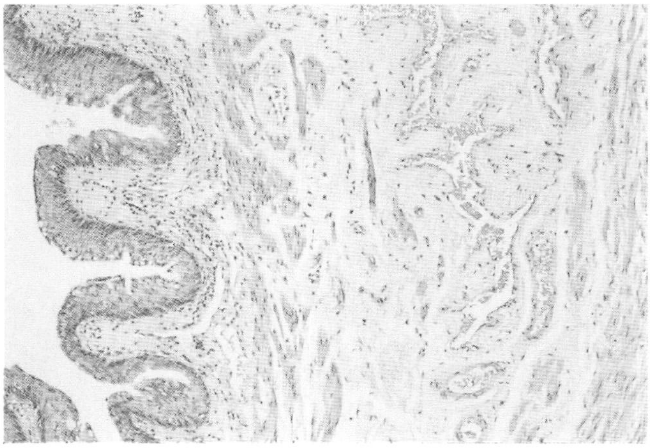

**FIG. 17.** Anal transitional zone: vascular spaces located between fibers from the muscularis mucosae (*left*) and the musculus submucosae ani (*right*) (H&E).

### *Intersphincteric Longitudinal Muscle*

The intersphincteric longitudinal muscle is situated between the internal and external sphincters (Fig. 7). Its thickness varies and its exact function is unknown (47). An excellent review on the various opinions on the anatomy and purpose of the longitudinal muscle was published a few years ago (48). According to Shafik (49), it consists of three layers, whereas others regard it as a conjoined coat (19). It contains unstriped fibers from the longitudinal muscle coat of the rectum and striped fibers from the levator ani muscles. At the lower end of the internal sphincter it breaks up into a number of septae, which diverge fanwise through the subcutaneous part of the external sphincter to end in the corium, thus forming the characteristic corrugation of the perianal skin. These bands are, therefore, referred to as the corrugator cutis ani muscle, although there is not complete agreement over the number of muscle fibers.

### *External Sphincter*

The striated anal sphincter is traditionally described as a circular muscle, which can be divided into a deep part and a superficial part that surround the internal sphincter and a subcutaneous part below these muscles (Fig. 7). Most investigators have been unable to find a clear separation between these three parts (26,30,47). The puborectalis muscle is situated above the external sphincter. There are two prevailing theories about the arrangement of these muscles.

Shafik (49) has described three U-shaped loops, with their convexity directed backward, forward, and backward, respectively. The top loop comprises the deep part and the puborectalis muscle, which is attached to the lower part of the symphysis; the intermediate loop is formed by the superficial part and is attached by a fibrous tendon to the dorsal part of the tip of the coccyx; the base loop is formed by the subcutaneous part, which is attached anteriorly to the perianal skin and is split from the longitudinal muscle by the above-mentioned fibers.

Oh and Kark (50) described a double-loop theory according to which the puborectalis is directed anteriorly and most of the external sphincter posteriorly. This is in accordance with recent endosonographical studies (47).

Anal endosonography also has demonstrated hitherto unknown fiberlike structures radiating from the external anal sphincter into the anterolateral plane. The finding has been confirmed by dissection, but the function of the fibers remains unknown (51).

The superficial and subcutaneous parts differ from normal striated musculature. They consist of relatively small muscle fibers, in the adult predominantly of the slow switch type (type I) (52), separated by delicate strands of connective tis-

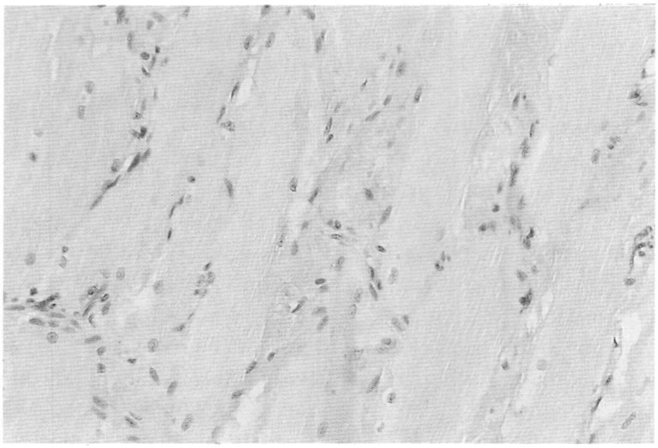

**FIG. 18.** The striated external anal sphincter with delicate strands of connective tissue between individual muscle fibers (H&E).

sue (Fig. 18) (53). There is a study indicating that the internal sphincter is innervated by the pudendal nerves (S2–4), whereas the puborectalis muscle is innervated by direct branches from S3 to S4, a possibility that should be taken into account during surgery in this area (54).

## Blood Supply

The arterial supply to the anal canal is considerably greater than would be necessary for metabolism alone. The branching pattern described by Miles (55) has not been reproducible by others. Branches from the superior rectal artery reach the ATZ in nearly all cases, but the middle and inferior rectal arteries often also make substantial contributions (39).

The terminal branches of the arteries split up into small tortuous vessels, some of which form tiny arteriovenous anastomoses with the submucosal venous plexus. This plexus consists of small convoluted vessels with discrete dilatations, which may be fusiform, saccular, or serpentine. Connective tissue fibers and fibers from the musculus submucosae ani are situated between the vessels, thus anchoring them to the internal sphincter (Fig. 17). The picture is more complex above the DL, whereas the dilatations are fewer and often larger below it. The drainage is mainly cranial to the superior rectal vein, but branches of the superior, middle, and inferior veins communicate freely below as well as through the internal sphincter (39).

Some investigators have described so-called anal glomeruli, in which groups of small convoluted vessels were surrounded by connective tissue, which separated them from the surrounding loose tissue (Fig. 19). Such structures probably represent thrombosed vessels with recanalization. The whole system has been referred to as the corpus cavernosum recti (although it is situated in the anal canal) and is more pronounced in the areas corresponding to the anal cushions (40).

### *Hemorrhoids*

According to this new understanding of anal vasculature, hemorrhoids or hemorrhoidal disease should be defined as enlargement or prolapse of the anal cushions, in some cases followed by bleeding and thrombosis (56,57). However, it is still debated whether the term "hemorrhoid" or "hemorrhoidal tissue" should be used to describe the normal anatomical structure (58,59).

The pathogenesis of symptomatic hemorrhoids (Greek *haema,* blood, and *rhoos,* flowing) is under debate. A low-fiber diet, constipation, and prolonged straining have been named as important factors (60). Other investigators have found that patients with hemorrhoids are not necessarily constipated but more often complain of diarrhea and are obese (56). They tend to have abnormal anal pressure profiles with elevated maximal resting anal pressure and decrease in anal compliance (61). It has been suggested that the high anal pressure in patients with hemorrhoids is due to hypertension in the anal cushions (62). Hereditary (63) and hormonal factors (64) may be involved. Portal hypertension in itself is not accompanied by increased frequency of hemorrhoids, but severe bleeding may occur due to the elevated portal venous pressure and possibly to coagulation defects (65).

Deterioration of the supporting and anchoring connective tissue and degenerative changes of the collagen fibers, together with replacement of muscle tissue by collagen, which begins in the third decade, make the structures less stable. The result is venous stasis and dilatation and sliding down of the anal cushions, sometimes followed by prolapse. Damage to the surface may lead to bleeding of arteriolar origin. Inflammation and focal pressure may be followed by further stasis, edema, and thrombosis.

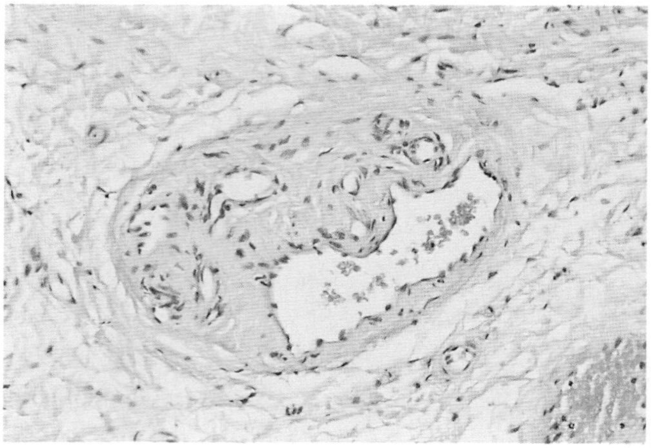

**FIG. 19.** So-called anal glomerulus (H&E).

This new understanding harmonizes well with the histologic picture of tissue from hemorrhoidectomies. The specimens most often consist of connective tissue stroma with scattered fibers of smooth muscle. The stroma contains many blood vessels and larger vascular spaces that vary in size and configuration and are often less than 2 to 3 mm in diameter. Inflammatory changes and signs of recent or past thrombosis may be present, as may stromal fibromuscular hyperplasia and elastic fiber proliferation (57). Neuronal hyperplasia is common (66). The surface lining depends on the degree of descent of the cushion and of course the extent of the surgical excision. It therefore may show colorectal, ATZ, or squamous epithelium, as well as perianal skin. The mucosa may show inflammatory reaction or frank erosion or may be the site of regenerative, metaplastic, or keratotic reactions. The so-called fibrous anal polyp is assumed to represent an end stage of a prolapsed cushion (67).

### *Other Vascular Changes*

There are a few differential diagnoses to chronic hemorrhoidal disease. Perianal thrombosis, formerly referred to as perianal hematoma, is an acute dark hard lesion arising under the squamous zone of the anal canal or the perianal skin. It represents a thrombus lying in the larger venous dilatations (67,68). Rectal varices are a result of portal hypertension and represent dilated submucosal veins formed when the communicating veins that connect the superior with the middle and inferior hemorrhoidal veins become enlarged. They extend above the level of hemorrhoids and occasionally downward to reach the buttock, perineum, or upper thigh (69,70). Diffuse cavernous hemangioma of the rectosigmoid is a vascular malformation consisting of vascular channels of variable size and thickness, which may involve the whole bowel wall and mesentery or perirectal tissue and may extend down to the DL (71).

A variant of the course of the inferior rectal artery has been blamed for a reduced perfusion of the posterior commissure and thereby of significance in the pathogenesis of anal fissure (72). Using Doppler laser flow cytometry, it has been shown that the blood flow in the posterior quadrant of the anal canal and perianal skin is significantly lower than in the anterior left and right quadrant. In addition, the higher the anal pressure, the lower the perfusion (73). These observations have led to the hypothesis that anal fissures are ischemic ulcers.

## Nerves

Ganglion cells in the rectum are found in three separate plexuses: the superficial, deep submucous, and myenteric. In the anal canal, ganglion cells belonging to these plexuses are absent or sparse in the first centimeter above the DL, which should be taken into account when examining biopsy specimens from patients with suspected Hirschsprung's disease (74).

The sensory innervation (75) of the lower part of the anal canal is accomplished by the inferior rectal nerves. The lining contains free nerve endings as well as organized endings (Meissner's corpuscles, Krause's endbulbs, Golgi-Mazzoni bodies, and genital corpuscles). It is sensitive to touch, pain, heat, and cold.

Sensitivity also can be demonstrated just above the DL in the ATZ, where the same endings can be found just above the anal valves. Thus, pain occasionally can be felt from injections given just above the DL. The ATZ is well supplied with intraepithelial nerve fibers and endings (76). Both types of nerve endings cease abruptly at the transition to the colorectal zone, where only a poorly defined dull sensation is present. However, discrimination seems not to be impaired by excision of the ATZ after restorative proctocolectomy (77).

Patients with hemorrhoids have a mild anal sensory deficit, probably due to the mucosal descent (78). Surgical specimens of hemorrhoids and their end stage, the fibrous polyp, may show proliferation of peripheral nerves without increased terminal density (66) (Fig. 20).

## Lymphatics

Lymphoid follicles are present in the anal canal from the DL and upward in approximately the same number as in the rectum (about 25/cm$^2$) (79).

The lower part of the anal canal (below the DL) and the perianal skin are drained to the superficial inguinal nodes. The drainage of the upper part is more complex, and varying results have been obtained from injection studies. Most investigators agree that an indirect or intramural system connects lymphatics in the anal canal to the lymphatic plexuses of the rectum (80). Other more direct lymphatics follow the

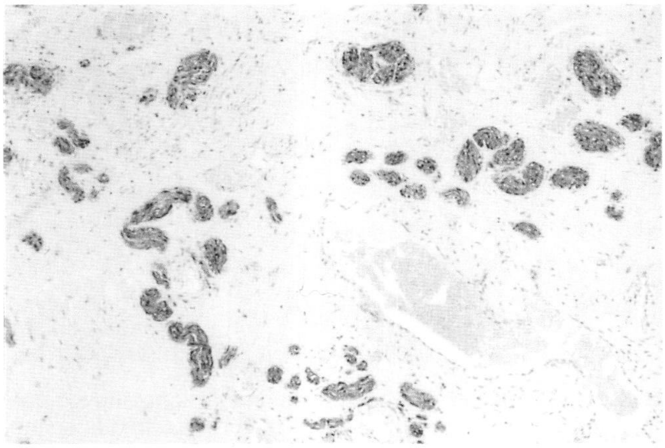

**FIG. 20.** Neuromatous hyperplasia in the anal canal. Squamous epithelium appears in upper left corner (S-100 protein).

inferior or medial rectal vessels to end in the hypogastric, obturator, and internal iliac nodes, or follow the superior rectal vessels to end in nodes in the sigmoid mesocolon and near the origin of the inferior mesenteric artery (81). Occasional connections also have been demonstrated to the common iliac, middle and lateral sacral, lower gluteal, external iliac, and deep inguinal nodes (82).

Lymphatic metastases from carcinoma of the anal canal are most often found in the inguinal, femoral, pararectal, and iliac nodes, and eventually in the mesenteric or paraaortical nodes. Hematogenous metastases are most often located in the liver and lungs (81,83,84).

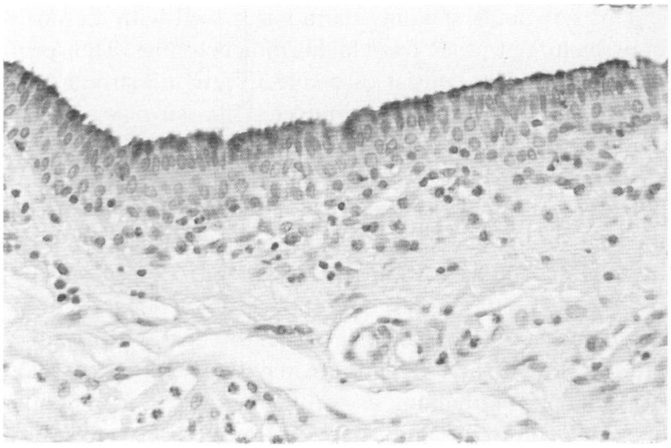

**FIG. 22.** Anal transitional zone: ATZ epithelium with columnar surface cells and scanty mucin production [alcian blue pH 2.7, periodic acid-Schiff (PAS)].

## LIGHT MICROSCOPY

### Colorectal Zone

The mucosa of the upper, colorectal zone is a continuation of the rectal mucosa, and no line of demarcation marks the transition to the anal canal. However, some shortening and irregularity of the crypts often are found in the area closest to the ATZ (Fig. 16).

### Anal Transitional Zone

As stated above, the upper border of the ATZ is defined by the appearance of other epithelial types. In one third of cases, the upper part of the ATZ consists of a small rim of mature squamous epithelium (Figs. 9 and 21) (16). Many epithelial variants can be found in the ATZ, the most prominent being the so-called ATZ epithelium.

The term "ATZ epithelium" (85) is not generally accepted but can be used until an exact classification is established. It consists of four to nine cell layers. The basal cells are small, and their nuclei are arranged perpendicular to the basement membrane. The surface cells can be columnar (Fig. 22), cuboidal or polygonal (Fig. 23), or flattened (Fig. 24). Small areas can show umbrella-shaped surface cells and more distinct cell borders (Fig. 25).

Other epithelial types are often present in the ATZ. Small areas of mature squamous epithelium may be present, especially at the upper border. Scattered crypts of colorectal type and small areas of simple columnar epithelium also may be found (Fig. 26). The anal glands open in the ATZ (Fig. 9).

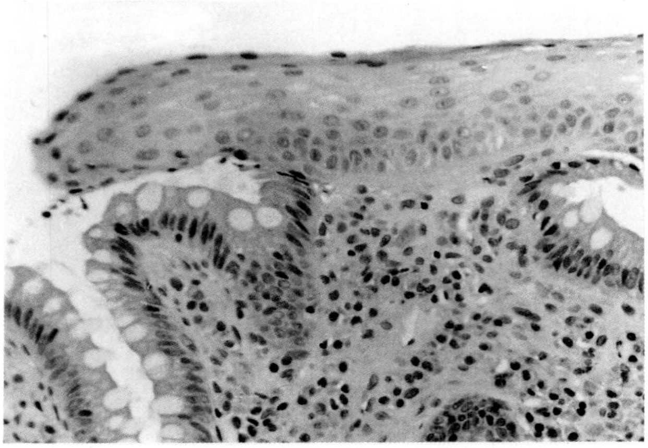

**FIG. 21.** Transition between the colorectal zone and the anal transitional zone, showing area of mature squamous epithelium. Such areas are present in nearly one third of sections (H&E).

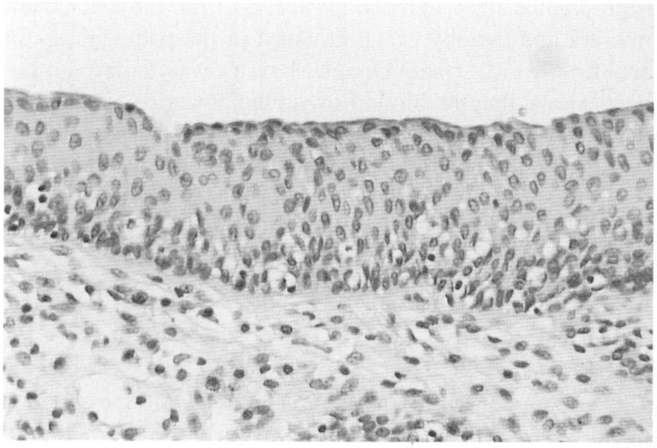

**FIG. 23.** Anal transitional zone: ATZ epithelium with cuboidal or polygonal surface cells (H&E).

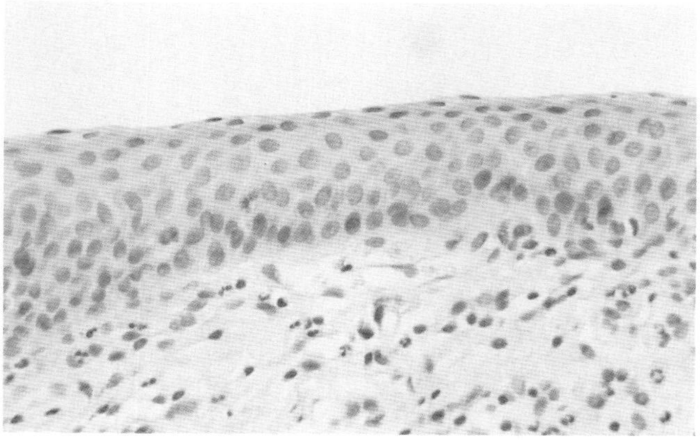

**FIG. 24.** Anal transitional zone: ATZ epithelium with flattened surface cells and resemblance to squamous epithelium (H&E).

### Squamous Zone

The transition to uninterrupted squamous epithelium usually takes place at the level of the DL. The squamous epithelium is unkeratinized with short or no papillae (Fig. 27). Melanocytes increase in number as the perianal skin is approached and the epithelium may contain Langerhans' cells (66) (Fig. 28) and Merkel cells (86) (Fig. 29). Langerhans' cells also may be present in squamous metaplasia covering hemorrhoids. Glands or skin appendages are never present.

### Perianal Skin

Keratinization becomes apparent at the lower end of the anal canal, and the squamous zone gradually merges into the perianal skin with sweat glands, hairs, and sebaceous glands

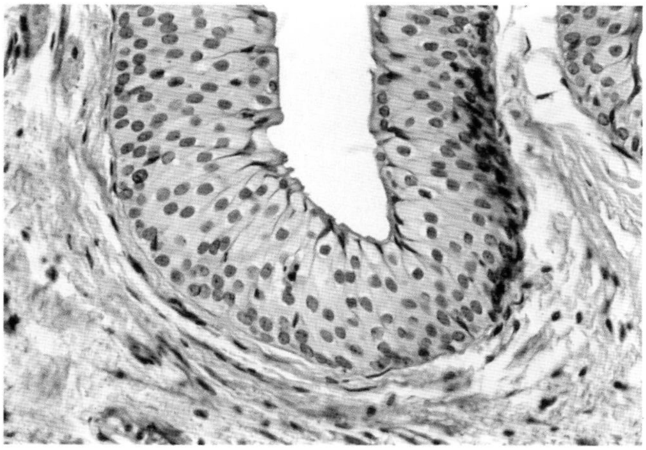

**FIG. 25.** Anal transitional zone: ATZ epithelium with umbrella-shaped surface cells resembling urothelium. The surface cells are small (H&E).

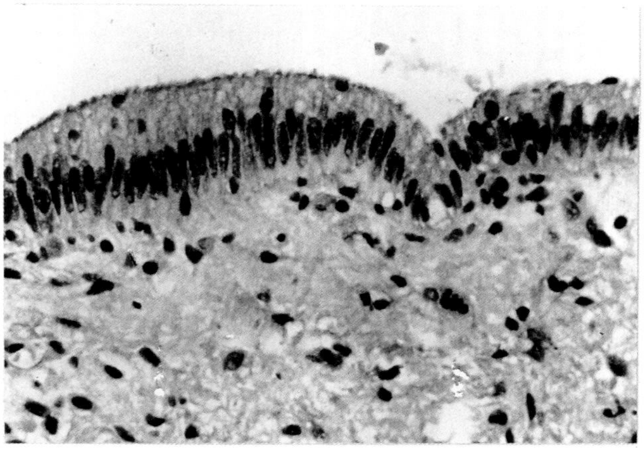

**FIG. 26.** Anal transitional zone: area covered with columnar epithelium (H&E).

(Fig. 30). A characteristic finding is the presence of apocrine glands in the subcutaneous tissue (Fig. 31).

### Anal Glands

The anal (intramuscular) glands seem to be present in all anal canals and arise from the anal sinuses in the ATZ (87). The median number is six, with a range of three to ten. Four of five are only present in the submucosa, but the rest extend into the internal sphincter and a few percent reach the intersphincteric space or even penetrate the external sphincter (88) (Fig. 9). The epithelial lining and mucin production are similar to the ATZ epithelium (89), and endocrine cells are occasionally present (90). A characteristic feature is the presence of intraepithelial microcysts (Fig. 32) and occasionally goblet cell metaplasia (Fig. 33). The epithelium is surrounded by one or two cell layers of myoepithelial cells

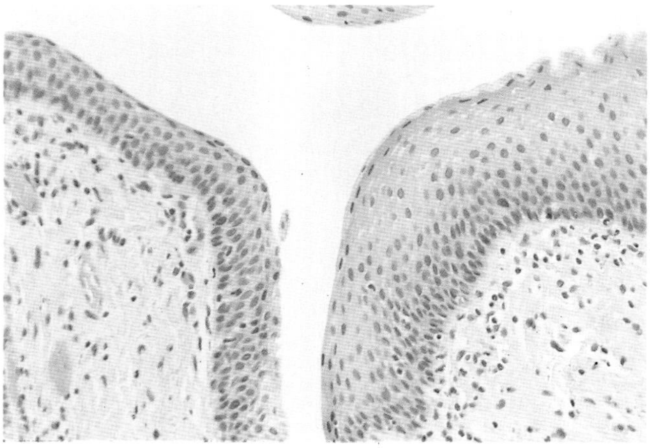

**FIG. 27.** Transition from ATZ epithelium (*left*) to squamous zone (*right*) (H&E).

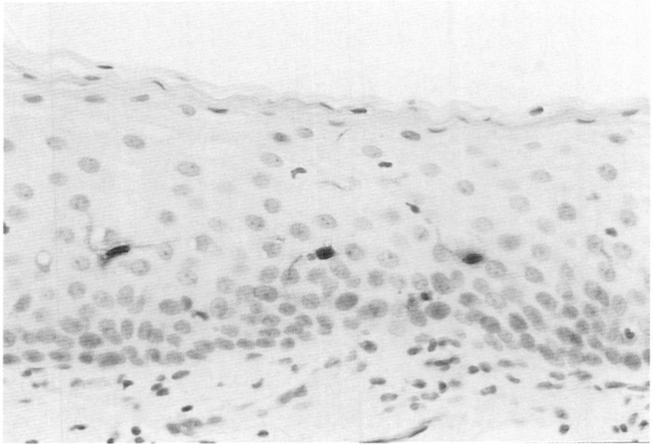

**FIG. 28.** Langerhans' cells in the squamous zone (S-100).

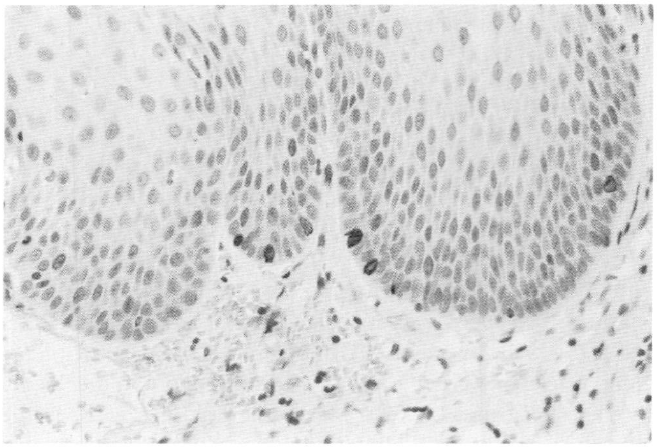

**FIG. 29.** Merkel cells in the squamous zone (CK20).

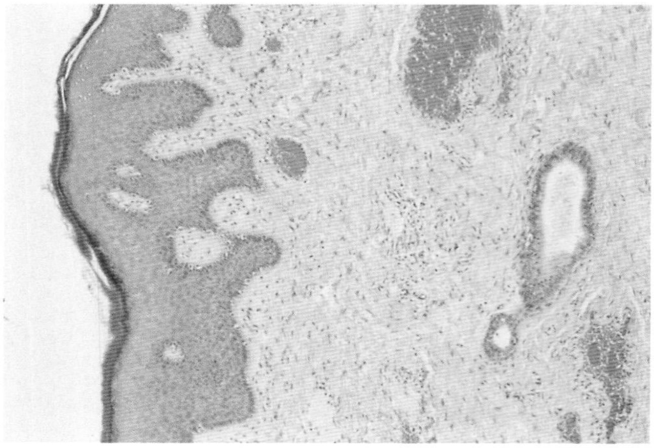

**FIG. 30.** Perianal skin with keratinized squamous epithelium and an underlying apocrine gland (H&E).

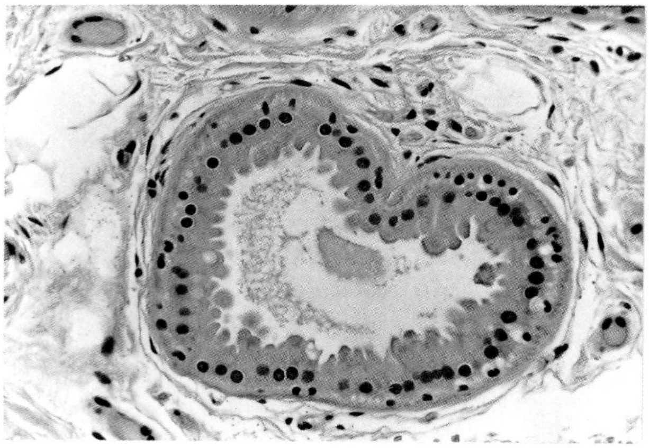

**FIG. 31.** Detail of apocrine gland with the characteristic eosinophilic cells with apocrine secretion (H&E).

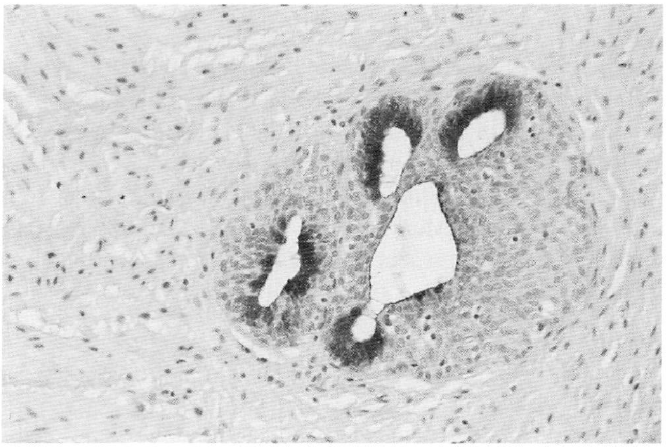

**FIG. 32.** Anal gland in the submucosa of the ATZ, situated among fibers from the musculus submucosae ani. Intraepithelial microcysts with scanty mucin production (alcian blue pH 2.7, PAS).

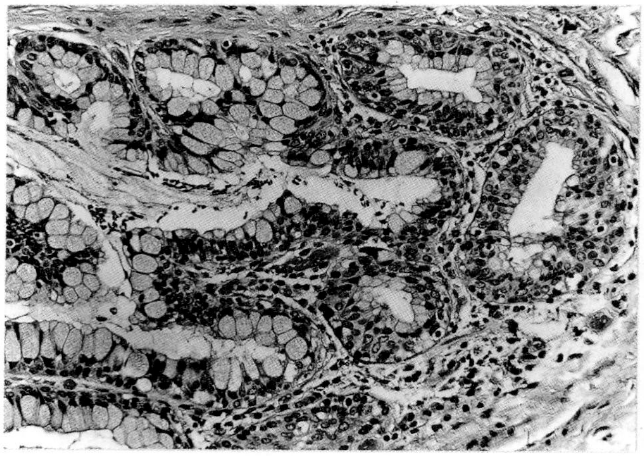

**FIG. 33.** Anal gland showing pronounced goblet cell metaplasia (H&E).

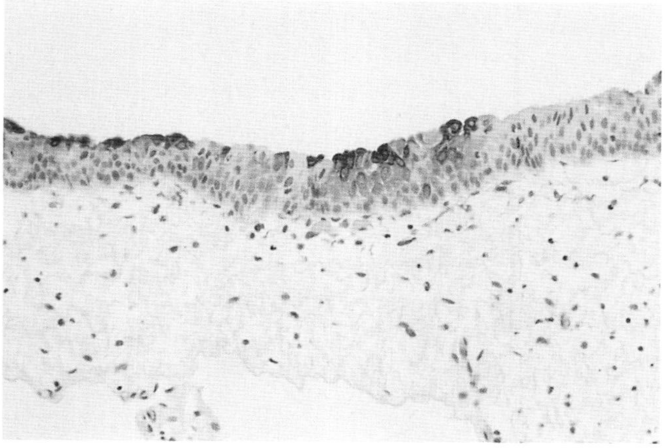

**FIG. 34.** ATZ epithelium with varying cytokeratin expression (CK7).

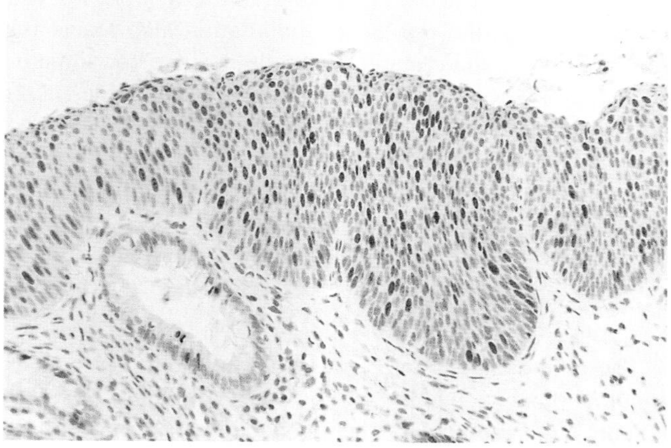

**FIG. 36.** Anal intraepithelial neoplasia (AIN). Proliferative activity (MIB 1).

that stain positive for smooth muscle actin (88). The glands are often surrounded by groups of lymphocytes. It is believed that the anal glands may take part in the formation of fistulas. Cysts are usually due to trauma and inflammation. Well-documented cases of anal gland carcinoma are rare (89).

## SPECIAL TECHNIQUES

### Cytokeratin Polypeptides

Two studies have addressed the expression of cytokeratin polypeptides in the normal anal epithelium. Together these studies have shown that the ATZ and anal glands have the same profile, with expression of cytokeratins typical for nonkeratinizing squamous epithelia (CK4, 13, and 16) as well as for secretory and complex epithelia (CK7, 8, 17, 18, and 19) (91,92). The coexpression of CK4 and 13 has also been observed in the transitional epithelium of the urinary bladder.

The reaction for CK7 varies in the ATZ epithelium, sometimes being very strong throughout all layers, sometimes being absent in the basal layer or the whole epithelium (Fig. 34). The ATZ epithelium is unvariably negative for CK20, a cytokeratin typical for gastrointestinal epithelium.

The proliferative marker MIB-1 for Ki 67 is positive in a layer of cells immediately above the basal layer and may be quite pronounced, especially in cases of hemorrhoids and prolapse (Fig. 35). However, the reaction still differs from that seen in anal intraepithelial neoplasia (AIN) (Fig. 36).

### Neuroendocrine Markers

The characteristic epithelia of the ATZ and anal glands contain a large and heterogeneous population of endocrine cells (85,90), which all show positive reaction for chromogranin A (Fig. 37). The cells have slender processes that ap-

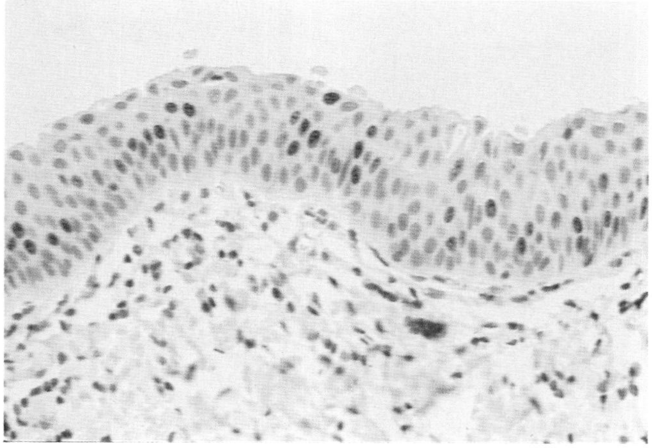

**FIG. 35.** ATZ epithelium. Proliferative activity (MIB 1).

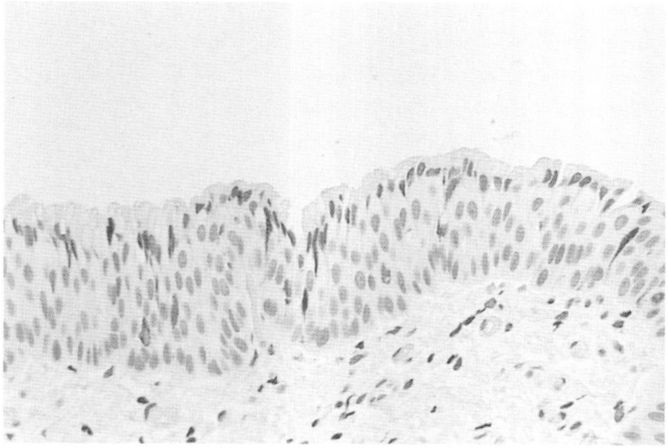

**FIG. 37.** ATZ epithelium. Endocrine cells (chromogranin).

proximate the surface and a fine granular cytoplasm. The number varies, and the largest population also reacts for serotonin and pancreastatin, but cells positive for somatostatin, peptide tyrosine tyrosine, glucagonlike peptide 1, calcitonin gene–related peptide, protein gene product 9.5, and neurotensin are occasionally present. The pattern is a mixture of products typical for colorectal epithelium and for Merkel cells in the squamous epithelium (86,93).

### Mucin Histochemistry

The columnar variant of the ATZ epithelium produces small amounts of mucin that consist of a mixture of sulfomucins and sialomucins, characterized by a scarcity of O-acylated sialic acids, in contrast to the colorectal-type mucosa above (94).

### Melanin-Containing Cells

A few melanocytes are also occasionally present in the ATZ (90,95,96). These are positive for S-100 protein and HMB-45 (Fig. 38). The corresponding malignant melanoma may be amelanotic and positive for polyclonal but not monoclonal carcinoembryonic antigen (CEA) (97).

### Flow Cytometric Microscopy and Electron Microscopy

Flow cytometric DNA analyses of the ATZ epithelium have shown a dominating diploid population with a small hyperdiploid peak (Fig. 39), resembling the picture of metaplastic epithelium (98). Transmission electron microscopy has not shown asymmetric unit membranes. In scanning electron microscopy the surface cells show distinct cell borders and short microvilli (Fig. 40) (85).

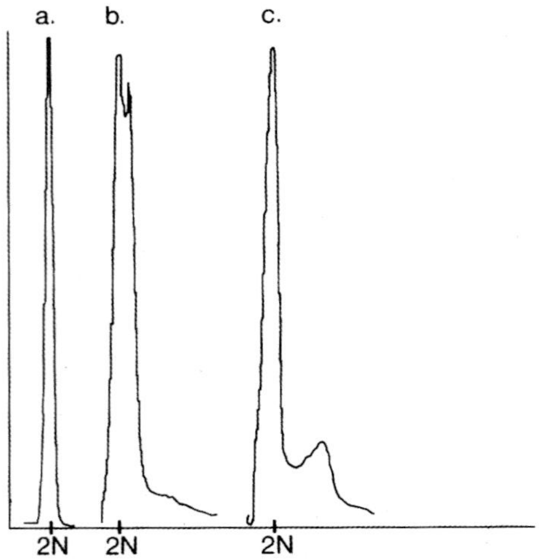


**FIG. 39.** Frequency distribution of nuclear DNA content. N, diploid DNA content. About 50,000 cells were analyzed. Curve a, normal human lymphocytes; curve b, normal ATZ epithelium; curve c, squamous carcinoma of the anal canal. [Reprinted with permission (44).]

## METAPLASIA AND HETEROTOPIA

Other epithelial types may be present and sometimes indicate pathologic conditions. Occasionally, colorectal-type crypts in the ATZ may contain Paneth's cells (Fig. 41) or show pyloric metaplasia (Fig. 42), probably as a result of mucosal damage, as in longstanding colitis. Keratinization of the squamous zone can be found in cases of prolapse (Fig. 43).

I have seen a single example of fundic gastric mucosa in the anal canal (Fig. 44). Such areas, rarely found in the rectum, are histochemically almost identical to their orthotopic

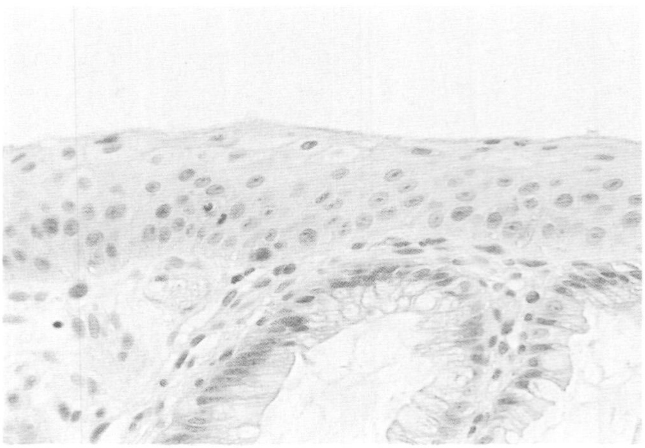

**FIG. 38.** ATZ. Three melanin-containing cells in the surface epithelium (HMB-45).

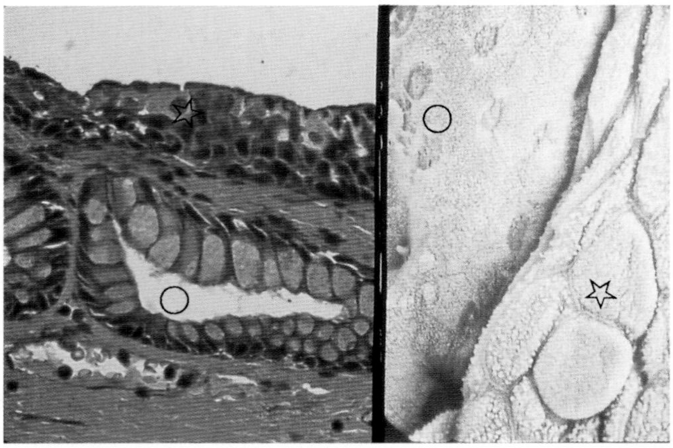

**FIG. 40.** Anal transitional zone: colorectal crypt (○) and ATZ epithelium (✶). Same area in H&E and SEM, original magnification ×**1500**. Reprinted with permission (40).

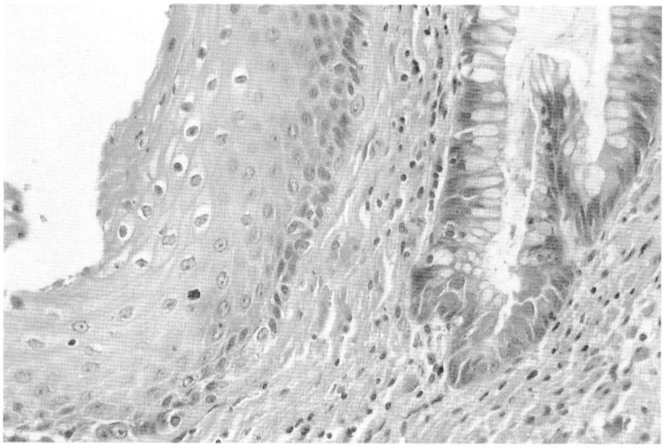

**FIG. 41.** Anal transitional zone: area with squamous epithelium covering a colorectal-type crypt with Paneth's cell metaplasia (H&E).

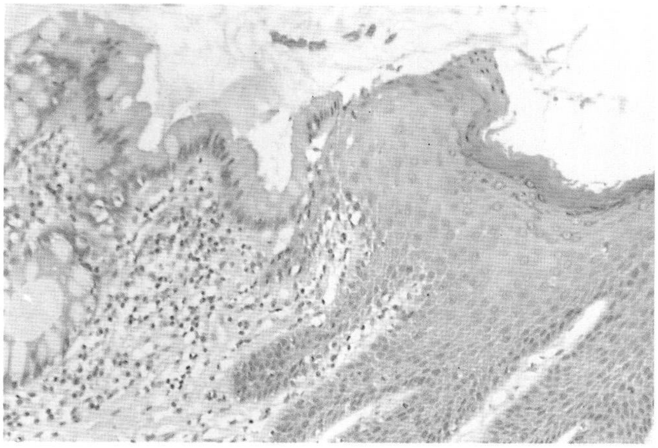

**FIG. 43.** Anal transitional zone: keratinizing squamous epithelium extending up to the colorectal zone, as is typical in cases of prolapse (H&E).

counterpart (99). Probably *Helicobacter pylori* can turn up in the anal canal as it has done in body-type gastric epithelium in the rectum (100). A unique case has been reported showing ectopic prostatic tissue in the lower anal canal (101).

## VIRAL AND NEOPLASTIC CHANGES

Cytomegalovirus, which occasionally infects the rectum, is rarely seem in the anal canal histiocytes (102). Herpesvirus-induced changes are more commonly found in the squamous epithelium (Fig. 45), and koilocytotic changes due to papillomavirus can be found as high up as in the ATZ (Fig. 46).

Dysplasia or AIN is not uncommon and may be present in the squamous zone as well as in the ATZ and in minor surgical as well as in resection specimens (Figs. 36 and 47) (103,104). AIN is particularly common among homosexuals and HIV-infected individuals, and HPV is often found in these lesions (105–107). There is considerable interobserver variation in the grading of AIN (108), and the risk of developing a subsequent carcinoma is unknown but probably low (36,109).

A wide variety of tumors may be found in the anal canal. A summary of the normal epithelial types and their possible neoplastic counterparts is given in Table 3. However, there is substantial overlap of the histologic features found in these tumors (110), and the reproducibility of the histologic classification is rather low here also (111).

Finally, it should be remembered that the anal area is a common site of extramammary Paget's disease and that many of these patients have a synchronous or metachronous malignant tumor. The Paget's cells are nearly always positive for mucins and CEA (Fig. 48) (112).

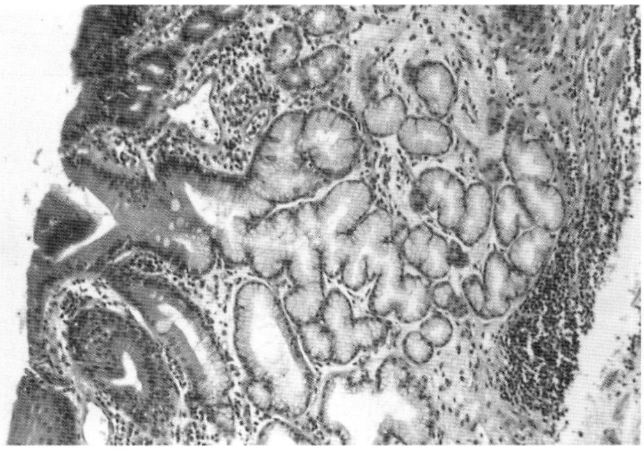

**FIG. 42.** Anal transitional zone: area with group of pyloric-type glands (H&E).

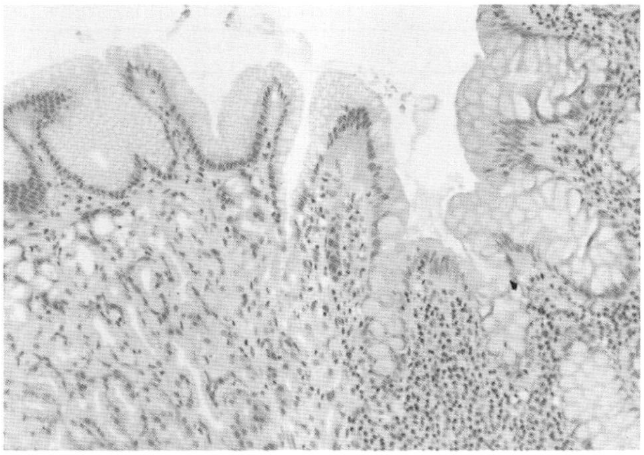

**FIG. 44.** Anal transitional zone: area with colorectal-type crypt and fundic gastric glands with parietal cells (H&E).

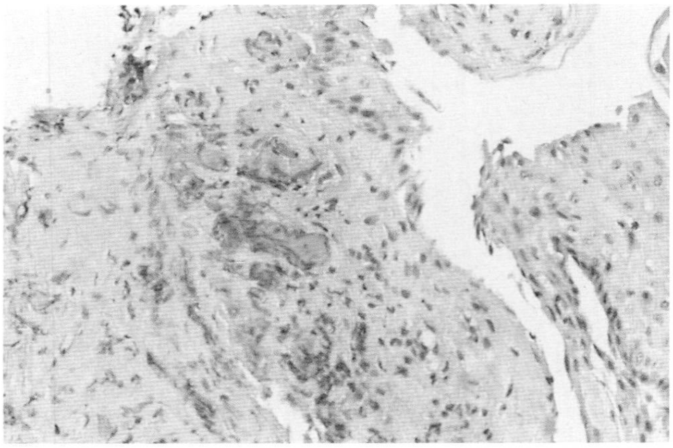

**FIG. 45.** Herpes-induced epithelial changes in the squamous zone below the DL (H&E).

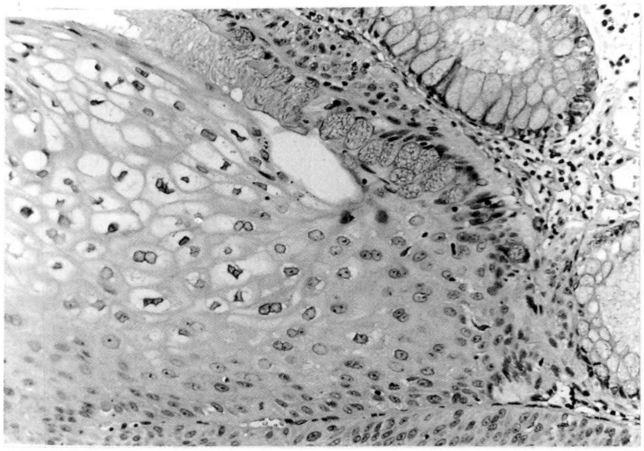

**FIG. 46.** Anal transitional zone: area with squamous epithelium showing koilocytotic changes. Colorectal-type crypts appear to the right (H&E).

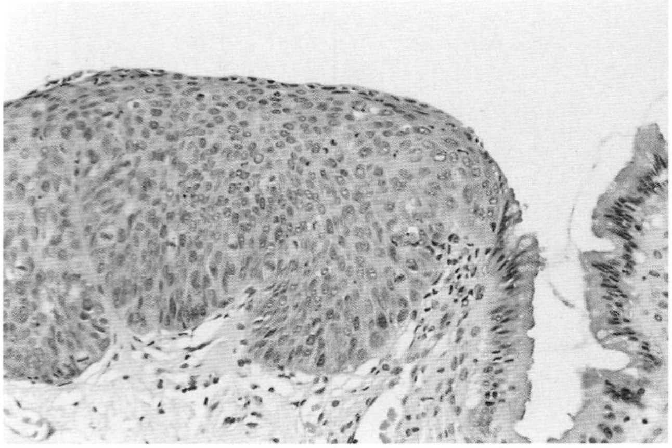

**FIG. 47.** Anal transitional zone: area with severe dysplasia (ACIN III) (H&E).

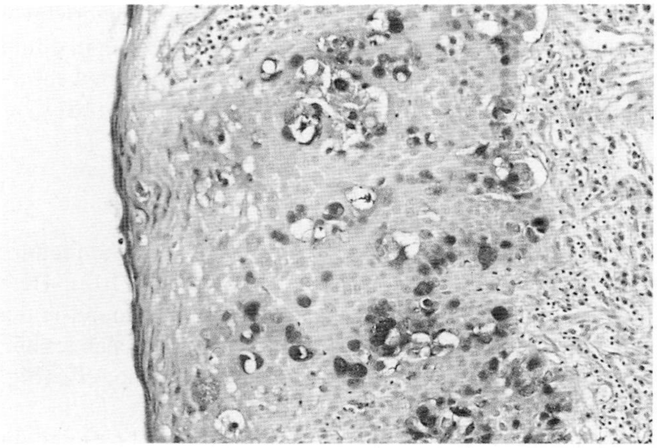

**FIG. 48.** Squamous zone. Paget cells (alcian blue pH 2.6, PAS).

**TABLE 3.** *Anal canal zones: epithelial types and neoplastic counterparts*

| Zone | Epithelium | Neoplasia |
|---|---|---|
| A. Colorectal | Colorectal | As in colon and rectum |
| B. ATZ | ATZ epithelium | Basaloid carcinoma? |
| | Squamous epithelium | Squamous carcinoma variants |
| | Colorectal epithelium | Adenocarcinoma |
| | Endocrine cells | Endocrine tumor |
| | Melanocytes | Malignant melanoma |
| | Anal glands | Adenocarcinoma |
| C. Squamous zone | Nonkeratinizing squamous epithelium | Squamous carcinoma |
| | Melanocytes | Malignant melanoma |
| D. Perianal skin | Keratinizing squamous epithelium | Squamous carcinoma, basal cell carcinoma |
| | Melanocytes | Malignant melanoma |
| | Apocrine glands | Apocrine tumors |
| | Skin appendages | As in skin |

## FUNCTION

The function of the anal canal recently was reviewed extensively (41). The normal function is obtained by a contribution from the rectum, the puborectalis, levator ani, external and internal sphincter muscles, mucosa, and the anal cushions. Continence is maintained by a combination of factors, the relative importance of which is still under discussion. The most important factor seems to be the angulation between the rectum and anal canal, provided by continuous activity in the puborectalis muscles (113). Other factors may be the triradiate slitlike configuration of the canal and the action of the internal sphincter, mainly on the DL. The external sphincter provides additional support, possibly via a double- or triple-loop system. The sphincter thus provides a higher pressure in the anal canal than in the rectal ampulla (114). Further support may be provided by the musculus submucosae ani in combination with the vascular system (43). Thus in vivo and in vitro studies have shown that the internal anal sphincter cannot close the anal canal completely but leaves an intersphincteric gap of at least 7 to 8 mm in diameter (115). This gap is filled up by the anal cushions.

Defecation starts with the feeling of need to defecate, probably released by stretch receptors in the puborectalis muscle when the rectum is distended. If defecation takes place, the levator ani and puborectalis muscles relax and the anorectal angle is increased from a mean of 92° at rest to a mean of 111 to 137° during straining, most in a squatting position. The external sphincter relaxes, and contraction of the longitudinal muscle leads to shortening and widening of the anal canal and eversion of the anal orifice (48).

## GENDER AND AGING

There is little information on differences in the anal canal between the two sexes and as a result of aging. The surgical anal canal is a few millimeters shorter in females (4.4 cm vs. 4.0 cm in males) (38), and the external sphincter is also shorter, particularly its anterior part (47,51). With aging the collagen fiber deposition increases in the internal sphincter (45). The resting pressure in the anal canal is lower in women and decreases with age in both sexes (114).

The mucosal surface is often more smooth in the elderly, and the papillae may be more pronounced (Fig. 6). The underlying connective tissue becomes less stable, which may result in descent of the anal cushions and subsequent squamous metaplasia of the ATZ (57). The number of lymphoid follicles does not change with age (79).

## SPECIMEN HANDLING

In minor surgical specimens it is often possible to identify the smooth gray–brown squamous zone from the gray–blue more glistening anal mucosa. The tissue always should be cut and embedded along the longitudinal axis in order to describe the lesions (i.e., AIN) in relation to the different epithelial zones.

**TABLE 4.** *Panel for typing of anal canal tumors*

| Question | Reaction |
|---|---|
| Carcinoma | Cytokeratins |
| Adenocarcinoma? Paget? | Mucin stains, CEA |
| Local Paget? | Gross cystic fluid disease protein |
| Malignant melanoma | HMB-45, S-100 protein |
| Endocrine tumor? | Chromogranin and others |
| Small (oat) cell carcinoma | Neuron-specific enolase |
| Lymphoma? | Lymphoma markers |
| Condyloma? | Human papilloma virus |

Local excisions should be provided by the surgeon with a suture at the proximal end, pinned up on a plate and sectioned in the same way with special attention to resection lines. Larger surgical specimens are rare nowadays where anal carcinoma often is treated nonsurgically. They should also be pinned up, and multiple sections may be necessary to find or exclude residual tumor tissue.

Normally most diagnoses can be established without the use of special stains, but occasionally a panel of immunohistochemical reactions is useful (Table 4).

## REFERENCES


1. Fenger C. The anal transitional zone [Thesis]. *Acta Pathol Microbiol Immunol Scand [A]* 1987;95(suppl 289):1–42.
2. Parks AG. De haemorrhois. A study in surgical history. *Guys Hosp Rep* 1955;104:135–156.
3. Braun WO. *Untersuchungen über das Tegument der Analöffnung [inaugural dissertation].* Königsberg: R Leopold, 1901.
4. Glisson F. Tractatus de ventriculo et intestinis. In: Clerici D, Mangeti JJ, eds. *Bibliotheca anatomica sive thesaurus. 2nd ed.* Vol 1. Geneva: Chouët et Ritter, 1699. (Quoted in Braun, ref. 3.)
5. Morgagni GB. Adversaria anatomica omnia. Advers III Animadv. VI. Patavii, Italy: Josephus Cominus; 1717:10–11.
6. Heister L. *Compendium anatomicum. 3rd ed.* Altorf et Norimbergae; 1727:344.
7. Winslöw JB. Exposition anatomique de la structure de corps humain. Nouvelle Edition, Tome III. Amsterdam: Tourneisen, 1752:346, 351.
8. Robin CP, Cadiat LO. Sur la structure et les rapports des teguments au niveau de leur jonction dans les regions anale, vulvaire et du col utérin. *J Anat Physiol* 1874;10:589–620.
9. Gay A. Die Circumanaldrüsen des Menschen. *S K Akad Wiss Wien* 1871;43:329–333.
10. Chiari H. Über die analen Divertikel der Rectumschleimhaut und ihre Beziehung zu den Analfisteln. *Med Jahrbücher* 1878;8:419–427.
11. Hermann G, Desfosses L. Sur la muquese de la region cloacale de rectum. *C R Acad Sci* 1880;90:1301–1302.
12. Hilton J. In: Jacobsen WHA, ed. *Rest and pain. 3rd ed.* London: Bell & Sons, 1880:288.
13. Stroud BB. The anatomy of the anus. *Ann Surg* 1896;24:1–15.
14. Ewing MR. The white line of Hilton. *Proc R Soc Med* 1954;47: 525–530.
15. Parks AG. Modern concepts of the anatomy of the anorectal region. *Postgrad Med J* 1958;34:360–366.
16. Fenger C. The anal transitional zone. Location and extent. *Acta Pathol Microbiol Scand* [A] 1979;87:379–386.
17. Fenger C, Nielsen K. Stereomicroscopic investigation of the anal canal epithelium. *Scand J Gastroenterol* 1982;17:571–575.
18. Symington J. The rectum and anus. *J Anat Physiol* 1888;23:106–115.

19. Morgan CN, Thompson HR. Surgical anatomy of the anal canal: with special reference to the surgical importance of the internal sphincter and conjoint longitudinal muscle. *Ann R Coll Surg Engl* 1956;19: 88–114.
20. Buie LA. *Practical proctology.* Philadelphia: WB Saunders, 1937: 40–50.
21. Tourneux F. Sur le premiers développements du cloaque du tubercle genitale et de l'anus chez l'embryon de mouton. *J Anat (Paris)* 1888; 24:503–517.
22. Retterer E. Sur l'origine et l'evolution de la region anogenitale des mammiferes. *J Anat (Paris)* 1890;26:126–216.
23. Politzer G. Über die Entwicklung des Dammes beim Menschen. *Z Anat* 1931;95:734–768.
24. Van der Putte SCJ. Normal and abnormal development of the anorectum. *J Pediatr Surg* 1986;21:434–440.
25. Johnson FP. The development of the rectum in the human embryo. *Am J Anat* 1914;16:1–57.
26. Jit I. Prenatal and postnatal structure of the anal canal and development of its sphincters. *J Anat Soc India* 1974;23:37–56.
27. de Vries PA, Friedland GW. The staged sequential development of the anus and rectum in human embryos and fetuses. *J Pediatr Surg* 1974; 9:755–769.
28. Morgado PJ, Sùarez JA, Gomez LG, Morgado PJ Jr. Histoclinical basis for a new classification of hemorrhoidal disease. *Dis Colon Rectum* 1988;31:474–480.
29. Santulli TV, Kiesewetter WB, Bill AH Jr. Anorectal anomalies: a suggested international classification. *J Pediatr Surg* 1970;5:281–287.
30. Goligher J. *Surgery of the anus, rectum and colon. 5th ed.* London: Bailliére Tindall, 1984.
31. Lewin KJ, Riddell RH, Weinstein WM. The anal canal. In: *Gastrointestinal pathology and its clinical implications.* New York: Igaku-Shoin, 1992.
32. International Anatomical Nomenclature Committee. *Nomina anatomica. 6th ed.* Edinburgh: Churchill Livingstone, 1989.
33. Fenger C. The anal transitional zone. A method for macroscopic demonstration. *Acta Pathol Microbiol Scand* [A] 1978;86:225–230.
34. Morson BC, Dawson IMP. *Gastrointestinal pathology. 3nd ed.* London: Blackwell,; 1990.
35. Jass JR, Sobin LH. *Histological typing of intestinal tumours. 2nd ed.* World Health Organization: International Histological Classification of Tumours. Berlin: Springer Verlag, 1989.
36. Fenger C, Nielsen VT. Intraepithelial neoplasia in the anal canal. The appearance and relation to genital neoplasia. *Acta Pathol Microbiol Immunol Scand* [A] 1986;94:343–349.
37. Wright VC, Chapman WB. Colposcopy of intraepithelial neoplasia of the vulva and adjacent sites. *Obstet Gynecol Clin North Am* 1993;20: 231–255.
38. Ninatvongs S, Stern HS, Fryd DS. The length of the anal canal. *Dis Colon Rectum* 1981;24:600–601.
39. Thomson WHF. The nature of haemorrhoids. *Br J Surg* 1975;62: 542–552.
40. Stelzner F, Staubesand J, Machleidt H. Das Corpus Cavernosum Recti-die Grundlage der inneren Hämorrhoiden. *Langenbecks Arch Klin Chir* 1962;299:302–312.
41. Rasmussen Ø. Anorectal function. *Dis Colon Rectum* 1994;37: 386–403.
42. Treitz W. Über einen neuen Muskel am Duodenum des Menschen, über elastische Sehnen, und einige andere anatomische Verhältnisse. *Viertel-Jahrschrift für die Praktische Heilkunde* 1853;37:113–144.
43. Hansen HH. Die Bedeutung des Musculus canalis ani für die Kontinenz und anorectale Erkrankungen. *Langenbecks Arch Chir* 1976; 341:23–37.
44. Wattchow DA, Furness JB, Coste M. Distribution and coexistence of peptides in nerve fibers of the external muscle of the human gastrointestinal tract. *Gastroenterology* 1988;95:32–41.
45. Klosterhalfen B, Offner F, Topf N, Vogel P, Mittermayer C. Sclerosis of the internal anal sphincter—a process of aging. *Dis Colon Rectum* 1990;33:606–609.
46. Speakman CTM, Hoyle CHV, Kamm MA, et al. Abnormal internal anal sphincter fibrosis and elasticity in fecal incontinence. *Dis Colon Rectum* 1995;38:407–410.
47. Sultan AH, Kamm MA, Hudson CN, Nicholls JR, Bartram CI. Endosonography of the anal sphincters: normal anatomy and comparison with manometry. *Clin Radiol* 1994;49:368–374.
48. Lunnis PJ, Phillips RKS. Anatomy and function of the anal longitudinal muscle. *Br J Surg* 1992;79:882–884.
49. Shafik A. A concept of the anatomy of the anal spincter mechanism and the physiology of defecation. *Dis Colon Rectum* 1987;30: 970–982.
50. Oh C, Kark AE. Anatomy of the external anal sphincter. *Br J Surg* 1972;59:717–723.
51. Eckardt VF, Jung B, Fischer B, Lierse W. Anal endosonography in healthy subjects and patients with idiopathic fecal incontinence. *Dis Colon Rectum* 1994;37:235–242.
52. Lierse W, Holschneider AM, Steinfeld J. The relative proportions of type I and type II muscle fibers in the external sphincter ani muscle at different ages and stages of development—observations on the development of continence. *Eur J Pediatr Surg* 1993;3:28–32.
53. Schrøder HD, Reske-Nielsen E. Fiber types in the striated urethral and anal sphincters. *Acta Neuropathol (Berl)* 1983;60:278–282.
54. Percy JP, Swash M, Neill ME, et al. Electrophysiological study of motor nerve supply of pelvic floor. *Lancet* 1981;1:16–17.
55. Miles WE. Observations upon internal piles. *Surg Gynecol Obstet* 1919;29:497–506.
56. Johanson JF, Sonnenberg A. Constipation is not a risk factor for hemorrhoids: a case control study of potential etiological agents. *Am J Gastroenterol* 1994;89:1981–1986.
57. Kaftan SM, Haboubi NY. Histopathological changes in haemorrhoid associated mucosa and submucosa. *Int J Colorect Dis* 1995;10:15–18.
58. Haas PA, Haas GP, Schmaltz S, et al. The prevalence of hemorrhoids. *Dis Colon Rectum* 1983;26:435–439.
59. Haas PA. The prevalence of confusion in the definition of hemorrhoids. *Dis Colon Rectum* 1992;35:290–291.
60. Burkitt DP. Varicose veins, deep vein thrombosis and haemorrhoids: epidemiology and suggested aetiology. *Br Med J* 1972;2:556–561.
61. Gibbons CP, Bannister JJ, Read NW. Role of constipation and anal hypertonia in the pathogenesis of haemorrhoids. *Br J Surg* 1988;75: 656–660.
62. Sun WM, Peck RJ, Shorthouse AJ, Read NW. Haemorrhoids are associated not with hypertrophy of the internal anal sphincter, but with hypertension of the anal cushions. *Br J Surg* 1992;79:592–594.
63. Brondel H, Gondran M. Facteurs prédisposants liés à l'heredité et à la profession dans la maladie hémorrhoidaire. *Arch Fr Mal App Dig* 1976;65:541–550.
64. Saint-Pierre A, Treffot MJ, Martin PM. Hormone receptors and haemorrhoidal disease. *Coloproctology* 1982;4:116–120.
65. Jacobs DM, Bubrick MP, Onstad GR, et al. The relationship of hemorrhoids to portal hypertension. *Dis Colon Rectum* 1980;23:567–569.
66. Fenger C, Schrøder HD. Neuronal hyperplasia in the anal canal. *Histopathology* 1990;16:481–485.
67. Thomson H. The anal cushions—a fresh concept in diagnosis. *Postgrad Med J* 1979;55:403–405.
68. Brearley S, Brearley R. Perianal thrombosis. *Dis Colon Rectum* 1988; 31:403–404.
69. Johansen K, Bardin J, Orloff MJ. Massive bleeding from hemorrhoidal varices in portal hypertension. *JAMA* 1980;244:2084–2085.
70. McCormack TT, Bailey HR, Simms JM, et al. Rectal varices are not piles. *Br J Surg* 1984;71:163.
71. Aylward CA, Orangio GR, Lucas GW, et al. Diffuse cavernous hemangioma of the rectosigmoid—CT scan, a new diagnostic modality, and surgical management using sphincter-saving procedures. Report of three cases. *Dis Colon Rectum* 1988;31:797–802.
72. Klosterhalfen B, Vogel P, Rixen H, et al. Topography of the inferior rectal artery: a possible cause of chronic, primary anal fissure. *Dis Colon Rectum* 1989;32:43–52.
73. Schouten WR, Briel JW, Auwerda JJA. Relationship between anal pressure and anodermal blood flow. the vascular pathogenesis of anal fissures. *Dis Colon Rectum* 1994;37:664–669.
74. Aldridge RT, Campbell PE. Ganglion cell distribution in the normal rectum and anal canal. A basis for the diagnosis of Hirschsprung's disease by anorectal biopsy. *J Pediatr Surg* 1968;3:475–490.
75. Duthie HL, Gairns FW. Sensory nerve-endings and sensation in the anal region of man. *Br J Surg* 1960;47:585–595.
76. Lassmann G. Histologie und Innervation der analen Ductus und Glandulae. *Coloproctology* 1983;4:232–235.
77. Keighley MRB, Winslet MC, Yoshioka K, et al. Discrimination is not impaired by excision of the anal transition zone after restorative proctocolectomy. *Br J Surg* 1987;74:1118–1121.

78. Miller R, Bartolo DC, Roe A, et al. Anal sensation and the continence mechanism. *Dis Colon Rectum* 1988;31:433–438.
79. Langman JM, Rowland R. Density of lymphoid follicles in the rectum and at the anorectal junction. *J Clin Gastroenterol* 1992;14:81–84.
80. Blair JB, Holyoke EA, Best RR. A note on the lymphatics of the middle and lower rectum and anus. *Anat Rec* 1950;108:635–644.
81. Paradis P, Douglas HO, Holyoke ED. The clinical implications of a staging system for carcinoma of the anus. *Surg Gynecol Obstet* 1975; 141:411–416.
82. Caplan I. The lymphatic vessels of the anal region—a study and investigation of about 50 cases. *Folia Angiol* 1976;24:260–264.
83. Junghanns K, Ott G, Knickel A. Das analcarcinom in TNM-System. *Langenbecks Arch Chir* 1969;326:62–71.
84. Kuehn PG, Eisenberg H, Reed JF. Epidermoid carcinoma of the perianal skin and anal canal. *Cancer* 1968;22:932–938.
85. Fenger C, Knoth M. The anal transitional zone. A scanning and transmission electron microscopic investigation of the surface epithelium. *Ultrastruct Pathol* 1981;2:163–173.
86. Hörsch D, Fink T, Göke B, Arnold R, Büchler M, Weihe E. Distribution and chemical phenotypes of neuroendocrine cells in the human anal canal. *Regul Pept* 1994;54:527–542.
87. McColl I. The comparative anatomy and pathology of anal glands. *Ann R Coll Surg Engl* 1967;40:36–67.
88. Seow-Choen F, Ho JMS. Histoanatomy of anal glands. *Dis Colon Rectum* 1994;37:1215–1218.
89. Fenger C, Filipe MI. Pathology of the anal glands with special reference to their mucin histochemistry. *Acta Pathol Microbiol Immunol Scand [A]* 1977;85:273–285.
90. Fenger C, Lyon H. Endocrine cells and melanin-containing cells in the anal canal epithelium. *Histochem J* 1982;14:631–639.
91. Williams GR, Talbot IC, Northover JMA, Leigh IM. Cytokeratin expression in the normal anal canal [Abstract]. *J Pathol* 1994; 172(suppl):111.
92. Levy R, Czernobilsky B, Geiger B. Cytokeratin polypeptide expression in a cloacogenic carcinoma and in the normal anal canal epithelium. *Virchows Archiv [A] Pathol Anat* 1991;418:447–455.
93. Hörsch D, Fink T, Büchler M, Weihe E. Regional specificities in the distribution, chemical phenotypes, and coexistence patterns of neuropeptide containing nerve fibers in the human anal canal. *J Comp Neurol* 1993;335:381–401.
94. Fenger C, Filipe MI. Mucin histochemistry of the anal canal epithelium. Studies of normal mucosa and mucosa adjacent to carcinoma. *Histochem J* 1981;13:921–930.
95. Fetissof F, Dubois MP, Assan R, et al. Endocrine cells in the anal canal. *Virchows Arch [A]* 1984;404:39–47.
96. Clemmensen OJ, Fenger C. Melanocytes in the anal canal epithelium. *Histopathology* 1991;18:237–241.
97. Fenger C. Critical commentary to "CEA reactivity in amelanotic malignant melanoma of the anal canal." *Pathol Res Pract* 1993;189: 1077–1078.
98. Fenger C, Bichel P. Flow cytometric DNA analysis of anal canal epithelium and ano-rectal tumours. *Acta Pathol Microbiol Immunol Scand [A]* 1981;89:351–355.
99. Carlei F, Pietroletti R, Lomanto D, et al. Heterotopic gastric mucosa of the rectum—characterization of endocrine and mucin-producing cells by immunocytochemistry and lectin histochemistry. Report of a case. *Dis Colon Rectum* 1989;32:159–164.
100. Dye KR, Marshall BJ, Frierson HF, Pambianco DJ, McCallum RW. *Campylobacter pylori* colonizing heterotopic gastric tissue in the rectum. *Am J Clin Pathol* 1990;93:144–147.
101. Morgan MB. Ectopic prostatic tissue of the anal canal. *J Urol* 1992; 147:165–166.
102. Blackman E, Vimadalal S, Nash G. Significance of gastrointestinal cytomegalovirus infection in homosexual males. *Am J Gastroenterol* 1984;79:935–940.
103. Fenger C, Nielsen VT. Dysplastic changes in the anal canal epithelium in minor surgical specimens. *Acta Path Microbiol Scand [A]* 1981;89: 463–465.
104. Fenger C, Nielsen VT. Precancerous changes in the anal canal epithelium in resection specimens. *Acta Pathol Microbiol Immunol Scand [A]* 1986;94:63–69.
105. Carter PS, Ruiter de A, Whatrup C, et al. Human immunodeficiency virus infection and genital warts as risk factors for anal intraepithelial neoplasia in homosexual men. *Br J Surg* 1995;82:473–474.
106. Kiviat NB, Critchlow CW, Holmes KK, et al. Association of anal dysplasia and human papillomavirus with immunosuppression and HIV infection among homosexual men. *AIDS* 1993;7:43–49.
107. Duggan MA, Boras VF, Inoue M, et al. Human papilloma-virus DNA determination of anal condylomata, dysplasias, and squamous carcinomas with in situ hybridization. *Am J Clin Pathol* 1989;92:16–21.
108. Carter PS, Sheffield JP, Shepherd N, et al. Interobserver variation in the reporting of the histopathological grading of anal intraepithelial neoplasia. *J Clin Pathol* 1994;47:1032–1034.
109. Fenger C. Anal precancers: a challenge for surgeons and pathologists. *Acta Chir Aust* 1995;26:399–403.
110. Williams GR, Talbot IC. Anal carcinoma—a histological review. *Histopathology* 1995;25:507–516.
111. Fenger C, Frisch M, Jass JJ, Williams GT, Hilden J. Anal cancer reproducibility study. *Pathol Res Pract* 1995;1991:663.
112. Helm KF, Coellner JR, Peters MS. Immunohistochemical stains in extramammary Paget's disease. *Am J Dermatopathol* 1992;14:402–407.
113. Parks AG, Porter NH, Melzak J. Experimental study of the reflex mechanism controlling the muscles of the pelvic floor. *Dis Colon Rectum* 1962;5:401–414.
114. Poos RJ, Frank J, Bittner R, et al. Influence of age and sex on anal sphincters: manometric evaluation of anorectal continence. *Eur Surg Res* 1986;18:343–348.
115. Lestar B, Pennickx F, Rigauts H, Kerremans R. The internal anal sphincter cannot close the anal canal completely. *Int J Colorect Dis* 1992;7:159–161.

# Associated Intestinal Tract Organs

*Histology for Pathologists, second edition,*
Edited by Stephen S. Sternberg.
Lippincott-Raven Publishers, Philadelphia


# CHAPTER 25

# Liver

Swan N. Thung and Michael A. Gerber



The embryology, gross morphology, and histology of the normal human liver—the single largest organ in the human body—are described in this chapter. It is emphasized that liver biopsy specimens must be processed with special care in order to obtain optimal sections for diagnostic histologic evaluation. In many instances, immunohistologic studies of liver tissue have the potential to yield more information than electron microscopy. In surgical and autopsy liver specimens, nonspecific histologic alterations may be prominent, but they often have little significance. On the other hand, some morphologic changes, particularly in needle biopsy specimens, are frequently subtle but may be of diagnostic importance. The pathologist must be familiar with these histologic variations of and from the normal liver.

S. N. Thung: Lillian and Henry M. Stratton-Hans Popper Department of Pathology, Mount Sinai School of Medicine, New York, New York 10029.

M. A. Gerber: Chairman, Department of Pathology and Laboratory Medicine, Tulane University School of Medicine, New Orleans, Louisiana 70112.

## EMBRYOLOGY

The liver arises as the hepatic diverticulum from the endodermal lining of the most distal portion of the foregut during the 3rd to 4th week of gestation (1–3). In embryos 4 to 5 mm in length, the hepatic diverticulum differentiates cranially into proliferating hepatic cords and caudally into the gallbladder and extrahepatic bile ducts. The anastomosing cords of hepatic epithelial cells grow into the mesenchyme of the septum transversum. As the hepatic cords extend outward during the 5th week of gestation, they are interpenetrated by the inwardly growing capillary plexus, which arises from the vitelline veins in the outer margins of the septum transversum and forms the primitive hepatic sinusoids.

Scattered mesenchymal cells derived from the septum transversum lie between the endothelial wall of the sinusoids and the hepatic cords and form the connective tissue elements of the hepatic stroma, as well as the capsule, which is covered by a mesothelial layer. Hematopoietic tissue and Kupffer's cells also derive from splanchnic mesenchyme of the septum transversum. Once these structures are established, the liver grows rapidly to fill most of the embryonal abdominal cavity and by 9 weeks' gestation accounts for approximately 10% of the total weight of the embryo (4). The bile canaliculi appear in the 10-mm embryo as intercellular spaces between immature hepatocytes (hepatoblasts).

The epithelium of the intrahepatic bile ducts arises from the proximal part of the primitive hepatic cords. This process is largely determined by the progressive development and branching of the portal vein with its surrounding mesenchyme. First, the epithelial layer in direct contact with the mesenchyme around the portal vein transforms into bile duct-type cells. Then a second layer transforms into bile duct epithelial cells, resulting in a circular cleft in the shape of a cylinder around the portal vein and its enveloping mesenchyme (Fig. 1). This primitive channel duct in the 8-mm embryo (5 to 6 weeks of gestation) is termed the "ductal plate" (5), which then undergoes gradual remodeling to form the normal anastomosing system of bile ducts in the portal tracts (6,7). The differentiation of intrahepatic ducts is recognized in embryos of 22 to 30 mm. Despite the common ancestry of hepatic parenchymal cells and ductal epithelium, each cell type is structurally and functionally distinct. The walls of the terminal twigs of the biliary tree, the canals of Hering, which connect bile canaliculi to bile ducts, include both typical hepatocytes and bile duct cells, without intermediate forms.

Functionally, intrahepatic hematopoiesis begins during the 6th week, hepatocyte bile formation by the 12th week, and excretion of bile into the duodenum by the 16th week. The third trimester marks the cessation of hematopoiesis with a concomitant decrease in liver growth so that the liver accounts for approximately 5% of the newborn's body weight.

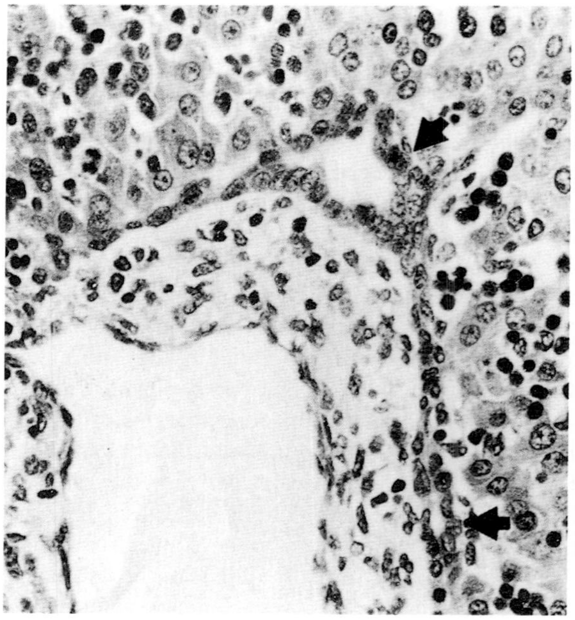

**FIG. 1.** Ductal plate (*arrows*) developing around the portal vein mesenchyme in the liver of a 10-week-old embryo. There is extramedullary hematopoiesis in the sinusoids.

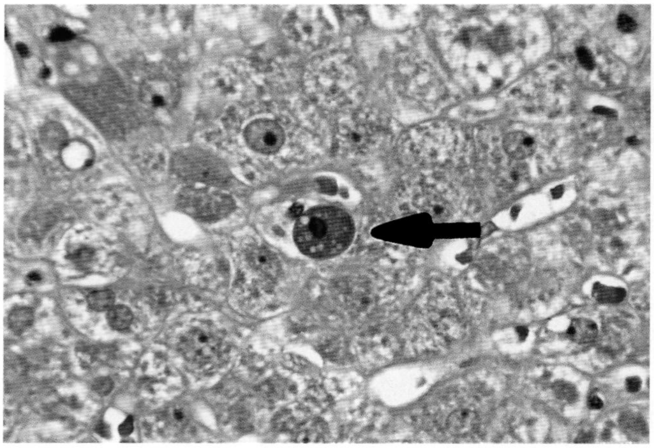

**FIG. 2.** A hepatocyte undergoing apoptosis (*arrow*).

## APOPTOSIS

Apoptosis occurs at all stages during fetal growth and development of ductal plates and hepatoblasts. There is a good correlation between the proliferative and the apoptotic activities in the ductal plate depending on the remodeling process (8). Involution of liver hyperplasia and neoplasia (9–12) also is controlled by apoptosis, which is induced by transforming growth factor-$\beta 1$ (11–13). In these regressing livers or tumors, scattered apoptotic bodies, rather than massive lytic necrosis, are observed. In viral infections, such as viral hepatitis B, apoptosis has been proposed as a mechanism of cell death. However, it is not clear if cell death in this system is mediated directly by the virus or by the host immune system through the release of cytokines such as tumor necrosis factor-$\alpha$ to the infected cells (14). In normal liver tissue, although rare, individual apoptotic bodies may be seen, which suggests that apoptosis is a physiological process in the liver (15) (Fig. 2).

## GROSS MORPHOLOGY

The liver of an adult weighs 1,400 to 1,600 g, comprising 2% of the body weight (3,16). The liver resides predominantly in the abdominal right upper quadrant and is completely protected by the rib cage. It extends from the right fifth intercostal space in the midclavicular line down to the right costal margin, and to the left as far as the left midclavicular line. It has the appearance of a wedge with the base to the right and measures about 10 cm in vertical span, 12 to 15 cm in thickness, and 15 to 20 cm in its greatest transverse diameter.

It is divided by deep grooves into two large lobes—the right (lateral to falciform ligament) and left (medial to falciform ligament)—and two smaller lobes—the caudate and quadrate lobes. This traditional division is only of topographical significance. Functionally, the division into eight segments, which do not correspond to the anatomical division into lobes (17), is more important. Each segment is served by its own vascular pedicle of arterial and portal venous blood supply and branch of the biliary tree. This segmental division is of critical importance, particularly when dissecting small space-occupying lesions from these areas or when removing segments of liver for transplantation. The superior, anterior, and lateral surfaces of the liver are smooth and almost completely covered by peritoneum, except for a small triangular area—the "bare area" below the diaphragm—which is surrounded by the reflections of the peritoneum forming the coronary ligaments. A thin layer of fibrous connective tissue, the Glisson's capsule, surrounds the liver and extends into the parenchyma to form extensions that support arterial and biliary structures. Anteriorly, the falciform and round ligaments, which during fetal life conducted the left umbilical vein, connect the liver to the abdominal wall. Through the posterior surface of the liver at the base of the bare area runs the inferior vena cava, to which two to four hepatic veins connect. The fossa of the gallbladder and the round ligament separate the quadrate lobe from the right and left liver lobes, respectively. The fossa of the ductus venosus (i.e., the connection of the left umbilical vein to the vena cava inferior) and the inferior vena cava separate the caudate lobe from the left and right lobes of the liver. The horizontal portal fissure or porta hepatis, which joins the upper ends of the gallbladder fossa and the groove of the round ligament, contains the branches of the hepatic artery, the portal vein, the hepatic nerve plexus, the hepatic ducts, and lymph vessels.

## ANATOMY

### Blood Supply and Drainage

The liver is nourished by a dual blood supply, approximately three fourths via the portal vein and the remainder via the hepatic arteries. Venous outflow is provided by the right, middle, and left hepatic veins. The right hepatic vein drains the right lobe, the middle hepatic vein drains primarily the middle portion of the left lobe and a variable portion of the right, and the left hepatic vein provides the principal drainage of the left lateral lobe. The middle and the left hepatic veins often join together to form a common trunk before entering the vena cava. In addition, there are short venous segments that drain the posterior surface of the liver directly into the inferior vena cava (18). The portal vein carries blood from the alimentary tract, including the pancreas, which is rich in nutrients, whereas the hepatic artery supplies most of the oxygen that the liver needs for survival.

### Bile Ducts

Bile ducts accompany the hepatic artery and portal vein while coursing through the liver. They are nourished by the hepatic arteries via a complex peribiliary plexus of capillaries, which supplies all structures within the portal tracts. Bile is formed in hepatocytes, steadily secreted into bile canaliculi and then to the intra- and extrahepatic bile ducts. The extrahepatic biliary tract consists of a gallbladder that ends in the cystic duct. The cystic duct joins the hepatic duct to form the common bile duct, which enters the second portion of the duodenum through its muscular structure, the sphincter of Oddi (19).

### Lymphatics

The capsule and the stroma of the liver is rich in lymphatic structures. The lymphatic plexus found in the capsule forms significant anastomoses with the intrahepatic lymphatics. The intrahepatic lymphatic system exists as fine, valved plexus associated with branches of hepatic artery in portal tracts. Hepatic lymph is most likely formed in the interstitial space of Disse, although lymphatic capillaries are not observed within the acini (20,21). Most of the hepatic lymphatics leave the liver at the porta hepatis and drain into hepatic nodes along the hepatic artery and into the celiac nodes. The liver represents the largest single source of lymph in the body, producing 15% to 20% of the overall total volume (22) and 25% to 50% of the thoracic duct flow (21).

### Nerve Supply and Innervation

The liver is innervated by two separate but intercommunicating plexuses around the hepatic artery and portal vein and are distributed with their branches (23). They include parasympathetic fibers from both vagi and sympathetic fibers, which receive their preganglionic connections from spinal segments T7 to T10 (24). The hilar plexuses also include afferent visceral and phrenic fibers. Besides their presence around vascular structures in portal tracts, nerve fibers, mostly sympathetic, are present in the parenchyma along the sinusoids. Release of neurotransmitters from the intrasinusoidal fibers modulate hepatocyte and perisinusoidal cell function. It controls in part carbohydrate and lipid metabolism and induces contraction of perisinusoidal cells, thereby regulating intrasinusoidal blood flow (25). However, neural mechanisms may have only a minor regulatory role because limited reinnervation in liver allografts does not seem to impair their function. Denervation probably explains the impaired normal response of the liver to ischemia, sinusoidal dilatation seen in liver allografts, and impaired metabolic function in cirrhosis (26,27).

## HISTOLOGY

The structural organization (16,28–31) of the liver into parenchymal, interstitial, vascular, and ductal elements is based on its many functions and its position between the digestive tract and the rest of the body. The functional unit of the liver is represented by the hepatic lobule or rather, as defined by Rappaport (3,32), the hepatic acinus (Fig. 3). The latter is a regular, three-dimensional structure in which blood flows from a central axis, formed by the terminal portal venule and terminal hepatic arteriole in the portal tract, into the acinar sinusoids and empties into several terminal hepatic venules at the periphery of the acinus (Fig. 4).

In contrast, the hepatic lobule consists of an efferent central vein with cords of hepatocytes radiating to several peripheral portal tracts (33). Therefore, in a two-dimensional view, the acinus occupies parts of several adjacent lobules. The acini measure 560 to 1,050 $\mu$m in length and 300 to 600 $\mu$m in width. The division of the hepatic parenchyma into the classic lobules, with lesions described as being centrilobular, midzonal, peripheral, or periportal, is still used as a convenient landmark. However, Rappaport's acinus has now come to be more generally accepted. The acinus is subdivided into zones 1, 2, and 3 with decreasing oxygenation (34). The hepatocytes in zone 1 are nearest to portal tracts and correspond to the peripheral area of the classic lobule. Zone 2 corresponds roughly to the midzonal area of a classic lobule, and zone 3 corresponds to parts of several centrilobular areas.

The terminal vascular branches, which bring substances for nutrition and metabolism into the acinus, run along the terminal bile ducts that drain the secretory products of the same acinus. The vessels form a vascular plexus around the bile ducts (35). Thus, as a result of the sinusoidal blood flow, structural, secretory, and functional unity is established in the acinus. The oxygen gradient, metabolic heterogeneity, and differential distribution of enzymes across the three zones of the acini (14) explain the zonal distribution of liver damage due to ischemia and toxic substances.

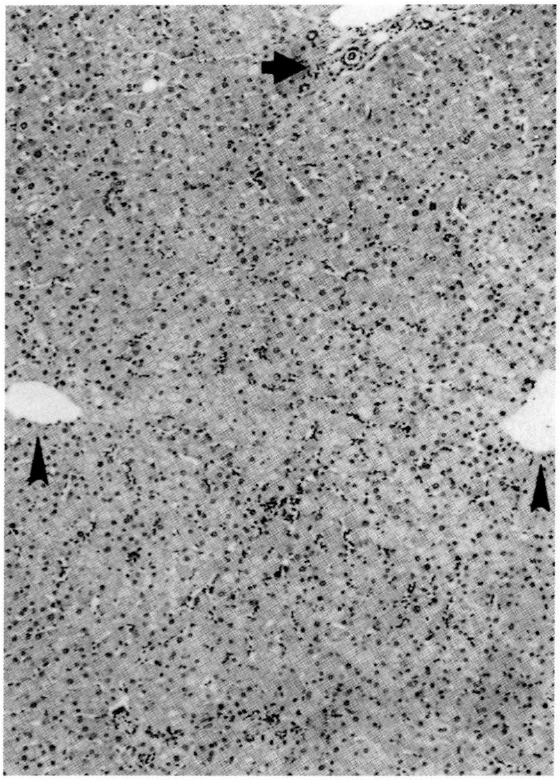

**FIG. 4.** Normal human liver showing a portal tract (*arrow*) and two terminal hepatic venules (*arrowheads*).

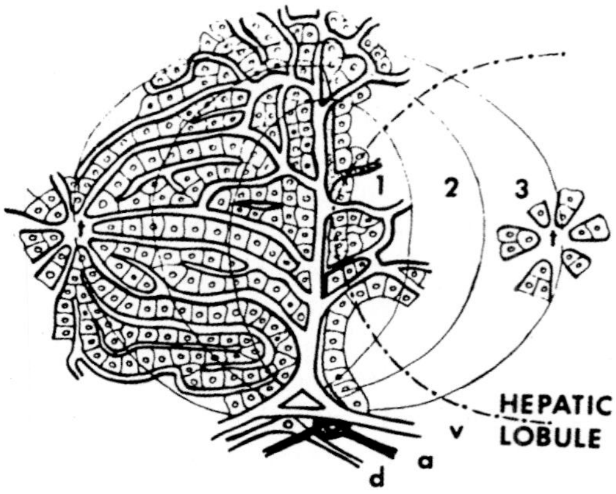


**FIG. 3.** Diagram comparing the hepatic acinus with zones 1, 2, and 3 to the hepatic lobule (*dotted line*). Portal tract contains portal venule (v), hepatic arteriole (a), and hepatic duct (d). t1, terminal hepatic venule.

### Hepatocytes and Bile Canaliculi

The hepatocytes are arranged in spongelike plates that in the adult are normally one cell layer thick and are separated by sinusoids along which blood flows from portal tracts to terminal hepatic venules (Fig. 5). In children up to 5 or 6 years of age, the liver cells are arranged in two-cell thick plates. The individual hepatocyte is a polygonal epithelial cell approximately 25 $\mu$m in diameter with a well-defined plasma membrane that is differentiated into basolateral (75%) and bile canalicular (15%) domains with different molecular, chemical, and antigenic compositions and functions.

The nucleus is centrally located, round, and contains one or more nucleoli. Although binucleate forms are not uncommon, mitotic activity is rare. Nuclei vary in size in the adult, and the great majority are diploid (36). Some nuclei are larger than others, indicating polyploidy, particularly in persons over 60 years of age (37) (Fig. 6, Table 1).

The abundant cytoplasm is eosinophilic and contains fine

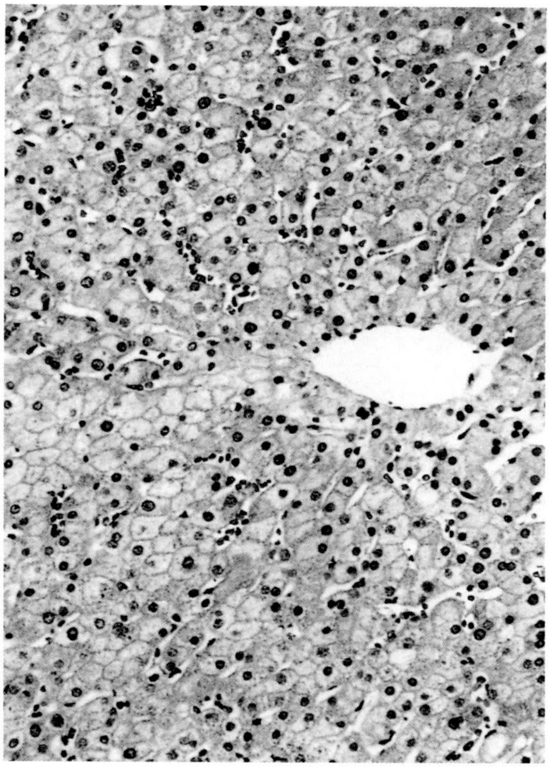

**FIG. 5.** Terminal hepatic venule surrounded by converging hepatocyte plates and sinusoids.

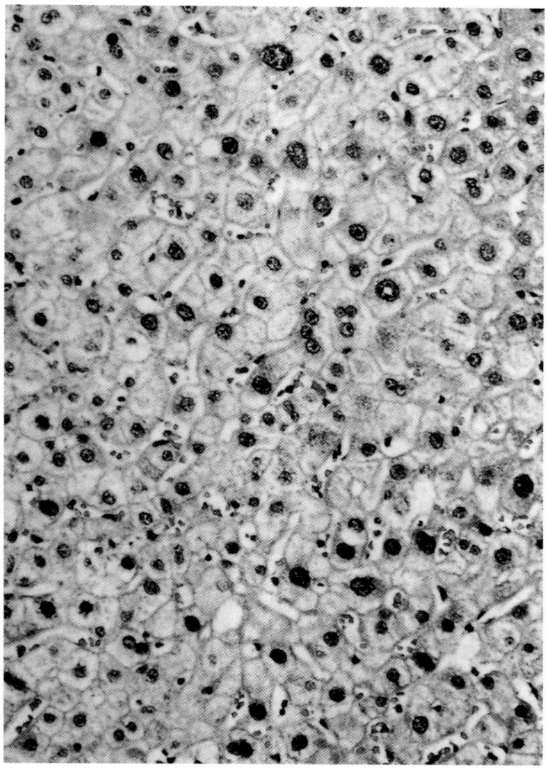

**FIG. 6.** Liver of a 65-year-old patient showing significant polyploidy of hepatocyte nuclei.

basophilic granules representing rough endoplasmic reticulum. Cytoplasmic glycogen is present and after proper fixation is stainable with periodic acid-Schiff (PAS) reagent. On hematoxylin and eosin (H&E) preparations, glycogen gives a fine, reticulated, foamy appearance to the cytoplasm. The amount and distribution of glycogen show diurnal and diet-related variations. Glycogen accumulation in hepatocytic nuclei around portal tracts produces a vacuolated appearance (Fig. 7) and is common in adolescents. In adults, such an appearance may be conspicuous in conditions such as diabetes mellitus, pancreatic carcinoma, and chronic heart failure but is usually of no diagnostic significance.

A few vacuoles and small amounts of stainable iron are common in normal hepatocytes, particularly in older individuals. Hemosiderin and copper are abundant in the cytoplasm of hepatocytes during the first week of life, then gradually disappear and should be absent at the age of 6 to 9 months.

Lipofuscin, the "wear and tear" pigment, is seen in varying amounts as fine, well-delineated, light brown, PAS-positive, diastase-resistant, partly acid-fast–positive granules in the cytoplasm of hepatocytes in zone 3, particularly at the canalicular pole (Fig. 8). There is a progressive increase of its amount in individual hepatocytes and in the number of cells involved in older individuals. It is rich in oxidized lipids accumulating in secondary lysosomes as a result of autophagy and uptake of exogenous substances. It may be difficult to distinguish lipofuscin from the pigment that accumulates in hepatocytes in large amounts in Dubin-Johnson syndrome.

In contrast, iron and copper are coarser, birefringent, and usually deposited in periportal hepatocytes. Intracellular bile is poorly defined and less granular than the other pigments and often forms thrombi in bile canaliculi in zone 3 (38) (Fig. 9). Isolated eosinophilic bodies as a result of coagulative necrosis, rare apoptotic bodies representing normal turnover of hepatocytes (15), and an occasional focal necrosis where chronic inflammatory cells replace a few necrotic hepatocytes are not unusual in otherwise apparently normal livers.

The bile canaliculus is an intercellular space with a diameter of approximately 1 $\mu$m, formed by the apposition of the edges of gutterlike hemicanals on adjacent surfaces of two or three neighboring hepatocytes. Bile canaliculi are not readily

**TABLE 1.** *Age-related variations of the histologic appearance of the normal liver*

| | Young children | Old adults |
|---|---|---|
| Hepatocytes | Small and regular | Variable in size and polyploid |
| | Double cell plates | Single cell plates |
| Portal tracts | Delicate | Sclerotic or fibrotic |
| Nuclear glycogen | Often present | Usually absent |
| Lipofuscin | Scanty | Increased |

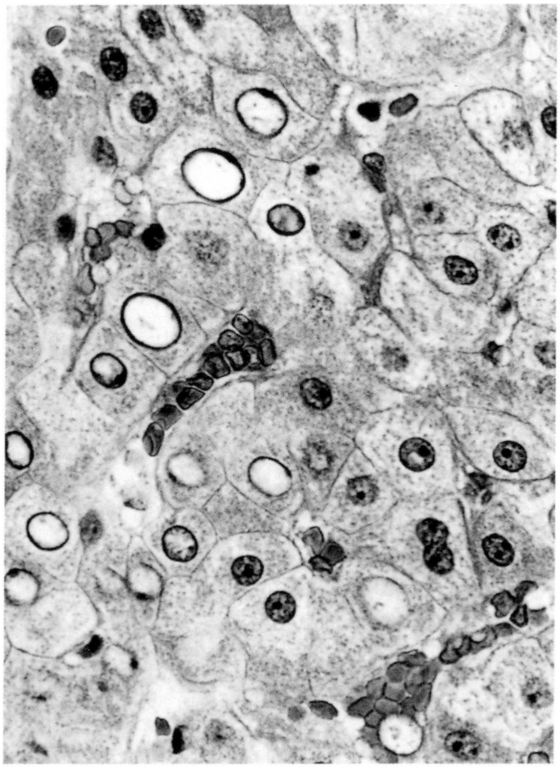

**FIG. 7.** Glycogen accumulation in hepatocyte nuclei resulting in clear, empty appearance.

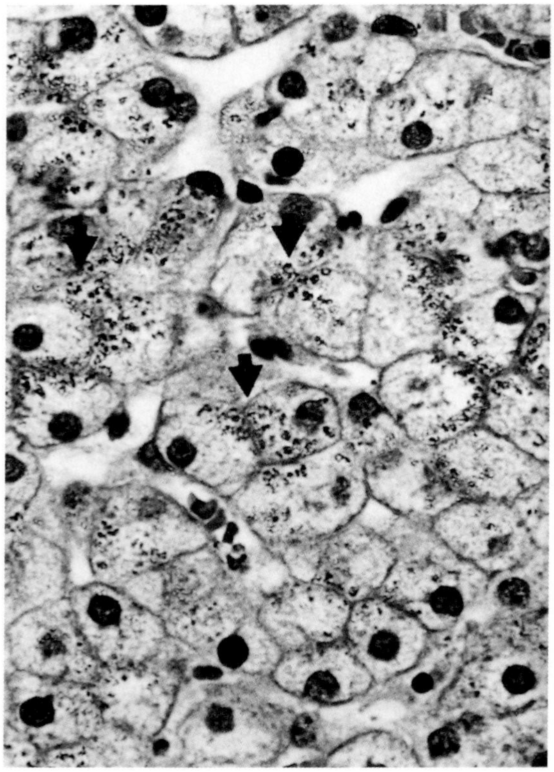

**FIG. 8.** Lipofuscin in hepatocytes of zone 3 of the acinus. The finely granular pigment accumulates along the bile canaliculi (*arrows*).

recognized under the light microscope unless distended in conditions with parenchymal cholestasis. They form a chicken wire–like network in the center of the hepatic plates, which can be demonstrated immunohistochemically with polyclonal anti–carcinoembryonic antigen (CEA). They connect to small portal bile ducts via canals of Hering.

### Sinusoidal Lining Cells

The hepatic sinusoids separate cords of hepatocytes and are lined by sinusoidal lining cells supported by reticulin fibers (Fig. 10). These cells, which include endothelial and Kupffer's cells and together constitute a coordinated defense system, are not conspicuous in normal biopsy specimens. The endothelial cells have thin, indistinct cytoplasm and small, elongated, darkly stained nuclei without nucleoli. The sievelike plates of the endothelial cytoplasm and the absence of a structurally defined basement membrane (in contrast to capillaries) facilitate exchange between blood and hepatocytes (20,39,40).

The Kupffer's cells have a bean-shaped nucleus and plump cytoplasm with star-shaped extensions (41). They are more numerous near the portal tracts. They belong to the mononuclear–phagocytic system and are derived in part from the bone marrow. They contain vacuoles and, particularly in the diseased liver, many diastase-resistant PAS (D-PAS)–positive lysosomes and phagosomes, as well as acid-fast granular aggregates of ceroid pigment. These cells respond actively to many types of injury with proliferation and enlargement. In normal liver biopsy specimens, the sinusoids are slitlike spaces that contain a few blood cells.

Between the endothelial cells and the hepatocytes lies the space of Disse, a zone of rapid intercellular exchange. It contains plasma, scanty connective tissue that constitutes the normal framework of the liver, and perisinusoidal cells such as lipocytes (Ito, interstitial fat-storing or hepatic stellate cells) and pit cells. The connective tissue fibers along the si-

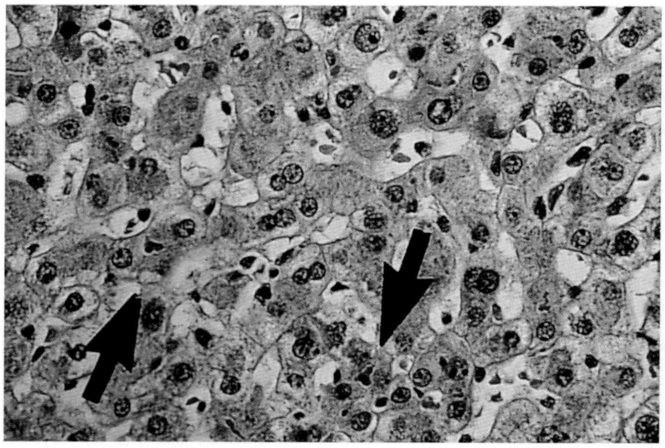

**FIG. 9.** Intracellular bile and canalicular bile thrombi (*arrows*) in zone 3 of the acinus.

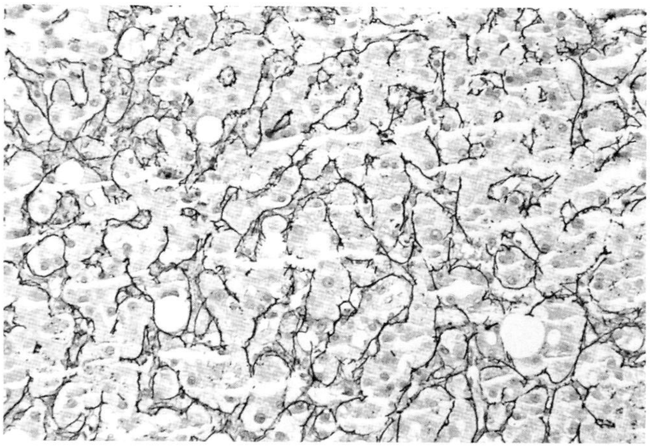

**FIG. 10.** Hepatic sinusoids lined by reticulin fibers in a normal liver (reticulin stain).

nusoids represent predominantly collagen type III, which stains black in silver impregnations (reticulin) and forms a regular network radiating from the center of the lobules. Elastic fibers and basement membranes are absent from normal sinusoids (42,43). The space of Disse is not discernible in well-fixed, normal liver biopsy material; but in postmortem liver, the hepatocytes shrink, pericellular edema develops, and the space becomes more conspicuous (Fig. 11).

On light microscopy, hepatic stellate cells (44) are difficult to differentiate from sinusoidal lining cells. They are modified resting fibroblasts that can store fat and vitamin A and produce hepatocyte growth factor (45) and collagen. They appear to play a significant role in hepatic fibrogenesis. When loaded with fat, such as in hypervitaminosis A, they may be recognized due to cytoplasmic fat droplets of rather uniform size with scalloping of the elongated nucleus (Fig. 12). When activated, these cells contain stainable desmin and actin in their cytoplasm (46), justifying their designation as myofibroblasts.

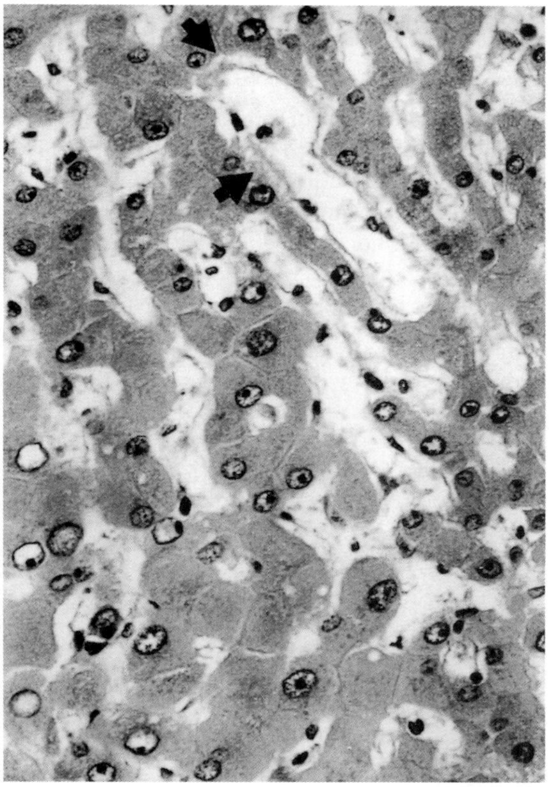

**FIG. 11.** Autopsy liver specimen exhibiting dilation of sinusoids and Disse's space (*arrows*) with prominent sinusoidal lining cells including endothelial and Kupffer's cells.

Pit cells (47,48) have not been characterized by light microscopy. Under the electron microscope, they have neurosecretory-like electron-dense granules and rod-cored vesicles. Recent evidence indicates that pit cells are not endocrine cells but correspond to the large granular lymphocytes and have natural killer cell activity (49). Occasional inflammatory cells, lymphocytes, or polymorphonuclear leukocytes may be present in the sinusoids. During the first few weeks after birth, the presence of foci of extramedullary hematopoietic cells in the sinusoids and wall of terminal hepatic venules is a normal feature.

### Hepatic Veins

The intrahepatic course of the valveless hepatic veins, which are embedded in a thin sheath of connective tissue, is straight to the inferior vena cava. The smaller branches, or sublobular veins, and the smallest efferent veins, or terminal hepatic venules, are in direct contact with the hepatic parenchyma. There is a defined spatial relationship between the terminal hepatic venules and the branches of the portal vein and hepatic artery in the portal tracts, which interdigitate but do not directly connect in the three-dimensional space.

The distance between two terminal hepatic venules represents the size of an acinus. The terminal hepatic venules have a very thin wall (Fig. 5) lined by endothelial cells, which is readily demonstrable after staining with trichrome for collagen or Victoria blue for elastic fibers, but they do not have an adventitia around their wall (50).

It has been suggested that perivenular sclerosis in alcoholic patients may be an index of progressive liver injury (50), although this has been disputed subsequently (51). Thickening of the wall of terminal hepatic venules is often part of pericellular fibrosis and central hyaline sclerosis in alcoholic liver disease (51). It may be seen focally in apparently normal individuals as well as in children up to 2 years of age.

### Portal Tracts

Each portal tract contains a bile duct and ductules, a hepatic artery branch, a portal vein branch, and lymphatic channels embedded in connective tissue (Fig. 13). The amount of connective tissue and the size of the intraportal structures depend on the size of the portal tract. Nerve fibers,

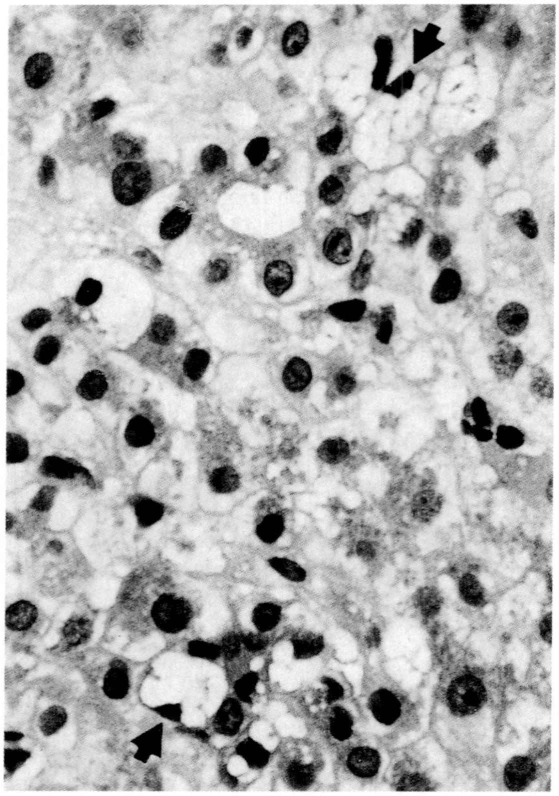

**FIG. 12.** Prominent lipocytes in liver biopsy specimen of patient with hypervitaminosis A. The nuclei of the lipocytes are scalloped (*arrows*) due to fat droplets in cytoplasm.

both sympathetic and parasympathetic for innervation of blood vessels and bile ducts, can be seen in large portal tracts. The largest portal tracts are round or triangular, the smaller ones are triangular or branching, and the smallest terminal divisions are round or oval. The size of a portal tract is approximately three to four times the diameter of the hepatic artery branch. They normally contain a few lymphocytes, macrophages, and mast cells, but no polymorphonuclear leukocytes or plasma cells. The number of inflammatory cells increases with age. However, their density varies from one portal tract to the next. The connective tissue consists mainly of collagen type I, which is seen as thick, deep blue fibers on the trichrome stain. Newly formed collagen type III appears as fine, light blue fibers. In the subcapsular region of the liver, the portal tracts contain more and denser connective tissue. Irregular extensions of fibrous tissue from Glisson's capsule into the parenchyma, sometimes connecting adjacent portal tracts, must not be interpreted as cirrhosis in wedge or superficial biopsy specimens of subcapsular parenchyma (52).

### Bile Ducts

The larger intrahepatic or septal bile ducts are lined by tall columnar epithelial cells measuring about 10 $\mu$m in diameter with basally situated, pale, oval nuclei and light

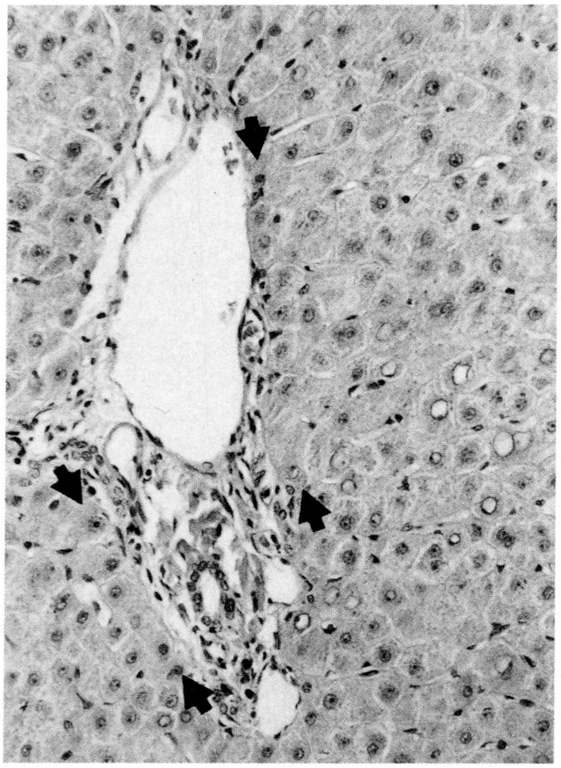

**FIG. 13.** Normal portal tract with bile duct, hepatic arteriole, portal venule, and clearly defined limiting plate (*arrows*).

eosinophilic cytoplasm (53,54) (Fig. 14). They have an internal diameter greater than 100 $\mu$m and a distinct basement membrane stainable with D-PAS. The larger bile ducts are located in the central part of the portal tracts and have more periductal fibrous tissue than the smaller ones. The collagen fibers are arranged in an irregular, circumferential, but not concentric, manner, as may be seen in biliary tract diseases such as sclerosing cholangitis and even as a sequela of cholecystitis.

The smaller or interlobular bile ducts are lined by cuboidal

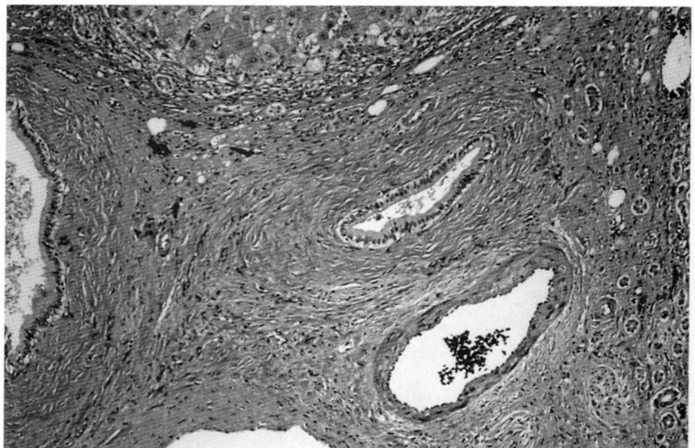

**FIG. 14.** A large portal tract containing an artery and a bile duct lined by columnar epithelial cells.

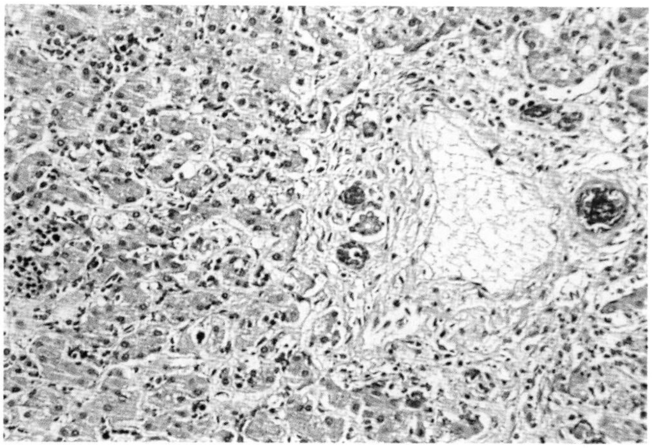

**FIG. 15.** Normal portal tract in a newborn with bile ducts and their corresponding hepatic arterioles of approximately the same diameter.

or low columnar epithelium. They have a basement membrane and a small amount of periductal connective tissue. One or more interlobular ducts may be present in a portal tract. Bile ducts are always accompanied by a portal vein and hepatic artery, the latter having approximately the same diameter as the bile ducts (external caliber ratio of bile duct to artery is 0.7:0.8) (54) (Fig. 15). The bile ducts are connected to the bile canaliculi by bile ductules and canals of Hering.

Bile ductules are located in the peripheral zone of the portal tracts and are smaller (lumen of less than 20 $\mu$m) than interlobular bile ducts (Fig. 16). They have a basement membrane and cuboidal epithelium and are accompanied by a portal vein but not by a hepatic artery branch. Proliferating bile ductules occur in a variety of chronic liver diseases and can be so extensive as to raise the question of adenocarcinoma (55). Canals of Hering are not discernible on routine sections of normal liver. They are lined partly by bile ductular cells and partly by hepatocytes. They can be demonstrated by staining for high-molecular-weight cytokeratin polypeptides, which are prominent in all cells of ductal origin.

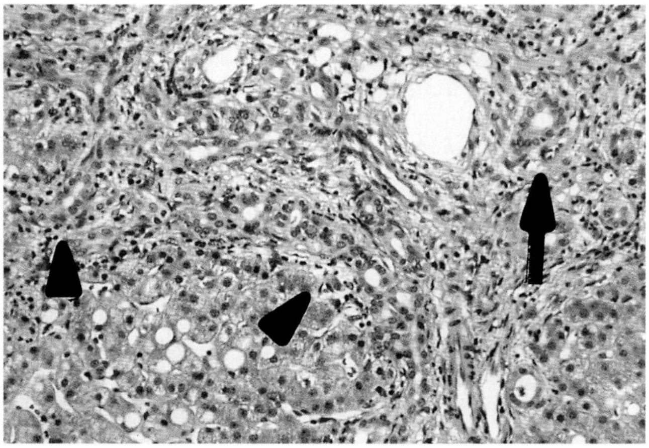

**FIG. 16.** Bile ductule (*arrowheads*) are located in the peripheral zone of the portal tract and are smaller than the bile duct (*arrow*).

### Portal Vein and Hepatic Artery

The lymphatic vessels in portal tracts drain the Disse spaces. The lymph flows in the same direction as the bile, opposite to that of the blood. The hepatic artery branches are intimately related to the corresponding portal veins. They may show thickening and hyalinization of the wall in older persons, although these changes are usually milder than in other organs. The terminal hepatic arterioles regulate the parenchymal blood supply with their muscular sphincter (56), whereas portal venous supply is controlled by mesenteric venous blood flow.

The portal veins are the largest vessels in the portal tracts and produce venules that empty into periportal sinusoids. In contrast to hepatocytes around the terminal hepatic venules, the hepatocytes bordering the portal tracts are joined together and form a distinct row called the "limiting plate" (57). Destruction of this limiting plate by necroinflammation is a hallmark of chronic hepatitis (piecemeal necrosis) (Fig. 17).

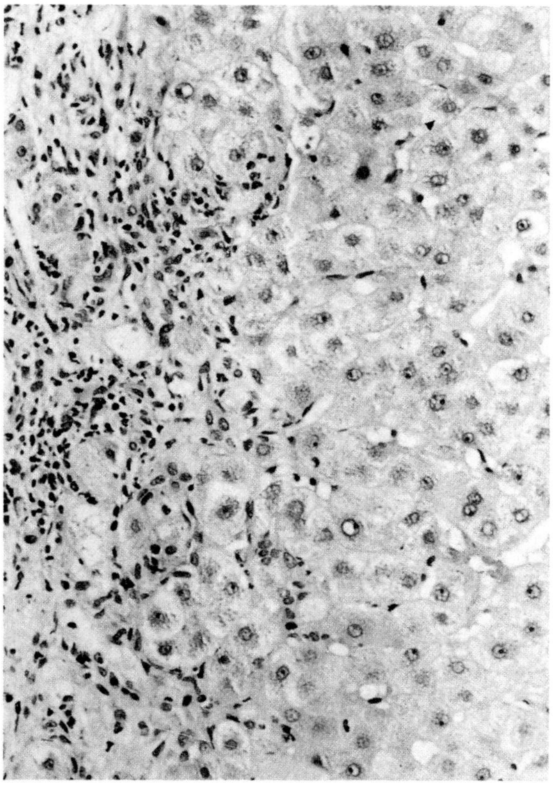

**FIG. 17.** Liver from a patient with chronic active hepatitis showing destruction of the limiting plate by extension of inflammatory cells from the portal tract (*left*) into the periportal parenchyma with necrosis of hepatocytes (piecemeal necrosis).

## EXTRACELLULAR MATRIX

Both interstitial and basement membrane collagens are present in the liver and play an important role not only as structural elements but also in hepatic function (58). Collagen I—the main component of the dense, birefringent connective tissue fibers—is seen mainly in portal tracts, walls of hepatic veins, and rarely in the normal parenchyma, whereas collagen III and IV are present along the sinusoids (5). Collagen I can be demonstrated with connective tissue stains; collagen III can be seen with silver impregnation for reticulin. Collagen II, characteristic of cartilage, is absent from the liver. Collagens IV and V, the basement membrane collagens, and laminin are seen in the basement membrane of vessels, bile ducts, and bile ductules but (except for some collagen IV) not along the sinusoids of normal human liver (42,58). Distribution of elastic fibers in the liver, as demonstrated by orcein, resorcin, or Victoria blue stains, seems to follow that of collagen I (43). Fibronectin, an extracellular matrix glycoprotein, is present diffusely along the sinusoidal surface of hepatocytes and in portal tracts together with the other collagens (59). All components of the extracellular matrix are visualized best by immunohistochemical staining using specific antibodies.

## METHODOLOGY

### Specimen Handling

After removal from the patient (60), the liver specimen should be handled as little as possible and with utmost care to avoid squeezing artifacts. If the case so indicates, small pieces of liver tissue may be frozen for histochemistry, immunohistochemistry, or chemical analysis and fixed in glutaraldehyde for electron microscopy. If required, cultures should be taken. Then the tissue should be transferred quickly into the appropriate fixative solution, usually 10% buffered formalin. Needle biopsy specimens may be arranged on a piece of card to prevent distortion and fragmentation. At this stage, the gross appearance of the liver specimen is noted. Particular attention should be paid to fragmentation, which suggests cirrhosis, and to the number, size, shape, and color of the fragments.

Needle biopsy specimens are fixed for at least 3 hr at room temperature, whereas wedge biopsy specimens, after sectioning into 2-mm thick slices, need longer fixation. In order to avoid shrinkage and hardening of the tissue, it is important to process liver specimens separately from other tissues and on a more rapid schedule in the automated tissue processor. More than 10 consecutive sections, 3 to 5 $\mu$m in thickness, can be cut without artifact from well-embedded specimens. Usually paraffin is used for embedding, but plastic embedding may be used to obtain thinner sections.

### Special Stains

The tissue is routinely stained with H&E, Masson's trichrome, or chromotrope-aniline blue for fibrous tissue; Victoria blue or orcein is used for hepatitis B surface antigen (HBsAg), elastic fibers, lipofuscin, ceroid, and copper-binding protein; D-PAS is used for glycoproteins, including $\alpha$1-antitrypsin inclusions, ceroid in macrophages, basement membranes of bile ducts, cytoplasmic inclusions of cytomegalovirus, and *Mycobacterium avium-intracellulare*; stains for reticulin and iron are also important. If it is not possible to perform all these stains, at a minimum a special stain for connective tissue or reticulin should be obtained in order to assess the lobular architecture and facilitate the diagnosis of cirrhosis.

It should be emphasized that an adequate and properly processed liver specimen without artifacts is an important prerequisite for the accurate evaluation by an experienced histopathologist, who should be supplied with all relevant clinical and laboratory data.

Microscopic examination should conform to a routine and include all tissue fragments and all structures of the liver (architecture, portal triads, limiting plate, hepatocytes, sinusoidal cells, and terminal hepatic venules). We usually start with careful examination of zone 3 of the acinus because many changes are found here (congestion, fat, necrosis, cholestasis, pigments, endophlebitis) and then move to the remainder of the parenchyma and portal tracts. Sampling error, particularly in focally or irregularly distributed disease processes, always must be taken into consideration. Squeezing of tissue during the biopsy procedure results in distortion of cells and elongation of nuclei, which makes cytologic evaluation of the specimen very difficult (for other artifacts, see section In the Liver at Autopsy below).

### Immunohistologic Studies

Recent progress in immunology, particularly the development of monoclonal antibodies and of highly sensitive immunohistochemical staining procedures (peroxidase-antiperoxidase and avidin-biotin-peroxidase complex methods), has made it possible to demonstrate many antigens in routinely processed (i.e., formalin-fixed and paraffin-embedded) tissue sections. Detection of some of these antigens is useful in the diagnostic evaluation of liver diseases, such as $\alpha$1-antitrypsin in D-PAS–positive intracytoplasmic globules in periportal hepatocytes of patients with $\alpha$1-antitrypsin deficiency (Fig. 18), alpha-fetoprotein in hepatocellular carcinoma, CEA, and Lewis blood group antigens in bile duct carcinoma, although CEA is also expressed in some hepatocellular and many metastatic carcinomas (61,62).

The presence or absence and distribution pattern of viral antigens are helpful in the diagnostic and prognostic evaluation of viral hepatitis, particularly hepatitis B surface (Fig. 19) and core antigens (Fig. 20), hepatitis A, C, and delta (D)

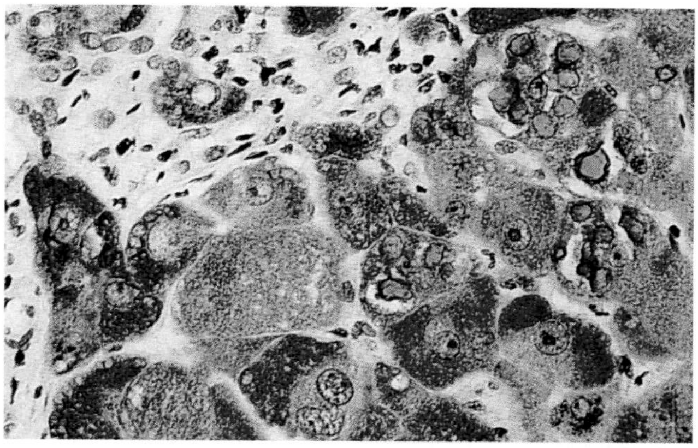

**FIG. 18.** $\alpha$1-Antitrypsin (AAT) granules and globules with peripheral staining only in hepatocytes of a patient with AAT deficiency (immunoperoxidase method using anti-AAT, counterstained with hematoxylin).

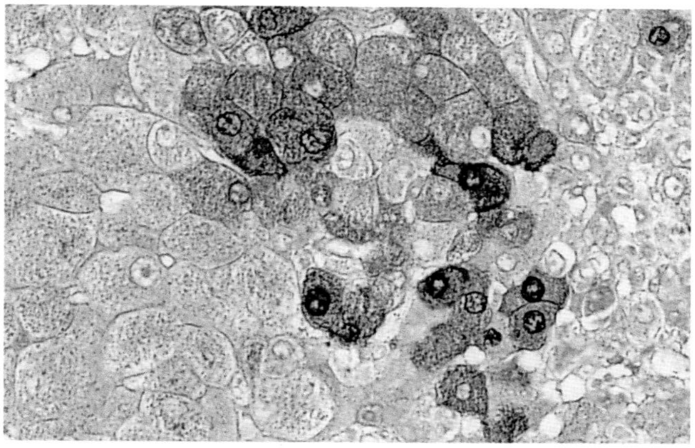

**FIG. 20.** Hepatitis B core antigen (HBcAg) in nuclei and cytoplasm of hepatocytes (immunoperoxidase method using anti-HBc, counterstained with methylene blue).

antigens, and herpes virus antigens (cytomegalovirus, herpes simplex virus, and Epstein-Barr virus) (63). Since the cloning and sequencing of the hepatitis C virus (HCV) genome in 1989, there have been a number of studies for the detection of HCV antigens in the liver. However, the reports are conflicting (64–66). The detection rate of positive cases varied, which may be related to tissue sampling and differences in sensitivity of various methods. Immunohistochemical studies on frozen sections appeared to demonstrate HCV antigens more reliably than on formalin-fixed, paraffin-embedded sections. Different as well as similar cytokeratin polypeptides are expressed by hepatocytes (45-, 52-, and 54-kDa polypeptides) (67) and bile ducts (40-, 54-, 57-, and 66-kDa polypeptides) (68) (Figs. 21 and 22) and may be altered in specific liver diseases such as alcoholic hepatitis with formation of alcoholic hyalin (69–71). The expression of the various components of extracellular matrix in the diseased liver is currently under intensive investigation. It is clear that development of additional monoclonal antibodies to other antigens will further expand the usefulness of immunohistologic staining for the diagnostic hepatopathologist.

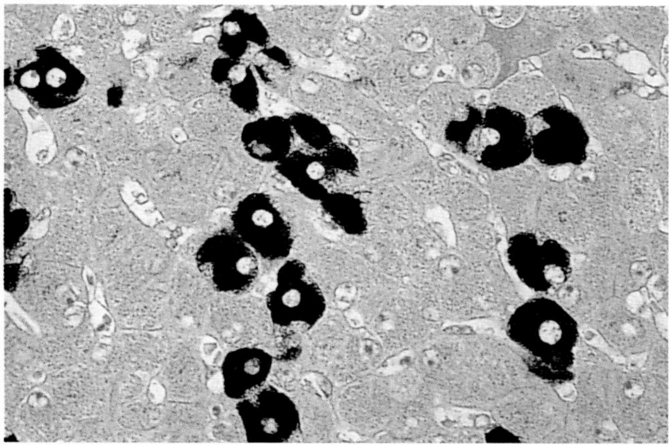

**FIG. 19.** Hepatitis B surface antigen (HBsAg) in cytoplasm of ground-glass hepatocytes (immunoperoxidase method using anti-HBs, counterstained with methylene blue).

## Molecular Studies

In situ hybridization for the detection of DNA or RNA may be performed on formalin-fixed, paraffin-embedded tis-

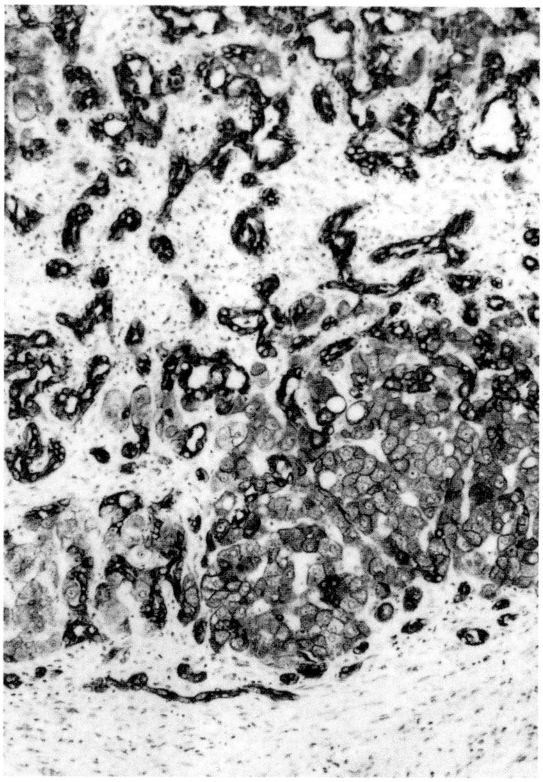

**FIG. 21.** Cytokeratin polypeptides expressed in both hepatocytes and bile ductal epithelium (immunoperoxidase stain using anti-45-, -52-, and -54-kDa cytokeratin polypeptides).

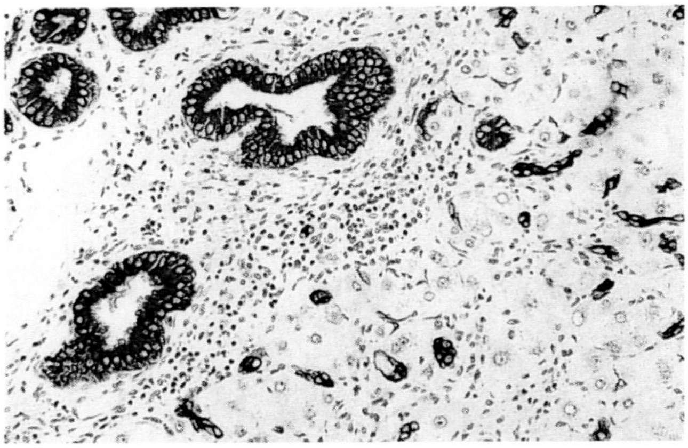

**FIG. 22.** Cytokeratin polypeptides expressed in bile ductal and bile ductular cells in a liver with cirrhosis. Hepatocytes are negative for these polypeptides (immunoperoxidase stain using anti-40-, -54-, -57-, and -66-kDa cytokeratin polypeptides).

sue sections. In liver biopsy evaluation, the detection of viral sequences such as those of Epstein-Barr virus and more recently of HCV by in situ hybridization appear to be more sensitive than by immunohistochemical methods (72–74). The sensitivity, especially in HCV infection, in which the number of virus in the liver is low, can be further increased by in situ polymerase chain reaction (75).

## AGING CHANGES

There are several changes in the liver related to aging. These are commonly seen in individuals 60 years of age and older. There is more variation in the size of the hepatocytes and their nuclei, similar to that seen in patients on methotrexate, due to increased polyploid cells (76). More abundant lipofuscin deposition is present in the centrilobular hepatocytes, and sometimes there are some iron pigments in the periportal hepatocytes. The portal tracts contain denser collagen and may exhibit a higher number of mononuclear inflammatory cells than in younger subjects. The arteries may have thickened walls (Fig. 23), even in normotensive individuals. These histologic changes of aging need to be kept in mind because they are often present in viable donors for which frozen sections are requested and should not be interpreted as pathologic. These aging-related findings are accompanied by alteration in the metabolic function of the liver, including the metabolism of toxins and drugs (77), and may increase the susceptibility of the liver to hypovolemia.

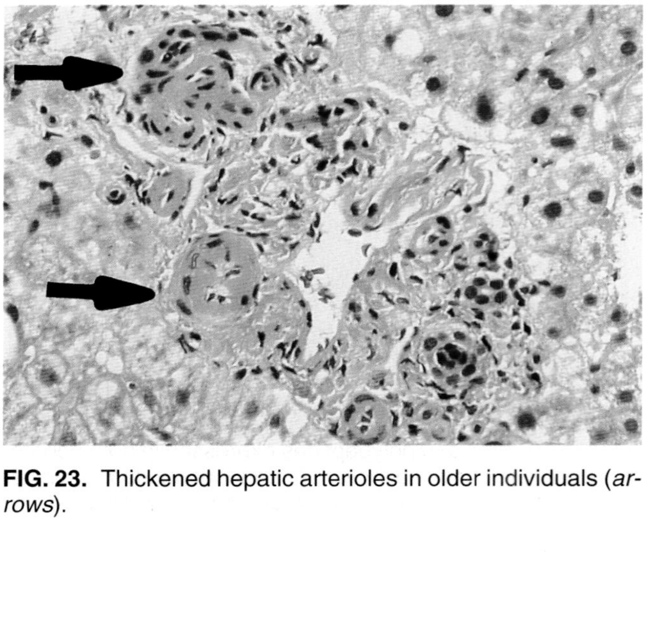

**FIG. 23.** Thickened hepatic arterioles in older individuals (*arrows*).

## FREQUENT HISTOLOGIC CHANGES OF LITTLE SIGNIFICANCE

### In the Liver at Autopsy

Liver tissue obtained at autopsy often shows changes that are usually not seen in liver biopsy specimens and therefore may cause difficulties in the evaluation: agonal loss of glycogen from hepatocytes causes increased density and eosinophilia of the cytoplasm. Poor fixation results in irregular staining of hepatocytes, particularly in the center of the specimen. This may result in striking differences in the appearance of liver cells in the peripheral versus the central part of the tissue.

Agonal necrosis, particularly of hepatocytes in zone 3 in patients with shock or heart failure, may not be reflected in elevated aminotransferase levels. Its terminal nature is recognized from the lack of any inflammatory response. Autolysis of hepatocytes, particularly in hepatitis and cholestasis resulting in loss of cellular detail and prominent sinusoidal lining cells, is often more pronounced than in other tissues because the liver is rich in proteolytic enzymes. Loss of inflammatory cells by autolysis may make the diagnosis of hepatitis in postmortem specimens difficult (78).

Dilatation of the sinusoidal and perisinusoidal spaces is of little significance in postmortem liver tissues (Fig. 11) as opposed to similar changes in well-preserved biopsy specimens. Focal accumulation of lymphocytes in scattered portal tracts is frequently seen in autopsy livers and does not justify the diagnosis of chronic hepatitis. Large tissue sections obtained at autopsy often include many large triangular portal tracts with abundant connective tissue that can be distinguished from true portal fibrosis by evaluation of the size of the intraportal structures. Increased fibrous tissue in portal tracts and parenchyma is a normal phenomenon in older individuals.

### In Surgical Liver Biopsy Specimens

Surgical biopsy specimens may have several features not seen in needle biopsy specimens that may cause diagnostic difficulties. If the surgeon removes a small, superficial wedge of liver tissue from the inferior margin, the triangular

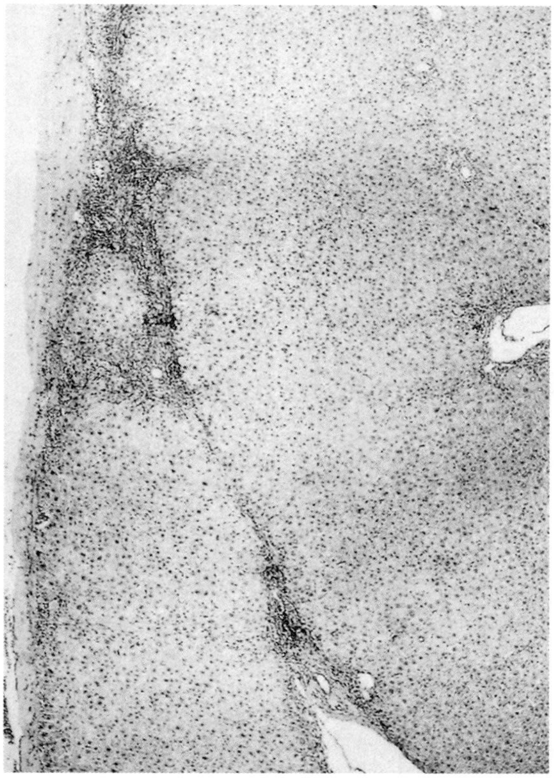

**FIG. 24.** Surgical liver biopsy specimen showing fibrous connections between the capsule and superficial portal tracts imitating the picture of cirrhosis.

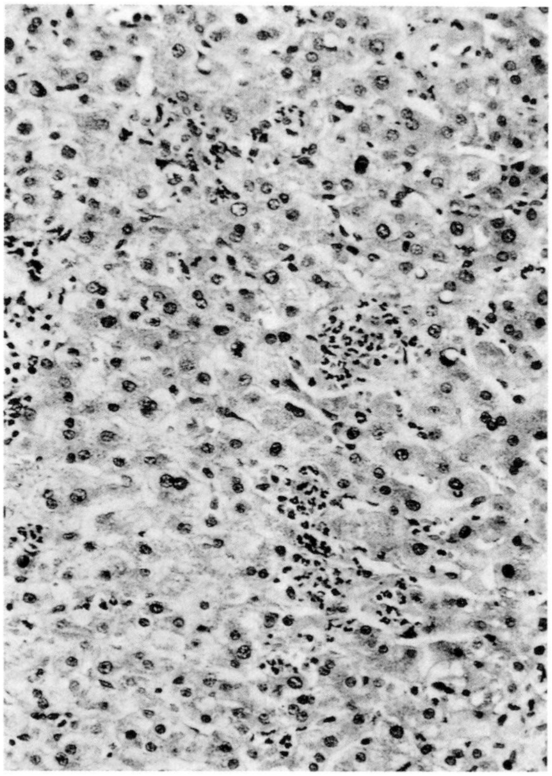

**FIG. 25.** Surgical liver biopsy specimen showing clusters of polymorphonuclear neutrophiles in sinusoids resembling microabscesses.

tissue fragment is covered on two sides by capsule. The fibrous connections between the superficial portal tracts and the capsule may imitate cirrhosis (31) (Fig. 24). However, these changes usually do not extend more than 2 mm into the liver parenchyma.

In biopsy specimens removed at the end of a long surgical procedure, clusters of polymorphonuclear neutrophils are seen, probably as a result of minor trauma in or under the capsule, in sinusoids, around terminal hepatic venules, in portal tracts, and in areas of small focal necroses resembling microabscesses (79) (Fig. 25). This characteristic lesion must be distinguished from inflammatory liver diseases such as cholangitis. Other "innocent" hepatic lesions include focal steatosis involving small groups of hepatocytes, fat globules, fat granulomas, sometimes mineral oil in portal tracts, undefined pigmentation, and unexplained mitoses of hepatocytes that normally have a life span of many years.

## MINOR, BUT SIGNIFICANT, HEPATIC ALTERATIONS

### Nonspecific Reactive Hepatitis

This poorly defined histologic change represents a reaction of the liver to a variety of extrahepatic, particularly febrile and gastrointestinal, diseases. Nonspecific reactive hepatitis must be differentiated from primary liver diseases such as mild chronic hepatitis and residual stages of acute viral hepatitis. The alterations consist of activation of sinusoidal lining cells with prominent Kupffer's cells, small foci of necrosis of isolated hepatocytes with accumulation of macrophages and other inflammatory cells, and infiltration of portal tracts by scattered mononuclear cells (Fig. 26). The inflammatory infiltrates in only slightly enlarged portal tracts are not as dense as in chronic hepatitis, usually do not involve all portal tracts, and are not accompanied by piecemeal necrosis or fibrosis (Fig. 27). Scattered hepatocytes also may contain microvesicular or macrovesicular fat globules.

Nonspecific reactive hepatitis with steatosis, increased variation in size, and staining quality of hepatocyte nuclei, sinusoidal dilatation, and poorly developed granulomata are often seen in the liver of patients with acquired immunodeficiency syndrome (AIDS) (80,81). The granulomata may be difficult to recognize, but special stains frequently show large numbers of microorganisms such as *M. avium-intracellulare.* Although patients with AIDS are often infected with cytomegalovirus, the characteristic intranuclear and cytoplasmic inclusions are sometimes not detected in the liver, but focal aggregates of polymorphonuclear leukocytes, so-called microabscesses may be seen in sinusoids and at sites

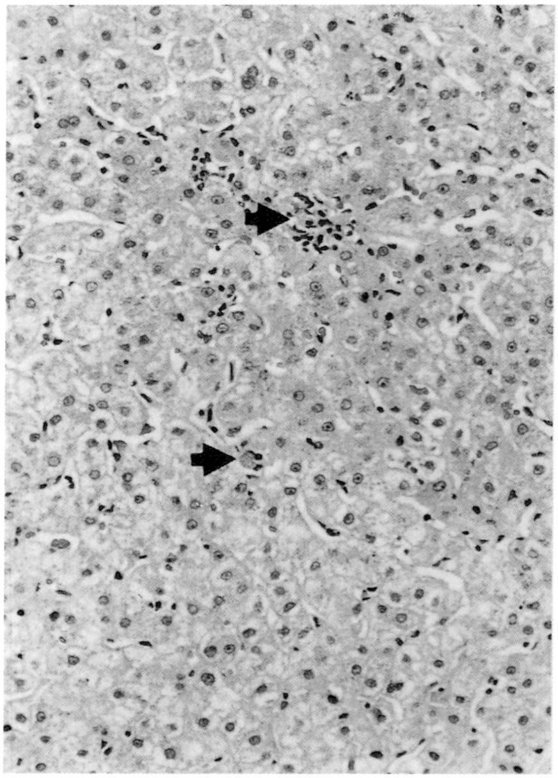

**FIG. 26.** Nonspecific reactive hepatitis characterized by activation of sinusoidal lining cells and focal necrosis (*arrows*).

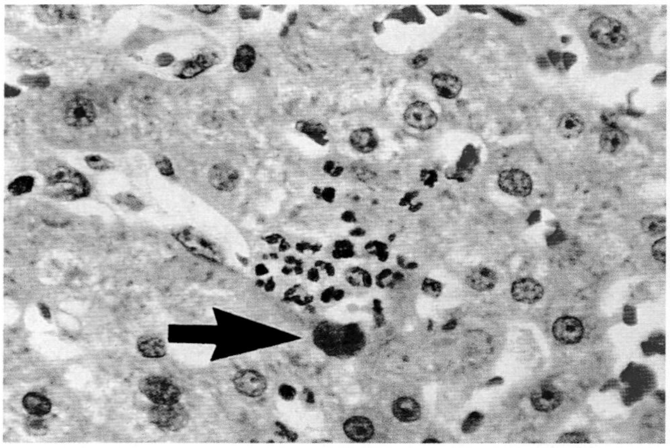

**FIG. 28.** Aggregates of polymorphonuclear leukocytes in sinusoid adjacent to a cytomegalovirus-infected cell (*arrow*).

of necrosis of single hepatocytes or sinusoidal lining cells (81,82) (Fig. 28).

### Vicinity of Space-Occupying Lesions

Nonspecific reactive changes are also seen in patients with space-occupying lesions (83) in the liver. Although the biopsy specimen may not include the neoplasm, abscess, or cyst, a characteristic histologic triad is often observed in the adjacent liver. These changes consist of proliferated and distorted bile ductules with irregular and even atypical epithelium, infiltration of scattered polymorphonuclear leukocytes in edematous portal tracts, and focal sinusoidal dilatation and congestion (Fig. 29). In contrast to large bile duct obstruction and other biliary tract diseases such as sclerosing cholangitis, cholestasis is usually absent. The liver cell plates may be compressed and distorted with atrophy of hepatocytes. These histologic changes are the result of focal obstruction of blood and bile flow by the expanding mass. They may be subtle and are usually focal with involvement of

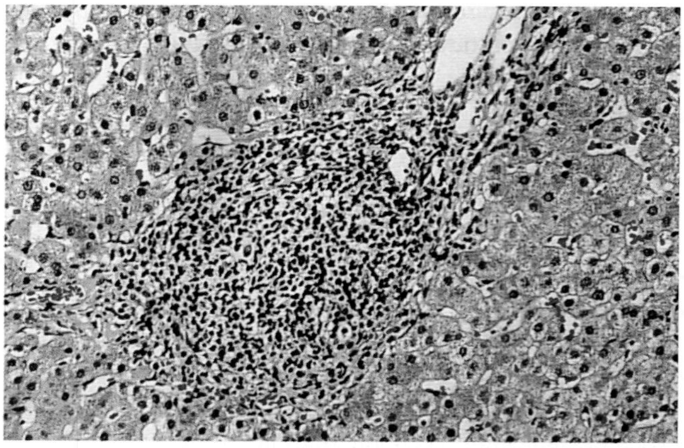

**FIG. 27.** Dense lymphocytic aggregate in a portal tract with chronic hepatitis without piecemeal necrosis.

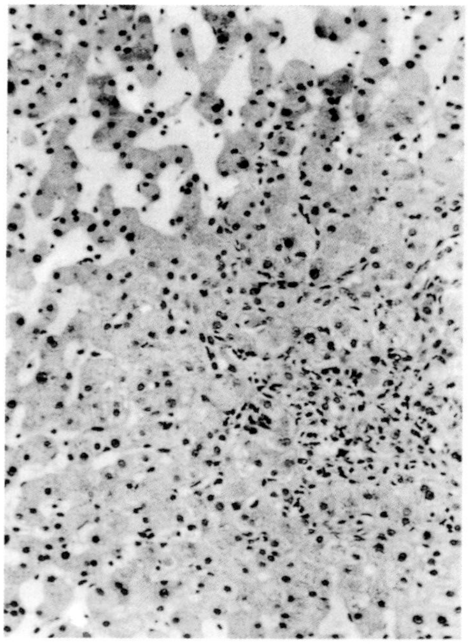

**FIG. 29.** Liver biopsy specimen of patient with metastatic carcinoma showing dilatation of sinusoids in zone 2, as well as proliferation of bile ductules and infiltration of portal tract by polymorphonuclear leukocytes. The specimen did not contain metastatic carcinoma, but the histologic changes are consistent with the vicinity of a space-occupying lesion.

small portal tracts. The described triad is characteristic for the vicinity of a space-occupying lesion, and its recognition in a liver specimen should lead to continued search for a neoplasm, cyst, or abscess.

### Sinusoidal Dilatation

Acute or chronic venous congestion with dilatation of sinusoids in Rappaport's zone 3 and of terminal hepatic venules is frequently seen at autopsy but also in biopsy specimens; it is usually a consequence of right-sided congestive heart failure, whereas irregular necrosis of hepatocytes in zone 3 is often caused by left-sided heart failure or shock (84). In more severe and chronic cases, there is also atrophy of hepatocytes with increased lipofuscin accumulation and scattered fat vacuoles, enlargement of Kupffer's cells with ceroid pigment, occasional cholestasis, and progressive fibrosis in the periphery of the acinus (rather than concentric around the central vein). Engorgement of sinusoids around terminal hepatic venules is also observed in patients with Budd-Chiari syndrome, venoocclusive disease, sepsis, malignant tumors, so-called collagen diseases, granulomatous diseases, Crohn's disease, and in patients with AIDS (80,85–87).

In contrast, dilatation of sinusoids in Rappaport's zone 1 has been observed in pregnancy, in renal transplant patients, after exposure to anabolic/androgenic or contraceptive steroids (88–90), and near space-occupying lesions (83). After exposure to vinyl chloride, thorotrast, arsenicals, and oral contraceptives, sinusoidal dilatation may be accompanied by hepatocellular and sinusoidal cell hypertrophy, hyperplasia, and dysplasia, increased reticulin fibers along sinusoids, and portal fibrosis (89–91).

## ACKNOWLEDGMENTS

The late Dr. Hans Popper reviewed the manuscript and offered invaluable constructive criticism. We also thank Elizabeth Vargas for secretarial help and Steve Mortillo for photographic assistance.

## REFERENCES

1. Clearfield HR. Embryology, malformations and malposition of the liver. In: Berk JE, Haubrich WS, Kalser MH, Roth JLA, Schaffner F, eds. *Bockus gastroenterology.* 4th ed. Philadelphia: WB Saunders; 1985:2659–2665.
2. MacSween RNM, Scothorne RJ. Developmental anatomy and normal structure. In: MacSween RNM, Anthony PP, Scheuer PJ, eds. *Pathology of the liver.* 2nd ed. Edinburgh: Churchill Livingstone; 1985:1–31.
3. Rappaport AM. Physioanatomic considerations. In: Schiff L, Schiff ER, eds. *Diseases of the liver.* 5th ed. Philadelphia: JB Lippincott; 1982:1–57.
4. Moore KL. *The developing human.* 3rd ed. Philadelphia: WB Saunders; 1982.
5. Hammar JA. Ueber die erste Entstehung der nicht kapillaren intrahepatischen Gallengange beim Menschen. *Z Mikrosk Anat Forsch* 1926; 5:59–89.
6. Desmet VJ. Intrahepatic bile ducts under the lens. *J Hepatol* 1985; 1:545–559.
7. Jorgensen MJ. The ductal plate malformation. *Acta Pathol Microbiol Immunol Scand* (Suppl) 1977;257:1–88.
8. Terada T, Nakanuma Y. Detection of apoptosis and expression of apoptosis-related proteins during human intrahepatic bile duct development. *Am J Pathol* 1995;146:67–74.
9. Columbano A, Ledda-Columbano GM, Coni PP, et al. Occurrence of cell death (apoptosis) during the evolution of liver hyperplasia. *Lab Invest* 1925;52:670–675.
10. Columbano A, Ledda-Columbano GM, Rao PM, Rajalakshmi S, Sarma DSR. Occurrence of cells death (apoptosis) in preneoplastic and neoplastic liver cells. *Am J Pathol* 1984;116:441–446.
11. Fukuda K, Kojiro M, Chiu JF. Induction of apoptosis by transforming growth factor-$\beta 1$ in the rat hepatoma cell line McA-RH7777: a possible association with tissue transglutaminase expression. *Hepatology* 1993;10:945–953.
12. Oberhammer F, Bursch W, Tiefenbacher R, et al. Apoptosis is induced by transforming growth factor-$\beta 1$ within 5 hours in regressing liver without significant fragmentation of the DNA. *Hepatology* 1993;18: 1238–1246.
13. Ohno K, Ammann P, Fasciati R, Maier P. Transforming growth factor-$\beta 1$ preferentially induces apoptotic cell death in rat hepatocytes cultured under pericentral-equivalent conditions. *Toxicol Appl Pharmacol* 1995;132:227–236.
14. Desmet VJ. Liver lesions in hepatitis B viral infection. *Yale J Biol Med* 1988;61:61–65.
15. Wyllie AH. Apoptosis: cell death in tissue regulation. *J Pathol* 1987; 153:313–316.
16. Schaffner F, Popper H. Structure of the liver. In: Berk JE, Haubrich WS, Kalser MH, Roth JLA, Schaffner F, eds. *Bockus gastroenterology.* 4th ed. Philadelphia: WB Saunders; 1985:2625–2658.
17. Bismuth H. Surgical anatomy and anatomical surgery of the liver. *World J Surg* 1982;6:3–9.
18. Emond JC, Renz JF. Surgical anatomy of the liver and its application to hepatobiliary surgery and transplantation. *Semin Liver Dis* 1994;14: 158–168.
19. Behar J. Anatomy and anomalies of the biliary tract. In: Haubrich WS, Schaffner F, Berk JE, eds. *Bockus gastroenterology.* 5th ed. Philadelphia: WB Saunders; 1995:2547–2553.
20. Henricksen JH, Horn T, Christoffersen P. The blood lymph barrier in the liver. A review based on morphological and functional concepts of normal and cirrhotic liver. *Liver* 1984;4:221–232.
21. Barrowman JA. Hepatic lymph and lymphatics. In: McIntyre N, Benhamou J-P, Bircher J, Rizetto M, Rodes J, eds. *Oxford textbook of clinical hepatology.* Oxford: Oxford University Press; 1991:37–40.
22. Witte MH, Witte CL. Lymphatic system in the liver. In: Abramson DI, Dobrin PB, eds. *Blood vessels and lymphatics in organ systems.* New York: Academic Press; 1984.
23. MacSween RNM, Scothorns RJ. Developmental anatomy and normal structure. In: MacSween RNM, Anthony PP, Scheuer PJ, Burt AD, Portmann BC, eds. *Pathology of the liver.* London: Churchill Livingstone; 1994:1–49.
24. Friedman JM. Hepatic nerve function. In: Arias IM, Popper H, Jakoby W, Schachter D, Schafritz DA, eds. *The liver, biology and pathology.* New York: Raven Press; 1988:949–959.
25. Dhillon AP, Sankey EA, Wang JH, et al. Immunohistochemical studies on the innervation of human transplanted liver. *J Pathol* 1992;167: 211–216.
26. Henderson JM, Mackay GJ, Lumsden AB, Alta HM, Brouillard R, Kutner MH. The effect of liver denervation on hepatic haemodynamics during hypovolemic shock in swine. *Hepatology* 1992;15:130–133.
27. Lee JA, Ahmed Q, Hines JE, Burt AD. Disappearance of hepatic parenchymal nerves in human liver cirrhosis. *Gut* 1992;33:87–91.
28. Hilden M, Christoffersen P, Juhl E, Dalgaard JB. Liver histology in a normal population—examinations of 503 consecutive fatal traffic casualties. *Scand J Gastroenterol* 1977;12:593–597.
29. Millward-Sadler GH, Jezequel AM. Normal histology and ultrastructure. In: Wright R, Millward-Sadler GH, Alberti KGMM, Karran S, eds. *Liver and biliary disease.* 2nd ed. London: Bailliere Tindall; 1985: 13–44.
30. Patrick RS, McGee JO. Normal liver pathology. In: *Biopsy pathology of the liver.* Philadelphia: JB Lippincott; 1980:4–14.
31. Scheuer P. The normal liver. In: *Liver biopsy interpretation.* 3rd ed. London: Bailliere Tindall; 1980:15–26.

32. Rappaport AM. The structural and functional unit in the human liver (liver acinus). *Anat Rec* 1958;130:673–689.
33. Elias H. A re-examination of the structure of the mammalian liver. I. Parenchymal architecture. *Am J Anat* 1949;84:311–333.
34. Gumucio JJ, Miller DL. Functional implications of liver cell heterogeneity. *Gastroenterology* 1981;80:393–403.
35. Terada T, Ishida F, Nakanuma Y. Vascular plexus around intrahepatic bile ducts in normal livers and portal hypertension. *J Hepatol* 1989; 8:139–149.
36. Ranek L, Keiding N, Jensen ST. A morphometric study of normal human liver cell nuclei. *Acta Pathol Microbiol Immunol Scand* 1975;83: 467–476.
37. Findor J, Perez V, Bruch Igartua E, Giovanetti M, Fioravanti N. Structure and ultrastructure of the liver in aged persons. *Acta Hepatogastroenterol* 1973;20:200–204.
38. Thung SN, Gerber AM. Differentiation of brown pigments in the liver. In: Thung SN, Gerber MA, eds. *Differential diagnosis in pathology. Liver disease.* New York: Igaku Shoin; 1995:34.
39. Jones EA. Hepatic sinusoidal cells: new insights and controversies. *Hepatology* 1983;3:259–266.
40. McCuskey RS. The liver sieve: considerations concerning the structure and function of endothelial fenestrae, the sinusoidal wall and the space of Disse. *Hepatology* 1985;5:683–692.
41. Wisse E, Knook DL. *Kupffer cells and other liver sinusoidal cells.* Amsterdam: Elsevier; 1977.
42. Bianchi FB, Bianini G, Ballardini G, et al. Basement membrane production by hepatocytes in chronic liver disease. *Hepatology* 1984; 4:1167–1172.
43. Thung SN, Gerber MA. The formation of elastic fibers in livers with massive hepatic necrosis. *Arch Pathol Lab Med* 1982;106:468–469.
44. Kent G, Gay S, Inouye T, Bahu R, Minick OT, Popper H. Vitamin A-containing lipocytes and formation of type III collagen in liver injury. *Proc Natl Acad Sci U S A* 1976;73:3719–3722.
45. Schirmacher P, Geerts A, Pietrangelo A, Dienes HP, Rogler CE. Hepatocyte growth factor/hepatopoietin A is expressed in fat-storing cells from rat liver but not myofibroblast-like cells derived from fat-storing cells. *Hepatology* 1992;15:5–11.
46. Ogawa K, Suzuki J-I, Mukai H, Mori M. Sequential changes of extracellular matrix and proliferation of Ito cells with enhanced expression of desmin and actin in focal hepatic injury. *Am J Pathol* 1986;125: 611–619.
47. Kaneda K, Kurioka N, Seki S, Wake K, Yamamoto S. Pit cell– hepatocyte contact in autoimmune hepatitis. *Hepatology* 1984;4:955–958.
48. Wisse E, van't Noordende JM, van der Meulen J, Daems WT. The pit cell: description of a new type of cell occurring in rat liver sinusoids and peripheral blood. *Cell Tissue Res* 1976;173:423–435.
49. Bouwens L, Wisse E. Tissue localization and kinetics of pit cells or large granular lymphocytes in the liver of rats treated with biological response modifiers. *Hepatology* 1988;8:46–52.
50. Van Waes L, Lieber CS. Early perivenular sclerosis in alcoholic fatty liver: an index of progressive liver injury. *Gastroenterology* 1977;73: 646–650.
51. Nasrallah SM, Nassar VH, Galambos JT. Importance of terminal hepatic venule thickening. *Arch Pathol Lab Med* 1980;104:84–86.
52. Petrelli M, Scheuer PJ. Variation in subcapsular liver structure and its significance in the interpretation of wedge biopsies. *J Clin Pathol* 1967; 20:743–748.
53. International Group. Histopathology of the intrahepatic biliary tree. *Liver* 1983;3:161–175.
54. Nakanuma Y, Ohta G. Histometric and serial section observations of the intrahepatic bile ducts in primary biliary cirrhosis. *Gastroenterology* 1979;76:1326–1332.
55. Thung SN, Gerber MA. Adenocarcinoma vs. proliferating bile ductules vs. ductular hepatocytes. In: Thung SN, Gerber MA, eds. *Differential diagnosis in pathology. Liver disorders.* New York: Igaku-Shoin; 1995: 120–129.
56. Yamamoto K, Sherman I, Phillips MJ, Fisher MM. Three-dimensional observations of the hepatic arterial terminations in rat, hamster and human liver by scanning electron microscopy of microvascular casts. *Hepatology* 1985;5:452–456.
57. Elias H. Anatomy of the liver. In: Rouler C, ed. *The liver: morphology, biochemistry, physiology.* Vol. 1. New York: Academic Press; 1963:41–52.
58. Popper H, Martin GR. Fibrosis of the liver: the role of the ectoskeleton. In: Popper H, Schaffner F, eds. *Progress in liver diseases.* Vol. 7. New York: Grune & Stratton; 1982:133–156.
59. Hahn E, Wick G, Pencev D, Timple R. Distribution of basement membrane proteins in normal and fibrotic human liver: collagen type IV, laminin and fibronectin. *Gut* 1980;91:63–71.
60. Thung SN, Schaffner F. Liver biopsy. In: MacSween RNM, Anthony PP, Scheuer PJ, Burt AP, Portmann BC, eds. *Pathology of the liver.* London: Churchill Livingstone; 1994:787–796.
61. Thung SN, Gerber MA, Sarno E, Popper H. Distribution of 5 antigens in hepatocellular carcinoma. *Lab Invest* 1979;41:101–105.
62. Gerber MA, Thung SN, Shen SC, Stromeyer FW, Ishak KG. Phenotypic characterization of proliferation: comparison of antigenic expression by proliferating epithelial cells in fetal liver, massive hepatic necrosis and nodular transformation of the liver. *Am J Pathol* 1983;110: 70–74.
63. Gerber MA, Thung SN. Diagnostic value of immunohistochemical demonstration of hepatitis viral antigens in the liver. *Hum Pathol* 1987; 18:771–774.
64. Blight K, Lesniewski RR, LaBrooy JT, Gowans EJ. Detection and distribution of hepatitis C specific antigens in naturally infected livers. *Hepatology* 1994;20:553–557.
65. Krawczynski K, Beach MJ, Bradley DW, et al. Hepatitis C virus antigen in hepatocytes: immunomorphologic detection and identification. *Gastroenterology* 1992;103:622–629.
66. Tsutsumi M, Urashima S, Takada A, Date, T, Tanaka Y. Detection of antigens related to hepatitis C virus RNA encoding the NS 5 region in the livers of patients with chronic type C hepatitis. *Hepatology* 1994; 19:265–272.
67. Cooper D, Schermer A, Sun T-T. Classification of human epithelia and their neoplasms using monoclonal antibodies to keratins: strategies, applications, and limitations. *Lab Invest* 1985;52:243–256.
68. Gown AM, Vogel AM. Monoclonal antibodies to human intermediate filament proteins. *Am J Pathol* 1984;114:309–321.
69. Franke WW, Denk H, Kalt R, Schmid E. Biochemical and immunological identification of cytokeratin proteins present in hepatocytes of mammalian liver tissue. *Exp Cell Res* 1981;131:299– 318.
70. Lai Y-S, Thung SN, Gerber MA, Chen M-L, Schaffner F. Expression of cytokeratins in normal and diseased livers and primary liver carcinomas. *Arch Pathol Lab Med* 1989;113:134–138.
71. Feldman G. The cytoskeleton of the hepatocyte structures and functions. *J Hepatol* 1989;8:320–386.
72. Negro F, Pacchioni D, Shimizu Y, et al. Detection of intrahepatic replication of hepatitis C virus RNA by in situ hypbridization and comparison with histopathology. *Proc Natl Acad Sci U S A* 1992;89:2247–2251.
73. Tanaka Y, Enomoto N, Kojima S, et al. Detection of hepatitis C virus RNA in the liver by insitu hybridization. *Liver* 1993;13:203–208.
74. Lones MA, Shintaku IP, Weiss LM, Thung SN, Nichols WS, Geller SA. Epstein-Barr virus in liver allograft biopsies; three methods compared [Abstract]. *Mod Pathol* 1994;7:134.
75. Nuovo GJ, Lidonnici K, MacConnell P, Lane B. Intracellular localization of polymerase chain reaction (PCR)-amplified hepatitis C DNA [Abstract]. *Am J Surg Pathol* 1994;7:134.
76. Watanabe T, Tanaka Y. Age-related alterations in the size of human hepatocytes. A study of mononuclear and binucleate cells. *Virchows Arch [B]* 1982;29:9–20.
77. Popper H. Aging and the liver. In: Popper H, Schaffer F, eds. *Progress in liver diseases.* Vol. VIII. Orlando: Grune & Stratton; 1986:659–683.
78. Gerber MA. Viral hepatitis in the autopsy specimen. *Virchows Arch [A]* 1971;354:285–292.
79. Christoffersen P, Poulsen H, Skei E. Focal liver cell necrosis accompanied by infiltration of granulocytes arising during operation. *Acta Hepatosplenol* 1970;17:240–245.
80. Lebovics E, Thung SN, Schaffner F, Radensky PW. The liver in the acquired immunodeficiency syndrome: a clinical and histologic study. *Hepatology* 1985;5:293–298.
81. Sieratzki J, Thung SN, Gerber MA, Ferrone S, Schaffner F. Major histocompatibility antigen expression in the liver in acquired immunodeficiency syndrome. *Arch Pathol Lab Med* 1987;111:1045–1049.
82. Bach N, Thung SN, Berk PD. The liver in acquired immunodeficiency syndrome (AIDS). In: Bianchi L, Gerok W, Maier KP, eds. *Infectious diseases of the liver.* Boston: Kluwer Academic; 1990:333–351).
83. Gerber MA, Thung SN, Bodenheimer HC, Kapelman B, Schaffner F.

Characteristic histologic triad in liver adjacent to metastatic neoplasm. *Liver* 1986;6:85–88.
84. Arcidi JD Jr, Moore GW, Hutchins GM. Hepatic morphology in cardiac dysfunction. A clinicopathologic study of 1,000 subjects at autopsy. *Am J Pathol* 1981;104:159–166.
85. Banks JG, Foulis AK, Ledingham I, MacSween RNM. Liver function in septic shock. *J Clin Pathol* 1982;35:1249–1252.
86. Bruguera M, Aranguibel F, Ros E, Rodes J. Incidence and clinical significance of sinusoidal dilatation in liver biopsies. *Gastroenterology* 1978;75:474–478.
87. Camilleri M, Schafler K, Chadwick VS, Hodgson HJ, Weinbren K. Periportal sinusoidal dilatation, Inflammatory bowel disease, and the contraceptive pill. *Gastroenterology* 1981;80:810–815.
88. Ishak KG. Hepatic lesions caused by anabolic and contraceptive steroids. *Semin Liver Dis* 1981;1:16–28.
89. Thung SN, Gerber MA. Precursor stage of hepatocellular neoplasm following long exposure to orally administered contraceptives. *Hum Pathol* 1981;12:472–475.
90. Winkler K, Poulsen H. Liver disease with periportal sinusoidal dilatation: a possible complication to contraceptive steroids. *Scand J Gastroenterol* 1975;10:699–704.
91. Popper H, Maltoni C, Selikoff IJ. Vinyl chloride-induced hepatic lesions in man and rodents. A comparison. *Liver* 1981;1:7– 20.

*Histology for Pathologists, second edition,*
Edited by Stephen S. Sternberg.
Lippincott-Raven Publishers, Philadelphia


CHAPTER 26

# Gallbladder and Extrahepatic Biliary System

Henry F. Frierson, Jr.



The diseased gallbladder is a common specimen submitted to the surgical pathology laboratory. The gallbladder is routinely examined for the presence of gallstones, inflammation, and the rare occurrence of a clinically unsuspected adenocarcinoma. Nonneoplastic changes such as intestinal and gastric metaplasia, hyperplasia, Rokitansky-Aschoff sinuses, and Luschka's ducts are usually ignored. Biopsy specimens from the cystic duct, hepatic ducts, common bile duct, and the papilla of Vater are infrequently submitted to the surgical pathology laboratory, and they are usually accompanied by a clinical diagnosis of adenocarcinoma. Complete, normal extrahepatic bile ducts can be studied only at autopsy, but autolysis of the biliary tree is rapid and hinders histologic examination. The choledochoduodenal junction can be examined in detail in Whipple resection specimens, but the normal Vaterian system is often distorted or obliterated by carcinoma or is affected by inflammation and fibrosis. For these reasons, the normal histology of the extrahepatic biliary system is difficult to study.

In this chapter, the gross anatomy, physiology, histology, immunohistochemistry, and ultrastructure of the normal gallbladder, extrahepatic bile ducts, structures of the Vaterian system, and minor papilla are reviewed.

H. F. Frierson, Jr.: Department of Pathology, University of Virginia Health Sciences Center, Charlottesville, Virginia 22908.

## GALLBLADDER

### Gross Anatomy

The gallbladder, the pear-shaped sac that lies in the depression on the posterior aspect of the right lobe of the liver, measures up to 10 cm long and 3 to 4 cm wide in normal adults. Its wall is approximately 1 to 2 mm thick and varies depending on whether the organ is relaxed or contracted. Its free surface is covered by serosa that continues over the hepatic surface. Subserosal connective tissue merges with the interlobular connective tissue of the liver. The gallbladder is composed of a blindly ending fundus, a large central body, and a narrow neck that joins the cystic duct. The body tapers to an infundibulum as it joins the neck. A peritoneal fold, the cholecystoduodenal ligament, attaches the infundibulum to the first portion of the duodenum. Hartmann's pouch, occurring as a small bulge at the infundibulum, probably results from chronic inflammation (1). The neck is S shaped, measures 5 to 7 mm long, and narrows as it connects with the cystic duct (2).

### Physiology

The gallbladder concentrates, stores, and releases bile. It also has a secretory role, liberating mucosubstances from the surface epithelial cells and neck mucous glands. Approximately 800 to 1,000 ml of bile flow daily into the gallbladder from the liver (3). Its filling is believed to be an active process, resulting from specific neural and hormonal stimulations that result in its relaxation and the closing of the sphincter of Oddi. Bile therefore enters the gallbladder when its intraluminal pressure is lower than that of the common bile duct. Although the gallbladder can store only 40 to 70 ml of bile, a much larger volume can be handled by effective concentration (3). The epithelial cells absorb water by the sodium-coupled transport of chloride, mediated by NaK-ATPase (4). The active transport of electrolyte into the lateral intercellular space creates an osmotic gradient for water, which ultimately flows through the basement membrane into the capillaries of the lamina propria. Contraction of the gallbladder smooth muscle and emptying occur when a fatty meal enters the duodenum. Cholecystokinin, released from the mucosa of the proximal small intestine, is the most important hormone that promotes gallbladder contraction. Motilin indirectly aids in interdigestive gallbladder contraction, whereas pancreatic polypeptide results in its relaxation (5). Somatostatin, when present in plasma levels similar to those in patients with somatostatinomas, inhibits gallbladder emptying that occurs after a meal is ingested, after cholinergic stimulation, or after intravenous administration of the octapeptide of cholecystokinin (6).

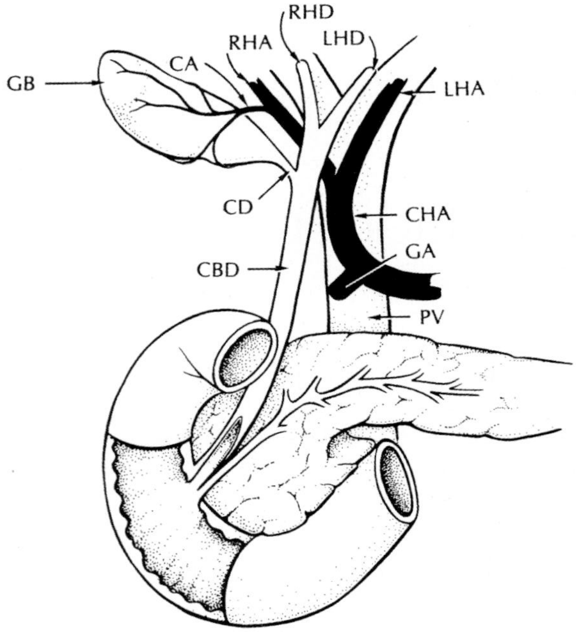


**FIG. 1.** Although variations are common, this diagram depicts the "usual" relationships of the extrahepatic bile ducts, portal vein, and branches of the common hepatic artery. PV, portal vein; GA, gastroduodenal artery; CHA, common hepatic artery; LHA, left hepatic artery; LHD, left hepatic duct; RHD, right hepatic duct; RHA, right hepatic artery; GB, gallbladder; CA, cystic artery; CD, cystic duct; CBD, common bile duct.

### Blood Supply and Lymphatic Drainage

The cystic artery supplies the gallbladder and usually arises from the proximal portion of the right hepatic artery. It is located superior to the cystic duct (Fig. 1). The artery branches to form superficial channels that lie over the gallbladder serosa and deep channels that lie between the gallbladder and its hepatic bed (2). In a study of the extrahepatic biliary tree in 250 cadavers, Moosman and Coller (7) noted a double cystic artery in 14% of their cases. Michels (8) found double cystic arteries in one quarter of 200 cadavers. Seventy-two percent of all cystic arteries in the Moosman and Coller (7) study arose from the right hepatic artery, and 13% arose from the superior mesenteric artery; the remainder originated from the common hepatic artery, left hepatic artery, gastroduodenal artery, celiac artery, or aorta. Seventy percent of all cystic arteries coursed to the right of the common hepatic duct, and 17% traveled anterior to the common hepatic duct. The remainder of the cystic arteries passed posterior to the common hepatic duct, anterior or posterior to the common bile duct, to the right and inferior to the cystic duct, or posterior to both hepatic ducts.

The venous drainage consists, in part, of small venous channels on the hepatic side of the gallbladder that lead directly into the liver. Other small veins flow toward the cystic duct and merge with channels from the common bile duct before terminating in the portal venous system. There is no single, large cystic vein (2).

Lymphatic channels lead to one or more lymph nodes at the gallbladder neck or cystic duct. In a recent study in which dye was injected directly into lymphatic vessels of the gallbladder, the dye flowed initially into the cystic node and pericholedochal nodes, then into lymph nodes posterior to the pancreas, portal vein, and common hepatic artery, and finally into interaortocaval nodes near the left renal vein (9). Ascending lymph flow to the hepatic hilum was not found in this study. However, lymphatic channels may lead superiorly to lymph nodes near the hepatic hilum or directly connect with those of the hepatic bed (2). Retrograde flow to the hepatic hilum occurs when there is blockage of lymphatic channels by cancer, inflammation, or surgical ligation (9).

### Nerve Supply

Afferent, sympathetic, and parasympathetic nerve fibers from the hepatic plexus supply the gallbladder (2). Nerve branches from the left trunk of the vagus join the hepatic plexus. Vagal stimulation results in interdigestive periodic contractions of the smooth muscle in the gallbladder wall (10). Neuropeptide Y nerve fibers are found in all layers of the gallbladder but form a particularly dense network in the lamina propria, running near the epithelium and paralleling the muscle bundles (11). The nerve fibers supply blood vessels present throughout the gallbladder. It is possible that neuropeptide Y participates in smooth muscle contraction, but its role in epithelial physiology is uncertain (11).

### Histology

The layers of the gallbladder include the surface epithelium, lamina propria, smooth muscle, perimuscular subserosal connective tissue, and serosa. The gallbladder lacks a muscularis mucosae and submucosa. The luminal folds are lined by columnar epithelium and have cores of lamina propria. The height and width of the folds are variable, and branching is characteristic (Fig. 2). The single row of tall columnar cells lies above a basement membrane (Fig. 3). The cells have pale or lightly eosinophilic cytoplasm with occasional small apical vacuoles. Nuclei, aligned at the cell base or more centrally, are oval, uniform, have fine chromatin, and smooth membranes. Nucleoli are absent or very small. A few columnar cells are narrow and have dark eosinophilic cytoplasm (1). These cells, dignified with the appellation "pencil-like" cells, appear little more than contracted columnar cells, although they have a few ultrastructural differences from the usual columnar cells. Basal cells are inconspicuous. Their nuclei lie just above and parallel to the basement membrane (1). Tubuloalveolar mucous glands, located only in the neck of the gallbladder (12), have cuboid or low columnar cells with abundant clear cytoplasm and round, basally oriented nuclei (Fig. 4). Their lectin-binding profile is dissimilar to that of the surface epithelial cells (13). The neck mucous glands also differ morphologically and histochemically from the antral-type metaplastic glands found in the fundus, body, or neck of chronically inflamed gallbladders or those that contain gallstones (12). Gastric metaplasia (foveolar-type epithelium or antral-type glands) and "intestinal" metaplasia (absorptive cells with prominent brush borders, endocrine cells, goblet cells, and Paneth's cells) are not observed in the normal gallbladder but commonly occur in chronic cholecystitis and cholelithiasis (1,14–20). Squamous metaplasia, rarely found in diseased gallbladders (1), is also absent in normal gallbladders. Melanocytes are not found in the normal epithelial lining. However, a few small lymphocytes often are seen between the surface columnar cells.

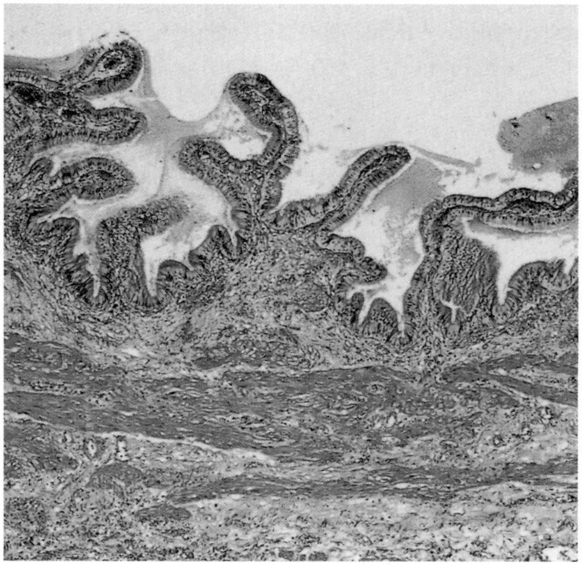

**FIG. 2.** The luminal folds of the gallbladder vary in height and contain a delicate core of lamina propria above the bundles of smooth muscle.

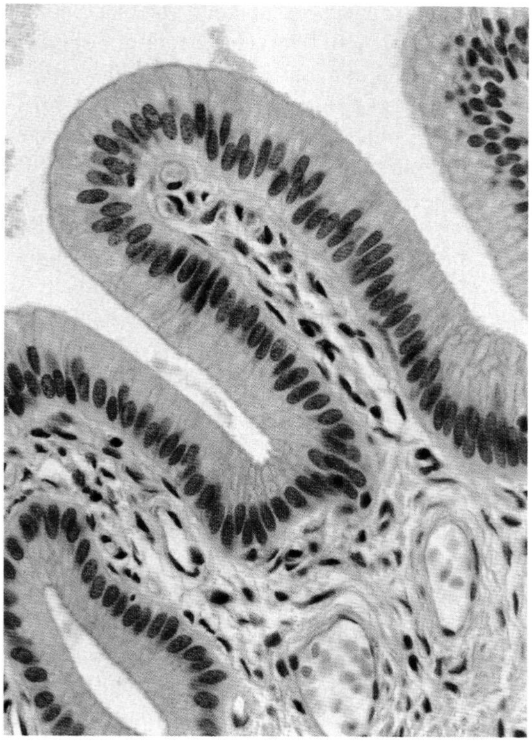

**FIG. 3.** The gallbladder is lined by a single layer of tall columnar cells with basally oriented nuclei.

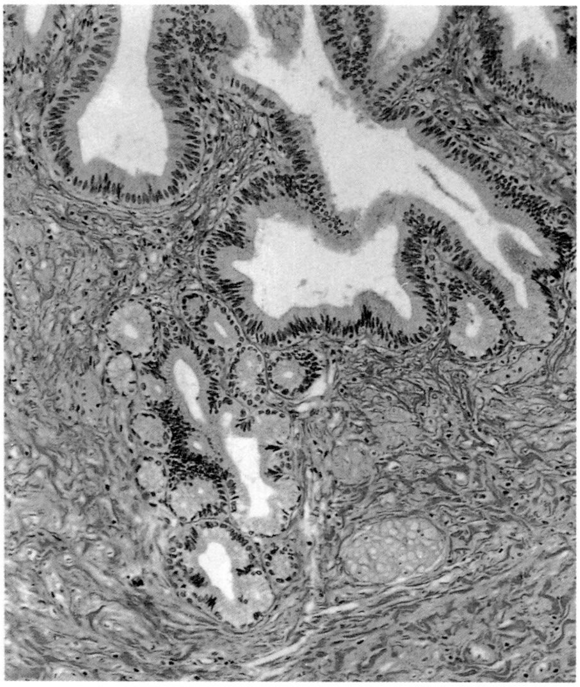

**FIG. 4.** Mucous glands are present only in the neck of the normal gallbladder.

The lining cells and neck mucous glands contain chiefly sulfated acid mucin with very small quantities of nonsulfated acid mucin (17). In contrast, metaplastic cells (goblet cells, superficial gastric-type cells, antral-type glands) contain nonsulfated acid mucin and neutral mucin, but little sulfated acid mucin. Immunohistochemically, pepsinogens I and II, present in pyloric gland metaplasia, are not seen in normal gallbladder epithelium (19). Lysozyme is also absent in the normal columnar cells but may be found in metaplastic glands (20,21). Alpha-1-antitrypsin and alpha-1-antichymotrypsin are present in both normal and metaplastic epithelia (21). Immunohistochemical staining for carcinoembryonic antigen (CEA) (polyclonal; unabsorbed) shows focal weak positivity along the apices of some lining cells (22). In contrast to the results using monoclonal antibodies to CEA, inflamed epithelium usually shows immunostaining with polyclonal antisera (23). Absorption of at least one polyclonal antibody with human liver powder abolishes the immunoreactivity because there is removal of the CEA-related glycoproteins nonspecific cross-reacting antigen (NCA) and biliary glycoprotein (BGP) (23). Weak immunoreactivity for secretory component may be observed in normal gallbladder epithelium (20). The surface epithelium and neck mucous glands are strongly immunoreactive for epithelial membrane antigen and low-molecular-weight keratin (CAM 5.2 antibody) (Fig. 5). The CAM 5.2 antibody also stains some smooth muscle fibers in the gallbladder wall. Because endocrine cells are not found in the normal epithelium of the fundus or body, immunohistochemical staining for neuron-specific enolase and chromogranin A is absent. A few argentaffin (enterochromaffin) cells are present in the mucous glands of the neck (24); these cells are readily detected by an antibody to chromogranin A. Normal gallbladder mucosa lacks immunoreactivity for estrogen receptor, whereas in six of 31 cases of cholelithiasis a few immunoreactive cells were observed chiefly in metaplastic mucous glands (pseudo-pyloric glands) (25).

The lamina propria contains loose connective tissue, elastic fibers, nerve fibers, small blood vessels, and lymphatic channels. Mast cells and macrophages may be seen in small numbers, and it has been noted that these cells are more numerous in "normal" or minimally inflamed gallbladders than in those with overt chronic cholecystitis (26). Polymorphonuclear leukocytes normally are not present in the lamina propria, but small numbers of lymphocytes and plasma cells are usual. Plasma cells that contain immunoglobulin (Ig)A occur chiefly in the lamina propria, whereas IgM-containing cells are more frequent in the smooth muscle layer (27). A few IgG-containing plasma cells also may be present. The smooth muscle consists of loosely arranged bundles of circular, longitudinal, and oblique fibers that do not form well-developed layers. Fibrovascular connective tissue often separates the muscle bundles. The muscle fibers sometimes extend high in the lamina propria, just beneath the epithelial basement membrane. The thickness of the muscle layer is quite variable, relating to the state of contraction or relaxation. Ganglion cells are found in the lamina propria, between smooth muscle bundles, and in the subserosal connective tissue (Fig. 6). The subserosal tissue contains loose collagen fibers, fibroblasts, elastic fibers, adipocytes, blood vessels, nerves, and lymphatics. Small aggregates of lymphocytes may occur around vessels. Uncommonly, a lymph node is found in the subserosal connective tissue (28). Para-

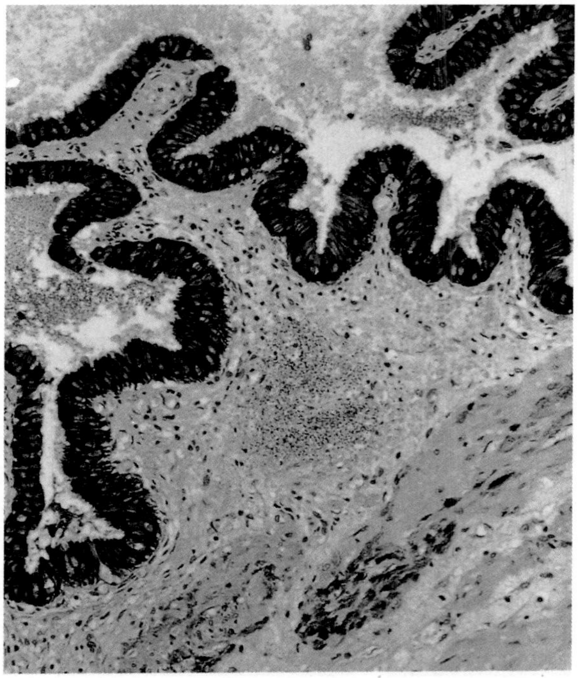

**FIG. 5.** The epithelial lining of the gallbladder is strongly immunoreactive for low-molecular-weight keratin (CAM 5.2 antibody). The smooth muscle bundles may also show positivity (immunoperoxidase technique).

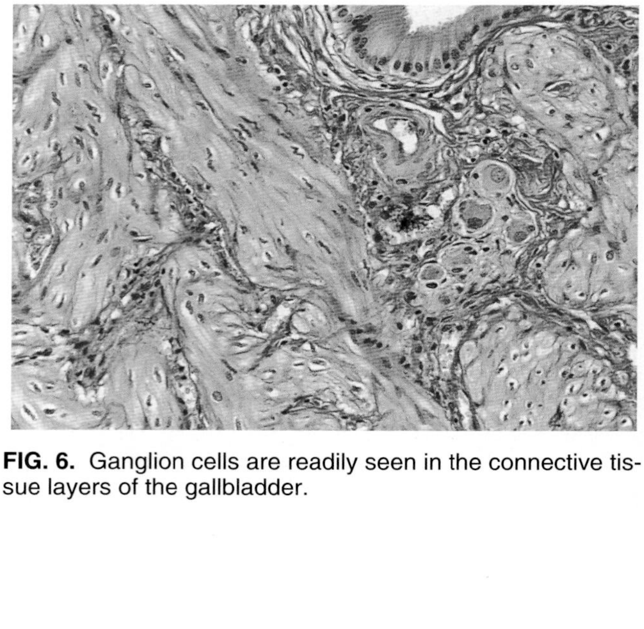

**FIG. 6.** Ganglion cells are readily seen in the connective tissue layers of the gallbladder.

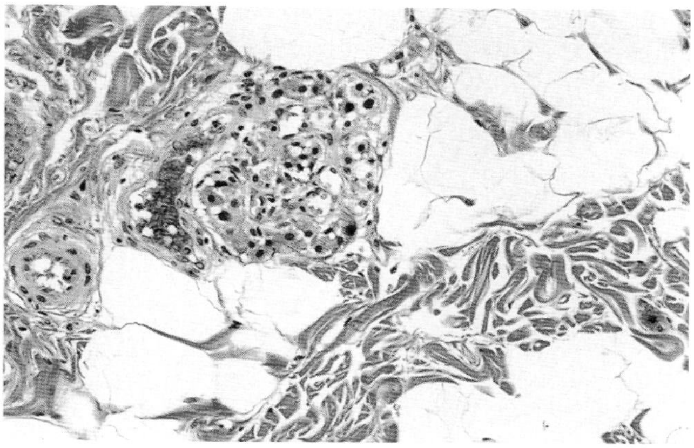

**FIG. 7.** Paraganglia are located in the subserosal connective tissue of the normal gallbladder.

ganglia, infrequently seen in routine sections, are found adjacent to blood vessels and small nerves (Fig. 7). Examining serial blocks and subserial sections of gallbladders, the investigators of one study found one to five paraganglia in the subserosal tissue of nine of ten cholecystectomy specimens (29).

Rokitansky-Aschoff sinuses represent herniations of epithelium into the lamina propria, smooth muscle, or subserosal connective tissue (Fig. 8). In a series of 125 cholecystectomy specimens that were inflamed or contained gallstones, 86% had Rokitansky-Aschoff sinuses, almost 90% of which penetrated into or through the smooth muscle (30). The sinuses also occur in grossly and microscopically normal gallbladders, having been observed in 42% of 112 gallbladders examined at autopsy (31). When present in normal gallbladders, they tend to be few and superficial, confined to the lamina propria, with infrequent penetration of the smooth muscle. The sinuses are not found in gallbladders from fetuses, but a few superficial outpouchings may be observed in organs from infants (32). The diameters of the sinuses are variable, and flask-shaped formations are usual. Although the exact mechanism for their formation is unknown, herniation of the epithelium may result from overdistension (with increased intraluminal pressure) and extreme contractions of the gallbladder with subsequent weakening of its wall (32).

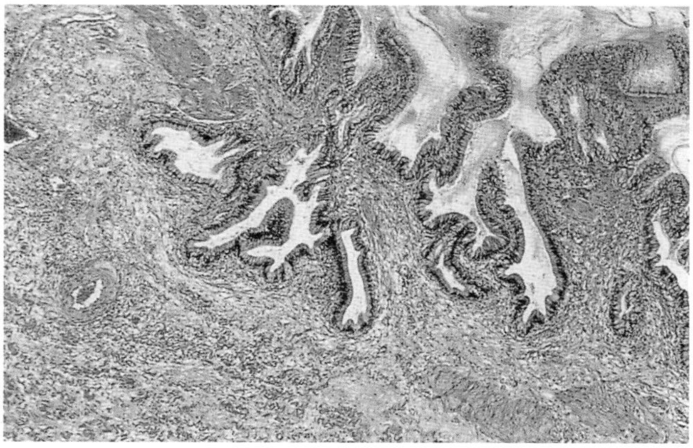

**FIG. 8.** Rokitansky-Aschoff sinuses occur in the normal gallbladder but uncommonly penetrate through the smooth muscle bundles.

Luschka's ducts are small, usually microscopic, bile ducts that lie in the subserosal connective tissue on the hepatic side of the gallbladder (Fig. 9). Occasionally, a few ducts are present in the subserosal connective tissue on the peritoneal side. The ducts have been found in 10% to 12% of routine sections from cholecystectomy specimens, occurring in both normal and diseased organs (31,32). They have been observed in gallbladders from infants, adolescents, and adults (32). Luschka's ducts may represent embryonic remnants. Some have been shown to communicate with intrahepatic bile ducts (30,32), and those located beneath the serosa possibly open into the peritoneal cavity. There is little evidence that the ducts drain into the gallbladder lumen, although Beilby reported that some ducts communicated with the lumen of the neck in a few specimens with strictures (33). The ducts are solitary or multiple. They are present in small groups and are surrounded by a distinctive ring of connective tissue. In serial sections, they sometimes are seen as a system of anastomosing channels. The diameters of their lumina vary from several microns up to a few millimeters. They are lined by cells similar to those of the intrahepatic bile ducts. In some instances, small foci of hepatic parenchyma are located adjacent to the ducts (32). Luschka's ducts are distinct from Rokitansky-Aschoff sinuses. There is never communication between the ducts and sinuses.

At surgery and by cholangiography, larger accessory ducts (up to several millimeters long) sometimes are seen in the gallbladder bed. They may be mistaken grossly for small veins or thin strands of fibrous tissue (34). Absence of ligation during surgery sometimes results in leakage of bile, which typically ceases spontaneously. In one study, 9% of 204 patients with randomly selected cholecystectomies had bile leaks from the drain tube; some of these were considered to be due to a divided subvesical duct (35). Although these ducts lie in the gallbladder wall, they usually do not drain into the lumen of the fundus but communicate with the cystic or hepatic ducts (36,37). In a study of 20 autopsy dissections from patients without biliary disease, six subvesical ducts were found, five of which were placed centrally in the gallbladder bed and one in the lateral peritoneal reflection (35). Five led to the right hepatic duct, and one entered the common hepatic duct.

Ectopic hepatic (38), pancreatic (39), and adrenal (40) tissues have been reported in the gallbladder. Gastric and thyroid ectopic tissues also have been described (41). Ectopic hepatic and adrenal tissues are typically incidental findings, whereas ectopic pancreatic or gastric tissues may lead to symptoms related to their secretions (38).

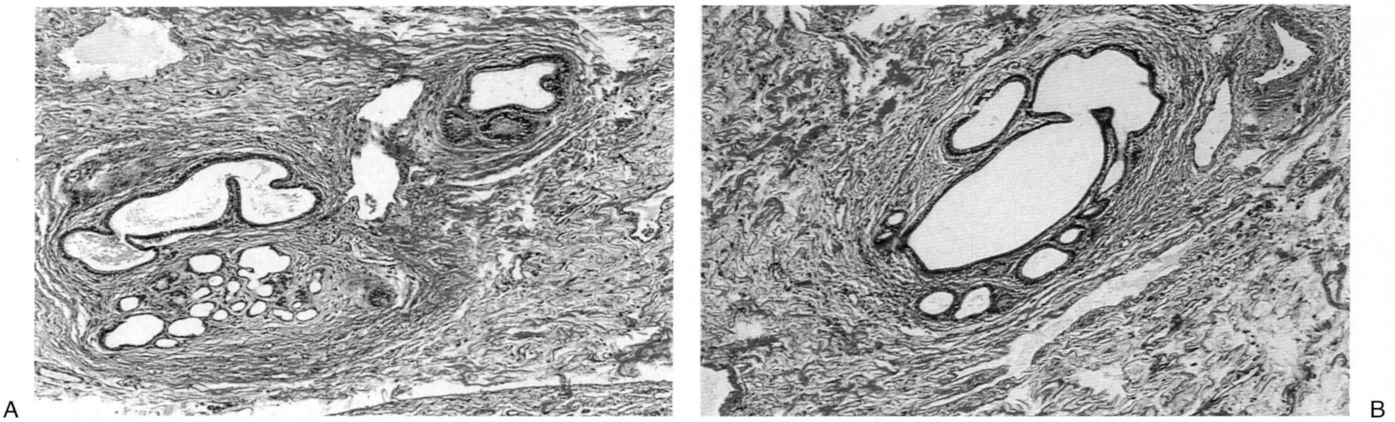


**FIG. 9.** Luschka's ducts consist of groups of small ducts having lumina of various caliber. They are surrounded by condensed connective tissue.

### Ultrastructure

The surface columnar (clear) cells, measuring 15 to 25 $\mu$m in height and 2.5 to 7.0 $\mu$m in width (42) and resting on a basement membrane, have numerous apical microvilli with filamentous glycocalyx and core rootlets (Fig. 10). The microvilli are shorter and more variable in size and density than those of the intestinal epithelium. Pinocytotic vesicles are formed from the intervillous portions of the cell membrane. The lateral cell membranes are straight at the apex and connected by junctional complexes. Below this boundary, the cell membranes have complex interdigitations that surround lateral intercellular spaces (Fig. 10). The diameter of the intercellular space varies depending on the state of fluid transport (43). It is collapsed when there is no water transport but is distended during influx of electrolytes and water. The nuclei are oval, have prominent euchromatin, and occasional small nucleoli. The cytoplasm contains rough endoplasmic reticulum, mitochondria, glycogen, filaments, Golgi apparatus, mucous granules, vesicles, and lysosomes. Pencil (dark) cells have slender outlines, narrow nuclei, and dense cytoplasm that is packed with organelles. At the base of the pencil cell, cytoplasmic extensions project into the basement membrane, unlike that for the typical columnar cell (44). However, microvilli and lateral membrane interdigitations are similar for the pencil cell. The basal cell measures 10 to 15 $\mu$m in diameter (42), has an irregular nucleus, and has cytoplasmic organelles that include rough and smooth endoplasmic reticulum, mitochondria, vacuoles, and ring-shaped osmiophilic inclusions (42,44). They have a cytoplasmic extension that runs parallel to the basement membrane, changes direction to run perpendicularly, and then branches toward the lumen (42). The branches are variable in length, delicate, and complex. Throughout the lining epithelium there are intraepithelial nerve endings that originate from the nerve submucosal plexus and are associated with the small basal cells (42).

Capillaries are found just below the epithelial basement membrane, and their lumina change in size according to the state of fluid transport. The epithelial cells of the glands in the gallbladder neck have a few short microvilli, relatively even lateral membranes, secretory granules, and round nuclei (12).

## CYSTIC DUCT

The cystic duct, located in the right free edge of the lesser omentum, usually joins the right lateral portion of the common hepatic duct approximately 2 cm from the union of the right and left hepatic ducts. In one study, the mean length of the cystic duct was 30 mm and the range was 4 to 65 mm (7). The mean collapsed diameter was 4 mm. It has been stated that in most cases the cystic duct drains laterally and at an angle into the common bile duct (45). For instance, in almost 70% of cases in one study, the cystic duct joined the right side of the common hepatic duct at an acute angle (7). In 10%, it formed an angular junction with either the anterior or posterior aspect of the common hepatic duct. A short cystic duct parallel to the common hepatic duct was present in 15% of cases, and a long cystic duct was seen in 4%. Rarely, the cystic duct was spiral and joined the common hepatic duct anteriorly or posteriorly. In a recent cholangiographic study involving large numbers of patients, however, the cystic duct drained laterally into the common bile duct in only 17% of the cases, whereas in 35% it drained in a spiral form, in 41% posteriorly, and in 7% parallel (45). In rare instances, the cystic duct may join the right and left hepatic ducts, forming a trifurcation. The cystic duct usually passes inferiorly to the cystic artery and to the right of the right hepatic artery.

The lining of the cystic duct is pleated, and in some areas there are short folds of varying width and height. The surface cells are identical microscopically (46) and immunohistochemically to those of the gallbladder. Groups of mucous glands are embedded in the dense, collagenous lamina pro-

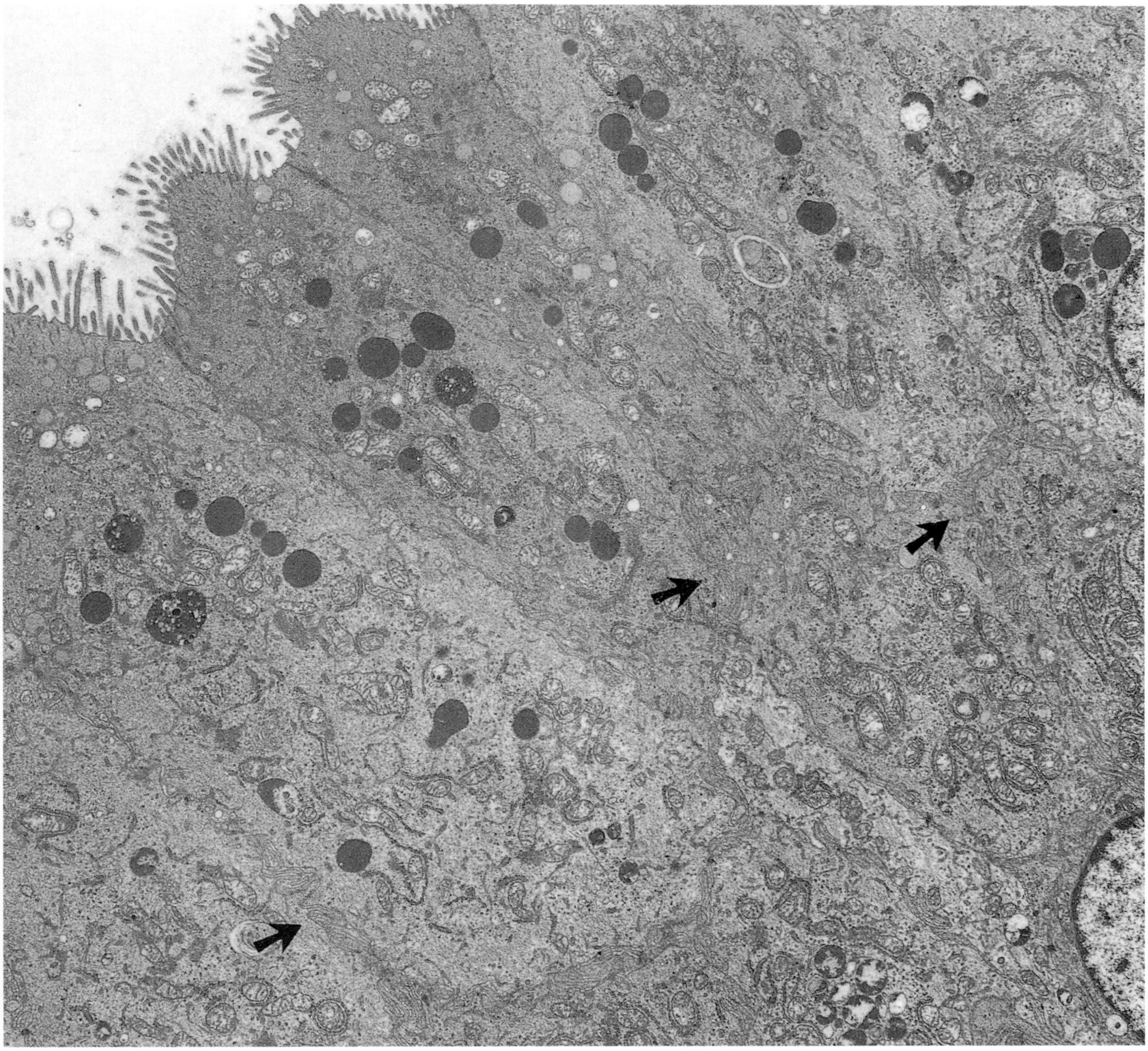

**FIG. 10.** Ultrastructurally, the apical portion of the columnar cells of the gallbladder contains abundant microvilli with core rootlets, mitochondria, Golgi apparatus, mucous granules, lysosomes, and a few strands of rough endoplasmic reticulum. The lateral cell membranes form complex interdigitations (*arrows*).

pria. Lectin-binding patterns of the lining cells are similar to those for the surface epithelial cells of the gallbladder body and neck, whereas the lectin-binding profiles for the glands of the cystic duct are indistinguishable from those of the glands at the gallbladder neck (13). Enterochromaffin cells containing serotonin have been described in cystic ducts from patients with pancreaticobiliary disease (47). In this same group of patients, a few intramural gland cells have shown immunoreactivity for somatostatin.

The connective tissue of the large, oblique folds, grossly visible in the cystic duct at the junction with the gallbladder neck, contains thin groups of smooth muscle fibers (spiral valve of Heister) (Fig. 11). The smooth muscle is believed to prevent both overdistention and collapse of the cystic duct when it is subjected to changes in pressure (2). Abundant collagen and some elastic fibers, nerve fibers, and ganglion cells are intermixed with the smooth muscle. Nerve fibers showing immunoreactivity for vasoactive intestinal peptide (VIP) have been described in the wall (47). The loose subserosal connective tissue contains adipose tissue, nerves with occasional ganglion cells, large blood vessels, and lymphatic channels. Lymphocytes and plasma cells are sparse or absent.

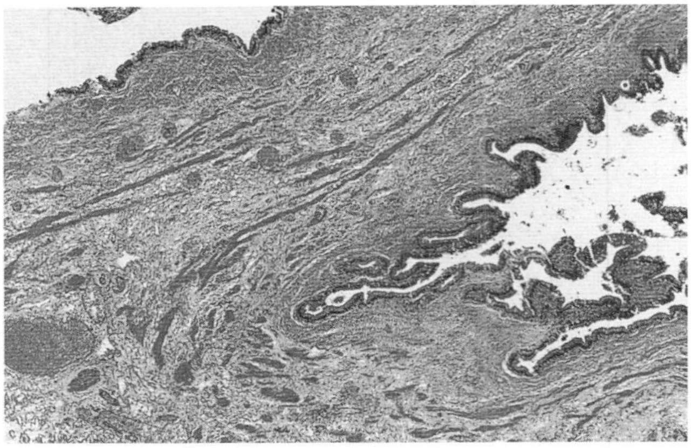

**FIG. 11.** The stroma of the spiral valve of Heister contains thin strands of smooth muscle fibers.

## RIGHT AND LEFT HEPATIC DUCTS, COMMON HEPATIC DUCT, AND COMMON BILE DUCT

### Gross Anatomy

The right and left hepatic ducts, common hepatic duct, and common bile duct are embedded between the serous layers of the hepatoduodenal ligament (the right free border of the lesser omentum). The hepatic ducts emerge from the liver and, in most instances, unite in the hilum approximately 1 cm from the liver to form the common hepatic duct. In 10 to 30% of cases, two large segmental ducts drain the right hepatic lobe and join separately with the left hepatic duct, common hepatic duct, or cystic duct; it is incorrect to label one of these ducts the right hepatic duct and the other "accessory" (48). In a dissection of 100 autopsy specimens, the mean length of the right hepatic duct was 0.8 cm (range 0.2–2.5) and that of the left hepatic duct 1.0 cm (range 0.2–3.5) (49). The usual diameter of each hepatic duct is 3 to 4 mm. The length of the common hepatic duct ranges from 0.8 to 5.2 cm (mean 2.0) (49). Its diameter ranges from 0.2 to 0.8 cm (50). The diameter of the common hepatic duct and its number of elastic fibers increase with age (50). The common bile duct, resulting from the union of the cystic duct and common hepatic duct, can be divided into supraduodenal, retroduodenal, pancreatic, and intraduodenal segments. It is usually about 1 mm thick and 5 cm long, but its length is quite variable (range 1.5–9.0) (49). The diameter at its midpoint ranges from 0.4 to 1.3 cm (mean 0.66) (49), and its lumen narrows approximately 50% after entering the duodenal window (51). In an autopsy study of 100 selected subjects who ranged in age from 15 to 102 years, lacked a history of biliary tract disease, and had completely intact biliary tracts, the outer diameters of the upper portions of the common bile ducts ranged from 0.4 to 1.2 cm (mean 0.74) (52). The outer diameters increased with age but were not related to body weight or length (52). The pits in the surface epithelium (sacculi of Beale) are conspicuous in the extraduodenal portion of the common bile duct and the hepatic ducts. At approximately 2 mm from the duodenal wall, the wall of the common bile duct thickens (due to an increase in muscle), resulting in the abrupt narrowing of the duct's lumen.

### Arterial Supply, Venous Drainage, and Relationship to Bile Ducts

The common hepatic artery arises from the celiac trunk and divides into right and left hepatic branches (Fig. 1). Variations in the origins of the right and left hepatic arteries and their relationships to the extrahepatic bile ducts are typical (53). In one study, almost 42% of 200 cadavers had "aberrant" hepatic arteries (either replaced or accessory) (8). Most often, the right hepatic artery is dorsal to the common hepatic duct and right hepatic duct. The common hepatic and left hepatic arteries lie to the left of the extrahepatic bile ducts and ventral to the portal vein. The gastroduodenal artery lies to the left of the common bile duct, and a branch, the superior pancreaticoduodenal, traverses the duct either dorsally or ventrally (2).

The major arteries that supply branches to the common hepatic duct and the common bile duct include the retroduodenal, right and left hepatic, common hepatic, cystic, gastroduodenal, and retroportal arteries. The most important branches travel along the lateral borders of the common bile duct (54).

The portal vein, formed by the union of the splenic and superior mesenteric veins, lies dorsal to the bile ducts (Fig. 1). The mean length is 6.4 cm (range 4.8–8.8) and its mean diameter is 0.9 cm (range 0.64–1.21) (55). Venous channels that drain the superior portion of the common bile duct enter the liver directly, and those from the inferior portion lead to the portal vein.

### Lymphatic Drainage

Lymphatic channels from the common bile duct drain into lymph nodes located along the duct and then into a group of nodes near the porta hepatis. Other channels lead to deep pancreatic nodes. The ultimate drainage is to the celiac lymph nodes (2).

### Nerve Supply

The nerve supply to the cystic and hepatic ducts derives from the anterior portion of the hepatic plexus, whereas nerves that supply the common bile duct arise from the posterior segment of the hepatic plexus. The nerve of the common bile duct, lying dorsally, is the right portion of the posterior hepatic plexus. Smaller branches from the posterior hepatic plexus travel inferiorly along the common bile duct and accompany the duct to the major duodenal papilla (2). Neuropeptide Y–containing nerve fibers have the same pattern of distribution in the common bile duct as in the gallbladder (11).

**Histology**

The extrahepatic bile ducts, serving as conduits for the flow of bile, are lined by a single layer of tall columnar cells surrounded by a dense connective tissue layer (Fig. 12). The surface of the epithelium is relatively flat or pleated. The columnar cells have basally oriented nuclei that are oval and uniform. Nucleoli are absent or very small. Goblet cells are absent. The epithelium dips into the stroma to form shallow depressions or deeper pits—the sacculi of Beale. In some sections, the deeper sacculi appear isolated from the surface epithelium (Fig. 12), but additional sections show their connections. Surrounding the sacculi are unevenly distributed lobules of glands that empty into the sacculi (Fig. 13). These glands have been termed diverticula, crypts, parietal sacculi, deep glands, biliary glands, periductal glands, and extrahepatic peribiliary glands (56). When located in the more peripheral connective tissue, the glands are encircled by condensed stroma. The peribiliary tubular glands are branched or, occasionally, simple (56). Although they are found in all parts of the extrahepatic bile duct system, they are less frequent in the central portion of the common bile duct and in the intrapancreatic portion than around the bile duct at the ampulla. They are lined by low-columnar or cuboid cells, many of which are filled with mucus (Fig. 14). With inflammation and fibrosis, the sacculi and glands may be distorted, mimicking well-differentiated adenocarcinoma with desmoplastic stroma. In small biopsy specimens and especially frozen sections, the distinction between adenocarcinoma and distorted benign glands may be impossible. The lack of a lobular arrangement and the presence of marked nuclear atypia and perineural invasion are diagnostic of adenocarcinoma (57). Hence, a haphazard growth pattern and cells whose nuclei vary in size and have irregular nuclear membranes are characteristic of adenocarcinoma. Benign glands of the extrahepatic bile ducts have not been reported to invade nerves.

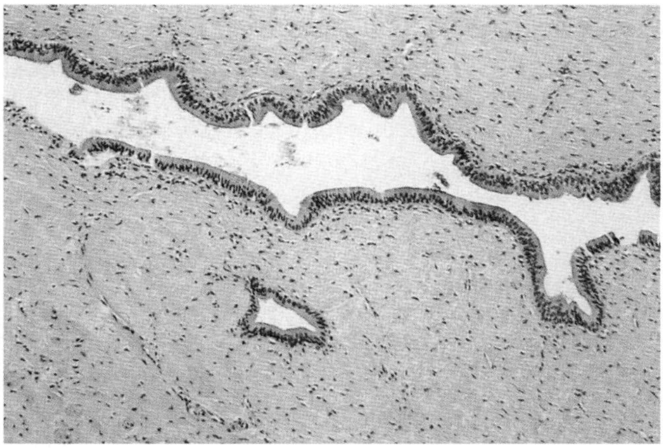

**FIG. 12.** Intrapancreatic segment of common bile duct. The extrahepatic bile ducts are lined by a single layer of tall columnar cells overlying dense, collagenous connective tissue. In segments of the common bile duct away from the duodenum, a few small groups of smooth muscle fibers are sometimes found in the outer half of the wall.

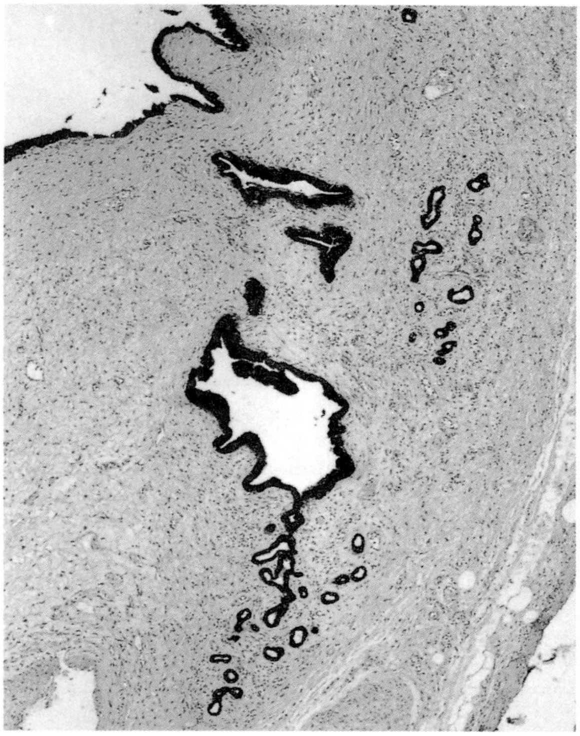

**FIG. 13.** Groups of small glands in the wall of the extrahepatic bile ducts drain into the sacculi of Beale (immunoperoxidase technique for low-molecular-weight keratin).

The surface epithelial cells contain smaller quantities of mucin than the cells that line the gallbladder (58). The former also contain sulfated acid mucin, whereas metaplastic and dysplastic cells primarily contain nonsulfated acid mucin and smaller quantities of sulfated and neutral mucins. The normal lining epithelium stains similarly to that of the gallbladder for epithelial membrane antigen and low-molecular-weight keratin (CAM 5.2 antibody) (Fig. 13). CEA may be absent (using absorbed polyclonal antibody) (59) or appear as focal weak staining along the apices of some cells (using unabsorbed polyclonal antibody). Cytoplasmic staining using either polyclonal or monoclonal anti-CEA antibodies is typically absent (60). Secretory component has been detected in the cells of the surface epithelium and glands (59). Immunoreactivity for lysozyme has been found in the cytoplasm of the cells in the glands, whereas staining of the surface epithelial cells is absent or very weak (59). In addition, cells of the peribiliary glands are usually im-

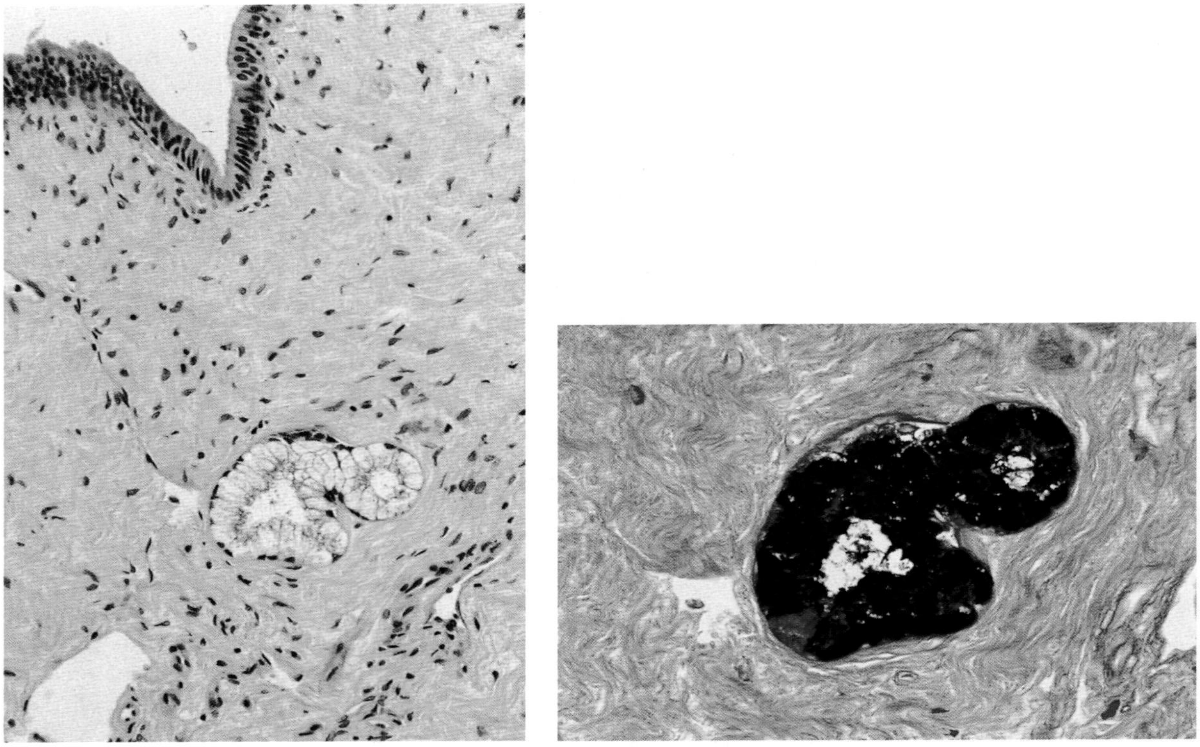

A B

**FIG. 14. A:** Glands embedded in the subepithelial collagenous stroma of the extrahepatic bile ducts typically contain cells with mucin-filled cytoplasm. **B:** Alcian blue–periodic acid-Schiff (PAS) stain from the same field.

munoreactive for pancreatic and salivary alpha-amylase, trypsin, and lipase (56). The surface epithelium of the common bile duct also shows immunoreactivity for these enzymes.

Gastric metaplasia and intestinal metaplasia are sometimes found in inflamed and fibrotic extrahepatic bile ducts that harbor carcinoma (16,58). Scattered endocrine cells, including cells immunoreactive for somatostatin, have been seen in the glands of the hepatic ducts and common bile duct in patients with pancreaticobiliary disease (47,61,62). In resections for pancreatic carcinoma, I have seen scattered benign epithelial cells that are immunoreactive for chromogranin A in the sacculi and glands of the intrapancreatic segment of the common bile duct (Fig. 15). It is unknown at this time whether endocrine cells are present normally in the extrahepatic bile ducts of adults without pancreaticobiliary disease or whether these cells represent partial intestinal metaplasia.

The stroma directly beneath the surface epithelium is dense and contains abundant collagen and elastic fibers and some small vessels (Fig. 12). Lymphocytes are sparse. Pancreatic acini and ducts may be seen in the wall of the intrapancreatic portion of the common bile duct (63). Small pancreatic ducts sometimes empty into this segment of the duct. The peripheral stroma of the common bile duct is less dense than the inner connective tissue and contains large blood vessels, lymphatics, nerves and ganglion cells, elastic fibers, and smooth muscle fibers. This stroma merges with the connective tissue of the hepatoduodenal ligament. The frequency of finding smooth muscle fibers in the wall of the common bile duct, excluding the portion at or near the choledochoduodenal junction, differs in published series. Burden (64), in an early study of 100 necropsies, found that groups of smooth muscle fibers were present almost always in the supraduodenal portion of the duct, typically in its outermost

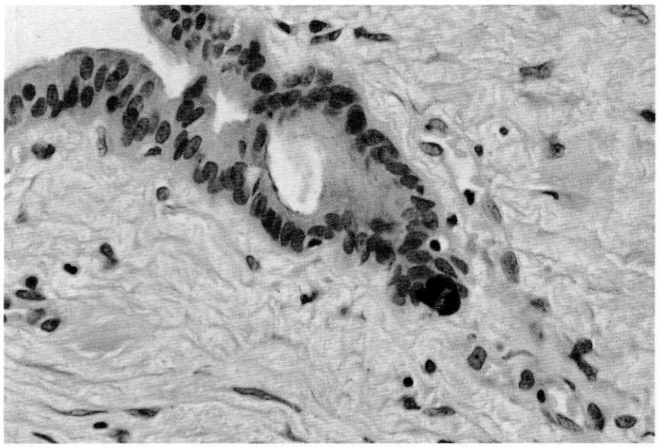

**FIG. 15.** In this Whipple resection specimen for carcinoma of the pancreas, sacculi of the intrapancreatic segment of the common bile duct had rare cells that were positive for chromogranin A (immunoperoxidase technique).

wall. However, in a later autopsy study that included 100 patients without hepatobiliary disease, Mahour et al. (65) observed that 88% of the common bile ducts (the examined portions of which were located in the lesser omentum) lacked smooth muscle fibers in their walls, whereas 12% had varying amounts of muscle. The muscle fibers, when present, are circular or, more frequently, longitudinal and tend to be scanty, discontinuous, and intermixed with collagen and elastic fibers. In contrast, smooth muscle bundles are prominently and characteristically found in the intrapancreatic (a few millimeters from the duodenal wall) and intraduodenal portions of the common bile duct (sphincter choledochus). Nerve fibers showing immunoreactivity for VIP are present beneath the epithelium and in muscle fibers (47).

## VATERIAN SYSTEM AND MINOR PAPILLA

### Gross Anatomy

The Vaterian system is composed of the segments of the common bile duct and major pancreatic duct (occurring either separately or as a common channel) at the duodenum, major papilla, and the sphincteric musculature. It also includes the extraduodenal portion of the common bile duct and major pancreatic duct that join to form a common channel outside the duodenal wall (49). It is a complex structural unit composed of a highly developed mucosa, musculature, and nerve supply that regulates the flow of bile and pancreatic secretions. Its sphincteric function (sphincter of Oddi) is a part of the overall gastrointestinal motility system and is subject to regulation by myogenic, neural, and gastrointestinal hormonal elements (66).

The major pancreatic duct of Wirsung drains many small channels in its course from the tail of the pancreas to the duodenal ostium. It typically inserts into the duodenal window caudal or a little lateral to the common bile duct. Its lumen narrows at the duodenal wall. The minor duct of Santorini, usually present, joins the major pancreatic duct at a variety of angles and locations in the pancreas. Uncommonly, the duct of Wirsung is smaller than the duct of Santorini and the latter may be the chief conduit for drainage of the pancreas (67). The duct of Santorini leads into the minor papilla, but the former may end blindly in at least 10% to 20% of cases (67,68). The luminal pressure of the major pancreatic duct is nearly always higher than that for the common bile duct. The pressure of the latter briefly exceeds that of the former when the gallbladder empties shortly after a meal (69).

The relationship of the common bile duct and duct of Wirsung at the papilla is complex. The ducts may have separate openings into the duodenum, an interposed septum, or a common channel (sometimes forming an ampulla) (Fig. 16). An ampulla, defined strictly, is a dilated, juglike conduit resulting from the union of the common bile duct and major pancreatic duct. In various studies of the pancreaticoduodenal junction, the frequency for separate openings into the duodenal lumen ranged from 12% to 54% and for a common channel, 36% to 88% (49,67,68,70–74). In most studies, more than two thirds of the patients had a common channel. In a detailed gross and radiographic study, DiMagno et al. (70) examined 390 pancreaticoduodenal specimens at autopsy and found that 74% of the patients had a common channel, 19% had separate openings for the pancreatic duct and common bile duct, and 7% had an interposed septum. Twenty-five percent of their specimens had a well-defined ampulla, 18% had a long common channel (defined as a channel greater than 3 mm long in the absence of an ampulla), and 31% had a short common channel (defined as a channel less than 3 mm in length). For those specimens with an interposed septum, the two ducts emptied together at the ostium of the papilla. For the ducts that opened separately into the duodenal lumen, their ostia were located from 1 mm to several centimeters apart. On occasion, the ducts unite before the duodenal wall is breached, forming an extended common channel. In one study, the length of the extended common channel ranged from 0.9 to 3.3 cm (mean 2.2) (75). This lengthy common channel occurred in 13.8% of patients with carcinoma of the biliary tract (18 of 130 cases) and in those with congenital biliary dilatation (four of four cases)

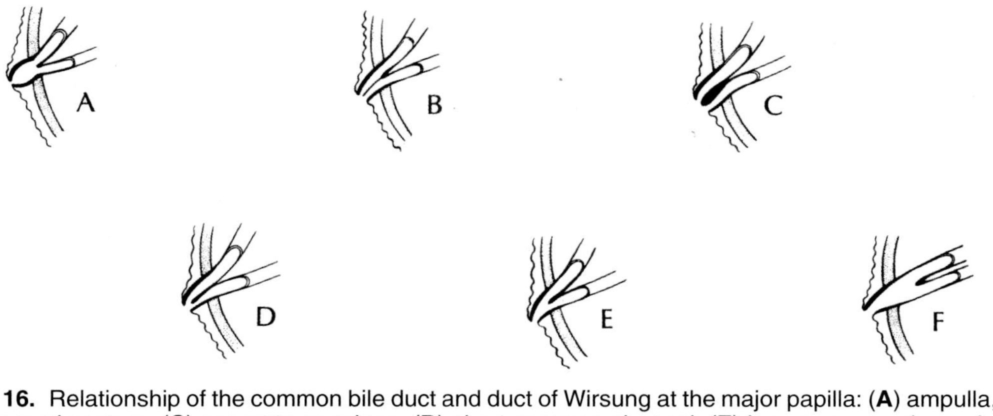


**FIG. 16.** Relationship of the common bile duct and duct of Wirsung at the major papilla: (**A**) ampulla, (**B**) interposed septum, (**C**) separate openings, (**D**) short common channel, (**E**) long common channel, and (**F**) extended common channel.

but was absent in a control group of 30 cases (75). This confluence of the pancreatic and bile ducts outside of the duodenal wall has been increasingly described in association with congenital dilatation of the bile duct or choledochal cyst (76).

The major papilla, a cylindrical protuberance housing the terminations of the common bile duct and major pancreatic duct or a common channel, is situated medially at the midportion of the second part of the duodenum. It is usually covered by a triangular fold of duodenal mucosa completely or partially (77); a longitudinal mucosal fold projects from the caudal portion of its base, forming a frenulum, which was absent in about one quarter of the cases in one study (77). In one series, the mean length of the papilla was 11.7 mm and its width was 5.2 mm (72). Rarely, the major papilla is located at or just below the level of the duodenal mucosa or is absent. Mucosal reduplications (valves of Santorini) (78) at the ostium of the major papilla consist of columnar-shaped protrusions and traverse leaflike flaps of ductal mucosa (79). In one study, the columnar-shaped projections, arising from the terminal common bile duct, numbered one to four per specimen and ranged from 1 to 5 mm in length (79). They were found in approximately one third of adults but were not observed in fetuses. Leaflike flaps, present in the caudal wall of the common channel in over 90% of fetuses and adults, were separated by small cul-de-sacs of varying size and depth. The flaps sometimes extended into the major pancreatic duct. In cases in which a common channel was absent, the leaflike flaps were found only at the orifice of the duct of Wirsung. It has been postulated that the flaps flatten during the flow of pancreatic juice into the duodenum; when the cul-de-sacs are filled, the ostium is blocked and regurgitation is prevented (79).

The sphincter of Oddi consists of the intrinsic circular and longitudinal musculature of the Vaterian system. It is embryologically and functionally distinct from the musculature of the duodenal wall. However, the muscle fibers from the duodenal wall aid in anchoring the Vaterian system in place in the duodenal window. In a study of the structure of the dense connective tissue around the major duodenal papilla, the papilla and duodenal wall were noted to form both a morphologic and a functional unit (80). Connective tissue fibers spread from the papilla orifice to the circular duodenal musculature and cross at different angles from the orifice to the distal common bile duct. The arrangement and amount of muscle bundles that form the sphincter are highly complex and variable. Important fibers are those around the intrapancreatic (near the duodenal wall) and intraduodenal portions of the common bile duct (sphincter choledochus) (81). In one study, accumulation of circular muscle fibers extended up the common bile duct to a mean distance of 13.6 mm from the pore of the papilla (77). Smooth muscle fibers are also present in the wall of the common channel, around the duct of Wirsung, and near the ostium of the papilla. It is controversial whether the smooth muscle bundles around the pancreatic duct above the common channel have important sphincteric function, but the finding of a sustained pancreatic duct high-pressure zone with phasic contractions after sphincterotomy is evidence that the sphincter of Oddi extends above the common channel to include portions of the pancreatic duct (81–83). Muscle fibers have been found to extend up the pancreatic duct a mean of 7.3 mm from the papillary pore (77). The tunica muscularis of the duodenum may not have a primary role in managing the flow of bile and pancreatic juice at the choledochoduodenal junction.

The sphincter of Oddi serves to inhibit the flow of bile into the duodenum, pumps bile into the duodenum when necessary, and likely precludes the entry of duodenal contents into the common bile duct or major pancreatic duct (66). Manometric studies have shown that the control of the flow of bile during fasting results from the phasic contractions of the sphincter of Oddi (84). These contractions result in the liberation of small volumes of bile. The flow of pancreatic juice is also regulated. The contractions are in addition to the steady basal pressure of the sphincter of Oddi, which is several mm Hg higher than that for the common bile and pancreatic ducts (85). The high pressure zone measures 4–6 mm long, and the phasic contractions may be antegrade, retrograde, or simultaneous (83). Cholecystokinin has been found to inhibit the phasic contractions of the sphincter and decrease the basal pressure, allowing the flow of large quantities of bile into the duodenum (84). Manometric and contractility studies of the effects of various hormones on the sphincter of Oddi in humans and animals have been summarized (66,83). Glucagon-like cholecystokinin decreases sphincteric pressure, whereas gastrin and secretin elevate basal pressure (83). The phasic contractions and basal tone of the sphincter can be increased or decreased by exogenous drugs. For instance, most narcotics increase sphincteric pressure, whereas atropine decreases it (83).

The minor papilla is nearly always present but may be difficult to locate grossly (68). Its size is variable (86). It is usually situated 2 cm proximal to the major papilla (68).

### Vascular and Nerve Supply and Lymphatic Drainage

The intraduodenal portion of the common bile duct is supplied by vessels from the anterior and posterior superior pancreaticoduodenal arteries (2). Venous drainage occurs via small veins that lead to the portal vein. The fine venous architecture of the major papilla has been described in detail (87). Lymphatics from the pancreaticoduodenal junction drain into the anterior and posterior pancreaticoduodenal lymph nodes and to the superior and inferior lymph nodes at the head of the pancreas (88). The Vaterian system is innervated extrinsically by parasympathetic nerve fibers in the vagal nerve and by sympathetic nerve fibers in the splanchnic nerves (66). Although little is known regarding the role of these nerve fibers in regulating the motility of the sphincter of Oddi, some evidence indicates that its motility is inhibited by vagal activation (66). Three separate ganglia cell groups provide intrinsic innervation. These are found at the base of the papilla in the duodenal wall, within the musculature of the papilla, and within the submucosa (66). This intrinsic innervation appears to provide tonic inhibition and is similar to that for other gastrointestinal sphincters, including the lower esophageal, pyloric, and internal anal sphincters.

## Histology

The epithelial lining of the duct of Wirsung is identical to that of the common bile duct. The cytoplasm of the columnar cells also contains sulfated acid mucin (89). The epithelium sometimes undergoes hyperplastic or metaplastic changes, including mucinous cell hypertrophy, papillary hyperplasia, adenomatous hyperplasia, squamous metaplasia, and pyloric gland metaplasia (88). Surrounding the normal epithelium is a dense fibrous layer with abundant collagen and elastic fibers. A few ganglion cells may be seen in the outer half of the fibrous wall. Small pancreatic ducts draining acini traverse the dense fibrous layer. At the orifice of the papilla, the epithelium of Wirsung's duct is thrown into folds (mucosal reduplications) that have cores of fibrovascular stroma. Goblet cells are found interspersed between the columnar lining cells within the papilla. Numerous small accessory pancreatic ducts drain into the ductal lumen near the ostium, and pancreatic acini are sometimes present just beneath the lining of the duct (Fig. 17). A few lymphocytes may be seen within the ductal epithelium, and lymphocytes, plasma cells, and mast cells sparsely populate the fibrovascular cores. Circular smooth muscle bundles are present around the duct as it penetrates the duodenal wall (86).

The epithelium of the terminal portion of the common bile duct and common channel (if present) covers long, slender papillary fronds or valvules that in some respects resemble the fimbriae of the fallopian tube (Fig. 18). They correspond to the mucosal reduplications seen grossly. These papillary formations are considerably larger than the duodenal villi, which are few or absent at the surface of the papilla. The valvules may branch and sometimes project beyond the ostium of the papilla (51), shorter fronds at the periphery and longer ones centrally (90). The columnar lining cells have eosinophilic cytoplasm and basal nuclei. Interspersed goblet cells are more numerous near the ostium. The stroma forming the cores of the fronds contains a few lymphocytes, mast cells, and plasma cells. Muscle fibers, present at the base of the fronds, are occasionally found in the stroma of the fronds. The smooth muscle, forming the sphincter choledochus, becomes apparent in the wall of the duct several millimeters before the duct enters the duodenal window. About 5 mm from the duodenal wall, longitudinal muscle fibers are present around two thirds of the common bile duct; at 2 mm from the duodenal musculature, circular muscle fibers increase and completely surround the duct (86). These intrinsic muscle fibers are separated from the muscularis propria of the duodenum by connective tissue and, at times, pancreatic tissue (86). Variable amounts of circular and longitudinal muscle fibers also surround the common channel. Before forming a common channel, the common bile duct is set apart from the pancreatic duct by a septum that eventually loses its muscle fibers, becoming a thin connective tissue membrane (86). Interspersed between areas of smooth muscle around the common bile duct or common channel are collagen, elastic fibers, small nerves, and ganglion cells. When the common bile duct and duct of Wirsung are separate within the papilla, they are distinguishable by light microscopy because the common bile duct is larger, has more prominent fronds, a greater amount of enveloping smooth muscle, and bile in its lumen.

A bewildering assortment of glands and ducts of various caliber surround the common bile duct at the papilla. Frequently, it is only possible to distinguish mucous glands from the terminations of accessory pancreatic ducts by studying serial sections (63). Mucous glands drain into the

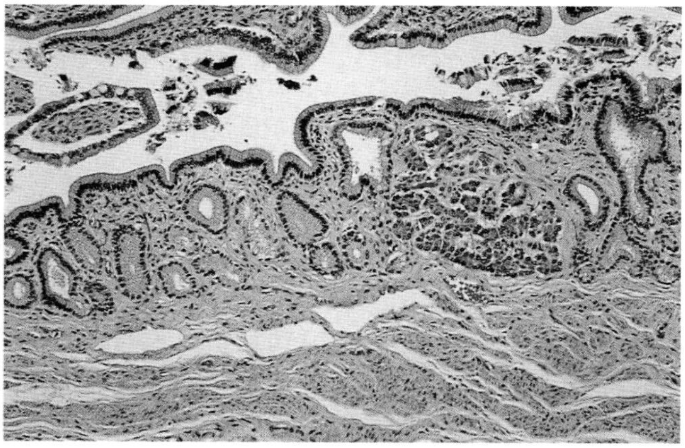

**FIG. 17.** The duct of Wirsung at the papilla of Vater is lined by a single layer of tall columnar cells with occasional interspersed goblet cells. Accessory pancreatic ducts and acini are also observed.

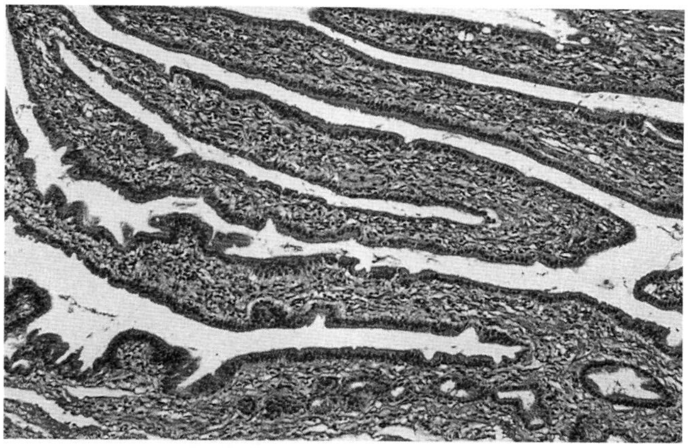

**FIG. 18.** Near the ostium of the major papilla, the epithelium of the common bile duct lines prominent papillary fronds (valvules).

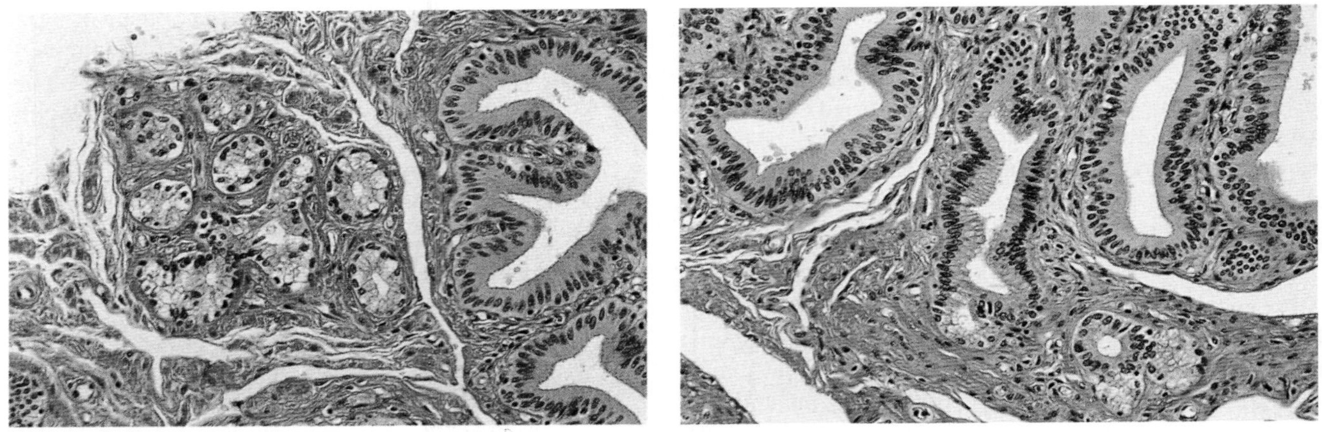


**FIG. 19.** Mucous glands are present around the common bile duct at the papilla and drain into recesses between the papillary fronds.

shallow or deep recesses between the papillary fronds (Fig. 19). The number of these glands and their distribution are variable. Glands near the surface of the papilla may be distended with mucus (90). Some may even represent dilated accessory pancreatic ducts. The number and distribution of accessory pancreatic ducts within the major papilla are also inconstant. These small accessory pancreatic channels, having been studied in serial sections and by camera lucida drawings (91), empty into the common bile duct (Fig. 20), duct of Wirsung, common channel, surface of papilla, or through the duodenal mucosa near the papilla (63). They are sometimes numerous and may cause obstruction of the common bile duct, duct of Wirsung, or common channel. In such instances, a diagnosis of accessory duct hyperplasia is appropriate (90). In an autopsy study, accessory pancreatic ducts were absent in only two of 100 major papillae (91). The ducts drain small lobules of pancreatic acini located within or, more often, near the papilla. In one study, pancreatic acini were found in 8% of 145 major papillae, whereas pancreatic islets were not seen in any of the major papillae (92). The ducts appear as packets of multiple lumens of small caliber encircled by a cellular fibrovascular stroma (Fig. 21). Within a group of ducts, the larger central duct is surrounded by smaller branches. Groups of ducts are sometimes seen penetrating the duodenal smooth muscle. Small groups of heterotopic pancreatic acini and ducts also occur in the submucosa of the duodenum away from the major papilla (Fig. 22).

Immunohistochemically, the cells lining the common bile duct and the duct of Wirsung at the papilla are positive for low-molecular-weight keratin (CAM 5.2 antibody) and epithelial membrane antigen. There may be linear apical staining for CEA (unabsorbed polyclonal antibody). The adjacent mucous glands and accessory pancreatic ducts have the same immunoreactivity for keratin and epithelial membrane antigen. A few scattered cells lining the large ducts within the pancreas are positive for neuron-specific enolase, chromogranin A, insulin, and glucagon (93). Chromogranin-positive cells are sometimes located in the lining epithelium of the duct of Wirsung and common bile duct within the papilla. Mucous glands and accessory pancreatic ducts also contain scattered cells immunoreactive for neuron-specific enolase and chromogranin A (Fig. 23). In patients with pancreaticobiliary disease, a few cells lining the lumen of the papilla and in adjacent mucous glands have been found to be im-

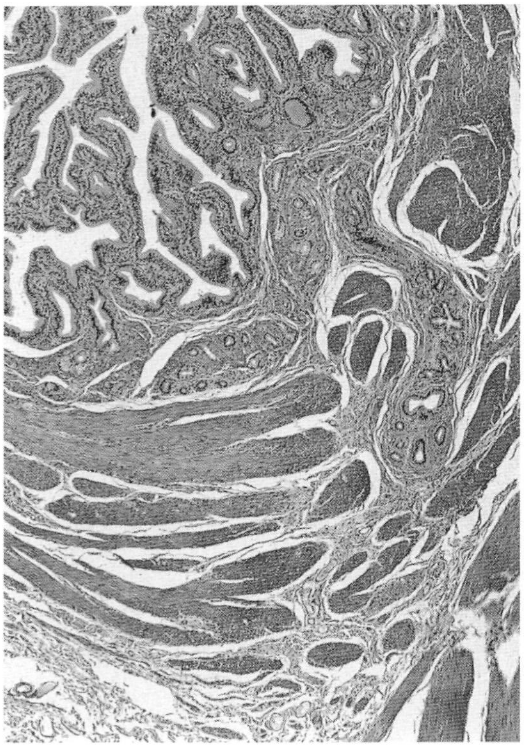

**FIG. 20.** Accessory pancreatic ducts pierce the large smooth muscle bundles to empty into the lumen of the common bile duct.

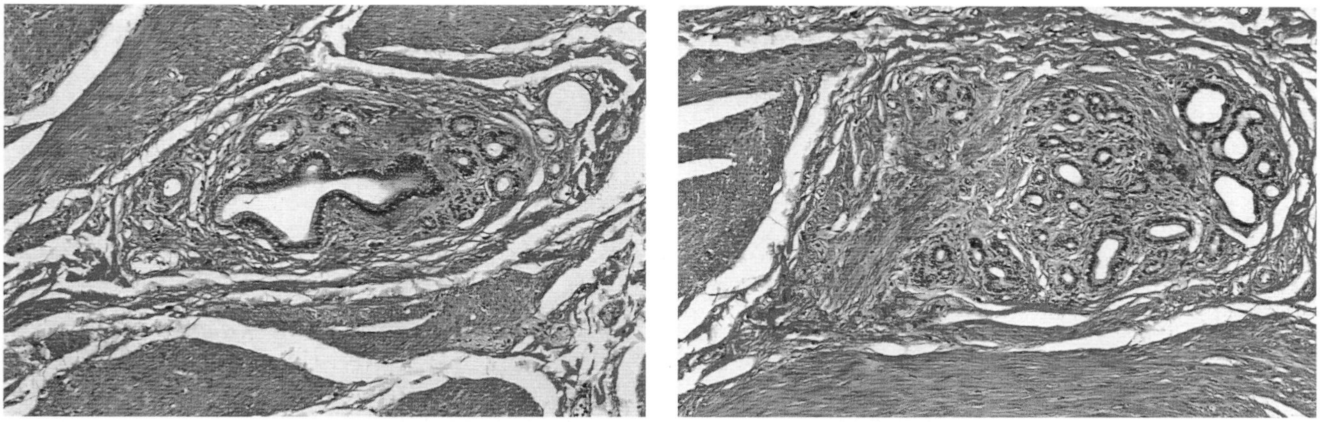

A B

**FIG. 21.** Accessory pancreatic ducts that penetrate the smooth muscle bundles at the choledochoduodenal junction are surrounded by a fibrovascular stroma.

munoreactive for somatostatin (47,61). Although usually absent, endocrine cell micronests may be scattered singly or are grouped in the stroma adjacent to pancreatic ducts, ductules, or accessory glands but not around the common bile duct (92). They have been found in about 3% of major papillae. They consist of round, oval, trabecular, or ribbonlike groups of cells that immunohistochemically are distinct from those of pancreatic islets. They are typically scattered, rarely nodular, and immunohistochemically stain for somatostatin and pancreatic polypepide. It is unclear whether they are a normal finding or represent a metaplastic/hyperplastic or neoplastic condition. The functional role of these endocrine cells in the papilla of Vater is unknown.

At the minor papilla, the pancreatic duct of Santorini contains papillary fronds that are lined by simple columnar epithelium with some goblet cells (Figs. 24 and 25). Small pancreatic ducts open into the lumen of the duct of Santorini at the minor papilla or separately into the duodenum (68). Small lobules of pancreatic acini may be present within the connective tissue of the minor papilla (Fig. 26). They were seen in 77% of 167 minor papillae in a study by Noda et al., who noted that 14% of the papillae also contained well-

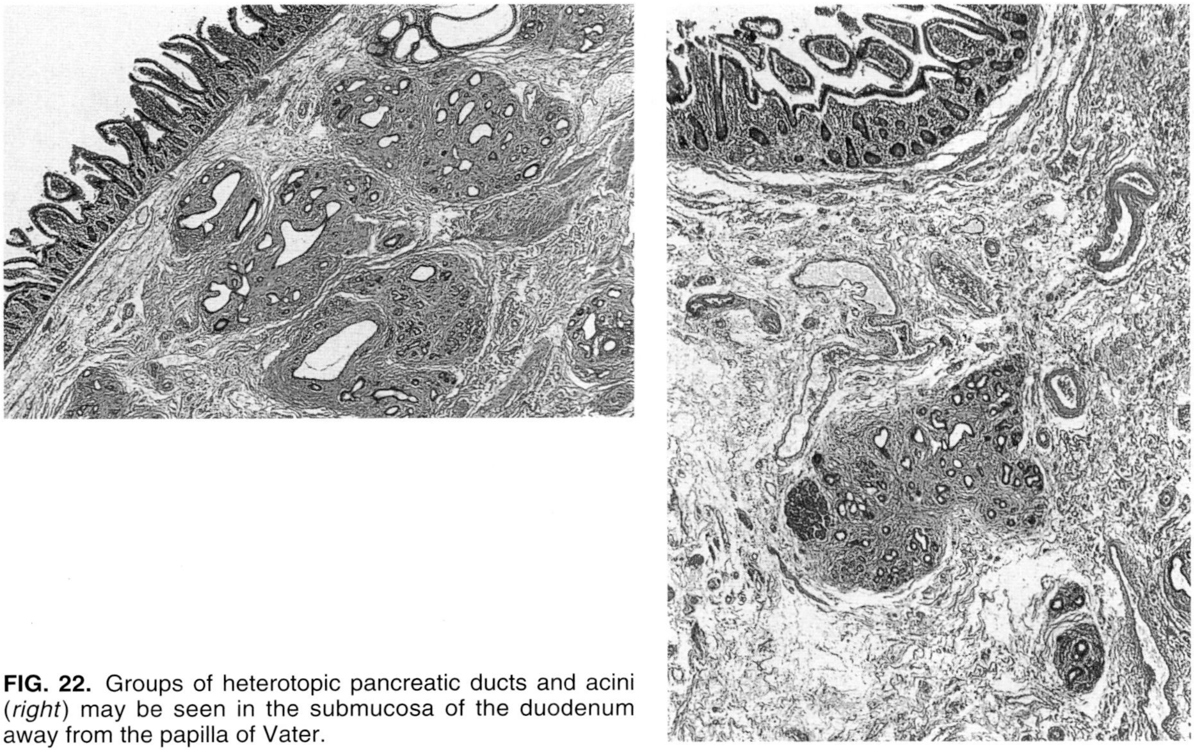

A B

**FIG. 22.** Groups of heterotopic pancreatic ducts and acini (*right*) may be seen in the submucosa of the duodenum away from the papilla of Vater.

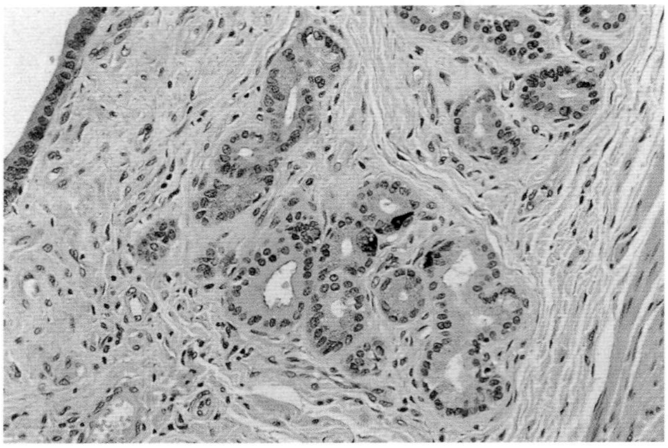

**FIG. 23.** Some of the small ducts around the duct of Wirsung at the major papilla contain a few cells that are immunoreactive for chromogranin A (immunoperoxidase technique).

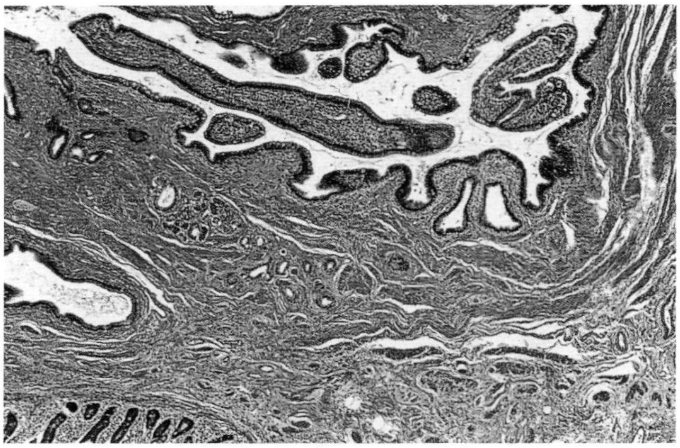

**FIG. 24.** The duct of Santorini at the minor papilla contains papillary fronds and is surrounded by muscle bundles.

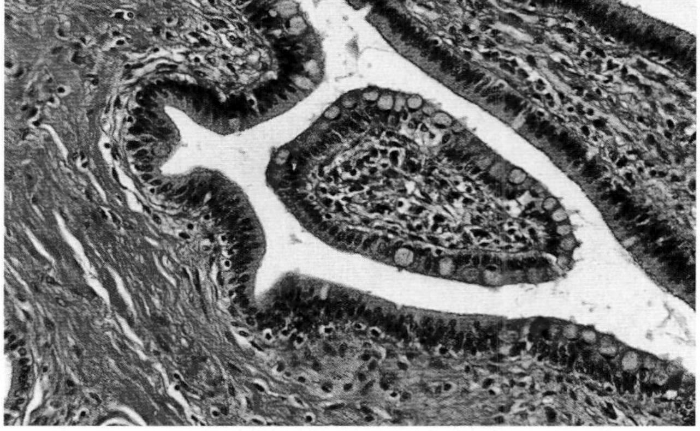

**FIG. 25.** The duct of Santorini at the minor papilla is lined by tall columnar cells with interspersed goblet cells.

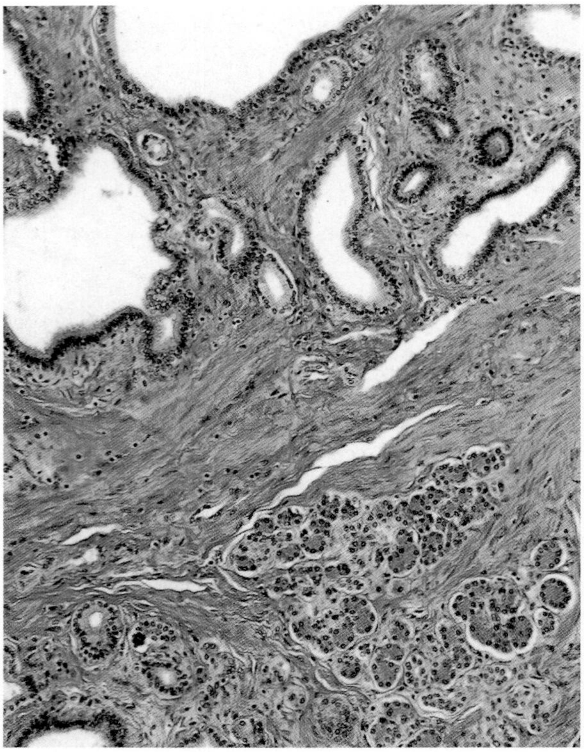

**FIG. 26.** Pancreatic acini and small ducts may be found near the lumen of the duct of Santorini at the minor papilla.

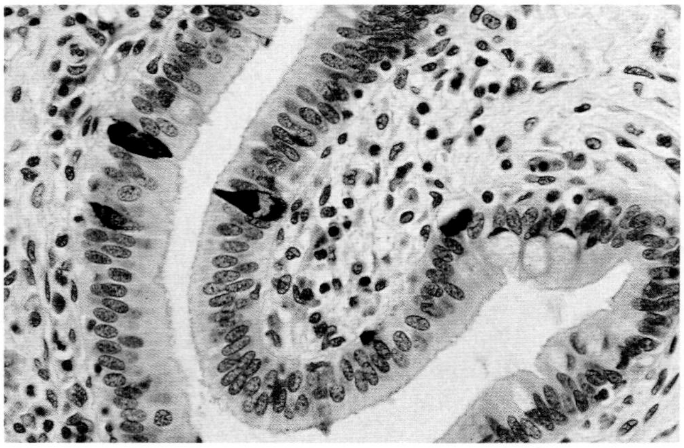

**FIG. 27.** A few cells that line the duct of Santorini at the minor papilla are flask shaped and immunoreactive for chromogranin A (immunoperoxidase technique).

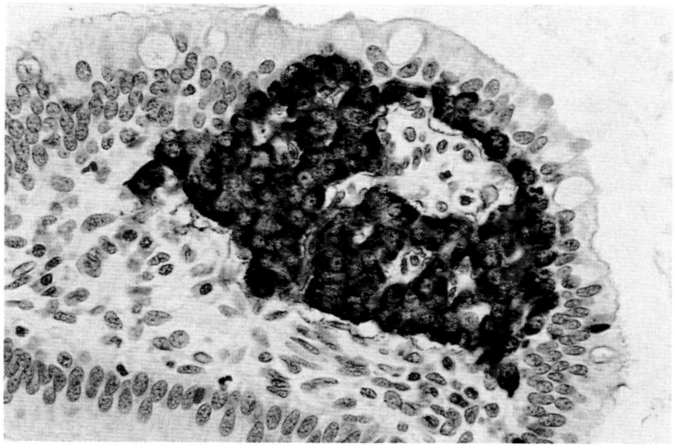

**FIG. 28.** A group of cells below the lining epithelium of the duct of Santorini at the minor papilla is immunoreactive for chromogranin A (immunoperoxidase technique).

formed pancreatic islets (92). Atrophic or poorly formed islets are present uncommonly. Smooth muscle bundles separated by collagen, small nerves, and ganglion cells surround the duct. The bundles of muscle occasionally are continuous with those of the muscularis mucosae of the duodenum, but in many instances continuity between the groups of muscle fibers is lacking (68). The lining epithelial cells and those of the small pancreatic ducts stain strongly for low-molecular-weight keratin (CAM 5.2 antibody) and weakly for CEA (unabsorbed polyclonal antibody). A few cells within small ducts and some that line the lumen of the duct of Santorini are flask shaped and immunoreactive for neuron-specific enolase and chromogranin A (Fig. 27). Small groups of neuroendocrine cells may extend below the epithelial lining (Fig. 28). In the above-mentioned study of 167 minor papillae, 16% contained endocrine micronests (92), which were predominantly scattered and rarely nodular. They were usually immunoreactive for somatostatin and pancreatic polypeptide and lacked staining for insulin and glucagon. It is possible that some of these micronests represent metaplasia/hyperplasia or neoplasia.

## ACKNOWLEDGMENTS

I thank Nancy Kriigel and Tijuana Battle for secretarial support, Ursula Bunch for photographic assistance, Linda Hamm for artwork, and Joyce Nash for performing the immunoperoxidase technique.

## REFERENCES

1. Albores-Saavedra J, Henson DE. Tumors of the gallbladder and extrahepatic bile ducts. In: *Atlas of tumor pathology. Fascicle 22, 2nd series.* Washington DC: Armed Forces Institute of Pathology; 1986: 3–16,130–150.
2. Lindner HH. Embryology and anatomy of the biliary tree. In: Way LW, Pellegrini CA, eds. *Surgery of the gallbladder and bile ducts.* Philadelphia: WB Saunders; 1987:3–22.
3. Guyton AC. The liver and biliary system. In: *Textbook of medical physiology. 5th ed.* Philadelphia: WB Saunders; 1976:936–944.
4. Frizzell RA, Heintze K. Transport functions of the gallbladder. In: Javitt NB, ed. *Liver and biliary tract physiology I. International review of physiology., Vol 21.* Baltimore: University Park Press; 1980: 221–247.
5. Pomeranz IS, Davison JS, Shaffer EA. In vitro effects of pancreatic polypeptide and motilin on contractility of human gallbladder. *Dig Dis Sci* 1983;28:539–544.
6. Fisher RS, Rock E, Levin G, Malmud L. Effects of somatostatin on gallbladder emptying. *Gastroenterology* 1987;92:885–890.
7. Moosman DA, Coller FA. Prevention of traumatic injury to the bile ducts. A study of the structures of the cystohepatic angle encountered in cholecystectomy and supraduodenal choledochostomy. *Am J Surg* 1951;82:132–143.
8. Michels NA. The hepatic, cystic and retroduodenal arteries and their relations to the biliary ducts. With samples of the entire celiacal blood supply. *Ann Surg* 1951;133:503–524.
9. Shirai Y, Yoshida K, Tsukada K, Ohtani T, Muto T. Identification of the regional lymphatic system of the gallbladder by vital staining. *Br J Surg* 1992;79:659–662.
10. Magee DF, Naruse S, Pap A. Vagal control of gall-bladder contraction. *J Physiol (Lond)* 1984;355:65–70.
11. Ding W-G, Fujimura M, Mori A, Tooyama I, Kimura H. Light and electron microscopy of neuropeptide Y-containing nerves in human liver, gallbladder, and pancreas. *Gastroenterology* 1991;101:1054–1059.
12. Laitio M, Nevalainen T. Gland ultrastructure in human gallbladder. *J Anat* 1975;120:105–112.
13. Karayannopoulou G, Damjanov I. Lectin binding sites in the human gallbladder and cystic duct. *Histochemistry* 1987;88:75–83.
14. Albores-Saavedra J, Nadji M, Henson DE, Ziegels-Weissman J, Mones JM. Intestinal metaplasia of the gallbladder: a morphologic and immunocytochemical study. *Hum Pathol* 1986;17:614–620.
15. Kozuka S, Hachisuka K. Incidence by age and sex of intestinal metaplasia in the gallbladder. *Hum Pathol* 1984;15:779–784.
16. Kozuka S, Kurashina M, Tsubone M, Hachisuka K, Yasui A. Significance of intestinal metaplasia for the evolution of cancer in the biliary tract. *Cancer* 1984;54:2277–2285.
17. Laitio M. Morphology and histochemistry of non-tumorous gallbladder epithelium. A series of 103 cases. *Pathol Res Pract* 1980;167:335–345.
18. Yamamoto M, Nakajo S, Tahara E. Endocrine cells and lysozyme immunoreactivity in the gallbladder. *Arch Pathol Lab Med* 1986;110: 920–927.
19. Tatematsu M, Furihata C, Miki K, et al. Complete and incomplete pyloric gland metaplasia of human gallbladder. *Acta Pathol Jpn* 1987;37: 39–46.
20. Tsutsumi Y, Nagura H, Osamura Y, Watanabe K, Yanaihura N. Histochemical studies of metaplastic lesions in the human gallbladder. *Arch Pathol Lab Med* 1984;108:917–921.
21. Aroni K, Kittas C, Papadimitriou CS, Papacharalampous NX. An immunocytochemical study of the distribution of lysozyme, alpha-1-antitrypsin and alpha-1-antichymotrypsin in the normal and pathological gallbladder. *Virchows Arch [A]* 1984;403:281–289.
22. Albores-Saavedra J, Nadji M, Morales AR, Henson DE. Carcinoembryonic antigen in normal, preneoplastic and neoplastic gallbladder epithelium. *Cancer* 1983;52:1069–1072.
23. Maxwell P, Davis RI, Sloan JM. Carcinoembryonic antigen (CEA) in benign and malignant epithelium of the gallbladder, extrahepatic bile ducts, and ampulla of Vater. *J Pathol* 1993;170:73–76.
24. Delaquerriere L, Tremblay G, Riopelle J-L. Argentaffin cells in chronic cholecystitis. *Arch Pathol Lab Med* 1962;74:142–151.
25. Yamamoto M, Nakajo S, Tahara E. Immunohistochemical analysis of estrogen receptors in human gallbadder. *Jpn Soc Pathol* 1990;40: 14–21.
26. Hudson I, Hopwood D. Macrophages and mast cells in chronic cholecystitis and "normal" gallbladders. *J Clin Pathol* 1986;39:1082–1087.
27. Green FHY, Fox H. An immunofluorescent study of the distribution of immunoglobulin-containing cells in the normal and the inflamed human gallbladder. *Gut* 1972;13:379–384.
28. Weedon D. *Pathology of the gallbladder.* New York: Masson; 1984.
29. Fine G, Raju UB. Paraganglia in the human gallbladder. *Arch Pathol Lab Med* 1980;104:265–268.
30. Elfving G. Crypts and ducts in the gallbladder wall. *Acta Pathol Microbiol Immunol Scand (Supp)* 1960;49:1–45.
31. Robertson HE, Ferguson WJ. The diverticula (Luschka's crypts) of the gallbladder. *Arch Pathol Lab Med* 1945;40:312–333.
32. Halpert B. Morphological studies on the gall-bladder. II. The "true

Luschka ducts" and the "Rokitansky-Aschoff sinuses" of the human gallbladder. *Bull Johns Hopkins Hosp* 1927;41:77–103.
33. Beilby JOW. Diverticulosis of the gallbladder. The fundal adenoma. *Br J Exp Pathol* 1967;48:455–461.
34. Moosman DA. Accessory bile ducts. Their significance during cholecystectomy. *Mich Med* 1964;63:355–358.
35. Foster JH, Wayson EE. Surgical significance of aberrant bile ducts. *Am J Surg* 1962;104:14–19.
36. McQuillan T, Manolas SG, Hayman JA, Kune GA. Surgical significance of the bile duct of Luschka. *Br J Surg* 1989;76:696–698.
37. Goor DA, Ebert PA. Anomalies of the biliary tree. Report of a repair of an accessory bile duct and review of the literature. *Arch Surg* 1972;104: 302–309.
38. Tejada E, Danielson C. Ectopic or heterotopic liver (choristoma) associated with the gallbladder. *Arch Pathol Lab Med* 1989;113:950–952.
39. Mutschmann PN. Aberrant pancreatic tissue in the gallbladder wall. *Am J Surg* 1946;72:282–283.
40. Busuttil A. Ectopic adrenal within the gallbladder wall. *J* Pathol 1974; 113:231–233.
41. Curtis LE, Sheahan DG. Heterotopic tissues in the gallbladder. *Arch Pathol Lab Med* 1969;88:677–683.
42. Kaye GI, Wheeler HO, Whitlock RT, Lane N. Fluid transport in the rabbit gallbladder. A combined physiological and electron microscopic study. *J Cell Biol* 1966;30:237–268.
43. Gilloteaux J, Pomerants B, Kelly TR. Human gallbladder mucosa ultrastructure: evidence of intraepithelial nerve structures. *Am J Anat* 1989;184:321–333.
44. Evett RD, Higgins JA, Brown AL Jr. The fine structure of normal mucosa in human gallbladder. *Gastroenterology* 1964;47:49–60.
45. Berci G. Biliary ductal anatomy and anomalies. The role of intraoperative cholangiography during laparoscopic cholecystectomy. *Surg Clin North Am* 1992;72:1069–1075.
46. Repassy G, Schaff Z, Lapis K, Marton T, Jakab F, Sugar I. Mucosa of the Heister valve in cholelithiasis. Transmission and scanning electron microscopic study. *Arch Pathol Lab Med* 1978;102:403–405.
47. Dancygier H. Endoscopic transpapillary biopsy (ETPB) of human extrahepatic bile ducts—light and electron microscopic findings, clinical significance. *Endoscopy* 1989;21:312–320.
48. Northover JMA, Terblanche J. Applied surgical anatomy of the biliary tree. In: Blumgart LH, ed. *The biliary tract. Clinical surgery international. vol 5.* Edinburgh: Churchill Livingstone; 1982:1–16.
49. Dowdy GS Jr, Waldron GW, Brown WG. Surgical anatomy of the pancreatobiliary ductal system. *Arch Surg* 1962;84:229–246.
50. Takahashi Y, Takahashi T, Takahashi W, Sato T. Morphometrical evaluation of extrahepatic bile ducts in reference to their structural changes with aging. *Tohoku J Exp Med* 1985;147:301–309.
51. Baggenstoss AH. Major duodenal papilla. Variations of pathologic interest and lesions of the mucosa. *Arch Pathol Lab Med* 1938;26: 853–868.
52. Mahour GH, Wakim KG, Ferris DO. The common bile duct in man: its diameter and circumference. *Ann Surg* 1967;165:415–419.
53. Benson EA, Page RE. A practical reappraisal of the anatomy of the extrahepatic bile ducts and arteries. *Br J Surg* 1976;63:853–860.
54. Northover JMA, Terblanche J. A new look at the arterial supply of the bile duct in man and its surgical implications. *Br J Surg* 1979;66: 379–384.
55. Douglass BE, Baggenstoss AH, Hollinshead WH. The anatomy of the portal vein and its tributaries. *Surg Gynecol Obstet* 1950;91:562–576.
56. Terada T, Kida T, Nakanuma Y. Extrahepatic peribiliary glands express alpha-amylase isozymes, trypsin and pancreatic lipase: an immunohistochemical analysis. *Hepatology* 1993;18:803–808.
57. Qualman SJ, Haupt HM, Bauer TW, Taxy JB. Adenocarcinoma of the hepatic duct junction. A reappraisal of the histologic criteria of malignancy. *Cancer* 1984;53:1545–1551.
58. Laitio M. Carcinoma of extrahepatic bile ducts. A histopathologic study. *Pathol Res Pract* 1983;178:67–72.
59. Nagura H, Tsutsumi Y, Watanabe K, et al. Immunohistochemistry of carcinoembryonic antigen, secretory component and lysozyme in benign and malignant common bile duct tissues. *Virchows Arch [A]* 1984; 403:271–280.
60. Davis RI, Sloan JM, Hood JM, Maxwell P. Carcinoma of the extrahepatic biliary tract: a clinicopathological and immunohistochemical study. *Histopathology* 1988;12:623–631.
61. Dancygier H, Klein U, Leuschner U, Hubner K, Classen M. Somatostatin-containing cells in the extrahepatic biliary tract of humans. *Gastroenterology* 1984;86:892–896.
62. Yamamoto M, Nakajo S, Tahara E, Miyoshi N. Endocrine cell carcinoma of extrahepatic bile duct. *Acta Pathol Jpn* 1986;36:587–593.
63. Cross KR. Accessory pancreatic ducts. Special reference to the intrapancreatic portion of the common duct. *Arch Pathol Lab Med* 1956;61: 434–440.
64. Burden VG. Observations on the histologic and pathologic anatomy of the hepatic, cystic, and common bile ducts. *Ann Surg* 1925;82: 584–597.
65. Mahour GH, Wakim KG, Soule EH, Ferris DO. Structure of the common bile duct in man: presence or absence of smooth muscle. *Ann Surg* 1967;166:91–94.
66. Allescher HD. Papilla of Vater: structure and function. *Endoscopy* 1989;21:324–329.
67. Millbourn E. On the excretory ducts of the pancreas in man, with special reference to their relations to each other, to the common bile duct and to the duodenum. A radiological and anatomical study. *Acta Anat (Basel)* 1950;9:1–34.
68. Baldwin WM. The pancreatic ducts in man, together with a study of the microscopical structure of the minor duodenal papilla. *Anat Rec* 1911; 5:197–228.
69. Parry EW, Hallenbeck GA, Grindlay JH. Pressures in the pancreatic and common ducts. Values during fasting, after various meals, and after sphincterotomy: an experimental study. *Arch Surg* 1955;70: 757–765.
70. DiMagno EP, Shorter RG, Taylor WF, Go VLW. Relationships between pancreaticobiliary ductal anatomy and pancreatic ductal and parenchymal histology. *Cancer* 1982;49:361–368.
71. Howard J, Jones R. The anatomy of the pancreatic ducts. The etiology of acute pancreatitis. *Am J Med Sci* 1947;214:617–622.
72. Newman HF, Weinberg SB, Newman EB, Northup JD. The papilla of Vater and distal portions of the common bile duct and duct of Wirsung. Surg *Gynecol Obstet* 1958;106:687–694.
73. Stamm BH. Incidence and diagnostic significance of minor pathologic changes in the adult pancreas at autopsy: a systematic study of 112 autopsies in patients without known pancreatic disease. *Hum Pathol* 1984;15:677–683.
74. Sterling JA. The common channel for bile and pancreatic ducts. *Surg Gynecol Obstet* 1954;98:420–424.
75. Suda K, Matsumoto Y, Miyano T. An extended common channel in patients with biliary tract carcinoma and congenital biliary dilatation. *Surg Pathol* 1988;1:65–69.
76. Okada A, Nakamura T, Higaki J, Okumura K, Kamata S, Oguchi Y. Congenital dilatation of the bile duct in 100 instances and its relationship with anomalous junction. *Surg Gynecol Obstet* 1990;171: 291–298.
77. Flati G, Flati D, Porowska B, Ventura T, Catarci M, Carboni M. Surgical anatomy of the papilla of Vater and biliopancreatic ducts. *Am Surgeon* 1994;60:712–718.
78. Suarez CV. The Santorini valves. *Mt Sinai J Med* 1981;48:149–157.
79. Brown JO, Echenberg RJ. Mucosal reduplications associated with the ampullary portion of the major duodenal papilla in humans. *Anat Rec* 1964;150:293–302.
80. Dziwisch L, Lierse W. Three-dimensional arrangement of dense connective tissue around the human major duodenal papilla. Including the ampullary region and the distal choledodal duct. *Acta Anat* 1989;135: 231–235.
81. Boyden EA. The anatomy of the choledochoduodenal junction in man. *Surg Gynecol Obstet* 1957;104:641–652.
82. Suarez CV. Structure of the major duodenal papilla. *Mt Sinai J Med* 1982;49:31–37.
83. Goff JS. The human sphincter of Oddi. Physiology and pathophysiology. *Arch Intern Med* 1988;148:2673–2677.
84. Toouli J, Hogan WJ, Geenen JE, Dodds WJ, Arndorfer RC. Action of cholecystokinin-octapeptide on sphincter of Oddi basal pressure and phasic wave activity in humans. *Surgery* 1982;92:497–503.
85. Coelho JCU, Moody FG. Certain aspects of normal and abnormal motility of sphincter of Oddi. *Dig Dis Sci* 1987;32:86–94.
86. Hand BH. An anatomical study of the choledochoduodenal area. *Br J Surg* 1963;50:486–494.
87. Biazotto W. The fine venous architecture of the major duodenal papilla in human beings. *Anat Anz* 1990;171:105–108.
88. Cubilla AL, Fitzgerald PJ. Tumors of the exocrine pancreas. In: *Atlas*

*of tumor pathology. Fascicle 19, 2nd series.* Washington, DC: Armed Forces Institute of Pathology; 1984:31–42,71–89.

89. Kozuka S, Sassa R, Taki T, et al. Relation of pancreatic duct hyperplasia to carcinoma. *Cancer* 1979;43:1418–1428.
90. Edmondson HA. Tumors of the gallbladder and extrahepatic bile ducts. In: *Atlas of tumor pathology. Fascicle 26.* Washington, DC: Armed Forces Institute of Pathology; 1967:121–167.
91. Loquvam GS, Russell WO. Accessory pancreatic ducts of the major duodenal papilla. Normal structures to be differentiated from cancer. *Am J Clin Pathol* 1950;20:305–313.
92. Noda Y, Watanabe H, Iwafuchi M, et al. Carcinoids and endocrine cell micronests of the minor and major duodenal papillae. Their incidence and characteristics. *Cancer* 1992;70:1825–1833.
93. Alpert LC, Truong LD, Bossart MI, Spjut HJ. Microcystic adenoma (serous cystadenoma) of the pancreas. A study of 14 cases with immunohistochemical and electron-microscopic correlation. *Am J Surg Pathol* 1988;12:251–263.

*Histology for Pathologists, second edition,*
Edited by Stephen S. Sternberg.
Lippincott-Raven Publishers, Philadelphia
© 1997.

# CHAPTER 27

# Pancreas

David S. Klimstra



The pancreas is an unpaired secretory organ situated in the left superior retroperitoneum. It is composed of exocrine elements, including acini and ducts, endocrine elements largely in the form of islets of Langerhans, and scanty connective tissue elements, which comprise the interstitium. There are relatively few opportunities for pathologists to study the normal histology of the pancreas because of the relative inaccessibility of the organ, the clinical consequences associated with biopsy of the pancreas, and the rapid onset of autolysis in the postmortem period or after excision. For this reason, minor clinically insignificant alterations may be misinterpreted as neoplastic changes.

## ANATOMIC CONSIDERATIONS

### Location and Relationship to Other Structures

Located within the retroperitoneum posterior to the omental bursa at the level of the second and third lumbar vertebrae, the pancreas extends from the duodenal loop at the right of the midline across the posterior abdominal wall to the left toward the spleen (Fig. 1) (1). The head of the gland is intimately attached to the second and third portions of the duodenum. The neck of the gland lies inferior to the pylorus. The posterior wall of the stomach overlies the body, and the proximal jejunum immediately distal to the ligament of Treitz passes inferior to the body. The distal portion of the common bile duct passes through the posterosuperior head of the pancreas to enter the duodenum at the ampulla of Vater. The left lobe of the liver lies anterior to the head. The posterior aspect of the body approximates the left adrenal gland and kidney (2). The tail gradually tapers to a blunt end within several centimeters of the splenic hilus. The anterior aspect of the pancreas as well as the superior surfaces of the neck, body, and tail are covered by a free peritoneal surface, part of the posterior aspect of the lesser sac (3).

Because of the proximity of the pancreas to several organs and other anatomic structures, tumors of these sites may be difficult to distinguish radiographically. Pancreatic masses may be confused with tumors of the left adrenal gland, the superior poles of either kidney, the spleen, the left lobe of the liver, the duodenum, the greater curve of the stomach, the root of the mesentery, and the superior retroperitoneum.

A number of major blood vessels are closely opposed to the pancreas (3,4). The body and tail rest on the aorta. The celiac artery arises from the aorta superior to the neck of the pancreas and gives off the hepatic artery as well as the tortuous splenic artery, which runs along the superior pancreatic tail. The superior mesenteric artery arises posterior to the junction of the neck and body, and the adjacent superior mesenteric vein passes through a groove between the head and the neck, with a portion of the head (the uncinate process) extending around the superior mesenteric vessels to lie anterior to the aorta. The splenic vein accompanies the splenic artery along the superior aspect of the tail, joining the superior mesenteric vein to form the hepatic portal vein near the posterosuperior border of the head. The head of the gland also rests on the inferior vena cava, the right renal vessels,

D. S. Klimstra: Department of Pathology, Memorial Sloan-Kettering Cancer Center, New York, NY 10028.

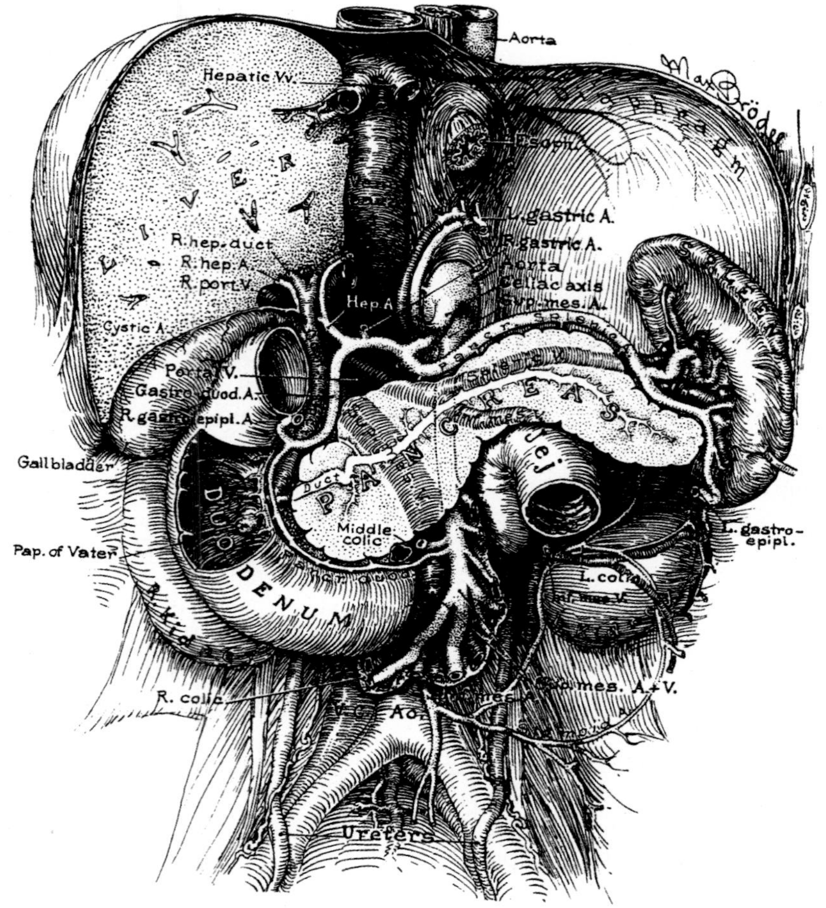


FIG. 1. Anatomic relationships of the pancreas. The anterior aspect of the upper abdominal viscerae is shown after removal of the stomach and omentum. Note the close relationship of the pancreas to the duodenum, jejunum, spleen, and major vessels. [Drawing by M. Brodell. Reprinted with permission (161).]

and the left renal vein. The celiac and superior mesenteric arteries ultimately provide the blood supply to the pancreas via the anterior and posterior pancreatoduodenal arteries, the dorsal pancreatic artery, and the inferior pancreatic artery, branches of the splenic artery supplying the tail (2,5). Anastomoses between the arteries supplying the pancreas are commonly present. Venous drainage occurs ultimately through the hepatic portal vein. Lymphatic vessels follow the course of the blood vessels. Lymph nodes may be closely opposed to the periphery of the gland or even embedded within its substance, especially along the inferior and superior borders and in the anterior and posterior pancreatoduodenal regions. Many lymph nodes are also found around the celiac axis, adjacent to the common bile duct, and at the splenic hilus (6).

Innervation of the pancreas is from the vagus nerve (parasympathetic) and the splanchnic nerves (sympathetic) via the celiac and superior mesenteric plexi (2,3). The course of the nerves accompanies the vasculature (5).

**Gross Anatomy**

In adults the pancreas usually measures 15 to 20 cm in length and weighs 85 to 120 g, being slightly larger in men (4,7). The weight of the gland gradually decreases after 40 years of age to a mean of 70 g in the ninth decade of life (7).

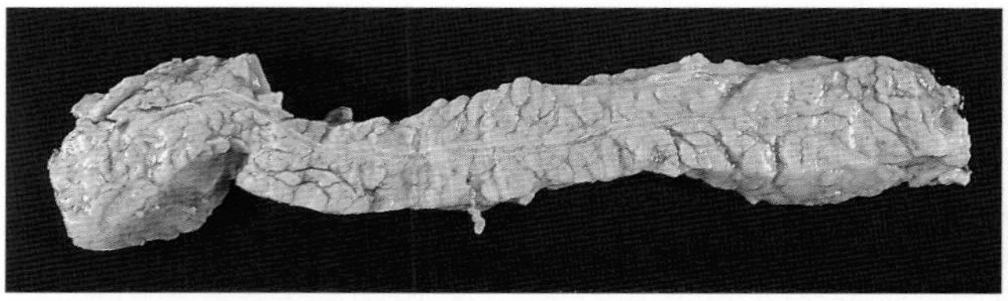

FIG. 2. Gross appearance of the normal pancreas. The bulbous head (left) is connected to the neck, body, and tail, which merge imperceptibly. The parenchyma consists of distinctly lobulated pink–tan fleshy tissue. The pancreatic duct (opened longitudinally) is thin and smooth throughout its course.

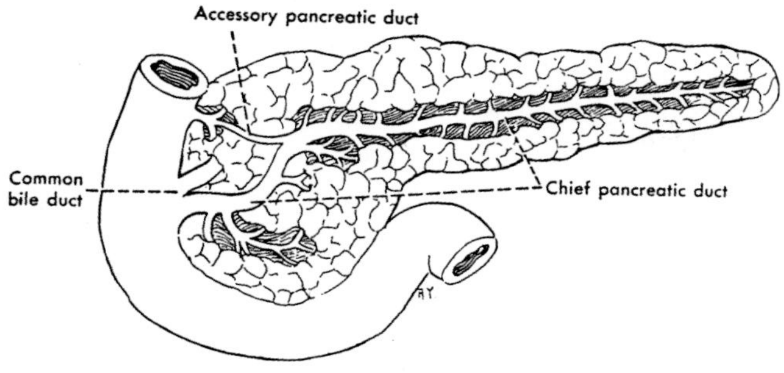


**FIG. 3.** Schematic diagram of the pancreas showing the pattern of the major ducts and their tributaries. In this example the accessory duct is patent at the duodenum through the minor papilla. [Reprinted with permission (10).]

In the newborn the pancreas weighs 2 to 3 g, reaching 7 g at 1 year of age (8).

The pancreas is composed of four anatomic regions that are not sharply separated from one another: the head, neck, body, and tail (Fig. 2). The bulk of the organ is composed of the head, including the uncinate process, which develops separately and may be anatomically separate in some individuals. The neck and body are somewhat triangular in cross section, whereas the tail is flat (2).

The normal pancreas is tan–pink to yellow and uniformly lobulated. The anterior surface is smooth and covered by a layer of peritoneum; the remaining surfaces are invested by a thin layer of loose fibroconnective tissue. No discrete capsule is present, and depending on the amount of parenchymal fat and the extent of any fibrotic changes, the interface with the surrounding retroperitoneal adipose tissue may be indistinct.

Cut sections of the pancreas show arborizing thin-walled white ducts extending into the well-demarcated lobules. The main pancreatic duct of Wirsung varies from 1.8 to 9.0 mm (average 3.0 mm) in diameter (9), gradually enlarging to 4.5 mm near the ampulla of Vater, through which it drains into the duodenum. Up to 50 secondary ducts drain into the main duct (10,11), entering alternately from either side in a herringbone pattern (Fig. 3) (4). The course of the major ducts is highly variable and depends on the pattern of fusion and atrophy of ducts which occurs during development. In general, the main pancreatic duct of Wirsung begins in the tail, collecting tributaries as it passes through the body and neck toward the head. The duct makes an acute turn inferiorly in the head of the gland, where it is joined by the accessory duct of Santorini from the superior head as well as the major duct from the uncinate lobe, ultimately exiting through the ampulla at the major papilla. The accessory duct generally does not communicate separately with the duodenum, although patency through the minor duodenal papilla is not uncommon.

The relationship of the main duct to the distal common bile duct is also highly variable. In some individuals the two ducts fuse to form a common channel within the wall of the duodenum, the prototypical ampulla. In many cases, however, length of the common channel is less than 3 mm. In others, the two ducts remain separate throughout their course, entering side by side at the major papilla or completely separately (Fig. 4) (5,7,12). In these individuals, a true ampulla (defined as a common channel) does not exist or is extremely short. In one study only 43% of individuals had a common channel greater than 3 mm in length (13). Villiform mucosal projections are present within the distal ducts; these valves of Santorini may prevent reflux of secretions (14,15). The intraduodenal portions of the pancreatic and bile ducts are surrounded by thin fascicles of smooth muscle known as the sphincter of Oddi.

## DEVELOPMENT

### Organogenesis

The pancreas forms from the distal embryonic foregut as dorsal and ventral buds during the fourth to fifth weeks of

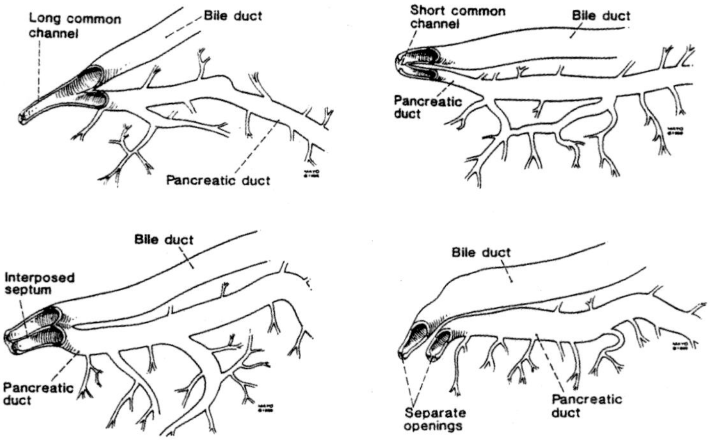


**FIG. 4.** Anatomic variations in the paths of the pancreatic and biliary ducts at the ampulla. A long common channel (the prototypical ampulla) is only present in some individuals. In others, the ducts fuse within only a few millimeters of the duodenum, resulting in a short common channel, or the two ducts enter separately. [Reprinted with permission (13).]

gestation (16,17). The dorsal bud forms opposite the hepatic diverticulum, whereas the ventral bud, which may be bilobed, forms adjacent to the hepatic diverticulum (11). Thus, the duct from the ventral pancreas is closely opposed to the common bile duct. During the sixth week the ventral pancreas is carried with the common bile duct circumferentially to the right around the posterior aspect of the duodenum to lie posterior and slightly inferior to the dorsal pancreas (Fig. 5). The two portions generally fuse during the seventh week. The dorsal portion makes up the superior head as well as the entire neck, body, and tail of the adult gland, and the ventral portion contributes the remainder of the head, including the uncinate process (17). The ductal systems of the two lobes also generally fuse, with connection of the dorsal duct to the duodenum being lost and the ventral duct providing the drainage for the exocrine secretions. Thus, the distal two thirds of the main pancreatic duct (of Wirsung) develop from the embryonic dorsal duct, whereas the proximal third forms from the ventral duct. The remaining proximal portion of the dorsal embryonic duct becomes the accessory duct of Santorini. The ampulla of Vater develops during the eighth week.

### Cytogenesis

The ducts develop as solid cords of cells that push by proliferation into the surrounding mesenchyme. The ducts branch progressively, and luminal spaces are formed. Both acinar and endocrine cells develop from these primitive ducts (18). The cells at the termini of the branches differentiate into acinar cells during the third month of gestation (18). The pancreatic lobules are formed by the accumulation of acinar units around ductular branches that are separated by layers of mesenchyme. The acinar cells contain zymogen granules by the fourth month (8). The earliest granules identified in acinar cells are elongated and angular, and the internal structure is somewhat fibrillar. These granules, along with small spherical granules, may be detected at 15 to 20 weeks (17,19,20). By 20 weeks, the granules resemble the zymogen granules of the adult pancreas. The nature of the elongate granules remains unclear, and enzymes have not yet been detected in them. However, it is interesting that although these granules are not present in the adult pancreas, similar granules have been repeatedly detected in pancreatic neoplasms with acinar differentiation (20–26).

Islet cells also develop from the ducts at 8 to 10 weeks, somewhat earlier than the acinar cells. Most of the islet cells appear to originate from the intralobular and interlobular ducts (10). In the third month, developing endocrine cell clusters bud off from the ducts and surround capillaries to form discrete islets (27,28). In even the earliest developing islets, differentiated alpha and beta cells can be recognized by special stains (28–30). At 16 weeks the alpha and beta cells are segregated at opposite ends of the islet; these bipolar islets are gradually replaced between 18 and 20 weeks by mantle islets having a central core of beta cells surrounded by a rim of alpha cells (18,28,30). Although the two cell types are more intermingled in the mature adult islets, the peripheral location of the alpha cells found in the mantle islets is roughly maintained.

During the third to fourth months the pancreatic tissue becomes increasingly organized around the branching ductal structures to form lobules (Fig. 6A and B). The characteristics of the ductal lining cells specific to their level within the ductal system become established during this period. The mesenchymal elements of the early pancreas are prominent.

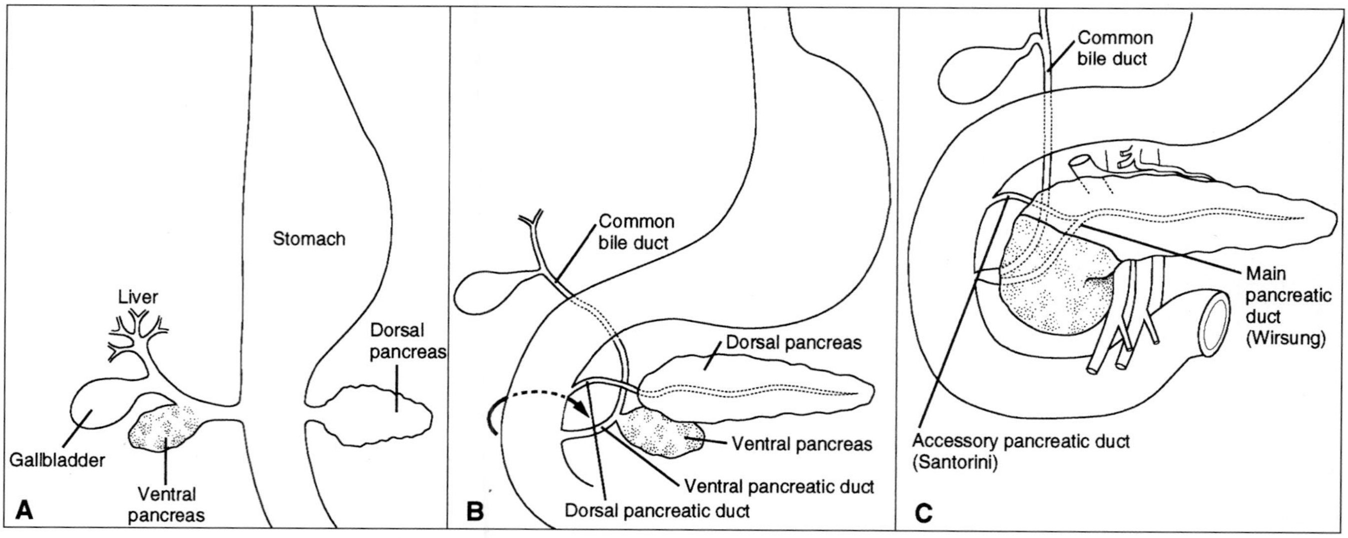


**FIG. 5.** Development of the pancreas. The dorsal and ventral buds form on opposite sides of the duodenum (**A**). During the sixth week, the ventral pancreas migrates posteriorly around the duodenum (**B**) to lie inferior to the dorsal pancreas, where it comprises much of the head of the gland (**C**). [Reprinted with permission (5).]

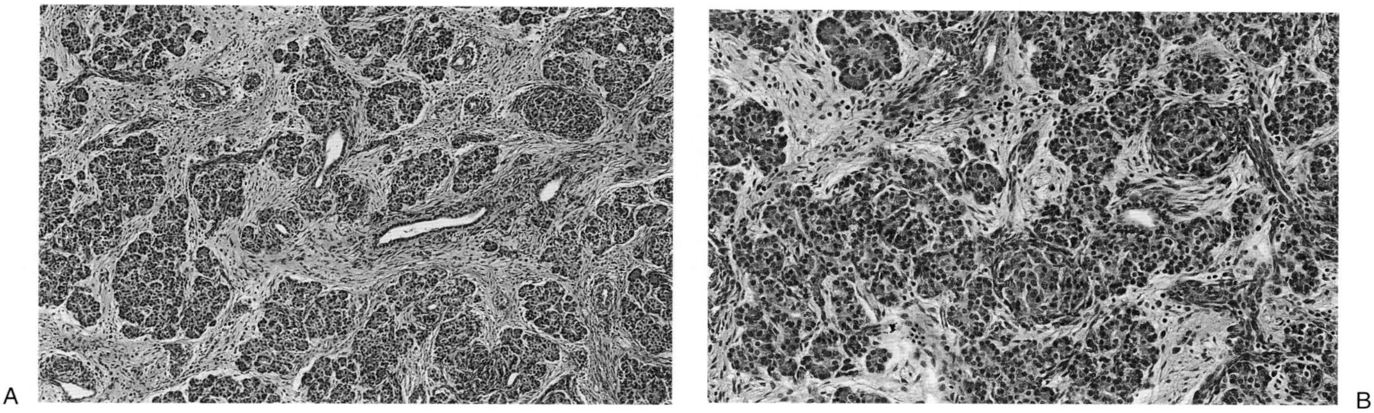

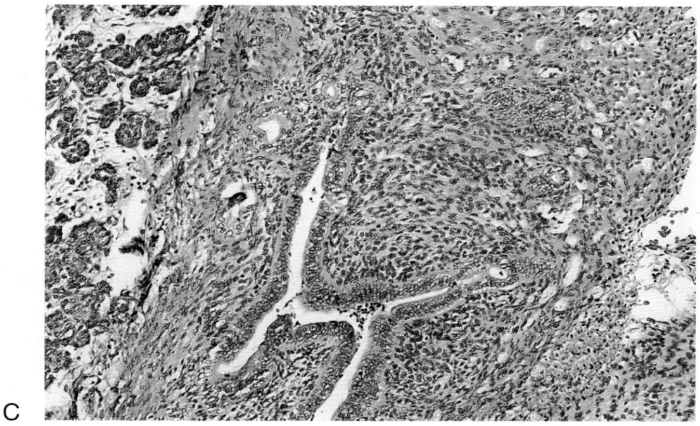

**FIG. 6.** The fetal pancreas at 18–20 weeks of gestation exhibits a well-developed lobular architecture (**A**). The loose connective tissue between the lobules is relatively abundant. Both acinar and endocrine elements are well developed (**B**) and are functioning at this stage. The mesenchyme surrounding the ducts is highly cellular (**C**), resembling the so-called ovarian-like stroma of mucinous cystic neoplasms.

The early periductal stroma is highly cellular (Fig. 6C), resembling the ovarian-like stroma that characterizes mucinous cystic neoplasms (31,32). As the pancreas develops, the mesenchyme becomes increasingly less abundant and less cellular, representing a relatively minimal component of the adult gland.

### Heterotopia and Developmental Anomalies

Pancreatic heterotopia is defined as pancreatic tissue located outside of the normal anatomic position of the gland (33). Heterotopic pancreatic tissue is found in portions of the upper gastrointestinal tract and its appendages in up to 15% of individuals at autopsy (34). The surgical incidence, however, is only 0.2% (35). Twenty-five percent to 50% of the cases detected during life are symptomatic (34,36). Although it is considered to be a congenital anomaly, most symptomatic cases present in adulthood (36). The duodenum and stomach are the most common locations of pancreatic heterotopia (5,37), most duodenal cases occurring in the second portion several centimeters proximal to the ampulla of Vater. In many of these cases the tissue is present subjacent to the minor duodenal papilla and represents remnants of the embryonic dorsal ductal system. Pancreatic heterotopia also may occur elsewhere in the duodenum and may involve the ampulla of Vater (38,39). Other sites of pancreatic heterotopia include the jejunum, Meckel's diverticulum, the large bowel, and the liver, where it is generally located around the bile ducts (40). A case of pancreatic heterotopia in a lymph node has been reported (41), as have many other unusual sites (5,33). In the tubular gastrointestinal tract, heterotopic pancreas appears as lobulated submucosal nodules of yellow to white firm tissue ranging from several millimeters to several centimeters in size. The overlying mucosa may be umbilicated in larger examples (Fig. 7A). Rarely heterotopic pancreatic tissue is present on the serosal surface. Microscopically there are submucosal aggregates of small ducts and lobules of ductules. Although most cases do show some acinar and endocrine elements, they may be a minor component (Fig. 7B). Interlacing smooth muscle fascicles also may be present, resulting in the appearance of so-called adenomyoma in cases lacking acinar and endocrine cells. Some duodenal foci of heterotopic pancreas exhibit acini with the features of Brunner's glands, emphasizing the embryologic relationship these glands have with the pancreas (10). The ductules surrounded by smooth muscle may resemble an infiltrating adenocarcinoma, but there is generally no cytologic atypia. One of the important reasons to recognize heterotopic pancreas is to avoid misinterpretation of these ductules as carcinoma; however, cases of adenocarcinoma arising in heterotopic pancreas have been described (42–44).

Acinar cells also may occur as a metaplastic change in the

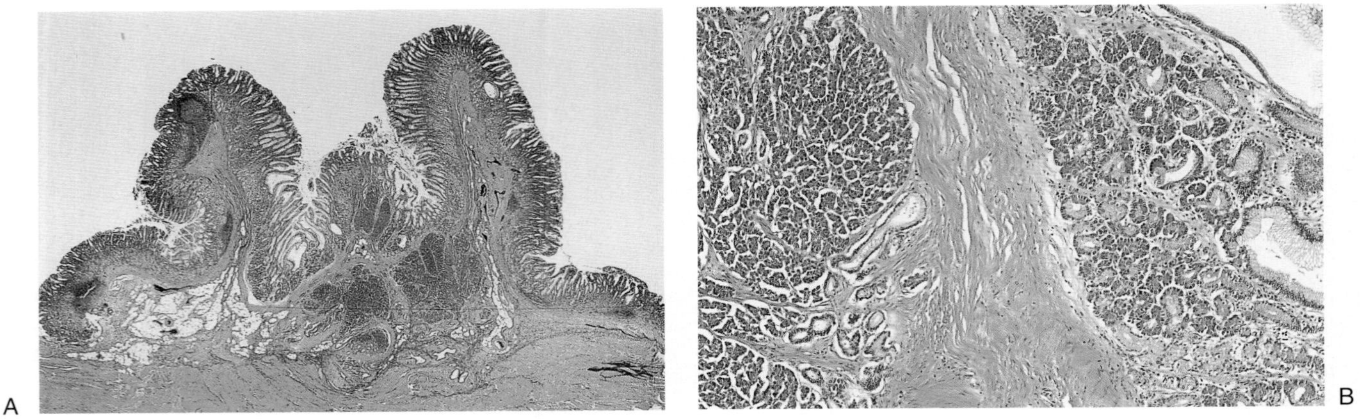

FIG. 7. Heterotopic pancreatic tissue in the stomach. At low power, a submucosal nodule of pancreatic tissue results in an umbilicated appearance (**A**). In this example, lobules of normal-appearing acinar and ductular structures are separated by bands of fibromuscular tissue (**B**). Islet cells are not evident by routine microscopy.

gastric mucosa or in Barrett's mucosa of the esophagus (45,46); this should not be confused with heterotopic tissue, which is generally submucosal.

Heterotopic tissues also may be found within the pancreas. Accessory splenic tissue may be found in the tail of the pancreas or more rarely in the head (47). In most cases the splenic tissue is small (less than 2 cm), dark red, and spherical.

There are many variations in the paths of the pancreatic ducts and their relationship to the bile duct (11,33). Failure of the communication between the dorsal pancreatic duct and the duodenum to obliterate occurs in up to 40% of adults (11,48) and results in a separate opening of the accessory duct (of Santorini) at the minor papilla, proximal to the opening of the main duct and bile duct at the major papilla. In such instances the dorsal duct may provide the main route of drainage for the gland and may be much larger in circumference than the ventral duct. This condition appears to be more prevalent in children, suggesting that obliteration of the accessory duct opening may continue to occur in adulthood (49). The two ducts also may fail to fuse entirely, resulting in two separate ductal systems, a condition known as pancreas divisum. Although this anomaly occurs in 5% to 10% of individuals (11,50), the pancreatic parenchyma of the two lobes is usually fused (17), and the abnormality may not be detected unless a careful study of the ductal system is performed. In this condition, the majority of pancreatic secretions drain from the dorsal duct at the minor papilla; the bile duct accompanies the smaller ventral duct through the major papilla. Patients with pancreas divisum seem to have a higher incidence of pancreatitis, especially when the opening of the dorsal duct at the minor papilla is small (33,50,51).

Anomalous junction of the main pancreatic duct with the distal common bile duct may occur within the head of the pancreas more than 2 cm proximal to the duodenum (11,33). This abnormality may be associated with choledochal cysts and carcinomas of the extrahepatic bile ducts or gallbladder (11,52,53). In a rare abnormality of the pancreatic duct, bifid pancreas, the main pancreatic duct bifurcates within the body of the pancreas (54).

Annular pancreas occurs when the ventral pancreas fails to properly migrate, resulting in a ring of pancreatic tissue encircling the duodenum (5,33,55,56). Pancreas divisum usually accompanies annular pancreas (57), and the condition affects only 0.015% of the population (58). Annular pancreas commonly causes duodenal obstruction which varies in severity and age of symptomatology, depending on the extent of luminal constriction. Some cases are also associated with duodenal atresia (33). The band of pancreatic tissue partially or completely encircling the duodenum is flattened and may be embedded within the muscularis propria. Histologically it contains all of the normal elements. Because the portion of pancreas encircling the duodenum is derived from the ventral pancreas, it is rich in pancreatic polypeptide-containing islets (59).

## MICROSCOPIC FEATURES

Microscopically the pancreas is arranged in 1- to 10-mm lobules (Fig. 8). The parenchyma within the lobules is highly cellular, consisting largely of the three epithelial components of the gland: the acini, the ducts, and the islets of Langerhans.

### Acini

Acinar cells make up roughly 85% of the mass of the pancreas and constitute the main exocrine secretory component of the gland. The prototypical arrangement of the acinar cells in routine histologic sections is a single layer of polygonal cells surrounding a minute central lumen, suggesting a spherical configuration (Fig. 9); however, the three-dimensional architecture of the pancreatic acini is much more com-

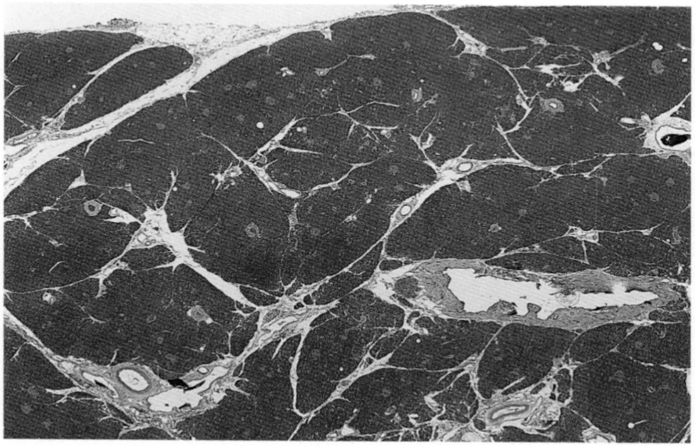

**FIG. 8.** At low power, the normal pancreas has a well-developed lobular arrangement of highly cellular glandular tissue.

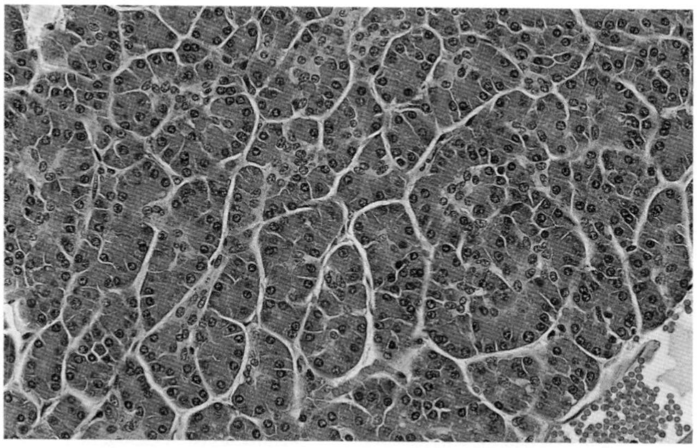

**FIG. 10.** Other acini have tubular configurations and exhibit interanastomosing loops when studied by serial sectioning.

plex (60). Indeed, tubular acini are commonly detected in histologic sections (Fig. 10). Also, not all acini are located at the terminal end of ductules. Acini may bud from the side of a ductule or may be situated between two ductules. Anastomosing loops of acini also may be found (60). Thus, the secretions of a given acinus may pass through a number of different pathways to reach the ductal system.

The individual acinar cells are polarized, with basally situated round nuclei and apical granular eosinophilic cytoplasm. The eosinophilia of the apical cytoplasm is due to the accumulation of numerous zymogen granules (Figs. 11 and 12), which contrast with the basophilic granules of salivary serous acini. The zymogen granule content is highly dynamic, depending on the secretory state of the pancreas, which is largely regulated by digestive hormones (1). The basal acinar cytoplasm is basophilic, reflecting the high concentration of ribonucleoproteins in the abundant rough endoplasmic reticulum (RER). There may be a clear cytoplasmic zone above the nucleus that contains the Golgi apparatus. The nuclei are uniform and frequently contain distinct central nucleoli; clumps of chromatin are generally present beneath the nuclear membrane.

Although the acinar cells from different regions of the pancreas are all morphologically and functionally similar, there are subtle differences in the size and zymogen granule content in the acinar cells immediately adjacent to islets compared with those distant from islets, perhaps as a reflection of regional variations in islet hormone levels (61,62).

Zymogen granules are positive with periodic acid-Schiff (PAS) stain, and the staining is resistant to diastase digestion (Fig. 13). Acinar cells also can be demonstrated using stains for butyrate esterase; because butyrate is a short chain fatty acid, the reaction is positive in the presence of lipase (22). Immunohistochemical stains for pancreatic enzymes such as trypsin, chymotrypsin, lipase, amylase, and elastase are positive in acinar cells (Fig. 14) and with the exception of amylase are also sensitive markers for acinar differentiation in pancreatic neoplasms (22–24,63). Each individual zymogen granule contains all of the various digestive enzymes, usually in a proenzyme form (64,65). Keratins detected by the Cam5.2 antibody are present in acinar cells; however, there is no staining with the AE1 and AE3 antibodies or antibodies against cytokeratins 7 and 20 (Fig. 15). Mucins are not produced, and immunohistochemical stains for glycoproteins such as DUPAN-2 and Ca19.9 are negative.

Ultrastructural examination shows a well-developed ex-

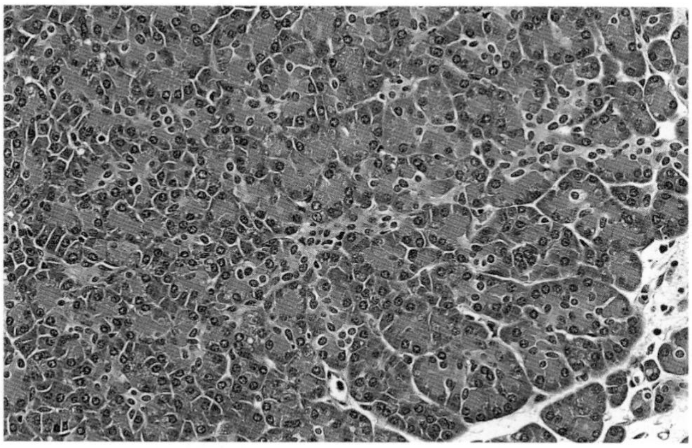

**FIG. 9.** Acini are tightly packed, most consisting of spherically arranged individual acinar cells.

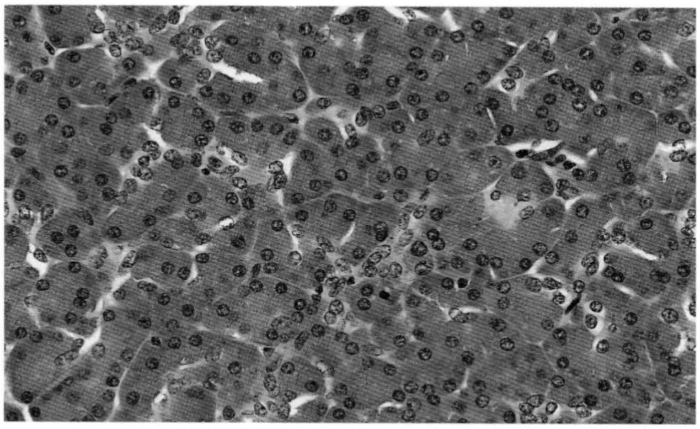

**FIG. 11.** Acinar cells contain abundant granular eosinophilic cytoplasm in the apical aspect, with basophilic basal cytoplasm. The nuclei are also basally located.

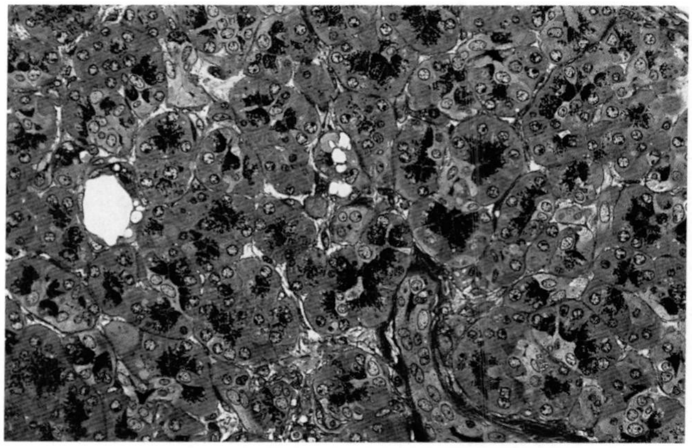

**FIG. 12.** Plastic-embedded semi-thin sections show the densely staining apical zymogen granules within the acinar cell cytoplasm.

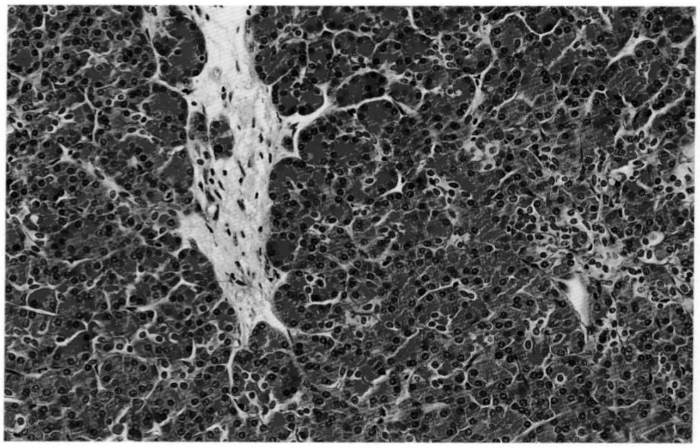

**FIG. 13.** Zymogen granules stain positively with periodic acid-Schiff's stain with diastase pretreatment.

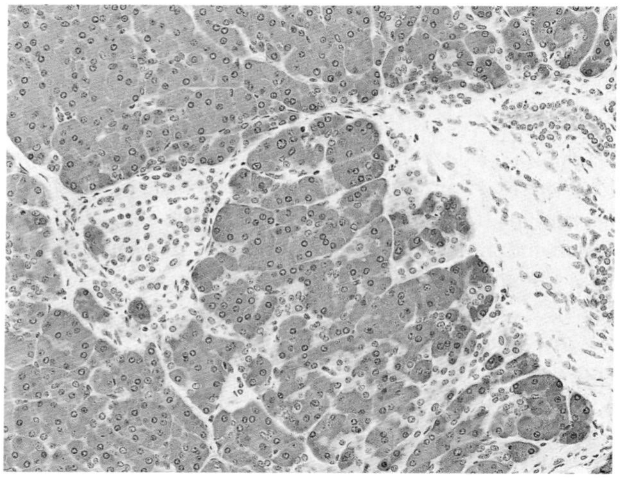

**FIG. 14.** Immunohistochemical staining for trypsin results in intense positivity of acinar cells with negative staining of ductal and islet cells. Faint luminal staining of ductal cells may be seen due to deposition of luminal enzymatic secretions on the apical cell surfaces (*upper right*).

A

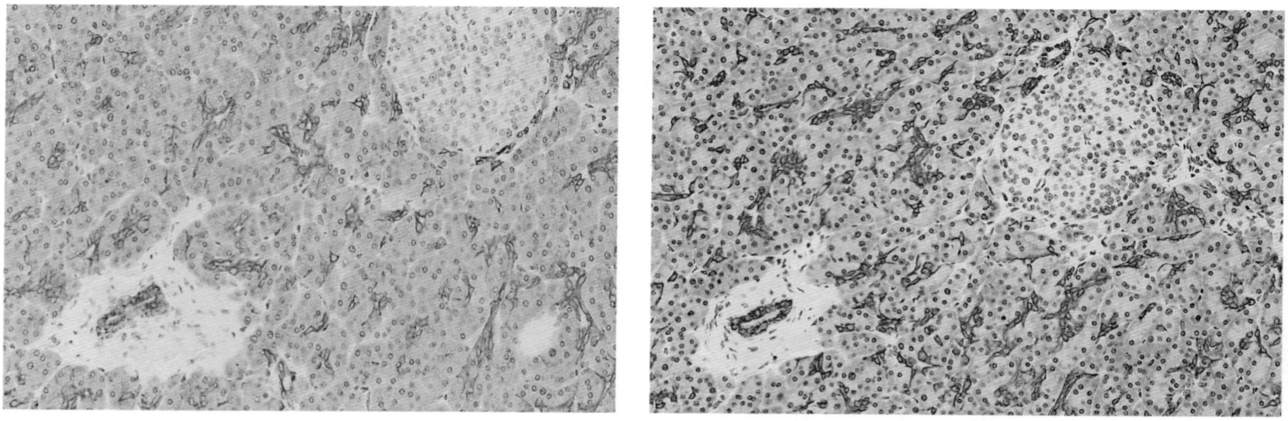

B

**FIG. 15.** Immunohistochemical staining for keratins. Staining with the Cam5.2 antibody shows diffuse staining of acinar cells and ductal cells, the latter being more intensely positive (**A**). The AE1/AE3 antibodies stain only ductal cells (**B**). Islet cells show only focal faint staining with any of these antibodies.

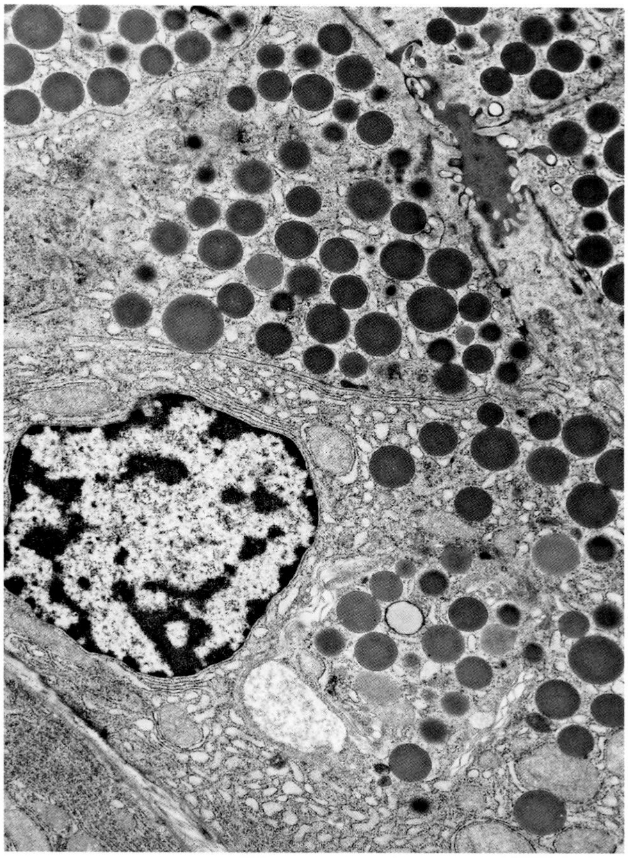

**FIG. 16.** The ultrastructural appearance of acinar cells. These polarized cells have abundant parallel stacks of rough endoplasmic reticulum with interspersed mitochondria in the basal cytoplasm. Homogeneous electron-dense zymogen granules are concentrated in the apical cytoplasm underlying the lumina.

ocrine secretory apparatus. The RER is arranged in parallel stacks and fills the basal cytoplasm (Fig. 16). Scattered mitochondria and free polyribosomes are present between RER cisternae (66). The Golgi apparatus is situated in the central region of the cytoplasm near the nucleus. Immature electron-dense zymogen granules emanate from the *trans* side of the Golgi apparatus. Larger round, homogeneous mature zymogen granules are present within the apical cytoplasm. They range in size from 250–1,000 nm and have limiting membranes closely opposed to the dense secretory content (Fig. 17). Upon stimulation, the membranes of the secretory granules fuse with the apical plasma membrane, expelling the contents into the lumen; the excess cell membranes are then recycled to the Golgi apparatus (67,68). Accumulated secretions are often present within the lumina, sometimes with crystal formation. The luminal membranes contain sparse, short microvilli containing inner microfilaments that are continuous with the terminal web of filaments beneath the apical membrane (66). Adjacent acinar cells are joined by apical junctional complexes composed of zonula occludens- and zonula adherens-type junctions, whereas desmosomes (macula adherens junctions) join cells along the basal aspects of their lateral membranes (8,66). Each acinus is surrounded by a continuous basement membrane. No basal cells or myoepithelial cells are present around the acini, in contrast to those of salivary glands.

### Ducts

The ductal system is subdivided into five portions: centroacinar cells, intercalated ducts, intralobular ducts, interlobular ducts (large and small), and main ducts (69). The ductal system begins with the centroacinar cells, which are small, relatively inconspicuous, flat to cuboidal cells with pale or lightly eosinophilic cytoplasm and oval central nuclei (Fig. 18). Centroacinar cells are located in the middle of the acini, where they border the acinar lumina along with the acinar cells, to which they are joined by tight junctions (Fig. 17). The lining of the acinus is incompletely bordered by centroacinar cells. Ultrastructurally the centroacinar cells have cytoplasm largely devoid of organelles, with only scattered mitochondria; no zymogen, neurosecretory, or mucigen granules are present. Relative to the acinar cells, the cytoplasm is less dense and rough endoplasmic reticulum is minimal (Fig. 17). The cell surfaces contain scattered short microvilli similar to those on the adjacent acinar cells. Adjacent cells are joined by abundant junctional complexes, and there are often complex interdigitations between them. Some centroacinar cells have more abundant granular oncocytic cytoplasm (Fig. 19) that reflects numerous mitochondria (69,70); the significance of this variation is unknown.

The lumen surrounded by acinar and centroacinar cells drains into the intercalated ducts, which are the smallest ducts outside the acini (Fig. 20). The cells lining the intercalated ducts resemble the centroacinar cells. They are low cuboidal and have central oval nuclei with indistinct nucleoli. Mucins are not detected with alcian blue or mucicarmine stains in centroacinar or intercalated duct cells. The intercalated ducts fuse to form the intralobular ducts, and the transition is imperceptible. The cells lining the intralobular ducts are essentially identical to those of the intercalated ducts, although the nuclei are round rather than oval (Fig. 20). Neither intercalated nor intralobular ducts have a significant collagenous matrix surrounding them.

Once the ducts leave the lobules, they become enveloped by a variably thick rim of collagen and are termed interlobular ducts (Fig. 21). The interlobular ductal cells have slightly more cytoplasm than those of the intralobular ducts and assume a low columnar shape in the larger ducts. As the interlobular ducts approach the main pancreatic ducts (of Wirsung or Santorini), they develop an increasingly thick collagenous wall within which lobular aggregates of small ductules may be seen, resembling the ductules of Beale that surround the major bile ducts (Fig. 22).

The main pancreatic ducts receive numerous tributaries of interlobular ducts (Fig. 23). The lining epithelium remains flat, without papillary projections, except in the very distal

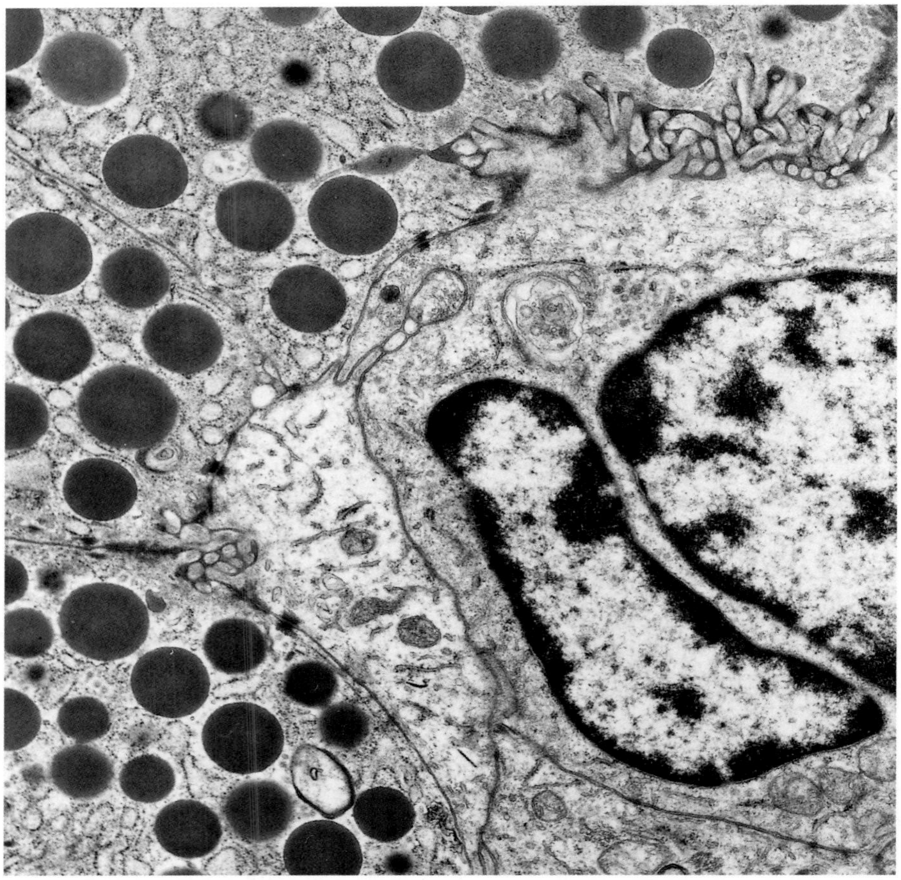

**FIG. 17.** At higher magnification, the zymogen granules lack a halo between the secretory content and the limiting membrane. The luminal spaces are lined by short microvilli. Adjacent acinar cells are joined to one another and to the centroacinar cells (*lower right*) by apical junctional complexes. The centroacinar cells have lucent cytoplasm devoid of secretory granules, with scattered mitochondria and individual lamellae of rough endoplasmic reticulum.

A 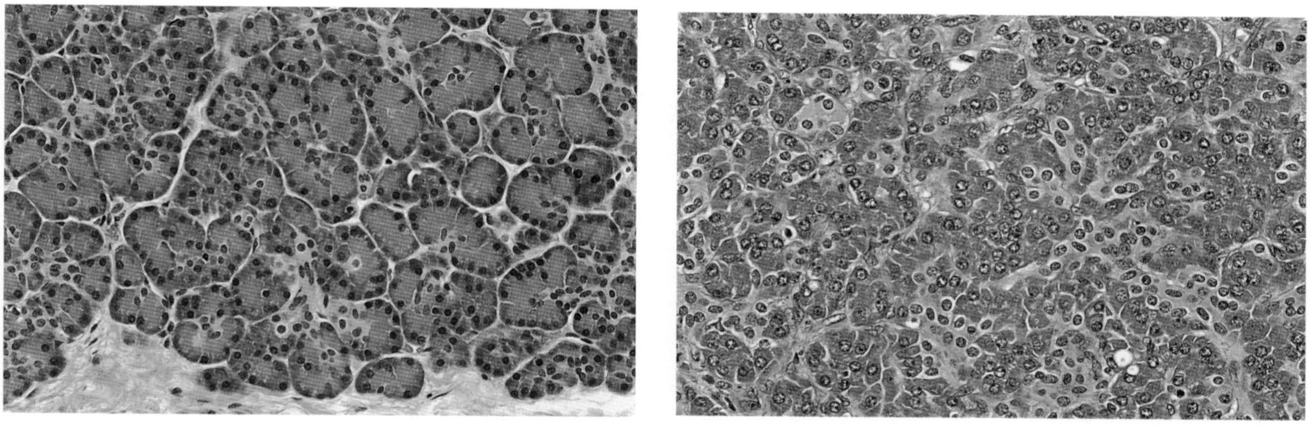 B

**FIG. 18.** Most centroacinar cells are inconspicuous small cells with minimal cytoplasm and oval nuclei situated in the center of the acini (**A**). In other regions the centroacinar cells may be more prominent, with more abundant lightly eosinophilic cytoplasm (**B**). Centroacinar cells constitute the beginning of the ductal system and convey the secretions of acinar cells to the intercalated ducts.

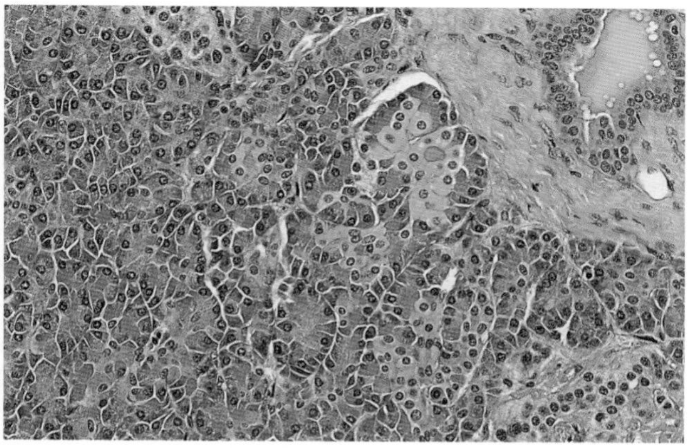

**FIG. 19.** Some centroacinar cells are enlarged and have oncocytic cytoplasm, a variation of uncertain significance.

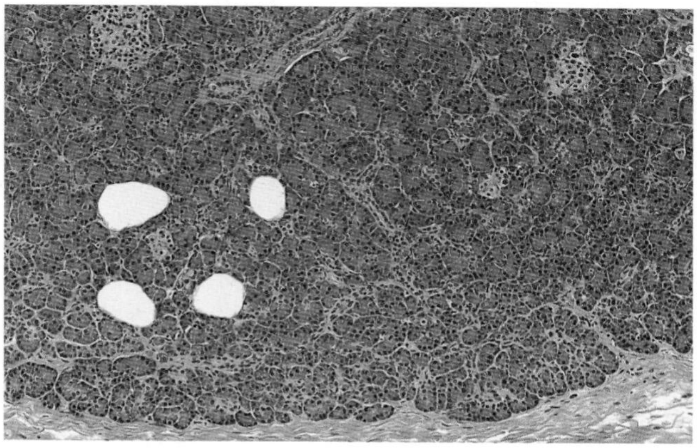

**FIG. 20.** The ductal system within the lobules consists of innumerable intercalated ducts that fuse to form intralobular ducts. The cytologic appearance of the intercalated and intralobular ductal cells resembles that of the centroacinar cells, and the transition from one to the next is imperceptible. Only minimal collagenized stroma surrounds the intralobular ducts (top).

A 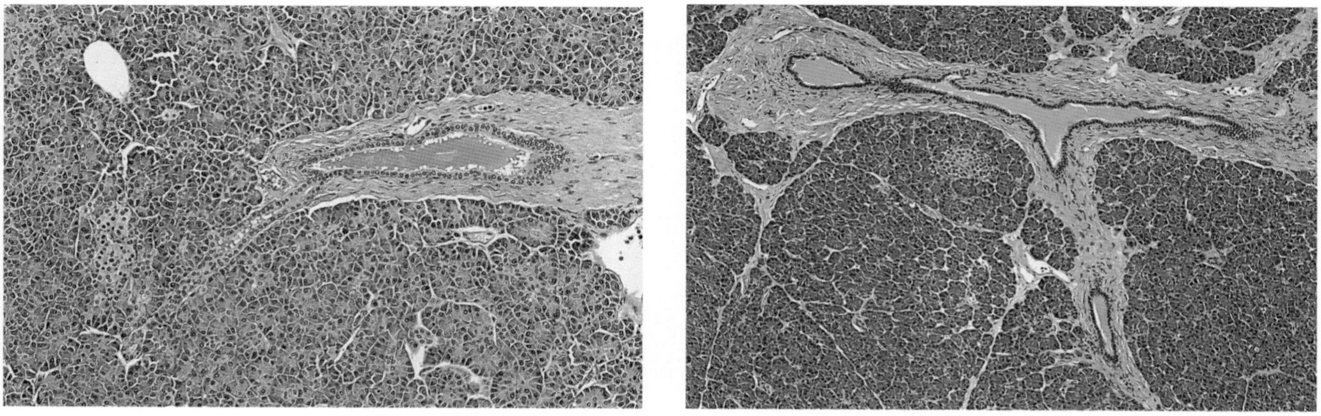 B

**FIG. 21.** Intralobular ducts come together to form interlobular ducts (**A**). The interlobular ducts are surrounded by a variably thick rim of dense fibrous tissue and carry the pancreatic secretions to the major ducts, receiving tributaries of small interlobular ducts as they pass through the connective tissue septa of the gland (**B**).

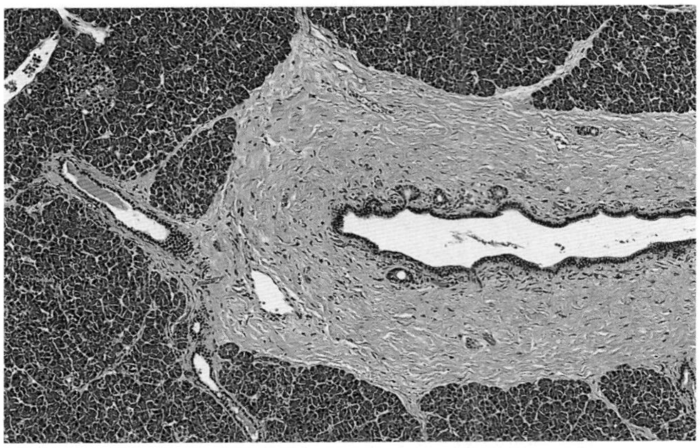
A

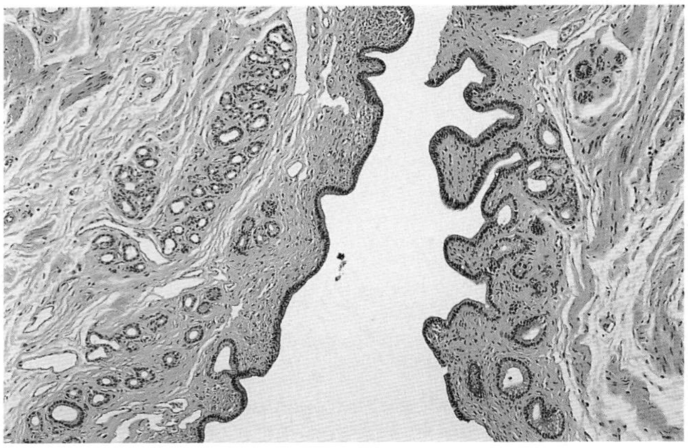
B

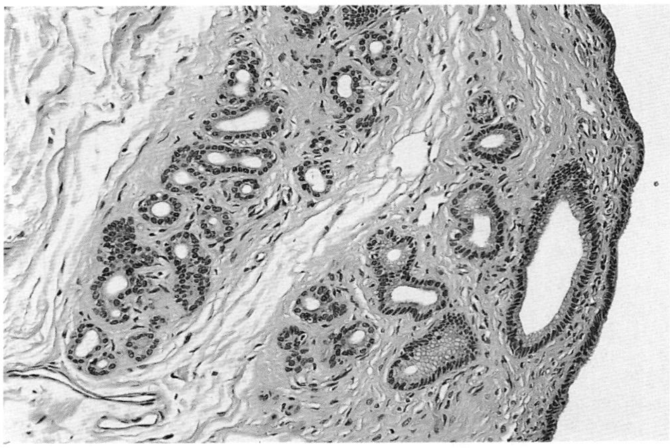
C

**FIG. 22.** The largest interlobular ducts are surrounded by a thick rim of collagen (**A**). Small lobular aggregates of ductules are present within the wall of the larger ducts (**B**). These resemble the ductules of Beale that surround the bile ducts; they are lined by simple cuboidal to low columnar epithelium similar to that lining the duct itself (**C**).

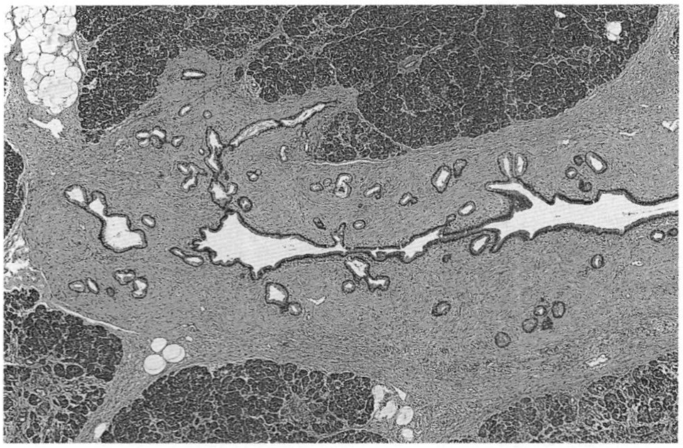

**FIG. 23.** Numerous interlobular ducts join the main pancreatic duct along its course.

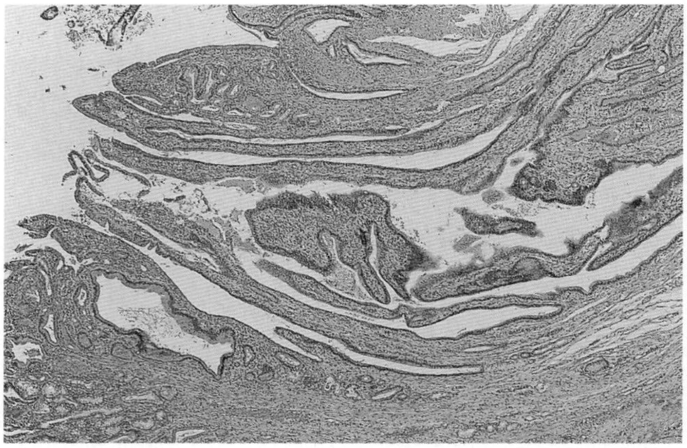

**FIG. 24.** As the main pancreatic duct enters the ampulla of Vater, the ductal epithelium forms broad, simple papillae known as the valves of Santorini.

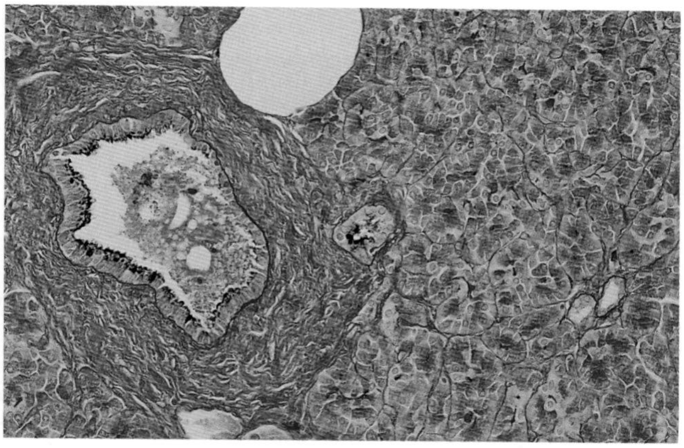
A

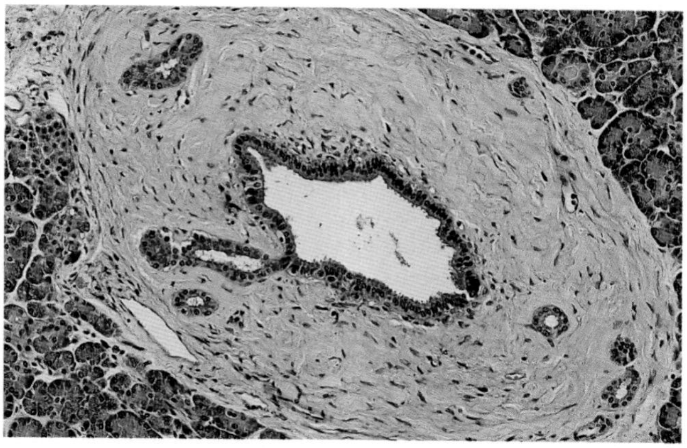
B

**FIG. 25.** The cells of the intralobular and smaller interlobular ducts contain mucin in the apical cytoplasm that stains positively with alcian blue/PAS (**A**). Staining with mucicarmine shows a similar distribution of mucin (**B**).

duct within the ampulla, where simple papillae are found (Fig. 24). The cells are low columnar with basal round nuclei. There may be apical cytoplasmic clearing, reflecting mucin that can be detected with mucicarmine and other histochemical stains or as mucigen granules by electron microscopy (69). The larger interlobular ducts accumulate more mucin within the apical cytoplasm, and pronounced mucin retention is a common minor alteration. The mucins of the intralobular and smaller interlobular ductal cells are predominantly sulphomucins and stain positively with alcian

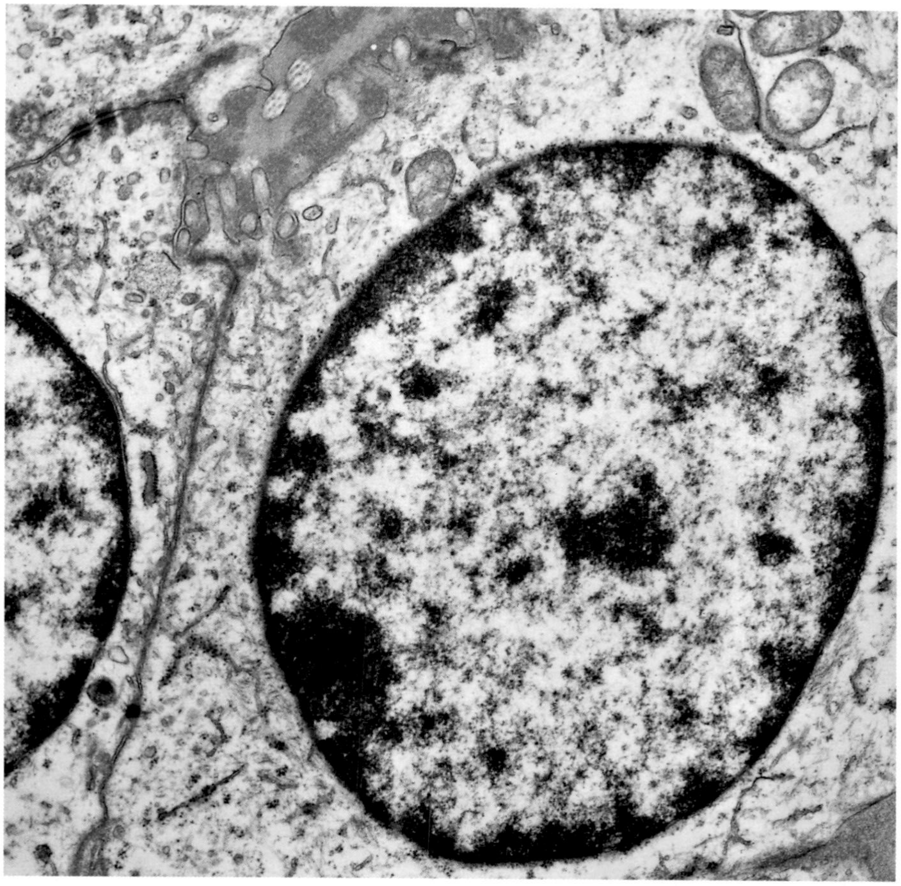

**FIG. 26.** Ultrastructural appearance of intralobular ductal cells. The cytoplasm resembles that of centroacinar cells, with an electron-lucent appearance and scattered mitochondria and rough endoplasmic reticulum. In the smaller ducts, mucigen granules are largely absent. The luminal surface exhibits short microvilli. In addition, scattered cilia are present, the cross section of which may be seen within the lumen (*top*).

blue at pH 1.0 (Fig. 25) (48,71). In the cells of the larger ducts there are fewer sulphomucins and more neutral mucins and sialomucins (71). Scattered goblet cells also may be seen in the main ducts. There is relatively frequent cell exfoliation in the main duct, perhaps reflecting a high turnover rate due to injury; degenerating cells may be observed within the epithelium by electron microscopy (66). The thick connective tissue wall contains numerous periductal ductules as well as fascicle of smooth muscle (1).

Other than the appearance of increasing numbers of mucigen granules and increased exocrine secretory apparatus (RER, mitochondria, and Golgi) in the larger ducts, the ultrastructural appearance of the ductal cells resembles that of the centroacinar cells (Figs. 26 and 27). In ductal cells from the level of the small interlobular ducts, single long kinocilia project from the cell surfaces (66,69); cross sections of these cilia may be observed within the lumina of the ducts (Fig. 26). The cilia are connected to basal bodies in the paranuclear cytoplasm and may function in mixing and propulsion of the pancreatic secretions (66).

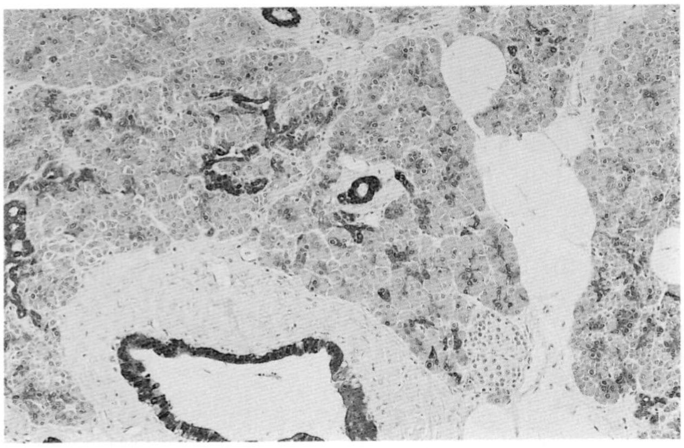

**FIG. 28.** Immunohistochemical staining for carbonic anhydrase. In this preparation, there is staining of ductal cells of all sizes, including centroacinar, intercalated duct, as well as intralobular and interlobular ductal cells.

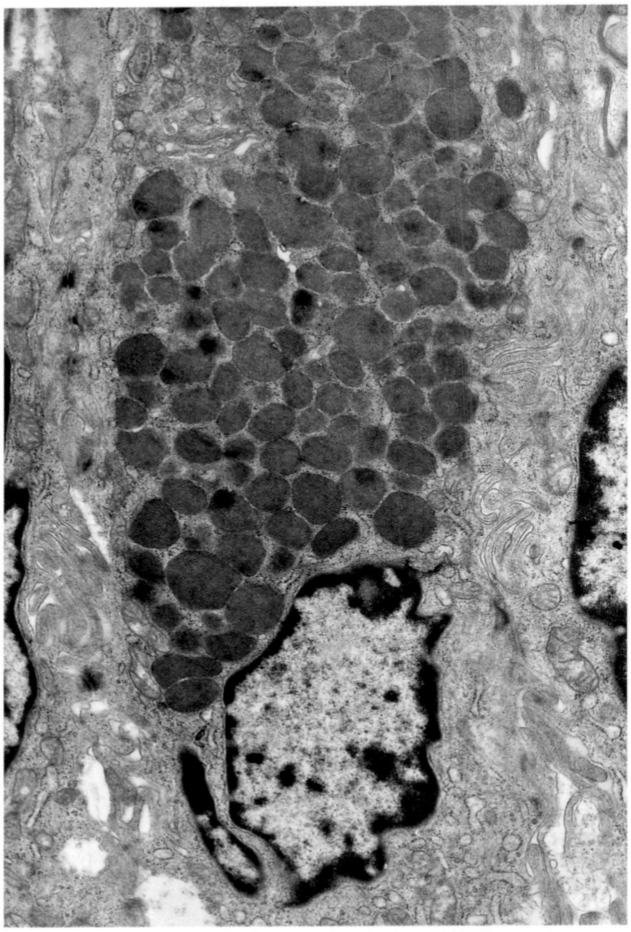

**FIG. 27.** In the larger ducts, more abundant mucigen granules accumulate within the apical cytoplasm. These granules vary in size and have irregular contours and heterogeneous, variably electron-dense secretory contents. There are complex interdigitations of the lateral membranes between adjacent cells.

Immunohistochemical staining shows strong expression of keratins AE1, AE3, Cam5.2, and CK7 in all ductal cells (Fig. 15), with negative staining for CK20. Enzyme and endocrine markers are also negative. Carbonic anhydrase is detectable in ductal cells, reflecting their role in fluid and ion transport (72); most is detected in intercalated and intralobular ducts (73), although ducts of larger caliber also may stain by immunohistochemistry (Fig. 28). Other markers of ductal cells include antibodies against CA19-9, DUPAN-2, cystic fibrosis transmembrane conductance regulator (CFTR), and N-terminal gastrin-releasing peptide (N-GRP) (74–78). Normal ducts are not stained for carcinoembryonic antigen when monoclonal antisera are used (79).

### Islets

The endocrine component of the pancreas constitutes only 1% to 2% of the volume of the adult gland (1,62); about 10% of the pancreas is endocrine in the newborn (48,80). The vast majority of endocrine cells are found in the over one million islets of Langerhans, first described by Paul Langerhans in 1869. Although islets are distributed throughout the pancreas, they are somewhat more numerous in the tail (81). Apparently random variations in islet concentration may occur from one lobule to the next, resulting in the appearance of plentiful islets in one area and sparse islets in an adjacent region (Fig. 29).

The apparent volume of islets observed in histologic sections also varies with the age of the individual and the presence and extent of exocrine atrophic changes. In the fetus and neonate the relative volume of endocrine cells far outmeasures that of the adult, especially in the portions derived from the dorsal lobe (Fig. 30) (82). In rats there is an increase in beta cell mass during pregnancy to accomodate the increased insulin needs. After parturition, the beta cells par-

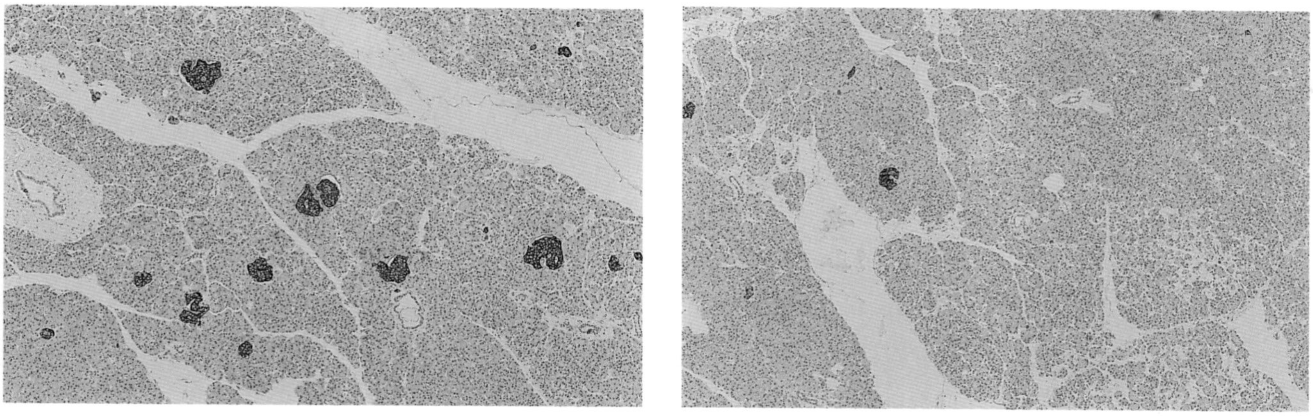
A B

**FIG. 29.** As highlighted by immunohistochemical staining for chromogranin, the concentration of islets varies considerably from one lobule (**A**) to the next (**B**).

tially involute through reduced cell proliferation, apoptosis, and decreased individual cell volume until the normal beta cell mass is reached (83). However, this observation has not yet been extended to humans.

Two types of islets occur. Most (90%) are sharply circumscribed nests measuring 75 to 225 $\mu$m; islets as small as 50 $\mu$m or as large as 280 $\mu$m also may be found (84). These so-called compact islets are found predominantly in the body and tail of the gland, with lesser concentrations in the head. The second islet type, the diffuse islets, are essentially restricted to the posteroinferior head of the gland, which constitutes the derivation of the embryonic ventral lobe (85,86). These islets are much less numerous than the compact islets and may reach up to 450 $\mu$m in size. Despite the circumscribed appearance of the compact islets, they are actually composed of intertwining trabeculae that interdigitate to appear as small lobules of cells in cross section (84). Cytologically, the cells of the compact islets have uniform round nuclei with a coarsely clumped chromatin pattern and inconspicuous nucleoli (Fig. 31). The cytoplasm is pale and amphophilic. Occasional islet cells have nuclei two to four times the size of their neighbors, although no irregularities of shape or chromatin pattern are present (Fig. 32). These nuclei have a 4n or 8n DNA content and have been shown to occur exclusively in beta cells (87); there is no known pathologic significance. Mitotic figures are only rarely encountered in normal islets (88). The stroma of the islets is vascular, although the capillary-sized vessels are almost inapparent by light microscopy. Essentially all of the cells of the islets contact the vasculature. In contrast to those supplying the acinar tissue, the capillaries of the islets have a fenestrated endothelium (1). A thin layer of connective tissue separates the compact islets from the surrounding acinar tissue, but they are not truly encapsulated.

Diffuse islets have a trabecular appearance, with winding cords of cells intermingled among acini (Fig. 33A). Because they are less commonly encountered and have a pseudoinfiltrative appearance, they may be mistakenly regarded as a neoplastic proliferation, an occurrence even more likely in the setting of chronic pancreatitis. In addition to the archi-

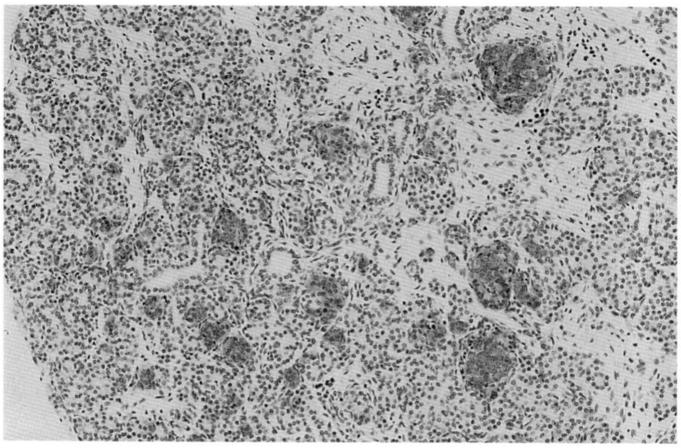

**FIG. 30.** A fetal pancreas stained immunohistochemically for chromogranin. Note the abundance of endocrine cells relative to acinar cells at this stage of development.

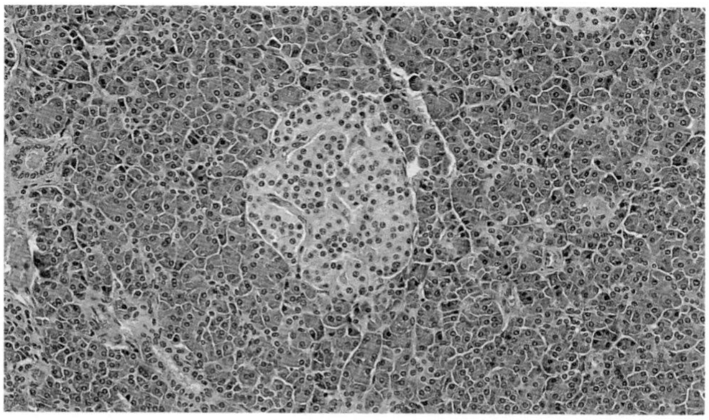

**FIG. 31.** Compact islets consist of round to oval, generally circumscribed collections of endocrine cells. Small capillaries separate the islet into lobules. The nuclei have a stippled chromatin pattern and there is moderate amphophilic cytoplasm.

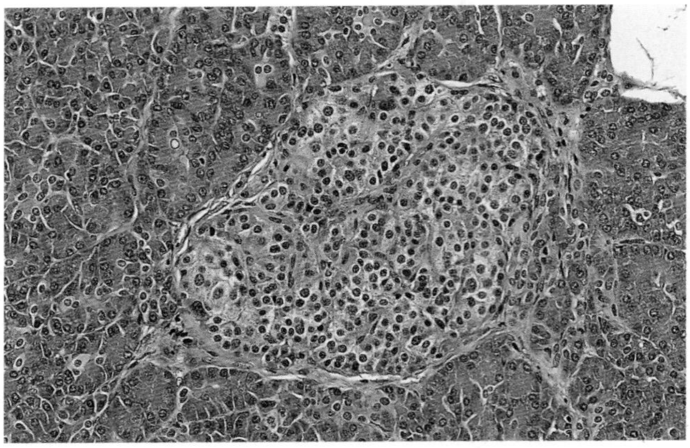

**FIG. 32.** Some islet cells contain enlarged nuclei several times the size of those in the neighboring cells. These nuclei have a tetraploid or octaploid DNA content.

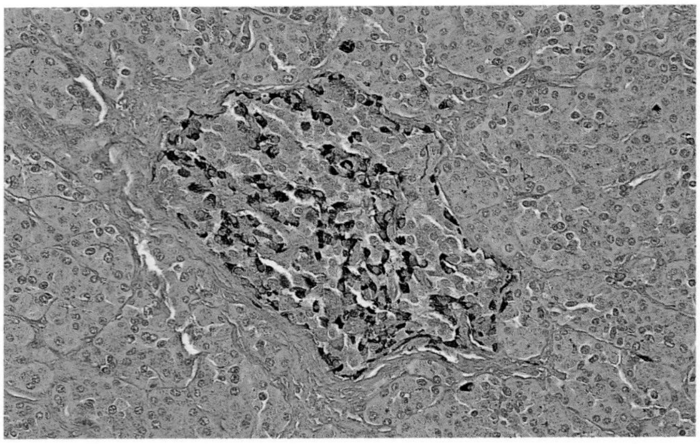

**FIG. 34.** The Grimelius silver stain reacts predominantly with the alpha cells.

tectural differences already mentioned, the diffuse islets exhibit columnar cells within the trabeculae. The cytoplasm is basophilic, the nuclei are somewhat hyperchromatic, and there may be more prominent nucleoli than in the compact islets (Fig. 33B).

Each endocrine cell synthesizes and secretes only one specific peptide. The four major peptides produced by islet cells are insulin, glucagon, somatostatin, and pancreatic polypeptide (89). Although some pancreatic endocrine neoplasms may produce ectopic peptides such as gastrin or vasoactive intestinal polypeptide, these are not found in normal islet cells. Classic histochemical staining has been used to distinguish the different cell types. The aldehyde-fuchsin stain is specific for insulin-secreting beta cells, whereas the Grimelius silver stain labels glucagon-secreting alpha cells (Fig. 34) and the Hellerstrom-Hellman silver preparation identifies somatostatin-secreting delta cells. Immunohistochemical staining with antibodies against insulin, glucagon, somatostatin, and pancreatic polypeptide (produced by PP cells) provides another more specific method to distinguish the cell types. There is a fairly consistent distribution of the cell types within the compact islets. The beta cells are more centrally located, whereas the alpha cells populate the periphery of the islets (Figs. 35 and 36). Beta cells make up 60% to 70% and alpha cells make up 15% to 20% of the compact islets, whereas the delta cells are much less numerous (84,90). Alpha cells are generally found in close contact with delta cells (27). PP cells are rare in the compact islets, being concentrated in the diffuse islets where they constitute the majority (70%) of the cells (Fig. 37) (91,92). The remaining cells of the diffuse islets are largely beta cells (20%), with minor components of alpha and delta cells (5% of each). The difference in proportion of cell types between the compact and diffuse islets reflects their different embryologic origin (85,86). The relative proportion of the different peptide-producing cells also varies with age; for instance, the ratio of beta to delta cells in the compact islets is manyfold higher in adults than in infants, in whom delta cells constitute one third of the islet cell population (80,93). All of the islet cells are also positive for general endocrine markers

A

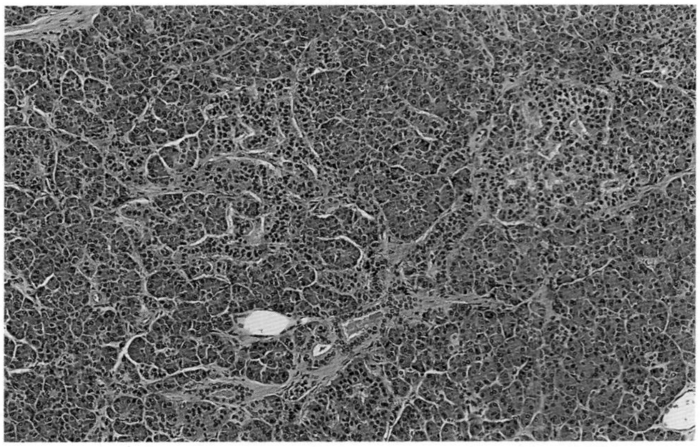

B

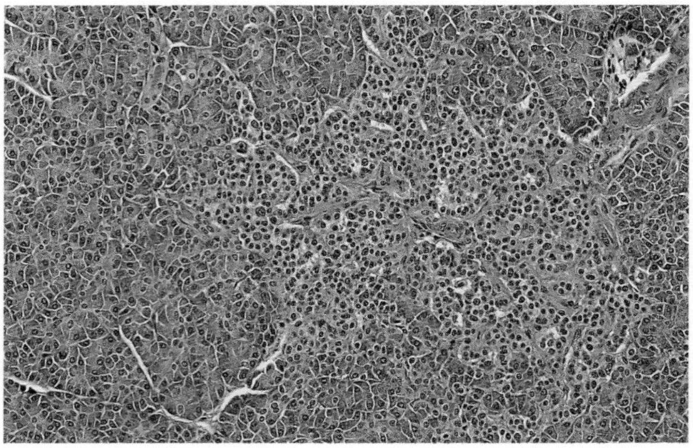

**FIG. 33.** Diffuse islets are composed of trabeculae of endocrine cells interspersed between adjacent acini (**A**). The borders of the diffuse islets are ill-defined (**B**). The cells have somewhat basophilic cytoplasm.

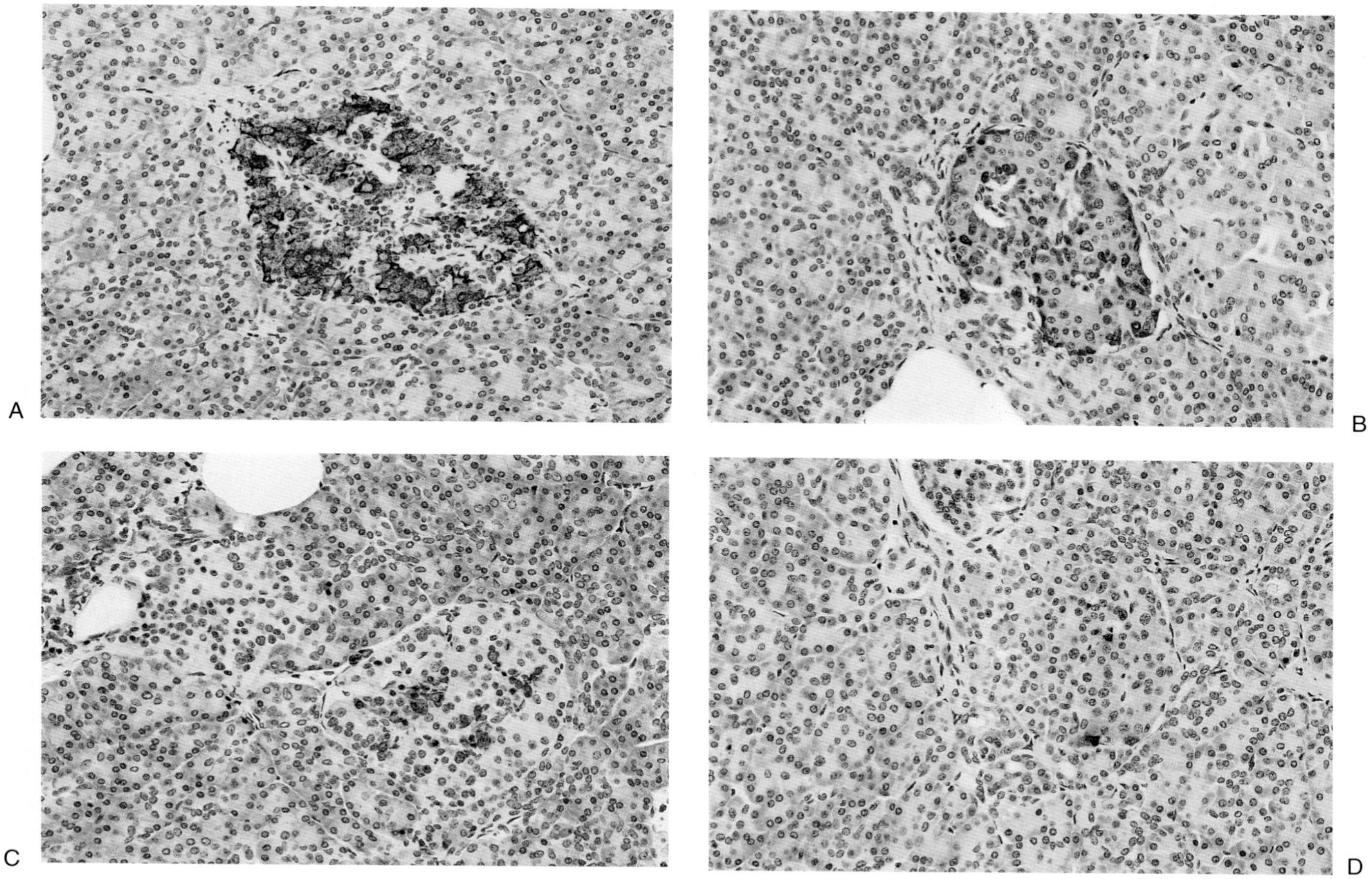


**FIG. 35.** The distribution of the different peptide-producing cells within the islets of Langerhans. Beta cells (stained for insulin) are the most numerous (**A**) and are situated in the central regions of the islet. Alpha cells (stained for glucagon) are generally arranged around the periphery (**B**). Delta cells (stained for somatostatin) (**C**) and PP cells (stained for pancreatic polypeptide) (**D**) are much less numerous and do not display an obvious pattern of arrangement.

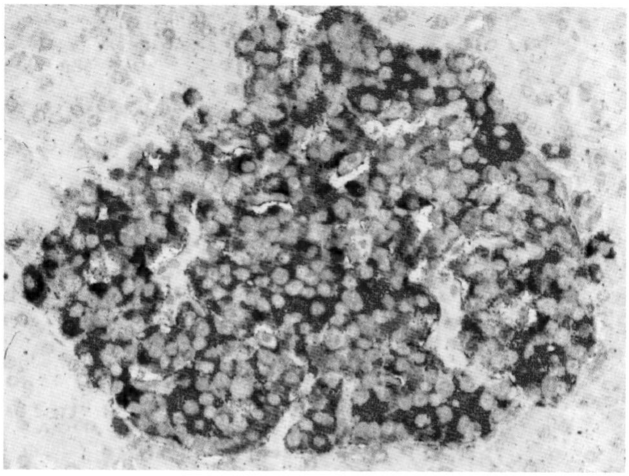

**FIG. 36.** Triple immunohistochemical labeling of a compact islet for insulin (red–brown reaction product), glucagon (violet reaction product), and somatostatin (green reaction product) shows the characteristic distribution of the different cell types.

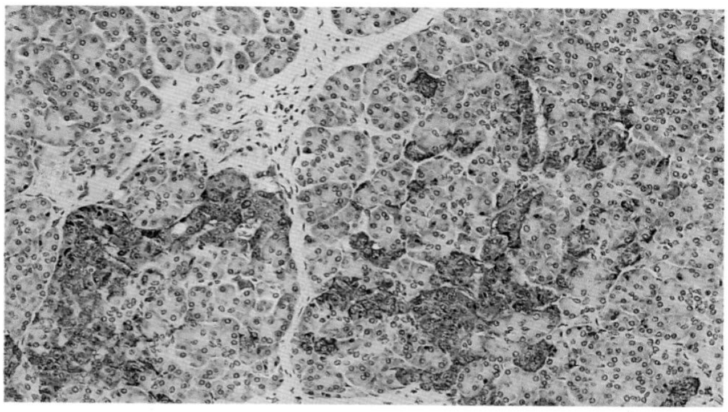

**FIG. 37.** Immunohistochemistry for pancreatic polypeptide shows positive staining in most of the cells in the diffuse islets.

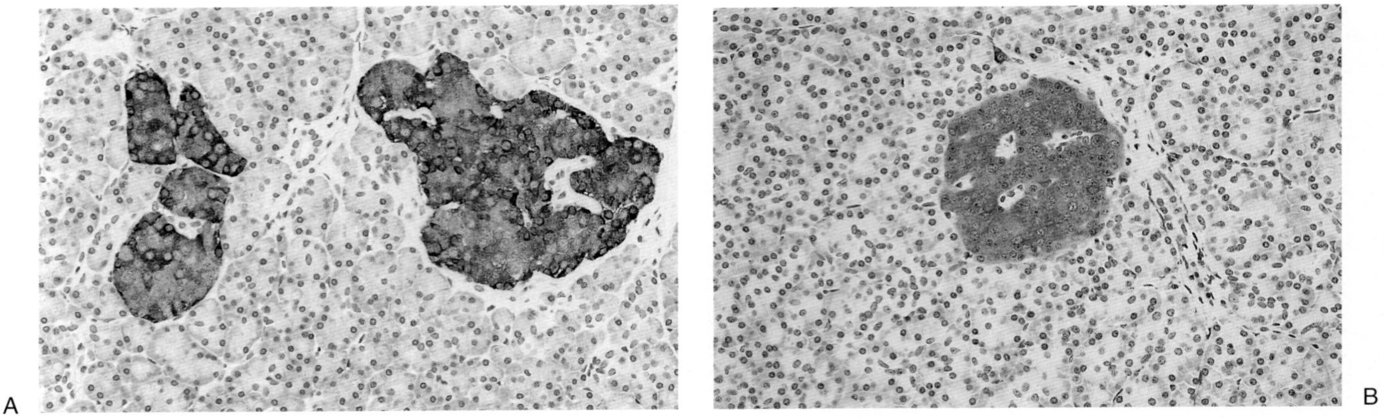


**FIG. 38.** Alpha cells stain more intensely for chromogranin than do beta cells (**A**), whereas all of the islet cells stain uniformly for synaptophysin (**B**).

such as neuron-specific enolase, synaptophysin, and chromogranin (Fig. 38). The last marker is expressed more intensely in alpha cells than in beta cells, and the pattern of staining also reflects the characteristic distribution of the cell types in the compact islets.

Keratins are generally not detected in islet cells by immunohistochemistry, although there may be some faint staining for Cam5.2. Enzymes are also not detectable. The Ewing's sarcoma/PNET antibody O13 stains normal islets as well as pancreatic endocrine neoplasms (94,95).

Ultrastructural examination of the islets shows polygonal cells joined by tight and gap junctions, suggesting that there is electronic or metabolic coupling between adjacent cells (27,84). Scattered desmosomes are also present. The cytoplasm contains all of the organelles necessary for protein synthesis, including RER, mitochondria, and Golgi apparatus; however, the abundant parallel arrays of RER characterizing acinar cells are absent (Fig. 39). The granules are also more randomly distributed within the cytoplasm, with some concentration in the basal cytoplasm adjacent to the capillaries into which they are secreted. The granule size and morphology differ substantially from that of zymogen granules and are also relatively specific for each cell type (89,96). Alpha cell granules measure 200 to 300 nm and contain an eccentrically located, dense core within a less dense outer region that is separated from the limiting membrane by a thin halo (Fig. 40A). Beta cells contain 225- to 375-nm granules with either a finely granular or a crystalline core surrounded by a wide halo underlying the limiting membrane (Fig. 40B). There is considerable variation in the shape of the crystalline core from one granule to another. Cytoplasmic lipid inclusions (or ceroid bodies) are often found in beta cells (Fig. 39A) (27). Delta cell granules are slightly smaller (170 to 220 nm) than alpha cell granules and have a uniformly dense core (Fig. 40C). Delta cells have cytoplasmic processes extending toward the alpha and beta cells, presumably allowing local paracrine release of somatostatin in addition to systemic release into the bloodstream (84). Delta cells are generally located in close proximity to capillaries and tend to be contiguous with other delta cells (84). The PP cells of the ventrally derived portion of the pancreas have 180- to 220-nm granules of variable shape and density, whereas the PP cell granules of the remainder of the pancreas are smaller (120 to 150 nm) and more homogeneous (Fig. 40D) (48). The cells are separated from the fenestrated endothelial cells of the capillaries only by the basement membranes of both cells and minimal interstitial material (27).

### Extrainsular Endocrine Cells

In addition to the pancreatic endocrine cells arranged in islets of Langerhans, there are small numbers of individual endocrine cells within the ducts and scattered among the acini (Fig. 41). These extrainsular endocrine cells are especially abundant during infancy, but they constitute less than 10% of the total pancreatic endocrine cell population in the adult (48). The ductal endocrine cells are most commonly detected in the main and larger interlobular ducts and are rare in the smaller ducts (69,97). Some of them border the lumina and are joined to neighboring ductal cells by tight junctions (98), whereas others are situated between the ductal cells and the basement membrane. It has been speculated that they may secrete peptides directly into the pancreatic ducts, accounting for their detection in pancreatic juice (98). Specific peptides may be found, especially insulin, somatostatin, and pancreatic polypeptide (97,99). Some of the extrainsular endocrine cells in the larger ducts also produce serotonin (99); these cells may be the origin of the extremely rare true carcinoid tumors of the pancreas (100,101). A wide variety of other neurosecretory granule types may be found in the ductal endocrine cells by electron microscopy (69); some of these cells may represent precursors to endocrine cell proliferations (including tumors), which may develop from the

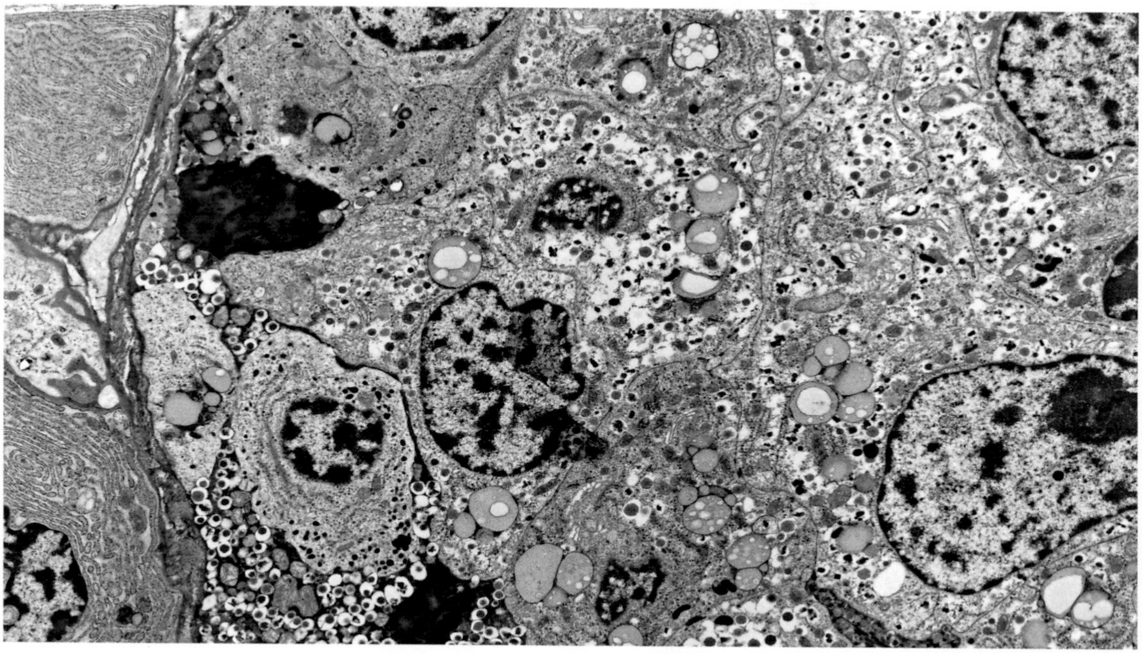

A

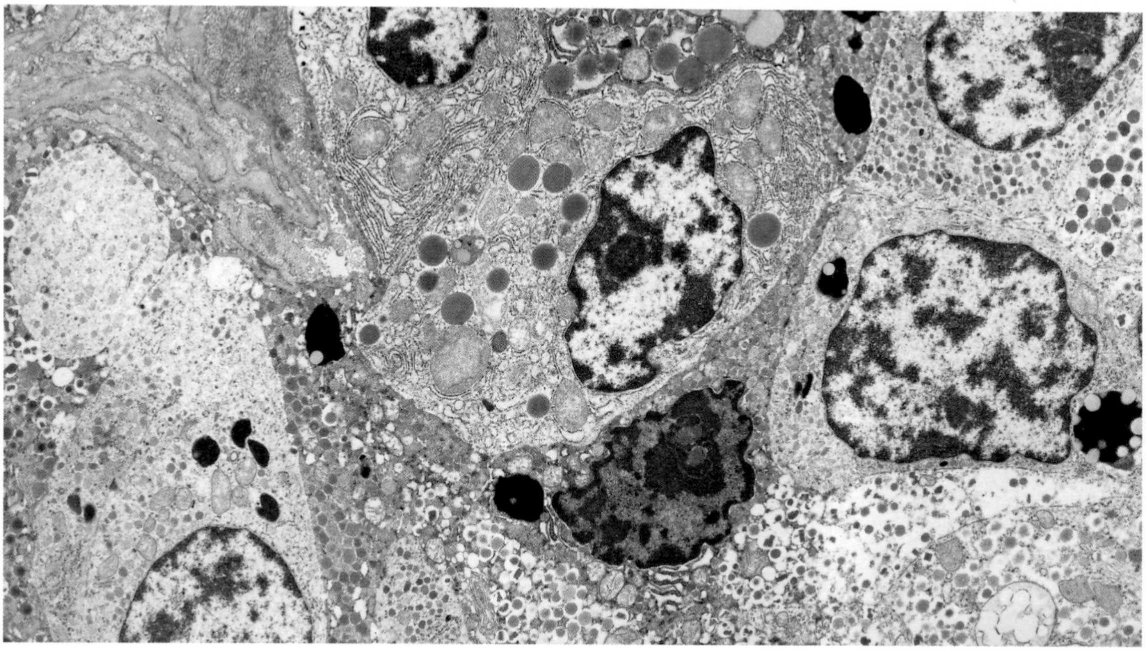

B

**FIG. 39.** Ultrastructural appearance of islets of Langerhans. The compact islets (**A**) are circumscribed and separated from the adjacent acinar cells (*left*). The peptide granules are randomly distributed within the cytoplasm. Lipid inclusions (ceroid bodies) are found within the beta cells. The diffuse islets (**B**) partially encircle clusters of acinar cells (*center*).

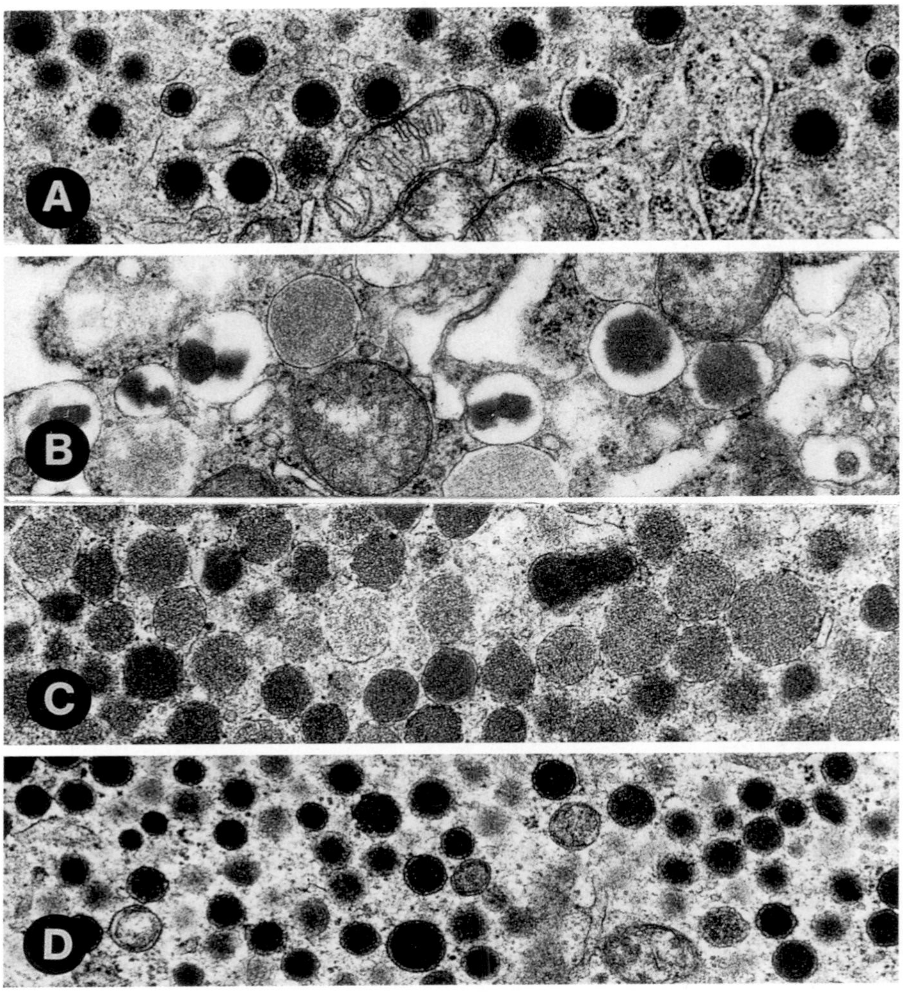


**FIG. 40.** Ultrastructural appearance of islet cell granules. Alpha cell granules (**A**) are round and contain an eccentric electron-dense core within a less dense peripheral region. There is a thin halo beneath the limiting membrane. Beta cell granules (**B**) are polymorphous and contain crystalline cores with a wide halo beneath the limiting membrane. Delta cell granules (**C**) are round with a moderately dense core surrounded by a very thin halo. The granules of PP cells (**D**) are smaller and have homogenous hyperdense cores. [Reprinted with permission (96).]

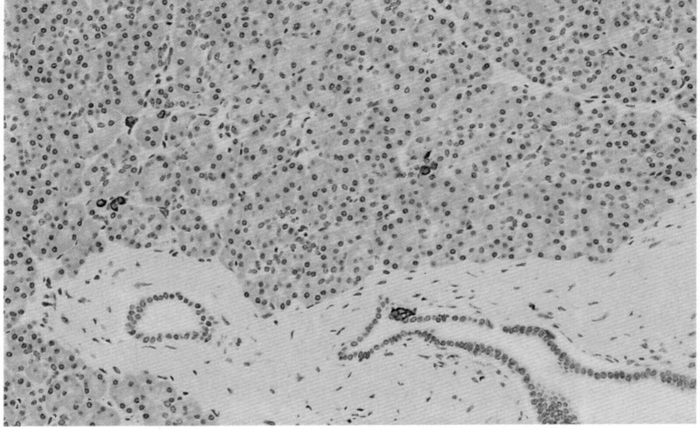

**FIG. 41.** Extrainsular endocrine cells within the ducts and between the acini are only detectable with immunohistochemical staining for chromogranin.

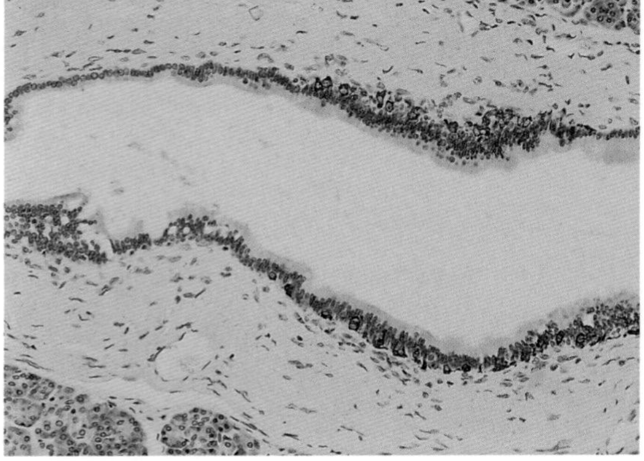

**FIG. 42.** The number of ductal endocrine cells is increased in areas showing hyperplasia of the ductal epithelium (*right*).

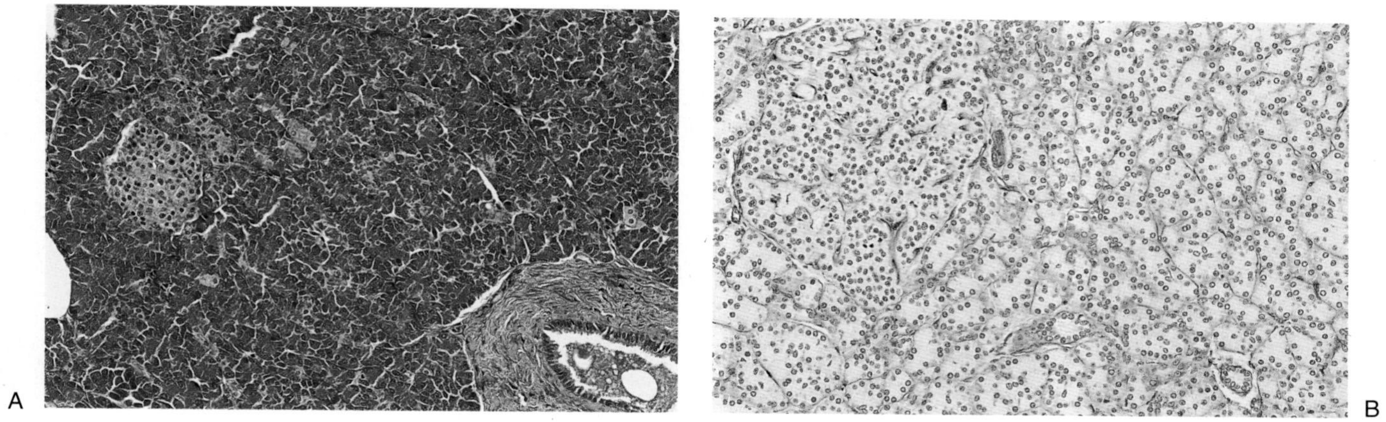

**FIG. 43.** Connective tissues are minimal within the pancreas. Collagen is largely restricted to the tissues surrounding the interlobular ducts, with only thin bands extending into the lobules, as demonstrated with a trichrome stain (**A**). Immunohistochemical staining for type IV collagen (**B**) shows that an extensive network of basement membranes surrounds each acinus and duct and accompanies the capillaries within the islets (*upper left*).

ducts under certain conditions (69,102). The number of ductal endocrine cells also appears to increase in the presence of hyperplasia of the ductal epithelium (Fig. 42) (97).

### Connective Tissues

In the normal adult pancreas there is little connective tissue between the lobules and almost none within them. In the neonatal pancreas, mesenchymal tissue comprises nearly 30% of the volume of the gland (Fig. 6A); there is a gradual decrease during infancy (80). The acini are surrounded by basement membranes, but very little other collagen is present (Fig. 43). Small portal vessels exist that deliver hormonal secretions from the islets directly to the exocrine elements of the gland (61,62,103,104). A complex capillary network surrounds the acini, and accompanying nerve fibers may be found. The acini and ducts are innervated by bundles of unmyelinated nerves that travel through the interlobular connective tissues. In most cases the nerve endings are separated from the acinar or ductal cells by the basement membrane, although in some cases direct contact with the basal cell membrane of acinar cells may be seen (69). Islets are innervated by both sympathetic and parasympathetic fibers; in addition, there are peptidurgic fibers from the autonomic ganglia. Some of the periacinar nerves produce neuropeptide Y, whereas vasoactive intestinal polypeptide-containing nerves are found within islets and adjacent to ducts (105). Other peptides found in pancreatic nerves include substance P, cholecystokinin, and calcitonin gene–related peptide (105). Small autonomic ganglia are located between clusters of acini (Fig. 44). Paraganglia also may be found occasionally in the peripancreatic tissues. The interlobular connective tissue contains the larger vessels as well as nerves and interlobular and major ducts.

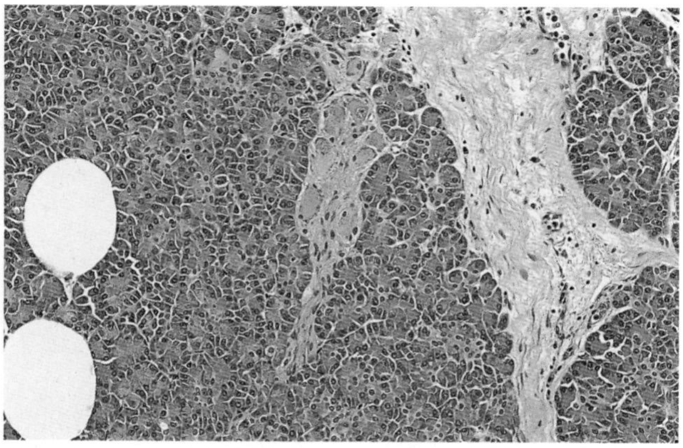

**FIG. 44.** Small autonomic ganglia are located within lobules of acinar tissue.

In almost every individual there are some adipocytes within the pancreas (Fig. 20). The proportion of the gland composed of fat varies from 3% to 20% (4). The amount of adipose tissue in the pancreas varies with the nutritional state and the age of the individual, older or overweight individuals having more intrapancreatic fat (106). The portions of the gland derived from the dorsal lobe may have more intraparenchymal fat than those from the ventral lobe (107,108).

## MINOR ALTERATIONS

A number of minor alterations may affect various components of the pancreas because of physiologic changes, response to injury, or aging. In some cases these changes are so minimal that they may be overlooked, whereas in other instances they may be confused with a neoplastic process. Recognition of these potential diagnostic pitfalls is essential for the accurate interpretation of biopsy results and is complicated by the fact that many of these pseudoneoplastic alterations may accompany pancreatic tumors.

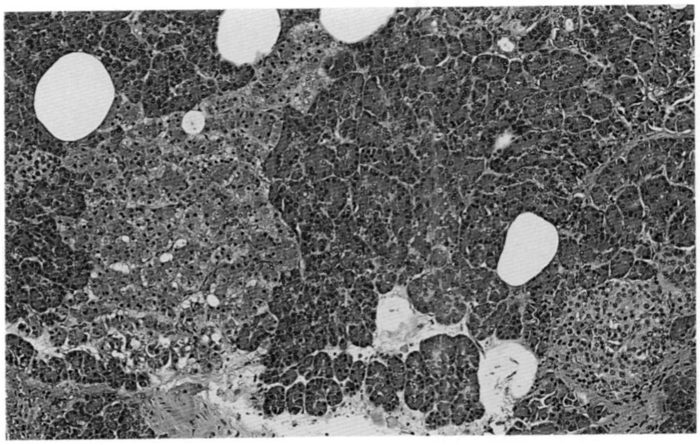

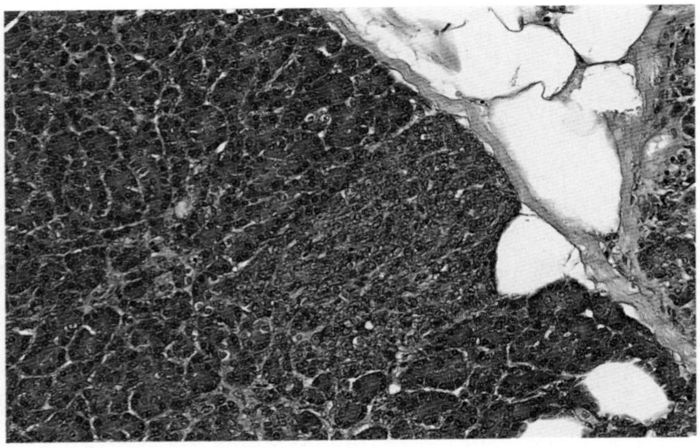

A B

**FIG. 45.** Atypical acinar cell nodules. The eosinophilic type (**A**) is more common and consists of a collection of acini showing loss of basophilia in the basal cytoplasm and hyperchromasia of the nuclei. The eosinophilic granules within the apical cytoplasm are maintained. An islet of Langerhans, with which these lesions may be confused, is present at lower right. The basophilic type of atypical acinar cell nodule (**B**) exhibits an increased nucleus to cytoplasm ratio with loss of eosinophilic granularity of the apical cytoplasm. Some degree of nuclear atypia is also present.

### Acinar Cells

Atypical acinar cell nodules are common incidental findings consisting of circumscribed clusters of acini showing cytoplasmic or nuclear differences from the surrounding acini (109,110). Alternative terms include "focal acinar transformation," "eosinophilic degeneration," and "focal acinar cell dysplasia" (7,48,111,112). The latter term implies some preneoplastic significance to the lesion, and atypical acinar cell nodules are indeed common in the pancreata of rats treated with azaserine, a compound that also induces acinar cell carcinomas in those animals (113). However, there has not been any proven preneoplastic significance to atypical acinar cell nodules in humans, where they are found in nearly half of nontumorous pancreata (114). The lesions are more prevalent in adults, suggesting that they are acquired (111). Although sometimes larger, atypical acinar cell nodules are often similar in size to compact islets, with which they may be confused. Two types of atypical acinar cell nodules exist (110). The more common is the eosinophilic type, which appears as an abnormally pale, eosinophilic cluster of acini (Fig. 45A). At higher power, the cells are larger than the adjacent normal acinar cells, and the deep basophilia of the basal cytoplasm is lacking. The cytoplasm also may be vacuolated. The nuclei appear normal or hyperchromatic. This change is due to dilatation of the rough endoplasmic reticulum (115) and may be a result of localized hypoxia or other degenerative phenomena. The other less common type of atypical acinar cell nodule, the basophilic type, exhibits a loss of the eosinophilic zymogen granules from the apical cytoplasm as well as an increased nucleus-to-cytoplasm ratio (Fig. 45B). Nuclear enlargement, mild atypia, and prominent nucleoli also may be seen. The reason for such localized depletion of zymogen granules is unclear.

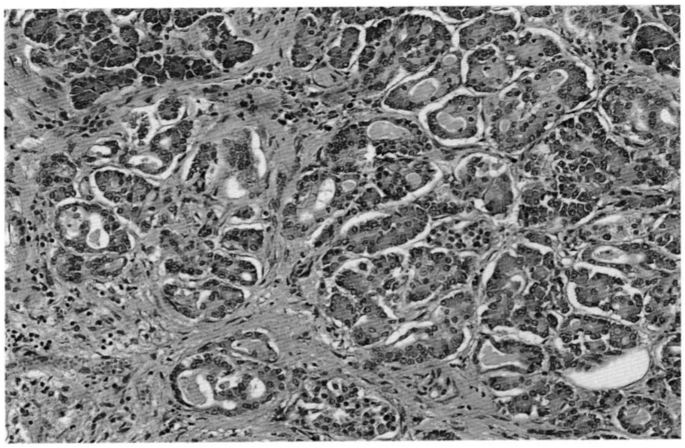

**FIG. 46.** In acinar ectasia, the acinar lumina are dilated and filled with eosinophilic secretions. The lining cells have a flattened appearance, often resembling small ductules cells more than acinar cells.

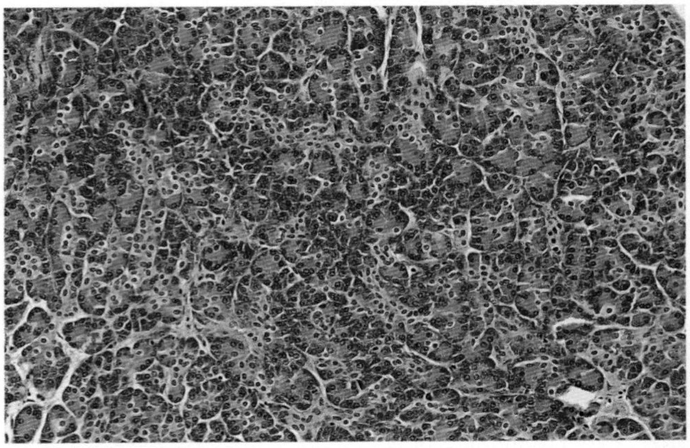

**FIG. 47.** Apparent proliferation of centroacinar cells.

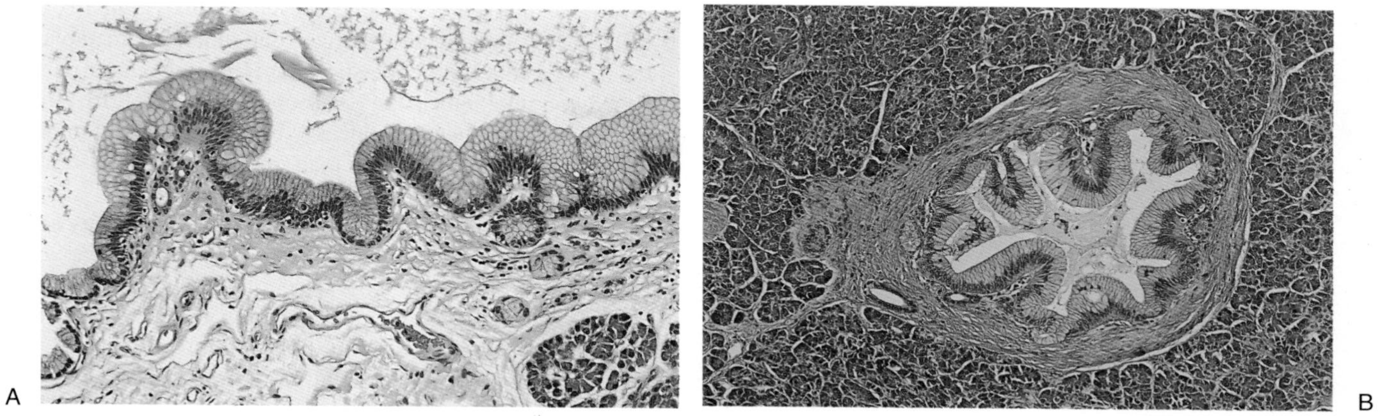

**FIG. 48.** Mucinous metaplasia of the ducts. In simple mucinous metaplasia (**A**) the normal cuboidal to low columnar ductal epithelial cells are replaced by tall columnar cells containing abundant apical mucin. The nuclei remain basally located and show minimal pseudostratification. Superimposed papillary hyperplasia may also be present (**B**).

Acinar lumina may become somewhat dilated during active secretion (1) or due to ductal obstruction (112). This acinar ectasia is also a relatively common finding at autopsy, where it is associated with premortem uremia, septicemia, and dehydration (7,116,117). Acinar ectasia often involves an entire lobular unit. The ectatic acini resemble small ductules, with flattened lining cells, but some of the cells are still recognizable as acinar cells that have lost most of their zymogen granules (Fig. 46). Centroacinar cells also line the dilated lumina and may proliferate (117). Retention of eosinophilic secretory material within the lumina is often found.

Metaplastic changes involving the acini are less common than those involving the ducts; they include replacement by mucinous cells or squamous cells (118). Proliferating centroacinar cells may appear to replace the acinar cells (Fig. 47), especially in the presence of early atrophy (112). The possibility that acinar cells may transform into centroacinar or ductular cells remains speculative (119).

### Ductal Cells

Metaplastic changes that may affect the pancreatic ducts include mucinous, squamous, oncocytic, goblet cell, and acinar metaplasia. Mucinous metaplasia (also known as mucous cell hypertrophy or pyloric gland metaplasia) is a common alteration in ductal cells and may affect ducts of any size (120–122). The change is present in 60% to 90% of nontumorous pancreata (7,10,112,121,123) and is usually more prevalent in the head of the gland (123). The normal cuboidal cells are replaced by tall columnar cells with abundant apical mucin (Fig. 48A) resembling gastric foveolar or pyloric gland cells. The ductal epithelium may remain flat, or there may be superimposed hyperplastic changes, with formation of micropapillae or true papillae with fibrovascular cores (Fig. 48B). The lesion may involve a single ductal profile or may extend into clusters of ductules adjacent to larger ducts. The latter circumstance results in the appearance of collections of small back-to-back tubules of muci-

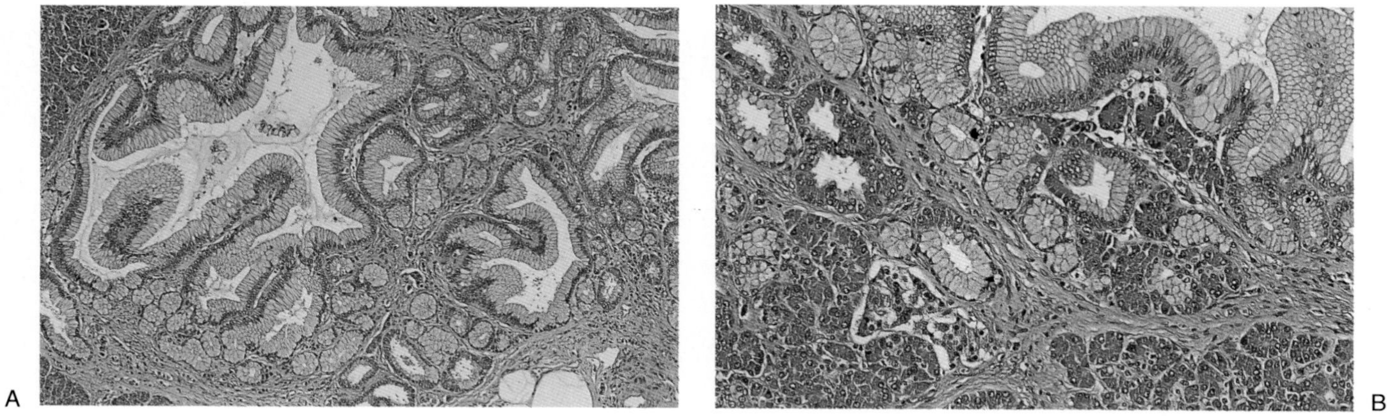

**FIG. 49.** Mucinous metaplasia may involve aggregates of small ductules around larger ducts resulting in clusters of mucinous glands (**A**). Because the smallest components of the ductal system are involved, the metaplastic mucinous cells may abut adjacent acinar cells (**B**).

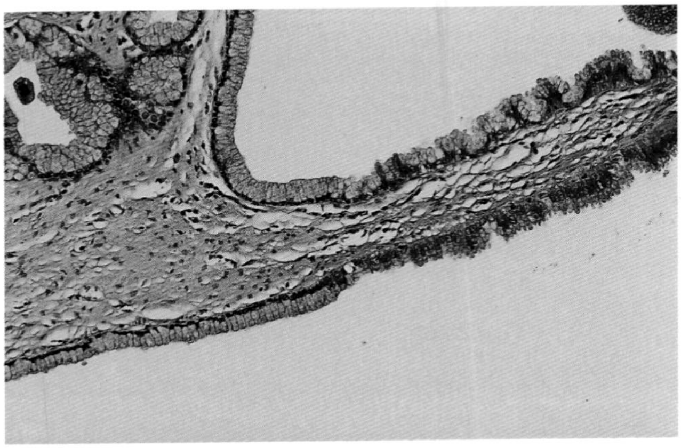

**FIG. 50.** The transition between an area of mucinous metaplasia and hyperplasia. The simple metaplastic epithelium (*left*) shows a single row of basally located nuclei with no cytologic abnormalities. In the hyperplastic regions (*right*) the nuclei are enlarged and pseudostratified.

nous cells and has been termed "adenomatous hyperplasia" (120); it is particularly associated with areas of chronic pancreatitis (Fig. 49). The cells of mucinous metaplasia produce largely neutral mucins and sialomucins; sulphomucins are less abundant than in normal ductal cells (48). The histochemical and immunohistochemical profile of the mucins in these cells resembles that of the superficial gastric mucosa in some cases or of the pyloric glands in others (78,122). Because there is little morphologic difference between these two mucin-producing cells types, pyloric gland metaplasia may not be distinguishable from gastric foveolar metaplasia by routine microscopy. The nuclei in areas of simple mucinous metaplasia are small, hyperchromatic, and confined to the basal cytoplasm by the abundant apical mucin (Fig. 50). When hyperplastic changes are also present, however, the nuclei are enlarged, mildly atypical, and pseudostratified, with prominent nucleoli (Fig. 50). The significance of mild nuclear atypia in mucinous metaplasia and the relationship of this lesion to atypical hyperplasia and carcinoma is unclear (124). Some studies suggest that mucinous metaplasia itself may have preneoplastic significance because of the finding of mutations in the K-*ras* oncogene (125,126). However, the lesion does not appear to be more prevalent in pancreata harboring carcinomas than in the nontumorous gland (121).

Squamous metaplasia also may involve ducts of any size. Up to 45% of pancreata exhibit squamous metaplasia (10,112,127). Although it may occur in the larger interlobular and main ducts, it is most common in the intercalated ducts, and metaplastic cells may extend into the center of the acini (Fig. 51). It is exceptional for squamous metaplasia to exhibit keratinization or a granular cell layer. For this reason, the term "multilayered metaplasia" has been suggested for this lesion (112). Histologically, the stratified squamous epithelium appears immature, with only minimal flattening of the superficial layers. There may be retention of a luminal mucinous cell layer. In the smaller ducts and ductules, the metaplastic epithelium may fill the lumen, virtually obliterating it. In most instances squamous metaplasia is associated with chronic inflammation; there is no known preneoplastic significance.

Oncocytic changes are common in centroacinar cells, and oncocytic metaplasia may affect intercalated and intralobular ducts as well (70,128,129). The oncocytic cells have abundant granular eosinophilic cytoplasm (reflecting the accumulation of mitochondria), and the nuclei may be enlarged with prominent nucleoli (Fig. 52). Involvement of clusters of small ductules may occur in a similar distribution to that of so-called adenomatous hyperplasia. Like mucinous and squamous metaplasia, oncocytic metaplasia may be associated with chronic inflammatory processes or it may occur in the absence of other specific abnormalities (10,130).

Goblet cells may be found within the ductal epithelium, especially in the main ducts near the ampulla of Vater (1,71). In addition, isolated goblet cells may appear in smaller ducts, presumably as a metaplastic change (112,118). In contrast to

A

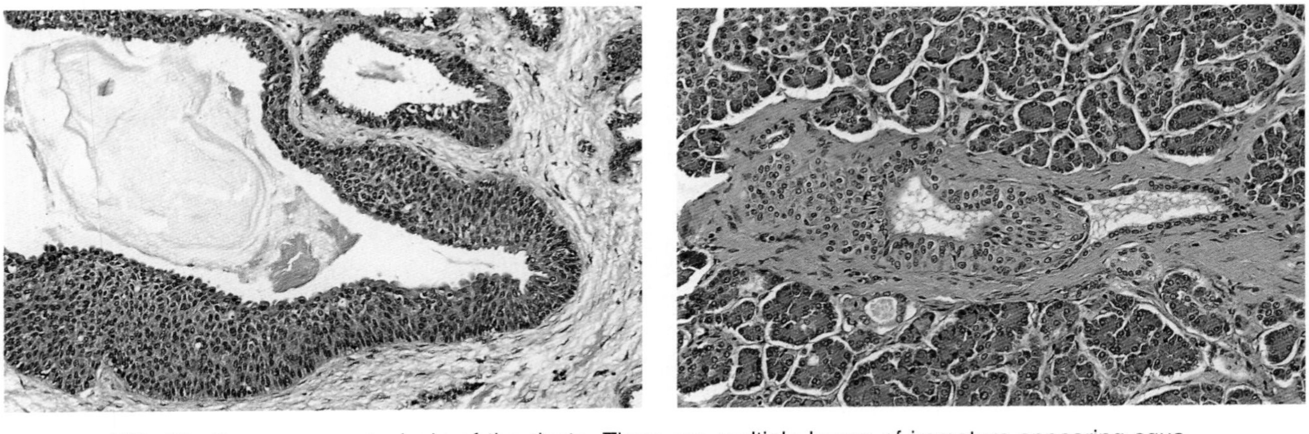

B

**FIG. 51.** Squamous metaplasia of the ducts. There are multiple layers of immature-appearing squamous cells without keratinization. The process may involve larger ducts (**A**). In this example (**B**) there is partial involvement of a small interlobular duct.

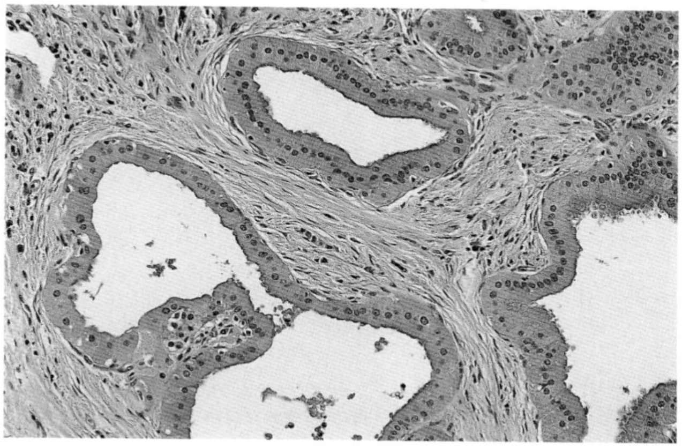

**FIG. 52.** Oncocytic changes involving small ducts. In this example there is associated fibrosing pancreatitis.

mucinous metaplasia, the mucin-containing goblet cells occur singly and are more flask-shaped. Presumably they reflect an intestinal metaplastic phenotype rather than the gastric phenotype of typical mucinous metaplasia.

Acinar metaplasia of the ducts has not been widely recognized but occasionally may be seen in the smaller ducts. The acinar cells occur singly or in clusters and exhibit the same appearance as their normally situated counterparts (Fig. 53). Immunohistochemical staining for trypsin or chymotrypsin may facilitate identification of acinar metaplasia, although the granular apical cytoplasmic staining of true acinar cells must be distinguished from the staining of deposited intraluminal enzyme secretions on the surface of ductal cells (Fig. 14).

In addition to metaplasia, the ducts may exhibit proliferative changes ranging from simple hyperplasia to papillary or micropapillary hyperplasia to atypical hyperplasia to carcinoma in situ (120,121,127,131,132). A full discussion of these changes is beyond the scope of this chapter. There appears to be a continuum of atypia within this spectrum, and at what point the lesion acquires significant preneoplastic potential is unclear (124). Proliferative changes of all types have been associated with invasive ductal adenocarcinomas (77,120,121), although the frequency and time course of progression of the various lesions to carcinoma is unknown. Increasing evidence suggests that there is accumulation of genetic abnormalities in atypical hyperplasia and carcinoma in situ (126,133,134). The various proliferative lesions tend to coexist within the same pancreas, with gradual transitions from one to the next. Furthermore, as already discussed, mucinous metaplasia often coexists with hyperplastic changes, especially those with lesser degrees of atypia. In simple hyperplasia there is an increase in the thickness of the flat epithelial layer, generally with pseudostratification of elongated, slightly enlarged nuclei. Mucinous metaplasia is commonly present (Fig. 50). In papillary hyperplasia there may be papillary or micropapillary formations, but the nuclei remain uniform in size and basally located or slightly pseudostratified (Fig. 48B). The chromatin is evenly distributed, and there are no macronucleoli. Papillary hyperplasia is found in 10% to 20% of normal pancreata when thoroughly examined (7,121). Atypical hyperplasia and carcinoma in situ are generally found in pancreata also harboring an invasive ductal adenocarcinoma (120,121), although they have also rarely been observed in pancreata without an invasive carcinoma. Atypical hyperplasia is characterized by loss of polarity, mild to moderate variation in nuclear shape and size, and some chromatin abnormalities; there is no complete loss of polarity, increased mitoses, or severe nuclear atypia (Fig. 54). In carcinoma in situ there is marked loss of polarity, often with budding of cell clusters into the lumen. The nuclei vary considerably from cell to cell, and irregular chromatin patterns and macronucleoli may be seen (Fig. 55). Mitotic figures are easily found, often with the superficial layer of the epithelium. Architectural alterations such as cribriforming may be present but often are not seen.

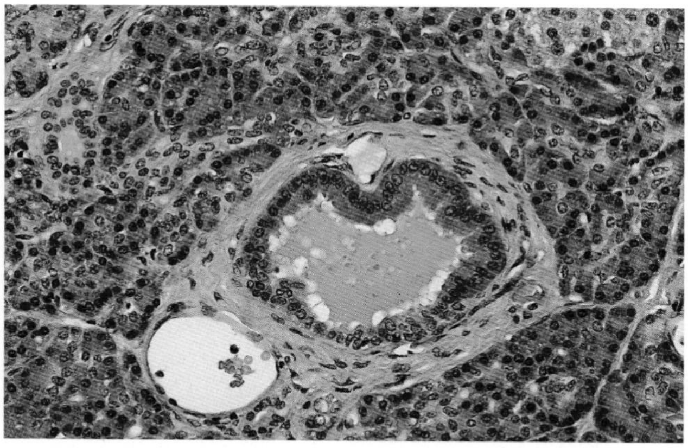

**FIG. 53.** This small interlobular duct shows partial acinar metaplasia, with slightly enlarged acinar cells having granular eosinophilic apical cytoplasm replacing the normal cuboidal ductal epithelium.

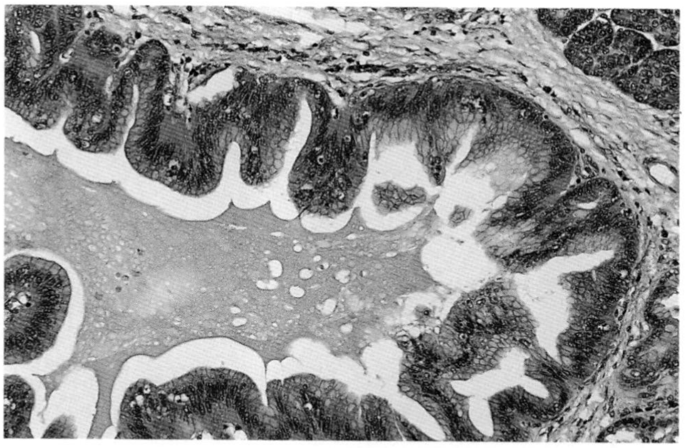

**FIG. 54.** Atypical hyperplasia of the ducts is characterized by pseudostratified nuclei showing focal loss polarity. Although there is nuclear atypia and prominent nucleoli there is not complete loss of uniformity to the cytologic appearance.

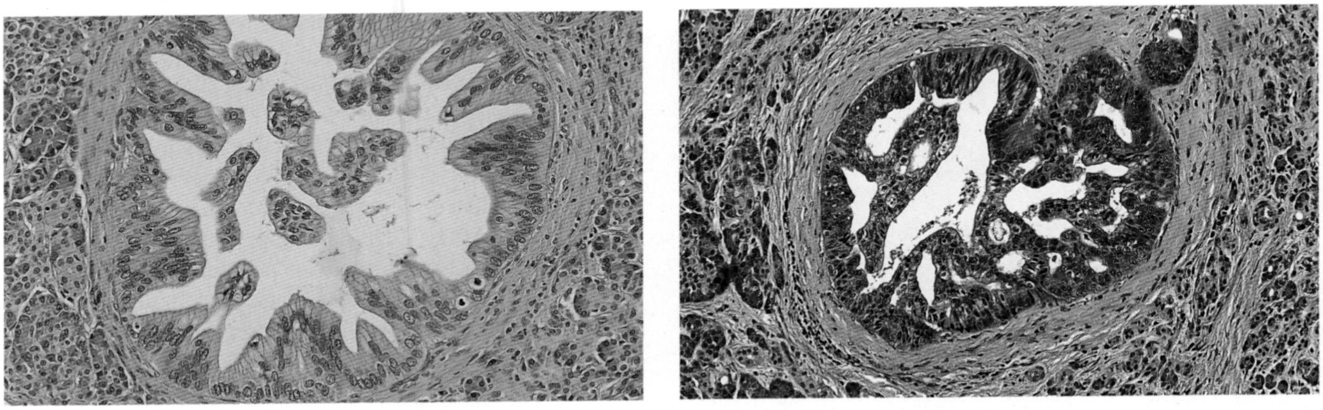
A B

**FIG. 55.** In carcinoma in situ there is complete loss of polarity, with budding of disorganized cellular clusters into the ductal lumen. The nuclei are markedly irregular and vary in morphology between adjacent cells. Increased mitoses are present (**A**). In another focus (**B**), architectural abnormalities include cribriforming, and there is extreme nuclear atypia.

Centroacinar and intercalated duct cells appear to proliferate in various conditions, including uremia, dehydration, hypergastrinemia, and ductal obstruction, as well as with insulin-producing neoplasms (112).

Another frequent alteration of the ducts is ectasia. Ectatic ducts are generally (but not invariably) found in association with chronic pancreatitis in older patients (7,10,135). The ectatic ducts range up to several millimeters in size and occasionally are recognizable grossly. Dilatation of the main pancreatic duct to more than 4 mm is found in 16% of patients at autopsy (7). Because ectatic ducts are often tortuous and the dilatation may be localized, they may appear as single or multiple small cysts (retention cysts) in cross section. Careful study of serial sections shows the continuity with the ductal system. The lining epithelium often displays mucinous metaplasia and may show hyperplastic or atypical changes as well (Fig. 56). Larger ectatic ducts with more significant proliferative changes merge histologically with the tumorous entity of intraductal papillary-mucinous neoplasm (136–138). In fact, a clinical term used for the latter entity is "mucinous duct ectasia" (139,140), reflecting the radiographic appearance that often accompanies the intraductal neoplasm. In simple duct ectasia, the lesion is incidentally detected, and there are minimal proliferative changes. Intraductal papillary mucinous neoplasms commonly have exuberant papillary formations with a range of cytoarchitectural atypia, and the patients come to medical attention because of pancreatitis-like symptoms. However, there is no sharp dividing line between the two lesions, and it is tempting to speculate that intraductal papillary–mucinous neoplasms begin as simple ectatic ducts.

## Islet Cells

Islet hyperplasia is defined as an absolute increase in the size or number of islets relative to the normal islet volume at a given age. Thus, some objective assessment of islet volume must be made for a diagnosis of islet hyperplasia, rather than just a casual observation of "a lot" of islets. Conditions as-

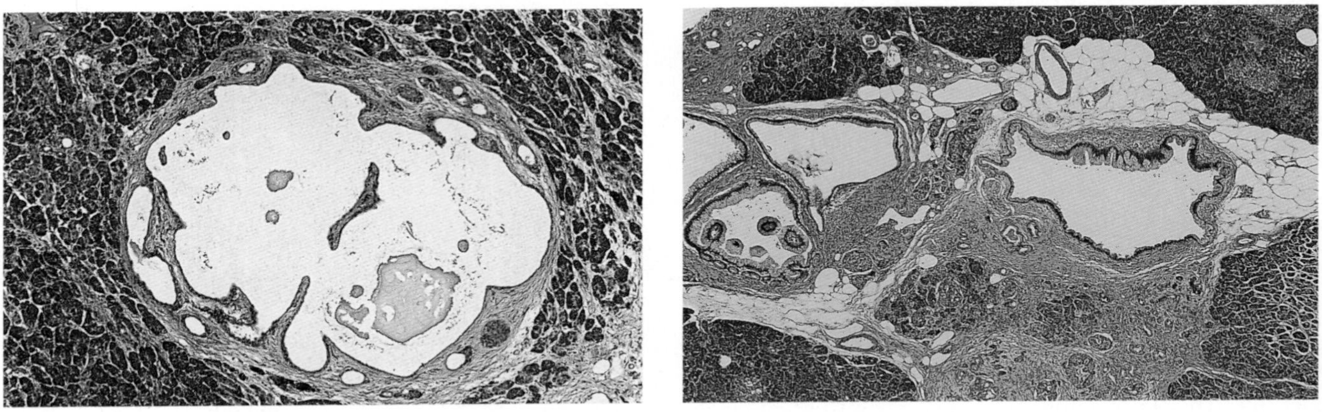
A B

**FIG. 56.** Duct ectasia. The dilated ducts may be lined by a flattened cuboidal epithelium resembling normal ductal epithelium (**A**) or there may be mucinous metaplasia or proliferative changes (**B**). In the latter circumstance, the lesion merges morphologically with intraductal papillary–mucinous neoplasm.

sociated with islet hyperplasia in infancy include Beckwith-Wiedemann syndrome, maternal diabetes, erythroblastosis fetalis, and hyperinsulinemic hypoglycemia (48); cases have also been described in adults with hyperinsulinism (141). Islet hyperplasia may occur either by proliferation of islet cells or by neoformation of islet cells from progenitors within the ductal epithelium (27). Usually there are enlarged islets with diameters exceeding 250 μm (142). Although the distribution of the different cell types is usually maintained, there may be a relative increase in the number of beta cells, some of which may show hypertrophy.

One specific condition that involves islet hyperplasia is nesidioblastosis. The term "nesidioblastosis" refers to the neogenesis (or budding off) of endocrine cells from the pancreatic ducts, resulting in ductuloinsular complexes. There is usually an associated abnormal distribution of hyperplastic endocrine cells throughout the exocrine regions of the gland (Fig. 57). Both localized and diffuse types are described (143). The term was originally applied to describe the appearance of the endocrine pancreas in cases of persistent neonatal hyperinsulinemic hypoglycemia, and the ductuloinsular complexes and other abnormally distributed islet cells in this disease appeared to reflect an increase in beta cells responsible for the excess insulin secretion (144). However, comparative studies of normal neonatal pancreata have found a similar morphologic appearance to the endocrine elements, raising questions whether the morphologic lesions designated as "nesidioblastosis" are truly abnormal and responsible for the clinical syndrome (80,142). Instead, it may be an abnormal relative proportion of beta cells or an abnormal relationship between beta and delta cells that is resposible for the clinical syndrome (145,146). In the adult, rare cases of hyperinsulinemic hypoglycemia have been associated with similar histologic findings in the absence of a discrete insulinoma (141,147). Although such symptomatic cases may represent nesidioblastosis in the adult, the isolated histologic finding of ductuloinsular complexes is not uncommon in asymptomatic individuals, especially associated with chronic pancreatitis (90,148) (Fig. 58). Although the term "nesidioblastosis" may be descriptively applied to such incidental findings, it does not reflect significant clinical implications to the lesions and probably should be avoided.

The apparent increase in number of islets that occurs secondary to exocrine atrophy has been termed "islet aggregation" and is not necessarily a result of hyperplasia. Islet aggregation is discussed more fully below.

The appearance of dilated blood-filled spaces within the islets (Fig. 59) has been referred to as peliosis insulis. Although reported in a pancreas from a patient with multiple endocrine neoplasia-I (MEN-I) also harboring multiple pancreatic endocrine neoplasms (149), peliosis insulis usually occurs in otherwise normal pancreata. It is of unclear etiology and significance. The blood-filled spaces are not observed to be endothelium lined by electron microscopy.

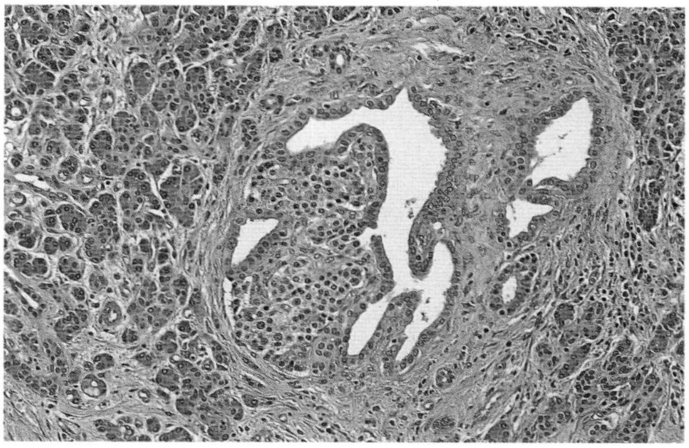

**FIG. 58.** A ductuloinsular complex in an adult with mild chronic pancreatitis. Small ductules are surrounded by nests of endocrine cells, a finding that does not necessarily reflect true islet cell hyperplasia.

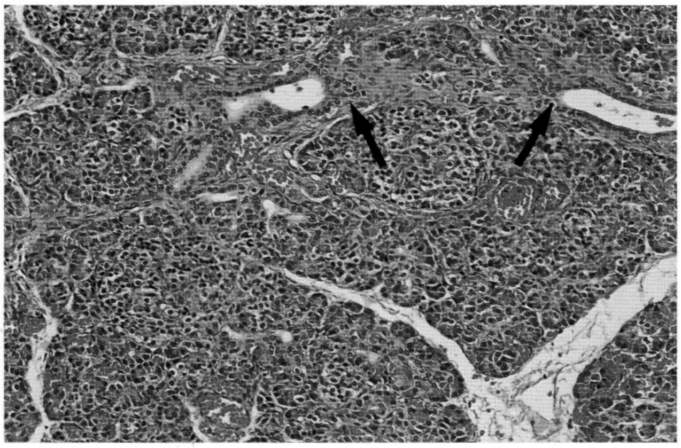

**FIG. 57.** The pancreas from an infant with persistent neonatal hyperinsulinemic hypoglycemia shows nesidioblastosis. There is a diffuse increase in endocrine cells throughout the lobules. Endocrine cells are also seen budding from the smaller ducts (*arrows*).

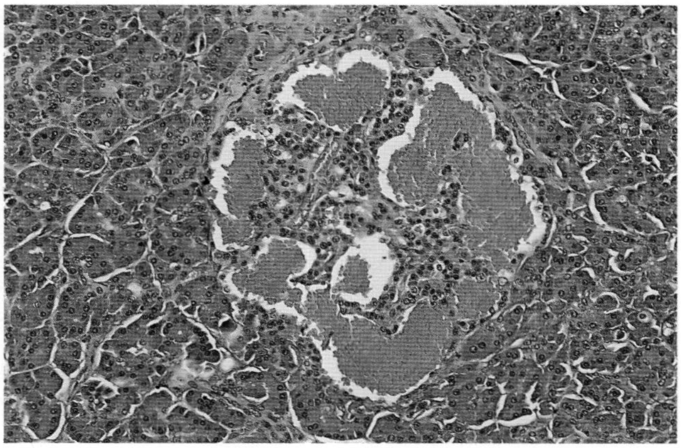

**FIG. 59.** The appearance of dilated, blood-filled spaces within the islets has been called peliosis insulis. It is probably of no clinical significance.

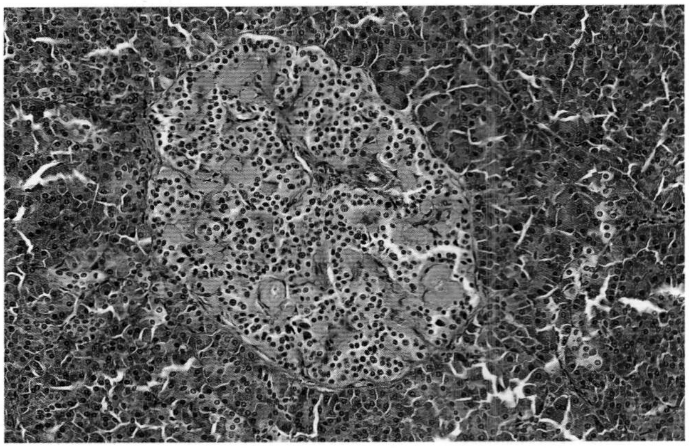

**FIG. 60.** Amyloid-like hyalinization of the perivascular tissue may be seen in the islets, especially in older patients with type II diabetes. The surrounding acinar tissue is not fibrotic.

Perivascular deposition of amyloid or amyloid-like material may be seen in older patients (Fig. 60), especially in association with non–insulin-dependent (type II) diabetes mellitus (150). Insular amyloid is biochemically different from systemic amyloid, and there is no association between insular amyloidosis and systemic amyloidosis. In insular amyloidosis, the hyalinized stroma is limited to the islets. In patients with generalized fibrosis of the pancreatic parenchyma due to chronic pancreatitis or other causes, the islets also may be involved (insular fibrosis); however, the hyalinized stroma in these cases has no ultrastructural features of amyloid (150).

### Chronic Pancreatitis, Atrophy, and Fibrosis

An entire chapter devoted to chronic pancreatitis would probably still provide inadequate discussion of this complex topic. Several different types of chronic pancreatitis exist, with etiologies including chronic alcoholism, ductal obstruction, autoimmune disorders, or genetic predisposition (151,152). Although the distribution of the disease within the pancreas varies with the different types, the histologic features are similar, especially at the end stages when fibrosis and atrophy are prominent (10). In fact, some degree of fibrosis and atrophy (pathologic chronic pancreatitis) are common incidental pathologic findings in pancreatic resection specimens or at autopsy, and the pathologic findings often reported as chronic pancreatitis are only loosely related to the clinical disease of chronic pancreatitis. Clinically, chronic pancreatitis may mimic pancreatic carcinoma, and the resultant morphologic patterns also frequently simulate neoplasia pathologically. Early in the process the fibrosis is

A

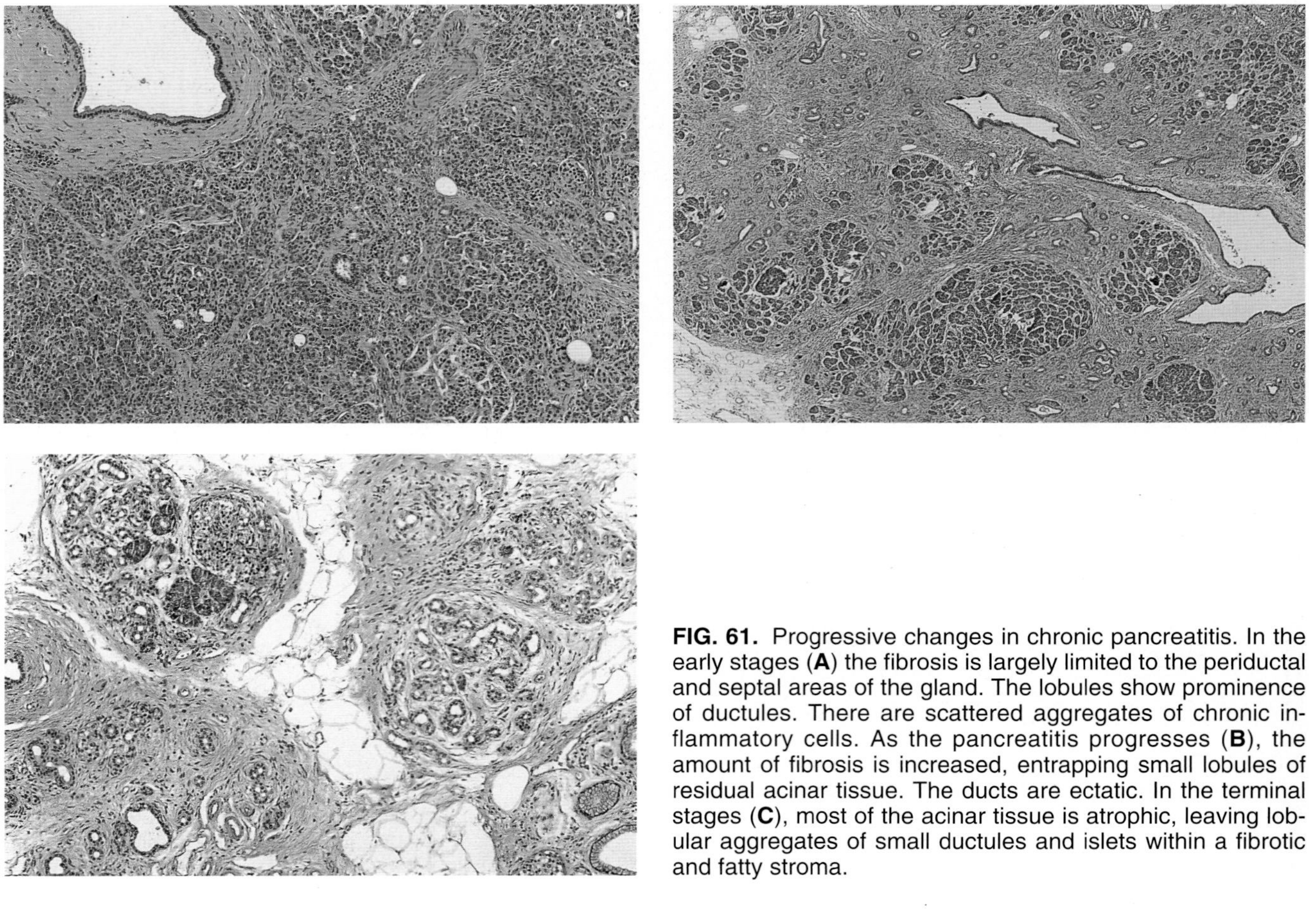

B

C

**FIG. 61.** Progressive changes in chronic pancreatitis. In the early stages (**A**) the fibrosis is largely limited to the periductal and septal areas of the gland. The lobules show prominence of ductules. There are scattered aggregates of chronic inflammatory cells. As the pancreatitis progresses (**B**), the amount of fibrosis is increased, entrapping small lobules of residual acinar tissue. The ducts are ectatic. In the terminal stages (**C**), most of the acinar tissue is atrophic, leaving lobular aggregates of small ductules and islets within a fibrotic and fatty stroma.

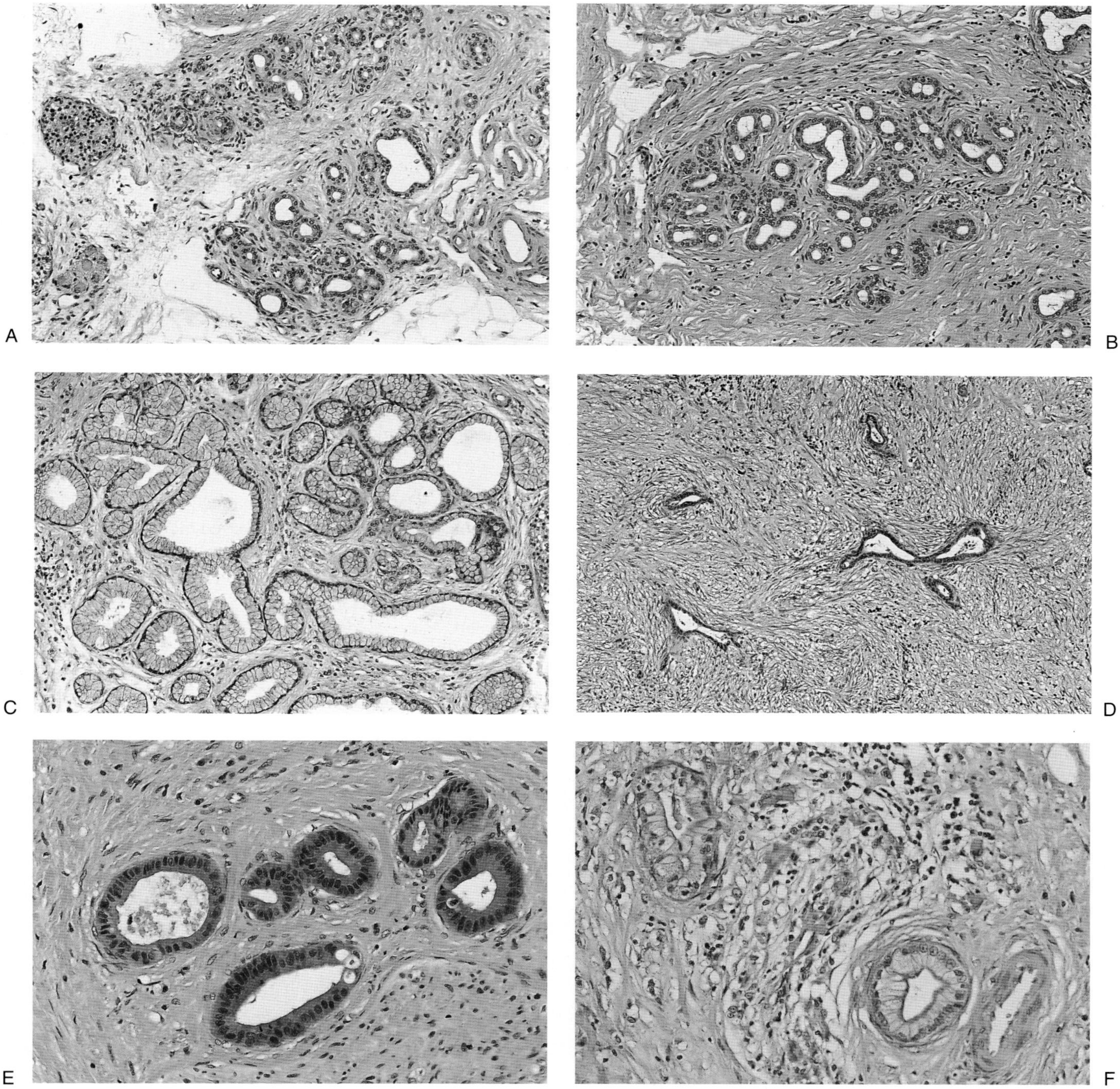


**FIG. 62.** Comparison of ductules in atrophic chronic pancreatitis with well-differentiated ductal adenocarcinoma. In chronic pancreatitis, there is often a preservation of the lobular arrangement of small ductules (**A**) with larger branching ductules surrounded by collections of smaller tubular glands. Some residual islets of Langerhans are also present. At higher power (**B**) the cells are generally uniform, with round nuclei having a similar cytologic appearance from cell to cell. In areas showing mucinous metaplasia (**C**), there may not be a lobular arrangement. However, the glands retain a benign cytologic appearance and have uniformly basally oriented nuclei. In infiltrating adenocarcinoma (**D**), the lobular arrangement of the glands is lost. There is a haphazard configuration of angulated glands within a desmoplastic stroma. In some instances (**E**) there may not be significant stromal desmoplasia and the glands may retain rounded contours. However, there is variability in cytologic appearance from one cell to the next, with occasional macronucleoli, loss of polarity, and mitotic figures. Some individual glands of infiltrating carcinoma may be almost impossible to distinguish from benign ductules (**F**). This remarkably well differentiated gland (*lower right*) contrasts with an adjacent gland showing marked loss of nuclear polarity.

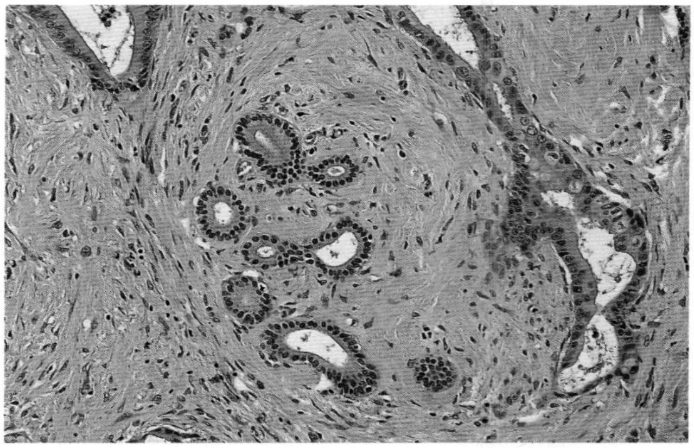

**FIG. 63.** It is helpful to identify two populations of cells in specimens harboring an infiltrating adenocarcinoma. In this example, a lobular collection of benign ductules contrasts with irregularly shaped glands of adenocarcinoma.

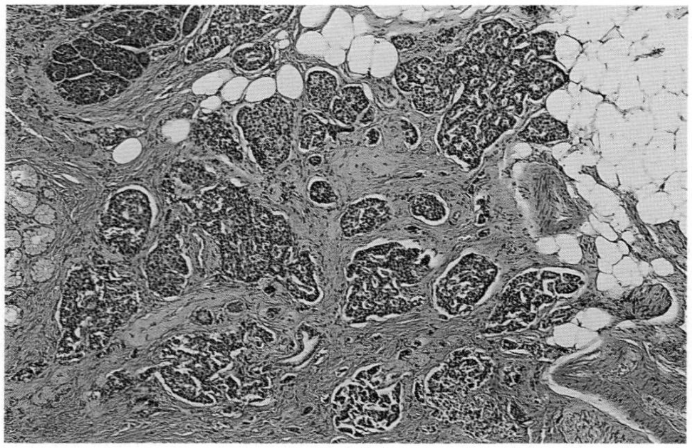

**FIG. 65.** When advanced atrophy of exocrine elements occurs, aggregation of the remaining endocrine elements may simulate a neoplasm. The nests of cells may be poorly circumscribed and separated by bands of fibrous tissue, with extension into peripancreatic adipose tissue.

largely around the periphery of the lobules, there is minimal acinar atrophy, and chronic inflammatory cells are evident (Fig. 61A). The gland may be enlarged. However, as chronic pancreatitis progresses, the fibrosis involves the entire lobule, with marked distortion of the architecture. There is marked (or even complete) acinar atrophy, and the ducts become ectatic and irregularly shaped (Fig. 61B). In experimental pancreatitis induced by duct ligation, acinar atrophy occurs by apoptosis (153,154), resulting in closely packed lobules of ductular structures. Small ductules and islets remaining after acinar atrophy become entrapped and distorted by the fibrous tissue (Fig. 61C), often acquiring a pseudoinfiltrative appearance. As the gland becomes replaced by fibrous tissue, it decreases in size and acquires a woody consistency. Inflammatory cells are sparse at this stage and may be aggregated around small nerves (112). Calcification and intraductal calculi may occur (155). The ducts may show metaplastic or hyperplastic changes, although these may not be increased in comparison with pancreata without chronic pancreatitis when they are systematically studied (121). It is also not clear that there is an increased incidence of atypical hyperplasia or carcinoma in situ in chronic pancreatitis (121), and other than the congenital type, chronic pancreatitis per se is only associated with a small increased risk for pancreatic cancer (156). It is likely that the foci of chronic pancreatitis that commonly accompany ductal adenocarcinomas are secondary to ductal obstruction by the tumor rather than a preexisting condition.

Biopsy samples of pancreata affected by chronic pancreatitis may be difficult to distinguish from those affected by infiltrating ductal adenocarcinoma. The distorted ducts and ductules in areas of fibrosis closely resemble the pattern of ductal adenocarcinoma, and the fibrotic stroma may simulate the desmoplastic stroma often accompanying carcinoma. Features that support the interpretation of chronic pancreatitis include a retention of the lobular architecture of the small collections of ductules, a lack of two cell populations (one

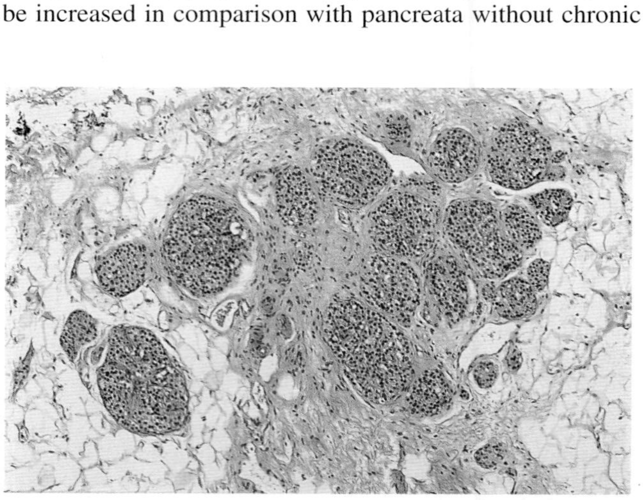

**FIG. 64.** With extreme atrophy, only residual islets of Langerhans remain, often surrounded by scanty fibrous stroma and adipose tissue.

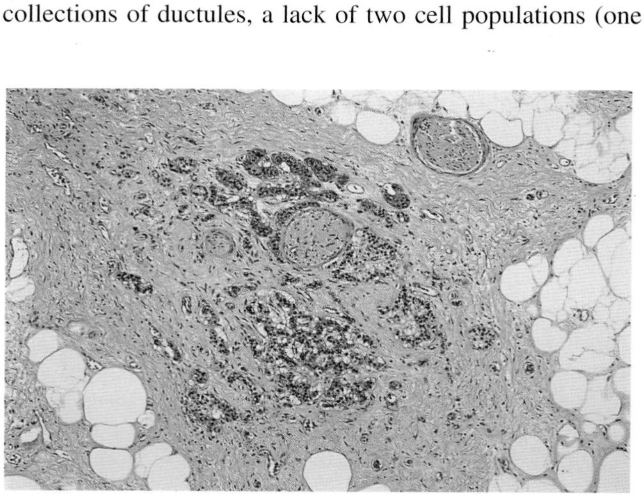

**FIG. 66.** Exocrine atrophy in areas containing diffuse-type islets results in a pseudoinfiltrative pattern of individual cells and trabeculae.

malignant, the other benign) within the same biopsy, uniformity of nuclear morphology from one cell to the next, and branching glands (Fig. 62A–C). Features that conversely favor the diagnosis of carcinoma include individual angulated glands infiltrating the stroma, "naked" glands in fat unsupported by connective tissue, two different populations of ductular structures (one with more atypical or enlarged nuclei), variation in shape and size of nuclei from one cell to the next, macronucleoli, loss of nuclear polarity, perineural invasion by glandular elements, markedly irregularly shaped glands, and individual cells or small cell clusters (Figs. 62D–F and 63). Unfortunately, biopsy samples of the pancreas are frequently small, and it is uncommon for all of the characteristic features to be present. Even if carcinoma is present, it may only be represented by two or three glands. Furthermore, needle biopsy samples are frequently subjected to frozen section examination, which may introduce artifacts complicating the interpretation. Even for the experienced observer, there may be cases having rare atypical glands that cannot be confidently diagnosed as benign or malignant. Performance of serial sections sometimes reveals additional diagnostic features.

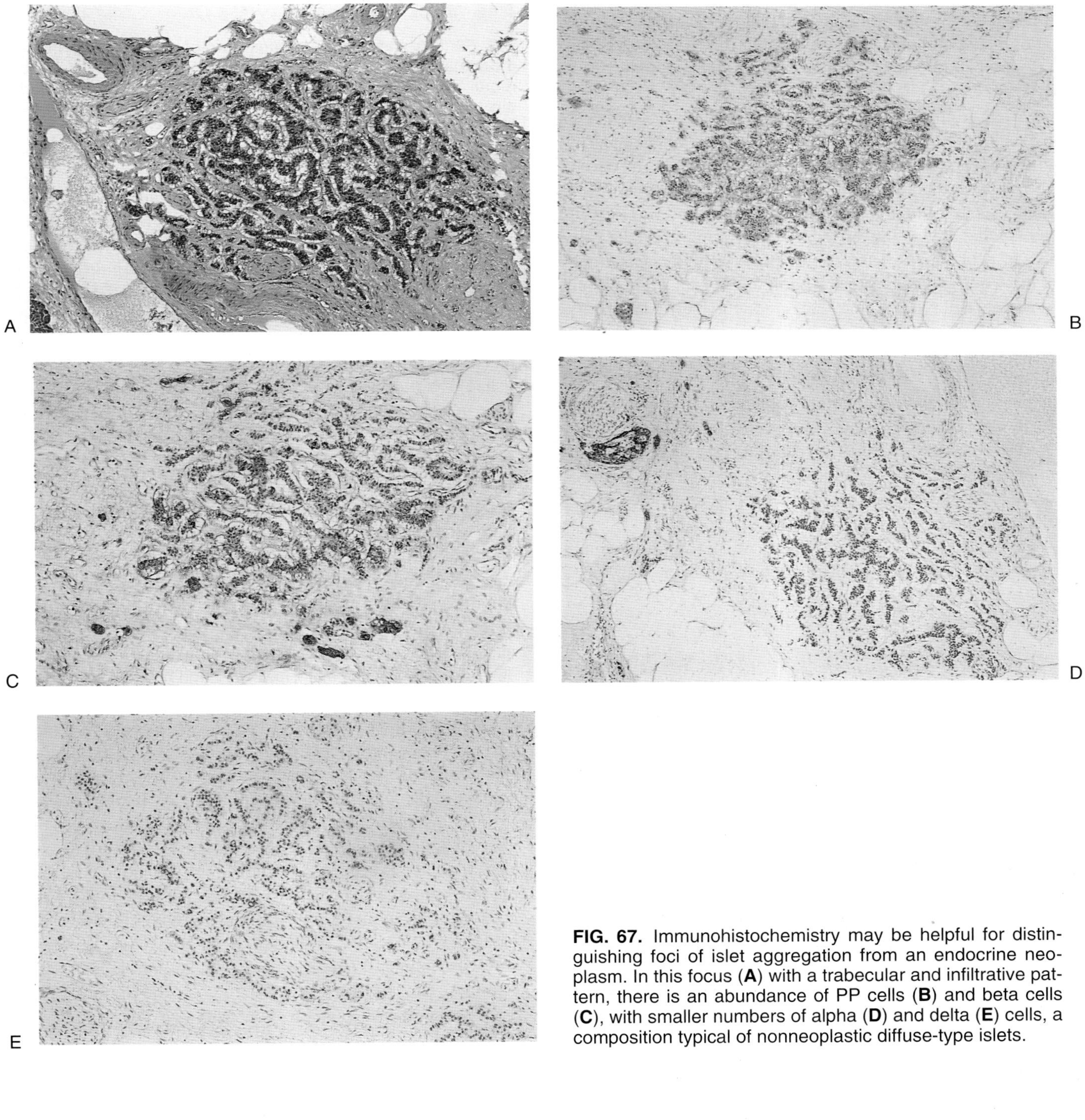


**FIG. 67.** Immunohistochemistry may be helpful for distinguishing foci of islet aggregation from an endocrine neoplasm. In this focus (**A**) with a trabecular and infiltrative pattern, there is an abundance of PP cells (**B**) and beta cells (**C**), with smaller numbers of alpha (**D**) and delta (**E**) cells, a composition typical of nonneoplastic diffuse-type islets.

Eventually in chronic pancreatitis even the ducts become atrophic, leaving only residual islets embedded in fibrous or adipose tissue (Fig. 64) (119). The clustering together of islets that results from atrophy of the exocrine elements has been termed "islet aggregation." In addition, some degree of islet cell proliferation may occur (157); however, islet aggregation should be distinguished from true islet cell hyperplasia, where there is an absolute increase in the volume of endocrine tissue as determined morphometrically. The clustering of islets found in regions of severe atrophy may result in the appearance of a solid tumorlike process with a nesting pattern, reminiscent of a pancreatic endocrine neoplasm (Fig. 65). Individual islets may extend into the peripancreatic adipose tissue, simulating invasion. The appearance of infiltration is even more marked when the process involves the regions of the head of the pancreas containing the diffuse islets; these islets lack the insular arrangement of the compact islets from the tail and appear as small clusters, trabeculae, and individual cells when the acinar elements undergo atrophy (Fig. 66). In contrast to most pancreatic endocrine neoplasms, the border of foci of islet aggregation is ill defined. The surrounding pancreas often exhibits areas of pancreatitis that are less advanced, with incomplete acinar atrophy. In problematic cases, immunohistochemical staining for the specific peptides may be helpful. In islet aggregation, the normal cell types are present, in roughly normal numbers and distribution, although the relative proportions of alpha and PP cells may be increased (90,157). Although more than one peptide may be expressed in endocrine neoplasms, it is exceptional for all of the normal peptides to be found in normal numbers, and there may be expression of ectopic peptides (vasoactive intestinal polypeptide or gastrin) not found in normal islets. Bear in mind that the diffuse islets have a different normal peptide cell constitution (abundance of PP cells) from that of the compact islets (Fig. 67).

Another pseudoneoplastic property of islet cells in chronic pancreatitis is the ability of perineural invasion (Fig. 68).

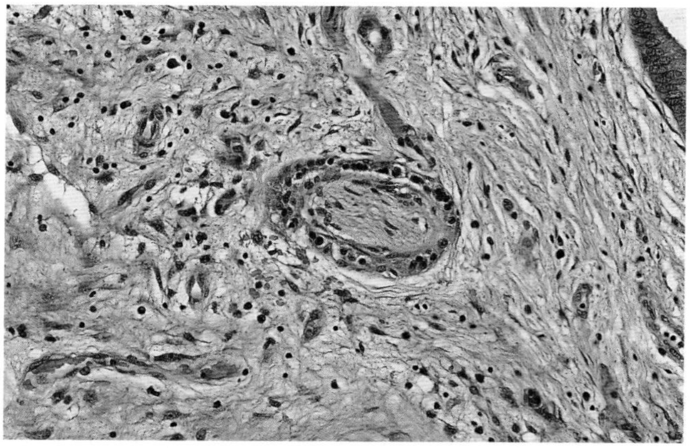

**FIG. 68.** Perineural invasion by islet cells in chronic pancreatitis may simulate carcinoma.

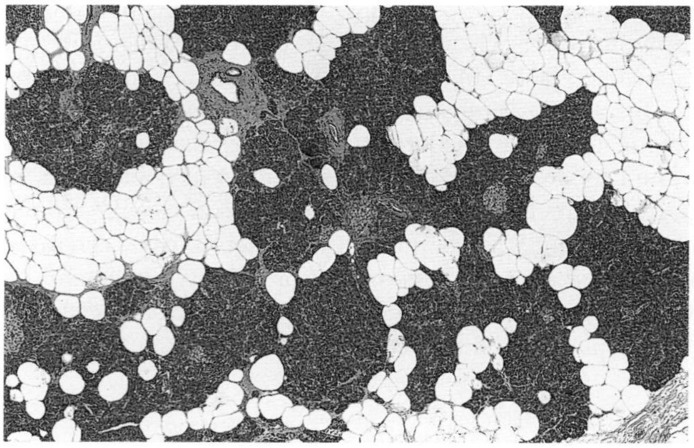

**FIG. 69.** In pancreatic lipomatosis, adipose tissue comprises more than 25% of the volume of the gland. As in this case, the remaining parenchyma may not necessarily show changes of atrophic chronic pancreatitis.

Small clusters of islet cells may extend along nerves, simulating the perineural invasion that is so common in pancreatic adenocarcinoma. Fortunately, benign glands do not exhibit perineural invasion. Thus, immunohistochemical staining for chromogranin may be used to distinguish benign perineural invasion by islet cells from adenocarcinoma.

Although atrophy and fibrosis generally occur as a result of chronic pancreatitis, they probably also occur through other mechanisms (112). By the time fibrosis is well established, the mechanism underlying it may be impossible to determine. Some degree of fibrosis is found in approximately two thirds of pancreata at autopsy (158). Pancreatic fibrosis has been related to increasing age (7), as well as to type II diabetes mellitus (158). Fibrosis may be largely periductal or may involve the pancreatic interstitium. Coexistent acinar atrophy, mucinous metaplasia of the ducts and ductules, and chronic inflammation are commonly found (158,159), and many observers regard such foci of pancreatic fibrosis to likely represent healed areas of pancreatitis.

Atrophy of pancreatic parenchyma due to long-standing ductal obstruction is often associated with infiltration by adipose tissue. Only rare islets may be found between lobules of fat in extreme cases (Fig. 64). A rare primary form of fatty infiltration is Shwachman's syndrome or lipomatous pseudohypertrophy, which affects children (160). Lipomatous pseudohypertrophy may result in an enlarged gland, but the amount of parenchymal tissue is reduced and exocrine insufficiency is present (10). The term "lipomatosis" has been applied to pancreata containing more than 25% adipose tissue (Fig. 69). The distribution of the adipose tissue is generally not uniform. Lipomatosis is generally associated with a degree of parenchymal atrophy and is more common in older individuals (7). Other associations include adult-onset diabetes and generalized atherosclerosis, conditions that are also more prevalent in the elderly. Pancreatic lipomatosis is not associated with generalized obesity (7).

## REFERENCES


1. Fawcett DW. *Bloom and Fawcett. A textbook of histology*. 12th ed. New York: Chapman & Hall; 1994.
2. Moore KL. *Clinically oriented anatomy*. Baltimore: Williams & Wilkins; 1980.
3. Pansky B. Anatomy of the pancreas. Emphasis on blood supply and lymphatic drainage. *Int J Pancreatol* 1990;7:101–108.
4. Bockman DE. Anatomy of the pancreas. In: Go VLW, Brooks FP, DiMagno EP, Gardner JD, Lebenthal E, Scheele GA, eds. *The exocrine pancreas. Biology, pathobiology, and diseases*. New York: Raven Press; 1986:1–7.
5. Skandalakis LJ, Rowe JS, Gray SW, Skandalakis JE. Surgical embryology and anatomy of the pancreas. *Surg Clin North Am* 1993;73: 661–697.
6. Cubilla AL, Fortner J, Fitzgerald PJ. Lymph node involvement in carcinoma of the head of the pancreas area. *Cancer* 1978;41:880–887.
7. Stamm BH. Incidence and diagnostic significance of minor pathologic changes in the adult pancreas at autopsy: a systematic study of 112 autopsies in patients without known pancreatic disease. *Hum Pathol* 1984;15:677–683.
8. Heitz PU, Beglinger C, Gyr K. Anatomy and physiology of the exocrine pancreas. In: Kloppel G, Heitz PU, eds. *Pancreatic pathology*. New York: Churchill-Livingstone; 1984:3–21.
9. Birstingl MA. Study of pancreatography. *Br J Surg* 1959;47:128–139.
10. Cubilla AL, Fitzgerald PJ. Tumors of the exocrine pancreas. In: Hartmann WH, Sobin LH, eds. *Atlas of tumor pathology*. 2nd series, fascicle 19. Washington, DC: Armed Forces Institute of Pathology; 1984.
11. Kozu T, Suda K, Toki F. Pancreatic development and anatomic variation. *Pancreatography* 1995:5;1–30.
12. Baggenstoss AH. Major duodenal papilla. Variations of pathologic interest and lesions of the mucosa. *Arch Pathol* 1938;26:853–868.
13. DiMagno EP, Shorter RG, Taylor WF, Go VLW. Relationships between pancreatobiliary ductal anatomy and pancreatic ductal and parenchymal histology. *Cancer* 1982;49:361–368.
14. Flati G, Flati D, Porowska B, Ventura T, Catarci M, Carboni M. Surgical anatomy of the papilla of Vater and biliopancreatic ducts. *Am Surg* 1994;60:712–718.
15. Frierson HF. The gross anatomy and histology of the gallbladder, extrahepatic bile ducts, Vaterian system, and minor papilla. *Am J Surg Pathol* 1989;13:146–162.
16. Corliss CE. *Patten's human embryology. Elements of clinical development*. New York: McGraw-Hill; 1976.
17. Lebenthal E, Lev R, Lee PC. Prenatal and postnatal development of the human exocrine pancreas. In: Go VLW, Brooks FP, DiMagno EP, Gardner JD, Lebenthal E, Scheele GA, eds. *The exocrine pancreas. Biology, pathobiology, and diseases*. New York: Raven Press; 1986:33–43.
18. Conklin JL. Cytogenesis of the human fetal pancreas. *Am J Anat* 1962; 111:181–189.
19. Chong JM, Fukayama M, Shiozawa Y, et al. Fibrillary inclusions in neoplastic and fetal acinar cells of the pancreas. *Virchows Arch* 1996; 428:261–266.
20. Laitio M, Lev R, Orlic D. The developing human fetal pancreas: an ultrastructural and histochemical study with special reference to exocrine cells. *J Anat* 1974;117:619–634.
21. Hassan MO, Gogate PA. Malignant mixed exocrine-endocrine tumor of the pancreas with unusual intracytoplasmic inclusions. *Ultrastruct Pathol* 1993;17:483–493.
22. Klimstra DS, Heffess CS, Oertel JE, Rosai J. Acinar cell carcinoma of the pancreas. A clinicopathologic study of 28 cases. *Am J Surg Pathol* 1992;16:815–837.
23. Klimstra DS, Rosai J, Heffess CS. Mixed acinar-endocrine carcinomas of the pancreas. *Am J Surg Pathol* 1994;18:765–778.
24. Klimstra DS, Wenig BM, Adair CF, Heffess CS. Pancreatoblastoma. A clinicopathologic study and review of the literature. *Am J Surg Pathol* 1995;19:1371–1389.
25. Kuopio T, Ekfors TO, Nikkanen V, Nevelainen TJ. Acinar cell carcinoma of the pancreas. Report of three cases. *APMIS* 1995;103:69–78.
26. Tucker JA, Shelburne JBD, Benning TL, Yacoub L, Federman M. Filamentous inclusions in acinar cell carcinoma of the pancreas. *Ultrastruct Pathol* 1994;18:279–286.
27. Kloppel G, Lenzen S. Anatomy and physiology of the endocrine pancreas. In: Kloppel G, Heitz PU, eds. *Pancreatic pathology*. New York: Churchill-Livingstone; 1984:133–153.
28. Robb P. The development of the islets of Langerhans in the human fetus. *Q J Exp Physiol* 1961;46:335–343.
29. Clark A, Grant AM. Quantitative morphology of endocrine cells in human fetal pancreas. *Diabetologia* 1983;25:31–35.
30. Grasso S, Palumbo G, Fallucca F, Lanzafame S, Indelicato B, San-Filippo S. The development and function of the endocrine pancreas of fetuses and infants born to normal and diabetic mothers. *Acta Endocrinol* 1986;112(suppl 277):130–135.
31. Albores-Saavedra J, Gould EW, Angeles-Angeles A, Henson DE. Cystic tumors of the pancreas. *Pathol Annu* 1990;25:19–50.
32. Compagno J, Oertel JE. Mucinous cystic neoplasms of the pancreas with overt and latent malignancy (cystadenocarcinoma and cystadenoma). *Am J Clin Pathol* 1978;69:573–580.
33. Newman BM, Lebenthal E. Congenital abnormalities of the exocrine pancreas. In: Go VLW, Brooks FP, DiMagno EP, Gardner JD, Lebenthal E, Scheele GA, eds. *The exocrine pancreas. Biology, pathobiology, and diseases*. New York: Raven Press; 1986:773–782.
34. Pang L-C. Pancreatic heterotopia: a reappraisal and clinicopathologic analysis of 32 cases. *South Med J* 1988;81:1264–1275.
35. Barbosa J, Dockerty MB, Waugh JM. Pancreatic heterotropia: surgical cases. *Proc Mayo Clin* 1946;21:246–255.
36. Lai ECS, Tompkins RK. Heterotopic pancreas. Review of 26 year experience. *Am J Surg* 1986;151:697–700.
37. Dolan RV, ReMine WH, Dockerty MB. The fate of heterotopic pancreatic tissue. A study of 212 cases. *Arch Surg* 1974:109:762–765.
38. Laughlin EH, Keown ME, Jackson JE. Heterotopic pancreas obstruction the ampulla of Vater. *Arch Surg* 1983;118:979–980.
39. Tsunoda T, Eto T, Yamada M, et al. Heterotopic pancreas: a rare cause of bile duct dilatation. Report of a case and review of the literature. *Jpn J Surg* 1990;20:217–220.
40. Seifert G. Congenital anomalies. In: Kloppel G, Heitz PU, eds. *Pancreatic pathology*. New York: Churchill-Livingstone; 1984:22–26.
41. Murayama H, Kikuchi M, Imai T. A case of heterotopic pancreas in lymph node. *Virchows Arch [A]* 1978;377:175–179.
42. Goldfarb WB, Bennett D, Monafo W. Carcinoma in heterotopic gastric pancreas. *Ann Surg* 1963;158:56–58.
43. Persson GE, Boiesen PT. Cancer of aberrant pancreas in jejunum. Case report. *Acta Chir Scand* 1988;154:599–601.
44. Tanimura A, Yamamoto H, Shibata H, Sano E. Carcinoma in heterotopic gastric pancreas. *Acta Pathol Jpn* 1979;29:251–257.
45. Doglioni C, Laurino L, Dei Tos A, et al. Pancreatic (acinar) metaplasia of the gastric mucosa: histology, ultrastructure, immunocytochemistry and clinicopathologic correlation of 101 cases. *Am J Surg Pathol* 1993;17:1134–1143.
46. Krishnamurthy S, Dayal Y. Pancreatic metaplasia in Barrett's esophagus: an immunohistochemical study. *Am J Surg Pathol* 1995;19: 1172–1180.
47. Landry MM, Sarma DP. Accessory spleen in the tail of the pancreas. *Hum Pathol* 1989;20:497.
48. Solcia E, Capella C, Kloppel G. Tumors of the pancreas. In: Rosai J, Sobin LH, eds. *Atlas of tumor pathology*. 3rd series, fascicle. Washington, DC: Armed Forces Institute of Pathology; 1996.
49. Dawson W, Langman J. An anatomical–radiological study on the pancreatic duct pattern in man. *Anat Rec* 1961;139:59–68.
50. Cotton PB. Pancreas divisum. *Pancreas* 1988;3:245–247.
51. Leese T, Chiche L, Bismuth H. Pancreatitis caused by congenital anomalies of the pancreatic ducts. *Surgery* 1989;105:125–130.
52. Kimura K, Ohto M, Saisho H, et al. Association of gallbladder carcinoma and anomalous pancreatobiliary ductal union. *Gastroenterology* 1985;89:1258–1265.
53. Kinoshita H, Nagata E, Hirohashi K, Sakai K, Kobayashi Y. Carcinoma of the gallbladder with anomalous connection between the choledochus and the pancreatic duct. *Cancer* 1984;54:762–769.
54. Krishnamurty VS, Rajendran S, Korsten MA. Bifid pancreas. An unusual anomaly associated with acute pancreatitis. *Int J Pancreatol* 1994;16:179–181.
55. Kiernan PD, ReMine SG, Kiernan PC, ReMine WH. Annular pancreas: Mayo clinic experience from 1957 to 1976 with review of the literature. *Arch Surg* 1980;115:46–50.
56. Lloyd-Jones W, Mountain JC, Warren KW. Annular pancreas in the adult. *Ann Surg* 1972;176:163–170.
57. England RE, Newcomer MK, Leung JW, Cotton PB. Case report: annular pancreas divisum—a report of two cases and review of the literature. *Br J Radiol* 1995;68:324–328.

58. Ravitch MM, Woods AC. Annular pancreas. *Ann Surg* 1950;132: 1116–1127.
59. Dowsett JF, Rode J, Russell RCG. Annular pancreas: a clinical, endoscopic, and immunohistochemical study. *Gut* 1989;30:130–135.
60. Akao S, Bockman DE, Lechene De La Porte P, Sarles H. Three-dimensional pattern of ductuloacinar associations in normal and pathological human pancreas. *Gastroenterology* 1986;90:661–668.
61. Henderson JR, Daniel PM, Fraser PA. The pancreas as a single organ: the influence of the endocrine upon the exocrine part of the gland. *Gut* 1981;22:158–167.
62. Williams JA, Goldfine ID. The insulin-acinar relationship. In: Go VLW, Brooks FP, DiMagno EP, Gardner JD, Lebenthal E, Scheele GA, eds. *The exocrine pancreas. Biology, pathobiology, and diseases*. New York: Raven Press; 1986:347–360.
63. Hoorens A, LeMoine NR, McLellan F, et al. Pancreatic acinar cell carcinoma: an analysis of cell lineage markers, p53 expression, and K-ras mutation. *Am J Pathol* 1993;143:685–698.
64. Bendayan M, Roth J Perrelet A, Orci L. Quantitative immunocytochemical localization of pancreatic secretory proteins in subcellular compartment of the rat acinar cells. *J Histochem Cytochem* 1980;28: 149–160.
65. Krahenbuhl JP, Racine L, Jamieson JD. Immunohistochemical localization of secretory proteins in bovine pancreatic exocrine cells. *J Cell Biol* 1977;72:406–423.
66. Kern HF. Fine structure of the human exocrine pancreas. In: Go VLW, Brooks FP, DiMagno EP, Gardner JD, Lebenthal E, Scheele GA, eds. *The exocrine pancreas. Biology, pathobiology, and diseases*. New York: Raven Press; 1986:9–19.
67. Palade GE. Intracellular aspects of the process of protein secretion. *Science* 1975;189:347–358.
68. Romagnoli P. Increases in apical plasma membrane surface paralelling enzyme secretion from exocrine pancreatic acinar cells. *Pancreas* 1988;3:189–192.
69. Kodama T. A light and electron microscopic study on the pancreatic ductal system. *Acta Pathol Jpn* 1983;33:297–321.
70. Greider MH. Oxyphil cells of the human pancreas. *Anat Rec* 1967; 157:251.
71. Roberts PF, Burns J. A histochemical study of mucins in normal and neoplastic human pancreatic tissue. *J Pathol* 1972;107:87–94.
72. Schulz I. Electrolyte and fluid secretion in the exocrine pancreas. In: Johnson LR, ed. *Physiology of the gastrointestinal tract*. New York: Raven Press; 1981:795–819.
73. Spicer SS, Sens MA, Tashian RE. Immunocytochemical demostration of carbonic anhydrase in human epithelial cells. *J Histochem Cytochem* 1982;30:864–873.
74. Atkinson BF, Ernst CS, Herlyn M, Steplewski Z, Sears HF, Koprowski H. Gastrointestinal cancer–associated antigen in immunoperoxidase study. *Cancer Res* 1982;42:4820–4823.
75. Borowitz MJ, Tuck FL, Sindelar WF, Fernsten PD, Metzgar RS. Monoclonal antibodies against human pancreatic adenocarcinoma: distribution of DU-PAN2 antigen on glandular epithelia and adenocarcinomas. *J Natl Cancer Inst* 1984;72:999–1003.
76. Haglund C, Lindgren J, Roberts PJ, Nordling S. Gastrointestinal cancer–associated antigen CA 19-9 in histological specimens of pancreatic tumours and pancreatitis. *Br J Cancer* 1986;53:189–195.
77. Klimstra DS, Hameed MR, Marrero AM, Conlon KC, Brennan MF. Ductal proliferative lesion associated with infiltrating ductal adenocarcinoma of the pancreas. *Int J Pancreatol* 1994;16:224–225.
78. Sessa F, Bonato M, Frigerio B, et al. Ductal cancers of the pancreas frequently express markers of gastrointestinal epithelial cells. *Gastroenterology* 1990;98:1655–1665.
79. Kim J-H, Ho SB, Montgomery CK, Kim YS. Cell lineage markers in human pancreatic cancer. *Cancer* 1990;66:2134–2143.
80. Rahier J, Wallon J, Henquin JC. Cell populations in the endocrine pancreas of human neonates and infants. *Diabetologia* 1981;20:540–546.
81. Wittingen J, Frey CF. Islet concentration in the head, body, tail, and uncinate process of the pancreas. *Ann Surg* 1974;179:412–414.
82. Stefan Y, Grasso S, Perrelet A, Orci L. A quantitative immunofluorescent study of the endocrine cell populations in the developing human pancreas. *Diabetes* 1983;32:293–301.
83. Scaglia L, Smith EE, Bonner-Weir S. Apoptosis contributes to the involution of beta cell mass in the post partum rat pancreas. *Endocrinology* 1995;136:5461–5468.
84. Grube D, Bohn R. The microanatomy of human islets of Langerhans, with special reference to somatostatin (D-) cells. *Arch Histol Jpn* 1983;46:327–353.
85. Malaisse-Lagae F, Stefan Y, Cox J, Perrelet A, Orci L. Identification of a lobe in the adult human pancreas rich in pancreatic polypeptide. *Diabetologia* 1979;17:361–365.
86. Stefan Y, Grasso S, Perrelet A, Orci L. The pancreatic polypeptide-rich lobe of the human pancreas: definitive identification of its derivation from the ventral pancreatic primordium. *Diabetologia* 1982;23: 141–142.
87. Ehrie MG, Swartz FJ. Diploid, tetraploid and octaploid beta cells in the islets of Langerhans of the normal human pancreas. *Diabetes* 1974;23:583–588.
88. LeCompte PM, Merriam JC. Mitotic figures and enlarged nuclei in the islands of Langerhans in man. *Diabetes* 1962;11:35–39.
89. Pelletier G. Identification of four cell types in the human endocrine pancreas by immunoelectron microscopy. *Diabetes* 1977;26: 749–756.
90. Bommer G, Friedl U, Heitz PU, Kloppel G. Pancreatic PP cell distribution and hyperplasia. Immunocytochemical morphology in the normal human pancreas, in chronic pancreatitis and pancreatic carcinoma. *Virchows Arch [A]* 1980;387:319–331.
91. Orci L, Baetens D, Ravazzola M, Stefan Y, Malaisse-Lagae F. Pancreatic polypeptide and glucagon: non-random distribution in pancreatic islets. *Life Sci* 1976;19:1811–1816.
92. Orci L, Malaisse-Lagae F, Baetens D, Perrelet A. Pancreatic-polypeptide–rich regions in human pancreas. *Lancet* 1978;2:1200–1201.
93. Orci L, Stefan Y, Malaisse-Lagae F, Perrelet A. Instability of pancreatic endocrine cell populations throughout life. *Lancet* 1979; 1:615–616.
94. Fellinger EJ, Garin-Chesa P, Triche TJ, Huvos AG, Rettig WJ. Immunohistochemical analysis of Ewing's sarcoma cell surface antigen p30/32MIC2. *Am J Pathol* 1991;139:317–325.
95. Weidner N, Tjoe J. Immunohistochemical profile of monoclonal antibody O13: antibody that recognizes glycoprotein p30/32MIC2 and is useful in diagnosing Ewing's sarcoma and peripheral neuroepithelioma. *Am J Surg Pathol* 1994;18:486–494.
96. Kloppel G. Endokrines pankreas und diabetes mellitus. In: Doerr W, Seifert G, eds. *Spezielle pathologische anatomie*. Vol. 14. Berlin: Springer; 1981:523–728.
97. Chen J, Baithun SI, Pollock DJ, Berry CL. Argyrophilic and hormone immunoreactive cells in normal and hyperplastic pancreatic ducts and exocrine pancreatic carcinoma. *Virchows Arch [A]* 1988;413: 399–405.
98. Bendayan M. Presence of endocrine cells in pancreatic ducts. *Pancreas* 1987;2:393–397.
99. Oertel JE, Heffess CS, Oertel YC. Pancreas. In: Sternberg SS, ed. *Histology for pathologists*. New York: Raven Press; 1992:657–668.
100. Patchefsky AS, Solit R, Phillips LD, et al. Hydroxyindole-producing tumors of the pancreas. Carcinoid-islet cell tumors and oat cell carcinoma. *Ann Intern Med* 1972;77:53–61.
101. Wilson RW, Gal AA, Cohen C, DeRose PB, Millikan WJ. Serotonin immunoreactivity in pancreatic endocrine neoplasms (carcinoid tumors). *Mod Pathol* 1991;4:727–732.
102. Creutzfeldt W. Pancreatic endocrine tumors—the riddle of their origin and hormone secretion. *Israel J Med Sci* 1975;11:762–776.
103. Chey WY. Hormonal control of pancreatic exocrine secretion. In: Go VLW, Brooks FP, DiMagno EP, Gardner JD, Lebenthal E, Scheele GA, eds. *The exocrine pancreas. Biology, pathobiology, and diseases*. New York: Raven Press; 1986:301–313.
104. Henderson JR, Daniel PM. A comparative study of the portal vessels connecting the endocrine and exocrine pancreas, with a discussion of some functional implications. *Q J Exp Physiol* 1979;64:267–275.
105. Adeghate E, Donath T. Distribution of neuropeptide Y and vasoactive intestinal polypeptide immunoreactive nerves in normal and transplanted pancreatic tissue. *Peptides* 1990;11:1087–1092.
106. Olsen TS. Lipomatosis of the pancreas in autopsy material and its relation to age and overweight. *Acta Pathol Microbiol Immunol Scand [A]* 1978;86:367–373.
107. Orci L, Stefan Y, Malaisse-Lagae F, Perrelet A, Patel Y. Pancreatic fat. *N Engl J Med* 1979;301:1292.
108. Suda K, Mizuguchi K, Hoshino A. Differences of the ventral and dorsal anlagen of pancreas after fusion. *Acta Pathol Jpn* 1981;31: 583–589.
109. Shinozuka H, Lee RE, Dunn JL, Longnecker DS. Multiple atypical acinar cell nodules of the pancreas. *Hum Pathol* 1980;11:389–390.
110. Tanaka T, Mori Williams GM. Atypical and neoplastic acinar cell lesions of the pancreas in an autopsy study of Japanese patients. *Cancer* 1988;61:2278–2285.

111. Longnecker DS, Hashida Y, Shinozuka H. Relationship of age to prevalence of focal acinar cell dysplasia in the human pancreas. *J Natl Cancer Inst* 1980;65:63–66.
112. Oertel JE. The pancreas. Nonneoplastic alterations. *Am J Surg Pathol* 1989;13(suppl 1):50–65.
113. Longnecker DS. Lesions induced in rodent pancreas by azaserine and other pancreatic carcinogens. *Environ Health Perspect* 1984;56: 245–252.
114. Longnecker DS, Shinozuka H, Dekker A. Focal acinar cell dysplasia in human pancreas. *Cancer* 1980;45:534–540.
115. Kodama T, Mori W. Atypical acinar cell nodules of the human pancreas. *Acta Pathol Jpn* 1983;33:701–714.
116. Baggenstoss AH. The pancreas in uremia: a histopathologic study. *Am J Pathol* 1948;24:1003.
117. Walters MN-I. Studies on the exocrine pancreas. I. Non-specific pancreatic ductular ectasia. *Am J Pathol* 1964;44:973–981.
118. Walters MN-I. Goblet cell metaplasia in ductules and acini of the exocrine pancreas. *J Pathol* 1965;89:569–572.
119. Bockman DE, Boydston WR, Anderson MC. Origin of tubular complexes in human chronic pancreatitis. *Am J Surg* 1982;144:243–249.
120. Cubilla AL, Fitzgerald PJ. Morphological lesions associated with human primary invasive nonendocrine pancreas cancer. *Cancer Res* 1976;36:2690–2698.
121. Kloppel G, Bommer G, Ruckert K, Seifert G. Intraductal proliferation in the pancreas and its relationship to human and experimental carcinogenesis. *Virchows Arch [A]* 1980;387:221–233.
122. Roberts PF. Pyloric gland metaplasia of the human pancreas. A comparative histochemical study. *Arch Pathol* 1974;97:92–95.
123. Allen-Mersh TG. Pancreatic ductal mucinous hyperplasia: distribution within the pancreas, and effect of variation in ampullary and pancreatic duct anatomy. *Gut* 1988;29:1392–1396.
124. Klimstra DS, Longnecker DS. K-*ras* mutations in pancreatic ductal proliferative lesions [Letter]. *Am J Pathol* 1994;145:1547–1548.
125. DiGiuseppe JA, Hruban RH, Offerhaus GJA, et al. Detection of K-*ras* mutations in mucinous pancreatic duct hyperplasia from a patient with a family history of pancreatic carcinoma. *Am J Pathol* 1994;144: 889–895.
126. Yanagisawa A, Ohtake K, Ohashi K, et al. Frequent c-Ki-*ras* oncogene activation in mucous cell hyperplasias of pancreas suffering from chronic inflammation. *Cancer Res* 1993;53:953–956.
127. Pour PM, Sayed S, Sayed G. Hyperplastic, preneoplastic, and neoplastic lesions found in 83 human pancreases. *Am J Clin Pathol* 1982; 77:137–152.
128. Tasso F, Picard D. Sur les oncocytes du pancréas humain. *C R Soc Biol (Paris)* 1969;163:1855–1858.
129. Tasso F, Sarles H. Canalicular cells and oncocytes in the human pancreas. Comparative study on the normal condition and in chronic pancreatitis. *Ann Anat Pathol (Paris)* 1973;18:277–300.
130. Frexinos J, Ribet A. Oncocytes in human chronic pancreatitis. *Digestion* 1972;7:294–301.
131. Kozuka S, Sassa R, Taki T, et al. Relationship of pancreatic duct hyperplasia to carcinoma. *Cancer* 1979;43:1418–1428.
132. Mukada T, Yamada S. Dysplasia and carcinoma in situ of the exocrine pancreas. *Tohoku J Exp Med* 1982;137:115–124.
133. Boschman CR, Stryker S, Reddy JK, Rao MS. Expression of p53 protein in precursor lesions and adenocarcinoma of human pancreas. *Am J Pathol* 1994;145:1291–1295.
134. Hameed M, Marrero AM, Conlon KC, Brennan MF, Klimstra DS. Expression of p53 nucleophosphoprotein in *in situ* pancreatic ductal adenocarcinoma [Abstract]. *Mod Pathol* 1994;7:132.
135. Komatsu K. Pancreatographical and histopathological study of dilations of the pancreatic ductules with special references to cystic dilatation. *Juntendoo Med J* 1974;19:250–269.
136. Nagai E, Ueki T, Chijiiwa K, Tanaka M, Tsuneyoshi M. Intraductal papillary mucinous neoplasms of the pancreas associated with so-called "mucinous ductal ectasia." Histochemical and immunohistochemical analysis of 29 cases. *Am J Surg Pathol* 1995;19:576–589.
137. Nishihara K, Fukuda T, Tsuneyoshi M, Kominami T, Maeda S, Saku M. Intraductal papillary neoplasm of the pancreas. *Cancer* 1993;72: 689–696.
138. Sessa F, Solcia E, Capella C, et al. Intraductal papillary-mucinous tumours represent a distinct group of pancreatic neoplasms: an investigation of tumour cell differentiation and K-*ras*, p53 and c-*erb*B-2 abnormalities in 26 patients. *Virchows Arch* 1994;425:357–367.
139. Agostini S, Choux R, Payan M, Sastre B, Sahel J, Clement JP. Mucinous pancreatic duct ectasia in the body of the pancreas. *Radiology* 1989;170:815–816.
140. Tian F, Myles J, Howard JM. Mucinous pancreatic ductal ectasia of latent malignancy: an emerging clinicopathologic entity. *Surgery* 1992; 111:109–113.
141. Weidenheim KM, Hinchey WW, Campbell WG. Hyperinsulinemic hypoglycemia in adults with islet cell hyperplasia and degranulation of exocrine cells of the pancreas. *Am J Clin Pathol* 1983;79:14–24.
142. Jaffe R, Hashida Y, Yunis EJ. Pancreatic pathology in hyperinsulinemic hypoglycemia of infancy. *Lab Invest* 1980;42:356–365.
143. Gossens A, Gepts W, Saudubray JM, et al. Diffuse and focal nesidioblastosis: a clinicopathological study of 24 patients with persistent neonatal hyperinsulinemic hypoglycemia. *Am J Surg Pathol* 1989;13: 766–775.
144. Heitz PU, Kloppel G, Hacki WH, Polak JM, Pearse AGE. Nesidioblastosis: the pathologic basis of persistent hyperinsulinemic hypoglycemia in infants: morphologic and quantitative analysis of seven cases based on specific immunostaining and electron microscopy. *Diabetes* 1977;26:632–642.
145. Gould VE, Memoli VA, Dardi LE, Gould NS. Nesidiodysplasia and nesidioblastosis of infancy: ultrastructural and immunohistochemical analysis of islet cell alterations with and without associated hyperinsulinemic hypoglycemia. *Scand J Gastroenterol* 1981;16(suppl 70):129–142.
146. Witte DP, Greider MH, DeSchryver-Kecskemeti K, Kissane JM, White NH. The juvenile human endocrine pancreas: normal v. idiopathic hyperinsulinemic hypoglycemia. *Semin Diagn Pathol* 1984; 1:30–42.
147. Gould VE, Chejfec G, Shah K, Paloyan E, Lawrence AM. Adult nesidiodysplasia. *Semin Diagn Pathol* 1984;1:43–53.
148. Karnauchow PN. Nesidioblastosis in adults without insular hyperfunction. *Am J Clin Pathol* 1982;78:511–513.
149. Kovacs K, Horvath E, Asa SL, Murray D, Singer W, Reddy SSK. Microscopic peliosis of pancreatic islets in a woman with MEN-1 syndrome. *Arch Pathol Lab Med* 1986;110:607–610.
150. Kloppel G. Islet histopathology in diabetes mellitus. In: Kloppel G, Heitz PU, eds. *Pancreatic pathology*. New York: Churchill-Livingstone; 1984:154–192.
151. Kloppel G, Maillet B. Pathology of acute and chronic pancreatitis. *Pancreas* 1993;8:659–670.
152. Lilja P, Evander A, Ihse I. Hereditary pancreatitis. A report on two kindreds. *Acta Chir Scand* 1978;144:35–37.
153. Abe K, Watanabe S. Apoptosis of mouse pancreatic acinar cells after duct ligation. *Arch Histol Cytol* 1995;58:221–229.
154. Walker NI. Ultrastructure of the rat pancreas after experimental duct ligation. I. The role of apoptosis and intraepithelial macrophages in acinar cell deletion. *Am J Pathol* 1987;126:439–451.
155. Gyr K, Heitz PU, Beglinger C. Pancreatitis. In: Kloppel G, Heitz PU, eds. *Pancreatic pathology*. New York: Churchill-Livingstone; 1984: 44–72.
156. Lowenfels AB, Maisonneuve P, Cavallini G, et al. Pancreatitis and the risk of pancreatic cancer. *N Engl J Med* 1993;328:1433–1437.
157. Bartow SA, Mukai K, Rosai J. Pseudoneoplastic proliferation of endocrine cells in pancreatic fibrosis. *Cancer* 1981;47:2627–2633.
158. Shimizu M, Hayashi T, Saitoh Y, Itoh H. Interstitial fibrosis in the pancreas. *Am J Clin Pathol* 1989;91:531–534.
159. Olsen TS. The incidence and clinical relevance of chronic inflammation in the pancreas in autopsy material. *Acta Pathol Microbiol Scand [A]* 1978;86:361–365.
160. Seifert G. Lipomatous atrophy and other forms. In: Kloppel G, Heitz PU, eds. *Pancreatic pathology*. New York: Churchill-Livingstone; 1984:27–31.
161. Tremble IR, Parsons JW, Sherman CP. A one stage operation for the cure of carcinoma of the ampulla of vater and of the head of the pancreas. *Surg Gynecol Obstet* 1941;73:711.

# Hematopoietic and Lymphoid System

*Histology for Pathologists, second edition,*
Edited by Stephen S. Sternberg.
Lippincott-Raven Publishers, Philadelphia


# CHAPTER 28

# Reactive Lymph Nodes

Paul van der Valk and Chris J. L. M. Meijer



The function of the lymph nodes is to deal with antigen. This complex process requires uptake and processing of the antigen, eventually leading to its destruction (1). Because this function is crucial to the survival of the individual, lymph nodes are found throughout the body and are especially numerous in areas draining organs with environmental contact.

Thus, the respiratory and digestive tracts have large groups of draining lymph nodes: the hilar and mediastinal and the mesenteric lymph nodes, respectively. Likewise, the skin has groups of lymph nodes draining one or several areas (cervical, inguinal, axillary). The respiratory and digestive tracts also have structures resembling lymph nodes directly underneath their epithelium, the so-called mucosa-associated lymphoid tissue (MALT) (2–4). [These structures, which probably have a damping influence on some immunologic reactions (5), are not discussed here.] The whole system of draining lymph node groups (mediastinal, mesenteric, superficial and deep inguinal, axillary, cervical, etc.) converges onto a single lymphatic—the thoracic duct—which in turn drains into the bloodstream, creating an effective filtering system for purging unwanted substances.

P. van der Valk and C. J. L. M. Meijer: Department of Pathology, Free University Hospital, Amsterdam, The Netherlands.

It is this important role in reacting to antigens—that is, the immune response—that makes the lymph node such an intriguing organ. Because we encounter an enormous variety of antigenic challenges from our environment, the immune response must be a process of considerable complexity and adaptability. Thus, the immune system reacts to some classes of antigens differently than it does to others. For instance, reactions to certain macromolecules with repetitive features in their overall structure, such as lipopolysaccharides, are mediated by B-lymphocytes independent of T-lymphocytes, whereas reactions to most soluble antigens are T cell dependent; in addition, some reactions to particulate antigens require primarily T-lymphocytes (6). This is all reflected in lymph node histology, and this gives a normal, functioning lymph node its protean character.

## EMBRYOLOGY/PRENATAL CHANGES

Relatively little is known of the development of the lymph nodes in the embryonic period, but they arise from the lymphatic sacs, which in turn develop from the venous system. From these sacs a lymphatic plexus forms and in the first trimester small collections of lymphoblasts can be found in association with these plexus (7). In the second trimester the differentiation in a cortex and medulla takes place, gradually making recognizable the familiar compartmentalized structure of the lymph node parenchyma, probably also under the influence of appearing hematopoietic cells, such as macrophages and interdigitating cells (IDCs), and mesenchymally derived cells, i.e., dendritic and fibroblastic reticulum cells (FRCs).

After compartmentalization is completed, no specific changes take place other than those that follow antigenic challenge, and they are dependent on the type of antigen and not dependent on the developmental stage of the individual.

## APOPTOSIS

In the immune system, and therefore in the lymph node, apoptosis plays an important role. Through this mechanism the immune system removes cells (or cell clones) that are redundant or potentially dangerous (autoreactive immunocompetent cells). In the lymph node apoptosis is important in selecting cell clones that have maximum avidity, i.e., cells that produce the antibody with the best possible "fit" for any given antigen. With a suboptimal fit, *bcl-2* expression is not induced, and this eventually leads to activation of the apoptotic pathway and the death of the cell (8). Thus, only cells producing antibodies with high avidity are selected to survive and go on to produce antibodies, or become memory cells. The *bcl*-2 gene product is instrumental in this process, and under normal circumstances expression of this protein is low in the area where this selection process takes place, the follicle (Fig. 1). In follicular lymphomas the *bcl*-2 gene on chromosome 18 is translocated to chromosome 14, bringing it under control of the immunoglobulin gene promotor, leading to *bcl*-2 overexpression. This overexpression blocks apoptosis, causing follicle center cells to accumulate, thus contributing to lymphomagenesis. In several reactive conditions, massive apoptosis takes place, including follicular hyperplasia (a physiologic response in selecting high-avidity antibodies), histiocytic necrotizing lymphadenitis (Kikuchi's disease), and some viral infections.

## GROSS FEATURES

Reactive lymph nodes are mostly small structures, round or reniform. If they are detectable, it usually means there is some enlargement through immunologic reactivity/stimulation. Normally they do not exceed a diameter of 1 cm, but during immune reactions they can become much larger. A diameter of more than 3 cm is relatively uncommon and should raise suspicions of an underlying malignant condition. Their cut surfaces normally are pinkish and homogenous. A white cut surface or distinct nodular changes are suspicious. Sometimes they resemble fatty tissue, especially in fixed axillary dissection preparations or in mesenteric fat. In those cases, however, their resistance to the palpating finger gives them away.

## ANATOMY

### Blood Supply

Arteries enter the lymph node at the hilus, then branch and form a capillary network in the parenchyma, both in the paracortex and the follicles. Subtle differences in the basal membrane of the capillaries at these two locations exist, with exclusive expression of kalinin (i.e. type 5 laminin) in the follicular capillary basal membrane (9). These compartment-specific differences probably play a role in positioning lym-

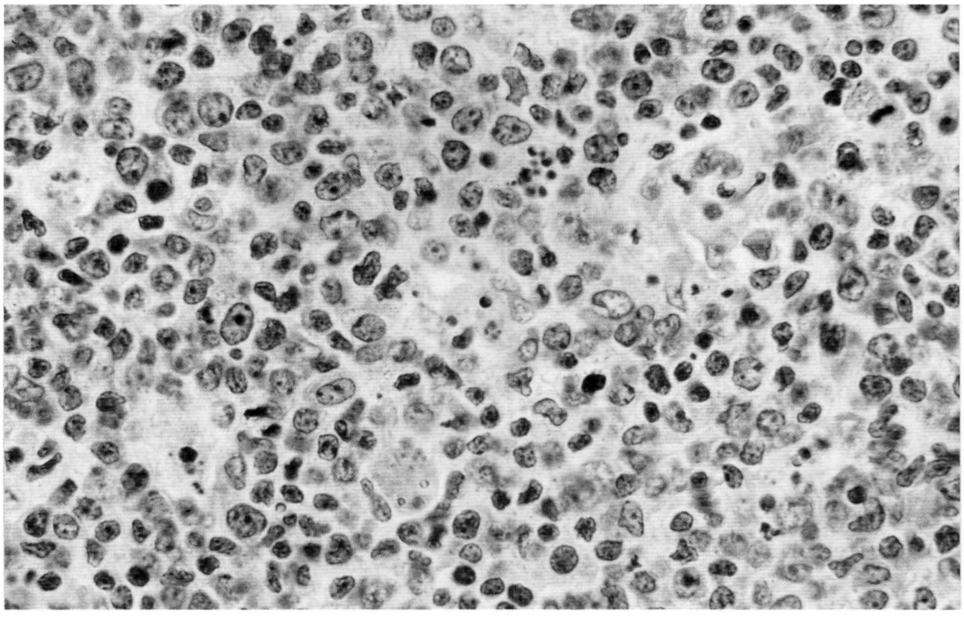

**FIG. 1.** Apoptosis in follicle center (H&E-stained paraffin section). Numerous small, dark and round bodies are seen, indicating a high rate of apoptosis in this area.

phocytes in the different compartments. Venous drainage accompanies the arteriolar route, and the vein leaves the lymph node in the hilus. The postcapillary venules have a specific function in the lymph node because they are the gate of entry of circulating lymphocytes into the lymph node parenchyma. These venules are discussed in more detail later.

### Lymphatics

Afferent lymphatics enter the lymph node in the subcapsular sinus. This sinus has an endothelial layer, but the system of branching sinuses that arises from it, and eventually drains into the efferent lymph vessels in the hilus, has no endothelial lining.

## LIGHT MICROSCOPY

Examination of a lymph node section at low power shows four compartments (Fig. 2A); most obvious are the round structures surrounded by a darker rim, the follicles. The germinal center may have a mottled appearance. Follicles usually are found near the capsule (the area of the cortex) but also may be present deeper in the lymph node substance. Between the follicles and extending to the deeper layers is a

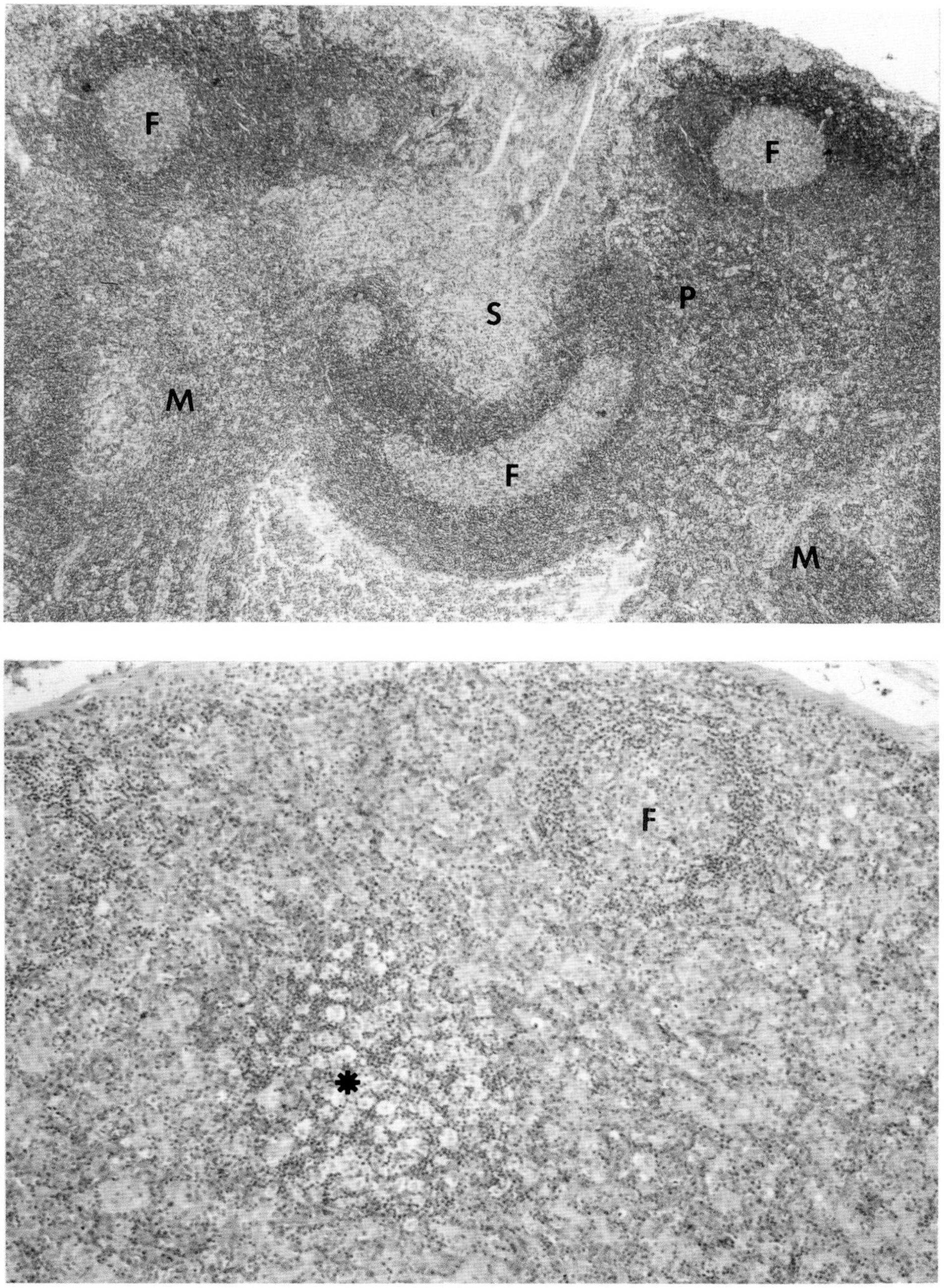


A

B

**FIG. 2. A:** Low-power view of lymph node [periodic acid-Schiff (PAS)-stained, paraffin-embedded section] illustrating the four different compartments of the lymph node. Note follicular hyperplasia (F), small paracortical areas (P), and, in the center, medullary cords (M) and sinuses (S). **B:** Low-power view of lymph node (H&E-stained, paraffin-embedded section). There is a considerable influx of macrophages and IDC. The typical mottling of the paracortex is seen in the center of the figure (*asterisk*).

less well-defined zone, mostly dark staining, but occasionally showing a mottling not unlike that seen in the follicle center (Fig. 2B), although usually not as pronounced. One feature of this area is the presence of epithelioid or postcapillary venules, which are lined with a plump, swollen endothelium. This area is known as the paracortical area or paracortex.

The third area is found in the medullary region of the lymph node. Here, between sinuses filled with macrophages, sheets of dark-staining cells with no mottling are found; in Giemsa-stained sections, occasional mast cells are seen. These sheets make up the medullary cords. The fourth compartment, the sinuses, are predominantly seen in the medullary region but also are present in the cortical area; an important sinus—the subcapsular sinus—is located directly beneath the capsule.

These four areas can be identified via low-power field screening (Fig. 2A), but their representation in each specimen is variable. For instance, medullary cords often are scarcely represented in specimens. This scarcity may be attributable to sampling error or may be physiologic in nature. Because we are in constant contact with antigens, a lymph node should always demonstrate some degree of stimulation. Depending on the kind of antigenic challenge, one (or more) of the compartments is stimulated, which results in an increase in the volume of that compartment (Fig. 3) or a shift in its cellular composition. In the latter instance, an increase in blast cells is often seen. Because blasts represent the proliferative phase of a reaction (10), their increase leads to expansion of the entire compartment.

This adaptability to the challenging antigen explains the variability in normal lymph node histology. As we have already indicated, most "normal" lymph nodes are stimulated to some degree.

Each of the four areas—follicles, medullary cords, paracortex, and sinuses—is discussed separately.

### Follicles

Distinction must be made between primary and secondary follicles. Primary follicles are aggregates of small, dark-

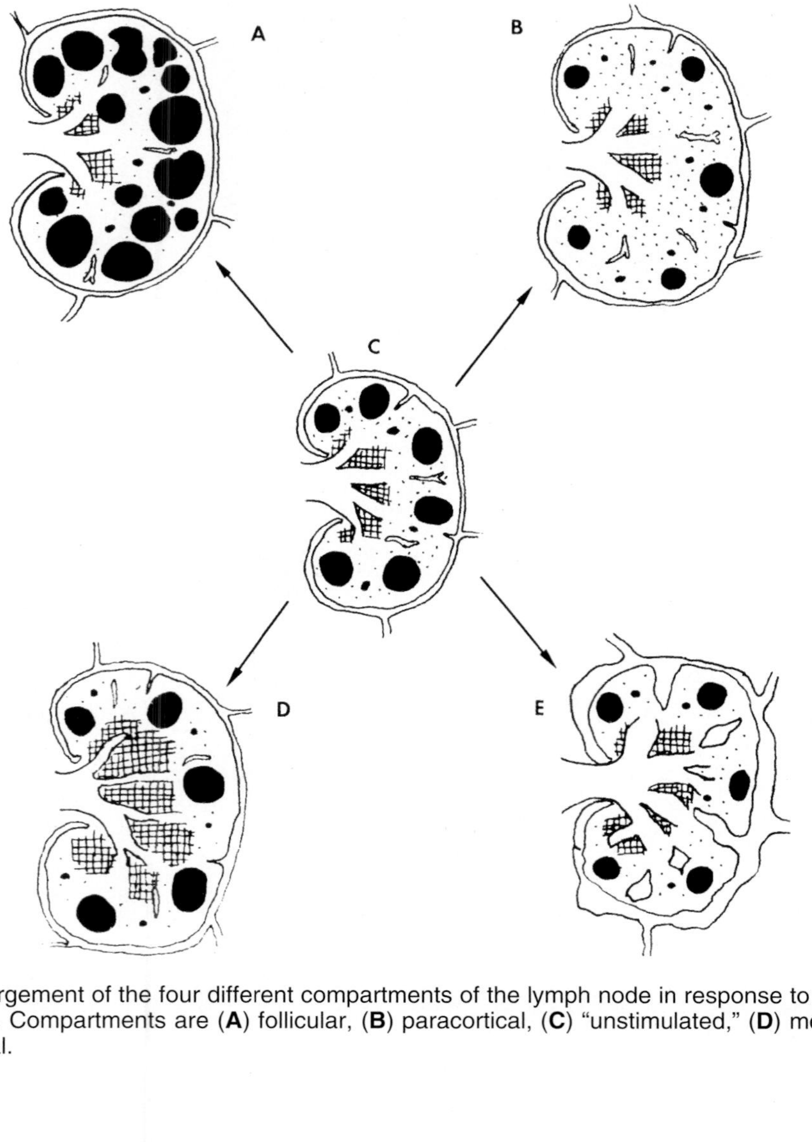


**FIG. 3.** Enlargement of the four different compartments of the lymph node in response to various antigenic stimuli. Compartments are (**A**) follicular, (**B**) paracortical, (**C**) "unstimulated," (**D**) medullary, and (**E**) sinusoidal.

staining lymphoid cells. When a (germinal) center develops in a primary follicle, it becomes a secondary follicle. The mantle zone around the follicle center thus has the same characteristics as the primary follicle. The outer layers of the mantle zone are somewhat less densely packed and, as in the spleen, this outer rim has been called the marginal zone (11). However, in the lymph node this marginal zone is more difficult to distinguish as its splenic counterpart.

In the follicle center, and thus in the follicle center cell reaction that takes place there, dendritic reticulum cells (DRCs), lymphoid cells, and tingible body macrophages all cooperate (Fig. 4A and B).

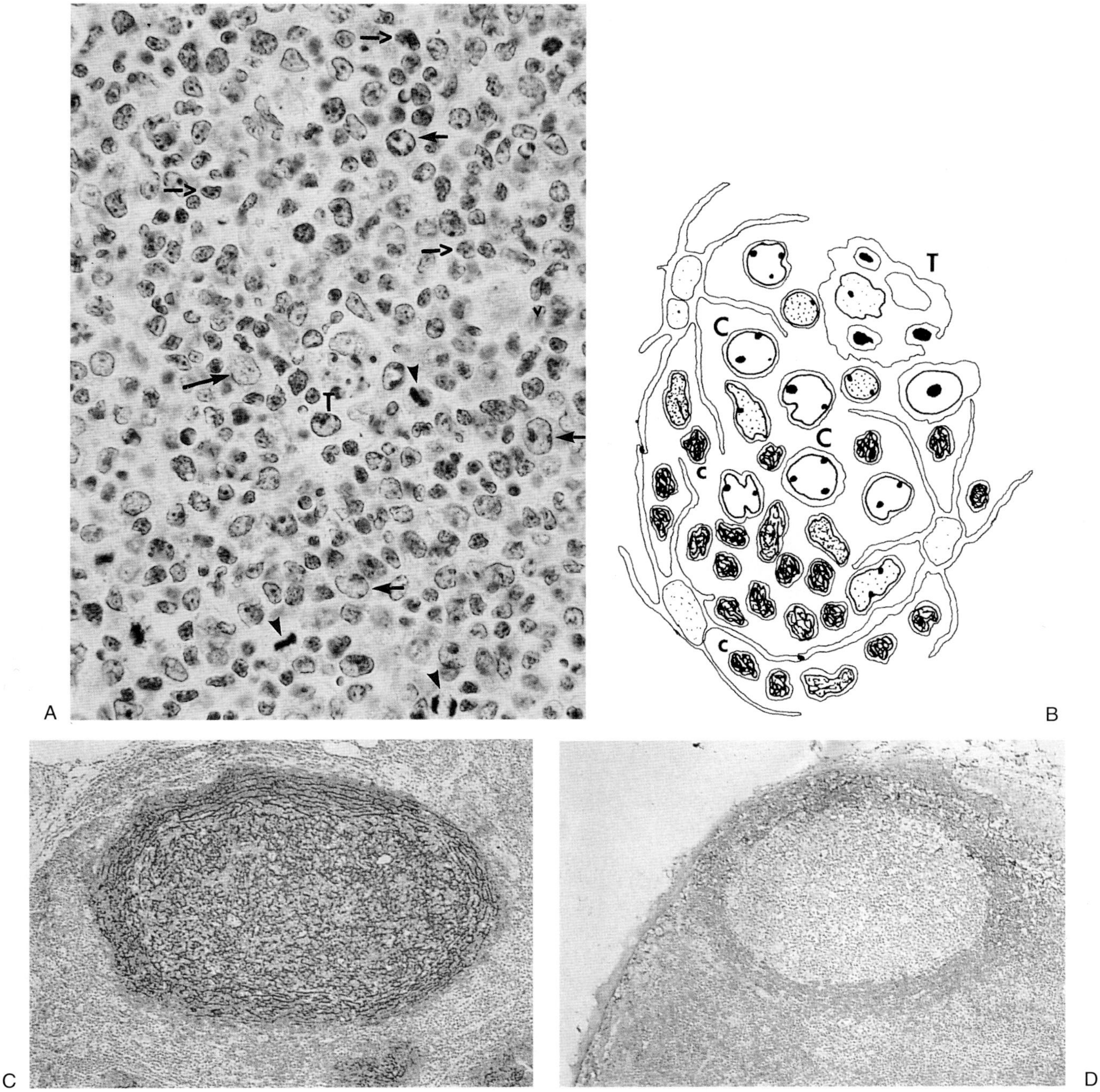


**FIG. 4. A:** Plastic-embedded, Giemsa-stained section. All typical elements are present: mitotic figures (*arrowheads*), a tingible body macrophage (T) with phagocytized debris (staining intensely black), large (*short arrows*) and small (*open arrows*) follicle center cells, and a DRC (*long arrow*). Note the elongation of several of the lymphoid cells. **B:** Diagrammatic representation of a follicle with the various elements. Note the DRC's protrusions. T, tingible body macrophage; c, small (cleaved) FCC; C, large (noncleaved) FCC. **C:** Frozen section stained with CD35 (anti–C3b receptor). Note the coarse staining of the DRC lattice. **D:** Frozen section stained for IgD. Cells in the mantle zone are clearly positive. Counterstained with hematoxylin.

### *Dendritic Reticulum Cells*

DRCs trap antigens on their surface, process/modulate them, and present them to B cells (12). Because these cells retain antigen on their surface, they can provide a long-lasting reaction to that antigen, which may be important in immune memory (13). DRCs, difficult to recognize in light microscopic sections, were first characterized by electron microscopy (12) and later by enzyme and immunohistochemistry (14–16). They have a medium-sized to large nucleus, often elongated, with a very fine chromatin pattern and an inconspicuous nucleolus. Occasionally the nucleus is binucleated. The cytoplasm is invisible with the light microscope. In immunohistochemical staining, it has many long and slender cytoplasmic protrusions (Fig. 4C). These are linked to the protrusions of other DRCs via (hemi)desmosomes (17), with which they form a network, and are thus also responsible for the typical structure of the follicle. Their origin is still a matter of debate, but an origin from (peri)vascular tissue as opposed to a derivation from the mononuclear phagocyte system (18) has been proposed (19).

### *Lymphoid Cells*

The lymphoid cells of the primary follicle and mantle zone have small, round to slightly irregular nuclei with a dark-staining, condensed chromatin. They have scanty cytoplasm. [The cells of the marginal zone may be slightly larger (11).] These cells are B cells, reacting with monoclonal antibodies directed against B cells (CD20, CD22, CD24). They express immunoglobulin (Ig)M and IgD on their surface (Fig. 4D) and are largely alkaline phosphatase positive (16,20–23). In the germinal center, distinctive B cells can be found:

1. Large noncleaved follicle center cells (FCCs) or centroblasts are large cells with large round or slightly irregular, vesicular nuclei with one to three small but conspicuous nucleoli located at the periphery of the nucleus (Fig. 4A and B). The cells have a narrow rim of basophilic cytoplasm. They are the proliferative cells of the follicle center; mitotic figures abound in areas where large noncleaved FCCs predominate (14).
2. Large and small cleaved FCCs or centrocytes probably develop from the large noncleaved FCCs, as morphologic and experimental (14) studies have shown. The large cleaved FCCs have medium-sized to large nuclei with mostly inconspicuous, marginal nucleoli and a finely dispersed chromatin. Small cleaved FCCs have small, irregular nuclei with small clefts or an angular appearance with condensed chromatin. Cleaved FCCs often show elongated nuclei and have little cytoplasm.
3. Small noncleaved FCCs or lymphoblasts are scarcer than the other cell types; they have a medium-sized nucleus with absent or inconspicuous nucleoli and very little but intensely basophilic cytoplasm.
4. Other lymphoid cells include occasional plasma cells and immunoblasts as well as small lymphocytes with dark-staining, irregular nuclei. The latter probably represent T-lymphocytes. The number of these various lymphoid elements varies considerably. Thus, sometimes plasma cells can be quite numerous; likewise, occasionally many T-cells can be found.

### *Tingible Body Macrophages*

Tingible body macrophages are large cells with abundant cytoplasm containing phagocytized debris and apoptotic bodies. Their nuclei are mostly medium sized to large and rather inconspicuous. Because nuclear size is fairly constant, these nuclei can be used to measure the nuclear size of other cells, especially in lymphomas. Because their cytoplasm is clear in most histologic stains, their presence causes white spots in the tissue (mottling), the so-called starry sky pattern. The cellular composition of a germinal center is dependent on its phase of development. Initially (i.e., about 4 days after antigenic challenge), only large noncleaved FCCs are found (24). Then macrophages appear, producing the mottled or starry sky appearance of the follicle. Then centrocytes and larger numbers of DRCs follow, creating the polymorphic histologic picture well known to histologists and pathologists. In this phase, zonation of the follicles may be observed: a dark zone (containing the large noncleaved FCCs) and a light zone (containing the small cleaved FCCs and DRCs). In a typical case the light zone is found closest to the capsule of the lymph node; the darker zone is directed to the medullary region (14,24,25). This zonation and orientation of the follicles is not always seen; it is, of course, largely dependent on the way the lymph node specimen happens to be cut. In the end, follicles can undergo hyalinization. In most reactive lymph nodes, such atrophic, hyalinized follicles are rare, but in Castleman's disease they are found more frequently. Sometimes they appear to be infiltrated by small lymphocytes—progressive transformation of the follicle center (14). This obscures the follicular structure and may cause an alarming histology, but because progressive transformation usually involves only a minority of the follicles in a lymph node, the presence of normal follicles is reassuring.

All different phases (with or without zonation) may be seen in a single specimen.

## Medullary Cords

The medullary cords are found in the hilar region of the lymph node, between the sinuses. The cellular composition of this reaction and this compartment is described next (Fig. 5A and B).

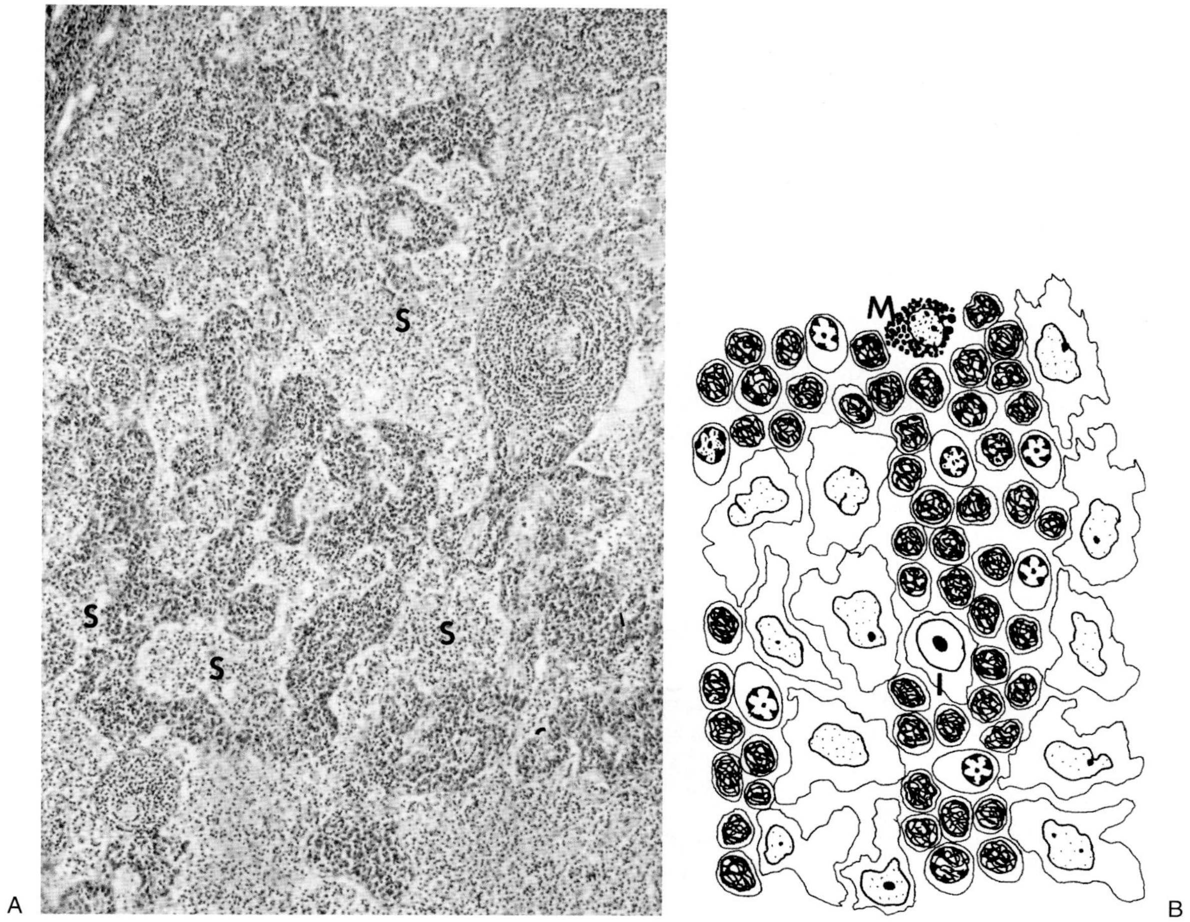


**FIG. 5.** Medullary cords. **A:** H&E-stained, paraffin-embedded section. A sheet of fairly dark-staining (basophilic) cells, mostly plasma cells, is flanked by less cellular areas, the medullary sinuses (S). **B:** Schematic representation also depicting an immunoblast (I). M, mast cell.

### *Lymphoid Cells*

Small lymphocytes make up the majority of cells in the medullary cords. They have small, more or less round nuclei and usually scant to moderate amounts of cytoplasm. In some cells the chromatin is clumped and peripherally distributed, similar to the plasma cell nucleus, although the typical "spoke wheel" chromatin pattern is not seen. Cells with this kind of nucleus tend to have more cytoplasm and a perinuclear hof; they are called plasmacytoid lymphocytes or lymphoplasmacytoid cells. The cells with less cytoplasm and more irregular nuclei are T-lymphocytes—necessary to modulate the process of antibody formation. Immunoblasts are scarce but have a striking morphology; they have large, vesicular, and round nuclei with a large central nucleolus and ample basophilic cytoplasm. Occasionally a similar cell may be found that has a slightly smaller nucleus and one to three paracentrally located nucleoli, and a perinuclear hof in its cytoplasm: the plasmablast. Both cells are proliferative phases in the plasma cell reaction. Plasma cells are present in varying numbers. They demonstrate the typical spoke wheel chromatin: small clumps of chromatin on the nuclear membrane in an otherwise clear (and round) nucleus. The cells have abundant cytoplasm, and a clear hof is easily seen in the Giemsa stain. Periodic acid-Schiff (PAS) staining sometimes shows PAS-positive globules in their cytoplasm, the so-called Russell bodies.

### *Macrophages*

Macrophages, which are scarce, have medium-sized to large nuclei, slightly irregular and vesicular. Their cytoplasm is abundant. They are not as avidly phagocytic as the tingible body macrophages from the germinal center, perhaps because their function is more directed at antigen presentation than at phagocytosis.

### *Other Cell Types, Including Mast Cells*

Mast cells are, in the lymph node, most frequently found in the medullary region. They are moderately sized cells and best visualized with metachromic dyes such as Giemsa or toluidine blue, in which they show their characteristic purple granulation. Occasional eosinophilic and neutrophilic granulocytes also may be seen.

## Paracortex

The paracortex was the last area to be described and named (26), probably because it is best seen and appreciated in "hard" (acidic) fixative such as Zenker or B5 and these fixatives were not standardly used. Also, it lacks the typical structure or form of the follicle. Nevertheless, it is easily recognizable because of its location and its typical structural elements—the epithelioid venules and the IDCs (Fig. 6).

### *Epithelioid (or Postcapillary or High Endothelial) Venules*

These highly distinctive vessels are found only in the paracortex; they are lined with plump, cuboidal to cylindrical endothelial cells with fairly large oval nuclei with small nucleoli. There is a moderate amount of cytoplasm. Sometimes the lumina of these vessels appear to be obliterated by the endothelium. They function as a gate of entry for lymphocytes from the peripheral blood to the lymph node parenchyma (27,28). Therefore, they play a crucial part in the recirculation, distribution, and homing of lymphocytes in the different lymphoid organs, a process mediated by specific homing receptors on the lymphocyte surface (29–31), which react with organ-specific ligands, also called vascular addressins, on the endothelial cell surface (Fig. 7).

### *Interdigitating Cells*

An IDC is a large cell with a large and bizarre nucleus with deep clefts and folds. The chromatin pattern is delicate, almost transparent, and nucleoli are inconspicuous. The cytoplasm is abundant, clear and pale, with ill-defined borders (Fig. 6C). With electron microscopy, they are shown to have broad cytoplasmic protrusions that are sometimes veil-like

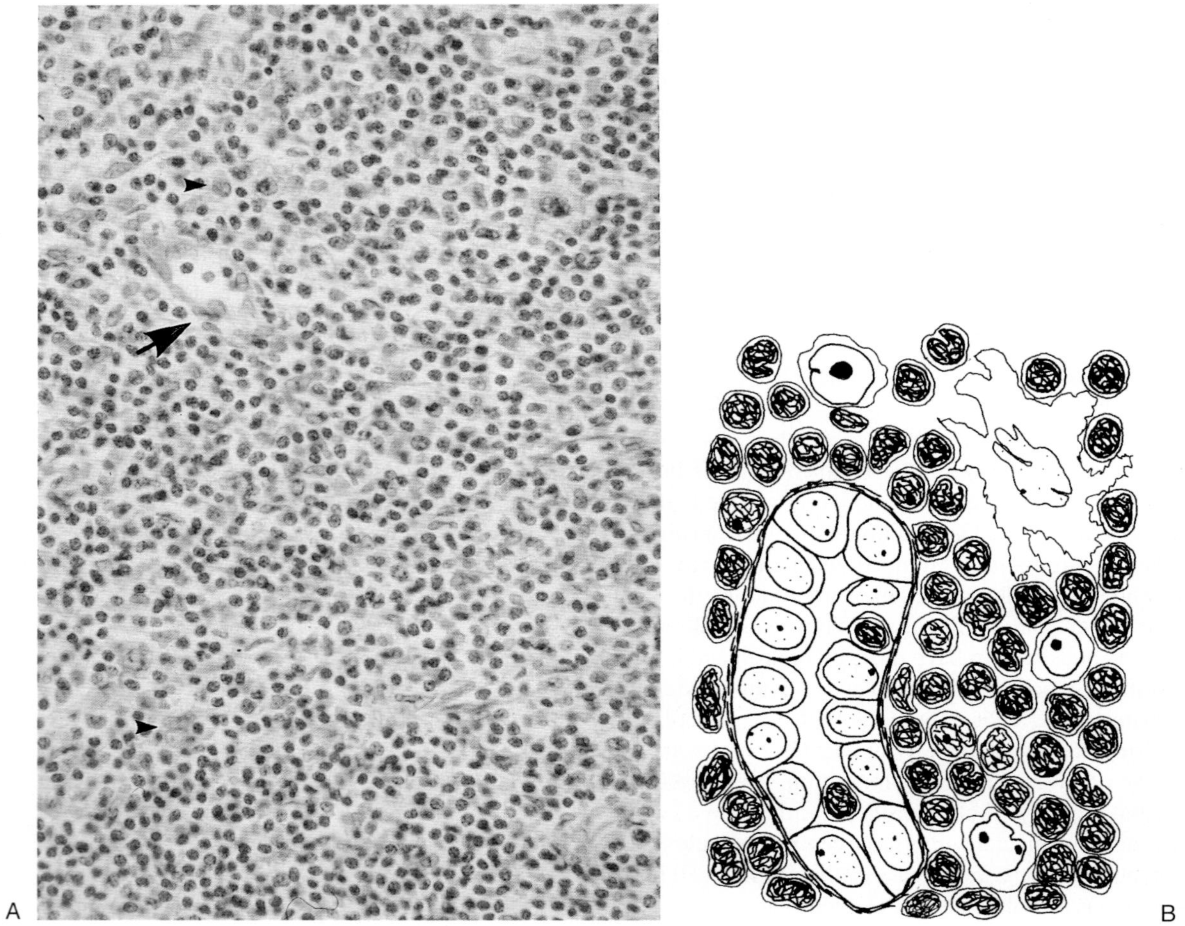


**FIG. 6. A:** H&E-stained, paraffin-embedded section. An epithelioid venule is seen (*arrow*). Small cells predominate, with occasional blasts. IDCs with characteristically irregular nuclei (*arrowheads*). **B:** Schematic representation. Note the typical IDC. **C:** Giemsa-stained, plastic-embedded section demonstrating an increase in the number of IDCs. Their morphologic characteristics can be seen clearly, with the nuclear irregularity and abundant cytoplasm (lymph node showing dermatopathic lymphadenopathy).

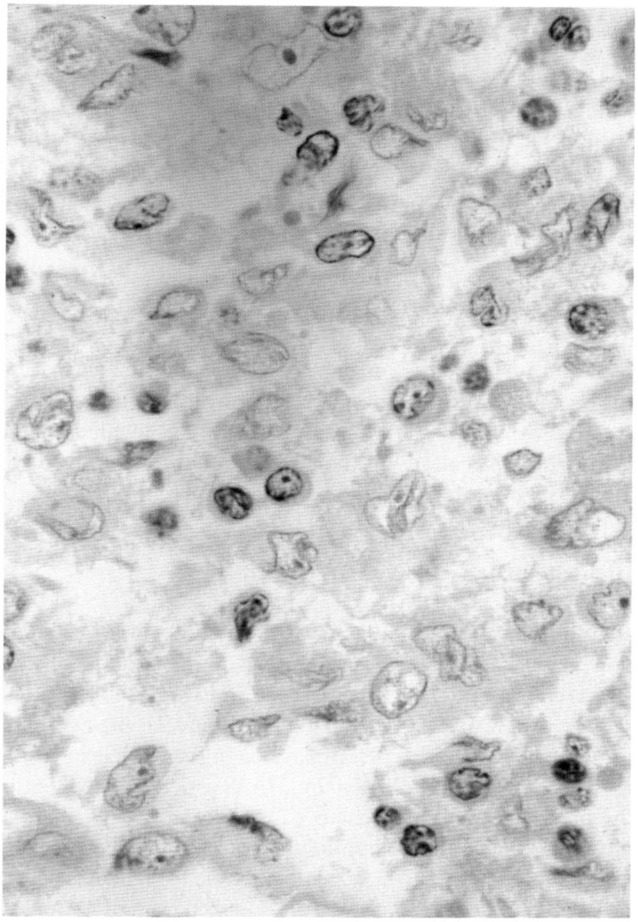

C

**FIG. 6.** *Continued.*

and that interdigitate, although without the anchoring desmosomes the DRCs have. Furthermore, they have a typical organelle of undetermined function: the tubulovesicular system (14). When present in large numbers, the IDCs cause the mottled aspect of the paracortex. IDCs are bone marrow derived, possibly via a circulating monocyte or a macrophage (16,32,33). They are intimately related to the Langerhans' cells of the skin, both morphologically and functionally (34,35). They probably initially present antigens to lymphoid cells, thus playing a crucial role in initiating an immune response (36).

### *T-Lymphocytes*

Most of the paracortical cells are small T-lymphocytes. They have small, irregular or round nuclei with dark, condensed chromatin and little cytoplasm. Occasionally, blastic cells are seen; they sometimes resemble B-immunoblasts, with a single central nucleolus, but more often they show irregular nuclei with two or more marginal nucleoli. The cytoplasm is moderately abundant and mostly indifferent. All these different forms are rather indiscriminately referred to as T-immunoblasts. Whether these different morphologies represent different cell types (helper cell blasts, suppressor cell blasts, blasts of cytokine-producing T cells, etc.) is an open question (37). Thus, although not striking at low power, the paracortex can be recognized easily.

Another cell that warrants mention here is the FRC. It is not exclusively found in the paracortical area, but appears often at the margins of the T-cell areas (14). They form reticular fibers that are involved in the transport of cytokines and/or antigens through the lymph node parenchyma, the so-called FRC conduit system (38), an effective means of spreading important activating molecules through the entire node.

### Sinuses

The sinuses are the structures carrying the lymph from the afferent lymphatics through the lymph node to the efferent lymph vessels. The afferent lymphatics drain into the subcapsular sinus. This sinus is at least partially lined by endothelium. As the sinuses traverse the node toward the hilus (where they are called medullary sinuses), they lose their endothelial lining and acquire a "lining" of macrophages (39).

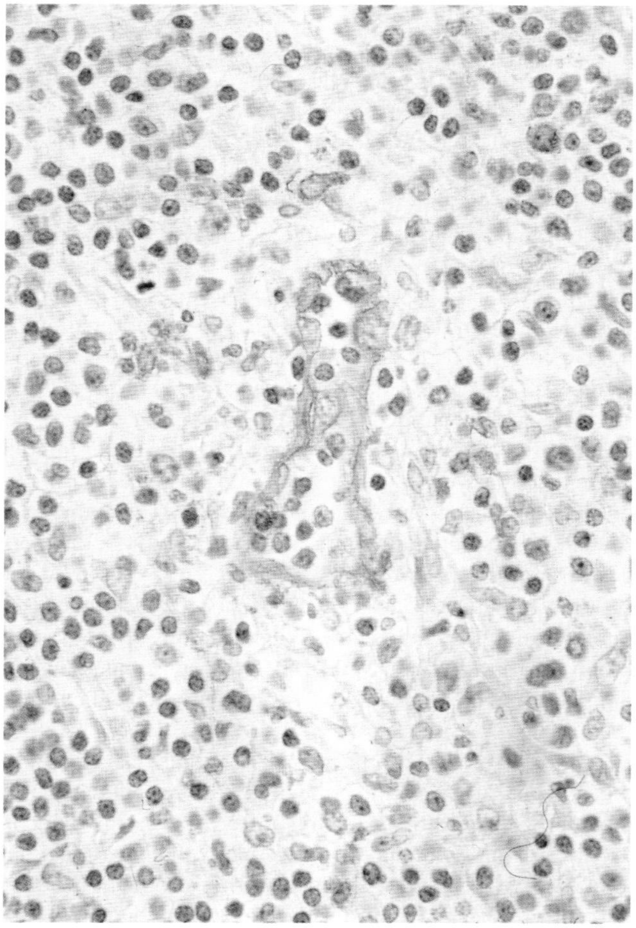

**FIG. 7.** HECA 452 staining. Epithelioid venule is clearly highlighted. Lymphocytes are seen adhering to the endothelium and passing through the vessel wall.

Additionally, small lymphocytes are also found in the sinuses (Figs. 5A and 8A).

The macrophages in the sinuses are similar to macrophages elsewhere: a low nucleus-to-cytoplasm ratio, irregular vesicular nuclei, and signs of phagocytosis. In some reactive conditions, large numbers of typical cells having a somewhat monocytoid appearance with medium-sized, often reniform nuclei, and moderately abundant cytoplasm can be observed in the sinuses. They are probably always present, but usually in numbers too small to be easily discerned. They are often found in toxoplasma lymphadenitis and were first called (incorrectly) "immature sinus histiocytes" (Fig. 8B, C) (40). However, immunologic investigation has since shown the B-cell nature of these cells (41,42).

## FUNCTION

Each of the four different compartments recognized in the lymph node harbors its own immunologic reaction; together these reactions make up an individuals immunologic integrity. These four specific compartments of the lymph node are the follicles, the medullary cords, the paracortex, and the sinuses, and in each a typical reaction pattern may be observed:

1. In the follicle is found the germinal center cell reaction, which leads to the formation of precursors of antibody-forming cells and of memory B cells (20,25,43). As was discussed under Apoptosis, selection of high-avidity clones occurs in the follicles; several cell clones can be found in a single follicle. That is, a follicle develops from more than one cell (oligoclonal development) (44). This process of selection involves further changes of the already rearranged immunoglobulin genes, a process called hypermutation; in this process small changes are made in the genes, leading to changes in the protein. These changes cause conformational adaptation to the antigen structure, leading to a better fit between antigen and antibody. Selected cells can either migrate to the medullary cords and develop into plasma cells directly or can recirculate to other lymph nodes and to the bone marrow, thereby spreading immunocompetence for "their" antigen throughout the body.

2. In the medullary cords, the plasma cell reaction leads to the formation of antibody-secreting (B) cells. The antibody production in the lymph node does not contribute substantially to the level of circulating antibodies but may be locally important.

3. In the paracortex, the specific cellular response takes place, generating antigen-specific T cells and probably memory T cells (29). The cellular processes in the paracortex are still poorly understood. It is likely that reactions such as memory T-cell formation, cytokine production, and a number of other reactions also take place in the paracortex, but little is known about this. In any case, the paracortex plays a central role in the cellular immune response. Its role in contact sensitivity (a T-cell–mediated process) is well recognized (26).

4. In the sinuses, macrophages clear the lymph through which the antigens pass to the lymph nodes. Besides dendritic cells, macrophages are probably also involved in processing antigens because they are the first cells to come into contact with lymph-borne antigen. Thus, they also may have an antigen-presenting function, but little is known about this.

## SPECIAL TECHNIQUES AND PROCEDURES

In many instances, a careful morphologic evaluation shows the benign or malignant nature of a lymph node lesion. However, in doubtful cases, additional techniques are invaluable, and although their role should not be overestimated, without them diagnostic accuracy would be limited.

### Histochemistry

Apart from a routine hematoxylin and eosin (H&E) section, Giemsa, PAS with and without diastase pretreatment, and a reticulin stain are invaluable to assess morphology. The reticulin stain shows clear differences between the two most prominently represented compartments: the follicles and the paracortex. The follicles contain little reticulin, whereas in the paracortical area a coarse network of reticulin fibers is present. Expansion of the follicular compartment compresses this paracortical network, accentuating the follicular structure because the follicular structures, whether benign or malignant, always contain few fibers. If necessary, a methyl green pyronine stain can be performed to facilitate identification of cells with active protein synthesis (i.e., among others, dividing cells). However, in our opinion this staining is not absolutely necessary. In case of a suspected infectious lymphadenopathy, stains such as Ziehl-Neelsen, Warthin-Starry, or Grocott's methenamine silver stain can be used.

### Immunohistochemistry

Immunohistochemistry is an important additional technique in studying lymph node specimens, benign or malignant (45–47). It is used primarily for demonstrating the presence or absence of clonality, as well as the presence or absence of (normal) compartmentalization. Because all compartments have a specific function with a specific morphology, they also have a typical immune profile, and they can be clearly recognized in immunohistochemical stains.

#### *Follicle*

Immunohistology shows the follicle to be a B-cell area. The DRCs stain with monoclonal antibodies directed against DRCs (15) as well as with antibodies against receptors for complement components C3b (CD35) (16) and C3d (Fig.

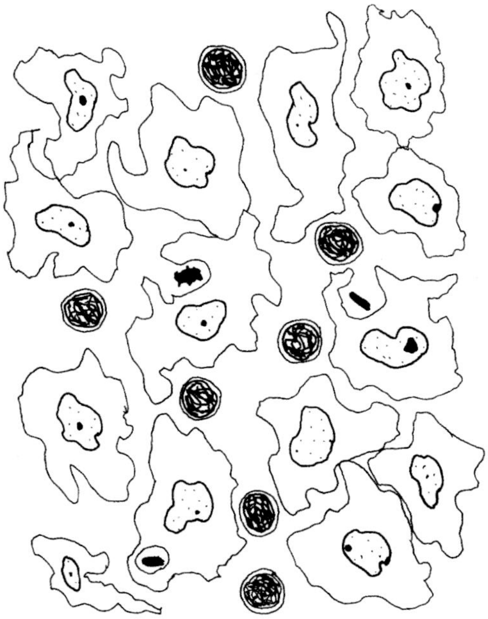

A

FIG. 8. **A:** Schematic representation of sinuses. **B:** Immature sinus histiocytosis (low-power view) recognizable as the pale area next to the follicle. **C:** Detail of **B**, showing intermediate-sized cells with ample cytoplasm.

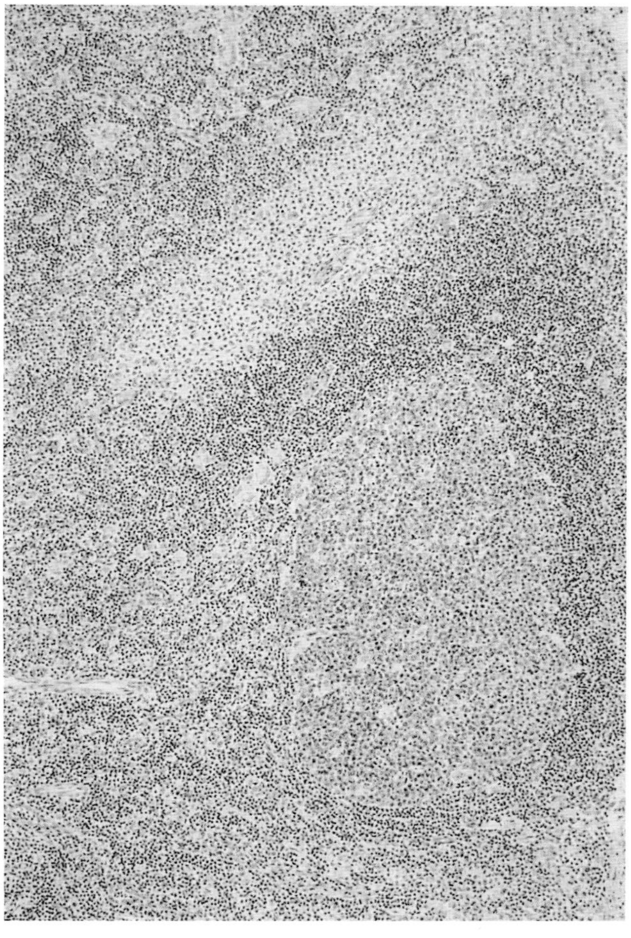

B

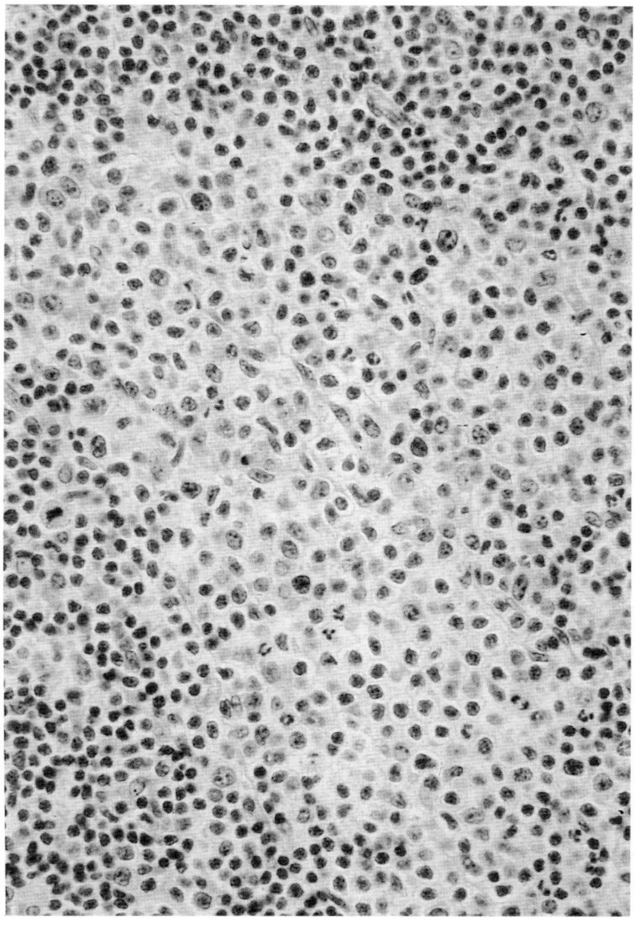

C

4C). With immunoglobulin stains, especially with IgM, the lattice formed by the DRCs stands out clearly (48). DRCs are 5′-nucleotidase-positive (14). The FCCs are B-lymphocytes as proved by their reactivity with B cell–specific antibodies CD19, 20, and 22 and their surface immunoglobulins, although the latter can be present in quantities too low to be detected with a routine immunoperoxidase technique (16,22,48). The immunoglobulin expressed is mostly IgM. To a much lesser degree IgG and IgA are found. IgD is not present in normal germinal centers but is found on follicle mantle cells (Fig. 4D). In addition to this, FCCs express CD10, the common acute lymphoblastic leukemia antigen. Another important point is the absence of the bcl-2 protein from these cells (49), not surprising given the high rate of apoptosis in normal follicles and bcl-2's role in blocking apoptosis.

If they are present, plasma cells—and often immunoblasts as well—can be shown to contain cytoplasmic immunoglobulin. The small lymphocytes are mostly T-lymphocytes. They are present in varying numbers, and sometimes they are quite numerous. The CD45RO stain, reactive with activated and memory T cells, demonstrates follicular T cells particularly well. Cells of the helper/inducer phenotype (CD4 positive) usually dominate over the suppressor/cytotoxic phenotype (CD8 positive) in a ratio of approximately 3:1 (16,50,51).

Tingible body macrophages have many characteristics of other histiocytes/macrophages: coarsely granular anti-(chymo)- trypsin (52), acid phosphatase, and nonspecific esterase (53), as well as reactivity with monoclonal antibodies such as CD11b, CD35, and CD68 (21).

### *Medullary Cords*

Immunohistochemically, the medullary cords are a B-cell area. Reactivity with the different B-cell markers can thus be found, but it must be said that with terminal differentiation into plasma cells B cells gradually lose their surface markers. Thus, CD20 is absent from plasma cells (45) and may be absent or only weakly expressed on lymphoplasmacytoid cells. There are also a fair number of T-lymphocytes present, mostly of the helper/inducer phenotype (50). Plasma cells, plasmablasts, immunoblasts, and (rarely) lymphoplasmacytoid cells show intracytoplasmic immunoglobulins of various classes (20), though IgD and IgE are not found. Of course, in the normal situation both kappa and lambda light chain positive cells will be found, in a ratio of approximately 2:1. Some variation in this ratio is possible, but if it exceeds 4:1 or gets reversed, an underlying malignancy or immune disturbance must be considered.

### *Paracortex*

Immunologically, the T cells predominate here (Fig. 9A), with a majority of T-helper/inducer cells (ratio of helper to suppressor cells is 2–3:1) (20,21,23,54). Normal paracortical T-lymphocytes express all or most mature T-cell markers, such as CD2, CD3, CD5, and CD7. Some scattered B cells are also found (48). According to most studies, nearly all T cells are HLA-DR negative.

High endothelial venules can be stained with a specific antibody, HECA 452 (Fig. 7). This antibody also stains IDCs and a subset of T cells (55,56). The antigen recognized by HECA 452 on T cells is the cutaneous homing receptor; its presence on HEV and the importance of these vessels for recirculation suggest a function of the HECA-recognized molecule in homing.

The IDCs can be recognized with S-100 antibodies in paraffin sections (57), with monoclonal antibodies such as HLA-DR and CD24 (16,54), and with IDC-specific antibodies (58). The HLA-DR staining is typical: a coarse, thick reaction product in a stellate pattern (Fig. 9B). It allows dis-

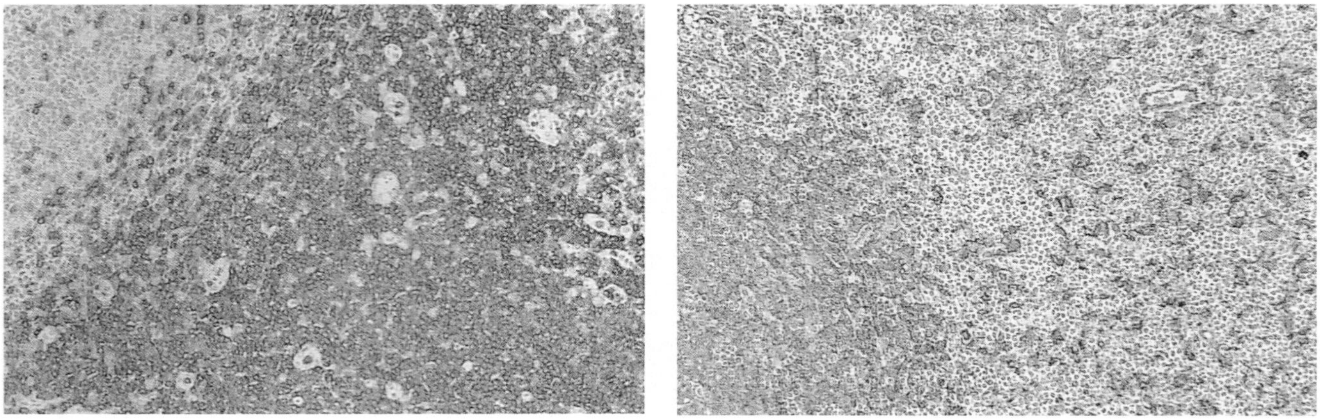

A B

**FIG. 9. A:** Frozen section stained with anti-CD3 antibody (leu 4). A follicle (*upper left*) is not stained. Amid the positive cells, small white spots (IDCs) and somewhat larger white areas (epithelioid venules) are seen. **B:** Frozen section stained with HLA-DR. The IDCs are the darker and fairly large, positive cells at the left. At the left is a follicle whose B cells stain positive with HLA-DR.

tinction of B and T cells and IDCs in frozen sections. IDCs also exhibit adenosinetriphosphatase (ATPase) activity (14).

### *Sinuses*

Immunohistochemistry shows the macrophages to be positive with histiocytic markers: lysozyme, $\alpha$1-anti-(chymo)trypsin, acid phosphatase, CD68, and so on (52,59). S-100 protein–positive cells in the sinuses can be dendritic cells, but some macrophages also express this marker, in the sinuses as well as in the parenchyma.

With immunohistochemistry, especially using markers on paraffin sections, the compartmentalization is beautifully illustrated; it shows which compartment is proliferating. This is important because lesions that show proliferation (mitoses, blast cells identified with markers) of more than one compartment/cell type are rarely malignant.

### Molecular Biologic Techniques

Molecular biology is primarily applied in the demonstration of clonality, but demonstration of certain specific translocations [t(14;18)] and viral genomes are also important applications.

Only one of these techniques is a morphologic technique: in situ hibridization. Others are nonmorphologic, and of these, special mention must be made of the Southern blotting technique, as used to demonstrate gene rearrangement of the immunoglobulin and T-cell receptor genes. The genes of the immunoglobulin chains and the chains of the T-cell receptor for antigen are made operational by rearranging them (60). That is, from a variety of variable (V), diversity (D), joining (J), and constant (C) gene segments, an appropriate choice is made and the chosen segments are brought together with deletion of the interjacent gene segments. Demonstration of such a rearrangement is accomplished by digesting DNA with restriction enzymes (enzymes that split DNA on specific loci); the resulting fragments are subjected to electrophoresis and then incubated with a (radioactive-) labeled probe (a piece of single-stranded DNA identical to the DNA segment under investigation, here an immunoglobulin or T-cell receptor gene segment). Unrearranged DNA, called germline DNA, shows a certain pattern of bands; but a previous rearrangement of the DNA alters the number of sites of DNA cleavage, and with that the number and size of the DNA fragments and thus the pattern of bands after the electrophoresis and incubation with the probe. Because only B cells use (and thereupon rearrange) immunoglobulin genes and only T cells use the T-cell receptor genes, rearrangement of either gene is proof of cell lineage. Furthermore, if a proliferation is clonal, the cells in this proliferation will all have the same rearrangement. This shows up in the electrophoresis pattern. A germline pattern shows one or more distinct bands; a polyclonal process, having many different rearrangements, shows a smear (the many different-sized fragments do not result in distinct bands but form a blurred smear), but a monoclonal process shows distinct bands again, only on different places when compared with the germline bands.

This technique (Fig. 10) already has proved its diagnostic worth (60,61). Theoretically, this method promises absolute lineage specificity. In practice, however, this is not the case. Rare nonlymphoid tumors show rearrangements of immunoglobulin genes (62,63); not infrequently, cells in a B-cell lymphoma show a rearrangement of a gene encoding for one of the chains of the T-cell receptor (64,65), and likewise immunoglobulin gene rearrangement can be found in T-cell lymphomas (66,67). We have seen occasional mismatches in immunophenotype and gene rearrangement studies. Care must be taken with the interpretation of genotypic data.

At this time, the method is still time consuming, labor intensive, rather difficult, and expensive, and requires a fairly large amount of freshly frozen material; in the context of this chapter, most problems can be solved with immunohistochemistry, but in a fairly small but distinct number of cases molecular biology is the only technique that can help, especially with the T-cell proliferations and rare follicular lesions.

Gene rearrangements also can be demonstrated using a polymerase chain reaction (PCR) approach. The problem here is the choice of the primers in this PCR; with the enormous variability in the genetic changes, it is difficult to select a primer set for the PCR that encompasses all potential rearrangements. Using several primer pairs can circumvent this problem at least partially, and with the use of three primer sets the technique approaches or matches Southern blotting. A PCR approach decreases the amount of material drastically, an important advantage.

## ARTIFACTS

### Technical Artifacts

Lymph node tissue is vulnerable and easily damaged in processing. Undue pressure on a specimen can cause considerable crushing artifact, to the point of obliterating morphology completely. Specimens with extensive crushing artifact should not be evaluated; morphologic differences are already subtle and no chance should be taken with poor material.

A second disturbing artifact is fixation related and occurs especially in larger specimens. If fixation in formalin is too short, only the outer edge of the specimen is formalin fixed. The central part is fixed in the alcohol series used to dehydrate the specimen. This causes a marked difference in the morphology of the outer and inner segments. The central parts often show a loss of cohesion and cells appear smaller, with darker, more condensed chromatin (Fig. 11). Great care should be taken when evaluating specimens like this.

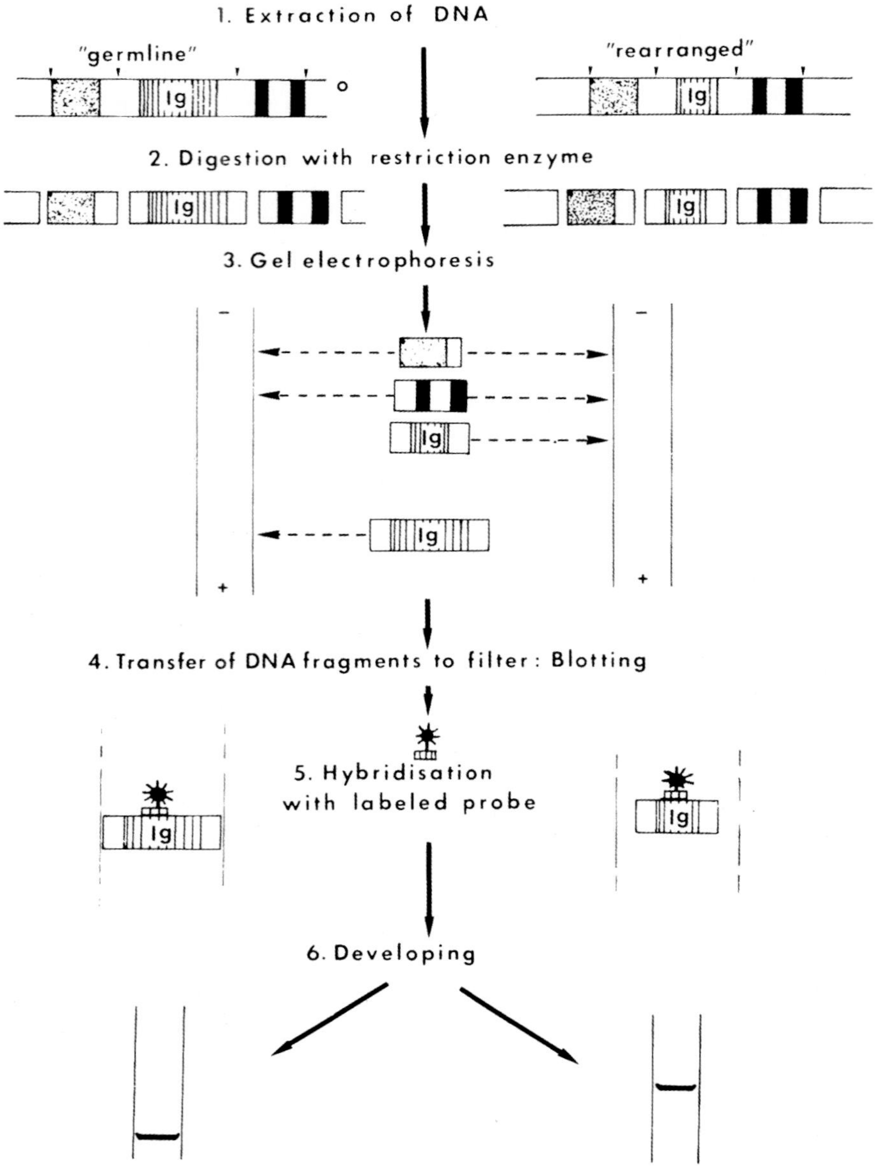


**FIG. 10.** Demonstration of gene rearrangement by Southern blotting, schematically represented.

### "Intrinsic" Artifacts

Although the above-described structure of the lymph node is the same in nodes from all parts of the body, nodes from some areas can have special features. Most important here are the inguinal nodes. In practice, all kinds of curious changes can be found in inguinal lymph nodes, especially fibrotic reactions that occasionally distort the normal architecture. This should always be kept in mind when evaluating such a specimen. Somewhat similar is the frequent presence of sclerotic or hyaline deposits in parailiac and paraaortic lymph nodes.

## DIFFERENTIAL DIAGNOSIS: BENIGN VERSUS MALIGNANT

The differential diagnosis of benign and malignant lesions is important in the discussion of "normal" lymph node histology for two principal reasons: (a) it is naturally of the utmost importance for the surgical pathologist to decide between benign and malignant, and (b) it is often difficult to distinguish between benign and malignant changes. The first goes without saying; the second can be clarified somewhat.

Recently, through careful morphologic and immunologic studies, a link was made between normal lymph node histology and malignant lymphomas. We have now come to re-

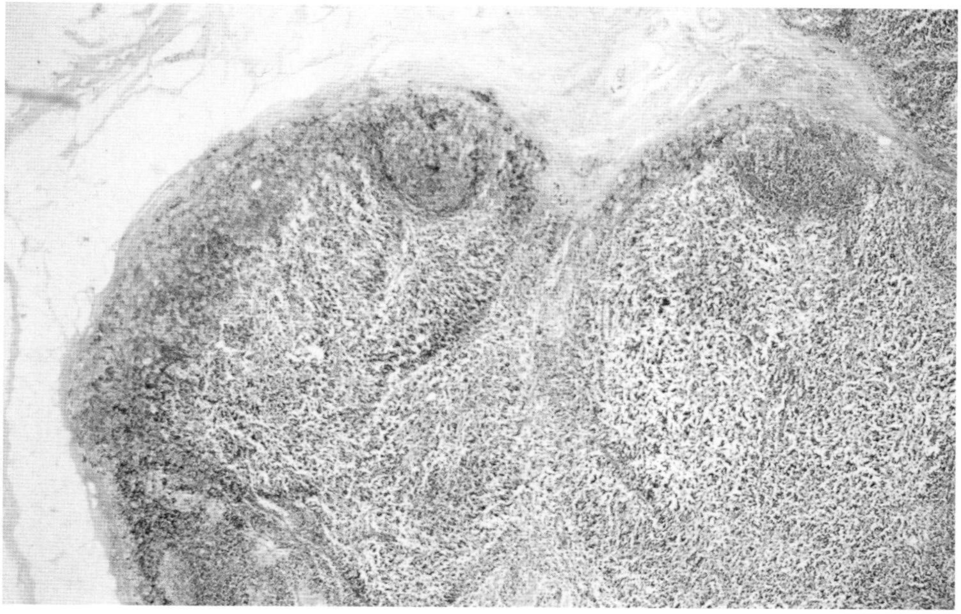

**FIG. 11.** Fixation artifact. Edge of the specimen is properly fixed, the center shows loss of tissue structure.

gard the (non-Hodgkin's) lymphomas as malignant counterparts of the normal immunologic reactions to antigens in the lymphoid tissue (14,68–70). The lymphoma cells thus have similar morphologic, immunologic, and functional characteristics when compared with normal cells. This makes it understandable why a malignant process can so closely resemble a benign one.

Table 1 shows some of the benign variations in normal histology opposite malignant counterparts. Because so many excellent articles have been written on the subject of differential diagnosis and this chapter deals with normal histology, we will discuss this matter briefly.

### Changes in the Follicular Compartment

Most important here (and most difficult) is the distinction between follicular hyperplasia and a follicle center cell lymphoma. The term "follicular hyperplasia" is used here as a collective noun. It is seen in a number of conditions of known and unknown origin: (a) in lymph nodes in the vicinity of (bacterial) inflammation (e.g., cervical lymphadenopathy accompanying tonsillitis); (b) associated with conditions such as rheumatoid arthritis (71) and syphilis (72); (c) in several "idiopathic" conditions (73) such as (multicentric) giant lymph node hyperplasia or Castleman's disease (74), reactive lymph node hyperplasia with giant follicles (75), and multicentric angiofollicular lymph node hyperplasia (76) (it is by no means clear whether these conditions are all separate entities); and (d) in the recently recognized cause of follicular hyperplasia caused by infection with human immunodeficiency virus (HIV) (Fig. 12A) (77,78). The pattern of hyperplasia here is not specific (79), although typically the follicles in HIV lymphadenopathy are variable in shape and signs of follicular desintegration (also of the DRC network) (Fig. 12B) are common. The diagnosis of HIV infection on the lymph node specimen can be made using immunohistochemistry with the p24 antibody (80) but in rare instances may require demonstration of virus particles in the germinal centers with electron microscopy (81).

Because the follicles are not essentially different (apart, perhaps, from changes in vasculature) in these conditions, they are considered together here. The most important morphologic criteria arguing for a benign lesion that are mentioned in the literature (14,73,82–86) are as follows:

1. Cellular pleomorphism of the germinal center.
2. Presence of tingible body macrophages.
3. High number of mitotic figures.
4. Well-defined mantle zone.

**TABLE 1.** *Benign compartmental enlargements and their malignant counterparts*

| Compartment | Benign | Malignant |
|---|---|---|
| Follicle | Follicular hyperplasia | FCC lymphomas |
| Paracortex | Paracortical hyperplasia | T-NHL |
| | Dermatopathic lymphadenopathy | Early mycosis fungoides |
| Medullary cords | Medullary hyperplasia | Lymphoplasmacytoid lymphoma |
| | Reactive plasmacytosis | Plasmacytoma |
| Sinuses | Sinus histiocytosis (with massive lymphadenopathy) | Malignant histiocytosis |

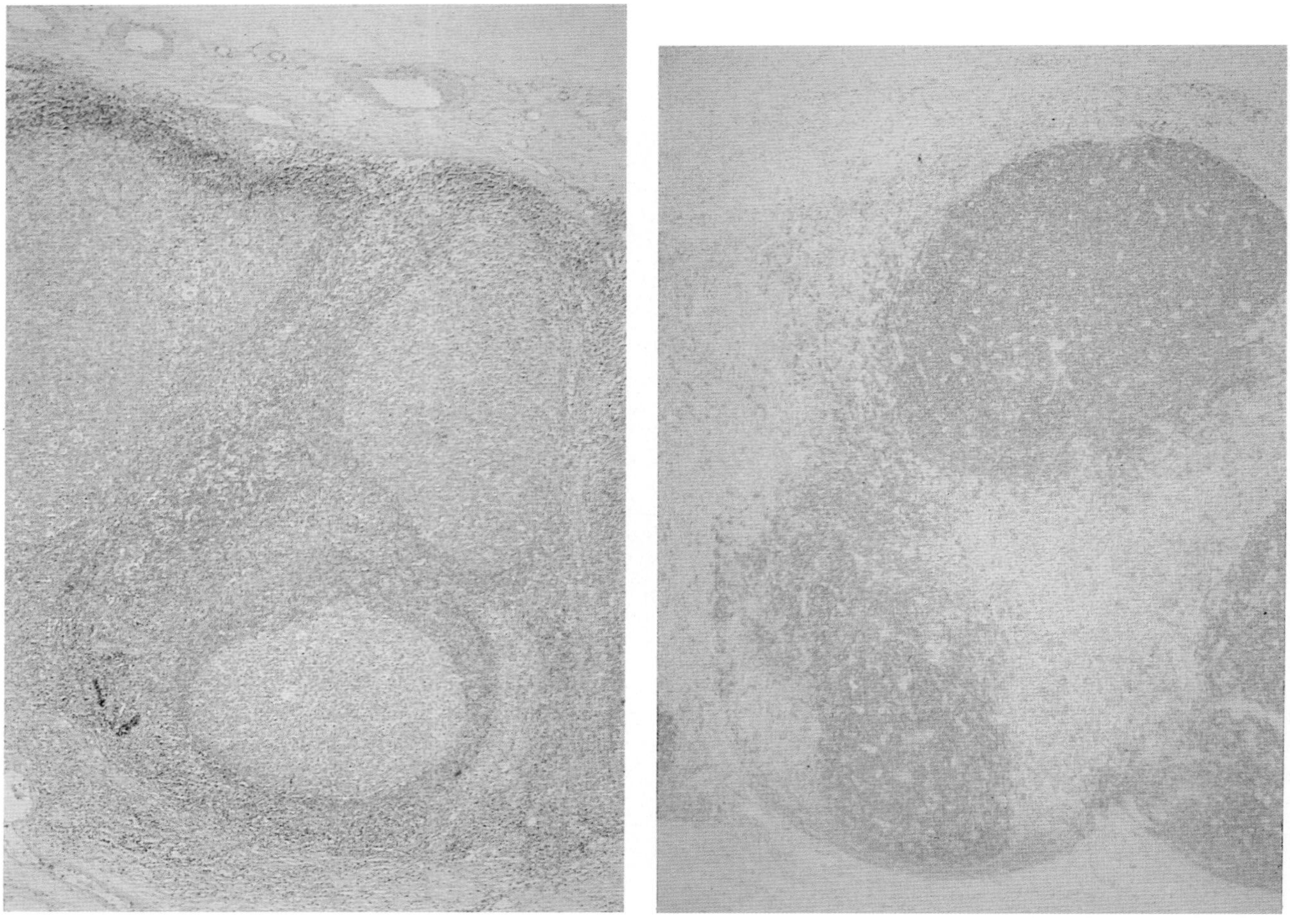

A B

**FIG. 12. A:** H&E-stained, paraffin-embedded section. HIV-induced follicular hyperplasia. Huge, irregularly shaped follicles are present. **B:** CD20 staining, showing two follicles with ragged borders (follicular desintegration).

5. Differences in size and shape of the follicles.
6. Low number of follicles per surface area of lymph node parenchyma and predominant cortical localization.
7. High number of DRCs and a well-developed and intact meshwork formed by the DRCs.

Despite this impressive list of criteria, it may not be possible—at least for the less experienced pathologist—to distinguish between benign and malignant on morphology alone. Here, marker studies are essential. Therefore, in addition there are a number of immunohistochemical criteria (87):

1. Demonstration of clonality by means of showing light chain restriction (follicular cells express either/or). In follicular lesions this is considered proof of malignancy.
2. Clear expression of immunoglobulin heavy chains (in the absence of light chains), mostly IgM.
3. A well-defined rim of cells (mantle) staining with IgD antibody (Fig. 4D) (a benign sign).
4. Expression of bcl-2 in the follicle centers of malignant lesions.

Unfortunately all three mentioned characteristics are only reliably demonstrable in frozen sections because it concerns membrane-bound immunoglobulin only and there is too little of it to be demonstrable after fixation. However, even with marker studies, a 100% certainty cannot be reached because some lymphomas are immunoglobulin negative. Fortunately, this is rare in FCC lymphomas (48,88).

It should be remembered that a lymph node can be partially involved. Careful study of the entire section is important in such cases.

## Changes of the Medullary Cords

The following two distinctions are important. First is reactive plasmacytosis (Fig. 13) versus plasmacytoma. A preserved lymph node architecture and presence of plasma cell precursors favor the diagnosis of reactive plasmacytosis (14). In doubtful cases, marker studies can be used to demonstrate either polyclonality (benign) or monoclonality (malig-

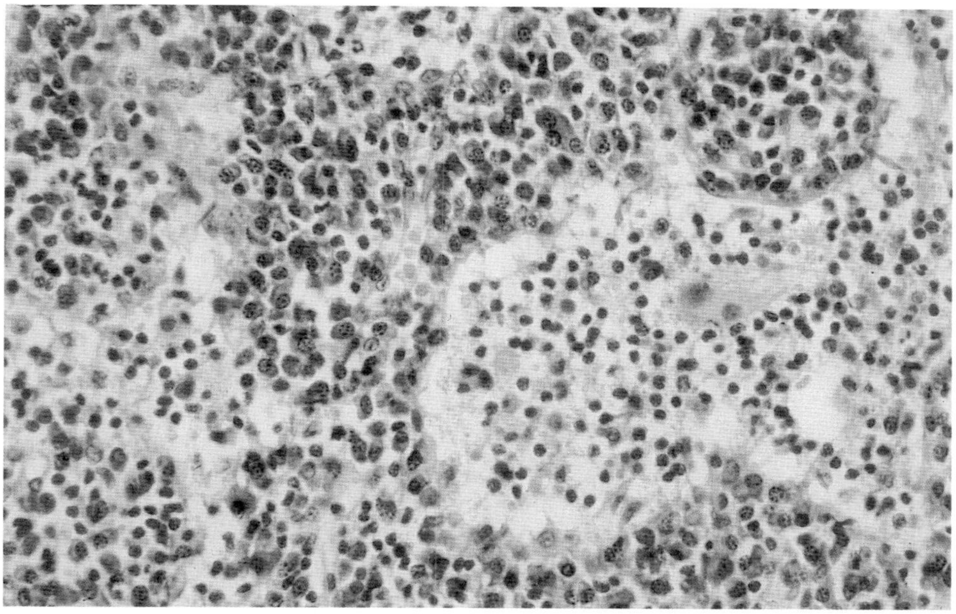

**FIG. 13.** H&E-stained, paraffin-embedded section. Reactive plasmacytosis. Medullary cords consist almost entirely of plasma cells. Sinuses are patent, sign of a preserved lymph node structure.

nant) of the plasma cells (in this case, of intracytoplasmic immunoglobulins and therefore demonstrable in paraffin sections).

Second is the expansion of the medullary cords versus plasmacytoid lymphocytic lymphoma/lymphoplasmacytoid immunocytoma. The latter condition usually involves the lymph node diffusely, leaving no or little residual normal lymphoid tissue. However, we have observed rare cases of lymphoma that mimic normal lymph node histology closely, with mast cells, occasional blasts, patent (even distended) sinuses, a remaining paracortical area, and rare follicles. Problems do not arise frequently, mostly due to the rarity of such a pattern, but when sections show that the medullary cords take up a disproportionate part of the lymph node, and lymphoplasmacytoid cells predominate, marker studies are necessary (surface and intracytoplasmic immunoglobulins).

Demonstration of clonality in paraffin sections may be difficult due to diffusion artifacts. If a specimen is not promptly fixed, proteins from the extracellular fluid can diffuse into the cell; subsequent fixation traps these proteins in the cell, where they can be demonstrated with immunohistochemistry. Because the extracellular fluid also contains immunoglobulins (polyclonal), this may cause interpretative problems.

## Changes in the Paracortical Compartment

Paracortical hyperplasia can show three patterns, each with differential diagnostic considerations.

### *Increase in Small Lymphocytes and Epithelioid Venules*

Here the composition of the compartment does not change drastically, but the paracortex is enlarged. This reactive change must be distinguished from T-cell non-Hodgkin's lymphomas (T-NHL), especially the small lymphocytic variants (14,89). Distinctive features are cellular monotony and signs of destruction of the lymph node architecture in instances of lymphoma. Marker studies can be of (limited) value here. Two features can be helpful:

1. A predominance of cells with helper/inducer phenotype (CD4-positive) over suppressor/cytotoxic cells (CD8-positive) or vice versa, in our experience, meaning a CD4:CD8 ratio of either greater than 10:1 or less than 1:3. Quantitation of these cells can be difficult, especially when a lot of histiocytic cells are present. These cells stain positive with CD4 as well, and their presence alone makes difficult the accurate assessment of the percentages of T-cell subsets. We have seen an occasional reactive lesion, for instance, a dermatopathic lymphadenopathy, with a ratio of more than 10:1, so this criterion is of limited value.
2. Loss of markers argues for malignancy (90). T-cell neoplasms fairly often show loss of markers for mature (i.e., peripheral) T cells. CD7, CD5, CD4, or CD8 are usually the first markers to go; CD2 and CD3 are lost only occasionally (90). Clearly, this obviates the use of a fairly extensive number of antibodies, and, as said earlier, it is no proof of a malignant lymphoma because they cannot offer proof of clonality. Loss of markers is indicative of lymphoma, but only

molecular biology can bring actual proof by demonstrating clonal T-cell receptor gene rearrangement(s).

### *Expansion of the Paracortex with Increase of Blasts*

This pattern can be caused by vaccinations, viral infections, or drugs (e.g., dilantin, penicillin, griseofulvin) (83,91,92). Additionally, an influx of eosinophils, neutrophils, or histiocytes can be seen (83,93). Occasionally these changes may exhibit a nodular pattern (94). In a typical condition, called Kikuchi's disease or histiocytic necrotizing lymphadenitis (95–97), small foci of necrosis also are observed, notably lacking neutrophils. Some of these conditions are difficult to distinguish from a malignant lymphoma.

Two types of lymphoma must be excluded. The first is Hodgkin's disease. With the presence of a pleomorphic infiltrate with eosinophils, plasma cells, histiocytes, and blasts, Hodgkin's disease is a serious consideration. Of course Reed-Sternberg cells in a characteristic background of cell types effacing the nodal architecture are diagnostic for Hodgkin's disease. The fact that Reed-Sternberg–like cells can be found in reactive conditions such as toxoplasmosis and mononucleosis does not simplify things. Immunohistochemistry is only marginally helpful here. The marker for Reed-Sternberg cells (CD30) also stains the atypical cells in the reactive conditions. Leu M1 (CD15) usually is not found in reactive conditions and sometimes is not expressed by genuine Reed-Sternberg cells.

The second type of lymphoma to exclude is a peripheral T-NHL. Given the histologic variety in T-NHL (37,89, 98–101), any reactive paracortical condition may resemble a peripheral T-NHL, or vice versa. Distinction of the two should rest on clinical data, morphologic features (preservation of lymph node architecture, presence of neutrophils, and a normal or increased number of epithelioid venules argue for a benign lesion), and marker studies (marker loss argues for malignancy), including genotyping (molecular biology). The combination of all data is all important (73).

### *Dermatopathic Lymphadenopathy*

Dermatopathic lymphadenopathy represents an increase primarily of IDCs (Fig. 6C). This pattern is frequently seen in lymph nodes draining an itching skin disorder (102,103). It is a benign disorder but must be mentioned here because patients with a cutaneous T-NHL (i.e., mycosis fungoides, Sézary syndrome) often show dermatopathic lymphadenopathy, and in these cases, involvement of the lymph node by the T-NHL may be present. Marker studies are not helpful here (104,105). Instead, a careful search for the so-called cerebriform lymphocytes with a nuclear diameter of 7.5 $\mu$m or more (in buffered formalin-fixed sections) must be made. These large cerebriform cells are not found in chronic benign skin disorders and are, therefore, diagnostic of early involvement by cutaneous T-NHL (106). Although Colby et al. (107) reported that "atypical" lymphocytes were present in benign skin disorders, their report makes no mention of size. Furthermore, preliminary findings on evaluation of the criteria reported by Scheffer et al. (106) indicate their validity. Molecular biology can be helpful, but if the number of cerebriform lymphocytes is low, below 2% to 5%, the sensitivity of most techniques is insufficient.

## Sinusoidal Changes

Sinus histiocytosis is a common finding of undefined significance in lymph node specimens; it is easily recognized. Lymph nodes in draining areas of inflammation and tumors often show sinus histiocytosis. In one rare condition, the sinus histiocytosis has a typical feature: the benign-appearing histiocytes show many lymphocytes in their cytoplasm. This is the clinicopathologic entity known as sinus histiocytosis with massive lymphadenopathy (108,109).

Langerhans' cell histiocytosis also causes a (probably) benign sinus histiocytosis (83,110). The cells appear benign, and eosinophils are present. Because these cells are identical to the cells of the Langerhans' cell/IDC lineage [Birbeck granules, reactivity with CD1 antibodies (111,112)], involvement of the paracortical area can be expected. In rare instances, Langerhans' cell histiocytosis–like changes may accompany a malignant lymphoma (113). Of course Langerhans' cell histiocytosis is easily demonstrated with an S-100 stain. Although not only Langerhans' cells stain with this marker, in combination with the characteristic morphology, the diagnosis can be made with a fair amount of certainty, with proof from additional CD1 staining or electron microscopy.

All these benign conditions must be distinguished from malignant sinusoidal lesions: malignant histiocytosis/histiocytic sarcoma (114–116) (CD 68, lysozyme stains), occasional large-cell lymphoma of B- (117) or T-cell type (118) (CD45), and metastatic carcinoma (keratin antibodies) and melanoma (melanin stain, S-100, HMB 45). The recently described large-cell anaplastic lymphoma, characteristically expressing CD30 antigen (119), also can show sinusoidal lymph node involvement, but it rarely if ever is mistaken for a reactive condition and is not discussed here further. Differential diagnosis between a reactive sinus histiocytosis and the other malignancies mentioned rarely is problematic, but if it is, marker studies can be helpful (120).

As mentioned earlier, there may be sinusoidal expansion by the so-called monocytoid B-cells or immature sinus histiocytes. Recent reports of malignant lymphomas of these cells (121,122) stressed that immature sinus histiocytes also have a malignant counterpart: monocytoid B cell or marginal zone B-cell lymphoma. Another term for this tumor is parafollicular lymphoma (123) due to its pronounced orientation around follicles. Whether this is a sinusoidal or a marginal zone location (as the term marginal zone B-cell lymphoma implies) is not completely clear. Distinction between benign and malignant immature sinus histiocytosis may be difficult; morphologic distinction between benign immature sinus histiocytosis and the aforementioned malignant tumors is not.

A sinusoidal pattern also can be found in a condition called vascular transformation of the sinuses or nodal angiomatosis (124). In this condition the sinuses show vascular proliferation and some degree of fibrosis. The histologic picture can vary markedly from a delicate vascular pattern to more solid spindle cell proliferations (resembling Kaposi's sarcoma). It can occur as a result of vascularization problems or secondary to some malignancies in the lymph node (metastatic carcinoma, Hodgkin's disease).

### Combined Patterns

Follicular, paracortical, medullary, and sinusoidal enlargements often occur simultaneously; any combination of these patterns is possible. Interestingly, combined patterns are relatively rare in malignant lesions and thus argue strongly for a reactive lesion. Most frequent is a combination of follicular and paracortical hyperplasia, whereas sinus histiocytosis is often accompanied by either follicular or paracortical hyperplasia (or vice versa). Toxoplasma and Epstein-Barr virus infections, for instance, show a combination of patterns. For the distinction of malignancy, the same criteria as described previously would be applied to combined lesions.

### Other Lesions

This chapter does not aspire to completeness in discussing benign lymph node lesions; it is primarily concerned with normal lymph node histology. Therefore, conditions not resembling a benign disorder—for instance, angioimmunoblastic lymphadenopathy (125)—are not addressed.

Neither are granulomatous inflammations discussed separately. Granulomas are found in many conditions, including tuberculosis (necrosis), sarcoidosis, berylliosis, Hodgkin's disease, toxoplasmosis, and in lymph nodes draining carcinomas (126,127). Granulomas develop mostly in the T-cell–dependent area and thus usually are accompanied by some degree of paracortical hyperplasia or by a combined pattern (toxoplasmosis); again, criteria for distinction between benign and malignant lesions are the same as described previously.

## HANDLING OF THE LYMPH NODE SPECIMEN

Morphologic differences between cell types are subtle in the lymphoid tissue. Indeed, the differences can be so subtle that only marker studies can bring them out. Therefore, specimens must always be handled with great care. Because it is best to divide the tissue into several parts, excision of a complete node is to be preferred to incision biopsy. Furthermore, it is important to avoid squeezing of the tissue because undue pressure on the specimen can cause changes in histology that completely obscure subtle morphologic differences. After excision, the specimen should be sent to the pathology laboratory in a plastic bag, preferably on ice. If the specimen is to be processed upon arrival, it can be transported dry—for instance, in a Petri dish—or wrapped in gauze soaked in physiologic saline solution. Contact with water or dry gauze should be scrupulously avoided. At the pathology laboratory the specimen should be carefully bisected across the long axis to allow evaluation of the macroscopic aspects of the node. Use of a sharp (i.e., new) scalpel blade avoids undue pressure. Then different parts can be divided for the various techniques (Table 2):

1. One part of the node should be snap-frozen in liquid nitrogen for immunoperoxidase, immunofluorescence, or enzyme histochemistry.
2. One part should be set in a fixative especially suited for immunoperoxidase on paraffin sections, such as B5 or sublimate-formol.
3. One part may be used for fixation in buffered formalin and paraplast embedding. Some elements in lymph node histology are seen more easily in routinely fixed material (e.g., lacunar cells of Hodgkin's disease).
4. One part may be used for plastic embedding. Specimens 1 to 4 may be of equal size; they should not be smaller than 0.5 × 0.5 × 0.5 cm.
5. A few tiny pieces may be cut for electron microscopy (use of a sharp blade is vital here). These should be set in a special fixative—glutaraldehyde or a glutaraldehyde–formaldehyde mixture.
6. A cell suspension may be made, if desired.
7. Touch imprints of one of the parts should be made. They can be very helpful.

If circumstances so indicate, a piece of tissue may be sent to the microbiology department for culture; one of the poles of the lymph node can be used for that purpose. When the cut surface is homogeneous, any part of the node can be used for the various techniques. Needless to say, if macroscopic inspection indicates a process partially involving the node, special care must be taken in sampling.

Not infrequently, a specimen is too small to allow all techniques. In this case, a choice will have to be made. It is always best to ensure material for specimens 1 and 2; at the present time, most membrane-bound antigens can only be demonstrated in frozen sections, although an increasing

**TABLE 2.** *Dividing a lymph node specimen*

| Part of specimen | Prefixation procedure | Fixation method | Embedding | Procedure | Demonstration of: |
|---|---|---|---|---|---|
| 1 | — | Snap-freezing | — | Immunoperoxidase, immunofluorescence, enzyme histochemistry | Any membrane-bound antigen, enzyme activity |
| 2 | — | Fixative especially for immunoperoxidase on paraffin sections (B5, sublimate-formol, Bouin's solution, etc.) | Paraffin | Histology, immunoperoxidase | Morphology, cytoplasmic antigens, few membrane-bound antigens |
| 3 | — | Formalin (buffered) | Paraffin | Histology | Morphology |
| 4 | — | Any of two or three | Resin | Histology, morphometry (immunoperoxidase) | High-quality morphology, cytoplasmic antigens |
| 5 | Make small pieces of tissue | Glutaraldehyde–formaldehyde | Resin | Electron microscopy | Ultrastructural detail |
| 6 | Cell suspension | Snap-freezing or acetone | — | Immunoperoxidase, immunofluorescence | Membrane-bound antigens |
| 7 | Touch imprints | Air-drying or wet fixation (acetone) | — | Cytology | Cytologic features |

number of useful markers do work in paraffin-embedded material (128–132). These markers allow diagnosis in a considerable number of cases. Nevertheless, frozen sections are still necessary in some cases, so sampling procedures are required. Methods have been described that allow detection of membrane-associated antigens in paraffin sections (133) and plastic sections (134); however, the tissue cannot be processed in a routine manner, and separate sampling remains necessary. With a protocol as described here, optimal evaluation of a lymph node specimen is possible; it allows recognition of normal and abnormal lymph node histology in almost all cases.

Certainly with a question as vitally important as the distinction between benign or malignant, the investment in (some of) these techniques is worthwhile. Immunohistochemistry, molecular biology, and electron microscopy are the most important additional techniques widely used. There are others, for instance, quantitative techniques such as morphometry and flow cytometry, but they generally are not used in the diagnosis of lymph node lesions. Of the three techniques mentioned, electron microscopy cannot, in this field, be considered a routine technique, and its use is limited to special questions (e.g., demonstration of Birbeck granules).

## REFERENCES


1. Hall JG. The functional anatomy of lymph nodes. In: Stansfeld AG, ed. *Lymph node biopsy interpretation.* Edinburgh: Churchill Livingstone, 1985:1–25.
2. Parrott DMV. The gut as a lymphoid organ. *Clin Gastroenterol* 1976; 5:211–228.
3. McDermott MR, Bienenstock J. Evidence for a common mucosal immunologic system. I. Migration of B-immunoblasts into intestinal, respiratory and genital tissues. *J Immunol* 1979;122:1892–1898.
4. Sminia T, Plesch BEC. An immunohistochemical study of cells with surface and cytoplasmic immunoglobulins in situ in Peyer's patches and lamina propria of rat small intestine. *Virchows Arch [B]* 1982;40: 181–189.
5. Brown WR. Immunology. In: Kermijn F, Blum AL, eds. *Gastroenterology annual 2.* Amsterdam: Elsevier, 1984:190–213.
6. Roitt IM, Brostoff J, Male DK. *Immunology.* Edinburgh: Churchill Livingstone, 1985.
7. O'Rahilly R, Müller F. *Human embryology and teratology.* New York: Wiley-Liss, 1992.
8. Janeway CA Jr, Travers P. The humoral immune response. In: *Immunobiology. The immune system in health and disease.* Oxford: Blackwell Scientific, 1994:8.1–8.58.
9. Jaspars LJ, van der Linden JC, Scheffer GL, Scheper RJ, Meijer CJLM. Monoclonal antibody 4C7 recognizes an endothelial basement membrane component that is selectively expressed in capillaries of lymphoid follicles. *J Pathol* 1993;170:121–128.
10. Taylor CR. Classification of lymphoma. "New thinking" on old thoughts. *Arch Pathol Lab Med* 1978;102:549–554.
11. van den Oord JJ, deWolf-Peeters C, Desmet VJ. The marginal zone of the human reactive lymph node. *Am J Clin Pathol* 1986;86: 475–479.
12. Nossal GJV, Abbot A, Mitchell J, Lummus Z. Antigens in immunity. XV. Ultrastructural features of antigen capture in primary and secondary follicles. *J Exp Med* 1968;127:277–290.
13. Donaldson SL, Kosco MH, Szakal AK, Tew JG. Localization of antibody-forming cells in draining lymphoid organs during long-term maintenance of the antibody response. *J Leukoc Biol* 1986;40:147–157.
14. Lennert K. Malignant lymphomas, other than Hodgkin's disease. In: *Handbuch der speziellen pathologischen Anatomie und Histologie I/3/B.* Berlin: Springer-Verlag, 1978.
15. Naiem M, Gerdes J, Abdulaziz Z, Stein H, Mason DY. Production of a monoclonal antibody reactive with human dendritic reticulum cells and its use in the immunohistological analysis of lymphoid tissue. *J Clin Pathol* 1983;36:167–175.
16. van der Valk P, van der Loo EM, Jansen J, Daha MR, Meijer CJLM. Analysis of lymphoid and dendritic cells in human lymph node, tonsil and spleen. A study using monoclonal and heterologous antibodies. *Virchows Arch* [B] 1984;45:169–185.
17. Kojima M, Imai Y. Genesis and function of germinal centers. In: *Gann monograph on cancer research. Vol 15.* Tokyo: University of Tokyo Press, 1973:1–24.

18. Gerdes J, Stein H, Mason DY, Ziegler A. Human dendritic reticulum cells of lymphoid follicles: their antigenic profile and their identification as multinucleated giant cells. *Virchows Arch [B]* 1983;42:161–172.
19. Beranek JT, Masseyeff R. [Commentary]. Hyperplastic capillaries and their possible involvement in the pathogenesis of fibrosis. *Histopathology* 1986;10:543–546.
20. Stein H, Bonk A, Tolksdorf G, Lennert K, Rodt H, Gerdes J. Immunohistologic analysis of the organization of normal lymphoid tissue and non-Hodgkin's lymphomas. *J Histochem Cytochem* 1980;28: 746–760.
21. Hsu SM, Cossman J, Jaffe ES. Lymphocyte subsets in normal human lymphoid tissue. *Am J Clin Pathol* 1983;80:21–30.
22. Hsu SM, Jaffe ES. Phenotypic expression of B-lymphocytes. I. Identification with monoclonal antibodies in normal lymphoid tissues. *Am J Pathol* 1984;114:396–402.
23. Janossy G, Thomas JA, Pizzolo G. The analysis of lymphoid subpopulations in normal and malignant tissues by immunofluorescence technique. *J Cancer Res Clin Oncol* 1981;101:1–11.
24. van den Oord JJ. *The immune response in the human lymph node. A morphological, enzyme, and immunohistochemical study* [Thesis]. Leuven, Belgium: University of Leuven, 1985.
25. Veldman JE. *Histophysiology and electron microscopy of the immune response* [Ph.D. thesis]. Groningen, The Netherlands: State University of Groningen, 1970.
26. Oort J, Turk JL. A histological and autoradiographic study of lymph nodes during the development of contact sensitivity in the guinea pig. *Br J Exp Pathol* 1964;46:147–154.
27. Gowans JL, Knight EJ. The route of recirculation of lymphocytes in the rat. *Proc R Soc Biol* 1964;159:257–282.
28. Chin YH, Carey GD, Woodruff JJ. Lymphocyte recognition of lymph node high endothelium. IV. Cell surface structures mediating entry into lymph nodes. *J Immunol* 1982;129:1911–1915.
29. Stevens SK, Weissman IL, Butcher EC. Differences in the migration of B and T lymphocytes: organ-selective localization in vivo and the role of lymphocyte-endothelial cell recognition. *J Immunol* 1982;128: 844–851.
30. Butcher EC, Scollay RG, Weissman IL. Organ aspecificity of lymphocytic migration: mediation by highly selective lymphocyte interaction with organ-specific determinants on high-endothelial venules. *Eur J Immunol* 1980;10:556–561.
31. Pals ST, Kraal G, Horst E, de Groot A, Scheper RJ, Meijer CJLM. Human lymphocyte-high endothelial venule interaction: organ selective binding of T and B lymphocyte populations to high endothelium. *J Immunol* 1986;137:760–763.
32. Kamperdijk EWA, Raaymakers EM, de Leeuw JHS, Hoefsmit EChM. Lymph node macrophages and reticulum cells in the immune response. I. The primary response to paratyphoid vaccine. *Cell Tissue Res* 1978;192:1–23.
33. Groscurth P. Non-lymphatic cells in the lymph node cortex of the mouse. I. Morphology and distribution of the interdigitating cells and the dendritic reticular cells in the mesenteric lymph node of adult ICR mouse. *Pathol Res Pract* 1980;169:212–234.
34. Thorbecke GJ, Silberberg-Sinakin I, Flotte TH. Langerhans' cells as macrophages in skin and lymphoid organs. *J Invest Dermatol* 1980; 75:32–43.
35. Hoefsmit EChM, Duyvestijn AM, Kamperdijk EWA. Relation between Langerhans' cells, veiled cells, and interdigitating cells. *Immunobiology* 1982;161:255–265.
36. Niewenhuis P, Keuning FJ. Germinal centres and the origin of the B cell system. II. Germinal centres in the rabbit spleen and popliteal lymph nodes. *Immunology* 1974;26:509–519.
37. van der Valk P, Willemze R, Meijer CJLM. Peripheral T-cell lymphomas: a clinicopathological and immunological study of 10 cases. *Histopathology* 1986;10:235–249.
38. Anderson AO, Shaw S. T-cell adhesion to endothelium: the FRC conduit system and other anatomic and molecular features which facilitate the adhesion cascade in lymph nodes. *Semin Immunol* 1993; 5:271–282.
39. Forkert PG, Thliveris JA, Bertalanfy FD. Structure of sinuses in the human lymph node. *Cell Tissue Res* 1977;183:115–130.
40. Lennert K. Diagnose und Atiologie der Piringerschen Lymphadenitis. *Verh Dtsch Ges Pathol* 1959;42:203–208.
41. De Almeida PC, Harris NH, Bhan AK. Characterization of immature sinus histiocytes (monocytoid cells) in reactive lymph nodes by use of monoclonal antibodies. *Hum Pathol* 1984;15:330–335.
42. Sheibani K, Fritz RM, Winberg CD, Burke JS, Rappaport H. "Monocytoid" cells in reactive follicular hyperplasia with and without multifocal histiocytic reactions: an immunohistochemical study of 21 cases including suspected cases of toxoplasmic lymphadenitis. Am *J Clin Pathol* 1984;81:453–458.
43. Nieuwenhuis P, Keuning FJ. Germinal centres and the origin of the B-cell system. II. Germinal centres in the rabbit spleen and popliteal lymph nodes. *Immunology* 1974;26:509–519.
44. Kroese FGM. *The generation of germinal centers* [Ph.D. thesis]. Groningen, The Netherlands: State University of Groningen, 1987.
45. Knowles DM, Chadburn A, Inghirani G. Immunophenotypic markers useful in the diagnosis and classification of hematopoietic neoplasms. In: Knowles DM, ed. *Neoplastic hematopathology*. Baltimore: Williams & Wilkins, 1992.
46. Taylor CR. Immunomicroscopy: a diagnostic tool for the surgical pathologist. In: *Major problems in pathology*. Philadelphia: WB Saunders, 1986.
47. Jenette JC, Wick MR. Immunohistochemical techniques. In: Jenette JC, ed. *Immunohistology in diagnostic pathology*. Boca Raton, FL: CRC Press, 1989:2–28.
48. Stein H. The immunologic and immunochemical basis for the Kiel classification. In: Lennert K, ed. *Malignant lymphomas, other than Hodgkin's disease*. Berlin: Springer-Verlag, 1978.
49. Pezzella F, Tse AGD, Cordell JL, Pulford KAF, Gatter KC, Mason DY. Expression of the bcl-2 oncogene protein is not specific for the 14;18 chromosomal translocation. *Am J Pathol* 1990;137:225–232.
50. Poppema S, Bhan AK, Reinherz EL, McCluskey RT, Schlossman SF. Distribution of T cell subsets in human lymph nodes. *J Exp Med* 1981; 153:30–41.
51. Dvoretsky P, Wood GS, Levy R, Warnke RA. T-lymphocyte subsets in follicular lymphomas compared with those in non-neoplastic lymph nodes and tonsils. *Hum Pathol* 1982;13:618–625.
52. Papadimitriou CS, Stein H, Papacharalampoulos NX. Presence of $\alpha$1-antichymotrypsin and $\alpha$1-antitrypsin in hematopoietic and lymphoid tissue cells as revealed by the immunoperoxidase method. *Pathol Res Pract* 1980;169:287–297.
53. Crocker J. The enzyme histochemistry of lymphoid and non-lymphoid cells of the human palatine tonsil: A basis for the study of lymphomas. *J Pathol* 1981;134:81–95.
54. Janossy G, Tidman N, Selby WS, et al. Human T-lymphocytes of inducer and suppressor type occupy different microenvironments. *Nature* 1980;287:81–84.
55. Duijvestijn AM, Horst E, Pals ST, et al. High endothelial differentiation in human lymphoid and inflammatory tissues defined by monoclonal antibody HECA 452. *Am J Pathol* 1988;130:147–155.
56. Picker LJ, Terstappen LWMM, Rott LS, Streeter PR, Stein H, Butcher EC. Differential expression of homing-associated adhesion molecules by T-cell subsets in man. *J Immunol* 1990;145:3247–3255.
57. Nakajima T, Watanabe S, Sato Y, Shimosato Y, Motoi M, Lennert K. S100 protein in Langerhans' cells, interdigitating reticulum cells and histiocytosis X cells. *Gann* 1982;73:429–432.
58. Poulter LW, Campbell DA, Munro C, Janossy G. Discrimination of human macrophages and dendritic cells by means of monoclonal antibodies. *Scand J Immunol* 1986;24:351–357.
59. Crocker J, Williams M. An enzyme histochemical study of the sinuses of reactive lymph nodes. *J Pathol* 1984;142:31–38.
60. Korsmeyer SJ. Immunoglobulin and T-cell receptor genes reveal the clonality, lineage and translocations of lymphoid neoplasms. In: DeVita VT, Hellman S, Rosenberg SA, eds. *Important advances in oncology*. Philadelphia: JB Lippincott, 1987:3–25.
61. O'Connor NTJ, Gatter KC, Wainscoat JS, et al. Practical value of genotypic analysis for diagnosing lymphoproliferative disorders. *J Clin Pathol* 1987;40:147–150.
62. Ha K, Minden M, Hozumi N, Gelfland EW. Immunoglobulin gene rearrangement in acute myelogenous leukemia. *Cancer Res* 1984;44: 4658–4660.
63. Rovigatti U, Mirro J, Kitchingman G, et al. Heavy chain immunoglobulin gene rearrangement in acute non-lymphocytic leukemia. *Blood* 1984;63:1023–1027.
64. Waldmann TA, Davis MA, Bongiovanni KF, Korsmeyer SJ. Rearrangement of genes for the antigen receptor on T-cells as markers of lineage and clonality in human lymphoid neoplasms. *N Engl J Med* 1985;313:776–783.
65. Asou N, Matsuoka M, Hattori T, et al. T-cell gamma gene rearrangements in hematologic neoplasms. *Blood* 1987;69:968–970.

66. Zuniga M, D'Eustachio P, Ruddle NH. Immunoglobulin heavy chain gene rearrangement and transcription in murine T-cell hybrids and T-lymphomas. *Proc Natl Acad Sci U S A* 1982;79:3015–3019.
67. Ha-Kawa K, Hara J, Keiko Y, et al. Kappa-chain rearrangement in an apparent T-lineage lymphoma. *J Clin Invest* 1986;78:1439–1442.
68. Lennert K. Follicular lymphoma. A tumor of the germinal centers. In: Akanaki K, Rappaport H, Bernard CW, Bennett JM, Ishikawa E, eds. *Gann monograph on cancer research. Vol 15.* Tokyo: University of Tokyo Press, 1973:217–231.
69. Lukes RJ, Collins RD. A functional approach to the classification of malignant lymphomas. *Recent Results Cancer Res* 1974;46:18–30.
70. Mann RB, Jaffe ES, Bernard CW. Malignant lymphomas—a conceptual understanding of morphologic diversity. *Am J Pathol* 1979:94; 104–191.
71. Nosanchuk JS, Schnitzer B. Follicular hyperplasia in lymph nodes from patients with rheumatoid arthritis. *Cancer* 1969;24:334–354.
72. Evans N. Lymphadenitis of secondary syphilis: its resemblance to giant follicular lymphadenopathy. *Arch Pathol* 1944;37:175–179.
73. Schnitzer B. Reactive lymphoid hyperplasia. In: Jaffe ES, ed. *Surgical pathology of the lymph nodes and related organs.* Philadelphia: WB Saunders, 1985:22–56.
74. Keller AR, Hochholzer L, Castleman B. Hyaline-vascular and plasma cell types of giant lymph node hyperplasia of the mediastinum and other locations. *Cancer* 1972;29:670–683.
75. Osborne BM, Butler JJ, Variakojis D, Kott M. Reactive lymph node hyperplasia with giant follicles. *Am J Clin Pathol* 1982;78:493–499.
76. Weisenburger DD, Nathwani BN, Winberg CD, Rappaport H. Multicentric angiofollicular lymph node hyperplasia: a clinicopathologic study of 16 cases. *Hum Pathol* 1985;16:162–172.
77. Ioachim HL, Lerner CW, Tapper ML. The lymphoid lesions associated with the acquired immunodeficiency syndrome. *Am J Surg Pathol* 1983;7:543–553.
78. Ewing EP, Chandler FW, Spira TJ, Byrnes RK, Chan WC. Primary lymph node pathology in AIDS and AIDS-related lymphadenopathy. *Arch Pathol Lab Med* 1985;109:977–981.
79. Stanley MW, Frizzera G. Diagnostic specificity of histologic features in lymph node biopsy specimens from patients at risk for the acquired immunodeficiency syndrome. *Hum Pathol* 1986;17:1231–1239.
80. Schuurman HJ, Krone WJA, Broekhuizen R, Goudsmit J. Expression of RNA and antigens of human immunodeficiency virus type-1 (HIV-1) in lymph nodes from HIV-1 infected individuals. *Am J Pathol* 1988; 133:516–524.
81. Le Tourneau A, Audouin J, Diebold J, Marche C, Tircottet V, Reynes M. LAV-like viral particles in lymph node germinals centers in patients with the persistent lymphadenopathy syndrome and the acquired immunodeficiency syndrome–related complex. An ultrastructural study of 30 cases. *Hum Pathol* 1986;17:1047–1053.
82. Rappaport H. Tumors of the hematopoietic system. In: *Atlas of tumor pathology. 3rd series, Fascicle 8.* Washington, DC: Armed Forces Institute of Tumor Pathology, 1966.
83. Dorfman RF, Warnke R. Lymphadenopathy simulating the malignant lymphomas. *Hum Pathol* 1974;5:519–550.
84. Nathwani BN, Winberg CD, Diamond LW, Bearman RM, Kim H. Morphologic criteria for the differentiation of follicular lymphoma from florid reactive follicular hyperplasia. A study of 80 cases. *Cancer* 1981;48:1794–1806.
85. Mann RB. Follicular lymphoma and lymphocytic lymphoma of intermediate differentiation. In: Jaffe ES, ed. *Surgical pathology of the lymph nodes and related organs.* Philadelphia: WB Saunders, 1985: 165–202.
86. Rademakers LHPM, Peters JPJ, van Unnik JAM. Histiocytic and dendritic reticulum cells in follicular structures of follicular lymphoma and reactive hyperplasia. A quantitative electron microscopical analysis. *Virchows Arch [B]* 1983;44:85–98.
87. Harris NL, Ferry JA. Follicular lymphoma and related disorders (germinal center lymphomas). In: Knowles DM, ed. *Neoplastic hematopathology.* Baltimore: Williams & Wilkins, 1992.
88. Stein H, Lennert K, Feller AC, Mason DY. Immunohistological analysis of human lymphoma: correlation of histological and immunological categories. *Adv Cancer Res* 1984;42:67–147.
89. Lennert K, Feller AC, Gödde-Salz E. Morphologie, Immunohistochemie und Genetik peripherer T-zellen-Lymphome. *Onkologie* 1986;9:97–107.
90. Picker LJ, Weiss LM, Medeiros LJ, Wood GS, Warnke RA. Immunophenotypic criteria for the diagnosis of non-Hodgkin's lymphoma. *Am J Pathol* 1987;128:181–201.
91. Saltzstein SL, Ackerman LV. Lymphadenopathy induced by anticonvulsant drugs and mimicking clinically and pathologically malignant lymphoma. *Cancer* 1959;12:164–182.
92. Hartsock RJ. Postvaccinial lymphadenitis. Hyperplasia of lymphoid tissue that simulates malignant lymphomas. *Cancer* 1968;21: 632–649.
93. Audouin J, Diebold J. Modifications histologiques des ganglions lymphatiques au cours des réactions de stimulation immunocytaire. *Ann Pathol* 1986;6:85–98.
94. van den Oord JJ, de Wolf-Peeters C, Desmet VJ, Takahashi K, Ohtsuki Y, Akagi T. Nodular alteration of the paracortical area. An in situ immunohistochemical analysis of primary, secondary and tertiary T nodules. *Am J Pathol* 1985;120:55–66.
95. Kikuchi M, Yoshizumi T, Nakamura H. Necrotizing lymphadenitis: possible acute toxoplasmic infection. *Virchows Arch [A]* 1977;376: 247–253.
96. Chan JKC, Saw D. Histiocytic necrotizing lymphadenitis (Kikuchi's disease). A clinicopathologic study of 9 cases. *Pathology* 1986;18: 22–28.
97. Dorfman RF. Histiocytic necrotizing lymphadenitis of Kikuchi and Fujimoto. *Arch Pathol Lab Med* 1987;111:1026–1029.
98. Knowles DM, Hapler JP. Human T-cell malignancies. Correlative clinical, histopathologic, immunologic and cytochemical analyses of 23 cases. *Am J Pathol* 1982;106:187–203.
99. Lennert K, Stein H, Feller AC, Gerdes J. Morphology, cytochemistry and immunohistology of T-cell lymphomas. In: *B and T cell tumors.* New York: Academic Press, 1982:9–28.
100. Grogan TM, Fielder K, Rangel C, et al. Peripheral T-cell lymphoma: aggressive disease with heterogenous immunotypes. *Am J Clin Pathol* 1985;83:279–288.
101. Knowles DM II. The human T cell leukemias: clinical, cytomorphologic, immunophenotypic and genotypic characteristics. *Hum Pathol* 1986;17:14–33.
102. Rausch E, Kaiserling E, Goos M. Langerhans' cells and interdigitating reticulum cells in the thymus-dependent region in human dermatopathic lymphadenitis. *Virchows Arch [B]* 1977;25:327–343.
103. van den Oord JJ, de Wolf-Peeters C, de Vos R, Desmet VJ. The cortical area in dermatopathic lymphadenitis and other reactive conditions of the lymph node. *Virchows Arch [B]* 1984;45:289–299.
104. Burke JS, Sheibani K, Rappaport H. Dermatopathic lymph adenopathy. An immunophenotypic comparison of cases associated and unassociated with mycosis fungoides. *Am J Pathol* 1986;123:256–263.
105. Willemze R, Scheffer E, Meijer CJLM. Immunohistochemical studies using monoclonal antibodies on lymph nodes from patients with mycosis fungoides and Sézary's syndrome. *Am J Pathol* 1986;120: 46–54.
106. Scheffer E, Meijer CJLM, von Vloten WA. Dermatopathic lymphadenopathy and lymph node involvement in mycosis fungoides. *Cancer* 1980;45:137–148.
107. Colby TV, Burke JS, Hoppe RT. Lymph node biopsy in mycosis fungoides. *Cancer* 1981;47:351–359.
108. Rosai J, Dorfman RF. Sinus histiocytosis with massive lymphadenopathy. A newly recognized benign clinicopathological entity. *Arch Pathol* 1969;87:63–70.
109. Rosai J, Dorfman RF. Sinus histiocytosis with massive lymphadenopathy: pseudolymphomatous benign disorder. Analysis of 34 cases. *Cancer* 1972;30:1174–1180.
110. Callihan TR. The surgical pathology of the differentiated histiocytoses. In: Jaffe ES, ed. *Surgical pathology of the lymph nodes and related organs.* Philadelphia: WB Saunders, 1985:357–380.
111. Favara BE, McCarthy RC, Mierau GW. Histiocytosis X. *Hum Pathol* 1983;14:663–676.
112. Schuler G, Stingl G, Aberer W, Stingl-Gazze LA, Höningsmann H, Wolff K. Histiocytosis X cells in eosinophilic granuloma express Ia and T6 antigens. *J Invest Dermatol* 1983;80:405–409.
113. Brown WR. Immunology. In: Kermijn F, Blum AL, eds. *Gastroenterology annual 2.* Amsterdam: Elsevier, 1984:190–213.
114. Byrne GE, Rappaport H. Malignant histiocytosis. In: Akanaki K, Rappaport H, Bernard CW, Bennett JM, Ishikawa E, eds. *Gann monograph on cancer research. Vol 15.* Tokyo: University of Tokyo Press, 1973:145–162.
115. Warnke R, Kim H, Dorfman RF. Malignant histiocytosis (histiocytic

medullary reticulosis). I. Clinicopathologic study of 29 cases. *Cancer* 1975;35:215–230.
116. van der Valk P, Meijer CJLM, Willemze R, van Oosterom AT, Spaander PJ, Te Velde J. Histiocytic sarcoma (true histiocytic lymphoma). A clinicopathological study of 20 cases. *Histopathology* 1984; 8:105–123.
117. Osborne BM, Butler JJ, Mackay B. Sinusoidal large cell (histiocytic) lymphoma. *Cancer* 1980;46:2484–2491.
118. Kadin ME, Kamoun M, Lamberg J. Erythrophagocytic T$\tau$ lymphoma. A clinicopathologic entity resembling malignant histiocytosis. *N Engl J Med* 1981;304:648–653.
119. Delsol G, Al Saati T, Gatter KC, et al. Coexpression of epithelial membrane antigen (EMA), Ki-1, and interleukin-2 receptor by anaplastic large-cell lymphomas. Diagnostic value in so-called malignant histiocytosis. *Am J Pathol* 1988;130:59–70.
120. Meijer CJLM, Willemze R, Mullink H, Henzen-Logmans SC, van der Valk P. Monoclonal antibodies in the histopathological diagnosis of non-Hodgkin's lymphomas. *Neth J Med* 1985;28:138–141.
121. Sheibani K, Sohn CC, Burke JS, Winberg CD, Wu A, Rappaport H. Monocytoid B-cell lymphoma. A novel B-cell neoplasm. *Am J Pathol* 1986;124:310–318.
122. Cousar JB, McGinn DL, Glick AD, List AF, Collins RD. Report of an unusual lymphoma arising from parafollicular B-lymphocytes (PBL) or so-called "monocytoid" lymphocytes. *Am J Clin Pathol* 1987;87: 121–128.
123. Lukes RJ, Collins RD. Tumors of the hematopoietic system. In: *AFIP atlas of tumor pathology. Fascicle 28,* Armed Forces Institute of Pathology, Washington, DC. 1992.
124. Chan JKC, Warnke RA, Dorfman RF. Vascular transformation of sinuses in lymph nodes. A study of its morphological spectrum and distinction from Kaposi's sarcoma. *Am J Surg Pathol* 1991;15:732–743.
125. Frizzera G, Moran EM, Rappaport H. Angioimmunoblastic lymphadenopathy. Diagnosis and clinical course. *Am J Med* 1975;59: 803–818.
126. Robb-Smith AHT, Taylor CR. *Lymph node biopsy: a diagnostic atlas.* London: Miller-Heyden, 1981.
127. Ioachim HL. *Lymph node biopsy.* Philadelphia: JB Lippincott, 1982.
128. Marder RJ, Variakojis D, Silver J, Epstein AL. Immunohistochemical analysis of human lymphomas with monoclonal antibodies to B-cell and Ia antigens reactive in paraffin sections. *Lab Invest* 1985;52: 497–504.
129. Linder J, Armitage JO, Weisenburger DD. B-cell monoclonal antibodies in paraffin and frozen tissue [Abstract]. *Lab Invest* 1986;54:37.
130. West KP, Warford A, Fray L, Allen M, Campbell AC, Lauder I. The demonstration of B-cell, T-cell and myeloid antigens in paraffin sections. *J Pathol* 1986;150:89–101.
131. Linder J, Ye Y, Harrington DS, Armitage JO, Weisenburger DD. Monoclonal antibodies marking T-lymphocytes in paraffin-embedded tissue. *Am J Pathol* 1987;127:1–8.
132. Poppema S, Hollema H, Visser L, Vos H. Monoclonal antibodies (MT1, MT2, MB1, MB2, MB3) reactive with leukocyte subsets in paraffin-embedded tissue sections. *Am J Pathol* 1987;127:418–429.
133. Sato Y, Mukai K, Watanabe S, Goto M, Shimosato Y. The AMeX method. A simplified technique of tissue processing and paraffin embedding with improved preservation of antigens for immunostaining. *Am J Pathol* 1986;125:431–435.
134. Casey TT, Cousar JB, Collins RD. A simplified plastic embedding and immunohistologic technique for immunophenotypic analysis of human hematopoietic and lymphoid tissue. *Am J Pathol* 1988;131: 183–189.

*Histology for Pathologists, second edition,*
Edited by Stephen S. Sternberg.
Lippincott-Raven Publishers, Philadelphia
© 1997.

# CHAPTER 29

# Spleen

J. Han J. M. van Krieken and Jan te Velde



For a long time, the human spleen received attention from poets as a producer of melancholy. Galen (131–201 A.D.) called the human spleen an enigmatic organ, and this qualification still holds. In the 17th century Malpighi described macroscopically the splenic lymph follicles, the white pulp against a background of red pulp. In 1857 Billroth published one of the first histologic studies of the human spleen in which he divided the red pulp into cord tissue and venous sinuses (1). Still, until the second half of this century, the spleen was considered a rather useless reservoir for blood cells and was hardly studied. The invention of the electron microscope enabled Weiss to elucidate the fine structure of the organ, which gave insight into red pulp function (2,3). In the 1970s Nieuwenhuis, Ford, and Keuning performed immunologic function studies on rat spleen (4–6), and Veerman published a detailed description of the white pulp of the rat spleen (7).

Nevertheless, there is still much confusion surrounding the histology and function of the human spleen. There are several reasons for this confusion. The organ is extremely vulnerable to autolysis, which often makes findings in postmortem specimens difficult to interpret and of limited value for detailed study. Surgically removed spleens are suitable, but they must be processed without delay.

Another source of misunderstanding with respect to the structure of the human spleen is in the terminology and definitions used. As a rule, these terms and definitions originate from studies on animal spleens, but the human spleen does not have an identical architecture. For example, in the human spleen the periarteriolar lymphocyte sheath and the marginal sinus as described in the rat and mouse spleen are not present. Furthermore, certain definitions, for example of the marginal zone, vary widely from author to author (8,9).

The next problem is the large variations that occur in the "normal" spleen. Stimulation of one of the many functions of the spleen can lead to morphologic changes in the compartment that is responsible for that function. The normal spleen therefore shows wide variation. As we have already shown in previous studies, it is essential to define a normal control population if one undertakes histologic studies in the spleen in specific disorders (10). For example, a morphometric analysis showed that spleens removed incidentally during abdominal surgery (i.e., for highly selective vagotomy or early gastric cancer) differed from traumatically ruptured spleens; we therefore excluded the latter from our control group. All these problems sometimes make it difficult to differentiate physiologic from pathologic changes.

J. Han J. M. van Krieken and J te Velde: Department of Pathology, Leiden University Hospital, 2300 RC Leiden, The Netherlands.

Part of this chapter is based on our findings in the study of methylmethacrylate sections of more than 400 surgically removed human spleens and immunohistochemical studies conducted on frozen tissue (11,12).

## PRENATAL AND DEVELOPMENTAL CHANGES

During embryogenesis the spleen can be recognized from about the fifth week of gestation and blood vessels appear at week nine. Red and white pulp cannot be distinguished until the ninth month. The role of the spleen during prenatal development varies widely from that of the adult spleen, and this is reflected in the microscopic anatomy of the organ. Hematopoiesis was considered to take place in the fetal spleen (and liver) and to contribute largely to blood cell formation in the fetus until the sixth month of gestation, but it has been shown that in fact the spleen functions as a site of maturation for hematopoietic precursors from the peripheral blood (13,14). In adults one may see occasionally hematopoietic cells in the spleen in sepsis, as well as in disorders of the bone marrow leading to fibrosis.

The immune system develops during fetal growth, and this development continues after birth (15). This functional maturation is reflected by the morphology: until birth the splenic white pulp does not contain follicles and marginal zones. There are immature B cells in clusters and T cells scattered throughout the organ. Their numbers increase with the developmental age of the fetus, and from the end of the second semester on, B- and T-cell areas can be recognized (16,17). Phagocytosis can be demonstrated at the 12th week of gestation (13,14).

Developmental changes of the spleen are very familiar. The presence of accessory spleens (so-called splenculi, small extra pieces of spleen tissue with the complete and normal histology of the red and white pulp) can be found in at least 25% of autopsies. In disorders being treated with splenectomy, these splenculi may lead to recurrence of the disease.

Rare but well known is the polysplenia associated with immotile cilia syndrome (18). In this syndrome left–right orientation of thoracal and abdominal organs may be abnormal, and the spleen at the right side is often divided into many small pieces, generally having normal function. This is not to be confused with acquired splenosis, in which many small fragments of spleen are present after trauma. Congenital asplenia, which is exceedingly rare, is associated with abnormalities of the cardiovascular system.

## APOPTOSIS

In the development of the spleen, apoptosis does not seem to play an important role, but the lymphoid compartment, as in other lymphoid tissues, shows extensive apoptosis, especially in the germinal centers of the B-cell follicles. This is illustrated in Fig. 1, where the "starry sky" phenomenon can be observed. The starry sky cells are macrophages that phagocytose remnants of lymphocytes that are dying through apoptosis, generally because they have an unsuccessful gene rearrangement of the antigen receptor or because of the fact that the produced immunoglobulin recognizes autoantigen. This physiologic process is important in the protection against autoimmune diseases. The bcl-2 protein that protects against certain forms of apoptosis (see Chapter one), which is expressed in most B and T cells, is lacking in germinal center B cells, rendering them susceptible for apoptosis. In follicular lymphoma the t(14;18) translocation leads to aberrant expression of bcl-2 in the tumor cells. This is sometimes helpful in the recognition of follicular lymphoma in the spleen for the following reasons. Because the spleens of patients above about 20 years of age contain only rarely active germinal centers, the distinction between a primary follicle and follicular lymphoma can be difficult. Furthermore, the involvement of the spleen by follicular lymphoma is often nodular but does not lead to the disturbance of the architecture that is so noticeable in the lymph nodes involved by follicular lymphoma. Because spleens are often received after fixation, immunoglobulin clonality assessment is not possible by immunohistochemistry or immunofluorescence.

## GROSS FEATURES/ORGAN WEIGHT

The human spleen is a bean-shaped organ surrounded by a smooth capsule covered by the peritoneum. In contrast to several species, the capsule does not contain smooth muscle and therefore does not function as a reservoir that can increase rapidly the amount of circulating blood cells like it does in cats and dogs. The surface may be covered with fibrotic or even calcified plaques the cause of which is unknown. It is not uncommon to find several grooves at the outer surface that have no clinical significance. The weight of the spleen is highly variable (19). In adults the spleen generally weighs 150 to 250 g, but in the elderly the spleen is often substantially smaller, even when there is no apparent hypofunction.

On the cut surface, the red and white pulp can be discerned, the latter consisting of small (≤2-mm) nodules. It is important to realize that involvement of the spleen in malignant lymphoma often is observed foremost in the white pulp (20) which becomes enlarged but often not to a great extent. Therefore, the spleen should be cut up into small sections (≤5 mm).

## ANATOMY

### Blood Supply

Blood reaches the spleen via the splenic artery, a large branch from the celiac artery, and enters the spleen through four to six branches, but these latter branches are highly variable in number and location. Venous outflow occurs via the four to six venous branches, which combine in the lienorenal ligament to form the splenic vein, which discharges in the

A

B

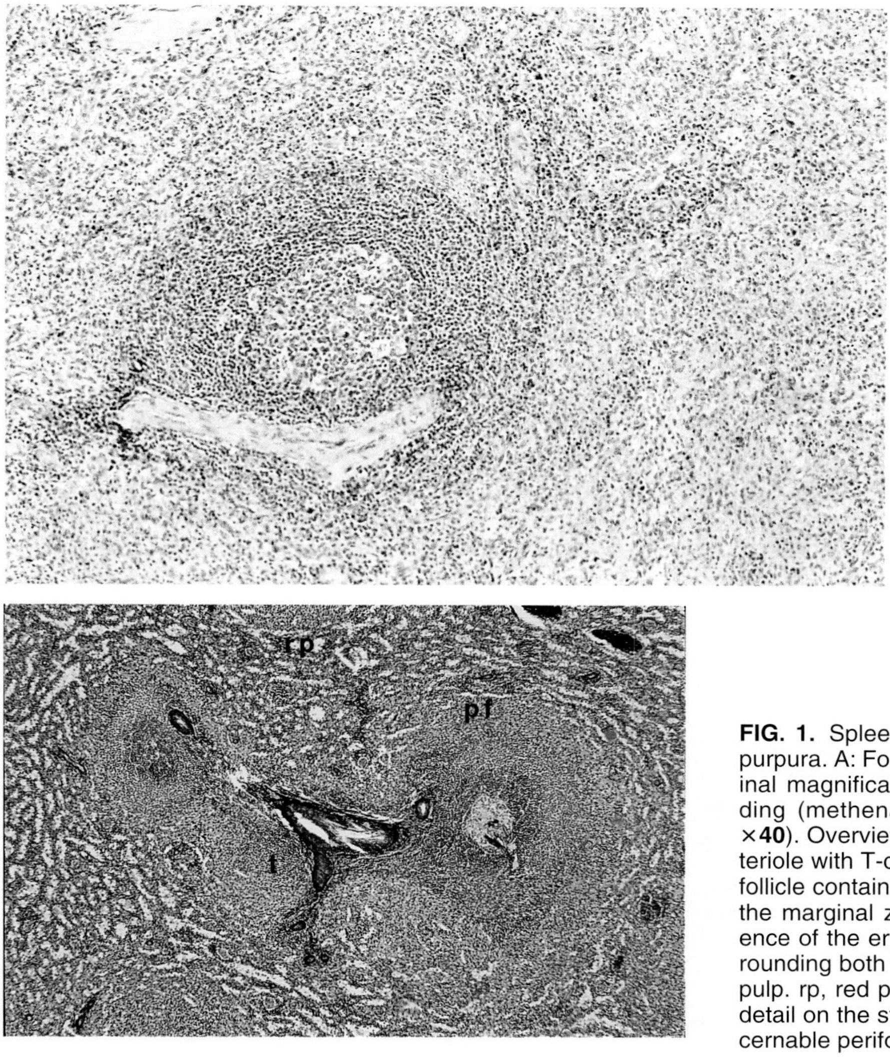


**FIG. 1.** Spleen removed in idiopathic thrombocytopenic purpura. A: Formalin-fixed paraffin embedding (H&E, original magnification ×**40**). B: Methylmethacrylate embedding (methenamine–silver/H&E, original magnification ×**40**). Overview of red and white pulp showing central arteriole with T-cell area, a primary follicle and a secondary follicle containing a germinal center. Note the absence of the marginal zone around the T-cell area and the presence of the erythrocyte-rich (pink) perifollicular zone surrounding both the T- and B-cell compartment of the white pulp. rp, red pulp; pf, perifollicular zone. Note the lack of detail on the structure of the red pulp and the difficult discernable perifollicular zone in standard H&E section.

portal vein (21). This is the reason for splenomegaly in portal hypertension. The blood flow within the spleen is highly specialized and relates to the different functions of the spleen.

### Nerves

The spleen is innervated by nonmyelinated fibers from the major splanchnic nerves and the celiac plexus (22). These nerve fibers run along the splenic artery. Innervation in human spleens is less extensive than in cat and dog spleens, and this might be related to the important reservoir function of the spleen in these animals.

### Lymphatics

The lymph drainage of the spleen occurs via hilar lymph nodes and lymph nodes in the gastrosplenic ligament. The lymph then flows through lymphatics along the splenic artery to the celiac lymph nodes along the celiac artery. The lymphatics in the spleen are described below.

## LIGHT MICROSCOPY

### Vascular Tree

After entering at the hilus, the splenic artery branches like a tree (23). In the splenic tissue the arteries are accompanied by veins and lymph vessels and surrounded by collagenous fibers. These fibrous structures are usually referred to as septa, but serial sections show that this term is inaccurate because they are arranged as cuffs. Real, albeit short, septa are connected to the capsule; they lack vessels and only impinge superficially on the splenic tissue. Focal condensations of reticular fibers without vessels are found in direct continuity with the reticular meshwork of the surrounding red pulp; they seem to be formed after collapse or involution of red pulp tissue (Fig. 2).

Arteries branch to form arterioles that are no longer accompanied by veins and are surrounded not by a collagenous cuff but rather by lymphatic tissue. This lymphatic compartment is present around the vessels and becomes smaller toward the capillary ending. The arterioles are usually de-

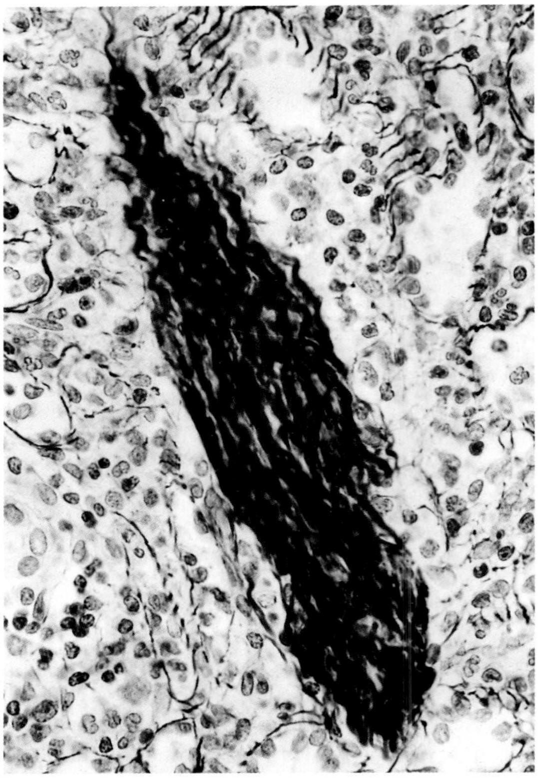

**FIG. 2.** Spleen removed during gastric surgery for highly selective vagotomy. Methylmethacrylate embedding (methenamine–silver/H&E, original magnification ×**250**). Condensed reticulum. Note the continuity with the reticular fibers of red pulp tissue and the circular layers of sinusoidal basal membrane.

scribed as branching into penicilliary arteries, which run in parallel. In humans, however, this phenomenon seems to be restricted to involuted specimens in which the disappearance of tissue between arterioles has left them lying close to each other.

Branching of arterioles and capillaries often occurs at right angles, as can frequently be seen in sections. Reconstructions based on serial sections have shown that the terminal end of the capillary forms a peculiar and specifically splenic structure (24,25) (Figs. 3 and 4). These structures are known by several names, determined partly by the species in which they have been studied, for example, sheathed capillaries, Hülsekapillaren, ellipsoids, or periarteriolar macrophage sheaths. In humans they are present in the red pulp and the perifollicular zone and are generally referred to as sheathed capillaries. The sheathed capillaries are composed solely of mononuclear phagocytes. The endothelial lining of the capillary ends abruptly in a string of concentrically arranged macrophages. Blood cells leaving the capillary have to pass through this sheathed capillary on their way to the lumen of the sinus, which they reach through the stroma of the cord tissue and the slits in the basement membrane of the sinus (3,26). There is no direct opening into the sinusoidal meshwork, which is part of the venous tree. Because autolysis is so rapid, visualization of the sheathed capillaries in particular is dependent on adequate tissue processing. The localization and shape of the sheathed capillaries at the end of the arterial tree seem perfect for a function as the filtering unit of the spleen.

Within the sinusoidal meshwork there are large sinuses that show alkaline phosphatase activity and open directly

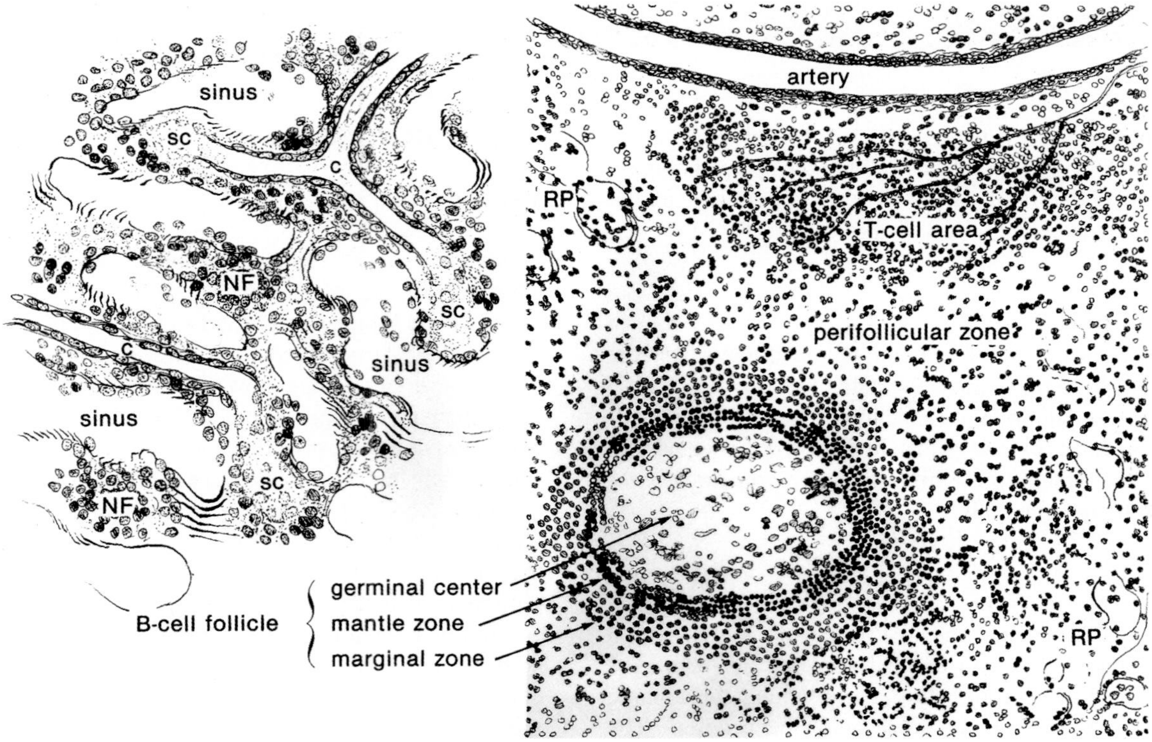

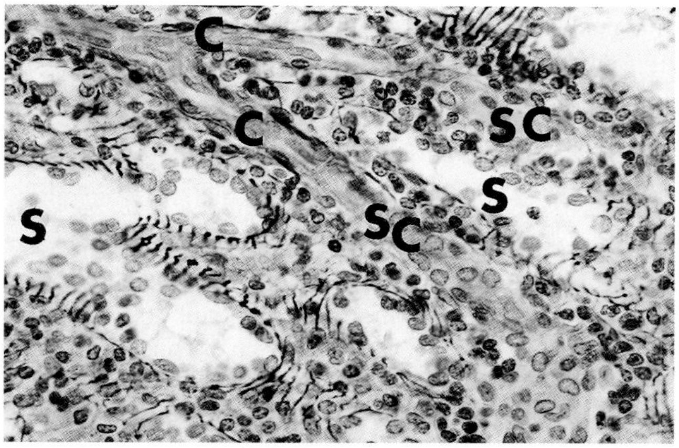

A

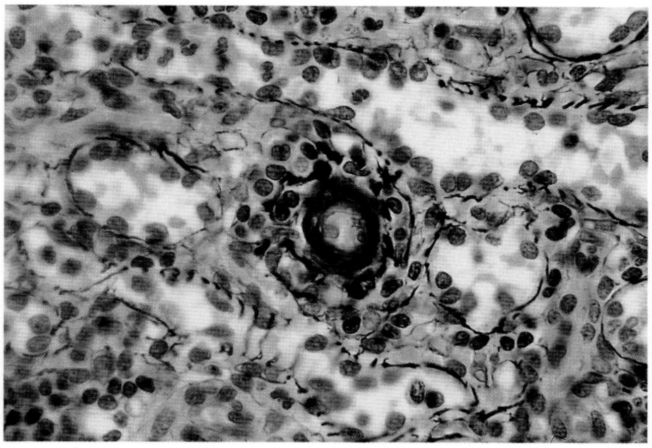
B

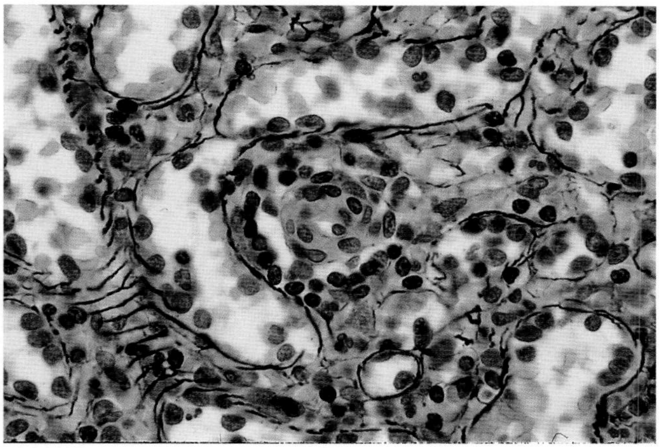
C

**FIG. 4. A:** Traumatic ruptured spleen. Methylmethacrylate embedding (methenamine–silver/H&E, original magnification ×**400**). Capillary transitioning into sheathed capillary. Note the proximity to, but lack of connection with, the sinuses. C, capillary (unsheathed); SC, sheathed capillary; S, sinus. **B:** Same specimen as in A (original magnification ×**1,000**). Detail of unsheathed capillary. **C:** Same specimen as in A (original magnification ×**1,000**). Detail of sheathed capillary.

into veins running along the arteries in the collagenous cuff.

Small lymph vessels can be found in the T-lymphocyte compartment of the white pulp in about two thirds of the spleens. They are not seen in the surrounding perifollicular zone. Figure 5 shows an exceptional example with expanded lymph vessels in a T-cell area along an arteriole. A reconstruction from serial sections showed that these lymph vessels form a network around arterioles and eventually follow the arterial tree to the hilar region (8,27).

## Red Pulp

Seventy-five percent of the volume of the spleen is made up of red pulp (25). The two-dimensional picture given by sections suggests that the red pulp is composed of true cords between vascular spaces, but serial sections show the red pulp to be a loose reticular tissue rich in capillaries and penetrated by venous sinuses (Fig. 6). The sinuses account for about 30% of the red pulp (25). They are surrounded by almost circular strands of basal membrane that are interconnected. In direct continuity with these strands, fibers running through the pulp cords form a reticular network. The sinuses themselves form a meshwork with many interconnections but also with bulblike extensions with blind ends projecting into the cord tissue [see Fig. 4 of van Krieken et al. (25)].

The sinuses are lined by elongated, flat endothelial cells with typical bean-shaped nuclei having a longitudinal cleft. Immunoperoxidase studies have shown positivity for endothelial markers (factor VIII, *Ulex europeus),* but also for other markers such as Leu 2a (CD8) and often Leu 3a (CD4). Parts of the endothelial lining react with a monoclonal antibody against high endothelial venules in the lymph node (van Krieken JHJM, *unpublished observation*).

The red pulp is usually reported to be associated with the filtering function only. In sections one might notice that a

◄

**FIG. 3.** Schematic impression of red **(left)** and white **(right)** pulp, showing the main compartments and structures of the human spleen. The magnifications are the same as in Figs. 6 and 7. The capillaries (c) end as sheathed capillaries (sc) without direct communication with the sinuses. The nonfiltering areas (NF) are bordered by sinuses and are devoid of (sheathed) capillaries. The perifollicular zone surrounds the white pulp (follicle and T-cell area) and lacks fully developed sinuses. Note the zoning in the B-cell, not in the T-cell, compartment. The T-cell area contains a lymphatic plexus.

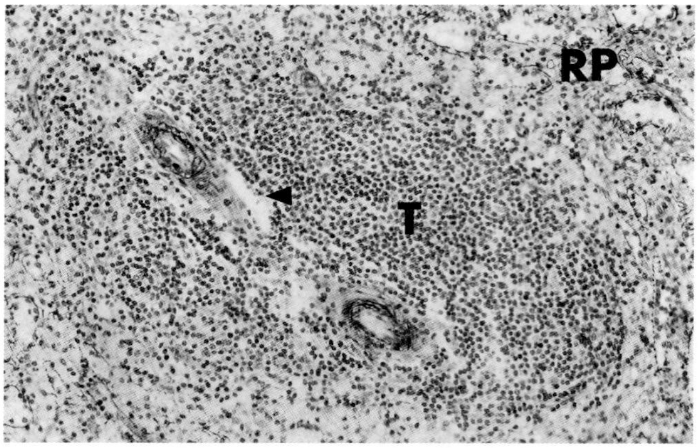


**FIG. 5.** Same specimen as in Fig. 1 (original magnification ×**100**). T-cell area containing exceptionally large lymph vessels in relation to arteriole. *Arrowhead,* lymph vessel; T, T-cell area; RP, red pulp.

fair amount of the red pulp tissue does not include capillary endings or, especially, sheathed capillaries. Serial sections show that these areas are surrounded only by sinuses. Small aggregates of lymphocytes (both B and T) and mononuclear phagocytes are present (Figs. 3 and 6), which means that these nonfiltering areas should be regarded as a part of the lymphoid compartment of the spleen, in addition to the white pulp. Morphometrically, the size of this lymphoid, nonfiltering red pulp compartment seems to equal that of the white pulp (25). Blood cells can only reach these areas by passing through large stretches of red pulp tissue or, which seems more likely, via influx from the sinus by passing through the sinus endothelium. A return of lymphocytes from the sinus lumen back into the splenic tissue is known for the rat spleen, where lymphocytes migrate through the walls of what is called the marginal sinus in the white pulp. This type of sinus is histologically not discernable in the white pulp of the human spleen. In humans, the role played in the rat by the marginal sinus in the exchange of lymphocytes between the sinusoidal circulation and the splenic lymphoid compartment might be taken up by the bulblike extensions of the red pulp sinuses, probably the parts of the sinus endothelium with high endothelial venule characteristics. This hypothesis is supported by the observation that in humans splenic follicles are surrounded by the perifollicular zone, which has a structure similar to that of red pulp cord tissue that is extended by the influx and local proliferation of lymphoreticular cells within pulp cords. New white pulp follicles might thus be formed within the red pulp from the small aggregates in the nonfiltering areas.

## White Pulp

The white pulp consists of B- and T-cell compartments (10) (Fig. 1). The B-cell follicles are composed of a germinal center (only found in secondary follicles) directly surrounded by a ring of small lymphocytes, called the mantle zone or corona, which in turn is surrounded by the marginal zone consisting of medium-sized lymphocytes (Fig. 7). Apart from morphologic differences, the mantle zone and marginal zone lymphocytes can be differentiated by immunophenotyping: the mantle zone lymphocytes are IgD and KiB3 positive and alkaline phosphatase negative, whereas the marginal zone lymphocytes show the opposite (28). In the rat spleen the mantle and marginal zones are separated by a marginal sinus that can easily be seen by light microscopic examination. It plays an essential role in the splenic immune function as the site of entry of lymphocytes and antigen (29). This dividing sinus is not discernible in humans via only light microscopy. Recently, by using electron microscopy, a marginal sinuslike structure was described (30), although it seems to be absent in active follicles (31).

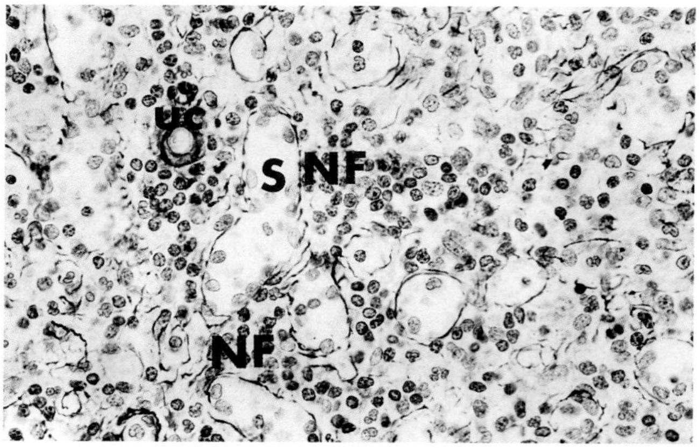


**FIG. 6.** Same specimen as in Fig. 3 (original magnification ×**250**). Detail of the red pulp showing sinuses in cord tissue. Note the nonfiltering areas devoid of capillaries and completely surrounded by sinuses. Uc, unsheathed capillary; S, sinus; NF, nonfiltering area.

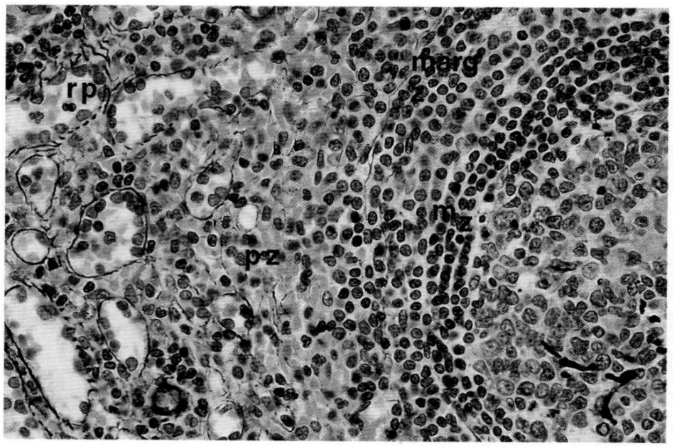


**FIG. 7.** Same specimen as in Fig. 3 (original magnification ×**100**). Secondary follicle (germinal center to the right) bordering the red pulp. mz, mantle zone; margz, marginal zone; pz, perifollicular zone; rp, red pulp.

However, neither the exact location nor functional properties of this structure are known. The light microscopic differences with rodent spleens has led to confusion in the definition of follicular structures.

The term *marginal zone* has been used with different meanings (10,32–34). Some investigators use the term to refer to the ring of medium-sized lymphocytes; others include the mantle zone of small cells or the bordering area between the red and white pulp, and sometimes even the zone surrounding the T-cell areas. We prefer to reserve the term *marginal zone* for the unique splenic structure that is always and exclusively present around the small IgD- and IgM-positive lymphocytes of the mantle zone or primary follicle. We refer to the bordering area between the red and white pulp as the perifollicular zone. The same definitions are used in the extensive Japanese literature on the histology of the human spleen. However, the Japanese investigators call our marginal zone the inner marginal zone. They refer to the perifollicular zone as the outer marginal zone. Because of the totally different architecture and cell population of these two structures, we find it preferable to use different names.

The T-cell areas lie around arterioles but are not as regularly arranged as in the periarteriolar lymphocyte sheath in the rodent spleen (Fig. 5). In humans, they are irregular areas occupied by small polymorphic lymphocytes, most of which stain immunohistochemically with antibodies of the CD4 cluster (T-helper/inducer lymphocytes). Around the T-cell areas too there is a perifollicular zone. The arterioles are not surrounded solely by these T-cell areas because they can be seen traversing follicles and even germinal centers. The follicles sometimes border T-cell areas, with which they share a common perifollicular zone.

### Perifollicular Zone

Around the white pulp follicles and the T-cell areas a zone of splenic reticular tissue is found, the perifollicular zone. In this area the fibers are more widely spaced than in the red pulp cord tissue (Figs. 3 and 7). Here there are capillaries, sheathed capillaries, and considerable numbers of erythrocytes and leukocytes. At the outer border of this area sinuses are more widely spaced.

This zone surrounding the white pulp stands out in silver-stained sections but is usually difficult to recognize in routine hematoxylin and eosin (H&E) sections (Fig. 1A). It is indicated by the presence of a large number of erythrocytes surrounding the densely packed lymphocytes of the T- and B-cell areas. These erythrocytes are distributed more regularly in the perifollicular zone than in the red pulp, where sinuses appear to be emptier than cord tissue is. In silver-stained plastic sections this area can be identified by the absence of the normal sinus distribution of the red pulp and the paucity of strands of basal membranes. The perifollicular zone, which makes up about 8% of the spleen, contains a mixture of blood cells comparable with that of the peripheral blood. It has been suggested that this area is responsible for the slow passage of about 10% of the blood, which is known to have a retarded flow (10).

## ULTRASTRUCTURE

Electron microscopy, especially scanning electron microscopy, including the use of microcasts from the vasculature, has eluded largely the functional microanatomy of the spleen. These studies have shown the routes that blood cells take through the spleen and have illustrated beautifully the fitting function of the spleen by the sinusoids. In surgical pathology of the spleen there is hardly if ever the necessity of using ultrastructural studies.

## FUNCTION

The human spleen has several functions but splenectomy generally does not lead to impaired health. Except for the presence of Howell-Jolly bodies in the peripheral blood, the only well-known health problem in asplenic individuals is the increased risk of overwhelming postsplenectomy infections often caused by pneumococcal sepsis. The reason for this apparent discrepancy is the fact that many functions of the spleen, at least in adults, can be taken over by other organs. In humans the spleen is involved in the primary immune response to blood-borne antigens and polysaccharide antigens; it also acts as a regulator of immune reactions elsewhere in the body. It contains a specific environment for the binding of antibody and antigen; cells or microorganisms coupled with (auto)antibody are trapped and destroyed in the spleen, as are erythrocytes that have decreased flexibility and lowered osmotic resistance (1,35–41). Each of these functions takes place in a specific environment and even under physiologic conditions these compartments change rapidly in size and composition. The main functions therefore to be considered are the filter function, the immunologic function, hematopoiesis, and reservoir function.

### Filter Function

The location of the spleen and the specialized anatomy is especially suitable for its function as a filter of the blood. Normal blood cells pass the barrier of macrophages of the sheathed capillary and the red pulp cord tissue as well as the sinus endothelium (the filtering unit of the spleen) at a speed comparable with the flow in the capillary bed of other organs. If the flexibility of the blood cells is diminished, for example, by aging, intoxication, or congenital defects, the macrophages can ingest the abnormal cells. In addition, bacteria, antigens, and immune complexes are readily taken up by the macrophages of the spleen.

### Immunologic Function

The spleen plays a role in the immune system that is especially important in development, but in adults the spleen is a large producer of B- and T-lymphocytes. The marginal zone is a component of the B-cell follicle and is remarkably large in the spleen, but the exact role is not clear (34). There is possibly a recirculation between the gut-associated lymphoid tissue and the marginal zone of the spleen, which has led to the concept of mucosa-associated lymphoid tissue (MALT) lymphomas as a special entity and which has been the denominator of marginal zone lymphoma (42,43).

The most important role in the immune system is the early response. Because (especially blood-borne) antigens are rapidly trapped in the spleen and brought directly in contact with immunocompetent cells, the spleen is well situated for the early response.

### Hematopoiesis

In rodents the spleen has a large hematopoietic function, but this is not the case in humans. As described above, the hematopoietic function is only small in the fetal spleen and in the adult spleen hematopoiesis occurs only under pathologic conditions.

### Reservoir Function

The spleen contains about 300 ml of blood. This is a relatively small amount, in contrast to dog or cat spleens. Cat and dog spleens function as a reservoir and in situations where more blood is needed can rapidly contract, after which the amount of circulating blood cells increases significantly. This function is not important in humans. There is also not a capsule with a large component of smooth muscle present. The spleen does function as a reservoir for factor VIII, platelets, granulocytes, and iron.

## SPECIAL TECHNIQUES AND PROCEDURES

The spleen is received only rarely for diagnostic purposes. Staging laparotomy is no longer part of the diagnostic workup of a patient with Hodgkin's disease. Therefore, findings of importance are generally incidental. Splenic lymphoma is the most important incidental finding, and for lymphoma diagnosis it is often necessary that frozen tissue be available. Clonality assessment by immunohistochemistry for immunoglobulins is the most important special technique, although this might be done using polymerase chain reaction on paraffin tissue as well. Immunohistochemistry on paraffin-embedded tissue often can be necessary when tumors are found, primary or metastatic, although this situation is rare. In storage disorders such as Gaucher's disease, electron microscopy can be of additional value, although biochemical analysis generally is much easier and more specific.

## AGING DIFFERENCES

In infancy and childhood the immune system is not yet fully developed, and this is reflected in the histology of the spleen containing one of the major lymphoid tissues. The marginal zone is observed as a separate compartment not before four months of age, and the marginal zone B cells in the spleen of infants have a different phenotype (lack of CD21; IgD and IgM positive) compared with adult marginal zones cells (44). An age influence found in our material was the regular occurrence of germinal centers in spleens of patients younger than 20 years; older patients have been shown to have few secondary follicles (8). The often mentioned age-dependent atrophic change has only been documented in patients in the eighth decade (10).

Hyalinization of vessels in the spleen is seen frequently, even in very young children, and is, therefore, an unreliable marker for disease (45).

## ARTIFACTS

Routine paraffin embedding leads to shrinkage and loss of cellular detail. Because routine H&E staining does not yield sufficient information, the use of appropriate histotechniques, for example, plastic embedding (46) and methenamine-silver/H&E (47) or at least periodic acid-Schiff (PAS) staining, is necessary for the study of the splenic architecture (Fig. 8).

## DIFFERENTIAL DIAGNOSIS

In the spleen, a large amount of compartmentalized lymphoid tissue is interwoven by the filtering red pulp. Each

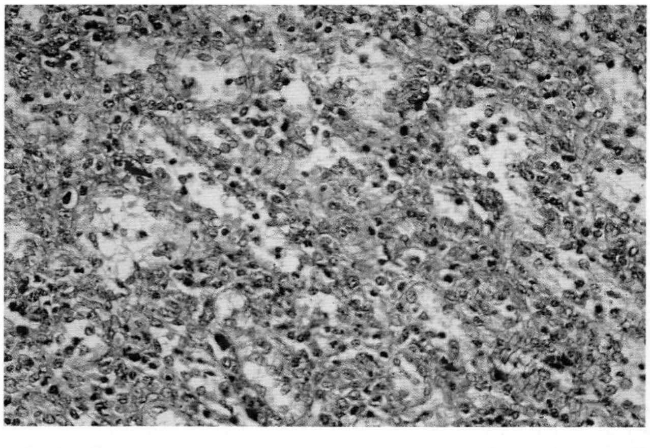

**FIG. 8.** Same specimen as in Fig. 1 (original magnification ×**200**; parafin embedding, PAS stain). Detail of red pulp showing with some difficulty the structure of the sinuses.

compartment reacts to external stimuli with physiologic changes in its composition and histology. As in the lymph node, the line between pathologic and impressive but essential physiologic reactions is vague. The amount of white pulp for instance varied from 5% to 22% in the control group (10).

Normal blood cells pass the barrier of macrophages of the sheathed capillary and the red pulp cord tissue as well as the sinus endothelium (the filtering unit of the spleen) at a speed comparable with the flow in the capillary bed of other organs. If the flexibility of the blood cells is diminished, for example, by aging, intoxication, or congenital defects, the macrophages can ingest the abnormal cells. In this process, the sheathed capillaries seem to breakup; the phagocytes spread out in the surrounding red pulp or enter the sinuses to be transported to the liver. In chronic stimulation of the filtering function, it can be demonstrated that the amount and length of the capillaries increase with the hypertrophy of the red pulp, whereas the sheathed capillaries are less readily seen in the sections (25). In idiopathic thrombocytopenic purpura (ITP), remnants of phagocytosed thrombocytes can be seen as PAS-positive fragments in macrophages. If blood cells are covered by immunoglobulins or complexes, parts of the cell membrane can be removed in a similar fashion as nuclear remnants by the sinus endothelium (pitting and culling), giving rise to spherocytes (14).

Lymphoplasmacytoid and plasma cells occur just around the arteries and arterioles and extend along red pulp capillaries. Their presence is not sufficient for the diagnosis of splenitis. This rim also may contain some macrophages or small epithelioid granulomas, the significance of which is unclear.

In septicemia, the filtering compartment may show all the signs of chronic or acute hemolysis, possibly induced by the amount of circulating complexes, fragmented cells, or coated cells. In patients dying in these conditions with fever, postmortem autolysis of the activated macrophages can lead to early disintegration of the red pulp cells and stroma. The septic spleen at autopsy thus probably represents an artifact that can be the result of, but is not specific for, sepsis; it especially should not be diagnosed as splenitis. True splenitis, in which the spleen contains an inflammatory response to a local noxious agent such as in typhoid fever or tropical diseases, is rare in the Western hemisphere. The presence of plasma cells along the capillary tree is normal and by no means diagnostic for splenitis, nor is the diffuse influx of granulocytes throughout the red pulp in specimens resected during prolonged surgery.

The effects of chronic venous congestion are not clear. In our preliminary studies in patients dying with chronic cardiac disease, the so-called effect of chronic cardiac congestion on the lymphoid and filtering compartments appears more likely to be the effect of accompanying infections and therapy. In venous congestion due to portal hypertension, the sinuses are normal in size but contain fewer buds and appear rigid. The amount of cord tissue per section and the amount of capillaries are decreased; in the cord tissue, an increase of fibers is seen (25). We have not yet been able to study the effects of venous congestion on the composition of the lymphoid compartment of the red pulp.

Infarcts in the splenic tissue are microscopically more irregularly defined and poorly demarcated than could be expected macroscopically due to the intricate arborization of the splenic vessels. In three-dimensional reconstructions, capillaries from different arterioles are seen to cross each other with overlapping territories.

Primary tumors of the spleen are rare. Metastatic carcinoma seems especially to occur in neuroendocrine tumors, including small cell carcinoma of the lung, with a conspicuous tendency for outgrowth into the sinus lumina. Malignant lymphoma exhibits in the spleen a homing pattern to specific compartments dependent on the type of lymphoma, similar to the spread in other lymphoid tissues (20). In hematopoietic cancers with spread to the spleen, the distribution is similar to the pattern in the bone marrow: erythropoiesis and megakaryopoiesis are found primarily along and in the sinuses, whereas myelomonopoiesis is found along the capillaries in the cord tissue. The blasts in acute leukemia can be found anywhere in the spleen. In massive or diffuse involvement of the spleen by malignancy, the architecture of the compartments may be totally disrupted; but with the PAS or methenamine-silver stains, remnants of splenic tissue can still be found, and these remnants may be helpful in the differential diagnosis at autopsy.

## SPECIMEN HANDLING

The spleen is quite vulnerable, and due to the large numbers of macrophages and granulocytes there is rapid autolysis. Proper and rapid fixation is therefore important, and this goal is not reached when the entire organ is put into formalin. For proper handling the specimen has to be received fresh and handling has to be rapid. The organ is weighed and the surface examined. After that the organ is cut into small slices of 0.5 cm and the cut surface is inspected carefully for nodules larger than normal white pulp. Ideally pieces should be frozen for immunohistochemistry. When no abnormalities are seen, three or four pieces are taken out randomly for microscopic examination. Apart from H&E staining, a PAS stain is helpful for examining the structure of the red pulp.

## CONCLUSION

The human spleen is still an enigmatic organ. Studies of its histology must be based on carefully selected, surgically excised "normal" spleens. The organ should be processed immediately and appropriately for optimal results.

The human spleen differs from animal spleen in too many structural aspects to permit extrapolation of animal studies to humans.

Our study of a large series of spleens with adequate histotechniques and with reconstruction based on serial sections

**TABLE 1.** *Summary of histology, function, and relation to lymph node compartments of the lymphoid compartments of the spleen*

| Spleen compartment | Description | Function/composition | Equivalent in lymph node |
|---|---|---|---|
| White pulp | | | |
| T-cell area | Irregular area of small lymphocytes containing lymph vessels bordering arteries | Predominant CD4 lymphocytes | Paracortex |
| B-cell follicle | Round area of small lymphocytes syrrounded by medium-sized lymphocytes (a germinal center may be present) | Production of Ig-producing cells and probably memory cells | Follicle |
| Perifollicular zone | Area between white and red pulp containing many erythrocytes and lacking a normal sinusoidal structure | Place of retarded blood flow with interaction of blood cells, antigen, and antibody | Medulla (?) |
| Red Pulp | | | |
| Sinuses/cord tissue with sheathed capillaries | Tissue containing a meshwork of sinuses (with interrupted basement membrane) and capillaries, partly sheathed | Removal of particles from blood cells. Possible place of interaction of new antigens with reticulum cells | Sinus: partly high endothelial venule<br>Sheathed capillary: medullary sinus |
| Nonfiltering area | Area of red pulp tissue lacking capillaries and containing lymphocytes | Probably place of onset of immune reaction | Medulla or compartment of primary follicles |
| Perivascular rim | Small area along the vessel tree containing lymphocytes and plasma cells | Probably connected to lymphatics | Medulla (?) |

shows that the spleen is a highly compartmentalized organ (Table 1). Each compartment has its own structure and cell population and therefore may have a separate function. The old division into red and white pulp is probably oversimplified and should be expanded.

## REFERENCES


1. Crosby WH. The spleen. In: Wintrobe MM, ed. *Blood pure and eloquent.* New York: McGraw-Hill; 1980:96–138.
2. Chen L, Weiss L. Electron microscopy of the red pulp of human spleen. *Am J Anat* 1972;134:425–458.
3. Weiss L. The spleen. In: Greep RO, Weiss L, eds. *Histology. 3rd ed.* New York: McGraw-Hill; 1973:545–573.
4. Nieuwenhuis P, Keuning FJ. Germinal centres and the origin of the B-cell system II germinal centres in the rabbit spleen and popliteal lymph nodes. *Immunology* 1974;26:509–519.
5. Nieuwenhuis P, Ford WL. Comparative migration of B- and T-lymphocytes in the rat spleen and lymph nodes. *Cell Immunol* 1976;23: 254–267.
6. Ford WL. Lymphocyte migration and immune responses. *Prog Allergy* 1975;19:1–59.
7. Veerman AJP. White pulp compartments in the spleen of rats and mice. *Cell Tissue Res* 1975;156:417–441.
8. van Krieken JHJM, te Velde J, Kleiverda K, Leenheers-Binnendijk L, van der Velde CJH. The human spleen; A histological study in splenectomy specimens embedded in methylmethacrylate. *Histopathology* 1985;9:571–585.
9. Scothorne RJ. The spleen: structure and function. *Histopathology* 1985; 9:663–669.
10. van Krieken JHJM, te Velde J, Hermans J, Cornelisse CJ, Welvaart K, Ferrari M. The amount of white pulp in the spleen: a morphometrical study done in methylmethacrylate-embedded splenectomy specimens. *Histopathology* 1983;7:167–182.
11. van Krieken JHJM. *The architecture of the human spleen* [Academic thesis]. Pijnacker, The Netherlands: Dutch Efficiency Bureau, 1985.
12. van Krieken JHJM, te Velde J. Immunohistology of the human: an inventory of the localization of lymphocyte subpopulations. *Histopathology* 1986;10:285–294.
13. Wolf BC, Luevano E, Neiman RS. Evidence that the human fetal spleen is not a hematopoietic organ. *Am J Clin Pathol* 1983;80:140.
14. Wolf BC, Neiman RS. *Disorders of the spleen.* Philadelphia: WB Saunders, 1989
15. Timens W, Rozeboom-Uiterwijk T, Poppema S. Fetal and neonatal development of human spleen: an immunohistological study. *Immunology* 1987;60:603–609.
16. Jones JF. Development of the spleen. *Lymphology* 1983;16:83–89.
17. Namikawa R, Mizuno T, Matsuoka H, et al. Ontogenic development of T and B cells and non-lymphoid cells in the white pulp of human spleen. *Immunology* 1986;57:61–69
18. Moller JH, Nakib A, Anderson RC, Edwards JE. Congenital cardiac disease associated with polysplenia. A developmental complex of bilateral "leftsidedness." *Circulation* 1967;36:789.
19. Myers J, Segal RJ. Weight of the spleen. I. Range of normal in a nonhospital population. *Arch Pathol* 1974;98:33.
20. van Krieken JHJM, Feller AC, te Velde J. The distribution of non-Hodgkin's lymphoma in the lymphoid compartments of the human spleen. *Am J Surg Pathol* 1989;13:757–765.
21. Seufert RM. *Chirurgie der Milz.* Stuttgart, Germany: Enke Verlag, 1983.
22. Tischendorf F. *Blutgefäss- und Lympfgefässapparat Innersekretorische Drusen. Die Milz.* Berlin: Springer Verlag, 1969.
23. Snook T. A comparative study of the vascular arrangements in mammalian spleens. *Am J Anat* 1950;87:31–65.
24. Buyssens N, Paulus G, Bourgeois N. Ellipsoids in the human spleen. *Virchows Arch [A]* 1984;403:27–40.
25. van Krieken JHJM, te Velde J, Hermans J, Welvaart K. The splenic red pulp: a histomorphometrical study in splenectomy specimens embedded in methylmethacrylate. *Histopathology* 1985;9:401–416.
26. Heusermann U, Stutte HJ. Comparative histochemical and electron microscopic studies of the sinus and venous walls of the human spleen with special reference to the sinus–venous connections. *Cell Tissue Res* 1975;163:519–533.

27. Fukuda T. Deep lymphatics of the spleen. *Tohoku J Exp Med* 1963;79: 281–292.
28. van Krieken JHJM, Von Schilling C, Kluin PhM, Lennert K. Splenic marginal zone cells and related cells in the lymph node: a morphologic and immunohistochemical study. *Hum Pathol* 1989;20:320–325.
29. Sasou S, Satodate R, Katsura S. The marginal sinus in the perifollicular region of the rat spleen. *Cell Tissue Res* 1976;172:195–203.
30. Schmidt EE, MacDonald IC, Groom AC. Microcirculatory pathways in normal human spleen, demonstrated by scanning electron microscopy of corrosion casts. *Am J Anat* 1988;181:253–266.
31. Schmidt EE, MacDonald IC, Groom AC. Changes in microcirculatory pathways in chronic idiopathioc thrombocytopenic purpura. *Blood* 1991;78:1485–1489.
32. Takasaki S. Light microscopic, scanning and transmission electron microscopic, and enzyme histochemical observations on the boundary zone between the red pulp and its surroundings in human spleens. *Tokyo Yikekai Med J* 1979;94:553–568.
33. Yamamoto K, Arimasa N, Yamamoto T, Tokuyama K, Kobayashi T, Itoshima T. Scanning electron microscopy of the perimarginal cavernous sinus plexus of the human spleen. *Scanning Microsc* 1979; 3:763–768.
34. Kraal G. Cells in the marginal zone of the spleen. *Int Rec Cyt* 1992;132: 31–74
35. Koyama S, Aoki S, Deguchi K. Electron microscopic observations of the splenic red pulp with special reference to the pitting function. *Mie Med J* 1964;14:143–165.
36. Sampson D, Grotelueschen C, Kauffman HM. The human splenic suppressor cell. *Transplantation* 1975;20:362–367.
37. Videbaek A, Christensen BE, Jonsson V. *The spleen in health and disease.* Chicago: Year Book Medical; 1983.
38. Wyler DJ. The spleen in malaria. In: *Malaria and the red cell.* London: Pitman; 1983.
39. Van Krieken JHJM, Breedveld FC, te Velde J. The spleen in Felty's syndrome: A histological, morphometrical, and immunohistochemical study. *Eur J Haematol* 1988;40:58–64.
40. Claassen E. Histological organization of the spleen: implications for immune functions in different species (38th forum in immunology). *Res Immunol* 1991;142:315–372.
41. Van Rooijen N, Claassen E, Kraal G, Dijkstra C. Cytological basis of immune functions of the spleen. *Prog Histochem Cytochem* 1989;19: 1–69.
42. Harris NL, Jaffe ES, Stein H, et al. A revised European–American classification of lymphoid neoplasms: A proposal from the international lymphoma study group. *Blood* 1998;84:1361–1392.
43. Isaacson PG, Wright DH. Malignant lymphoma of the mucosa-associated lymphoid tissue. *Cancer* 1983;52:1410–1416.
44. Timens W, Boes A, Rozeboom-Uiterwijk T, Poppema S. Immaturity of the human splenic marginal zone in infancy: Contribution to the deficient infant immune response.
45. Lindey RP. Splenic arteriolar hyalin in children. *J Pathol* 1986;148: 321–326.
46. te Velde J, Burckhardt R, Kleiverda K, Leenheers-Binnendijk L, Sommerfeld W. Methyl-methacrylate as an embedding medium in histopathology. *Histopathology* 1977;1:319–330.
47. Jones DB. Nephrotic glomerulonephritis. *Am J Pathol* 1975;33: 313–323.

*Histology for Pathologists, second edition,*
Edited by Stephen S. Sternberg.
Lippincott-Raven Publishers, Philadelphia
© 1997.

# CHAPTER 30

# Thymus

Saul Suster and Juan Rosai



The thymus is a prototypical lymphoepithelial organ. As such, it is composed of intimately admixed epithelial and lymphoid elements that act in concert to perform their assigned roles. In addition, the thymus harbors other cellular constituents, such as a variety of mesenchymal-derived elements, scattered neuroendocrine cells, and presumably germ cells, all of which may take part in the development of neoplastic and nonneoplastic processes of this organ. Although much progress has been made in the immunohistochemical characterization of the cellular components of the thymus, the diagnosis of thymic lesions still remains largely dependent on the light microscopic interpretation of the findings by the pathologist.

## EMBRYOLOGY

The thymus is derived from the third and, to a lesser extent, the fourth pharyngeal pouches, which contain elements derived from all three germinal layers. During the sixth week of gestation, the endodermal lining of the ventral wing of the third pharyngeal pouch forms a pronounced sacculation, which subsequently detaches from the pharyngeal wall, giving rise to the thymic primordia (1,2). It is postulated that, at approximately the same time, the cervical sinus (an ectodermal structure that results from the fusion of the second, third, and fourth branchial clefts) attaches to the thymic primordia, investing them with a layer of ectodermal cells (1,3). As development continues, the thymic primordia migrate in a caudal and medial direction along with the lower parathyroid glands. During the eighth week, these primordia enlarge toward their lower ends, forming two epithelial bars that fuse along the midline to occupy their definitive position within the anterosuperior mediastinum. During this descent, the tail portion of the organ becomes thin and elongated and breaks up into small fragments that usually disappear but that may persist in the soft tissues of the neck, often in intimate connection with the lower parathyroid gland and sometimes embedded within the thyroid gland (see section on Developmental Abnormalities) (1,4). After migration has been completed, the thymic endodermal-derived epithelial cells develop into stellate elements, forming a reticular meshwork. The surrounding mesenchymal elements form a capsule around it, and as a result of ingrowth of the capsule, trabeculae form that divide the organ into numerous lobules. By the tenth week, small lymphoid cells originating in the fetal liver and bone marrow populate the thymus, and the organ differentiates into a cortex and a medulla (5). Small, tubular structures composed of epithelial cells (sometimes referred

S. Suster: Department of Pathology, Mount Sinai Medical Center of Greater Miami, and the University of Miami School of Medicine, Miami Beach, Florida 33140.
J. Rosai: Department of Pathology, Memorial Sloan-Kettering Cancer Center, New York, New York 10021.

to as medullary duct epithelium) also make their appearance at this time and later give rise to Hassall's corpuscles (6). The thymus progressively enlarges until puberty and from then on begins to involute, although persisting in an atrophic state into old age.

## DEVELOPMENTAL ABNORMALITIES

Disturbances in the embryologic development of the thymus may give rise to a series of congenital anomalies. One of the anomalies most frequently encountered is the presence of parathyroid gland tissue within the thymus (7) (Fig. 1). Such ectopically located tissue is most frequently encountered within the thymic capsule or in close proximity to it (8). This abnormality is easily explained by the close developmental relationship that exists between the two organs, as described in the section on embryology. The thymus itself also may be found in ectopic locations; this usually results from failure of the organ to migrate to its final destination during embryonic development. Undescended thymuses most often are located in the lateral neck, in close association with or even buried within the parathyroid or thyroid glands (9). These rests have a tendency to undergo cystic changes (9). They also may give rise to thymomas, ectopic examples of which have been described in submandibular (10), paratracheal (11,12), and intratracheal locations (13), as well as within the thyroid gland (14,15). A morphologically distinctive lesion of the thymus displaying combined features of neoplasia and hamartoma occurring in the lower neck has also been recognized (16). Ectopic nodules composed of thymic tissue have been reported in several other locations, including the pulmonary hilus at the root of the bronchus (17), and the base of the skull (18).

Ectopic sebaceous glands have been reported in the thymus (19) and are felt to be related to the contribution of the ectodermally derived cervical sinus to the developing thymus. Mature-appearing salivary gland tissue also may be present in the thymus (Fig. 2) and has been reported as a component of an intrathoracic cyst that contained within its walls normal thymus and parathyroid tissue (20). It was postulated that this finding could be related to a developmental malformation whereby salivary gland anlagen had been incorporated into the uppermost portion of the third pharyngeal pouch during embryogenesis.

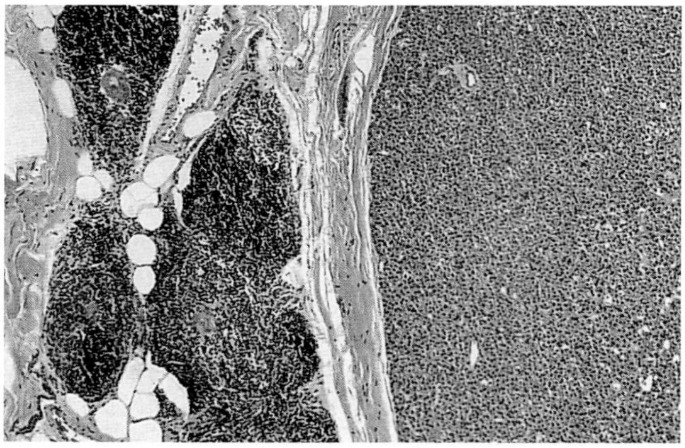

**FIG. 1.** Ectopic parathyroid tissue adjacent to normal thymic gland.

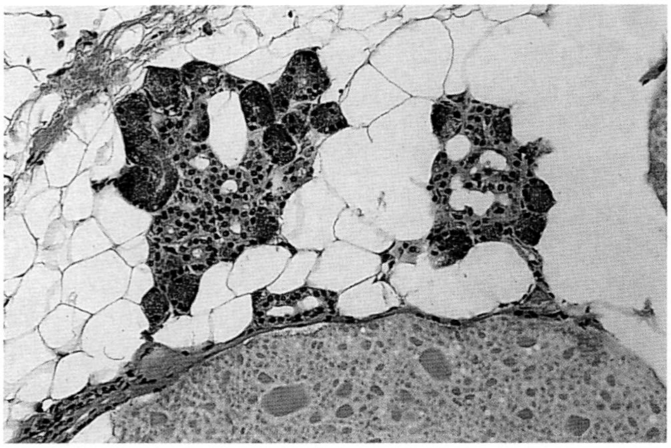

**FIG. 2.** Mature-appearing salivary gland acini are seen adjacent to cystically dilated Hassall's corpuscle.

Morphologic abnormalities of the thymus characterized by an embryonal appearance, with a predominance of small spindle epithelial cells adopting a lobular configuration and lacking small lymphocytes and Hassall's corpuscles, have been observed in association with combined immunodeficiency syndromes and T-cell defects (21). Such morphologic alterations have been termed thymic dysplasias and are believed to represent disturbances of normal development. In conditions such as reticular dysgenesis, Swiss-type hypogammaglobulinemia, thymic alymphoplasia, and ataxia–telangiectasia, the immune deficit is accompanied by aplasia or hypoplasia of the thymus with dysplastic changes (22–24). In DiGeorge's syndrome, which is believed to result from an arrest in development of the third and possibly fourth branchial arches, there is a vestigial but normal thymus associated with absence or hypoplasia of the parathyroid glands (25). In Nezelof's syndrome (26), the thymic abnormality is similar to that of DiGeorge's syndrome except that the parathyroids are normal. The failure of development is thus thought to involve only that part of the branchial entoderm that will differentiate into thymic epithelium. Histologic changes in the thymus similar to those of thymic dysplasia of primary immunodeficiency disease have been observed in infants as a consequence of graft-versus-host disease after blood transfusions (27). A case of congenital aplasia of the parathyroid glands and thymus in the newborn also has been described (28).

## APOPTOSIS

Apoptosis is the name that has been given to the process of physiologic (programmed) cell death. Most thymic lymphocytes die in situ by such a process. During T-cell ontogeny in the thymus, the T cells may undergo a process of positive or negative selection. The accumulated evidence appears to support that apoptosis plays a major role in the process of negative selection and that the vast majority of cortical thymocytes die by this mechanism. Autoreactive thymocytes or harmful cells in the thymus with injured DNA or alterations of their metabolism are also thought to be eliminated by the process of apoptosis at a specific stage of their differentiation (29,30). Therefore, it is believed that disturbances of the apoptotic process within the thymus can be responsible for the appearance of autoreactive cells in the circulation that may give rise to the development of autoimmune disease. In addition, failure of apoptosis also may play a role in carcinogenesis. On the other hand, massive induction of apoptosis within the thymus may lead to immunodeficiency due to a decrease in the number of lymphocytes. Thus, thymocyte apoptosis plays an integral role in the pathophysiology of the immune system.

The exact biochemical mechanism involved in thymocyte apoptosis has not yet been completely elucidated; however, it is known that various complex physiologic and nonphysiologic mechanisms can induce it (31). This has led many investigators to seek the genes and their products that are necessary for apoptosis. Several groups have noted that messenger RNA (mRNA) levels for various proteins are increased early in thymocytes after treatment with glucocorticoids or radiation, two agents known to induce massive apoptosis of cortical thymocytes (32,33). A number of genes also have been identified whose expression is increased in cells undergoing apoptosis. Among them, three protooncogene products have been shown to act as important regulators of the apoptotic process in mammals: *c-myc, bcl-2,* and *p53.* In thymocytes, *bcl-2* mRNA is present in the surviving mature thymocytes of the medulla and also in most immature ($CD4^+CD8^+$) thymocytes, although the majority of cortical thymocytes, most of which die by apoptosis, display no *bcl-2,* suggesting that this oncogene may be involved in the preservation of T cells (34). Alterations of the *p53* gene also have been shown to play a role in the process of thymocyte apoptosis. Malfunction of the tumor suppressor gene *p53* may promote carcinogenesis by permitting mutated cells to duplicate their DNA before it is repaired. In mice, *p53*-deficient thymocytes have been shown to display drastic resistance to the apoptotic effects of radiation (35). The latter observation suggests that the integrity of the *p53* gene, whose product is known to arrest cell proliferation, may be necessary for the normal apoptotic process in the thymus.

Another pathway of thymocyte apoptosis that has been the object of close scrutiny is the role of the T-cell receptor (TCR)/CD3 complex in this process. During thymocyte development, rearrangement of TCR genes leads to expression of unique, clonally expressed TCRs. Potentially autoreactive thymocytes bearing TCRs with high avidity for self undergo TCR-mediated, activation-induced apoptosis (negative selection), whereas thymocytes with TCRs of low avidity survive (positive selection) (36,37). Recent experiments have demonstrated that the activation of the CD3/TCR complex leads to the preferential elimination of immature ($CD4^+/CD8^+$) thymocytes (38). These and other studies have demonstrated that TCR-mediated signals are involved in cell death (apoptosis), and this phenomenon is strongly related to the mechanism of negative selection, although the precise in situ mechanism of apoptosis has not yet been elucidated (39,40).

## ANATOMY

The fully mature human thymus is an encapsulated midline structure predominantly located in the anterosuperior mediastinum and composed of two lobules joined in the midline by loose connective tissue and thymic parenchyma. The base of the organ lies on the pericardium and great vessels. The upper poles of each lobe extend into the lower neck and are closely applied to the trachea. The lower poles extend down over the pericardium for a variable distance, generally up to the level of the fourth costal cartilage. The anterior border of the gland is made up by the cervical fascia, strap muscles of the neck, sternum, costal cartilages, and intercostal muscles, and the lateral borders are covered by reflections of the parietal pleura.

The size and weight of the gland may vary considerably depending on the age of the person, although wide variations among individuals in the same age group have been observed (41). The mean weight at birth is about 20 g. The organ exhibits a continuous growth in size until puberty, when it reaches a mean weight of approximately 35 to 50 g; thereafter, it undergoes atrophy manifested by a decrease in weight and volume and progressive fatty replacement of the parenchyma.

The blood supply of the organ is derived from the internal mammary, superior and inferior thyroid arteries, and, to a lesser degree, the pericardiophrenic arteries. The arterial branches course along fibrous septa to the region near the corticomedullary junction, where they branch into the cortex and the medulla. The capillaries descend from the outer cortex toward the medulla to form postcapillary venules, and exit the thymus through the septa as interlobular veins. The venous system drains into the left brachiocephalic, internal thoracic, and inferior thyroid veins. There are no true thymic intraparenchymatous afferent lymphatics. Lymph vessels arise in the interstitium of the lobular septa and merge to form large lymph vessels that course alongside the arteries in the septa. The innervation of the organ is derived from branches of the vagus nerve and the cervical sympathetic nerves.

## HISTOLOGY

The basic structural unit of the thymus is the lobule. Each lobule is composed of two morphologically distinctive compartments, the cortex and the medulla, both of which are largely composed of varying proportions of epithelial cells and thymic lymphocytes (thymocytes) (Fig. 3). In the cortex, the sparse epithelial cells present are overshadowed by the numerous, closely packed small lymphocytes. The medulla, in contrast, contains a larger number of epithelial cells and fewer lymphocytes.

### Epithelial Cells

The epithelial cells of the thymus have traditionally been divided into cortical and medullary; some of the latter are arranged in round keratinized structures known as Hassall's corpuscles. In the active thymus of infancy, most epithelial cells are plump, with round or oval nuclei. Their cytoplasm (particularly in the case of the cortical cells) is endowed with numerous prolongations that join with those of adjacent cells to form a veritable network or reticulum. This feature (rather than the relationship with reticulin fibers or presumptive embryologic origin) has led to the alternative designation of reticuloepithelial cells. These various epithelial elements play an active role in promoting T-cell maturation in the thymus, either through the action of their humoral substances or through direct contact with thymocytes (42).

A subset of thymic epithelial cells that have predominantly localized to the cortex has been designated as nurse cells. They are characterized by having an abundant cytoplasm within which are engulfed numerous mature thymic T-lymphocytes. A ringlike staining pattern has been observed in these cells with antiepithelial cell antibodies by immunohistochemistry on sections of human thymus (43). It has been postulated that nurse cells may provide a specialized microenvironment for T-cell maturation, differentiation, and selection in the thymus (43,44).

### Hassall's Corpuscles

Hassall's corpuscles constitute the most readily identifiable feature of the thymus at the light microscopic level. They are restricted to the medulla and are characterized by a concentric pattern of keratinization, the keratin formed being of high-molecular-weight (epidermal) type (Fig. 4). These structures may show much variation in their morphologic appearance, mainly as a result of reactive changes secondary to inflammation. This includes cystic degeneration with accumulation of cellular debris, dystrophic calcification, and infiltration by lymphocytes, foamy macrophages, and eosinophils (Fig. 5). The thymic lesions known as Dubois's microabscesses and traditionally ascribed to congenital syphilis (45) represent an exaggeration of the cystic changes in Hassall's corpuscles as a result of infection. We believe that most so-called multilocular thymic cysts are not congenital abnormalities but rather the result of cystic enlargement of Hassall's corpuscles on the basis of acquired inflammatory changes in this organ (46). An additional change that can be seen in relation to cystic Hassall's corpuscles is the presence of glandular elements, as manifested by the appearance of columnar epithelium (sometimes ciliated- or of goblet-cell type) and the secretion of sulfated acid mucopolysaccharides in the lumen (47). It is likely that these glandular changes are related to the embryologic origin of Hassall's corpuscles (6).

### Thymic Lymphocytes (Thymocytes)

The predominant cell population of the thymic cortex is made up of lymphocytes that may be large, medium, or small. Large, mitotically active lymphoblasts comprise about 15% of the lymphoid cells and are found predominantly in the subcapsular portion of the outer cortex (48). These lymphocytes have a round or oval (occasionally convoluted) nucleus, one or two prominent nucleoli, and relatively abundant, strongly basophilic cytoplasm. A gradient of smaller, less mitotically active cells occurs from the outer cortex to the corticomedullary junction and to a lesser degree into the medulla of the normal thymus (Fig. 6). In

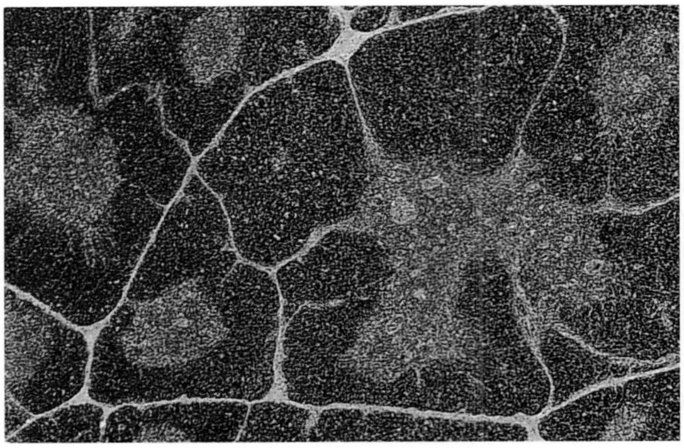

**FIG. 3.** Normal lobular architecture of the thymus demonstrating clear separation between cortex and medulla.

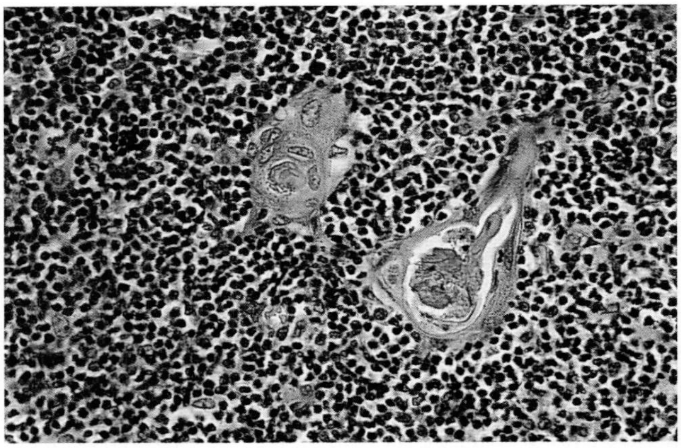

**FIG. 4.** Normal Hassall's corpuscles showing characteristic concentric arrangement of keratinizing epithelial cells.

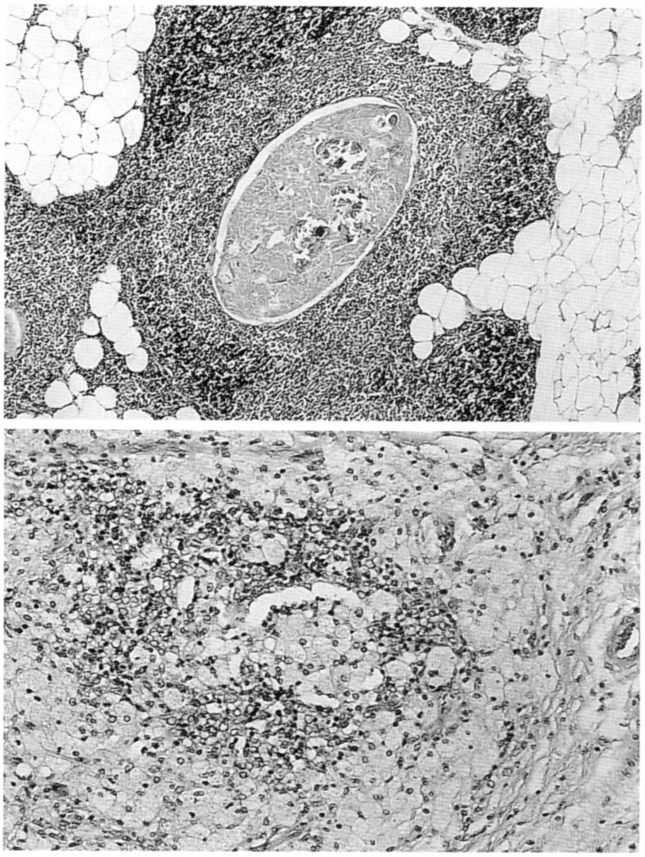

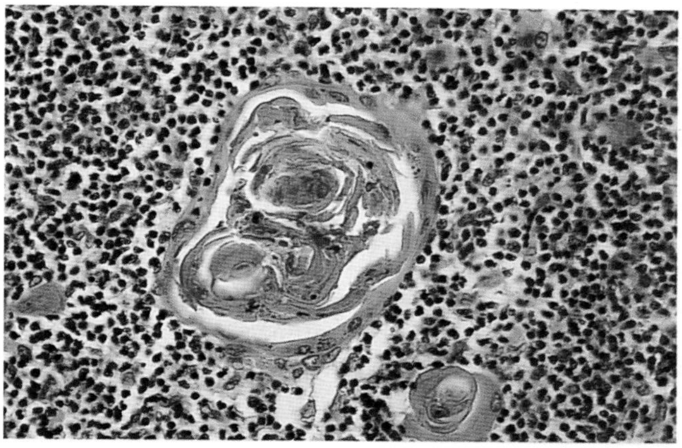

FIG. 5. Hassall's corpuscles showing (**A**) cystic dilatation with accumulation of cellular debris, (**B**) dystrophic calcification, and (**C**) accumulation of foamy macrophages.

the capsular region and deep cortex, the vast majority of thymic lymphocytes are short-lived and die in situ (49). This results in lympholysis and active phagocytosis, features that impart these areas with a prominent "starry sky" appearance and that become particularly prominent in accidental (stress) thymic involution (see section on Thymic Involution) (Fig. 7).

### Other Cell Types

In addition to epithelial cells and lymphocytes of T-cell lineage, the thymus contains an array of additional cell types. B-lymphocytes can be found aggregated as lymphoid follicles or scattered as individual cells. Lymphoid follicles with active germinal centers may be found in otherwise normal

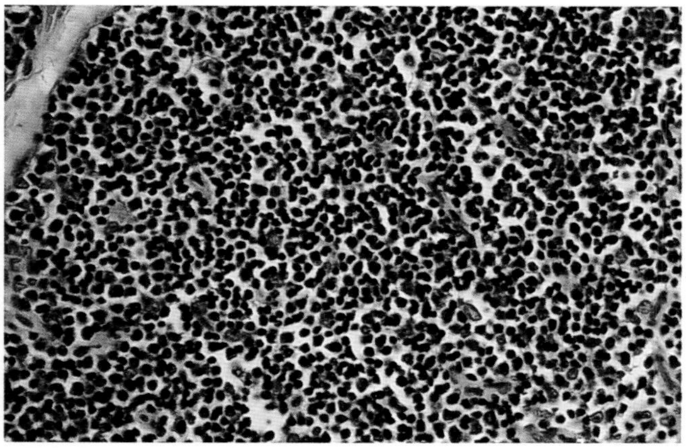

**FIG. 6.** Normal thymic cortex. There are numerous cortical thymocytes most of which have small nuclei with densely packed chromatin.

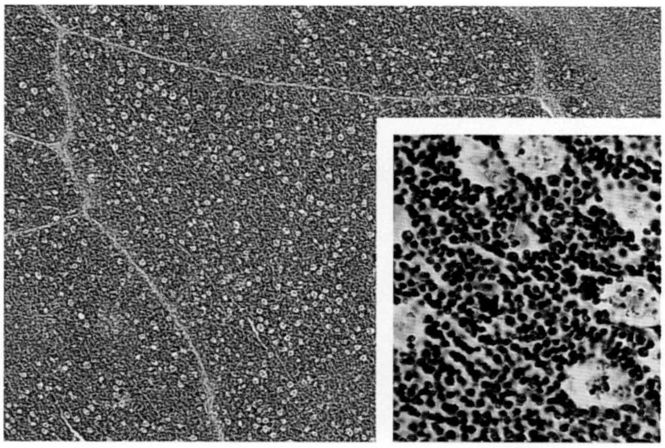

**FIG. 7.** Prominent starry sky appearance in the deep cortex of patient with accidental thymic involution. Note abundance of tingible-body macrophages (*inset*).

thymuses, especially in children and adolescents (Fig. 8) (49,50). The presence of such B-cell structures would seem difficult to reconcile with the fact that the thymus constitutes a predominantly T-cell organ. However, ultrastructural studies have indicated that germinal centers in the thymus arise within perivascular spaces, the latter being clearly separated from the thymic parenchyma by a basal lamina (51). This observation led to the proposal that the thymus may be divided into two major functional compartments: (a) the cortex and medulla (which constitute the true thymic parenchyma) and (b) the extraparenchymal compartment composed of the perivascular spaces (52). Germinal centers in the thymus could thus be explained as being derived from preexisting perivascular B cells in the extraparenchymal compartment. Germinal centers are well known to be prominent in patients with myasthenia gravis and other immune-mediated diseases (see section on Thymic Hyperplasia) (9), but their presence in an otherwise normal thymus should not necessarily be taken as an indicator of an underlying immune disorder. The incidence of germinal centers in the thymus of normal individuals without septicemia or disease of a presumed autoimmune cause has varied in published studies from 2.1% (53) to 40% (51). This wide variation may be related to a sampling factor or to the age of the patients; germinal centers would be expected to be less frequent in the older age groups. Also, stress has been shown to be a factor responsible for the decrease in the number of these formations (50). Determination of the incidence and number of germinal centers in normal human thymus glands still remains an unsettled issue.

Isolated B-lymphocytes are found in both fetal and normal adult thymuses distributed along the septa, in close proximity to small vessels at the corticomedullary junction and in the medulla (54). Intrathymic B-lymphocytes have been found to be significantly increased in patients with myasthenia gravis, a finding that some investigators consider to be a more specific change for this disorder than the presence of germinal centers (54,55). More recently, a population of intramedullary B-lymphocytes with a tendency to cluster around Hassall's corpuscles has been identified in the thymus gland from fetuses, newborn babies, children, and adults; these lymphocytes show evidence of activation and bear a distinctive immunophenotype (56). Unlike B cells of germinal centers and surrounding mantle zones, the medullary B cells are negative for CD21 and do not express surface/cytoplasmic immunoglobulins. It has been proposed that a significant proportion of non-Hodgkin's lymphomas of the B-cell type located in the anterior mediastinum arise from this intrathymic B-cell population. Additionally, a newly described type of mucosa-associated lymphoid tissue (MALT) lymphoma composed of monocytoid B cells recently was identified as arising from the thymus (57); this finding raises the possibility that monocytoid B cells may be another as yet unidentified cellular constituent of the normal thymus (58).

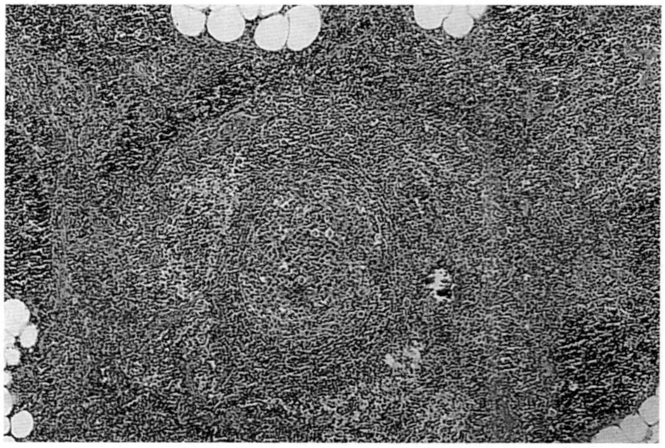

**FIG. 8.** Lymphoid follicle with germinal center in normal thymus.

Several other types of hematolymphoid cells are present in small number but constant fashion in the normal thymus (59–61). Macrophages are mainly located in the cortex, show phagocytic activity, are markedly alpha-naphtyl acetate esterase positive, acid phosphatase positive, HLA-DR negative, and are antigenically indistinguishable from macrophages of other organs (42,61). Interdigitating dendritic cells are mainly located in the medulla, are markedly HLA-DR positive, have little lysosomal enzyme activity, and show S-100 protein reactivity (62). Both of these cell types are thought to be involved in lymphocyte and epithelial cell interaction. Langerhans' cells also have been identified in the thymic medulla; both interdigitating dendritic cells and Langerhans' cells are said to be increased in the thymus of patients with myasthenia gravis (63). The latter cells provide the anatomic substrate for the development of Langerhans' cell granulomatosis (histiocytosis X) within the thymus (64). Eosinophils are usually present in the thymus of children, sometimes in large numbers (65). They appear in fetal life and persist until puberty, after which they become infrequent. They are found mainly in the connective tissue septa or within the medulla and may occasionally be present within Hassall's corpuscles. Mast cells are also normally present in human thymuses. They are usually found within and scattered parallel to the connective tissue septa, often in a perivascular location. The presence of mast cells can be a source of confusion in the course of immunohistochemical and other special stains of the thymus gland because of their propensity to react with a wide variety of reagents; they are easily identified by the use of metachromatic stains. Increased numbers of mast cells in the thymus have been observed in patients with severe combined immunodeficiency and thymic alymphoplasia (66), but the significance of this finding is not understood. Plasma cells are rare in the normal thymus; they are usually located in the connective tissue septa or, more rarely, in the medulla (67). Plasma cells may be numerous in the involuting thymus and also may be present in increased numbers in the thymus of patients with myasthenia gravis (68).

Neuroendocrine cells are now accepted as being a minor but constant component of the normal thymus (69). Peptide- and amine-producing neuroendocrine cells have been identified in the thymus glands of reptiles and avians (70–72) and, to a lesser degree, in mammalian (including human) thymuses. It has been postulated that some of these cells may be embryologically and functionally analogous to C cells of thyroid (73). The physiologic role of these various neuroendocrine elements in the thymus is not yet understood, but their presence has been offered as the probable substrate for the development of carcinoid tumors and other neuroendocrine neoplasms in this organ, including calcitonin-positive medullary carcinomas (74,75).

Myoid cells are located in the thymic medulla. They are common in reptilian and avian thymuses but also can be found (albeit with some difficulty) in human thymuses, particularly in infants. They have microscopic, immunohistochemical, and ultrastructural features of striated muscle cells (76,77). Their histogenesis remains a subject of debate, some studies pointing toward a derivation from the neural crest (78) and others showing the existence of shared epitopes with thymic epithelial cells (79). Myoid cells have been said to be increased in the thymus of patients with myasthenia gravis (54,80) and in patients with true thymic hyperplasia (81), suggesting that these cells may play a role in immunoregulatory mechanisms. Thymic neoplasms thought to represent the neoplastic counterpart of myoid cells also have been described (82).

Germ cells are another cellular element thought to be normally present in the thymus. It has been proposed that scattered germ cells reach the thymus during ontogenesis and that some of them persist into adult life. However, direct evidence of their presence in the normal thymus gland has never been demonstrated, and the only presumptive evidence of their occurrence is the fact that nearly all mediastinal germ cell tumors arise within the thymus (9). Rosai et al. (83) have recently proposed that germ cells in the thymus may develop into somatic cells, thus making their detection and identification difficult by conventional means. They further hypothesize that thymic myoid cells may be of germ cell origin and thus provide indirect evidence for the existence of the latter in this organ (83).

Connective tissue elements of the thymus include vessels, fibrous tissue, nerves, and fat. The vasculature of the thymus arises from arteries that enter the organ via fibrous trabeculae from the capsule. In contrast to other major lymphoid organs, the thymus lacks a hilus. The thymic vessels are ensheathed by a layer of thymic epithelial cells. This anatomic configuration, plus the failure of the thymus to produce antibodies against circulating antigen, led to the concept of the blood–thymus barrier (84). Raviola and Karnovsky (85), in an elaborate study using electron-opaque tracers of different molecular dimensions, demonstrated convincingly that, although some blood-borne macromolecules do penetrate the thymus, their distribution was limited to the medulla, thus pointing to the existence of a blood–thymus barrier operating at the level of the cortex. However, more recent studies have challenged the concept of the blood–thymus barrier by showing that the thymic cortex also may be permeable to immunoglobulin molecules present in the extravascular compartment (86).

The presence of a distinct anatomic compartment bound by the vessel wall and the sheath of epithelial cells has been postulated. It has further been suggested that it is through these perivascular spaces that the mature T-lymphocytes exit the thymus to colonize peripheral lymphoid organs once their maturation process is complete. The spaces are inconspicuous in the normal thymus; they may appear dilated in atrophic and involuting organs, but they acquire their greatest prominence in some thymomas (9).

## ULTRASTRUCTURE

Ultrastructurally, very elongated cytoplasmic processes can be appreciated in the epithelial cells of the thymic cortex, which are also covered by basal lamina material (Fig. 9) (87–89). Medullary epithelial cells are more densely packed and have blunted cytoplasmic projections (Fig. 10). A consistent feature of medullary epithelial cells is the greater frequency of desmosomes and the presence of dense tonofilaments that often insert into desmosomes. This feature is particularly obvious in Hassall's corpuscles. Cortical epithelial cells may display a range of ultrastructural appearances depending on the electron density of their cytoplasm, including pale cells with electron-lucent cytoplasm, intermediate cells with variable electron density, and dark cells with electron-dense cytoplasm. The same range may be observed in medullary epithelial cells; in addition, the medulla contains undifferentiated epithelial cells with sparse cytoplasm (90).

Thymic myoid cells display ultrastructural features of skeletal muscle, including myofilaments with dense patches (Fig. 11). Some investigators have identified cells displaying both tonofilaments and myofilaments by electron microscopy, and in some instances myoid cells have been observed to display desmosomal connections with epithelial cells (91).

## IMMUNOHISTOCHEMISTRY

### Thymic Epithelial Cells

Immunohistochemical studies have demonstrated that thymic epithelial cells may express a variety of distinctive differentiation antigens. Currently, at least four antigenically distinctive types of epithelial cell are recognized in the normal thymus: subcapsular cortical, inner cortical, medullary, and the cells of Hassall's corpuscles (Table 1) (92–95). Inner cortical epithelium, in addition to exhibiting keratin positiv-

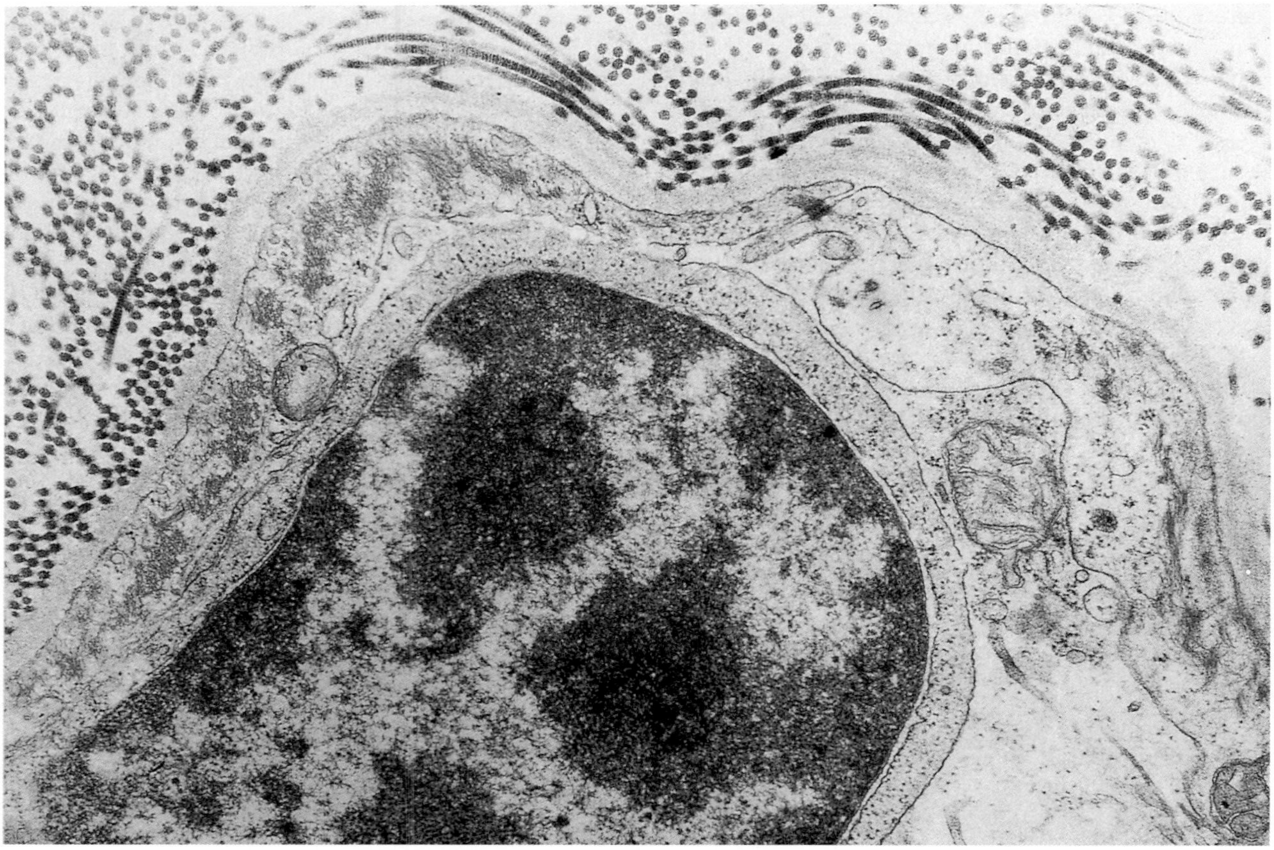

**FIG. 9.** Ultrastructural detail of normal cortical epithelial cells showing large cytoplasmic processes joined by a desmosome and wrapped around a small lymphocyte. A thick basal lamina separates the epithelial cells from the surrounding collagen. [Reprinted with permission (9).]

ity, strongly reacts with TE-3, a murine monoclonal antibody raised against human thymic stroma (96). Subcapsular cortical epithelial cells and medullary epithelial cells react strongly with TE-4 monoclonal antibody. Both of these cells also label with A2B5, a monoclonal antibody directed against a complex neuronal ganglioside found on the cell surface of neurons and neuroendocrine cells (97). Another marker of subcapsular cortical epithelium and medullary epithelium in normal thymus is that detected with anti-p19, an antibody that defines the structural core protein of the human T-cell lymphoma virus and that is believed to be acquired during normal thymic ontogeny. In the normal human thymus, the antigen defined by anti-p19 is found to parallel the reactivity of A2B5 antibody in epithelial cells (98). Interestingly, a recent study on thymomas has demonstrated that the expression of the p19 antigen is lost with malignant transformation (99). Subcapsular cortical, inner cortical, and medullary epithelial cells also have been found to express class I and class II major histocompatibility antigens (94,100). However, recent studies using double immunolabeling have shown that HLA-DR expression is absent in medullary epithelial cells and that the positivity reported in previous studies may have been the result of diffusion of the stain from surrounding interdigitating dendritic cells (101). A recent study has demonstrated that the epithelial cells in the normal thymus and in thymomas also express epithelium-associated glycoprotein H (tissue blood group O antigen), peanut agglutinin receptor antigen (PNA-r), and Saphora Japonica agglutinin receptor antigen (SJA-r), which are detectable by lectin binding (102). Recent studies also have demonstrated expression of the epidermal growth factor receptor and transforming growth factor alpha in subcapsular, cortical, and medullary epithelial cells, suggesting that this substance plays a role in the growth and differentiation of these cells (103). Subcortical epithelial cells lining the boundaries between the thymic parenchyma and its surrounding fibrous tissue also demonstrate positivity for Leu 7, a differentiation antigen found in human null/killer cells and neuroendocrine cells (104). The cells of Hassall's corpuscles show the strongest keratin positivity of all thymic epithelial cells and react particularly strongly with the high-molecular-weight keratin AE-2 antibody, which is considered a marker of terminal epithelial maturation (105). Conversely, they are unreactive for the other antigens mentioned above.

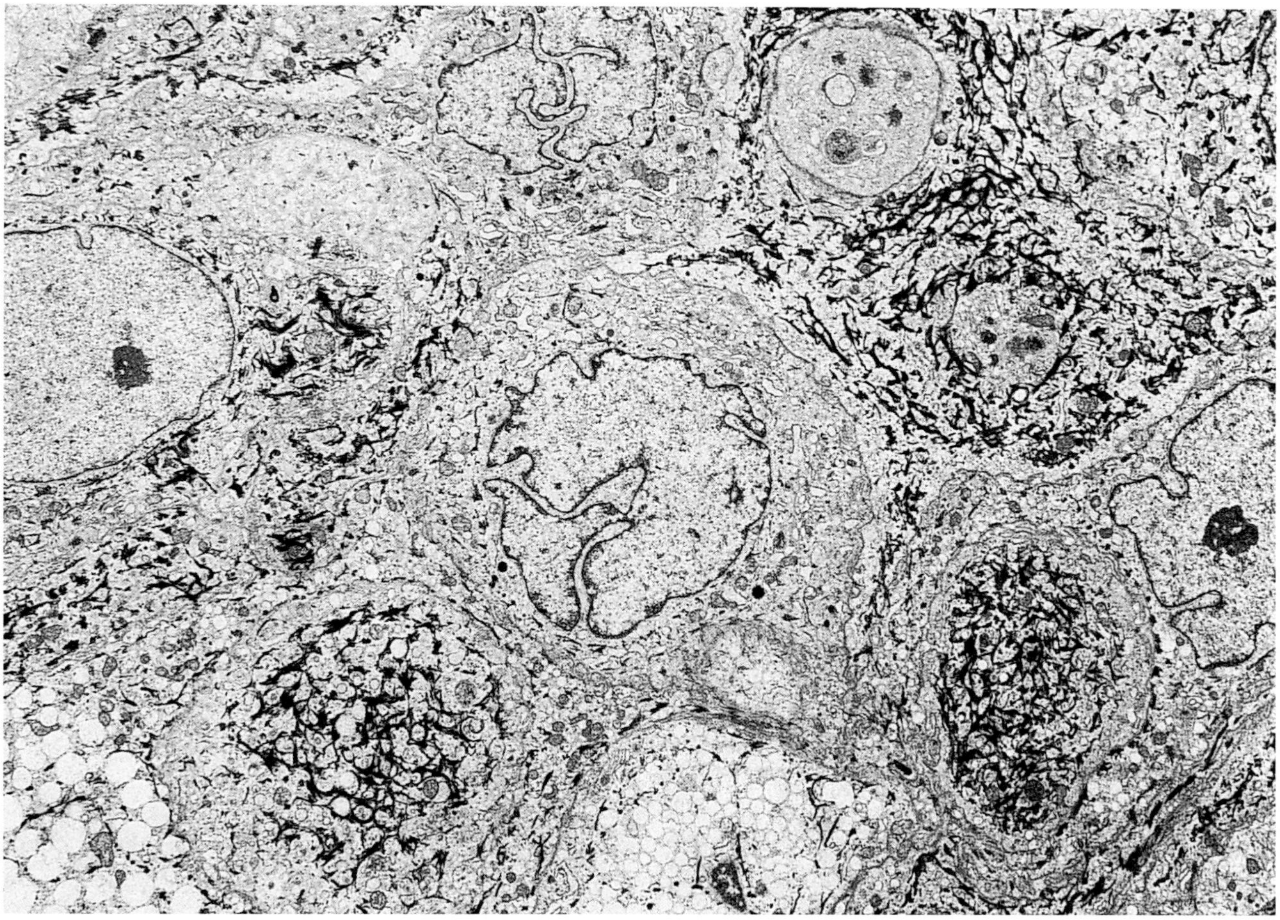

**FIG. 10.** Ultrastructural detail of medullary epithelial cells showing compact arrangement and blunted cytoplasmic projections. [Reprinted with permission (9).]

### Thymic Lymphocytes

The normal lymphoid population of the thymus has been shown to exhibit marked immunophenotypic heterogeneity, reflective of their functional status. The very term "thymocyte," which was originally introduced to designate all thymic lymphocytes, has acquired a more specific immunologic meaning and is now restricted to immature thymic lymphocytes of T-cell lineage (with the exclusion of pre–T-cell lymphocytes). Thymocytes can be divided into three types in accordance with their different stages of intrathymic maturation (19,106–108) (Table 2). The earliest stage of differentiation is found in subcapsular thymocytes, which are characterized by a Leu $1^+$ (T1), Leu $2a^+$ (T8), Leu $3a^+$ (T4), Leu $4^+$ (T3), Leu $5^+$ (T11), Leu $6^+$ (T6), Leu $9^+$ (T2), $Tdt^+$, and $T200^+$ phenotype (Fig. 12A). The next stage in maturation is seen in cortical thymocytes, which comprise the majority of thymic lymphocytes (60–70%) and are characterized by a Leu $1^+$ (T1), Leu $2a^+$ (T8), Leu $3a^+$ (T4), Leu $4^+$ (T3), Leu $5^+$ (T11), Leu $6^+$ (T6), Leu $9^+$ (T2), Leu M3, OKT 10 (T10), $Tdt^+$, and $T200^+$ phenotype. The last stage of intrathymic maturation is seen in medullary thymocytes, which show a Leu $1^+$ (T1), Leu $4^+$ (T3), Leu $5^+$ (T11), Leu $9^+$ (T2), and $T200^+$ phenotype (Fig. 12B). Antigens Leu 2a and Leu 3a are present in only one third to two thirds of these cells, respectively (54,106). Of the above markers, the ones that may distinguish specifically between cortical and medullary thymocytes are Leu 6 (T6/CD1), OKT 10 (CD38), Leu M3 (CD14), and Tdt. Recent studies on thymomas have attempted to correlate the degree of T-cell maturation with the morphologic appearance of the tumor (104,109–111). It has been well established that the lymphoid cell population in thymomas is made up of immature T-lymphocytes (110,112,113). In lymphocyte-rich thymomas, the lymphocytes have the phenotypic markers of cortical thymocytes; it has, therefore, been proposed that these tumors are attempting to recapitulate the structure and function of the cortical compartment of the normal thymus (111,114,115). In the better-differentiated examples, the analogy with the normal thymus is accentuated by the presence of foci of medullary differentiation. These findings support the originally proposed theory that, in thymomas, prothymocytes from the

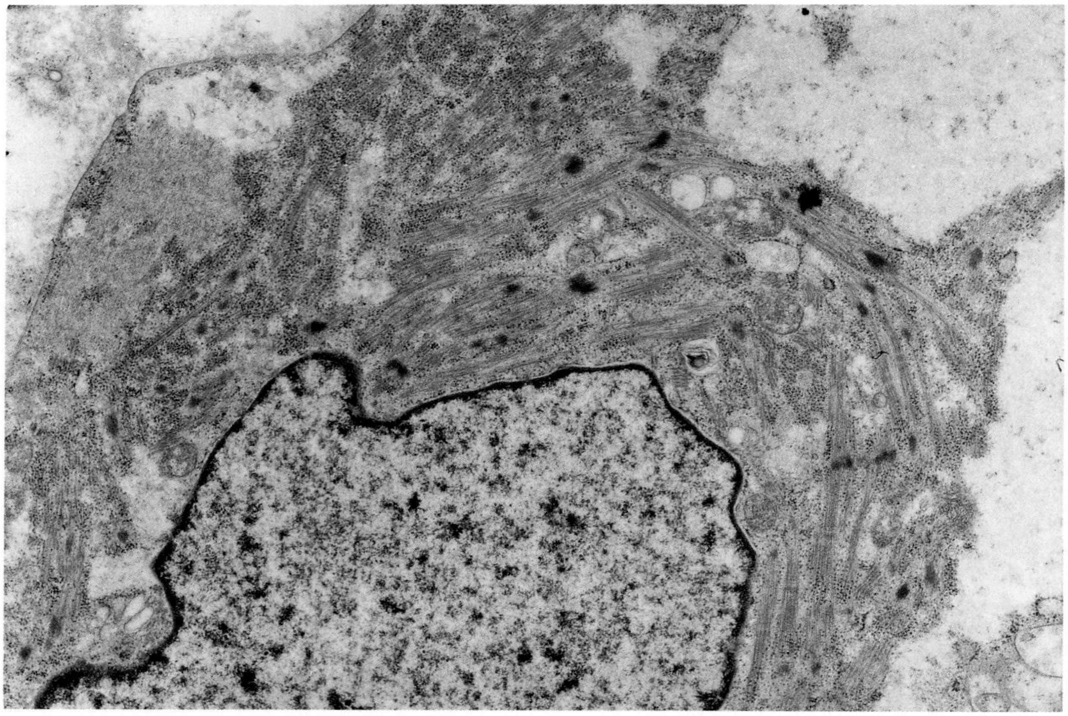

**FIG. 11.** Ultrastructural appearance of myoid cell in the thymus. Note bundles of actin and myosin myofilaments with clearly discernible Z lines in the cytoplasm.

stem cell compartment undergo a series of maturational events induced by the neoplastic thymic epithelial cells analogous to those that take place in the normal thymus, the lymphoid elements in these tumors thus being an environmental rather than a neoplastic component (9). This contention, which was initially based solely on light microscopic observations of thymomas, has recently gained support from studies with DNA hybridization for T-cell receptor genes that showed that the lymphoid elements in thymomas lacked gene rearrangements that would denote a clonal proliferation of T-lymphocytes (116). As already indicated, such interaction is thought to be mediated by thymic hormones produced by thymic epithelial cells.

## MOLECULAR BIOLOGY

Molecular studies have demonstrated the presence of rearrangement and expression of T-cell antigen receptors (TCRs) in thymic lymphocytes. Expression of the TCR represents a critical step in the development of T cells in the thymus (117,118). The TCR molecules are heterodimeric proteins analogous in structure to the immunoglobulin molecules. Rearrangement and expression of the TCRs are needed for the T cell to recognize antigen in association with self–major histocompatibility complex (MHC) antigens. There are two major types of TCRs: one type contains alpha and beta polypeptide chains, and the other contains gamma and delta chains. The alpha-beta TCR is expressed in nearly all T cells, whereas the gamma-delta TCR is expressed in only about 2% of T cells. Immature thymic lymphocytes (CD4/CD8 negative) have been shown to contain mRNA only for the beta chain of the TCR. Mature thymic lymphocytes ($CD4/CD8^+$), on the other hand, contain mRNA for both beta and alpha chains (119).

## FUNCTION

The thymus plays a central role in cell-mediated immunity. In early embryonic development, prothymocytes enter the thymus from the bone marrow and migrate to the outer

**TABLE 1.** *Summary of main antigenic determinants found in epithelial cells of the normal thymus*

| Cells | Keratin | TE-3 | TE-4 | A2B5 | Anti-p19 | Anti-thymosin $\alpha 1$ | Anti-thymopoietin | HLA/Ia |
|---|---|---|---|---|---|---|---|---|
| Inner cortical epithelium | + | + | − | − | − | − | − | + |
| Subcapsular cortical epithelium | + | − | + | + | + | + | + | + |
| Medullary epithelium | + | − | + | + | + | + | − | − |
| Hassall's corpuscles | ++ | − | − | − | − | − | − | − |

**TABLE 2.** *Sequence of maturation in thymic lymphocytes*

| | | | |
|---|---|---|---|
| Stage I | Leu 1 (CD5)<br>Leu 2a (CD8)<br>Leu 3a (CD4)<br>Leu 4 (CD3)<br>Leu 5 (CD2)<br>Leu 6 (CD1)<br>Leu 9 (CD7)<br>T200 | 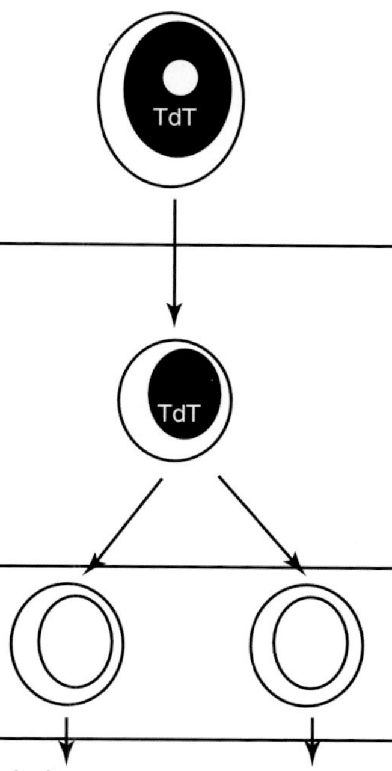 TdT | Large thymic blast<br>(0.5–5%) |
| Stage II | Leu 1 (CD5)<br>Leu 2a (CD8)<br>Leu 3a (CD4)<br>Leu 4 (CD3)<br>Leu 5 (CD2)<br>Leu 6 (CD1)<br>Leu 9 (CD7)<br>Leu M3 (CD14)<br>OKT-10 (CD38)<br>T200 | TdT | Common cortical thymocyte<br>(60–80%) |
| Stage III | Leu 1 (CD5)<br>Leu 4 (CD3)<br>Leu 5 (CD2)<br>Leu 9 (CD7)<br>T200 | | Mature medullary thymocyte<br>(15–20%) |
| | | inducer suppressor<br>peripheral T lymphocytes | |

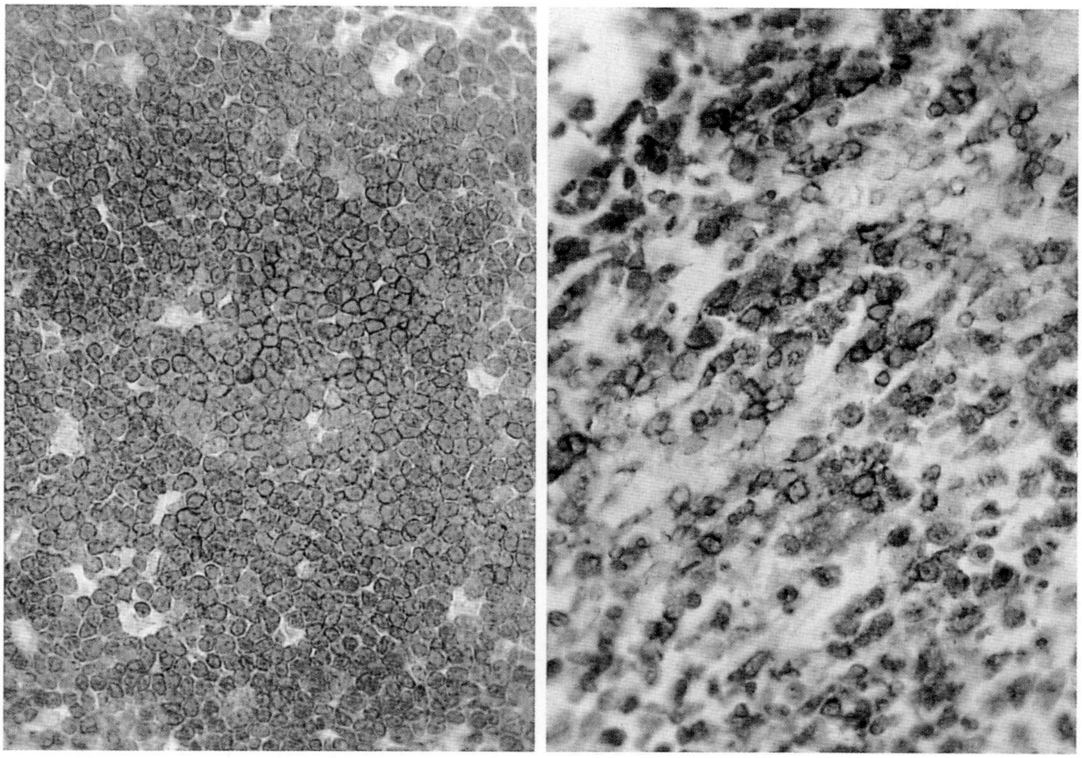

A B

**FIG. 12. A:** Immunoperoxidase stain of cortical thymocytes on fresh frozen tissue with Leu 1 (CD5) antibody. **B:** Medullary thymocytes showing focal Leu 3a (CD4) positivity on fresh frozen tissue.

cortex, where they undergo a process of maturation. Mature thymocytes move from the outer cortex to the medulla, from whence they migrate into the peripheral circulation where they function as mature T-cells. During their sojourn in the thymus, T cells learn to distinguish self from nonself and acquire the ability to recognize antigens bound to cell surface molecules encoded by the major histocompatibility complex (MHC). Circulating helper ($CD4^+$) and suppressor ($CD8^+$) thymus-derived T cells play a variety of roles in cell-mediated immunity, including the induction of cytotoxicity, delayed-type hypersensitivity reactions, and transplant rejection.

A controversial aspect of thymic function is that related to the production of thymic hormones, which are thought to play a role in the induction of differentiation of early T-cell precursors in the thymus. Four distinct types of thymic hormones have been identified: thymopoietin, thymosin $\alpha 1$, thymulin (formerly known as facteur thymique serique), and thymic humoral factor (119–121). Thymopoietin and thymulin are said to be produced only by thymic epithelium, whereas thymosins are a family of peptides that are synthesized in many organs. The production of thymic hormones by thymic epithelial cells has been an extremely interesting but highly contested subject. At the immunohistochemical level, studies using polyclonal and monoclonal antibodies claim to have demonstrated the presence of thymulin, thymosin $\alpha 1$, and thymopoietin in the cytoplasm of murine and human thymic epithelial cells (121–124). In some studies, the hormone localization has been found to be restricted to $A2B5^+$ cells, that is, subcapsular cortical and medullary epithelial cells (125). This finding has led to the suggestion that these two cell subtypes represent the functional (secretory or endocrine) portion of the thymus, as contrasted with the nonsecretory epithelium of the inner cortical region and of Hassall's corpuscles. In a murine system, thymic hormones also have been described in a subtype of medullary epithelial cell characterized ultrastructurally by numerous cytoplasmic membrane–bound vacuoles containing amorphous material (126). A study by Hirokawa et al. (127) using rabbit antisera against synthetic thymosin $\alpha 1$ and bovine thymosin $\beta 3$ in 45 cases of human thymomas and normal thymus of newborns described reactivity of the tumor cells and normal thymic epithelial cells with these antibodies in 80% and 89% of cases, respectively. The thymosin-containing cells were said to be predominantly localized to the medulla and the subcapsular cortex, and the reaction was most intense in the lymphocyte-rich thymomas. These reactions appeared to be specific for thymic tumors because neither thymosin $\alpha 1$ nor thymosin $\beta 3$ could be detected in other epithelial malignancies tested, including gastric, pulmonary, and hepatic carcinomas. So far, however, sufficiently reliable specific antibodies have not become available for routine use in diagnostic pathology.

In addition to thymic hormones, thymic epithelial cells may contain a wide variety of neuropeptides such as oxytocin, vasopressin, beta-endorphin, somatostatin, and other anterior pituitary hormones (128–130), as well as produce various cytokines and growth factors, including interleukin-1, interleukin-6, and granulocyte-monocyte colony-stimulating factor (131,132).

## AGE-RELATED AND OTHER TROPHIC CHANGES

### Thymic Involution

The thymus undergoes a slow physiologic process of involution with age. This process starts at puberty, at which time the organ reaches its maximum absolute weight. From then on, it undergoes gradual and progressive atrophic changes (133–135). This process of aging, also known as physiologic involution, is accompanied by gradual changes in thymocyte populations relative to different rates of involution of the cortical and medullary epithelium. In its early stages, the changes consist primarily of a decrease in the number of cortical thymocytes with relative sparing of the epithelial elements (136). In the more advanced stages, the parenchyma of the thymus reverts to a more primitive appearance and is replaced by islands of epithelial cells depleted of lymphocytes, with partly cystic, closely aggregated Hassall's corpuscles and abundant intervening adipose tissue (137). It should be realized that, whereas thymic involution can proceed to a point where no thymic tissue can be appreciated grossly, microscopic thymic remnants are probably always present. The best way to locate them is to examine microscopically the preepicardial fat in a subserial fashion.

A type of change not related to senescence that must be distinguished from the normal physiologic type of involution is accidental or stress involution. This condition results from the dramatic response of the thymus gland to episodes of severe stress, in which the sudden release of corticosteroids from the adrenal cortex leads to rapid depletion of thymic cortical lymphocytes (138). Microscopically, there is prominent karyorrhexis of lymphocytes with active phagocytosis by macrophages, which creates a prominent starry sky appearance characteristically confined to the cortex. If the stimulus persists, a loss of corticomedullary distinction ensues, with accentuation of the epithelial elements, cystic dilatation of Hassall's corpuscles, and the emergence of elongated, epithelium-lined cystic spaces that recapitulate the early stages of Hassall's corpuscle formation. With further loss of thymocytes, the lobular architecture collapses and fibrosis ensues. The thymus is thus transformed into a mass of adipose tissue containing scattered islands of parenchyma with a few lymphocytes. Acute thymic involution in infancy and childhood has been observed to significantly correlate with the duration of acute illness, and it has been proposed that morphologic parameters such as the presence of abundant macrophages in the cortex, increase of interlobular fibrous tissue, and lymphoid depletion of the cortex may enable the pathologist to estimate the duration of acute disease before death (139). A precocious type of thymic involution manifested by epithelial injury also has been observed in

**TABLE 3.** *Weight and volume of normal human thymuses*

| Age (years) | *n* | Weight (g)[a] | Volume ($cm^3$)[a] |
|---|---|---|---|
| 0–1 | 6 | 27.3 ± 16.4 | 26.8 ± 16.1 |
| 1–4 | 4 | 28.0 ± 19.3 | 27.9 ± 10.4 |
| 5–9 | 7 | 22.1 ± 9.2 | 21.5 ± 8.8 |
| 10–14 | 5 | 21.5 ± 6.1 | 21.1 ± 6.4 |
| 15–19 | 9 | 20.2 ± 10.3 | 19.3 ± 10.1 |
| 20–24 | 18 | 21.6 ± 9.5 | 23.0 ± 10.6 |
| 25–29 | 9 | 23.1 ± 11.8 | 23.7 ± 11.9 |
| 30–34 | 5 | 25.5 ± 9.9 | 27.6 ± 11.2 |
| 35–44 | 17 | 21.9 ± 9.2 | 22.2 ± 10.5 |
| 45–54 | 14 | 24.8 ± 12.8 | 26.5 ± 12.4 |
| 55–64 | 15 | 21.3 ± 9.5 | 23.5 ± 10.4 |
| 65–84 | 17 | 23.8 ± 16.1 | 25.6 ± 17.0 |
| 85–90 | 5 | 18.2 ± 5.4 | 20.4 ± 6.8 |
| 91–107 | 5 | 12.4 ± 6.9 | 13.4 ± 7.2 |
| Total | 136 | 22.8 ± 12.5 | 23.4 ± 11.9 |

From ref. 135.
[a] Values are means ± SD.

both children and adult patients with acquired immunodeficiency syndrome (140,141). These changes have been interpreted by some as an indication that the thymus may constitute a primary target organ in human immunodeficiency virus infection (142), whereas others have considered these changes as an expression of stress involution (141,143).

### Thymic Hyperplasia

True thymic hyperplasia is defined as an enlargement of the thymus gland (as determined by weight or volume) beyond that considered as the upper limit of normal for that particular age group (144). The existence of true thymic hyperplasia has been questioned in the past, largely because of the diagnostic excesses committed with the much abused concept of status thymicolymphaticus. The latter is probably a myth, but true thymic hyperplasia is currently accepted as a distinct entity (145–147). In order to establish the diagnosis of true thymic hyperplasia, reference must be made to standard weight charts of normal thymus glands for comparison. The first extensive studies on the normal weights of the thymus were made in fresh autopsy specimens by Hammar in 1906 (148), whose studies remained for many years the standard. More recently, several workers have updated these studies; the most comprehensive of these is that of Steinman (135), who examined the weight and volume of human thymuses in 136 healthy individuals (Table 3). He concluded that determination of the volume of the gland, as measured by the displacement of a physiologic saline solution, was more reliable than weighing the gland and constitutes the optimal parameter for this type of evaluation.

Thymic hyperplasia has been recognized as a complication of chemotherapy for Hodgkin's disease in children (149,150) and germ cell tumors in adults (151,152) and has been interpreted as the expression of an immunologic rebound phenomenon. A similar enlargement of the thymus also has been observed in children recovering from thermal burns (153) and after cessation of administration of corticosteroids in infants (154).

True thymic hyperplasia must be distinguished from lymphoid hyperplasia. In the latter condition the thymus is usually not enlarged, the term *hyperplasia* referring to the presence of an increased number of lymphoid follicles in the medullary region of the gland. The problems in establishing the presence of lymphoid hyperplasia vis-à-vis the occurrence of lymphoid follicles in the normal thymus has already been discussed.

Lymphoid hyperplasia of the thymus most commonly has been associated with myasthenia gravis but also has been observed in several other immune-mediated disorders, including systemic lupus erythematosus, rheumatoid arthritis, scleroderma, allergic vasculitis, and thyrotoxicosis.

## ARTIFACTS AND OTHER POTENTIAL PITFALLS IN DIFFERENTIAL DIAGNOSIS

Microscopic changes related to involution may be a source of considerable confusion in the interpretation of thymic biopsies. Such changes are primarily related to the distribution, architectural arrangement, and cytologic appearance of the epithelial cells (Fig. 13). Some of these cells may acquire a spindle, mesenchyma-like appearance, whereas others can arrange themselves in rosettelike formations devoid of central lumina (Fig. 14). The fact that both of these appearances also are found with some frequency in thymic dysplasia and thymoma (but not in the normal active gland of infancy) suggests that they represent regressive and functionally inactive states of the epithelial cells (9). Sometimes thymic remnants are almost exclusively formed of epithelial elements, arranged in well-defined round nests that may simulate neuroendocrine growths (155) (Fig. 15). A particularly distinctive appearance is that of thin, elongated strands of thymic epithelium composed of a single or double cell layer, surrounded by or circumscribing dense connective tissue in a fibroepitheliomatous fashion. These thin, elongated epithelial strands may often be flanked by small lymphocytes and may occasionally exhibit an antlerlike, branching configuration (Fig. 16A). They may be seen by themselves or at the periphery of thymic cysts, thymomas, thymic lymphomas, and other thymic neoplasms. In the case of thymic lymphomas and seminomas, these strands can be present not only around but also within the tumor, surrounded and infiltrated by the neoplastic elements. Their presence, whether detected at the hematoxylin and eosin (H&E) level or with the more sensitive techniques of ultrastructure and immunohistochemistry, can be interpreted erroneously as evidence supporting an epithelial nature for the lesion (Fig. 16B). As a matter of fact, in our experience these formations constitute the single most important cause of misdiagnosis in cases of large cell lymphoma of the thymus.

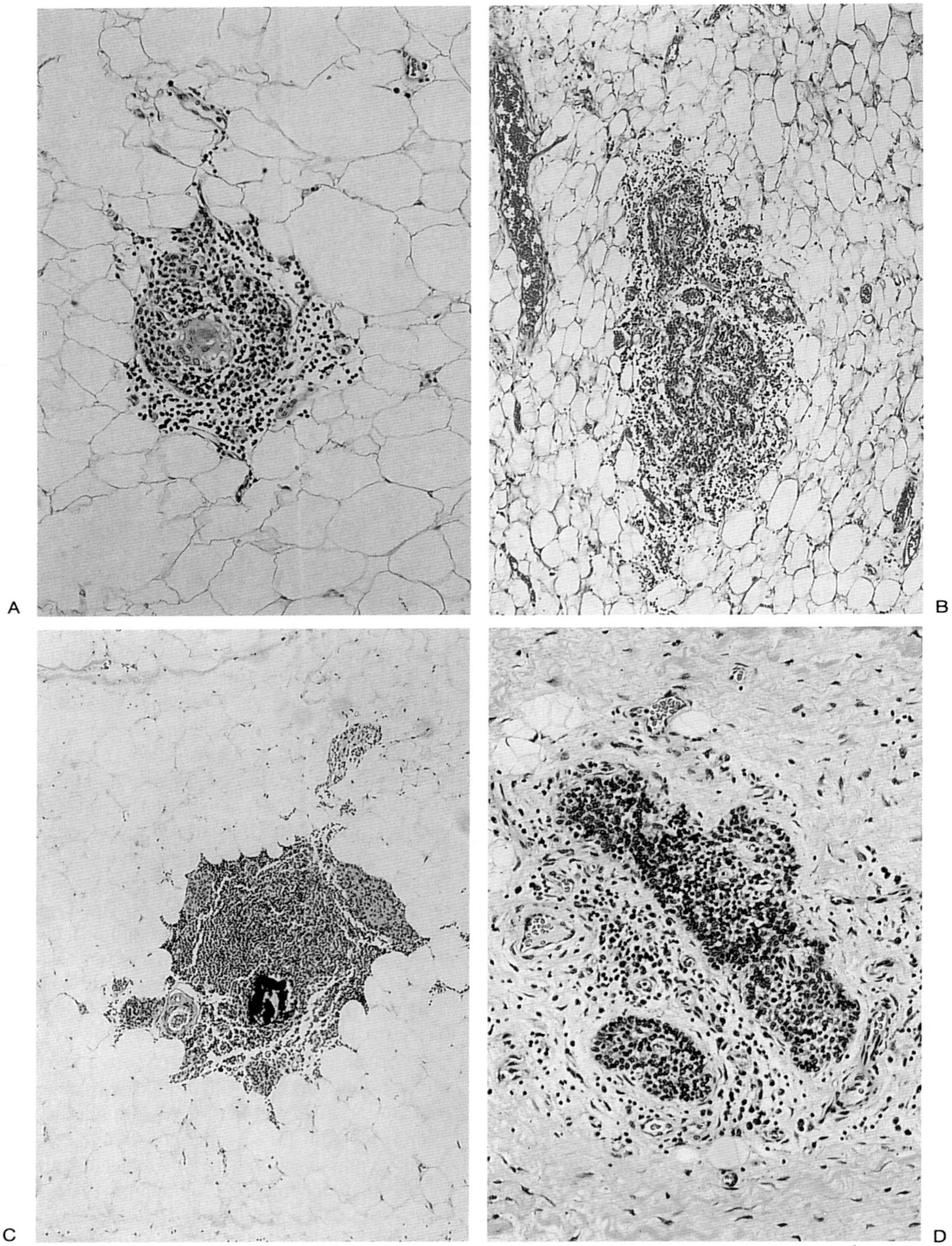


**FIG. 13.** Epithelial remnants in involuting thymus. **A:** Abortive Hassall's corpuscle surrounded by small lymphocytes and scattered epithelial cells. **B:** Anastomosing strands of epithelial cells surrounded by small lymphocytes embedded within the preepicardial fat. **C:** Residual thymic island with predominance of lymphocytes, small solid epithelial cell clusters at the periphery, and calcified Hassall's corpuscle. **D:** Anastomosing strands of epithelial cells admixed with small lymphocytes embedded within a collagenized stroma.

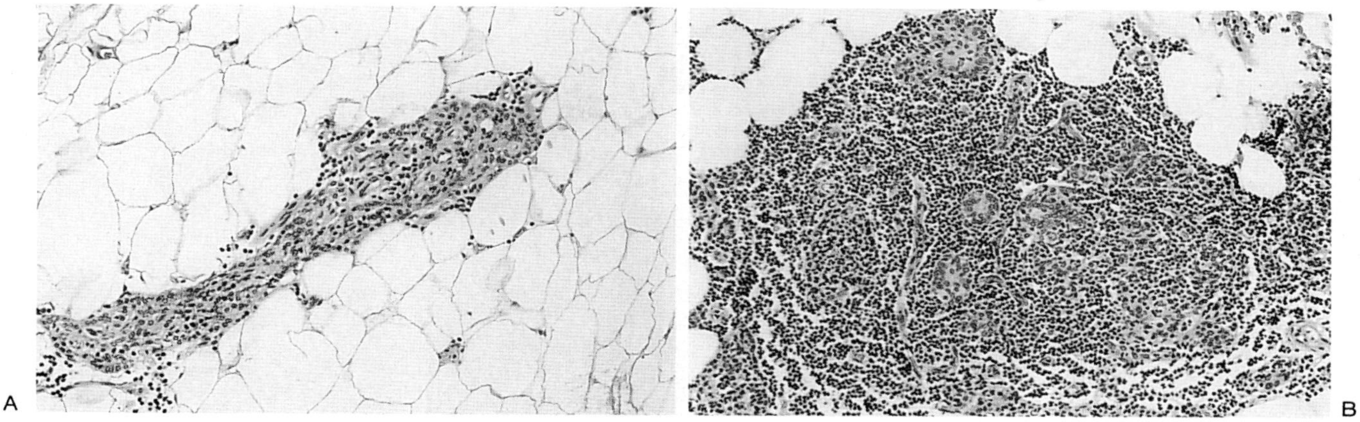

FIG. 14. **A:** Thymic remnant showing elongated configuration with prominent spindling of the cells. **B:** Involuting thymus with epithelial rosettes.

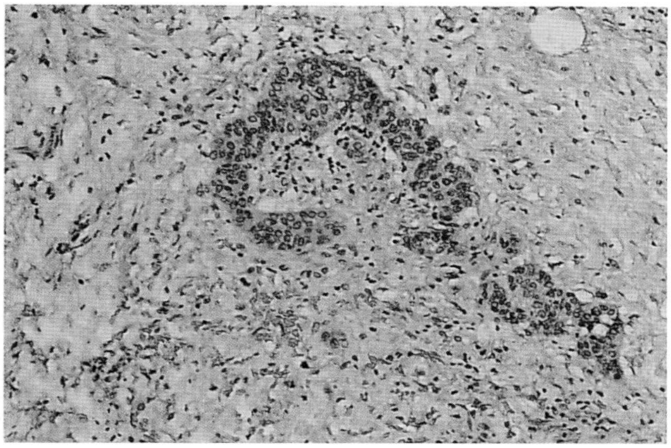

FIG. 15. Strands of residual thymic epithelium arranged in small nests resembling neuroendocrine growths.

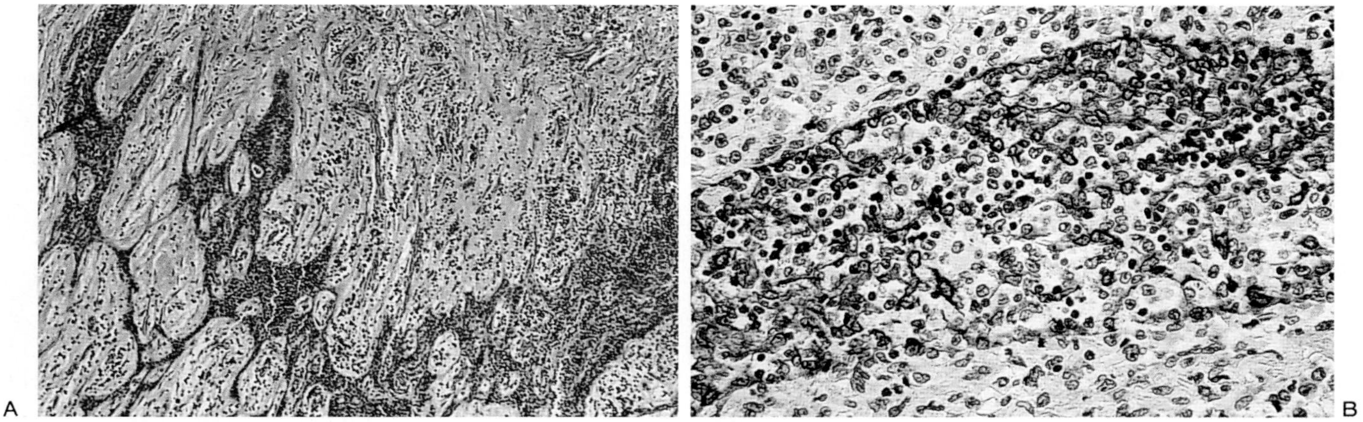

FIG. 16. **A:** Wall of thymic cyst showing branching strands of thymic epithelial cells surrounded by a fibrous stroma. **B:** Entrapped thymic epithelial elements within anterior mediastinal malignant lymphoma. The strong keratin positivity seen in these cells may lead to an erroneous diagnosis of thymic carcinoma.

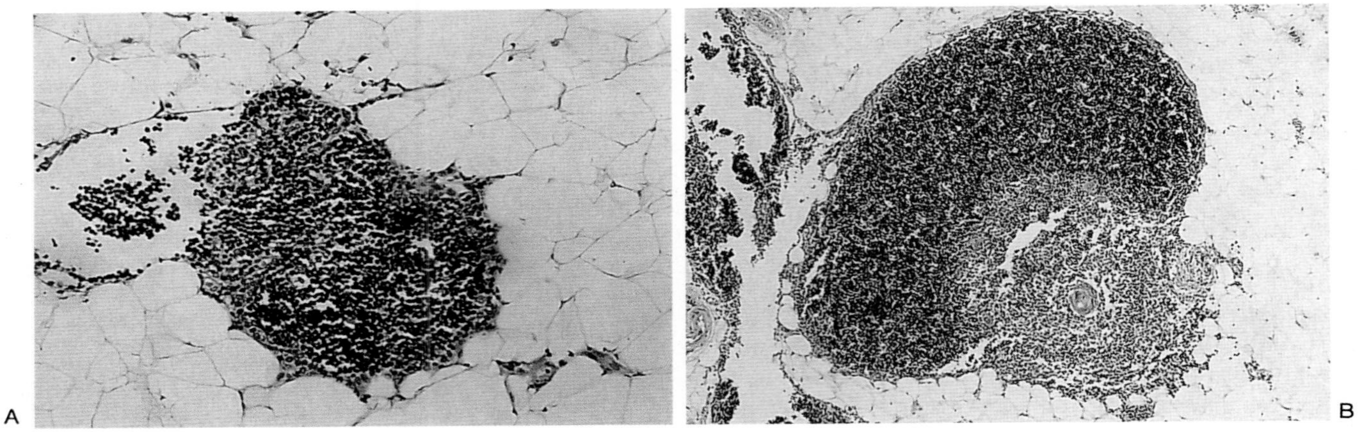


**FIG. 17. A:** Thymic remnant composed predominantly of small lymphocytes simulating a lymphoid nodule. Note the single row of flattened epithelial cells at the periphery (*arrows*). **B:** Thymic remnant composed of cortical and medullary portion, the latter containing a small Hassall's corpuscle (*bottom half*).

Conversely, some thymic remnants (perhaps the majority) are made up almost exclusively of lymphocytes, thus simulating lymph nodes. A clue to their real nature should be sought at the very periphery, in which epithelial cells can sometimes be identified encircling the nests, perhaps representing the residual coat of subcapsular cortical cells of the normal organ (Fig. 17).

Certain patterns of tissue response to injury in the thymus may also constitute a major source of confusion in the interpretation of biopsies of this organ (156). A common form of response of this organ to injury, particularly in cases associated with inflammation, is cystic degeneration of thymic epithelium. The cystic degeneration in such cases is thought to be the result of an acquired process, which in its fullest expression will lead to the formation of a multilocular thymic cyst (157). The main histologic features of such cysts include the formation of large cavities lined by squamous, columnar, or cuboidal epithelium, often in continuity with remnants of normal thymic epithelium within the cyst walls; severe acute and chronic inflammation accompanied by fibrovascular proliferation, necrosis, hemorrhage and cholesterol granuloma formation; and reactive lymphoid hyperplasia with the formation of prominent germinal centers. In some instances, the cyst lining may show a moderate degree of cytologic atypia with features of pseudoepitheliomatous hyperplasia that can be easily misinterpreted for malignancy (158). In the majority of cases the cystic structures are closely associated with Hassall's corpuscles, many of which show marked dilatation and may be found to be in continuity with the lining of the cystic cavities (Fig. 18). We believe that this type of reaction is the result of an exaggerated response of medullary duct epithelium-derived structures of the thymus to an underlying inflammatory process (157). However, it is important to point out that seemingly identical changes may take place in uninvolved thymic parenchyma in cases of Hodgkin's disease, mediastinal seminoma, and (less commonly) thymoma, to the extent that the neoplastic elements may be overshadowed by the cystic/inflammatory process (159,160). Other primary thymic neoplasms, which also may be closely associated with prominent cystic changes, al-

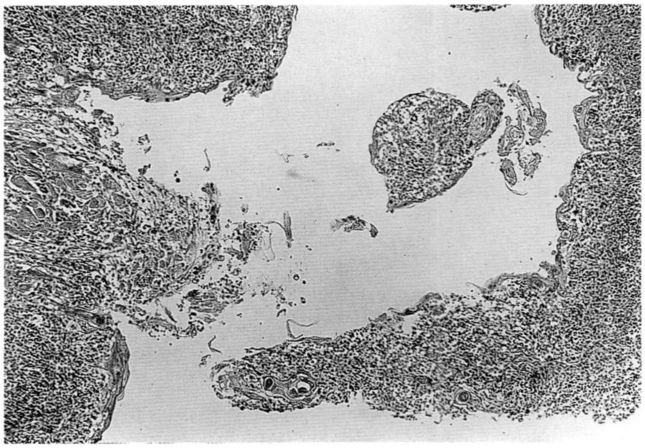

**FIG. 18.** Cystic dilatation of Hassall's corpuscle. Notice dense inflammatory infiltrate within the wall of the cyst.

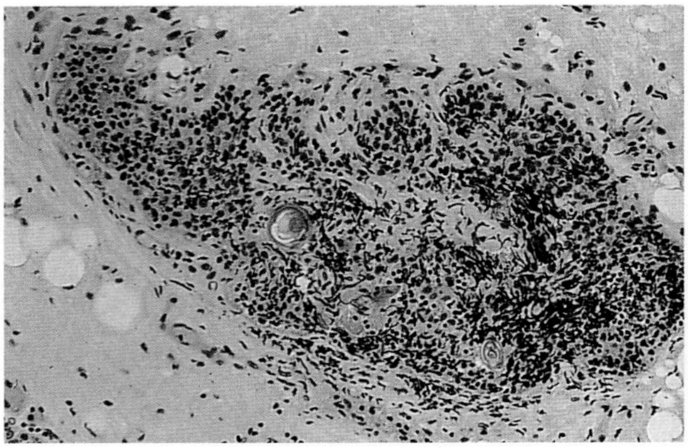

**FIG. 19.** Extensive crush artifact is seen in this thymic remnant obtained through mediastinoscopic biopsy.

though to a lesser extent, include basaloid carcinoma and mucoepidermoid carcinoma (161,162). Careful search and extensive sampling must therefore be undertaken in cystic mediastinal lesions for proper identification of the diagnostic neoplastic areas.

Another form of tissue response to injury of the thymus that may introduce difficulties for diagnosis is that of stromal fibrosis. Fibrous overgrowth of the stroma may be the result of various mechanisms in a variety of nonneoplastic conditions, including a specific stimulus such as ionizing radiation or fungal infection (163,164), or of undetermined etiology, such as in idiopathic sclerosing mediastinitis (165,166). In addition, a variety of malignant conditions of this organ also may be accompanied by prominent fibrous changes of the stroma, including primary diffuse large cell lymphoma of the mediastinum, Hodgkin's disease, and thymic seminoma (156). In many such instances, the gland may show extensive sclerosis with entrapment of a few scattered foci harboring the diagnostic atypical cells. Such cases may prove literally impossible to diagnose in small mediastinoscopic biopsies and will require extensive sampling of the mass to identify the diagnostic areas. The surgeon must be informed of the need for obtaining additional tissue for diagnosis at the time of frozen section examination.

Another potential pitfall for diagnosis is given by the high cellularity, immaturity, and mitotic activity of the normal thymic cortex, which can pose great diagnostic difficulties in mediastinoscopic biopsies and result in a mistaken diagnosis of malignant lymphoma, particularly of the lymphoblastic type. The paucity or absence of cells with convoluted nuclei and the identification (morphologically or immunohistochemically) of epithelial cells regularly scattered throughout the lymphoid population should point toward the correct interpretation. Finally, an additional source of difficulty for diagnosis lies in the presence of biopsy-induced artifacts, one of the most common being the crush artifact, leading to marked nuclear elongation reminiscent of that seen in small cell carcinoma (Fig. 19).

## REFERENCES


1. Norris EH. The morphogenesis and histogenesis of the thymus gland in man: in which the origin of the Hassall's corpuscles of the human thymus is discovered. *Contrib Embryol Carnegie Inst* 1938;27: 193–207.
2. Weller GL Jr. Development of the thyroid, parathyroid and thymus gland in man. *Contrib Embryol Carnegie Inst* 1933;24:95–138.
3. Cordier AC, Haumont SM. Development of thymus, parathyroids and ultimobranchial bodies in NMRI and nude mice. *Am J Anat* 1980;157: 227–263.
4. Gilmour JR. The embryology of the parathyroid glands, the thymus and certain associated rudiments. *J Pathol Bacteriol* 1937;45: 507–522.
5. Jotereau FV, Hounaint E, Le Douarin NM. Lymphoid stem cells homing to the early thymic primordium of the avian embryo. *Eur J Immunol* 1980;10:620–627.
6. Shier KJ. The thymus according to Schambacher: medullary ducts and reticular epithelium of the thymus and thymomas. *Cancer* 1981;48: 1183–1199.
7. Gilmour JR. Some developmental abnormalities of the thymus and parathyroid glands. *J Pathol Bacteriol* 1941;52:213–218.
8. Nathaniels EK, Nathaniels AM, Wang CA. Mediastinal parathyroid tumors: a clinical and pathological study of 84 cases. *Ann Surg* 1970; 171:165–170.
9. Rosai J, Levine GD. Tumors of the thymus. In: *Atlas of tumor pathology. 2nd series, fascicle 13.* Washington, DC: Armed Forces Institute of Pathology, 1976.
10. Domaniewski J, Ukleja Z, Rejmanowski T. Problemy immunologiczne I kliniczne w grasiczakach ektopicznych. *Otolaringol Pol* 1975; 29:579–585.
11. Martin JME, Rundhawa G, Temple WJ. Cervical thymoma. *Arch Pathol Lab Med* 1986;110:354–357.
12. Yamashita H, Murakami N, Noguchi S, et al. Cervical thymoma and incidence of cervical thymus. *Acta Pathol Jpn* 1983;33:189–194.
13. Wadon A. Thymoma intratracheale. *Zentralbl Allg Pathol* 1934;60: 308–312.
14. Harach RR, Day ES, Fransilla KG. Thyroid spindle cell tumor with mucous cyst: an intrathyroid thymoma? *Am J Surg Pathol* 1985; 9:525–530.
15. Miyauchi A, Kuma K, Matsuzuka F, Matsubayashi A, Tamai H, Katayama S. Intrathyroid epithelial thymoma: an entity distinct from squamous cell carcinoma of the thyroid. *World J Surg* 1985; 9:128–135.
16. Rosai J, Limas C, Husband EM. Ectopic hamartomatous thymoma: a distinctive benign lesion of the lower neck. *Am J Surg Pathol* 1984; 8:501–513.
17. Castleman B. Tumors of the thymus gland. In: *Atlas of tumor pathology. 1st series, fascicle 19.* Washington, DC: Armed Forces Institute of Pathology, 1955.
18. Gagens EW. Malformation of the auditory apparatus in the newborn associated with ectopic thymus. *Arch Otolaryngol* 1932;15:671–680.
19. Wolff M, Rosai J, Wright DH. Sebaceous glands within the thymus. Report of 3 cases. *Hum Pathol* 1984;15:341–343.
20. Becklet IA, Johnston DG. Choristoma of the thymus. *Am J Dis Child* 1956;92:175–178.
21. Landing BH, Yutuc IL, Swanson VL. Clinicopathologic correlation in immunologic deficiency diseases of children, with emphasis on thymic histologic patterns. In: *Proceedings of the International Symposium on Immunodeficiency.* Tokyo: Tokyo University Press, 1976: 3–33.
22. Blackburn WR, Gordon DS. The thymic remnant in thymic alymphoplasia. Light and electron microscopic studies. *Arch Pathol* 1967;84: 363–375.
23. Hoyer JR, Cooper MD, Gabrielson AE, Good RA. Lymphopenic forms of congenital immunologic deficiency states. *Medicine (Baltimore)* 1968;47:201–226.
24. Peterson RDA, Kelly WD, Good RA. Ataxia–telangiectasia. Its association with a defective thymus, immunological-deficiency disease and malignancy. *Lancet* 1964;1:1189–1193.
25. Cooper MD, Petersen RDA, Good RA. A new concept of the cellular basis of immunity. *J Pediatr* 1965;67:907–908.
26. Nezeloff C, Jammet M-L, Lortholary P, Labrune R, Lamy M. L'hypoplasie hereditaire du thymus. *Arch Fr Pediatr* 1964;21:897–920.
27. Seemayer TA, Bolande RP. Thymus involution mimicking thymic dysplasia: a consequence of transfusion-induced graft-versus-host disease in a premature infant. *Arch Pathol Lab Med* 1980;104:141–144.
28. Huber J, Cholnoky P, Zoethout HE. Congenital aplasia of parathyroid glands and thymus. *Arch Dis Child* 1967;42:190–192.
29. Fowlkes BJ, Pardoll DM. Molecular and cellular events of T-cell development. *Adv Immunol* 1989;44:207–264.
30. MacDonald HR, Lees RK. Programmed death of autoreactive thymocytes. *Nature* 1990;343:642–644.
31. Kizaki HO, Tadakuma T. Thymocyte apoptosis. *Microbiol Immunol* 1993;37:917–925.
32. Colbert RA, Young DA. Glucocorticoid-induced messenger ribonucleic acids in rat thymic lymphocytes: rapid primary effects specific for glucocorticoids. *Endocrinology* 1986;119:2598–2605.
33. Domashenko AD, Nazarova LF, Umansky SR. Comparison of the spectra of protein synthesis in mouse thymocytes after irradiation or hydrocortisone treatment. *Int J Radiat Biol* 1990;57:315–329.
34. Korsmeyer SJ. Bcl-2: a repressor of lymphocyte death. *Immunol Today* 1992;13:285–288.
35. Lowe SW, Schmitt EM, Smith SW, Osborne BA, Jacks T. p53 is re-

quired for radiation-induced apoptosis in mouse thymocytes. *Nature* 1993;362:847–849.
36. Smith CA, Williams GI, Kinsgton R, Jenkins EJ, Owen JJT. Antibodies to CD3/T-cell receptor complex induce death by apoptosis in immature T cells in thymic cultures. *Nature* 1989;337:181–184.
37. von Boehmer H. Positive selection of lymphocytes. *Cell* 1994;76:219.
38. Shi Y, Bissonnette RP, Parfrey N, Szalay M, Kubo RT, Green DR. *In vivo* administration of monoclonal antibodies to the CD3 T-cell receptor complex induces cell death (apoptosis) in immature thymocytes. *J Immunol* 1991;146:3340–3346.
39. Blackman M, Kappler J, Marrack P. The role of the T cell receptor in positive and negative selection of developing T cells. *Science* 1990; 248:1335–1341.
40. Mountz JD, Zhou T, Wu J, Wang W, Su X, Cheng J. Regulation of apoptosis in immune cells. *J Clin Immunol* 1995;15:1–16.
41. Hammar JA. Die Menschen Thymus in Gesundheit und krankheit. *Z Mikrosk Anat Forsch* 1926;6(suppl):107–208.
42. Lobach DF, Haynes BF. Ontogeny of the human thymus during fetal development. *J Clin Immunol* 1987;7:81–97.
43. Dipasquale B, Tridente G. Immunohistochemical characterization of nurse cells in normal human thymus. *Histochemistry* 1991;96: 499–503.
44. von Gaudeker B. Functional histology of the human thymus. *Anat Embryol* 1991;183:1–15.
45. Ribbert H. Die Entwicklungsstorung der Thymusdruse bei kongenitaler Lues. *Frankfurt Z Pathol* 1912;11:209–218.
46. Suster S, Rosai J. Multilocular thymic cyst: an acquired reactive process. Study of 18 case. *Am J Surg Pathol* 1991;15:388–398.
47. Henry K. Mucin secretion and striated muscle in the human thymus. *Lancet* 1966;1:183–185.
48. Cantor H, Weisman I. Development and function of subpopulations of thymocytes and T lymphocytes. *Prog Allergy* 1976;20:1–64.
49. Everett NB, Tyler RW. Lymphopoiesis in the thymus and other tissues: functional implications. *Int Rev Cytol* 1967;22:205–237.
50. Middleton G. The incidence of follicular structures in the human thymus at autopsy. *Aust J Exp Biol Med Sci* 1967;45:189–199.
51. Vetters JM, Barclay RS. The incidence of germinal centers in the thymus glands of patients with congenital heart disease. *J Clin Pathol* 1973;26:583–591.
52. Levine GD, Rosai J. Electron microscopy of the human thymus. In: Johannenssen JV, ed. *Electron microscopy* in human medicine. Vol 5. New York: McGraw-Hill, 1980.
53. Goldstein G, Mackay IR. The thymus in systemic lupus erythematosus. A quantitative histopathologic analysis and comparison with stress involution. *Br Med J* 1967;2:475–478.
54. Palestro G, Tridente G, Micca FB, Novero D, Valente G, Godia L. Immunohistochemical and enzyme histochemical contributions to the problem concerning the role of the thymus in the pathogenesis of myasthenia gravis. *Virchows Arch [B]* 1983;44:173–186.
55. Shirai T, Miyota M, Nakase A, Itoh T. Lymphocyte subpopulations in neoplastic and non-neoplastic thymus and in blood of patients with myasthenia gravis. *Clin Exp Immunol* 1976;26:118–123.
56. Isaacson PG, Norton AJ, Addis BJ. The human thymus contains a novel population of B-lymphocytes. *Lancet* 1987;2:1488–1492.
57. Isaacson PG, Chan JKC, Tang C, Addis BJ. Low-grade B-cell lymphoma of mucosa-associated lymphoid tissue arising in the thymus: a thymic lymphoma mimicking myoepithelial sialadenitis. *Am J Surg Pathol* 1990;14:342–351.
58. De Almeida PC, Harris NH, Bhan AK. Characterization of immature sinus histiocytes (monocytoid cells) and reactive lymph node by use of monoclonal antibodies. *Hum Pathol* 1984;15:330–335.
59. Duijvestin AM, Schuute R, Kohler YG, Korm C, Hoefsmit ECM. Characterization of the population of phagocytic cells in thymic cell suspension. A morphologic and cytochemical study. *Cell Tissue Res* 1983;231:313–323.
60. Kaiserling E, Stein H, Muller-Hermelink HK. Interdigitating reticulum cells in normal thymus and thymoma: an immunohistochemical study. *Histopathology* 1989;14:37–45.
61. Ruco LP, Rosati S, Monardo F, Pescarmona E, Rendina EA, Baroni CD. Macrophage and interdigitating reticulum cells in normal thymus and thymoma: an immunohistochemical study. *Histopathology* 1989; 14:37–45.
62. Lauriola L, Michetti F, Stolfi VM, Tallini G, Cocchia D. Detection by S-100 immunolabeling of reticulum cells in human thymomas. *Virchows Arch [B]* 1984;45:187–195.
63. Bofill M, Janossy G, Willcox N, Chilosi M, Trejdosiewicz LK, Newson-Davis J. Microenvironments in the normal thymus and the thymus in myasthenia gravis. *Am J Pathol* 1985;119:462–473.
64. Siegal GP, Dehner LP, Rosai J. Histiocytosis-X (Langerhans' cell granulomatosis) of the thymus. *Am J Surg Pathol* 1985;9:117–124.
65. Bhathal PS, Campbell PE. Eosinophil leukocytes in the child's thymus. *Aust Ann Med* 1965;14:210–214.
66. Wise WS, Still WJS, Joshi VV. Severe combined immunodeficiency with thymic mast cell hyperplasia. *Arch Pathol Lab Med* 1976;100: 283–286.
67. Goldstein G. Plasma cells in the human thymus. *Aust J Exp Biol Med Sci* 1966;44:695–698.
68. Henry K. The human thymus in disease, with particular emphasis on thymitis and thymoma. In: Kendall MD, ed. *The thymus gland.* London: Academic Press, 1981:85–111.
69. Moll VM, Lane BL, Robert F, Green V, Legros JJ. The neuroendocrine thymus. Abundant occurrence of oxytocin-, vasopressin-, and neurophysin-like peptides in epithelial cells. *Histochemistry* 1988;89: 385–390.
70. Ciaccio C. Contributo all istochimica delle cellule cromaffini. II. Cellule cromaffini del timo di Gallum domesticus. *Bull Soc Ital Biol Sper* 1942;17:619–620.
71. Hakanson R, Larsson L-I, Sundler F. Peptide and amine producing endocrine-like cells in the chicken thymus. A chemical, histochemical and electron microscopic study. *Histochemistry* 1974;39:25–34.
72. Vialli M, Sacati C. Sulla presenza di cellule enterocromaffini del timo dei rettili. *Riv Histochem Norm Pat* 1958;4:343.
73. Vialli M. Elementi del systema delle cellule enterocromaffini e cellule C nel timo. *Ann Histochem* 1973;18:3–7.
74. Rosai J, Higa E. Mediastinal endocrine neoplasm of probable thymic origin, related to carcinoid tumor: clinicopathologic study of 8 cases. *Cancer* 1972;29:1061–1074.
75. Wick MR, Rosai J. Neuroendocrine neoplasms of the thymus. *Pathol Res Pract* 1988;183:188–199.
76. Drenkhan D, von Gaudeker B, Muller-Hermelink HK. Myosin and actin containing cells in the human postnatal thymus: ultrastructural and immunohistochemical findings in normal thymus and myasthenia gravis. *Virchows Arch [B]* 1979;32:33–45.
77. Hayward AR. Myoid cells in the human fetal thymus. *J Pathol* 1972; 106:45–48.
78. Nakamura H, Ayer-Le-Lievre C. Neural crest cell and thymic myoid cells. *Curr Top Dev Biol* 1986;20:111–115.
79. Dardenne M, Savino W, Bach JF. Thymomatous epithelial cells and skeletal muscle share a common epitope defined by a monoclonal antibody. *Am J Pathol* 1987;126:194–198.
80. Van de Velde RL, Friedman NB. Thymic myoid cells and myasthenia gravis. *Am J Pathol* 1970;59:347–361.
81. Judd RL, Welch SL. Myoid cell differentiation in true thymic hyperplasia and lymphoid hyperplasia. *Arch Pathol Lab Med* 1988;112: 1140–1144.
82. Murakami S, Shamoto M, Miura K, et al. A thymic tumor with massive proliferation of myoid cells. *Acta Pathol Jpn* 1984;34: 1375–1383.
83. Rosai J, Parkash V, Reuter VE. The origin of mediastinal germ cell tumors in men. *Int J Surg Pathol* 1994;2:73–78.
84. Marshall AHE, White RG. The immunological reactivity of the thymus. *Br J Exp Pathol* 1961;42:379–385.
85. Raviola E, Karnovski MJ. Evidence for a blood–thymus barrier using electron-opaque tracers. *J Exp Med* 1972;136:466–498.
86. Stet RJM, Wagenaar-Hilbers JPA, Niauwenhuis P. Thymus localization of monoclonal antibodies circumventing the thymus–blood barrier. *Scand J Immunol* 1987;25:441–446.
87. Bearman RM, Levine GD, Bensch KG. The ultrastructure of the normal human thymus. A study of 36 cases. *Anat Rec* 1978;190:755–781.
88. Hirokawa K. Electron microscopic observations of the human thymus of the fetus and the newborn. *Acta Pathol Jpn* 1969;19:1–13.
89. Pinkel D. Ultrastructure of the human fetal thymus. *Am J Dis Child* 1968;115:222–238.
90. van de Wijngaert FP, Kendall MD, Schuurman H-J, Rademakers LHPM, Kater L. Heterogeneity of epithelial cells in human thymus: An ultrastructural study. *Cell Tissue Res* 1984;237:227–237.
91. Henry K. The human thymus in disease with particular emphasis on thymitis and thymoma. In: Kendall MD, ed. *The thymus gland.* London; Academic Press, 1981:85–111.
92. De Maagd RA, McKenzie WA, Schuurman HJ, et al. Human thymus

microenvironment: heterogeneity detected by monoclonal antiepithelial cell antibodies. *Immunology* 1985;54:745–754.
93. Haynes BF. The human thymic microenvironment. *Adv Immunol* 1984;36:87–142.
94. Janossy G, Thomas JA, Bollum FJ, et al. The human thymic microenviroment. An immunohistologic study. *J Immunol* 1980;125:202–212.
95. Van Ewijk W. Immunohistology of the lymphoid and non-lymphoid cell in the thymus in relation to T-lymphocyte differentiation. *Am J Anat* 1984;170:330–331.
96. McFarland EJ, Scearse RM, Haynes BF. The human thymic microenvironment: cortical thymic epithelium is an antigenically distinct region of the thymic microenvironment. *J Immunol* 1984;133: 1241–1249.
97. Eisenbarth GS, Shimizu K, Bowring MA, Wells S. Expression of receptor for tetanus toxin and monoclonal antibody A2B5 by pancreatic islet cells. *Proc Natl Acad Sci U S A* 1982;79:5066–5070.
98. Haynes BF, Robert-Guroff M, Metzgar RS, et al. Monoclonal antibodies against human T cell leukemia virus p19 defines a human thymic epithelial antigen acquired during ontogeny. *J Exp Med* 1983; 157:907–920.
99. Savino W, Berrih S, Dardenne M. Thymic epithelial antigen acquired during ontogeny and defined by the anti-p19 monoclonal antibody, is lost in thymoma. *Lab Invest* 1984;51:292–296.
100. Bhan AK, Rheinherz EL, Poppema S, McCluskey RT, Schlossman JF. Location of T-cell and major histocompatibility antigens in the human thymus. *J Exp Med* 1980;152:771–782.
101. Bofill M, Janossy G, Willcox N, Chilosi M, Trejdosiewicz LK, Newson-Davis J. Microenvironments in the normal thymus and the thymus in myasthenia gravis. *Am J Pathol* 1985;119:462–473.
102. Wiley EL, Noral JM, Freeman RG. Immunohistochemical demonstration of H antigen, peanut agglutinin receptor and Saphora Japonica receptor expression in infant thymuses and thymic neoplasia. *Am J Clin Pathol* 1990;93:44–48.
103. Le PT, Lazorick S, Whichard LP, et al. Regulation of cytokine production in the human thymus: epidermal growth factor and transforming growth factor alpha regulate mRNA levels of interleukin 1 alpha (IL-1 alpha), IL-1 beta, and IL-6 in human thymic epithelial cells at a post-transcriptional level. *J Exp Med* 1991;174:1147–1157.
104. Chan WC, Zaatari GS, Tabei S, Bibb M, Byrnes RK. Thymoma: an immunohistochemical study. *Am J Clin Pathol* 1984;82:160–166.
105. Lobach DF, Scearse RM, Haynes BF. The human thymic microenvironment. Phenotypic characterization of Hassall's bodies with the use of monoclonal antibodies. *J Immunol* 1985;134:250–257.
106. Hsu S-M, Jaffe ES. Phenotypic expression of T lymphocytes in thymus and peripheral lymphoid tissue. *Am J Pathol* 1985;121:69–78.
107. Janossy G, Bofill M, Trejdosiewicz LK, Wilcox HNA, Chilosi M. Cellular differentiation of lymphoid subpopulations and their microenvironments in the human thymus. In: Muller-Hermelink HK, ed. *The human thymus. Histophysiology and pathology.* Berlin: Springer-Verlag, 1986:89–125.
108. Tidman N, Janossy C, Bodger M, Granger S, Kung PC, Goldstein G. Delineation of human thymocyte differentiation pathways utilizing double staining techniques with monoclonal antibodies. *Clin Exp Immunol* 1981;45:457–467.
109. Chilosi M, Iannucci AM, Pizzolo G, Menestrina F, Fiore-Donati L, Janossy G. Immunohistochemical analysis of thymoma. Evidence of medullary origin of epithelial cells. *Am J Surg Pathol* 1984; 8:309–318.
110. Mokhtar N, Hsu S-M, Lad RP, Haynes BF, Jaffe ES. Thymoma: lymphoid and epithelial components of thymoma mirror the phenotype of normal thymus. *Hum Pathol* 1984;15:378–384.
111. Sato Y, Watanabe S, Mukai K, Kodama T, Upton MP, Goto M, Shimosato Y. An immunohistochemical study of thymic epithelial tumors. II. Lymphoid component. *Am J Surg Pathol* 1986;10:862–870.
112. Lauriola L, Maggiano N, Marino M, Carbone A, Piantelli M, Musiani P. Human thymoma: Immunologic characterization of the lymphocyte component. *Cancer* 1981;48:1992–1995.
113. van der Kwast TH, van Vliet E, Cristen E, van Ewijk W, van der Heul RO. An immunohistologic study of the epithelial and lymphoid components of six thymomas. *Hum Pathol* 1985;16:1001–1008.
114. Eimoto T, Teshima K, Shirakusa T, et al. Heterogeneity of epithelial cells and reactive components in thymomas: an ultrastructural and immunohistochemical study. *Ultrastruct Pathol* 1986;10:157–173.
115. Shirai T, Miyota M, Nakase A, Itoh T. Lymphocyte subpopulations in neoplastic and non-neoplastic thymus and in blood of patients with myasthenia gravis. *Clin Exp Immunol* 1976;26:118–123.
116. Katzin WE, Fishleder AJ, Linden MD, Tubbs RR. Immunoglobulin and T-cell receptor genes in thymomas: genotypic evidence supporting the non-neoplastic nature of the lymphocytic component. *Hum Pathol* 1988;19:323–328.
117. Swerdlow SH, Angermeier PA, Hartman AL. Intrathymic ontogeny of the T cell associated CD3 (T3) antigen. *Lab Invest* 1988;58:421–427.
118. Nikolic-Zugic J. Phenotypic and functional stages in the intrathymic development of alpha beta T cells. *Immunol Today* 1991;12:65–70.
119. Bach JF, Dardenne M, Pleau JM, Rosa J. Biochemical characteristics of a serum thymic factor. *Nature* 1976;266:55–56.
120. Goldstein AL, Low TLK, McAdoo M, et al. Thymosin alpha-1. Isolation and sequential analysis of an immunologically active thymic polypeptide. *Proc Natl Acad Sci U S A* 1977;74:725–729.
121. Goldstein G. The isolation of thymopoietin (thymin). *Ann NY Acad Sci* 1975;249:177–185.
122. Fabien N, Auger C, Morier JC. Immunolocalization of thymosin alpha 1, thymopoietin and thymulin in mouse thymic epithelial cells at different stages of culture: a light and electron microscopic study. *Immunology* 1988;63:721–727.
123. Jambon B, Montague P, Bene MC, Brayer MP, Faure G, Duheille J. Immunohistologic localization of facteur thymique serique (FTS) in human thymic epithelium. *J Immunol* 1981;127:2055–2059.
124. Savino W, Dardenne M. Thymic hormone–containing cells. VI. Immunohistologic evidence for the simultaneous presence of thymin, thymopoietin and thymosin alpha 1 in normal and pathological human thymuses. *Eur J Immunol* 1984;14:987–991.
125. Haynes BF, Warren RW, Buckley RH, et al. Demonstration of abnormalities in expression of thymic epithelial surface antigen in severe cellular immunodeficiency disease. *J Immunol* 1983;130:1182–1188.
126. Clark SL Jr. The thymus in mice of strains 129/J, studied with the electron microscope. *Am J Anat* 1963;112:1–32.
127. Hirokawa K, Utsuyama M, Morizumi E, Hashimoto T, Masaoka A, Goldstein AL. Immunohistochemical studies in human thymoma. Localization of thymosin and various cell markers. *Virchows Arch [B]* 1988;55:371–380.
128. Geenen V, Robert F, Defresne M-P, Boniver J, Legros J-J, Franchimont P. Neuroendocrinology of the thymus. *Horm Res* 1989;31: 81–84.
129. Jevremovic M, Terzic M, Kartaljevic G, Popovic V, Rosic B, Filipovic S. The determination of immunoreactive beta-endorphin concentration in the human fetal and neonatal thymus. *Horm Metab Res* 1991;23:623–624.
130. Batanero E, de Leeuw F-E, Jansen GH, van Wichen DF, Huber J, Schuurman H-J. The neural and neuroendocrine components of the human thymus. II. Hormone immunoreactivity. *Brain Behav Immun* 1992;6:249–264.
131. Le PT, Lazorick S, Whichard LP, et al. Human thymic epithelial cells produce IL-6, granulocyte-monocyte-CSF, and leukemia inhibitory factor. *J Immunol* 1990;145:3310–3315.
132. Wainberg MA, Numazaki K, Destephano L, Wong I, Goldman H. Infection of human thymic epithelial cells by human cytomegalovirus and other viruses: effect on secretion of interleukin-1–like activity. *Clin Exp Immunol* 1988;72:415–421.
133. Hirokawa K. Age related changes of the thymus. Morphological and functional aspects. *Acta Pathol Jpn* 1978;28:843–856.
134. Simpson JG, Gray ES, Beck JS. Age involution in the normal adult thymus. *Clin Exp Immunol* 1975;19:261–265.
135. Steinman GG. Changes in the human thymus during aging. In: Muller-Hermelink HK, ed. *The human thymus. Histophysiology and pathology.* Berlin: Springer-Verlag, 1986:43–88.
136. Steinman GG, Klaus B, Muller-Hermelink HK. The involution of the aging human thymic epithelium is independent of puberty. A morphometric study. *Scand J Immunol* 1985;22:536–575.
137. Smith SM, Ossa-Gomez LJ. A quantitative histologic comparison of the thymus in 100 healthy and diseased adults. *Am J Clin Pathol* 1981; 76:657–665.
138. Selye H. Thymus and adrenals in the response of the organism to injuries and intoxications. *Br J Exp Pathol* 1936;17:234–248.
139. Van Baarlen J, Schuurman H-J, Huber J. Acute thymus involution in infancy and childhood: a reliable marker for duration of acute illness. *Hum Pathol* 1988;19:1155–1160.
140. Joshi VV, Oleske JM, Saad S, Gadol C, Connor E, Bobila R, Minefor AB. Thymus biopsy in children with acquired immunodeficiency syndrome. *Arch Pathol Lab Med* 1986;110:837–842.
141. Seemayer TA, Laroche AC, Russo P, et al. Precocious thymic involu-

tion manifest by epithelial injury in the acquired immunodeficiency syndrome. *Hum Pathol* 1984;15:469–474.
142. Grody WW, Fligiel S, Naeim F. Thymus involution in the acquired immunodeficiency syndrome. *Am J Clin Pathol* 1985;84:85–95.
143. Schuurman H-J, Krone WJA, Broekhuizen R, et al. The thymus in acquired immune deficiency syndrome. Comparison with other types of immunodeficiency diseases, and presence of components of human immunodeficiency virus type 1. *Am J Pathol* 1989;134:1329–1338.
144. Kendall MD, Johnson HRM, Singh J. The weight of the human thymus gland at necropsy. *J Anat* 1980;131:485–499.
145. Lack EE. Thymic hyperplasia with massive enlargement. Report of two cases with review of diagnostic criteria. *J Thorac Cardiovasc Surg* 1981;81:786–790.
146. Katz SM, Chatten J, Bishop HD, Rosenblum H. Massive thymic enlargement. Report of a case of gross thymic hyperplasia in a child. *Am J Clin Pathol* 1977;68:786–790.
147. Judd RL. Massive thymic hyperplasia with myoid cell differentiation. *Hum Pathol* 1987;18:1180–1183.
148. Hammar JA. Uber Gewicht Involution und Persistenz der Thymus im Postfotalleben der Menschen. *Arch Anat Physiol Anat Abt* 1906; (suppl);91–182.
149. Durkin W, Durant J. Benign mass lesions after therapy for Hodgkin's disease. *Arch Intern Med* 1979;139:333–336.
150. Shin MS, Ho KT. Diffuse thymic hyperplasia following chemotherapy for nodular sclerosis Hodgkin's disease. *Cancer* 1983;51:30–33.
151. Carmosino L, DiBennedetto A, Feller S. Thymic hyperplasia following successful chemotherapy. A report of 2 cases and review of the literature. *Cancer* 1985;56:1526–1528.
152. Due W, Dieckman K-P, Stein H. Thymic hyperplasia following chemotherapy of a testicular germ cell tumor. Immunohistochemical evidence for a simple rebound phenomenon. *Cancer* 1989;63: 446–449.
153. Gelfland DW, Goldman AS, Law AJ. Thymic hyperplasia in children recovering from thermal burns. *J Trauma* 1972;12:813–817.
154. Caffey J, Sibley R. Regrowth and overgrowth of the thymus after atrophy induced by oral administration of corticosteroids to human infants. *Pediatrics* 1960;26:762–770.
155. Croxatto OC. Cordones epiteliales con aspecto endocrino observado en restos timicos del adulto. *Medicina (B Aires)* 1972;32:203–208.
156. Suster S, Moran CA. Malignant thymic neoplasms that may mimic benign conditions. *Semin Diagn Pathol* 1995;12:98–104.
157. Suster S, Rosai J. Multilocular thymic cyst: an acquired reactive process. Study of 18 cases. *Am J Surg Pathol* 1991;15:388–398.
158. Suster S, Barbuto D, Carlson G, Rosai J. Multilocular thymic cysts with pseudoepitheliomatous hyperplasia. *Hum Pathol* 1991;22: 455–460.
159. Suster S, Rosai J. Cystic thymomas. Clinicopathologic study of 10 cases. *Cancer* 1992;69:92–97.
160. Moran CA, Suster S. Mediastinal seminomas with prominent cystic changes. A clinicopathologic study of 10 cases. *Am J Surg Pathol* 1995;19:1047–1053.
161. Suster S, Rosai J. Thymic carcinoma. A clinicopathologic study of 60 cases. *Cancer* 1991;67:1025–1032.
162. Moran CA, Suster S. Mucoepidermoid carcinomas of the thymus. A clinicopathologic study of six cases. *Am J Surg Pathol* 1995;19: 826–834.
163. Penn CRH, Hope-Stone HF. The role of radiotherapy in the management of malignant thymoma. *Br J Surg* 1972;59:533–539.
164. Goodwin RA, Nickell JA, Des Pres RM. Mediastinal fibrosis complicating healed primary histoplasmosis and tuberculosis. *Medicine* 1972;51:227–256.
165. Light AM. Idiopathic fibrosis of the mediastinum: a discussion of three cases and a review of the literature. *J Clin Pathol* 1978;31: 78–82.
166. Sobrino-Simoes MA, Saleiro JV, Waagensvoort CA. Mediastinal and hilar fibrosis. *Histopathology* 1981;5:53–58.

*Histology for Pathologists, second edition,*
Edited by Stephen S. Sternberg.
Lippincott-Raven Publishers, Philadelphia
© 1997.

# CHAPTER 31

# Bone Marrow

S. N. Wickramasinghe



The bone marrow is a large and complex organ that is distributed throughout the cavities of the skeleton. The total mass of the bone marrow of an adult has been estimated to be 1,600 to 3,700 g, exceeding that of the liver. About half this mass consists of hematopoietically inactive fatty marrow (which appears yellow) and the remainder of hematopoietically active marrow (which appears red). Although essentially hematopoietically inactive, even fatty marrow contains a few scattered microscopic foci of hematopoietic cells. The functions of the hematopoietic marrow include (a) the formation and release of various types of blood cells (hematopoiesis), (b) the phagocytosis and degradation of circulating particulate material such as microorganisms and abnormal or senescent red cells and leukocytes, and (c) antibody production. The nonhematopoietic marrow serves as a large store of reserve lipids. The various functions of hematopoietic marrow are based on a high degree of structural organization. However, this organization is labile, altering rapidly in response to many stimuli.

S. N. Wickramasinghe: Department of Haematology, St. Mary's Hospital Medical School, Imperial College of Science, Technology and Medicine, London W2 1PG, England.

## TECHNIQUES FOR STUDYING THE MARROW

The microscopic structure of the human bone marrow can be studied during life by performing a trephine biopsy of the posterior superior iliac spine or anterior iliac crest. This provides a core of bone and associated marrow. The biopsy specimen may be fixed in neutral buffered formalin for at least 18 h, in Zenker's solution for a minimum of 4 h, or in B5 (formalin and mercury chloride) for 4 h and decalcified in 10% formic acid and 1% formalin or in one of a number of other decalcifying reagents. It is then processed in the usual manner and embedded in paraffin (1,2). Decalcification and paraffin embedding result in some shrinkage of marrow tissue, loss of the activity of cellular enzymes, and, sometimes, blurring of nuclear staining. In addition, certain decalcification procedures cause leaching of the iron stores (i.e., of the hemosiderin present within macrophages). However, the reactivity of some antigens with antibody is retained.

Histologic studies also can be performed on aspirated marrow. Two methods are in use. The first is to allow the marrow to clot, before fixation and subsequent processing to paraffin. The clot sections obtained usually show only a few marrow fragments within a large mass of clotted blood. The second approach is to concentrate the marrow fragments by filtration or some other procedure, before processing. This approach yields better preparations than do clot sections.

Sections of paraffin-embedded marrow fragments or decalcified bone cores are cut to a thickness of 3 to 5 μm and are routinely stained with hematoxylin and eosin (H&E), with the Giemsa stain, by a silver impregnation technique for reticulin, and by Perls' acid ferrocyanide method for hemosiderin (Prussian blue reaction). They may also be stained by the periodic acid-Schiff (PAS) reaction for glycogen or glycoprotein. A Leder stain for chloroacetate esterase may be performed on sections of marrow fragments but works poorly on decalcified specimens (1). A limited range of antibodies can be used for immunohistochemical studies on formalin- or B5-fixed, paraffin-embedded sections of trephine biopsy specimens, using an immunoalkaline phosphatase or immunoperoxidase method. The most useful antibodies and the cell types they recognize are given in Table 1 (3–9).

The cores obtained by trephine biopsy also may be fixed in a mixture containing formaldehyde, methanol, and glucose phosphate and embedded in methyl methacrylate without decalcification (10–13). Semithin sections (1–3 μm thick) of the undecalcified methyl methacrylate–embedded material then may be cut using a special heavy-duty microtome. Such sections show cellular features in much greater detail than do paraffin-embedded sections but have no antigenic or enzymic reactivity. On the other hand, if the core is appropriately fixed and embedded in glycol methacrylate (a water-miscible plastic) or a mixture of methyl and glycol methacrylate, a number of antigen epitopes and enzyme activities are preserved (14–16).

Methyl methacrylate–embedded semithin sections may be stained after removing the methacrylate, with H&E or gallamine blue–Giemsa for cellular detail, Gomori's stain for reticulin fibers, PAS stain, Berlin blue stain for iron, and Ladewig's and Goldner's stains for osteoid, calcified bone, and connective tissue (12,13,17–19). Trephine biopsy cores that are embedded in a mixture of methyl methacrylate and glycol methacrylate may be used for the demonstration of chloroacetate esterase, acid phosphatase, peroxidase, nonspecific esterase, and alkaline phosphatase, as well as for the immunohistochemical detection of some antigens (14,15).

For immunohistochemical studies with the widest range of antibodies, frozen sections of trephine biopsy cores must be used (20,21). However, such sections show less cytologic detail than paraffin-embedded sections and tend to become distorted, making interpretation difficult. The distortion when cutting frozen sections can be reduced using a special supporting medium such as Histocon (Polysciences, Warrington, Pennsylvania), which does not impair antigenic reactivity.

The trephine biopsy core can be used to prepare several imprints by gently touching it with glass slides before fixation for histology. The imprints so obtained are used for de-

**TABLE 1.** *Some monoclonal and polyclonal antibodies which can be used in immunohistochemical studies on sections of decalcified, paraffin-embedded trephine biopsies of the marrow*

| Antibody | Antigen | Cellular specificity in normal tissue |
|---|---|---|
| Anti-CD34 | CD34 | Hematopoietic stem cells |
| Leu-M1 | CD15 | Neutrophil granulocyte series[a], monocytes |
| Anti-lysozyme | Lyosozyme | Neutrophil granulocyte series[a], monoblasts, monocytes, macrophages |
| Leu-M3 | CD14 | Monocytes, macrophages, granulocytes |
| NP57 | Elastase | Neutrophil promyelocytes and myelocytes (strong), neutrophil metamyelocytes and granulocytes (weak), monocytes |
| Anti-myeloperoxidase | Myeloperoxidase | Neutrophil granulocyte series* |
| Anti-lactoferrin | Lactoferrin | Neutrophil myelocytes to granulocytes |
| PG-M1 | CD68 | Monocytes, macrophages |
| Anti-glycophorin A or C | Glycophorin A or C | Erythroid series |
| Anti-hemoglobin A | Hemoglobin A | Erythroid series |
| UEA | | Erythroid series, megakaryocytes, endothelial cells |
| Anti-factor-VIII-related antigen | von Willebrand factor | Megakaryocytes, endothelial cells |
| Y2/51 | CD61, GP IIIa | Megakaryocytes, platelets |
| PD7/26, 2B11, anti-leucocyte common antigen | CD45 | T- and B-lymphocytes, macrophages, granulocytes (weak) |
| MT1, Leu 22 | CD43 | T-lymphocytes, granulocytes, monocytes, macrophages |
| UCHL 1 | CD45RO | T-lymphocytes |
| pT3 | CD3 | T-lymphocytes |
| L26 | CD20 | B-lymphocytes, activated B-lymphocytes |
| MB2 | | B-lymphocytes, endothelial cells |
| LN2 | CD74 | B-lymphocytes macrophages |
| Anti-Ig light chain (κ or λ) | Light chain | Plasma cells, immunoblasts, B-lymphocytes |
| Anti-Ig heavy chain | Heavy chain | Plasma cells, immunoblasts, B-lymphocytes |
| Leu 7 | CD57 | Natural killer cells |
| AA1 | Mast cell tryptase | Mast cells |

[a] Other than myeloblasts

tailed investigations into the morphology and other characteristics of individual marrow cells. However, such studies are best performed on smears of aspirated marrow. In adults, marrow is aspirated from the sternum at the level of the second intercostal space or from the posterior superior iliac spine or the iliac crest. In children, marrow is usually aspirated from the posterior superior iliac spine and, in the case of patients less than 1 year of age, also from the upper end of the medial surface of the tibia just below and medial to the tibial tuberosity. The imprints from the trephine biopsy core and marrow smears are usually stained by a Romanowsky method such as the May-Grünwald-Giemsa (MGG) stain and also by Perls' acid ferrocyanide method. The smears also may be briefly fixed under conditions that preserve enzyme activity and antigenic sites and used to perform cytochemical and immunocytochemical studies. The details of these techniques and their value in hematologic diagnosis have been discussed by Hayhoe and Quaglino (22). Antibodies useful in immunocytochemical studies of appropriately fixed smears include those listed in Table 1 as well as several others such as those against CD2 (a pan-T marker), CD19 (a pan-B marker), and CD41 or CD42b (megakaryocyte lineage markers).

A thorough study of the marrow requires examination of both marrow smears and tissue sections. Marrow smears are undoubtedly the best preparations for the study of cellular detail but provide little information on intercellular relationships and the organization of the marrow. Histologic sections provide this information and are therefore superior to marrow smears for the detection of tumor infiltration, granulomas, amyloidosis, and necrosis of the marrow. They are essential for studying the distribution and quantity of extracellular reticulin and collagen fibers and may show vascular lesions (e.g., in thrombotic thrombocytopenic purpura and polyarteritis nodosa).

When electron microscopic studies are to be performed, an aliquot of a marrow aspirate is mixed with heparinized Hanks' solution. A few marrow fragments are then removed without delay and placed in a solution of 2.5% to 4% glutaraldehyde in 0.1 M phosphate buffer (pH 7.3). Alternatively, 1-mm pieces of the trephine biopsy core are fixed in glutaraldehyde for 1 h, after which the marrow is gently teased out of the bone using a dissecting microscope.

In this chapter, unless otherwise stated, the descriptions of cells in marrow smears apply to smears stained by a Romanowsky method. The electron microscopic data relate to ultrathin sections stained with uranyl acetate and lead citrate. Such sections were prepared from marrow fragments that were fixed in glutaraldehyde and postfixed in osmium tetroxide.

## GENERAL FEATURES OF HEMATOPOIESIS

Blood cells are produced in the embryo and fetus and throughout postnatal life. In the developing fetus and growing child, the total number of hematopoietic cells and blood cells increases progressively with time. By contrast, the hematopoietic systems of healthy adults are examples of steady-state cell renewal systems. In such systems, a relatively constant rate of loss of mature blood cells from the circulation is balanced by the production of new blood cells at the same rate. The number of hematopoietic cells and blood cells therefore remains constant.

New blood cells are eventually derived from a small number of hematopoietic stem cells (23). These cells have two properties: (a) the ability to mature into several types of blood cell and (b) an extensive capacity to generate new stem cells and thus to maintain their own number. The most primitive hematopoietic stem cells are pluripotent (23–25) and give rise to lymphoid stem cells and multipotent myeloid stem cells. The lymphoid stem cells mature into all types of lymphocytes. The myeloid stem cells mature into neutrophil, eosinophil, and basophil granulocytes, monocytes, erythrocytes, platelets, mast cells, and osteoclasts. The immediate progeny of the lymphoid and myeloid stem cells are usually termed hematopoietic progenitor cells. The myeloid progenitor cells are committed to one, two, or a few hematopoietic differentiation pathways (i.e., are unipotent, bipotent, or oligopotent) and have only a limited capacity for self-renewal. The most immature of the myeloid progenitor cells are oligopotent. Such cells undergo a progressive restriction of their differentiation potential such that the most mature progenitor cells are committed to only a single line of differentiation. Human stem cells and hematopoietic progenitor cells have been identified and characterized by their ability to form colonies containing cells of one or more hematopoietic lineages in vitro and are therefore called colony-forming units (CFUs) or colony-forming cells (CFC). Myeloid stem cells generate colonies containing a mixture of granulocytes, erythroblasts, macrophages, and megakaryocytes and are, therefore, termed CFU-GEMM. There is some indirect evidence for the presence of tripotent hematopoietic cells (CFU-E mega baso) that give rise to erythroblasts, megakaryocytes, and basophil granulocytes. Bipotent hematopoietic progenitor cells that give rise to colonies containing granulocytes and macrophages are termed CFU-GM. There are also bipotent progenitor cells generating colonies containing a mixture of erythroblasts and megakaryocytes (CFU-E mega). The unipotent progenitor cells that give rise to neutrophil granulocytes, eosinophil granulocytes, basophil granulocytes, macrophages, erythroblasts, and megakaryocytes are described as CFU-G, CFU-eo, CFU-baso, CFU-M, CFU-E, and CFU-mega, respectively. These develop into the most immature of the morphologically recognizable blood cell precursors in the marrow. Thus, CFU-G develop into myeloblasts, CFU-eo into eosinophil promyelocytes, CFU-baso into basophil promyelocytes, CFU-M into monoblasts, CFU-E into pronormoblasts, and CFU-mega into megakaryoblasts. The stem cells and progenitor cells are found in both the blood and the marrow but cannot be identified on morphologic criteria. The characteristics of the various types of morphologically recognizable hematopoietic cell found in the marrow are described later in this chapter. The relationships between

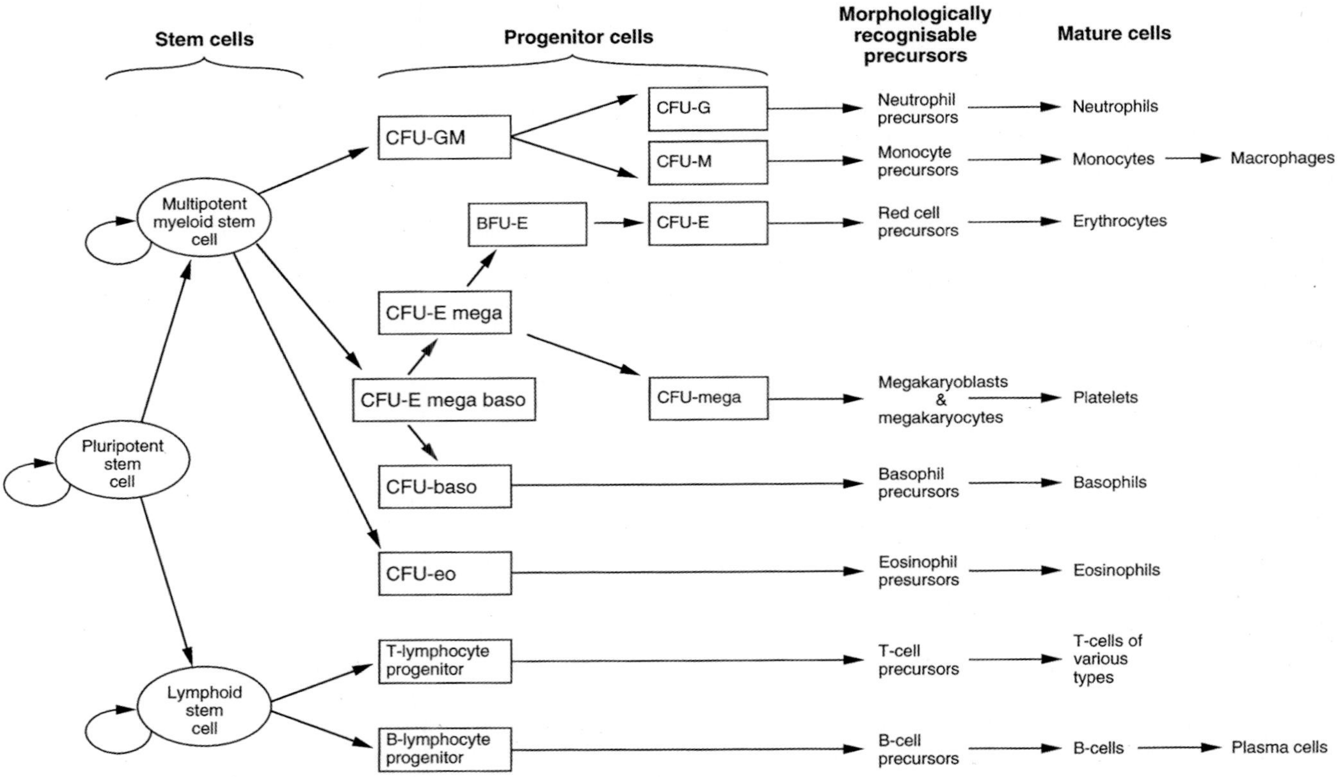


**FIG. 1.** Model of hematopoiesis showing the relationships between the various types of stem cell, progenitor cell, and morphologically recognizable precursor cell. BFU, burst-forming units; CFU, colony-forming units; E, erythroblasts; GM, granulocytes and macrophages; eo, eosinophil granulocytes; baso, basophil granulocytes; mega, megakaryocytes; G, neutrophil granulocytes; M, macrophages. The existence of CFU-E mega baso is postulated on the basis of the expression of the transcription factor GATA 1 only in cells of these three lineages.

the different categories of cell involved in hematopoiesis are illustrated in Fig. 1.

Two processes are involved in the formation of all types of blood cells. These are the progressive acquisition of the morphologic, biochemical, and functional characteristics of the particular cell type (i.e., cytodifferentiation or maturation) and cell proliferation. The latter results in the production of a large number of mature cells from a single cell committed to one or more differentiation pathways. Cytodifferentiation occurs at all stages of hematopoiesis, and cell proliferation occurs in the hematopoietic stem cells and progenitor cells and, except in the megakaryocytic lineage, in the more immature morphologically recognizable precursor cells. The nearly mature blood cells seem to enter the circulation mainly by passing through the endothelial cells of the marrow sinusoids.

## REGULATION OF HEMATOPOIESIS

Bone marrow stromal cells (e.g., macrophages, nonphagocytic reticular or fibroblastoid cells, adipocytes, endothelial cells, and T-lymphocytes) play a major role in the regulation of hematopoiesis not only by providing sites of attachment for stem cells and their progeny but also by their involvement in the secretion of various stimulatory hematopoietic growth factors and inhibitory cytokines (26,27).

The regulation of the stem cells and the early hematopoietic progenitor cells depends on (a) intimate contact with certain stromal cells and with components of the extracellular matrix and (b) interaction of specific cell surface receptors with multilineage hematopoietic growth factors. The latter include stem cell factor (Steel factor, kit ligand), interleukin-1 (IL-1) and IL-6 for the pluripotent stem cells and stem cell factor, IL-3 and granulocyte-macrophage colony stimulating factor (GM-CSF) for the multipotent myeloid stem cells. The regulation of later progenitor cells and the morphologically recognizable hematopoietic cells is dependent both on multilineage growth factors and lineage-specific growth factors such as G-CSF, MCSF, IL-5 (influencing CFU-eo), thrombopoietin (influencing CFU-mega), and erythropoietin. The growth factors influencing lymphocyte progenitor cells and precursors include IL-2, IL-4, IL-5, IL-6, and IL-11 for the B-lineage and IL-2, IL-3, IL-4, and IL-10 for the T-lineage.

Hematopoietic growth factors are glycoproteins and influence the survival, proliferation, and differentiation of their target cells via second messengers. In their absence the target cells undergo programmed cell death (apoptosis). Some growth factors such as G-CSF and GM-CSF not only regulate hematopoiesis but also enhance the function of the mature cells. Most hematopoietic growth factors are produced by bone marrow stromal cells either constitutively (e.g., M-CSF production by fibroblastoid cells and endothelial cells) or after their activation by various signals. Thus, fibroblastoid cells and endothelial cells that have been activated by macrophage-derived IL-1 or tumor necrosis factor (TNF) and endotoxin-stimulated macrophages produce M-CSF, GM-CSF, G-CSF, IL-6, and stem cell factor. IL-1– or antigen-activated T cells produce IL-3, IL-5, and GM-CSF.

The main organ of erythropoietin production in postnatal life is the kidney, and the probable site of synthesis appears to be peritubular cells. About 10% of the erythropoietin is produced in the liver, which is the main organ of synthesis in the fetus. The production of erythropoietin by the kidney is inversely proportional to the degree of oxygenation of renal tissue. A limited amount of data suggest that there also may be paracrine or autocrine erythropoietin production in the bone marrow.

In addition to the stimulatory cytokines mentioned above, inhibitors (negative regulators) of hematopoiesis are produced by macrophages, fibroblastoid cells, and endothelial cells. These include transforming growth factor-$\beta$1 (TGF-$\beta$1), which inhibits multilineage progenitor cells, early erythroid progenitors, and megakaryocytes; TNF-$\alpha$, which inhibits the proliferation of granulocyte precursors; interferon-$\alpha$, which inhibits megakaryocyte progenitors; and macrophage inflammatory protein-1$\alpha$ (MIP-1$\alpha$), which inhibits the proliferation of stem cells.

## HEMATOPOIESIS IN THE EMBRYO AND FETUS: DEVELOPMENT OF THE BONE MARROW

Studies in experimental animals have shown that hematopoietic stem cells develop in the yolk sac and subsequently circulate and colonize the fetal liver and other fetal tissues (28).

In the human embryo, erythropoietic cells first appear within the blood islands of the yolk sac about 19 days after fertilization (29,30). A few megakaryocytes are found in these blood islands during the sixth and seventh weeks of gestation. Yolk sac erythropoiesis is megaloblastic and results in the production of nucleated red cells (Fig. 2) containing three embryonic hemoglobins (23), namely, hemoglobins Gower I ($\zeta_2\epsilon_2$), Gower II ($\alpha_2\epsilon_2$), and Portland I ($\zeta_2\gamma_2$), and, in later embryos, hemoglobin F ($\alpha_2\gamma_2$).

Hematopoietic foci develop in the hepatic cords during the sixth week of gestation, and the liver becomes the major site of erythropoiesis in the middle trimester of pregnancy (31,32). During this period, about half the nucleated cells of the liver consist of erythropoietic cells (Fig. 3). A few granulocytopoietic cells and megakaryocytes also are found in this organ. Fetal hepatic erythropoiesis is normoblastic and gives rise to nonnucleated red cells containing hemoglobin F. These red cells are considerably larger than the red cells of adults. The number of erythropoietic cells in the liver decreases progressively after the seventh month of gestation; a few cells persist until the end of the first postnatal week.

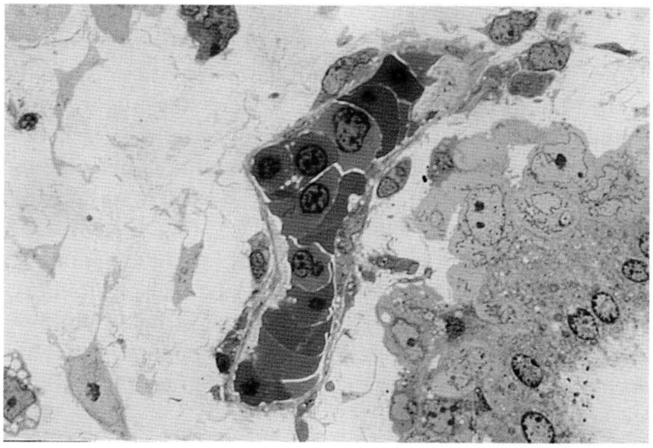

**FIG. 2.** Semithin section of a plastic-embedded chorionic villus biopsy sample obtained at 7 weeks of gestation, showing a blood vessel containing nucleated embryonic red cells. Toluidine blue.

Marrow cavities are formed as a result of the erosion of bone or calcified cartilage by blood vessels and cells from the periosteum (30). The first marrow cavity to develop is that of the clavicle (at about 2 months). After the formation of the marrow cavities, the vascular connective tissue present within them becomes colonized by circulating hematopoietic stem cells. The latter generate erythropoietic

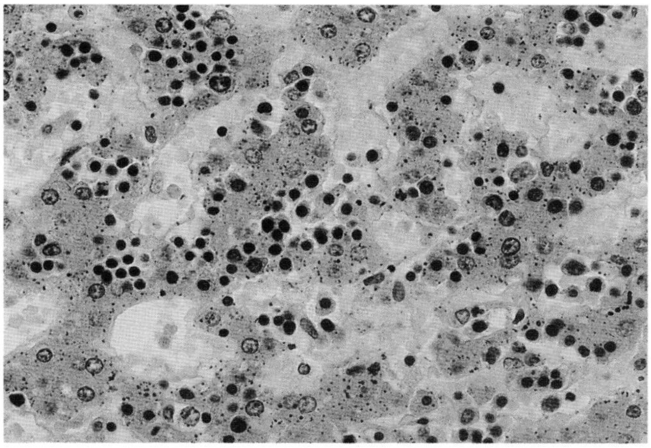

**FIG. 3.** Fetal liver tissue obtained postmortem showing erythropoietic activity. The erythroblasts are found extravascularly both within the hepatic cords and between the cords and the sinusoidal endothelial cells. The brown material within hepatocytes is formalin pigment, a comon postmortem fixation artifact. Hematoxylin and eosin.

cells during the third and fourth months of gestation, the order of appearance of erythropoietic cells being the same as the order of formation of the marrow cavities. After the sixth month, the bone marrow becomes the major site of hematopoiesis. Erythropoiesis in fetal bone marrow is normoblastic and results in the production of nonnucleated red cells, which contain hemoglobins F and A ($\alpha_2\beta_2$) and which are larger than adult red cells. The fetal bone marrow is the predominant site of intrauterine granulocytopoiesis and megakaryocytopoiesis. In this tissue, the myeloid/erythroid ratio (i.e., the ratio of the number of neutrophil precursors plus neutrophil granulocytes to the number of erythroblasts) remains constant at about 1:4 after 6½ months of gestation (33).

## POSTNATAL CHANGES IN THE DISTRIBUTION OF RED MARROW AND IN THE TYPE OF HEMOGLOBIN

At birth all the marrow cavities contain red, hematopoietic marrow. Furthermore, the red marrow contains only a few fat cells. After the first 4 years of life, an increasing number of fat cells appears between the hematopoietic cells, particularly in certain regions of the marrow, and these regions eventually become yellow and virtually devoid of hematopoietic cells (34,35). Zones of yellow, fatty marrow are found just below the middle of the shafts of the long bones between the ages of 10 and 14 years and, subsequently, extend in both directions, distal spread being more rapid than proximal spread. By the age of about 25 years, hematopoietic marrow is confined to the proximal quarters of the shafts of the femora and humeri, the skull bones, ribs, sternum, scapulae, clavicles, vertebrae, pelvis, and the upper half of the sacrum. Although the distribution of hematopoietic marrow remains essentially unaltered throughout adult life, its fat cell content increases slightly with increasing age and more substantially after the age of 70 years, in association with a gradual expansion of the volume of the marrow cavities.

The percentages of hemoglobins F and A in the blood of full-term neonates are, respectively, 50% to 85% and 15% to 50%. The proportion of hemoglobin F decreases postnatally at different rates in different individuals, but adult levels of less than 1% are reached in nearly all children by the age of 2½ years.

Because young children have red marrow containing few fat cells in virtually all their marrow cavities, a rapid increase in hematopoietic tissue in this age group is presumably accommodated mainly by a reduction in the proportion of marrow space occupied by sinusoids. If the increase in the rate of hematopoiesis is substantial and prolonged (e.g., in congenital hemolytic anemias), there is an increase in the total volume of the marrow cavities and the reestablishment of extramedullary hematopoiesis in organs such as the liver, spleen, and lymph nodes (36). The expansion of the marrow cavities leads to skeletal abnormalities, such as frontal and parietal bossing, dental deformities, and malocclusion of the teeth. It also causes thinning of the cortex, which may lead to fractures after minor trauma. In adults, increased hematopoiesis is initially associated with the replacement of fat cells in red marrow by hematopoietic cells and also with the spread of red marrow into marrow cavities normally containing yellow marrow (36). If the increase in hematopoiesis is gross (e.g., in beta-thalassemia intermedia), extramedullary hematopoiesis may develop.

## STRUCTURAL ORGANIZATION OF HEMATOPOIETIC MARROW

The marrow cavities of most bones contain trabeculae of cancellous bone. The inner surface of the cortex and the outer surfaces of the trabeculae are lined by the endosteum, which consists of a single layer of cells supported on a delicate layer of reticular connective tissue. In most areas of the endosteum, the cells consist of very flat bone-lining cells, but in some areas they consist of osteoblasts or osteoclasts. The marrow, which is located between the trabeculae, is supplied with an extensive microvasculature and some myelinated and nonmyelinated nerve fibers. It does not have a lymphatic drainage (37). The space between the small blood vessels contains a few reticulin fibers and a variety of cell types. The latter include fat cells, precursors of red cells, granulocytes, monocytes and platelets, lymphocytes, plasma cells, macrophages (phagocytic reticular cells), nonphagocytic reticular cells, and mast cells.

### Blood Supply

One or more nutrient canals penetrate the shafts of the long bones obliquely. Each canal contains a nutrient artery and one or two nutrient veins. After entering the marrow, the nutrient artery divides into ascending and descending branches, which coil around the central longitudinal vein, the main venous channel of the marrow. The ascending and descending arteries give off numerous arterioles and capillaries that travel radially toward the endosteum and often open into a plexus of sinusoids (23). The sinusoids drain through a system of collecting venules and larger venous channels into the central longitudinal vein, which in turn drains mainly into the nutrient veins. In the diaphyses of long bones containing yellow fatty marrow, the nutrient artery gives off relatively few branches until it reaches the lower edge of the red marrow, where it breaks up into numerous vessels that penetrate the hematopoietic tissue. Many blood vessels of various sizes supply the marrow within flat and cuboidal bones, entering the marrow cavity via one or more large nutrient canals as well as through numerous smaller canals.

There are interconnections between the blood supply of the bone marrow and bone through an endosteal network of blood vessels. This network communicates both with the pe-

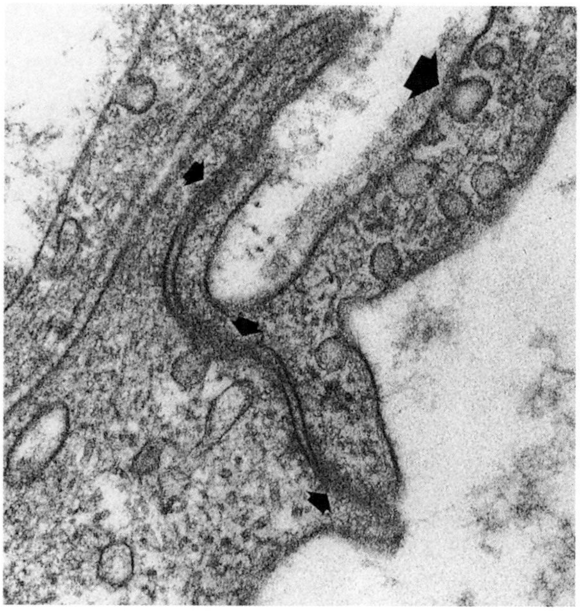

**FIG. 4.** Electron micrograph of part of the wall of a sinusoid from normal bone marrow. There are three tight junctions (*small arrows*) at the area of contact between two adjacent endothelial cells. Several pinocytotic vesicles (*large arrow*) are present both at the luminal and abluminal surface of one of the endothelial cells, and a single pinocytotic vesicle is present at the outer surface of the adventitial cell.

riosteal vessels via fine veins passing through the bone and with branches of the nutrient artery. Furthermore, studies in experimental animals have shown that many capillaries derived from the nutrient artery enter haversian canals but swing back into the marrow and open into sinusoids or venules (38,39). There has been much speculation as to whether blood reaching the marrow from the bone contains one or more hematopoietic factors derived from the bone or endosteal cells. This question has not yet been settled, but recent studies have indicated that mouse bone marrow–derived osteogenic cells secrete M-CSF, GM-CSF, and IL-6 (40).

The sinusoids of human bone marrow have thin walls consisting of an inner complete layer of flattened endothelial cells with little or no underlying basement membrane and an outer incomplete layer of adventitial cells (41). The endothelial cells are characterized by the presence of numerous small pinocytotic vesicles along both their luminal and abluminal surfaces (Fig. 4). The nucleus is flattened and contains moderate quantities of nuclear membrane–associated condensed chromatin. The cytoplasm also contains ribosomes, rough endoplasmic reticulum (RER), mitochondria, some microfilaments, a few lysosomes, and occasional fat droplets. Adjacent endothelial cells overlap and may interdigitate extensively. These areas of contact are characterized by (a) a strictly parallel alignment of the membranes of the interacting cells with a narrow gap between the opposing membranes and (b) short stretches in which the membranes fuse together, forming tight junctions (not true desmosomes). There is an increased electron density of the cytoplasm immediately adjacent to and on both sides of the tight junctions (Fig. 4). Some endothelial cells show alkaline phosphatase activity. Endothelial cells contain no stainable iron except when the iron stores are increased.

Adventitial cells project long peripheral cytoplasmic processes, which may be closely associated with some extracellular reticulin fibers. Some of these processes lie along the sinusoidal surface and others protrude outward between hematopoietic cells. Thus, adventitial cells are a type of reticular cell (i.e., form part of the cytoplasmic network or reticulum of the marrow stroma). The cytoplasm of adventitial cells contains ribosomes, RER, some pinocytotic vesicles, a few electron-dense lysosomes, occasional fat globules, and numerous microfilaments that are often arranged in bands. The latter are usually situated within the peripheral cytoplasmic processes. The cytoplasm of some adventitial cells appears very electron lucent. Adventitial cells stain strongly for alkaline phosphatase.

### Nerve Supply

In the case of a long bone, the nerve supply enters the bone marrow mainly via the nutrient canal but also through a number of epiphyseal and metaphyseal foramina. Bundles of nerve fibers travel together with the nutrient artery and its branches and supply the smooth muscle in such vessels or, occasionally, terminate between hematopoietic cells (42).

### Extracellular Connective Tissue

Normal marrow contains a scanty incomplete network of fine branching reticulin fibers between the parenchymal cells (Fig. 5). A higher concentration of thicker fibers is

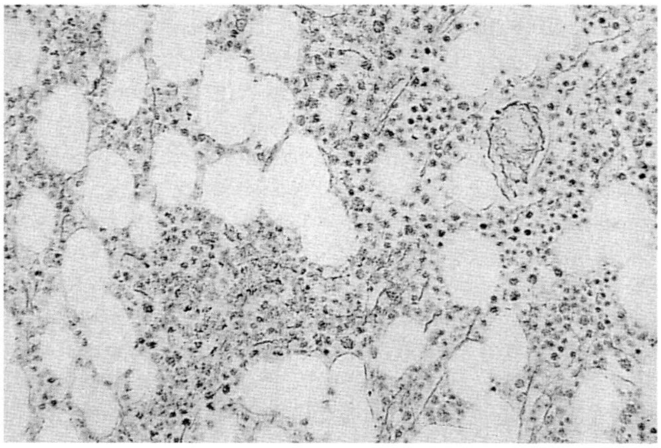

**FIG. 5.** Section of a decalcified, paraffin-embedded trephine biopsy core from a hematologically normal adult, showing a scant network of fine reticulin fibers. The upper right-hand quadrant of the photomicrograph shows a circular arrangement of fibers associated with a blood vessel. Silver impregnation of reticulin.

found in and around the walls of the larger arteries and near the endosteum; such fibers are continuous with the fibers in the parenchyma.

### Nonhematopoietic Cells (Stromal Cells)

These are cells that do not develop into blood cells and that are not found in normal blood. However, some of them are end cells derived from hematopoietic stem cells, and some appear to be intimately involved in the regulation of hematopoiesis.

#### *Osteoblasts and Osteoclasts*

Osteoblasts are present in the endosteum in areas of deposition of osseous matrix (osteoid). In histologic sections, osteoblasts are cuboidal or pyramidal and have eccentric nuclei. Their cytoplasm is markedly basophilic and contains a large round pale zone. Osteoblasts are frequently found in a continuous layer, usually one or two cells thick, and appear like an area of epithelium. They become surrounded by the osteoid they produce and thus eventually become osteocytes. Osteoclasts are large multinucleate cells involved in bone resorption and are often found in shallow excavations on the surface of the bone, termed Howship's lacunae. Osteoblasts are not derived from the hematopoietic stem cells but arise from the bone-lining cells of the endosteum. Osteoclasts originate from the myeloid hematopoietic stem cells. The relationship between the osteoclast progenitor cell and other hematopoietic progenitor cells (e.g., CFU-GEMM, CFU-GM, CFU-M) is not yet clear (43).

Romanowsky-stained normal marrow smears may contain groups of osteoblasts or individual osteoclasts. In such preparations, osteoblasts have an oval or elongated shape and are 20 to 50 $\mu$m in diameter. They have abundant basophilic cytoplasm, often with somewhat indistinct margins, and a single small eccentric nucleus with only small quantities of condensed chromatin and with one to three nucleoli. The cytoplasm contains a rounded pale area corresponding to the Golgi apparatus, which often is situated some distance from the nucleus (Fig. 6). Osteoblasts stain positively for alkaline phosphatase activity. They superficially resemble plasma cells, but the latter are smaller, contain heavily stained clumped chromatin, and have a Golgi zone situated immediately adjacent to the nucleus. Osteoclasts appear as giant multinucleate cells with abundant pale blue cytoplasm containing many azurophilic (purple–red) granules (Fig. 7). The individual nuclei are rounded in outline, uniform in size, contain a single prominent nucleolus, and do not overlap. Osteoclasts are strongly acid phosphatase positive. They must be distinguished from the other polyploid giant cells in the marrow, the megakaryocytes. These are usually not multinucleate but contain a single large lobulated nucleus.

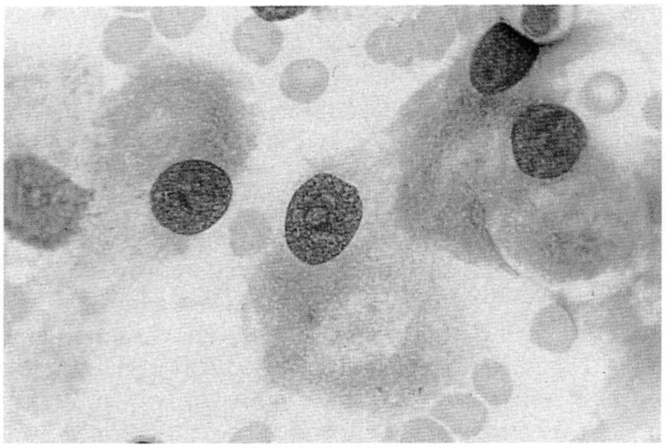

**FIG. 6.** Group of osteoblasts from an MGG-stained smear of normal bone marrow.

#### *Fat Cells*

The number of fat cells in hematopoietic bone marrow varies markedly with age (44,45). In normal adults, 30% to 70% of the area of a histologic section of hematopoietic marrow consists of fat cells (Figs. 8 and 9). Fat cells are the largest cells in the marrow, and sections of such cells have average diameters of about 85 $\mu$m. Ultrastructural studies show that these cells have a single large fat globule at their center and a narrow rim of cytoplasm at their periphery. This cytoplasmic rim contains a flattened nucleus, several small lipid droplets, ribosomes, strands of endoplasmic reticulum, and several mitochondria. The fat cells of the bone marrow only have small quantities of reticulin and collagen fibers around them. They are in intimate contact with vascular channels, macrophages, and all types of hematopoietic cells. Marrow fat cells seem to be formed by the accumulation of lipid within adventitial cells, other nonphagocytic reticular cells, and, possibly, sinus endothelial cells. Whenever there is an increase or decrease in the number of hematopoietic cells in bone marrow, there is a corresponding decrease or

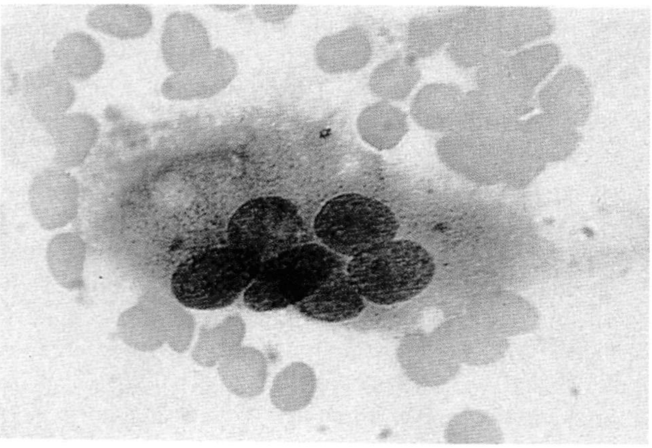

**FIG. 7.** A multinucleate osteoclast from an MGG-stained smear of normal bone marrow.

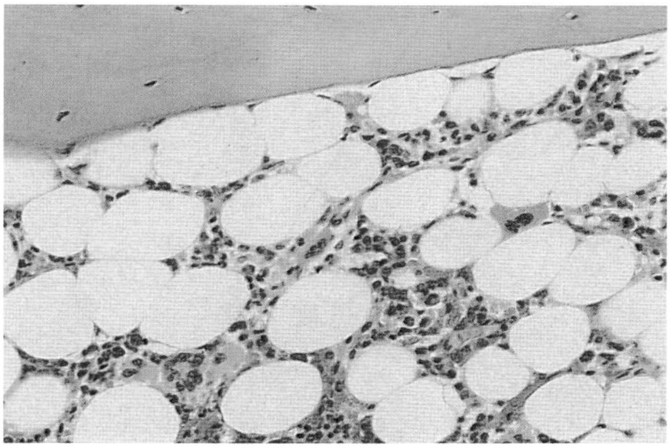

**FIG. 8.** Section of a decalcified, paraffin-embedded trephine biopsy core from a hematologically normal adult. About 70% of the area of marrow tissue in this photomicrograph is occupied by fat cells. There may be a substantial variation in cellularity in different parts of the same section. Hematoxylin and eosin.

increase, respectively, of the number of fat cells so that the intersinusoidal space within marrow cavities is always fully occupied by cells. The mechanisms underlying this inverse relationship between the mass of fat cells and hematopoietic cells in the marrow are uncertain. In severe anorexia nervosa or cachexia secondary to chronic disorders such as tuberculosis or carcinoma, there is a marked reduction in fat cells, often together with a reduction in hematopoietic tissue. In these conditions, the space normally occupied by cells is filled with a gelatinous extracellular substance composed of acid mucopolysaccharide (46).

### *Macrophages (Phagocytic Reticular Cells)*

The bone marrow contains many macrophages. The frequency of this cell type is best appreciated in sections of trephine biopsies stained for an antigen found in macrophages such as CD68 (Fig. 10) or in electron micrographs of ultrathin sections of marrow fragments rather than in smears of aspirated bone marrow. In H&E-stained sections of trephine biopsies, macrophages appear as moderately large cells with abundant cytoplasm. In Romanowsky-stained marrow smears, they appear as irregularly shaped cells 20 to 30 $\mu$m in diameter and have a round or oval nucleus with pale, lacelike chromatin and one or more large nucleoli. The cytoplasm is voluminous, stains pale blue, and contains azurophilic granules, vacuoles, and variously sized inclusions consisting of phagocytosed material (Fig. 11A). Macrophages are derived from monocytes and, therefore, eventually from the hematopoietic stem cells.

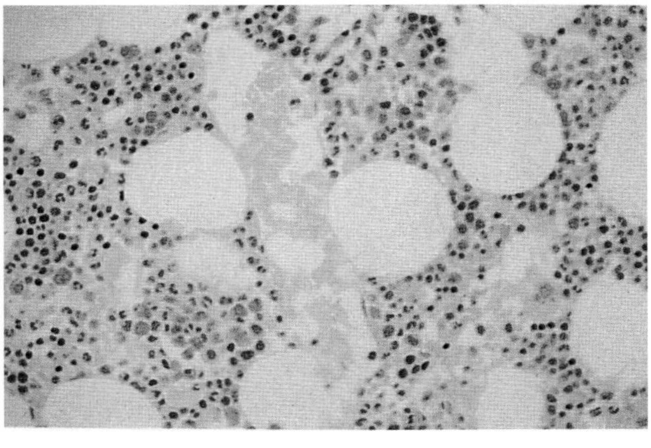

**FIG. 9.** Semithin section of an undecalcified, plastic-embedded trephine biopsy core from a hematologically normal adult. A wide sinusoid containing red cells is seen passing vertically between some fat cells. Hematoxylin and eosin.

In unstained smears and sections of normal marrow and in Giemsa- or H&E-stained sections, macrophages may show refractile yellow–brown hemosiderin-containing intracytoplasmic inclusions, which vary between 0.5 and 4 $\mu$m in diameter. These appear as blue or blue–black granules when stained by Perls' acid ferrocyanide method. This stain also may color the entire cytoplasm a diffuse pale blue (Fig. 12). The amount of iron-positive granules within the marrow fragments on a marrow smear (Fig. 13) or the amount in a histologic section of a trephine biopsy sample may be assessed semiquantitatively and is a useful guide to the total iron stores in the body (47). Stainable iron is absent or virtually absent in iron deficiency (with or without anemia) and increased in conditions such as idiopathic hemochromatosis or transfusion-induced hemosiderosis. Macrophages contain PAS-positive material and are strongly positive for alpha-naphthyl acetate esterase (Fig. 11B, C) and acid phosphatase. They do not stain for alpha-naphthol AS-D chloroacetate esterase activity (48), and most do not stain with Sudan black. Some macrophages appear to stain positively for alkaline phosphatase activity.

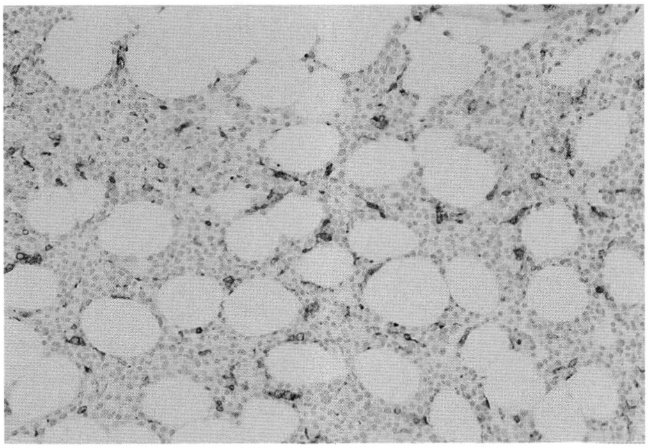

**FIG. 10.** Immunohistochemical demonstration of macrophages in a section of a paraffin-embedded trephine biopsy core from a hematologically normal subject. The section was reacted with the monoclonal antibody PG-M1 (against CD 68) and the reaction visualized using an immunoperoxidase technique.

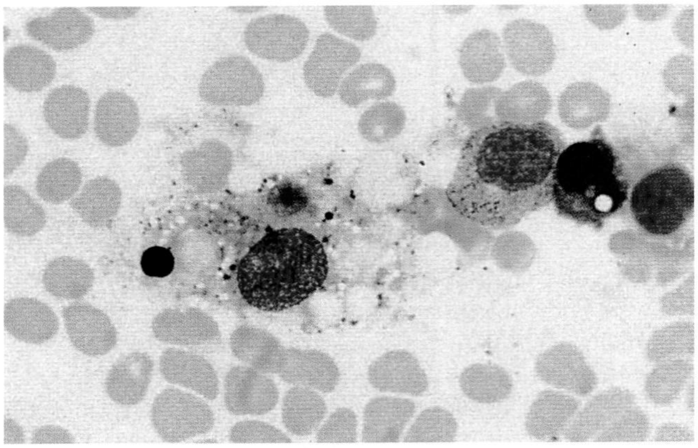
A

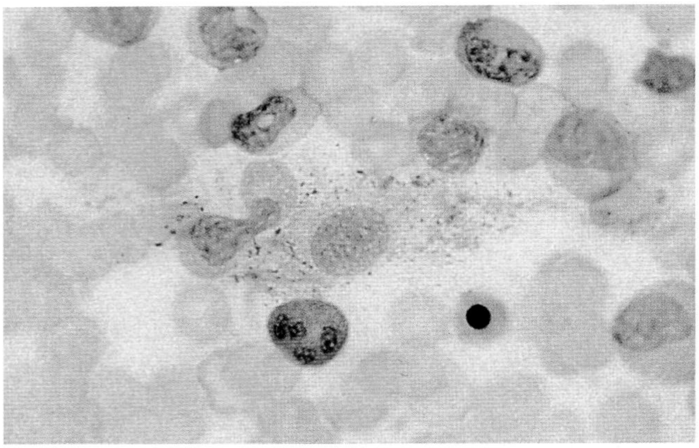
B

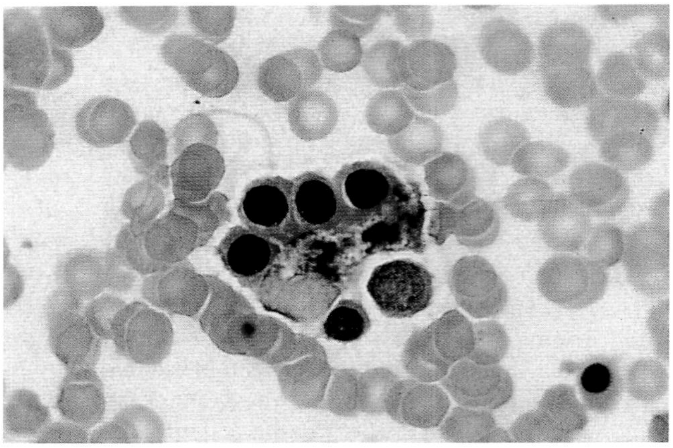
C

**FIG. 11.** Macrophages from normal bone marrow smears. **A:** Macrophage containing a black extruded erythroblast nucleus and several intracytoplasmic inclusions of various shapes, sizes, and staining characteristics. The large pale rounded inclusions may represent degraded red cells (MGG stained). **B:** Macrophage containing several PAS-positive cytoplasmic granules, together with a PAS-negative late erythroblast and several PAS-positive neutrophil myelocytes and granulocytes. **C:** Macrophage showing strong alpha-naphthyl acetate esterase activity, surrounded by six unreactive erythroblasts. The diazonium salt of fast blue BB was used as the capture agent.

Ultrastructural studies of marrow fragments show that macrophages form long cytoplasmic processes at their periphery and that such processes extend for considerable distances between various types of hematopoietic cells (Fig. 14). Some cytoplasmic processes protrude through the endothelial cell layer into the sinusoidal lumen (Fig. 15) and appear to be involved in recognizing and phagocytosing senescent or damaged erythrocytes and granulocytes and circulating microorganisms. The nucleus often has an irregular outline and contains small to moderate quantities of nuclear membrane–associated condensed chromatin. The cytoplasm has many strands of RER, scattered ferritin molecules, a well-developed Golgi apparatus, several mitochondria, a number of small or medium-sized homogeneous electron-

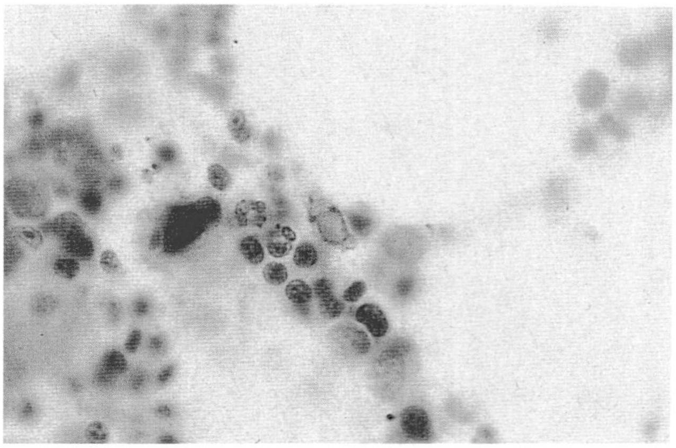

**FIG. 12.** Section of a paraffin-embedded normal marrow fragment (*clot section*). The macrophage in the center shows blue hemosiderin-containing intracytoplasmic granules and a diffuse bluish coloration of the cytoplasm. Perls' acid ferrocyanide reaction.

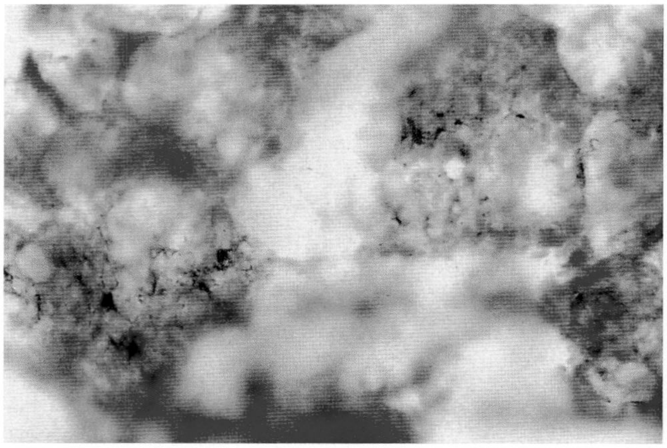

**FIG. 13.** Marrow fragment from a normal marrow smear stained by Perls' acid ferrocyanide reaction. The dark blue granular material represents hemosiderin within macrophages.

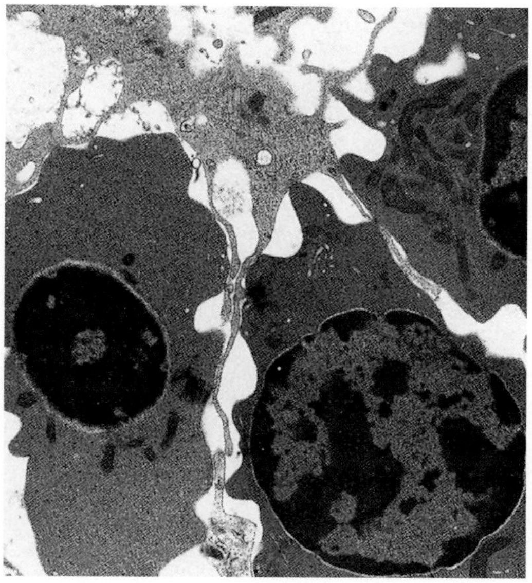

**FIG. 14.** Electron micrograph of three erythroblasts from a normal marrow showing fine processes of macrophage cytoplasm extending between the cells.

dense primary lysosomes of variable shape, and a number of large inclusions. Some of the latter have a complex ultrastructure with both electron-dense and electron-lucent areas and myelin figures and may contain numerous ferritin and hemosiderin molecules; these appear to represent secondary lysosomes with residual material from phagocytosed cells (Fig. 16). Other large inclusions can be recognized readily as granulocytes (Fig. 17), extruded erythroblast nuclei, and erythrocytes at various stages of degradation. A few reticulin fibers may be found in contact with parts of the cell surface.

Macrophages are present within erythroblastic islands (Fig. 11C), plasma cell islands, and lymphoid nodules but also may occur elsewhere in the marrow parenchyma. Some are found immediately adjacent to the endothelial cells of sinusoids, forming part of the adventitial cell layer. Bone marrow macrophages not only function as phagocytic cells but also generate various hematopoietic growth factors (e.g., IL-1 and GM-CSF) and are thus involved in short-range regulation of lymphopoiesis and myelopoiesis. They presumably also are involved in antigen processing.

### *Nonphagocytic Reticular Cells*

In Romanowsky-stained marrow smears, nonphagocytic reticular cells have an irregular or spindle shape and resemble macrophages except that they lack large intracytoplasmic inclusions. Light microscope cytochemical and histochemical data indicate that these cells are PAS negative, strongly positive for alkaline phosphatase, negative for acid phosphatase, negative or only weakly positive for alpha-naphthyl acetate esterase, and negative for stainable iron. Thus, there seems to be some overlap between the cytochemical characteristics of nonphagocytic reticular cells and macrophages (48,49). In the case of mice and rats, however, light and electron microscopic cytochemical data have clearly established the existence of two distinct types of reticular cells in the marrow stroma: (a) fibroblast-like nonphagocytic reticular cells that have cell membrane–associated alkaline phosphatase and no acid phosphatase and (b) macrophage-like phagocytic reticular cells that are positive for acid phosphatase but not for alkaline phosphatase (50).

Electron microscopic studies of nonphagocytic reticular cells in human bone marrow (41,51,52) have shown that, like macrophages, these cells extend branching cytoplasmic processes between hematopoietic cells and are in contact with extracellular reticulin fibers (Fig. 18). However, unlike macrophages, they do not have secondary lysosomes or have only an occasional secondary lysosome. They may contain variable numbers of filaments or a few small fat globules in their cytoplasm. A rare profile contains a cilium. The intracytoplasmic filaments sometime occur in bundles, and the cells are then ultrastructurally indistinguishable from adventitial cells. It is possible that the nonphagocytic reticular cells comprise a number of different cell types including fibroblasts, adventitial cells, and cells whose functions have not yet been defined.

At least some of the nonphagocytic reticular cells are probably not derived from the hematopoietic stem cells but may arise from a cell capable of giving rise to colonies of fibroblast-like cells in vitro. As mentioned earlier, nonphagocytic reticular cells appear to play an important role in the microenvironmental regulation of hematopoiesis, both by binding to primitive hematopoietic cells (53) and by producing certain hematopoietic growth factors both constitutively and in response to stimulation by monokines (54). In mice and presumably also in humans, they synthesize collagen (types I and III) and fibronectin.

### *Mast Cells*

Mast cells tend to be found in association with the periphery of lymphoid follicles and the adventitia of small arteries and adjacent to the endosteal cells of bone trabeculae and the endothelial cells of sinusoids.

It is now known that the hematopoietic stem cells generate morphologically unrecognizable progenitors of mast cells within the bone marrow (55) and that the most mature of these cells enter the blood (56,57). The circulating cells, which still lack mast cell granules, migrate into the tissues where they proliferate and mature into mast cells. It is not yet certain whether mast cells and basophils share a common early progenitor cell (57,58).

Unlike the granules of basophils, which are very water soluble, those of mast cells are much less so. Nevertheless, mast cells are not easily recognized in sections of marrow stained with hematoxylin and eosin. By contrast, they are readily identified in sections stained with the Giemsa stain.

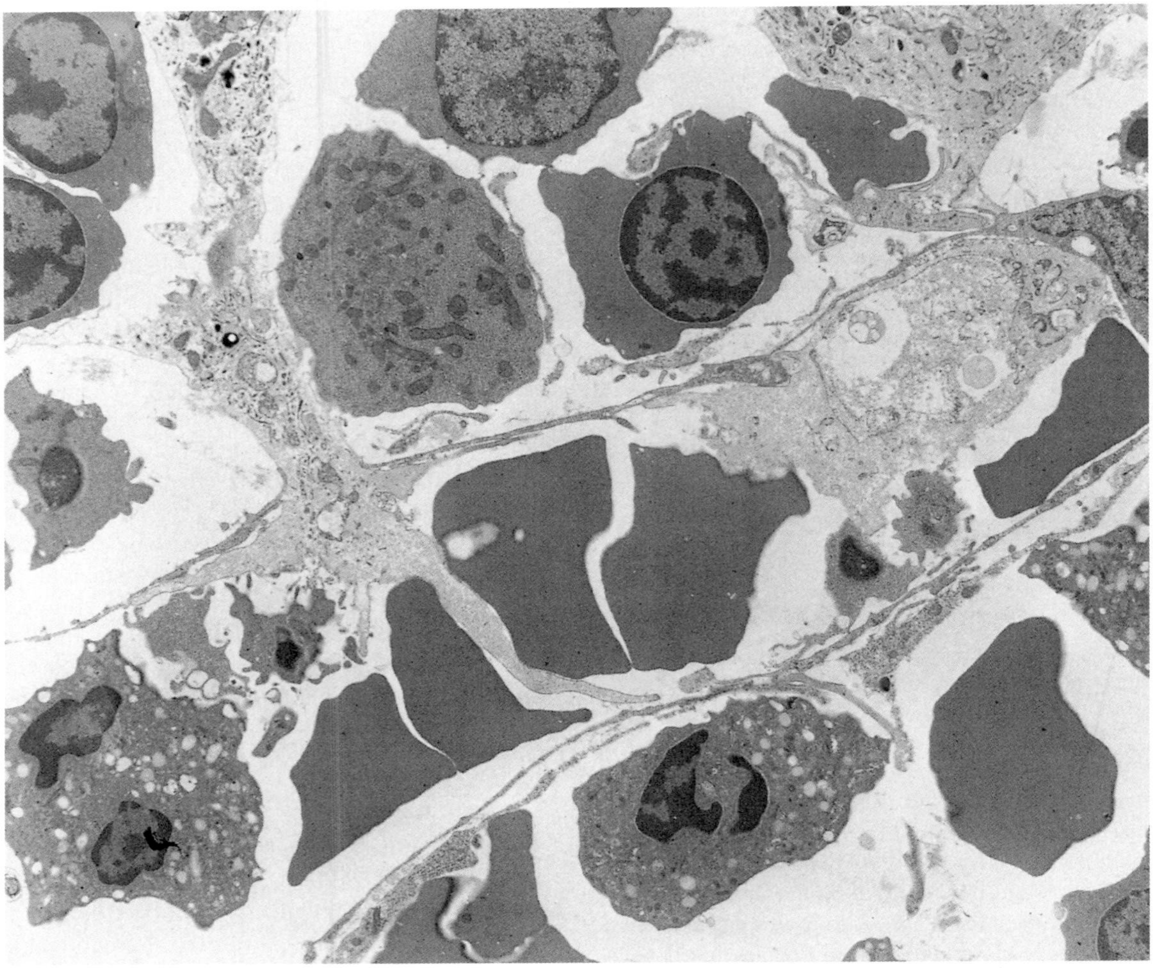

**FIG. 15.** Electron micrograph of a sinusoid from a normal bone marrow. A process of macrophage cytoplasm is seen protruding through the lining endothelial cell into the sinusoidal lumen. Serial sectioning of this sinusoid showed that the mass of macrophage cytoplasm occupying the right-hand side of the sinusoidal lumen connected transendothelially with a second extrasinusoidal cytoplasmic process. Both processes arose from the same macrophage.

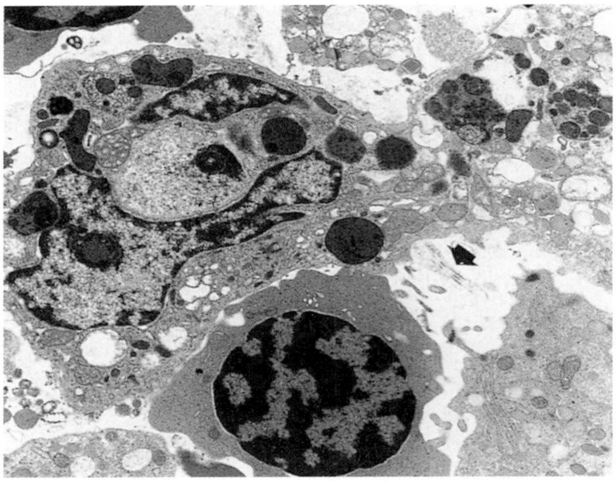

**FIG. 16.** Electron micrograph of a macrophage lying next to an early polychromatic erythroblast in a normal bone marrow. The nucleus of the macrophage is irregular in outline and its cytoplasm contains several inclusions and vacuoles. Some of the inclusions are ultrastructurally complex and probably represent secondary lysosomes. There are some reticulin fibers (*arrow*) near the macrophage.

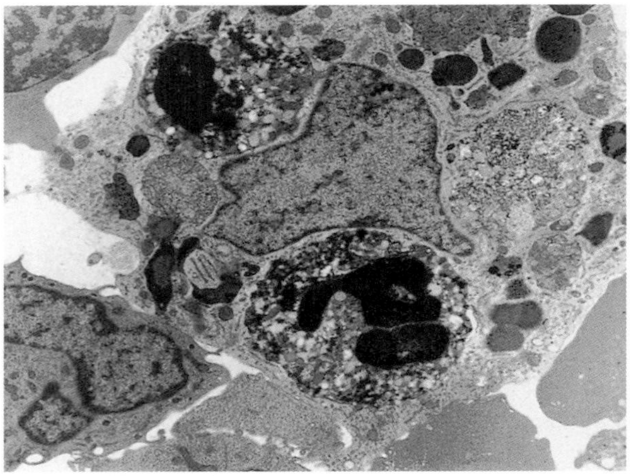

**FIG. 17.** Electron micrograph of a macrophage from normal bone marrow. The cytoplasm contains two phagocytosed neutrophils and a large number of other inclusions of varying size, shape, and appearance.

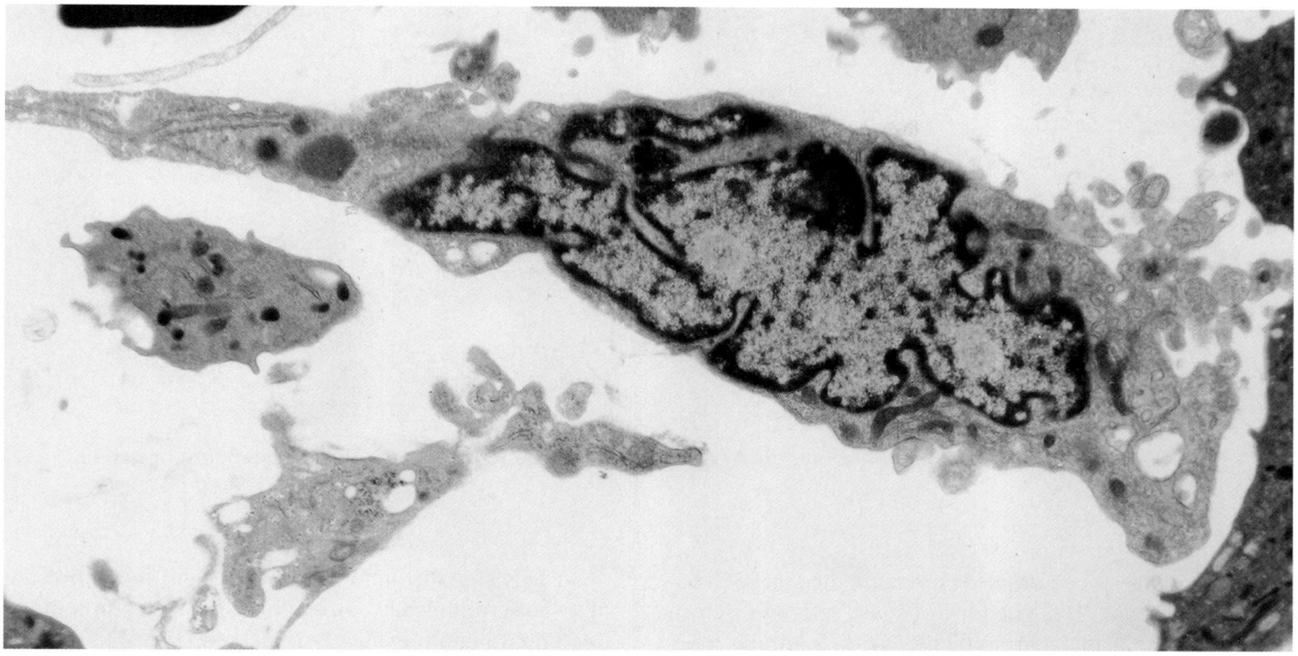

A

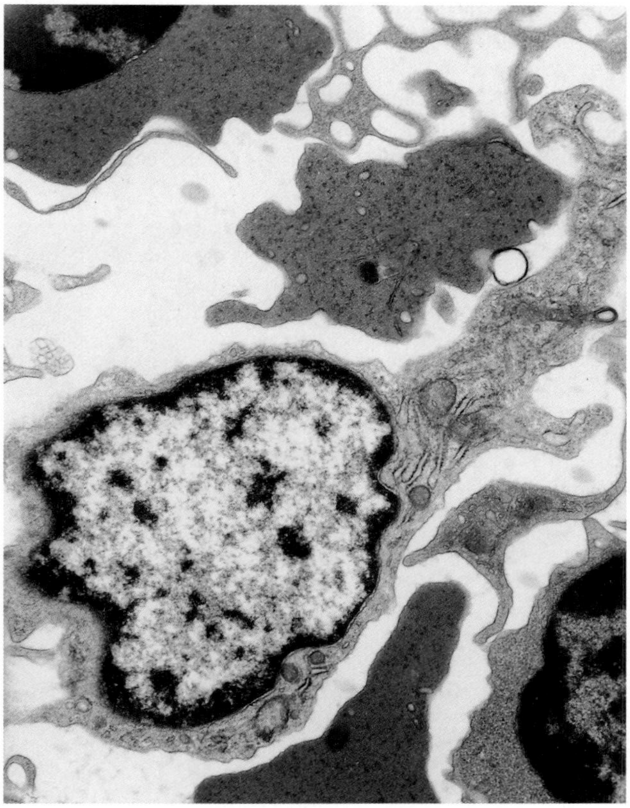

B

**FIG. 18.** Electron micrographs of two nonphagocytic reticular cells from normal bone marrow. The nuclear outline of one of these cells (**A**) shows several deep clefts and that of the other (**B**) is less irregular.

In such sections, mast cells have round, oval, or spindle-shaped outlines and many dark purple cytoplasmic granules. The nucleus is often oval and may be situated eccentrically. Immunochemical staining can be performed using the antibody AA1, which reacts with mast cell tryptase (8) and does not cross-react with basophils. In Romanowsky-stained marrow smears, mast cells vary between 5 and 25 $\mu$m in their long axis and tend to have an ovoid or elongated shape (Fig. 19A, B). The cytoplasm is packed with coarse purple–black to red–purple granules, but unlike in basophil granulocytes, the granules seldom overlie the nucleus. The nucleus is small, round or oval, and either centrally or eccentrically lo-

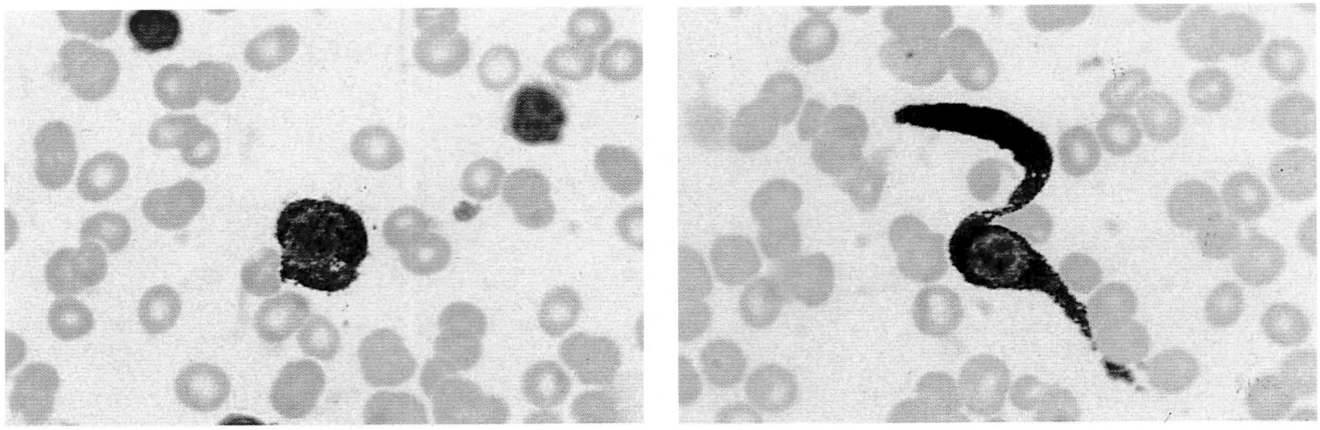


**FIG. 19.** Two mast cells, one rounded (**A**) and one elongated (**B**) from MGG-stained smears of bone marrow.

cated. It contains less condensed chromatin than that of a basophil granulocyte. The granules of mast cells are rich in heparin and stain metachromatically with toluidine blue. Mast cells are also peroxidase negative, PAS positive, acid phosphatase positive, and alpha-naphthol AS-D chloroacetate esterase positive. Unlike basophil granulocytes, mast cells are capable of mitosis.

In the electron microscope, the granules of mast cells vary considerably in appearance. They may be homogeneously electron dense, have areas of increased electron density at their centers, or contain parallel arrangements, whorls, or scrolls of a crystalline or fibrillar structure (Figs. 20 and 21). The nucleus contains moderate quantities of condensed chromatin. In addition to the numerous granules, the cytoplasm contains some mitochondria, a few short strands of endoplasmic reticulum, occasional lipid droplets, and some fibrils.

## Hematopoietic Cells

### *Lymphocytes and Plasma Cells*

Histologic sections of normal marrow show nodules of small lymphocytes that are 0.08 to 1.2 mm in diameter and contain occasional reticular cells (59) (Fig. 22A), as well as much smaller lymphoid aggregates; these nodules and aggregates rarely are found immediately adjacent to trabeculae. About 20% of the lymphoid nodules are irregular in outline, poorly circumscribed, and often contain several fat cells and a few eosinophils between the lymphocytes; they do not contain germinal centers, and their reticulin content is normal for marrow or only slightly increased. The remaining 80% are rounded or oval, well circumscribed, and compact, and they have a follicular structure with blood vessels at their center and some plasma cells and mast cells toward their periphery. Well-developed germinal centers are seen in about 5% of the sections of lymphoid nodules. Lymphocytes extend between surrounding fat cells, and the entire nodule may be surrounded by eosinophils. The reticulin content of a lymphoid nodule is clearly increased (Fig. 22B). Immunohistochemical studies indicate that the lymphocytes within such nodules are of both B and T phenotypes and contain a mixture of $\kappa$ and $\lambda$ light chain–positive B-lymphocytes.

B- and T-lymphocytes and plasma cells also are found unassociated with lymphoid nodules. Lymphocytes are found scattered between hematopoietic cells, and plasma

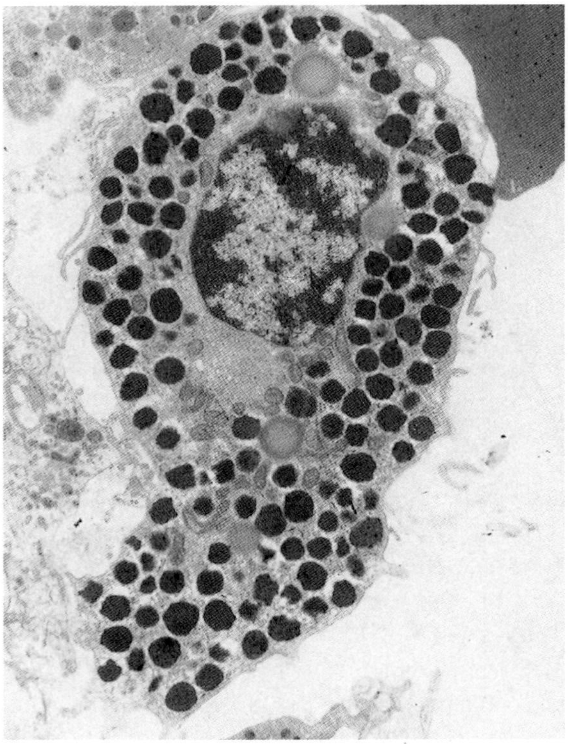

**FIG. 20.** Electron micrograph of a mast cell from normal bone marrow. The cytoplasm is packed with granules and contains four lipid droplets.

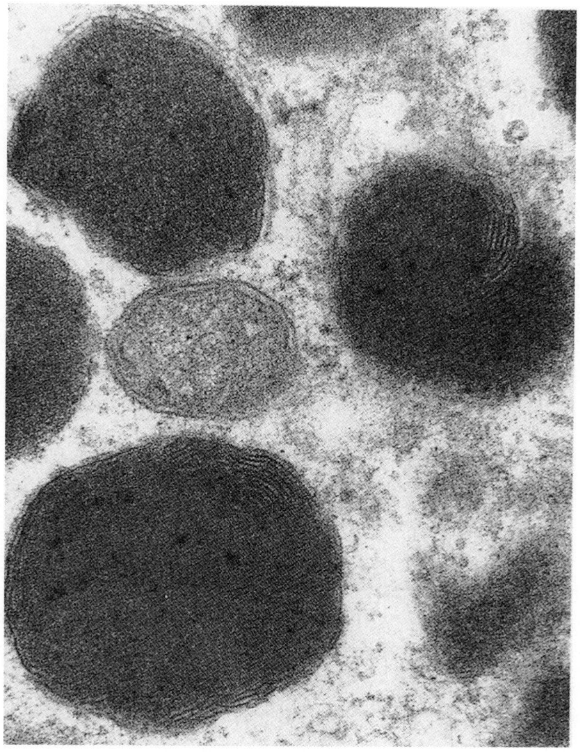

FIG. 21. Granules from a normal mast cell at high magnification showing parallel lamellae.

cells are often present in small groups, surrounding a central macrophage or sheathing some small blood vessels.

### *Precursors of Red Cells, Granulocytes, Monocytes, and Platelets*

The early granulocytopoietic cells (myeloblasts and promyelocytes) mainly are found near the surfaces of bone trabeculae and the adventitial aspects of arterioles. Maturing granulocyte precursors radiate outward from these sites, and the neutrophil granulocytes often are found adjacent to sinusoids. A few promyelocytes and myeloctyes are present singly or in small clusters at sites away from bone trabeculae and blood vessels. The erythroblasts occur in one or two layers surrounding one or two central macrophages; the late erythroblasts and marrow reticulocytes usually are situated next to sinusoids. The megakaryocytes often lie astride sinusoids and protrude cytoplasmic processes into their lumina; these processes discharge platelets directly into the microcirculation.

## HEMATOPOIETIC CELLS: CHARACTERISTICS IN MARROW SMEARS AND ULTRASTRUCTURE

### Neutrophil Precursors

The earliest morphologically recognizable neutrophil precursor is termed the myeloblast. The successive cytologic classes through which myeloblasts mature into circulating neutrophil granulocytes are termed neutrophil promyelocytes, neutrophil myelocytes, neutrophil metamyelocytes, juvenile neutrophils, and marrow neutrophil granulocytes (Figs. 23 and 24). Cell division occurs in myeloblasts, promyelocytes, and myelocytes but not in more mature cells.

A myeloblast is 10 to 20 $\mu$m in diameter. It has a large rounded nucleus with finely dispersed chromatin and two to five nucleoli. The nucleus-to-cytoplasm ratio is moderately high, and the cytoplasm is basophilic and nongranular. It is likely that only some myeloblasts mature into neutrophil promyelocytes and that others mature into eosinophil or basophil promyelocytes.

Neutrophil promyelocytes are larger than myeloblasts and have basophilic cytoplasm containing a few to several purple–red (azurophilic) granules. The nuclear chromatin pat-

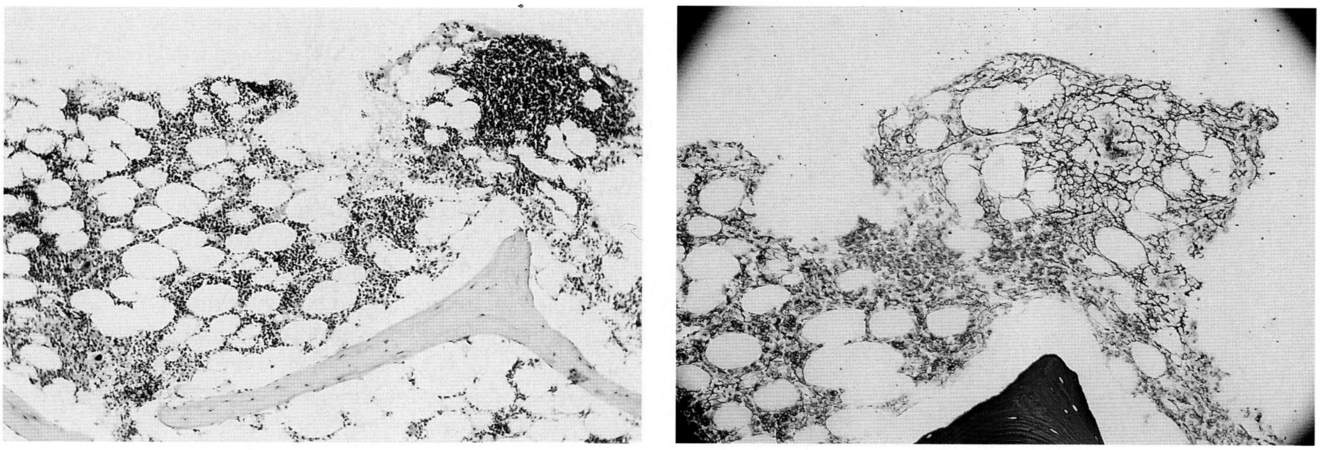


FIG. 22. Lymphoid nodule in a paraffin-embedded trephine biopsy core from a woman without any evidence of a lymphoproliferative disorder. **A:** Section stained with hematoxylin and eosin showing a nodule (*top right*) incorporating fat cells at its periphery. **B:** Parallel section stained by a silver impregnation technique, showing increased reticulin in the nodule (photographed at higher magnification than **A**).

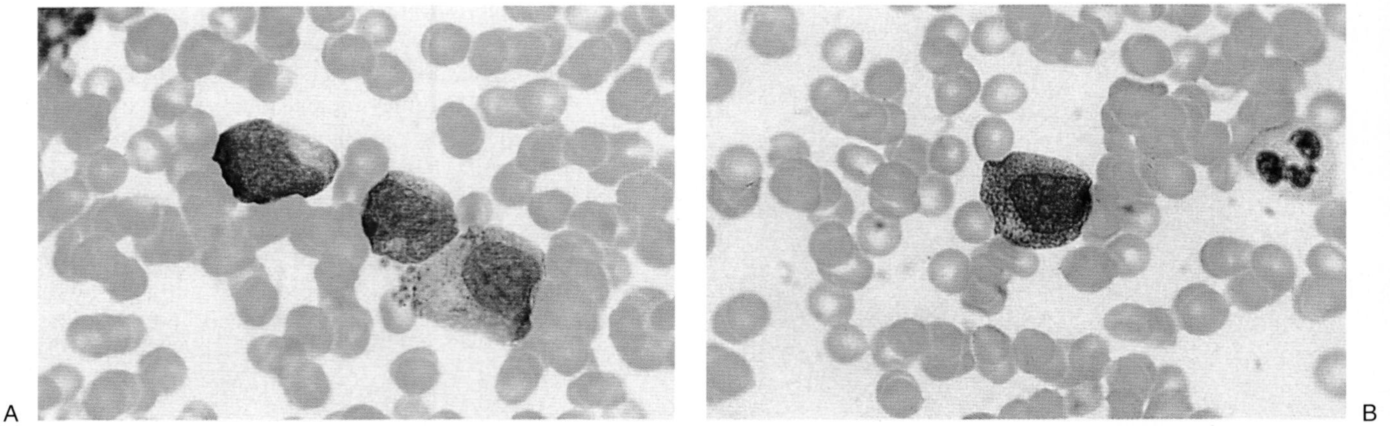

FIG. 23. Neutrophil precursors from an MGG-stained normal marrow smear. A: A myeloblast, an early promyelocyte, and a late promyelocyte/early myelocyte. B: A promyelocyte and a neutrophil granulocyte.

tern is slightly coarser than in myeloblasts, and there may be prominent nucleoli. The neutrophil myelocytes are characterized by the presence in their cytoplasm of many fine light pink (neutrophilic) granules in addition to some azurophilic granules; the neutrophilic granules also are termed *specific granules*. The nucleus is often eccentric and is round, oval, or slightly indented. The nuclear chromatin is coarsely granular, and the nucleoli are indistinct. The cytoplasm occupies a larger fraction of the cell volume than in promyelocytes; it initially appears pale blue but subsequently becomes predominantly pink. The progressive reduction of cytoplasmic basophilia during the maturation of a myeloblast to a mature myelocyte results largely from a reduction of blue-staining cytoplasmic RNA. The neutrophil metamyelocyte has a C-shaped nucleus and an acidophilic cytoplasm containing numerous fine neutrophilic granules. Few or no azurophilic granules are seen. Juvenile neutrophils (also called band or stab forms) have U-shaped or long relatively narrow band-like nuclei that are often twisted into various configurations.

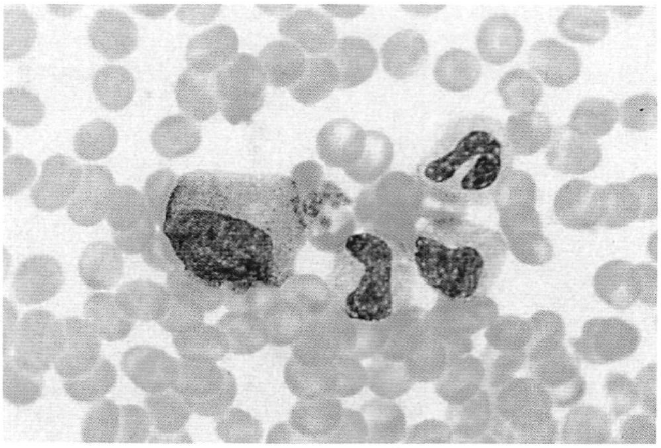

FIG. 24. Two neutrophil myelocytes (one large and one small), a neutrophil metamyelocyte, and a juvenile neutrophil (stab form) from a normal marrow smear.

The nuclei contain large clumps of condensed chromatin and may show one or more partial constrictions along their length. These constrictions become progressively more complete and eventually develop into the fine strands of chromatin that are typical of the segmented nuclei of marrow and blood neutrophil granulocytes. Most neutrophil granulocytes have two to five nuclear segments that are joined together by such strands. Some of the neutrophil granulocytes of females have a drumsticklike nuclear appendage (representing an inactivated X chromosome) attached to one of the nuclear segments.

### *Cytochemistry* (22,60–62)

When stained by the PAS reaction, myeloblast cytoplasm shows a diffuse, pale red–purple tinge, sometimes with fine granules of the same color. Myeloblasts either do not stain with Sudan black or show a few small sudanophilic granules near the nucleus. They are also peroxidase negative and, usually, alpha-naphthol AS-D chloroacetate esterase negative. The cytoplasm of neutrophil promyelocytes and more mature cells of the neutrophil series stain positively with the PAS reagent, with Sudan black, and with reactions for peroxidase and alpha-naphthol AS-D chloroacetate esterase activity. A granular staining pattern is produced with all these cytochemical reactions (Fig. 25). The intensity of staining increases in cell classes of increasing maturity with the PAS reaction and, to a lesser extent, with Sudan black. Promyelocytes and neutrophil myelocytes, but not neutrophil granulocytes, stain for alpha-naphthyl acetate esterase activity and, more weakly, for alpha-naphthyl butyrate esterase activity. Acid phosphatase activity is present in cells at and after the promyelocyte stage; this activity is strongest in the immature cells and weak in neutrophil granulocytes. A few neutrophil metamyelocytes stain weakly for alkaline phosphatase activity, and segmented neutrophil granulocytes

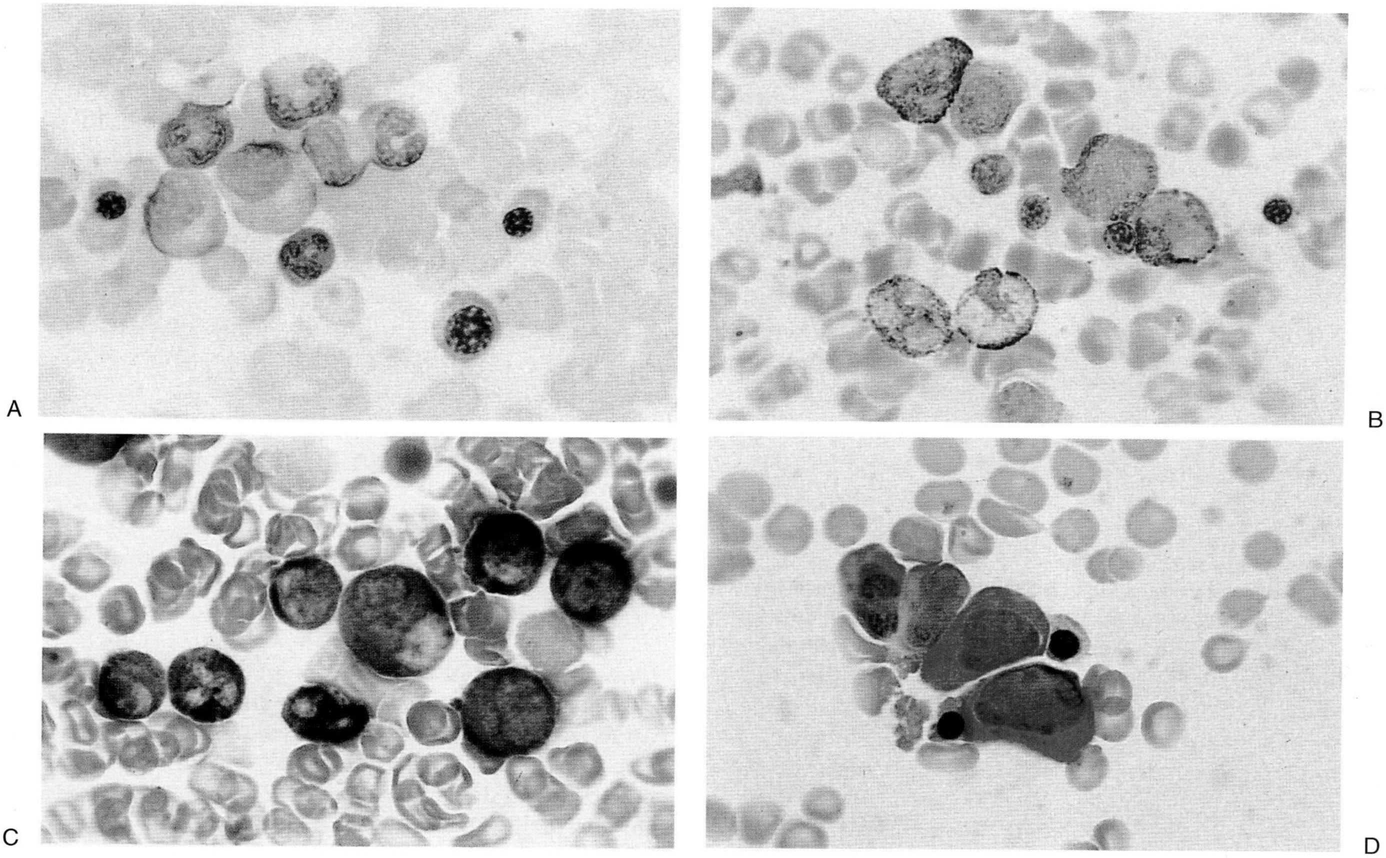

**FIG. 25.** Cytochemical reactions of neutrophil precursors and neutrophil granulocytes. **A:** Faint PAS positivity in neutrophil myelocytes and stronger positivity in neutrophil granulocytes. The three erythroblasts are PAS negative. **B:** Sudan black positivity in two neutrophil myelocytes, one eosinophil myelocyte, a neutrophil metamyelocyte, and a neutrophil granulocyte. The lymphocytes and erythroblasts are sudanophobic. **C:** Strong peroxidase positivity in neutrophil myelocytes and granulocytes. p-Phenylene diamine and catechol were used as the substrate. **D:** Alpha-naphthol AS-D chloroacetate esterase positivity in three neutrophil myelocytes and a neutrophil granulocyte. The two erythroblasts have not stained. The diazonium salt of fast violet-red LB was used as the capture agent.

stain with a variable intensity (weak to strong). Immunocytochemical studies indicate that both lysozyme (muramidase) and elastase are present in promyelocytes and all of the more mature cells of the neutrophil series and that lactoferrin is present in neutrophil myelocytes, metamyelocytes, and granulocytes.

### *Ultrastructure*

Myeloblasts show no special ultrastructural features (63–66). The nucleus has one or more well-developed nucleoli and shows only slight peripheral chromatin condensation. The cytoplasm contains many ribosomes but only a few strands of endoplasmic reticulum and a poorly developed Golgi apparatus. By contrast, the cytoplasm of a promyelocyte is much more complex, being rich in ribosomes, RER, and mitochondria. It also contains a highly developed Golgi apparatus. During the maturation of a promyelocyte to a neutrophil granulocyte, there is a progressive increase in the degree of condensation of nuclear chromatin; a progressive reduction in the quantity of ribosomes, RER, and mitochondria; a diminution of the Golgi apparatus after the myelocyte stage; and the accumulation of large quantities of glycogen at the metamyelocyte and granulocyte stages. The cytoplasm of a promyelocyte characteristically contains a variable number of immature and mature primary granules. Mature primary granules are elliptical, measure 0.5 to 1.0 $\mu$m in their long axis, are electron dense, and contain peroxidase, lysozyme, elastase, $\alpha$1 antitrypsin, and sulphated mucosubstances. Some have a core with a linear periodic substructure. Ultrastructurally different granules, the secondary granules, are found in addition to primary granules at the neutrophil myelocyte stage (Figs. 26 and 27). Secondary granules are larger and less electron dense than primary granules, have rounded outlines, tend to undergo a variable degree of extraction, and are only peroxidase positive if a high concentration of diaminobenzidine is used at alkaline

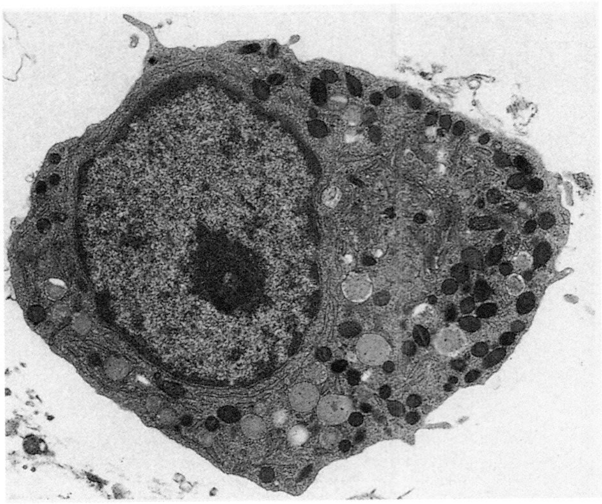

FIG. 26. Electron micrograph of an immature neutrophil myelocyte from normal bone marrow. The nucleus contains a prominent nucleolus and a small quantity of nuclear membrane–associated condensed chromatin. The cytoplasm contains several strands of endoplasmic reticulum, a prominent paranuclear Golgi apparatus, and two ultrastructurally distinct types of granules.

pH. They contain lysozyme and vitamin $B_{12}$ binding protein. Another variety of granule, known as tertiary granules, is present at and after the metamyelocyte stage. These granules are small (0.2 to 0.5 $\mu$m in their long axis), pleomorphic (including rounded, elongated, or dumbbell-shaped forms), and peroxidase negative. Their electron density is usually between that of primary and secondary granules (Fig. 28). Other electron microscopic cytochemical studies have

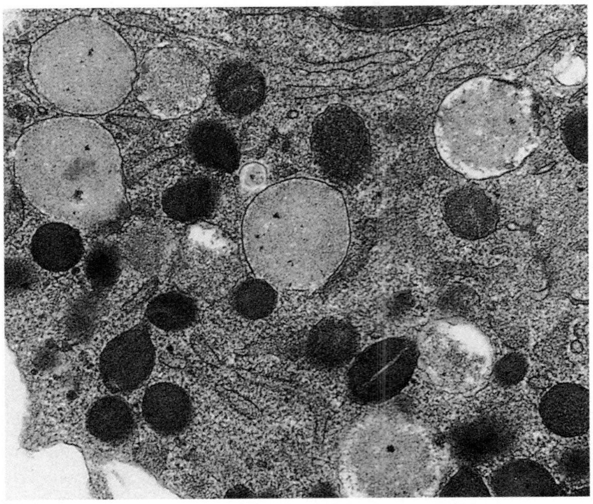

FIG. 27. Part of the cytoplasm of the cell in Fig. 26 at higher magnification. Two types of granules can be clearly recognized. These are (a) rounded or elliptical, very electron-dense primary granules (formed at the promyelocyte stage) and (b) larger, rounded, less electron-dense secondary granules (formed at the myelocyte stage).

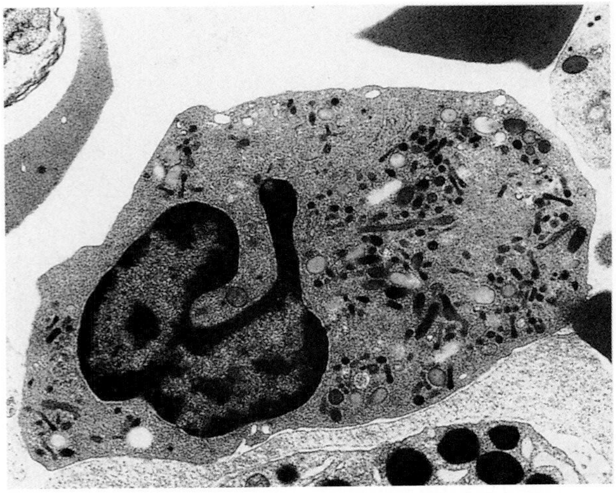

FIG. 28. Electron micrograph of a neutrophil granulocyte from a normal bone marrow. In addition to some primary and secondary granules, the cytoplasm contains several small pleomorphic tertiary granules.

shown that acid phosphatase is present in primary granules but not in secondary or tertiary granules. The above data on the distribution of peroxidase and acid phosphatase suggest that secondary and tertiary granules do not arise from the modification of primary granules but are synthesized de novo at the myelocyte and metamyelocyte stages, respectively (63). Immunoelectron microscopy has demonstrated that lactoferrin is only found in some of the granules at and after the neutrophil myelocyte stage. The alkaline phosphatase activity in neutrophil granulocytes is present within small membrane-bound intracytoplasmic vesicles called phosphosomes.

The primary granules observed with the electron microscope correspond to the azurophilic granules seen in Romanowsky-stained smears, and the secondary and tertiary granules correspond to the neutrophilic or specific granules. Although primary granules are present in all granule-containing cells of the neutrophil series, they lose their azurophilic property and are therefore not detectable by light microscopy at and after the metamyelocyte stage.

### Eosinophil and Basophil Precursors

The eosinophil and basophil granulocytes develop through stages that are essentially similar to those through which the neutrophil granulocytes develop. The earliest morphologically recognizable precursors are cells in which a few eosinophil or basophil granules have formed, that is, the eosinophil promyelocytes and basophil promyelocytes. Eosinophil promyelocytes have rounded nuclei with dispersed chromatin and nucleoli and contain two types of granules: large red–orange (eosinophilic) granules and large bluish granules. Eosinophil myelocytes (Fig. 29), metamyelocytes, and granulocytes have only large eosinophilic gran-

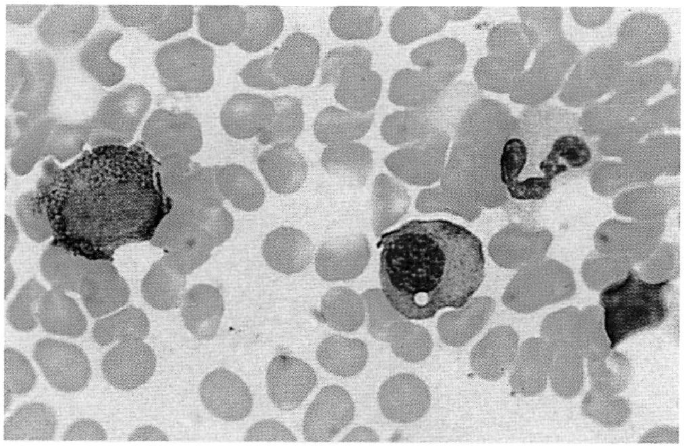

**FIG. 29.** Cells from an MGG-stained normal bone marrow smear. The cell types shown are, from left to right, an eosinophil myelocyte, a plasma cell, a neutrophil granulocyte, and a lymphocyte.

ules. Basophil myelocytes, metamyelocytes, and granulocytes are characterized by the presence of large, round, deeply basophilic granules that often overlie the nucleus (Fig. 30); the more mature granules stain metachromatically with toluidine blue. The majority of circulating eosinophil and basophil granulocytes have two nuclear segments.

### *Cytochemistry*

The granules of eosinophil and basophil granulocytes and their precursors do not stain by the PAS reaction (22,67). However, PAS-positive deposits are found between the specific granules in both cell lineages. The periphery of the eosinophil granules of all cells of the eosinophil series stains strongly with Sudan black, and the core stains weakly or not at all. Basophil granules are strongly sudanophilic in basophil promyelocytes and myelocytes, but the degree of sudanophilia decreases with increasing maturity; in mature basophils, the granules either do not stain or stain metachromatically (reddish). Peroxidase and acid phosphatase but not lysozymes are demonstrable in the eosinophil granules in all eosinophil precursors and eosinophils. Human eosinophil peroxidase is biochemically and immunochemically distinct from myeloperoxidase, the type of peroxidase present in the neutrophil series. In the basophil series, the granules are strongly positive for peroxidase in basophil promyelocytes and myelocytes, weakly positive in basophil metamyelocytes, and almost negative in basophil granulocytes. Basophil granules stain positively for acid phosphatase. Basophil and eosinophil granulocytes are essentially negative for alpha-naphthol AS-D chloroacetate esterase and alpha-naphthyl butyrate esterase.

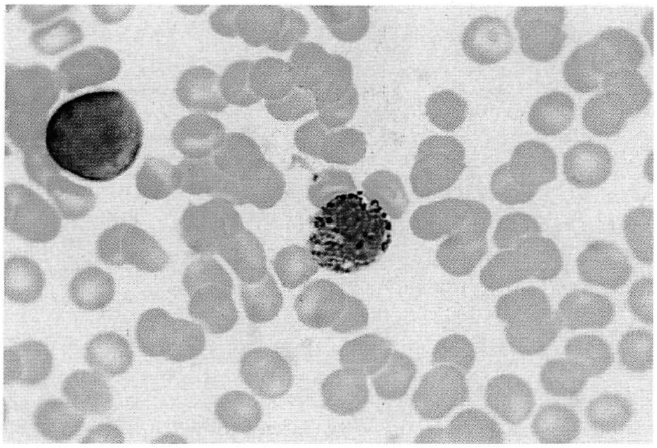

**FIG. 30.** Basophil granulocyte from an MGG-stained normal marrow smear.

Eosinophil granules contain eosinophil cationic proteins and an arginine- and zinc-rich major basic protein that are involved in the killing of metazoan parasites. The major basic protein also stimulates basophils and mast cells to release histamine. Other constituents of eosinophil granules include histaminase and arylsulfatase, which are involved in the modulation of immediate-type hypersensitivity reactions. Basophil granules contain chondroitin sulfate and heparin sulfate, which account for their property of staining metachromatically (red–violet) with toluidine blue. They also contain histamine, one of the substances released when immunoglobulin E (IgE)-coated basophils react with specific antigen.

### *Ultrastructure*

On the basis of their electron microscopic features, two types of eosinophil granules, termed primary and secondary granules, are recognized (63,66,68). Primary granules are large, rounded, homogeneous, and electron dense, and secondary granules contain a central electron-dense crystalloid inclusion consisting largely of polymerized major basic protein. It is generally held that the primary granules mature into secondary granules. Early eosinophil promyelocytes contain only primary granules, but more mature promyelocytes contain many primary and a few secondary granules. Eosinophil myelocytes contain some primary and several secondary granules (Fig. 31). By contrast, the majority of the granules in eosinophil metamyelocytes and granulocytes are secondary granules (Fig. 32). The primary granules of eosinophil promyelocytes are larger and more rounded than the primary granules of neutrophil promyelocytes and promonocytes.

Cells of the basophil series contain characteristic basophil granules, which are prone to undergo varying degrees of extraction during processing for electron microscopy (Fig. 33). Basophil granules are made up of numerous, closely packed, fine rounded particles (Fig. 34); the particles are about 20 nm in diameter in mature basophils and slightly smaller in basophil promyelocytes and myelocytes (58).

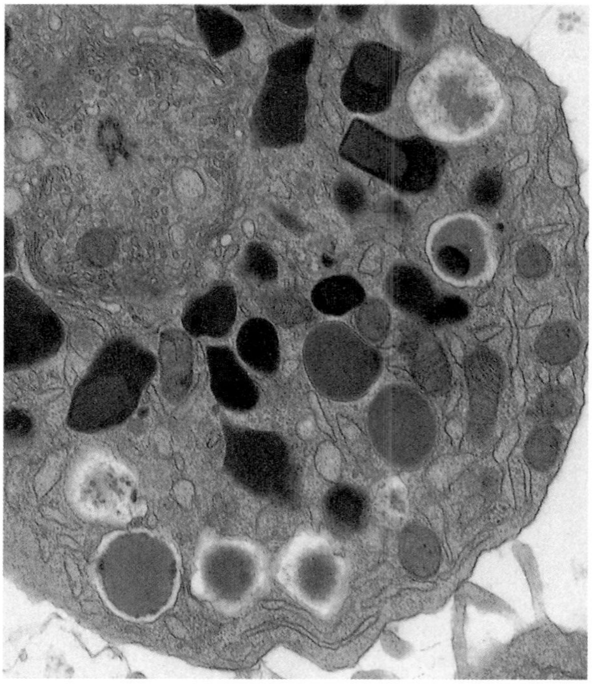

**FIG. 31.** Electron micrograph of part of the cytoplasm of an early eosinophil myelocyte. A centriole surrounded by well-developed Golgi saccules, several strands of rough endoplasmic reticulum, and a number of large granules are seen. Some of the granules are homogeneously electron dense (primary granules) but others have a central crystalloid (secondary granules).

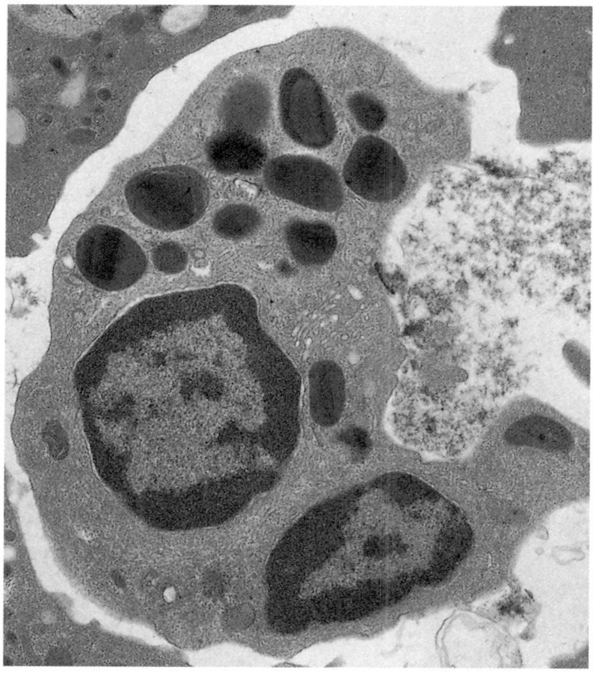

**FIG. 32.** Electron micrograph of an eosinophil granulocyte from normal bone marrow. The majority of the cytoplasmic granules are crystalloid-containing secondary granules. Note that the uppermost granule is unusual in that its crystalloid stains more lightly than the surrounding granule matrix.

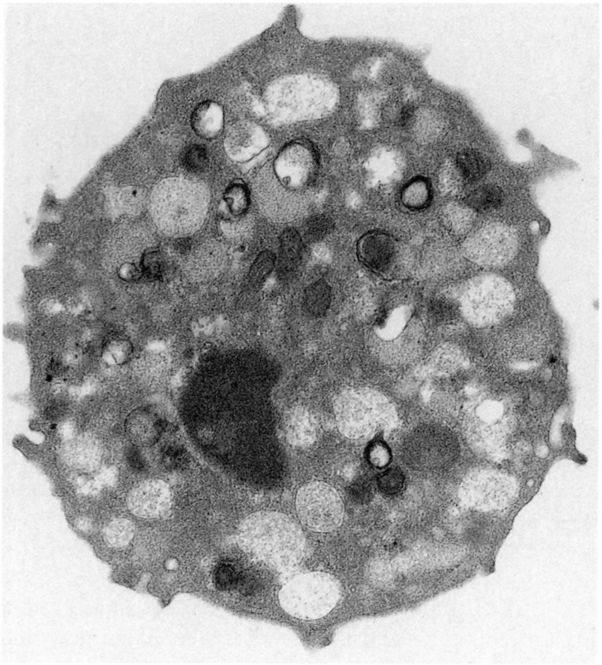

**FIG. 33.** Electron micrograph of a basophil granulocyte from a normal bone marrow. The granules have been markedly extracted during processing, but the characteristic closely packed rounded particles can still be recognized in several of the granules.

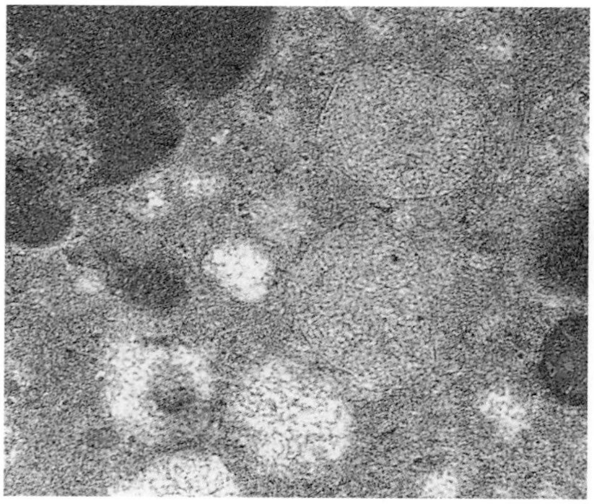

**FIG. 34.** Electron micrograph illustrating the particulate ultrastructure of basophil granules at high magnification.

## Monocyte Precursors

The morphologically recognizable cells belonging to the monocyte series are the monoblasts, promonocytes, marrow monocytes, and blood monocytes. The blood monocytes are not end cells but develop further in the tissues to become macrophages. Certain data suggest that macrophages and osteoclasts have a common progenitor. All these cells are considered to constitute the mononuclear phagocyte system. In this system, cell division occurs mainly in the monoblasts and promonocytes.

Monoblasts are similar in appearance to myeloblasts except that their nuclei may be slightly indented or lobulated. They have small quantities of agranular deeply basophilic cytoplasm and can only be reliably distinguished from other types of blast cells by cytochemical and other special techniques (Fig. 35). Promonocytes are larger, have a lower nucleus-to-cytoplasm ratio, and contain less basophilic cytoplasm than monoblasts; their cytoplasm contains a few azurophilic granules. Promonocytes usually have a large, rounded, cleft or lobulated nucleus with the chromatin appearing as a fine network. Nucleoli may or may not be visible.

Marrow monocytes and blood monocytes have a lower nucleus-to-cytoplasm ratio ($<1$), a less basophilic cytoplasm, and a larger number of azurophilic granules than promonocytes. The cytoplasm is pale gray–blue, has a ground glass appearance, and may contain vacuoles. The nucleus is eccentrically placed and may be oval, kidney shaped, horseshoe shaped, or lobulated; the chromatin has a skeinlike or lacy appearance.

### *Cytochemistry*

Some normal monocytes show several fine or moderately coarse PAS-positive granules and sudanophilic granules and a few peroxidase-positive granules scattered in their cytoplasm (22,62,69). Monocytes do not stain for alkaline phosphatase but stain strongly for acid phosphatase. They contain lysozyme.

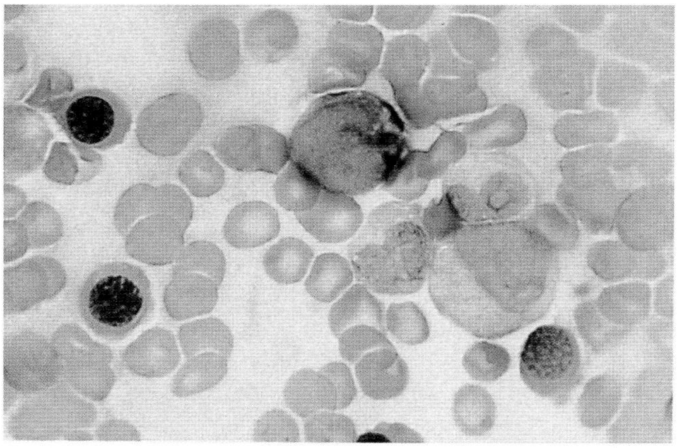

**FIG. 35.** A cell with strong alpha-naphthyl acetate esterase activity from a normal marrow smear (the diazonium salt of fast blue BB was used as the capture agent). This cell has a slightly convoluted nucleus and relatively little cytoplasm and is most probably a monoblast or early promonocyte.

Monocytes are alpha-naphthol AS-D chloroacetate esterase negative but are alpha-naphthyl acetate esterase (nonspecific esterase) positive. Alpha-naphthyl acetate esterase activity is present not only in monocytes and macrophages but also in other myeloid cells, including neutrophil promyelocytes and myelocytes, megakaryocytes, and immature red cell precursors. Alpha-naphthyl butyrate esterase activity is stronger than alpha-naphthyl acetate esterase activity in monocytes and macrophages and is much weaker in the other types of myeloid cells mentioned above. Both the alpha-naphthyl acetate and the alpha-naphthyl butyrate esterase activities of monocytes are inhibited by fluoride; in granulocytes and their precursors, these enzyme activities are fluoride insensitive.

### *Ultrastructure*

The earliest monocyte precursor that can be identified on ultrastructural criteria (63,66) is the promonocyte. The nucleus of this cell has only small quantities of nuclear membrane–associated condensed chromatin and has one or more nucleoli. The cytoplasm contains many ribosomes, a moderate number of mitochondria, several strands of RER, bundles of fibrils, a prominent Golgi apparatus, and a few characteristic cytoplasmic granules. The strands of endoplasmic reticulum are shorter and less abundant than in neutrophil promyelocytes. Two types of cytoplasmic granules are seen in promonocytes: (a) immature granules, which have a central zone of flocculent electron-dense material and a clear peripheral zone, and (b) mature granules, which are smaller than the immature granules, vary considerably in size and shape, and are homogeneously electron dense (Figs. 36 and 37). The maturation of promonocytes first into marrow monocytes and then into blood monocytes is associated with some increase in the quantity of condensed chromatin in the nucleus, a progressive reduction in the number of ribosomes, RER, and fibrils in the cytoplasm, and an increase in the number of cytoplasmic granules. Most or all of the granules of marrow monocytes and all the granules of blood monocytes are of the mature type. Ultrastructural cytochemical studies have shown that some large round granules have acid phosphatase activity and that such granules are more frequent in promonocytes than monocytes. All the promonocyte granules and some of the monocyte granules are peroxidase positive.

## Red Cell Precursors

In this chapter, the term *erythroblast* is used to describe any nucleated red cell precursor, normal or pathologic, and the term *normoblast* to describe all cells that have the mor-

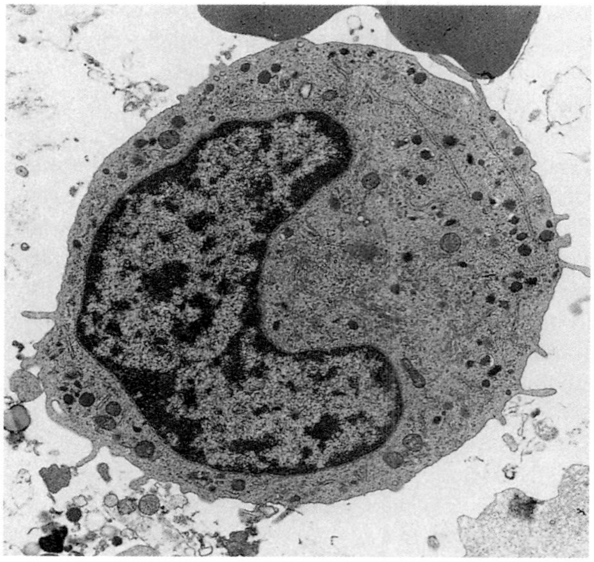

**FIG. 36.** Electron micrograph of an immature monocyte from normal bone marrow. The cytoplasm contains many small mature granules and a few immature granules (see Fig. 37). Several short cytoplasmic processes can be seen at the periphery of the cell.

phologic characteristics of the erythroblasts found in normal bone marrow. The terms used to describe various classes of normal red cell precursor are, in order of increasing maturity, pronormoblast, basophilic normoblast, early polychromatic normoblast, late polychromatic normoblast, marrow reticulocyte, and blood reticulocyte (Fig. 38). Cell division occurs only in the first three of these cytologic classes. Marrow samples containing normoblasts are said to show normoblastic erythropoiesis.

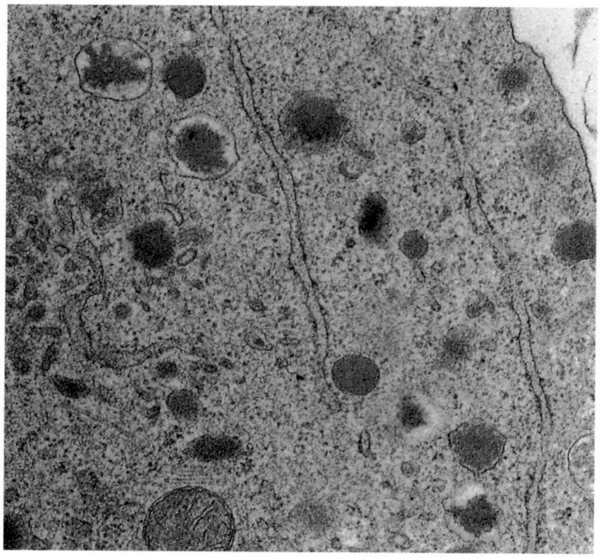

**FIG. 37.** A higher-power view of part of the cytoplasm of the cell in Fig. 36 showing a few immature-looking granules with an electron-dense central zone and an electron-lucent peripheral zone. There are also some small, uniformly electron-dense mature granules.

Pronormoblasts are large cells with a diameter of 12 to 20 μm. They have rounded nuclei and moderate quantities of agranular cytoplasm that stains intensely basophilic except for a pale area (corresponding to the Golgi apparatus) adjacent to the nucleus. The nuclear chromatin has a finely stippled or fine reticular appearance, and there are one or more prominent nucleoli. The basophilic normoblasts resemble pronormoblasts except that their nuclear chromatin is slightly more condensed and consequently has a coarsely granular appearance. The early polychromatic normoblasts are smaller than basophilic normoblasts and have a smaller nucleus and a lower nucleus-to-cytoplasm ratio. The cytoplasm is polychromatic and agranular, and the nucleus contains several medium-sized clumps of condensed chromatin, particularly adjacent to the nuclear membrane. The polychromasia results from the presence of moderate quantities of cytoplasmic RNA, which stains blue, as well as of hemoglobin, which stains red. Late polychromatic normoblasts are even smaller and show a further reduction in the ratio of the area of the nucleus to the area of the cytoplasm. The cytoplasm is predominantly orthochromatic but still has a grayish tinge (i.e., is faintly polychromatic). The nucleus is small and eccentric and contains large clumps of condensed chromatin. The nuclear diameter is less than about 6.5 μm. When mature, late polychromatic normoblasts extrude their nuclei and become marrow reticulocytes; the extruded nuclei are rapidly phagocytosed and degraded by adjacent macrophages. The marrow reticulocyte is irregular in outline and has faintly polychromatic cytoplasm. It is motile and soon enters the marrow sinusoids. When marrow and blood reticulocytes are stained supravitally with brilliant cresyl blue, the ribosomal RNA responsible for their polychromasia precipitates into a basophilic reticulum (hence the term reticulocyte). Reticulocytes circulate in the blood for 1 to 2 days before becoming mature red cells. The average volume of blood reticulocytes is 20% larger than that of red cells. The latter are circular, biconcave, and acidophilic (i.e., stain red) and in dried, fixed smears have an average diameter of 7.2 μm (range 6.7–7.7 μm).

### *Cytochemistry*

Normal erythroblasts are PAS negative. They also fail to stain with Sudan black and are peroxidase negative. Most nucleated red cells are alpha-naphthol AS-D chloroacetate esterase negative, but occasional cells show a few positive granules. A few alpha-naphthol butyrate esterase–positive granules are seen in some nucleated red cells of all degrees of maturity; the positive granules are sometimes seen at the nuclear margin. Coarse acid phosphatase–positive paranuclear granules are frequently present in all types of erythroblasts.

In normal bone marrow smears stained by Perls' acid ferrocyanide method, 20% to 90% of the polychromatic erythroblasts contain one to five small blue–black granules

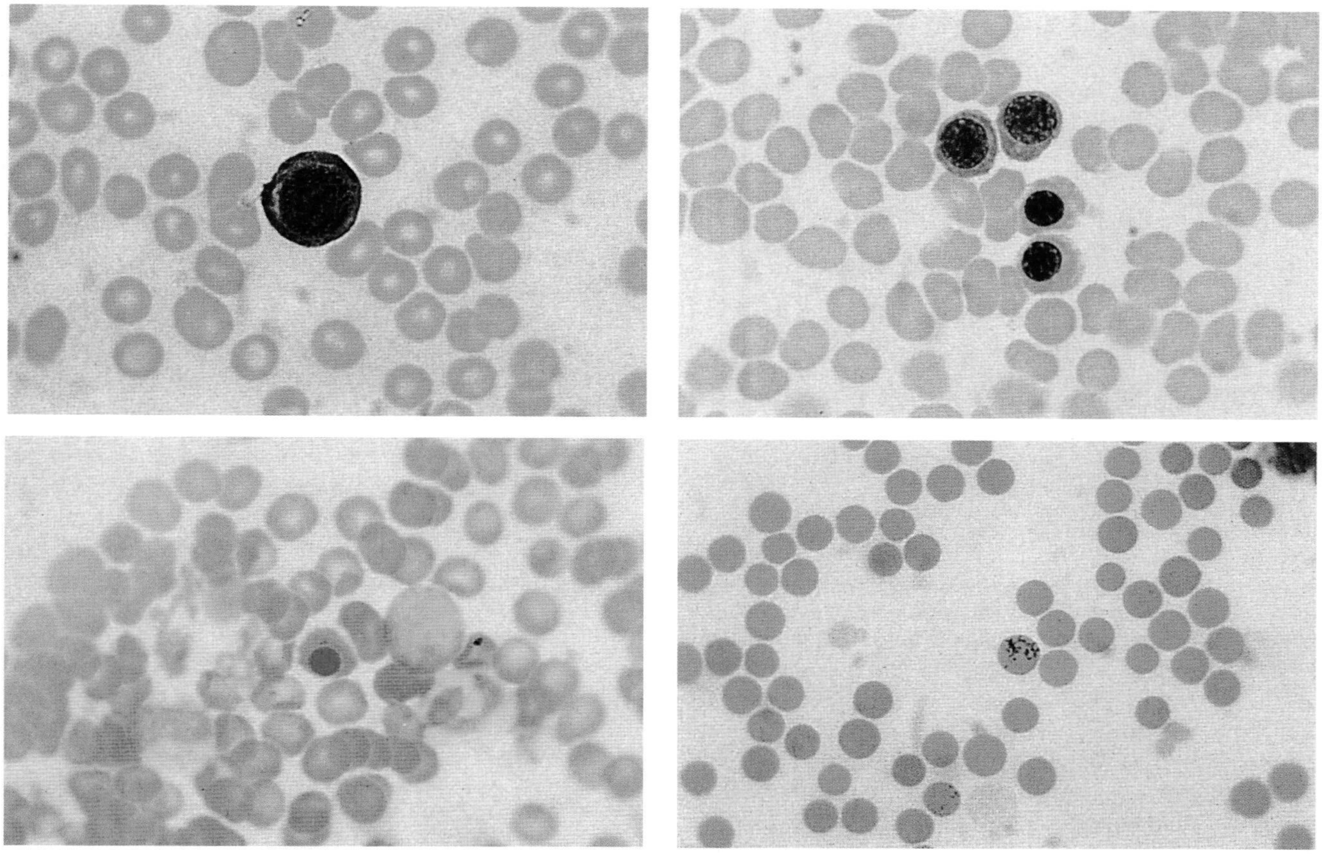


**FIG. 38.** Red cell precursors from a normal bone marrow smear (**A–C**) and a reticulocyte from normal peripheral blood (**D**). **A:** Pronormoblast. **B:** Two early polychromatic normoblasts and two late polychromatic normoblasts. **C:** A sideroblast showing a fine, barely visible blue siderotic granule. (A) and (B) MGG stain; (C) Perls' acid ferrocyanide reaction; (D) supravital staining with brilliant cresyl blue.

that are usually just visible at high magnification (Fig. 38C). These iron-containing (siderotic) granules are randomly distributed within the cytoplasm and correspond to the siderosomes seen under the electron microscope. Erythroblasts containing siderotic granules are termed *sideroblasts.* In iron deficiency anemia and, to a lesser extent, in the anemia of chronic disorders, the percentage of sideroblasts is decreased. In conditions associated with an increased percentage saturation of transferrin (e.g., hemolytic anemias), the average number of siderotic granules per cell and the average size of such granules are increased.

### *Ultrastructure*

All nucleated red cell precursors are characterized by the presence of small surface invaginations that develop into intracytoplasmic vesicles (rhopheocytotic vesicles) (63,66) (Fig. 39). The nucleus of the pronormoblast has a small quantity of nuclear membrane–associated condensed chromatin (Fig. 40). The cytoplasm is of low-electron density and contains numerous ribosomes, a moderately well-developed Golgi apparatus, several mitochondria, some strands of endoplasmic reticulum, and small numbers of scattered fer-

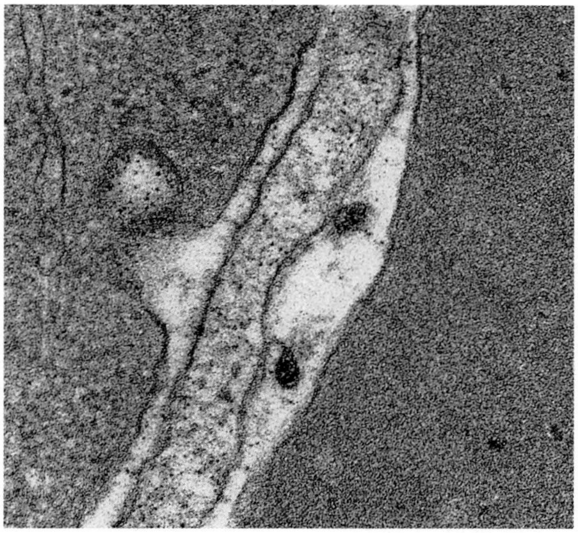

**FIG. 39.** Part of an early polychromatic erythroblast showing a rhopheocytotic surface invagination with a few adherent ferritin molecules. A rhopheocytotic vesicle containing several ferritin molecules is closely apposed to the surface invagination. A narrow process of ferritin-containing macrophage cytoplasm is present between the erythroblast displaying rhopheocytosis and the adjacent cell.

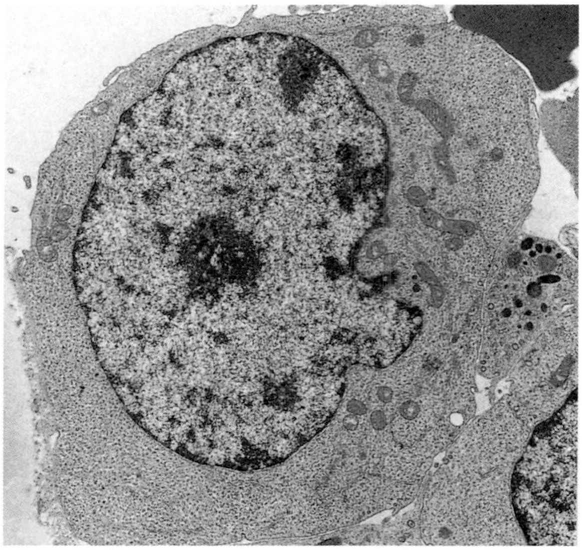

FIG. 40. Electron micrograph of a pronormoblast from normal bone marrow. The nucleus contains very small quantities of condensed chromatin and has a prominent nucleolus. The cytoplasm is relatively electron lucent and rich in polyribosomes.

ritin molecules. It also contains a few pleomorphic electron-dense acid phosphatase–positive lysosomal granules, which are usually arranged in a group near the Golgi saccules. During the maturation of a pronormoblast into a late polychromatic normoblast (Fig. 41), the following changes are seen: (a) a steady increase in the quantity of condensed chromatin, (b) a gradual increase in the electron density of the cytoplasmic matrix due to the synthesis of increasing quantities of hemoglobin, (c) a progressive reduction in the number of ribosomes in the cytoplasm, (d) a reduction in the number and size of the mitochondria, and (e) an increasing tendency for some of the intracytoplasmic ferritin molecules to aggregate and form siderosomes (Figs. 42 and 43). Small autophagic vacuoles are found in 22% and slight to substantial degrees of myelinization of the nuclear membrane in 12% of erythroblast profiles (70). Other data shown by electron microscopic studies of the erythron are (a) that part of the cell's cytoplasmic membrane and a narrow rim of hemoglobin-containing cytoplasm completely surrounds the extruded erythroblast nucleus (Fig. 44), (b) that the marrow reticulocytes enter the sinusoids by passing through, rather than between, endothelial cells (Fig. 45), and (c) that whereas reticulocytes contain ribosomes and mitochondria, mature red cells do not.

### *Dyserythropoiesis and Ineffective Erythropoiesis*

Most of the erythroblasts in normal bone marrow are uninucleate and do not display any unusual morphologic features. However, when 400 to 1,000 consecutive erythroblasts (excluding mitoses) were studied in bone marrow smears from each of 10 healthy volunteers with stainable iron in the bone marrow, 0% to 0.57% (mean 0.31%) were found to be binucleate, 0.7% to 4.8% (mean 2.4%) showed intererythroblastic cytoplasmic bridges, 0% to 0.9% (mean 0.24%) showed cytoplasmic stippling, and 0% to 0.7% (mean 0.39%) showed cytoplasmic vacuolation. In addition, 0% to 0.55% (mean 0.22%) had markedly irregular nuclear outlines or karyorrhectic nuclei, and 0% to 0.39% (mean 0.18%) contained Howell-Jolly bodies (micronuclei), a marker of chromosome breaks (71) (Fig. 46). In another study of 15 healthy males in which 5,000 erythroid cells (including mitoses) were assessed per subject, 0.14% ± 0.04% (SD) were found to be binucleate or multinucleate cells or to be pluripolar mitoses (72). A number of other unusual morphologic features are seen in some erythroblast profiles when the marrow is examined with the electron microscope. These include short stretches (250–910 nm) of duplication of the nuclear membrane in 2% of the profiles, short (260–520 nm) intranuclear clefts in 1.7%, and iron-laden mitochondria in less than 0.2% (70). The above-mentioned light and electron microscopic features are sometimes described as dyserythropoietic changes, with the implication that they are morphologic manifestations of a minor disturbance of proliferation or maturation in the affected cells. In many congenital or acquired disorders characterized by grossly disordered erythropoiesis, the proportion of erythroblasts showing these dyserythropoietic changes is increased, and some erythro-

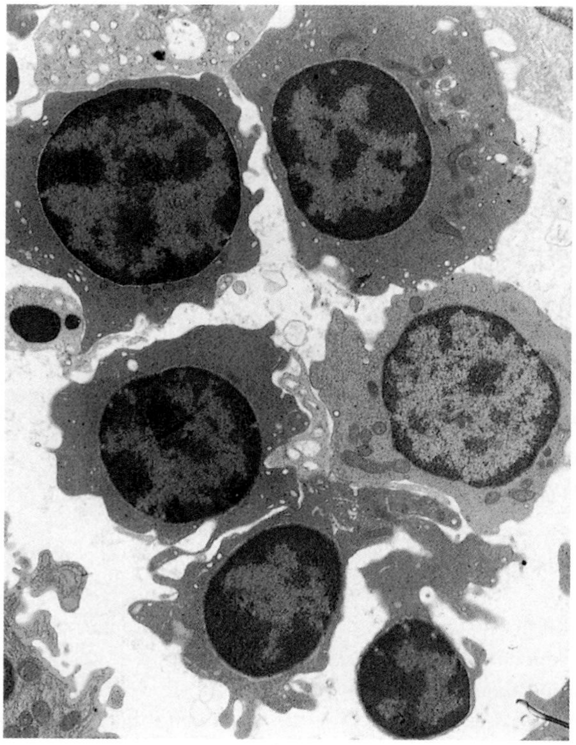

FIG. 41. Electron micrograph of a group of six erythroblasts at various stages of maturation. Note that maturation is associated with an increase in the electron density of the cytoplasm. The lowermost cell is a late erythroblast about to extrude its nucleus.

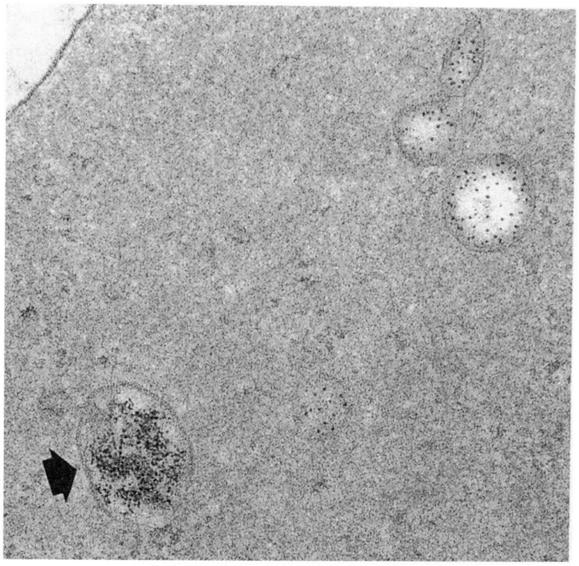

**FIG. 42.** Electron micrograph of part of the cytoplasm of a polychromatic erythroblast from normal bone marrow. The cytoplasm shows a membrane-bound accumulation of ferritin and hemosiderin (siderosome) (*arrow*) and a few ferritin-containing rhopheocytotic vesicles.

blasts show various dyserythropoietic changes not seen in normal marrow (36). The latter include nonspecific abnormalities such as large autophagic vacuoles and extensive intranuclear clefts, as well as abnormalities that are specific for certain diseases or groups of diseases.

The phrase ineffective erythropoiesis is used to describe the loss of potential erythrocytes due to the destruction of developing erythroblasts within the bone marrow. The extent of ineffective erythropoiesis in normal bone marrow is small (23). However, there is a significant ineffectiveness in hemoglobin production during normal erythropoiesis because some hemoglobin is lost around each extruded erythroblast nucleus. In a number of conditions such as homozygous beta-thalassemia and the megaloblastic anemias, there is a gross increase in the ineffectiveness of erythropoiesis. In such conditions, erythroblasts at various stages of

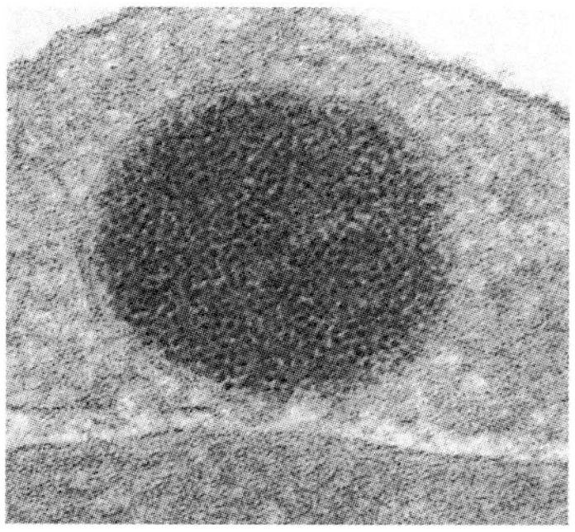

**FIG. 43.** Part of a polychromatic erythroblast from a normal marrow showing a membrane-bound siderosome that is much more densely packed with ferritin and hemosiderin molecules than the siderosome in Fig. 42.

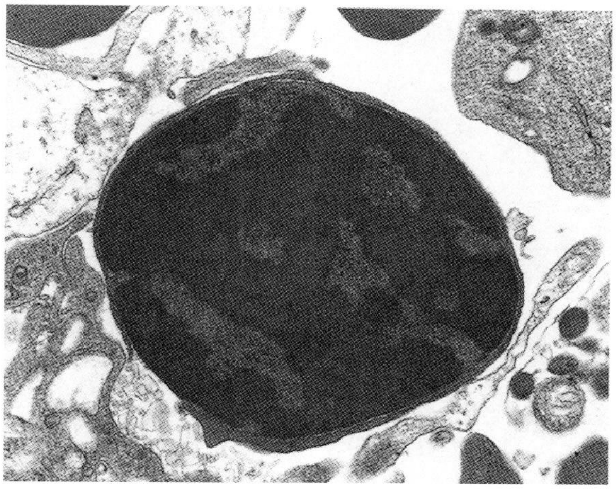

**FIG. 44.** Electron micrograph of an extruded erythroblast nucleus. Note that the nucleus is surrounded by a rim of hemoglobin-containing cytoplasm and lies in close contact with processes of macrophage cytoplasm.

degradation may be recognized within marrow macrophages both by light and electron microscopy.

### Megakaryocytes

The majority of the cells of the megakaryocyte series are larger than other hematopoietic cells and have polyploid DNA contents. The earliest morphologically recognizable cells in this series are called megakaryoblasts. These are 20

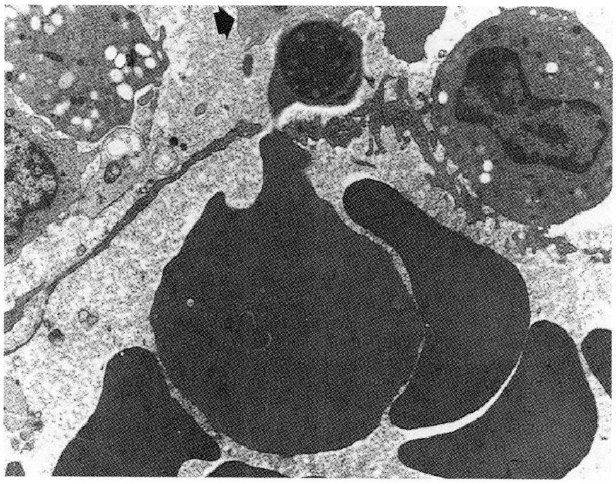

**FIG. 45.** Electron micrograph illustrating an uncommon mechanism of formation of a reticulocyte. Whereas nuclear expulsion often occurs extravascularly and the resulting reticulocytes then enter a sinusoid, the cytoplasm of the late erythroblast shown has passed through the endothelial cell of the sinusoid before nuclear expulsion. The nucleus of this erythroblast has not passed through the narrow passage in the endothelial cell and presumably will be severed from the rest of the cell and phagocytosed by the macrophage (*arrow*) lying in contact with it. Thus, in this erythroblast, nuclear expulsion appears to occur during entry of the future reticulocyte into the sinusoid.

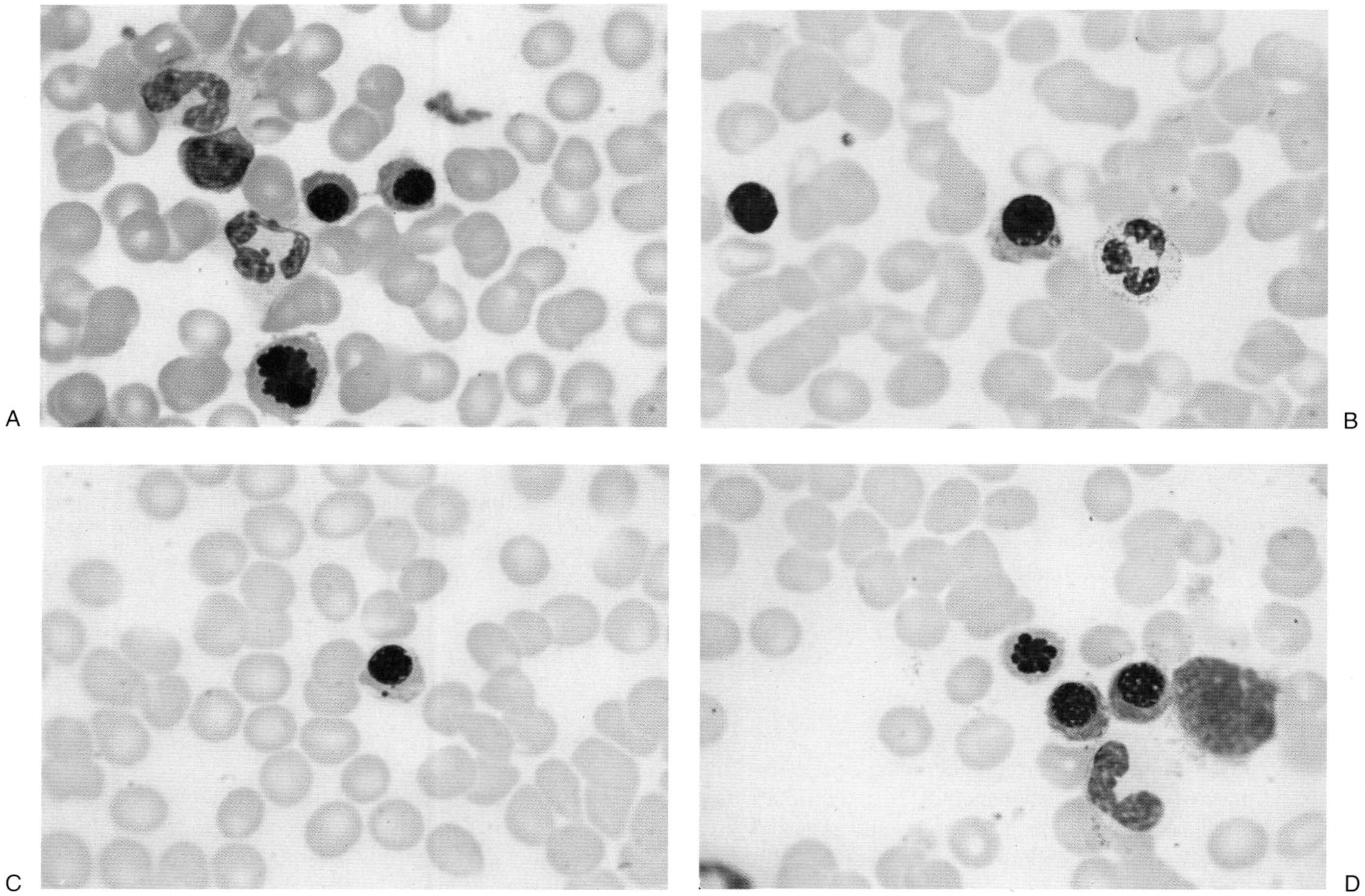

**FIG. 46.** Morphologic evidence of dyserythropoiesis in bone marrow smears from healthy volunteers. **A:** Intererythroblastic cytoplasmic bridge. **B:** Large Howell-Jolly body in an early polychromatic erythroblast. **C:** Two smaller Howell-Jolly bodies in a late polychromatic erythroblast. **D:** Karyorrhexis in a late polychromatic erythroblast.

to 30 $\mu$m in diameter and have a single large, oval, kidney-shaped, or lobed nucleus that is surrounded by a narrow rim of intensely basophilic agranular cytoplasm. The nucleus contains several nucleoli. Megakaryoblasts (group I megakaryocytes) mature into promegakaryocytes (group II megakaryocytes), which in turn develop into granular megakaryocytes (group III megakaryocytes). Promegakaryocytes are larger than megakaryoblasts and have a larger volume of cytoplasm relative to that of the nucleus. They possess a single large multilobed nucleus with the overlapping lobes arranged in a C-shaped formation. The cytoplasm is less basophilic than that of megakaryoblasts and contains a few azurophilic granules that are usually grouped within the concavity formed by the overlapping nuclear lobes. The granular megakaryocytes (Fig. 47) are up to 100 $\mu$m in diameter and have abundant pale-staining cytoplasm containing many azurophilic granules. The nucleus has multiple lobes, and these become fairly tightly packed together before the shedding of platelets. The nuclear chromatin has a coarse-grained appearance. Platelets are formed by the fragmentation of cytoplasmic processes of the mature granular megakaryocytes. When platelet formation is completed, a bare nucleus remains.

Mature platelets are usually 2 to 3 $\mu$m in diameter and are irregular in outline. The cytoplasm stains pale blue and has a number of azurophilic granules at its center. Newly formed platelets are slightly larger than mature ones.

About 40% of megakaryoblasts, 20% of promegakaryocytes, and 2% of granular megakaryocytes synthesize DNA (73). However, cell division is probably uncommon in megakaryoblasts and is not seen in the other two cell types. The occurrence of cycles of DNA replication without cytokinesis results in the characteristic polyploidy of these cells. The total DNA contents of megakaryoblasts range between 4c and 32c and of promegakaryocytes and granular megakaryocytes between 8c and 64c (1c = the haploid DNA content). There is a positive correlation between the nuclear area and DNA content of megakaryocytes.

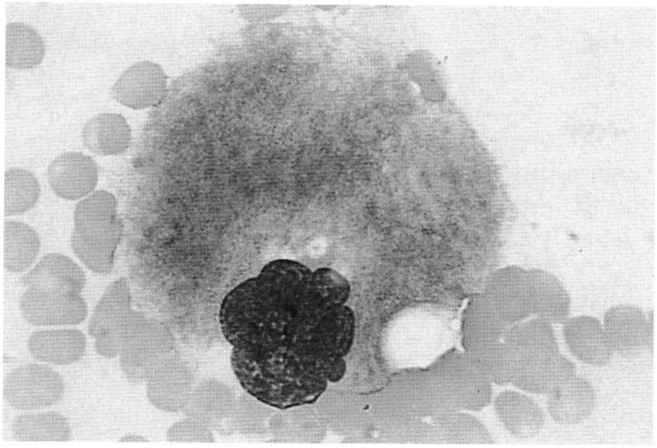

**FIG. 47.** Granular megakaryocyte from an MGG-stained normal bone marrow smear.

### *Cytochemistry*

When stained by the PAS reaction, megakaryocytes show a diffuse and finely granular positivity over both the nucleus and the perinuclear and intermediate zones of the cytoplasm (22,60–62). These positive areas also contain varying numbers of densely positive blocks (Fig. 48). A narrow peripheral zone of the cytoplasm is often PAS negative, and this may be surrounded by clumps of positive granules within attached platelets. PAS-positive material within platelets appears as scattered, lightly staining fine granules at the periphery and as clumps of darkly staining coarse granules at the center. Megakaryocytes and platelets are usually unstained by Sudan black, but occasional megakaryocytes may show a diffuse positivity with fine positive granules scattered both in the cytoplasm and over the nucleus. Megakaryocytes and platelets display strong acid phosphatase activity.

Peroxidase activity cannot be demonstrated in megakaryocytes by light microscopy but can be demonstrated in a characteristic distribution using the electron microscope.

Megakaryocytes show no alpha-naphthol AS-D chloroacetate esterase activity. However, they have substantial alpha-naphthyl acetate esterase activity (Fig. 49) and weaker alpha-naphthyl butyrate esterase activity; the latter generates many coarse or fine positive granules in the cytoplasm and over the nucleus.

### *Ultrastructure*

The nucleus of a megakaryoblast has two or more lobes, very little condensed chromatin, and prominent nucleoli (63,66,74,75). The cytoplasm contains large numbers of ribosomes, scattered RER, several mitochondria, and a few membrane-lined vesicles representing the beginning of the demarcation membrane system (DMS). The cytoplasm also contains a well-developed Golgi apparatus within a deep nuclear indentation. A few immature alpha granules and a few lysosomal vesicles containing acid phosphatase and arylsulfatase are present near the Golgi apparatus. The maturation of megakaryoblasts into promegakaryocytes and granular megakaryocytes (Fig. 50) is accompanied by a progressive increase in the quantity of nuclear membrane–associated condensed chromatin, an increase in the number of alpha granules, a progressive development of the DMS, and a reduction in the number of ribosomes, RER, and mitochondria. Megakaryocyte maturation also is accompanied by the formation of increasing quantities of glycogen in the cytoplasm; the glycogen particles often are found in large clumps. The DMS is an extensive system of membrane-lined cytoplasmic sacs, which arises as invaginations of the surface membrane; it demarcates areas of cytoplasm that eventually become platelets (Fig. 51).

Three zones can be recognized in the extensive cytoplasm of a granular megakaryocyte (Fig. 50): (a) a narrow perinuclear zone containing the Golgi apparatus, and some of the

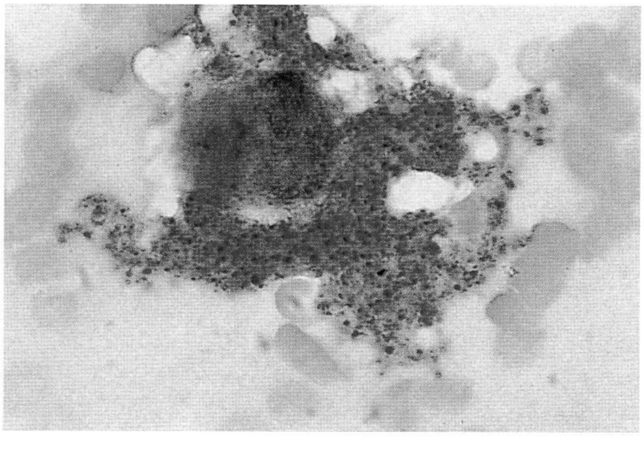

**FIG. 48.** Megakaryocyte from a normal bone marrow smear showing large quantities of PAS-positive material.

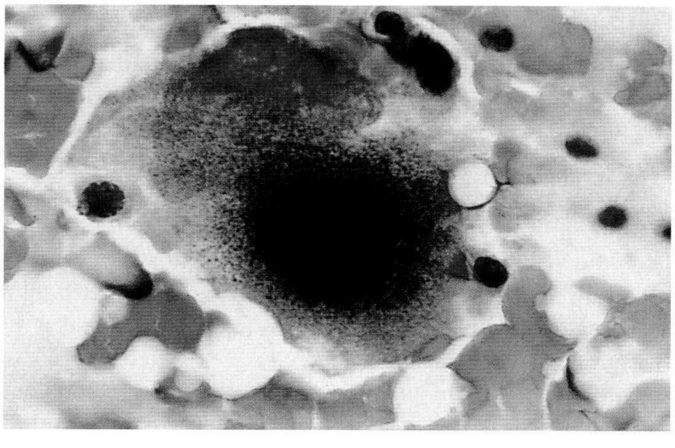

**FIG. 49.** Strong alpha-naphthyl acetate esterase activity in a normal megakaryocyte.

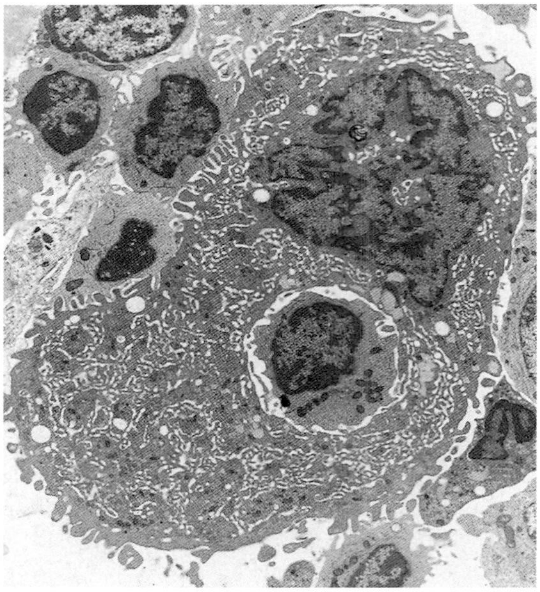

**FIG. 50.** Electron micrograph of a granular megakaryocyte from normal bone marrow. The cytoplasm contains a lymphocyte that appears to be traveling through the megakaryocyte (emperipolesis).

ribosomes, RER, and mitochondria, (b) a wide intermediate zone containing many ovoid, electron-dense alpha granules, numerous sacs of the DMS, lysosomal vesicles, ribosomes, RER, and mitochondria, and (c) a narrow outer zone that is devoid of organelles. Mature granular megakaryocytes protrude cytoplasmic processes that lie near to or within marrow sinusoids. Platelets are formed by the fragmentation of these processes, the platelet membranes being made up of membranes of the DMS.

Ultrastructural cytochemical studies of the oxidation of 3,3′-diaminobenzidine have demonstrated a platelet peroxidase (PPO) in the endoplasmic reticulum and perinuclear space but not in the Golgi apparatus of megakaryoblasts and megakaryocytes and in the dense bodies and dense tubular system of platelets (76). A few small rounded cells present in normal marrow also have PPO activity in the endoplasmic reticulum and perinuclear space and have been identified as promegakaryoblasts (77). PPO appears to be distinct from myeloperoxidase.

Some normal megakaryocytes display the phenomenon of emperipolesis (78,79). This term is used to describe the movement of one cell type within the cytoplasm of another. The cytoplasm of an affected megakaryocyte may contain one or more cells of a number of types, including neutrophil and eosinophil granulocytes and their precursors, and lymphocytes, erythroblasts, and red cells (Fig. 50). The physiologic relevance of megakaryocyte emperipolesis is uncertain; one suggestion has been that certain marrow cells may enter the circulation via the processes of megakaryocyte cytoplasm that protrude into marrow sinusoids.

Nonactivated platelets are biconvex and have a smooth surface. Their shape is maintained by an equatorial bundle of microtubules situated below the cell membrane as well as by microfilaments found between various organelles. Other structures found in the cytoplasm include various types of granules, mitochondria, a surface-connected canalicular system, the dense tubular system, and many glycogen particles, which may occur singly or in clumps (Fig. 52).

Four types of cytoplasmic granule are recognized, namely, the alpha granules, lambda granules (lysosomal granules), delta granules, and peroxisomes (66,80,81). The alpha and lambda granules are moderately electron dense and can be distinguished from each other only by ultrastructural cytochemistry; for example, lambda granules have acid phosphatase activity and alpha granules do not. Substances present in alpha granules include beta-thromboglobulin, platelet factor 4, platelet-derived growth factor, fibrinogen, fibronectin, von Willebrand factor, and thrombospondin. In addition to acid phosphatase, the lambda granules contain $\beta$-glucuronidase and arylsulfatase. The delta granules (dense granules) are smaller and much more electron dense than alpha granules and often have a peripheral electron-lucent zone, which gives them a bull's-eye appearance. They contain serotonin, calcium, and the storage pool of ADP and ATP. The peroxisomes are smaller than the alpha and lambda granules; they are moderately electron dense and contain catalase.

The surface-connected canalicular system is an extensive system of electron-lucent intracytoplasmic canaliculi and

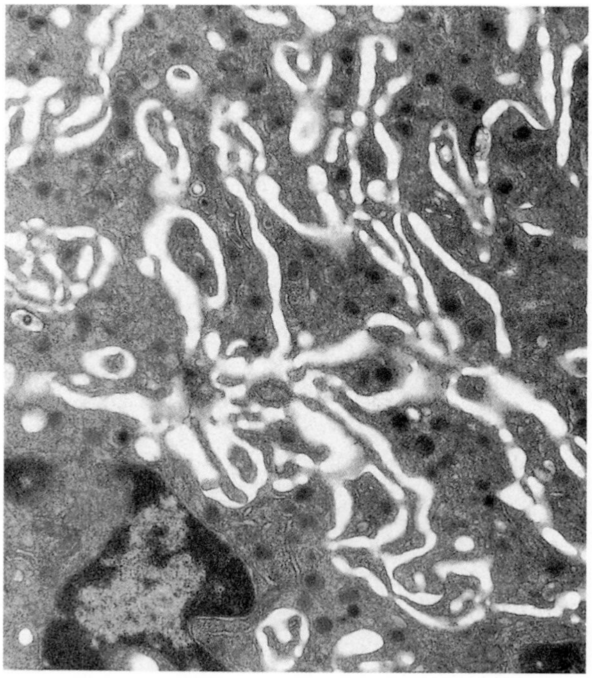

**FIG. 51.** Electron micrograph of a part of the intermediate zone of the cytoplasm of a granular megakaryocyte, showing the extensive demarcation membrane system, demarcating granule–containing future platelet areas.

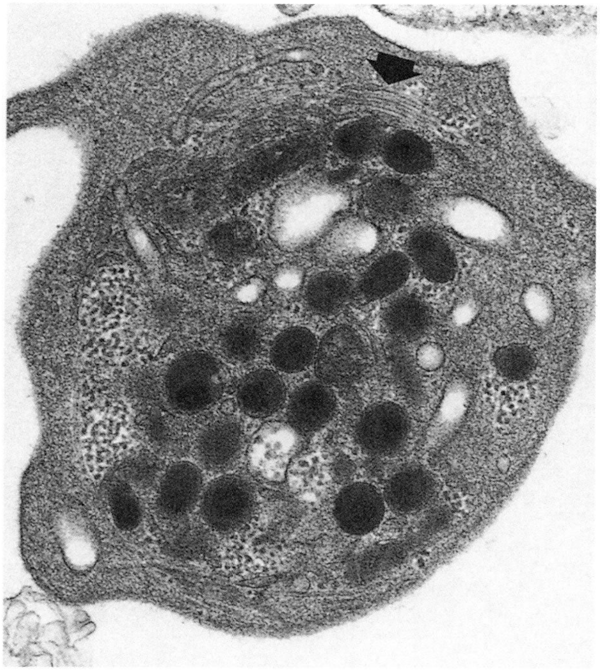

**FIG. 52.** Electron micrograph of a platelet from normal blood. The platelet has been sectioned near, rather than at, the equatorial plane and, consequently, shows only part of the circumferential band of microtubules (*arrow*). The section also shows the electron-lucent vesicles of the surface-connected canalicular system, several platelet granules, a few mitochondria, and numerous clumps of glycogen molecules.

saccules that open to the exterior at multiple sites on the cell membrane. This canalicular system provides a large surface through which various substances, including granule contents, could be discharged extracellularly. The channels of the dense tubular system are shorter and narrower than those of the surface-connected canalicular system and contain material with an electron density similar to that of the cytoplasm. The dense tubular system contains platelet peroxidase and seems to be derived from the endoplasmic reticulum of megakaryocytes. It is an important site of synthesis of thromboxane $A_2$, which is involved in the release of granule contents. It is also rich in calcium and may regulate various calcium-dependent reversible reactions such as the activation of actomyosin and the polymerization of tubulin.

## Lymphocytes and Plasma Cells

All lymphocytes are eventually derived from the lymphoid stem cells present in the marrow, which are in turn derived from the pluripotent hematopoietic stem cells. The lymphoid stem cells generate both B-cell progenitors and T-cell progenitors. The former mature through a number of antigen-independent intermediate stages into B cells; this maturation occurs within the microenvironment of the marrow. The newly formed B cells travel via the blood into the B-cell zones of peripheral lymphoid tissue. Either the lymphoid stem cells or early T-cell progenitors migrate from the marrow through the blood into the thymus. Here, these cells undergo antigen-independent maturation into T cells, and those T cells that recognize self are deleted. The mature T cells then travel through the blood into the T-cell zones of the peripheral lymphoid organs. The mature B- and T-lymphocytes that enter the peripheral lymphoid tissue are triggered into division when they react with specific antigen in the presence of appropriate accessory cells. Their progeny develop into effector cells or memory cells. In the case of B cells, the effector cell is an antibody-secreting plasma cell. Some antigen-dependent proliferation of B cells does occur in the normal marrow and results in the presence of plasma cells in this tissue.

Flow cytometric studies of cells stained with various monoclonal antibodies have shown that an average of 10% of lymphocytes in trephine biopsy cores are B cells and 22% are T cells (82). Between 40% and 80% have neither B-cell nor T-cell markers; these presumably include T- and B-cell precursors, lymphoid progenitor cells, and stem cells. The light and electron microscopic appearances of bone marrow lymphocytes are indistinguishable from those of other lymphocytes in the body. Some T- and B-lymphocytes have fine or coarse PAS-positive granules arranged in one to four (usually one or two) rings around the nucleus, and occasional cells have large clumps of PAS-positive material. Lymphocytes are peroxidase negative and alpha-naphthol AS-D chloroacetate esterase negative, and over 99% of cells are alkaline phosphatase negative. Some lymphocytes show a positive paranuclear dot when stained for alpha-naphthyl butyrate esterase; this staining is unaffected by fluoride. A substantial proportion of normal lymphocytes show either a paranuclear dot or diffuse granular positivity when stained for acid phosphatase. A paranuclear dot is found in both T cells and B cells but more frequently in T cells.

### *Plasma Cells*

Plasma cells seen in smears of normal bone marrow vary considerably in size and appearance. Most are 14 to 20 $\mu$m in diameter and have deep blue cytoplasm. The cytoplasm has a pale paranuclear area corresponding to the Golgi apparatus and may contain one or more vacuoles (Fig. 53A, B). The nucleus is small relative to the volume of cytoplasm, contains moderate quantities of condensed chromatin, and is eccentrically located. Although most plasma cells are uninucleate, a few are binucleate or multinucleate. Some normal plasma cells have other features. For example, occasional cells may contain one or a few large rounded acidophilic, PAS-positive cytoplasmic inclusions (Russell bodies) or several smaller slightly basophilic rounded inclusions (Mott cells, grape cells, or morular cells). Some plasma cells have many pleomorphic cytoplasmic inclusions and, consequently, appear reticulated (Fig. 53C). Others have

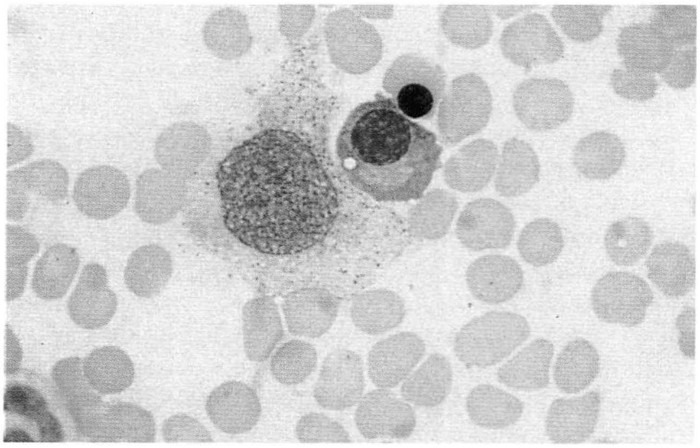

A

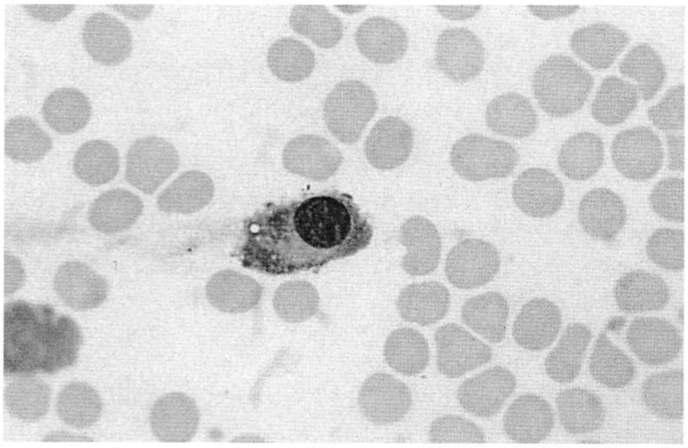

B

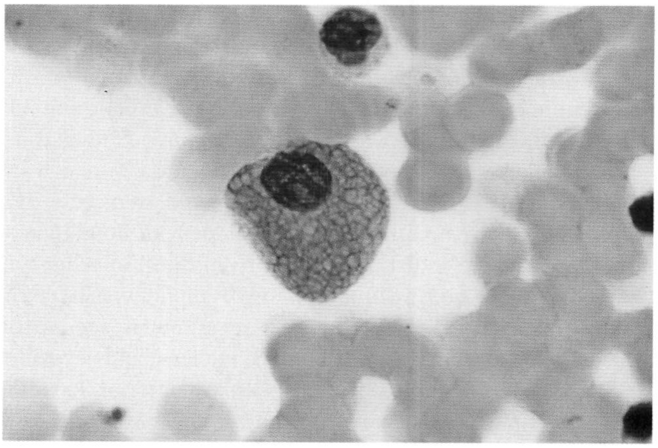

C

**FIG. 53.** Various appearances of plasma cells in a smear of normal bone marrow. A prominent pale paranuclear zone and cytoplasmic vacuoles are seen in (**A**) and (**B**). The cytoplasm in (**C**) has a reticular appearance. The other cells in (A) are a nonphagocytic reticular cell and a late polychromatic erythroblast.

eosinophilic cytoplasm, usually at the periphery, but sometimes in the entire cell (flaming cell); when the eosinophilia is confined to the periphery, it contrasts markedly with the intense basophilia of the rest of the cytoplasm. Occasional plasma cells have azurophilic rods that resemble Auer rods present in acute myeloid leukemia but that are PAS, Sudan black, and peroxidase negative. Plasma cells show strong acid phosphatase activity, particularly around the nucleus and over the Golgi zone. They do not stain for alpha-naphthol AS-D chloroacetate esterase.

The electron microscope shows that the eccentric rounded nucleus of a plasma cell contains a variable quantity of condensed chromatin (Figs. 54 and 55A) and a well-developed nucleolus (Fig. 55A). The presence of moderately large clumps of nuclear membrane–associated condensed chromatin gives the nuclei of mature plasma cells a cartwheel or clock face appearance in histologic sections (but not in marrow smears). The cytoplasm contains numerous long flattened sacs of RER that are arranged either parallel to each other (Fig. 56), concentrically, or spirally; the sacs are distended to varying extents with a granular, moderately electron-dense material, consisting mostly of immunoglobulin. The cytoplasm also contains mitochondria, a large Golgi apparatus situated immediately adjacent to the nuclear membrane (Fig. 54), and a few small or medium-sized membrane-bound electron-dense granules. The latter are often found near the Golgi complex, contain acid phosphatase, and appear to be primary lysosomes. Occasional cells contain larger cytoplasmic inclusions that vary markedly in size, electron density, and shape and are often lined by RER.

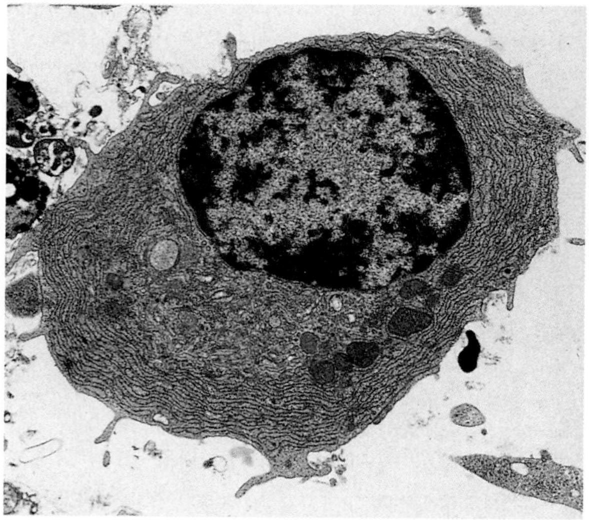

**FIG. 54.** Electron micrograph of a plasma cell from a normal bone marrow showing numerous parallel sacs of rough endoplasmic reticulum and a very prominent Golgi apparatus immediately adjacent to the nucleus. The nucleus has moderate quantities of condensed chromatin.

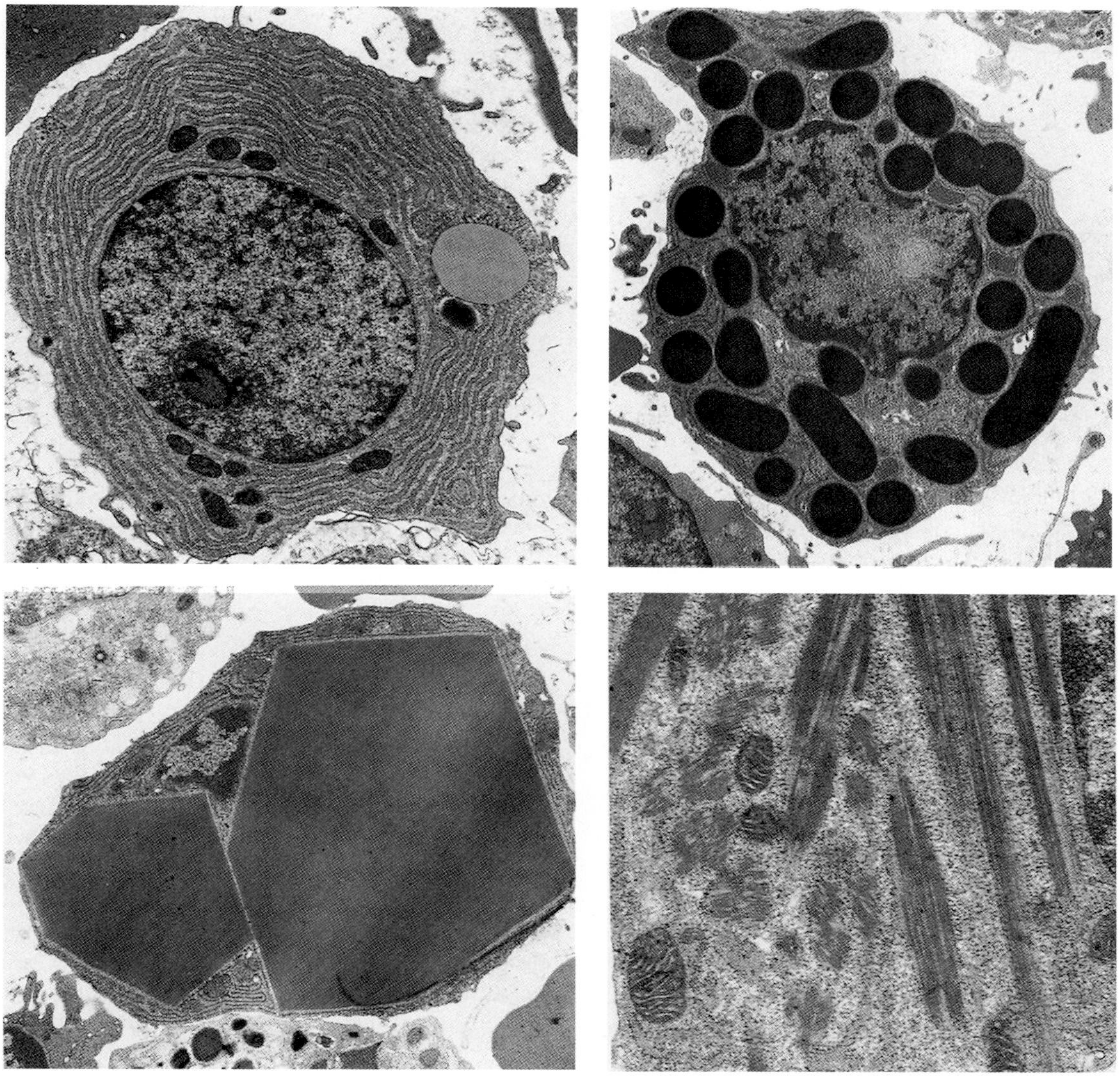

A B C D

**FIG. 55.** Different ultrastructural appearances of plasma cells from normal bone marrow. **A:** Cell with a prominent nucleolus, small quantities of condensed chromatin, several perinuclear mitochondria, some electron-dense material within all the sacs of rough endoplasmic reticulum (RER), and a single large, round, relatively electron-lucent intracytoplasmic inclusion lined by RER. **B:** Cell with multiple rounded or elliptical electron-dense intracytoplasmic inclusions lined by RER. **C:** Cell with two polygonal inclusions lined by RER. **D:** Cell with needlelike crystalline inclusions. The inclusions in (**A–C**) probably result from the accumulation of large quantities of altered immunoglobulin within sacs of RER.

Many of these inclusions are rounded, elliptical, or irregular in outline, but a few are rhomboidal or needlelike and have a crystalline structure (Fig. 55B–D). Thus, the various types of cytoplasmic inclusion seen under the light microscope appear to be formed by the accumulation of unusually large quantities of immunoglobulin within regions of the RER.

## HEMATOPOIETIC CELLS: CHARACTERISTICS IN HISTOLOGIC SECTIONS

In H&E-stained sections of formalin-fixed paraffin-embedded trephine biopsies, insufficient cytoplasmic basophilia and nuclear detail is seen to enable reliable distinction between myeloblasts, neutrophil promyelocytes, neutrophil myelocytes, and early erythroblasts. However, neutrophil metamyelocytes and band cells can be recognized by their C- or U-shaped nuclei and neutrophil granulocytes by the presence of two or more darkly staining nuclear lobes or segments lying close together (Fig. 57). In histologic sections, the fine chromatin strands that join the nuclear lobes of granulocytes usually are not seen. The cytoplasm of neutrophil myelocytes and metamyelocytes stains pale pink and that of neutrophil granulocytes a very pale pink. The granules contained within cells of the neutrophil series stain poorly and are usually difficult to see. Neutrophil promyelocytes and myelocytes can be reliably distinguished from immature cells belonging to other cell lineages by immunohis-

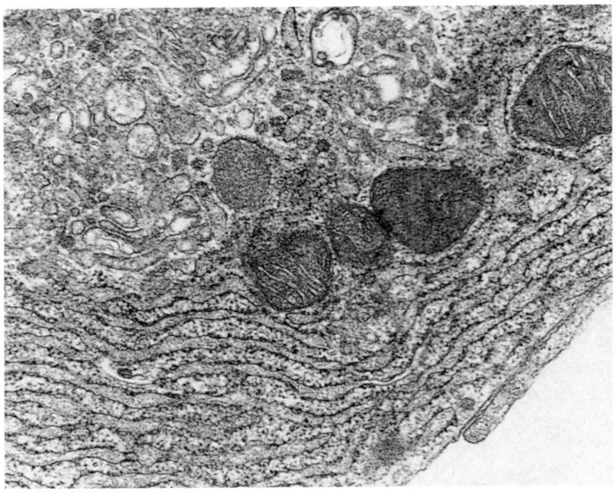

**FIG. 56.** Electron micrograph showing part of the Golgi apparatus and some of the sacs of RER from the plasma cell in Fig. 54, at higher magnification. Four mitochondria are also present.

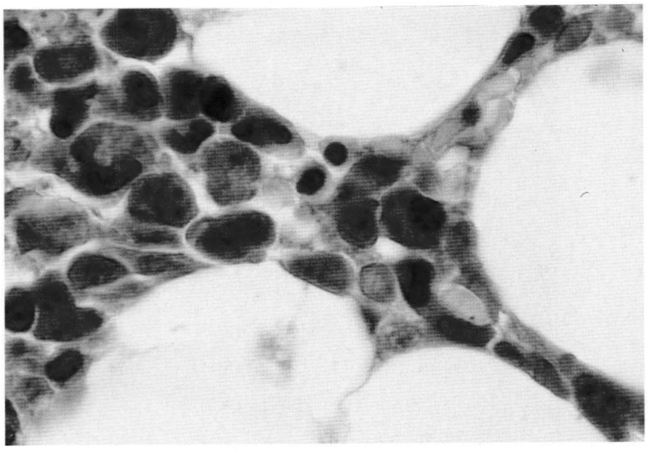

**FIG. 58.** Section of a paraffin-embedded marrow fragment from a hematologically normal subject showing cytoplasmic chloroacetate esterase activity in neutrophil promyelocytes/myelocytes and metamyelocytes but not in two erythroblasts. Leder's stain.

tochemical staining of neutrophil series–specific antigens such as neutrophil elastase (Table 1). In sections of paraffin-embedded marrow fragments, the neutrophil promyelocytes/myelocytes, metamyelocytes, and granulocytes are stained by Leder's stain for chloroacetate esterase (Fig. 58). These cells are also stained, both in sections of marrow fragments and trephine biopsy cores, by the PAS reaction (Fig. 59). Eosinophil myelocytes, metamyelocytes, and myelocytes can be readily recognized by their red–orange cytoplasm resulting from the presence of large eosinophilic granules (Fig. 57). Because basophil granules are water soluble, their contents become extracted during routine fixation for histologic studies. Consequently, basophil granulocytes cannot be seen in histologic sections processed in the usual way.

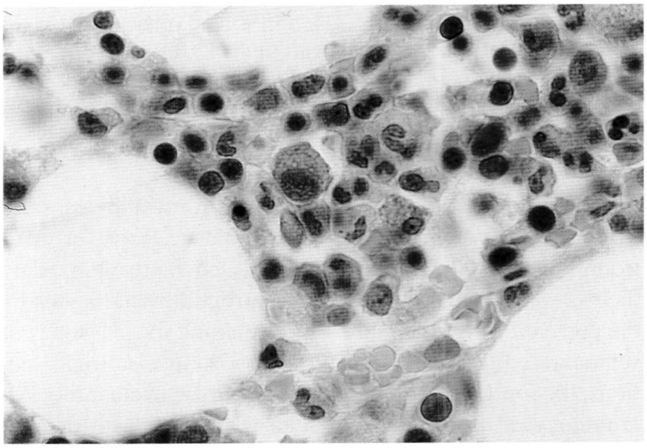

**FIG. 57.** Neutrophil promyelocytes/myelocytes, metamyelocytes, stab cells, and granulocytes in a section of a paraffin-embedded trephine biopsy core from a hematologically normal subject. The two cells with large orange granules belong to the eosinophil granulocyte series. Hematoxylin and eosin.

Erythroblasts of varying degrees of maturity are found in distinctive clumps. Pronormoblasts and basophilic normoblasts are large cells with rounded nuclei containing nucleoli. They only show slight cytoplasmic basophilia when stained by H&E and thus resemble early granulocyte precursors; their identification is therefore based largely on their association with groups of more mature erythroblasts. The late erythroblasts contain rounded heavily stained nuclei showing little structural detail and have moderate quantities of poorly staining cytoplasm, usually with a distinct cytoplasmic membrane. They may show clear halos around the nucleus as a consequence of the shrinkage of the cytoplasm (Fig. 60). Lymphocytes do not show this artifact. Erythroblasts can be reliably identified by immunohistochemical staining of glycophorins A and C and of hemoglobin A (Table 1).

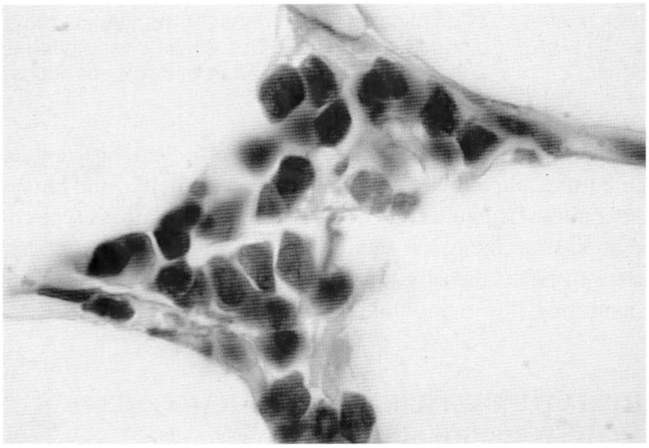

**FIG. 59.** Section of a paraffin-embedded trephine biopsy core showing PAS positivity in neutrophil granulocytes and their precursors.

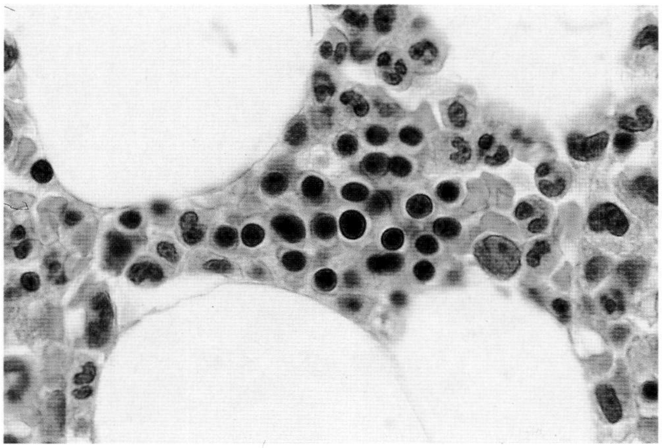

**FIG. 60.** Section of a paraffin-embedded trephine biopsy core from a hematologically normal adult showing a group of early and late polychromatic erythroblasts with halos around their nuclei. Hematoxylin and eosin.

The Giemsa stain is superior to H&E for identifying myeloblasts and promyelocytes as well as pronormoblasts and basophilic normoblasts, staining their cytoplasm blue. However, it is still not possible to reliably distinguish myeloblasts from promyelocytes. In Giemsa-stained sections, pronormoblasts have more basophilic cytoplasm than do other blasts and promyelocytes (Fig. 61).

Lymphocytes may be difficult to distinguish from late erythroblasts in histologic sections of paraffin-embedded trephine biopsy cores except when present in lymphoid nodules. They have a narrow rim of slightly basophilic (Giemsa) or poorly staining (H&E) cytoplasm, indistinct cytoplasmic margins, and a clumped nuclear chromatin pattern. The nuclei of lymphocytes are less perfectly rounded and more variable in size and shape and show more structural detail than those of late erythroblasts. In H&E-stained sections, plasma cells can be identified by the presence of slightly or moderately basophilic cytoplasm, an eccentric nucleus with a cartwheel or clock face chromatin pattern, and a pale paranuclear zone corresponding to the Golgi apparatus. In Giemsa-stained sections, the cytoplasm of many plasma cells stains a deep blue and, consequently, the pale Golgi zone is especially prominent.

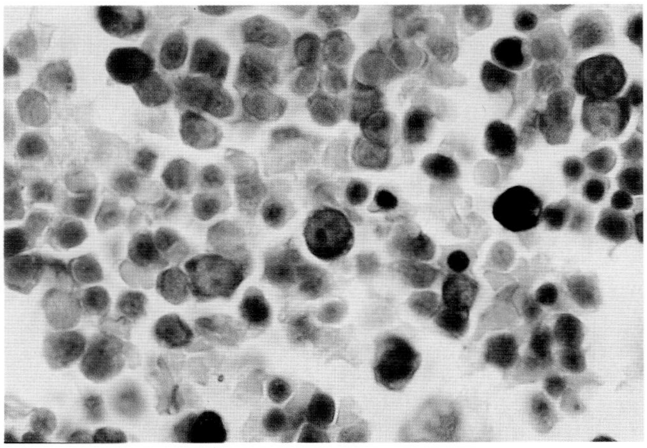

**FIG. 61.** Giemsa-stained section of a paraffin-embedded marrow fragment from a patient with erythroid hyperplasia due to a congenital dyserythropoietic state. The cell in the center with deep blue cytoplasm and prominent nucleoi is a proerythroblast. The photomicrograph also shows a few other proerythroblasts, several basophilic erythroblasts, and some early and late polychromatic erythroblasts.

Megakaryocytes are readily recognized by their large size, light or dark pink cytoplasm, and lobulated nucleus in sections stained either with hematoxylin and eosin or Giemsa (Fig. 62). In sections of normal bone marrow they are present in clusters of two to five cells and are usually not found in a paratrabecular position. Small numbers of bare megakaryocyte nuclei, with convoluted nuclei and a considerable quantity of condensed chromatin, also are seen.

B- and T-lymphocytes, plasma cells, and megakaryoctyes can be identified immunohistochemically, and megakaryoblasts can be reliably identified only in this way (Table 1). Using the monoclonal antibody Y2/51 which is directed against Gp IIIa, the mean value for the total number of megakaryocytes and megakaryoblasts in 15 normal subjects was 24/mm$^2$ (range 14–38) and for megakaryoblasts alone it was 2.8/mm$^2$ (range 1.2–4.9) (83).

As has already been mentioned, much more cytologic detail and especially nuclear detail can be seen in semithin sections of undecalcified plastic-embedded trephine cores (Fig. 63) than in conventional sections of decalcified paraffin-embedded cores (Fig. 62A).

## CELLULARITY OF THE MARROW

The term *marrow cellularity* usually is defined as the proportion of the area of a histologic section excluding bone occupied by hematopoietic cells (by cells other than fat cells). Cellularity is usually assessed by point counting using an eyepiece with a graticule (histomorphometry) or, more accurately, by computerized image analysis (84). The shrinkage of tissue subjected to decalcification and paraffin embedding results in the cellularity of paraffin-embedded sections being about 5% lower than in plastic-embedded sections (85).

In healthy subjects, cellularity varies with age (44,45). In neonates there are very few fat cells in the marrow, and the cellularity approaches 100%. Cellularity decreases steadily in the first three decades and stabilizes at 30% to 70% between the ages of 30 and 70 years. During the eighth decade of life, cellularity decreases further and may be less than 20%; this reduction is largely caused by a reduction in bone volume and a consequent increase in the volume of the marrow cavities.

In assessing cellularity it should be noted that cellularity varies markedly from one intertrabecular space to the next in a single biopsy specimen so that a reliable estimate requires the examination of at least five such spaces (i.e., a biopsy

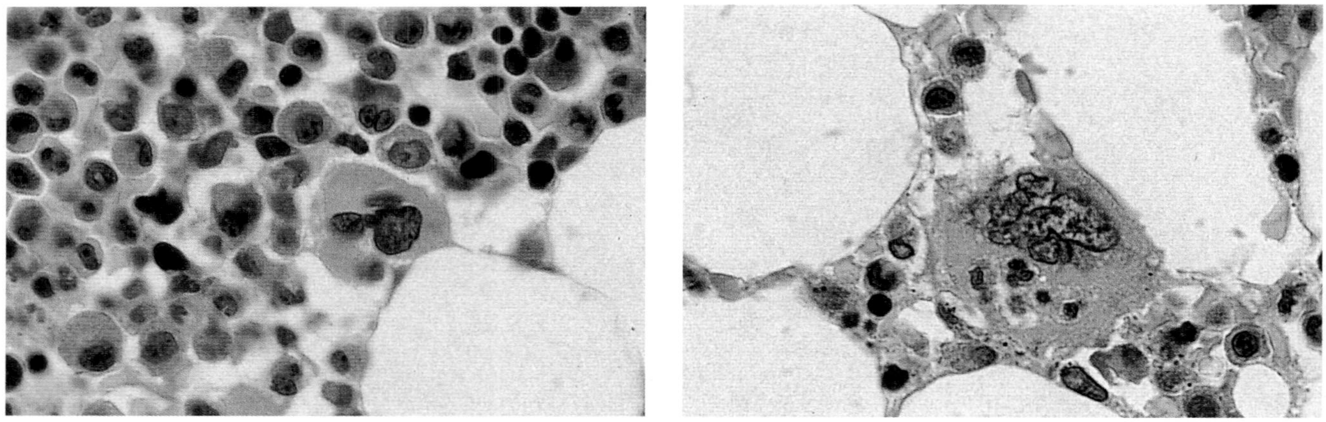


**FIG. 62.** Two megakaryocytes from a section of a paraffin-embedded sample of clotted normal marrow (*clot section*). The megakaryocyte in (**B**) displays emperipolesis. The cells in (**A**) showing a slight orange tinge are eosinophils and their precursors. Hematoxylin and eosin.

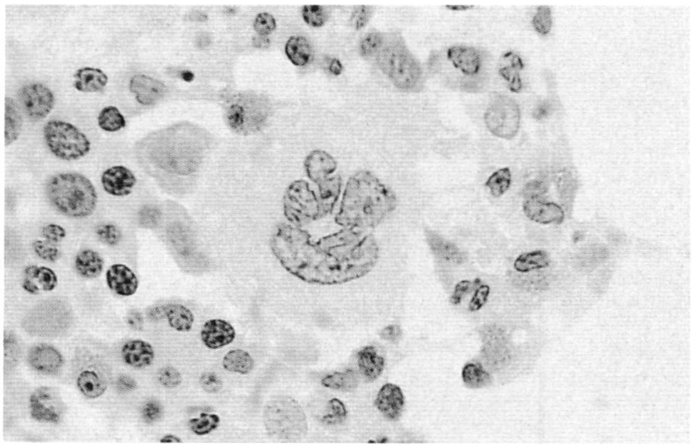

**FIG. 63.** Semithin section of an undecalcified, plastic-embedded trephine biopsy core showing a megakaryocyte and adjacent marrow cells. When compared with Fig. 62A, this semithin section shows considerably more cellular detail, especially nuclear detail. The cytoplasmic granules of cells of the eosinophil series are clearly seen; these are stained red–orange. Hematoxylin and eosin.

**TABLE 2.** *Differential counts[a] on marrow smears from 28 healthy adults aged between 20 and 29 years (92)*

| Cell type | Percentages | | |
|---|---|---|---|
| | Mean | 95% confidence limits | Observed range |
| Myeloblasts | 1.21 | 0.75–1.67 | 0.75–1.80 |
| Promyelocytes | 2.49 | 0.99–3.99 | 1.00–3.75 |
| Myelocytes | | | |
| Neutrophil | 17.36 | 11.54–23.18 | 12.25–22.65 |
| Eosinophil | 1.37 | 0–2.85 | 0.25–3.45 |
| Basophil | 0.08 | 0–0.21 | 0.00–0.25 |
| Metamyelocytes | | | |
| Neutrophil | 16.92 | 11.40–22.44 | 11.45–23.60 |
| Eosinophil | 0.63 | 0.07–1.19 | 0.25–1.30 |
| Juvenile neutrophil granulocytes (stab forms) | 8.70 | 3.58–13.82 | 4.85–13.95 |
| Granulocytes | | | |
| Neutrophil | 13.42 | 4.32–22.52 | 8.70–28.95 |
| Eosinophil | 0.93 | 0.21–1.65 | 0.45–1.55 |
| Basophil | 0.20 | 0–0.48 | 0.05–0.50 |
| Monocytes | 1.04 | 0.36–1.72 | 0.65–2.10 |
| Plasma cells | 0.46 | 0–0.96 | 0.10–0.95 |
| Lymphocytes | 14.60 | 6.66–22.54 | 9.35–25.05 |
| Basophilic erythropoietic cells | 0.92 | 0.40–1.44 | 0.50–1.60 |
| Early polychromatic normoblasts | 6.76 | 2.56–10.96 | 3.30–12.20 |
| Late polychromatic normoblasts | 11.58 | 6.16–17.0 | 7.85–19.55 |
| Reticular cells | 0.24 | 0–0.54 | 0.05–0.65 |

[a] Two thousand cells were studied in each individual.

core of greater than 2 cm). Furthermore, the immediate subcortical marrow of the ilium is frequently less cellular than deeper marrow. A study of postmortem biopsy samples from 100 normal subjects who died suddenly without evidence of bone or marrow disease showed only slight differences in the cellularity at different hematopoietic sites. The percentage cellularity ± SD in biopsies from the anterior iliac crest, posterior iliac crest, lumbar vertebrae, and sternum were, 60 ± 6, 62 ± 7, 64 ± 7, and 61 ± 8, respectively (86).

## MARROW DIFFERENTIAL COUNT

During the first day of life, the erythroblasts account for 18.5% to 65% (mean 40%) of the nucleated cells in a marrow smear. Over the next 8 to 10 days, this figure decreases progressively to 0% to 20.5% (mean 8%). After a period of erythroblastopenia lasting about 3 weeks, the percentage of erythroblasts increases again, reaching values of 6.5% to 31.5% (mean 16%) at the age of 3 months (87). These changes are caused by an increase in arterial oxygen saturation soon after birth and the consequent suppression of erythropoietin production. Erythropoietin production increases again 6 to 13 weeks later when the hemoglobin concentration in the blood decreases to about 11 g/dl. The proportion of granulocytes and their precursors ranges between 20 and 73% (mean 46%) of the nucleated marrow cells on the first day of life (87), increases during the next 3 weeks, and then decreases again to reach a stable value of about 55% after the second month. The average value for the proportion of lymphocytes in the marrow increases from 12% during the first 2 days of life, to 33% at 7 to 10 days, and 47% at 1 month. The lymphocyte percentage then remains stable until the end of the first year, after which it decreases slowly to 19% at 4 to 4.5 years, which is only slightly higher than the adult value of 15% (87–90). Plasma cells are infrequent in the neonate, accounting for 0% to 0.4% (mean 0.016%) of nucleated marrow cells (91). They gradually increase in number to reach adult values (mean 0.38%) by the age of 12 years.

The differential count in bone marrow smears from normal adults is given in Table 2. The mean and range for the myeloid/erythroid ratio in healthy adults are 3.1 and 2.0 to 8.3, respectively (93).

## REFERENCES


1. Rywlin AM. *Histopathology of the bone marrow.* Boston: Little, Brown; 1976.
2. Krause JR, ed. *Bone marrow biopsy.* Edinburgh: Churchill Livingstone; 1981.
3. Andrade RE, Wick MR, Frizzera G, Gajl-Peczalska KJ. Immunophenotyping of hematopoietic malignancies in paraffin sections. *Hum Pathol* 1988;19:394–402.
4. Pulford KAF, Erber WN, Crick JA, et al. Use of monoclonal antibody against human neutrophil elastase in normal and leukaemic myeloid cells. *J Clin Pathol* 1988;41:853–860.
5. Gatter KC, Cordell JL, Turley H, et al. The immunohistological detection of platelets, megakaryocytes and thrombi in routinely processed specimens. *Histopathology* 1988;13:257–267.
6. Kubic VL, Brunning RD. Immunohistochemical evaluation of neoplasms in bone marrow biopsies using monoclonal antibodies reactive in paraffin-embedded tissues. *Mod Pathol* 1989;2:618–629.
7. van der Valk P, Mullink H, Huijgens PC, Tadema TM, Vos W, Meijer CJLM. Immunohistochemistry in bone marrow diagnosis. Value of a panel of monoclonal antibodies on routinely processed bone marrow biopsies. *Am J Surg Pathol* 1989;13:97–106.
8. Walls AF, Jones DB, Williams JH, Church MK, Holgate ST. Immunohistochemical identification of mast cells in formaldehyde fixed tissue using monoclonal antibodies specific for tryptase. *J Pathol* 1990;162: 119–126.
9. Horny H-P, Wehrmann M, Steinke B, Kaiserling E. Assessment of the value of immunohistochemistry in the subtyping of acute leukemia on routinely processed bone marrow biopsy specimens with particular reference to macrophage-associated antibodies. *Hum Pathol* 1994;25: 810–814.
10. teVelde J, Burkhardt R, Kleiverda K, et al. Methyl-methacrylate as an embedding medium in histopathology. *Histopathology* 1977; 1:319–330.
11. Burkhardt R. Bone marrow histology. In: Catovsky D, ed. *Methods in hematology. The leukaemic cell.* Edinburgh: Churchill Livingstone; 1981:49–86.
12. Frisch B, Lewis SM, Burkhardt R, Bartl R. *Biopsy pathology of bone and bone marrow.* London: Chapman & Hall; 1985.
13. Frisch B, Bartl R. *Atlas of bone marrow pathology. Current histopathology.* Vol. 15. Dordrecht, The Netherlands: Kluwer Academic; 1990.
14. Beckstead JH, Halvarsen PS, Ries CA, Bainton D. Enzyme histochemistry and immunohistochemistry on biopsy specimens of pathologic human bone marrow. *Blood* 1981;57:1088–1098.
15. Beckstead JH. The bone marrow biopsy: a diagnostic strategy. *Arch Pathol Lab Med* 1986;110:175–179.
16. Archimbaud E, Islam A, Preisler HD. Immunoperoxidase detection of myeloid antigens in glycolmethacrylate-embedded human bone marrow. *J Histochem Cytochem* 1987;35:595–599.
17. Burkhardt R. Präparative Voraussetzungen zur klinischen Histologie des menschlichen Knochenmarks. I Mitteilung. *Blut* 1966;13:337–357.
18. Burkhardt R. Präparative Voraussetzungen zur klinischen Histologie von Knochenmark und Knochen. II Ein neues Verfahren zur histologischen Präparation von Biopsien aus Knochenmark und Knochen. *Blut* 1966;14:30–46.
19. Burkhardt R. *Bone marrow and bone tissue. Color atlas of clinical histopathology.* Berlin: Springer-Verlag; 1971.
20. Wood GS, Warnke RA. The immunologic phenotyping of bone marrow biopsies and aspirates: frozen section techniques. *Blood* 1982;59: 913–922.
21. Falini B, Martelli MF, Tarallo F, et al. Immunohistological analysis of human bone marrow trephine biopsies using monoclonal antibodies. *Br J Haematol* 1984;56:365–386.
22. Hayhoe FGJ, Quaglino D. *Haematological cytochemistry.* 2nd ed. Edinburgh: Churchill Livingstone; 1988.
23. Wickramasinghe SN. *Human bone marrow.* Oxford: Blackwell Scientific; 1975.
24. Gordon MY. Human haemopoietic stem cell assays. *Blood Rev* 1993; 7:190–197.
25. Ogawa M. Hematopoiesis. *J Allergy Clin Immunol* 1994;94:645–650.
26. Lord BI, Dexter TM, ed. Growth factors in haemopoiesis. *Baillieres Clin Haematol* 1992;5:.
27. Brenner M, ed. Cytokines and growth factors. *Baillieres Clin Haematol* 1994;7:.
28. Moore MAS, Metcalf D. Ontogeny of the haemopoietic system: yolk sac origin of in vivo and in vitro colony forming cells in the developing mouse embryo. *Br J Haematol* 1970;18:279–296.
29. Bloom W, Bartelmez GW. Hemopoiesis in young human embryos. *Am J Anat* 1940;67:21–44.
30. Kelemen E, Calvo W, Fliedner TM. *Atlas of human hemopoietic development.* Berlin: Springer-Verlag; 1979.
31. Gilmour JR. Normal haemopoiesis in intrauterine and neonatal life. *J Pathol Bacteriol* 1941;52:25–55.
32. Emura I, Sekiya M, Ohnishi Y. Two types of immature erythrocytic series in the human liver. *Arch Histol Jpn* 1983;46:631–643.
33. Kalpaktsoglou PK, Emery JL. Human bone marrow during the last three months of intrauterine life. A histological study. *Acta Haematol (Basel)* 1965;34:228–238.
34. Piney A. The anatomy of the bone marrow with special reference to the distribution of the red marrow. *Br Med J* 1922;2:792–795.

35. Custer RP, Ahlfeldt FE. Studies on the structure and function of bone marrow. II. Variations in cellularity in various bones with advancing years of life and their relative response to stimuli. *J Lab Clin Med* 1932; 17:960–962.
36. Wickramasinghe SN, ed. *Blood and bone marrow. Systemic pathology.* 3rd ed. Vol. 2. Edinburgh: Churchill Livingstone; 1986.
37. Munka V, Gregor A. Lymphatics and bone marrow. *Folia Morphol (Praha)* 1965;13:404–412.
38. Branemark PI. Bone marrow, microvascular structure and function. *Adv Microcirc* 1968;1:1.
39. de Bruyn PPH, Breen PC, Thomas TB. The microcirculation of the bone marrow. *Anat Rec* 1970;168:55–68.
40. Benayahu D, Horowitz M, Zipori D, Wientroub S. Hemopoietic functions of marrow-derived osteogenic cells. *Calcif Tissue Int* 1992;51: 195–201.
41. Wickramasinghe SN. Observations on the ultrastructure of sinusoids and reticular cells in human bone marrow. *Clin Lab Haematol* 1991;13: 263–278.
42. Miller MR, Kasahara M. Observations on the innervation of human long bones. *Anat Rec* 1963;145:13–17.
43. Chambers TJ. Regulation of osteoclast development and function. In: Rifkin BR, Gay CV, eds. *Biology and physiology of the osteoclast.* Boca Raton, FL: CRC Press; 1992:105–128.
44. Sturgeon P. Volumetric and microscopic pattern of bone marrow in normal infants and children. III. Histologic pattern. *Pediatrics* 1951; 7:774–781.
45. Harstock RJ, Smith EB, Petty CS. Normal variations with aging of the amount of hematopoietic tissue in bone marrow from the anterior iliac crest. A study made from 177 cases of sudden death examined by necropsy. *Am J Clin Pathol* 1965;43:326–331.
46. Tavassoli M, Eastlund DT, Yam LT, et al. Gelatinous transformation of bone marrow in prolonged self-induced starvation. *Scand J Haematol* 1976;16:311–319.
47. Gale E, Torrance J, Bothwell T. The quantitative estimation of total iron stores in human bone marrow. *J Clin Invest* 1963;42:1076–1082.
48. Trubowitz S, Masek B. A histochemical study of the reticuloendothelial system of human marrow—its possible transport role. *Blood* 1968; 32:610–628.
49. Burgio VL, Magrini U, Ciardelli L, Pezzoni G. An enzyme-histochemical approach to the study of the human bone-marrow stroma. *Acta Haematol (Basel)* 1984;71:73–80.
50. Westen H, Bainton DF. Association of alkaline-phosphatase-positive reticulum cells in bone marrow with granulocytic precursors. *J Exp Med* 1979;150:919–937.
51. Tanaka Y. An electron microscopic study of non-phagocytic reticulum cells in human bone marrow. I. Cells with intracytoplasmic fibrils. *Acta Haematol Jpn* 1969;32:275–286.
52. Biermann A, Graf von Keyserlingk D. Ultrastructure of reticulum cells in the bone marrow. *Acta Anat* 1978;100:34–43.
53. Tsai S, Patel V, Beaumont E, et al. Differential binding of erythroid and myeloid progenitors to fibroblasts and fibronectin. *Blood* 1987;69: 1587–1594.
54. Broudy VC, Zuckerman KS, Jetmalani S, et al. Monocytes stimulate fibroblastoid bone marrow stromal cells to produce multilineage hemopoietic growth factors. *Blood* 1986;68:530–534.
55. Kirshenbaum AS, Kessler SW, Goff JP, Metcalfe DD. Demonstration of the origin of human mast cells from CD34+ bone marrow progenitor cells. *J Immunol* 1991;146:1410–1415.
56. Zucker-Franklin D, Grusky G, Hirayama N, Schnipper E. The presence of mast cell precursors in rat peripheral blood. *Blood* 1981;58:544–551.
57. Denburg JA, Richardson M, Telizyn S, Bienenstock J. Basophil/mast cell precursors in human peripheral blood. *Blood* 1983;61:775–780.
58. Zucker-Franklin D. Ultrastructural evidence for the common origin of human mast cells and basophils. *Blood* 1980;56:534–540.
59. Rywlin AM, Ortega RS, Dominguez CJ. Lymphoid nodules of bone marrow: normal and abnormal. *Blood* 1974;43:389–400.
60. Rheingold JJ, Wislocki GB. Histochemical methods applied to hematology. *Blood* 1948;3:641–655.
61. Gibb RP, Stowell RE. Glycogen in human blood cells. *Blood* 1949; 4:569–579.
62. Rozenszajn L, Leibovich M, Shoham D, Epstein J. The esterase activity in megaloblasts, leukaemic and normal haemopoietic cells. *Br J Haematol* 1968;14:605–610.
63. Scott RE, Horn RG. Ultrastructural aspects of neutrophil granulocyte development in humans. *Lab Invest* 1970;23:202–215.
64. Bainton DF, Ullyot JL, Farquhar MG. The development of neutrophilic polymorphonuclear leukocytes in human bone marrow. Origin and content of azurophil and specific granules. *J Exp Med* 1971;134:907–934.
65. Cawley JC, Hayhoe FGJ. *Ultrastructure of haemic cells. A cytological atlas of normal and leukaemic blood and bone marrow.* London: WB Saunders; 1973.
66. Bessis M. *Living blood cells and their ultrastructure.* Berlin: Springer-Verlag; 1973.
67. Parwaresch MR. *The human blood basophil.* Berlin: Springer-Verlag; 1976.
68. Scott RE, Horn RG. Fine structural features of eosinophil granulocyte development in human bone marrow. *J Ultrastruct Res* 1970;33:16–28.
69. Leder LD. The origin of blood monocytes and macrophages. *Blut* 1967; 16:86.
70. Wickramasinghe SN, Hughes M. Globin chain precipitation, deranged iron metabolism and dyserythropoiesis in some thalassaemia syndromes. *Haematologia (Budap)* 1984;17:35–55.
71. Wickramasinghe SN. *Unpublished observations.*
72. Nêmec J, Polák H. Erythropoietic polyploidy. I. The morphology of polyploid erythroid elements and their incidence in healthy subjects. *Folia Haematol (Leipz)* 1964;84:24–40.
73. Queisser U, Queisser W, Spiertz B. Polyploidization of megakaryocytes in normal humans, in patients with idiopathic thrombocytopenia and with pernicious anaemia. *Br J Haematol* 1971;20:489–501.
74. Jean G, Lambertenghi-Deliliers G, Ranzi T, Poirier-Basseti M. The human bone marrow megakaryocyte. An ultrastructural study. *Haematologia* 1971;5:253–264.
75. Breton-Gorius J, Reyes F. Ultrastructure of human bone marrow cell maturation. *Int Rev Cytol* 1976;46:251–321.
76. Breton-Gorius J. The value of cytochemical peroxidase reactions at the ultrastructural level in haematology. *Histochem J* 1980;12:127–137.
77. Breton-Gorius J, Gourdin MF, Reyes F. Ultrastructure of the leukemic cell. In: Catovsky D, ed. *Methods in hematology. The leukemic cell.* Edinburgh: Churchill Livingstone; 1981:87–128.
78. Larsen TE. Emperipolesis of granular leukocytes within megakaryocytes in human hemopoietic bone marrow. *Am J Clin Pathol* 1970;53: 485–489.
79. Rozman C, Vives-Corrons JL. On the alleged diagnostic significance of megakaryocytic "phagocytosis" (emperipolesis). *Br J Haematol* 1981; 48:510.
80. White JG. Current concepts of platelet structure. *Am J Clin Pathol* 1979;71:363–378.
81. Berndt MC, Castaldi PA, Gordon S, et al. Morphological and biochemical confirmation of gray platelet syndrome in two siblings. *Aust N Z J Med* 1983;13:387–390.
82. Clark P, Normansell DE, Innes DJ, Hess CE. Lymphocyte subsets in normal bone marrow. *Blood* 1986;67:1600–1606.
83. Thiele J, Wagner S, Wenste R, et al. An immunomorphometric study of megakaryocyte precursor cells in bone marrow tissue from patients with chronic myeloid leukemia (CML). *Eur J Haematol* 1990;44; 63–70.
84. Al-Adhadh AN, Cavill I. Assessment of cellularity in bone marrow fragments. *J Clin Pathol* 1983;36:176–179.
85. Kerndrup G, Pallensen G, Melsen F, Mosekilde L. Histomorphometrical determination of bone marrow cellularity in iliac crest biopsies. *Scand J Haematol* 1980;24:110–114.
86. Bartl R, Frisch B. *Biopsy of bone in internal medicine. Current histopathology.* Vol. 21. Dordrecht, The Netherlands: Kluwer Academic; 1993.
87. Gairdner D, Marks J, Roscoe JD. Blood formation in infancy. Part I. The normal bone marrow. *Arch Dis Child* 1952;27:128–133.
88. Glaser K, Limarzi LR, Poncher HG. Cellular composition of the bone marrow in normal infants and children. *Pediatrics* 1950;6:789–824.
89. Diwany M. Sternal marrow puncture in children. *Arch Dis Child* 1940; 15:159–170.
90. Rosse C, Kraemer MJ, Dillon TL, et al. Bone marrow cell populations of normal infants: the predominance of lymphocytes. *J Lab Clin Med* 1977;89:1225–1240.
91. Steiner ML, Pearson HA. Bone marrow plasmacyte values in childhood. *J Pediatr* 1966;68:562–568.
92. Jacobsen KM. Untersuchungen über das Knockenmarkspunktat bei normalen Individuen verschiedener Altersklassen. *Acta Med Scand* 1941;106:417–446.
93. Young RH, Osgood EE. Sternal marrow aspirated during life. Cytology in health and in disease. *Arch Intern Med* 1935;55:186–203.

# Heart and Blood Vessels

*Histology for Pathologists, second edition,*
Edited by Stephen S. Sternberg.
Lippincott-Raven Publishers, Philadelphia


# CHAPTER 32

# Normal Heart

Margaret E. Billingham



With the advent of cardiopulmonary bypass, surgical pathologists found themselves dealing more and more with cardiac specimens. For many years this consisted of explanted valves, pericardiectomy specimens, aneurysectomies, and myomectomy specimens from outflow tract obstructions. It was not until cardiac transplantation began in 1968 that the surgical pathologist began dealing with entire heart specimens. Worldwide, more than 36,500 hearts have been explanted in the process of heart and heart–lung transplantation (1). More recently, neonatal and children's hearts are being transplanted more frequently (1). The explanted hearts from infants and children are often those with complicated congenital heart lesions. Therefore, surgical pathologists need to have some expertise in end-stage heart disease of all types. Beginning in the early 1970s, endomyocardial biopsies began to be performed on a regular basis. Like other biopsies, these also fell into the realm of the surgical pathologist. From these comments it is obvious that it is now necessary for surgical pathologists to know more about cardiac anatomy and histology than was true before 1960. The purpose of this chapter is to review normal cardiac anatomy and histology. The histology of the great vessels is described elsewhere in this book. For the most part, adult histology is described, but where there are important differences, the histology in infants and children is also addressed. Furthermore, the purpose is not to be all-encompassing, but rather to highlight those areas that are of practical importance to the surgical pathologist so that they may know what is normal from subtle myocardial pathology. For this reason, normal aging or gender differences also are described. The emphasis in this chapter is on the histology of the heart rather than the anatomy of the heart. As each of the major normal anatomic divisions of the heart are described,

M. E. Billingham: Stanford University School of Medicine, Stanford, California 94305.

mention is made of aging and gender changes, as well as of applied anatomy.

## HEART WEIGHTS

The adult heart weight is reached by age 17 to 20 years of age. Heart weight in children is related to age and body size. The weight of the adult human heart averages 325 ± 75 g in men and 275 ± 75 g in women. In the adult, the heart weight varies with age, sex, and body size so that in young athletic adults the heart weight may approach or exceed the upper limit of normal, whereas in the elderly it may approach or be slightly below the lower limit of normal. Age-related changes in cardiac weight and other cardiac measurements have been recorded and published previously for fetuses, infants, adolescents, and adults and are beyond the scope of this work. Descriptive tables may be found in the works of Silver and Freedom (2) and Kitzman, et al. (3), as well as in many other autopsy manuals.

## EMBRYOLOGY OF THE HEART

The embryology of the heart is complicated and is addressed in texts on embryology. The following is a brief review modified from the texts of Fitzgerald (4) and Moore (5). The heart has its origin in the splanchnic mesoderm in an area called the cardiogenic crescent. Heart development begins at around the third gestational week. The crescent gives rise to a pair of endothelial tubes that unite to form the primitive heart tube. The myocardium is also derived from the splanchnic mesoderm. As the heart tubes approach each other, they show dilatations of primitive heart chambers. The bulbus cordis, which is anterior and cephalad, gives rise to the truncus arteriosus. The second chamber forms the primitive ventricles, and the third turns cephalad to form the common atrium; the fourth chamber becomes the sinus venosus, which receives the umbilical, vitelline, and later the common cardinal veins. The lengthening heart tube bends and folds to accommodate itself within the forming pericardial sac. The atrioventricular (AV) canal is narrowed by the superior and inferior gelatinous subendocardial swellings or endocardial cushions. At this time, the septum primum grows down into the common atrium from the dorsal atrial wall and fuses with the endocardial cushions, leaving a foramen primum for passage of blood through the interatrial septum. As fusion of the atrial septum primum and endocardial cushions becomes complete, there is a breakdown of the septum primum to form the foramen secundum. Also at this time a septum secundum extends into the atrium on the right side, uniting partially with the septum primum to overlap the foramen secundum, forming a valvelike flap and the foramen ovale. The foramen ovale permits oxygenated blood from the placenta to bypass the unventilated lungs and pass into the systemic circulation in the fetus.

The primitive ventricle gives rise to the left ventricle and the bulbus cordis to the right ventricle. A ridge forms on the floor of the bulboventricular foramen or common ventricle that becomes the primitive interventricular septum. As the interventricular septum develops, the left and right ventricles communicate through the primary interventricular foramen. Both ventricles have access through the distal bulbs to the truncus arteriosus. The proximal bulbus forms the trabeculated part of the right ventricle, and the distal part forms the smoother wall of the infundibulum or outflow tract. The ventricular cavities continue to grow by downward extension. The endocardial cushions enlarge and form the leaflets of the tricuspid and mitral valves, which become separated. The interventricular septum fuses with the inferior cushion and forms the membranous septum, thus completing the interventricular septum and separating the two ventricles. The interventricular foramen usually closes by the seventh gestational week.

### Heart Valves

The subendocardial mesenchyme forms a thickening around each AV orifice, creating the leaflets of the tricuspid and mitral valves. The endocardial cushions also contribute to this structure.

The truncus arteriosus is divided longitudinally by the aorticopulmonary septum. Subendothelial swellings develop on the walls of the dividing truncus to make two of the six semilunar valves, whereas the other four develop on the opposite walls as the aortic and pulmonic trunk separate. The left and right coronary arteries grow outward from the corresponding cusps of the aortic semilunar valve.

The development of the outflow tract, aortic arches, and great vessels are addressed in textbooks on that subject.

After birth, myocardial hyperplasia is prominent and myocyte size increases up to 100 $\mu$m in length and to 20 to 30 $\mu$m in width. Cell volume (myocyte) increases with the numbers of mitochondria; the increase is most rapid after birth because of changes in myocardial metabolism.

## PRENATAL FETAL CIRCULATION

At which point during embryonal development the human heart begins to beat is uncertain, but it is thought to occur at about 21 days after fertilization. Well-oxygenated blood leaves the placenta via the umbilical vein, some of which passes through the hepatic sinusoids, and some bypasses the liver through the ductus venosus to the inferior vena cava. From the inferior vena cava the blood enters the right atrium of the heart together with an admixture of deoxygenated blood from the lower body in the inferior vena cava. Most of this blood is diverted through the ostium secundum (interatrial septum) into the left atrium, where it mixes with the small amount of deoxygenated blood returning from the lungs. The blood then passes into the left ventricle and leaves by the ascending aorta to supply the coronary arteries, brain, and upper limbs. Approximately 50% of the blood is returned to the placenta for reoxygenation by the umbilical arteries. The rest of the blood supplies the lower half of the body.

## POSTNATAL FETAL CIRCULATION

At birth, the circulation of fetal blood through the placenta ceases and the infant's lungs expand and begin to function, with an increase in pulmonary blood flow from the lowered pulmonary vascular resistance. The resulting increase in right atrial pressure presses the foramen ovale against the septum secundum and closes it, leaving the indentation called the fossa ovale. By the end of the first month after birth, the left ventricular wall becomes thicker because of increased hemodynamic load, and the right ventricular wall thins because of the decreased workload. The ductus arteriosus from the pulmonary to the aortic trunk becomes functionally closed about 15 h after birth, except in premature infants, because the hypoxia effects prostaglandin E, which is thought to keep the ductus arteriosus patent. Also, the umbilical veins constrict at birth.

## APOPTOSIS

It has been suggested that apoptosis or programmed cell (myocyte) death plays an important role during postnatal development of the heart (6). It has been postulated that the mechanical forces generated by alterations in cardiac hemodynamics may trigger apoptosis. Tanaka et al. also have shown that hypoxia induces apoptosis in neonatal cardiac myocytes in culture (7). It is known that programmed myocyte cell death also occurs during ischemia reperfusion injury in the myocardium, but to our knowledge it has not been shown to occur in the normal adult heart, although it probably also occurs in the normal aging heart. More detailed information on apoptosis may be found in this book on this subject.

## PERICARDIUM

The pericardium surrounds the heart and consists of a fibrous and a serous sac. The fibrous or parietal pericardium envelops the heart and is reflected off the great vessels, the ascending aorta, the pulmonary trunk, and the terminal 2 to 4 cm of the superior vena cava. In the normal state the fibrous pericardium is not attached to the visceral epicardial pericardium. The fibrous pericardium is composed of fibrous tissue or collagen (Fig. 1), which is inelastic and which, therefore, may result in cardiac tamponade if stretched with more than 250 ml of fluid, particularly if it develops acutely. The fibrous pericardium also may contain variable amounts of adipose tissue toward the apex of the heart. The parietal pericardium is lined by a thin layer of mesothelium on its inner surface.

The serous pericardium is also called the epicardium or the visceral pericardium. The serous pericardium is thin and covers the surface of the heart with a single layer of mesothelial cells continuous with that of the fibrous pericardium (Fig. 2). This delicate membrane covers the heart but also contains a variable amount of adipose tissue in which are embedded the coronary arteries, lymphatic vessels, nerves, fibroblasts, and macrophages (Fig. 3). The normal epicardium usually contains a few lymphocytes, and these are present from birth.

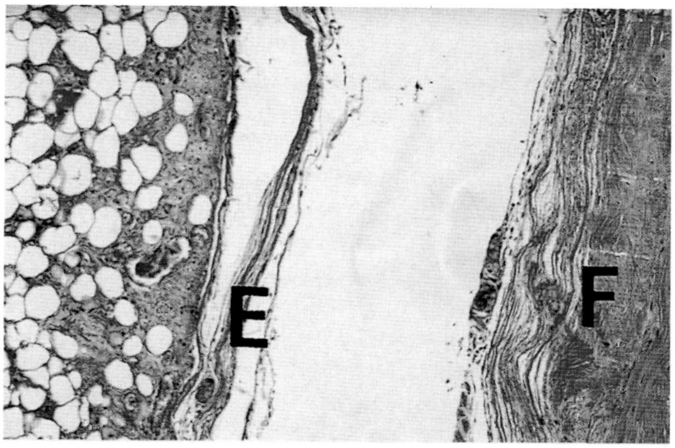


**FIG. 1.** Section showing fibrous pericardium (F) separated from the thinner epicardium (E) (elastic Van Giesen).

Between the two mesothelial layers of the fibrous pericardium and the epicardium is a potential space containing 1 to 30 ml of clear serous fluid that allows the surfaces to glide over one another in the normal state. The histology of the pericardium does not alter significantly with age and is similar in infants and children.

### Applied Anatomy

Surgical pathologists may receive pericardiectomy specimens in cases of constrictive pericarditis. In explanted

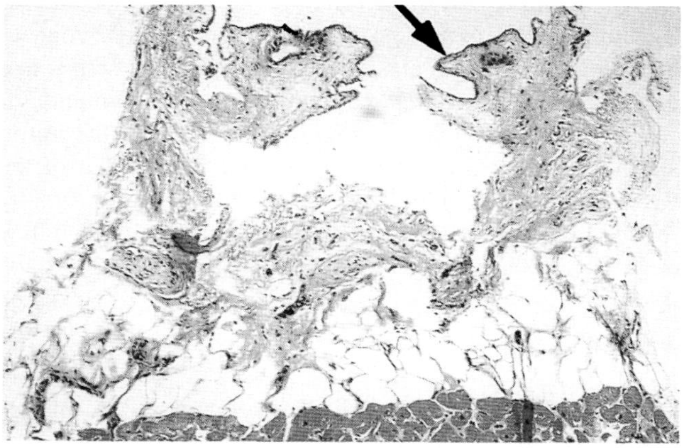

**FIG. 2.** Section showing the epicardium lined by mesothelial cells (*arrow*) covering the subepicardial adipose tissue and myocardium [hematoxylin and eosin (H&E)].

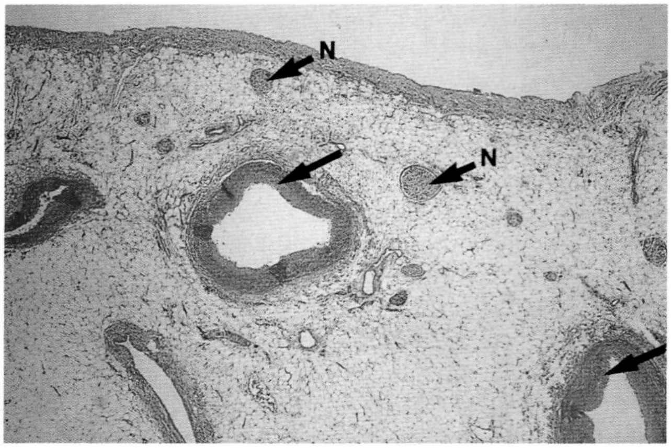


**FIG. 3.** Section of the epicardium showing the relationship of coronary vessels and nerves to the epicardium (H&E).

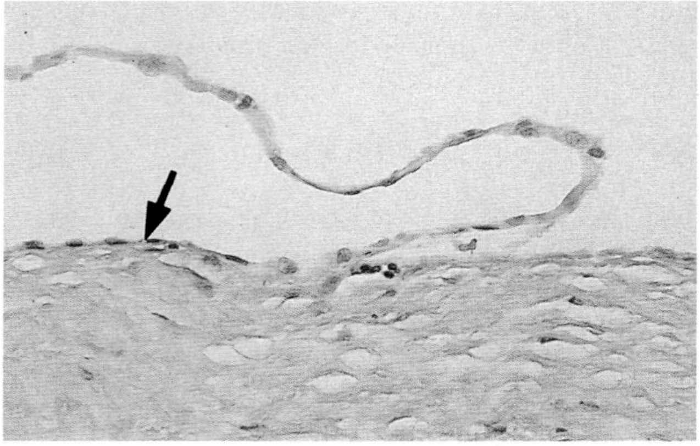

**FIG. 4.** Section showing a single layer of endothelial cells covering the myocardium (*arrow*) (H&E).

hearts, the pericardial surfaces may be thickened by previous disease states or previous surgery, in which case the epicardium and fibrous pericardium may adhere to one another. Occasionally, epicardial fat may be misinterpreted grossly as metastases. Congenital cysts of the pericardium also may be removed surgically but are rare.

### Aging Changes

In obese subjects there may be excessive epicardial depot fat. In cachectic states the epicardial depot fat may undergo serous atrophy, and only small gelatinous tissue tags will remain (8).

## CARDIAC SKELETON

The cardiac skeleton is the central supporting structure to which most of the muscle fibers of the myocardium are attached and with which the valves are also connected. The membranous septum, the fibrous trigone, and the fibrous annuli of the atrioventricular foramina are part of the fibrous skeleton (9). The fibrous skeleton consists of dense connective tissue with some elastic fibers. This dense connective tissue sometimes contains fat but consists predominantly of collagen bundles in layers. The fibrous tissue of the mitral and aortic valve rings is more substantial than that of the valves of the right side. Bone or cartilage are not normally found in the fibrous skeleton of human hearts, although they have been described in some animal species.

### Applied Anatomy

Portions of the cardiac skeleton may be seen in explanted valves. A separate mass of fibrous tissue (the conus ligament) joins the pulmonary ring to the aortic ring. The main bundle of His penetrates the central fibrous body. The membranous interventricular septum, although not strictly part of the fibrous skeleton, also comprises fibrous tissue and is in direct continuity with the aortic valve ring. The membranous septum appears as a triangle between the noncoronary and right coronary cusps of the aortic valve and can be viewed when the opened heart is held up to the light or is transilluminated. The continuity of the anterior cusp of the mitral valve and the left cusp of the aortic valve is both an important anatomic and radiologic relationship.

## INTERNAL STRUCTURE OF THE HEART

The wall of the heart in all chambers consists of three main layers: (a) the endocardium, (b) the intermediate portion or myocardium, and (c) the external portion or epicardium. Most investigators believe that the endocardium is homologous with the tunica intima of blood vessels, that the myocardium corresponds to the smooth muscle media of blood vessels, and that the external epicardium corresponds with the adventitia of vessels. The endocardium consists of a single layer of endothelial cells (Figs. 4 and 5) with a suben-

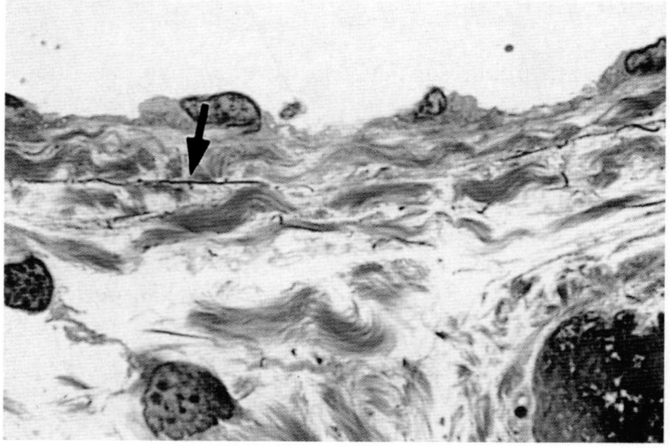

**FIG. 5.** One-micron thick section (plastic embedded) of the endothelium covering the fenestrated elastic fibers (*arrow*) and collagen fibers of the subendocardium (Toluidine blue).

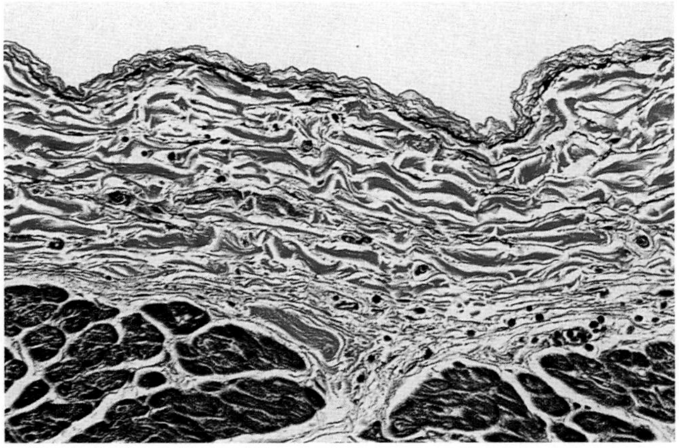

**FIG. 6.** Section of the endocardium showing the distribution of the elastic fibers (*black*) and the collagen bundles (*red*), as well as vessels and nerves in the subendocardial layer.

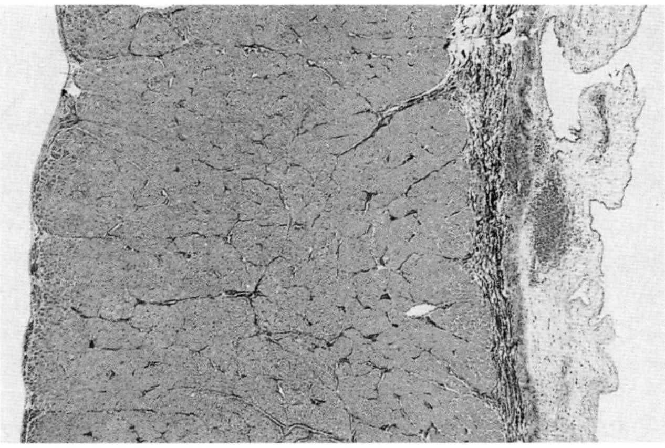

**FIG. 8.** Section through the right ventricular wall showing the distribution of collagen from the endocardium through the myocardium and to the epicardium in the normal heart (Masson's trichrome).

dothelial portion containing a loose elastic framework and collagen bundles as well as nerves and blood vessels (Fig. 6). All the changes of the heart are composed of these three layers, which vary only in thickness. A rudimentary layer of smooth muscle often is found in the endocardium of both atria and the ventricles (Fig. 7). The endocardium of the atria is thicker than that of the ventricles and usually contains smooth muscle, although the amount of smooth muscle is so small as to render questionable its functional significance. The myocardium consists of bundles of myocytes separated by fibrous bands (Fig. 8). The individual myocytes form a syncytium with end-to-end junctions called intercalated disks and sometimes side-to-side junctions. Individual myocytes contain a central ovoid nucleus with a clear zone at the poles (Fig. 9). The normal heart myocyte contains lipofuscin granules (lysosomes), which increase in quantity with age. The myocytes are filled with contractile myofibrils (actin and myosin). The myocardium of the atria also contains atrial dense-core bodies that can be seen only by electron microscopy (Fig. 10). The epicardial portion of the chamber walls was described earlier.

## Interatrial Septum

The interatrial septum separates the right and left atria. During development, the interatrial septum is formed from the embryonic septum primum and septum secundum, which are both incomplete. In the normal state, however, fusion of the two septae form a complete separation between the two atria, although the foramen ovale may remain anatomically open in approximately 31% of normal adult hearts (10,11). In the adult heart, traces of these two embryonic septa can be seen. The foramen ovale is closed by the septum secundum to form the fossa of the foramen ovale, which is about the size of a dime but is occasionally larger.

The thickness of the atrial septum varies considerably. The valve of the fossa ovale is a paper-thin translucent mem-

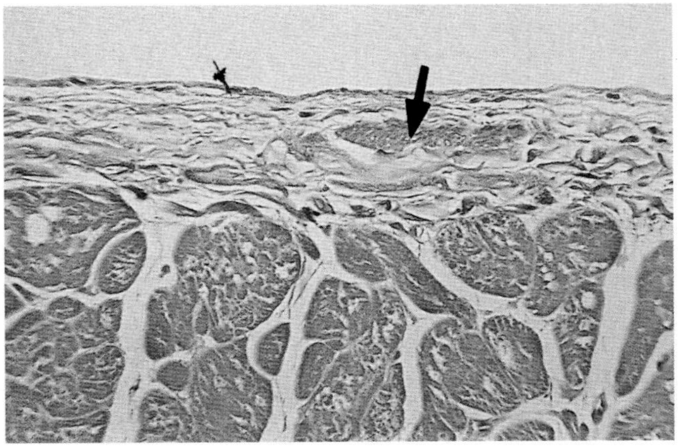

**FIG. 7.** Section of endocardium showing smooth muscle bundle (*arrow*) (Masson's trichrome).

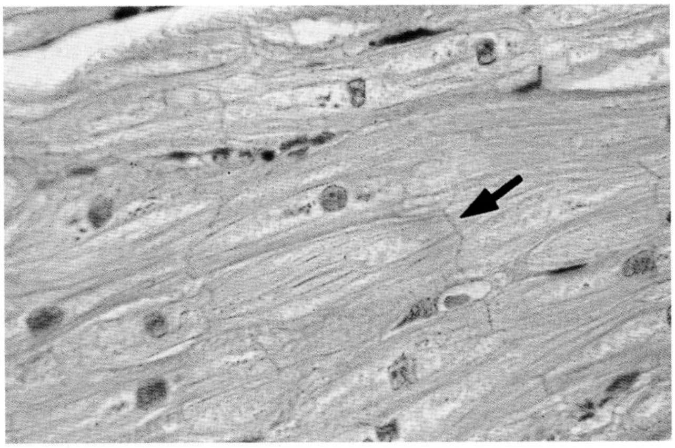

**FIG. 9.** Section of myocardium showing ovoid nuclei and intercalated disks (*arrow*) (H&E).

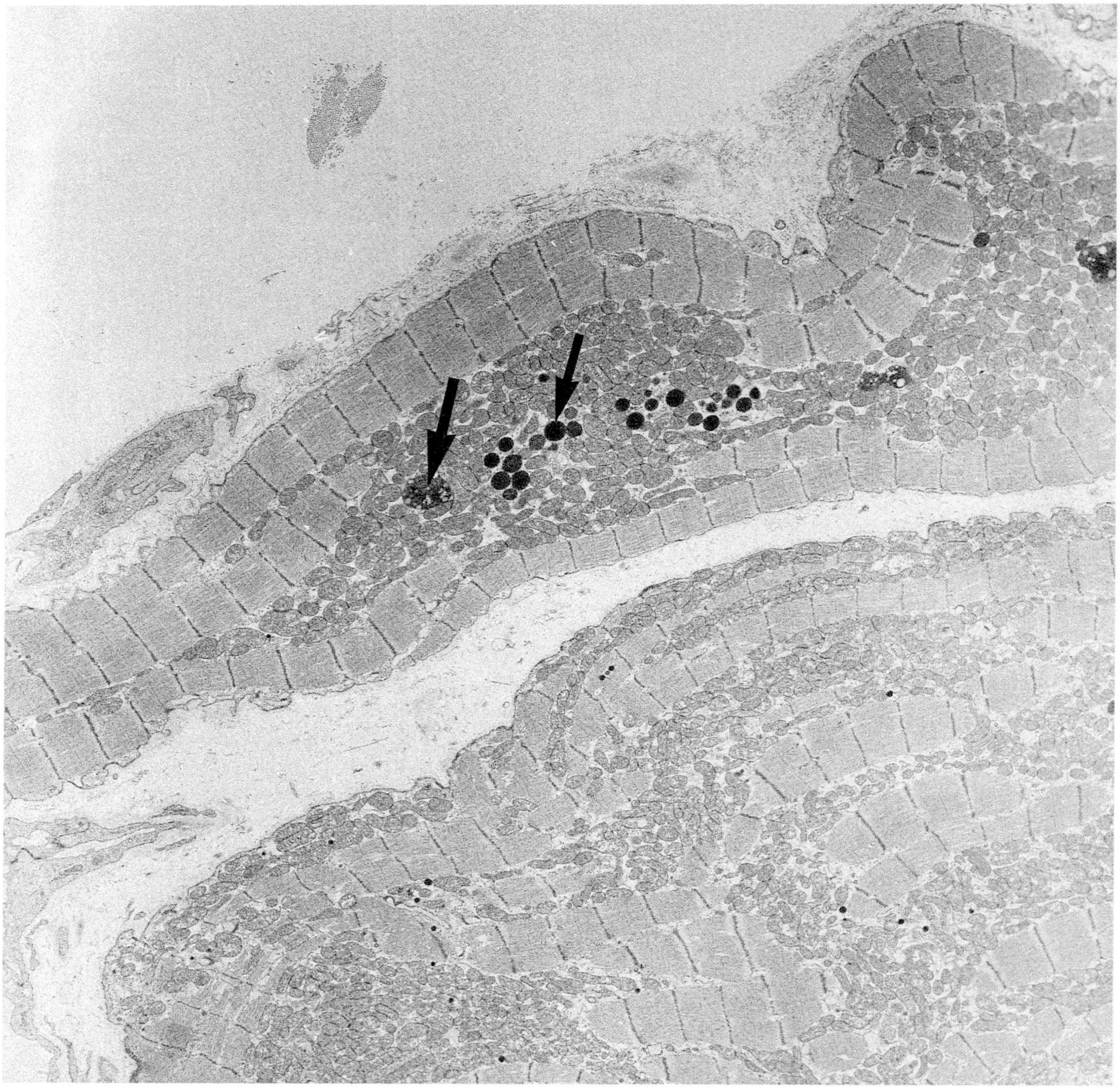

**FIG. 10.** Electron micrograph of atrial dense-care granules (*small arrow*) that can be differentiated from the lipofuscin granules (*large arrow*).

brane, but becomes more fibrotic with time and may achieve a thickness of 1 to 2 mm (8). Lipomatous hypertrophy may produce bulging of the interatrial septum. The histology of the interatrial septum, depending on where the sections are taken, shows varying amounts of atrial muscle, adipose tissue that often contains "brown fat," fetal adipose tissue, and fibrous tissue (Fig. 11).

## RIGHT ATRIUM

Venous return to the heart occurs via the inferior and superior vena cavae into the right atrium. The right atrium forms the right lateral cardiac border and is anterior to the left atrium as well as to the right of it. Anteromedially, the right atrial appendage protrudes from the right atrium and overlaps the aortic root (12). Extending between the right sides of the superior and inferior vena caval orifices is a prominent muscular ridge, the cristae terminalis, which underlies the sulcus terminalis. The interior of the right auricular appendage is trabeculated by muscular bands called the pectinate muscles. The portion of the right atrium lateral to the cristae terminalis is smooth and is derived embryologically from the sinus venosus (Fig. 11). The right atrial wall measures about 0.2 cm thick. The orifice of the superior vena cava has no valve. The orifice of the inferior vena cava has

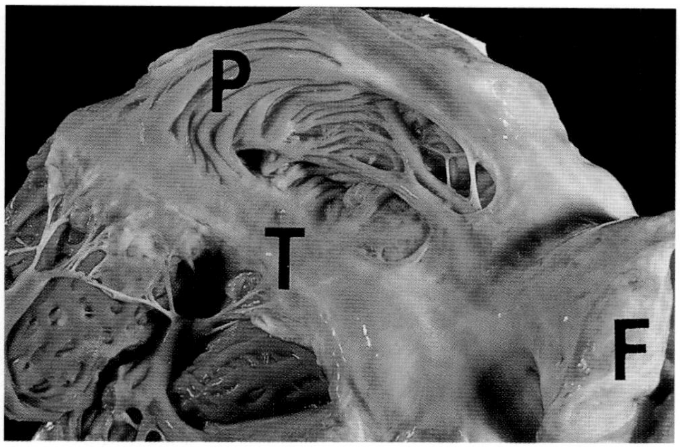


**FIG. 11.** The right atrium showing the pectinate muscles (P), the crista terminalis (T), and the interatrial septal fat (F).

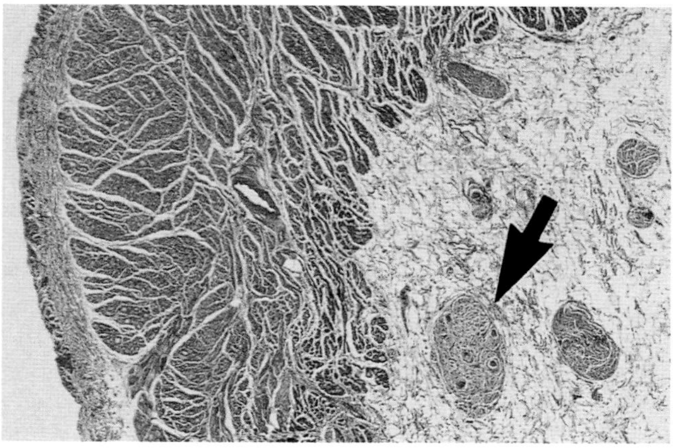

**FIG. 13.** Section through the right atrium showing the nerves and ganglion cells (*arrow*) in the overlying subepicardial adipose tissue (elastic Van Giesen).

an inconstant, rudimentary valve called the eustachian valve, which forms a crescentic fold. The coronary sinus opening located between the inferior vena cava and the tricuspid valve is also guarded by a rudimentary flap of tissue, the thebesian valve. These valves vary greatly in size and may be fenestrated or absent. A Chiari net, usually a lacelike veil of tissue, may be present in the normal heart, which represents a remnant of the right sinus venosus valve (Fig. 12). The left atrium is covered by endothelium, and in the subendocardium, elastic fibers pass into a typical fenestrated elastic membrane that contains blood vessels, nerves, and branches of the conducting system. In the spaces between the muscle bundles of the atria, the wall is so thin that the connective tissue of the endocardium blends with that of the epicardium. The epicardial surface of the atria is rich in nerves and ganglia (Fig. 13).

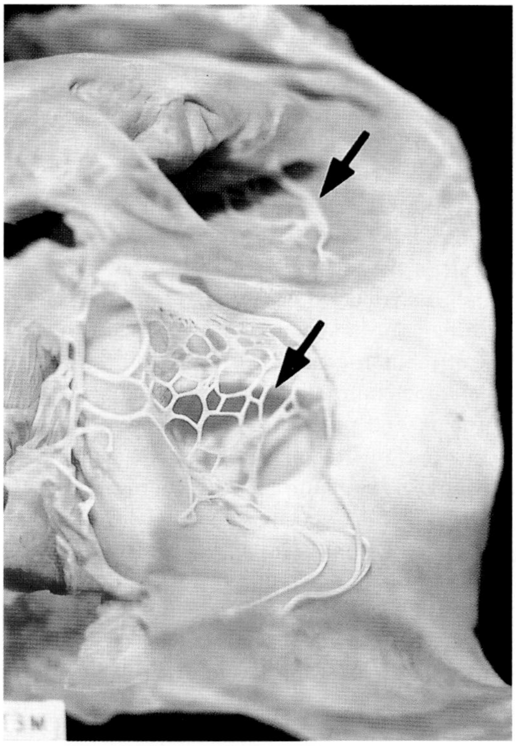

**FIG. 12.** Picture of the Chiari network or lacelike pattern of the remnants of the thebesian valve in the inferior vena cava opening into the right atrium.

## LEFT ATRIUM

The wall of the left atrium is 0.3 cm in average thickness and is slightly thicker than that of the right atrium (2). The luminal surface of the left atrium is smooth, being derived from the single pulmonary vein. The entrance of the four pulmonary veins and the entrance to the left atrial appendage open into the left atrium. The atrial appendage is lined by pectinate muscle similar to that of the right atrial appendage. The endothelium of the left atrium is thicker and more opaque than that of the right, thought to be due to the higher pressures of pulmonary veins emptying into the atrium. Sometimes a patch of thickened rough endocardium can be seen on the posterior wall superior to the mitral valve due to mitral regurgitation. This is called MacCullum's patch, but it is not usually seen in a normal heart. Two pulmonary veins enter posterolaterally on each side; there are no true valves at the junction of the pulmonary veins and the left atrium.

The atrial septum is smooth in the left atrium but may contain a central shallow area corresponding to the fossa ovale. The endocardium of the left atrium is thicker and contains more collagen than that of the right atrium, particularly near the entrance of the pulmonary valves. Otherwise the histology is similar to that on the right.

## RIGHT VENTRICLE

The right ventricle lies anterior to the other heart chambers. The anatomic right ventricle has an inflow portion (sinus) and an outflow portion (infundibulum conus) (13). The outflow tract is separated anatomically from the inflow tract by a muscular arch called the crista superventricularis. The luminal surface of the ventricle is coarsely trabeculated, and on sectioning the trabeculations form the inner two thirds of the ventricular wall. The septal surface of the right ventricle is deeply trabeculated with trabeculae carneae and a thick muscular column called the moderator band, which is present in many hearts and connects the distal portion of the septum to the free wall (Fig. 14). This band usually terminates in the area of the anterior papillary muscle. The right bundle branch travels through the muscular ventricular septum and courses down to end in the moderator muscle. The papillary muscles of the right ventricle are relatively constant, with an anterior papillary muscle on the anterior wall near its junction with its septum and a small papillary muscle arising under the crista superventricularis at the inferior border of the right ventricular outflow tract. In addition, there is an inconstant group of posterior papillary muscles rising from the diaphragmatic wall of the right ventricle. The histology of the right ventricle consists of a thin endocardial layer. In the adult this wall is thinner in comparison with that of the left ventricle, measuring only 4 to 5 mm in thickness. The endocardium is similar to that of the other chambers, except that the endocardial surface is variable in thickness, being slightly thicker on the septal wall. The subendocardial space includes the typical fenestrated elastic membrane, and bundles of smooth muscle may be found in this layer, particularly in the interventricular septum (Fig. 7). The interventricular septum also contains blood vessels, nerves, and the left bundle branch of the conducting system. The ventricular free wall has numerous vascular channels consisting of intertrabecular channels that lead into myocardial sinusoids and thebesian veins. Myocardial sinusoids are also found in the trabeculae. Arterioluminal vessels leading directly from the systemic coronary circulation into the capillary beds empty into the myocardial sinusoids. The myocardium is richly supplied with small vascular channels forming an intramural circulation (13). There is an extensive web of capillaries that course among the cardiac muscle fibers that are fed by branches of the coronary arteries and are drained in

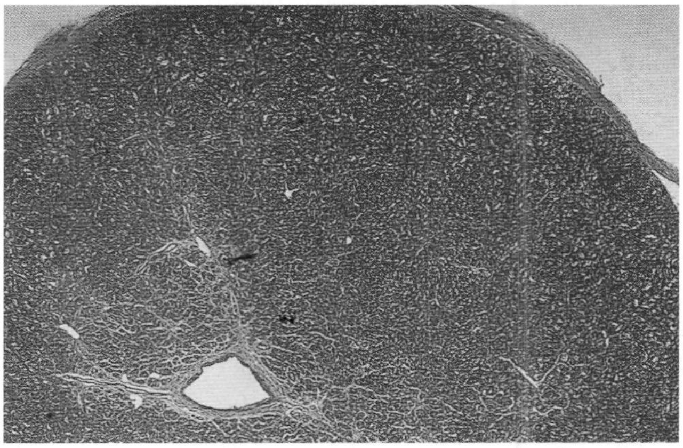

FIG. 14. A section of trabeculae carneae from the normal right ventricle.

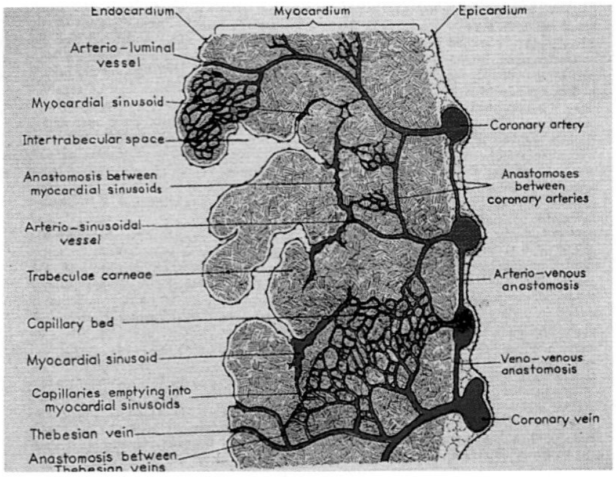


FIG. 15. Diagrammatic representation of the various intramural vascular channels. Reprinted with permission (13).

part by the coronary veins but also drain into the myocardial sinusoids and thence into the lumen of the heart. Deep within the myocardial musculature is, in addition to the capillary bed, a richly anastomosing network of irregular channels that have been called the myocardial sinusoids. These sinusoids receive vessels from the coronary arteries and the capillaries and communicate with coronary veins. The connections between the coronary arteries and the cardiac chambers are called arterioluminal vessels (Fig. 15).

## LEFT VENTRICLE

The left ventricle receives blood from the left atrium during ventricular diastole and ejects blood into the systemic arterial circulation through the aortic valve during ventricular systole. The left ventricle is somewhat bullet shaped, with the blunt tip directed anteriorly and inferiorly and to the left (12). The left ventricular chamber is surrounded by a thick muscular wall measuring 8 to 15 mm or approximately two to three times the thickness of the right ventricular wall. The medial wall of the left ventricle is the interventricular septum, which is shared with the right ventricle. The septum is roughly triangular in shape, with the base of the triangle at the level of the aortic cusps; it is entirely muscular, except for the small membranous septum located just below the right coronary and posterior cusps. The upper third of the septum, the outflow tract, is smooth endocardium. The inferior two thirds of the septum and remaining ventricular walls are composed of the trabeculae carneae. The free wall of the left ventricle is that portion that is exclusive of the septum. The histology of the left ventricle is similar to that of the right, although the endocardium is slightly thicker because of the higher hemodynamic pressures. The small arterioles subjacent to the endocardium have slightly thicker walls than those of the right ventricle, most likely due to the higher pressure in the left ventricle. The myocardium of the left ventricle is arranged in such a way that it appears to spiral inward from the superficial layers. The superficial layers run at right angles to the layers deeper in the wall. These layers are intimately interdigitated to prevent dissection into lamina structures. The attachment of the muscular layers is from the fibroskeleton at the base of the heart. The deeper muscle layers of the interventricular septum are composed of the deep bulbospiral muscle in the center of the septum originating from the septal portion of the atrial ventricular annulus. The fascicles of the deep bulbospiral and sinospiral muscles interdigitate in the muscular interventricular septum. The spiral muscle on contraction pulls the base of the ventricle toward the apex. The blood supply and histology of the left ventricle is similar to that of the right ventricle.

### Applied Anatomy

Portions of the left ventricular subaortic outflow tract may be submitted as myomectomy specimens in hypertrophic cardiomyopathy. Portions of the left ventricular free wall may be removed as aneurysectomy specimens or to insert left ventricular assist pumps. The intermediate bulbospiral muscle of the interventricular septum is that which is primarily involved in idiopathic hypertrophy subaortic stenosis (IHSS), and because it lies deep in the septum, the myocyte disarray associated with IHSS may not always be seen in the superficial myomectomy specimen.

## CARDIAC VALVES

### Semilunar Valves

The semilunar valves consist of the pulmonary valve and the aortic valve. The normal valve circumference for the aortic valve is 5.7 to 7.9 cm for women and 6.0 to 8.5 cm for men (2). The normal pulmonic valve circumference is 5.7 to 7.4 cm for women and 9.2 to 9.9 cm for men (2). Each semilunar valve consists of three semicircular cusps (9). Each cusp is attached by its semicircular border to the aortic or pulmonary ring. The three points of lateral attachment of adjacent cusps are the commissures (Fig. 16). The lines of cusp apposition are not at the free margin, but angulated lines extending from well below the point of attachment in the commissure to just below the midpoint of the free edge. In the aortic valve these lines (the linea alba) and the central nodules (the noduli arentii) can be seen (9). In the pulmonary valve these landmarks are less obvious because of the lower right-sided pressures. The lunulae are thin, delicate areas of cusp between the linear alba and the free edge. The semilunar aortic and pulmonary valves are similar in configuration, except that the aortic cusps are slightly thicker and they contain the coronary ostia. They are situated at the summit at the outflow tract of their corresponding ventricle, the pulmonary valve being anterior, superior, and slightly to the left of the aortic valve in the normal heart. The cusps that are often slightly unequal in width circle the inside of the respective vessel root (pulmonary artery or aorta). Behind each cusp, the vessel wall bulges outward, forming a pouchlike dilatation known as the sinus of Valsalva. The portion of the cusp adjacent to the rim is thin and may contain small perforations even in the normal situation. The noduli arentii meet in the center and contribute to the support of the leaflets. Because the plane of the aortic valve is oblique with the right posterior side lower than the left anterior side, the origin of the left coronary artery is slightly superior to that of the right coronary artery. The ostia of the coronary arteries are located in the upper third of their respective sinuses. The right coronary artery passes anteriorly and to the left. In some hearts, there is a separate ostium in the right coronary sinus for the conus artery, sometimes called the third coronary artery (12).

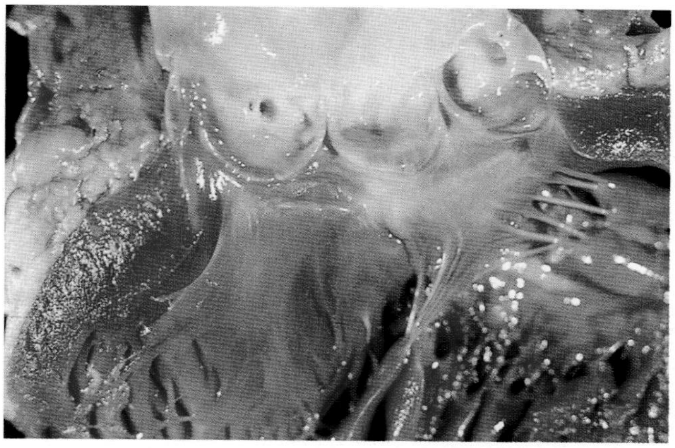

**FIG. 16.** Aortic valve from normal heart showing the cusps and the coronary ostia.

The histology of the semilunar valves is that of a well-defined layered structure. Three layers are recognizable: the fibrosa, the spongiosa, and the ventricularis. These layers are similar in distribution in the aortic and pulmonic valves but are thinner and more delicate in the pulmonic valve. The fibrosa is a layer of dense collagen that constitutes the major structural component of the cusp and extends to its free edge (14). The densely packed bundles of collagen blend into the collagen of the valvular ring in the region of the commissures. Some fibroblasts are present in this layer, as are some very fine elastic fibers. The spongiosa is subjacent to the fibrosa and occupies a central position in the thickness of the cusp (Fig. 17). It is best developed in the basal third of the cusp. It does not extend to the free edge, which is composed only of the fibrosis and ventricularis. The spongiosa is histologically similar to that of the atrioventricular valves, being composed of large amounts of proteoglycan, loosely arranged collagen fibrils and scattered fibroblasts, and poorly differentiated mesenchymal cells (14). The ventricularis is subjacent to the spongiosa and is in direct contact with the endothelial layer of the inflow surface of the cusp. The ventricularis is distinguished by its richness in elastic fibers, which are larger and more numerous than in the fibrosa. This feature is helpful in identifying the layers of excised aortic valvular cusps. The surface lining of the aortic cusps consists of a single layer of endothelial cells. The surface topography

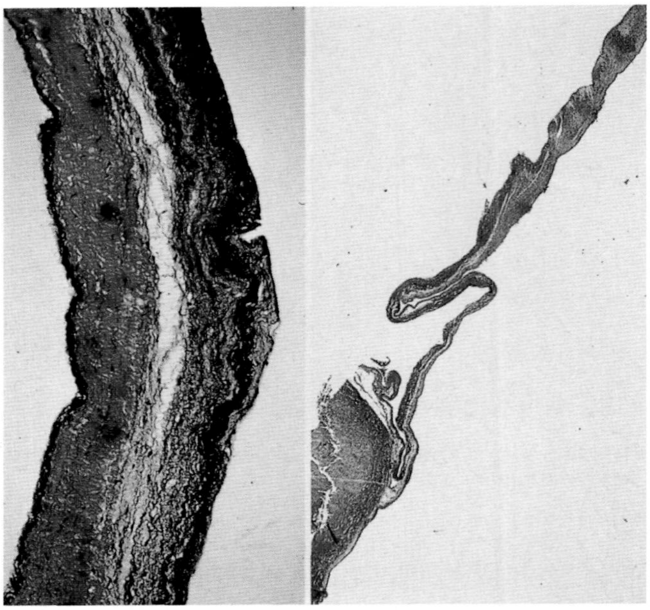

**FIG. 17.** High- and low-power views of a section of the aortic cusp showing the three distinct layers as described in the text.

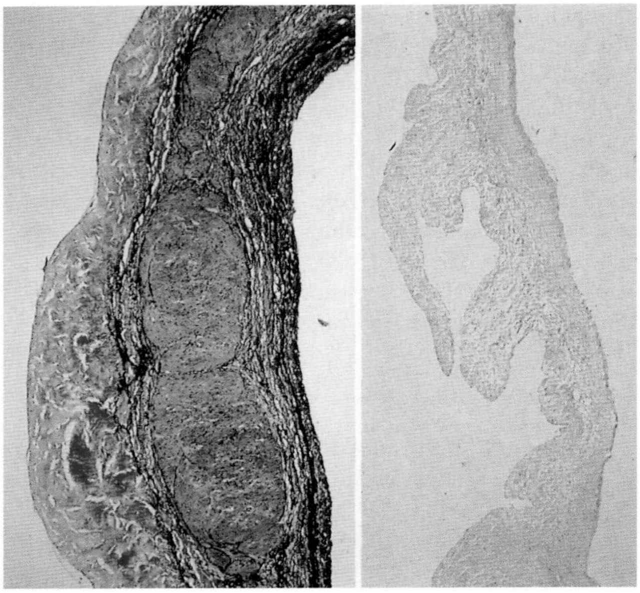

**FIG. 18.** High- and low-power views of a section of the mitral leaflet showing the three distinct layers with muscle in the central portion near the base of the valve.

of the aortic cusp varies according to its state of stress. The bundles are wavy, and the inflow surface is smoother in the stressed state and rougher in the relaxed state (14).

### Atrioventricular Valves

The atrioventricular valves consist of the mitral valve and the tricuspid valve. The normal circumference for the tricuspid valve is 10 to 11.1 cm in women and 11.2 to 11.8 cm in men (2). The normal valve circumference for the mitral valve is 8.2 to 9.1 cm for women and 9.2 to 9.9 cm for men (2). The mitral valvular apparatus is made up of the annulus, leaflets, chordae tendineae, and papillary muscles. The annulus is composed of a ring of circumferentially oriented collagen and elastic fibers with extensions into the ventricle and atrium. The artioventricular valves also are composed of three layers (Fig. 18). The collagen bundles of the annulus spread down into the cusp of the mitral valve and are known as the fibrosa, which continue on into the chordae tendineae and finally spread out into a network that covers the tip of the papillary muscles (Fig. 19). The ventricular aspect of the fibrosa is covered by the ventricularis and the ventricular surface endothelium. The ventricularis contains many elastic fibers and is immediately subjacent to the endothelium covering the ventricular outflow surface of the leaflet. Some of the elastic fibrils extend into the chordae tendineae. The atrial aspect of the fibrosa is covered by the spongiosa, which contains abundant proteoglycans, few elastic fibers, and some collagen fibrils and connective tissue cells (14). This layer extends through the entire length of the leaflet. The spongiosa in the anterior and posterior mitral leaflets contains cardiac muscle cells that are a direct extension of the left atrial myocardium (14) (Fig. 18). In the anterior mitral leaflet, this layer extends into the middle third; the posterior leaflet extends only into its proximal third. Neural elements can be found throughout the valve leaflets, as can lymphatics. The atrial aspect of the spongiosa is covered by the auricularis layer, which is directly subjacent to the endothelium of the atrial surface of the leaflet. The auricularis layer contains elastic fibers and smooth muscle cells and thins out in the distal third of the leaflet so that the distal portions of the leaflet are composed only of fibrosa and spongiosa. The endocardial endothelial cells on the atrial surface of the mitral and tricuspid leaflet are plump and have large irregular nuclei. The architecture of the tricuspid valve ap-

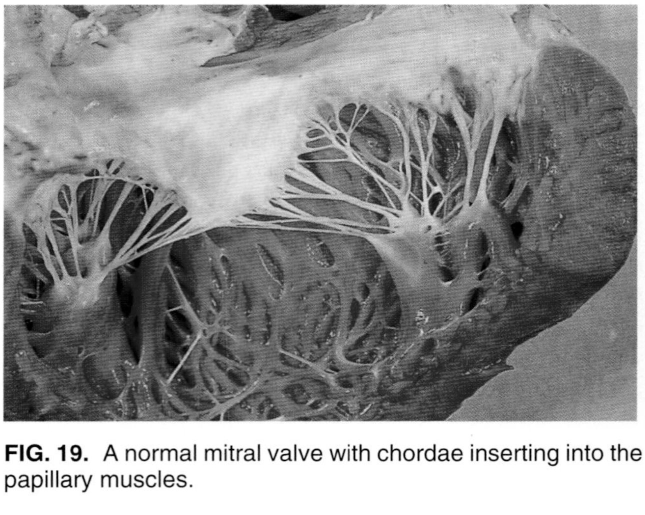

**FIG. 19.** A normal mitral valve with chordae inserting into the papillary muscles.

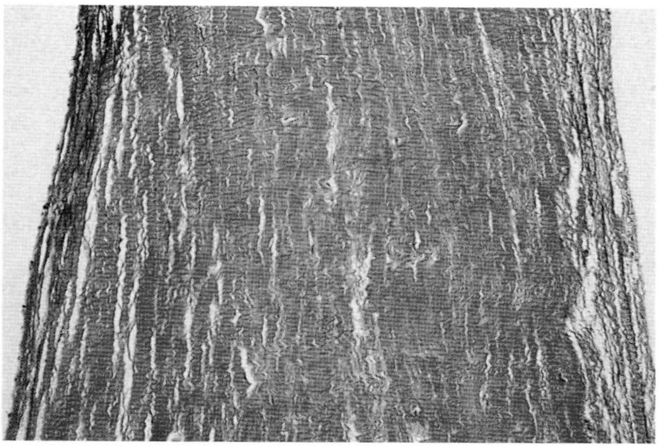

**FIG. 20.** Longitudinal section of chordae showing the relationships of elastic fibers on the surface and collagen in the center (elastic Van Giesen).

paratus and the layered arrangement of the tricuspid valve leaflets are generally similar to those in the mitral valve; however, the individual layers are thinner in the tricuspid valve. Cardiac muscle bundles insert fairly low into the base of the tricuspid leaflets but do not extend into the leaflet substance. In the posterior and septal leaflets the auricularis is thicker and contains more abundant smooth muscle cells.

### The Chordae Tendineae

The chordae in the normal state are thin fibrous cords that emanate in a fanlike shape from the broad leaflets of the tricuspid and mitral valves and insert into the papillary muscles (Fig. 19). The central cores of the chordae are composed of longitudinally oriented collagen fibrils. The core is surrounded more peripherally with more loosely arranged collagen fibrils and elastic fibers and is associated with proteoglycan material (14) (Fig. 20). Some chordae contain a small

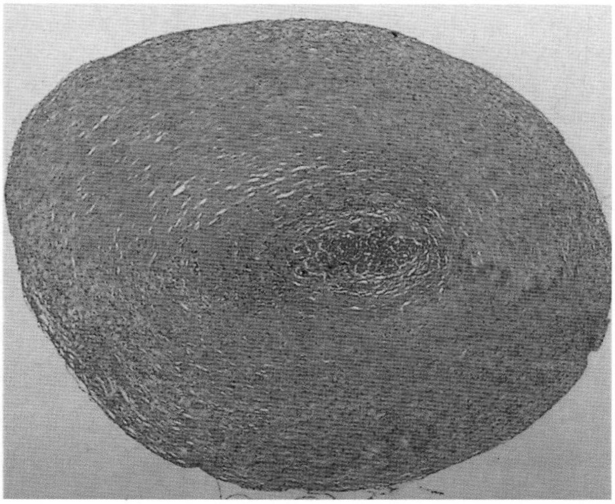

**FIG. 21.** Transverse section of chordae showing central core of muscle (H&E).

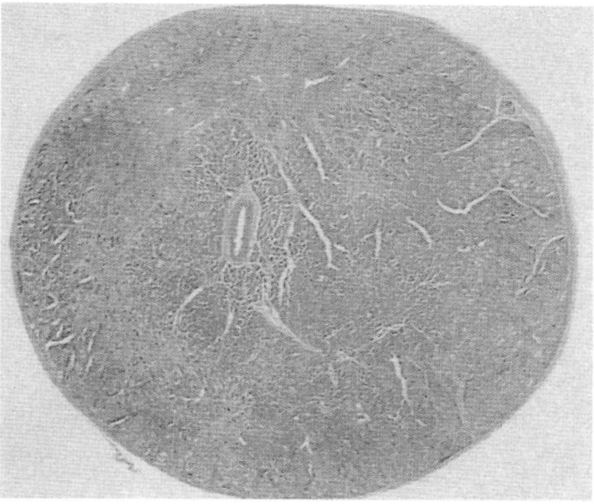

**FIG. 22.** Transverse section of a muscular chordae showing fibrous tissue, muscle, and small vessel within the chordae (Masson's trichrome).

central core of muscle (Fig. 21), although others contain blood vessels and collagen in variable amounts and are fleshier (Fig. 22). The endothelial cells on the ventricular surface and on the chordae tendineae have flattened ovoid nuclei.

### Applied Anatomy of Intracardiac Valves

Surgical pathologists get specimens of semilunar and atrioventricular valves for a variety of pathologic reasons. When removed the specimens usually contain chordae and portions of papillary muscle. Ruptured papillary muscles may become surgical specimens. Chordae and the leaflets may be involved with proliferation of central mucopolysaccharide material in floppy valve syndrome.

### Aging Changes of Intracardiac Valves

All the cardiac valves become thicker, more opaque, and less pliable with age. The collagen content is increased, and calcification may occur. The posterior leaflet of the mitral valves often shows yellow atheromatous changes. The mitral annulus may become calcified with age.

## PAPILLARY MUSCLES

Two papillary muscles of the right ventricle (anterior and conal) are relatively constant. There are also a group of inconstant posterior papillary muscles on the inferior wall. In the left ventricle there are two constant papillary muscles: the anterior and posterior. The papillary muscles receive the chordae. The papillary muscles are variable in shape and width and sometimes have multiple heads (Fig. 19).

The histology of the papillary muscles includes the fibrous

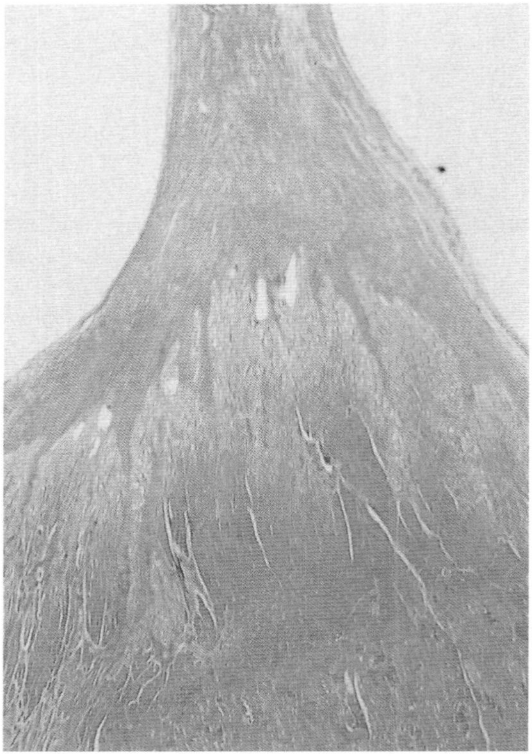

**FIG. 23.** Longitudinal section of papillary muscle showing the fibrous cap of the insertion of the chordae (Masson's trichrome).

cap, into which the chordae insert (Fig. 23). The papillary muscle arterioles are notable for the vessel wall thickness and irregularity as compared with other intracardiac small vessels (Fig. 24). The myocardium and endocardial covering is similar to that described elsewhere. In marked ventricular dilatation, the papillary muscles may become thinned and flattened.

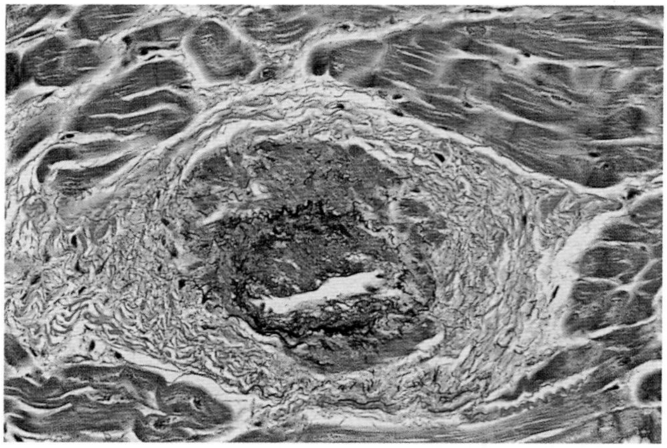

**FIG. 24.** Section of abnormally thickened arteriole within a papillary muscle (elastic Van Giesen).

## CONDUCTION SYSTEM

Mammalian myocardium contains two cell lines, the contractile myocardial fibers and myocardial fibers specialized for the initiation and conduction of an impulse for contraction (15). The conduction system is now recognized to be myogenic; nerves play only a subsidiary controlling function.

### Sinoatrial Node

It is now established that the primary pacemaker of the human heart having the highest inherent rate is the sinoatrial (SA) node (16). This node is situated at the junction of the superior vena cava and the lateral border of the right atrium. Its position is constant and marked by the apex of the crest of the atrial appendage. Histologic sectioning shows the node to be arranged around a central artery and to be immediately beneath the pericardium. The node is made up of dense connective tissue in which small muscle fibers are embedded. The muscle fibers contain sparse myofibrils, the striations are not prominent, and the whole mass has a pseudosyncytial appearance. Abundant nerve fibers run into the node. Several specialized bundles of conducting system cells conduct the impulse around the atrium. The anterior internodal tract runs anterior to the superior vena cava (Bachmann's tract). The remainder runs into the interatrial septum to join the atrioventricular (AV) node. The middle internodal tract passes behind the superior vena cava into the interatrial septum and the posterior tract and follows the crista terminalis to the AV node.

### Atrioventricular Node

The AV node lies on the right side of the interatrial septum just anterior to the opening of the coronary sinus and

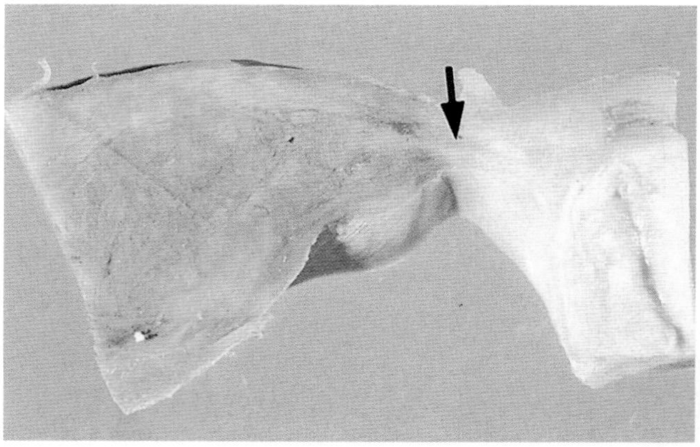

**FIG. 25.** Gross picture of the AV node (*arrow*) between the ventricle and atrium.

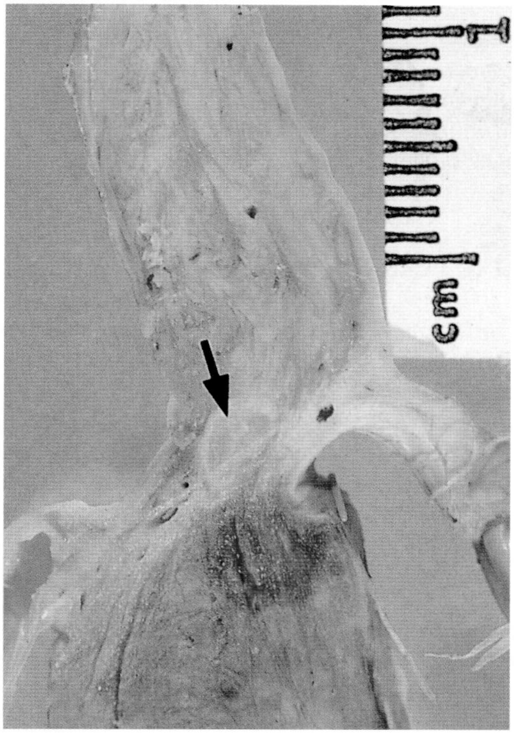


FIG. 26. Longitudinal section through the common bundle of His (*arrow*) and its relationship with the mitral and aortic valve.

posterior to the membranous intraventricular septum (16). The node is immediately subendocardial and lies above the insertion of the tricuspid valve (Fig. 25). The node is adjacent to the central fibrous body and is made up of a network of muscle fibers, with the superficial zone having fibers arranged in a parallel manner. In the anterior end of the AV node, the muscle fibers become arranged in parallel lines, forming the main bundle of His. To reach the ventricle, the main bundle pierces the central fibrous body of the heart and runs forward on the upper margin of the muscular ventricular septum. This penetrating portion of main bundle is surrounded by dense connective tissue and anatomically is closely related to the aortic and mitral valve rings (Fig. 26). The muscle fibers of the main bundle are arranged in parallel. The main bundle terminates as the left and right bundle branches (Fig. 27). The left fascicle runs downward over the endocardial surface of the interventricular septum, and the right bundle remains as a single discrete muscle bundle (Fig. 28) and runs downward and forward in the right ventricular septum to the base of the anterior papillary muscle and into the moderator band. Direct connection of both bundle branches to a complex ramifying system of subendocardial conduction fibers can be demonstrated in mammalian hearts. Light microscopy shows the fibers in the bundle of His and the conduction bundles to be small and contain few myofibrils (Fig. 29). Large Purkinje cells (transitional cells between ordinary contractile muscle cells and conducting muscle) are present only in small numbers. Purkinje cells are distin-

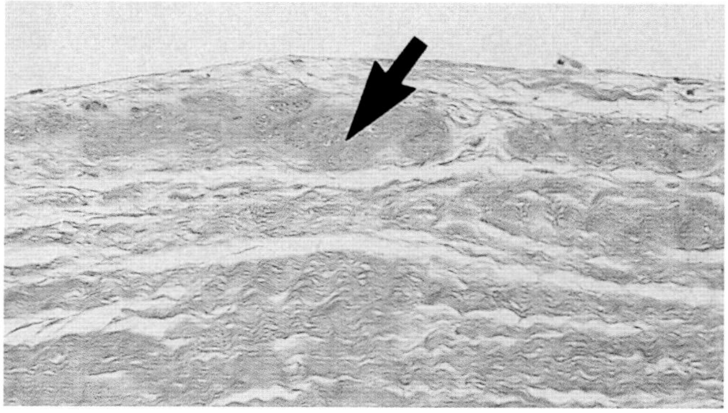

FIG. 28. Section showing the right bundle branch (*arrow*) in the subendocardium of the right ventricle (Masson's trichrome).

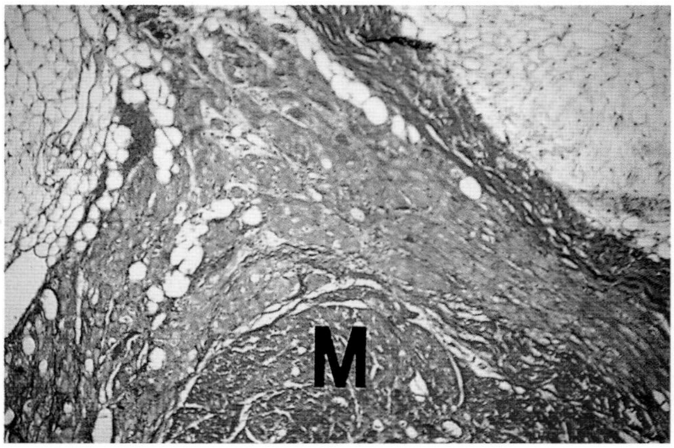


FIG. 27. Microscopic section showing the splitting of the common bundle into left and right bundles at the superior pole interventricular septum (M) (Masson's trichrome).

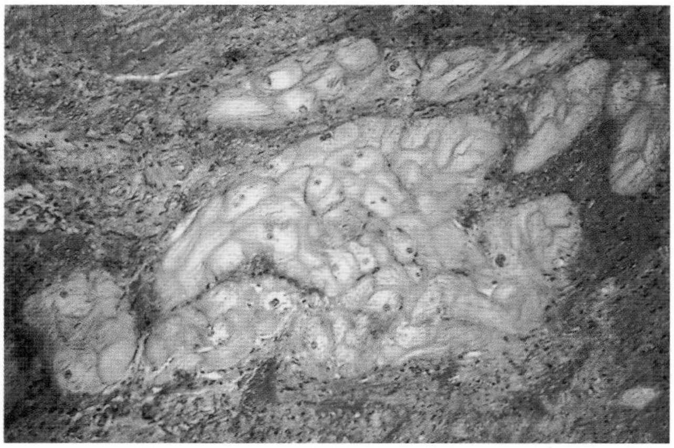

FIG. 29. Section showing the pale cells of the mammalian conducting system. These cells contain glycogen and only sparse myofibrils (Masson's trichrome).

guished from ventricular myocytes by their lack of t tubules on electron microscopy. The histology of the bundle branches is therefore inhomogeneous. No clear evidence exists on either a histochemical or ultrastructural level as to the mode of connection between the terminal Purkinje fibers and the contractile myocardial cells.

### Aging Changes in the Human Conduction System

With advancing age the SA node shows a progressive increase in fibrous tissue (16). In normal subjects over 70 years of age a significant loss of nodal muscle occurs and the internodal atrial tract shows similar changes. Significant loss with age has not been observed in the AV node. Similarly with advancing age, fibrous tissue increases in the upper portion of the interventricular septum, and these changes are associated with the loss of conduction fibers in the origin of the left bundle branch. Up to 50% of the left bundle origin may be lost in subjects over 60 years of age (16).

## CARDIAC INNERVATION

The nerve supply of the heart is autonomic, including both sympathetic and parasympathetic supply via both the effer-

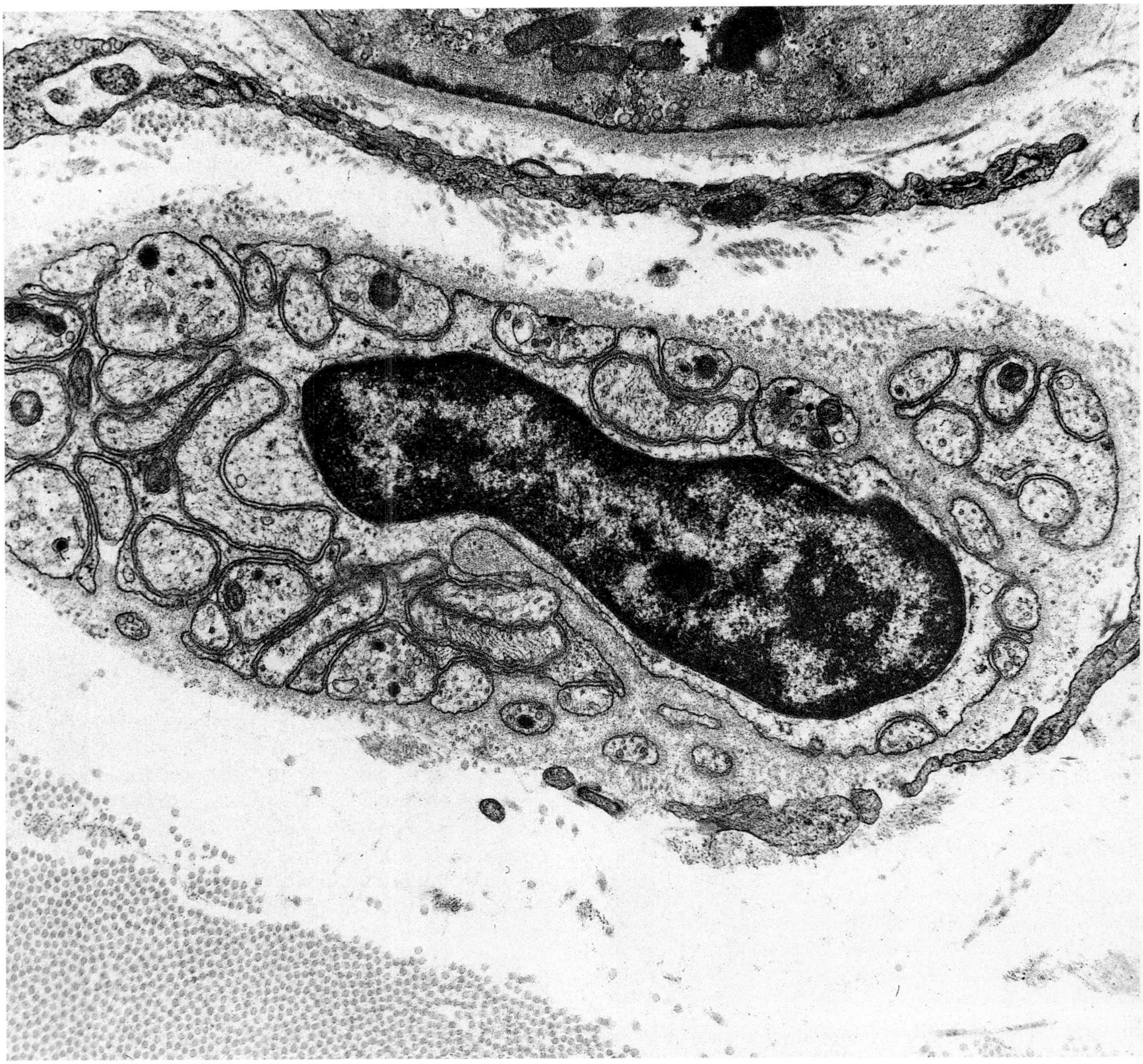

**FIG. 30.** Electron micrograph of sympathetic nerve showing dense-core granules in the myocardium (original magnification ×**22,500**).

ent and afferent fibers. Histologically, large nerves can be seen in the epicardium and adjacent to the coronary blood vessels. Small nerves within the myocardium are hard to see unless special stains are used. Myocardial nerves are best viewed using electron microscopic examination, via which the autonomic nerves can be distinguished. Cardiac ganglia (parasympathetic) can be found over the surface of the atria and in the AV groove (Fig. 13).

### Autonomic Nerves

Axonal varicosities occur at irregular intervals along autonomic fibers, and their morphology is considered useful in determining whether the nerve is adrenergic or cholinergic (14). In cholinergic nerves, the varicosities contain accumulations of agranular vesicles and a few mitochondria. In adrenergic nerves the varicosities contain vesicles that have electron-dense cores. Each of these cores is separated from the limiting membrane of the vesicle by an electron-lucent zone (Fig. 30). Presumptive sensory nerve terminals have large diameters and contain many mitochondria. They are located in perivascular regions and are surrounded by Schwann cells. A given Schwann cell may enclose adrenergic and cholinergic axons together with sensory axons (14). Autonomic ganglia are found in the subepicardial tissue of the atria, atrial appendages, and roots of the great vessels, along the interatrial and AV groove in the atrial septum and in the vicinity of the SA and AV nodes. Large nerves can be seen in the subepicardial layer adjacent to the epicardial coronary arteries.

## LYMPHATICS

There are two networks of lymphatics in the heart: (a) in the endocardium and (b) in the epicardium. The endocardial network drains through channels in the myocardium into the lymphatics of the epicardium. Epicardial meshwork of channels containing many valves drains toward the AV sulcus by means of several longitudinal channels that run for the most part parallel to the coronary veins in the anterior and posterior longitudinal sulci of the ventricles (14). Lymphatics leave the pericardial cavity to empty into one of the bronchial lymph nodes and join the lymphatic drainage system of the mediastinum. Lymphatics also are seen in the myocardial valves. The lymphatics also lie in the grooves of the coronary blood vessels.

### Histology

The lymph capillaries and larger lymphatic vessels accompany blood vessels in the myocardial interstitium. The walls of the myocardial lymphatics consist of extremely thin endothelial cells, the nuclei of which bulge into the lumen (Fig. 31). In contrast to endothelial cells of blood capillaries, those of the lymphatic capillaries do not have a well-defined external basal lamina. The endothelial cells of lymphatic capillaries may have Weibel Palade bodies and transport vesicles (14). The larger lymphatics are confined to the outer third of the myocardial wall and occasionally contain valves. These are flaplike structures consisting of a core of collagen embedded in microfibrils and covered by endothelial cells.

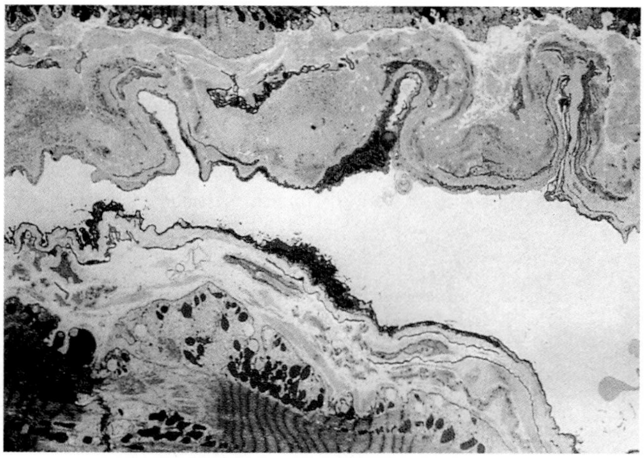

**FIG. 31.** Electron micrograph showing an intramyocardial lymphatic with thin walls and no basement membrane (original magnification ×**20,000**).

## SMALL INTRAMURAL CORONARY ARTERIES

The structure of the intramural coronary arteries is similar to that of the larger coronary arteries and consists of the endothelial, smooth muscle, and adventitia (Fig. 32). These smallest muscular arteries contain three or four layers of smooth muscle cells; with a further decrease in size they become arterioles (14). Arterioles have flat elongated endothelial cells that do not protrude into the lumen. Their internal elastic lamina is discontinuous. Metarterioles also are known as precapillary sphincters. The endothelial cells in metarterioles have numerous surface projections that bulge into the

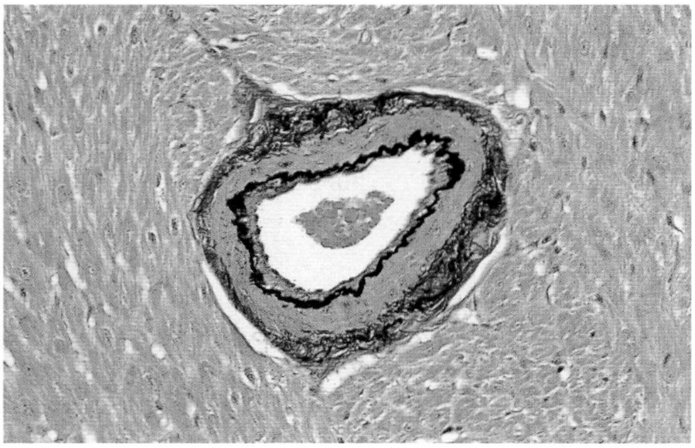

**FIG. 32.** Transverse section of intramyocardial arteriole (elastic Van Giesen).

lumen (14). Although the medial smooth muscle cells form a single discontinuous layer, it gradually disappears as capillaries begin. Capillaries are distinguished by the fact that their walls are composed of only a single layer of endothelial cells. They do not have smooth muscle cells but may have closely associated pericytes (14). Capillary endothelial cells may have microvilli and cytoplasmic processes (filopodia) (Fig. 33). The myocardium has a rich network of capillaries (14).

The capillaries branch and anastomose and eventually become venules that are thin walled and up to 100 $\mu$m in diameter.

**Veins and Venules**

Venules have thin, flat endothelial cells and characteristically contain a large amount of connective tissue in the vicinity of their external surface. Venules have collagen fibrils that approach the endothelial layer and are anchored on its outer surface (14). Venules gradually increase in size to become veins. Veins have larger lumens and are thinner walled than the corresponding arteries. Veins also have three layers: (a) the intima, (b) the media, and (c) the adventitia. The intima is thin, lacks smooth muscle, and has a poorly defined internal elastic lamina. The media is also thin and contains

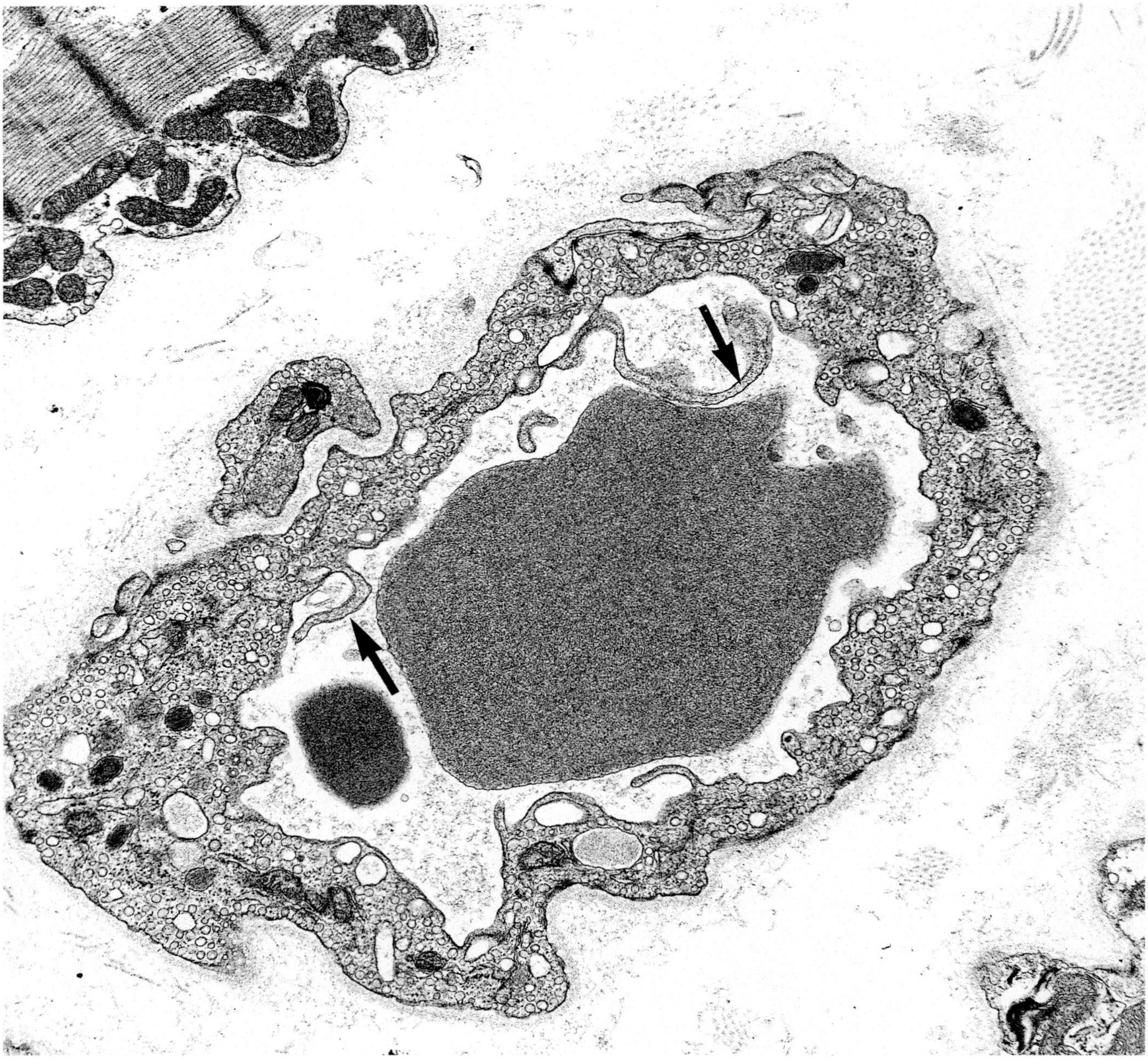

**FIG. 33.** Electron micrography of a capillary showing transport vesicles within the wall and filopodia (*arrows*) (original magnification ×**18,750**).

few smooth muscles and elastic fibers. The adventitia is thick and contains abundant collagen and fine elastic fibers.

## SPECIAL TECHNIQUES AND PROCEDURES

### Dissection Method for an Adult Heart

There are many good descriptions for opening the heart at autopsy included in most autopsy manuals (2,17). However, it is important that before cutting open the heart the prosector should take into consideration the expected lesion (in an abnormal or pathologic heart) so as to open the heart to provide the best exposure for that lesion and also not to damage or disturb important relationships (e.g., the position of an implanted cardiac pacemaker). Special procedures may be undertaken before opening the heart, such as plain radiography to show calcification in the coronary arteries or valve cusps or postmortem coronary angiography (2). Perfusion fixation (with controlled pressure) is effective for some congenital heart lesions or where documentation of chamber size is required. Examination of the conduction system also requires a different approach (15). The attachments of the vessels to the heart should be carefully examined to rule out congenital lesions (e.g., transposition of the great vessels), persistent ductus arteriosus, or anomalous venous return. Before excising the heart, a pericardial fluid sample for culture or cytology may be taken. If blood cultures are necessary, they should be taken from the right ventricle or inferior vena cava after searing. To remove the heart after the pericardium has been opened, it should be held up and toward the head while each of the vascular connections are severed (inferior vena cava, pulmonary veins, aorta and pulmonary artery) 2.0 cm above their valves. The superior vena cava should be severed last (2).

The external surface of the heart should be visualized carefully, as should the epicardial surface of the coronary arteries. To open the heart a cut should be made from the right atrium, through the tricuspid valve along the lateral wall of the right ventricle to the apex, then continued along the anterior interventricular septum wall through the pulmonary valve. This will display the right atrium, tricuspid valve, right ventricle chamber, outflow tract, pulmonary valve, and pulmonary artery, all of which can be examined.

The left side of the heart should be opened by making one transverse incision to expose the left atrial appendage and then another incision at right angles through the mitral valve along the posterior lateral wall of the left ventricle to the apex. From the apex an incision opening the left ventricular outflow tract should be made parallel and adjacent to the anterior interventricular septum through the aortic valve and up the left side of the aorta. The coronary arteries can now be examined. It is preferable to examine the coronaries by transverse sections through the vessels at 3-mm intervals either on or removed from the heart. The opened heart, with postmortem clot removed, can now be weighed, and measurements of ventricular and septal wall thickness, as well as of valvular rings, can be made. Useful tables on measurements and weights can be found in Ludwig's *Current Methods of Autopsy Practice* (17).

### Special Specimen Handling

Specimen handling depends very much on what is being looked for but some common examples are listed below:

1. Coronary artery specimens are best cut transversely and should be placed in a decalcification solution before processing if calcified (also calcified valves).
2. In sections of myocardium suspected of being ischemic, a fresh slice of myocardium can be incubated with tetrazolium salts (18).
3. If color photography is required, it can be performed on the fresh specimen or after fixing with Klotz solution to retain color. After fixation in formalin, if color restoration is required it may be obtained by fixing the specimen in alcohol. An excellent guide to photography of the heart is described by Edwards (19).
4. If a heart is to be stored as an anatomic specimen, it should be placed in Kaiserling III solution instead of 10% buffered formalin. Recipes for these solutions may be found in Ludwig's autopsy manual (17).
5. Specimens of heart also can be preserved via a plastination method (20). This has the advantage of easy storage, and the heart can be handled indefinitely without wear and tear.
6. Myocardium requiring electron microscopy (e.g., tumors, anthracycline or other cardiotoxicities, or mitochondrial abnormalities) should be freshly minced in 2- to 3-mm cubes and fixed immediately in 2% buffered glutaraldehyde for later plastic embedding. Because myocardium contracts, room temperature fixative is preferred.
7. In the event of microabscesses or other suspected infections, pieces of myocardium can be placed in culture medium and sent to the Infectious Disease Laboratory. Likewise, fresh (refrigerated or frozen) myocardium can be used to culture suspected viral infection. Staining fixed tissue with Gomori's silver stain is useful for fungal infections.
8. If a glycogen storage disease is expected, the myocardial sections should be fixed in Carnoy's medium to preserve the glycogen for histology.
9. If amyloid is suspected, obviously the tissue should be stained with Congo red or fresh frozen tissue with thioflavine T and viewed under ultraviolet light. Electron microscopy is the most reliable way to confirm amyloid in the heart. Light chain studies on frozen tissue also are sometimes required for amyloid-type distinction.
10. Nowadays, fresh frozen tissue should be set aside for studies requiring polymerase chain reaction or immunohistochemistry, although some of these studies can now be performed on formalin-fixed tissue.

11. In the case of a cardiac transplantation, the heart can be removed from the body in the same way as described above, making sure to include both donor and recipient myocardium around the suture lines. The heart should be examined carefully for opportunistic infection and graft coronary disease as well as for acute rejection.

In conclusion, normal development and knowledge of the gross anatomy of the human heart is necessary for all pathologists and cardiologists. The histopathology and knowledge of the ultrastructural profiles of the heart also are useful and important in a diagnostic sense. Newer techniques and better ways to examine the heart microscopically for genetic and other markers are emerging that promise to give new insights into the causes of myocardial diseases.

## REFERENCES


1. Hosenpud JD, Novick RJ, Green TJ, Keck B, Daily P. The Registry of the International Society for Heart and Lung Transplantation: 12th Official Report, 1995. *J Heart Lung Transplant* 1995;14:805–815.
2. Silver MM, Freedom RM. Gross examination and structure of the heart. In: Silver MM, ed. *Cardiovascular pathology.* 2nd ed. Vol. 1, New York: Churchill Livingston; 1991.
3. Kitzman DW, Scholz DG, Hager PT, Ilstrup DM, Edwards WD. Age-related changes in normal human hearts during the first 10 decades of life. Part II. Maturity: a quantitative anatomic study of 765 specimens from subjects 20 to 99 years old. *Mayo Clin Proc* 1988;63:137.
4. Fitzgerald MJT. Thoracic organs. In: Fitzgerald MJT, ed. *Human embryology. A regional approach.* London: Harper & Row; 1978.
5. Moore KL. The cardiovascular system. In: Moore KL, ed. *The developing human.* 4th ed. Toronto: WB Saunders; 1988.
6. Kajstura J, Mansukhani M, Cheng W, et al. Programmed cell death and the expression of the protooncogene Bcl-2 in myocytes during postnatal maturation of the heart. *Exp Cell Res* 1995;219:110–121.
7. Tanaka M, Itoh H, Adachi S, et al. Hypoxia induces apoptosis with enhanced expression of Fas antigen messenger RNA in cultured neonatal rat cardiomyocytes. *Circ Res* 1994;75:426–433.
8. Edwards WD. Applied anatomy of the heart. In: Brandenberg RO, et al., eds. *Cardiology: fundamentals and practice.* Chicago: Year Book Medical; 1987.
9. Davies MJ, Pomerance A, Lamb D. Techniques in examination and anatomy of the heart. In: Pomerance A, Davies MJ, eds. *Pathology of the heart.* Oxford: Blackwell Scientific; 1975.
10. Sweeney LJ, Rosenquest GC. The normal anatomy of the atrial septum in the human heart. *Am Heart J* 1979;98:194.
11. Tajik AJ, Seward JB, Hagler DJ, Mair DD. Two dimensional real time ultrasonic imaging of heart and great vessels. *Mayo Clin Proc* 1978;53:271.
12. James TN, Sherf L, Schlant RC, Silverman ME. Anatomy of the heart. In: Hurst JW, ed. *The heart.* New York: McGraw-Hill; 1982.
13. Barry A, Patten B. The structure of the adult heart. In: Gould SE, ed. *Pathology of the heart and blood vessels.* Springfield, IL: Charles C. Thomas; 1982.
14. Ferrans VJ, Thiedeman KU. Ultrastructure of the normal heart. In: Silver MD, ed. *Cardiovascular pathology.* New York: Churchill Livingstone; 1983.
15. Hudson REB. The conducting system: anatomy, histology, pathology in acquired heart disease. In: Silver MD, ed. *Cardiovascular pathology.* New York: Churchill Livingstone; 1983.
16. Davies MJ, Anderson RH. The pathology of the conducting system. In: Pomerance A, Davies MJ, eds. *Pathology of the heart.* Boston: Blackwell Scientific; 1975.
17. Ludwig J, Lie JT. In: *Current methods of autopsy practice.* 2nd ed. Philadelphia: WB Saunders; 1979.
18. Derias NW, Adam CWM. Nitro blue tetrazolium test: early gross detection of human myocardial infarcts. *Br J Exp Pathol* 1978;59:254.
19. Edwards WD. Photography of medical specimens—experiences from teaching cardiovascular pathology. *Mayo Clinic Proc* 1988;63:42.
20. Oostrom K. Plastination of the heart. *J Int Soc Klastination* 1987;1:12.

*Histology for Pathologists, second edition,*
Edited by Stephen S. Sternberg.
Lippincott-Raven Publishers, Philadelphia


# CHAPTER 33

# Blood Vessels

Patrick J. Gallagher



## GROSS AND LIGHT MICROSCOPIC FEATURES

The normal structure of vessels, particularly the aorta, elastic and muscular arteries, and the larger veins, changes progressively throughout life (Table 1). This is partly the result of a series of aging changes and partly because arteries and arterioles are often affected by common disorders such as atherosclerosis, hypertension, and diabetes (Table 2). Surgical pathologists must be fully aware not only of the nature and extent of these alterations, but also of their variation from site to site. Some of these changes have an important influence on the changes in cardiovascular physiology that accompany aging (1).

### Aorta and Arteries

The length and breadth of the aorta increase progressively throughout life. Although there are some variations in the rate of these changes, both between men and women and from decade to decade, the process continues well into the 70s and 80s (2). This enlargement produces the characteristic unfolding of the aorta so often seen in chest radiographs, and if the aortic valve annulus is also involved, aortic incompetence can result. Some atherosclerosis is almost inevitable in the abdominal aorta in the middle aged and elderly, but aging changes are independent of this phenomenon.

The principal components of all arteries are elastic and collagen fibers, smooth muscle cells, and the mucopolysaccharide-rich ground substance (3). In the media of the aorta and the carotid, innominate and proximal axillary arteries, elastic fibers predominate. Parallel lamellar units of elastin enclose smooth muscle nuclei, ground substance, and collagen. Interconnecting bands of collagen and elastin fibers provide strength, whereas the lamellar arrangement distributes stress evenly across the wall (4). Elastic fragmentation with associated foci of fibrosis are the most prominent aging changes and account for the weakening that leads to aortic dilatation (5,6). Techniques of in situ end labeling demonstrate apoptosis in smooth muscle cells of atheromatous plaques but not significantly in the normal aortic or arterial media (7,8). Calcification is a common complication, and although it is most frequent in atheromatous segments, it may occur in areas where the intima is virtually normal. The underlying causes of aortic and coronary arterial calcification remain poorly understood (9,10). Amyloid deposits are common in aortic atheromatous lesions of middle-aged and elderly subjects and may be derived from apolipoproteins (11,12). Cystic medial necrosis is a difficult concept, and many pathologists are unsure about the exact meaning of the term. Erdheim's original description encompassed both necrosis of smooth muscle cells and the accumulation of mu-

P. J. Gallagher: Department of Pathology, Southampton University Hospital, Southampton SO16 6YD, England.

**TABLE 1.** *Aging changes in blood vessels*

| | Major macroscopic and histologic features |
|---|---|
| Aorta | Progressive and linear increase in diameter with age. Eccentric or diffuse fibrous intimal thickening. Fragmentation of elastic lamellae with widening of interlamellar spaces. Focal amyloid deposits. Thickening of walls of vasa vasorum. |
| Muscular arteries | Progressive dilatation and tortuosity. Caliber of vessels usually less in females, especially coronary arteries. Intimal fibrosis, sometimes suggesting reduplication of the internal elastic lamella. Focal fragmentation and calcification of internal elastic lamella. Increased fibrosis and hyalinization of media. No significant inflammation in atheroma free segments. |
| Arterioles | Intimal thickening, usually as concentric layers of fibroelastic tissue. Hyalinization of media. |
| Capillaries | Basement membrane thicknening, approximately twofold increase in thickness from puberty to old age. |
| Venules and Veins | Few detailed studies of small veins. Larger veins show intimal fibrosis and hypertrophy of both circular and longitudinal bundles. |

**TABLE 2.** *Histologic changes in arteries and arteriols*

| Condition | Major histologic features |
|---|---|
| Normal adults | Minimal intimal thickening, may be eccentric or diffuse. Intact internal elastic lamella, occasional small breaks only. No significant inflammation. |
| Atherosclerosis | Eccentric fibrous intimal thickening, intimal and medial foam cell and lipid deposition; neovascularization with intimal and medial hemorrhage. Dystrophic calcification. Adventitial aggregates of plasma cells, lymphocytes and histiocytes. Intimal and medial aggregates of T-lymphocytes, especially at shoulders of lesion. The most important complication is rupture of fibrous cap of the lesion with associated thrombus formation. |
| Systemic hypertension | Concentric fibrous intimal thickening and medial hypertrophy, especially in arterioles; changes pronounced in accelerated or malignant phase, with fibrinoid necrosis; aneurysmal dilation of intracerebral arterioles and capillaries; increased atherosclerosis. |
| Diabetes mellitus | Hyaline change in arterioles; capillary microaneurysms with basement membrane thickening; loss of pericytes; retinal neovascularization. Increased atherosclerosis in arteries. |
| Active arteritis | Acute or chronic inflammatory cell inflammation of adventitia and media; mural edema, reactive intimal thickening, and endothelial necrosis; fibrinoid necrosis of wall, occasionally aneurysmal dilatation. |
| Healed arteritis | Bizarre patterns of disordered fibrous intimal thickening; medial scarring with patchy aggregates of chronic inflammatory cells; abnormally prominent medial blood vessels. |

coid material in the media. Most authorities now restrict the definition to the presence of cystic spaces within the elastic lamellar units. These cysts contain basophilic mucopolysaccharide, and because they have no true lining, their cystic appearance is largely a histologic artifact. In a study of 100 normal aortas, Schlatmann and Becker (13) found that 60% of aortas showed this change; in 6% it was graded as severe. In nonatheromatous segments of the aorta, some fibrous intimal thickening can usually be detected (Fig. 1). Although this increases with age, it is of no clinical consequence.

Aging changes are most prominent in the inner part of the media of the thoracic aorta. Elastic fragmentation and associated medial necrosis are the most common histologic findings in both ascending and thoracic aortic aneurysms (14,15). Aging changes are not obviously increased in patients with systemic hypertension or dissecting aneurysms (16). In Marfan's syndrome the histologic changes suggest exaggerated aging, but there are no features that allow a specific diagnosis to be made (Fig. 2). The underlying genetic abnormality involves a glycoprotein, fibrillin, which is closely associated with elastin fibers. The exact functions of fibrillin and other associated glycoproteins are uncertain, but they may act as a "scaffold" on which elastin fibers are laid down. There are a wide spectrum of clinical abnormalities in Marfan's syndrome, and certain clinical features, such as arachnodactyly or aortic dissection, are especially common in some families (17,18). As yet these have not been precisely linked with specific mutations, and because there are many of these, no simple screening test is available. Fibrillin has been demonstrated in tissue culture studies using immunofluorescence, but there are no commercial antibodies that can be used in diagnostic studies. Abnormalities in other connective tissue glycoproteins have been described, and these also may be implicated in Marfan's syndrome (19).

Traditionally, abdominal aortic aneurysms have been considered atheromatous in origin, but this may be an oversimplification (20). Some families have a predisposition to these aneurysms, and a number of genetic abnormalities have been identified, including mutations in the genes coding for collagen precursor proteins (21). Whether the atherosclerosis is the primary cause or a secondary complication, the inflammation and medial scarring that accompany all but the earliest stages of atheroma further damage a wall already weakened by normal aging. Patchy chronic inflammatory aggregates, including lymphocytes and plasma cells, are often present in the adventitia of atheromatous segments of the aorta and coronary arteries (22) (Fig. 3). Although the den-

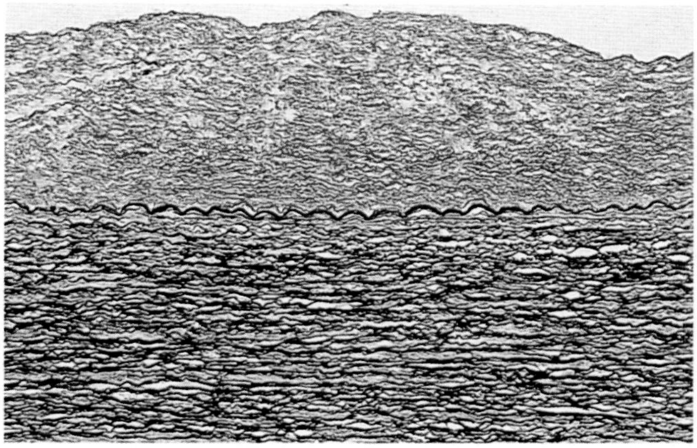

**FIG. 1.** Inner half of the aortic wall of a 62-year-old man. There is a moderate degree of fibrous intimal thickening. This has no immediate clinical relevance but may predispose to atherosclerosis. There was only slight fragmentation of the elastic lamellae; the overall appearance is well within normal limits for a patient of this age (elastic van Gieson).

sity of these infiltrates can be related to the severity of the atheromatous process, the role that they play in the initiation of the lesions or their complications is uncertain (23). In biopsies of the ascending aorta during repair of dissecting aneurysms or aortic reconstructions for root dilatation, these chronic adventitial infiltrates must not be mistaken as evidence of aortitis. In contrast, only small numbers of macrophages and mast cells can be detected in nonatheromatous intima or media, even if there is significant age-related intimal thickening (24). If appreciable numbers are present, aortitis should be suspected. In contrast, atheromatous plaques contain many macrophages, some with a foam cell appearance. T-lymphocytes can be identified immunohistochemically (25,26), and most have the $\alpha\beta$ receptor phenotype. They are especially prominent at the margins, or "shoulders," of lesions, and it is likely that they have complex interactions with other inflammatory cells within lesions (27–29). The release of macrophage enzymes, including metalloproteinases, may contribute to the weakening of the wall of atheromatous vessels and the progression of abdominal aortic aneurysms (30,31). In some abdominal aneurysms the inflammatory infiltrates are especially dense, and surgical repair may be difficult. The inflammation may be a reaction to ceroid pigment, and there can be associated retroperitoneal fibrosis (32,33).

Cardiac surgeons have several techniques for repairing aortic coarctations (34) and may submit samples of aorta, the narrowed aortic segment, the subclavian artery, or the ductus arteriosus (arterial duct) for histologic identification. The aorta around the coarctation may show reactive intimal thickening, even in neonates, but the underlying elastic structure is usually well preserved. The coarctation itself can

A

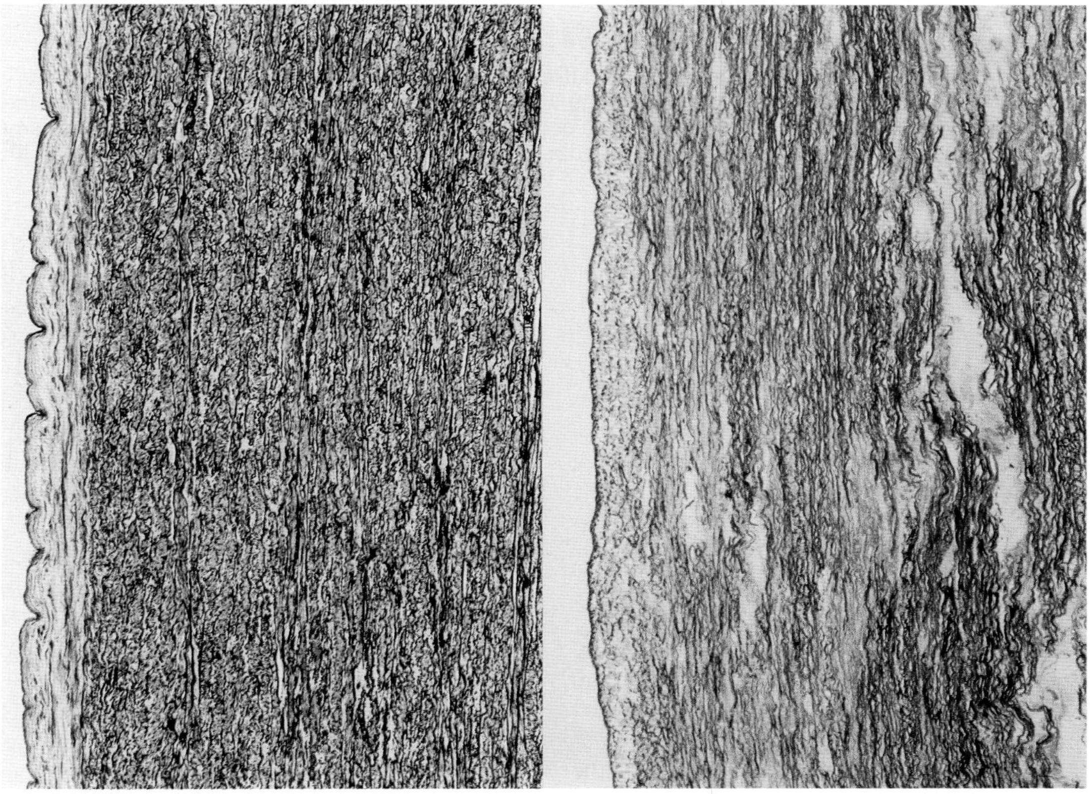

B

**FIG. 2. A:** The normal appearance of the aortic media of a 48-year-old man. There are many parallel lamellae of elastic tissue. There is no significant intimal thickening. **B:** The aortic wall of a 31-year-old man with Marfan's syndrome. The medial elastic tissue is extensively fragmented, and there is fibrosis and loose mucopolysaccharide-rich areas. Such extensive changes would be unusual even in an elderly patient (elastic van Gieson).

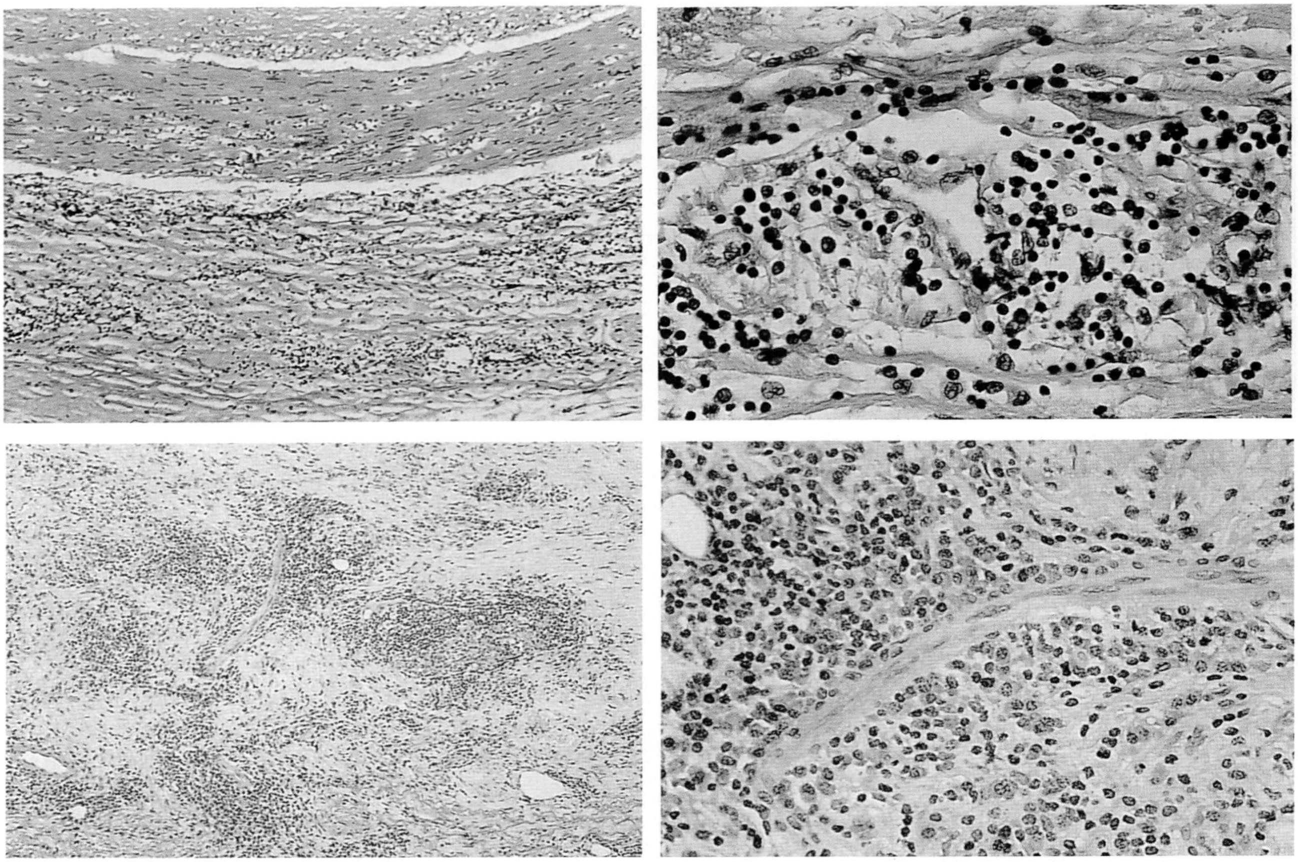

A B C D

**FIG. 3. A, B:** Adventitial chronic inflammatory infiltrates in the wall of an atheromatous coronary artery. A few inflammatory cells have infiltrated into the media. The magnified view on the right confirms that most of the inflammatory cells are lymphocytes or plasma cells. **C, D:** Marked lymphocytic and plasma cell infiltration of the adventitia of a syphilitic aorta. Note that the infiltrates are much denser than in the upper panels.

have a variety of appearances. In long-standing cases there may be dense intimal and medial fibrosis. In neonates the intima may have a distinctly irregular pattern of fibroelastic intimal thickening, resembling some forms of arterial dysplasia (Fig. 4). The structure of the arterial duct changes progressively during intrauterine growth and in the postnatal period (35) and can be influenced by prostaglandin treatment (36). Unlike the aorta and the proximal subclavian artery, which are elastic vessels, the arterial duct has a muscular media and a defined internal elastic lamella.

It is only in children and young adults that muscular arteries conform to the classical descriptions of textbooks. Arteries dilate and become more tortuous with increasing age, and this has a fortuitous antiocclusive effect. Cardiologists claim that the caliber of the coronary arteries in middle-aged and elderly women is less than that of men. This may make coronary artery surgery more difficult and contribute to the slightly poorer results recorded in women (37,38). If arterial dilatation is pronounced and irregular, as in so-called coronary artery ectasia, spontaneous thrombosis may result (39). Progressive intimal fibrosis affects nearly all arteries (Fig. 5), but in surgical pathology material it is especially noticeable in the spleen, myometrium, and thyroid (Fig. 6). Similarly, the fibrous tissue of the media also increases in amount throughout life. A committee of the American Heart Association has defined the intima and the early lesions of atherosclerosis in precise morphologic terms (24,40). They emphasize that a "thick but undiseased intima" is a physiologic adaptation to mechanical stress. When the process is eccentric, it is associated with arterial branches, orifices, and curvatures. Otherwise intimal and medial fibrosis is diffuse, affecting the full circumference of the vessels. The cause of this process is uncertain (41), but there is some experimental evidence that smooth muscle cells from aged animals have an increased synthetic activity and a more florid response to injury in comparison with younger controls (42). The turnover of endothelial and smooth muscle cells is increased in areas of intimal thickening (43). Low-density lipoprotein accumulates in areas of intimal thickening, probably through an interaction with arterial proteoglycans (44). Atherosclerotic lesions develop earlier and progress more rapidly in areas of intimal thickening, particularly if the process is eccentric.

As in the aorta, fragmentation of the elastic tissue, usually

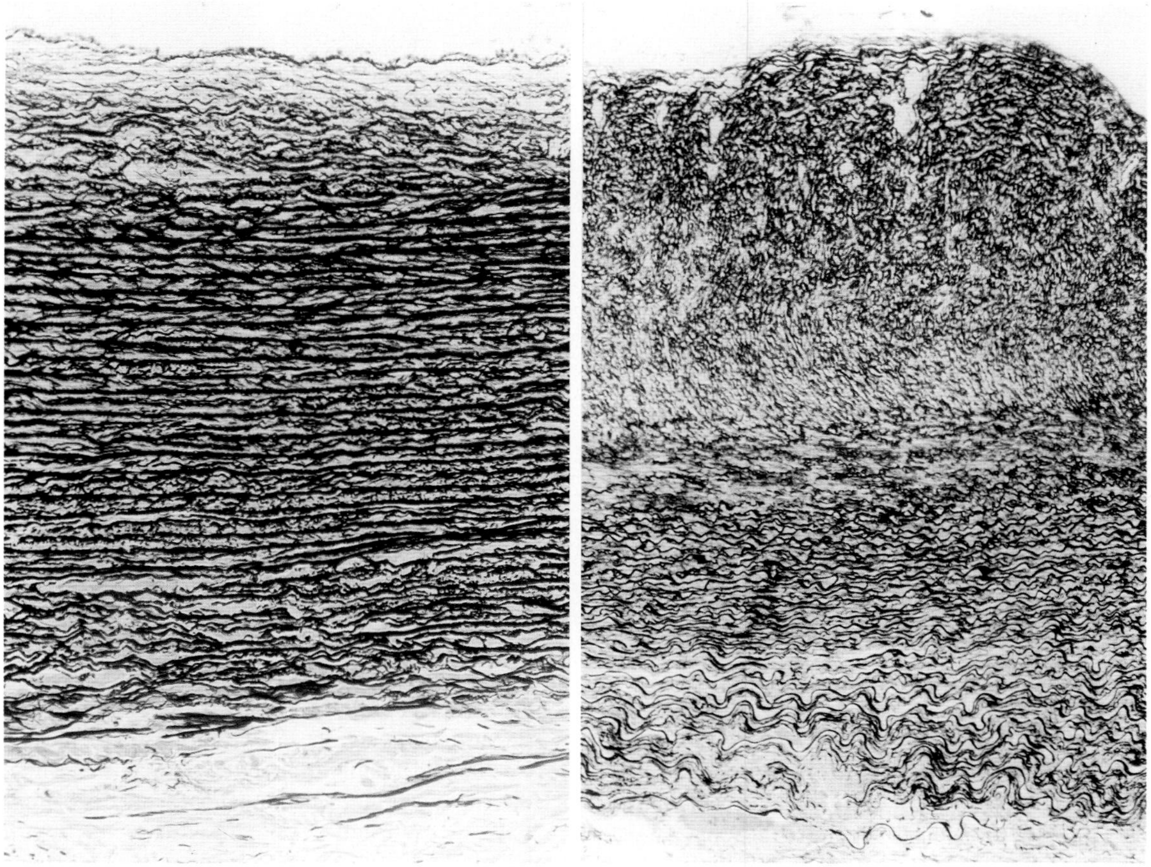

**FIG. 4.** Coarctation of the aorta. The **left** panel is the aortic wall distal to a coarctation in a 3-month-old child. There is slight intimal edema only. The **right** panel is the coarctation itself. Note the irregular arrangement of the intimal fibroelastic tissue (elastic van Gieson).

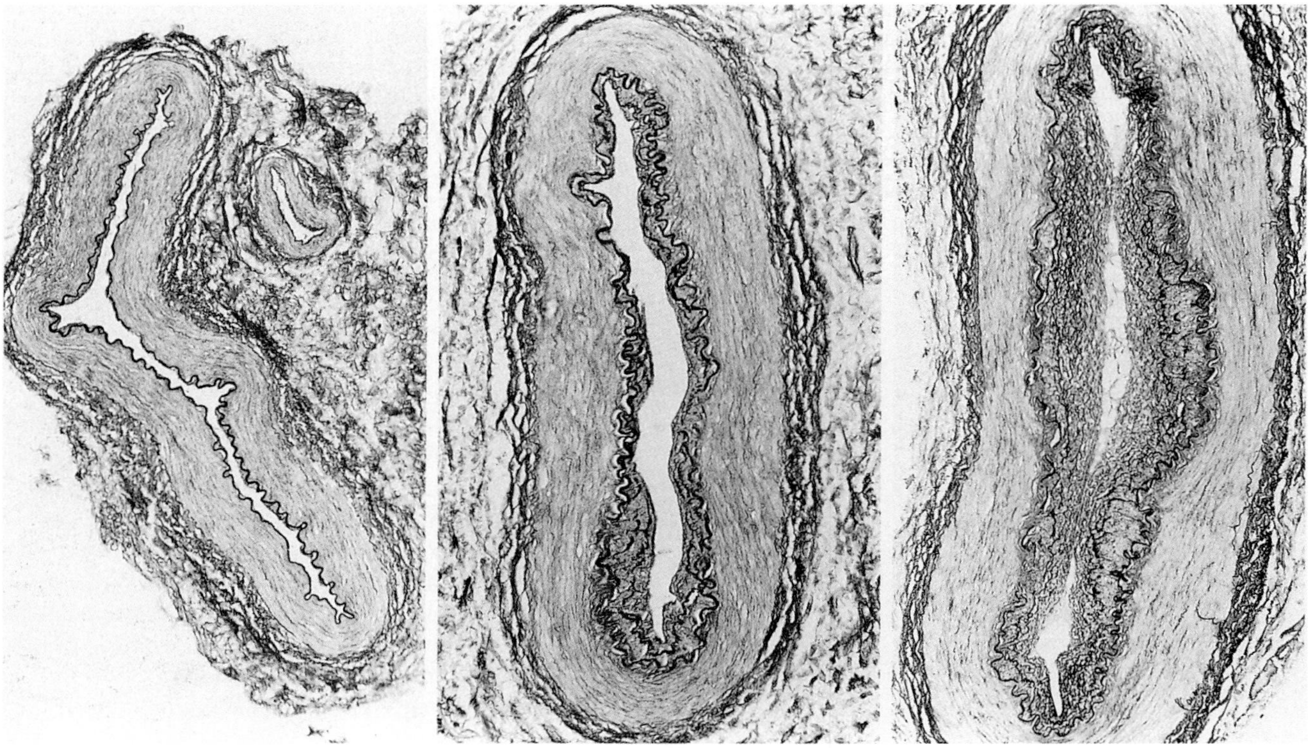

**FIG. 5.** Aging changes in muscular arteries. The **left** panel shows normal appearances in a 17-year-old girl. Note the progressive intimal fibrosis in the other panels taken from separate elderly males. In the **right** panel there is some reduplication of the internal elastic membrane (elastic van Gieson).

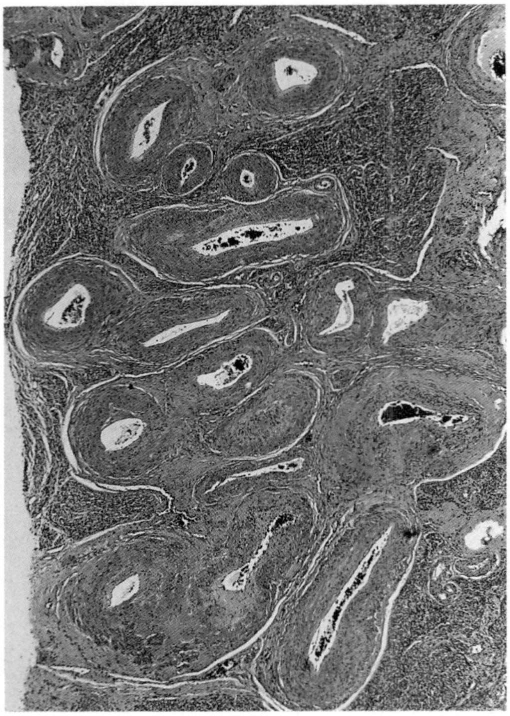

**FIG. 6.** A mass of thick-walled arteries close to the serosa of the myometrium in a 49-year-old woman. These have no importance and also can be seen in other biopsy samples, especially in thyroidectomy specimens.

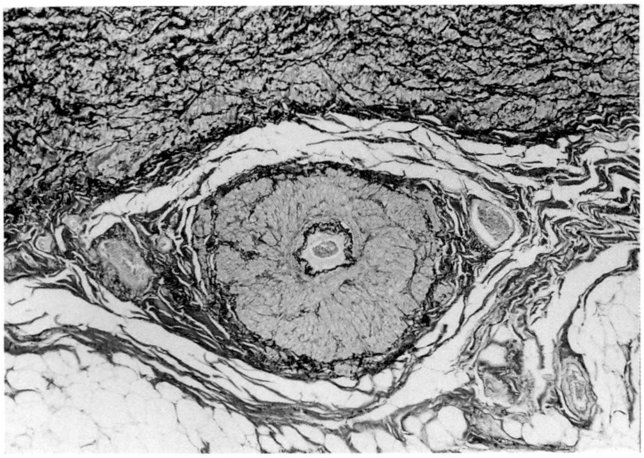

**FIG. 8.** The aortic adventitia containing a vasa vasorum. Thick-walled vessels, such as this, are not pathologic.

the internal elastic lamella, is common and is of no specific significance (Fig. 7). In some aging arteries the internal lamella appears to repeatedly reduplicate, producing a pattern of concentric intimal thickening (Fig. 5). Small foci of calcification can be identified in otherwise normal vessels, usually just to the medial aspect of the internal elastic lamella. These aging changes, often loosely termed arteriosclerosis, have been studied most extensively in the coronary arteries, where women generally show substantially less elastic fragmentation and intimal fibrosis than do men of the same age (45).

Nutrients reach the media of elastic or muscular arteries by direct diffusion through the intima or via small branches, the vasa vasorum, which reenter the media from the adventitial aspect. Small mammals with fewer than 20 parallel lamellar units have no demonstrable vasa. Even in humans and sheep, which have 35 to 70 elastic lamellae, a substantial proportion of the innermost media has no vasa vasorum and must survive by direct diffusion (46). Vasa are best seen in biopsy samples taken from the ascending aorta during root repairs and sometimes have remarkably thick muscular walls (Fig. 8). There is some experimental evidence that in systemic hypertension blood flow through the vasa in the thoracic aorta cannot increase physiologically (47). In contrast, in atheromatous vessels there is a marked increase in blood flow to the media, probably as a result of neovascular proliferation of small branches of these vessels (48).

Arteries in chronically inflamed tissues and coursing

A 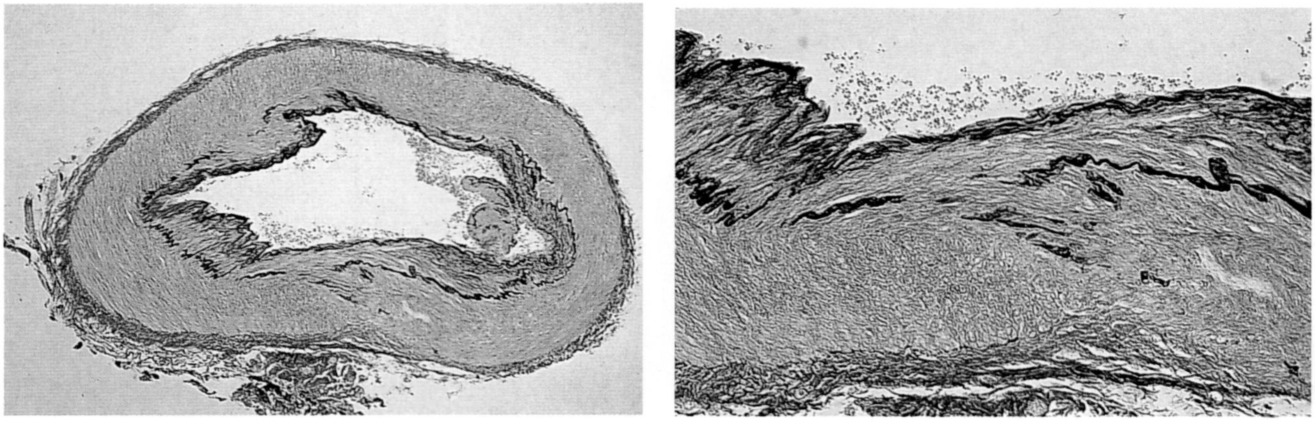 B

**FIG. 7. A, B:** Temporal artery from a 72-year-old woman who died suddenly from coronary heart disease. There was no past history of headache or temporal arteritis. Note the fragmentation of the elastic lamella with a little associated fibrosis (red coloration in B). Changes such as these are commonplace in the elderly and must not be interpreted as evidence of previous arteritis (elastic van Gieson).

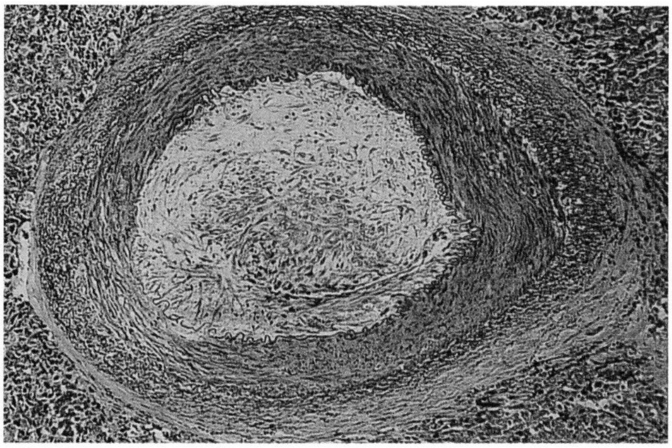

**FIG. 9.** A small muscular artery included in a biopsy sample of an undifferentiated blue cell tumor removed from the chest wall of a 6-year-old girl. Note the pronounced fibrous intimal thickening that has developed, presumably as a result of the surrounding tumor infiltrates.

through tumors often show pronounced fibrous intimal thickening, sometimes termed endarteritis obliterans. In the early stages of this process, the fibrous tissue has a loose histologic appearance and the ground substance may be basophilic (Fig. 9). Although inflammatory or tumor cells often closely surround the adventitia, they do not usually penetrate far into the muscular wall.

### Arterioles

There are no specific histologic features that accurately distinguish small arteries from larger arterioles, but for convenience arterioles are said to have a diameter of less than 100 $\mu$m. However, in biopsy material there is so much variation in the contours of these small vessels that accurate distinction is often impossible and probably unnecessary. Larger arterioles have an obvious media and an adventitial layer of connective tissue. In the smallest (terminal) arterioles the media may be only a few cells in thickness and an internal elastic lamella may not be identified. The muscular wall can be slightly attenuated just proximal to the capillary bed, forming the so-called precapillary sphincter.

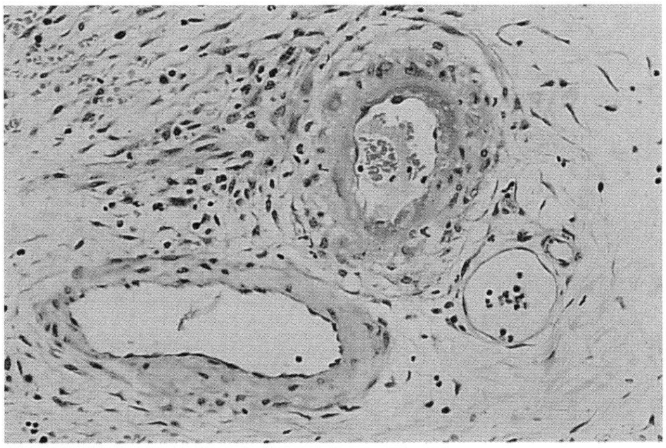

**FIG. 10.** Florid fibrinoid necrosis in a small intestinal vessel of a girl with systemic lupus erythematosus. Fibrinoid necrosis is not a feature of normal aging or uncomplicated hypertension. It always should be regarded as pathologic. In this case the involved vessel is probably an arteriole. Note small vein (*lower left*) and capillary (*lower right*).

Hyalinization is a common lesion of arterioles and small arteries and increases with age and in conditions such as hypertension and diabetes. The glassy uniform appearance is the result of accumulation of a variety of plasma proteins and small amounts of lipids. As in arteries, reduplication of elastic tissue and intimal fibrosis are common changes in the aged. In severe longstanding benign hypertension, and in the malignant phase, the arteriolar lumen can be substantially narrowed by concentric layers of fibrous tissue and smooth muscle cells, changes that are outside the normal range of aging (Table 1). Fibrinoid necrosis of the arteriolar media is the hallmark of malignant hypertension and some forms of acute vasculitis (Figs. 10 and 11). It must always be regarded as pathologic. In diabetes, arterioles and capillaries often show prominent basement membrane thickening, one of the earliest changes in diabetic microangiopathy (49). This thickening can be seen directly in renal and peripheral nerve biopsy samples but is probably generalized throughout the vascular system (50). The amounts of type IV collagen and laminin are increased, but the proteoglycan component of basement membrane is reduced (51,52). Albumin and immunoglobulins appear to attach preferentially to these abnormal basement membranes and also contribute to the overall eosinophilic appearance.

### Capillaries

In contrast to arterioles, capillaries have neither a muscular media nor an elastic lamella. A single but complete layer of endothelial cells lies on a basement membrane whose thickness varies from site to site. Basement membrane thickness increases with age, almost doubling in muscle capillaries from 10 to 70 years (53). There is no fibrous tissue support peripheral to this, but pericytes are present in and among the basement membrane. It is difficult to identify pericytes in routine sections but they are easily seen by electron microscopy. They provide structural support, and because they contain several forms of myosin (54), they may be able to regulate blood flow. It is likely that they are involved in the synthesis of vascular basement membrane and are capable of phagocytosis (55,56). It is generally accepted that the turnover of pericytes is increased in the capillaries of diabetics, and this may contribute to the development of microaneurysms (52,57).

In certain sites, such as the liver, pituitary, and bone marrow, the vessels that connect arterioles and venules are known as sinusoids rather than capillaries. With diameters of up to 30 to 40 $\mu$m, they are generally more distended than capillaries but retain a complete lining of endothelial cells.

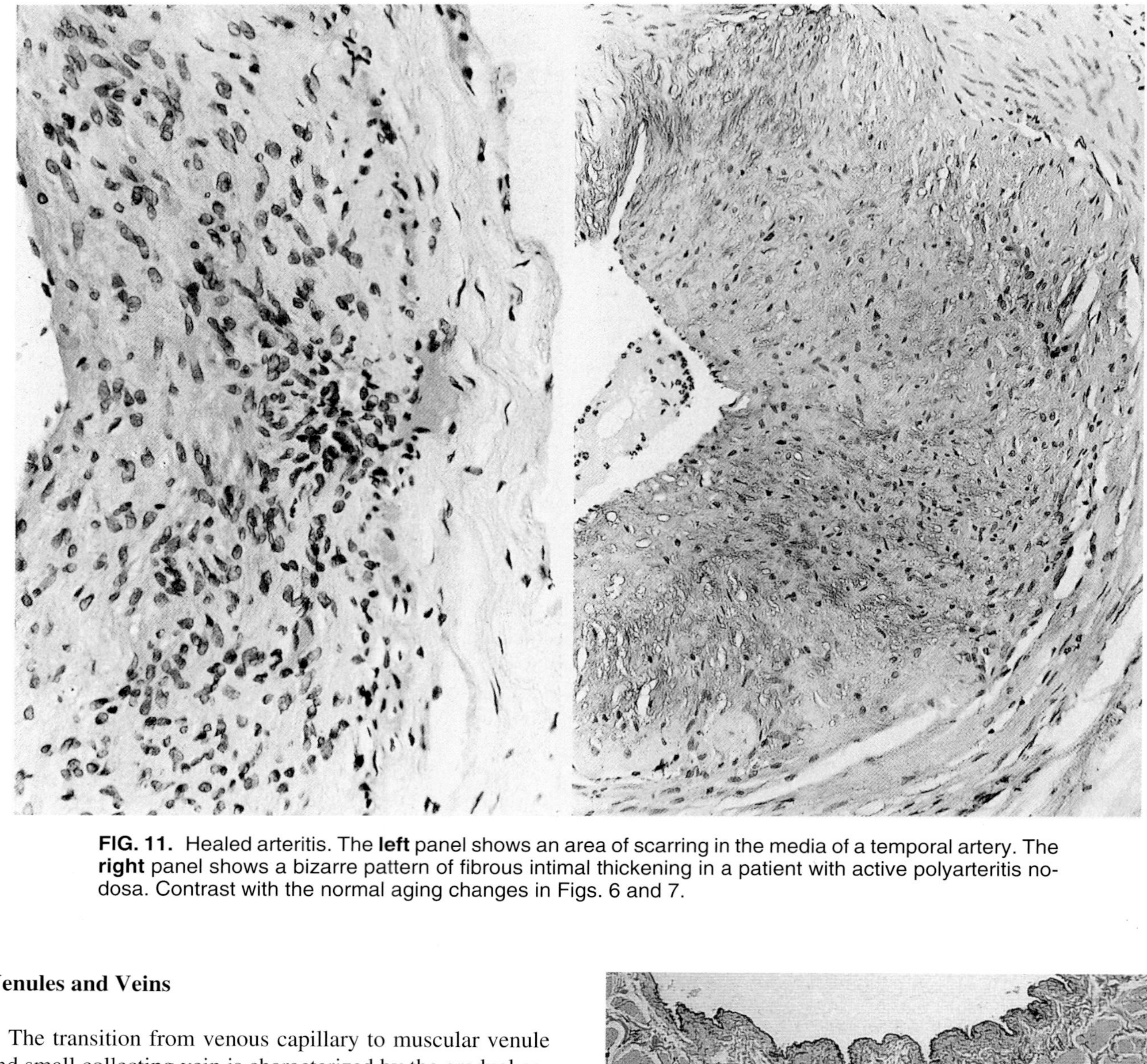

**FIG. 11.** Healed arteritis. The **left** panel shows an area of scarring in the media of a temporal artery. The **right** panel shows a bizarre pattern of fibrous intimal thickening in a patient with active polyarteritis nodosa. Contrast with the normal aging changes in Figs. 6 and 7.

### Venules and Veins

The transition from venous capillary to muscular venule and small collecting vein is characterized by the gradual acquisition of a muscular media. Even in medium-sized veins (Fig. 12) the internal elastic lamella is often incomplete and the muscle fibers are only poorly oriented into circular and longitudinal layers.

The paracortical or high endothelial venules of lymph nodes have an important role in lymphocyte recirculation, and their histologic and ultrastructural features have been studied in detail (58). There is convincing experimental evidence that T cells move from the vascular component to the lymph node paracortex by migrating between the endothelial cells of these venules and passing through the adjacent basement membrane. The endothelial cells of postcapillary venules have a prominent cuboidal or columnal appearance, usually with an ovoid nucleus and a single central nucleolus. In contrast to the endothelial cells of other small vessels, enzyme histochemistry demonstrates abundant nonspecific es-

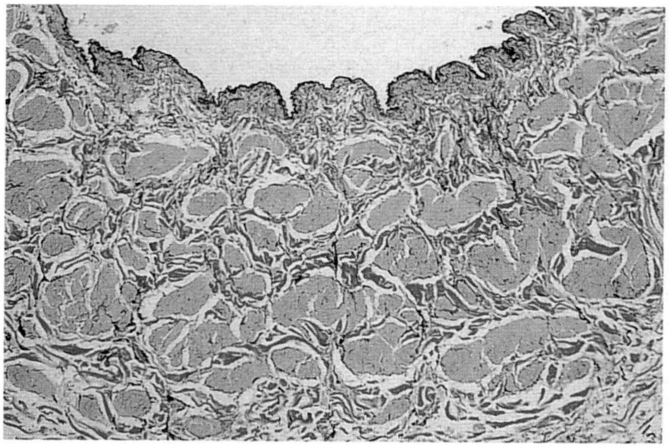

**FIG. 12.** A renal vein from a 58-year-old woman close to the junction with the inferior vena cava. There is no significant intimal thickening, and a thin internal elastic lamella can be identified. Note the thin layer of subendothelial collagen. The muscular wall is composed of coarse fascicles, which are not clearly arranged into circular and longitudinal layers (elastic van Gieson).

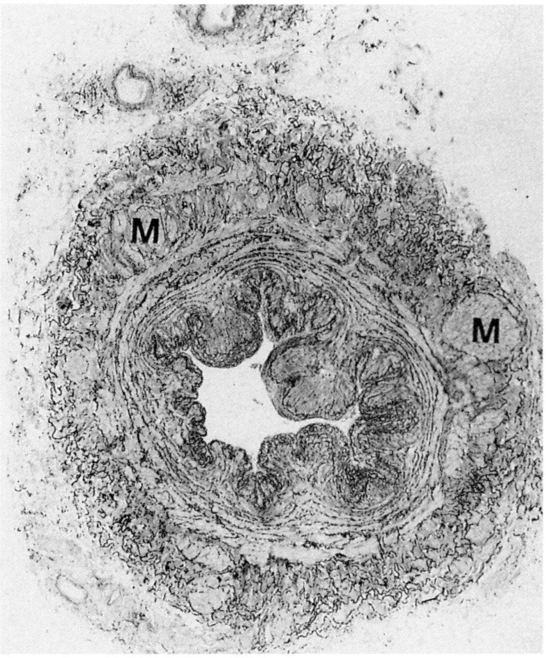


**FIG. 13.** A saphenous vein with a prominent third outer longitudinal muscular coat (M) (elastic van Gieson). [Reprinted with permission (60); copyright 1989 by John Wiley and Sons, Ltd.]

terase and $\beta$-glucuronidase. Acid phosphatase and succinic dehydrogenase are also expressed more strongly than in ordinary venules and capillaries. The increasing use of the saphenous vein as an arterial conduit has led to a greater understanding of the normal structure of larger veins and the changes that occur in them as a result of aging. The classical description states that large veins have a thin layer of subendothelial connective tissue with one or more incomplete elastic lamellae. Around this there is an inner longitudinal and outer circular smooth muscle coat. The connective tissue adventitia is often well developed. Surgical pathologists examining redundant segments of long saphenous vein often code these aging changes as phlebosclerosis. The major changes in these veins in middle-aged and elderly patients are intimal fibrosis and longitudinal and circular muscle hypertrophy with a substantial increase in medial connective tissue. Sometimes a prominent third outer longitudinal muscle layer (Fig. 13) forms between the circular coat and the adventitia (59,60). These changes must be carefully distinguished from the form of atherosclerosis that develops in vein bypass grafts.

## Lymphatics

At the light microscopic level, small lymphatics closely resemble capillaries. In general terms, lymphatics have a larger diameter and a less regular cross-sectional profile (61). They begin as dilated channels with closed ends and anastomose free. Although they are present in most tissues, they are rarely found in the epidermis, nails, cornea, articular cartilage, central nervous system, or bone marrow. Lymphatic channels have numerous valves and are often slightly distended at these sites, producing a slightly beaded appearance. Lymphatics with a diameter of more than 0.2 mm usually have a thin muscular media, with no clear division into circular or longitudinal coats, and a fibrous adventitia (62). A longitudinal muscular layer is present in the right lymphatic and thoracic ducts.

Surgical pathologists often attempt to distinguish lymphatics from capillaries or small veins, particularly when these are infiltrated by tumor deposits. Although lymphatics have a larger cross-sectional area than do capillaries, this is seldom of use in distinguishing isolated vascular channels in tissues whose normal structure has been distorted by nearby tumors (63,64). Small lymphatics have little basement membrane, but silver impregnation techniques do not reliably differentiate capillaries and lymphatics (65). At present, immunohistochemical stains with antibodies to type IV collagen, a major constituent of basement membrane, do not produce consistent results in paraffin-embedded tissue. Noncollagenous components of basement membrane, such as laminin, can be demonstrated in routinely processed material. There is considerable debate as to whether the absence of laminin staining can be used to identify lymphatics (66,67).

## Pulmonary Arteries and Veins

Although the basic histologic structure of pulmonary vessels resembles that of their systemic counterparts, there are differences that reflect the much lower pressure of the pulmonary circuit. The lumina of major pulmonary arteries are widely dilated in comparison with wall thickness. The intima is hardly discernible. In an adult the pulmonary arterial media is composed of only 10 to 15 parallel elastic lamellae, whereas even in a young child 30 aortic lamellae can be identified. The thickness of the pulmonary trunk is about 40% to 80% that of the aorta (Fig. 14).

In the systemic circulation the transition from elastic to muscular arteries is abrupt and is usually at the point of a major arterial orifice. In contrast, even pulmonary arteries as small as 0.5 to 1.0 mm in diameter are elastic vessels (68). Muscular pulmonary arteries and arterioles also have thin walls in relationship to their luminal diameter, but this may be difficult to appreciate unless special techniques of perfusion or fixation are used (69). In comparison with systemic arteries, there is usually a prominent internal and external elastic lamella. Arterioles give rise to a rich network of alveolar capillaries. Pericytes are not easily identified, and in places the endothelium and alveolar epithelium appear to share a common basement membrane. The walls of pulmonary veins are less structured than their systemic counterparts. The media is composed of a rather haphazardly ar-

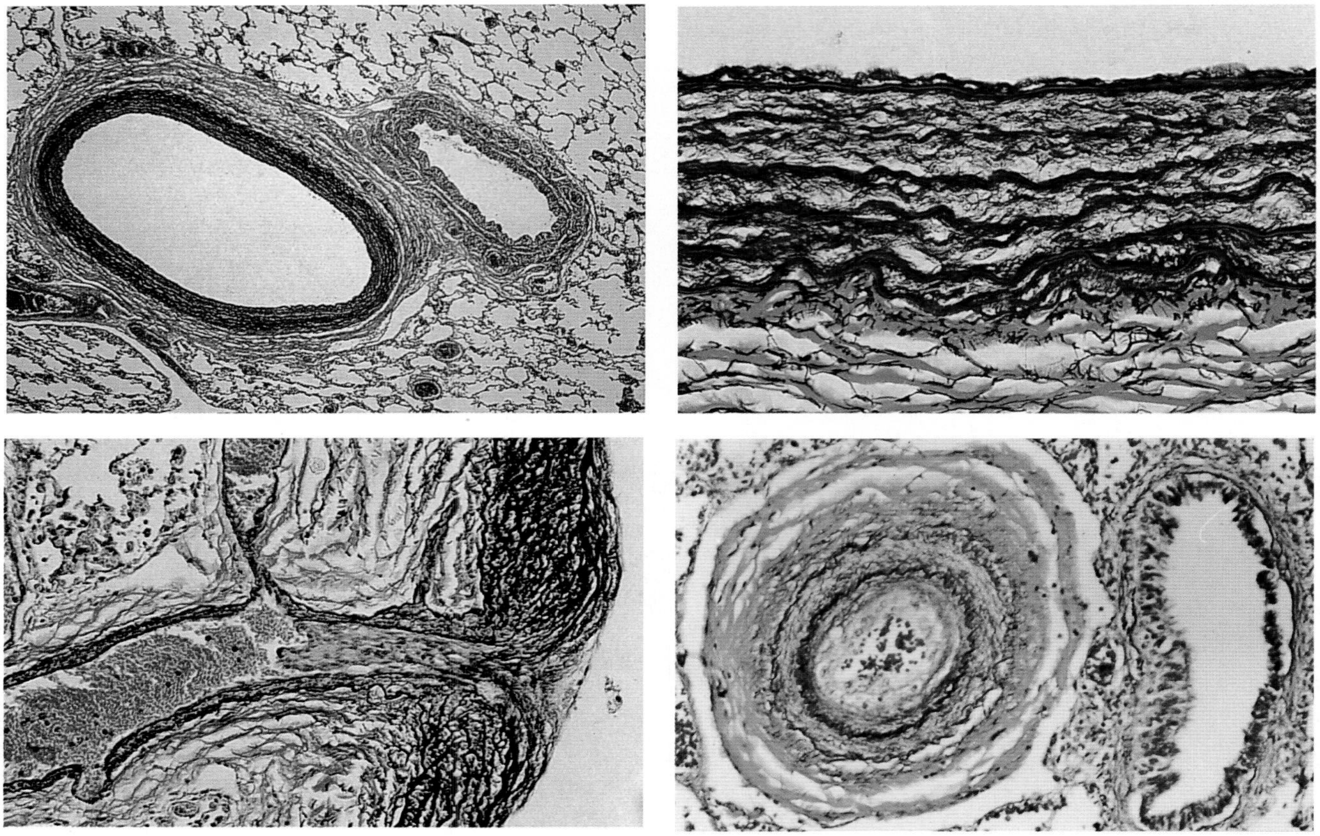

A B C D

**FIG. 14.** **A:** Elastic pulmonary artery from a 1-year-old child. The lung was inflated via the main pulmonary artery, which therefore appears much larger than the corresponding bronchus. **B:** A magnified view of the elastic wall (Gomori trichrome). **C:** The transition from elastic to muscular pulmonary arteries in a 73-year-old man. Note the larger number of elastic lamellae. There is slight fibrous intimal thickening only (elastic van Gieson). **D:** A small pulmonary artery from a a patient with longstanding pulmonary hypertension and chronic obstructive airways disease. There is hypertrophy of the muscular wall and pronounced fibrous intimal thickening (Gomori trichrome).

ranged but roughly circular layer of connective tissue and muscle. No distinct and continuous elastic lamellae are present, and valves are said to be absent (Fig. 15).

It can be difficult to distinguish the early vascular changes of pulmonary hypertension from those of normal aging (Table 3). The histologic changes have been described and comprehensively illustrated by Wagenvoort and Mooi (69) and Edwards (70). The initial changes in both conditions include intimal fibrosis and medial muscular hypertrophy and each of these features most prominent in muscular arteries and larger arterioles (71–73). The absence of significant changes in the larger arteries may be misleading. In longstanding pulmonary hypertension, the complex changes in muscular arteries include florid intimal thickening, marked medial hypertrophy, and prominent dilatation of small branches of parent vessels (Figs. 14D and 16). In the most extreme examples, angiomatoid malformations may develop, and occasionally there is fibrinoid necrosis of the vessel wall (69,70). There is debate about the value of open lung biopsy in the assessment of pulmonary hypertension in children with congenital heart disease (74–76) and adults with pulmonary hypertension (77). They are rarely performed in British centers.

Aging changes in pulmonary veins are seldom described in detail. In severe, longstanding cardiac failure, intimal fibrosis, medial hypertrophy, and hyalinization are prominent pulmonary venous abnormalities. Marked medial hypertrophy may confer an arterialized appearance to pulmonary veins, and they may appear to have an internal and external elastic lamina. Multiple levels should be taken and stained for elastin and a trichrome method. The elastic lamellae are seldom complete in these abnormal veins, and there is often more medial fibrosis than in corresponding pulmonary arteries. Even so, accurate distinction of abnormal pulmonary arteries and veins can be difficult.

### Anastomoses, Malformations, and Dysplasias

There is potential for anastomoses between many arteries and veins. These are especially developed in the skin, where

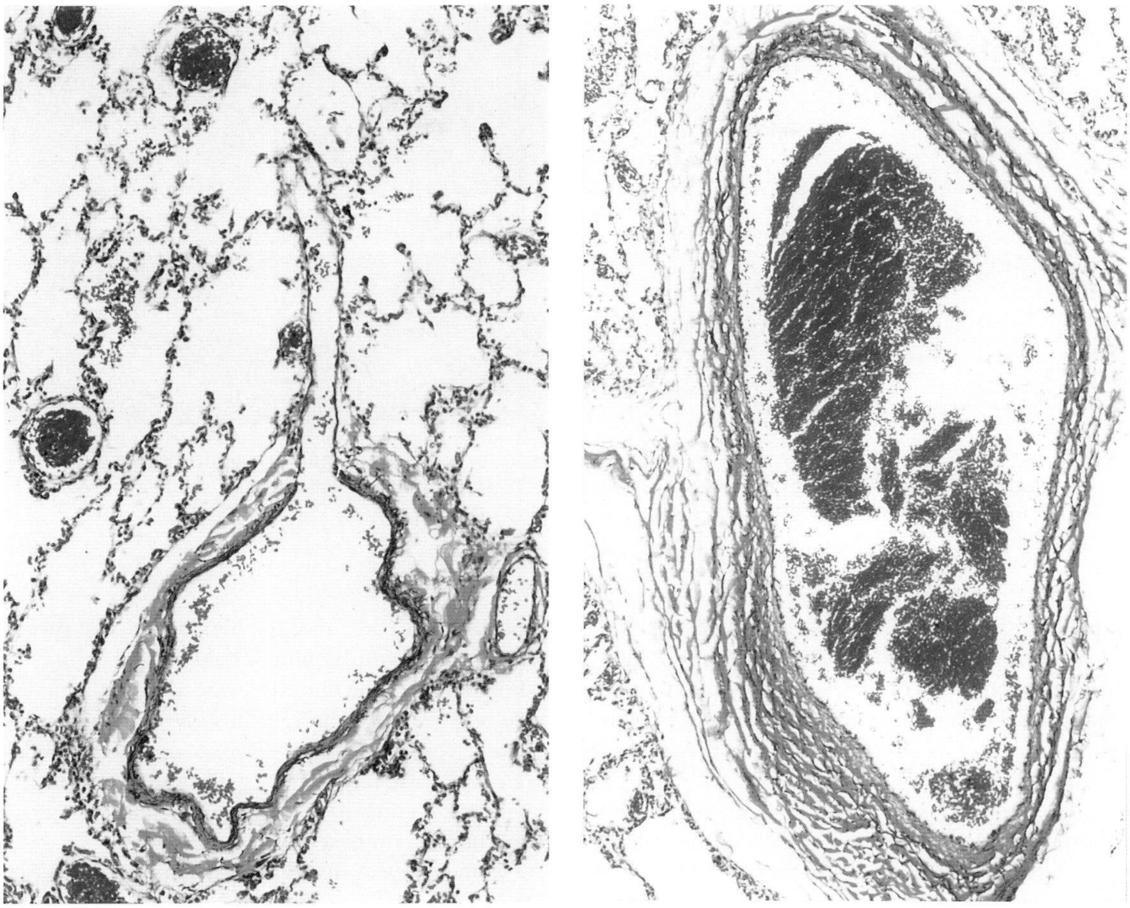


**FIG. 15.** Normal pulmonary veins. **A:** A pulmonary venule draining into a small vein. Very little muscle is present in the wall. **B:** A large pulmonary vein close to the hilum of the lung (Gomori trichrome).

they contribute to thermoregulation. They vary in size from about 200 to 800 $\mu$m and in some sites, such as the nail bed, have a complex structure (78). There are also anastomoses between pulmonary and bronchial veins and between the portal and systemic circulations. Peripheral glomus tumors almost certainly arise from supporting cells that surround the normal but rather complex anastomosing channels between digital arterioles and venules. Glomus cells do not express endothelial markers, such as Factor VIII, or react with *Ulex* agglutinin. Because they contain myosin and vimentin, they

**TABLE 3.** *Histologic features of pulmonary vessels*

| Vessel | Normal | Age changes | Pulmonary hypertension |
|---|---|---|---|
| Elastic arteries (>500 $\mu$m) | Widely patient lumen, media of 10 to 15 parallel lamellae of elastic tissue | Slight intimal fibrosis; increased medial thickness due to collagen deposition; occasional atheromatous plaques | Atherosclerosis and dilation of main pulmonary arteries; medial thickening due to hypertrophy of admixed muscular elements |
| Muscular arteries or arterioles | Thin muscular wall often with distinct internal and external elastic lamina | Increased muscular media, eccentric intimal fibrosis, especially in vessels less than 300 $\mu$m in diameter | Complex changes including florid intimal thickening, medial hypertrophy, dilation of small branches, angiomatoid (plexiform) lesions and fibrinoid necrosis |
| Veins | Thin media of irregularly arranged fibrous tissue and muscle. No distinct elastic lamella. No valves | Few detailed studies. The media may appear hyalinised | Intimal fibrosis, medial muscular hypertrophy—occasionally sufficient to mimic appearance of arteries. |

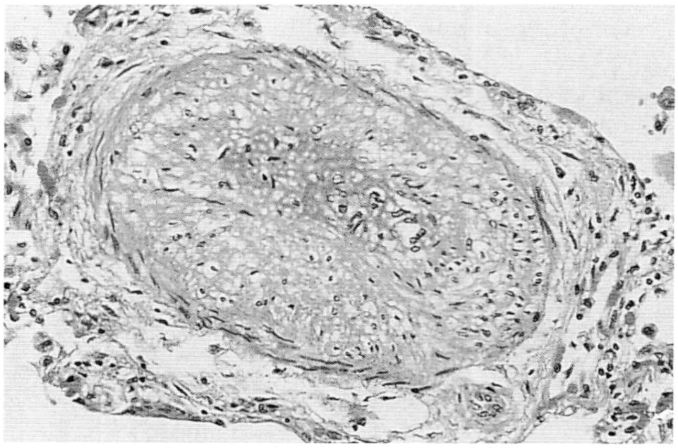

A

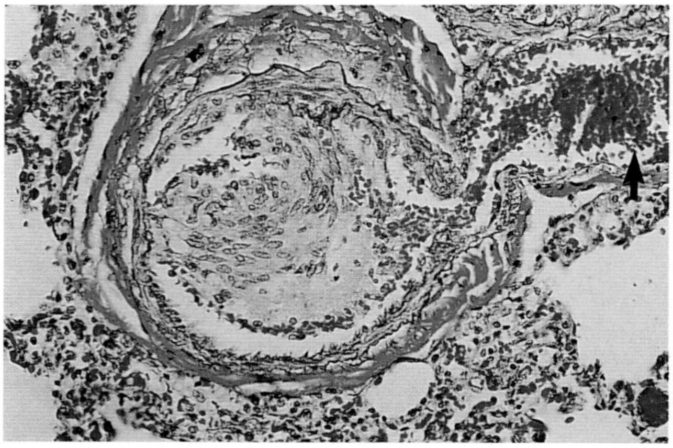

B

**FIG. 16. A, B:** Advanced pulmonary hypertensive changes. **A:** There is marked hypertrophy of the medial muscle in a small pulmonary artery. **B:** An early plexiform lesion with nearby dilated thin-walled branches (*arrow*) (Gomori trichrome).

may be related to vascular smooth muscle (79). The potential connections between the portal and systemic circulations, either in the submucosa of the esophagus or rectum, or in the periumbilical or diaphragmatic region, may be massively dilated in advanced hepatic disease (80). Biopsies are seldom performed surgically.

Surgical pathologists must be familiar with the normal vascular patterns of the cerebral meninges and the colonic submucosa if cerebral arteriovenous malformations and large intestinal angiodysplasia are to be accurately assessed. Each of these areas has a rich vascular supply with numerous, sometimes thick-walled, venous channels. Malformations or angiodysplasias must only be diagnosed if there is undoubted evidence of an abnormal vessel wall. Aging changes and atherosclerosis seldom involve the smaller leptomeningeal arteries. In arteries eccentric fibrous intimal thickening or disruption of the elastic lamellae (Fig. 17) support a diagnosis of a malformation. Veins in these malformations have irregular contours, the thickness of their muscular wall may vary markedly, and the wall can be uniformly fibrosed.

It is now accepted that angiodysplasia of the cecum and descending colon is a common cause of lower gastrointestinal hemorrhage. The lesions are usually present on the antimesenteric border of the cecum, often close to the ileocecal valve (81). They are not direct arteriovenous anastomoses but rather dilatations of preexisting, and previously normal, capillary rings and veins (Fig. 15). The dilatation of these vessels may be the result of increased colonic muscular pressure causing intermittent obstruction of draining vessels (82). Multiple blocks must be examined and the appearances contrasted with a control section of submucosa from a normal colon. Submucosal arteries of the large intestine may show pronounced age-related tortuosity, and this must not be interpreted as an abnormality. Some authorities suggest that the vascular pedicle of the hemicolectomy specimen should be injected with barium sulfate and the gross specimen radiographed or the mucosa stripped from the underlying muscle and viewed in a light box (83). If sufficient blocks are taken, vessel wall irregularities may well be demonstrated (Fig. 18). Nevertheless, a substantial proportion of cases with good clinical or radiologic evidence of angiodysplasia will not be confirmed histologically.

Some cases of massive gastrointestinal hemorrhage result from abnormally large submucosal arteries. This is most common in the stomach but also has been reported in the large and small intestine. Arteries in the submucosa of the proximal portion of the stomach can arise directly from omental vessels and may have a larger caliber than superficial arteries arising from a submucosal plexus, the so-called caliber-persistent artery or Dieulafoy lesion (84,85).

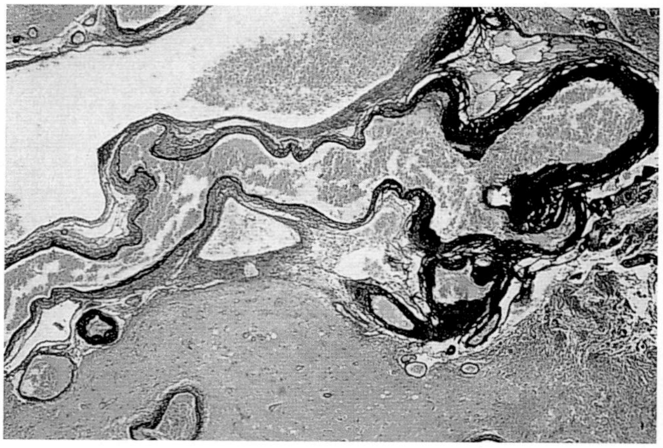

**FIG. 17.** Cerebral arteriovenous malformation. The involved vessels are irregularly distended, and there is fibrous and elastic intimal thickening (elastic van Gieson).

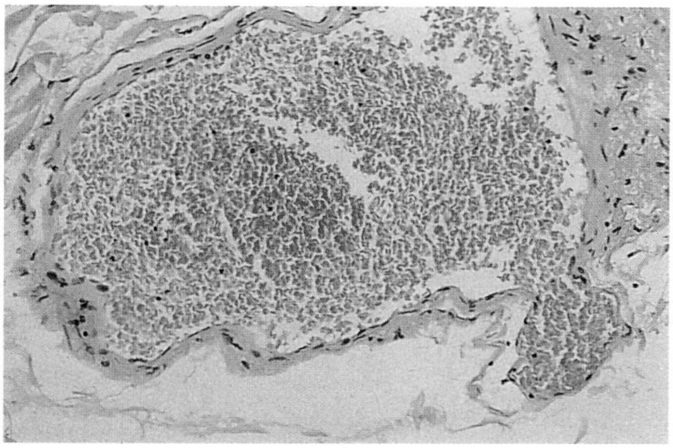

**FIG. 18.** Angiodysplasia of the colon. Note the irregular thinning of the wall of this medium-sized vein.

## Vascular Surgery

### *Endarterectomy*

Patency can be restored to a partially occluded artery by drawing out a proportion of the atherosclerotic intima. The procedure is usually applied to the carotid bifurcation, the iliac, femoral, or, occasionally, coronary arteries (86). Ideally, the surgeon should establish a plane between the innermost media and the intima, and the atheromatous material should be removed in its entirety. In practice, the ideal result is not always achieved, and the material removed may include internal elastic lamella and substantial amounts of muscular tissue as well as atheromatous debris and thrombus. Acute postoperative thrombus formation is the most important immediate complication of the procedure. At least 10% of successful endarterectomies are followed by restenosis (87), usually as a result of pronounced fibrous intimal proliferation. Some of these cases may be amenable to a second operation. The weakening of the arterial wall that follows endarterectomy predisposes to later aneurysmal dilatation (88).

### *Bypass Grafts*

The pathologic changes that occur in autologous saphenous vein bypass grafts have been extensively described (89,90). Care must be taken to distinguish these changes from those associated with normal aging (60). When subjected to arterial pressure, many vein grafts dilate and most develop some fibrous intimal thickening and medial muscular hypertrophy. In time many develop pronounced fibrous intimal thickening with areas of lipid deposition, intramural hemorrhage, and thrombosis (91). These appearances closely mimic atherosclerosis and are an important cause of graft failure. In one postmortem study in which saphenous vein conduits were sampled throughout their length, more than 75% narrowing was demonstrated in 11% to 26% of the segments examined (92). Grafts can be dilated by angioplasty, but some patients require reoperation.

In routine operations, occlusions of the left anterior descending coronary artery are usually bypassed with the left or sometimes the right internal mammary artery. Long-term patency rates are superior to saphenous vein grafts (93,94). The caliber of the normal internal mammary artery is similar to distal coronary arteries. Preexisting occlusive disease is present in fewer than 5% of patients (95,96), and only occasional grafts develop atheromatous obstructions (97). In

**TABLE 4.** *Pathologic changes after vascular surgery*

| Procedure | Spectrum of histologic change |
|---|---|
| Endarterectomy | *Acutely:* surface platelet and fibrin deposits on inner face of surgical dissection, occasionally progressing to occlusive thrombosis. *Chronically:* variable degrees of fibrous intimal hyperplasia, occasionally progressing to restenosis. "False" aneurysms formation. |
| Vein bypass grafting | *Acutely:* thrombosis, dissection at anastomosis site. *Chronically:* dilatation with fibrous intimal thickening and medial muscular hypertrophy (to be contrasted with preimplant state). Occasionally, marked intimal fibrosis with lipid deposition and hemorrhage, leading to occlusion ("vein atherosclerosis"). |
| Internal mammary artery grafting | *Acutely:* thrombosis and dissection at anastomosis site. *Chronically:* progressive dilatation. Few detailed accounts of long-term changes. As yet no evidence of "graft atherosclerosis." |
| Angioplasty | *Acutely:* dilatation of vessel lumen, cracking and fissuring of atheromatous intima with minimal medial dissection. *Chronically:* restenosis due to reactive fibrous intimal thickening. |
| Endovascular stenting | *Acutely:* thrombosis. *Chronically:* few detailed studies as yet. Experimental work suggests that fibrous intimal thickening will occur as in angioplasty. |
| Prosthetic vessels | *Acutely:* thrombotic occlusion. *Chronically:* extensive macrophage and giant cell infiltration of fabric wall. Formation of fibrin-rich pseudointima, occasionally progressing to partial or complete occlusion. Graft failure and thrombosis. |

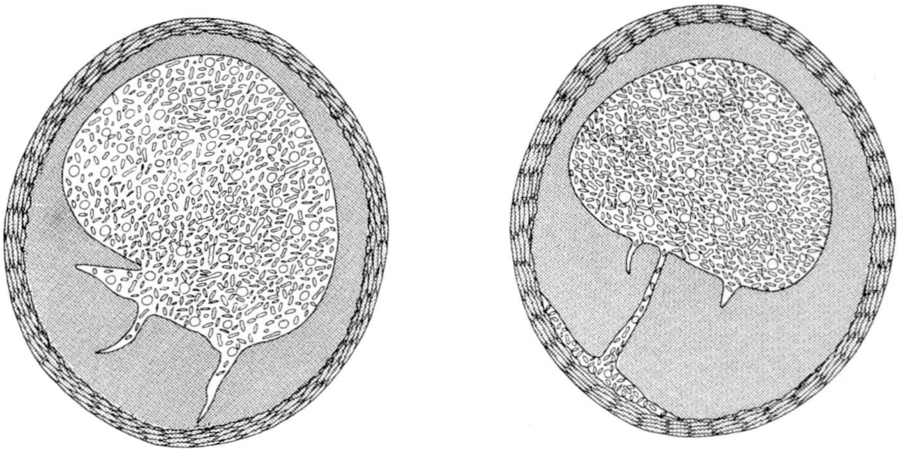

**FIG. 19.** A schematic drawing of the changes that follow coronary angioplasty. There is irregular cracking and fissuring of the atheromatous plaque **(left)**. Sometimes small dissections form (right).

its proximal portion the internal mammary is an elastic artery but the media is muscular from about the level of the fourth rib.

### *Angioplasty*

The technique of controlled dilatation (angioplasty) of peripheral limb vessels was described in the 1960s and applied to the coronary arteries in 1978. Percutaneous coronary angioplasty (PTCA) is now the treatment of choice for many proximal coronary stenoses (98,99) and may have a place in the treatment of unstable angina and in patients in shock after myocardial infarction (100). The mortality rate in most leading centers is now only 1% to 2%, and up to 95% of procedures are initially successful (101). In order to dilate the vessel, the heavily fibrous and focally calcified atheromatous plaque must be cracked open. Only when this has occurred can the deeper intima and underlying media be distended by the inflated balloon. Histologic studies of patients dying soon after angioplasty demonstrate a characteristic pattern of radial tears or splits, sometimes with dissections extending into the underlying media (101,102) (Fig. 19). There is some evidence that a minor degree of dissection is associated with a better long-term patency rate (103). However, if the dissection extends more widely, postoperative thrombus formation may occur. Occasional vessels have ruptured, and there may be a marked associated inflammatory reaction. Recurrent stenosis is usually the result of florid fibrous intimal proliferation (104–106). This may be modulated with antibodies to platelet membrane glycoprotein receptors (107,108) and often can be successfully treated by a second angioplasty (101).

Coronary arteries that are completely, or almost completely, occluded by atheroma may not be suitable for angioplasty. Devices that core through, or excise, the atheromatous material, or various forms of argon laser, are currently under evaluation (109). Metallic stents are increasingly used to maintain the patency of vessels after angioplasty (110,111). The full range of histologic appearances associated with these techniques are not yet clear (Table 4).

### *Prosthetic Vessels*

Various types of fabric graft are used for the treatment of peripheral vascular disease, for closing cardiac septal defects, or in other more complex procedures in children with congenital heart disease. Acute occlusion of prosthetic vessels is usually the result of surgical technique or poor flow rates. In time, prosthetic grafts develop a pseudointima. This has a jellylike consistency, may develop a partial, though not a complete, endothelial lining, and is composed of fibrin and enmeshed leukocytes (112). However, the most striking feature of these prosthetic vessels is the intense mononuclear and giant cell reaction that develops around the woven fibers of the graft. There is usually a moderate degree of adventitial fibrosis that binds the prosthesis to the surrounding tissues and reduces its elasticity. Long-term complications include thrombosis, particularly at flexures or surgical anastomoses, infection, and deterioration of the fibers of the graft (113,114).

## ELECTRON MICROSCOPY

### Endothelium

The entire vascular system is lined internally by a single layer of rather spindle-shaped endothelial cells. The overall appearance of endothelium, particularly on scanning electron microscopy, depends on whether pressure fixation was used (Fig. 20). In many areas, individual cells are oriented longitudinally with respect to the axis of the vessel wall. Individual cells measure up to 15 $\mu$m in width and 25 to 30 $\mu$m in length. Because they are very thin, their nuclei may produce bulges that protrude into the lumen.

Mature endothelial cells have many important synthetic and metabolic functions (115,116) but in comparison to some other cells and tissues have a low level of biochemical activity. This is reflected in the relatively sparse endoplas-

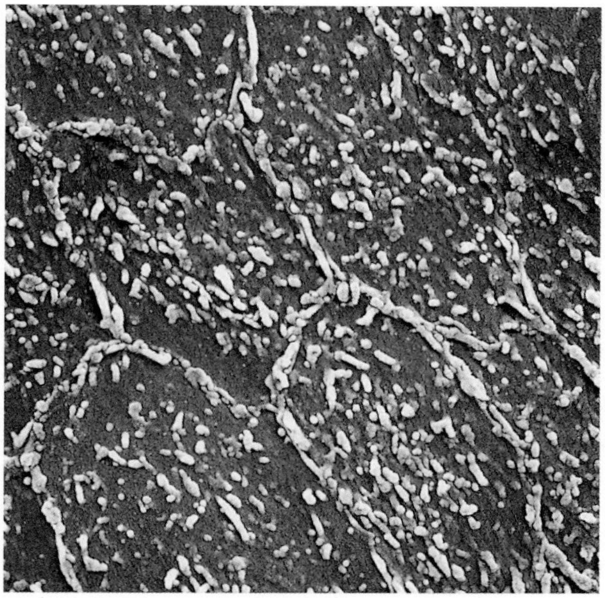

**FIG. 20.** Scanning electron microscopic appearances of the endothelium from an experimental animal perfused under pressure with fixative. The junctions between individual endothelial cells are clearly seen and in this preparation microvilli are particularly prominent (original magnification **×1,200**).

mic reticulum, small number of free ribosomes, and inconspicuous Golgi apparatus. However, in appropriate conditions in tissue culture, endothelial cells divide rapidly, forming an ordered monolayer of cuboidal rather than spindle-shaped cells.

The salient ultrastructural features of vascular tissue are listed as follows:

1. Despite a wide variety of biochemical functions, normal endothelium has poorly developed endoplasmic reticulum (ER) and relatively few ribosmal aggregates. Cultured endothelium (e.g., umbilical vein) shows greater evidence of synthetic activity.
2. Endothelial cells connected by tight, communicating (gap), and adherence junctions. Density of functions varies considerably from site to site. They are more numerous in arteries than in arterioles, capillaries, and other vessels.
3. Transendothelial channels characterize fenestrated endothelium (e.g., hepatic sinusoids, glomeruli, endocrine organs).
4. Cytoplasmic inclusions of endothelium include numerous plasmalemmal vesicles and Weibel-Palade bodies.
5. No significant media in small arterioles, capillaries, or lymphatics is present. Capillary endothelium is surrounded by basement membrane in which pericytes are embedded. There is very little basement membrane around lymphatic vessels. There are direct appositions between processes of pericytes and endothelium through gaps in the basement membrane.
6. Smooth muscle cells invested in basement membrane and are linked by communicating (gap) junctions. Elastin and collagen fibers may be closely opposed to the surfaces of smooth muscle cells.
7. In vivo smooth muscle cells of normal media are largely of the "contractile" phenotype. In culture and in certain physiologic and pathologic conditions, a "synthetic" phenotype may be assumed. This process may be mediated by T-cell cytokines.

In ideally fixed material, endothelial cells appear to overlap each other with flaps of cytoplasm producing something like the appearance of a tiled roof. These marginal flaps may disappear as the force of the pulse pressure is absorbed. The number and type of endothelial cell junctions varies in different parts of the vascular tree. There are many in large impermeable arteries but few in small capillaries and venules (117). Cerebral capillaries are particularly impermeable. Tight junctions effectively seal cells together, and the space between individual cells is seldom greater than 5 nm (118). This can prevent even the leakage of small molecules. Communicating (gap) junctions facilitate electrical or biochemical signaling from one endothelial cell to another, whereas adherence junctions leave a space of about 20 nm between endothelial cells. Specific classes of proteins characterize different types of junctions (119): for example, cadherins in adherence junctions and connexins in gap junctions.

Small fingerlike projections, the microvilli, may be seen on the surface of endothelial cells (Fig. 20). They usually measure 200 to 400 nm in length, but their exact function is uncertain. Their density varies from site to site and from species to species and they have been studied in detail in human atheromatous material (120). A thin polysaccharide layer, the glycocalyx, coats the luminal surface of the endothelium. This is up to 100 nm in thickness, but its exact function is uncertain.

**Inclusions of Endothelial Cells**

Lysosomes are readily identified in most endothelial cells and are involved in intracytoplasmic digestion of foreign debris and products of metabolism. In many areas of the vascular system membrane-bound vesicles measuring up to 80 to 90 nm can be identified (Fig. 21). They are most prominent on the abluminal surface of the endothelial cell. They were originally known as plasmalemmal vesicles but are now usually termed caveolae. Their functions include the sequestration and concentration of small molecules, potocytosis (121). Weibel-Palade bodies are characteristic inclusions of endothelium and measure up to 3 $\mu$m in maximum dimension. These membrane-bound structures contain up to 25 parallel tubular arrays. Immunologic studies have shown that Weibel-Palade bodies are sites of storage of von Willebrand protein (122). They are a useful marker of endothelial cells

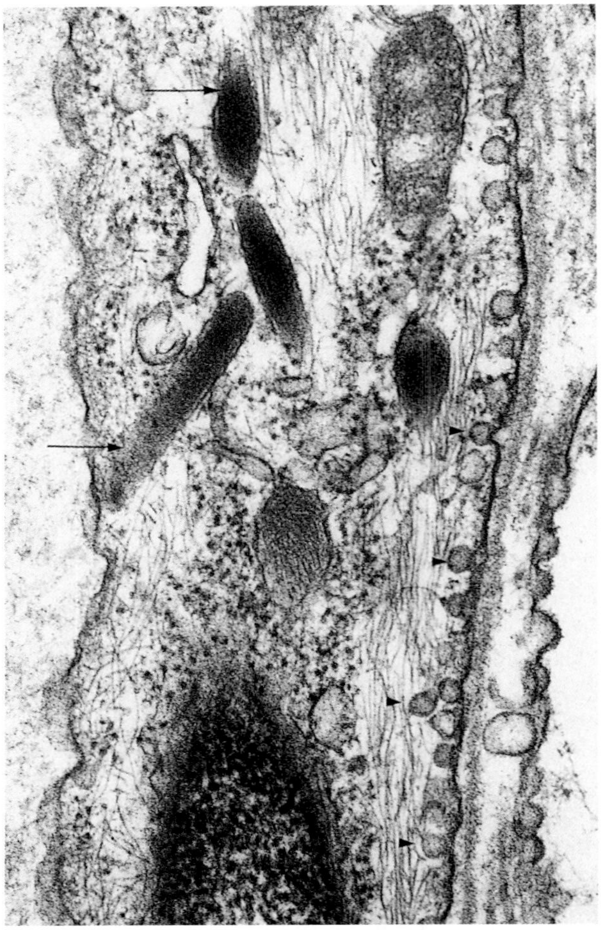

**FIG. 21.** Transmission electron micrograph of an endothelial cell from a small subcutaneous capillary. Plasmalemmal vesicles are present on the abluminal surface (*arrowheads*). There are conspicuous Weibel-Palade bodies (*arrows*). Only part of the endothelial cell nucleus is included (*lower part* of micrograph) (original magnification ×**15,000**).

but are seldom as conspicuous as in Fig. 21. A lengthy search of a number of tissue grids is sometimes necessary before they are detected.

The permeability of capillaries varies considerably from organ to organ. In some sites, such as the renal glomerulus, the hepatic sinusoids, the small intestine, and some endocrine glands, there is a rapid interchange between blood and the surrounding tissue. Some of these permeability differences are related to the exact nature of the junctions between endothelial cells, but endothelial fenestrae also have an important role in this respect. These fenestrations are in fact the openings of irregular, and sometimes incomplete, transendothelial channels, which allow the rapid interchange of fluid between the blood vessel lumen and the interstitium. There is a complex relationship between capillary endothelial cells, pericytes and their basement membranes (Figs. 22 and 23), which may be disordered in diabetes and hypertension (51,53).

### Media

In the human aorta, homogeneous parallel elastic lamellae alternate with layers containing smooth muscle cells and a variety of extracellular components. The interlaminar spaces are up to 25 μm in width, and the thickness of individual elastic bands is usually less than 2 μm (123). In animals, scanning electron microscopic studies have shown that individual lamellae anastomose with each other, forming a cylindrical elastic scaffold that imparts both strength and elasticity to the vessel wall (124,125). The internal elastic lamina of arteries usually consists of a single or double layer, but there are numerous fenestrae, often with a fishnet or sieve-like appearance. These fenestrae allow the passage of cells to and from the intima and media and sometimes contain cytoplasmic processes derived from endothelial cells. Larger fenestrations at branching points in the circle of Willis may be the sites at which berry aneurysms develop (126). When human aortic tissue obtained during cardiac surgery is examined by transmission electron microscopy, the structure of the elastic framework is more complex than in animals (123). In particular, smaller fragments of elastin are present in thin streaks forming bridges between the larger lamellae. The appearance of smooth muscle cells varies considerably under transmission electron microscopy (Fig. 24), although some of this is related to the angle in which individual cells are sectioned. Smooth muscle cell nuclei may appear lobated and have a wavy or crenated outline. The nucleolus is usually small and inconspicuous. Thin bands of elastic tissue appear to connect, or even anchor, smooth muscle cells to the larger elastic lamellae. This feature is thought to contribute to the vessel wall integrity during pulsatile distension of the aorta and arteries (127). Individual smooth muscle cells are often linked by communicating (gap) junctions, but, except in young animals, tight junctions are not seen. In the microcirculation and in some larger arteries and arterioles, there are gap junctions between the smooth muscle cells and the overlying endothelium (128). These myoendothelial junctions could have an important role in relaying physiologic or pharmacologic stimuli between the blood vessel lumen and the media.

Three types of filament can be identified in the cytoplasm. The thick myosin filaments measure up to 18 nm in diameter and may exceed 2 μm in length. In contrast, the thin actin filaments are only 6 to 8 nm in diameter but are far more numerous. As in many other cells, smooth muscle contains intermediate filaments measuring approximately 10 nm in diameter. Vimentin is the major intermediate filament in vascular smooth muscle and is often centered around electron-dense structures, dense bodies, which probably correspond to the Z bands of skeletal or cardiac muscle.

In tissue culture, arterial wall smooth muscle cells may adopt a rather different phenotype. The filamentous component is reduced, but there are comparatively larger amounts of endoplasmic reticulum, free ribosomes, and prominent

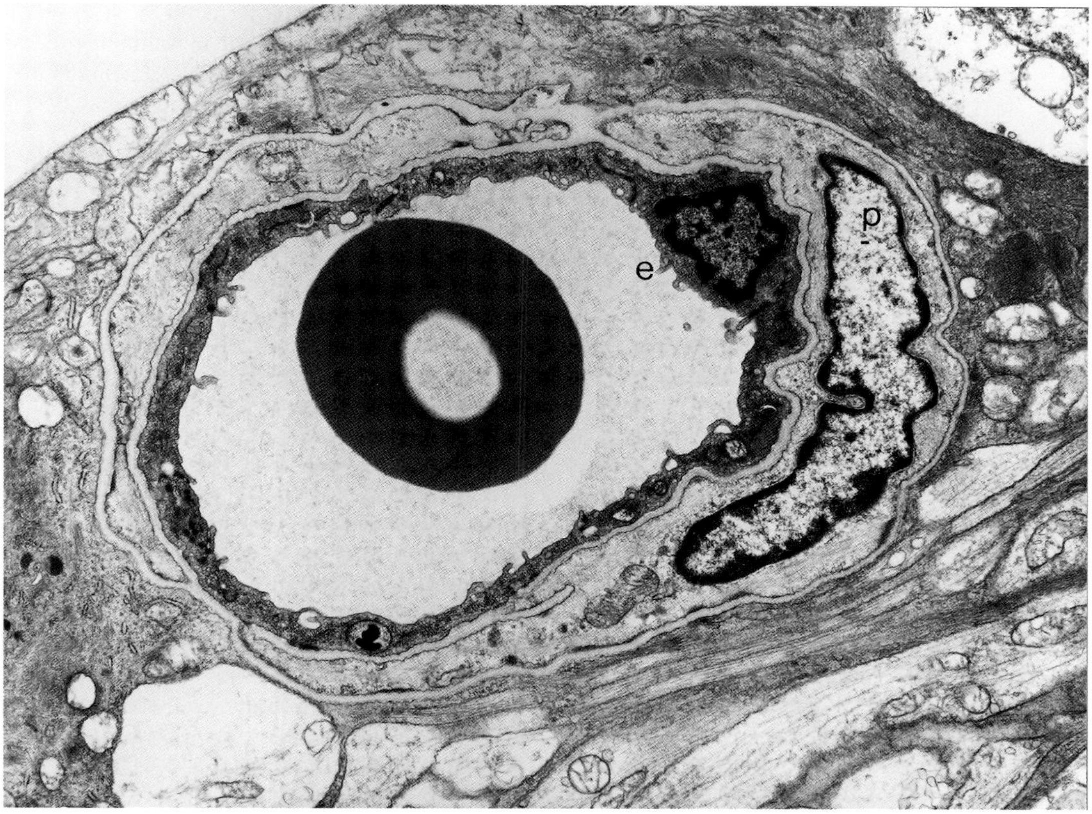


**FIG. 22.** Transmission electron micrograph of a superficial retinal capillary. Note that the basement membrane appears to split and envelope the pericyte proceses. e, endothelial cell nucleus; p, pericyte nucleus (original magnification ×**9,500**).

Golgi (27). Cells with this synthetic phenotype are thought to be responsible for the secretion of the connective tissue proteins that are present in the uterus in pregnancy and in atheromatous plaques.

### Adventitia and Supporting Cells

The adventitial layer consists almost entirely of collagen and elastic fibers. The thickness of this layer varies with the size of the vessel, and it may be continuous with the surrounding connective tissue. In some medium-sized veins it is particularly well developed but in cerebral arteries may be as thin as 80 $\mu$m (129). A layer of elastic tissue, the external elastic lamella, is present at the junction of the media and adventitia. In human material it is seldom as pronounced as the internal elastic lamella but is prominent in many other mammalian arteries. The pericytes that are present in and among the basement membrane of capillaries and small venules superficially resemble fibroblasts. The ultrastructural appearance of their cytoplasmic filaments suggests that they are contractile, and this is further evidence that they are of mesenchymal origin (56,130).

### Lymphatics and Veins

The smallest lymphatic vessels have wider lumina than blood capillaries and a discontinuous basement membrane. A variety of anchoring filaments bind the lymphatic endothelium to the surrounding collagenous tissues, perhaps providing the sort of support normally produced by basement membrane and enmeshed pericytes in capillaries (131). The ultrastructural appearances of venous capillaries, venules, and small veins mirror those seen at the light microscopic level (132).

## IMMUNOHISTOLOGY

### Technical Methods

Immunohistochemical methods have a long established role in experimental studies of arterial disease. In recent years particular attention has been directed to typing of cellular infiltrates (25,26), the distribution of apolipoproteins (133), oxidized lipoproteins (134), collagen subtypes (135), a variety of cytokines and cell adhesion molecules (136,137), and most recently to demonstrate apoptotic activ-

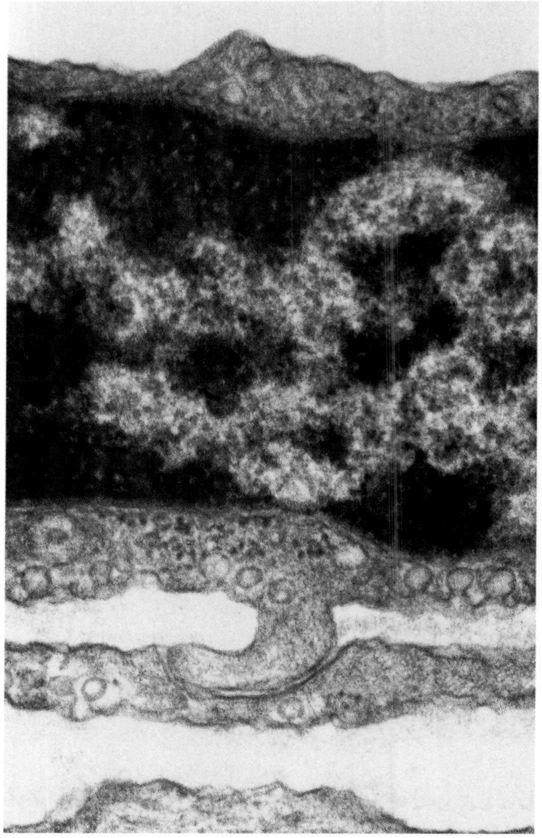

**FIG. 23.** Transmission electron micrograph showing direct contact between a process of an endothelial cell and a pericyte through a gap in basement membrane. The exact function of contacts between smooth muscle or pericytes and endothelial cells is unknown (original magnification ×**18,000**).

ity within lesions (7,8). Diagnostic histopathologists have sometimes questioned the value of immunohistochemistry in vascular disease. At first the range of antibodies was limited and, as in any tissue with a large connective tissue component, autofluorescence or background staining of collagen may obscure specific reaction products. These problems have been largely overcome, and there are now detailed schedules specifically designed for vascular tissue (138). Important technical aspects are summarized in the following list:

1. Most routine staining reactions can now be successfully applied to vascular tissue. Problems with background staining of collagen can usually be eliminated or reduced by careful attention to detail.
2. There is no entirely satisfactory marker of vascular endothelium. Factor VIII–related antigen is a reliable marker of normal endothelium. CD31 may be the best for the diagnosis of vascular tumors. It should be used with at least one other marker, such as Factor VIII, *Ulex,* or CD34. All of these have some cross-reactions with leukocytes, stromal cells, or malignant epithelial cells.
3. Alpha smooth muscle actin is an excellent marker of vascular smooth muscle in routinely processed sections.
4. No histologic or immunohistochemical method reliably distinguishes capillaries from lymphatics.

We use streptavidin biotin complexes (Dako K377) to detect both polyclonal and monoclonal primary antibodies. We routinely pretreat sections to be stained with polyclonal antibodies with trypsin, accepting that overtrypsinization enhances background staining (139). The staining of many monoclonal antibodies can be enhanced by pretreating sections in a microwave oven or pressure cooker. Careful titration of the primary antibody concentration, trypsin incubation, or heating times are essential before the best results can be obtained. We incubate all monoclonal and some polyclonal primary antibodies overnight at 4°C.

Although monoclonal primary antibodies usually produce excellent results, some nonspecific staining may occur. If sections are not pretreated, it is advisable to block with 1% bovine serum albumin for 30 minutes before applying the primary antibody. Occasionally, the brown reaction product of diamino benzidine may be confused with endogenous pigments such as hemosiderin or melanin. A variety of red and blue chromogens are now available and generally produce clear results, especially if sections are mounted in Crystal-Mount (Biomedia Corporation, Foster City, California).

## Antigen Expression of Normal and Neoplastic Vascular Tissue

### *Endothelium*

Despite the wide range of metabolic and synthetic reactions of the vascular wall (115,140), comparatively few immunologic methods have been developed to mark normal or neoplastic endothelium, at least in paraffin-embedded tissues (141). If it is important to identify endothelium or define the endothelial nature of a tumor staining with Factor VIII–related antigen, *Ulex* lectin and antibodies to CD31 and CD34 should be performed.

Factor VIII–related antigen is present in both normal lining and cultured human endothelium (115) and is probably stored in Weibel-Palade bodies (121,122). It can be detected in the subendothelium, stressing its role in the adhesion of platelets to deendothelialized surfaces (142). It was the first reliable marker of endothelium (143,144) and retains a useful role in diagnostic pathology. A granular cytoplasmic reaction product is characteristic. Megakaryocytes are also stained, but there are few, if any, troublesome cross-reactions. Background staining of serum is often noted. Renal glomerular endothelium may not stain, and the reaction may be weak or absent in solid areas of angiosarcomas (145–147).

The lectin *Ulex europaeus* 1 agglutinin binds to some $\alpha$-L-fucose–containing glycocompounds (148) and therefore to virtually all human endothelia. The staining pattern is some-

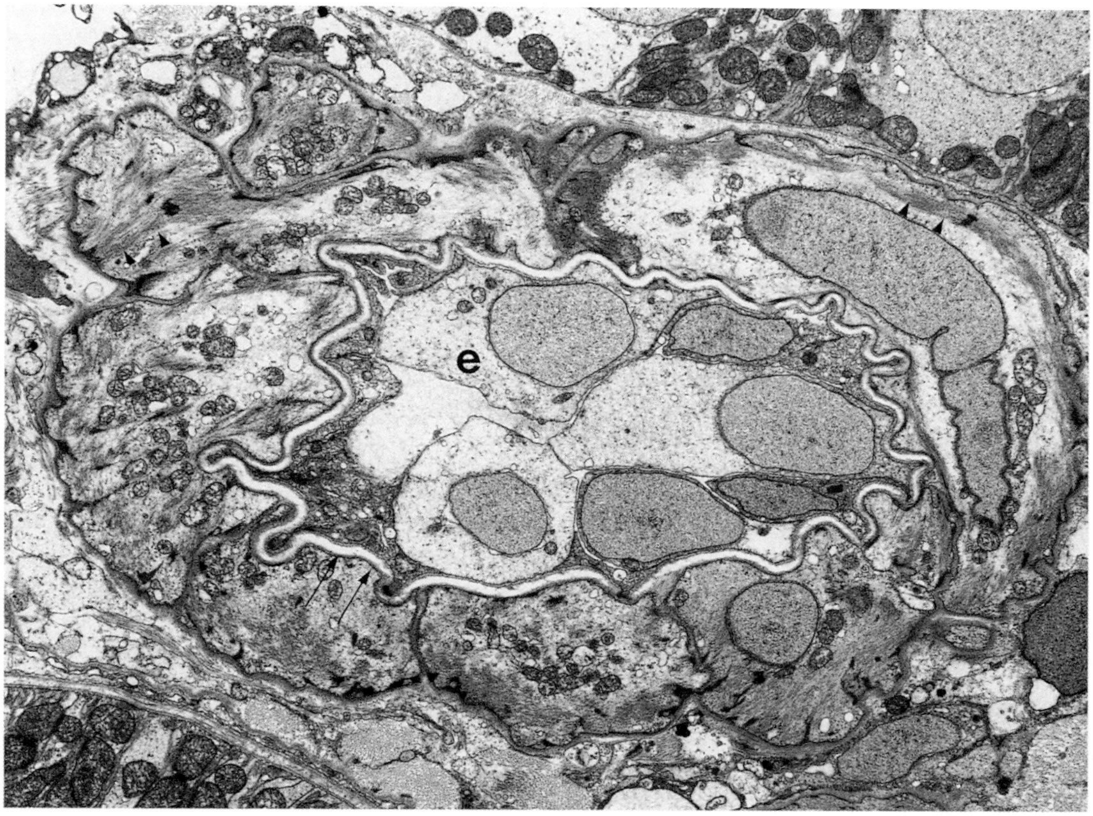


**FIG. 24.** Transmission electron micrograph of a small arteriole. Because of fixation artifact, the endothelial cells (e) have unusually clear cytoplasm. Note the prominent basement membrane (*arrows*) and the fibrils of smooth muscle cells (*arrowheads*) (original magnification ×**5,000**).

times more intense than with Factor VIII antibodies, especially in small vessels (149,150) (Fig. 25). Skin and skin appendage epithelia and some cutaneous tumors (151) also may stain with *Ulex,* but this is seldom a source of confusion.

CD31 and CD34 antibodies label endothelial cells and many vascular tumors in formalin-fixed, paraffin-embedded tissues. CD31 is a membrane glycoprotein and a member of the immunoglobulin superfamily (152,153). It may function as a minor histocompatibility antigen (154) and because of its role in facilitating leukocyte migration was originally

A 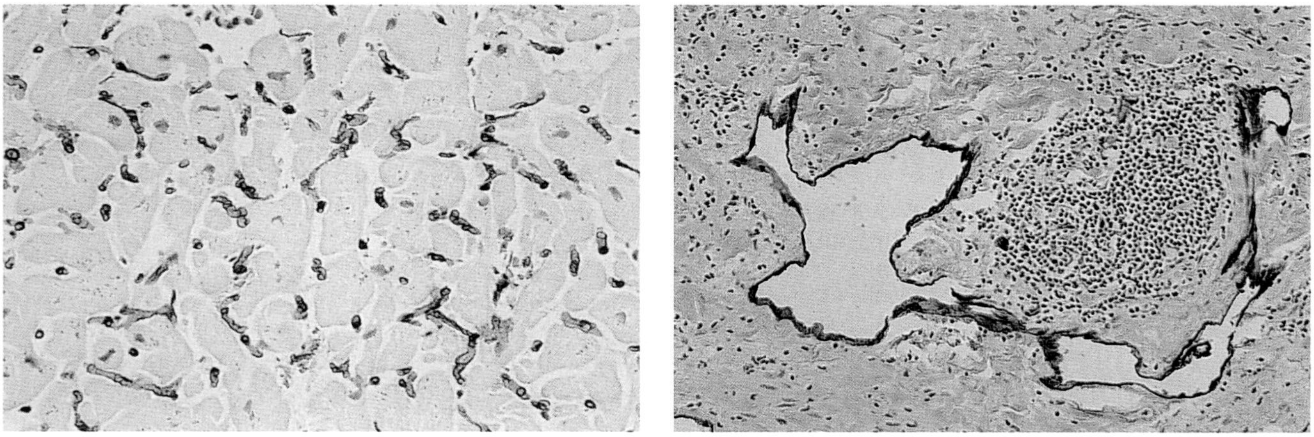 B

**FIG. 25. A, B:** *Ulex europaeus* lectin staining of endothelium. **A:** The normal myocardial capillary network is stained. **B:** Specimen from the axillary tail of a patient with breast carcinoma. A large and tortuous vascular channel has been stained by *Ulex,* but it is not clear whether this is a lymphatic or a small vein. Note the staining of small blood vessels within the lymphoid follicle. There is a moderate but acceptable degree of background staining.

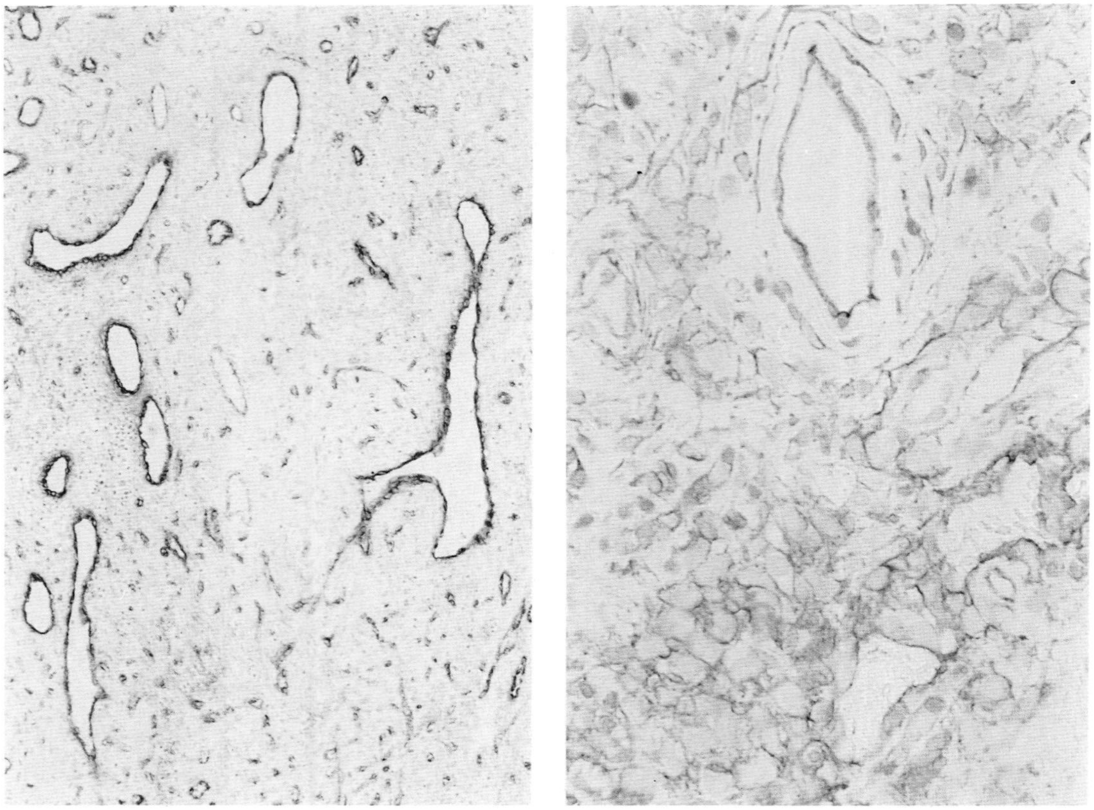

A B

**FIG. 26.** An epitheloid hemangioma stained with antibodies to Factor VIII–related antigen (**A**) and CD34 (**B**). Note the crisp staining of the endothelium of blood vessels with Factor VIII, but the tumor cells are negative. CD34 staining of endothelium is less prominent but the endothelial nature of the tumor cells is confirmed. In practice, Factor VIII is a satisfactory stain for normal vascular endothelium. If a tumor is thought to be of vascular origin, CD31 and CD34 also should be used.

designated platelet–endothelial cell adhesion molecule (PECAM-1). It is present on endothelial cells, bone marrow stem cells, platelets, and most circulating leukocytes, and the first monoclonal antibody to it was named JC70 (155). It is one of the best vascular markers (138,156) but also stains plasma cells, monocytes, and some other leukocytes and megakaryocytes. At present it is the most useful antibody for the identification of angiosarcomas (141,157). The CD34 antigen is a heavily glycosylated transmembrane protein expressed on a number of immature hematopoietic precursor cells (158). CD34 antibodies, sometimes known as QBEND 10, have important applications in the immunophenotyping of some leukemias. They also stain normal vascular endothelium and some vascular tumors (Fig. 26), especially Kaposi's sarcoma (159–161). Positive staining is obtained with some cutaneous tumors, occasional poorly differentiated carcinomas, and the stromal component of some tumors (162).

Other antibodies mark endothelial cells but, at present, are ineffective or inconsistent in paraffin sections. CD36 is associated with the thrombospondin receptor. It stains endothelial cells in most capillaries and many small vessels but not the endothelium of arteries and larger veins (138). Intercellular adhesion molecule 1 (ICAM-1; CD54) is present in normal endothelium and is upregulated in inflammation and in atheromatous lesions (137,163). Endothelial staining with antibodies to other cell adhesion molecules, such as E-selectin, is less consistent, and there is considerable variation in the expression of these molecules in different areas of the vascular tree (140). There are many recent reports of the distribution and expression of the different isoforms of nitric oxide synthase. Some of these have used biopsy material (164), and these antibodies may have a role in diagnostic histopathology in the future.

### *Smooth Muscle*

The immunochemical and immunohistologic studies of Gabbiani and Skalli et al. (165,166) have demonstrated that vascular smooth muscle has a distinctive component of contractile and intermediate filament proteins. In most smooth muscle, the gamma isoform of smooth muscle actin and desmin predominate. In contrast, in vascular tissue there is abundant alpha smooth muscle actin, and vimentin exceeds desmin. A monoclonal antibody directed against smooth

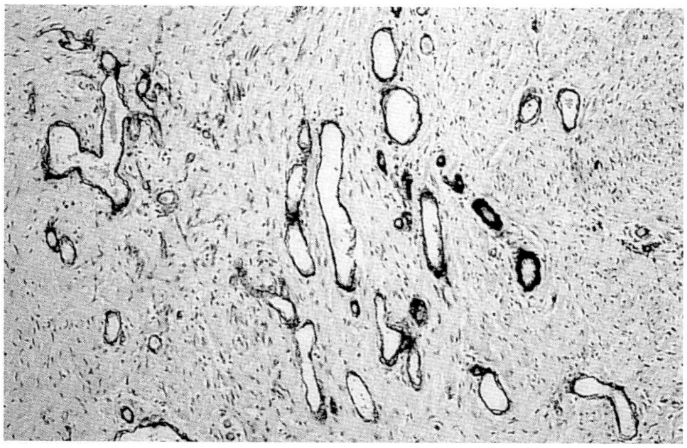

**FIG. 27.** Numerous blood vessels stained with an immunoperoxidase technique using a primary antibody to alpha smooth muscle actin.

muscle actin, which can be used in formalin-fixed tissue, is an excellent marker of medial muscle (166,167) (Fig. 27). It stains positively in glomus tumors and a variable proportion of benign and malignant smooth muscle tumors. Negative-staining results are usually obtained with rhabdomyosarcomas and hemangiopericytomas (167,168).

### *Capillaries and Lymphatics*

Because lymphatics lack a true basement membrane, they should, in theory, be distinguishable from capillaries by the lack of immunologic staining to antigens such as laminin or type IV collagen (66,67,169,170). In careful studies in which a retrograde injection of the thoracic duct was made, Hultberg and Svanholm (67) have confirmed that the smallest lymphatics do indeed give a negative, or at the most a weak, focal staining reaction in this way. However, larger lymphatics, including those within lymph nodes, stain with laminin, and it is doubtful whether laminin immunoreactivity can be used routinely for the identification of small vascular channels (66). Lymphangiomas are reported to stain strongly with laminin (171).

The identification of tumor emboli in vascular or lymphatic channels, rather than in artifactual tissue spaces, is of particular importance in the assessment of mammary carcinomas. There is a measure of agreement that staining with *Ulex* Factor VIII or basement membrane antibodies is useful in this respect (64,172). Nevertheless, not all small vascular channels will stain, and occasionally groups of malignant epithelial cells may react with *Ulex* lectins (65).

## REFERENCES


1. Lakatta EG, Mitchell JH, Pomerance A, Rowe GG. Human aging: changes in structure and function [Abstract]. *J Am Coll Cardiol* 1987; 10:42–47.
2. Gallagher PJ. The aging aorta. *Lancet* 1985;2:1402–1403.
3. Robins SP, Farquharson C. Connective tissue components of the blood vessel wall in health and disease. In: Stehbens W, Lie JT, eds. *Vascular* pathology. London: Chapman & Hall; 1995:89–127.
4. Clark JM, Glagov S. Transmural organisation of the arterial media. The lamellar unit revisited. *Arteriosclerosis* 1985;5:19–34.
5. Lie JT, Brown AL, Carter ET. Spectrum of aging changes in temporal arteries. Its significance in interpretation of biopsy of temporal artery. *Arch Pathol* 1970;90:278–285.
6. Bouissou H, Pieraggi MT, Julian M. Age related morphological changes of the arterial wall. In: Camilleri JP, Berry CL, Fiessinger JN, Bariety J, eds. *Diseases of the arterial wall.* London: Springer-Verlag; 1989:71–78.
7. Geng Y-J, Libby P. Evidence for apoptosis in advanced human atheroma. Co-localization with interleukin-1$\beta$–converting enzyme. *Am J Pathol* 1995;147:251–266.
8. Han DKM, Haudenschild CC, Hong MK, et al. Evidence for apoptosis in human atherogenesis and in a rat vascular injury model. *Am J Pathol* 1995;147:267–277.
9. Doherty TM, Detrand RC. Coronary artery calcification as an active process: a new perspective on an old problem. *Calcif Tissue Int* 1994; 54:224–230
10. Elliott RJ, McGrath LT. Calcification of the human thoracic aorta during ageing. *Calcif Tissue Int* 1994;54:268–273.
11. Westermark P, Mucchiano G, Marthin T, Johnson KH, Sletten K. Apolipoprotein A1 derived amyloid in human aortic atheromatous plaques. *Am J Pathol* 1995;147:1186–1192.
12. Mucchiano G, Cornwell GG Westermark P. Senile aortic amyloid. Evidence for two distinct forms of localised deposit. *Am J Pathol* 1992;140:871–877.
13. Schlatmann TJM, Becker AE. Histologic changes in the normal ageing aorta: implications for dissecting aortic aneurysm. *Am J Cardiol* 1977;39:13–20.
14. Pomerance A, Yacoub MH, Gula G. The surgical pathology of thoracic aortic aneurysms. *Histopathology* 1977;1:257–276.
15. Klima T, Spjut HJ, Coelho A, et al. The morphology of ascending aortic aneurysms. *Hum Pathol* 1983;14:810–817.
16. Leonard JC, Hasleton PS. Dissecting aortic aneurysms: a clinicopathological study. *Q J* Med 1979;49:55–63.
17. Tsipouras P, del Maestro R, Sarfarazi M, et al. Genetic linkage of the Marfan syndrome, ectopia lentis and contractural arachnodactyly to the fibrillin genes on chromosomes 15 and 5. *N Engl J Med* 1992;326: 905–909.
18. Edwards MJ, Challinder CJ, Colley PW, et al. Clinical and linkage study of a large family with simple ectopia lentis linked to FBNI. *Am J Med Gen* 1994;53:65–71.
19. Pan TC, Saski T, Zhang RZ, et al. Structure and expression of fibulin-2, a novel extracellular matrix protein with multiple EGF like repeats and concensus motifs for calcium binding. *J Cell Biol* 1993;123: 1269–1277.
20. Ernst CB Abdominal aortic aneurysms. *N Engl J Med* 1993;328: 1167–1172.
21. Kontusaari S, Trump G, Kuivaniemi H, Romanic AM, Prockop DJ. A mutation in the gene for type III procollagen (COL3A1) in a family with aortic aneurysm. *Clin Sci* 1990;86:1465–1473.
22. Mitchinson MJ. Chronic periaortitis and periarteritis. *Histopathology* 1984;8:589–600.
23. Stratford N, Britten K, Gallagher PJ. Inflammatory infiltrates in human coronary atherosclerosis. *Atherosclerosis* 1986;59:271–276.
24. Stary HC, Blankenhorn DH, Chandler AB, et al. A definition of the intima of human arteries and its atherosclerosis-prone regions. *Circulation* 1992;85:391–405.
25. Hansson GK, Jonasson L, Seifert PS, Stemme S. Immune mechanisms in atherosclerosis. Arteriosclerosis 1989;9:567–578.
26. Libby P, Hansson GK. Involvement of the immune system in human atherogenesis: current knowledge and unanswered questions. *Lab Invest* 1991;64:5–15
27. Rolfe BE, Campbell JH, Smith NJ, Cheong MW, Campbell GR. T lymphocytes affect smooth muscle cell phenotype and proliferation. *Arteriosclerosis Thromb Vasc Biol* 1995;15:1204–1210.
28. van der Wal AC, Becker AE, van der Loos CM, Das PK. Site of intimal rupture or erosion of thrombosed coronary atheromatous plaques is characterised by an inflammatory process irrespective of the damaged plaques morphology. *Circulation* 1994;89:36–43
29. Davies MJ, Richardson PD, Woolf N, Katz D, Mann J. Risk of thrombosis in human atherosclerotic plaques: role of extracellular lipid,

macrophage and smooth muscle cell content. *Br Heart J* 1993;69: 377–381.
30. Freestone T, Turner RJ, Coady A, Higman DJ, Greenhalgh RM, Powell JT. Inflammation and matrix metalloproteinases in the enlarging adbominal aortic aneurysm. *Arteriosclerosis Thromb Vasc Biol* 1995; 15:1145–1151.
31. Gallis ZS, Sukhova GK, Lark WW, Libby P. Increased expression of matrix metalloproteinases and matrix degrading activity in vunerable regions of human atherosclerotic plaques. *J Clin Invest* 1994;94: 2493–2503.
32. Ramshaw AL, Parums DV. The distribution of adhesion molecules in chronic periaortitis. *Histopathology* 1993;24:23.
33. Ramshaw AL, Roskell DE, Parums DV. Cytokine gene expression in aortic adventitial inflammation associated with advanced atherosclerosis (chronic periaortitis). *J Clin Pathol* 1994;47:721–727.
34. Kirklin JW, Barratt Boyes BS. *Cardiac surgery.* 2nd ed. New York: Churchill Livingstone; 1993:1276–1284.
35. Anderson RH, Becker AE. The arterial duct (ductus arteriosus). In: Anderson RH, Becker AE, Robertson WB, eds. *Systemic pathology. 3rd ed. Vol. 10. The Cardiovascular System. Part A.* Edinburgh: Churchill Livingstone; 1994:197–202.
36. Silver MM, Freedom RM, Silver MD, Olley PM. The morphology of the newborn ductus arteriosus: a reappraisal of its structure and closure with special reference to prostaglandin E therapy. *Hum Pathol* 1981;12:1123–1136.
37. Christakis GT, Weisel RD, Buth KJ, et al. Is body size the cause for poor outcomes of coronary artery bypass operation in women? *J Thorac Cardiovasc Surg* 1995;110:1344–1358.
38. O'Connor GT, Morton JR, Diehl MJ, et al. Differences between men and women in hospital mortality associated with coronary artery by pass graft surgery. Circulation 1993;88:2104–2110.
39. Hartnell GG, Parnell BM, Pridie RB. Coronary artery ectasia: its prevalence and clinical significance in 4993 patients. *Br Heart J* 1985; 54:392–395.
40. Stary HC, Chandler AB, Glagov S, et al. A definition of intima, fatty streak and intermediate lesions of atherosclerosis. *Arteriosclerosis Thrombosis* 1994;14:840–856.
41. Breton M, Picard J. Effects of "ageing" on arterial cells in vitro. In: Camilleri JP, Berry CL, Fiessinger JN, Bariety J, eds. *Diseases of the arterial wall.* London: Springer-Verlag; 1989:71–78.
42. Hariri RJ, Hajjar DP, Coletti D, et al. Aging and arteriosclerosis. Cell cycle kinetics of young and old arterial smooth muscle cells. *Am J Pathol* 1988;131:132–136.
43. Schwartz SM, Reidy MA. Common mechanisms of proliferation of smooth muscle cells in atherosclerosis and hypertension. *Hum Pathol* 1987;18:240–247.
44. Wagner WD, Edwards IJ, St Clair RW, Baraka J. Low density lipoprotein interactions with artery derived proteoglycan: the influence of LDL particle size and the relationship to atherosclerosis susceptibility. *Atherosclerosis* 1989;75:49–59.
45. Velican D, Velican C. Comparative study on age related changes and atherosclerotic involvement of the coronary arteries of male and female subjects up to 40 years of age. *Atherosclerosis* 1981;38:39–50.
46. Wolinsky H, Glagov S. Nature of species differences in the medial distribution of aortic vasa vasorum in mammals. *Circ Res* 1967;20: 409–421.
47. Marcus ML, Heistad DD, Armstrong ML, Abboud FM. Effects of chronic hypertension on vasa vasorum in the thoracic aorta. *Cardiovasc Res* 1985;19:777–781.
48. Heistad DD, Armstrong ML. Blood flow through vasa vasorum of coronary arteries in atherosclerotic monkeys. *Arteriosclerosis* 1988; 6:326–331.
49. Feingold KR, Browner WS, Siperstein MD. Prospective studies of muscle basement membrane width in prediabetics. *J Clin Endocrinol Metab* 1989;69:784–789.
50. Yarom R, Zirkin H, Stammler G, Rose AG. Human coronary microvessels in diabetes and ischaemia. Morphometric study of autopsy material. *J Pathol* 166;1992:265–270.
51. Merimee TJ. Diabetic retinopathy. A synthesis of perspectives. *N Engl J Med* 322;1990:978–983.
52. Timpe R, Dziadek M. Structure, development and molecular pathology of basement membranes. *Int Rev Exp Pathol* 1986;29:1–112.
53. Kilo C, Vogler N, Williamson JR. Muscle capillary basement membrane changes related to aging and to diabetes mellitus. *Diabetes* 1972;21:881–905.
54. Joyce NC, Haire MF, Palade GE. Contractile proteins in pericytes. II. Immunocytochemical evidence for the presence of two isomyosins in graded concentrations. *J Cell Biol* 1987;100:1387–1395.
55. Cancella PA, Baker RN, Pollock PS, Frommes SP. The reaction of pericytes of the central nervous system to exogenous protein. *Lab Invest* 1972;26:376–383.
56. Sims DE, Recent advances in pericyte biology—implications for health and disease. *Can J Cardiol* 1991;7:431–443.
57. Tilton RG, Hoffman PL, Kilo C, Williamson JR. Pericyte degeneration and basement membrane thickening in skeletal muscle capillaries of human diabetics. *Diabetes* 1981;30:325–334.
58. Freemont AJ, Jones CJP. Light microscopic, histochemical and ultrastructural studies of human lymph node paracortical venules. *J Anat* 1983;136:349–362.
59. Langes K. Hort W. Intimal fibrosis (phlebosclerosis) in the saphenous vein of the lower limb: a quantitative analysis. *Virchows Arch [A]* 1992;421:127–131.
60. Milroy CM, Scott DJA, Beard JD, Horrocks M, Bradfield JWB. Histological appearance of the long saphenous vein. *J Pathol* 1989;159: 311–316.
61. O'Morchol C, O'Morchol PJ. Differences in lymphatic and blood capillary permeability: ultrastructural–functional correlations. *Lymphology* 1987;20:205–209.
62. Boggon RP, Palfrey AJ. The microscopic anatomy of human lymphatic trunks. *J Anat* 1973;114:389–405.
64. Lee AKC, DeLellis RA, Silverman ML, Wolfe HJ. Lymphatic and blood vessel invasion in breast carcinoma. A useful prognostic indicator. *Hum Pathol* 1986;17:984–987.
65. Saigo PE, Rosen PP. The application of immunohistochemical stains to identify endothelial-lined channels in mammary carcinoma. *Cancer* 1987;59:51–54.
66. Listrom MB, Fenoglio Preiser CM. Does laminin immunoreactivity really distinguish between lymphatics and blood vessels. *Surg Pathol* 1988;1:71–74.
67. Hultberg BM, Svanholm H. Immunohistochemical differentiation between lymphangiographically verified lymphatic vessels and blood vessels. *Virchows Arch [A]* 1989;414:209–215.
68. Reid LM. The pulmonary circulation: remodelling in growth and disease. *Am Rev Respir Dis* 1979;119:531–546.
69. Wagenvoort CA, Mooi WJ. *Biopsy pathology of the pulmonary vasculature.* London: Chapman & Hall; 1989.
70. Edwards WD. Pulmonary hypertension and related vascular diseases. In: Stehbens WE, Lie JT, eds. *Vascular pathology.* London: Chapman & Hall; 1995:583–621.
71. Warnock ML, Kunzmann A. Changes with age in muscular pulmonary arteries. *Arch Pathol Lab Med* 1977;101:175–179.
72. Warnock ML, Kunzmann A. Muscular pulmonary arteries in chronic obstructive lung disease. *Arch Pathol Lab Med* 1977;101:180–186.
73. Hale KA, Niewoehner DE, Cosio MG. Morphologic changes in muscular pulmonary arteries: relationship to cigarette smoking, airway disease and emphysema. *Am Rev Respir Dis* 1980;122:273–278.
74. Wagenvoort CA. Open lung biopsies in congenital heart disease for evaluation of pulmonary vascular disease. Predictive value with regard to corrective operability. *Histopathology* 1985;9:417–436.
75. Haworth SG, Radley-Smith R, Yacoub M. Lung biopsy findings in transposition of the great arteries with ventricular septal defect; potentially reversible pulmonary vascular disease is not always synonymous with operability. *J Am Coll Cardiol* 1987;9:327–333.
76. Wilson NJ, Seear MD, Taylor GP, et al. The clinical value and risks of lung biopsy in children with congenital heart disease. *J Thoracic Cardiovasc Surg* 1990;99:460–468.
77. Nicod P, Moser KM. Primary pulmonary hypertension. The risks and benefit of lung biopsy. *Circulation* 80;1989:1486–1488.
78. Currie AE, Gallagher PJ. The pathology of clubbing; vascular changes in the nail bed. *Br J Dis Chest* 1988;82:382–385.
79. Miettinen M, Lehto VP, Virtanen I. Glomus tumour cells: evaluation of smooth muscle and endothelial cell properties. *Virchows Arch [B]* 1983;43:139–149.
80. Hobbs KEF. The surgery of portal hypertension. In: Millward-Sadler GH, Wright R, Arthur MJP, eds. *Liver and biliary disease.* 3rd ed. London: Bailliere Tindall; 1992:1323–1334.
81. Howard OM, Buchanan JD, Hunt RH. Angiodysplasia of the colon. Experience of 26 cases. *Lancet* 1982;2:16–19.
82. Boley SJ, Sammartano R, Brandt LJ, Sprayregen S. Vascular ectasias of the colon. *Surg Gynecol Obstet* 1979;149:353–359.

83. Thelmo WL, Vetrano JA, Wibowo A, et al. Angiodysplasia of the colon revisited: pathologic demonstration without the use of intravascular injection technique. *Hum Pathol* 1991;325:1086–1096.
84. Veldhuyzen van Zanten SJO, Bartlesman JFWM, Schipper MEI, Tytgat GNJ. Recurrent massive haematemesis from Dieulafoy vascular malformations—a review of 101 cases. *Gut* 1986;27:213–222
85. Miko TL, Thomazy VA. The caliber persistent artery of the stomach: a unifying approach to gastric aneurysm, Dieulafoy's lesion, and submucosal arterial malformation. *Hum Pathol* 1988;19:914–921.
86. Kragel AH, McIntosh CM, Roberts WC. Morphologic changes in coronary artery seen late after endarterectomy. *Am J Cardiol* 1989;63: 757–759.
87. Baker WH, Hayes AC, Manter D, Lettory FN. Durability of carotid endarterectomy. *Surgery* 1983;94:112–115.
88. Ehrenfeld WK, Hays RJ. False aneurysms after carotid endarterectomy. *Arch Surg* 1972;104:288–291.
89. Neitzel GF, Barboriak JJ, Pintar K, Qureshi I. Atherosclerosis in aortocoronary bypass grafts. Morphologic study and risk factor analysis 6–12 years after surgery. *Arteriosclerosis* 1986;6:594–600.
90. Garratt KN, Edwards WD, Kaufmann UP, Vietstra RE, Holmes DR. Differenial histopathology of primary atherosclerotic and stenotic lesions in coronary arteries and saphenous vein by pass grafts: analysis of tissue obtained by directional atherectomy. *J Am Coll Cardiol* 1991;17:442–448.
91. Dilley RJ, McGreachie JK, Prendergast FJ. A review of the histologic changes in vein to artery grafts with particular reference to intimal hyperplasia. *Ann Surg* 1988;123:691–696.
92. Kalan JM, Roberts WC. Morphologic findings in saphenous veins used as coronary arterial bypass conduits for longer than 1 year: necropsy analysis of 53 patients, 123 saphenous veins, and 1865 five millimetre segments of veins. *Am Heart J* 1990;119:1164–1173.
93. Cameron A, Davis KB, Green G, Schaff HV. Coronary artery grafts with internal–thoracic grafts—effects on survival over a 15 year period. *N Engl J Med* 1996;334:216–219.
94. Lewis MR, Dehmer GJ. Coronary bypass using the internal mammary artery. *Am J Cardiol* 1985;56:480–482.
95. Rainer WG, Sadler TR, Ligget MS. Internal mammary arteriography prior to coronary artery bypass surgery. *Chest* 1973;63:523–524.
96. Kay HR, Korns ME, Flemma RJ, Tector AJ, Lepley D. Atherosclerosis of the internal mammary artery. *Ann Thorac Surg* 1976;21: 504–507.
97. Stullman WS, Hilliard GK. Unrecognized internal mammary artery stenosis treated by percutaneous angioplasty after coronary bypass surgery. *Am Heart J* 1987;113:393–394.
98. Hamm CW, Reimers J, Ischinger T, et al. A randomised study of coronary angioplasty compared with bypass surgery in patients with symptomatic multi-vessel coronary disease. *N Engl J Med* 1994;331: 1037–1043.
99. King SB, Lembo WJ, Weintraub WS, et al. A randomised trial comparing coronary angioplasty with coronary by pass surgery. *N Engl J Med* 331;1994:1044–1050.
100. Lange RA, Hillis LD. Immediate angioplasty for acute myocardial infarction. *N Engl J Med* 1993;328:726–728.
101. Bittl JA. Medical progress: Advances in coronary angioplasty. *N Engl J Med* 1996;335:1290–1302.
102. Lee AHS, Dawkins KD, Gallagher PJ. Pathology of coronary angioplasty. *Lancet* 1989;2:423–424.
103. Matthews BJ, Ewels CJ, Kent KM. Coronary dissection: a predictor of restenosis. *Am Heart J* 1988;115:547–554.
104. Austin GE, Ratcliff NB, Hollman J, Tabei S, Phillips DF. Intimal proliferation of smooth muscle cells as an explanation for recurrent coronary artery stenosis after percutaneous transluminal angioplasty. *J Am Coll Cardiol* 1985;6:369–375.
105. Hirshfeld JW, Schwarz JS, Jugo R, et al. Restenosis after coronary angioplasty: A multivariate model to relate lesion and procedure variables to restenosis. *J Am Coll Cardiol* 1991;18:647–656.
106. Simons M, Leclerc G, Safian RD, et al. Relationship between activated smooth muscle cells in coronary artery lesions and restenosis after atherectomy. *N Engl J Med* 1993;328:608–614.
107. EPIC Investigators. Use of a monoclonal antibody directed against platelet glycoprotein IIb/IIIa receptor in high risk coronary angioplasty. *N Engl J Med* 1994;330:956–961.
108. Topol EJ. Prevention of cardiovascular ischaemic complications with new platelet glycoprotein IIb/IIIa inhibitors. *Am Heart J* 130:1995: 666–672.
109. Topol EJ, Leya F, Pinkerton CA, et al. A comparison of directional atherectomy with coronary angioplasty in patients with coronary artery disease. *N Engl J Med* 1993;329:221–227.
110. Kimura T, Yokoi H, Nakagawa Y, et al. Three year follow up of metallic coronary-artery stents. *N Engl J Med* 1996;334:561–566.
111. Rogers C, Edelman ER. Endovascular stent design dictates experimental restenosis and thrombosis. *Circulation* 1995;91:2995–3001.
112. Clowes AW, Kirkman TR, Reidy MA. Mechanisms of arterial graft healing. *Am J Pathol* 1986;123:220–230.
113. Walton KW, Slaney G, Ashton F. Atherosclerosis in vascular grafts for peripheral vascular disease. Part 2. Synthetic arterial prostheses. *Atherosclerosis* 1986;61:155–167.
114. Berger K, Sauvage LR. Late fibre deterioration in Dacron arterial grafts. *Ann Surg* 1981;193:477–491.
115. Pearson JD. The control of production and release of haemostatic factors in the endothelial cell. *Baillières Clin Haematol* 1993;6:629–651.
116. Davies MG, Hagen P-O The vascular endothelium. A new horizon. *Ann Surg* 1993;218:593–609.
117. Simionescu M, Simionescu N. Endothelial transport macromolecules: transcytosis and endocytosis. *Cell Biol Rev* 1991;25:5–80.
118. Schneeberger EE, Lynch RD. Tight junctions: their structure, composition and function. *Circ Res* 1984;55:723–733.
119. Lampugnami MG, Caveda L, Breviario F, del Maschio A, Dejana E. Endothelial cell to cell junctions. Structural characteristics and functional role in the regulation of vascular permeability and leukocyte extravasation. *Baillières Clin Haematol* 1993;6:539–558.
120. Haust MD. Endothelial cilia in human aortic atherosclerotic lesions. *Virchows Arch [A]* 1987;410:317–326.
121. Anderson RGW, Kamen BA, Rothberg KG, Lacey SW. Potocytosis: sequestration and transport of small molecules by caveolae. *Science* 1992;255:410–411.
122. Warhol MJ, Sweet JM. The ultrastructural localization of von Willebrand factor in endothelial cells. *Am J Pathol* 1984;117:310–315.
123. Dingemans KP, Jansen N, Becker AE. Ultrastructure of the normal human aortic media. *Virchows Arch [A]* 1981;392:199–216.
124. Wasano K, Yamamoto T. Tridimensional architecture of elastic tissue in the rat aorta and femoral artery—a scanning electron microscope study. *J Electron Microsc (Tokyo)* 1983;32:33–44.
125. Crissman RS. SEM observations of the elastic networks in canine femoral artery. *Am J Anat* 1986;175:481–492.
126. Campbell GJ, Roach MR. Fenestrations in the internal elastic lamina at bifurcations of human cerebral arteries. *Stroke* 1981;12:489–496.
127. Clark JM, Glagov S. Structural integration of the arterial wall. Relationships and attachments of medial smooth muscle cells in normally distended and hyperdistended aortas. *Lab Invest* 1979;40:587–602.
128. Spagnoli LG, Villaschi S, Neri L, Palmieri G. Gap junctions in myoendothelial bridges of rabbit carotid arteries. *Experientia* 1982;38: 124–125.
129. Sheffield AE, Weller RO. Age changes at cerebral artery bifurcations and the pathogenesis of berry aneurysms. *J Neurol Sci* 1980;46: 341–352.
130. Forbes MS, Rennels ML, Nelson E. Ultrastructure of pericytes in mouse heart. *Am J Anat* 1977;149:47–69.
131. Leak LV, Burke JF. Fine structure of the lymphatic capillary and the adjoining connective tissue area. *Am J Anat* 1966;118:785–809.
132. Rhodin JAG. Ultrastructure of mammalian venous capillaries, venules and small collecting veins. *J Ultrastruct Res* 1968;25:452–500.
133. Bocan TMA, Brown SA, Guyton JR. Human aortic fibrolipid lesions. Immunochemical localization of apolipoprotein B and apolipoprotein A. *Arteriosclerosis* 1988;8:499–508.
134. Hammer A, Kager G, Dohr G, Ghassemper I, Jurgens G. Generation, characterisation and histochemical application of monoclonal antibodies selectively recognising oxidatively modified apo-B containing serum lipoproteins. *Arteriosclerosis Thromb Vasc Biol* 1995;15: 704–713.
135. Katsuda S, Okada Y, Minamoto T, Oda Y, Matsui Y, Nakanishi I. Collagens in human atherosclerosis. Immunohistochemical analyses using collagen specific antibodies. *Arteriosclerosis Thrombosis* 1992; 12:494–502.
136. Jang J, Lincoff AM, Plow EF, Topol EJ. Cell adhesion molecules in coronary heart disease. *J Am Coll Cardiol* 1994;24:1591–1601.
137. van der Wal AC, Das PK, Tigges AJ, Becker AE. Adhesion molecules on the endothelium and mononuclear cells in human atherosclerotic lesions. *Am J Pathol* 1992;141;1427–1433.
138. Parums DV. Histochemistry and immunohistochemistry of vascular

disease. In: Stehbens WE, Lie JT, eds. *Vascular pathology*. London: Chapman & Hall; 1995:313–328.
139. Ordonez NG, Manning JT, Brooks TE. Effect of trypsinization on the immunostaining of formalin fixed, paraffin embedded tissues. *Am J Surg Pathol* 1988;12:121–129.
140. Page C, Rose M, Yacoub M, Pigott R. Antigenic heterogeneity of vascular endothelium. *Am J Pathol* 1992;141:673–683.
141. Kuzu I, Bicknell R, Harris AL, Jones M, Gatter KC, Mason DY. Heterogeneity of vascular endothelial cells with relevance to the diagnosis of vascular tumours. *J Clin Pathol* 1992;45:143–148.
142. Rand JH, Sussman H, Gordon RE, Chu SV, Solomon V. Localization of Factor VIII related antigen in human vascular subendothelium. *Blood* 1980;55:752–756.
143. Mukai K, Rosai J, Burgdorf WHC. Localisation of Factor VIII related antigen in vascular endothelial cells using an immunoperoxidase technique. *Am J Surg Pathol* 1980;4:273–276.
144. Selrested M, Hou Jensen K. Factor VIII related antigen as an endothelial cell marker in benign and malignant diseases. *Virchows Arch [A]* 1981;391:217–225.
145. Guarda LA, Ordonez NG, Smith L, Hanssen G. Immunoperoxidase localization of Factor VIII in angiosarcomas. *Arch Pathol Lab Med* 1982;106:515–516.
146. Alles JU, Bosslet K. Immunocytochemistry of angiosarcomas. A study of 19 cases with special emphasis on the applicability of endothelial cell specific markers to routinely prepared tissues. *Am J Clin Pathol* 1988;89:463–471.
147. Leader M, Collins M, Patel J, Henry K. Staining of Factor VIII–related antigen and Ulex europaeus agglutinin (UEA-1) in 230 tumours. An assessment of their specificity for angiosarcoma and Kaposi's sarcoma. *Histopathology* 1986;10:1153–1162.
148. Holtfhofer H, Virtanen I, Kariniemi AL, Hormia M, Linder E, Miettinen A. Ulex europaeus 1 lectin as a marker for vascular endothelium in human tissues. *Lab Invest* 1982;47:60–66.
149. Miettinen M, Holthofer H, Lehto V-P, Miettinen A, Virtanen I. Ulex europaeus 1 lectin as a marker for tumors derived from endothelial cells. *Am J Clin Pathol* 1983;79:32–36.
150. Ordonez NG, Batsakis JG. Comparison of Ulex europaeus 1 lectin and Factor VIII–related antigen in vascular lesions. *Arch Pathol Lab Med* 1984;108:129–132.
151. Heng MCY, Fallon-Friedlander S, Benett R. Expression of Ulex europaeus agglutinin I lectin binding sites in squamous cell carcinomas and their absence in basal cell carcinomas. *Am J Dermatopathol* 1992; 14:216–219.
152. Newman PJ, Berndt MC, Gorski J, et al. PECAM-1 (CD31) cloning and relation to adhesion molecules of the immunoglobulin gene superfamily. *Science* 1990;247:1219–1222.
153. DeLisser HM, Newman PJ, Aldelda SM. Molecular and functional aspects of PECAM-1/CD31. *Immunol Today* 1994;15:490–495.
154. Behar E, Chao NJ, Hiraki DD, et al. Polymorphism of adhesion molecule CD31 and its role in acute graft-versus-host disease. *N Engl J Med* 1996;334:286–291.
155. Parums DV, Cordell JL, Micklem K, Heryet AR, Gatter KC, Mason DY. JC 70. A new monoclonal antibody that detects vascular endothelium associated antigen on routinely processed tissue sections. *J Clin Pathol* 1990;43:752–757.
156. De Young R, Wick MR, Fitzgibbon JF, Sirgi KE, Swanson PE. CD31. An immunospecific marker for endothelial differentiation in human neoplasms. *Appl Immunohistochem* 1993;1:97–100.
157. Miettinen M, Lindenmayer AE, Chaubal A. Endothelial cell markers CD31, CD34, and BNH9 antibody to H- and Y-antigens. Evaluation of their specificity and sensitivity in the diagnosis of vascular tumours and comparison with von Willibrand factor. *Mod Pathol* 1994; 7:82–90.
158. Fina L, Molgaard HV, Robertson D, et al. Expression of the CD34 gene in vascular endothelial cells. *Blood* 1990;75:2417–2426.
159. Sirgi KE, Wick MR, Swanson PE. B72.3 and CD34 reactivity in malignant epitheloid soft tissue tumours. Adjuncts in the recognition of endothelial neoplasms. *Am J Surg Pathol* 1993;17:179–185.
160. Traweek ST, Kandalaft PL, Mehta P, Battifora H. The human hematopoietic progenitor cell antigen (CD34) in vascular neoplasia. *Am J Clin Pathol* 1991;96:25–31.
161. Fletcher C, Ramani P. QBEND 10: a useful but by no means specific marker of Kaposi's sarcoma. *J Pathol* 1990;162:273–277.
162. Poblet E, Jimenez-Acosta F, Rocamora A. QBEND 10 (anti-CD34 antibody) in external root sheath cells and hair tumours. *J Cutan Pathol* 1994;21:224–228.
163. Poston RN, Haskard DO, Coucher JR, Gall NP, Johnson-Tidey R. Expression of intercellular adhesion molecule-1 in atherosclerotic plaques. *Am J Pathol* 1992;140:665–673.
164. Giaid A, Saleh D. Reduced expression of endothelial nitric oxide synthase in the lungs of patients with pulmonary hypertension. *N Engl J Med* 1995;333:214–221.
165. Gabbiani G, Schmid E, Winter S. Vascular smooth muscle cells differ from other smooth muscle cells: Predominance of vimentin filaments and a specific type actin. *Proc Natl Acad Sci U S A* 1981;78:298–302.
166. Skalli O, Ropraz P, Trzeciak A, Benzonana G, Gillessen D, Gabbiani G. A monoclonal antibody against alpha smooth muscle actin. A new probe for smooth muscle differentiation. *J Cell Biol* 1986;103: 2787–2796.
167. Scharch W, Skalli O, Seemager TA, Gabbiani G. Intermediate filament proteins and actin isoforms as markers for soft tissue tumour differentiation and origin. 1. Smooth muscle tumors. *Am J Pathol* 1987; 128:91–103.
168. Jones H, Steart PV, du Boulay CEH, Roche WR. Alpha smooth muscle actin as a marker for soft tissue tumours: A comparison with desmin. *J Pathol* 1990;162:29–33
169. Barsky SH, Baker A, Siegal GP, et al. Use of antibasement membrane antibodies to distinguish blood vessel capillaries from lymphatic capillaries. *Am J Surg Pathol* 1983;7:667–677.
170. Kartunen T, Alavaikko M, Apaja-Sarkkinen M, Autio-Harmainen H. Distribution of basement membrane laminin and type IV collagen in human reactive lymph nodes. *Histopathology* 1986;10:841–850.
171. Autio-Harmainen H, Karttunen T, Apaja-Sarkkinen M, Dammert K, Ristell L. Laminin and type IV collagen in different histological stages of Kaposi's sarcoma and other vascular lesions of blood vessel or lymphatic vessel origin. *Am J Surg Pathol* 1988;12:469–476.
172. Bettelheim R, Mitchell D, Gusterson BA. Immunocytochemistry in the identification of vascular invasion in breast cancer. *J Clin Pathol* 1984;37:364–366.

# Urinary Tract

*Histology for Pathologists, second edition,*
Edited by Stephen S. Sternberg.
Lippincott-Raven Publishers, Philadelphia


CHAPTER 34

# Pediatric Kidney

J. Bruce Beckwith



The human kidney is structurally immature at the time of birth, and important morphologic changes occur during infancy and childhood. Pathologists not familiar with the histologic peculiarities of the pediatric kidney may mistake normal findings for abnormalities or fail to observe significant abnormalities of renal maturation. This chapter reviews aspects of renal morphology that are unique to early life, with emphasis on features susceptible to misinterpretation by pathologists who deal primarily with renal specimens from adults.

## FETAL DEVELOPMENT

Developmental changes occurring in the postnatal kidney represent a continuation of those occurring before birth. A brief outline of prenatal renal histogenesis is necessary in order to clarify certain aspects of postnatal anatomy. Detailed reviews of renal development during the embryonic and fetal periods should be consulted for more information (1–3).

The metanephric blastema, the precursor of nephronic and stromal elements of the definitive kidney, is derived from caudal portions of the intermediate mesoderm that condense around the ampullary end of the ureteral bud at embryonic stage 14, corresponding to day 32 of embryonic life (1). The ureteral bud, originating from the caudal end of the mesonephric duct, gives rise to the pelvicaliceal system and renal collecting ducts through an elaborate series of dichotomous branchings. Dilatation and effacement of the first three to five branches forms the renal pelvis, and the next three to five branches form the calces. Subsequent branchings involve the collecting ducts of the renal parenchyma, which are the most peripherally placed derivatives of the ureteral bud and the latest to appear. Induction of nephrons occurs with blastemal cells aggregated around the ampullary ends of the developing collecting ducts, with the first glomerulotubular structures appearing about the 8th gestational week. Potter's classic text presents in elegant fashion the complex process of ureteral bud branching, nephron induction, and glomerular differentiation and is indispensable for a clear understanding of this topic (1).

The cortex ultimately contains approximately nine to 11 generations of nephrons. These generations are added sequentially at the periphery of each lobe, beginning at about 8 weeks and continuing until week 32 to 36 of gestation. During the period of nephrogenesis, blastemal cells are concentrated at the lobar periphery. The blastemal layer is most obvious during mid-gestation, when it often forms a continuous layer outlining the cortical surface of each developing lobe (Fig. 1). Because of this centrifugal pattern of cortical development, position of a nephron within the renal cortex is directly related to developmental chronology. Nephronic units located near the medulla are necessarily older than those nearer the surface. This principle is fundamental to understanding postnatal structural changes in the kidney and is sometimes a useful clue to the timing of developmental disturbances in the cortex. For example, a disturbance during the early months of development may result in abnormality of the entire cortical thickness, whereas one that occurs in the last half of gestation may involve only the outermost layers of cortical nephrons.

J. B. Beckwith: Department of Pathology and Human Anatomy, Division of Pediatric Pathology, Loma Linda University, Loma Linda, California 92350.

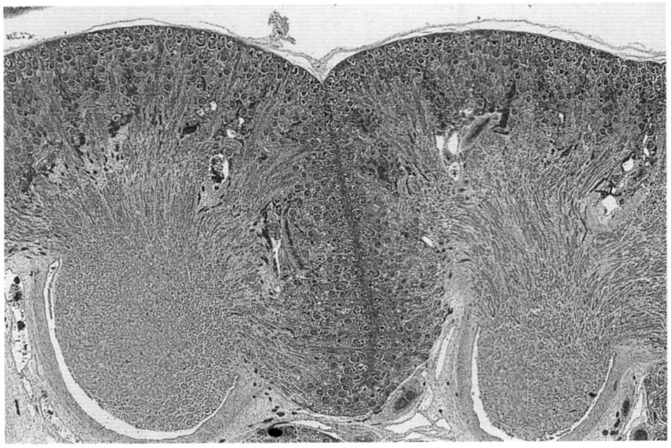

**FIG. 1.** Developing kidney at 21 weeks' gestation. Two medullary pyramids with portions of surrounding cortex. A thin layer of blastemal cells and glomerular neogenesis outlines the lobar periphery, both at the surface of the kidney and in the midplane of the cortical column of Bertin, between the two renal lobes.

Each nephron begins as a glomerular vesicle, formed from blastemal cap cells surrounding the ampullary end of a collecting duct. This vesicle becomes attached to the collecting duct via a short tubular connection. The connecting segment progressively elongates to form the tubular segments of the mature nephron, whereas the originally simple glomerular vesicle undergoes a complex process of invagination and ingrowth by capillaries and gradually evolves over many months into its complicated mature form (1). The zone within which the early stages of glomerular formation are occurring is known as the neogenic zone (Figs. 2 and 3). Neoformation of glomeruli and new nephrons ceases, and the neogenic zone disappears, between the 32nd and 36th weeks of gestation (Fig. 4). The presence or absence of a neogenic zone is one of the most useful histologic features distinguishing prematurely born from term or near-term infants in perinatal autopsies. This feature also can be helpful in evaluating fetal growth disturbances. For example, a term infant with growth retardation may have the same body weight and length as a normally grown premature infant, whereas the infant who is large for gestational age may have a body weight consistent with full term, but with a prominent neogenic zone indicating its immature developmental status.

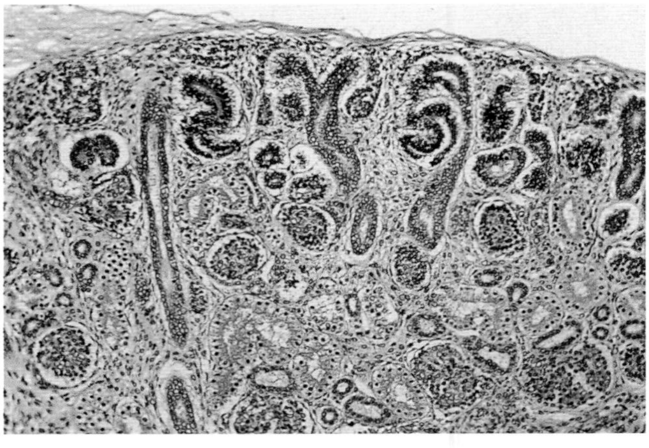

**FIG. 2.** Neogenic zone from a 26-week-old fetus showing several stages in glomerulogenesis.

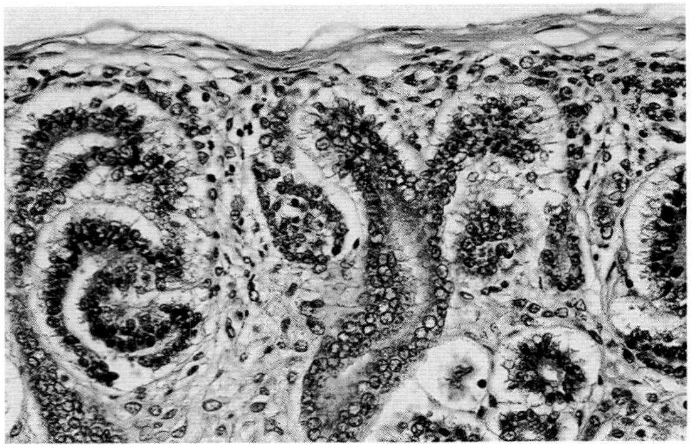

**FIG. 3.** Higher magnification of same field as in Fig. 2.

## GROSS ANATOMY

### Kidney Weight and Configuration

The data of Emery and Mithal (4) concerning the combined weight of the kidneys between birth and 10 years of age are shown in Table 1.

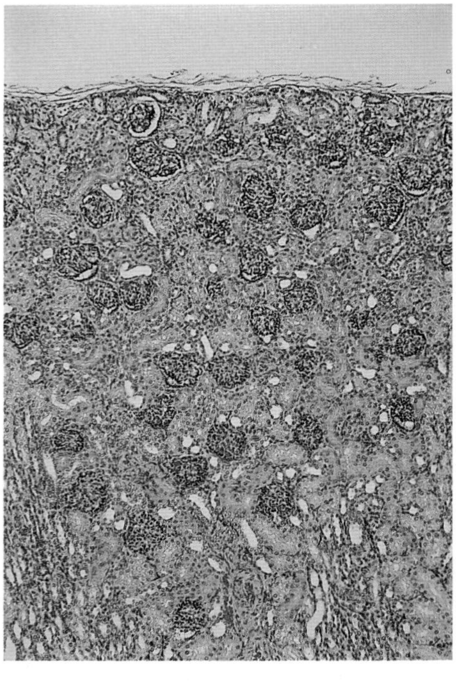

**FIG. 4.** Newborn kidney (40 weeks' gestation). Note absence of neogenic zone. Some glomeruli are near renal capsule.

**TABLE 1.** *Combined renal weight in infants and children*

| | | Percentiles | | | |
|---|---|---|---|---|---|
| Age | Mean | 5 | 25 | 75 | 95 |
| Birth | 26 | 13 | 22 | 34 | 44 |
| 1 mo | 32 | 16 | 26 | 38 | 50 |
| 2 | 36 | 18 | 29 | 42 | 54 |
| 3 | 39 | 21 | 33 | 46 | 60 |
| 4 | 44 | 24 | 36 | 50 | 65 |
| 5 | 48 | 27 | 40 | 54 | 70 |
| 6 | 51 | 30 | 43 | 58 | 76 |
| 7 | 56 | 32 | 46 | 63 | 82 |
| 8 | 60 | 35 | 50 | 68 | 88 |
| 9 | 62 | 38 | 54 | 72 | 95 |
| 10 | 67 | 40 | 58 | 78 | 100 |
| 11 | 69 | 43 | 63 | 85 | 109 |
| 12 | 78 | 48 | 68 | 92 | 118 |
| 2 yrs | 88 | 54 | 74 | 103 | 130 |
| 3 | 100 | 62 | 81 | 114 | 142 |
| 4 | 110 | 72 | 92 | 126 | 156 |
| 5 | 121 | 81 | 100 | 136 | 169 |
| 6 | 134 | 90 | 110 | 150 | 182 |
| 7 | 144 | 101 | 120 | 160 | 194 |
| 8 | 156 | 111 | 131 | 173 | 207 |
| 9 | 166 | 120 | 142 | 185 | 220 |
| 10 | 178 | 130 | 153 | 196 | 230 |

Modified from ref. 4.

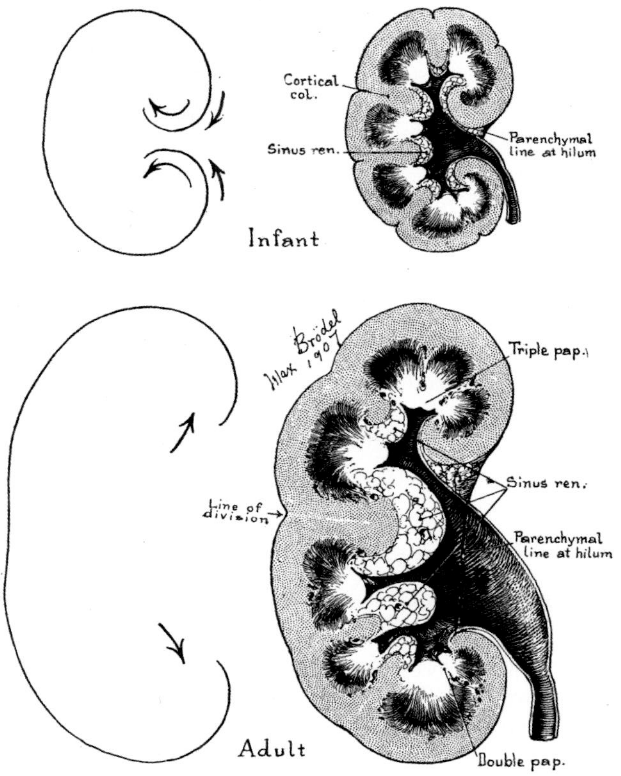


**FIG. 6.** Max Brödel's classic illustration of the process of unrolling of the kidney in postnatal life (5). The rounded configuration of the infantile organ becomes elongated as the upper and lower poles diverge and pelvicaliceal structures are partially everted from their original position within the renal sinus. The space thus created within the renal sinus is filled by fat, which is far more abundant in the adult kidney than in the infant kidney.

The newborn kidney has a shorter, more rounded configuration than that of the adult. The upper and lower poles project further medially, so the renal sinus is relatively deeper in the infant (Figs. 5 and 6) (5). The renal sinus of infants contains much less fat and connective tissue than in the adult, and the cortical columns of Bertin approach much closer to the pelvicaliceal system. Figure 6 illustrates the process of "unrolling" of the renal poles during childhood, as the kidney assumes the more elongated configuration observed in adults. This change in shape produces a shallower renal sinus with partial exteriorization of the pelvis. As the pelvicaliceal system assumes a more exterior position, it also becomes displaced further from the parenchyma lining the sinus. The additional space created between the pelvicaliceal system and the cortical columns of Bertin is normally filled by fat, which increases in amount as the kidney approaches maturity.

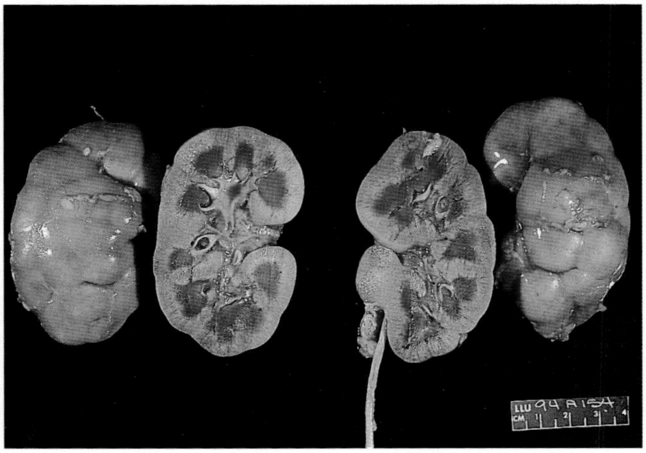

**FIG. 5.** Gross appearance of newborn kidneys. The rounded configuration with relatively deeper sinus, characteristic of the infantile kidney, is seen on the sectioned surface. Fetal lobations are prominent on the external surface.

## Fetal Lobations

The organizational unit of the mammalian metanephros is the renal lobe (Figs. 1 and 5), consisting of a medullary pyramid and its surrounding cortical mantle (5,6). Many mammals, including rodents, cats, and horses, have a unilobar kidney with a single papilla and medullary pyramid surrounded by cortex. The human kidney normally consists of a mean of nine to 10 lobes, when papillary count is used as the indicator of lobar number (7). Variable degrees of fusion of adjacent medullary pyramids, especially in the renal poles, result in the formation of compound lobes that contribute to the variability in lobar number.

The surface of the neonatal kidney is divided into polygons by prominent surface fissures that correspond roughly, although not precisely, to the lobar outlines (Fig. 5). These fetal lobations usually decrease in prominence with advancing age, persisting longer on the ventral than the dorsal surface of the organ. There is considerable individual variation in the chronology of their disappearance. Sykes (7) found one or more interlobar fissures in 51 of 100 adult kidneys. Peter (8) found extreme variation in the rate of disappearance, with deep fissures persisting in a 14-year-old child. The only valid generalization is that fetal lobations usually diminish in number and prominence in the first few years of life, but they remain apparent, especially on the ventral surfaces, in a significant proportion of adult kidneys. In adults and older children, it is important to distinguish persistent fetal lobations from cortical scars.

## HISTOLOGY

### Renal Cortex: General Structure and Organization

After the full complement of nephrons is attained by the fetus between the 32nd and 36th weeks of gestation, subsequent renal growth reflects elongation and maturation of nephrons. As nephrons elongate, they become interposed between glomeruli. The glomeruli in the outer cortex of newborns are crowded together (Fig. 4), whereas the older, more mature glomeruli deeper in the cortex are more widely separated. This process of tubular elongation not only separates glomeruli from one another, but it also tends to separate them from the lobar surface where they originally developed. In a normal term newborn, one normally sees many glomeruli in direct contact with the renal capsule (Fig. 4). By about 2 months of age, the process of nephron elongation has begun to separate the outermost glomeruli, with a narrow zone largely devoid of glomeruli beneath the renal capsule. This latter zone has been termed the cortex corticis (Fig. 7) (8). The cortex corticis becomes progressively wider during childhood (Fig. 8). Although it is normal to find an occasional glomerulus at the capsular surface in normal infants and children, the presence of numerous superficial glomeruli suggests defective renal growth during late fetal or early postnatal life. Abnormally crowded glomeruli also can be an important clue to defects in nephron growth and differentiation, which may involve only the outer cortex, or the entire cortical mantle.

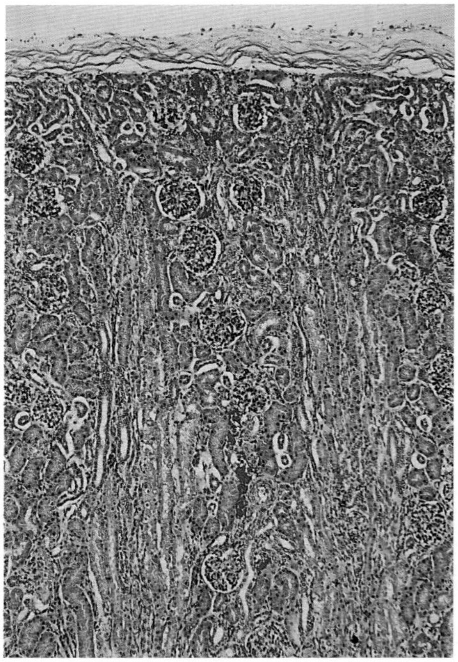

FIG. 7. Renal cortex at 2 months of age. Glomeruli in the outer cortex are becoming more widely spaced due to tubular elongation. Superficial glomeruli are beginning to separate from the renal capsule, the first indication of the cortex corticis.

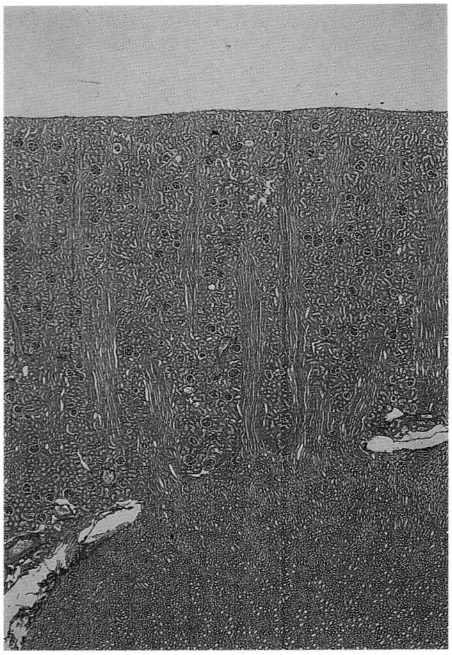

FIG. 8. Kidney at 21 months. Cortex corticis is well developed. This perpendicularly oriented section shows the full length of several medullary rays that extend from the outer medulla to a level near the cortex corticis. Each medullary ray marks the center of a cortical lobule.

Within the infantile renal cortex, the age discrepancy between the various levels is manifested by striking differences in glomerular structure. Deeper glomeruli are larger and more mature than those situated more superficially. The sequence of glomerular maturation is described in more detail below.

The cortex is subdivided into distinctly demarcated lobules by radially oriented groups of collecting ducts that extend from the medulla toward the cortex termed medullary rays (Fig. 8). The lobule is defined by most investigators as

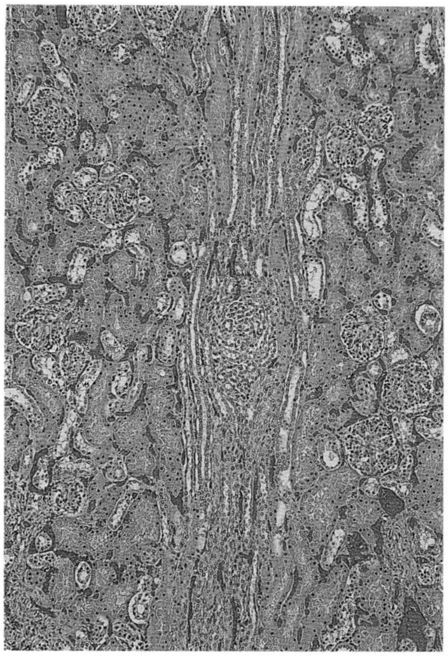

**FIG. 9.** Medullary ray nodule. In the center of the photograph a tangled cluster of collecting ducts forms a nodule near the midportion of a medullary ray. This structure is usually transitory, being uncommon in the first month of life, and extremely rare after 1 year.

that cortical domain surrounding a medullary ray. The term "fetal lobulation" is, therefore, anatomically misleading and should be replaced by the term "fetal lobation." Medullary rays usually extend to the cortical surface in infants, but not in older children. The presence of complete medullary rays is a good indicator that the plane of a given section is perpendicular and reflective of the true thickness of the cortex. Medullary ray nodules (9) are complex tangled tubular configurations commonly seen in the medullary rays of infants during the early months of life, being most prominent between 1 and 6 months of age (Fig. 9). These structures apparently represent a normal transitory developmental phenomenon of variable prominence, which is pathologic only when extreme.

### Glomerular Maturation and Growth

Newly formed glomeruli are structurally distinctive, and the evolution toward adult appearances is a gradual process. Because the period of glomerular development spans a 6- to 7-month period of fetal life, a progressive spectrum of maturational states is normally present in infant kidneys. This maturational spectrum is organized in an orderly fashion, with the most mature glomeruli in the deep cortex, followed by progressively earlier stages of maturation as one approaches the cortical surface. Familiarity with normal maturational processes can make possible a reasonably accurate assessment of renal developmental status in infants.

Figure 10 shows representative glomeruli from the midcortical region of infants and children from birth to 9 years of age, photographed at the same magnification, to illustrate the dramatic changes in glomerular structure and size through the early years of life. Figure 10A shows the characteristic appearance of a recently formed glomerulus from a term newborn infant. In addition to its small size, the most obvious distinction from mature glomeruli is the presence of a layer of cuboidal cells surfacing the visceral layer of Bowman's capsule. This layer apparently represents a germinal structure composed of precursors of the glomerular epithelium. The glomerular tuft is small and simple, with relatively few capillary loops. Ultrastructurally, these surface epithelial cells lack pedicles and are closely approximated to one another (Fig. 11A). Changes in thickness of the glomerular basement membrane during childhood are illustrated in Fig. 11. The data of Vogler et al. concerning changes in thickness of the basement membrane during childhood are presented in Fig. 12 (10).

A continuous layer of cuboidal cells exists only briefly; the cells become dispersed over the surfaces of developing capillary tufts and mature into podocytes, although Gruenwald and Popper (11) suggested that some of these cells may be sloughed into Bowman's space. The continuous cuboidal layer is soon represented only by small clusters of cells (Fig. 10B and C). After a glomerulus has been in existence for more than 12 months, remnants of the cuboidal layer are usually not seen in normally developed glomeruli. However, an occasional glomerulus with the small size and immature appearance of the neonatal glomerulus may be observed in older infants, especially in the outer third of the cortex (Fig. 13).

Glomerular growth during childhood has been evaluated quantitatively by several groups (12,13). Moore et al. found that the mean glomerular diameter in normal children dying suddenly increased from 112 to 167 $\mu$m between birth and 15 years of age, with a relatively linear increase averaging 3.6 $\mu$m per year during this period of life (12).

The maturational process in the first one or two generations of glomeruli is apparently accelerated because even in very young fetuses these juxtamedullary glomeruli rarely possess a cuboidal layer and are considerably larger than their slightly more superficially placed neighbors. Similar large juxtamedullary glomeruli were noted in the 48-mm fetal pig by Kampmeier (14), who noted that they disappeared subsequently, and suggested that they are transitory structures. Tsuda (15) observed that these glomeruli in human fetuses of 4 months' gestation have diameters similar to those of adult glomeruli. Emery and Macdonald (16) noted the disappearance of these enlarged glomeruli in the early months after birth, associated with the presence of scarred glomeruli in this same region. These findings support Kampmeier's suggestion that they represent a transitory population of nephrons. It is presumed that these precociously formed glomeruli are functionally important during fetal life and apparently disappear early in the postnatal period. Relatively little study has been made of these interesting structures.

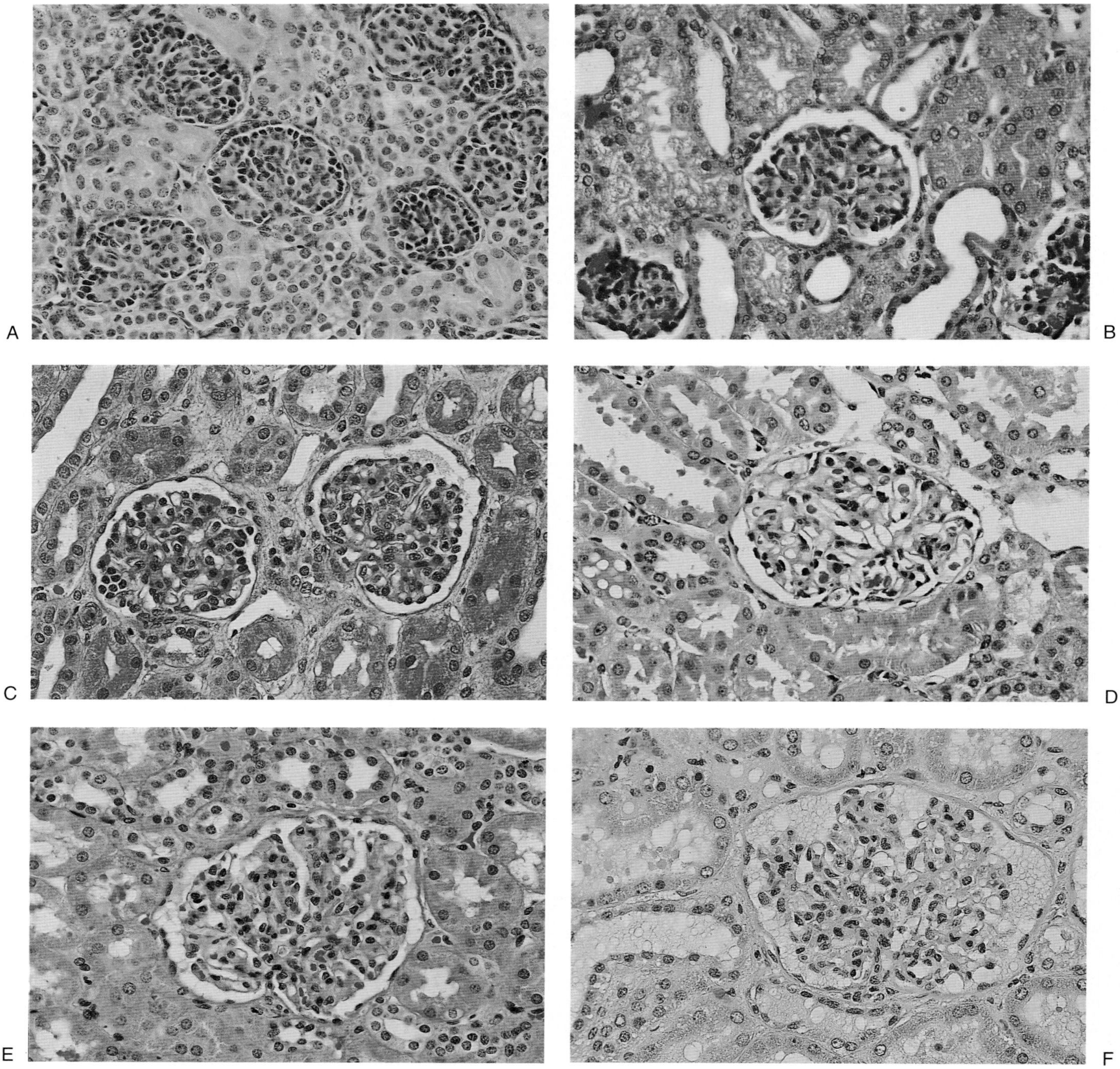

**FIG. 10.** Normal midcortical glomeruli of six infants and children from birth to 9 years of age. Photographs taken at identical magnification. **A:** Newborn. **B:** 6 months. **C:** 11 months. **D:** 21 months. **E:** 5 years. **F:** 9 years.

### *Infantile Glomerulosclerosis*

Glomerulosclerosis in infantile kidneys is a commonly observed and presumably normal phenomenon that must be distinguished from pathologic changes. Herxheimer in 1909 suggested that sclerotic glomeruli represented the defective formation of certain nephrons in otherwise normal kidneys and were not manifestations of a disease process (17). Other investigators have suggested that these sclerotic glomeruli might result from renal infection, excretion of toxic substances, and so forth.

Emery and Macdonald conducted quantitative studies of glomerulosclerosis (16). They counted 200 glomeruli in radially oriented fields (including the full cortical thickness) in 200 infants and children up to 15 years of age. They found one or more scarred glomeruli to be a frequent phenomenon,

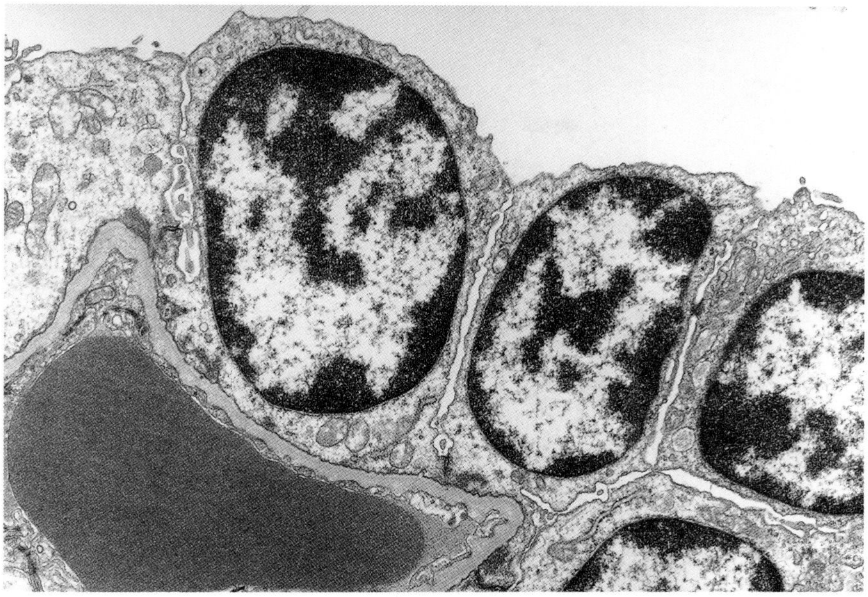

A

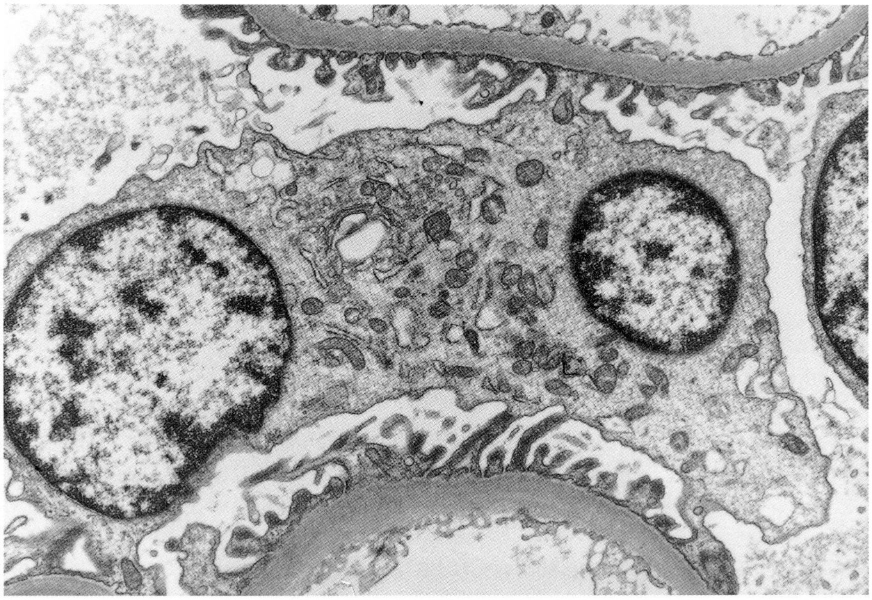

B

**FIG. 11.** **A:** Electron micrograph of a normal glomerulus from an infant 2 months of age. Note the continuous layer of epithelial cells lacking foot processes and the thin basement membrane. **B:** Mature glomerulus from a patient 16 years of age, taken at the same magnification as in **A**. Foot process development is prominent, spanning adjacent capillary loops, and the basement membrane is distinctly thicker than in the infant. (Photos kindly provided by Gary W. Mierau, Ph.D.)

involving 0.5% to 10% in most cases. Three infants with apparently normal kidneys had a higher proportion of sclerotic glomeruli, ranging up to 30%. Most counts fell into the 1% to 2% range.

In an expanded series of 475 cases included in the same report, Emery and Macdonald found that the percentage of infants having sclerotic glomeruli was age dependent. They occurred in 25% to 40% of kidneys from late fetal and newborn patients. They were found in 70% of cases by 3 months of age, remaining at this level throughout the second year. Their prevalence then declined rapidly, and they were found in only 10% of patients older than 6 years.

Emery and Macdonald found most sclerotic glomeruli to occur near the inner and outer cortical margins. The population of scarred glomeruli in the juxtamedullary zone was most prevalent in the first 6 months of life but was rare thereafter. Those in the outer cortex were most numerous in the latter half of the first year and into the second year of life. The prevalence of scarred glomeruli in the juxtamedullary zone coincided with the disappearance of the population of large glomeruli seen in this region during fetal life, as discussed above. A similar pattern of cortical distribution also was noted in the series of 800 infant kidneys reported by Thomas (18). Like most other investigators who have studied this phenomenon, Thomas considered a small percentage of sclerotic glomeruli in infant kidneys to be a statistically normal phenomenon, implying defective formation of a small proportion of the more than 1 million glomeruli that

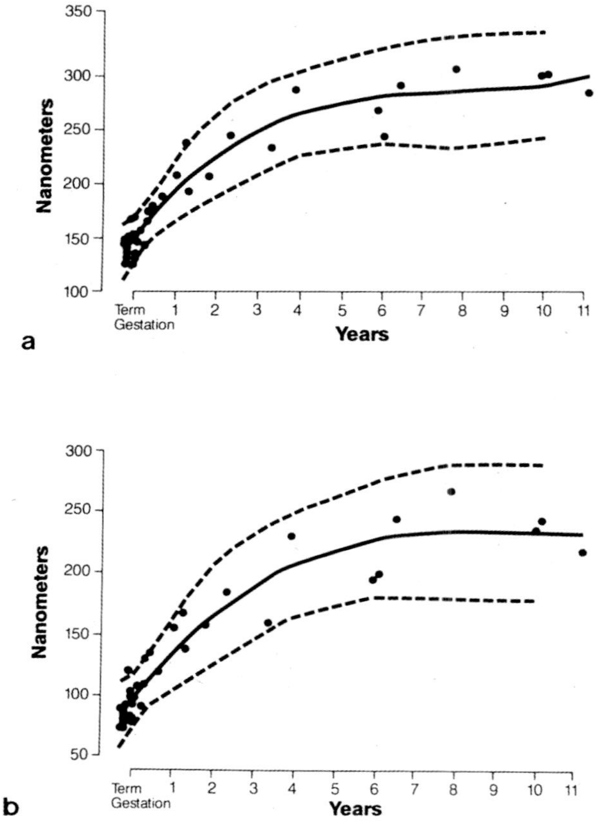


**FIG. 12.** Thickness of glomerular basement membrane in children. **a:** Total thickness of membrane. **b:** Thickness of lamina densa. Reproduced with permission (10).

develop in the human kidney. Their major significance for pathologists is that they not be interpreted as evidence of disease, unless their number is well above the usual range cited above.

A typical example of infantile glomerulosclerosis is

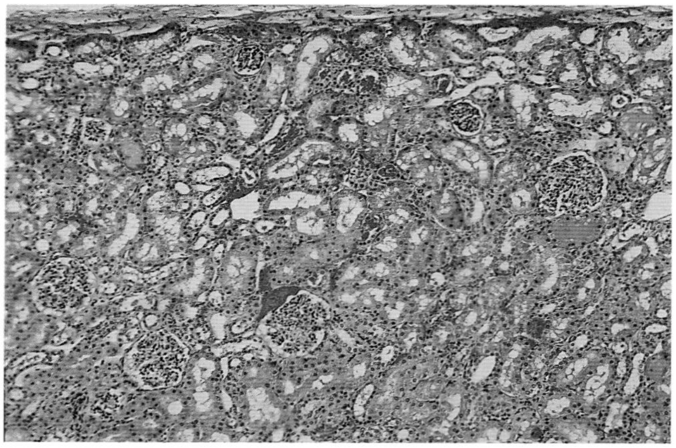

**FIG. 13.** Persistent immature glomeruli at 12 months. Two miniature glomeruli with cuboidal cells at the periphery of the tuft are present near the renal capsule. Small numbers of defective glomeruli can be found in most infant kidneys but are destined to undergo sclerosis and involution.

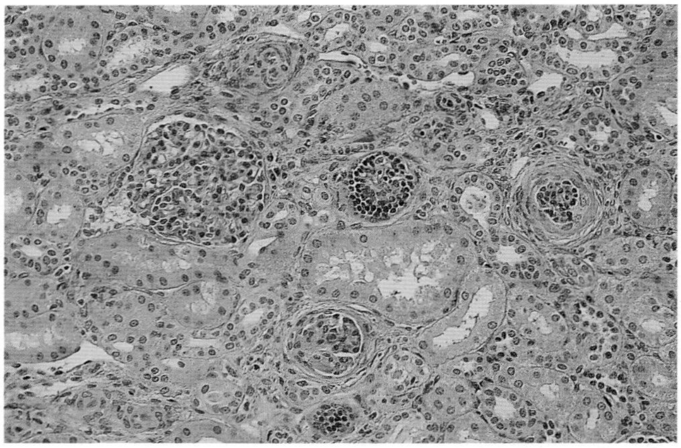

**FIG. 14.** Infantile glomerulosclerosis (9 months of age). One small, developmentally immature glomerulus is seen near the center, with two adjacent glomeruli undergoing involutional sclerosis.

shown in Fig. 14. These scarred glomeruli may occur in small groups or singly. They are usually smaller than normal, immature in appearance, and variably hyalinized. The afferent arteriole is often thickened, and periglomerular fibrosis may be present, often accompanied by chronic inflammatory cells. In later stages only a small globule of hyaline material in a minute focus of fibrous tissue is all that may be seen. The nephron supplied by these sclerotic glomeruli contains dense proteinaceous material and apparently disappears along with the glomerulus in most instances.

## Nephron Growth and Differentiation

Few studies have been made of tubular growth and differentiation between birth and adulthood. Osathanondh and Potter (19) have reviewed prenatal growth and maturation. Fetterman et al. (20) studied tubular growth by microdissection of kidneys from 23 subjects ranging from birth to 18 years, and Darmady et al. (cited in ref. 20) studied 24 specimens from birth to 14 years of age. The latter investigators found that mean proximal tubular length increased from 2 mm to 12.7 mm during this period. Fetterman et al. observed extreme variability in proximal tubular length in newborns but not in infants older than 1 month. This was thought to reflect the fact that specimens from the outer third of the cortex were appreciably shorter than those from deeper layers, a difference that was not consistently demonstrable after 1 month of age.

Fetterman et al. (20) noted a striking shift in ratio of proximal tubule volume to glomerular surface area in the first few months of life. These results are reflected in diminished proximal tubular function during the early months of postnatal life. The initial growth of proximal tubules was primarily a process of elongation, and thereafter growth was primarily due to increase in diameter.

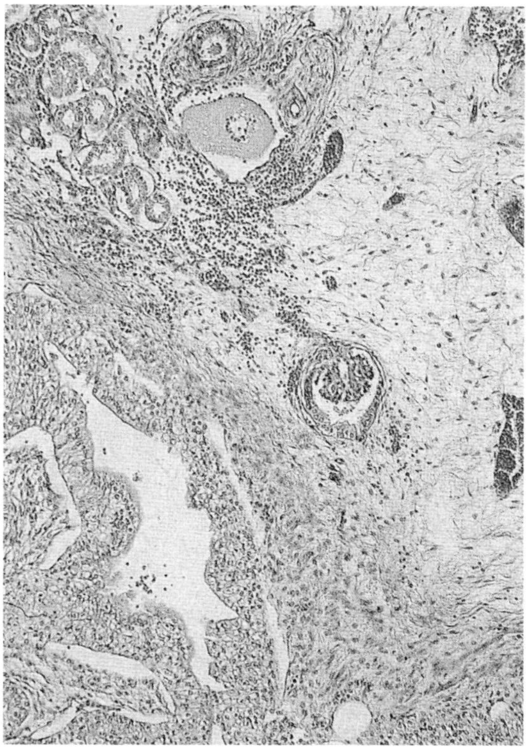

**FIG. 15.** Ectopic glomerulus in the renal sinus.

### Ectopic Nephrons

Sectioning of kidneys from fetuses and infants often shows nephrons outside the confines of the renal parenchyma, either in the renal sinus (Fig. 15) or in connective tissue around arcuate or other large vessels. These occur in several animal species as well as in human infants but usually appear to degenerate during early postnatal life (21). It has been suggested that some vessels supplying the renal pelvic mucosa may be derived from degenerated ectopic glomeruli (21).

## REFERENCES


1. Potter EL. *Normal and abnormal development of the kidney.* Chicago: Year Book; 1972.
2. Saxén L. *Organogenesis of the kidney.* Cambridge: Cambridge University Press; 1987.
3. Peter K. *Untersuchungen ueber Bau und Entwicklung der Niere.* Jena, Germany: Gustav Fischer; 1927.
4. Emery JL, Mithal A. The weights of kidneys in later intra-uterine life and childhood. *J Clin Pathol* 1960;12:490–493.
5. Kelly HA, Burnam CF. *Diseases of the kidneys, ureters, and bladder.* Vol. 1. New York: D Appleton; 1925:123.
6. Inke G. *The protolobar structure of the human kidney. Its biologic and clinical significance.* New York: Alan R Liss; 1988.
7. Sykes D. The correlation between renal vascularization and lobulation of the kidney. *Br J Urol* 1964;36:549–555.
8. Peter K. Harnorgane, Organe Uropoietica. In: Peter K, Wetzel G, Heiderich F, eds. *Handbuch der Anatomie des Kindes.* Vol. 2. Munich: JF Bergmann; 1938:1–41.
9. Benjamin DR, Beckwith JB. Medullary ray nodules in infancy and childhood. *Arch Pathol* 1973;96:33–35.
10. Vogler C, McAdams AJ, Homan SM. Glomerular basement membrane and lamina densa in infants and children: an ultrastructural evaluation. *Pediatr Pathol* 1987;7:527–534.
11. Gruenwald P, Popper H. The histogenesis and physiology of the renal glomerulus in early postnatal life: histological examinations. *J Urol* 1948;43:452–458.
12. Moore L, Williams R, Staples A. Glomerular dimensions in children under 16 years of age. *J Pathol* 1993;171:145–150.
13. Akaoka K, White RHR, Raafat F. Human glomerular growth during childhood: a morphometric study. *J Pathol* 1994;173:261–268.
14. Kampmeier OF. The metanephros or so-called permanent kidney in part provisional and vestigial. *Anat Rec* 1926;33:115–120.
15. Tsuda S. Histologic investigation of the foetal kidney. *Jpn J Obstet Gynecol* 1934;17:337–341.
16. Emery JL, Macdonald M. Involuting and scarred glomeruli in the kidneys of infants. *Am J Pathol* 1960;36:713–723.
17. Herxheimer G. Ueber hyaline Glomeruli der Neugeborenen und Saeuglinge. *Frankf Ztschr Pathol* 1909;2:138–152.
18. Thomas MA. Congenital glomerulosclerosis. *Pathology* 1969; 1:105–112.
19. Osathanondh V, Potter EF. Development of human kidney as shown by microdissection. IV. Development of tubular portions of nephrons. *Arch Pathol* 1966;82:391–402.
20. Fetterman GH, Shuplock NA, Philipp FJ, Gregg HS. The growth and maturation of human glomeruli and proximal convolutions from term to adulthood. Studies by microdissection. *Pediatrics* 1965;35: 601–619.
21. Moffat DB, Fourman J. Ectopic glomeruli in the human and animal kidney. *Anat Rec* 1964;149:1–7.

*Histology for Pathologists, second edition,*
Edited by Stephen S. Sternberg.
Lippincott-Raven Publishers, Philadelphia
© 1997.

# CHAPTER 35

# Adult Kidney

William L. Clapp and Byron P. Croker



The kidney has an intricate structure that underlies its diverse roles of excreting waste products, regulating body fluid and solute balance, regulating blood pressure, and secreting hormones. A familiarity with the basic structure of the kidney facilitates the evaluation and comprehension of diseases and functional disorders that can affect the kidney. The structure of the normal adult human kidney is considered in this chapter.

## GROSS ANATOMY

The kidneys lie within the retroperitoneum and extend from the 12th thoracic to the third lumbar vertebrae with the right kidney usually slightly more caudad. They are situated within the perirenal space, which contains abundant fat and is traversed by fine fibrous septae (1–3). Visualization of the renal fascia with radiologic procedures has been reported in normal individuals (4,5). Each kidney weighs 125 to 170 g in men and 115 to 155 g in women (6). If differences in body build are considered, kidney weight correlates best with body surface area, whereas age, sex, and race have less influence (7). Each kidney is 11 to 12 cm in length, 5 to 7.5 cm in width, and 2.5 to 3 cm in thickness. The left kidney tends to be slightly larger and may demonstrate irregularities of the lateral contour from compression by the spleen in 10% of normal individuals (8). A glistening tough fibroelastic capsule surrounds the kidney.

In the hilar region, the main renal artery branches to form anterior and posterior divisions (Fig. 1), which in turn divide into segmental arteries that supply the apical, upper, middle, lower, and posterior segmental regions of the parenchyma (9,10). No collateral circulation has been demonstrated between the segmental arteries. Some of the so-called accessory arteries actually represent normal segmental arteries with an early origin from the main-stem renal artery or aorta (10). Therefore, ligation of such a segmental artery in the belief that it is an accessory vessel results in necrosis of the corresponding segment. The intrarenal veins do not follow a segmental distribution, and there are numerous anastomoses of the veins throughout the kidney.

An outer pale region, the cortex, and an inner darker region, the medulla, can be distinguished on the cut surface of a bisected kidney (Fig. 2) The presence of glomeruli and convoluted tubules results in the cortex having a more granular appearance. The human kidney is a multipapillary type of mammalian kidney (11), with the medulla divided into eight to 18 striated conical masses called pyramids. The striated appearance reflects the parallel linear orientation of the loops of Henle and collecting ducts. The base of each pyramid is located at the corticomedullary junction, whereas the apex extends toward the renal pelvis, forming a papilla. The tip of each papilla is perforated by 20 to 70 small openings (12) that represent the distal ends of the collecting ducts (of

W. L. Clapp and B. P. Croker: Veterans Administration Medical Center and Department of Pathology, University of Florida College of Medicine, Gainesville, Florida 32610.

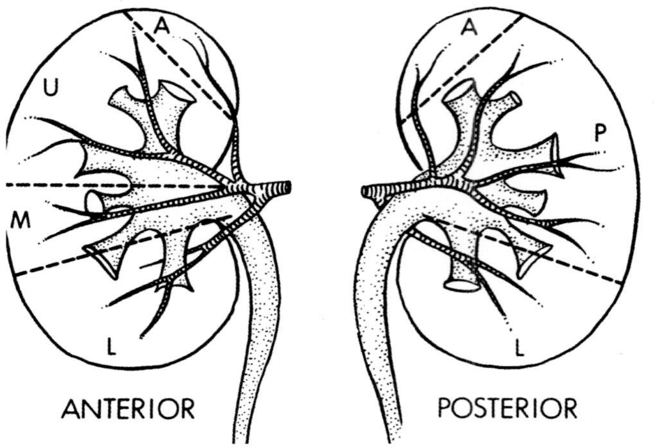


**FIG. 1.** Diagram of the vascular supply of the human kidney. The anterior division of the renal artery divides into three segmental branches that supply the upper (U) and middle (M) segments of the anterior surface and most of the lower segment (L). The small apical (A) segment is usually supplied by a branch from the anterior division. The posterior division of the renal artery supplies the posterior segment (P), which represents more than half of the posterior surface of the kidney. [Reprinted with permission (9).]

Bellini). The cortex is about 1 cm in thickness, encircles the base of each pyramid, and extends downward between pyramids to form the septa of Bertin. Despite well-described radiologic features (13,14), an enlarged septum of Bertin has on occasion been clinically mistaken for a renal tumor. Longitudinal striations extending from the base of the pyramids out into the cortex are termed the medullary rays (of Ferrein). Regardless of their name, they are actually part of the cortex and are formed by the straight segments of the proximal tubules (PSTs), the thick ascending limbs (TALs), and the collecting ducts. The medullary rays may be visualized during excretory urography in conditions with tubular fluid stasis (15).

A single pyramid with its surrounding cortical parenchyma constitutes a renal lobe (16), which is not generally regarded as a functional unit of the kidney (Fig. 3). The human kidney has an average of 14 lobes (17). During embryologic development, lobar fusion decreases the number of surface clefts, papillae, and calyces. A degree of persistent fetal lobation may be observed in some adult kidneys, and the mean number of calyces and papillae reported is 8.7 and 10.7, respectively (18). There is a greater degree of lobar fusion in the polar region than in the midpolar region of the kidney.

There are two main types of renal papillae (19). Simple papillae drain only one lobe and have convex tips containing small, often slitlike orifices. Compound papillae drain two or more adjacent fused lobes and have flattened, ridged, or concave tips with round, often gaping orifices. The distribution of papillae types within the kidney is related to the embryologic pattern of fusion involving the lobes, papillae, and calyces (Fig. 4). It is believed that the more open orifices of compound papillae are less capable of preventing intrarenal reflux (20), which may be associated with an increase in intrapelvic pressure. This concept is supported by the observation that pyelonephritic scars associated with intrarenal reflux are present more commonly in the renal poles, where the compound papillae predominantly occur.

The renal pelvis is the saclike expansion of the upper ureter. Two or three outpouchings or major calyces (infundibula) extend from the pelvis and divide into the minor calyces, into which the papillae protrude. In addition, elaborate leaflike extensions, termed fornices, extend from the minor calyces into the medulla, and secondary pouches increase the pelvic surface area (21). A detailed description of the gross anatomy of the kidney is provided elsewhere (22).

## NEPHRON

The structural and functional unit of the kidney is the nephron, which consists of the renal corpuscle (glomerulus and Bowman's capsule), proximal tubule, thin limbs, and distal tubule, all of which originate from the metanephric

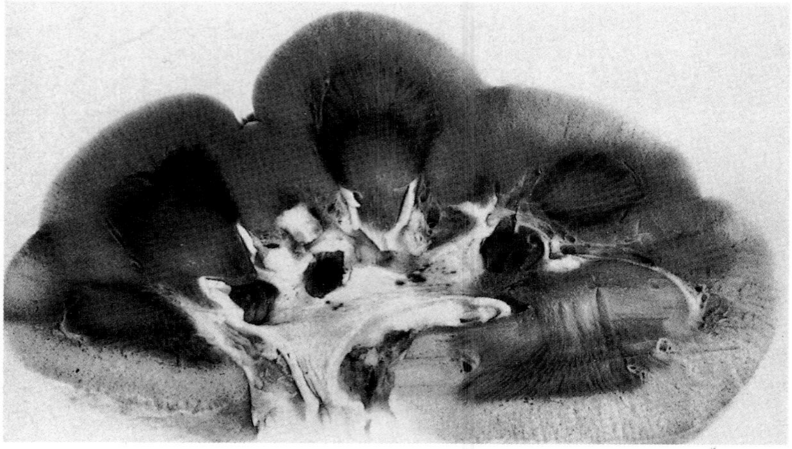

**FIG. 2.** Bisected kidney demonstrating the light-staining cortex and the dark-staining outer medulla. The inner medulla is lighter staining than the outer medulla. Septa of Bertin extend downward, separating the renal pyramids. [Reprinted with permission (203).]

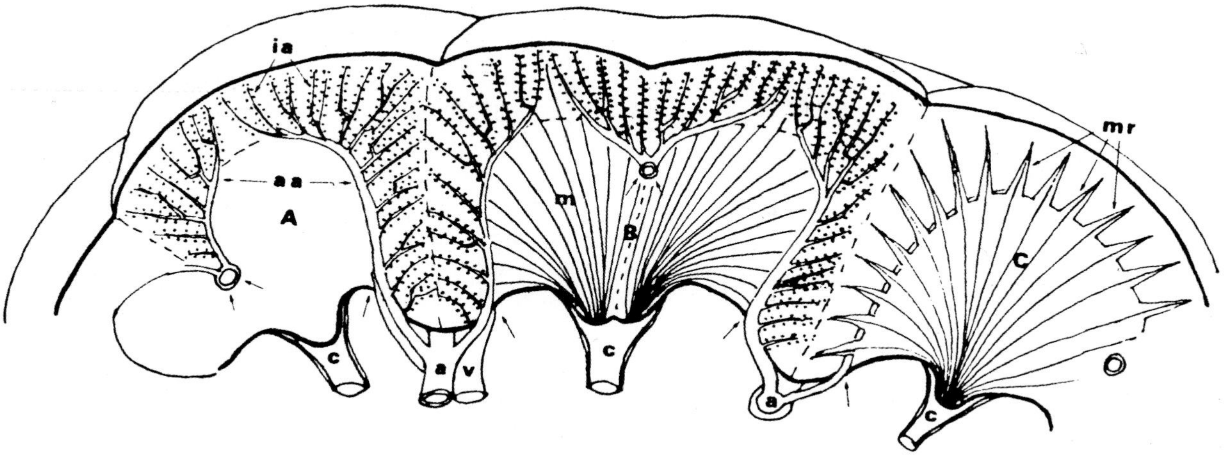


**FIG. 3.** Diagram of three renal lobes. **A:** Arcuate (aa) and interlobular (ia) arteries. **B:** Cortex and medulla are illustrated in a double lobe with fused double papillae. **C:** Lobe showing medullary rays (mr). *Small double arrows* in A and B indicate subsidiary septal arteries. *Single arrows* refer to where arcuate vessels enter the renal parenchyma. a, interlobar arteries; v, interlobar vein; c, calyces. A septum of Bertin represents the approximation of two layers of septal cortex from two adjacent lobes. [Reprinted with permission (204).]

blastema. Each human kidney contains about 800,000 to 1,200,000 nephrons (23,24).

Nephrons can be classified according to the position of their glomeruli in the cortex or the length of their loop of Henle (Fig. 5). In the former scheme, superficial, midcortical, and juxtamedullary nephrons are distinguished. Superficial nephrons have glomeruli located in the outer cortex, and their efferent arterioles usually ascend to the cortical surface. The glomeruli of juxtamedullary nephrons are located immediately above the corticomedullary junction in the inner cortex, and their efferent arterioles form the descending vasa recta. The glomeruli of midcortical nephrons are situated in the midcortex above the juxtamedullary region, but below the superficial nephrons. Glomeruli are normally located in the cortex. Ectopic glomeruli have been observed in the connective tissue surrounding interlobar blood vessels and in the pelvic septum of the neonatal kidney (25). In the more commonly used classification there are two main populations of nephrons: those with a short loop of Henle and those with a long loop. The length of the loop of Henle is generally related to the location of its parent glomerulus in the cortex. The short loops form their bend at various levels within the inner stripe of the outer medulla, whereas the long loops of Henle enter and turn back within the inner medulla. Although, there are numerous gradations between these two main types of nephrons, there are seven times more short than long loop nephrons (26). A correlation between the urinary concentrating ability and the relative length of the medulla has been established in several mammalian kidneys (27).

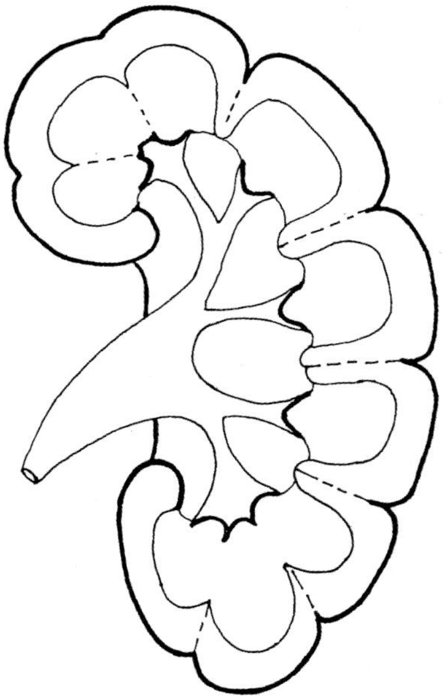

**FIG. 4.** Schematic representation of lobar architecture. In the polar regions, there is a greater degree of lobar fusion resulting in the formation of compound papillae and calyces and the loss of septal cortex. The individual lobes tend to be retained in the midpolar region, and the septal cortex extends between renal pyramids to the renal sinus. [Reprinted with permission (204).]

The connecting tubule, a transitional segment, joins the nephron to the collecting duct system, which originates from the ureteric bud. Although not correct in a strict anatomic sense, for practical considerations, the term nephron is commonly used to include the connecting segment and entire collecting duct. The collecting duct system can be divided into the cortical, outer medullary, and inner medullary collecting ducts (28,29). Structural and functional heterogene-

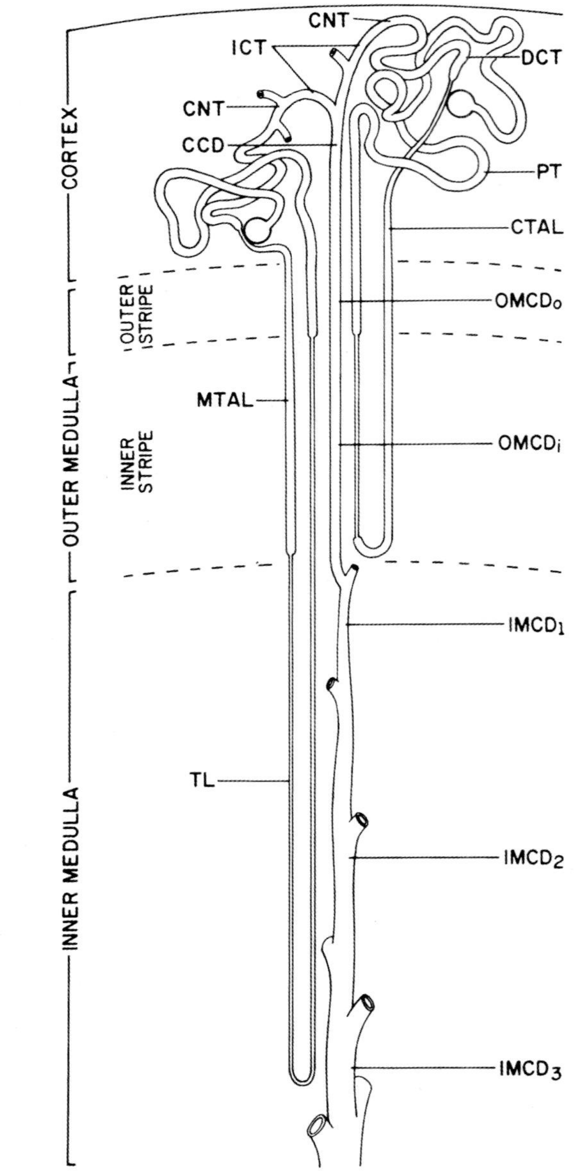


**FIG. 5.** Schematic drawing illustrating the segments of the nephron and the zones of the kidney. PT, proximal tubule; TL, thin limb of the Henle's loop; MTAL, medullary thick ascending limb; CTAL, cortical thick ascending limb; DCT, distal convoluted tubule; CNT, connecting tubule; ICT, initial collecting tubule; CCD, cortical collecting duct; $OMCD_O$, collecting duct in outer stripe of outer medulla; $OMCD_i$, collecting duct in inner stripe of outer medulla; $IMCD_1$, outer third of inner medullary collecting duct; $IMCD_2$, middle third of inner medullary collecting duct; $IMCD_3$, inner third of inner medullary collecting duct. (From ref. 28, with permission.)

ity exists along the nephron (30). Internephron heterogeneity refers to the differences between analogous segments in superficial and juxtamedullary nephrons. Intranephron or axial heterogeneity may be defined as the differences between early and successive later portions of an individual nephron segment.

## ARCHITECTURE

The renal cortex can be divided into lobules. A renal lobule consists of a centrally positioned medullary ray and its surrounding cortical parenchyma containing all nephrons draining into the collecting ducts of the medullary ray. In contrast to lobules of other organs, renal lobules are not distinctly separated by fine connective tissue septa; therefore, they are difficult to distinguish histologically. Furthermore, because it has been difficult to establish any structural–functional significance, the concept of the renal lobule is not commonly used.

The nephron segments and blood vessels in the cortex and medulla have a specific geometric arrangement (31). This intricate architecture allows for integration (axial) of complex transport functions along the length of a specific nephron

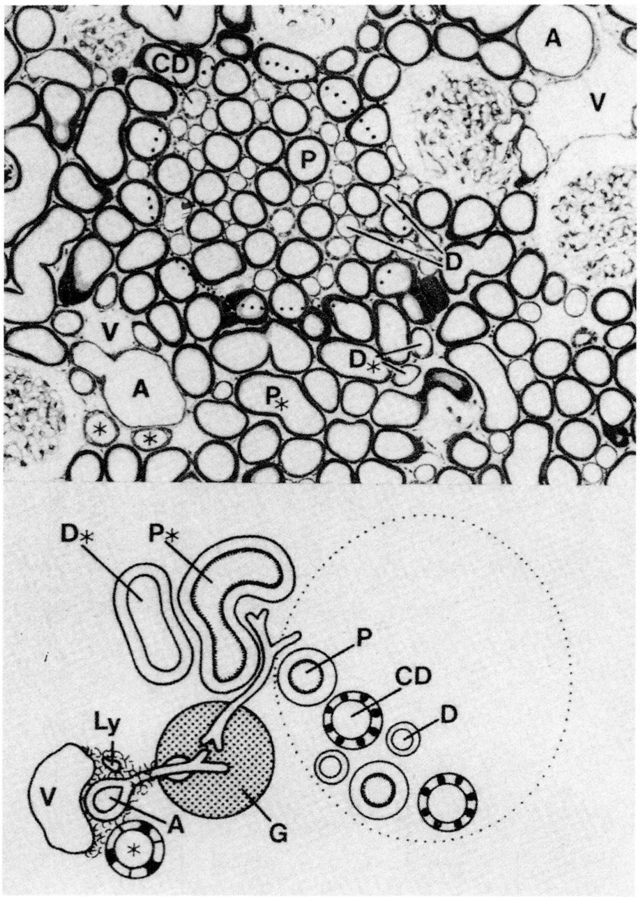


**FIG. 6.** Architectural regions of the renal cortex. **Top:** One-micron cross section. **Bottom:** Diagram illustrating a medullary ray, encircled by the dotted line, and the cortical labyrinth. The proximal straight (P) and distal straight thick ascending limb (D) tubules and the collecting ducts (CD) are located in the medullary ray. The adjacent cortical labyrinth contains the interlobular vessels. A, artery; V, vein; Ly, lymphatic, arcades (*) of connecting tubules, glomeruli (G), and the proximal (P*) and distal (D*) convoluted tubules. [Reprinted with permission (31).]

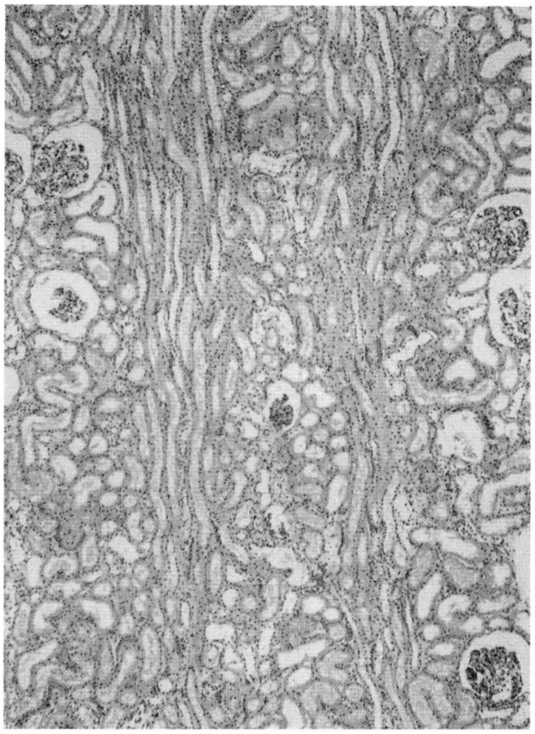

**FIG. 7.** Longitudinal section of cortex demonstrating two linear aggregates of tubules representing medullary rays (original magnification ×**50**).

segment, as well as integration (regional) between different nephron segments in a specific region or zone (32).

Two architectural regions of the renal cortex can be distinguished: the cortical labyrinth and the medullary rays (Fig. 6). The cortical labyrinth represents a continuous parenchymal zone that surrounds the regularly distributed medullary rays. Glomeruli, proximal and distal convoluted tubules, connecting tubules, initial collecting tubules, interlobular vessels, and a rich capillary network are situated in the cortical labyrinth. The large majority of convoluted tubule profiles are proximal tubules. Connecting tubules of juxtamedullary nephrons fuse and form so-called arcades within the cortical labyrinth. The medullary rays (Figs. 7 and 8) contain the proximal and distal straight tubules and collecting ducts, all of which enter into the medulla.

The localization of specific segments of the nephrons at various levels in the medulla account for the division of the medulla into an inner and outer zone, with the latter subdivided into an inner and outer stripe (Fig. 5). The relative tissue volumes for the cortex and the outer and inner medulla are 70%, 27%, and 3%, respectively (29).

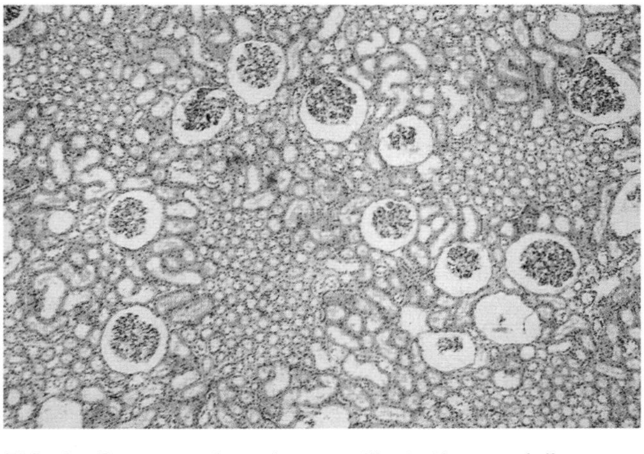

**FIG. 8.** Cross section of cortex illustrating medullary rays that are regularly distributed within the cortical labyrinth (original magnification ×**50**).

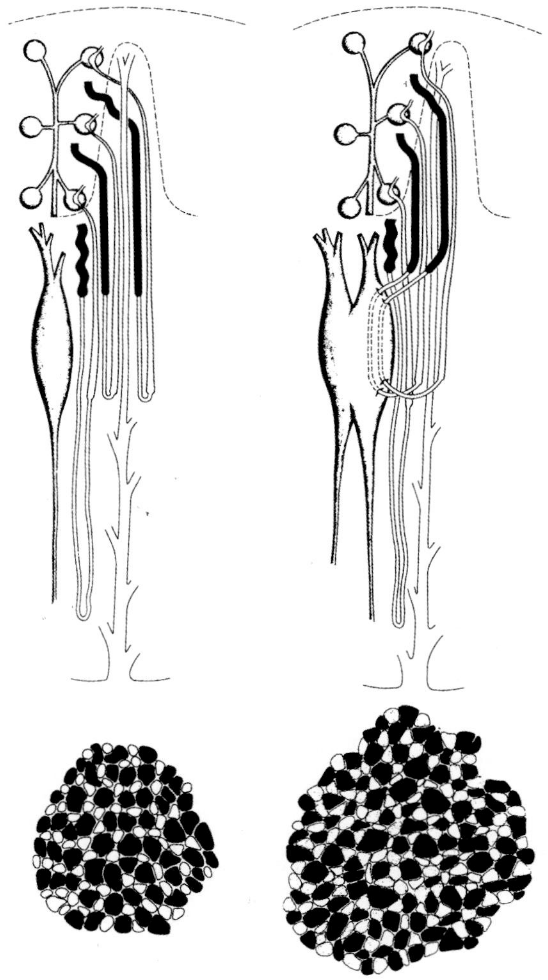

**FIG. 9.** Schematic diagram demonstrating the simple and complex types of medulla. **Upper left:** In the simple medulla, the loops of Henle remain separate from the vascular bundle. The vascular bundle itself (**lower left**) contains only descending (*black*) and ascending (*white*) vasa recta. **Upper right:** In the complex medulla, the descending thin limbs (DTLs) of short loops of Henle descend within the vascular bundles, which tend to fuse. Therefore, the complex bundles (**lower right**) contain the DTLs of short loops (*hatched*) in addition to descending (*black*) and ascending (*white*) vasa recta. [Reprinted with permission (29).]

The outer stripe of the outer medulla is relatively thin. It contains the terminal portions of the proximal straight tubules, the thick ascending limbs (TALs), and the collecting ducts. The outer stripe is also distinguished by the absence of thin limbs of Henle. In contrast to the outer stripe, the inner stripe of the outer medulla is thicker. It contains thin descending limbs, TALs, and collecting ducts. It is further characterized by the absence of the proximal straight tubules (PSTs). Aggregations of descending and ascending vasa recta known as vascular bundles develop in the outer stripe but are located predominantly in the inner stripe. Compared with the kidneys of some mammals with very high urine concentrating ability, the human kidney has a simple medulla (31). In contrast to the complex medulla, the vascular bundles of the simple medulla do not fuse to form larger vascular structures, and they do not incorporate descending thin limbs (DTLs) of short loops (Fig. 9). The inner medulla contains the thin descending and thin ascending limbs of long loops, as well as the collecting ducts. TALs are absent in the inner medulla.

## PARENCHYMA

An accurate morphologic evaluation of the kidney requires a detailed systematic examination of the glomeruli, tubules, interstitium, and blood vessels of the renal parenchyma. A detailed approach to the histopathologic evaluation of the kidney has been described (33), and a standard nomenclature for structures of the kidney exists (34). The following discussion emphasizes normal histologic aspects and structural–functional relationships in the kidney. Although the focus is on the human kidney, analogous renal structures in other mammalian species are discussed or illustrated when pertinent.

### Glomerulus

In 1666, Malpighi first described the glomeruli and demonstrated their continuity with the renal vasculature (35,36). About 175 years later, Bowman elucidated in detail the capillary architecture of the glomerulus and the continuity between its surrounding capsule and the proximal tubule (37,38). The renal corpuscle consists of a tuft of interconnected capillaries and an enclosing capsule named after Bowman. The term "glomerulus" is commonly used to refer to the glomerular capillary tuft and Bowman's capsule, although the term "renal corpuscle" is more accurate in a strict anatomic sense. The glomerulus does not simply represent a ball of capillaries. Providing structural support for the capillary tuft is a central region termed the mesangium, which contains cells and their surrounding matrix material. The capillaries are lined by a thin layer of endothelial cells, con-

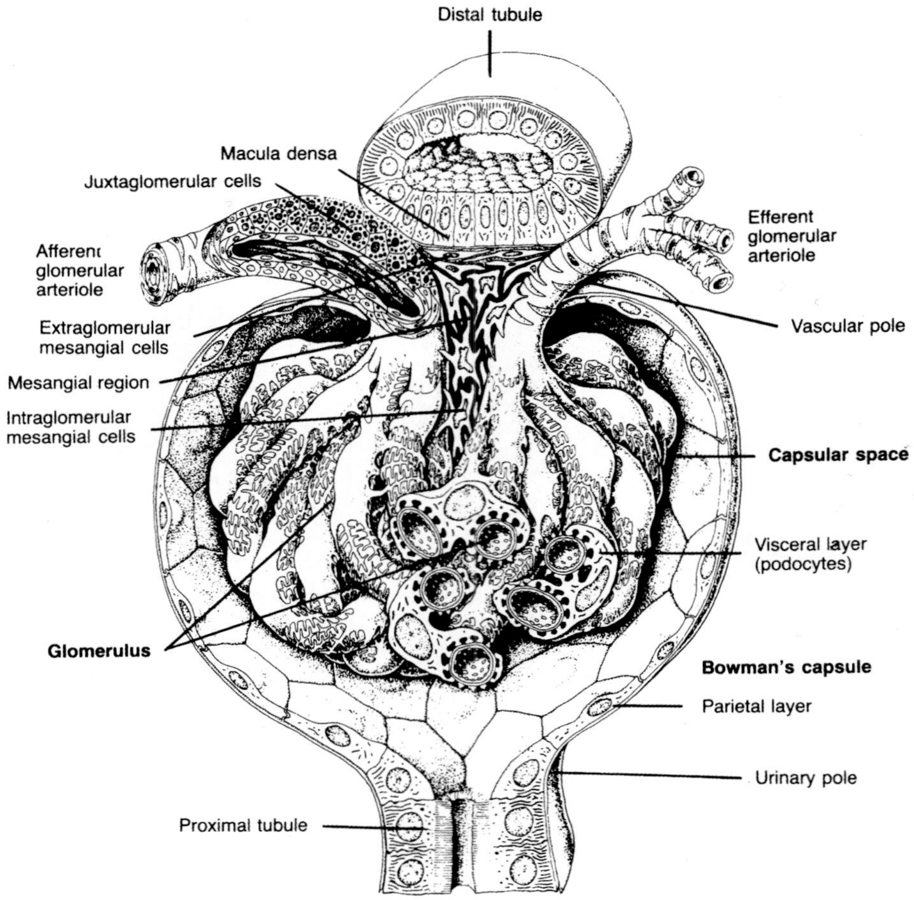


**FIG. 10.** Schematic three-dimensional representation of the glomerulus. [Reprinted with permission (205).]

tain a basement membrane, and are covered by epithelial cells that form the visceral layer of Bowman's capsule. The parietal epithelium is continuous with the visceral epithelium at the vascular pole where the afferent arteriole enters the glomerulus and the efferent arteriole exits. Therefore, the glomerulus resembles a blind-pouched extension (Bowman's capsule) of the proximal tubule invaginated by a tuft of capillaries (Fig. 10). The cavity situated between the two epithelial layers of Bowman's capsule is called Bowman's space or the urinary space. At the urinary pole, this space and the parietal layer of Bowman's capsule continue into the lumen and epithelium of the proximal tubule. The glomerular tuft originates from the afferent arteriole, which enters the glomerulus at the vascular pole and divides into four to eight lobules. Anastomoses are believed to exist between individual capillaries within a lobule as well as between lobules (31,39,40). The efferent arteriole is formed by rejoined capillaries and leaves the glomerulus at the vascular pole.

The glomerulus has a round configuration and an average diameter of 200 $\mu$m (23). The diameter of glomeruli from juxtamedullary nephrons is approximately 20% greater (40). It has been reported that the glomeruli in solitary functioning kidneys are significantly larger than those in control patients with two kidneys (41). Although the glomerulus has a lobular architecture, the lobulation is often inconspicuous in light microscopic sections. An accentuated degree of lobulation may be more prominent in autopsy kidneys than in biopsy specimens (33). An accurate assessment of glomerular cellularity requires histologic sections 2 to 4 $\mu$m thick (Fig. 11). An increase in the number of glomerular cells occurs with an increase in section thickness. Generally the presence of more than three cells in a mesangial area away from the vascular pole constitutes hypercellularity. The delicate character of the glomerular capillary walls can be observed on thin histologic and frozen sections (Fig. 12) (42).

A thin fenestrated endothelium lines the glomerular capillaries. By light microscopy, the endothelial cells have light eosinophilic cytoplasm and slightly oval nuclei. Their nuclei are present within the capillary lumina. The endothelial cells

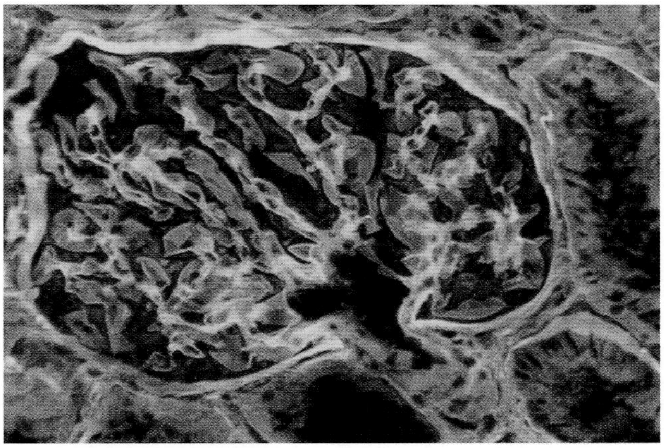

**FIG. 12.** Fluorescent micrograph of an H&E-stained frozen section. Note the delicate character of the glomerular capillary walls. (Courtesy of Dr. Stephen M. Bonsib.)

are extremely attenuated around the capillary lumen, and the thicker portions of the cells containing the nuclei lie adjacent to the mesangium away from the urinary space. The attenuated portion of endothelial cytoplasm is perforated by fenestrae 70 to 100 nm in diameter (39). The cytoplasm contains microtubules, microfilaments, and intermediate filaments (43). The endothelial cell surface carries a negative charge because of the presence of polyanionic glycoproteins and contributes to the charge selectivity of the glomerular capillary wall (44,45).

The mesangium, composed of mesangial cells and their surrounding matrix, is observed as a periodic acid-Schiff (PAS)- and methenamine silver–positive structural support for the glomerular capillary loops (Fig. 13). By light microscopy, the mesangial cells usually can be distinguished by their mesangial location and dark-staining nuclei. Ultrastructurally, they are irregular in shape and have elongated cytoplasmic processes that may extend between the endothelium and the glomerular basement membrane.

The mesangial cell contains actomyosin (46), has smooth

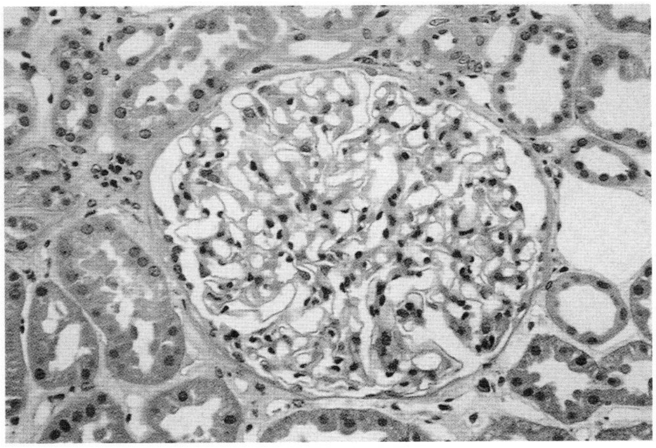

**FIG. 11.** Glomerulus exhibiting round configuration and normal cellularity (original magnification ×**250**).

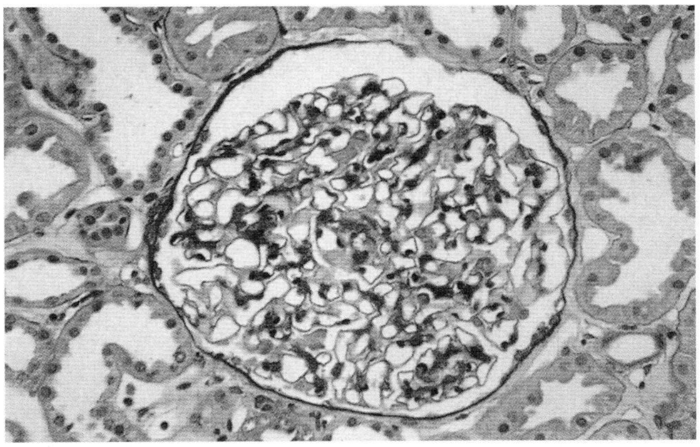

**FIG. 13.** PAS-stained normal glomerulus illustrating the PAS-positive mesangium within the central regions of the glomerular lobules (original magnification ×**250**).

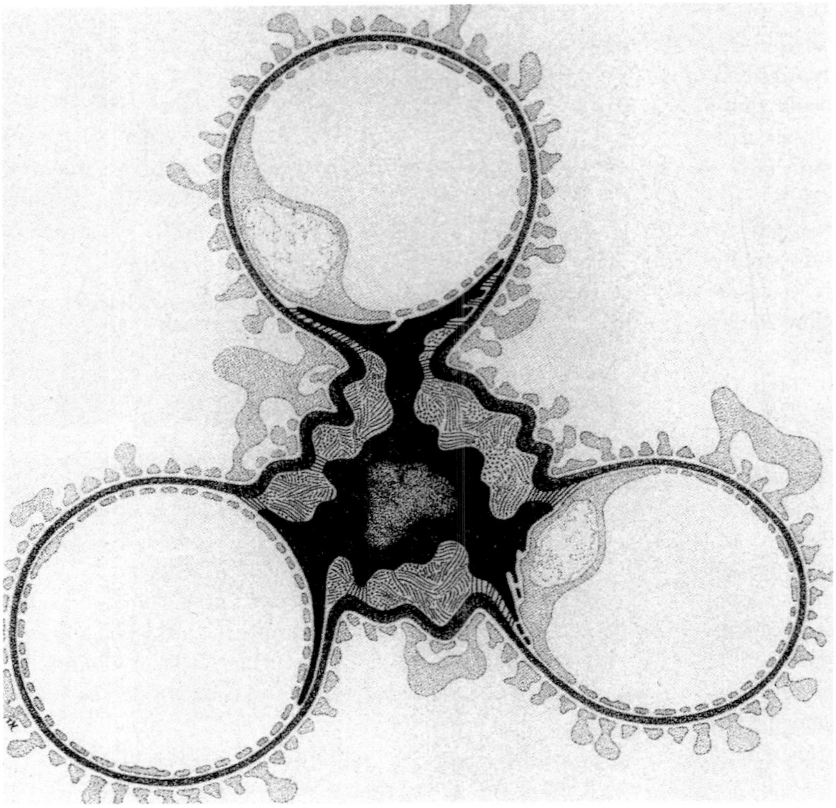

**FIG. 14.** Schematic diagram illustrating the relationship between the mesangium and the glomerular capillaries. The visceral epithelial cells and endothelial cell cytoplasm are light gray. Note that the glomerular basement membrane (*black*) encloses the mesangium and its attached capillaries. The central mesangial cell is represented as black, and the mesangial matrix is represented by the fibrillar texture. The cytoplasmic processes of mesangial cells are connected to the glomerular basement membrane directly or indirectly by microfibrils in the mesangial matrix. [Reprinted with permission (50).]

muscle contractile properties, and likely modulates glomerular filtration (47). Whereas the endothelium forms a continuous layer around the inner circumference of the glomerular capillary, the basement membrane and the visceral epithelial cell layer do not completely encircle the capillary but enclose the mesangial matrix and cells between the capillaries (Fig. 14). The presence of microfibril-mediated and direct attachments between glomerular basement membrane suggests that the mesangial cell and the glomerular basement membrane may represent a biomechanical functional unit (48,49). It has been proposed that the contractile apparatus of the mesangium appears to maintain the structure of the capillary walls by counteracting the distention caused by the capillary and mesangial interstitial pressure (50). The mesangial cell also has phagocytic capability and plays a role in the clearance of debris from the mesangium (51). Mesangial cells can respond to as well as generate a variety of molecules, including interleukin I, platelet-derived

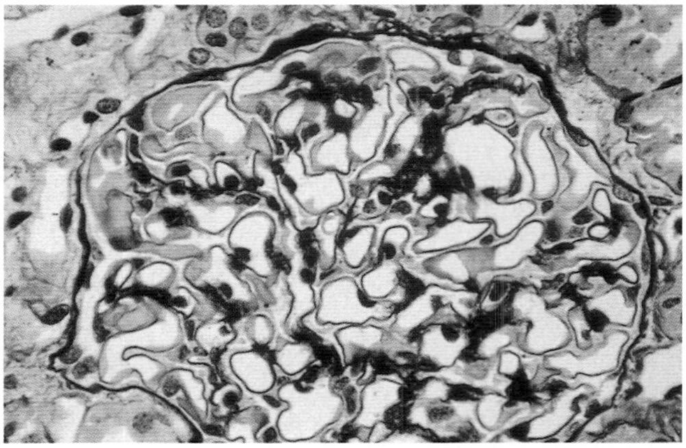

**FIG. 15.** Silver methenamine–stained normal glomerulus illustrating the silver-positive glomerular basement membranes and positive basement membrane of Bowman's capsule (original magnification ×**500**).

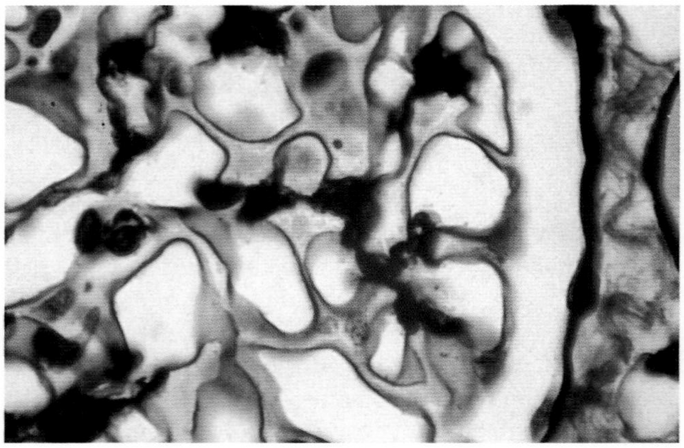

**FIG. 16.** Higher magnification micrograph demonstrating thin regular glomerular basement membranes of peripheral capillary loops. Silver methenamine stain (original magnification ×**1,250**).

growth factor, and arachidonic acid metabolites, which may play a central role in the response to glomerular injury (52). The mesangial matrix is structurally similar but not identical to the peripheral glomerular basement membrane.

The glomerular basement membrane can be demonstrated on light microscopy by PAS and methenamine silver stains (Fig. 15). The silver methenamine preparation is more specific; examination of a peripheral capillary loop away from the vascular pole and the mesangium shows a delicate basement membrane (Fig. 16). Hematoxylin and eosin (H&E) and even PAS may stain capillary luminal contents and the cytoplasm of the endothelial and visceral epithelial cell layers, resulting in an apparent thickening of the glomerular basement membrane. The basement membrane is situated between the endothelium and the visceral epithelial cells in the glomerular capillary wall. On ultrastructural examination, the glomerular basement membrane consists of a central dense layer, the lamina densa, and two surrounding thinner electron-lucent layers, the lamina rara interna and the lamina rara externa. In comparison with laboratory animals, the electron-lucent layers appear less prominent in the human glomerulus (Fig. 17). This may be due in part to differ-

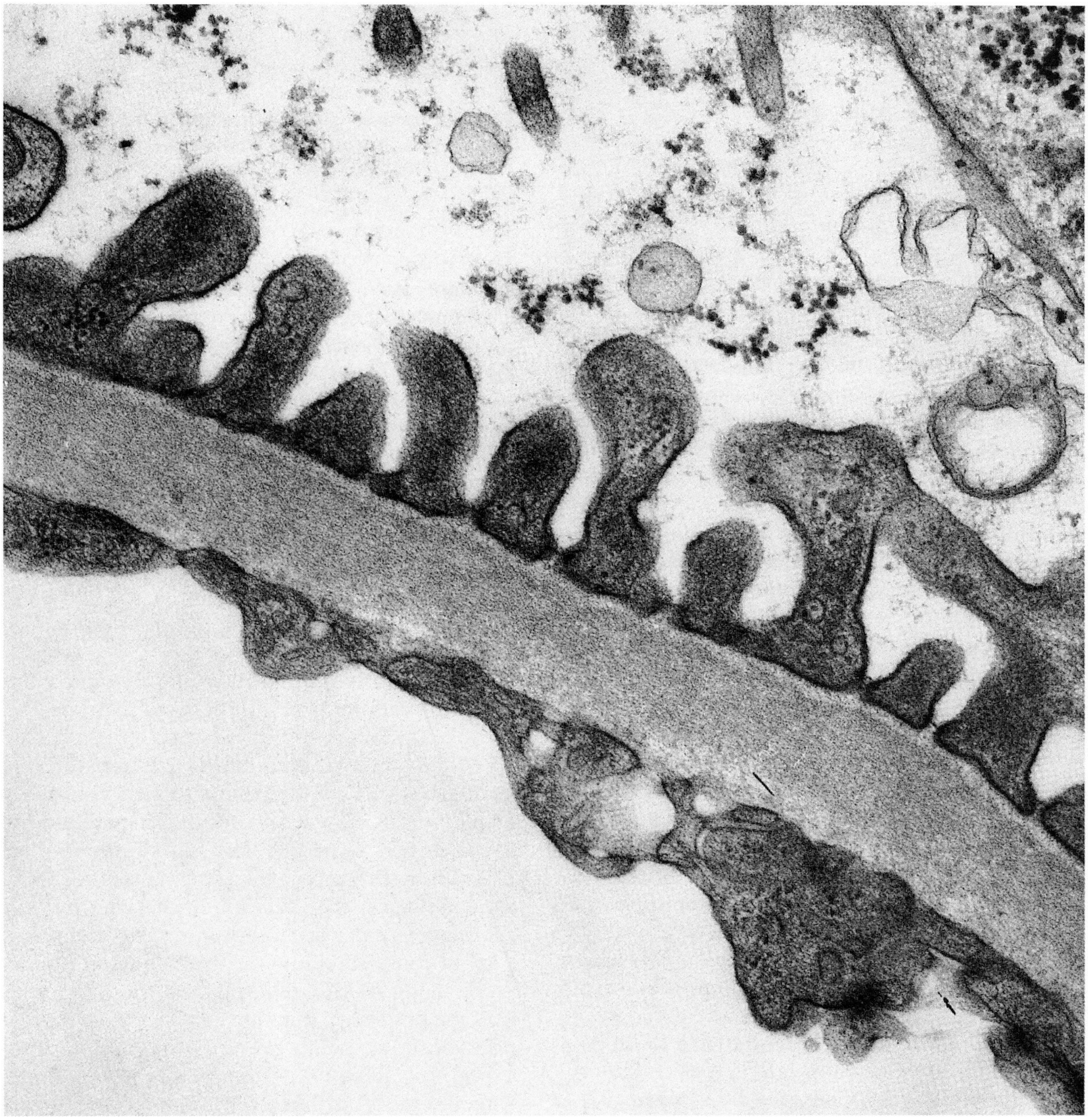

**FIG. 17.** Transmission electron micrograph of glomerulus. Bowman's space is above and the capillary lumen is below the glomerular capillary wall. Note the regular alignment of the foot processes of the visceral epithelial cells. The glomerular basement membrane consists primarily of the lamina densa, and the electron-lucent lamina rara interna and lamina rara externa are not prominent (original magnification **×48,000**).

ent fixation conditions. The glomerular basement membrane ranges between 310 and 380 nm in mean thickness (53–55). The glomerular basement membrane is significantly thicker in men (mean 373 nm) than in women (mean 326 nm) and increases in width until the fourth decade of life (56). Quantitative data on the normal glomerular capillary structure are available and include the following values: mean glomerular volume of $1.38 \times 10^6$ $\mu m^3$, average capillary diameter of 6.75 $\mu m$, and capillary filtration surface/glomerulus of $200 \times 10^3$ $\mu m^2$ (57).

The major components of the glomerular basement membrane are type IV collagen, heparan sulfate proteoglycans, and laminin, but other proteins, including fibronectin and nidogen, have been documented (58). A $\beta_1$-integrin receptor for fibronectin has been immunolocalized on the cell membranes of the endothelial cells and visceral epithelial cells that face the glomerular basement membrane (59). The glomerular basement membrane represents both a size-selective and a charge-selective barrier and is believed to be the principal structure responsible for ultrafiltration. Fixed negatively charged sites rich in heparan sulfate proteoglycans participate in establishing the charge barrier (60,61).

The visceral epithelial cells or podocytes are the largest cells in the glomerulus. By light microscopy, they are positioned on the outside of the glomerular capillary wall, often bulge into the urinary space, and have prominent nuclei and abundant light eosinophilic cytoplasm. Scanning electron microscopy shows that the visceral epithelial cells have long cytoplasmic ramifications, the primary processes that surround the glomerular capillaries and divide into individual foot processes or pedicles (Fig. 18) (62). The foot processes cover the capillary wall, directly contact the lamina rara externa of the glomerular basement membrane, and interdigitate with foot processes from different podocytes. By transmission electron microscopy, the cells have abundant rough endoplasmic reticulum, a well-developed Golgi apparatus, and prominent lyosomes. There are numerous microtubules, microfilaments, and intermediate filaments in the cytoplasm (43). The microfilaments are most abundant in the foot processes (63). Actin, myosin, and $\alpha$-actinin, the three major proteins of the contractile apparatus in muscle, have been immunolocalized to the foot processes, whereas vimentin and tubulin, the main proteins of intermediate filaments and microtubules, respectively, have been observed in the podocyte cell body but not in the foot processes (64,65). It has been suggested that this ultrastructural arrangement of contractile proteins may allow the podocytes to play an active role in modifying the glomerular filtration surface area (64).

The adjacent foot processes are separated by a 25- to 60-nm space termed the filtration slit, which is bridged by a 4- to 6-nm diaphragm called the filtration slit diaphragm. The diaphragm has an intricate zipperlike substructure consisting of a central filament that is connected by multiple rodlike subunits to the cell membrane of adjacent foot processes (66,67). The exact functional role of the filtration slit diaphragm remains unclear. The surface membranes of the visceral epithelial cells are covered with a negatively charged glycocalyx, which stains with colloidal iron or ruthenium red and is rich in sialic acid (68). The major sialoprotein, podocalyxin, is more abundant on the podocytes than the endothelial cells and has been demonstrated on the urinary sides but not the soles of the foot processes (69). Although the glomerular basement membrane is synthesized by both endothelial and visceral epithelial cells, the latter likely play a greater role (58).

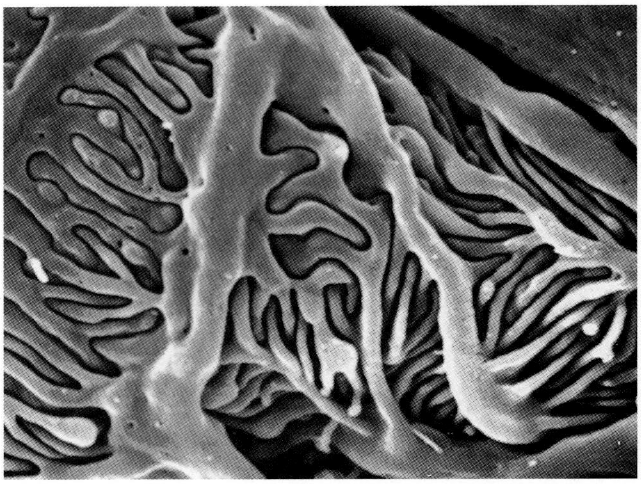

**FIG. 18.** Scanning electron micrograph of glomerulus illustrating the visceral epithelial cells and their multiple processes wrapping around the capillary loops. Note the interdigitation of the foot processes (original magnification ×**13,000**; courtesy of Dr. Jill W. Verlander).

The Wilms tumor suppressor gene, WT1, plays an indispensable role in the regulation of cell growth and differentiation during early nephrogenesis. Embyronic mice homozygous for a targeted mutation of WT1 fail to develop kidneys

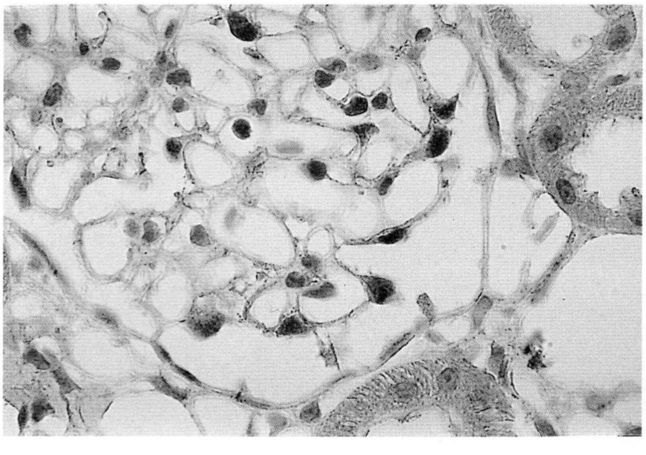

**FIG. 19.** Light micrograph demonstrating expression of the WT1 protein in podocyte nuclei of an adult glomerulus. WT1 immunoperoxidase (original magnification ×**210**).

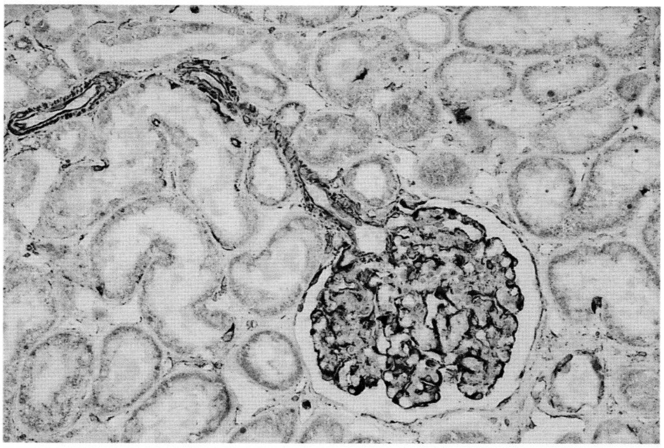

**FIG. 20.** Vascular structures including the glomerulus are heavily labeled with antibody to vimentin. Tubular and interstitial components show weaker and sparse labeling. Vimentin immunoperoxidase (original magnification ×**62**).

(70). Striking evidence also exists for the importance of WT1 in glomerular podocyte differentiation. During kidney development, WT1 expression is detected in the metanephric mesenchyme and becomes stronger in the renal vesicle, but highest levels occur during glomerulus formation within the podocyte cell layer (71,72). Expression of the WT1 protein, a transcription factor, in the nuclei of podocytes does not disappear with glomerular maturation but persists in the adult kidney (Fig. 19). Greater than 95% of patients with the Denys-Drash syndrome (nephrotic syndrome and genital anomalies and/or Wilms tumor), characterized by shrunken glomeruli with hypertrophied podocytes, have point mutations affecting the zinc finger DNA-binding domain of WT1 (73). These findings provide a functional link between a molecular defect of WT1 and podocyte pathology and suggest that WT1 has a role in maintenance of podocyte structure and function in the mature kidney.

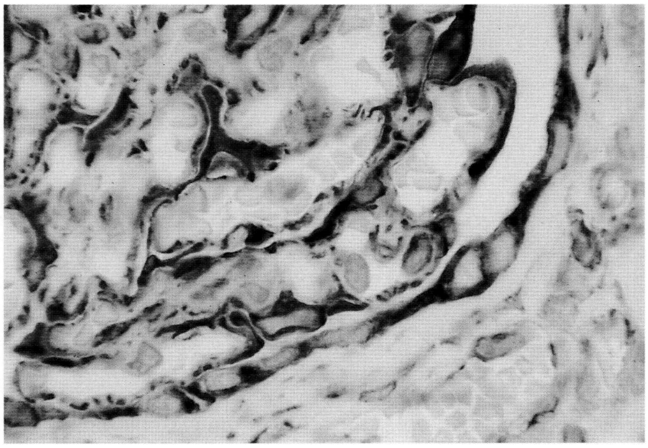

**FIG. 21.** Prominent expression of vimentin is seen in glomerular endothelium, podocytes, and parietal epithelium. Vimentin immunoperoxidase (original magnification ×**300**).

The parietal layer of Bowman's capsule is a simple squamous epithelium. Keratins, the intermediate filament proteins, have been demonstrated in these cells (65,74). The cells are 0.1 to 0.3 $\mu$m in height but may increase to 2 to 3.5 $\mu$m at the nucleus (39). The epithelium rests on the basement membrane of Bowman's capsule, which has been reported to range from 1,200 to 1,500 nm in thickness and may have a lamellated appearance (39). A peripolar cell situated between the visceral and parietal epithelial cell layers at the origin of the glomerular tuft in Bowman's space has been most commonly observed in sheep but also identified in humans (75–78). However, these cells have been detected only in approximately 1% of human glomeruli by light microscopy (76). Ultrastructurally, the peripolar cell contains multiple membrane-bound electron-dense secretory type granules. It has been proposed that this cell represents a component of the juxtaglomerular apparatus (75). The exact function of the peripolar cells is unknown, but they may have a secretory function and discharge their contents into Bowman's space.

The development of the glomerulus as a vascular structure distinct from the remainder of the nephron is reflected in the intrarenal distribution of intermediate filaments. Vimentin is present in glomerular endothelial and mesangial cells and podocytes (Figs. 20 and 21), whereas desmin expression is restricted to podocytes (74). The glomerular tuft does not stain for keratins, whereas the parietal epithelial cells express keratins 8, 18, and 19 of simple epithelium (Fig. 22) (79–81). Smooth muscle actin can be detected in the mesangium, and CD34 is present in the glomerular endothelium (Fig. 23). Occasional leukocytes are observed in the normal glomerulus and label with leukocyte common antigen (CD45 and CD45RB) staining (82–84). Although most of the leukocytes are present in the vascular spaces, macrophages are known to infiltrate the mesangium and play a role in immune responsiveness (Fig. 24) (85,86).

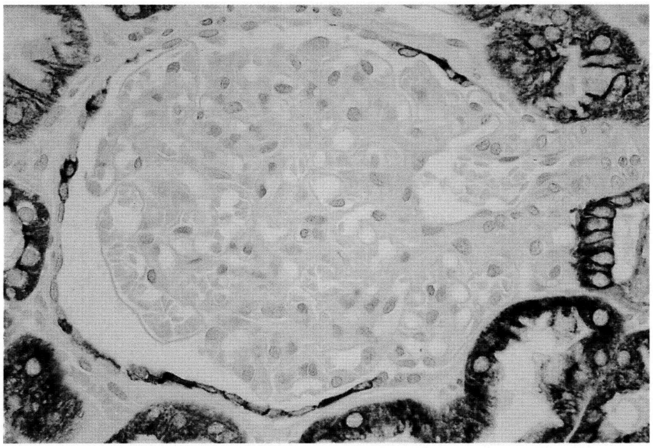

**FIG. 22.** Keratin expression is not observed in the glomerular tuft. The vascular pole is on the right and the macula densa (MD) (far right center) and other tubule segments are staining as are the parietal epithelial cells. CAM 5.2 immunoperoxidase (original magnification ×**120**).

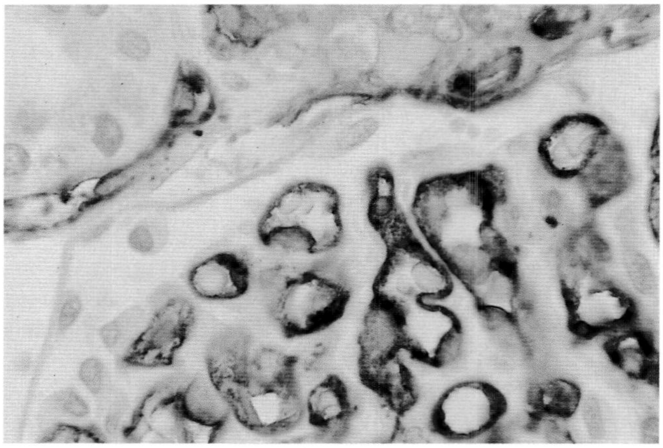

FIG. 23. Glomerular endothelium showing strong immunoreactivity for CD34. Several peritubular capillaries show staining along the upper border. CD34 immunoperoxidase (original magnification ×300).

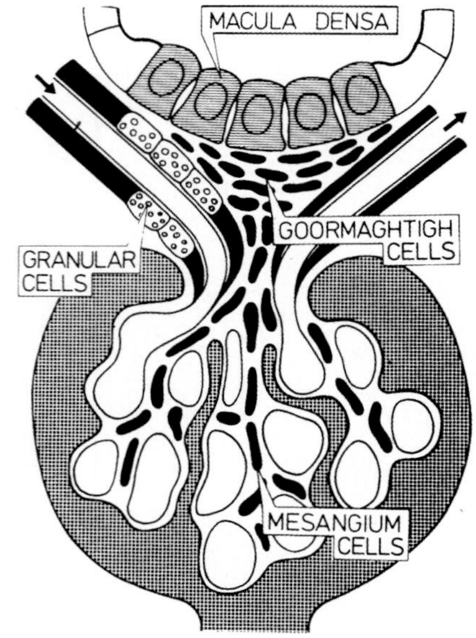


FIG. 25. The basic components of the juxtaglomerular apparatus. [Reprinted with permission (31).]

### Juxtaglomerular Apparatus

The juxtaglomerular apparatus, discovered by Golgi (87), is situated at the vascular pole of the glomerulus and includes the afferent and efferent arterioles, extraglomerular mesangial region, and macula densa (MD) (Fig. 25). Although the general outline of this anatomical unit usually can be observed in light microscopic sections (Fig. 26), histochemical or immunocytochemical methods are usually required to demonstrate the distinctive juxtaglomerular granular cells. These cells tend to occur in clusters and are most abundant in the wall of the afferent arteriole but are also found in the wall of the efferent arteriole and the extraglomerular mesangial region (88,89). Ultrastructural analysis shows the presence of myofilaments, attachment bodies, a well-developed endoplasmic reticulum and Golgi apparatus, and numerous membrane-bound granules (Fig. 27). The granules are variable in shape and size. It is believed that the smaller, often rhomboid-shaped granules with a crystalline substructure, called protogranules, observed in the Golgi region represent precursors that transform into larger amorphous mature granules. Renin and angiotensin II have been immunolocalized to the granules of these cells (90,91). The extraglomerular mesangium, also called the lacis or the cells of Goormaghtigh, is located between the afferent and efferent arterioles and has extensive contact with the basal surface of the MD. This extraglomerular region is continuous with the intraglomerular mesangium, and the Goormaghtigh cells are similar in ultrastructure to the mesangial cells. There are numerous gap junctions between the extraglomerular mesan-

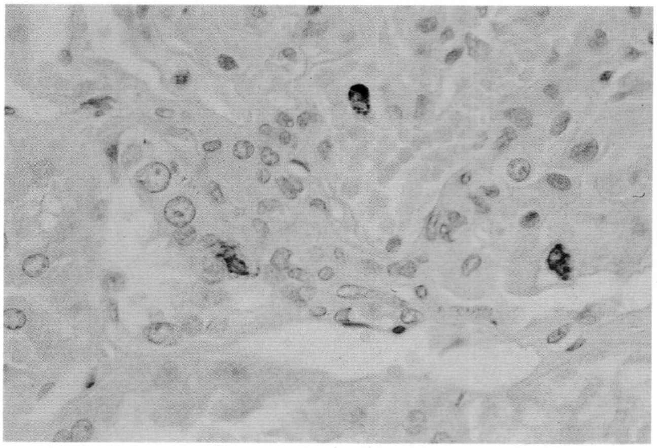

FIG. 24. KP-1 immunohistochemical stain illustrating that a small percentage of cells in the mesangium label as tissue monocytes. KP-1 immunoperoxidase (original magnification ×210).

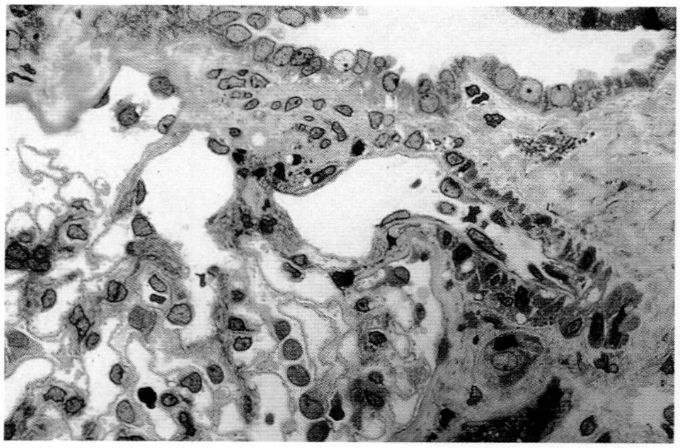

FIG. 26. Light micrograph depicting the juxtaglomerular apparatus. From the top to the bottom of the micrograph are the MD, extraglomerular mesangium, afferent arteriole, and glomerulus (original magnification ×750; courtesy of Dr. Luciano Barajas). [Reprinted with permission (89).]

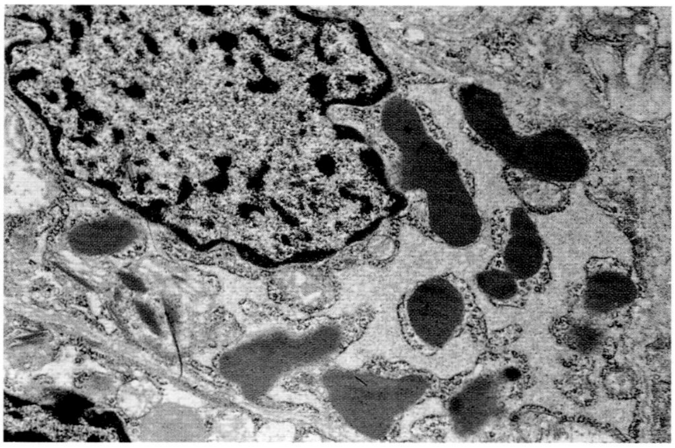

**FIG. 27.** Transmission electron micrograph of a juxtaglomerular granular cell. Note the prominent cytoplasmic membrane–bound granules (original magnification ×**19,000**; courtesy of Dr. Luciano Barajas). [Reprinted with permission (206).]

gial cells and the cells of the intraglomerular mesangium and glomerular arterioles (92,93). These morphologic features and the central position within the juxtaglomerular apparatus suggest that the extraglomerular mesangium may represent the structural–functional link between the MD and the glomerular arterioles and mesangium. The MD represents a plaque of specialized tubular cells within the cortical TAL of Henle adjacent to the hilus of the glomerulus. The cells are low columnar and may protrude into the tubular lumen (Fig. 28). By electron microscopy, they have apical nuclei, cellular organelles largely lateral to and beneath the nuclei, and basal cellular processes that interdigitate with the extraglomerular mesangial cells. The lateral intercellular spaces between the MD cells vary in width but usually are more dilated compared with the lateral intercellular spaces of other nephron segments (94). In contrast with contiguous portions of the TAL, there is evidence that the MD lacks epidermal

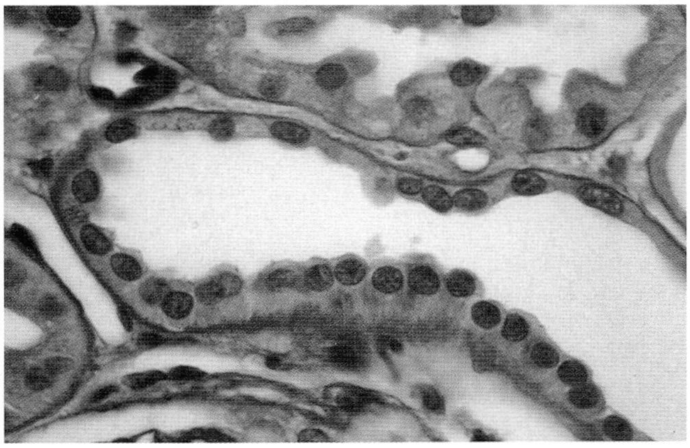

**FIG. 28.** MD characterized as a morphologically distinct plaque of low columnar cells with apically situated nuclei. PAS stain (original magnification ×**750**).

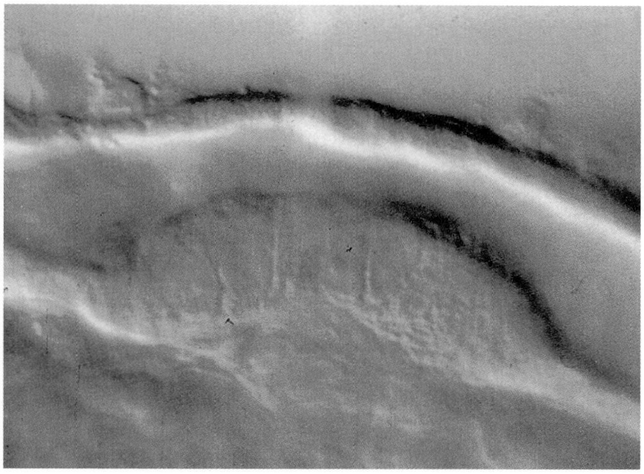

**FIG. 29.** Differential interference contrast image of an isolated TAL segment perfused in vitro. In response to a reduction in tubular luminal osmolality, there is dilatation of the lateral intercellular spaces in the MD, suggesting increased water flow (original magnification ×**1,250**) [Reprinted with permission (97).]

growth factor and Tamm-Horsfall protein but may be water permeable (Fig. 29) (95–97).

### Proximal Tubule

The proximal tubule is divided into an initial convoluted portion (PCT), the pars convoluta, and a straight portion (PST), the pars recta. The convoluted portion forms several coils around its parent glomerulus in the cortex and continues into the straight portion, which is located in the medullary ray. The human proximal tubule is approximately 14 mm in length (23). In histologic sections of the cortex, sectioned profiles of proximal convoluted tubules represent the major parenchymal component. The appearance of the cortex and especially the proximal tubules varies according to the method of fixation. A decrease in blood pressure results in decreased filtration and renal volume (98,99). After immersion fixation of excised pieces of renal tissue, the cortex has a more homogeneous compact appearance and there is collapse of the proximal tubular lumens (Fig. 30) (100). Free nuclei and vesicular membranous material may be observed in the proximal tubular lumens. Fixation of an experimental functioning kidney in situ by rapid freezing, dripping of fixative on the renal surface, or vascular perfusion results in more conspicuous intertubular interstitial spaces and widely open lumens of the proximal tubules. The cells of the proximal tubule are cuboidal to low columnar with eosinophilic, often granular cytoplasm and round nuclei situated in the center or near the base of the cells (Fig. 31). The lateral cell borders are indistinct because of extensive interdigitations of lateral cellular processes from adjacent cells (Fig. 32). In the basal part of the cells there are vertical striations that represent numerous elongated mitochondria. Cy-

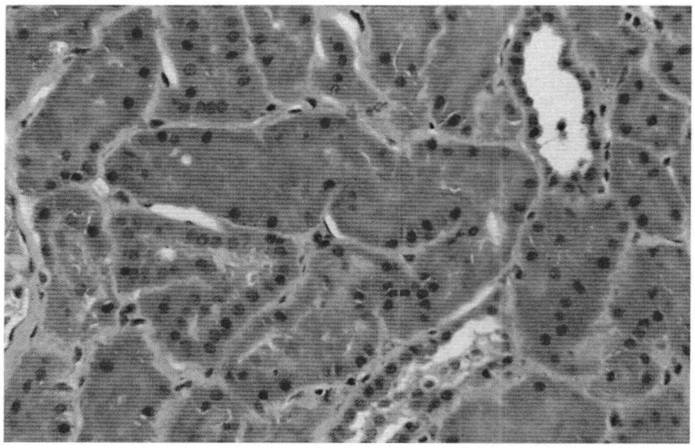

**FIG. 30.** Immersion fixed renal biopsy specimen demonstrating diffuse collapse of the proximal tubular lumens. Note the patent lumens of the distal nephron segments (original magnification ×**250**).

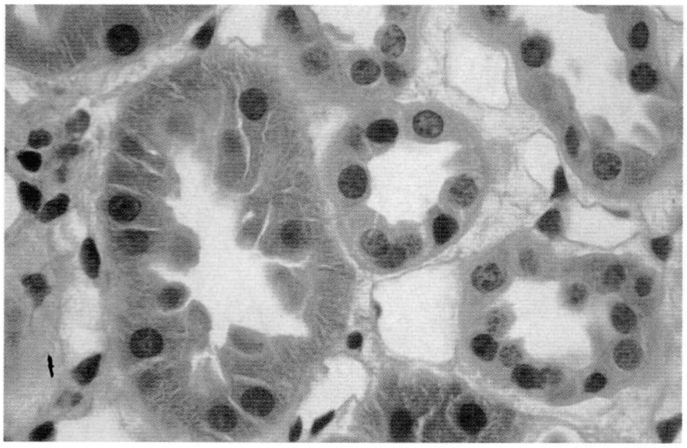

**FIG. 31.** Cross section of proximal tubule to the left of the center of the micrograph. The proximal tubular cells are taller and more eosinophilic than the cells of the distal nephron segments to the right (original magnification ×**750**).

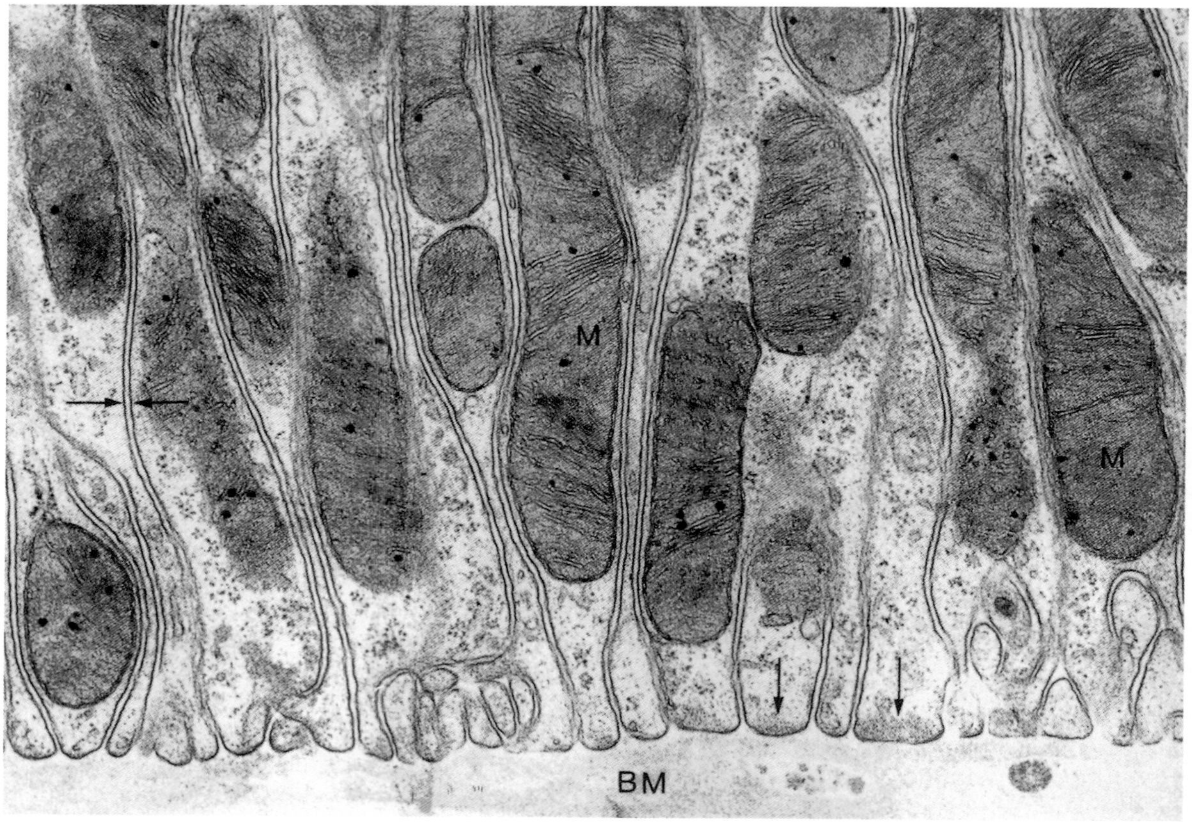


**FIG. 32.** Transmission electron micrograph illustrating extensive interdigitation of cellular processes in basal region of proximal tubular cells. The mitochondria (M) are elongated. The width of the extracellular space (*double arrows*) is constant, and there are bundles of cytoplasmic filaments (*single arrows*) adjacent to the basement membrane (BM) (original magnification ×**40,000**). [Reprinted with permission (104).]

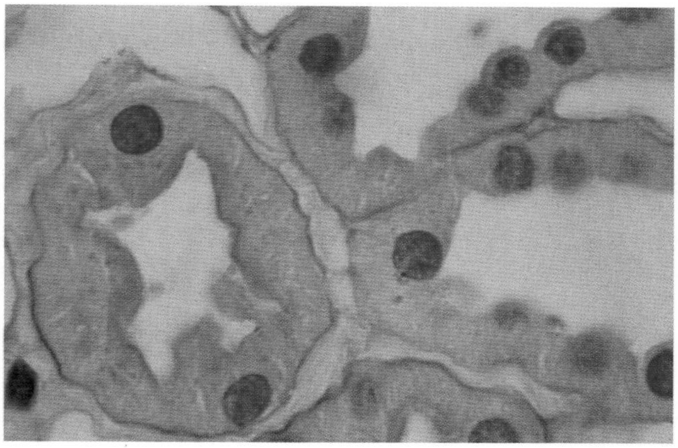

**FIG. 33.** PAS-stained cross section of proximal tubule to the left of the center of the micrograph. Note the prominent PAS-positive brush border (original magnification ×**1,250**).

toplasmic apical vacuoles and granules correspond to a well-developed endocytic–lysosomal apparatus. There is a prominent PAS-positive luminal brush border composed of the numerous densely packed long microvilli (Fig. 33). The brush border, apical cytoplasmic vacuoles, and basal striations are less prominent in the pars recta. Lectins have been used as selective probes to delineate renal tubular segments (101,102). Although a certain degree of nonspecificity has been reported, the lectin *Lotus tetragononolobus* has been used as a marker of proximal tubular epithelium (Fig. 34).

In most mammals, distinct segments of the tubule portion of the nephron can be distinguished by structural and functional differences. The structural differences have been characterized mainly on the ultrastructural level (103). However, these tubule segments often can be detected on light microscopy because of their known distribution within specific zones of the kidney (Fig. 5). In general, the degree of tubule segmentation has not been characterized in detail in the human kidney. In several mammals, the proximal tubule can be divided into three morphologically distinct segments (Fig. 35) (104). The $S_1$ segment originates at the glomerulus and constitutes one half to two thirds of the pars convoluta. The $S_2$ segment represents the remainder of the pars convoluta and the initial part of the pars recta. The $S_3$ corresponds to the remainder of the pars recta and is located in the inner cortex and outer stripe of the outer medulla. Although a pars convoluta and a pars recta have been described in the human kidney (105), the segmentation of the proximal tubule into three divisions has not been closely examined.

The cells in the $S_1$ segment have a tall brush border, a well-developed endocytic lysosomal apparatus, numerous

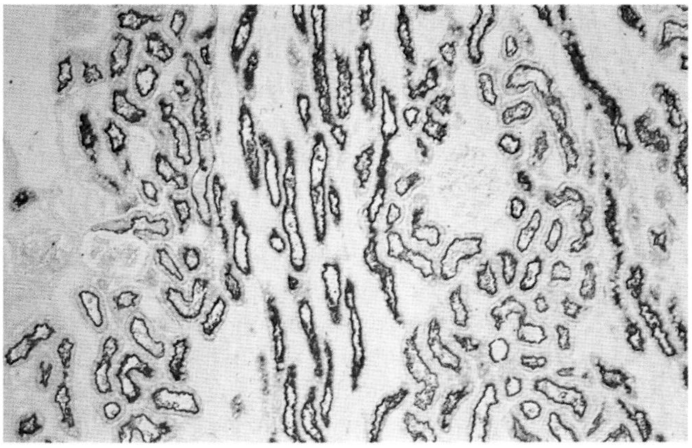

**FIG. 34.** Staining of the brush border of the proximal tubules with *Lotus tetragonolobus*. The distal nephron segments and glomeruli are negative. (Courtesy of Dr. Randolf A. Hennigar.)

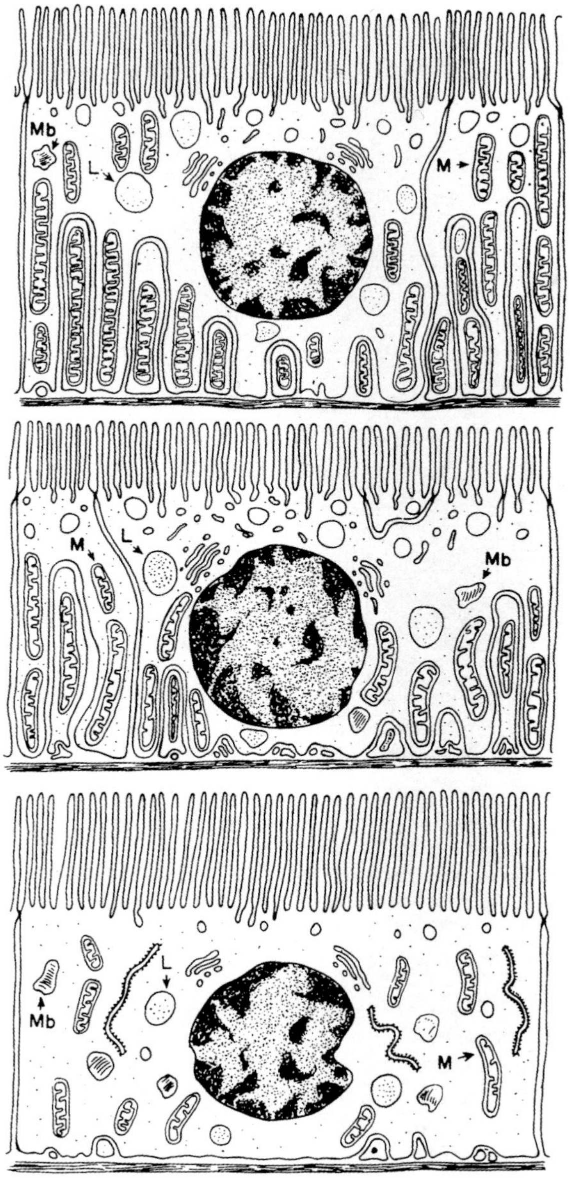


**FIG. 35.** Schematic diagram of the three segments of the proximal tubule: **upper**, $S_1$; **middle**, $S_2$; **lower**, $S_3$. Mb, microbody; M, mitochondrion; L, lysosome. [Reprinted with permission (104).]

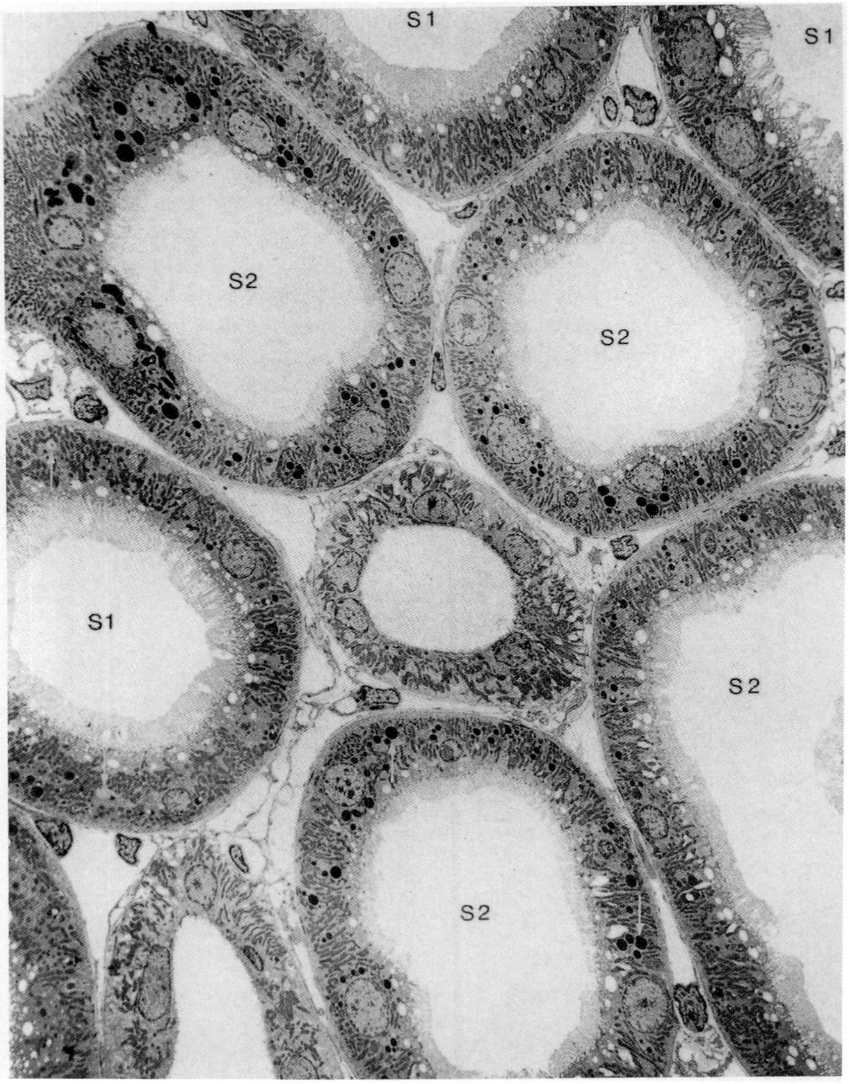


**FIG. 36.** Transmission electron micrograph of rat renal cortex. The cells in the $S_1$ segment are taller and have a more prominent brush border than the cells in the $S_2$ segment (original magnification ×**1,870**). [Reprinted with permission (104).]

elongate mitochondria, and extensive basolateral invaginations and interdigitations. The cells in the $S_2$ segment are similar to those in the $S_1$ segment; however, the brush border is shorter, and the endocytic organelles, mitochondria, and basolateral invaginations and interdigitations are less prominent (Fig. 36). The cells in the $S_3$ segment are more cuboidal and have relatively fewer endocytic organelles, small mitochondria, and inconspicuous membrane invaginations and interdigitations. The length of the brush border in the $S_3$ segment varies among species.

The proximal tubule is responsible for the reabsorption of about 60% of the glomerular ultrafiltrate. The reabsorption of chloride, bicarbonate, glucose, amino acids, and fluid is coupled to the active transport of sodium. An excellent correlation exists along the length of the proximal tubule between the elaborately developed basolateral membrane expressed as surface area (Fig. 37), the high $Na^+$,$K^+$ ATPase activities that are localized to the basolateral membrane, and the capacity to transport sodium and ions (106,107). The numerous mitochondria located in close proximity to the plasma membrane provide a source for the cellular energy required for active transport. In general, therefore, the intrinsic rates at which fluid and solutes are transported decrease along the proximal tubule from $S_1$ to $S_3$. The well-developed

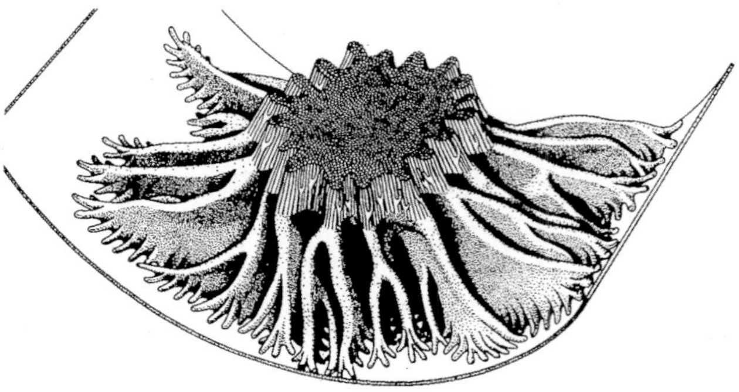

**FIG. 37.** Three-dimensional schematic diagram of the proximal convoluted tubule cell illustrating the complex basal and lateral processes that interdigitate with those from adjacent cells. [Reprinted with permission (207).]

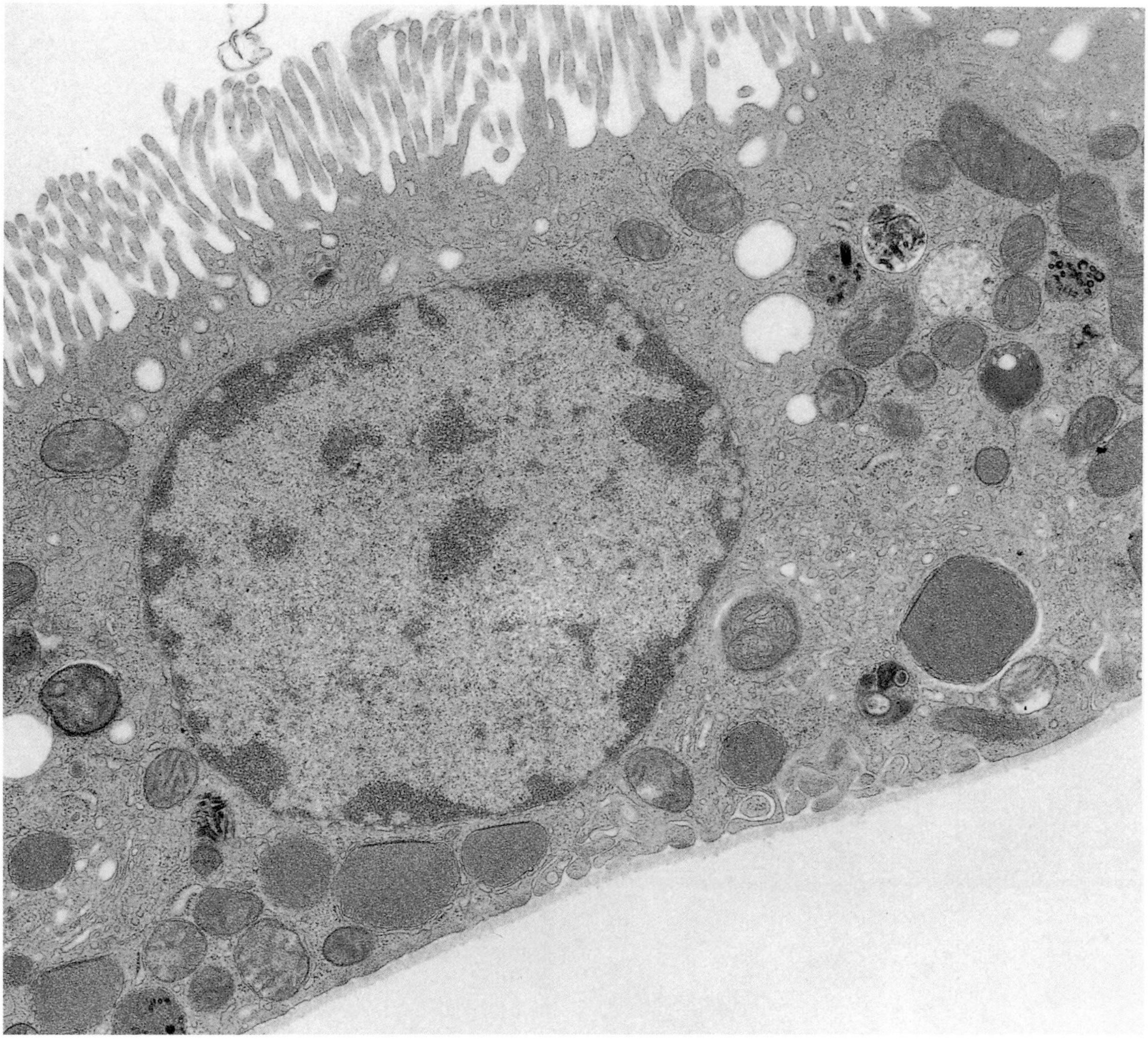

**FIG. 38.** Transmission electron micrograph illustrating an isolated perfused $S_2$ segment of the rabbit proximal tubule. Note the endocytic compartment consisting of coated pits and vesicles, apical tubules, small endocytic vesicles, and larger endocytic vacuoles. The lysosomes are heterogeneous and contain electron-dense material (original magnification ×**15,000**). [Reprinted with permission (208).]

endocytic–lysosomal apparatus in the proximal tubule (Fig. 38) plays an important role in reabsorption and degradation of albumin and low-molecular-weight proteins filtered by the glomerulus (108).

### Thin Limb of Henle's Loop

At the border between the outer and inner stripe of the outer medulla is an abrupt transition from the proximal tubule to the descending thin limb (DTL) of Henle's loop. Short-looped nephrons have only a short DTL located in the inner stripe of the outer medulla, whereas long-looped nephrons have both a long DTL and a long ascending thin limb (ATL). The long DTL traverses the inner stripe of the outer medulla and enters the inner medulla, whereas the long ATL resides entirely within the inner medulla. By light microscopy, the thin limb is lined with a flat, simple epithelium about 1 to 2 $\mu$m thick (Fig. 39). The lenticularly shaped nucleus bulges slightly into the lumen. Four types of epithelium have been described in the thin limb in several mammals (Fig. 40) (29,109). It is not known if four types exist in humans, but at least two different types of epithelium have been demonstrated (110). Type I is present in the DTL of short-looped nephrons. It is an extremely thin, simple epithelium with few cellular interdigitations and cell organelles. Type II epithelium lines the initial part of the DTL of long-looped nephrons located in the outer medulla. This epithelium exhibits species variation and is characterized by taller cells, short microvilli, and more prominent cell organelles than in the other epithelial types. In the rat and mouse the type II epithelium is complex and characterized

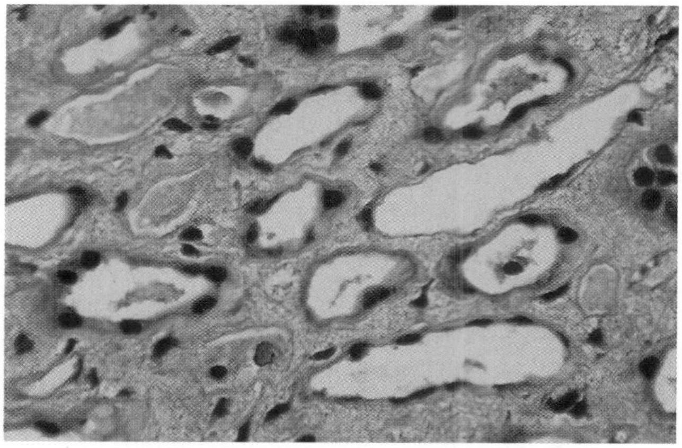

**FIG. 39.** Several thin limbs of Henle are depicted in the center of the light micrograph. The lining eithelium is extremely attenuated and the nuclei protrude into the lumens (original magnification ×**500**).

by extensive lateral interdigitations, whereas in the rabbit and human kidney the interdigitations are less prominent (29). Type III epithelium, found in the DTL of long-looped nephrons in the inner medulla, is composed of simple cells with few organelles and without lateral interdigitations. Type IV epithelium forms the bends of the long loops and lines the entire ATL in the inner medulla. It is characterized by low, flattened cells with few organelles and no microvilli, but abundant lateral interdigitations.

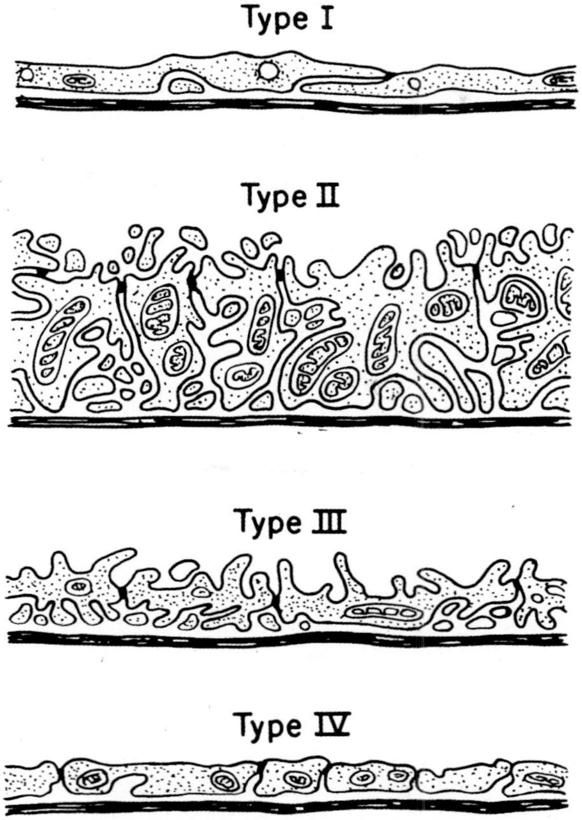


**FIG. 40.** The four types of epithelium in the thin limb of Henle's loop. [Reprinted with permission (203).]

The thin limb of Henle's loop plays an important role in the countercurrent multiplication component of urinary concentration. Physiologic studies have demonstrated that the DTL is permeable to water but has low permeability to sodium chloride, whereas the thin ascending limb is largely impermeable to water but has a high permeability to sodium chloride (29,111). In the passive model proposed by Kokko and Rector (112) and Stephenson (113), a hypertonic medullary interstitium concentrates sodium chloride in the DTL by extraction of water. The fluid that then enters the ATL has a higher sodium chloride concentration, resulting in passive salt absorption and dilution of the fluid of the ATL. Thus, the thin limb contributes to the maintenance of a hypertonic medullary interstitium and delivers a dilute fluid to more distal segments. The morphologic features of a simple epithelium with few organelles in the ATL are consistent with the lack of demonstrable active transport in this segment.

### Distal Tubule

The distal tubule consists of three distinct segments: the TAL of Henle's loop, the MD, and the distal convoluted tubule (DCT). At the border between the inner medulla and the inner stripe of the outer medulla is a transition from the thin limb to the TAL. The TAL can be divided into a medullary (MTAL) and a cortical segment (CTAL). The cells are eosinophilic and cuboidal, and the round nucleus tends to be located in the apical region and causes a bulge of the cell into the lumen (Fig. 41). Similar to the proximal tubule cells, the cells of the TAL have indistinct lateral cell borders because of elaborate basolateral membrane invaginations and interdigitations. They also have cytoplasmic

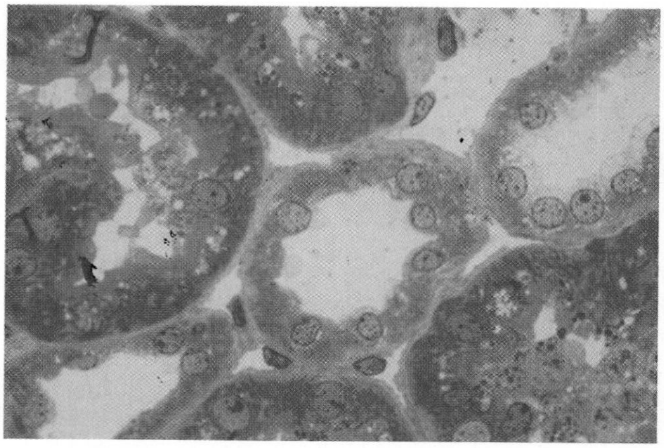

**FIG. 41.** Light micrograph demonstrating a cross section of a TAL in the center. There is no brush border and the cells are lower than adjacent proximal tubular cells. Toluidine blue–stained 1-$\mu$m Epon section (original magnification ×**750**).

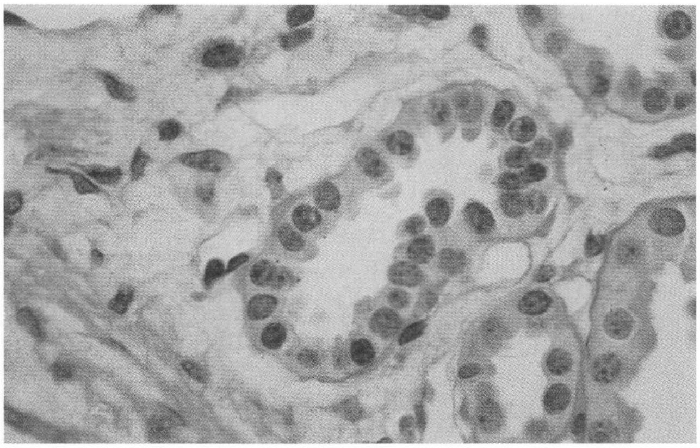

**FIG. 42.** Light micrograph showing a DCT. Note the absence of a brush border and the nuclei situated close to the lumen. PAS stain (original magnification ×**750**).

basal striations because of elongated mitochondria. These morphologic features are characteristic for epithelial cells involved in active transport. However, in contrast to the proximal tubule, the cells are lower and less eosinophilic and there is no brush border in the TAL. As the TAL ascends into the cortex, there is a gradual decrease in cell height, basolateral membrane area, and size of the mitochondria (114). Scanning electron microscopy has shown two luminal surface configurations of cells in the TAL (115). Cells with a relatively smooth surface are most commonly found in the medullary segment, whereas cells with a rough surface due to luminal microprojections and apical lateral membrane invaginations predominate in the cortical segment. The functional significance of these structural findings remains unexplained.

An important function of the TAL is the active reabsorption of sodium chloride. There is a correlation between structure and function in the ascending limb. The basolateral membrane surface area, the $Na^+$,$K^+$ ATPase activity, and the reabsorptive capacity for sodium chloride are all greater in the medullary segment than in the cortical segment of the TAL (106,114,116). This reabsorption of salt coupled with the water impermeability of the TAL results in a hypertonic interstitium and delivery of a hypotonic fluid to more distal tubular segments.

The DCT begins just beyond the MD in the cortex and represents the terminal part of the distal tubule. The cells of the DCT are similar to those of the TAL and contain numerous mitochondria; however, they are taller, characteristically have nuclei closer to the lumen, and lack lateral interdigitations in the apical region between adjacent cells (Fig. 42). In comparison with the proximal tubule, the cells of the DCT are lower and less eosinophilic, have a less prominent apical endocytic apparatus, and lack a brush border. More nuclei are observed in a cross section than in the proximal tubule, and the lumen is normally open. Morphologic and physiologic studies have provided evidence that the DCT, similar to the TAL, is relatively impermeable to water but responsible for the reabsorption of sodium chloride (117–119). In fact, biochemical studies have demonstrated that the DCT has a higher level of $Na^+$,$K^+$ ATPase activity than any other tubular segment (116).

### Connecting Tubule

The connecting tubule is a transitional segment that joins the DCT with the collecting duct system. In superficial nephrons, the connecting tubule (CS) continues directly into an initial collecting tubule (Fig. 43). In contrast, the connecting tubules of juxtamedullary nephrons join to form an arcade that ascends in the cortex before draining into an initial collecting tubule. Most nephrons empty individually into

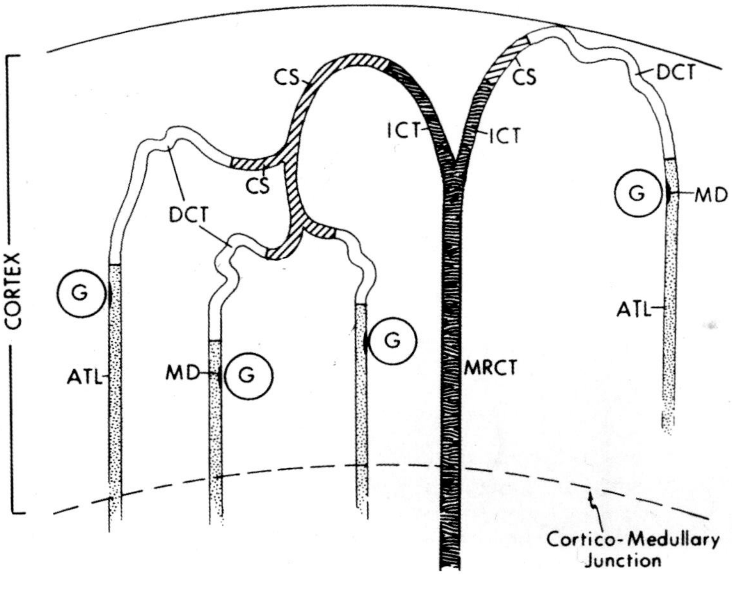


**FIG. 43.** The distal tubule in superficial and juxtamedullary nephrons and its various anatomic attachments by connecting segments (tubules) to a cortical collecting duct. G, glomerulus; ATL, ascending thick limb (of Henle); MD, macula densa; DCT, distal convuluted tubule; CS, connecting segment; ICT, initial collecting tubule; MRCT, medullary ray collecting tubule.

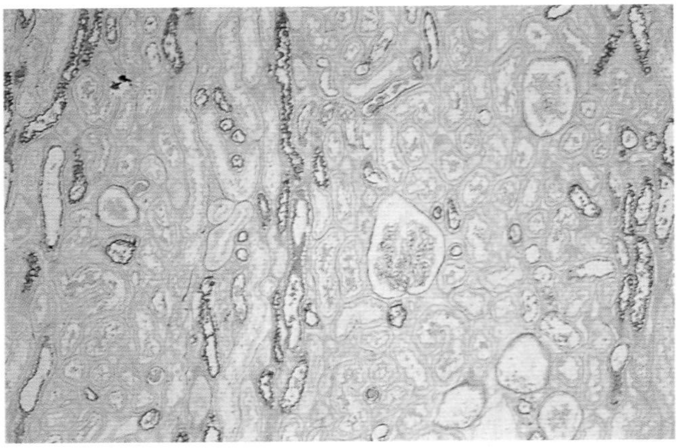

**FIG. 44.** Staining of the collecting ducts and TALs with *Arachis hypogaea*. The proximal tubules and glomeruli are negative. (Courtesy of Dr. Randolph A. Hennigar.)

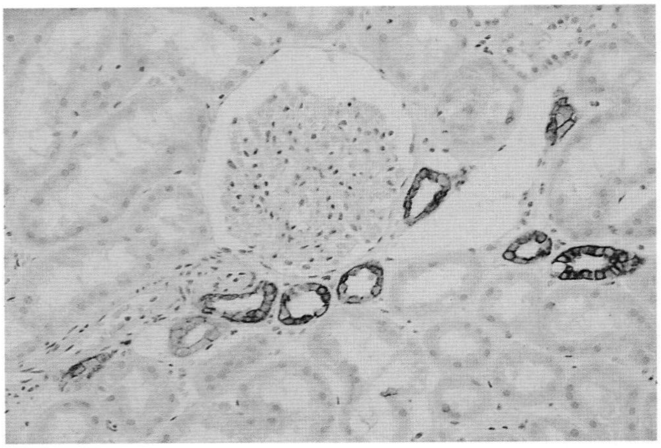

**FIG. 46.** Detection of keratin expression varies depending on the specificity and dilution of the antibody. In this micrograph there is prominent staining of the distal tubules and collecting ducts. 35$\beta$H11 immunoperoxidase (original magnification ×**62**).

initial collecting tubules (29). Fourteen percent of the nephrons are connected to arcades, and each arcade consists of about three nephron attachments (12). Each cortical collecting tubule receives an average of 11 nephrons (12). In most species (including humans) (120), the CS contains different cell types resulting from an intermixing of cells from the adjacent DCT and cortical collecting duct. The connecting tubule cell, intermediate in structure between the DCT cell and the principal cell of the collecting duct, is the most characteristic cell type of this transitional segment. The CS is an important site of potassium secretion (119).

### Collecting Duct

The collecting duct begins in the cortex and descends to the tip of the papilla, also called the area cribosa, where the inner medullary segments terminate as the ducts of Bellini. These terminal collecting duct segments were apparently described by Eustachio nearly 100 years before the observation of Bellini (121). During its course, there is an increase in diameter from the cortical portion to the terminal segments at the area cribosa. The collecting duct can be divided into the cortical, outer medullary (OMCD), and inner medullary collecting ducts (IMCD). Significant cellular heterogeneity exists along the collecting duct (28). Although there is a degree of nonspecificity, the lectins *Dolichos biflorus* and *Arachis hypogaea* have been used as markers for collecting duct epithelium (Fig. 44) (102). The distal tubules and collecting ducts show variable but generally more intense staining for keratins than the proximal tubules (Figs. 45 and 46).

The cortical collecting duct can be subdivided further into the initial collecting tubule and the medullary ray portion. By light microscopy, the epithelium of the cortical collecting duct consists of cuboidal cells with distinct lateral cell borders and central round nuclei (Fig. 47). The lumen is prominently open, and there is no brush border. The cortical collecting duct is composed of principal cells and intercalated

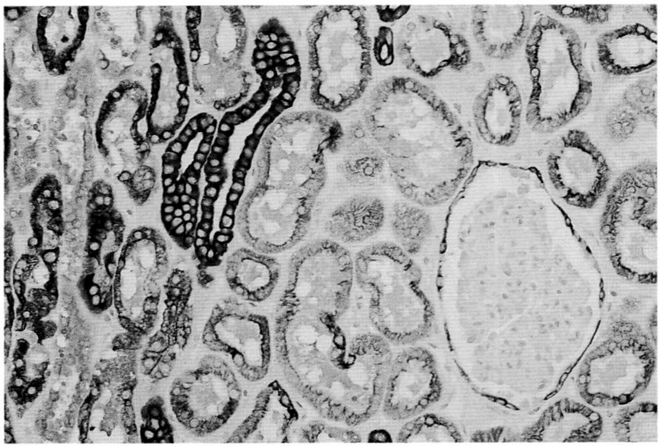

**FIG. 45.** Parietal epithelium lining Bowman's capsule, and distal tubules, collecting ducts, and proximal tubules showing expression of keratins. The distal tubules and collecting ducts label more intensely than the proximal tubules. CAM 5.2 immunoperoxidase (original magnification ×**62**).

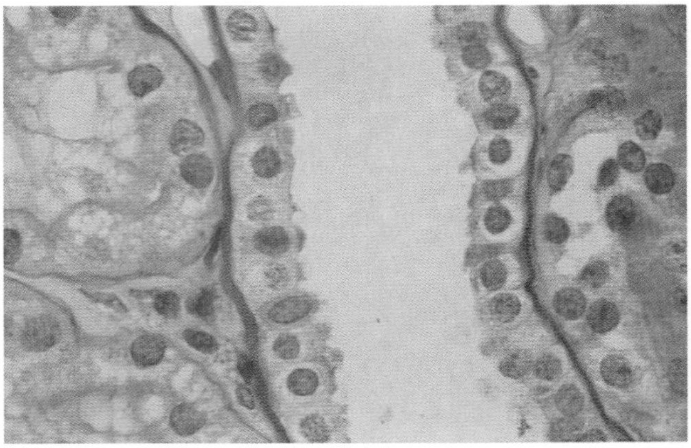

**FIG. 47.** Light micrograph illustrating a cortical collecting duct. Note the distinct lateral cell borders (original magnification ×**500**).

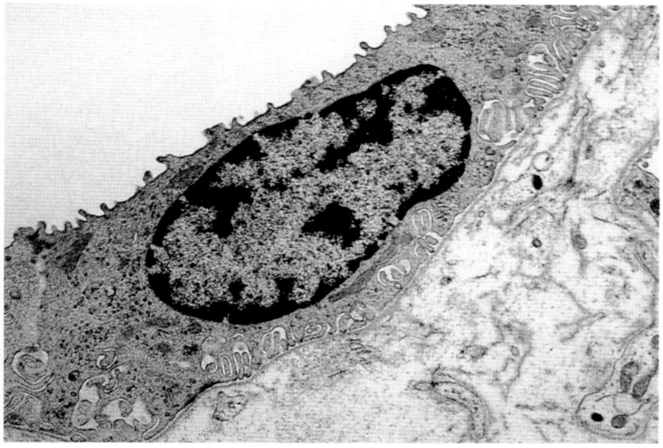

**FIG. 48.** Transmission electron micrograph of principal cell from the collecting duct. Note the relatively prominent infoldings of the basal plasma membrane (original magnification ×**12,500**).

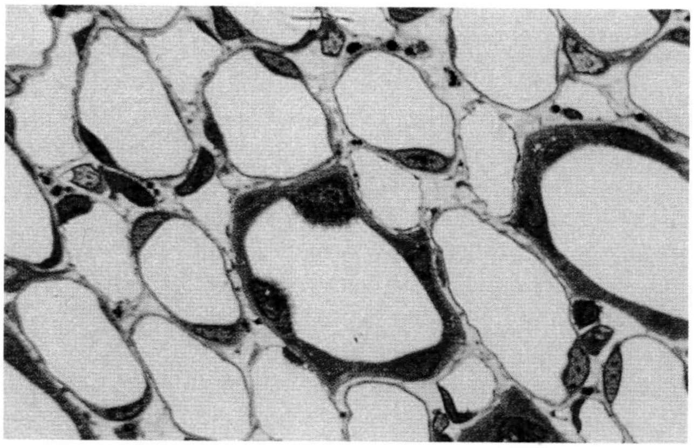

**FIG. 49.** Light micrograph of the medulla depicting intercalated cells in the collecting ducts. The intercalated cells exhibit a bulging apical surface covered with microprojections and dark-staining cytoplasm. One-micron toluidine blue–stained Epon section (original magnification ×**160**).

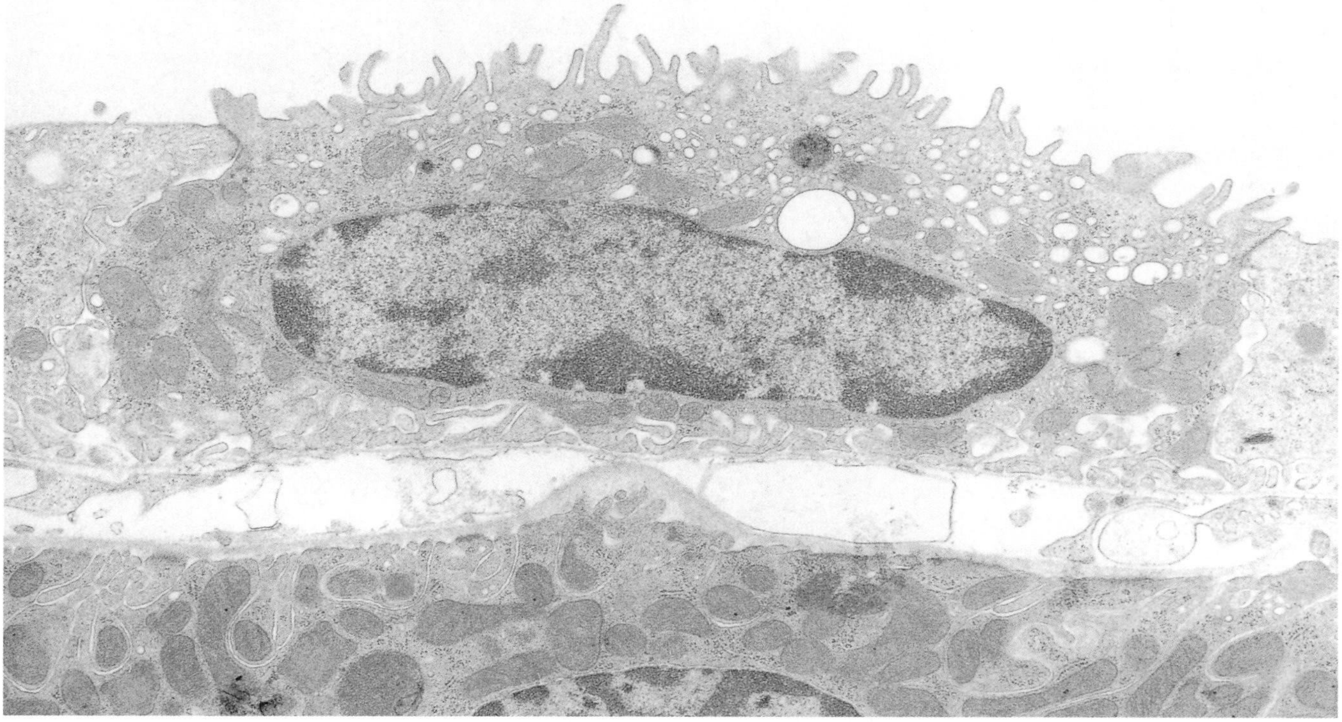

**FIG. 50.** Transmission electron micrograph of type A intercalated cell in the cortical collecting duct. Note the prominent tubulovesicular membrane compartment in the apical cytoplasm and the numerous microprojections on the luminal surface (original magnification ×**11,800**; courtesy of Dr. Jill W. Verlander).

cells. It is difficult to distinguish principal cells from intercalated cells on H&E paraffin sections. The principal cells on light microscopy have an extremely light or clear cytoplasm. By electron microscopy, the principal cells have relatively few cell organelles and no interdigitations of lateral cellular processes from adjacent cells, which accounts for the distinct cell borders observed on light microscopy (Fig. 48). However, there are prominent infoldings of the basal plasma membrane, which gives the basal region an accentuated clear appearance on light microscopy. The principal cell has a fairly smooth luminal surface with short microvilli and a single cilium by scanning electron microscopy (see Fig. 57). Experimental conditions of dietary potassium loading or mineralocorticoid stimulation have shown increases in potassium secretion and $Na^+,K^+$ ATPase activity in the cortical collecting duct along with an increase in the surface area of the basolateral membrane of the principal cells (122–126). These findings suggest that the principal cells are involved in potassium secretion in the cortical collecting duct.

The intercalated or "dark cells" are interspersed in the lining epithelia of the collecting duct. Intercalated cells represent 35% to 40% of the cells in the cortical collecting duct in some mammals (28,103). They are also present in the connecting segment. Intercalated cells are easily identified on 1-$\mu$m thick toluidine blue–stained Epon sections by their densely staining cytoplasm and their bulging convex luminal surface covered with numerous microprojections (Fig. 49). The darkly staining cytoplasm is due in part to the numerous mitochondria. Two distinct configurations of intercalated cells, types A and B, have been described in the cortical collecting duct of mammals (127,128). On ultrastructural examination, the type A intercalated cells have prominent microprojections of the apical membrane and extensive tubulovesicular structures in the apical cytoplasm (Fig. 50). In comparison with the type A cells, the type B intercalated

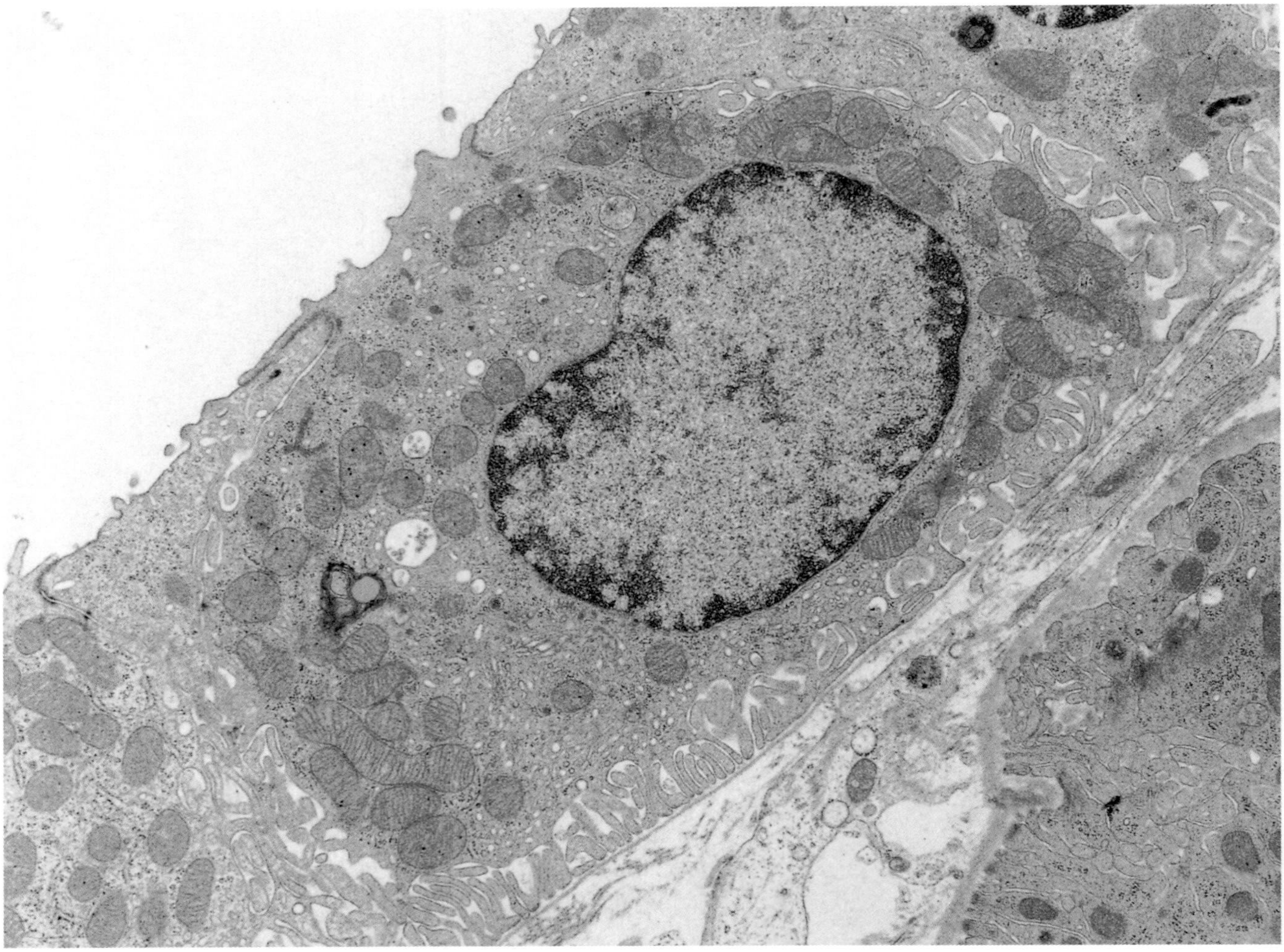

**FIG. 51.** Transmission electron micrograph of type B intercalated cell in the cortical collecting duct. There are numerous vesicles throughout the cytoplasm and the basolateral membrane is prominent. Note the paucity of microprojections on the luminal surface (original magnification ×**11,800**; courtesy of Dr. Jill W. Verlander).

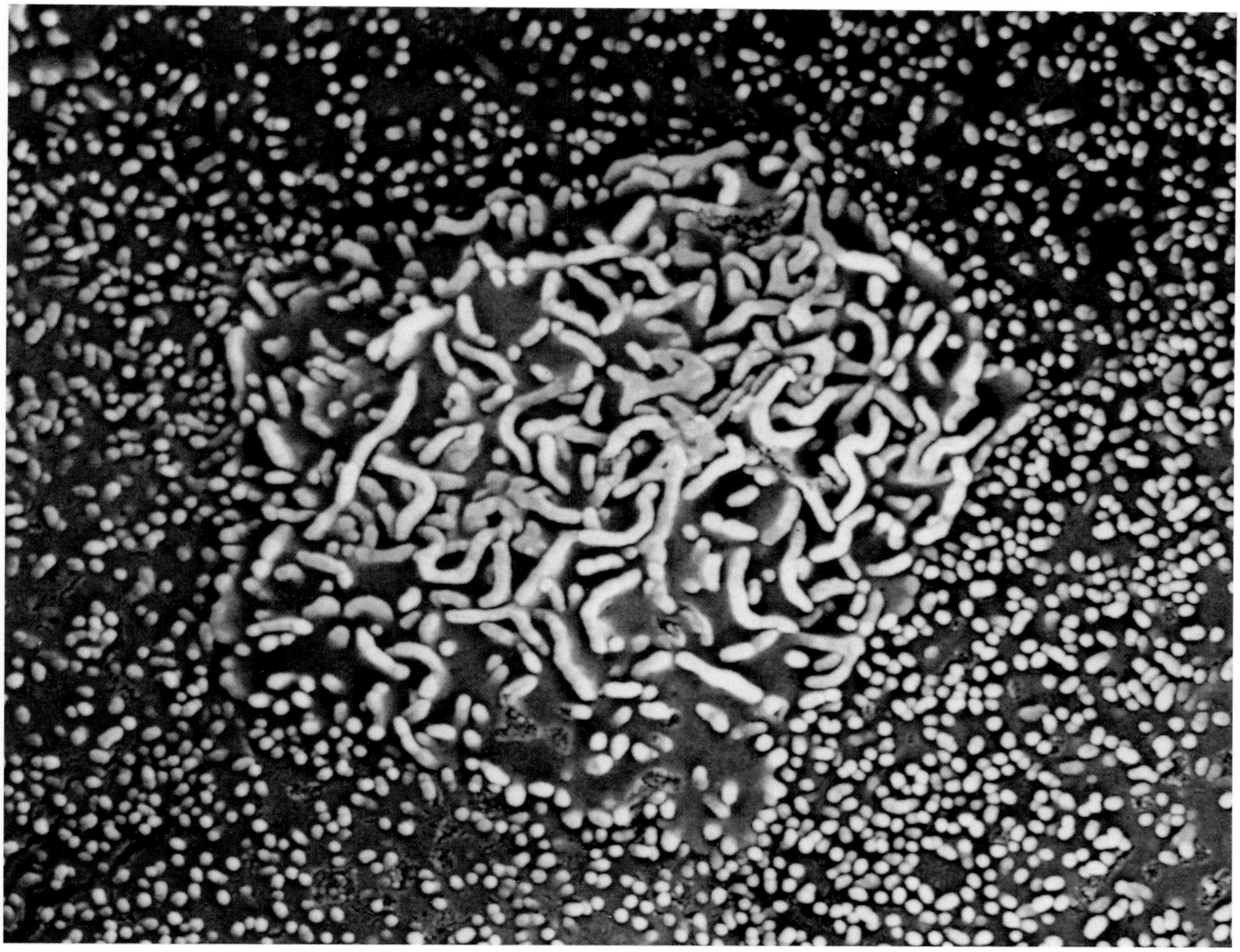

**FIG. 52.** Scanning electron micrograph of the luminal surface of a type A intercalated cell in the cortical collecting duct. The type A cell is well demarcated and has a large luminal surface covered primarily with microplicae but also microvilli (original magnification **×15,000**; courtesy of Dr. Jill W. Verlander).

cells have a denser cytoplasm, more mitochondria, a small number of microprojections on the apical surface, more spherical vesicular structures throughout the cytoplasm, and a larger basolateral membrane surface area (Fig. 51). By scanning electron microscopy, the type A cells have a large convex luminal surface covered with numerous complex microprojections called microplicae (Fig. 52), whereas the type B cells display a small angular luminal surface with small, relatively few microvilli (Fig. 53) (128). The type B intercalated cells may be inconspicuous on scanning electron microscopy.

Physiologic studies have demonstrated that the cortical collecting duct reabsorbs bicarbonate in acid-loaded animals (129) and secretes bicarbonate in alkali-loaded animals (130). The presence of high levels of carbonic anhydrase II, the enzyme that catalyzes the interconversion of $CO_2$ to $HCO_3$ in intercalated cells, suggests that these cells are involved in urine acidification (131). The type A intercalated cells have greater immunoreactivity for carbonic anhydrase II than the type B cells (132). In a study of experimental acute respiratory acidosis, there was a striking increase in the apical membrane surface area of the type A intercalated cells, whereas no morphologic changes were observed in the type B cells (128). Immunocytochemical studies have localized an $H^+$ ATPase in the apical membrane (133,134) and band 3, a chloride/bicarbonate exchanger in the basolateral membrane (135,136) of type A intercalated cells. These findings suggest that type A cells are responsible for hydrogen secretion in the cortical collecting duct. The immunolocalization of the $H^+$ ATPase to the basolateral membrane of type B cells (134,136) and the physiologic evidence for an apical chloride/bicarbonate exchange in these cells (137,138) suggest that B cells are involved in bicarbonate secretion. The type B intercalated cells are mainly localized to the collecting duct.

The collecting duct traverses the outer medulla without receiving tributaries. The outer medullary collecting duct is lined by principal cells and intercalated cells (Fig. 54). The

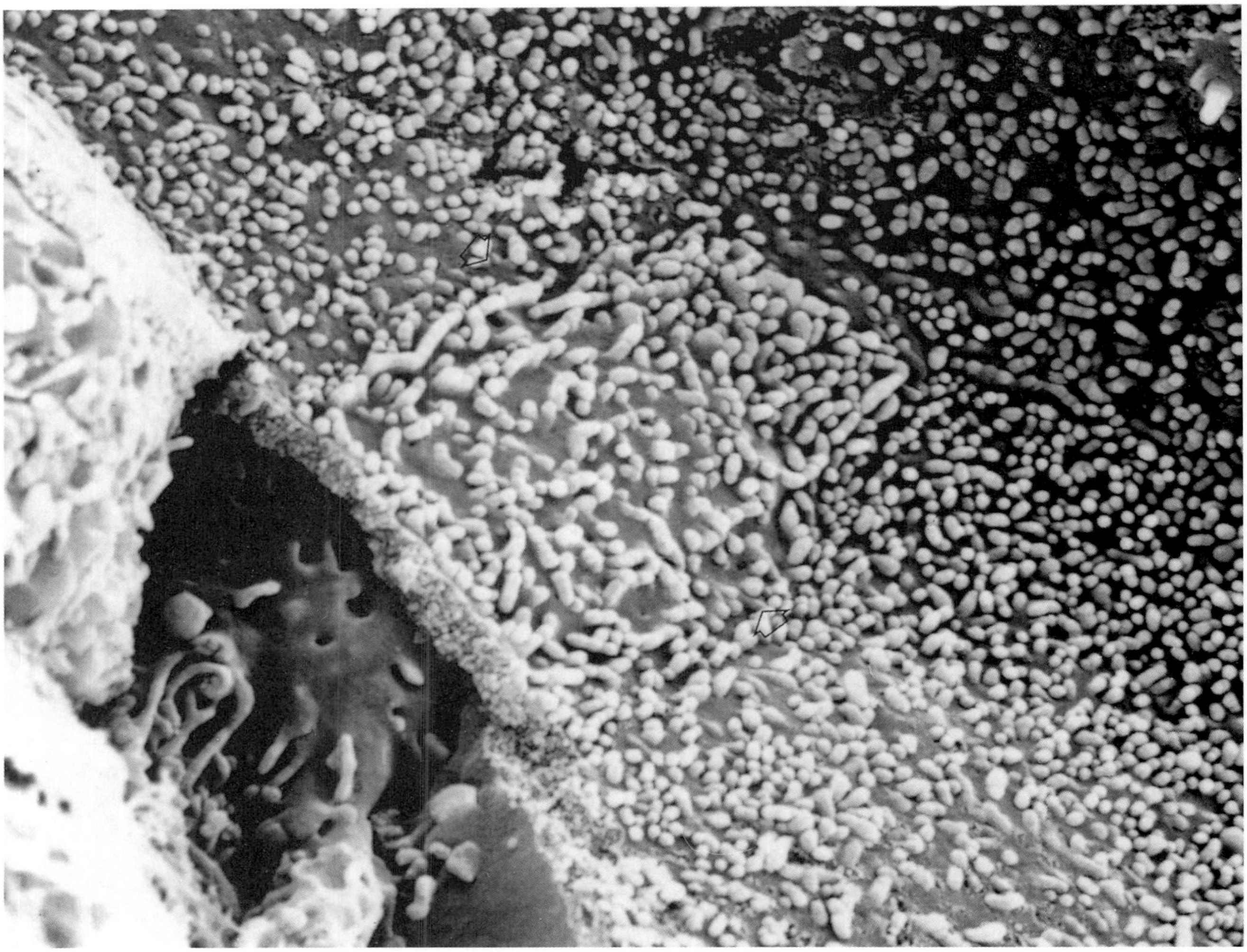

**FIG. 53.** Scanning electron micrograph of the luminal surface of a cortical collecting duct. A type B intercalated cell (*arrowheads*) displays a small angular luminal surface covered with short microprojections, mainly microvilli (original magnification ×**15,000**; courtesy of Dr. Jill W. Verlander).

principal cells in this segment are similar to those in the cortical collecting duct but are taller and have fewer organelles and basal membrane infoldings. The intercalated cells constitute 18% to 40% of the cells in the outer medullary collecting duct in some species and gradually decrease along this segment (139,140). The intercalated cells in the outer medullary collecting duct resemble the type A intercalated cells in the cortical collecting duct but are taller and have a less dense cytoplasm.

The outer medullary collecting duct plays a major role in urine acidification. An increase in the surface area of the apical plasma membrane of the intercalated cells in this segment has been demonstrated after hydrogen ion stimulation (141,142). The apical and basolateral membranes of these cells label with antibodies against the $H^+$ ATPase and the chloride/bicarbonate exchanger, respectively (133,135). These findings suggest that the intercalated cells in the outer medullary collecting duct are responsible for hydrogen ion secretion. In addition, this segment may be an important site of potassium reabsorption. The functional presence of $H^+,K^+$ ATPase activity in the outer medullary collecting duct (143,144) and the immunocytochemical localization of $H^+,K^+$ ATPase in the intercalated cells of this segment (145) indicate that these cells may be involved in potassium reabsorption in exchange for hydrogen ion secretion.

The IMCD represents the terminal portion of the collecting duct. Although the IMCD is often called the papillary collecting duct, only the inner two thirds of the IMCD are located in the papilla. Descending through the inner medulla, the collecting ducts join in successive fusions, which result in an arborescent architectural arrangement. There is a significant increase in diameter and height of the epithelium as the ducts descend (146). The height of the cells increases gradually from cuboidal to columnar (Fig. 55). However, in the terminal portion of the human inner medulla there is often an abrupt transition between collecting ducts lined with

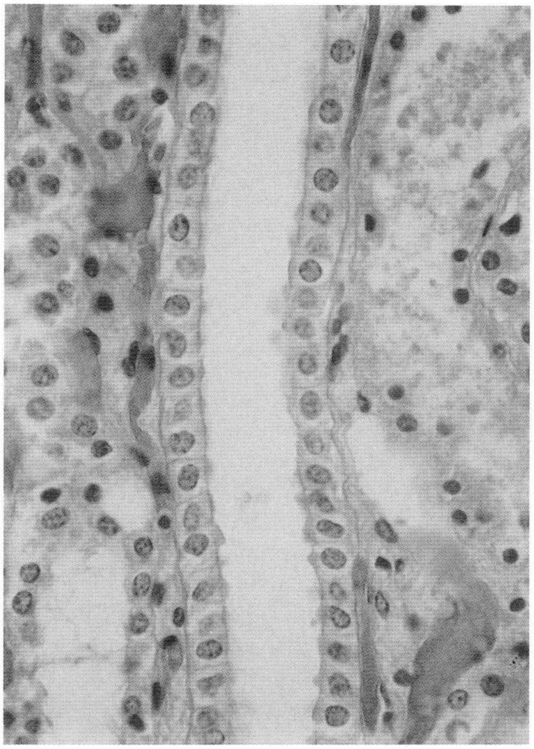

**FIG. 54.** Light micrograph illustrating longitudinal section of an outer medullary collecting duct (original magnification ×**250**).

cuboidal cells and the ducts of Bellini, which are composed of tall columnar cells (Fig. 56).

Structural and functional heterogeneity exists along the inner medullary collecting duct (146). It can be subdivided arbitrarily into three portions: the outer third ($IMCD_1$), middle third ($IMCD_2$), and inner third ($IMCD_3$). However, there is physiologic evidence for the division of the IMCD into two functionally distinct segments, which are termed the initial IMCD and the terminal IMCD (147,148). The initial IMCD is the outer segment and mainly corresponds to the $IMCD_1$, whereas the terminal IMCD includes most of the $IMCD_2$ and the $IMCD_3$. The initial IMCD consists mainly of principal cells that are similar in structure to the principal cells in the OMCD. In the rat, intercalated cells, similar to the type A intercalated cells in the OMCD, comprise approximately 10% of the cells in the initial IMCD (Fig. 57) (149). Intercalated cells are rare to absent in the initial IMCD of the human (120) and rabbit (139). The terminal IMCD is composed of mainly one cell type, the IMCD cell. Compared with principal cells, the IMCD cells are taller and have lighter staining cytoplasm containing numerous ribosomes, small lysosomes in the basal cytoplasm, and fewer infoldings of the basal plasma membrane (Fig. 58) (150). By scanning electron microscopy, the IMCD cells display more numerous small microvilli and lack the central cilium characteristic of principal cells (Fig. 59).

The inner medullary collecting duct has an important role in urinary concentration. The reabsorption of urea and water in this segment causes the formation of a concentrated urine. Physiologic studies demonstrated that urea and water per-

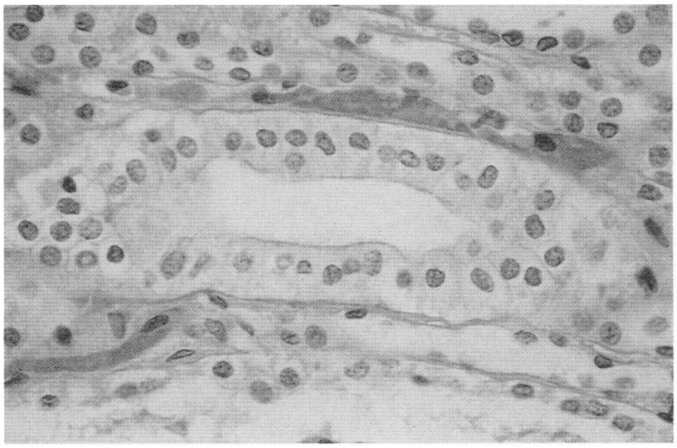

**FIG. 55.** Light micrograph illustrating columnar cells of the collecting duct in the inner medulla (original magnification ×**500**).

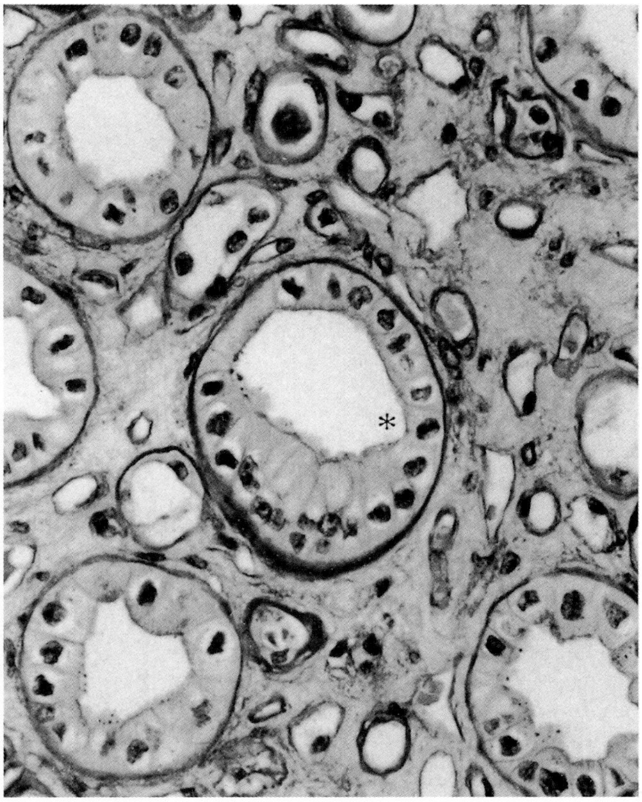

**FIG. 56.** Light micrograph of inner medulla demonstrating the inner medullary collecting ducts (IMCD). There is an abrupt transition (*) from the cuboidal epithelium of the IMCD to a duct of Bellini (original magnification ×**420**). [Reprinted with permission (146).]

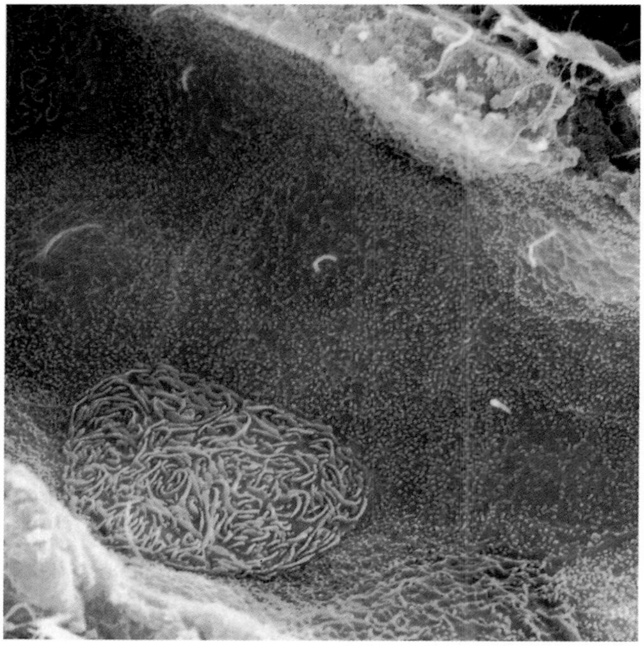

**FIG. 57.** Scanning electron micrograph of the rat $IMCD_1$. The intercalated cell is round and exhibits a convex luminal surface covered with prominent microplicae without cilia. The adjacent principal cells are characterized by short microvilli and a single central cilium on their luminal surface (original magnification ×**12,000**). [Reprinted with permission (150).]

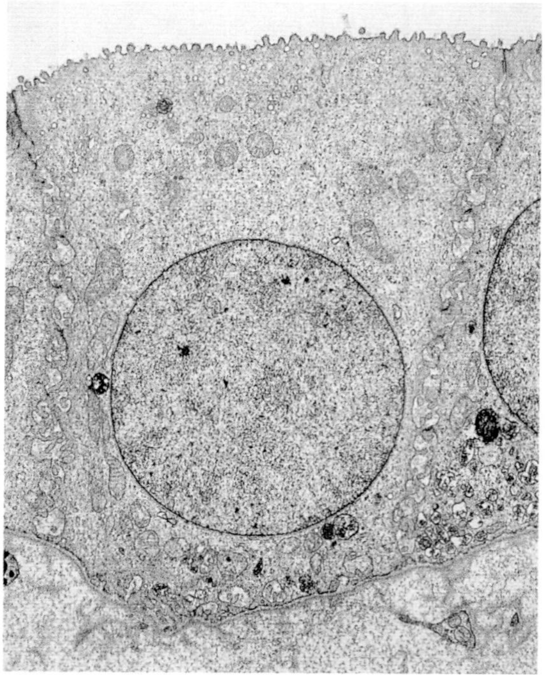

**FIG. 58.** Transmission electron micrograph of an IMCD cell. The cell is tall, has extensive lateral membrane, and exhibits small stubby apical microvilli. Infoldings of the basal plasma membrane are not prominent (original magnification ×**12,500**). [Reprinted with permission (150).]

meabilities are low in the initial IMCD and relatively high in the terminal IMCD (147,148). Vasopressin increases urea permeability only in the terminal IMCD, whereas water permeability is increased by vasopressin in both subsegments. There is evidence that the inner medullary collecting duct is also involved in urine acidification. Although the mechanism is not known, net acid secretion has been demonstrated in isolated perfused segments from this region (151).

### Interstitium

The renal interstitium consists of an extracellular matrix containing sulfated and nonsulfated glucosaminoglycans and interstitial cells (152). In humans, estimates of the relative cortical interstitial volume range from 5% to 20%, with a mean of 12% (24,153–155). A significant increase with age has been reported (155). The interstitial tissue in the normal cortex is inconspicuous on light microscopy, and the tubules and capillaries often have a back-to-back architectural appearance (Fig. 60). Types I and III collagen and fibronectin are present (156). Two types of cortical interstitial cells have been described: a fibroblast-like cell and a lymphocyte-like cell (152). Their function is unknown.

The relative volume of the renal interstitium increases

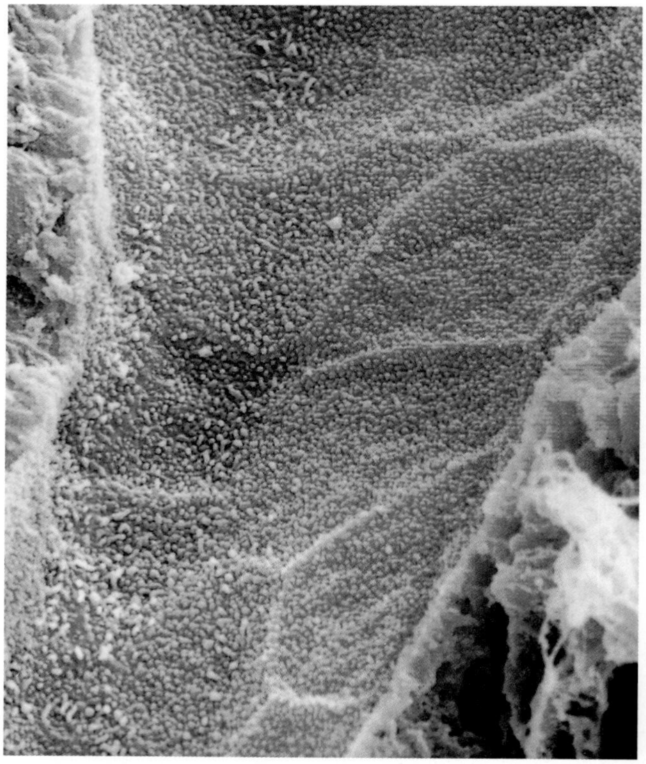

**FIG. 59.** Scanning electron micrograph of the terminal IMCD. The entire luminal surface of the IMCD cells is covered with abundant short microvilli. There is an absence of cilia (original magnification ×**12,500**). [Reprinted with permission (150).]

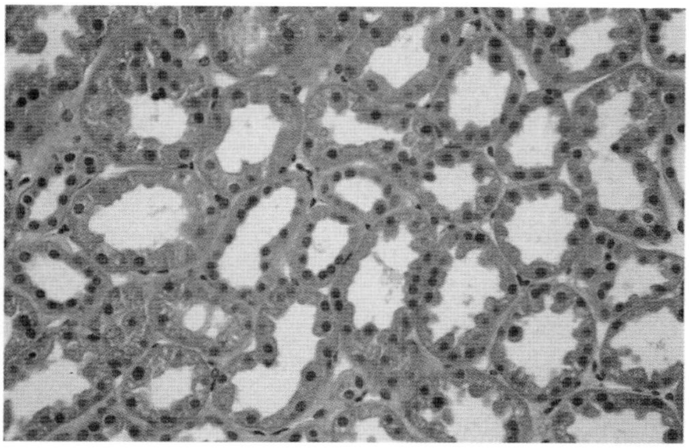

**FIG. 60.** Biopsy specimen of the cortex of a kidney donated for transplantation. Note the compact arrangement of the tubules and the limited amount of interstitial tissue (original magnification ×**250**).

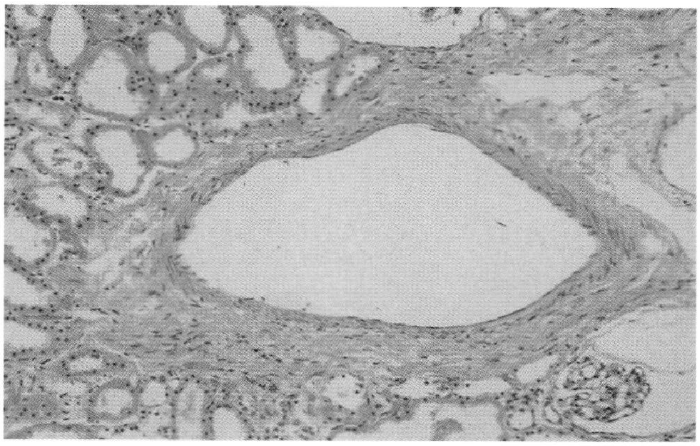

**FIG. 62.** Light micrograph of the corticomedullary junction illustrating an arcuate artery (original magnification ×**125**).

from the cortex to the tip of the papilla. The interstitial volume has been reported from 10% to 20% in the outer medulla to approximately 30% to 40% at the papillary tip in some species (157). The medullary interstitium has a gelatinous appearance on light microscopy (Fig. 61). The interstitial cells in the medulla include lymphocyte-like cells virtually identical to the ones in the cortex, pericytes situated near the descending vasa recta, and prominent lipid-containing cells mainly localized to the inner medulla (152). The latter, the renomedullary interstitial cells, are often arranged in rows between the loop of Henle and the vasa recta, have irregular, long cytoplasmic processes, and contain lipid inclusions. These cells can be observed on 1-$\mu$m thick toluidine blue–stained sections of the inner medulla. The lipid droplets contain mainly triglycerides that are rich in unsaturated fatty acids, including arachidonic acid, phospholipids, and cholesterol (152). In addition to the synthesis of the extracellular matrix of the interstitium, the renomedullary interstitial cells are believed to contribute to the endocrine-like antihypertensive function of the renal medulla (158).

### Vasculature

A detailed description of the renal vasculature is available (159). The segmental arteries, originating from the anterior and posterior divisions of the main renal artery, divide to form the interlobar arteries, which course toward the cortex along the septa of Bertin between adjacent renal pyramids. At the corticomedullary junction, the interlobar arteries give rise to the arcuate arteries, which follow a gently curved course along the base of the pyramids parallel to the kidney surface (Fig. 62). The interlobular arteries branch sharply from the arcuate arteries and ascend in the cortex in a radial fashion toward the renal surface. Because the renal lobules cannot be clearly distinguished, it has been recommended that the interlobular arteries be called cortical radial arteries (34,159). Most afferent arterioles originate from the inter-

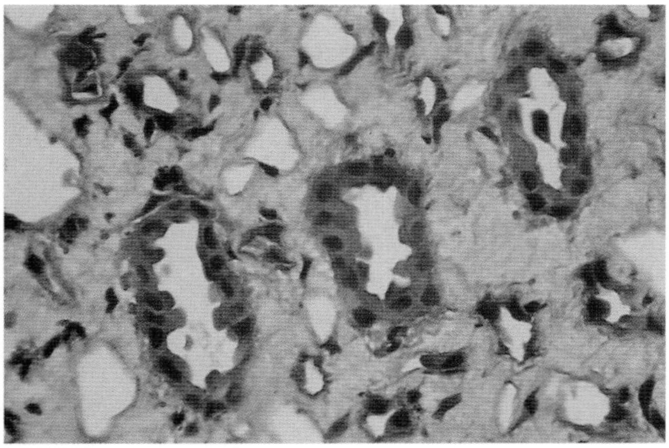

**FIG. 61.** Renal biopsy specimen illustrating the inner medulla. Note the prominent amount of interstitium surrounding the tubules (original magnification ×**500**).

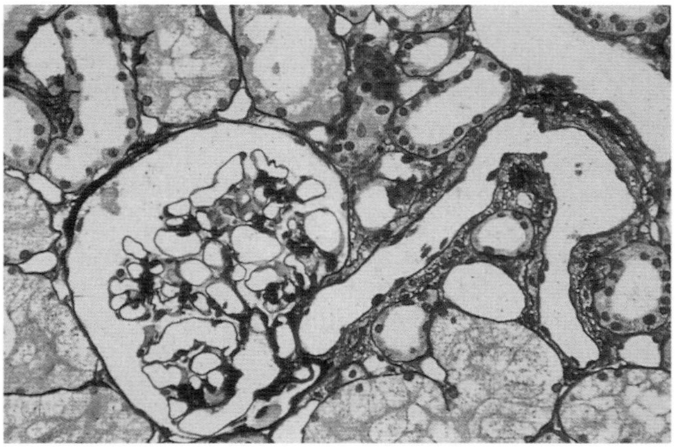

**FIG. 63.** Juxtamedullary glomerulus with a connected hilar arteriole. Note the recurrent angle of the arteriole. Silver methenamine stain (original magnification ×**250**).

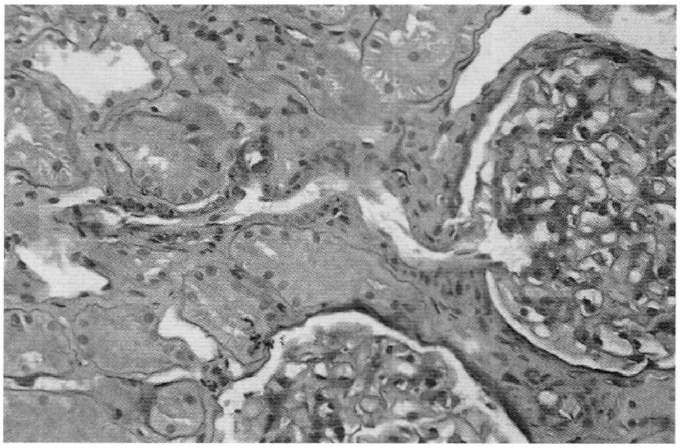

**FIG. 64.** Light micrograph depicting the transverse course of an afferent arteriole supplying a glomerulus. PAS stain (original magnification ×**250**).

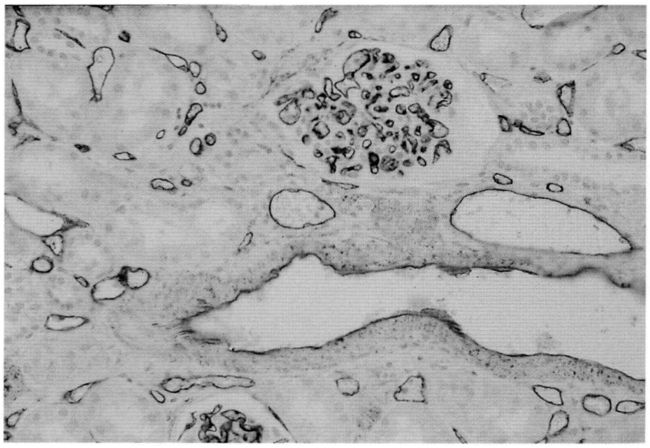

**FIG. 66.** CD34 immunoperoxidase staining demonstrates a greater variety of vascular structures that also label more intensely than with Factor VIII. In this micrograph, arteries, veins, glomeruli, and peritubular capillaries are labeled (original magnification ×**62**).

lobular arteries, and each supplies a single glomerulus. The angle of origin of the afferent arterioles becomes less recurrent and more open as the interlobular arteries extend to the outer cortex (Fig. 63) (160). The length of the afferent arterioles is variable; average values of 170 $\mu$m to 280 $\mu$m have been reported (Fig. 64) (161,162). Some rare branches of the intrarenal arteries that do not terminate in glomeruli, the so-called aglomerular vessels, may result from degeneration of the connected glomeruli (160). Aglomerular arterioles near the corticomedullary junction have been observed to enter the medulla, and shunt arterioles between afferent and efferent arterioles have been reported (163–165). The wall structure of the intrarenal arteries and the proximal portion of the afferent arterioles resembles that of blood vessels of the same size elsewhere in the body. The endothelium stains for Factor VIII–related antigen (Fig. 65) (166,167) and CD34 (Fig. 66) (168,169), whereas the muscularis stains for smooth muscle actin (Fig. 67) (170) and vimentin.

The efferent arterioles from the glomeruli branch to form a complex postglomerular microcirculation (Fig. 68). Although gradations exist, three basic types of efferent arterioles may be distinguished (171,172). The superficial or outer cortical efferent arterioles are fairly long and divide into extensive capillary networks that supply the convoluted tubules of the cortical labyrinth. These capillaries are readily identified by CD34 and smooth muscle actin staining (Figs. 67, 69 and 70). The midcortical efferent arterioles are variable in length and supply the cortical labyrinth as well as the straight tubules of the medullary rays. With the exception of the outer cortex, there is dissociation between the tubule seg-

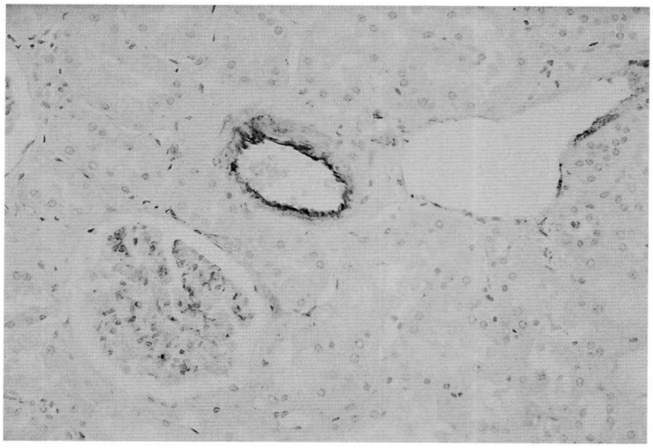

**FIG. 65.** Factor VIII is produced by endothelium. This micrograph shows Factor VIII immunoperoxidase staining of a medium-sized artery (*center*), vein (*right*), and glomerulus (*left*) (original magnification ×**62**).

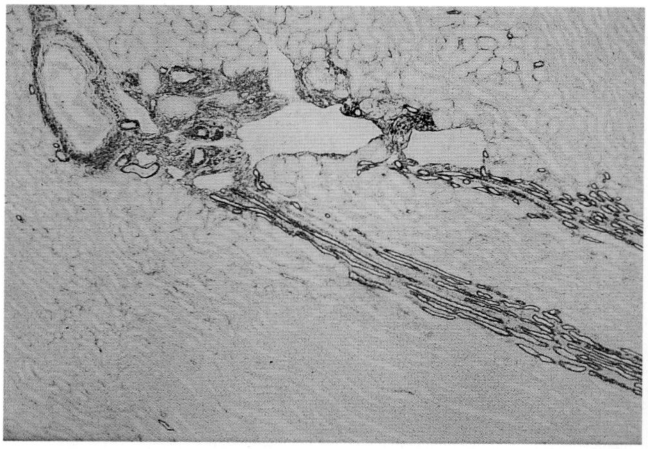

**FIG. 67.** Smooth muscle actin immunoperoxidase stain illustrating a labeled large artery (*left upper*) and arterioles at the corticomedullary junction and two positive-stained columns of vasa recta penetrating the medulla. Two venous profiles (*upper center*) have minimal muscularis (original magnification ×**11**).

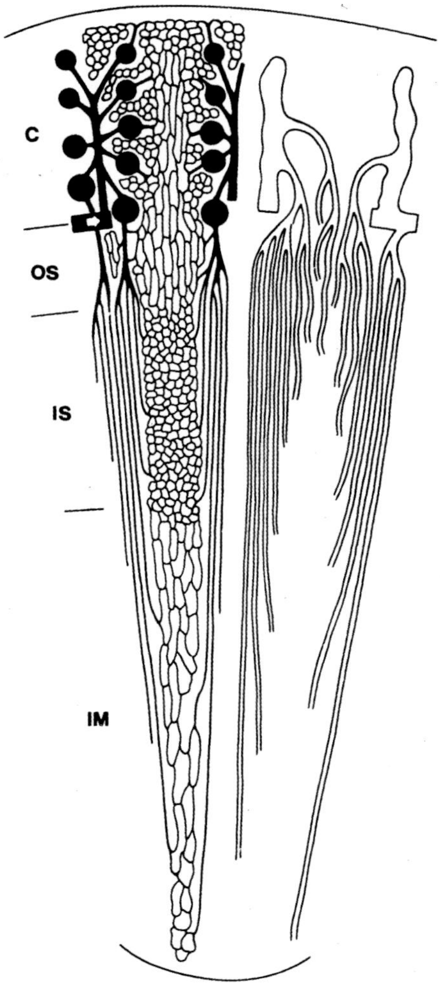


FIG. 68. The renal microvasculature. The left side illustrates the arterial vessels, glomeruli, and capillaries. An interlobular artery originates from an arcuate artery (*arrow*) and gives rise to the afferent arterioles, which supply the glomeruli. The efferent arterioles of the superficial and midcortical glomeruli supply the capillary plexuses of the cortical labyrinth and the medullary rays. The efferent arterioles of the juxtamedullary nephrons descend into the medulla and form the descending vasa recta, which supply the adjacent capillary plexuses. Note the prominence of the capillary plexus in the inner stripe. The right side, which may be superimposed on the left side, displays the venous system. The ascending vasa recta drain the medulla and empty into the arcuate and interlobular veins, which drain the cortex. The vasa recta from the inner medulla ascend within the vascular bundles, whereas most vasa recta from the inner stripe ascend between the bundels. C, cortex; OS, outer stripe; IS, inner stripe; IM, inner medulla. [Reprinted with permission (31).]

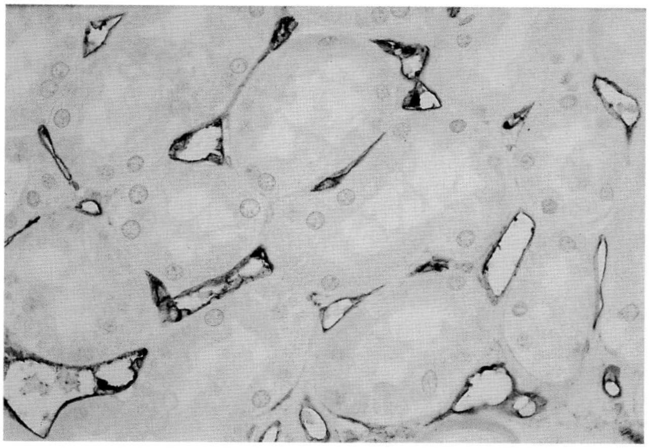

**FIG. 69.** The extensive cortical peritubular capillary network is shown by endothelial labeling with CD34 antibody. CD34 immunoperoxidase (original magnification ×**120**).

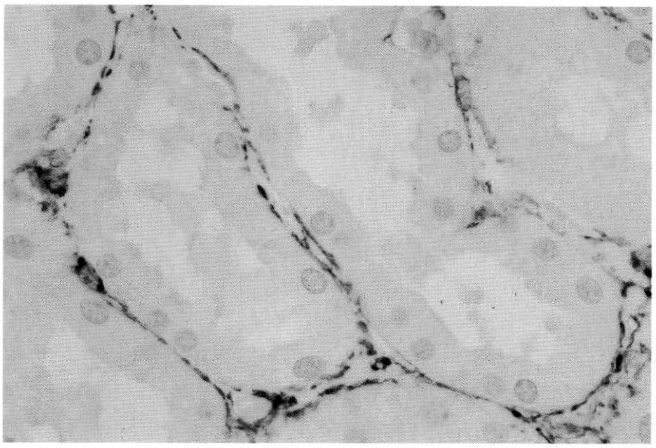

**FIG. 70.** Smooth muscle actin expression complements and parallels the CD34 expression in documenting the cortical peritubular capillaries. Smooth muscle actin immunoperoxidase (original magnification ×**120**).

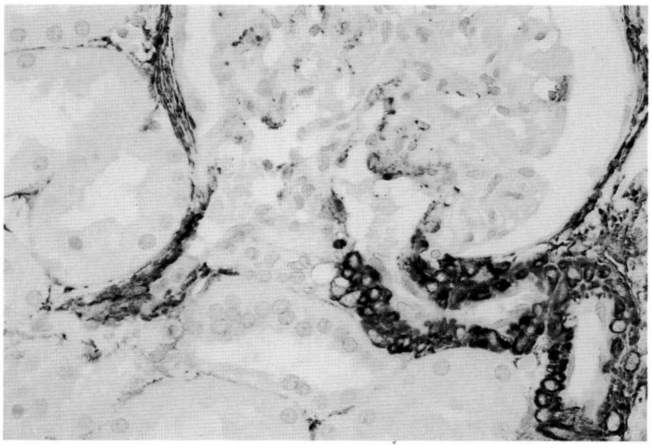

**FIG. 71.** Smooth muscle actin immunoperoxidase stain of a superficial glomerulus delineating the more prominent smooth muscle investment of the afferent arteriole (*right*) compared with the efferent arteriole (*left*) (Original magnification ×**120**).

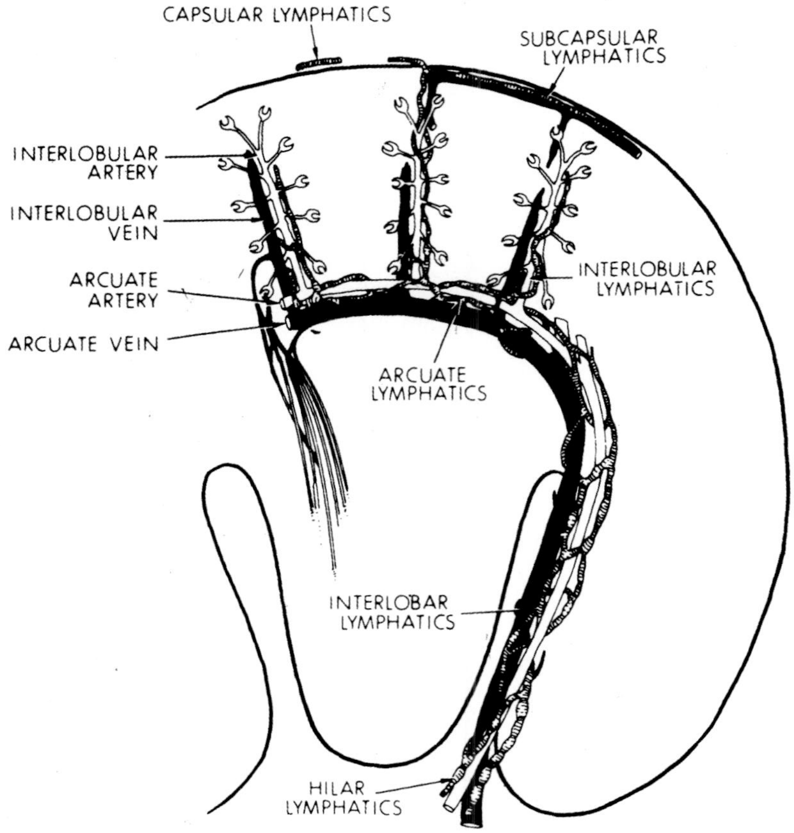


**FIG. 72.** The lymphatic vessels of the kidney. The arteries are indicated in *white*, the veins in *black*, and the lymphatics are *hatchmarked*. The lymphatics are primarily distributed in the cortex, although a subcapsular network is also present. Note the absence of lymphatics in the medulla. [Reprinted with permission (203).]

ments and the efferent arterioles of their parent glomeruli. In the midcortex and inner cortex, tubule segments are supplied by capillaries of efferent arterioles from other glomeruli (173,174). The efferent arterioles from juxtamedullary nephrons descend and supply the entire medulla. In contrast to the efferent arterioles of superficial and midcortical glomeruli (Fig. 71), those from juxtamedullary glomeruli are larger in diameter, display more layers of smooth muscle cells, and have more endothelial cells on cross sections (31,159). In the outer stripe of the outer medulla, the efferent arterioles of juxtamedullary nephrons divide to form the descending vasa recta that descend in the vascular bundles but at intervals leave the bundles to form capillary plexuses.

The ascending (or venous) vasa recta drain the renal

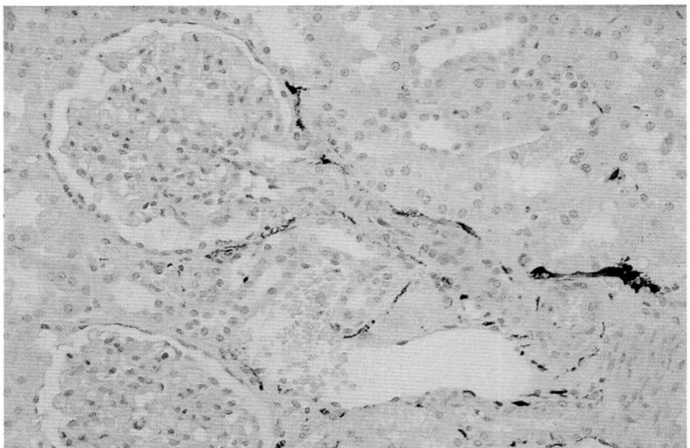

**FIG. 73.** S-100 immunoperoxidase stain demonstrating nerves extending along the afferent arteriole to the vascular pole of the glomerulus (original magnification ×**62**).

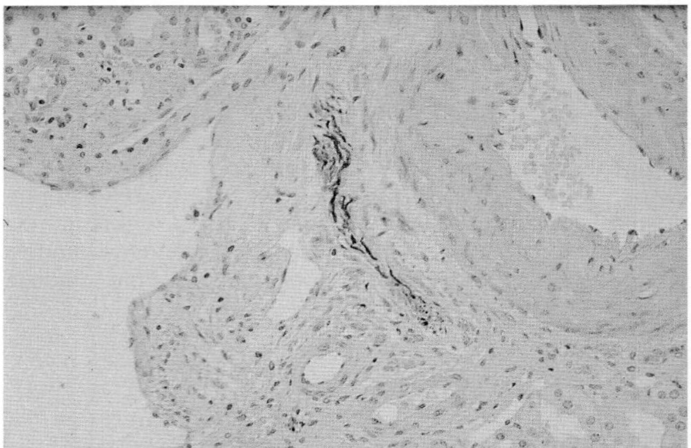

**FIG. 74.** Phosphoneurofilament (pNF) immunoperoxidase stain showing a nerve between an artery (*right*) and a vein (*left*) (original magnification ×**62**).

medulla. The ascending vasa recta from the inner medulla join the vascular bundles, whereas most from the inner stripe of the outer medulla ascend between the bundles (159). This architectural arrangement creates a functional separation of the blood flow to the outer and inner medulla. The close proximity of the arterial descending and venous ascending vasa recta within the vascular bundles allows for effective countercurrent exchange (31,159). The ascending vasa recta at the corticomedullary junction empty into the arcuate and interlobular veins (Fig. 67), which do form extensive anastomoses in contrast to the arcuate arteries. The interlobular veins, which accompany the interlobular arteries, drain the cortex and empty into the arcuate veins. In sections the intrarenal veins have less musculature than comparably sized veins in other organs (Fig. 67). The arcuate veins empty into the interlobar veins, which converge to form a single renal vein that exits at the hilus of the kidney.

## Lymphatics

The lymphatic vessels of the kidney are embedded in the loose periarterial connective tissue in the cortex (Fig. 72) (175–177). They are not prominent on routine histologic sections. The lymphatics originate as small vessels around the interlobular arteries and empty into arcuate and interlobar lymphatics, which finally drain into larger lymph vessels at the renal hilus. The interlobar and hilar lymphatics possess valves. Lymphatics are not believed to exist in the renal medulla (159,177). There is a less prominent subcapsular network of lymphatic vessels that appears to communicate with the major intrarenal lymphatics within the cortex (177). It has been proposed that the periarterial spaces and the lymphatics may function as a unit to allow exchange with the venous system and serve as a route for the intrarenal distribution of hormones and inflammatory cells (178).

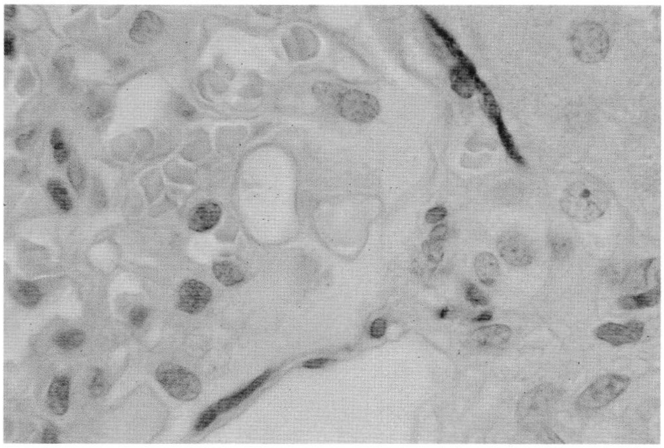

**FIG. 75.** Two axons are demonstrated in this view of the vascular pole of a glomerulus (*center*). One axon has a longitudinal profile (*upper right*), and the other is observed in cross-section as a dot approximately 24 μm (five nuclear diameters) below the first axon. pNF immunoperoxidase (original magnification ×**300**).

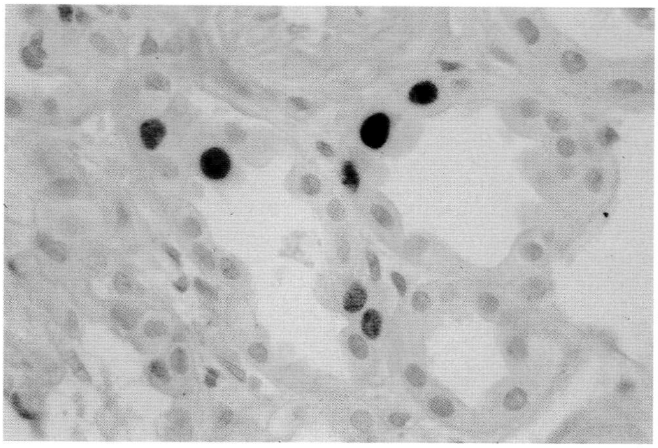

**FIG. 76.** Biopsy of kidney allograft with cyclosporine A toxicity. Normally there is sparse labeling for Ki-67, a nuclear protein expressed by proliferating cells. In this example, there is a prominent increase in labeling of tubular nuclei. Ki-67 immunoperoxidase (original magnification ×**210**).

## Nerves

The kidney is innervated by adrenergic fibers mainly derived from the celiac plexus (179). The nerve fibers generally accompany the arteries and arterioles in the cortex and outer medulla (180). Staining for myelin by S-100 (Fig. 73) or for peripheral axons with antibodies against phosphoneurofilament (pNF) (Fig. 74) demonstrates the nerve fibers (181–184). There is prominent innervation of the juxtaglomerular apparatus (Fig. 75) (185). The efferent arterioles and the descending vasa recta are accompanied by nerve fibers as long as they contain a surrounding smooth muscle layer (186). Although the direct relationship of nerve terminals to tubules is somewhat controversial, autoradiographic studies have provided evidence for monoaminergic innervation of cortical tubules (187,188).

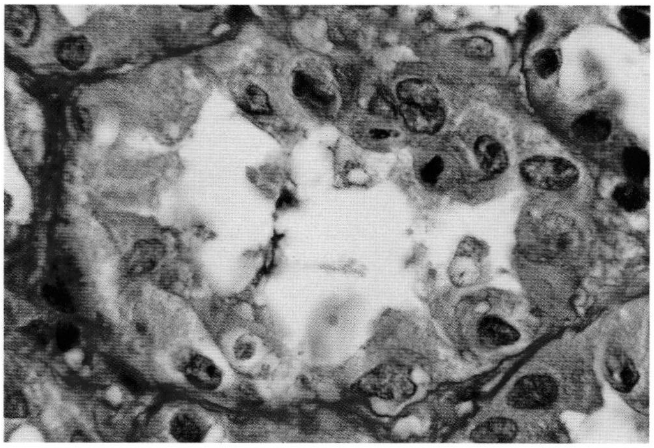

**FIG. 77.** Micrograph from same case as in Fig. 75. Several apoptotic nuclei are present (1–2 o'clock) in the tubular epithelium. PAS stain (original magnification ×**300**).

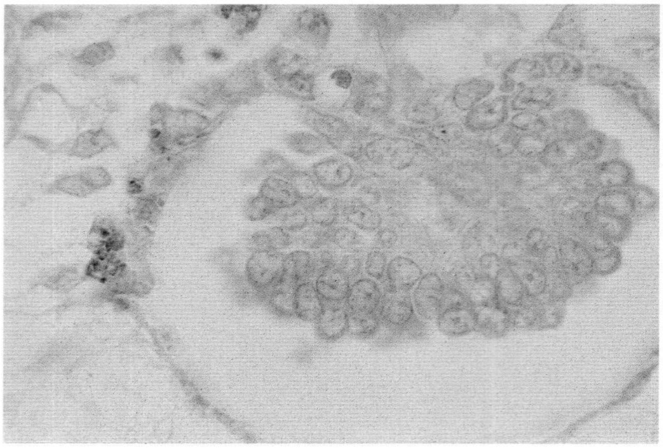

**FIG. 78.** Micrograph from cortical nephrogenic zone of a fetal kidney illustrating labeling for apoptosis in parietal epithelium of a developing glomerulus. Cells with fragmented DNA are identified by a Tdt-mediated dUTP-biotin nick end-labeling (TUNEL) immunoperoxidase method. (Courtesy of Dr. Jin Kim.)

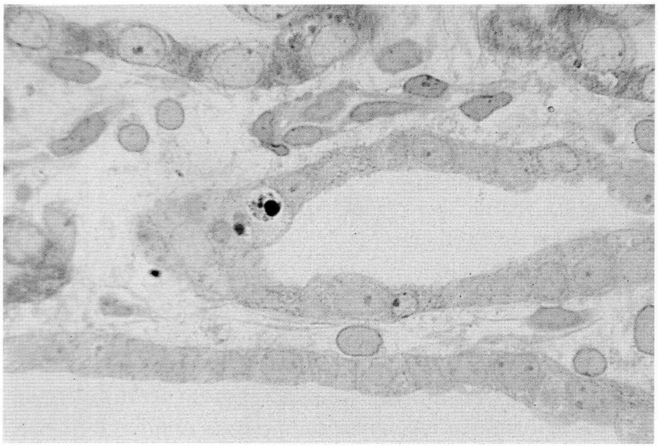

**FIG. 79.** Micrograph of a postnatal kidney demonstrating apoptotic bodies in the medullary collecting duct. After etching with sodium methoxide, the vital dye toluidine blue is removed from normal nuclei but remains in the nuclear fragments of apoptotic bodies (original magnification ×**300**; courtesy of Dr. Jin Kim).

## PROLIFERATION AND APOPTOSIS

The normal adult kidney has a relatively low rate of cell turnover, with little proliferation or apoptosis (189–191). However, renal cell turnover is accelerated during development of hypertrophy, and following injury. Histologic determination of proliferation can be made using a mitotic index or immunostaining with an antibody that detects proteins present during the cell cycle (192–194). During recovery after tubular injury, cell proliferation increases markedly (Fig. 76) (190,195).

Apoptosis has been documented in the adult kidney during the repair response to various forms of tubular injury, including hydronephrosis and ischemic and toxic insults (Fig. 77) (190,196–199). It is well documented that apoptosis plays an important role in embryologic remodeling of tissues. Apoptosis is prominent in the developing kidney and occurs primarily in the cortical nephrogenic zone and the medulla (200,201). In the fetal kidney, apoptosis is observed in uninduced metanephric mesenchyme as well as in the parietal epithelium of developing glomeruli (Fig. 78). At later stages of kidney development, apoptosis occurs in tubular epithelia. Intercalated cells are removed from the developing medullary collecting duct by two mechanisms: apoptosis followed by phagocytosis by neighboring cells (Figs. 79 and 80) and simple extrusion from the epithelium (202).

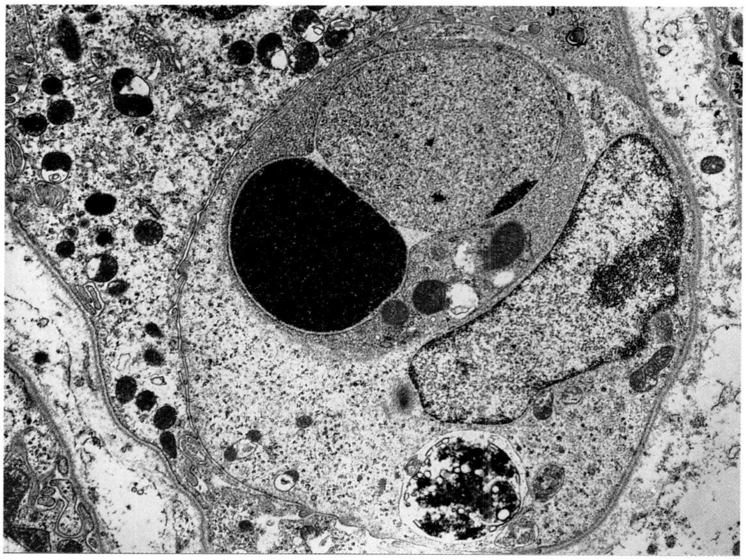

**FIG. 80.** Electron micrograph of a postnatal medullary collecting duct illustrating a phagocytosed apoptotic body composed of a nucleus with condensed chromatin and organelle remnants (original magnification ×**1,200**; courtesy of Dr. Jin Kim).

## REFERENCES


1. Raptopoulos V, Kleinman PK, Mark S, Snyder M, Silverman PM. Renal fascial pathway: posterior extension of pancreatic effusions within the anterior pararenal space. *Radiology* 1986;158:367–374.
2. Tobin CE. The renal fascia and its relation to the transversalis fascia. *Anat Rec* 1944;89:295–311.
3. Kunin M. Bridging septa of the perinephric space: anatomic, pathologic, and diagnostic considerations. *Radiology* 1986;158:361–365.
4. Kochkodan EJ, Hagger AM. Visualization of the renal fascia: a normal finding in urography. *AJR* 1983;140:1243–1244.
5. Parienty RA, Pradel J, Picard JD, Ducellier R, Lubrano JM, Smolarski N. Visibility and thickening of the renal fascia on computed tomograms. *Radiology* 1981;139:119–124.
6. Wald H. The weight of normal adult human kidneys and its variability. *Arch Pathol Lab Med* 1937;23:493–500.
7. Kaisiske BL, Umen AJ. The influence of age, sex, race, and body habitus on kidney weight in humans. *Arch Pathol Lab Med* 1986;110: 55–60.
8. Frimann-Dahl J. Normal variations of the left kidney. An anatomical and radiologic study. *Acta Radiol* 1961;55:207–216.
9. Graves FT. The anatomy of the intrarenal arteries and its application to segmental resection of the kidney. *Br J Surg* 1954;42:132–139.
10. Graves FT. *Anatomical studies for renal and intrarenal surgery.* Bristol, England: Wright; 1986.
11. Sperber I. Studies on the mammalian kidney. *Zool Bidrag Uppsala* 1944;22:249–431.
12. Oliver J. *Nephrons and kidneys: a quantitative study of development and evolutionary mammalian renal architectonics.* New York: Harper & Row; 1968.
13. Hodson CJ, Mariani S. Large cloisons. *AJR* 1982;139:327–332.
14. Lafortune M, Constantin A, Breton G, Vallee C. Sonography of the hypertrophied column of Bertin. *AJR* 1986;146:53–56.
15. Bigongiari LR, Patel SK, Appelman H, Thornburg JR. Medullary rays. Visualization during excretory urography. *AJR* 1975;125: 795–803.
16. Hodson CJ. The lobar structure of the kidney. *Br J Urol* 1972;44: 246–261.
17. Löfgren F. *Das topographische system der malpighischen pyramiden der menschenniere.* Lund, Sweden: Hakan Ohlssons Boktryckeri; 1949.
18. Sykes D. The morphology of renal lobulations and calices, and their relationship to partial nephrectomy. *Br J Surg* 1964;51:294–304.
19. Ransley PG, Risdon RA. Renal papillary morphology in infants and young children. *Urol Res* 1975;3:111–113.
20. Ransley PG. Intrarenal reflux. Anatomical, dynamic and radiologic studies—part I. *Urol Res* 1977;5:61–69.
21. Schmidt-Nielsen B. The renal pelvis. *Kidney Int* 1987;31:621–628.
22. Clapp WM, Abrahamson DR. Development and gross anatomy of the kidney. In: Tisher CC, Brenner BM, eds. *Renal pathology.* 2nd ed. Philadelphia: JB Lippincott; 1994:3–59.
23. Rouillier C. General anatomy and histology of the kidney. In: Rouillier C, Muller AF, eds. *The kidney: morphology, biochemistry, physiology.* New York: Academic Press; 1969:61–156.
24. Dunnill MS, Halley W. Some observations on the quantitative anatomy of the kidney. *J Pathol* 1973;110:113–121.
25. Moffat DB, Fourman J. Ectopic glomeruli in the human and animal kidney. *Anat Rec* 1964;149:1–12.
26. Oliver J. *Architecture of the kidney in chronic Bright's disease.* New York: Harper & Row, Hoeber Medical Division; 1939.
27. Schmidt-Nielsen B, O'Dell R. Structure and concentrating mechanism in the mammalian kidney. *Am J Physiol* 1961;200:1119–1124.
28. Madsen KM, Tisher CC. Structural–functional relationships along the distal nephron. *Am J Physiol* 1986;250:F1–F15.
29. Jamison RL, Kriz W. *Urinary concentrating mechanism: structure and function.* New York: Oxford University Press; 1982.
30. Jacobson HR, Kokko JP. Intrarenal heterogeneity: vascular and tubular. In: Seldin DW, Giebisch G, eds. *The kidney: physiology and pathophysiology.* New York: Raven Press; 1985:531–580.
31. Kriz W, Kaissling B. Structural organization of the mammalian kidney. In: Seldin DW, Giebisch G, eds. *The kidney: physiology and pathophysiology.* New York: Raven Press; 1985:265–306.
32. Knepper M, Burg M. Organization of nephron function. *Am J Physiol* 1983;244:F579–F589.
33. Pirani CL. Evaluation of kidney biopsy specimens. In: Tisher CC, Brenner BM, eds. *Renal pathology.* 2nd ed. Philadelphia: JB Lippincott; 1994:85–115.
34. Kriz W, Bankir L. A standard nomenclature for structures of the kidney. *Kidney Int* 1988;33:1–7.
35. Malpighi M. *De viscerum structura exercitatio anatomica.* Bonn, Germany: 1666.
36. Hayman JM Jr. Malpighi's "Concerning the structure of the kidneys." *Ann Med Hist* 1925;7:242–263.
37. Bowman W. On the structure and use of the Malpighian bodies of the kidney, with observations on the circulation through that gland. *Philos Trans R Soc Lond* 1842;132:57–80.
38. Fine LG. William Bowman's description of the glomerulus. *Am J Nephrol* 1985;5:437–440.
39. Jorgensen F. *The ultrastructure of the normal human glomerulus.* Copenhagan: Munksgaard; 1966.
40. Tisher CC, Brenner BM. Structure and function of the glomerulus. In: Tisher CC, Brenner BM, eds. *Renal pathology.* Philadelphia: JB Lippincott; 1994:143–161.
41. Newbold KM, Howie AJ, Koram A, Adu A, Michael J. Assessment of glomerular size in renal biopsies including minimal change nephropathy and single kidneys. *J Pathol* 1990;160:255–258.
42. Bonsib SM, Reznicek MJ. A fluorescent study of hematoxylin and eosin–stained sections. *Mod Pathol* 1990;3:204–210.
43. Vasmant D, Maurice M, Feldmann G. Cytoskeleton ultrastructure of podocytes and glomerular endothelial cells in man and in the rat. *Anat Rec* 1984;210:17–24.
44. Horvat R, Hovoka A, Dekan G, Poczewski H, Kerjaschki D. Endothelial cell membranes contain podocalyxin—the major sialoprotein of visceral glomerular epithelial cells. *J Cell Biol* 1986;102: 484–491.
45. Kerjaschki D, Sharkey DJ, Farquhar MG. Identification and characterization of podocalyxin—the major sialoprotein of the renal glomerular epithelial cell. *J Cell Biol* 1984;98:1591–1596.
46. Becker CG. Demonstration of actomyosin in mesangial cells of the renal glomerulus. *Am J Pathol* 1972;66:97–110.
47. Schlondorff D. The glomerular mesangial cell: an expanding role for a specialized pericyte. *FASEB J* 1987;1:272–281.
48. Mundel P, Elger M, Sakai T, Kriz W. Microfibrils are a major component of the mesangial matrix in the glomerulus of the rat kidney. *Cell Tissue Res* 1988;254:183–187.
49. Sakai T, Kriz W. The structural relationship between mesangial cells and basement membrane of the renal glomerulus. *Anat Embryol* 1987; 176:373–386.
50. Kriz W, Elger M, Lemley K, Sakai T. Structure of the glomerular mesangium: a biomechanical interpretation. *Kidney Int* 1990;38(suppl 30):2–9.
51. Michael AF, Keane WF, Raij L, Vernier RC, Mauer SM. The glomerular mesangium. *Kidney Int* 1980;17:141–154.
52. Sterzel RB, Lovett DH. Interactions of inflammatory and glomerular cells in the response to glomerular injury. In: Wilson CB, Brenner BM, Stein JH, eds. *Immunopathology of renal disease. Contemporary issues in nephrology.* New York: Churchill Livingstone; 1988;18: 137–173.
53. Jorgensen F, Bentzon MW. The ultrastructure of the normal human glomerulus. Thickness of glomerular basement membranes. *Lab Invest* 1968;18:42–48.
54. Osawa G, Kimmelstiel P, Seiling V. Thickness of glomerular basement membranes. *Am J Clin Pathol* 1966;45:7–20.
55. Osterby R. Morphometric studies of the peripheral glomerular basement in early juvenile diabetes. Development of initial basement membrane thickening. *Diabetologia* 1972;8:84–92.
56. Steffes MW, Barbosa J, Basgen JM, Sutherland DER, Najarian JS, Mauer SM. Quantitative glomerular morphology for the normal human kidney. *Lab Invest* 1983;49:82–86.
57. Ellis EN, Mauer M, Sutherland DER. Glomerular capillary morphology in normal humans. *Lab Invest* 1989;60:231–236.
58. Abrahamson D. Structure and development of the glomerular capillary wall and basement membrane. *Am J Physiol* 1987;253: F783–F794.
59. Kerjaschki D, Ojha PP, Susaui M, et al. A $\beta_1$-integrin receptor for fibronectin in human kidney glomeruli. *Am J Pathol* 1989;134: 481–489.
60. Farquhar MG. The glomerular basement membrane. A selective macromolecular filter. In: Hay ED, ed. *Cell biology of extracellular matrix.* 2nd ed. New York: Plenum; 1991:365–418.

61. Mahan JD, Sisson-Ross SS, Vernier RC. Anionic sites in the human kidney: ex vivo perfusion studies. *Mod Pathol* 1989;2:117–124.
62. Arakawa M. A scanning electron microscopy of the human glomerulus. *Am J Pathol* 1971;64:457–466.
63. Andrews PM, Bates SB. Filamentous actin bundles in the kidney. *Anat Rec* 1984;210:1–9.
64. Drenckhahn D, Franke R. Ultrastructural organization of contractile and cytoskeletal proteins in glomerular podocytes of chicken, rat and man. *Lab Invest* 1988;59:673–682.
65. Holthöfer H, Miettinen A, Lehto V, Lehtoven E, Virtanen I. Expression of vimentin and cytokeratin types of intermediate filament proteins in developing and adult human kidneys. *Lab Invest* 1984;50: 552–529.
66. Rodewald R, Karnovsky MJ. Porous substructure of the glomerular slit diaphragm in the rat and mouse. *J Cell Biol* 1974;60:423–433.
67. Schneeberger EE, Levey RH, McCluskey RI, Karnovsky MJ. The isoporous substructure of the human glomerular slit diaphragm. *Kidney Int* 1975;8:48–52.
68. Latta H, Johnston WH, Stanley TM. Sialoglycoproteins and filtration barriers in the glomerular capillary wall. *J Ultrastruct Res* 1975;51: 354–376.
69. Sawada H, Stukenbrok H, Kerjaschki D, Farquhar MG. Epithelial polyanion (podocalyxin) is found on the sides but not the soles of the foot processes of the glomerular epithelium. *Am J Pathol* 1986;125: 309–318.
70. Kreidberg JA, Sariola H, Loring JM, et al. WT1 is required for early kidney development. *Cell* 1993;74:679–691.
71. Pritchard-Jones K, Fleming S, Davidson D, et al. The candidate Wilms tumor gene is involved in genitourinary development. *Nature* 1990;346:194–197.
72. Mundlos S, Pelletier J, Darveau A, Bachmann M, Winterpacht A, Zabel B. Nuclear localization of the protein encoded by the Wilms tumor gene WT1 in embryonic and adult tissues. *Development* 1993; 119:1329–1341.
73. Pelletier J, Bruening W, Kashtan CE, et al. Germline mutations in the Wilms tumor suppressor gene are associated with abnormal urogenital development in Denys-Drash syndrome. *Cell* 1991;67:437–447.
74. Stamenkovic I, Skalli O, Gabliani G. Distribution of intermediate filament proteins in normal and diseased human glomeruli. *Am J Pathol* 1986;125:465–475.
75. Ryan GB, Coghlan JP, Scoggins BA. The granulated peripolar epithelial cell: a potential secretory component of the renal juxtaglomerular complex. *Nature* 1979;277:655–656.
76. Gall JAM, Alcorn D, Butkus A, Coghlan JP, Ryan GB. Distribution of glomerular peripolar cells in different mammalian species. *Cell Tissue Res* 1986;244:203–208.
77. Gardiner DS, Lindop GBM. The granular peripolar cell of the human glomerulus—a new component of the juxtaglomerular apparatus? *Histopathology* 1985;9:675–685.
78. Ryan GB, Alcorn D, Coghlan JP, Hill PA, Jacobs R. Ultrastructural morphology of granule release from juxtaglomerular myoepithelioid and peripolar cells. *Kidney Int* 1982;22(suppl 12):3–8.
79. Makin CA, Bobrow LG, Bodmer W. Monoclonal antibody and cytokeratin for use in routine histopathology. *J Clin Pathol* 1984;37: 975–983.
80. Hall PA, d'Ardenne AJ, Stansfeld AG. Paraffin section immunohistochemistry. I. Non-Hodgkin's lymphoma. *Histopathology* 1988;13: 149–160.
81. Moll R, Franke WW, Schiller DL, Geiger D, Krepler R. The catalog of human cytokeratins: patterns of expression in normal epithelia, tumors, and cultured cells. *Cell* 1982;31:11–24.
82. Streuli M, Morimoto C, Schrieber M, Schlossman SF, Saito H. Characterization of CD45 and CD45R monoclonal antibodies using transfected mouse cell lines that express individual human leukocyte common antigens. *J Immunol* 1988;141:3910–3914.
83. Hall PA, d'Ardenne AJ, Stansfeld AG. Paraffin section immunohistochemistry. I. Non-Hodgkin's lymphoma. *Histopathology* 1988;13: 149–160.
84. Pulido R, Cebrian M, Acevedo A, De Landazuri MO, Sanchez-Madrid F. Comparative biochemical and tissue distribution study of four distinct CD45 antigen specificities. *J Immunol* 1988;140:3851–3857.
85. Schreiner GF, Kiely JM, Cotran RS. Characterization of resident glomerular cells in the rat expressing Ia determinants and manifesting genetically restricted interactions with lymphocytes. *J Clin* Invest 1981;68:920–937.
86. Falini B, Flenghi L, Pileri S, et al. PG-M1: a new monoclonal antibody directed against a fixative-resistant epitope on the macrophage-restricted form of the CD68 molecule. *Am J Pathol* 1993;142: 1359–1372.
87. Golgi C. Annotazioni intorno all'istologia dei reni dell'uomo e di altri mammiferi e sull'istogenesi: dei canalicoli oriniferi. *Atti R Accad Naz Lincei Rendiconti* 1889;5:337–342.
88. Barajas L. Anatomy of the juxtaglomerular apparatus. *Am J Physiol* 1979;237:F333–F343.
89. Barajas L, Salido EC, Smolens P, et al. Pathology of the juxtaglomerular apparatus including Bartter's syndrome. In: Tisher CC, Brenner BM, eds. *Renal pathology.* Philadelphia: JB Lippincott; 1994: 948–978.
90. Cantin M, Gutkowska J, Lacasse J, et al. Ultrastructural immunocytochemical localization of renin and angiotensin II in the juxtaglomerular cells of the ischemic kidney. *Am J Pathol* 1984;115:212–224.
91. Taugner R, Mannek E, Nobiling R, et al. Coexistence of renin and angiotensin II in epithelioid cell secretory granules of rat kidney. *Histochemistry* 1984;81:39–45.
92. Pricam C, Humbert F, Perrelet A, Orci L. Gap junctions in mesangial and lacis cells. *J Cell Biol* 1974;63:349–354.
93. Taugner R, Schiller A, Kaissling B, Kriz W. Gap junctional coupling between the JGA and the glomerular tuft. *Cell Tissue Res* 1978;186: 279–285.
94. Kaissling B, Kriz W. Variability of intercellular spaces between macula densa cells: a transmission electron microscopic study in rabbits and rats. *Kidney Int* 1982;22(suppl):9–17.
95. Salido EC, Barajas L, Lechago J, Laborde NP, Fisher DA. Immunocytochemical localization of epidermal growth factor in mouse kidney. *J Histochem Cytochem* 1986;34:1155–1160.
96. Sikri KL, Foster CL, MacHugh N, Marshall RD. Localization of Tamm-Horsfall glycoprotein in the human kidney using immunofluorescence and immuno-electron microscopical techniques. *J Anat* 1981;132:597–605.
97. Kirk KL, Bell PD, Barfuss DW, Ribadeneira M. Direct visualization of the isolated and perfused macula densa. *Am J Physiol* 1985; 248:F890–F894.
98. Swann HG. The functional distention of the kidney: A review. *Tex Rep Biol Med* 1960;18:566–596.
99. Hodson CJ. Physiological changes in size of the human kidney. *Clin Radiol* 1961;12:91–94.
100. Parker MV, Swann HG, Sinclair JG. The functional morphology of the kidney. *Tex Rep Biol Med* 1962;20:424–458.
101. Farraggiana F, Malchiodi F, Prado A, Churg J. Lectin–peroxidase conjugate reactivity in normal human kidney. *J Histochem Cytochem* 1982;30:451–458.
102. Hennigar RA, Schulte BA, Spicer SS. Heterogeneous distribution of glycoconjugates in human kidney tubules. *Anat Rec* 1985;211: 376–390.
103. Madsen KM, Brenner BM. Structure and function of the renal tubule and interstitium. In: Tisher CC, Brenner BM, eds. *Renal pathology.* 2nd ed. Philadelphia: JB Lippincott; 1994:661–698.
104. Maunsbach AB. Ultrastructure of the proximal tubule. In: Orloff J, Berliner RW, eds. *Handbook of physiology. Section 8: Renal physiology.* Baltimore: Williams & Wilkins; 1973:31–79.
105. Tisher CC, Bulger RE, Trump BF. Human renal ultrastructure. I. Proximal tubule of healthy individuals. *Lab Invest* 1966;15: 1357–1394.
106. Burg MB. Renal handling of sodium, chloride, water, amino acids and glucose. In: Brenner BM, Rector FC Jr, eds. *The kidney.* 3rd ed. Philadelphia: WB Saunders; 1986:145–175.
107. Welling LW, Welling DJ. Relationship between structure and function in renal proximal tubule. *J Electron Microsc Tech* 1988; 9:171–185.
108. Maack T, Park CH, Camargo MJF. Renal filtration, transport, and metabolism of proteins. In: Seldin D, Giebisch G, eds. *The kidney: physiology and pathophysiology.* New York: Raven Press; 1985: 1773–1803.
109. Dieterich HJ, Barrett JM, Kriz W, Billhoff JP. The ultrastructure of the thin loops of the mouse kidney. *Anat Embryol* 1975;147:1–13.
110. Bulger RE, Tisher CC, Myers CH, Trump BF. Human renal ultrastructure. II. The thin limb of Henle's loop and the interstitium in healthy individuals. *Lab Invest* 1967;16:124–141.
111. Knepper MA, Rector FC Jr. Urinary concentration and dilution. Brenner BM, Rector FC Jr, eds. *The kidney.* 4th ed. Philadelphia: WB Saunders; 1991:445–482.

112. Kokko JP, Rector FC Jr. Countercurrent multiplication system without active transport in inner medulla. *Kidney Int* 1972;2:214–223.
113. Stephenson JL. Concentration of urine in a central core model of the renal counterflow system. *Kidney Int* 1972;2:85–94.
114. Kone BC, Madsen KM, Tisher CC. Ultrastructure of the thick ascending limb of Henle in the rat kidney. *Am J Anat* 1984;171:217–226.
115. Allen F, Tisher CC. Morphology of the ascending thick limb of Henle. *Kidney Int* 1976;9:8–22.
116. Garg LC, Knepper MA, Burg MB. Mineralocorticoid effects on Na-K-ATPase in individual nephron segments. *Am J Physiol* 1981; 240:F536–F544.
117. Woodhall PB, Tisher CC. Response of the distal tubule and cortical collecting duct to vasopressin in the rat. *J Clin Invest* 1973;52: 3095–3108.
118. Gross JB, Imai M, Kokko JP. A functional comparison of the cortical collecting tubule and the distal convoluted tubule. *J Clin Invest* 1975; 55:1284–1294.
119. Kaissling B. Structural aspects of adaptive changes in renal electrolyte excretion. *Am J Physiol* 1982;243:F211–F226.
120. Myers CH, Bulger RE, Tisher CC, Trump BF. Human renal ultrastructure. IV. Collecting duct of healthy individuals. *Lab Invest* 1966; 15:1921–1950.
121. Fine LG. Eustachio's discovery of the renal tubule. *Am J Nephrol* 1896;6:47–50.
122. Stanton BA, Biemesderfer D, Wade JB, Giebisch G. Structural and functional study of the rat nephron. Effects of potassium adaptation and depletion. *Kidney Int* 1981;19:36–48.
123. Petty KJ, Kokko JP, Marvery D. Secondary effect of aldosterone on Na-K-ATPase activity in the rabbit cortical collecting tubule. *J Clin Invest* 1981;68:1514–1521.
124. Mujais SK, Chekal MA, Jones WJ, Hayslett JP, Katz AI. Regulation of renal Na-K-ATPase in the rat: role of the natural mineral- and glucocorticoid hormones. *J Clin Invest* 1984;73:13–19.
125. Kaissling B, Lehir M. Distal tubular segments of the rabbit kidney after adaptation to altered Na- and K- intake. I. Structural changes. *Cell Tissue Res* 1982;224:469–492.
126. Wade JB, O'Neil RG, Pryor JL, Boulpaep EL. Modulation of cell membrane area in renal collecting tubules by corticosteriod hormones. *J Cell Biol* 1979;81:439–445.
127. Schuster VL, Bonsib SM, Jennings ML. Two types of collecting duct mitochondria-rich (intercalated) cells: lectin and band 3 cytochemistry. *Am J Physiol* 1986;251:C347–C355.
128. Verlander JW, Madsen KM, Tisher CC. effect of acute respiratory acidosis on two populations of intercalated cells in the rat cortical collecting duct. *Am J Physiol* 1987;253:F1142–F1156.
129. McKinney TD, Burg MB. Bicarbonate absorption by rabbit cortical collecting tubules in vitro. *Am J Physiol* 1978;234:F141–F145.
130. McKinney TD, Burg MB. Bicarbonate secretion by rabbit cortical collecting tubules in vitro. *J Clin Invest* 1978;61:1421–1427.
131. Lönnerholm G. Histochemical demonstration of carbonic anhydrase activity in the human kidney. *Acta Physiol Scand* 1973;88:455–468.
132. Kim J, Tisher CC, Linser PJ, Madsen KM. Ultrastructural localization of carbonic anhydrase II in subpopulations of intercalated cells of the rat kidney. *J Am Soc Nephrol* 1990;1:245–256.
133. Brown D, Gluck S, Hartwig J. Structure of the novel membrane-coating material in proton-secreting epithelial cells and identification as an $H^+$ATPase. *J Cell Biol* 1987;105:1637–1648.
134. Brown D, Hirsh S, Gluck S. An H-ATPase in opposite plasma membrane domains in kidney epithelial cell subpopultaions. *Nature* 1988; 331:622–624.
135. Verlander JW, Madsen KM, Low PS, Allen DP, Tisher CC. Immunocytochemical localization of band 3 protein in the rat collecting duct. *Am J Physiol* 1988;255:F115–F125.
136. Alper SL, Natale J, Gluck S, Lodish HF, Brown D. Subtypes of intercalated cells in rat kidney collecting duct defined by antibodies against erythroid band 3 and renal vacuolar $H^+$ATPase. *Proc Natl Acad Sci U S A* 1989;86:5429–5433.
137. Schwart GJ, Barasch J, Al-Awquati Q. Plasticity of functional epithelial polarity. *Nature* 1985;318:368–371.
138. Weiner ID, Hall LL. Regulation of intracellular pH in the rabbit cortical collecting tubule. *J Clin Invest* 1990;85:274–281.
139. LeFurgey A, Tisher CC. Morphology of rabbit collecting duct. *Am J Anat* 1979;115:111–124.
140. Hansen GP, Tisher CC, Robinson RR. Response of the collecting duct to disturbances of acid-base and potassium balance. *Kidney Int* 1980; 17:326–337.
141. Madsen KM, Tisher CC. Cellular response to acute respiratory acidosis in rat medullary collecting ducts. *Am J Physiol* 1983;245: F670–F679.
142. Madsen KM, Tisher CC. Response of intercalated cells of rat outer medullary collecting duct to chronic metabolic acidosis. *Lab Invest* 1984;51:268–276.
143. Garg LC, Narang N. Ouabain-insensitive $K^+$adenosine triphosphatase in distal nephron segments of the rabbit. *J Clin Invest* 1988;81: 1204–1208.
144. Wingo CS. Active proton secretion and potassium absorption in the rabbit outer medullary collecting duct: functional evidence of $H^+K^+$ATPase. *J Clin Invest* 1989;84:361–365.
145. Wingo CS, Madsen KM, Smolka A, Tisher CC. $H^+K^+$ATPase immunoreactivity in cortical and outer medullary collect duct. *Kidney Int* 1990;38:985–990.
146. Madsen KM, Clapp WL, Verlander JW. Structure and function of the inner medullary collecting duct. *Kidney Int* 1988;34:441–454.
147. Sands JM, Knepper MA. Urea permeability of mammalian inner medullary collecting duct system and papillary surface epithelium. *J Clin Invest* 1987;79:138–147.
148. Sands JM, Nonoguchi H, Knepper MA. Vasopressin effects on urea and $H_2O$ transport in inner medullary collecting duct subsegments. *Am J Physiol* 1987;253:F823–F832.
149. Clapp WL, Madsen KM, Verlander JM, Tisher CC. Intercalated cells of the rat inner medullary collecting duct. *Kidney Int* 1987;31: 1080–1087.
150. Clapp WL, Madsen KM, Verlander JW, Tisher CC. Morphologic heterogeneity along the rat inner medullary collecting duct. *Lab Invest* 1989;60:219–230.
151. Wall SM, Sands JM, Flessner MF, Nonoguchi H, Spring KR, Knepper MA. Net acid transport by isolated perfused inner medullary collecting ducts. *Am J Physiol* 1990;258:F75–F84.
152. Bohman SO. The ultrastructure of the renal medulla and the interstitial cells. In: Cotran RS, ed. *Tubulo-interstitial nephropathies.* New York: Churchill Livingstone; 1983:1–34.
153. Hestbech J, Hansen HE, Amdisen A, Olsen S. Chronic renal lesions following long-term treatment with lithium. *Kidney Int* 1977;12: 205–213.
154. Bohle A, Grund KE, MacKensen S, Tolon M. Correlations between renal interstitium and level of serum creatinine. Morphometric investigations of biopsies in perimembranous glomerulonephritis. *Virchows Arch* [A] 1977;373:15–22.
155. Kappel B, Olsen S. Cortical interstitial tissue and sclerosed glomeruli in the normal human kidney, related to age and sex. A quantitative study. *Virchows Arch* [A] 1980;387:271–277.
156. Mounier F, Foidart JM, Gubler MC. Distribution of extracellular matrix glycoproteins during normal development of human kidney: an immunohistochemical study. *Lab Invest* 1986;54:394–401.
157. Pfaller W. Structure function correlation in rat kidney. Quantitative correlation of structure and function in the normal and injured rat kidney. *Adv Anat Embryol Cell Biol* 1982;70:1–106.
158. Muirhead EE. Antihypertensive functions of the kidney. *Hypertension* 1980;2:444–464.
159. Lemley KV, Kriz W. Structure and function of the renal vasculature. In: Tisher CC, Brenner BM, eds. *Renal pathology.* 2nd ed. Philadelphia: JB Lippincott; 1994:981–1026.
160. Fourman J, Moffat DB. *The blood vessels of the kidney.* Oxford, England: Blackwell Scientific; 1971.
161. More RH, Duff GL. The renal arterial vasculature in man. *Am J Pathol* 1951;27:95–117.
162. Edwards JG. Efferent arterioles of glomeruli in the juxtamedullary zone of the human kidney. *Anat Rec* 1956;125:521–529.
163. Casellas D, Mimran A. Shunts in renal microvasculature of the rat. A scanning electron microscopic study of corrosion casts. *Anat Rec* 1981;201:237–248.
164. Ljungqvist A. Ultrastructural connection between afferent and efferent arterioles in juxtamedullary glomerular units. *Kidney Int* 1975; 8:239–244.
165. Ljungqvist A. Fetal and postnatal development of the intrarenal arterial pattern in man. *Acta Paediatr* 1963;52:443–464.
166. Mukai K, Rosai J, Burgdorf WH, Localization of factor VIII related antigen in vascular endothelial cells using an immunoperoxidase technique. *Am J Surg Pathol* 1980;4:273–276.
167. Sanfilippo F, Pizzo SV, Croker BP. Immunohistochemical studies of cell differentiation in a juxtaglomerular tumor. *Arch Pathol Lab Med* 1982;106:604–607.

168. Fina L, Molgard HV, Robertson D, et al. Expression of the CD34 gene in vascular endothelial cells. *Blood* 1990;75:2417–2425.
169. Civin CL, Trischmann TM, Fackler MJ, et al. Summary of CD34 cluster workshop section. In: Knapp W, ed. *Leucocyte typing IV.* London: Academic Press; 1989:818–825.
170. Gabbiani G, Schmid E, Winter S, et al. Vascular smooth muscle cells differ from other smooth muscle cells: Predominance of vimentin filaments and a specific α-type actin. *Proc Natl Acad Sci U S A* 1981;78: 298–302.
171. Rollhäuser H, Kriz W, Heinke W. Das gefäss—system der rattenniere. *Z Zellforsch* 1964;64:381–403.
172. Kriz W, Barrett JM, Peter S. The renal vasculature: anatomical–functional aspects. In: Thurau K, eds. *Kidney and urinary tract physiology II.* Baltimore: University Park Press; 1976:1–21.
173. Beeuwkes R, Bonventre JV. Tubular organization and vascular–tubular relations in the dog kidney. *Am J Physiol* 1975;229:695–713.
174. Beeuwkes R. Vascular–tubular relationships in the human kidney. In: Leaf A, Giebisch G, Bolis L, Gorini S, eds. *Renal pathophysiology.* New York: Raven Press; 1980:155–163.
175. Pierce EC. Renal lymphatics. *Anat Rec* 1944;90:315–335.
176. Bell RD, Keyl MJ, Shrader FR, Jones EW, Henry LP. Renal lymphatics: the internal distribution. *Nephron* 1968;3:454–463.
177. Kriz W, Dieterich HJ. Das lymphagefäss system der niere bei einigen säugetieren: Licht-und elektronenmikroskipische untersuchungen. *Z Anat Entwickl Gesch* 1970;131:111–147.
178. Kriz W. A periarterial pathway for intrarenal distribution of renin. *Kidney Int* 1987;31(suppl 20):551–556.
179. Mitchell GAG. The nerve supply of the kidneys. *Acta Anat* 1950;10: 1–37.
180. Gosling JA. Observations on the distribution of intrarenal nervous tissue. *Anat Rec* 1969;163:81–88.
181. Stefansson K, Wollmann RL, Jerkovic M. S-100 protein in soft tissue tumors derived from Schwann cells and melanocytes. *Am J Pathol* 1982;106:261–268.
182. Nakajima T, Uatanabe S, Sato Y, Kamega T, Hirota T, Shimosato Y. An immunoperoxidase study of S-100 protein distribution in normal and neoplastic human tissues. *Am J Surg Pathol* 1982;6:715–727.
183. Trojanowski JQ, Lee VMY, Schlaepfer WW. An immunohistochemical study of human central and peripheral nervous system tumors, using monoclonal antibodies against neurofilaments and glial filaments. *Hum Pathol* 1984;15:248–257.
184. Lee VMY, Carden MJ, Schlaepfer WW. Structural similarities and differences between neurofilament protiens from five different species as revealed using monoclonal antibodies. *J Neurosci* 1986; 6:2179–2186.
185. Barajas L. Innervation of the renal cortex. *Fed Proc* 1978;37: 1192–2001.
186. Fourman J. The adrenergic innervation of the efferent arterioles and the vasa recta in the mammalian kidney. *Experientia* 1970;26: 293–294.
187. Barajas L, Powers K, Wang P. Innervation of the renal cortical tubules: a quantitative study. *Am J Physiol* 1984;247:F50–F60.
188. Barajas L, Powers KV. Innervation of the thick ascending limb of Henle. *Am J Physiol* 1988;255:F340–F348.
189. Savill J. Apoptosis and the kidney. *J Am Soc Nephrol* 1994;5:12–21.
190. Olsen S, Solez K. Acute tubular necrosis and toxic renal injury. In: Tisher CC, Brenner BM, eds. *Renal pathology.* 2nd ed. Philadelphia: JB Lippincott; 1994:769–809.
191. Droz D, Zachar D, Charbit L, Gogusev J, Chretien Y, Iris L. Expression of the human nephron differentiation molecules in renal cell carcinomas. *Am J Pathol* 1990;137:895–905.
192. Gerdes J, Becker MHG, Key G, Cuttoretti G. Immunohistochemical detection of tumour growth fraction (Ki-67 antigen) in formalin fixed and routinely processed tissues. *J Pathol* 1992;168:85–87.
193. Celio JE, Bravo R, Larsen PM, Fey ST. Cyclin: a nuclear protein whose level correlates directly with the proliferative state of normal as well as transformed cells. *Leuk Res* 1984;8:143–157.
194. Pelosi G, Bresaola E, Manfrin E, Rodella S, Schiavon I, Iannucci A. Immunocytochemical detection of cell proliferation–related antigens in cytologic smears of human malignant neoplasms using PC10, reactive with proliferating cell nuclear antigen, and Ki-67. *Arch Pathol Lab Med* 1994;118:510–516.
195. Kliem V, Johnson RJ, Alpers CE, et al. Mechanisms involved in the pathogenesis of tubulointerstitial fibrosis in 5/6-nephrectomized rats. *Kidney Int* 1996;49:666–678.
196. Gobé GC, Axelsen RA. Genesis of renal tubular atrophy in experimental hydronephrosis in the rat. Role of apoptosis. *Lab Invest* 1987; 56:273–281.
197. Gobé GC, Axelsen RA, Searle JW. Cellular events in experimental unilateral ischemic renal atrophy and in regeneration after contralateral nephrectomy. *Lab Invest* 1990;63:770–779.
198. Schumer M, Colombel MC, Sawczuk IS, et al. Morphologic, biochemical and molecular evidence of apoptosis during the reperfusion phase after brief periods of renal ischemia. *Am J Pathol* 1992;140: 831–838.
199. Schimizu A, Yamanaka N. Apoptosis and cell desquamation in repair process of ischemic tubular necrosis. *Virchows Arch [B]* 1993;64: 171–180.
200. Koseki C, Herlinger D, Al-Awqati Q. Apoptosis in metanephric development. *J Cell Biol* 1992;119:1327–1333.
201. Coles HSR, Burne JF, Raff MC. Large-scale normal cell death in the developing rat kidney and its reduction by epidermal growth factor. *Development* 1993;118:777–784.
202. Kim J, Cha J-H, Tisher CC, Madsen KM. Role of apoptotic and non-apoptotic cell death in removal of intercalated cells from developing rat kidney. *Am J Physiol* 1996;270:F575–F592.
203. Tisher CC, Madsen KM. Anatomy of the kidney. In: Brenner BM, Rector FC Jr, eds. *The kidney.* 3rd ed. Philadelphia: WB Saunders; 1986:3–60.
204. Hodson CJ. The renal parenchyma and its blood supply. *Curr Probl Diagn Radiol* 1978;7:5–32.
205. Geneser F. *Textbook of histology.* Philadelphia: Lea & Febiger; 1986.
206. Barajas L, Bloodworth JMB Jr, Hartroft PM. Endocrine pathology of the kidney. In: Bloodworth JMB Jr, ed. *Endocrine pathology.* 2nd ed. Baltimore: Williams & Wilkins; 1982:723–766.
207. Welling LW, Welling DJ. Shape of epithelial cells and intercellular channels in the rabbit proximal nephron. *Kidney Int* 1976;9:385–394.
208. Clapp WL, Park CH, Madsen DM, Tisher CC. Axial heterogeneity in the handling of albumin by the rabbit proximal tubule. *Lab Invest* 1988;58:549–558.

*Histology for Pathologists, second edition,*
Edited by Stephen S. Sternberg.
Lippincott-Raven Publishers, Philadelphia


# CHAPTER 36

# Urinary Bladder, Ureter, And Renal Pelvis

Victor E. Reuter



The ureters are epithelium-lined muscular tubes designed to transport urine from the kidneys to the urinary bladder with the aid of peristalsis. The renal pelvis represents the expanded proximal end of the ureter and serves to collect the urine excreted from the kidney and transport it to the ureter proper. The urinary bladder is an epithelium-lined muscular viscus that has the ability to distend and accommodate up to 400 to 500 ml of urine without a change in intraluminal pressure. In addition, it is able to initiate and sustain a contraction until the organ is empty. Interestingly, micturition may be initiated or inhibited voluntarily despite the involuntary nature of the organ.

## EMBRYOLOGY

The cloaca is divided by the urorectal septum into a dorsal rectum and a ventral urogenital sinus (1,2). It is this urogenital sinus that gives rise to the majority of the urinary bladder, aided by the caudal migration of the cloacal membrane, which closes the infraumbilical portion of the abdominal wall. The caudal portions of the mesonephric ducts become dilated and eventually fuse with the urogenital sinus in the midline dorsally, contributing to the formation of the bladder trigone. Although these ducts contribute initially to the formation of the mucosa of the trigone, this is subsequently entirely replaced by endodermal epithelium of the urogenital sinus. The gradual absorption of the mesonephric ducts bring about the separate opening of the ureters into the urinary bladder in the area of the trigone. During embryologic development, the allantois regresses completely, forming a thick, epithelium-lined tube, the urachus, which extends from the umbilicus to the apex (dome) of the bladder (1). Before or shortly after birth, the urachus involutes further, becoming simply a fibrous cord. Pathologists commonly refer to this fibrous cord that extends from the dome of the bladder to the umbilicus as the urachal remnant. In fact, it is called the median umbilical ligament because the term "urachal remnant" refers to remnants of the epithelial lining of the urachus that occasionally persist within the median umbilical ligament. Normally, the epithelial lining of the urachus is similar to that of the urinary bladder and ureter, but it frequently undergoes metaplastic change, mostly glandular.

The epithelium of the urinary bladder is endodermally derived from the cranial portion of the urogenital sinus, in continuity with the allantois. The lamina propria, muscularis propria, and adventitia develop from the adjacent splanchnic mesenchyme. These facts are important in understanding the histogenesis and nomenclature of lesions arising from the epithelial surface as well as the bladder wall. For example, glandular features within benign (cystitis glandularis, nephrogenic adenoma) and malignant (adenocarcinoma) urothelium is not due to mesodermal or müllerian rests within the trigone but come about through a process of metaplasia and is a reflection of histologic multipotentiality of the urothelium. Because the mesonephric ducts involute totally during embryologic development, it is wrong to refer to mixed carcinomas and sarcomas arising in the bladder ep-

V. E. Reuter: Memorial Sloan-Kettering Cancer Center, New York, New York 10021.

ithelium as mesodermal mixed tumors. They are, in fact, endodermal mixed tumors and usually called carcinosarcomas.

The ureters develop by branching and elongation of the ureteric bud (metanephric diverticulum), which begins as a dorsal bud from the mesonephric duct (1,2). The stalk of the ureteric bud becomes the ureter, whereas the cranial end forms the renal pelvis as well as the calyces and the collecting tubules. The epithelium of the ureter and renal pelvis, although histologically identical to that of the bladder, is of mesodermal derivation.

## ANATOMICAL CONSIDERATIONS

### Bladder

In the adult, the empty urinary bladder lies within the anteroinferior portion of the pelvis minor, inferior to the peritoneum. In infants and children, it is located in part within the abdomen, even when empty (3). It begins to enter the pelvis major at about 6 years of age and is not found entirely within the pelvis minor until after puberty. Nevertheless, as the bladder fills in adults, it distends, ascending into the abdomen, at which time it may reach the level of the umbilicus.

The bladder lies relatively free within the fibrofatty tissues of the pelvis, except in the area of the bladder neck, where it is firmly secured by the pubovesical ligaments in the female and the puboprostatic ligaments in the male (3,4). The relative freedom of the rest of the bladder allows for expansion superiorly as the viscus fills with urine.

The adult empty bladder has the shape of a four-sided inverted pyramid and is enveloped by the vesical fascia (3). The superior surface faces superiorly and is covered by the pelvic parietal peritoneum (Figs. 1 and 2). The posterior surface, also known as the base of the bladder, faces posteriorly and inferiorly. It is separated from the rectum by the uterine cervix and the proximal portions of the vagina in females and by the seminal vesicles and the ampulla of the vasa deferentia in males. These posterior anatomic relationships are important clinically. Because the majority of vesicle neoplasms arise in the posterior wall adjacent to the ureteral orifices, invasive tumor may extend into adjacent soft tissue and organs (Fig. 3A). The intimate relationships to the previously mentioned organs explain why hysterectomy and partial vaginectomy are indicated at the time of radial cystectomy in women. Similarly, we know that perivesical and seminal vesical involvement is a bad prognostic sign in bladder carcinoma in men (5–7), a reflection of high pathologic stage. It is important to note that seminal vesicles may contain carcinoma without invasion, and this occurs in cases of in situ urothelial carcinoma involving prostatic as well as ejaculatory ducts and extending into the seminal vesicle epithelium. The latter is a rare occurrence, but patients thus affected do not appear to have a similarly bad prognosis. The two inferolateral surfaces of the bladder face laterally, inferiorly, and anteriorly and are in contact with the fascia of the levator ani muscles. The most anterosuperior point of the bladder is known as the apex, and it is located at the point of contact of the superior surfaces and the two inferolateral surfaces. The apex (dome) marks the point of insertion of the median umbilical ligament and consequently is the area where urachal carcinomas are located (Figs. 1 and 2).

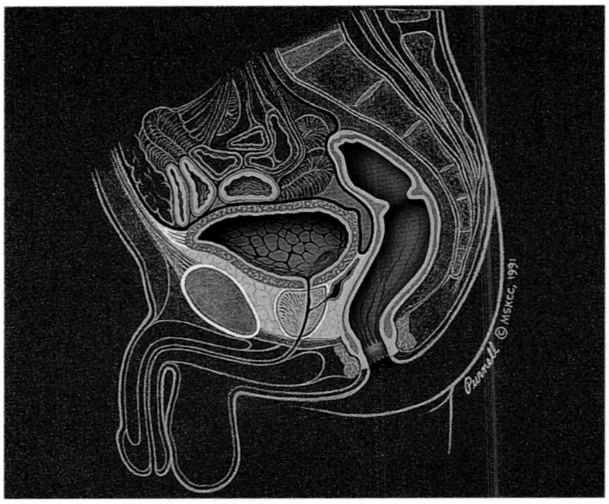


**FIG. 1.** Anatomical relationships of the urinary bladder in males. [Reprinted with permission (65).]

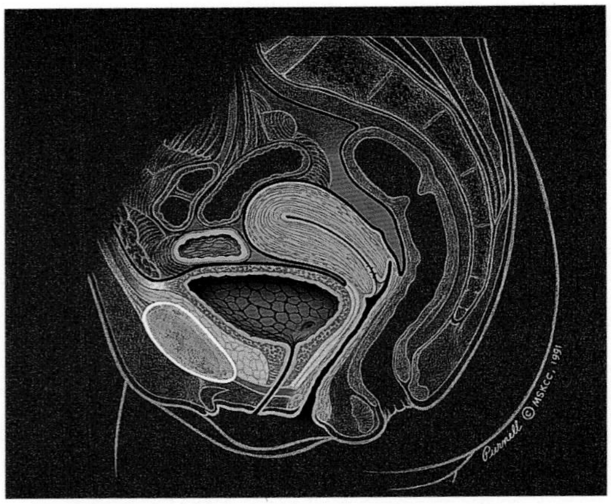


**FIG. 2.** Anatomical relationships of the urinary bladder in females. [Reprinted with permission (65).]

The trigone is a complex anatomic structure located at the base of the bladder and extending to the posterior bladder neck. In the proximal and lateral aspects of the trigone, the ureters enter into the bladder (ureteral orifices) obliquely. The muscle underlying the mucosa in this region is a combination of smooth muscle of the longitudinal layer of the intramural ureter and detrusor muscle (8–12). The intramural ureter is surrounded by a fibromuscular sheath (Waldeyer's sheath), which is fused into the ureteral muscle. This fibromuscular tissue fans out in the area of the trigone and mixes with the detrusor muscle, thus fixing the intramural ureter to the bladder. As the bladder distends, the surrounding musculature exerts pressure on the obliquely oriented intramural ureter, producing closure of the ureteral lumen and thus avoiding reflux of urine. The most distal portion of the blad-

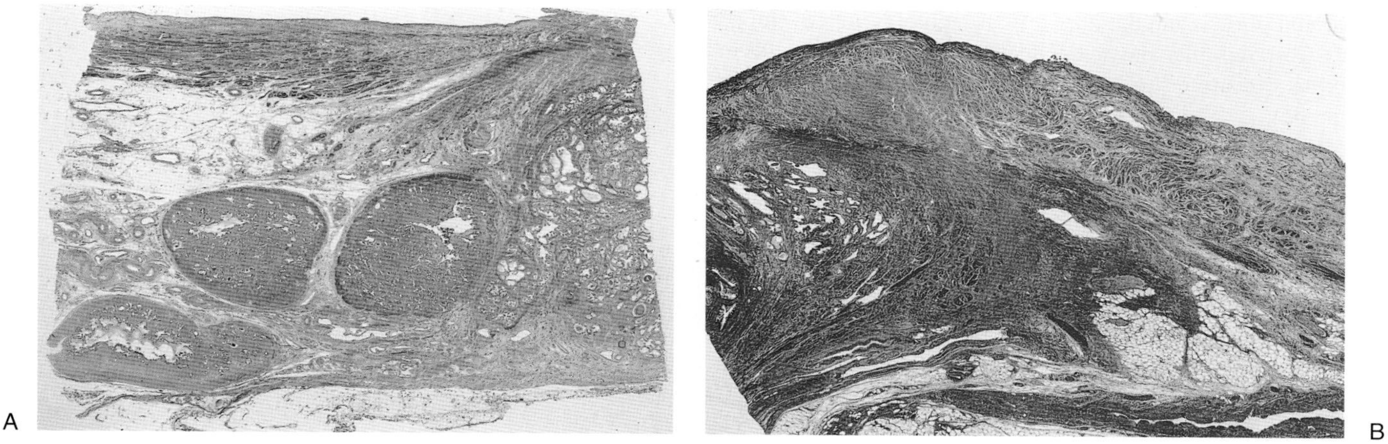


**FIG. 3.** Bladder neck and distal trigone. **A:** The seminal vesicles are separated from the muscularis propria of the trigone by a scant amount of soft tissue. **B:** The muscularis propria merges with the prostate in the bladder neck area. The central (circular) fibers predominate in this area and form the internal sphincter. The outer longitudinal layer contributes somewhat to the formation of the prostate musculature.

der is called the bladder neck, and it is marked by the area where the posterior and inferolateral walls converge and open into the urethra. In the male, the bladder neck merges with the prostate gland, and one may occasionally observe several prostatic ducts present in this area. It is important to recognize the existence of these ducts because their involvement by carcinoma should not be mistaken with invasive carcinoma. The bladder neck is formed with contributions from the trigonal musculature (inner longitudinal ureteral muscle and Waldeyer's sheath), the detrusor musculature, and the urethral musculature (8–13). The internal sphincter is located in this general area, with major contributions from the middle circular layer of the detrusor muscle (Fig. 3B).

The bladder bed (structures on which the bladder neck rests) is formed posteriorly by the rectum in males and vagina in females (Figs. 1 and 2). Anteriorly and laterally it is formed by the internal obturator and levator ani muscles as well as the pubic bones. These structures may be involved in advanced tumors occupying the anterior, lateral, or bladder neck regions and render the patient inoperable.

The main arterial blood supply of the bladder comes from the inferior vesical arteries, which are branches of the internal iliac arteries (3,14). The umbilical arteries, through their branches, the superior vesical arteries, also supply the bladder, as do the obturator and inferior gluteal arteries and, in females, the uterine and vaginal arteries. The veins of the urinary bladder drain into the internal iliac veins and form the vesical venous plexus. In the male, this plexus envelops the bladder base, prostate, and seminal vesicles and connects with the prostatic venous plexus. In females, it covers the bladder neck and urethra and communicates with the vaginal plexus. Lymphatic drainage is through the external and internal lymph nodes, although drainage of portions of the bladder neck region may occur via the sacral or common iliac nodes.

The urinary bladder is supplied by both sympathetic and parasympathetic nerves, which form the vesical nerve plexus (3,14). The former are derived from T11–L2 nerves and play no role in micturition. On the other hand, the parasympathetic nerves come from S2–4 and travel to the bladder via the pelvic nerve and inferior hypogastric plexus. These nerves are important to micturition because they contract the fibers of the muscularis propria, which in turn produce traction on the bladder neck, opening the internal sphincter of the bladder. In fact, it is believed that micturition is initiated by voluntary relaxation of the perineal muscles and the striated muscle of the external sphincter located along the urethra. This action decreases urethral resistance and triggers contraction of the smooth muscle of the trigone and remaining bladder, closing the ureteral orifices and increasing the hydrostatic pressure within the viscus (4,15). Astute observers now understand why it is difficult to "start a stream while you whistle a tune." The bladder also contains sensory nerves that travel along the pelvic and hypogastric nerves and account for the sensation of pain as the bladder becomes too distended.

## Ureters

The ureters measure approximately 30.0 cm in length, equally divided between the abdomen (retroperitoneum) and pelvis (16–21). The abdominal ureter takes a vertical course downward and medial on the anterior surface of the psoas muscle, covered by adventitia, which is in fact an extension of Gerota's fascia. The pelvic ureter can be subdivided into a longer parietal and a shorter intravesical portion. The parietal portion is intimately related to the peritoneum. It descends posterolaterally, and as it approaches the bladder base, it becomes medially directed to reach the urinary bladder. The ureters enter the base of the bladder obliquely and empty into the bladder at the ureteral orifices. The distal parietal portion and the intravesical segments are enveloped in a fibromuscular sheath (Waldeyer's sheath), which aids in fixing the ureter to the bladder (see description of the trigone).

The ureteral blood supply is quite diverse (3,16). Depending on the anatomic level, it receives blood from branches of the renal, abdominal aortic, gonadal, hypogastric, vesical, and uterine arteries, which form a richly intercommunicating plexus of vessels surrounding the tube. Venous drainage is variable but tends to follow a pattern similar to the arterial distribution. Lymphatic drainage is also complex. The upper portions drain into the lateral aortic lymph nodes. The middle portion drains into the common iliac lymph nodes, whereas the inferior portion drains into either the common, external, or internal iliac lymph nodes.

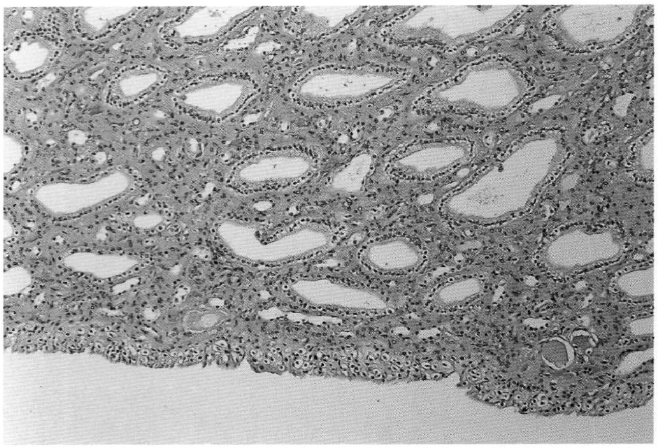

**FIG. 5.** Renal papilla. Distal collecting ducts open into the urothelium covering the papillae.

### Renal Pelvis

As previously mentioned, the renal pelvis has its origin in the cranial portion of the ureteric bud, together with the calyces and collecting ducts. The renal pelvis lies primarily within the renal hilum, a space formed medially when one draws a vertical plane through the medical aspects of the upper and lower poles of the kidney (Fig. 4). Within the hilum is the renal sinus, a space within the medial and antral portion of the kidney occupied by the renal pelvis, renal vessels and nerves, renal calyces, and fat. The fibrous capsule that lines the kidney passes over the lips of the hilum and lines the renal sinus, becoming continuous with the renal calyces. Within the renal sinus, the renal pelvis divides into two and rarely three major calyces, which in turn divide into 7 to 14 minor calyces. Urine from the distal collecting ducts within the renal medulla (ducts of Bellini) flows into the minor calyces at the tips of the renal papillae (area cribosa) (Fig. 5). The blood supply of the renal pelvis comes from branches of the renal arteries, and the venous drainage follows a similar distribution. Its lymphatic drainage is into the renal hilar lymph nodes.

## MICROSCOPIC ANATOMY

The urinary bladder, ureter and renal pelvis have a similar composition, the innermost layer being an epithelial lining and, extending outward, a lamina propria, smooth muscle (muscularis propria), and adventitia. The superior surface of the bladder comes in contact with parietal peritoneum and hence has a serosa. The anatomic landmarks are used clinically and pathologically to stage (i.e., choose therapy and es-

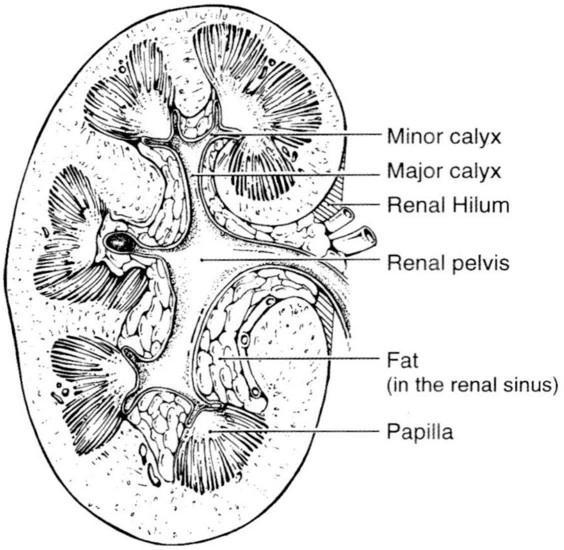


**FIG. 4.** Anatomical relationships of the renal pelvis. Notice that the pelvis is mostly within the renal hilum (medial shaded area) and the renal sinus.

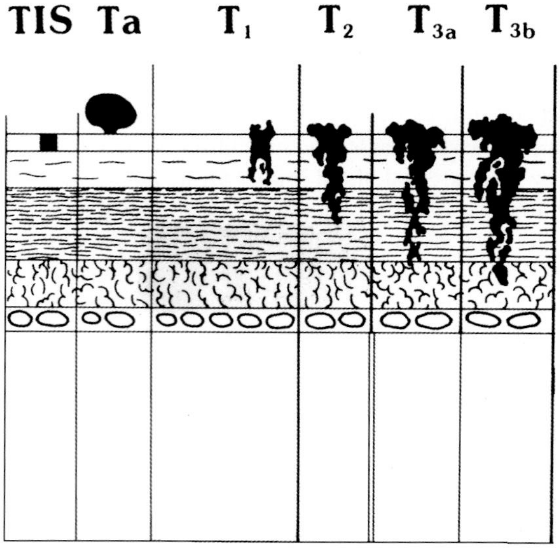


**FIG. 6.** Pathologic staging of bladder cancer. This classification follows the recommendations of the American Joint Committee on Cancer (AJCC). In addition, prostatic stromal invasion is considered stage pT4.

timate the survival of) patients with urothelial cancer (Fig. 6). For this reason, it is important to accurately identify these landmarks microscopically.

## Urothelium

The urinary bladder, ureters, and renal pelvis are lined by so-called transitional epithelium. This name was chosen because the histologic appearance of the epithelium was transitional between nonkeratinizing squamous and pseudostratified columnar epithelium. Many histologists and pathologists have suggested "urothelium" as a more appropriate term.

The thickness of the urothelium varies according to the degree of distension and anatomical location. It may be only two- or three-cell layers thick along the minor calyces. In the contracted bladder, it is usually six to seven cells thick and in the ureter three to five cells thick. One can identify three regions: the superficial cells (which are in contact with the urinary space), the intermediate cells, and the basal cells (which lie on a basement membrane) (22,23) (Fig. 7). In the distended viscus, the urothelium may be only two to three cells thick and flattened with their long axis horizontal to the basement membrane. In practice, the thickness of the urothelium is dependent not only on the degree of distension but also on the plane on which the tissue is cut. If the cut is tangential to the basement membrane, it is possible to generate an artificially thick mucosa. For these and other reasons, we feel that urothelial thickness is of marginal or no utility in the assessment of urothelial neoplasms.

Superficial cells are in contact with the urinary space. They are large, elliptical cells that lie umbrella-like over the smaller intermediate cells (22–25). They may be binucleated and have abundant eosinophilic cytoplasm (Fig. 8). In the distended bladder, they become flattened and barely discernible. Although the presence of these cells is taken as a sign of normalcy of the urothelium, one must be aware that they may become detached during manipulation or processing of biopsy or surgical material. Conversely, it is possible to see umbrella cells overlying frank carcinoma. In summary, the presence or absence of superficial cells cannot be used as a determining factor of malignancy. Ultrastructural studies have shown the superficial urothelial cells to be unique. The luminal surface is lined by a cytoplasmic membrane that is three layers thick: two electron-dense layers and a central lucent layer (Fig. 9A). The two dense layers are said to be of unequal thickness; for this reason the membrane is known as the asymmetric unit membrane (AUM) (23–27). In reality, although the trilaminar arrangement of the cytoplasmic membrane can be readily observed, it is difficult to see the asymmetry of the dense layers. The membrane contains frequent invaginations, giving it a scalloped appearance. The superficial (luminal) cytoplasm contains vesicles that are also lined by AUM (Fig. 9B). During the process of distention, these invaginations and vesicles are incorporated into the surface membrane, thus increasing the surface area and maintaining the structural integrity of the urothelium.

The intermediate cell layer may be up to five cells thick in the contracted bladder, where they are oriented with the long axis perpendicular to the basement membrane. The nuclei are oval and have finely stippled chromatin with absent or minute nucleoli. There is ample cytoplasm, which may be vacuolated. The cytoplasmic membranes are distinct, and these cells are attached to each other by desmosomes. In the distended state, this layer may be inconspicuous or only one cell thick and flattened. The basal layer is composed of cuboidal cells, which are evident only in the contracted bladder and which lie on a thin but continuous basement membrane composed of a lamina lucida, lamina densa, and anchoring fibrils (28). All normal urothelial cells may contain glycogen, but only the superficial cells are occasionally mucicarminophilic.

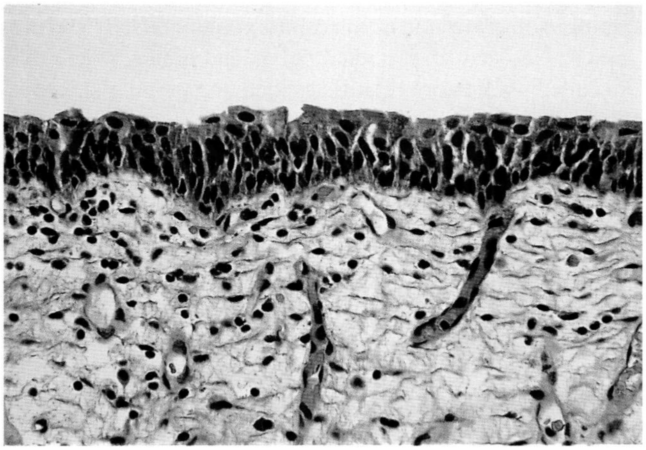

**FIG. 7.** Normal urothelium. **A:** The mucosa may be up to seven cells thick in the bladder, but thickness varies as a consequence of distension and other factors. The superficial (umbrella) cells have ample eosinophilic cytoplasm.

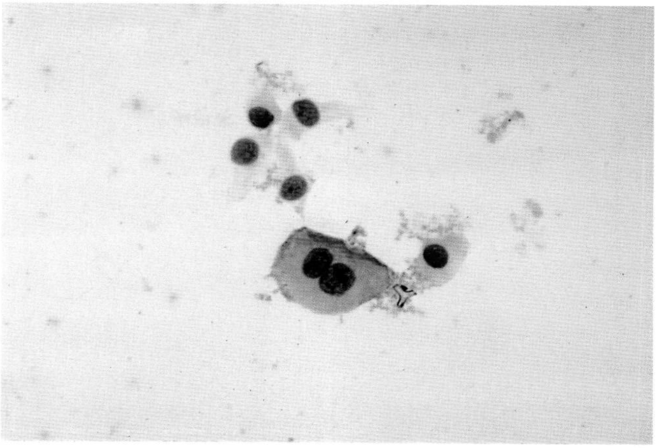

**FIG. 8.** Urine cytology preparation stained with monoclonal antibody BG-7 (Signet Laboratories). A large, binucleated umbrella cell expresses the antigen identified by this antibody, whereas other normal urothelial cells do not.

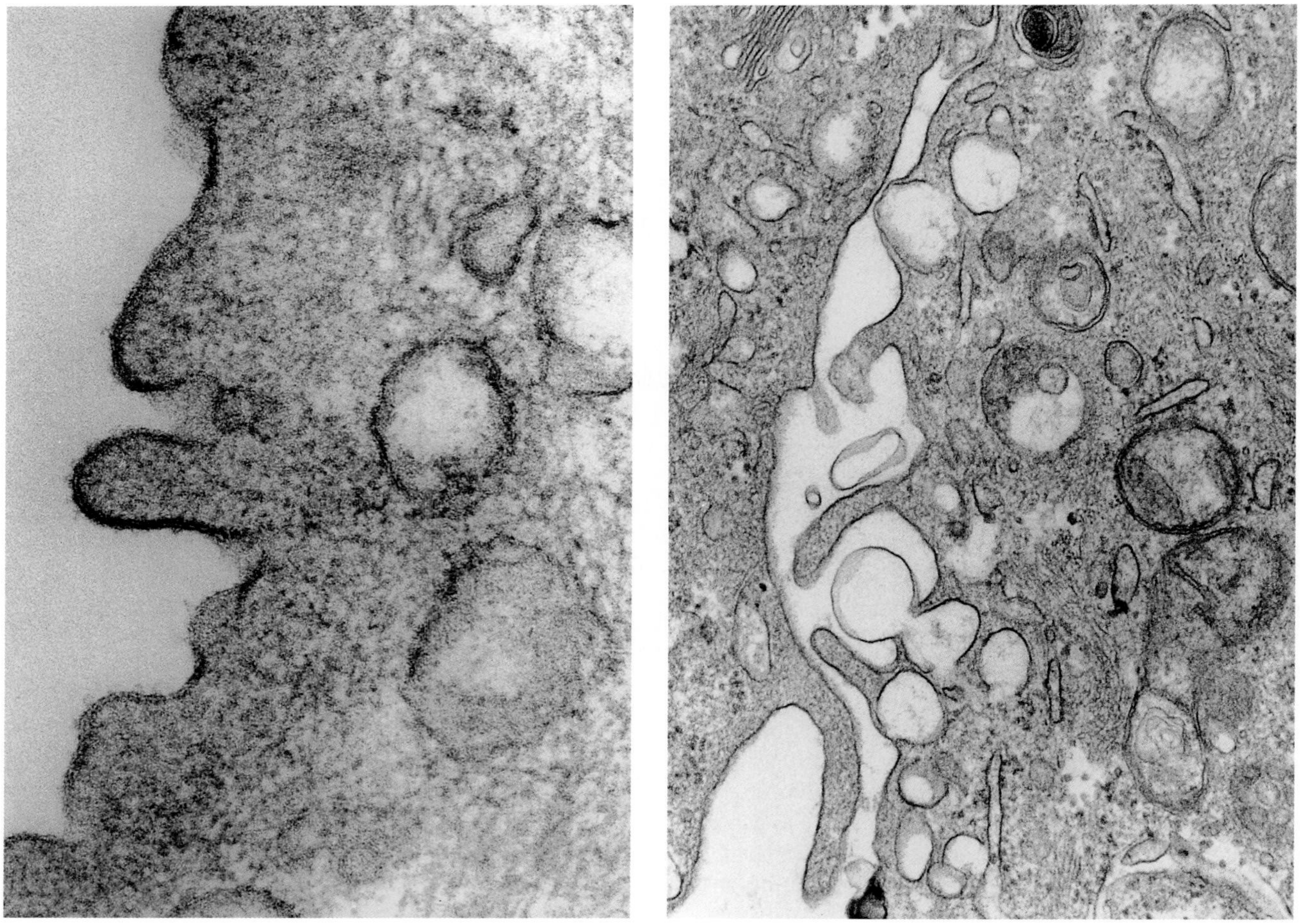


**FIG. 9.** Ultrastructure of the urothelium. **A:** Detail of the luminal surface of a urothelial cell from a 1-year-old infant. The trilaminar cell membrane does not appear to be asymmetric (original magnification ×136,000). **B:** Vesicles communicating with the apical/lateral surface of a urothelial cell (original magnification ×54,000).

### Urothelial Variants and Benign Urothelial Proliferations

Although the above microscopic and ultrastructural features describe normal urothelium, we know that there are many benign morphologic variants. Koss studied 100 grossly normal bladders obtained postmortem (29). Of these, 93% had either Brunn's nests, cystitis cystica, or squamous metaplasia.

The most common urothelial variant is the formation of Brunn's nests, which represent invaginations of the surface urothelium into the underlying lamina propria (Fig. 10). In some cases these solid nests of benign-appearing urothelium may lose continuity with the surface and are isolated within the lamina propria, where they become cystic because of an accumulation of cellular debris or mucin. The term "cystitis cystica" is used to describe this phenomenon. The lining epithelium of these small cysts is composed of one or several layers of flattened transitional or cuboidal epithelium. In some cases the epithelial lining undergoes glandular metaplasia, giving rise to what is called cystitis glandularis (Fig. 10). The cells become cuboidal or columnar and mucin secreting; some are transformed into goblet cells. These processes also occur in the renal pelvis and ureter, where they are called pyelitis or ureteritis cystica or glandularis, respectively.

Brunn's nests, cystitis cystica, and cystitis glandularis represent a continuum of proliferative or reactive changes seen along the entire urothelial tract, and it is common to see all three in the same tissue sample. Most investigators believe that they occur as a result of local inflammatory insult (29–31). Nevertheless, these proliferative changes are seen in the urothelium of patients with no evidence of local inflammation, so it is possible that they also represent either normal histologic variants or the residual effects of old inflammatory processes (32,33). The high incidence of these proliferative changes in the normal bladder suggests that they are not likely to be premalignant changes and that there is no cause-and-effect relationship between their presence and the appearance of bladder cancer. It is true that one or all

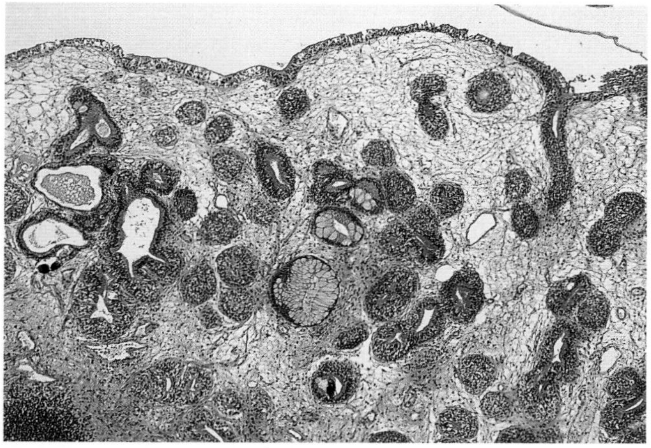

**FIG. 10.** Bladder urothelium exhibiting proliferative changes, including Brunn's nests and cystitis glandularis.

of these changes are commonly present in biopsy specimens containing bladder cancer, but the coexistence may be coincidental or the cancer itself may be producing the local inflammatory insult that causes them. The fact that exceptional cases may occur in which carcinoma clearly arises within the epithelium of these reactive lesions does not alter this assertion (34,35).

Metaplasia refers to a change in morphology of one cell type into another that is considered aberrant for that location. Transitional epithelium frequently undergoes either squamous or glandular metaplasia, presumably as a response to chronic inflammatory stimuli such as urinary tract infection, calculi, diverticula, or frequent catheterization (30,33).

Squamous metaplasia, particularly in the area of the trigone, is a common finding in women, responsive to estrogen production. This type of squamous metaplasia is characterized by abundant intracytoplasmic glycogen and lack of keratinization, making it histologically similar to vaginal or cervical squamous epithelium (Fig. 11). Under other conditions, the metaplastic squamous epithelium undergoes keratinization and may exhibit parakeratosis and even a granular layer. This metaplastic epithelium is not preneoplastic per se but, under some circumstances, may precede squamous carcinoma (36).

The most common site of glandular metaplasia of the urothelium is the bladder, in the form of cystitis glandularis. Nevertheless, it also may occur within surface urothelium elsewhere in the urinary tract, usually as a response to chronic inflammation or irritation and also in cases of bladder exstrophy (37,38). The epithelium is composed of tall columnar cells with mucin-secreting goblet cells (Fig. 12), strikingly similar to colonic or small intestinal epithelium in which one might identify even Paneth's cells. As with squamous metaplasia, glandular metaplasia is not of itself a precancerous lesion but may eventually undergo neoplastic transformation in exceptional cases (38).

So-called nephrogenic adenoma is a distinct metaplastic lesion characterized by aggregates of cuboidal or hobnail cells with clear or eosinophilic cytoplasm and small discrete nuclei without prominent nucleoli (39). These cells line thin papillary fronds on the surface or form tubular structures within the lamina propria of the bladder (Fig. 13). The tubules are often surrounded by a thickened and hyalinized basement membrane. Variable numbers of acute and chronic inflammatory cells are commonplace within the bladder wall.

Nephrogenic adenoma is thought to be secondary to an inflammatory insult or local injury (39–43). It was originally described in the trigone and given its name because it was thought to arise from mesonephric rests. We now know that nephrogenic adenoma may occur anywhere in the urothelial tract, although it is most common in the bladder. It is important in that it may present as an exophytic mass, mimicking carcinoma grossly and suggesting adenocarcinoma microscopically. The benign histologic appearance of the cells arranged in characteristic tubules surrounded by a prominent basement membrane should provide the correct diagnosis.

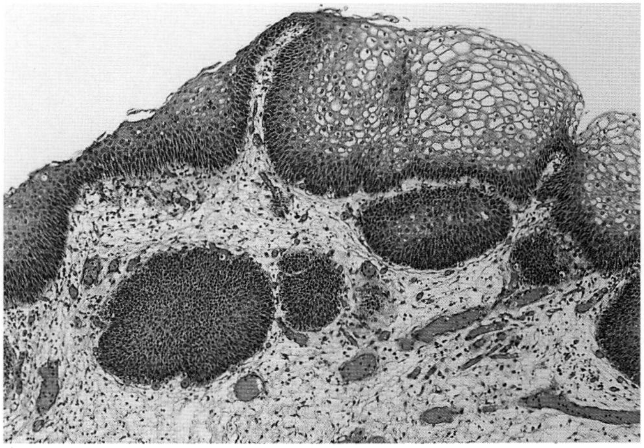

**FIG. 11.** Squamous metaplasia. This change is most commonly seen in the area of the trigone in women.

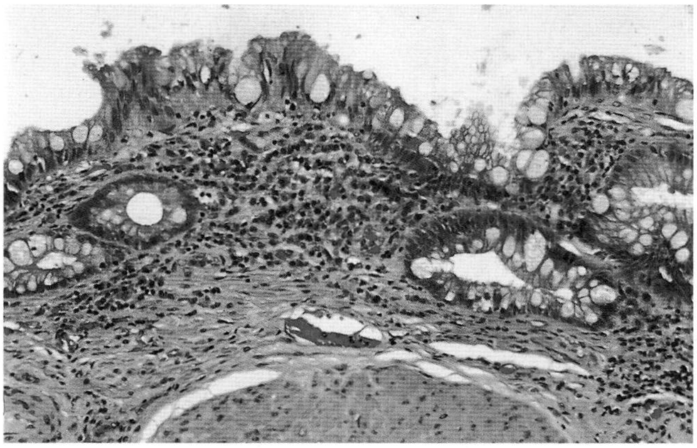

**FIG. 12.** Intestinal metaplasia. The individual cells are morphologically identical to intestinal-type epithelium, even at the electron microscopic level.

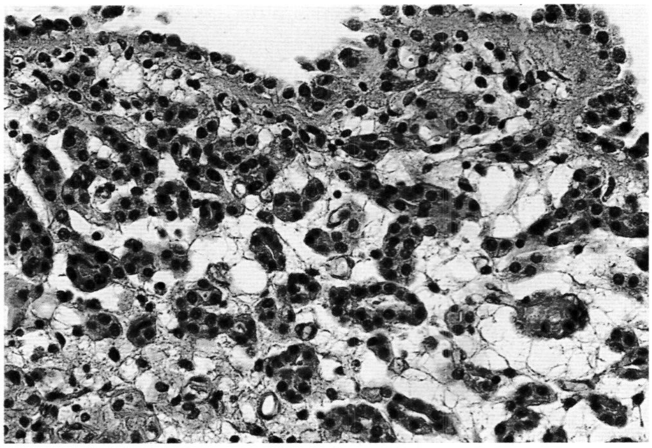

FIG. 13. Nephrogenic adenoma. This proliferative urothelial lesion is characterized by aggregates of cuboidal cells with scant eosinophilic cytoplasm forming small tubules within the lamina propria. It may exhibit an exophytic, papillary growth.

Inverted papillomas are relatively rare lesions that may occur anywhere along the urothelial tract and may be confused clinically and pathologically with transitional cell carcinoma (44,45). In order of decreasing frequency, they occur in the bladder, renal pelvis, ureter, urethra, and renal pelvis (46–52). Patients usually present with hematuria. Cytoscopically, the lesions are polypoid and either sessile or pedunculated. The mucosal surface is smooth or nodular without villous or papillary fronds. Microscopically, the surface transitional epithelium is compressed but otherwise unremarkable. It is undermined by invaginated cords and nests of transitional epithelium that occupy the lamina propria (Fig. 14). The accumulation of these endophytic growths gives the lesion its characteristic polypoid gross appearance. The urothelial cells forming the cords are benign, exhibiting normal maturation and few mitoses. They are similar to the cells of bladder papillomas, differing only in that the epithelial cords are endophytic and consequently more closely packed. Frequently the cells are oval or spindle shaped. Epithelial nests may become centrally cystic, dilated, and even lined by cuboidal epithelium.

These cords of transitional epithelium in the lamina propria represent invagination, not invasion. As such, there are no fibrous reactive changes within the stroma. Although mitotic figures can be seen, they are rare, regular, and located at or near the basal layer of the epithelium. Inverted papillomas are discrete lesions and do not exhibit an infiltrative border (46,47). One must be careful not to confuse a nested type of urothelial carcinoma infiltrating lamina propria with an inverted papilloma.

The etiology of rare lesions is unclear. Most investigators feel that, similar to other proliferative lesions such as Brunn's nests and cystitis cystica, they are a reactive, proliferative process secondary to a noxious insult. They are not premalignant, although in exceptional cases they have been associated with carcinoma (48–50). Given the rarity of this association, we consider it incidental.

### Lamina Propria

The lamina propria lies between the mucosal basement membrane and the muscularis propria. It is composed of dense connective tissue containing a rich vascular network, lymphatic channels, sensory nerve endings, and a few elastic fibers (14,22,23). In the deeper aspects of the lamina propria, urinary bladder, and ureter, the connective tissue is loose, allowing for the formation of thick mucosal folds when the viscus is contracted (Figs. 15 and 16). Its thickness varies with the degree of distention and is generally thinner in the areas of the trigone and bladder neck. In fact, in patients with urinary outflow obstruction (i.e., prostatic hyperplasia) the bladder neck may contain muscularis propria directly beneath the mucosa with the lamina propria being virtually

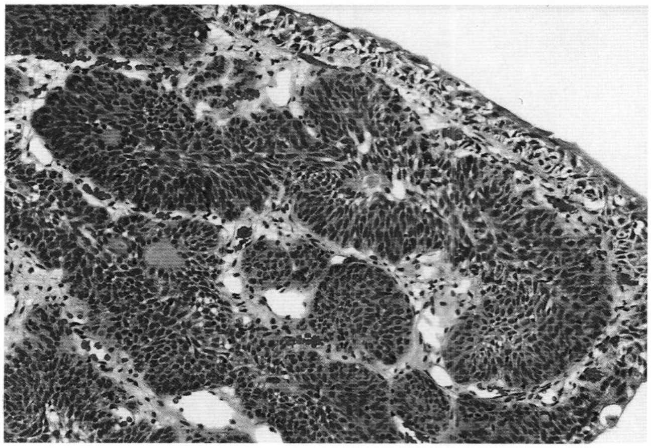

FIG. 14. Inverted papilloma. This proliferative urothelial lesion is characterized by invaginated cords and nests of transitional epithelium within the lamina propria.

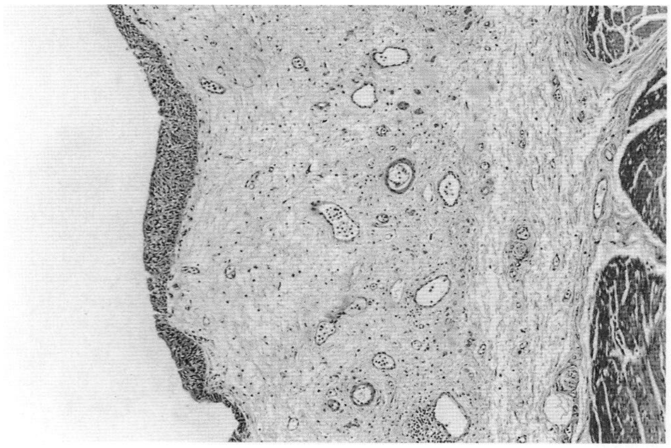

FIG. 15. Lamina propria is composed of connective tissue, vascular structures, sensory nerves, and elastic fibers. Notice that the superficial connective tissue is more dense than the deep portion.

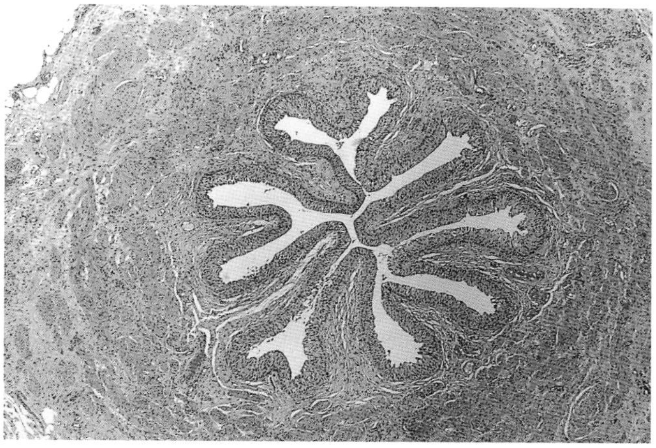

**FIG. 16.** Cross section of mid-ureter. The elastic fibers and loose connective tissue within the lamina propria impart a festooned appearance to the urothelium. Notice that the different layers of the muscularis propria are indiscernible.

indiscernible (Fig. 3B). Lamina propria is also absent beneath the urothelium lining the renal papillae in the renal pelvis and is quite thin along the minor calyces (Fig. 17). In the mid-portion of the lamina propria of the bladder lie intermediate-sized arteries and veins. Wisps of smooth muscle are commonly found in the lamina propria, usually associated with these vessels (53,54) (Fig. 18A, B). These fascicles of smooth muscle are not connected to the muscularis propria and appear as isolated bundles but may form a discontinuous thin layer of muscle. The anatomic relationship of these fibers to the overlying urothelium can be severely disrupted by inflammation or prior therapeutic intervention, when they may be seen juxtaposed to the basement membrane (Fig. 18C). Uncommonly, these muscle fibers may present as a continuous layer of muscle within the lamina propria, thus forming a true muscularis mucosae (54). In

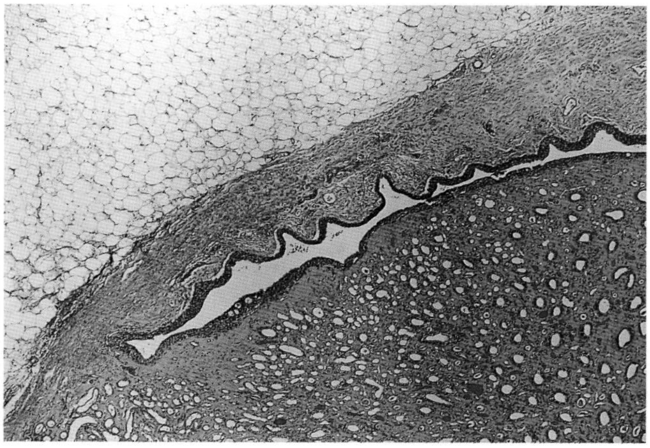

**FIG. 17.** Junction of the renal papilla with the minor calyx. Notice the absence of the lamina propria along the papilla and a very thin lamina propria and muscularis propria along the minor calyx.

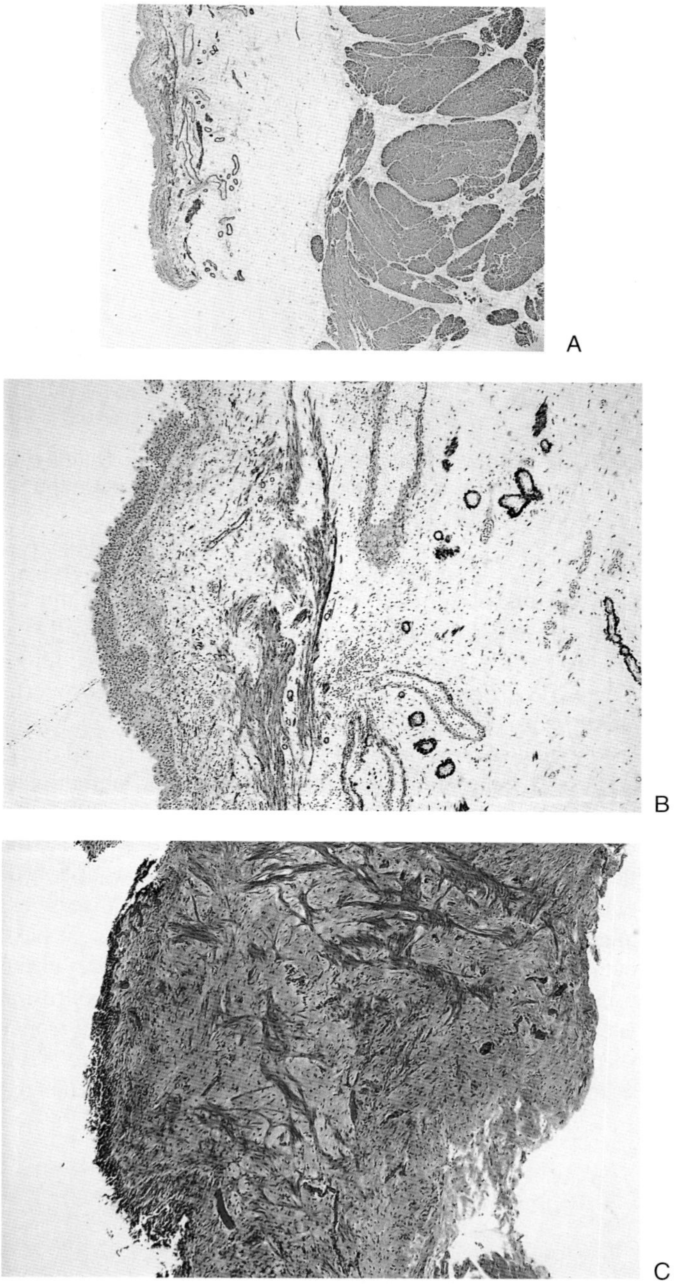


**FIG. 18.** Lamina propria of the urinary bladder. **A,B:** Discontinuous smooth muscle fascicles adjacent to intermediate-sized vessels within the lamina propria (antiactin monoclonal antibody). **C:** Disorganized wisps of superficial smooth muscle directly beneath the urothelium at the site of a prior biopsy. TURB specimen.

evaluating surgical and biopsy material, every effort should be made to distinguish these superficial muscle fascicles from muscularis propria because failure to do so will lead to errors in tumor staging and treatment. A pathologist should not sign out a biopsy sample as "transitional cell carcinoma invading muscle" because he or she is not giving useful information as to the depth of invasion. In fact, many urolo-

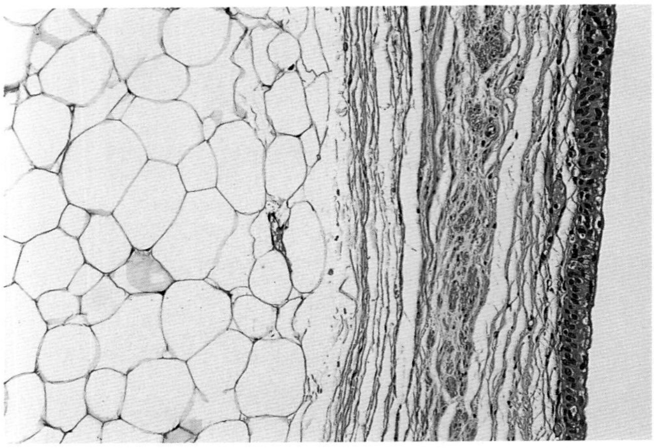

**FIG. 19.** Urothelial wall along the minor calices. Thin layers of lamina propria and muscularis propria are surrounded by fat within the renal sinus.

gists are unaware of the existence of a superficial muscle layer (muscularis mucosae), so the above diagnosis will lead the urologist to treat the patient as a deeply invasive tumor (stage pT2 or greater) when in fact the patient has superficially invasive disease (stage pT1).

Pathologists are surprised to learn that, in terms of prognosis and treatment, urologists and urologic oncologists lump noninvasive (Ta) and superficially invasive (T1) into a single category. It is my opinion that this is greatly due to the fact that we as pathologists do not agree as to what constitutes lamina propria invasion. Many cases of pT1 disease are unequivocal, but in an equal number invasion is, at best, questionable. Pathologists' interpretation in the latter group is inconsistent and not reproducible. Although this confusion is partly due to the lack of orientation of transurethral biopsy specimens and to disruption of the normal histologic architecture by tumor or prior therapy, it is clear that better parameters are needed to make this distinction. Furthermore, these parameters should be heeded by all pathologists. Studies evaluating the biologic differences between pTa and clear-cut pT1 lesions would be interesting and very informative.

## Muscularis Propria

The muscularis propria is said to be composed of three smooth muscle coats: inner and outer longitudinal layers and a central circular layer. In fact, these layers can only be identified consistently in the area of the bladder neck. In other areas, the longitudinal and circular layers mix freely and have no definite orientation. In the ureter, the muscularis propria is thicker distally and the proximal portion contains only two layers (55). In the renal pelvis the muscularis propria becomes thinner along the major and minor calyces, and no orientation of the muscle fibers is evident. No muscular fibers are evident between the urothelium and the renal medulla at the level of the renal papillae (Fig. 17). Within the renal sinus, the muscularis propria is surrounded by variable amounts of fat (Fig. 19). This fact is rarely remembered by pathologists at the time of evaluating urothelial tumors arising in the renal pelvis. Many cases are signed out as "invading renal hilar fat" or "invading perirenal fat" when in fact the invasion is solely into the fat within the renal sinus.

In the contracted bladder, the muscle fibers are arranged in relatively coarse bundles that are separated from each other by moderate to abundant connective tissue containing blood vessels, lymphatics, and nerves. Infrequently, one may see nests of paraganglia, usually associated with neural or vascular structures (Fig. 20A). The cells are arranged in discrete nests or cords and have clear or granular cytoplasm with round or vesicular nuclei. They should not be confused with invasive carcinoma. Immunohistochemical stains are negative for cytokeratins but positive for chromogranin (Fig. 20B).

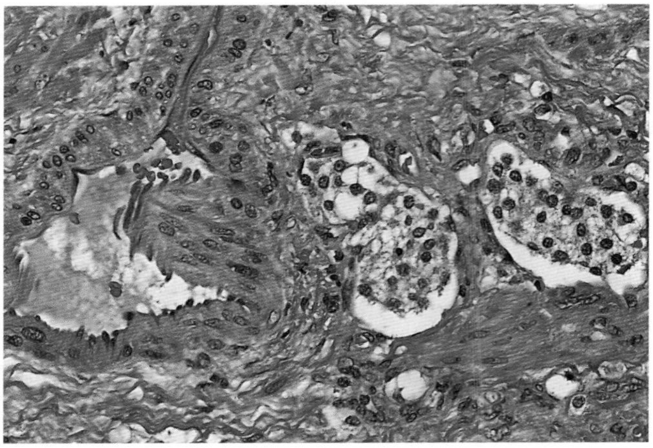

A

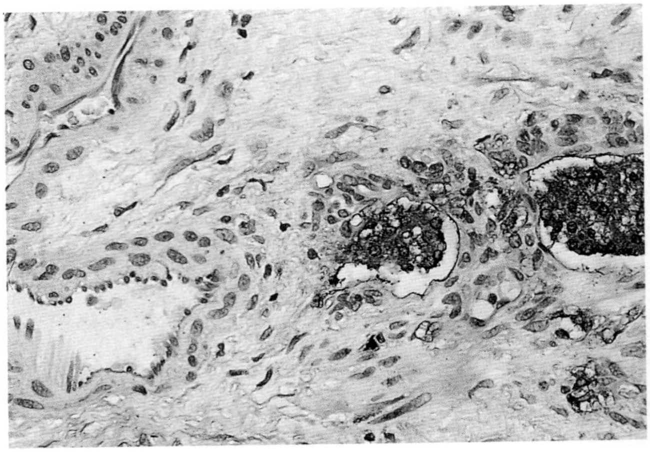

B

**FIG. 20.** Nests of paraganglia within the bladder wall. **A:** The cells are small, have vesicular nuclei and clear cytoplasm, and are seen adjacent to neural or vascular structures. They should not be confused with invasive carcinoma. **B:** Immunostain for chromogranin A can clarify the issue.

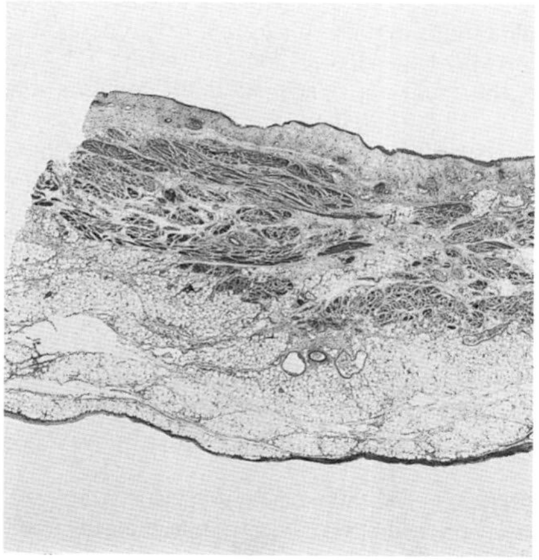

A

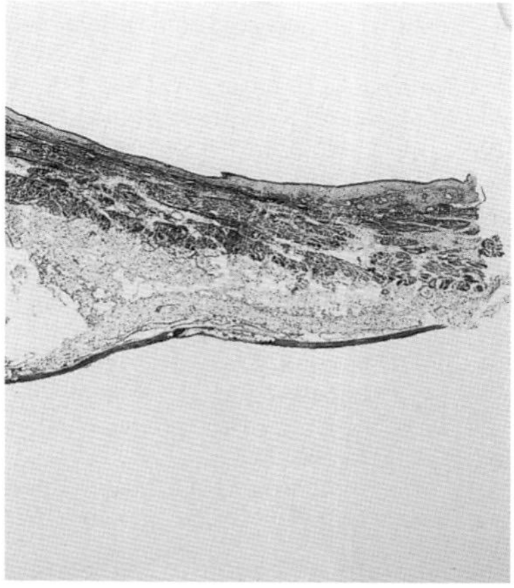

B

**FIG. 21.** Full-thickness section of the bladder. **A:** Notice the irregular thickness of the lamina propria. The three layers of muscle comprising the muscularis propria cannot be clearly defined. In contradistinction to the muscularis propria of the gut in the bladder, there are ample amounts of soft tissue between muscle bundles. **B:** Cross section of distended bladder. The overall thickness of the viscus is diminished as compared with the contracted bladder (4A). Both the lamina propria and muscularis propria become more condensed.

Similar to other layers, the thickness of the muscularis propria varies from patient to patient, with age, and with the degree of distention (Fig. 21A, B). In fact, Jequier et al. (56) performed sonographic measurements of the bladder wall thickness in 410 urologically normal children and 10 adults. They found that the bladder wall thickness varied mostly with the state of bladder filling and only minimally with age and gender. The bladder wall had a mean thickness of 2.76 mm when empty and 1.55 mm when distended.

For staging purposes, the muscularis propria has been divided into two segments, superficial and deep (T2 and T3a, respectively) (Fig. 6). No anatomical landmarks can be used to make this distinction so that it must be done by measuring the thickness of the muscle layer.

Bladder diverticula are relatively common, yet their etiology remains controversial. Most investigators agree that they occur secondary to increased intravesical pressure as a result of obstruction distal to the diverticulum (57–59). The obstruction brings about compensatory muscle hypertrophy and eventual mucosal herniation in areas of weakness. Others feel that at least some diverticula are a consequence of congenital defects in the bladder musculature, citing as evidence cases of diverticula in young patients without evidence of obstruction (59–61). The most common sites of diverticula are (a) adjacent to the ureteral orifices, (b) the bladder dome (probably related to a urachal remnant), and (c) the region of the internal urethral orifice. Grossly, one sees distortion of the external surface of the bladder. The diverticula may be widely patent but are usually narrow in symptomatic patients. The mucosa adjoining the diverticulum is usually hyperemic or ulcerated. There may be epithelial hyperplasia and hypertrophy of the muscularis propria. Commonly inflammation involves the lamina propria and muscularis. The wall of the diverticulum itself consists of urothelium and underlying connective tissue, similar to the bladder mucosa with lamina propria (Fig. 22). Few, if any, muscle fascicles are identified in the majority of cases of acquired diverticula. The true congenital diverticulum contains a thinned outer muscle layer. Infrequently the epithelium lining the sac undergoes squamous or glandular metaplasia due to local irritation associated with urine stasis, infection, or stone. In these cases it is not unusual for the diverticular wall to become extensively fibrotic.

Major complications of bladder diverticula include infection, lithiasis, and carcinoma. It is believed that 2% to 7% of patients with bladder diverticula develop an associated neoplasm, presumed secondary to the chronic inflammatory stimuli mentioned above (62,63). Ureteral diverticula are rare, and asymptomatic if uncomplicated (64). They are not seen in the renal pelvis.

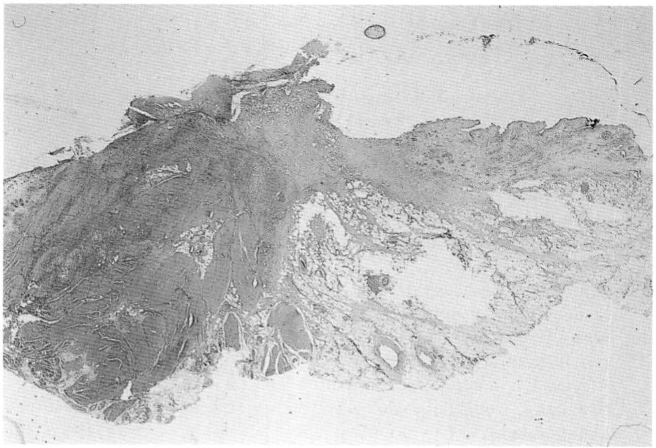

**FIG. 22.** Bladder diverticulum. To the left is the inflamed but anatomically normal bladder wall, whereas in the center and to the right one sees total absence of the muscularis propria. Perivesicular soft tissue comes in contact with the inflamed, fibrotic, and thickened lamina propria.

## REFERENCES


1. Moore KL. The urinary and genital systems. *The developing human*. 3rd ed. Philadelphia: WB Saunders; 1982:256–270.
2. Kissane JM. Development and structure of the urogenital system. In: Murphy WM, ed. *Urological pathology*. 1st ed. Philadelphia: WB Saunders; 1989:12–16.
3. Moore KL. The perineum and pelvis. *Clinically oriented anatomy*. 2nd ed. Baltimore: Williams & Wilkins; 1985:298–387.
4. Tanagho EA. Anatomy of the lower urinary tract. In: Walsh PC, Gittes RF, Perlmutter AD, Stamey TA, eds. *Campbell's urology*. 5th ed. Philadelphia: WB Saunders; 1986:46–58.
5. Mahadevia PA, Koss LG, Tar IJ. Prostatic involvement in bladder cancer: prostate mapping in 20 cystoprostatectomy specimens. *Cancer* 1986;58:2096–2102.
6. Utz DC, Farrow GM, Rife CC, et al. Carcinoma in situ of the bladder. *Cancer* 1980;45:1842–1848.
7. Ro JY, Ayala AG, el-Naggar A, Wishnow KI. Seminal vesicle involvement by in situ and invasive transitional cell carcinoma of the bladder. *Am J Surg Pathol* 1987;11:951–958.
8. Tanagho EA, Smith DR, Neyers FH. The trigone: anatomical and physiological considerations. 2. In relation to the bladder neck. *J Urol* 1968; 100:633–639.
9. Tanagho EA, Meyers FH, Smith DR. The trigone: anatomical and physiological considerations. 1. In relation to the ureterovesical junction. *J Urol* 1968;100:623–632.
10. Shehata R. A comparative study of the urinary bladder and the intramural portion of the ureter. *Acta Anat* 1977;98:380–395.
11. Politano VA. Ureterovesical junction. *J Urol* 1972;107:239–242.
12. Elbadawi A. Anatomy and function of the ureteral sheath. *J Urol* 1972; 107:224–279.
13. Tanagho EA, Smith DR. The anatomy and function of the bladder neck. *Br J Urol* 1966;38:54–71.
14. Bulger RE. The urinary system. Weiss L, ed. In: *Cell and tissue biology*. 6th ed. Baltimore: Urban & Schwarzenberg; 1988:844–848.
15. Fletcher TF, Bradley WE. Neuroanatomy of the bladder–urethra. *J Urol* 1978;119:153–160.
16. Olson CA. Anatomy of the upper urinary tract. In: Walsh PC, Gittes RF, Perlmutter AD, Stamey TA, eds. *Campbell's urology*. 5th ed. Philadelphia: WB Saunders; 1986:26–45.
17. Hanna MK, Jeffs RD, Sturgess JM, Barkin M. Ureteral structure and ultrastructure. Part I. The normal human ureter. *J Urol* 1976;116: 718–724.
18. Kaye KW, Goldberg ME. Applied anatomy of the kidney and ureter. *Urol Clin North Am* 1982;9:3–13.
19. Motola JA, Shahon RS, Smith AD. Anatomy of the ureter. *Urol Clin North Am* 1988;15:295–299.
20. Notley RG. Ureteral morphology: anatomic and clinical consideration. *Urology* 1978;12:8–14.
21. Crelin ES. Normal and abnormal development of the ureter. *Urology* 1978;12:2–7.
22. Koss LG. Tumors of the urinary bladder. In: *Atlas of tumor pathology*. Fascicle II, 2nd series. Washington, DC: Armed Forces Institute of Pathology; 1985.
23. Fawcett DW. The urinary system. In: *A textbook of histology*. 12th ed. Philadelphia: WB Saunders; 1994:758–764.
24. Hicks RM. The function of the golgi complex in transitional epithelium. Synthesis of the thick cell membrane. *J Cell Biol* 1966;30: 623–643.
25. Battifora H, Eisenstein R, McDonald JH. The urinary bladder mucosa. An electron microscopic study. *Invest Urol* 1964;1:354–361.
26. Koss LG. The asymmetric unit membranes of the epithelium of the urinary bladder of the rat. An electron microscopic study of a mechanism of epithelial maturation and function. *Lab Invest* 1969;21:154–168.
27. Newman J, Antonakopoulos GN. The fine structure of the human fetal urinary bladder. Development and maturation. *J Anat* 1989;166: 135–150.
28. Alvoy J, Gould VE. Epithelial–stromal interface in normal and neoplastic human bladder epithelium. *Ultrastruct Pathol* 1980;1:201–210.
29. Koss LG. Mapping of the urinary bladder: its impact on the concepts of bladder cancer. *Hum Pathol* 1979;10:533–548.
30. Mostofi FK. Potentialities of bladder epithelium. *J Urol* 1954;71: 705–714.
31. Morse HD. The etiology and pathology of pyelitis cystica, ureteritis cystica, and cystitis cystica. *Am J Pathol* 1928;4:33–50.
32. Goldstein AMB, Fauer RB, Chinn M, Kaempf MJ. New concepts on formation of Brunn's nests and cysts in the urinary tract mucosa. *Urology* 1978;11:513–517.
33. Weiner DP, Koss LG, Sablay B, Freed SZ. The prevalence and significance of Brunn's nests, cystitis cystica, and squamous metaplasia in normal bladders. *J Urol* 1979;122:317–321.
34. Edwards PD, Hurm RA, Jaeschke WH. Conversion of cystitis glandularis to adenocarcinoma. *J Urol* 1972;108:568–580.
35. Lin JI, Tseng CH, Choy C, Yong HS, Marsidi PS, Pilloff B. Diffuse cystitis glandularis associated with adenocarcinomatous change. *Urology* 1980;15:411–415.
36. Tannenbaum M. Inflammatory proliferative lesion of the urinary bladder: squamous metaplasia. *Urology* 1976;7:428–429.
37. Engel RM, Wilkinson HA. Bladder exstrophy. *J Urol* 1970;104: 699–704.
38. Nielsen K, Nielson KK. Adenocarcinoma in exstrophy of the bladder—the last case in Scandinavia? A case report and review of literature. *J Urol* 1983;130:1180–1182.
39. Bagharan BS, Tiamson EM, Wenk RE, Berger BW, Hamamoto G, Eggleston JC. Nephrogenic adenoma of the urinary bladder and urethra. *Hum Pathol* 1981;12:907–916.
40. Navarre RJ, Loening SA, Narayana A, Culp DA. Nephrogenic adenoma: a report of nine cases and review of the literature. *J Urol* 1982; 127:775–779.
41. Molland EA, Trott PA, Paris MI, Blandy JP. Nephrogenic adenoma: a form of adenomatous metaplasia of the bladder. A clinical and electron microscopical study. *Br J Urol* 1976;48:453–462.
42. Ford TF, Watson GM, Cameron KM. Adenomatous metaplasia (nephrogenic adenoma) of urothelium: an analysis of 70 cases. *Br J Urol* 1985;57:427–433.
43. Satodate R, Koike H, Sasou S, Ohori T, Nagare Y. Nephrogenic adenoma of the ureter. *J Urol* 1984;131:332–334.
44. DeMeester LT, Farrow GH, Utz DS. Inverted papilloma of the urinary bladder. *Cancer* 1975;36:505–513.
45. Henderson DW, Allen PW, Bourne AJ. Inverted urinary papilloma—report of five cases and review of the literature. *Virchows Arch [A]* 1975;336:177–186.
46. Caro DJ, Tessler A. Inverted papilloma of the bladder: a distinct urological lesion. *Cancer* 1978;42:708–713.
47. Anderstrom C, Johansson S, Pettersson S. Inverted papilloma of the urinary tract. *J Urol* 1982;127:1132–1134.
48. Lazarevic B, Garret R. Inverted papilloma and papillary transitional cell carcinoma of the urinary bladder: report of four cases of inverted papilloma, one showing papillary malignant transformation and review of the literature. *Cancer* 1978;42:1904–1911.
49. Whitesel JA. Inverted papilloma of the urinary tract: malignant potential. *J Urol* 1982;127:539–540.
50. Stein BS, Rosen S, Kendall R. The association of inverted papilloma and transitional cell carcinoma of the urothelium. *J Urol* 1984;131: 751–752.
51. Assor D. Inverted papilloma of the renal pelvis. *J Urol* 1976;116:654.
52. Lausten GS, Anagnostaki L, Thomsen OF. Inverted papilloma of the upper urinary tract. *Eur Urol* 1984;10:67–70.
53. Dixon JS, Gosling JA. Histology and fine structure of the muscularis mucosae of the human urinary bladder. *J Anat* 1983;136:265–271.
54. Ro JY, Ayala AG, El-Naggar A. Muscularis mucosa of urinary bladder: importance for staging and treatment. *Am J Surg Pathol* 1987;11: 668–673.
55. Notley RG. The musculature of the human ureter. *Br J Urol* 1970;40: 724–727.
56. Jequier S, Rousseau O. Sonographic measurements of the normal bladder wall in children. *AJR* 1987;149:563–566.
57. Miller A. The aetiology and treatment of diverticulum of the bladder. *Br J Urol* 1958;30:43–56.
58. Kertschmer HL. Diverticula of the urinary bladder. A clinical study of 236 cases. *Surg Gynecol Obstet* 1940;71:491–503.
59. Fox, M, Power RF, Bruce AW. Diverticulum of the bladder. Presentation and evaluation of treatment of 115 cases. *Br J Urol* 1962;34: 286–298.
60. Schiff M, Lytton B. Congenital diverticulum of the bladder. *J Urol* 1970;104:111–115.
61. Barrett DW, Malek RS, Kelalis PP. Observations on vesical diverticulum in childhood. *J Urol* 1976;116:234–236.

62. Abeshouse BS, Goldstein AE. Primary carcinoma in a diverticulum of the bladder. A report of four cases and a review of the literature. *J Urol* 1943;49:534–547.
63. Faysal MH, Freiha FS. Primary neoplasia in vesical diverticula: a report of 12 cases. *Br J Urol* 1978;53:141–143.
64. Corchran ST, Waisman J, Barbaric ZL. Radiographic and microscopic findings in multiple ureteral diverticula. *Diagn Radiol* 1980;137: 631–636.
65. Reuter VE, Melamed MR. The lower urinary tract. In: Sternberg S, Antonioli DA, Carter D, eds. *Diagnostic surgical pathology*. 2nd ed. Philadelphia: Lippincott–Raven; 1996:1768.

# Female Genital System

*Histology for Pathologists, second edition,*
Edited by Stephen S. Sternberg.
Lippincott-Raven Publishers, Philadelphia


# CHAPTER 37

# Vulva

Edward J. Wilkinson and Nancy S. Hardt



## CLINICAL PERSPECTIVE

Vulvar symptoms are a common cause of clinical visits to gynecologists and family practitioners. Complaints may include pruritis, burning, external dyspareunia, and a visible or palpable mass (1,2). The majority of sexually transmitted diseases, as well as many granulomatous and dermatologic diseases, may involve the vulva (2–4). The vulva (pudendum femininum) is also a crucial area for examination in cases of reported rape or sexual abuse. Ambiguous genitalia or genital anomalies challenge the clinician and demand critical examination of the patient and the external genitalia. Clitoral enlargement in the newborn resulting from adrenal genital syndrome, maternal exposure to exogenous androgens, maldevelopment of the clitoris, benign tumors, and other conditions, such as the Lawrence-Seip syndrome (3,5,6), may result in ambiguous-appearing external genitalia.

## SPECIAL TECHNIQUES IN CLINICAL EVALUATION

Examination of the vulva requires adequate illumination and is enhanced by the use of a ring light or magnifying glass (7). The use of higher magnification, using a colposcope, enhances the identification of small condyloma acuminatum, vestibular papillae, and vulvar intraepithelial neoplasia. In cases in which condyloma acuminatum or vulvar intraepithelial neoplasia is suspected, the use of 3% acetic acid (white vinegar) is of value. Gauze sponges soaked in acetic acid are applied for approximately 5 minutes, followed by prompt examination (8). The principle of this technique is that abnormal epithelium, especially condyloma acuminatum and vulvar intraepithelial neoplasia, becomes white immediately after exposure to acetic acid. This is related to poorly understood differences between normal epithelium and human papillomavirus–associated lesions. The color change to white after the dilute acetic acid is referred to as aceto-whitening, and the epithelium so changed is referred to as aceto-white epithelium. This procedure has gained wide acceptance in the evaluation of the cervical transformation zone during colposcopic examination to enhance identification of cervical intraepithelial neoplasia and carcinoma. However, its use on the vulva has two serious limitations. First, when ulcers or fissures are present on the vulva, the application of 3% acetic acid may be associated with pain and thus is unacceptable to the patient. Second, the vulvar vestibular epithelium is normally somewhat aceto-white. The inexperienced clinician may misinterpret this aceto-whitening as abnormal or as condyloma acuminatum. A biopsy is then performed of the vestibular epithelium and submitted as condyloma acuminatum. The vestibular epithelium in women of reproductive age is normally glycogenated (see section on Vulvar Vestibule) and can be misinterpreted by the unwary pathologist as koilocytosis suggestive of

E. J. Wilkinson: Section of Surgical Pathology, Department of Pathology and Laboratory Medicine, College of Medicine, University of Florida, Gainesville, Florida 32610.
N. S. Hardt: Department of Pathology and Laboratory Medicine, College of Medicine, University of Florida, Gainesville, Florida 32610.

condyloma acuminatum, resulting in both improper diagnosis and improper therapy for the patient. Inflammation within the vestibule may be associated with epithelial spongiosis, which also may be confused with koilocytosis.

The use of 1% toluidine blue O also has been used to assist in the recognition of areas requiring biopsy when invasive carcinoma is suspected (7). A solution of 1% toluidine blue O is applied to the areas in question, which then are rinsed with 1% acetic acid. Areas with ulceration, parakeratosis, and carcinomas without a keratinized surface retain the blue stain. In principle, toluidine blue O is a DNA stain, and as such it is retained where cell nuclei are present (3,7). This test has limited usefulness in that false-positive staining patterns occur, usually due to benign superficial ulceration or fissures. The test may be falsely negative when the carcinoma or intraepithelial neoplasm has a keratinized surface.

From the pathologist's perspective, the majority of vulvar specimens that are examined are either diagnostic biopsies, excisional biopsies, or partial or total vulvectomy specimens submitted as treatment for vulvar intraepithelial neoplasia, Paget's disease, carcinoma, melanoma, and other diseases (3). An understanding of the normal histology of the vulva enhances interpretive skills and prevents inappropriate diagnosis.

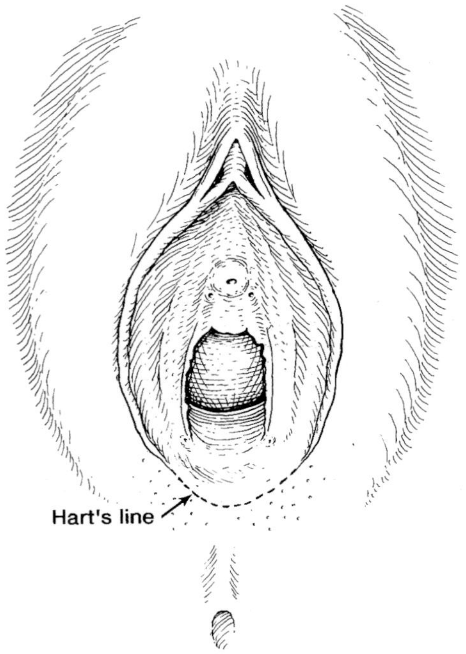


**FIG. 2.** The vulvar vestibule and the position of Hart's line. Hart's line can be found on the medial aspect of the labia majora, extending in a curvilinear manner from the most inferior posterior portion of the labia minora to the vaginal fourchette.

## ANATOMY

The female external genitalia can be defined as that portion of the female anatomy external to the hymen, extending anteriorly to include the mons pubis, posteriorly to the anus, and laterally to the inguinal–gluteal folds. Included are the mons pubis, clitoris, labia minora, labia majora, vulvar vestibule and vestibulovaginal bulbs, urethral meatus, hymen, Bartholin's and Skene's glands and ducts, and vaginal introitus (Fig. 1). The anterior investment of the clitoris includes the prepuce, which represents the anterior fusion of the labia minora and overlays the clitoris anteriorly, and the frenulum, which passes posteriorly and ends in its attachment to the flattened posterior aspect of the clitoris. Posteriorly, the labia minora end in the fourchette, or frenulum of the labia. The labia majora lie lateral to the intralabial sulcus and medial to the inguinal–gluteal fold. Anteriorly, the hair-bearing lateral aspects of the labia majora blend with the mons pubis, and posteriorly, the labia majora end in the perineal body. The hair follicles of the labia majora are absent in its medial portion; however, the sebaceous gland elements are retained medial and posterior to the labia minora at the junction with the vulvar vestibule at Hart's line (9,10) (Fig. 2). These sebaceous gland elements open directly to the epithelial surface in this portion of the vulva and can be observed as small, slightly pale to yellow elevations of the epithelium, known as Fordyce spots.

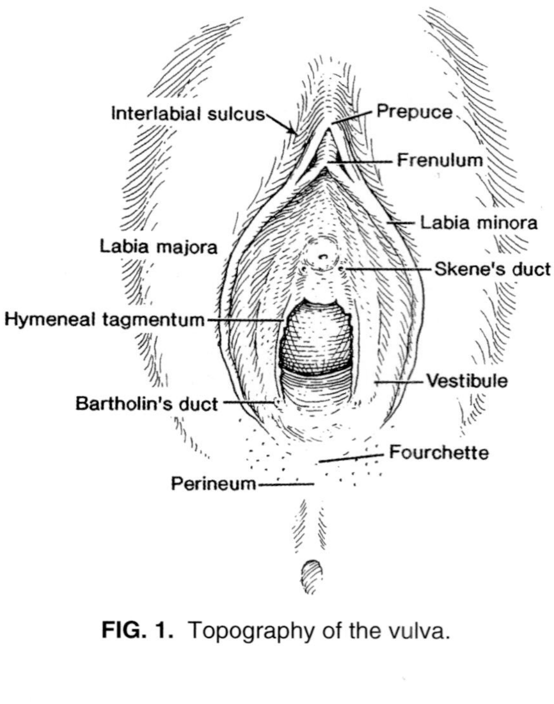


**FIG. 1.** Topography of the vulva.

The vulvar epithelium, especially that of the lateral labia minora, labia majora, and perineal body, contains melanocytes that are distributed among the basal cells of the epithelium in a ratio from 1:5 to 1:10 basal keratinocytes (11). Increased pigmentation of these areas during pregnancy relate to increased melanin production secondary to the effects of gestational hormones.

Langerhans cells are present in the suprabasal layers of vulvar epithelium in a ratio of approximately 18.7 Langerhans cells per 100 squamous cells (12). In the vulva, Langerhans cells are present in keratinized and nonkeratinized epithelia as well as within skin appendages. These cells are of bone marrow derivation and are associated with immunity through activation of T-lymphocytes (13) and also are believed to be associated with control of keratinocytic maturation (14).

Merkel cells are neuroendocrine cells that are present in vulvar epithelium as well as most other skin sites. These cells are involved in paracrine regulation of skin function (15). Merkel cell tumors of the vulva have been reported (16).

Lymphocytes are also commonly found in the dermis and submucosal areas of the vulva in small numbers, located pri-

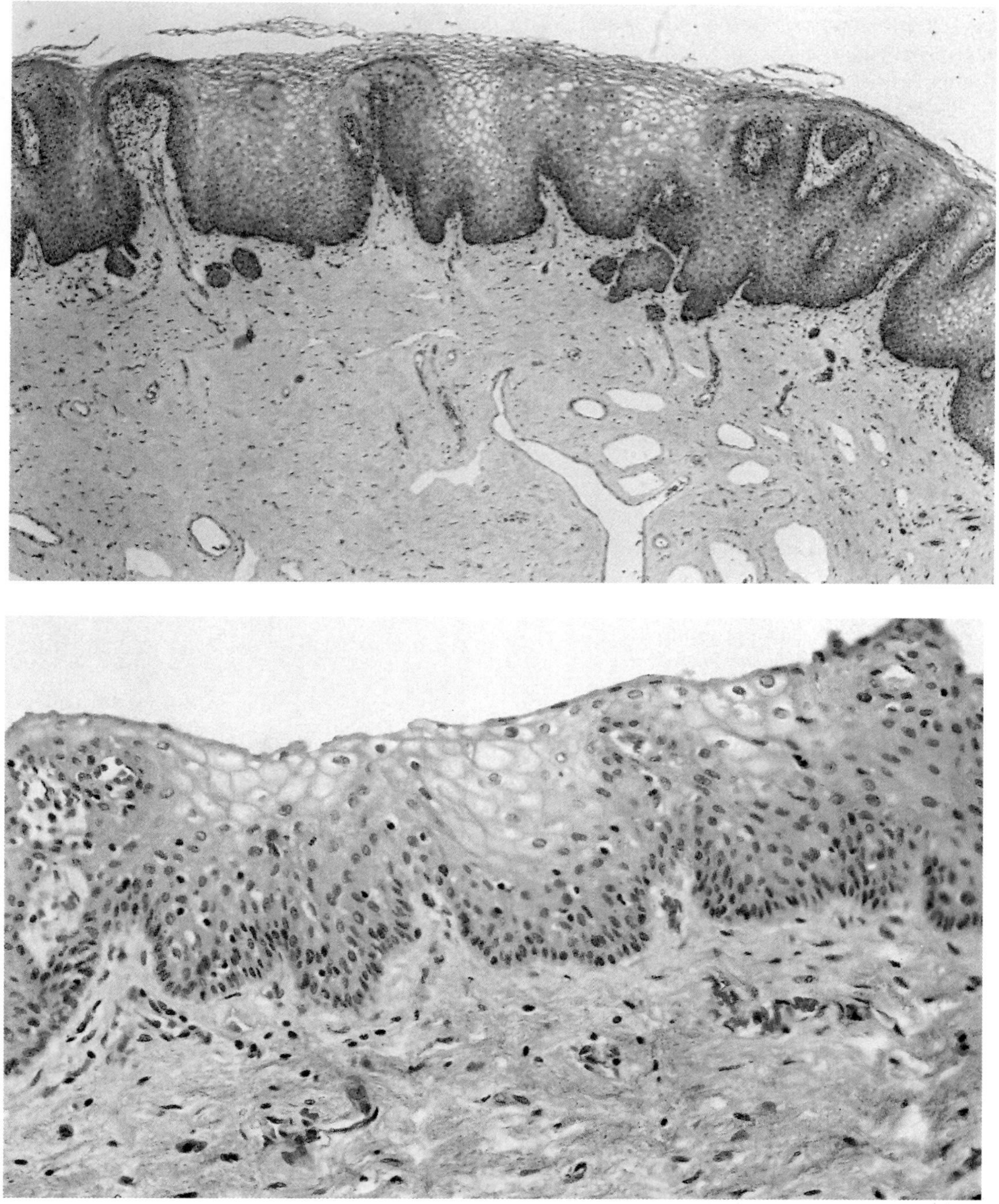

A

B

**FIG. 3. A:** Vulvar vestibule with adjacent prominent vascular submucosa. Superficial thin-walled vessels are prominent and are found within the delicate fibrous stroma. A few lymphocytes are seen scattered in the superficial submucosa. **B:** Epithelium of the vulvar vestibule of a 27-year-old woman. Note that the epithelium is stratified squamous and that the superficial cells have cytoplasmic clearing, reflecting the glycogen-rich epithelium.

marily in a perivascular area within the superficial tissues. Intraepithelial lymphocytes are infrequently seen in normal vulvar epithelium (12).

### Vulvar Vestibule

The vulvar vestibule is defined as that portion of the vulva that extends from the exterior surface of the hymen to the frenulum of the clitoris anteriorly, the fourchette posteriorly, anterolaterally to the labia minora, and posterolaterally to Hart's line, on the medial aspects of the labia majora (Figs. 1 and 2). The vestibular fossa (fossa navicularis) is that posterior portion of the vestibule, from the hymen to the fourchette, that is somewhat concave as compared with the remainder of the vestibule. Unlike the remainder of the vulvar epithelium, which is of ectodermal origin, the epithelium of the vulvar vestibule is of endodermal origin. One exception is the portion of the vulvar vestibular epithelium anterior to the urethra, which some think is of ectodermal origin (17). The vulvar vestibule is predominantly nonkeratinized stratified squamous epithelium, which peripherally blends with the thinly keratinized squamous epithelium of the labia minora, the medial labia majora at Hart's line, the prepuce, and the fourchette. Although the vestibular epithelium has an embryonic origin similar to that of the distal urethra of the male, the epithelium is not of a typical transitional type with associated surface umbrella cells. Rather, it is a stratified squamous epithelium that is rich in glycogen in women of reproductive age, similar to the mucosa of the vagina and ectocervix (Fig. 3).

Both the vaginal opening and the urethral orifice are within the vestibule. Also within the vulvar vestibule are gland openings from both the major and minor vestibular glands, as well as the paired opening of the periurethral Skene's ducts. Skene's ducts are the homologues of the male prostate gland. The major vestibular gland, or Bartholin's gland (glandula vestibularis major), is of ectodermal origin and consists of bilateral tubuloalveolar glands located beneath the hymen, labia minora, and labia majora in the posterior lateral area of the vulva. Bartholin's gland corresponds to the male bulbourethral glands, or Cowper's glands. The epithelial cells of Bartholin's gland acini consist of mucus-secreting columnar cells (18,19) (Fig. 4). The secretion of these acini empty into Bartholin's duct, which measures approximately 2.5 cm in length and enters the vestibule immediately exterior (distal) and adjacent to the hymen in a posterolateral location. Bartholin's duct is lined by transitional epithelium that is adjacent to columnar epithelium as it arises from the gland (Fig. 5) to adjoin the nonkeratinized stratified squamous epithelium of the vulvar vestibule in the distal end of the duct (19) (Fig. 6). Within the Bartholin duct epithelium, argentaffin cells also can be identified, predominantly concentrated within the transitional epithelial cell area and

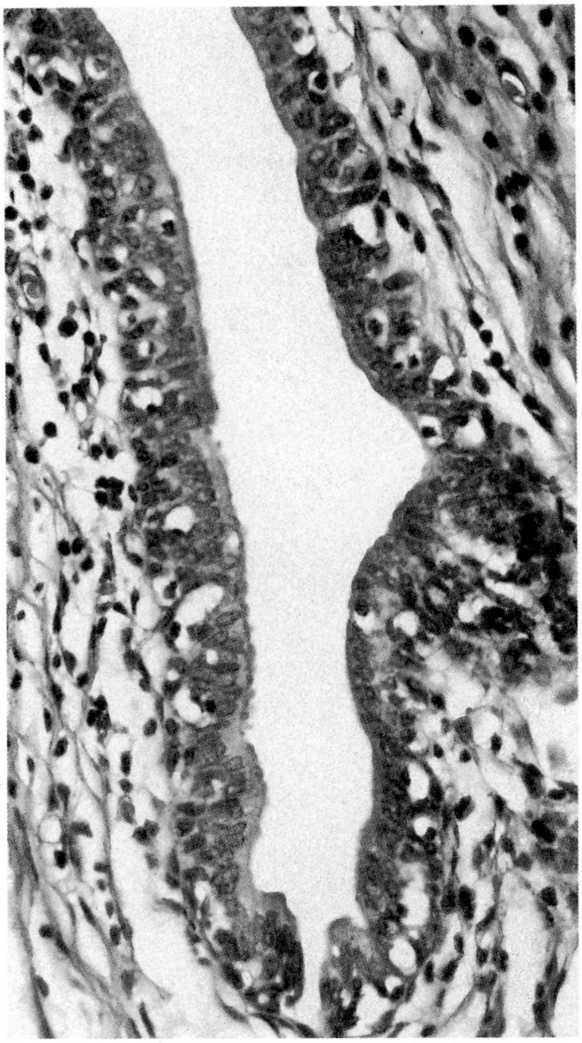

**FIG. 5.** Bartholin's duct near the gland. Bartholin's duct has a transitional-like epithelial lining, with columnar cells near the surface, similar to the columnar cells lining the gland acini.

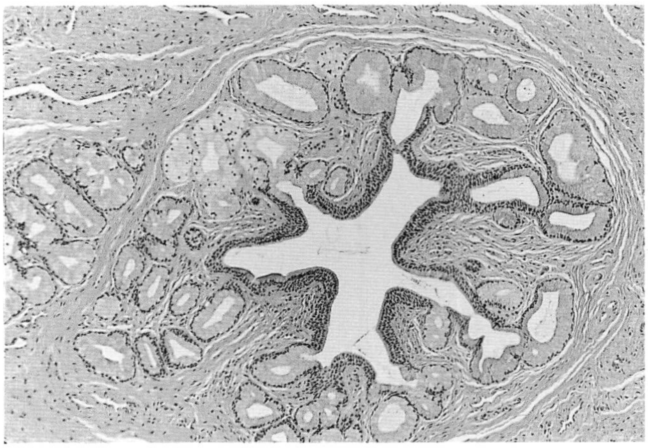

**FIG. 4.** Bartholin's gland acini are lined with a columnar epithelium. The adjacent branching Bartholin's duct is present adjacent to the gland.

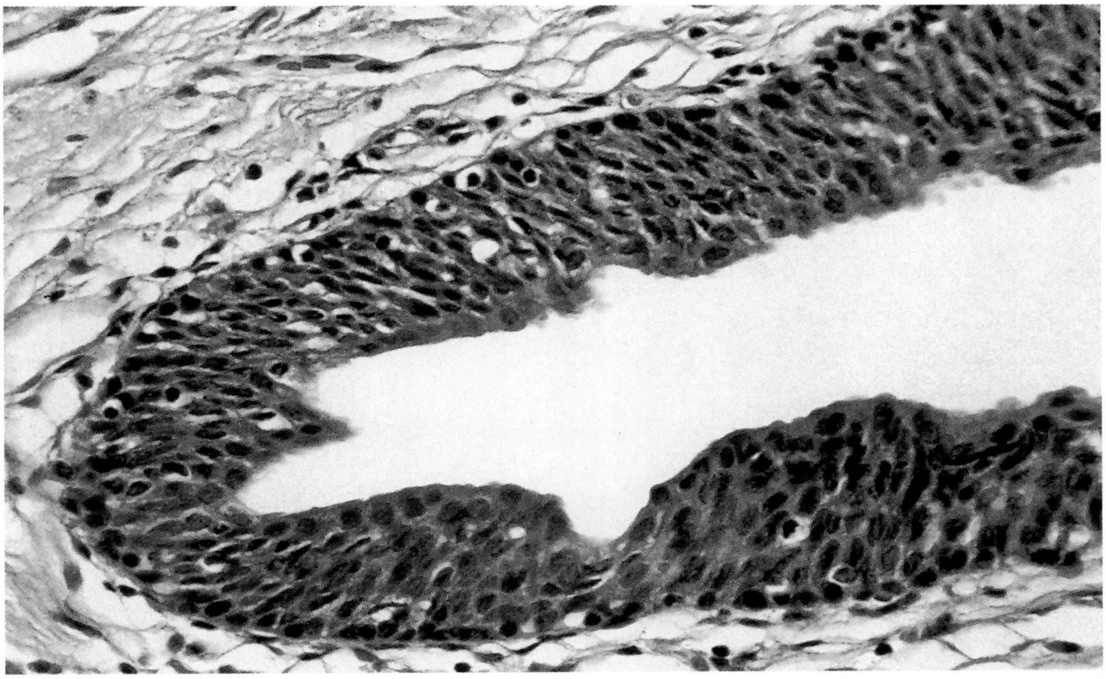

**FIG. 6.** Bartholin's duct near its exit to the vulvar vestibule. At this location the duct is lined by stratified squamous epithelium, without surface columnar cells.

absent in the gland area (20). Cysts that arise in the area of Bartholin's gland are primarily a result of dilation of Bartholin's duct (3,21).

The periurethral, or Skene's, glands also enter the vulvar vestibule as paired gland openings found immediately adjacent to and posterolateral to the urethra. These glands, with their adjacent ducts, are generally not more than 1.5 cm in length. These periurethral glands are analogous to the male prostate gland and are lined with a pseudostratified mucus-secreting columnar epithelium. The ducts of Skene's glands are lined with transitional-type epithelium that joins with the stratified squamous epithelium of the vestibule at the gland orifices. A cyst of Skene's duct may result from obstruction of the duct.

The minor vestibular glands (glandulae vestibulare minores) consist of simple tubular glands that enter directly to the mucosal surface of the vestibule (Fig. 7). They are analogous to the glands of Littre of the male urethra (17). Minor vestibular glands are small and shallow, with a maximum depth of 2.27 mm (22). These glands are lined with a mucus-secreting columnar epithelium that merges with the stratified squamous epithelium of the vestibule (22–24). Robboy et al. (24) identified minor vestibular glands within the vestibule in 47% of women studied in an autopsy-related series. We found minor vestibular glands in vulvar vestibulectomy specimens for vestibulitis in 66% of our cases (22). In the women with identifiable minor vestibular glands, Robboy et al. (24) found that the number ranged from one to over 100, with the majority having two to 10 identifiable minor vestibular glands. Although these glands were found to be distributed throughout the vestibule, they were found in greater numbers in the posterior vestibule, just anterior to the fourchette. Minor vestibular glands have been described as having ducts composed of transitional epithelium; however, this epithelium is essentially the same epithelium and borders that of the adjacent vulvar vestibule, which is stratified squamous epithelium without surface umbrella cells. Minor vestibular glands may undergo squamous metaplasia, similar to that seen within the endocervix, where the mucus-secret-

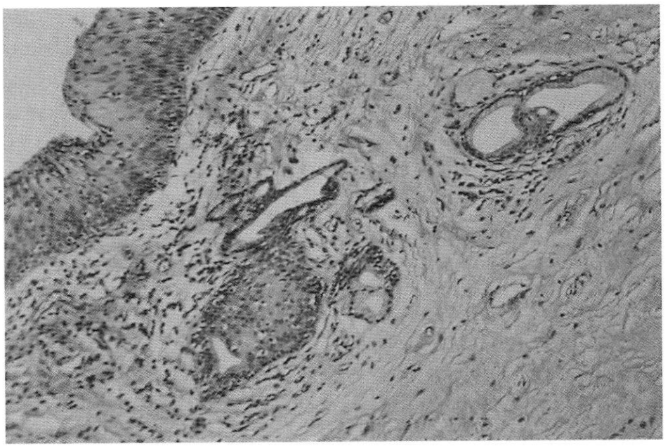

**FIG. 7.** Minor vestibular glands of the vulvar vestibule. The vulvar vestibular glands are simple glands with a mucus-secreting columnar epithelial lining. Near their exit at the vestibular surface the glands have a stratified squamous epithelium. Vascular vestibular stroma surrounds the superficial gland elements.

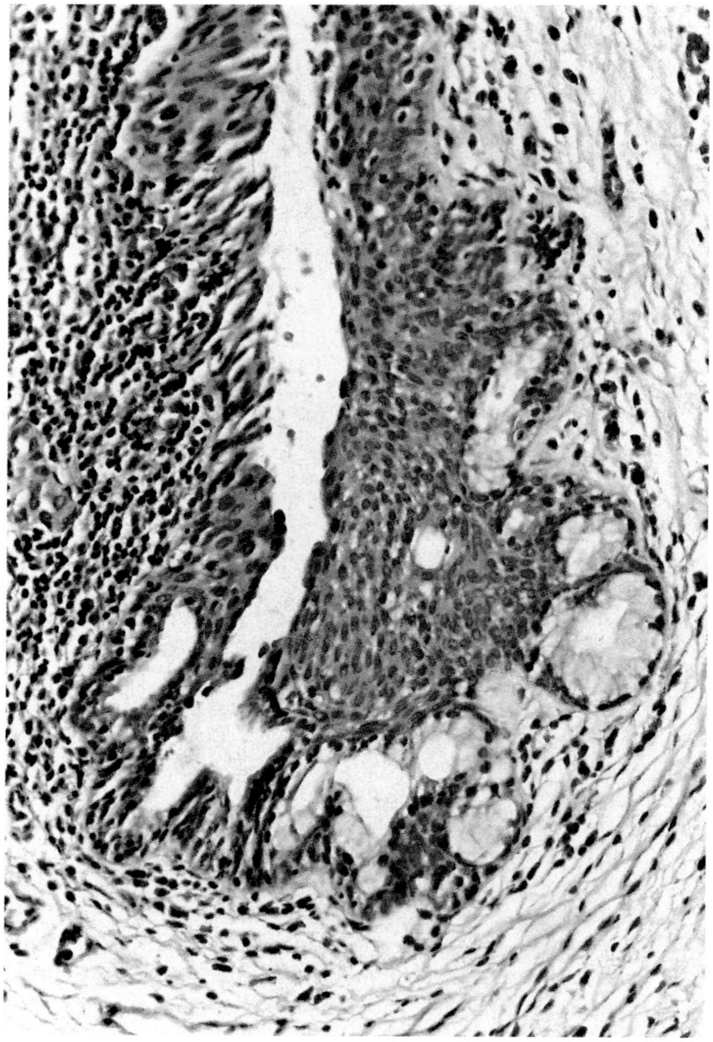

**FIG. 8.** Vestibular gland with squamous metaplasia near the vestibular surface. Moderate chronic inflammation, consisting predominantly of lymphocytes, is seen adjacent to the gland, consistent with vulvar vestibulitis.

ing epithelial cells lining the glandular epithelium are replaced by stratified squamous epithelium (Fig. 8). This metaplastic epithelium may completely replace the glandular epithelium, resulting in the formation of a vestibular cleft (22) (Fig. 9). Obstruction of a minor vestibular gland associated with this metaplastic process may result in accumulation of mucous secretion within the simple tubular gland, leading to the formation of a vulvar mucous cyst (22–24). Vestibular adenomas have been described arising from these minor vestibular glands (25,26). Severe external dyspareunia may be associated with inflammation of the vulvar vestibule, a poorly understood condition referred to as vulvar vestibulitis (1,22,27).

### Urethral Orifice (Meatus Urinarius)

The urethra has a transitional epithelial lining that merges with the stratified squamous epithelium at the urethral orifice. The periurethral glands of Huffman enter into the urethra throughout most of its length (28). Obstruction or inflammation of these periurethral glands may result in a urethral diverticulum or periurethral abscess. Partial prolapse of the urethra results in a polypoid mass, often referred to as a urethral caruncle. The mucosa may become ulcerated, and the underlying stroma may become inflamed with vascular dilation and engorgement; however, it otherwise retains the normal histology of the urethra.

### Hymen

The hymen marks the distalmost extent of the vagina and the most proximal boundary of the vulvar vestibule. The hymen may be imperforate, round, annular, septate, cribriform, or porous (2). On the vaginal surface, the hymen has a nonkeratinized stratified squamous epithelium, which is glycogenated upon estrogen exposure, as seen in women of reproductive age, newborn female infants, and postmenopausal women receiving estrogen therapy. On the vul-

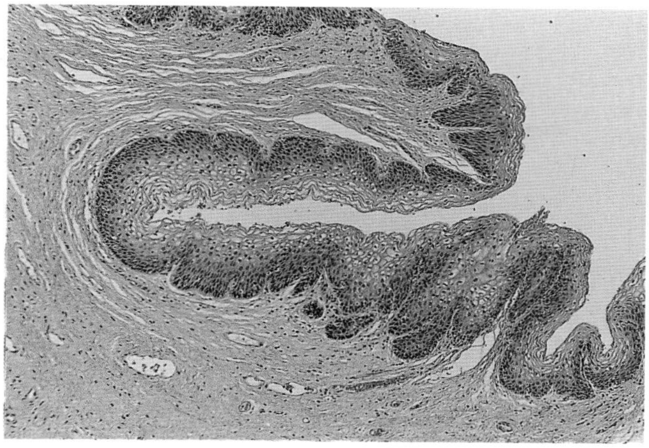

**FIG. 9.** Vulvar vestibular cleft. The vulvar vestibular cleft has a stratified squamous epithelial lining, similar to the vulvar vestibule. These clefts appear to arise as a result of squamous metaplasia of vestibular glands.

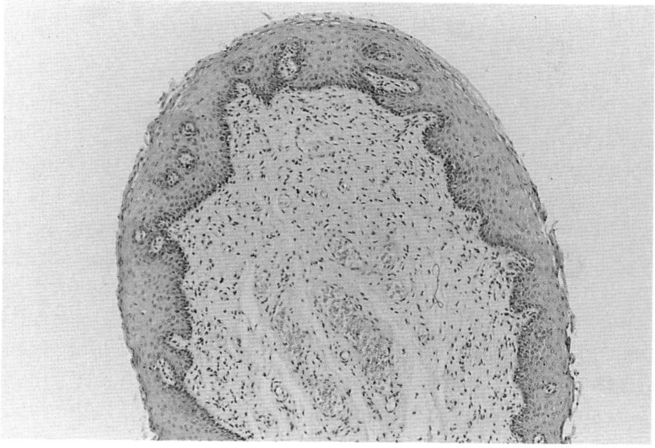

**FIG. 11.** Vulvar vestibular papillae. The papillae have a stratified squamous epithelial surface and fibrovascular stalks.

var surface the vestibular epithelium appears similar to the vaginal epithelium in women of reproductive age (Figs. 3 and 10).

The hymenal ring contains some Merkel tactile disks for touch and moderate numbers of free nerve endings, which are pain receptors; the hymenal ring lacks other receptors that are present in the labia majora (29,30).

In rare cases of imperforate hymen, the hymen lacks its normal opening. This leads to accumulation of menstrual exodus in the vagina, resulting in vaginal distension (1) with menstrual products, a condition referred to as hematocolpos. Coitus, or the routine use of intravaginal tampons, results in tears in the hymen, which result in small soft hymenal tags referred to as carunculae hymenales, or carunculae myrtiformes (13,31). On the external hymen and on the vulvar vestibule, small papillae may be identified, which are referred to as vestibular papillae. Multiple papillae are seen in the condition known as vestibular papillomatosis (32). Such papillae within the vestibule are infrequently associated with human papillomavirus. Solitary or isolated asymptomatic papillae on the hymen usually represent a normal anatomic variant (33) (Fig. 11).

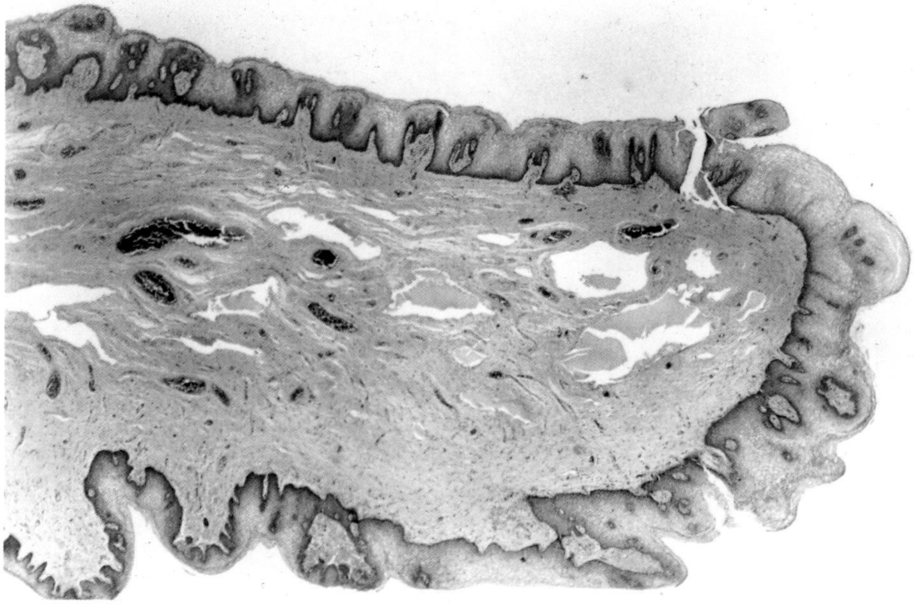

**FIG. 10.** Cross-section of the hymen of a 26-year-old woman. The epithelium of the vaginal (*upper*) as well as the vestibular (*lower*) surfaces of the hymen is a stratified squamous epithelium, which is nonkeratinized and glycogen rich. The fibrovascular component of the hymen supports the epithelium.

## Clitoris

The clitoris is the descendant of the embryonic phallus, homologous to the corpus cavernosum of the male penis. It is immediately anterior to the frenulum, at the junction of the labia minora, and it is enfolded by the prepuce. The clitoris measures approximately 2 cm in its long axis and consists of two crura and a glans clitoridis. The crura are composed of erectile tissue similar to that in the corpora cavernosa of the male (3,4). They consist of cavernous veins surrounded by longitudinal smooth muscle, as well as small centrally placed muscular arteries, enveloped by the tunica albuginea. The tunica albuginea is composed of wavy collagen fibers and straight elastic fibers. Peripheral to the tunica albuginea is the loose connective tissue that supports the nerves and receptors of this area. The glans clitoridis is covered with squamous mucosa without glands, retia, or papillae (18,30,34). The cavernous tissue of the corpus spongiosum of the male does not have its counterpart in the clitoris; it is found instead in the vascular erectile tissue of the labia minora (Fig. 12). The clitoris contains nerve endings in lesser amount than seen in the labia majora, although pacinian corpuscles are abundant. Peritrichous nerve endings for touch reception are absent. The other receptors are present, although their distribution is highly variable (30). Other touch receptors, namely, Meissner corpuscles and Merkel tactile disks, are present in reduced numbers in the clitoris, as compared with the labia majora or mons pubis. Pacinian corpuscles, for pressure reception, are present in large numbers (30). The free nerve endings for pain reception are found throughout the vulva and in relatively high concentrations in the clitoris, labia majora, and mons pubis (30). Ruffini and Dogiel-Krause corpuscles, which may be associated with temperature or sexual sensation, are found throughout the vulva, but not in the hymenal ring (30).

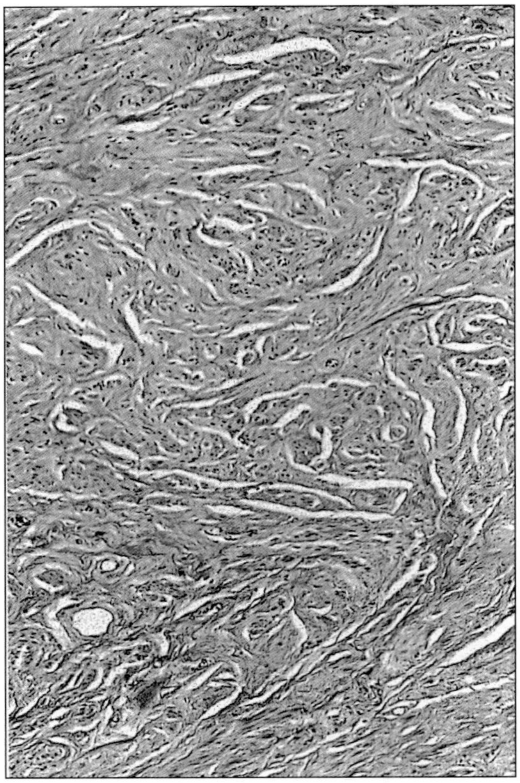

**FIG. 12.** Erectile tissue of the labia minora.

## Labia Minora

The bilateral labia minora derive from the embryonic medial folds (genital folds) and lie lateral to the vulvar vestibule and medial to the labia majora, bounded by the intralabial sulcus. The epithelium of the labia minora is of ectodermal origin. The labia minora have their male embryologic counterpart in the penile corpus spongiosum (13). The minora measure approximately 5 cm in length and 0.5 cm in thickness; however, their length can vary considerably. The epithelium of the labia minora is of the stratified squamous type and is not keratinized on its vestibular surface but has a thin keratin layer laterally. In many individuals the labia minora do not contain skin appendages; however, in some individuals the lateral labia minora contain both sweat and sebaceous glands (34). The epithelium of the labia minora may be somewhat pigmented, especially in lateral and posterior areas (Fig. 13). Beneath the epithelium is highly vascular, loose connective tissue, which is rich in elastic fibers. Posterior and deep to the labia minora are the vestibular bulbs (bulbi vestibuli), which are composed of erectile tissue and are invested by the bulbocavernous muscles. The labia minora contain erectile tissue and thus are highly vascular, yet they lack adipose tissue. The vessels and erectile tissue are supported by a rich elastic fiber component. The nerve endings within the labia majora are similar to those found within the clitoris, yet Meissner corpuscles and Merkel tactile disks occur in larger numbers than usually identified within the clitoris (30).

Congenital enlargement of the labia minora may occur and may be asymmetrical. Enlargement also may be secondary to irritation or minor trauma. Surgical reduction of the labia minora or local excision for therapeutic reasons does not appear to impede normal sexual function or response; however, excision of the labia minora for female circumcision has been associated with keratinous cysts of the vulva as well as sexual and urinary dysfunction (13,35).

## Labia Majora

The labia majora arise from the embryonic lateral folds (genital folds, labial folds), which arise lateral to the cloacal plate and do not fuse (17). The epithelium is ectodermally derived from the urogenital sinus. The endodermally derived epithelium of the vestibule joins with the ectodermally derived epithelium of the medial labial majora. This junction is apparently at Hart's line, where the epithelium of the medial (inner) labia majora joins the nonkeratinized squamous ep-

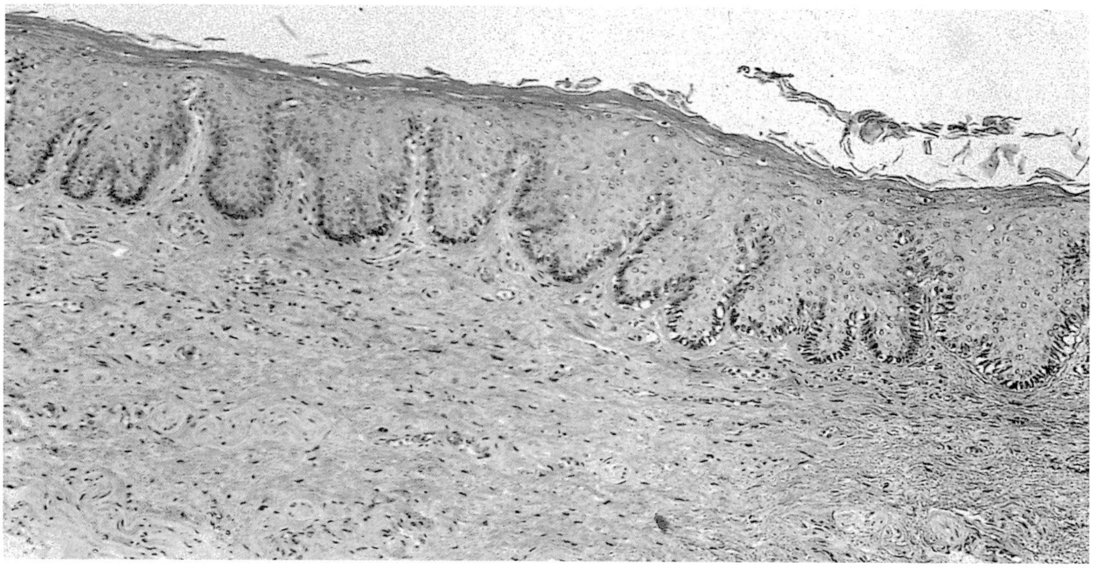

**FIG. 13.** Lateral labia minora biopsy from a 27-year-old white woman. Within this area, the labia minora contain no skin appendages. The epithelium is pigmented, and melanocytes and pigmented basal epithelial cells are seen in the basal layer. The stratified squamous epithelium has a thinly keratinized surface. Beneath the epithelium, there is an elastic fiber–rich stroma without fat or skin appendages. Moderate numbers of small vessels can be seen. Deeper tissue is demonstrated in Fig. 12.

ithelium of the vestibule (9,10). In the male the labial (scrotal) folds fuse to form the scrotum. This fusion usually occurs by 74 days of gestation (crown–rump length approximately 71 mm) (16). In the female, the labia majora merge with the mons pubis anteriorly and with the perineal body posteriorly. The labia majora lie immediately lateral and parallel to the labia minora, separated by the intralabial sulcus. In the medial posterior positions the labia majora are bounded by the vulvar vestibule. Laterally, they merge with the inguinal–gluteal folds, which separate the labia from the medial aspect of the thighs. Although minor asymmetry of the labia majora is considered to be normal, marked asymmetry may be early evidence of neurofibromatosis (36). Chronic inflammation, varicosities, edema, Bartholin's cysts, and benign or malignant tumors also may be associated with asymmetry of the labia majora.

### *Aging Changes*

The labia majora increase in size with puberty, primarily related to increased fat within the labia. In addition, there are dramatic changes in hair growth during puberty (see mons pubis discussion) (37). After menopause there is a progressive loss of hair follicles and consequent loss of labial hair (38) as well as shrinkage of the labia majora. This is primarily related to loss of fat within the labia (13). In addition to age-related changes, changes occur in the labia majora that are related to parity. During gestation, the influence of gestational hormones, especially progesterone, results in vascular dilation and stasis within the labia (30). These gestational changes may result in the development of vulvar venous varicosities (39).

Similar to other hair follicles, each follicle of the vulva has a hair root surrounded by the dermal root sheath, which invests the root sheath of the hair follicle. The inner root sheath is composed of an external clear epithelial cell layer (Henle's layer) and an inner granular epithelial cell layer (Huxley's layer). The hair matrix matures to the formed hair of the hair shaft, where the hair has an outer cuticle with a cortex and medulla. The hair papilla is found at the base of the hair root, protruding into and partially surrounded by the matrix of the hair. The papilla is supported by the dermal root sheath (18,34,40,41). Hair follicles are a portion of the pilosebaceous unit, which includes sebaceous glands.

In the labia majora, sebaceous glands can be found with and without associated hair follicles. The sebaceous glands are alveolar and arranged in a lobular manner, vested by collagen fibers. The cells of the sebaceous glands secrete in a holocrine manner, with the more mature cells accumulating sebaceous secretion (sebum) within their cytoplasm. The secretion is released as the cells undergo necrosis. The secretion may be released adjacent to the hair shaft in the pilosebaceous unit or directly to the surface when no hair shaft is present. There are two types of sweat gland: apocrine and merocrine (18,34,40,41). Apocrine glands are tubular and have a columnar secretory epithelium characterized by a

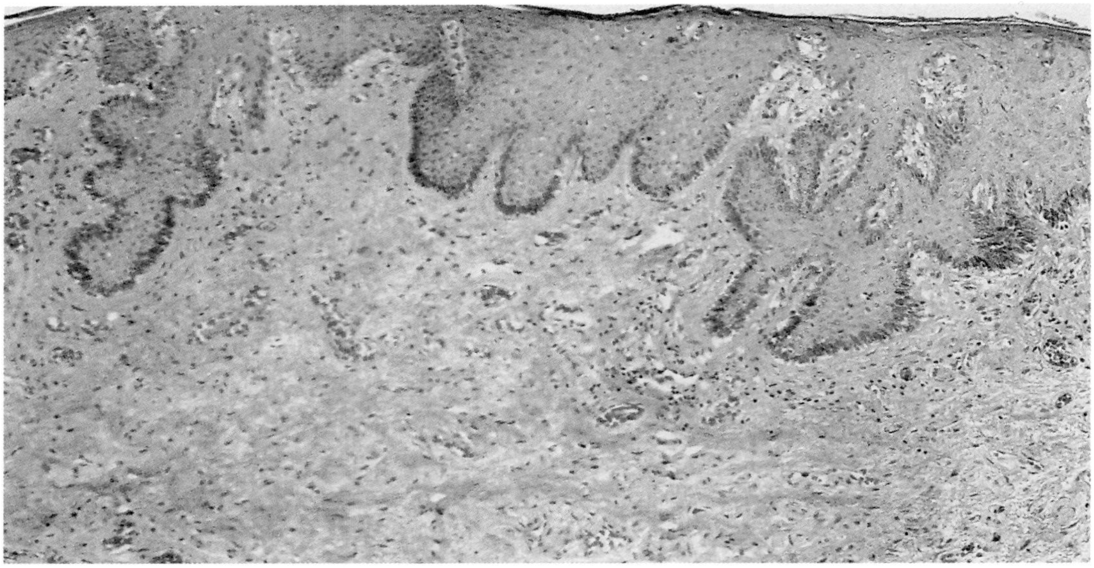

**FIG. 14.** Posterior medial labia majora of a 27-year-old white woman peripheral to Hart's line. This pigmented portion of the labia majora has a stratified squamous epithelium with a thin keratinized surface. The epithelium has deeper rete ridges than seen in the minora. The dermis is elastic fiber rich and moderately vascular. Sebaceous gland–bearing skin was immediately adjacent to this area and has a moderately vascular dermis.

prominent eosinophilic granular cytoplasm. These glands secrete by release of cytoplasmic secretion and are associated with scent production. The scent associated with these sudoriferous glands is related to bacterial growth supported by the secretory products (34,40). Beneath the epithelial layer, myoepithelial cells are identified. These myoepithelial cells are arranged about the periphery of the gland and their contraction promotes expression of the secretory contents from the gland lumen. The ducts of the apocrine glands are similar to those of the merocrine glands but may secrete into the

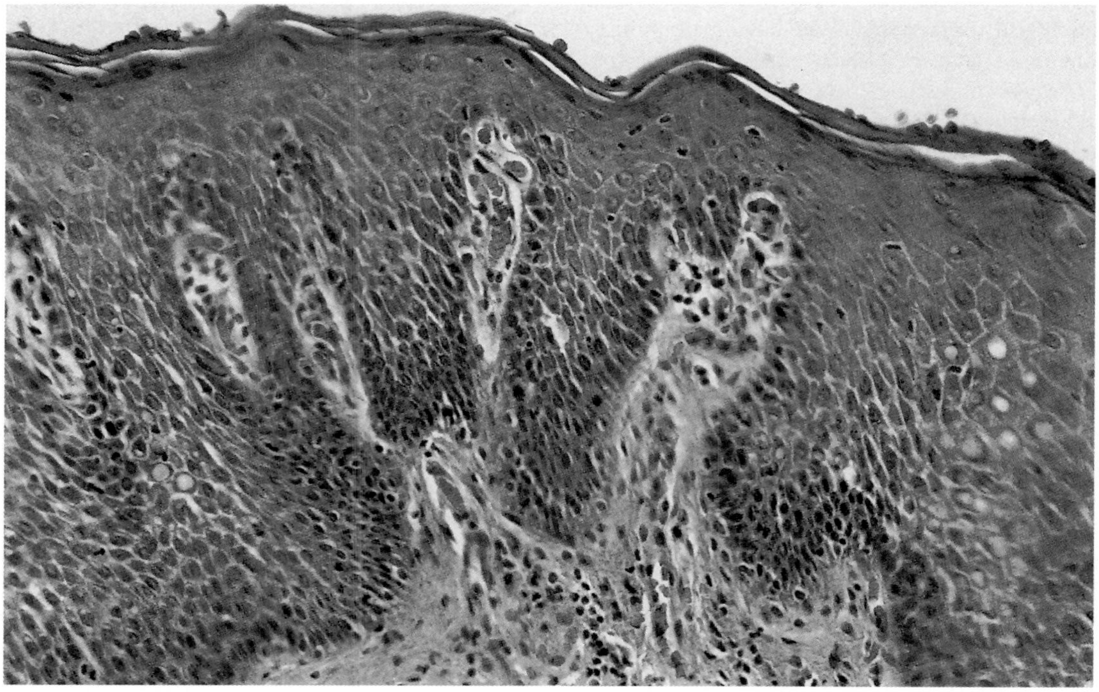

**FIG. 15.** Posterior vulvar vestibule at the fourchette. In the fourchette, the epithelium shows a moderately deep rete with a thinly keratinized surface. Some inflammatory cells are seen within the superficial dermis, consisting predominantly of lymphocytes.

upper hair follicle rather than to the skin surface when present in hair-bearing skin.

The merocrine glands are eccrine glands that produce clear watery sweat. The secretory cells have a pale slightly granular cytoplasm and an outer layer of myoepithelial cells. The glands are simple and coiled and are found deep to the reticular dermis. The sweat duct is lined by cuboidal epithelium two cells thick, and the double epithelial cell layer is lost as it joins with the stratified epithelial surface. Unlike sebaceous and apocrine glands, merocrine glands are not significantly stimulated by the sex hormones. [For further discussion on the histology of the skin elements, the reader is referred to Chapter 2 in this volume and to texts on histology (17,34,40,41).]

The epithelium of the posterolateral aspects of the labia majora, peripheral to Hart's line, is thinly keratinized and pigmented (Fig. 14). At the posterior fourchette, the retia are relatively deeper than in the posterior lateral area (Fig. 15). Pigmented cells are seen at the basal layer in this area (Fig. 16). A granular layer may be present immediately beneath the keratinized surface (stratum corneum). The granular layer arises from the underlying prickle cell (spinous cell) layer of the stratified squamous epithelium, with the stratum malpighii overlying the basal layer. The basal layer (stratum germinativum) is present immediately adjacent to the basement membrane (14,42). The medial hairless surfaces of the labia majora contain an abundance of sebaceous glands, which end at Hart's line. These glands are not associated with hair-bearing pilosebaceous units and open directly onto the epithelial surface, with a short nonkeratinized epithelium-lined duct joining with the keratinized epithelial surface (Fig. 17). Sebaceous glands within the labia majora may have a depth of up to 2.03 mm (43). Keratinous (epithelial) cysts may be associated with these sebaceous gland elements (3,35). Sebaceous glands are not found medial to Hart's line (Fig. 1). At the midportion of the labia majora, hair follicles are associated with the sebaceous gland elements. Hair follicles within the labia majora may be as deep as 2.38 mm (43) (Figs. 18 and 19). Apocrine and eccrine sweat glands are found associated with the hair-bearing areas of the vulva but

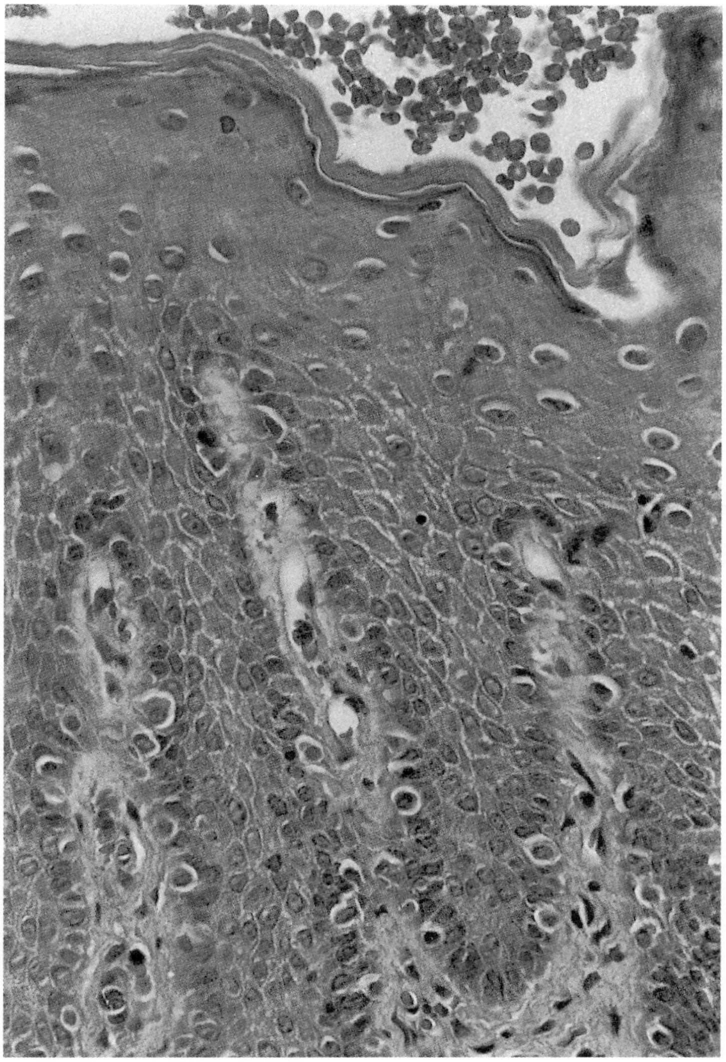

**FIG. 16.** Posterior perineal body of a 27-year-old white woman. The skin at the perineal body is pigmented and melanocytes and pigmented keratinocytes are present within the basal layer. The epithelium is stratified squamous epithelium, which has a thin keratin layer. The perinuclear halos present within the epithelial cells are normally seen and should not be confused with koilocytosis. Small clear cells are seen in the epithelial stromal junction within many of the retia.

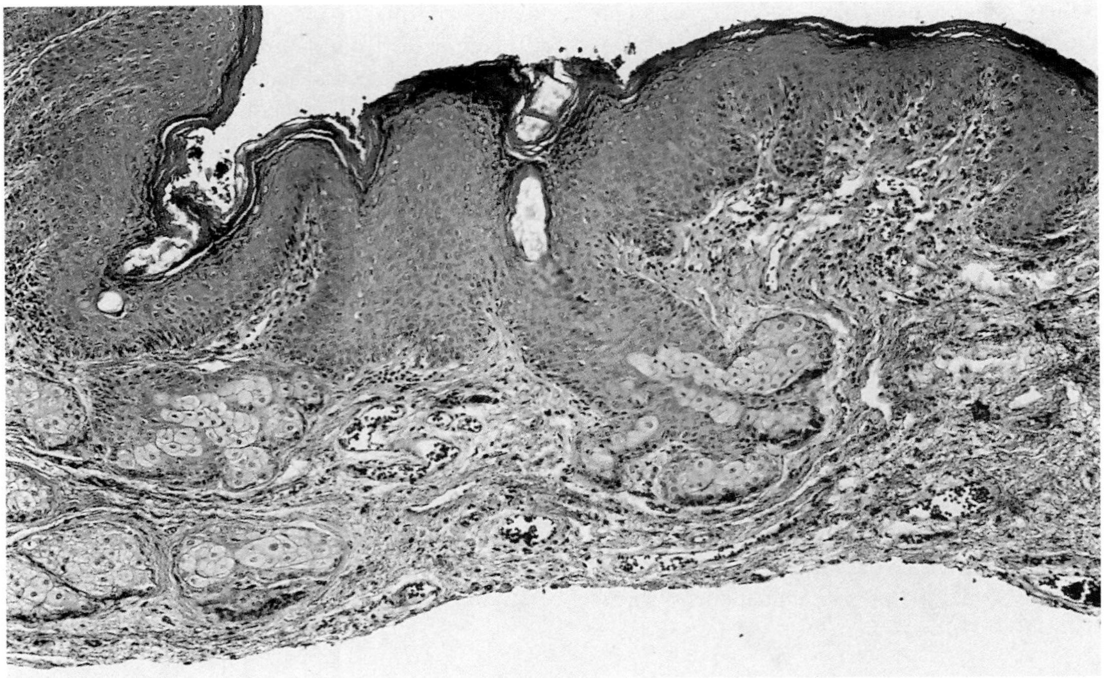

**FIG. 17.** Labia majora, medial portion, with sebaceous gland elements exiting directly to the skin surface. The epithelium of the medial labia majora has a thin keratin and granular layer. The sebaceous glands may be seen clinically as Fordyce spots.

are generally absent in the vestibule and medial non–hair-bearing areas of the medial labia majora (Fig. 20). Deeper within the dermis of the labia majora, a delicate muscle layer (tunica dartos labialis) is present. Beneath this layer is a fascial layer that has a prominent elastic fiber component (30). The fascial layer is associated with a prominent adipose layer in women of reproductive age.

Within the deep anterior labia majora, immediately adjacent to the inguinal canal, the round ligament joins with the deep longitudinal smooth muscle layer (cremaster muscle) of the labia majora (30). The round ligament may include entrapped peritoneum (processus vaginalis), which can become cystically dilated, resulting in a cyst of the canal of Nuck (3). These peritoneum-lined cysts are typically encountered in the anterior portion of the labia majora, adjacent to or within the inguinal canal.

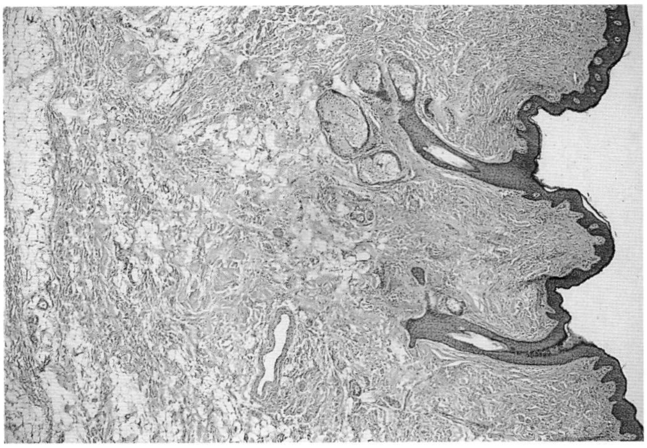

**FIG. 18.** Labia majora, midportion, with underlying dermis and deep fatty tissue. The thickness of the dermis can be seen in this section of the labia majora. A few deep hair follicles can be seen within the elastic fiber–rich dermis. The dermal junction with the deep fatty tissue is irregular.

The epithelium of the labia majora is rich in nerve endings and contains touch receptors, including Meissner corpuscles, Merkel tactile disks, and peritrichous nerve endings (30). Pacinian corpuscles for pressure sensation are present within the fatty layer of the labia majora, as well as within the labia minora, clitoris, and mons pubis. Free nerve endings for pain reception are also present within the epithelium, as well as within muscle cells and blood vessels (29,30). Ruffini corpuscles are seen throughout the subcutaneous tissue of the labia majora, labia minora, clitoris, and mons pubis. They are absent in the hymen. Their exact function in the vulva is uncertain; however, they may be temperature receptors and/or receptors for sexual stimuli (30). Dogiel-Krause receptors have a distribution similar to that of Ruffini corpuscles; however, they are present in a relatively smaller concentration in the mons pubis and labia majora (30).

Medial to the labia majora, within the sulcus between the labia majora and minora (sulcus interlabialis), anogenital mammarylike glands are present that may give rise to cysts within the intralabial sulcus, which also may involve the medial aspect of the labia majora. These glands, and the cyst de-

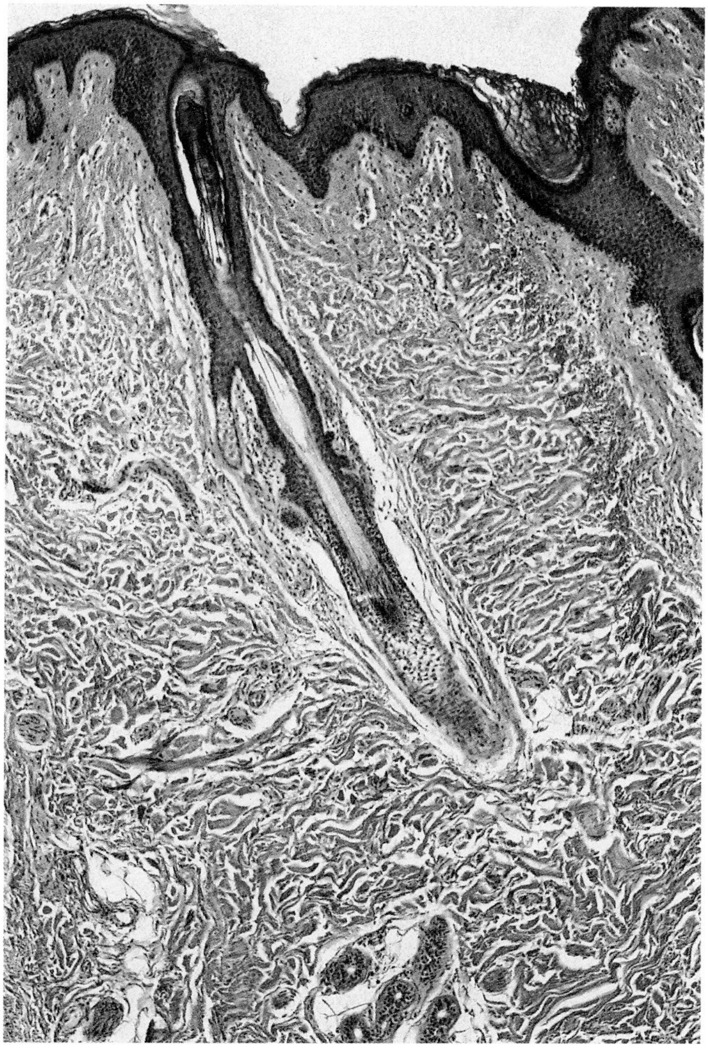

**FIG. 19.** Labia majora, lateral, with hair follicle and sweat gland elements. The sweat gland duct is seen adjacent to the portion of the hair follicle.

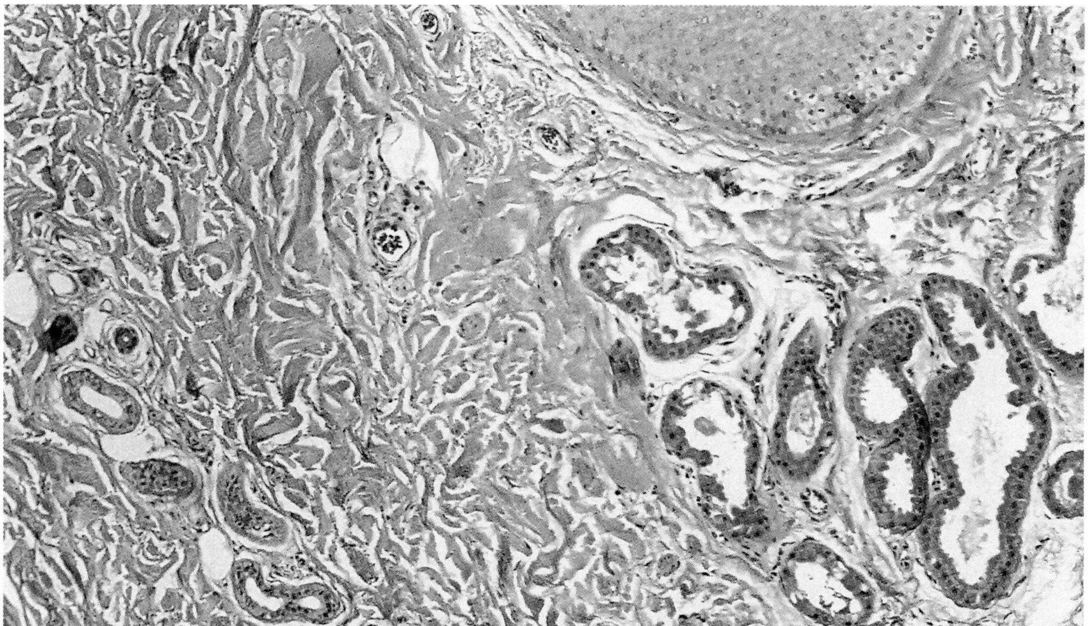

**FIG. 20.** Labia majora with apocrine glands and sweat ducts adjacent to a hair follicle. Moderate vascularity of the collagen-rich dermis of the labia majora surrounds these sweat gland elements.

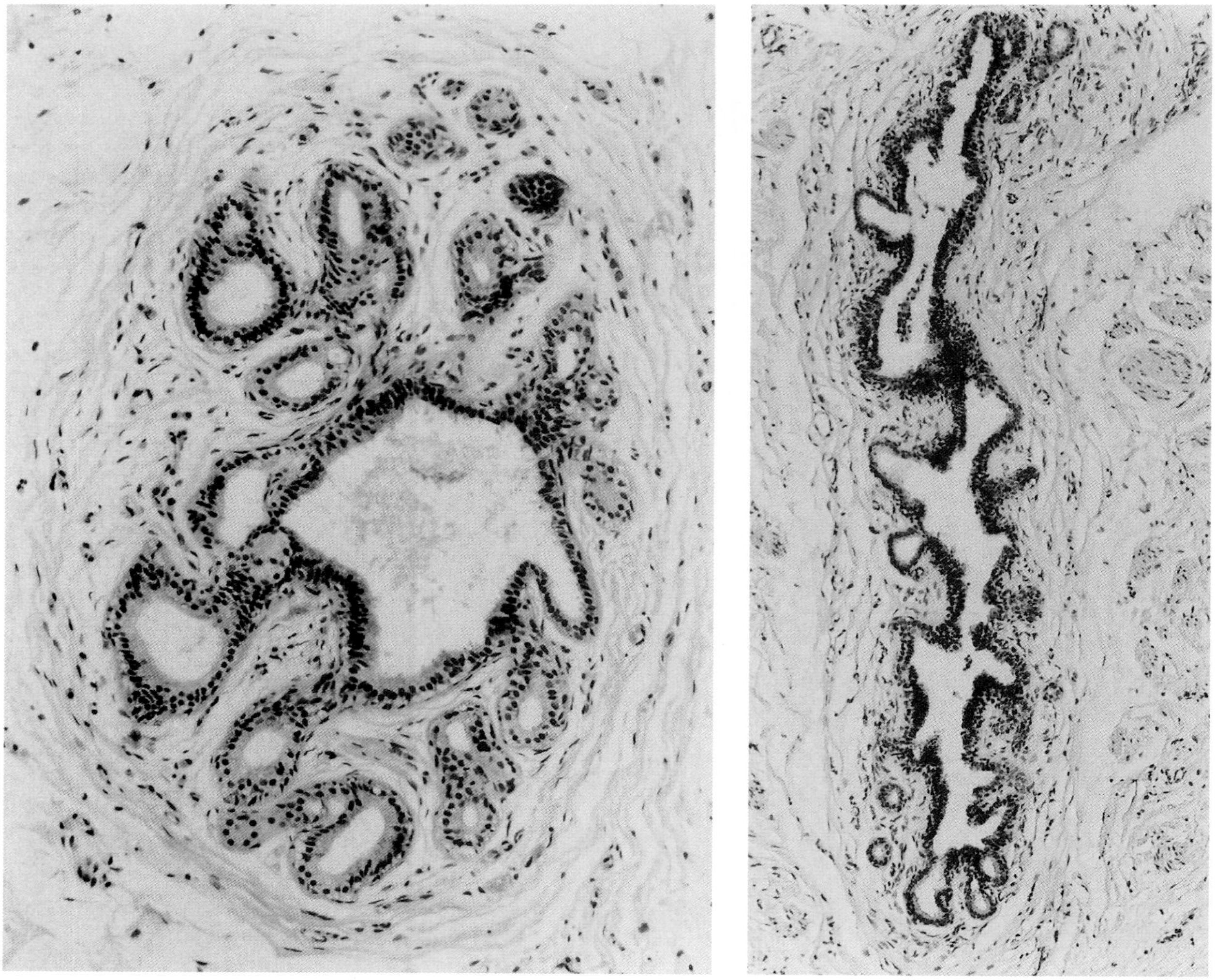

A B

**FIG. 21.** Mammarylike anogenital gland with main duct (**A** and **B**) and small small acini (A). The epithelial lining is composed of a two-layered epithelium with underlying myoepithelial cell layer and a low columnar epithelial luminal epithelium. [Reprinted with permission (48).]

scribed, are lined with a cuboidal to columnar epithelium with an underlying myoepithelium. The myoepithelial cells are immunoreactive for smooth muscle actin and S100 antigen, as well as low-molecular-weight keratin. The superficial luminal epithelial cells are of an apocrine type, with visible "snouts" (Fig. 21). These cells are immunoreactive for low-molecular-weight keratin as well as human milk fat globule antigen. Individual cells are also immunoreactive for carcinoembryonic antigen and S100 antigen. Estrogen and progesterone receptors have been detected in these cells. Mucus-containing or ciliated cells are not present, distinguishing them (cysts of anogenital mammarylike glands) from vestibular mucous cysts, müllerian-related cysts or ciliated cysts, or Bartholin gland. The lack of a stratified squamous epithelium or transitional epithelium distinguishes them from Bartholin duct cysts, keratinous cysts, or vestibular glandular cysts that have undergone squamous metaplasia (44). There is evidence that these glands are the origin of fibroadenoma, hidradenoma papilliferum, milk cysts, and apparent ectopic breast tissue that have been described in the vulva, rather than being from ectopic breast tissue (45) .

## Mons Pubis (Mons Veneris)

The mons pubis has its origin in the embryonic genital medial cranial swellings (16). The subcutaneous tissue of mons pubis becomes more prominent with the onset of puberty, when there is a progressive increase in fat tissue beneath the mons. There is also a dramatic increase in hair growth of the mons pubis and labia majora.

### *Aging Changes*

The hair growth changes have been summarized and staged by Tanner in the following sequence (37). Stage 1 is characterized by no visible pubic hair growth. In stage 2 a small amount of pubic-type hair is seen on the midportion of the mons pubis, and some similar hair may be seen on the labia majora. In stage 3 the mons pubis hair growth is more prominent, both in the amount of hair and the coarseness of the hair. In stage 4 the hair growth over the mons pubis is similar to the adult, with the exception that the upper lateral corners of hair growth are lacking. Stage 5 characterizes the adult pubic hair pattern (37). The adult hair growth distribution is reached between the ages of 12 and 17 years of age (13). There can be substantial variability in the amount and character of the pubic hair (escutcheon) related to racial and genetic factors; however, pubic-type hair growth generally does not extend above a horizontal line drawn between, and 2 cm above, the uppermost limits of the genitofemoral folds (38,46). Hair follicle depth within the vulva is greatest in the mons pubis, where hair follicle depth has been measured up to 2.72 mm (43). The mons veneris is richly endowed with nerve receptor types that were previously described for the labia majora (30).

### Lymphatic Drainage

The vulvar tissues drain to lymph nodes in the femoral and inguinal lymph node chains. The anterior labia minora and clitoris drain through channels anterior and superior to these structures to join lymphatics from the prepuce and labia majora. These channels course laterally to inguinal and femoral nodes (47). In some cases, lymphatic channels from a lateral site may drain to the contralateral node group, which has clinical relevance in planning therapy for malignancies of the vulva. The most common site of metastasis from vulvar malignancies are the superficial inguinal nodes. In general eight to 10 nodes are found in this area, with superior oblique (above the ligament of Poupart) and inferior ventral (between the ligament of Poupart and the saphenous vein and fascia lata) divisions.

Midline structures such as the clitoris and the midline perineum drain bilaterally. A second path of lymphatic drainage from the clitoris involves urethral lymphatics and lymphatics draining the dorsal vein of the clitoris. These channels lead inferior to the symphysis pubis through the anogenital diaphragm to join the lymphatic plexus of the anterior bladder surface. Ultimately these channels terminate in the interiliac and obturator nodes or course superiorly to the femoral and internal iliac nodes. Deep pelvic nodes are not generally involved unless the superficial inguinal nodes are involved.

### Arterial Supply

The major arterial supply of the vulva originates with the superficial and deep external pudendal arteries, which branch from the femoral artery, and the internal pudendal arteries, which branch from internal iliac arteries. The pudendal artery has anterior and posterior labial branches. Circulation to the clitoris is separate and emanates from the deep arteries of the clitoris. The anterior vaginal artery supplies the vestibule and Bartholin gland areas (3).

### Nerve Supply

The major nerves of the vulva are from the anterior and posterior labial nerves. The anterior nerve is a branch of the ilioinguinal nerve, and the posterior labial branch is from the pudendal nerve. The clitoral nerve supply is from the dorsal nerve of the clitoris and the cavernous nerves of the clitoris. The vestibule shares the clitoral nerve supply (3,29).

## REFERENCES


1. McKay M. Subsets of vulvodynia. *J Reprod Med* 1988;33:695–698.
2. Kaufman RH, Friedrich EG, Gardner HL. *Benign diseases of the vulva and vagina.* 3rd ed. Chicago: Year Book Medical; 1989.
3. Wilkinson EJ. Benign diseases of the vulva. In: Kurman RJ, ed. *Blaustein's pathology of the female genital tract.* 4th ed. New York: Springer-Verlag; 1994:31–86.
4. Ridley CM. *The vulva.* New York: Churchill Livingstone; 1988:1–69.
5. Janakiv JR, Dremalatha S, Raghuveera N, Thambiah AS. Lawrence-Sep syndrome. *Br J Dermatol* 1980;103:693.
6. Seely JR, Bley R Jr, Altmiller CJ. Localized chromosomal mosaicism as a cause of dysmorphic development. *Am J Hum Genet* 1984;36:899.
7. Wilkinson EJ, Stone IK. *Atlas of vulvar disease.* Baltimore: Williams & Wilkins; 1995.
8. Reid R, Greenberg MD, Daoud Y, Selvaggi S, Husain M, Wilkinson EJ. Colposcopic findings in women with vulvar pain syndromes: a preliminary report. *J Reprod Med* 1988;33:523–532.
9. Hart DB. *Selected papers in gynaecology and obstetrics.* Edinburgh, Scotland: W&AK Johnston, 1893.
10. Dickinson RL. *Human sex anatomy.* 2nd ed. Baltimore: Williams & Wilkins; 1949.
11. Hu F. Melanocyte cytology in normal skin. In: Ackerman AB, ed. *Masson monographs in dermatology-1.* New York: Masson; 1981.
12. Edwards JNT, Morris HB. Langerhans cells and lymphocyte subsets in the female genital tract. *Br J Obstet Gynecol* 1985;92:974–982.
13. McLean JM. Anatomy and physiology of the vulvar area. In: Ridley CM, ed. *The vulva.* New York: Churchill Livingstone; 1988:39–65.
14. MacKie RM. Milne's dermatopathology. 2nd ed. London: Arnold; 1984.
15. Gould VE, Moll R, Moll I, Lee I, Franke WW. Biology of disease. Neuroendocrine (Merkel) cells of the skin: hyperplasias, dysplasias, and neoplasms. *Lab Invest* 1985;52:334–352.
16. Bottle K, Lacey CG, Goldberg J, et al. Merkel cell carcinoma of the vulva. *Obstet Gynecol* 1984;63:61.
17. Robboy SJ, Bernhardt PF, Parmley T. Embryology of the female genital tract and disorders of abnormal sexual development. In: Kurman RJ, ed. *Blaustein's pathology of the female genital tract.* 4th ed. New York: Springer-Verlag; 1994:3–29.
18. Bloom W, Fawcett DW. *A textbook of histology.* 10th ed. Philadelphia: WB Saunders; 1975:904–905.
19. Rorat E, Ferenczy A, Richart RM. Human Bartholin gland, duct, and duct cyst. *Arch Pathol* 1975;99:367–374.
20. Fetissof F, Berger G, Dubois MP, et al. Endocrine cells in the female genital tract. *Histopathology* 1985;9:133–145.
21. Word B. Office treatment of cyst and abscess of Bartholin's gland duct. *South Med J* 1968;61:514–518.
22. Pyka R, Wilkinson EJ, Friedrich EG Jr, Croker BP. The histology of vulvar vestibulitis syndrome. *Int J Gynecol Oncol* 1988;7:249–257.
23. Friedrich EG Jr, Wilkinson EJ. Mucous cysts of the vulvar vestibule. *Obstet Gynecol* 1973;42:407.
24. Robboy SJ, Ross JS, Prat J, Keh PC, Welch WR. Urogenital sinus origin of mucinous and ciliated cysts of the vulva. *Obstet Gynecol* 1978; 51:347–351.
25. Fowler WC, Lawrence H, Edelman DA. Paravestibular tumor of the female genital tract. *Am J Obstet Gynecol* 1981;139:109–111.
26. Axe S, Parmley T, Woodruff JD, Hlopak B. Adenomas in minor vestibular glands. *Obstet Gynecol* 1986;68:16–18.
27. Friedrich EG Jr. Vulvar vestibulitis syndrome. *J Reprod Med* 1987;32: 110–114.
28. Huffman JW. The detailed anatomy of the paraurethral ducts in the adult human female. *Am J Obstet Gynecol* 1948;55:86.

29. Krantz KE. Innervation of the human vulva and vagina. *Obstet Gynecol* 1958;12:382.
30. Krantz KE. The anatomy and physiology of the vulva and vagina. In: Philipp EE, Barnes J, Newton M, eds. *Scientific foundation of obstetrics and gynaecology.* 2nd ed. London: Heinemann; 1977:65–78.
31. Novak ER, Woodruff JD. *Gynecologic and obstetric pathology.* Philadelphia: WB Saunders; 1974.
32. Growdon WA, Fu Y, Lebherz TB, Rapkin A, Mason GD, Parks G. Pruritic vulvar squamous papillomatosis: evidence for human papillomavirus etiology. *Obstet Gynecol* 1985;66:564–568.
33. Bergeron C, Ferenczy A, Richart RM, Guralnick M. Micropapillomatosis labialis appears unrelated to human papillomavirus. *Obstet Gynecol* 1990;76:281–286.
34. Amenta PS. *Elias-Pauly's histology and human microanatomy.* 5th ed. New York: John Wiley; 1987:502–503.
35. Junaid TA, Thomas SM. Cysts of the vulva and vagina: a comparative study. *Int J Gynecol Obstet* 1981;19:239–243.
36. Friedrich EG Jr, Wilkinson EJ. Vulvar surgery for neurofibromatosis. *Obstet Gynecol* 1985;65:135–138.
37. Tanner JM. *Growth at adolescence.* 2nd ed. Oxford: Blackwell; 1962.
38. Barmann JM, Astore J, Pecoraro V. The normal trichogram of people over 50 years. In: Montagna W, Dobson RL, eds. *Advances in biology of skin.* Vol. IX. Hair growth. Oxford, England: Pergamon Press; 1969.
39. Gallagher PG. Varicose veins of the vulva. *Br J Sex Med* 1986;13:12–14.
40. Geneser F. *Textbook of histology.* Philadelphia: Munksgaard/Lea & Febiger; 1986:616–617.
41. Leeson CR, Leeson TS, Paparo AA. *Textbook of histology.* Philadelphia: WB Saunders; 1985:485–486.
42. Zellickson AS. *Electron microscopy of skin and mucous membranes.* Springfield, IL: Charles C Thomas; 1963.
43. Shatz P, Bergeron C, Wilkinson EJ, Arseneau J, Ferenczy A. Vulvar intraepithelial neoplasia and skin appendage involvement. *Obstet Gynecol* 1989;74:769–774.
44. van der Putte SCJ, Van Gorp HM. Cysts of mammary-like glands in the vulva. *Int J Gynecol Pathol* 1995;14:184–188.
45. van der Putte SCJ. Mammary-like glands of the vulva and their disorders. *Int J Gynecol Pathol* 1994;13:150–160.
46. Lunde O. A study of body hair density and distribution in normal women. *Am J Phys Anthropol* 1984;64:179–184.
47. Parry-Jones E. Lymphatics of the vulva. *J Obstet Gynaecol Br Commonw* 1963;70:751–765.
48. van der Putte SCJ. *Am J Dermatopathol* 1991;13:557–567.

*Histology for Pathologists, second edition,*
Edited by Stephen S. Sternberg.
Lippincott-Raven Publishers, Philadelphia
© 1997.

# CHAPTER 38

# Vagina

Stanley J. Robboy and Rex C. Bentley



Tissue from the vagina is infrequently examined via biopsy. Excluding the vaginal cuff removed for cervical disease, most biopsies and surgical operations are for infection, small intramural growths, intrauterine exposure to diethylstilbestrol (DES), or, in older women, squamous cell cancer and its precursors. This chapter addresses the gross, microscopic, and ultrastructural anatomy of the normal vagina. The embryologic discussion focuses on developmental perturbations, which provide insights into normal and microscopic anatomy.

## EMBRYOLOGIC CHANGES

The paired müllerian (paramesonephric) ducts appear about the 37th day postconception as funnel-shaped openings of celomic epithelium (1,2). These develop into paired, undifferentiated tubes that later grow caudally, using the already formed wolffian (mesonephric) ducts as a guidewire to reach the level of the future hymen (Fig. 1). At about day 54, the paired müllerian ducts fuse, becoming a straight uterovaginal canal (primordia of uterine corpus, cervix, and vagina), the lining of which is an immature columnar (müllerian) epithelium (Fig. 2) (3). The above changes occur in both female and male embryos.

If the fetus is a male, the indifferent gonads become anatomically distinct testes at around day 44. The testis is important for two products it makes. One, müllerian inhibiting substance (MIS), affects the future of the müllerian ducts. The other, testosterone, affects the future of the wolffian ducts. Shortly after the testes become distinct, Sertoli cells begin to produce MIS, a protein in the large transforming growth factor-beta family, in amounts effective to cause the müllerian ducts to regress through a process of programmed cell death (4,5). If the embryo is female, testes do not develop. Because there is then no MIS, the müllerian ducts are not inhibited from developing and thus grow without impedance to become the fallopian tubes, uterus, and vagina.

In contradistinction to MIS, which acts as an inhibitor, testosterone stimulates and is required to promote wolffian duct growth. In the male, the critical period for testosterone stimulation begins early in the 10th week (circa day 71) and causes the embryonic wolffian ducts to differentiate into epididymis, seminal vesicle, and vas deferens. If there are no testes, as in the female, and testosterone stimulation has not occurred by the close of the critical window (circa day 84), the wolffian ducts wither and become vestigial remnants, which in the adult are found deep in the vaginal wall.

Until near the end of week 10 (to about day 66) the uterovaginal canal, with its solid tip already in contact with the urogenital sinus, continues to elongate caudally, still re-

S. J. Robboy: Department of Pathology and Obstetrics and Gynecology, Duke University Medical Center, Durham, North Carolina 27710.

R. C. Bentley: Department of Pathology, Duke University Medical Center, Durham, North Carolina 27710.

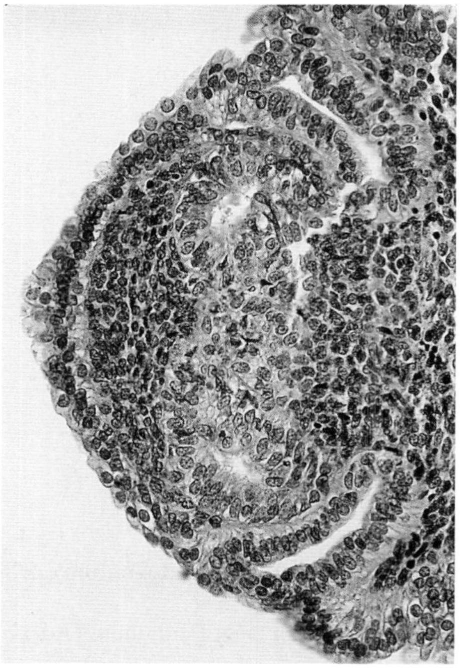

FIG. 1. Region of urogenital sinus disclosing the tips of two central müllerian ducts that have grown down the (outer) paired wolffian ducts. The cytologic features of the cells comprising both types of duct are indistinguishable on light microscopy at early stages of development. Circa day 54. [Reprinted with permission (29).]

maining as a simple tube lined by columnar epithelium (Fig. 2). Beginning in the 11th week, the epithelium stratifies, becoming several layers thick. The squamous cells are believed to derive from the urogenital sinus, invading the common tube from below and growing up the muscular scaffold to completely replace the müllerian epithelium to the level of the external cervical os (6). The transition from müllerian to squamous epithelium occurs at about the time when nuclear estrogen receptors appear in the vaginal stroma (7).

Stratification of the squamous epithelium lining the uterovaginal canal heralds formation of the so-called vaginal plate (circa the 11th week). The proliferation progressively occludes the canal beginning caudally and extending cranially (8). Studies with latex-injected specimens indicate that even the lateral wings of the vaginal plate may become occluded, but a central lumen persists, especially in the upper vagina (9).

During the 13th week (91 days), cervical glands develop; they exhibit a wavy architectural appearance but cytologically are minimally differentiated. By the 14th week, the caudal vagina increases markedly in size (Fig. 3). During the 15th week, the solid epithelial anlage of the anterior and posterior vaginal fornices appears. Starting with the 16th week, the squamous epithelium lining the vagina and the exocervix begins to mature, thus resembling the lining of the adult vagina. The epithelium thickens and glycogenates, features

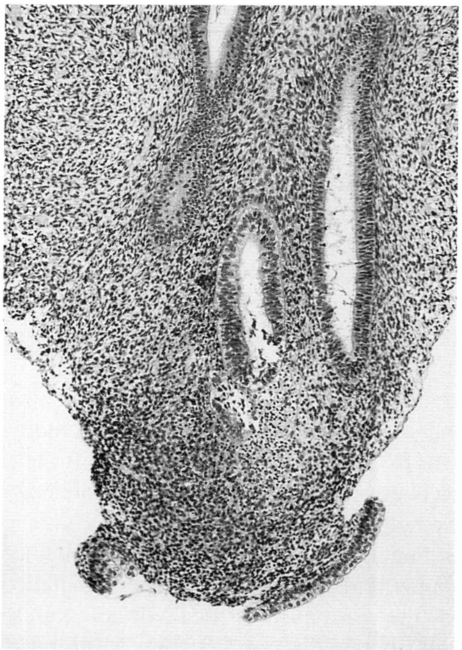

FIG. 2. Single müllerian tube flanked by two wolffian ducts. The cytologic features of the cells comprising both types of duct are indistinguishable on light microscopy at early stages of development. Circa day 67. [Reprinted with permission (29).]

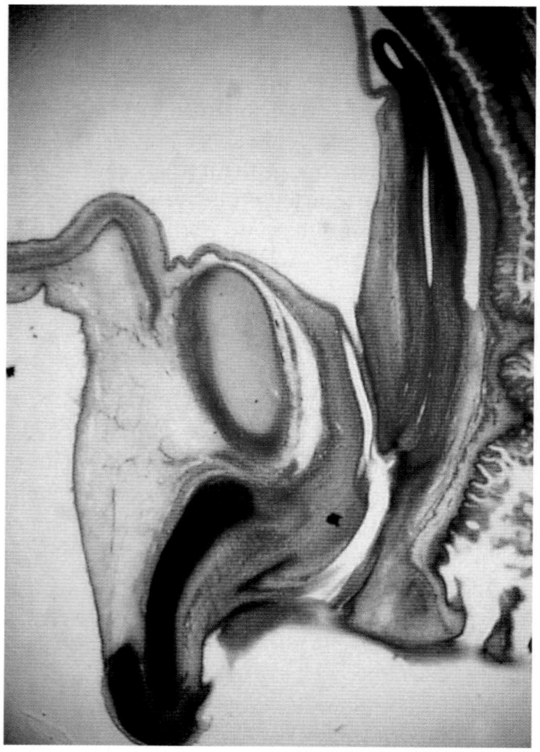

FIG. 3. Sagittal section of pelvis at 16 weeks, showing vagina, bladder, urethra, and urogenital sinus. The lower genital tract is a straight longitudinal tube, and at this stage the vagina and cervix cannot be distinguished.

most likely related to increased maternal and hence fetal estrogen levels. As the cells mature, they lose cellular adhesiveness and desquamate, heralding the canalization of the vaginal plate and thus the onset of the final gross adult structure of the vagina. By the 18th to 20th week, the development of the vagina is complete.

Why columnar epithelium with an embryonic appearance should initially line the müllerian system and later be replaced by squamous epithelium remains of teleologic interest. The answer to the mechanism may lie in the vaginal wall stroma. Prior work in the mouse has shown that lower genital tract epithelium differentiates dependent on the stroma on which it grows (10). For example, uterine epithelium, when grown intermingled with neonatal vaginal stroma, develops histotypic features of vagina. In contrast, vaginal epithelium, if grown with neonatal uterine stroma, develops a uterine phenotype. The final epithelium has cytosolic proteins characteristic of the induced rather than original epithelial source.

Additional evidence that the vaginal stroma plays a key role in epithelial differences comes from embryologic appearance of estrogen receptors. Among various body organs tested, the receptors are detected only in the genital tract. They appear in the mesenchyme at the 10th week, just before the müllerian epithelium is normally replaced by squamous epithelium (7) of sinus origin. Epithelial labeling appears later (16th week), at the time when the sinus (squamous) epithelium begins to mature and accumulate large quantities of glycogen. Interestingly, recent work has also suggested that the stroma plays a key role in the action of MIS as well; the receptor for MIS has been characterized and has been found to be located in the stroma surrounding the müllerian duct rather than in the müllerian epithelium (11).

From current evidence, both the developmental morphology of the vaginal mucosa and the inductive properties of the stroma supporting the vaginal mucosa are complex and have yet to be fully understood. For example, a hitherto unrecognized band of subepithelial stroma was described in 1973 that extended from the endocervix to the vulva (12) (Fig. 4). It is 0.5 to 5 mm thick in mature females and most prominent in the endocervix. It has been suggested that it is from this zone that fibroepithelial polyps arise, an entity of no apparent physiologic function, but which clinically should not be confused with malignant tumor (13,14).

In the event that the squamous epithelium described above fails during the critical weeks of embryonic life to replace the original columnar cells lining the vagina, the columnar cells remain in an arrested state of development until sometime around puberty, when they may further differentiate into the adult- type epithelium usually seen in biopsy material. It is conjectured that the tuboendometrial type of epithelium is the basic form of epithelium supported by the vaginal mesenchyme. In fact, it may be that this type of epithelium is the basic type of müllerian epithelium supported

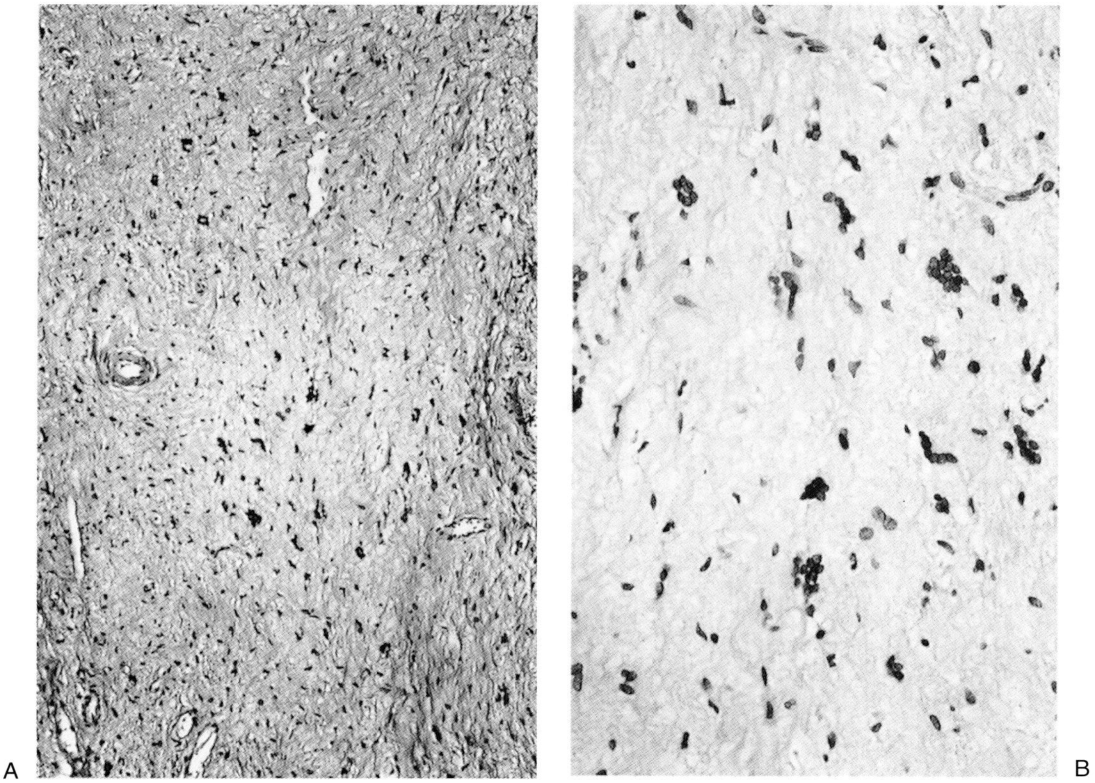


**FIG. 4.** Bandlike area composed of loose connective tissue and multinucleated cells running the length of the vagina. **A:** Low-power view. **B:** High-power view. [Reprinted with permission (30).]

throughout the female genital tract, manifesting as serous cells in the fallopian tube, endometrioid cells in the uterine corpus, and tuboendometrial cells in the vagina—cells that are quite similar. In the cervix, a tuboendometrial layer of epithelium also lies deep to and as a cuff about the luminal layer of mucinous epithelium (15); the tuboendometrial layer, which is continuous with the lining of the corpus, is readily observed in hysterectomy specimens but is located too deep to be detected on biopsy. In fetuses where the vaginal lining has become squamous (>10 weeks), the inner stromal zone is obvious in the fallopian tube, endometrium, and endocervix and tapers, appearing to end at the squamocolumnar junction of the cervix and vagina. Part of this layer may correspond to the most superficial stromal layer in the adult vagina described above (12). The original tuboendometrial layer is the origin of glandular remnants in the vagina of adults (adenosis).

## GROSS FEATURES

The vagina, from the Latin for "sheath," extends from the vestibule of the vulva to the uterus, lying posterior (dorsal) to the urinary bladder and anterior (ventral) to the rectum. Its axis averages 30° with the vertical and more than 90° with the uterus (Fig. 5). The ventral wall averages 8 cm in length and the dorsal wall 11 cm. In early life, the vagina is constricted distally, dilated in the middle, and narrowed proximally. It surrounds the exocervix and forms vaultlike fornices between its cervical attachment and the lateral wall. In the adult the anterior and posterior walls are slack and remain in contact with each other, whereas the lateral walls remain fairly rigid and separated. This gives an H-shaped appearance to the vaginal canal on cross-section.

Posteriorly, the upper fourth of the vagina is related to the rectouterine space, that is, the cul-de-sac or pouch of Douglas, which is covered with peritoneum. The middle half of the vagina is closely apposed to the rectum, separated only by fibrofatty adventitia and the rectovaginal septum. The lower fourth of the vagina is separated from the anal canal by anal and rectal sphincters, as well as the interposing perineal body, which contains the origin of the bulbocavernous and superficial transverse perineal muscles.

The urinary bladder and urethra lie anterior to the vagina. The urethra courses approximately one third of its length on the vagina and then enters into the vaginal wall to become an inseparable part of it, finally terminating with its external meatus at the introitus. The ureters course along both sides of the upper third of the vagina until entering the bladder wall.

The vagina opens into the vestibule formed from the urogenital sinus. The vestibule lies beneath the urethra and between the inner margins of the labia minora. The vagina, urethra, and ducts of Bartholin's glands open into the vestibule. The size and shape of the vaginal orifice are related to the state of the hymen. When the inner edges of the hymen are apposed, the vaginal opening resembles a cleft. When stretched, the hymen may persist in the form of a ringlike structure about the readily recognized vaginal orifice. (The reader is referred to Chapter 37 for the anatomy of the hymenal region.)

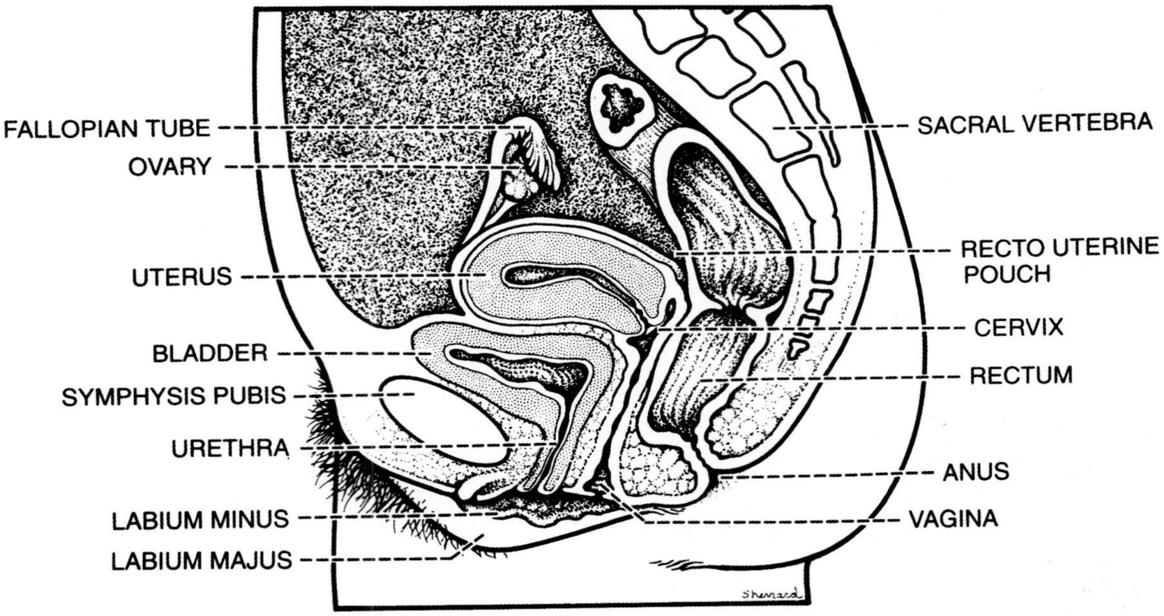


**FIG. 5.** Structural relationships of the vagina. Its axis forms an angle of more than 90° with the uterus. [Reprinted with permission (31).]

## ANATOMY

### Ligaments

The vaginal supports are intimately related to the uterus, urethra, bladder, and rectum (16). The lateral supports are called cardinal ligaments, the posterior supports sacrouterine ligaments. They originate where the isthmus of the uterine cervix and the uterine corpus meet and course outward, fanlike to the lateral and posterior pelvic walls. The isthmic fibers turn upward onto the uterus and downward onto the vagina. These ligaments, the connective tissues surrounding the vessels on the lateral vaginal walls, and the close proximity of the rectum, bladder, and urethra all contribute to support the vagina within the pelvis.

### Blood Supply

The blood supply to the vagina is complex, with extensive anastomoses maintaining an adequate blood supply to all areas of the vagina in the event that injury restricts any single route of supply. The internal iliac (hypogastric) artery is the principal source of blood cranially as branches of the uterine arteries, and caudally, as branches of the middle hemorrhoidal arteries and pudendal arteries. Beginning cranially, the uterine artery gives off a descending branch, the cervicovaginal artery. Several branches supply the cervix. Lower branches supply the vagina. The vaginal arteries, which lie lateral to the vagina, send branches to both the anterior and posterior surfaces. The lower vagina receives its supply from ascending branches of the middle hemorrhoidal arteries and pudendal arteries, which also divide to send rami to the anterior and posterior vaginal walls. In toto, the extensive rami form a plexus around the vagina from which arise the median arteries, the azygos vaginal arteries on the anterior and posterior walls. A rich venous plexus also surrounds the vagina and communicates with the vesicle, pudendal, and hemorrhoidal venous plexuses, which empty into the internal iliac veins.

### Nerves

The autonomic system of the pelvis originates in the superior hypogastric plexus (17). The middle hypogastric plexus, which passes into the pelvis, divides at the level of the sacral vertebra S1 into branches that pass to both sides of the pelvis and initiate the inferior hypogastric plexus. The inferior hypogastric plexus, a divided continuation of the middle hypogastric plexus, the superior hypogastric plexus, and the presacral nerve, descends into the pelvis in a position posterior to the common iliac artery and anterior to the sacral plexus; it curves laterally and finally enters the sacrouterine ligament. The medial segment of the primary division of the sacral nerves (S2–5), as it sends fibers into the pelvic plexus located within the sacrouterine folds, appears to contain both sympathetic (inferior hypogastric plexus) and parasympathetic (nervi erigentes) components. An extension of this plexus located in the base of the broad ligament and supplied by the middle vesical artery contains many ganglia. Most nerves enter the uterus near the isthmus. A lesser number descend along the lateral vagina, a pattern similar to the arteries that supply the vagina.

### Lymphatic Drainage

The vaginal lymphatic system, despite the simplified view given here, is highly variable (Fig. 6) (18). The lymphatics begin as a delicate plexus of small channels involving the entire mucosa and lamina propria and then drain into a deep muscular network. They terminate in a perivaginal plexus from which arise collecting trunks, which themselves coalesce into several larger channels.

The lymph drainage follows patterns that reflect functionally diverse geographic regions. The lymphatics of the upper anterior wall join those of the cervix, where they follow the cervical vessels to the uterine artery and accompany it to terminate in the medial chain of the external iliac nodes. The lymph from the posterior vagina drains into deep pelvic, rectal, and aortic nodes. The lymphatics of the lower vagina, which include also the hymenal region, follow two distinct courses. One passes to the interiliac nodes in company with the upper vaginal discharge. The other traverses the paravesical space, carrying lymph to the deepest portions of the pelvis, draining into the inferior gluteal nodes near the origin of the vaginal or internal pudendal artery. The channels that anastomose with those of the vulva drain to the superficial il-

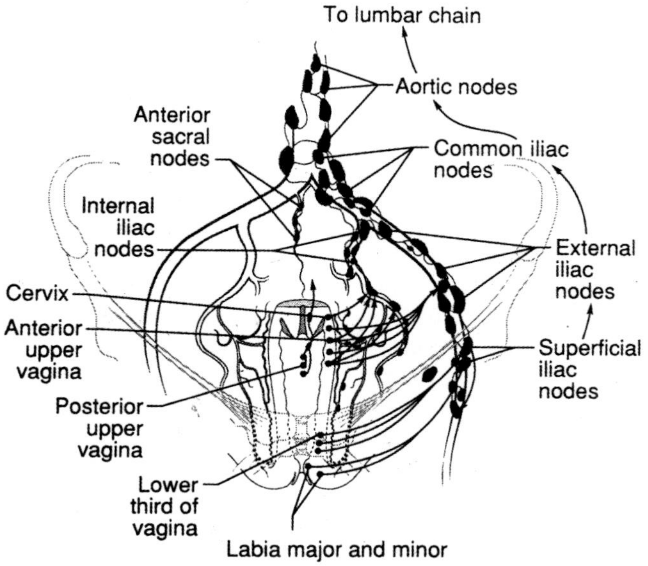


**FIG. 6.** Lymphatic drainage of the vagina. [Reprinted with permission (18).]

iac nodes. In summary, as a practical matter, one can generalize that tumors in the upper vagina will spread like cervical carcinoma to involve obturator and both internal and external iliac nodes. In contrast, tumors in the lower vagina will tend to involve superficial iliac (inguinal) and deep pelvic nodes, similar to vulvar cancer.

## LIGHT MICROSCOPY

### Epithelium

The vaginal wall consists of three principal layers: mucosa (epithelial and submucosal stroma), muscle, and adventitia. The epithelium is about 0.4 mm thick and, on gross examination, exhibits a characteristic pattern of folds or rugae separated by furrows of variable depth. There are two longitudinal (anterior and posterior) and multiple transverse furrows. The rugal pattern of the vaginal mucosa produces an undulating appearance on microscopic examination in contrast to the flat surface of the cervix. The rugae, which are more prominent in nulliparous than multiparous women, reinforce the gripping effect of the levator ani and vaginal constrictor muscles during intercourse. The luminal surface is lined with nonkeratinized squamous epithelium, similar to cervical epithelium. The normal vaginal mucosa lacks glands. Its surface is lubricated both by fluids that pass directly through the mucosa and by cervical mucus.

The mature, stratified squamous epithelium can be subdivided into several layers, typical of squamous epithelia elsewhere in the body (Fig. 7). From the base to the surface, they are the deep, intermediate, and superficial zones. The deep zone contains the basal cell layer and above this the parabasal layer. Both are the active proliferative compartments or germinal beds. The basal cell layer consists of a single layer of columnar-like cells, approximately 10 $\mu$m thick, the long axis of which is vertically arranged. The cells have a basophilic cytoplasm and relatively large oval nuclei. Mitoses may be present. Occasional melanocytes also are found.

The parabasal layer is poorly demarcated from the overlying cell layers. It consists usually of about two layers of small polygonal cells, having a total 14 $\mu$m thickness, often with intercellular bridges. The cells have basophilic cytoplasm, a relatively large, centrally placed, round nucleus, and occasional mitoses.

The intermediate cell layer is of variable thickness. The cells have prominent intercellular bridges, a naviculate configuration, and a long cell axis paralleling the surface. The cytoplasm is basophilic, although some glycogen may be present. The nuclei are round, oval, or irregular, with finely granular chromatin. This layer of cells has about 10 rows of cells of about 100 $\mu$m thickness.

The superficial layer is also of variable thickness. The cells are polygonal when viewed from above and flattened when viewed in cross-section. The cytoplasm is acidophilic,

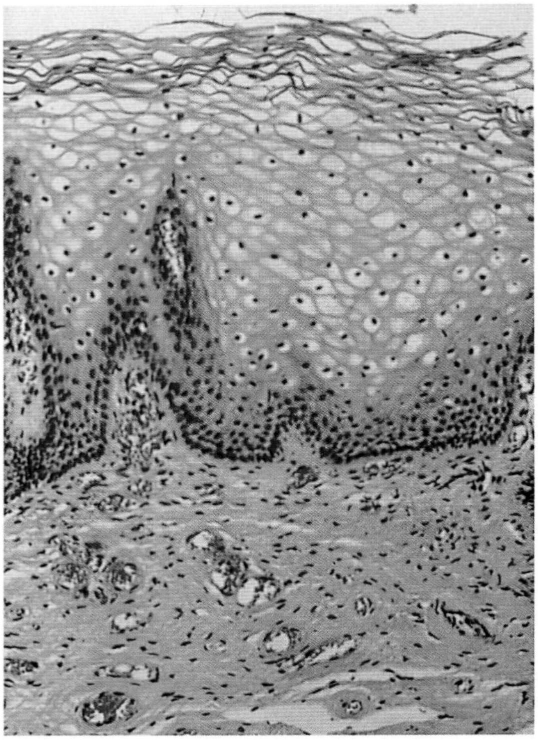

**FIG. 7.** Mucosa of the adult vagina. Mature cells with glycogenic cytoplasm and pyknotic nuclei occupy most of the epithelial thickness. There is a single layer of dark basal cells and three to four layers of intermediate cells.

and the nuclei are centrally located, small, round, and pyknotic. Keratohyalin granules are sometimes seen in the cytoplasm. This layer also contains about 10 rows of squamous cells.

### Epithelial Response to Hormones

Vaginal epithelial cells proliferate and mature in response to stimulation by ovarian or exogenous estrogenic hormones. Hence, the total number of squamous cell layers varies greatly during the normal menstrual cycle and as a woman passes through the various stages of the life cycle, that is, birth, childhood, reproduction, and the postmenopausal years (19). The high occurs at ovulation (average 45 layers). It builds up slowly during the proliferative phase and is 22 on day 10. After ovulation, the number recedes to 33 on day 19 and to 23 on day 24.

Without hormonal stimulation the cells atrophy (Fig. 8). At the peak of estrogenic activity, that is, just before ovulation, the vaginal epithelium attains its maximum thickness. Superficial cells with abundant intracytoplasmic glycogen predominate, both on histologic section and in smears (Fig. 9). Lactobacilli metabolize the glycogen normally present in the vagina to lactic acid, which maintains an acid vaginal pH (pH 4 to 5).

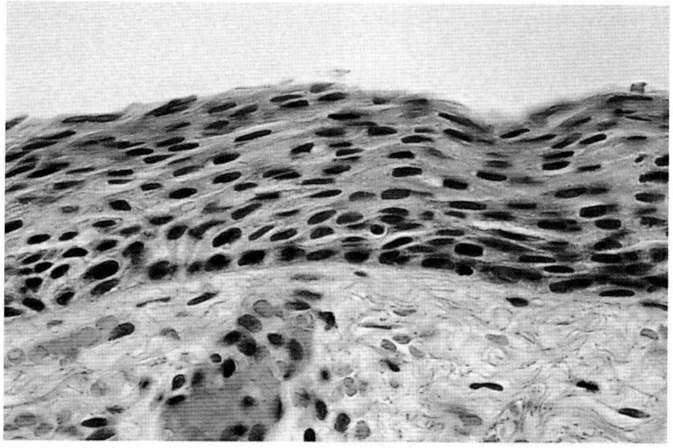

FIG. 8. Atrophic vagina with many mucosal layers of parabasal cells.

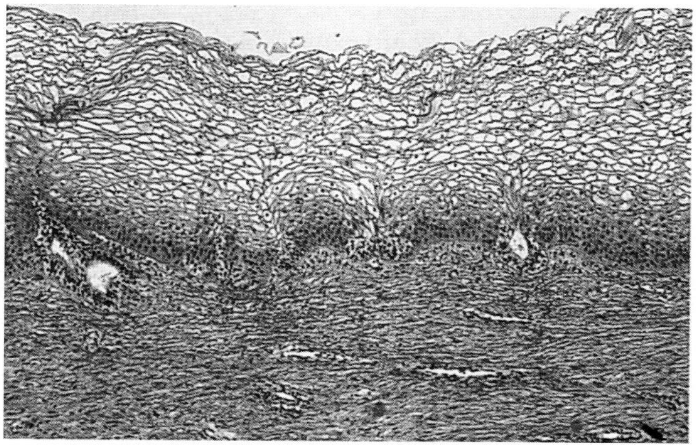

FIG. 10. Vaginal mucosa of a near-term fetus. Mature cells predominate and cannot be distinguished from that of the adult (compare with Fig. 7). In addition, two adenotic glands of the embryonic type are present.

Progesterone inhibits maturation of the vaginal epithelium. Consequently, intermediate cells predominate when the circulating levels of progesterone are high, for example, during the postovulatory phase of the menstrual cycle or during pregnancy. Estrogenic activity is low or absent before puberty and after the menopause; the vaginal epithelium fails to mature and hence remains thin. Parabasal and intermediate cells predominate in the vaginal smear. In the newborn child, the vaginal epithelium is frequently mature because of the influence of placental estrogens (Fig. 10). Quantitative studies measuring the rate of change in the maturation index in the infant's vagina from birth to the atrophic state indicate that vaginal cells replace themselves in less than 2 weeks, that is, the time required for basal cells to work their way up and become desquamated superficial cells (20). Studies of the exocervix indicate that turnover there is also rapid (21).

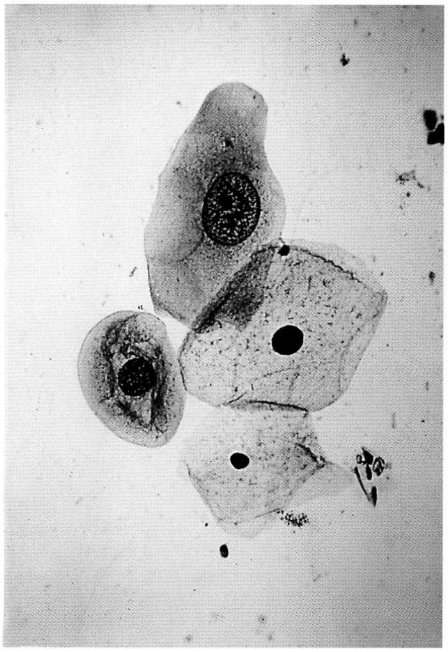

FIG. 9. Vaginal smear, showing basal cell, two intermediate cells, and a superficial cell (Papanicolaou stain). [Reprinted with permission (29).]

The submucosa, or lamina propria, lies beneath the squamous epithelium. It contains elastic fibers and a rich venous and lymphatic network. Sometimes the superficial lamina propria discloses a bandlike zone of loose connective tissue that contains atypical polygonal to stellate stromal cells with scant cytoplasm (Fig. 4). Many cells are multinucleated or have multilobulated hyperchromatic nuclei. Few are mononucleate. Mitoses are not observed. These atypical stromal cells are thought to give rise to fibroepithelial polyps, which have been observed within the cervix, vagina, and vulva (13,14). They have been shown to be fibroblastic in origin.

### Vaginal Wall and Adventitia

The vaginal musculature is continuous with that of the uterus. The outer layers of muscle of both the uterus and vagina run longitudinal to pass out onto the lateral pelvic wall to form the superior and inferior surfaces, respectively, of the cardinal ligaments. The longitudinal muscle fibers continue to course the length of the vagina to the region of the hymenal ring, where they gradually disappear in the connective tissue. On the anterior vaginal wall the longitudinal muscle fibers are displaced more by the urethra than diminished in number. The inner muscle layer of the vagina forms a spiral-like course, appearing in microscopic sections as somewhat circular in direction.

The adventitia is a thin coat of dense connective tissue adjoining the muscularis. The connective tissue of the adventitia merges with the stroma, connecting the vagina to the adjacent structures. This layer contains the many veins, lymphatics, nerve bundles, and small groups of nerve cells.

## ULTRASTRUCTURE

On ultrastructural examination, the component layers are not sharply demarcated from each other. Rather, they may be somewhat difficult to distinguish because each layer has ill-defined limits and displays gradual changes in structure (22). In general the ultrastructural changes observed by transmission electron microscopy resemble those of the exocervix and mucosal squamous cells and are not further covered herein.

On scanning electron microscopic examination, the superficial cells appear large (50 μm in greatest dimension) and polygonal. The intercellular edges are narrow and dense and protrude slightly. The pattern of fine webbing and anastomotic intercellular bridges typifies nonkeratinized squamous epithelium, such as that observed in buccal mucosa. The key structure on the cell surface is the microridge, or in reality myriad microridges, which are interanastomotic longitudinal elevations of the plasma membrane 0.2 nm long and 0.1 nm high (Fig. 11). Arranged in dense convolutions, they tie one cell to another, operating in a zipper-fastener principle. They are thought to provide surface adhesion. Desmosomes are prominent in these areas.

Microridge formation depends on the topographic configuration of disulfide-rich keratin or keratin precursors, which are absent in immature precursor cells, such as intermediate cells and young metaplastic squamous cells. From midcycle and early in the luteal phase, intercellular grooves widen. Porelike widening (porosites) of the intercellular crevices takes place where several cells interconnect. This porosity is thought to enhance continuity of the intercellular space system of the vaginal epithelium and the vaginal surface, thus permitting free passage of vaginal lubricating fluid.

## DIFFERENTIAL DIAGNOSIS AND SPECIAL ANATOMY

### Wolffian Ducts

The wolffian duct, known otherwise as the mesonephric duct or Gartner's duct, is vestigial in the adult female (Fig. 12). It begins to irreversibly wither if not stimulated to develop by testosterone before the 13th week postconception. This paired duct is most commonly situated in the lateral vaginal walls, although we have encountered it in all areas. Where encountered by chance in a radical vaginectomy specimen, the ducts are virtually always invisible grossly. Mitoses are absent. Usually it is a small duct or clusters of smalls glands about a duct. The lumen is filled frequently with a deeply eosinophilic, hyalinized secretion. The single layer of cells lining the duct is primarily nucleus. The cytoplasm is scant, relatively translucent, and lacks cilia. The nuclei frequently overlap. The chromatin is strikingly bland. On a clinical basis individual ducts occasionally become cystic and macroscopically visible. In the cervix, these ducts rarely appear diffusely throughout the wall and appear as mesonephric hyperplasia or even adenoma (23). We also have seen rare cases where the neoplasm present appeared to be a true wolffian duct carcinoma.

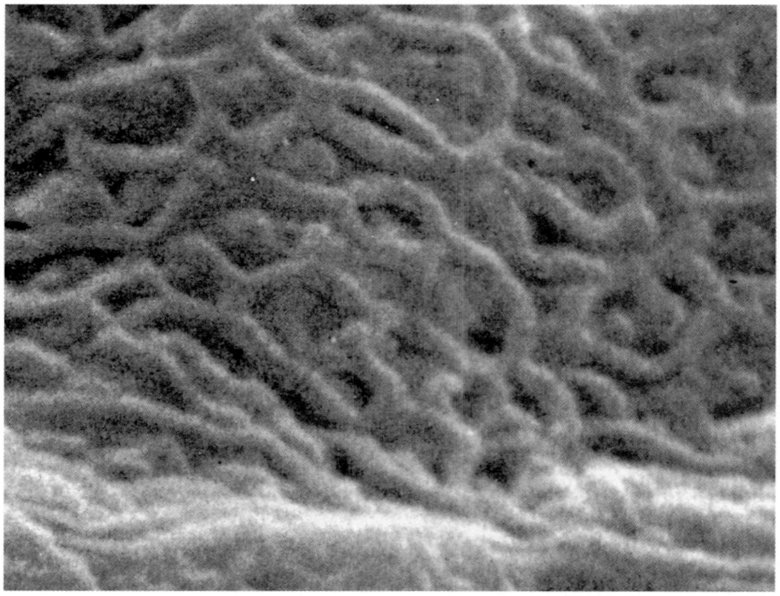

**FIG. 11.** Intricate network of microridges on surface plasma membrane of most superficial squamous cells living in the normal vaginal lumen. Scanning electron microscopy (original magnification ×**10,000**). [Reprinted with permission (22).]

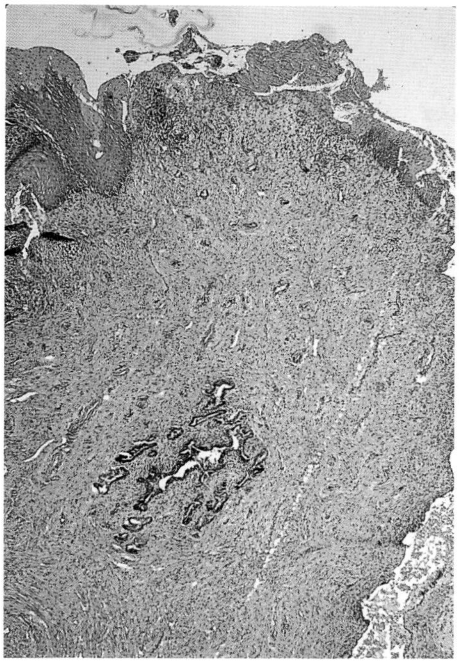

A

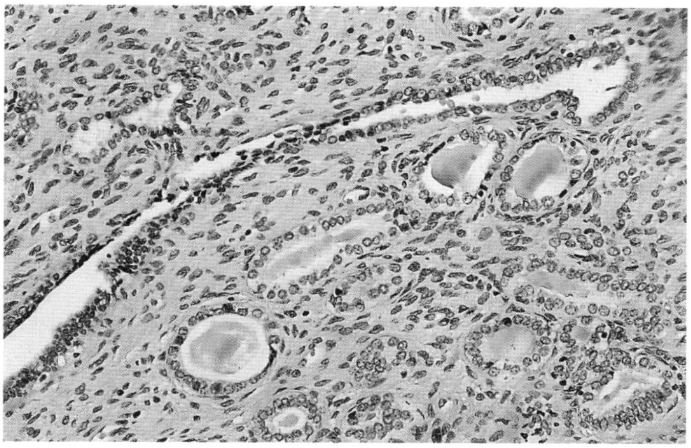

B

**FIG. 12.** **A:** Vestigial wolffian duct remnants, deep in wall. **B:** Detail of central duct and arborized ductal terminals with eosinophilic secretions. [Reprinted with permission (29).]

**Remnants of Müllerian Duct Epithelium (Adenosis)**

The DES story began in 1938 when this nonsteroidal estrogen was synthesized and then gained popularity for the treatment of high-risk pregnancy. By 1971, up to two million women had taken the drug, at which time it was linked to the extremely rare development of clear cell adenocarcinoma of the vagina in young female offspring. Subsequently, about one third of the exposed young women were found to have adenosis (presence of glandular tissue in the vagina). Both retrospective and prospective studies have shown that adenosis can be found in nonexposed women also, albeit rarely. In both exposed and nonexposed women, the adenosis is related to embryonic müllerian tissue that has remained entrapped and not been replaced by squamous epithelium during fetal life.

Adenosis appears in three forms. One type, the embryonic form, is exceedingly rare. The other two are the adult and common forms. In adenosis found during fetal life and in stillborns, but only rarely in adults, the glands are embryonic in character (24) (Figs. 10 and 13). They are small, usually at the epithelial–stromal interface, and are characterized by individual cells with small basal nuclei and copious bland cytoplasm that does not stain with either periodic acid-Schiff or mucicarmine.

It is believed that adenosis takes on its adult forms in women some time during puberty (25,26). Mucinous columnar cells, which by light and electron microscopy resemble those of the normal endocervical mucosa, comprise the glandular epithelium most frequently encountered as adenosis (62% of biopsy specimens with vaginal adenosis). This epithelium, because it frequently lines the surface of the vagina, is the type most commonly observed by colposcopy. Commonly, the mucinous columnar cells also line glands embedded in the lamina propria. This form of epithelium gives rise to the progestin-stimulated lesion, microglandular hyperplasia of the vagina (27).

Dark cells and light cells, often ciliated and resembling the lining cells of the fallopian tube and endometrium, are found in 21% of specimens in the upper vagina with adenosis. This form of adenosis has been called tuboendometrial, although serous might be equally appropriate. The cells are usually found in glands in the lamina propria and not on the vaginal surface. Although adenosis in the lower vagina is rare in absolute number, the percentage of biopsy specimens with adenosis that exhibits tuboendometrial rather than mucinous cells increases markedly in frequency in comparison with the more cranial aspects of the vagina. The tuboendometrial cell, which is benign, is the cell that we believe is related to clear cell adenocarcinoma, possibly through atypical adenosis, a transitional form (15,28). Mucinous glands and mucinous pools or droplets are encountered frequently in the same biopsy specimen; mucinous and tuboendometrial cells are found together only occasionally in biopsy material. The tuboendometrial form of adenosis is the instrumental type of glandular cell induced by all regions of the müllerian duct, be it fallopian tube, uterus, or vagina, whereas the mucinous cell is generally specific to the endocervix or, after DES exposure, to the deformed region of the cervix, which becomes ill-defined and includes what appears to be the upper vagina.

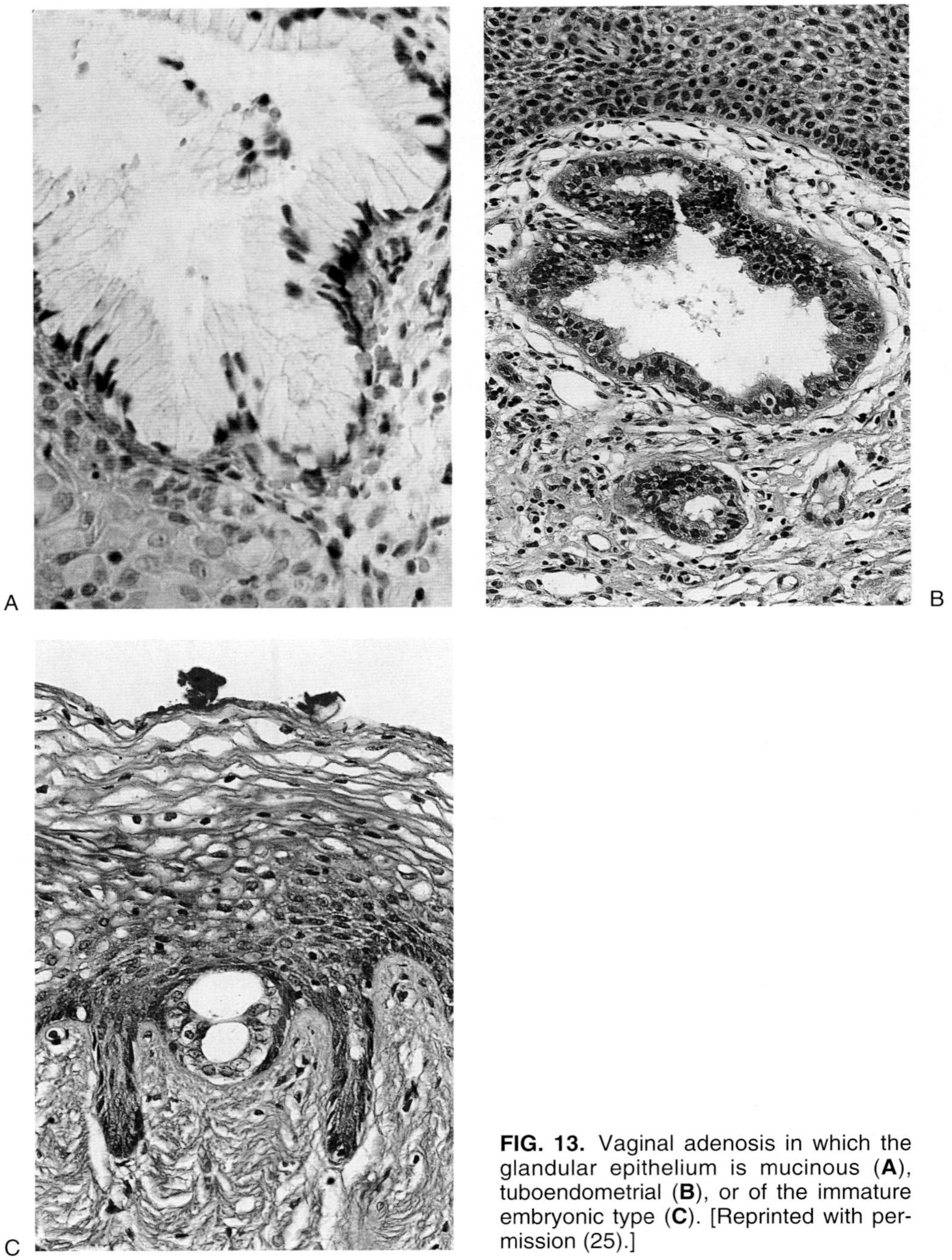


**FIG. 13.** Vaginal adenosis in which the glandular epithelium is mucinous (**A**), tuboendometrial (**B**), or of the immature embryonic type (**C**). [Reprinted with permission (25).]

## REFERENCES

1. Forsberg JG, Kalland T. Embryology of the genital tract in humans and rodents. In: Herbst AL, Bern HA, eds. *Developmental effects of diethylstilbestrol (DES) in pregnancy.* New York: Thieme-Stratton; 1981:4–25.
2. Robboy SJ, Taguchi O, Cunha GR. Normal development of the human female reproductive tract and alterations resulting from experimental exposure to diethylstilbestrol. *Hum Pathol* 1982;13:190–198.
3. Lawrence DW, Whitaker D, Sugimura Y, Cunha GR, Dickersin GR, Robboy SJ. An ultrastructural study of the developing urogenital tract in early human fetuses. *Am J Obstet Gynecol* 1992;167:185–193.
4. Taguchi O, Cunha GR, Lawrence WD, Robboy SJ. Timing and irreversibility of müllerian duct inhibition in the embryonic reproductive tract of the human male. *Dev Biol* 1984;106:394–398.
5. Behringer RR. The in vivo roles of müllerian-inhibiting substance. *Curr Top Dev Biol* 1994;29:171–187.
6. Ulfelder H, Robboy SJ. The embryological development of the human vagina. *Am J Obstet Gynecol* 1976;126:769–776.
7. Taguchi O, Cunha GR, Robboy SJ. Expression of nuclear estrogen binding sites within developing human fetal vagina and urogenital sinus. *Am J Anat* 1986;177:473–480.
8. Forsberg JG. Development of the human vaginal epithelium. In: Hafez ESE, Evans TN, eds. *The human vagina.* New York: North-Holland; 1978:3–20.
9. Terruhn V. A study of impression moulds of the genital tract of female fetuses. *Arch Gynecol* 1980;229:207–217.

10. Donjacour AA, Cunha GR. Stromal regulation of epithelial function. *Cancer Treat Res* 1991;53:335–364.
11. di Clemente N, Wilson C, Faure E, et al. Cloning, expression, and alternative splicing of the receptor for anti-müllerian hormone. *Mol Endocrinol* 1994;8:1006–1020.
12. Elliot GB, Elliot JDA. Superficial stromal reactions of lower genital tract. *Arch Pathol* 1973;95:100–101.
13. Abdul-Karim FW, Cohen RE. Atypical stromal cells of lower female genital tract. *Histopathology* 1990;17:249–253.
14. al-Nafussi AI, Rebello G, Hughes D, Blessing K. Benign vaginal polyp: a histological, histochemical and immunohistochemical study of 20 polyps with comparison to normal vaginal subepithelial layer. *Histopathology* 1992;20:145–150.
15. Robboy SJ, Welch WR, Young RH, Truslow GY, Herbst AL, Scully RE. Topographic relation of adenosis, clear cell adenocarcinoma and other related lesions of the vagina and cervix in DES exposed progeny. *Obstet Gynecol* 1982;60:546–551.
16. Mostwin JL. Current concepts of female pelvic anatomy and physiology. *Urol Clin North Am* 1991;18:175–195.
17. Clemente CD, ed. *Gray's anatomy.* 30th ed. Philadelphia: Lea & Febiger; 1985.
18. Moore TR, Reiter RC, Rebar RW, Baker VV. *Gynecology and obstetrics. A longitudinal approach.* London: Churchill Livingstone; 1993: 677.
19. Steger RW, Hafez ESE. Age associated changes in vagina. In: Hafez ESE, Evans TN, eds. *The human vagina.* New York: North-Holland; 1978:95–108.
20. Parker CE, Johnson FC. The effect of maternal estrogens on the vaginal epithelium of the newborn. *Clin Pediatr (Phila)* 1963;2:374.
21. Linhartova A. The height and structure of the cervical squamous epithelium in foetuses, newborns, and girls. *Cervix Low Female Genital Tract* 1989;7:37–48.
22. Ferenczy A, Richart RM. *Female reproductive system: dynamics of scan and transmission electron microscopy.* New York: John Wiley; 1974.
23. Ferry JA, Scully RE. Mesonephric remnants, hyperplasia, and neoplasia in the uterine cervix. A study of 49 cases. *Am J Surg Pathol* 1990; 14:1100–1111.
24. Robboy SJ, Hill EC, Sandberg EC, Czernobilsky B. Vaginal adenosis in women born prior to the diethylstilbestrol (DES) era. *Hum Pathol* 1986;17:488–493.
25. Robboy SJ. A hypothetic mechanism of diethylstilbestrol (DES)-induced anomalies in prenatally exposed women. *Hum Pathol* 1983;14: 831–833.
26. Robboy SJ, Kaufman RH, Prat J, et al. Pathologic findings in young women enrolled in national cooperative diethylstilbestrol adenosis (DESAD) project. *Obstet Gynecol* 1979;53:309–317.
27. Robboy SJ, Welch WR. Microglandular hyperplasia in vaginal adenosis associated with oral contraceptives and prenatal diethylstilbestrol (DES) exposure. *Obstet Gynecol* 1977;49:430–434.
28. Robboy SJ, Young RH, Welch WR, Truslow GY, Prat J, Herbst AL, Scully RE. Atypical (dysplastic) adenosis: forerunner and transitional state to clear cell adenocarcinoma in young women exposed in utero to diethylstilbestrol. *Cancer* 1984;54:869–875.
29. Robboy SJ. *Kodachrome atlas of gynecologic pathology.* 2nd ed. Durham, NC: Gyn-Path Assoc; 1996.
30. Fu YS, Reagan JW. *Pathology of the uterine cervix, vagina, and vulva.* Philadelphia: WB Saunders; 1989:397.
31. Zaino R, Robboy SJ, Bentley R, Kurman R. Vagina. In: Kurman RT, ed. *Blaustein's pathology of the female genital tract.* 4th ed. New York: Springer Verlag; 1994:131–185.

*Histology for Pathologists, second edition,*
Edited by Stephen S. Sternberg.
Lippincott-Raven Publishers, Philadelphia


# CHAPTER 39

# Normal Histology of the Uterus and Fallopian Tubes

Michael R. Hendrickson and Richard L. Kempson



The fallopian tubes and uterus in many ways constitute a natural anatomic and functional unit. They both derive embryologically from the müllerian duct. Taken together they provide the locations for the fusion of the descending egg and the ascending spermatozoon, the implantation of the resulting blastocyst, and the incubation of the developing gestation, and they ultimately provide the mechanism for the delivery of the conceptus at term. They have a common anatomic organization and share common responses to a changing steroidal milieu. Looking beyond normal structure and function to pathology, the fallopian tube and the uterus, together with the ovarian surface epithelium, comprise what has been termed the extended müllerian system (1), which gives rise to a common set of neoplasms and non-neoplastic metaplastic epithelial changes.

This chapter emphasizes those aspects of normal histology relevant to the diagnostic pathologist and focuses on those features of the normal uterus and fallopian tubes that, because of their striking appearance or unfamiliarity, raise the issue of pathologic alterations.

Accounts of conventional light microscopic appearance of the fallopian tube and uterus have not changed substantially over the past several decades. This is in sharp contrast to the impressive gains in our knowledge of the biochemical and physiologic details of the normal function of these organs. Parallel advances have been made in microsurgery and radiologic imaging techniques. Increasing use of in vitro fertilization and embryo transfer technology has exploited these advances, and that in turn has prompted a return to many

M. R. Hendrickson and R. L. Kempson: Department of Pathology, Stanford University Medical Center, Stanford, California 94305.

ancient questions: Why do women menstruate? What exactly does the endometrium do? Does it have an endocrine function? What are the functions of the many endometrial secretion products? Which of these endometrial contributions are essential to initiating and successfully sustaining a gestation? There has been an explosion of knowledge concerning the hormonal control of the reproductive system, fueled in large part by efforts to induce ovulation with pharmacologic agents. This has led in recent decades to a much more extensive knowledge of the neuroendocrine regulation of the menstrual cycle, the detailed anatomy and endocrinology of ovarian folliculogenesis, ovulation and corpus luteum function, the mechanism of action and genetics of steroid receptors, and the mechanisms responsible for normal menstrual bleeding. Paradoxically, most of this information is currently not of direct relevance to diagnostic pathologists. The practical orientation of this work notwithstanding, to ignore this knowledge would impart a distinctly dated character to this chapter. Therefore, we include a rough outline of some of this information and direct the interested reader to sources with a more detailed treatment of these issues.

This chapter first discusses the embryology and gross anatomy of the uterus and the fallopian tubes and then turns to the normal histology of the cervix, endometrium, myometrium, fallopian tube, and broad ligament.

## EMBRYOLOGY

The uterus and fallopian tubes have a complex developmental history (2–8). For poorly understood reasons, precursors of both male and female internal genitalia are laid down early in each embryo in a manner analogous to the initial development of the bipotential gonad. This is known as the indifferent stage of genital development. Upon completion of this indifferent stage, definitive female differentiation is accompanied by regression of the male anlage, whereas male differentiation is accompanied by regression of the female anlage. Topographically, both of these systems are intimately related to the developing urinary tract, and, not surprisingly, anomalous development of the internal genitalia is often accompanied by anomalies of the urinary tract. Fetal sexual differentiation is completed during the first half of gestation; the last half is marked primarily by growth of the newly established genitalia. Relevant milestones have been summarized by Ramsey (341) (Fig. 1).

| AGE | GLANDS | URINARY TRACT | ♂ DUCTS | ♀ DUCTS | EXTERNAL GENITALIA |
|---|---|---|---|---|---|
| 3-4 weeks | PRIMORDIAL GERM CELLS | PRONEPHROS (nonfunctional) Tubules and Ducts | PRONEPHRIC | | |
| 4-9 weeks | | MESONEPHROS or WOLFFIAN BODY (temporary function) Tubules and Ducts | MESONEPHRIC or WOLFFIAN | | CLOACA |
| 5th week | UROGENITAL RIDGE | | | | |
| 6th week | INDIFFERENT GONAD: GERMINAL AND CORE EPITHELIUM | METANEPHROS or KIDNEY (permanent) Tubules and Ducts | PARAMESONEPHRIC or MÜLLERIAN | | CLOACA SUBDIVIDES<br>GENITAL TUBERCLE |
| 7th week | MALE TYPE CORDS | | | | ANAL AND URETHRAL MEMBRANES RUPTURE |
| 8th week | TESTIS AND OVARY | | | | URETHRAL AND LABIOSCROTAL FOLDS, PHALLUS AND GLANS |
| 9th week | | | MÜLLERIAN DUCTS FUSE AT TUBERCLE | | |
| 10th week | | | MÜLLERIAN DUCTS DEGENERATE | WOLFFIAN DUCTS DEGENERATE | |
| 11th week | | | SEMINAL VESICLES, EPIDIDYMIS, VAS DEFERENS | | |
| 12th week | OVARY DESCENT COMPLETE | | | WALLS FORM | SEX DISTINGUISHABLE |
| 5 months | TESTIS AT INGUINAL RING | | | SINUS EPITHELIUM GROWS IN VAGINAL CLEFT | |
| 8 months<br>TERM | TESTIS DESCENT COMPLETE | | | RAPID UTERINE GROWTH | |

**FIG. 1.** Chart showing interrelations and time sequence of events in development of genitourinary system. Reprinted with permission (341).

### The Indifferent Stage

By the 6th week of fetal life the urogenital sinus and the mesonephric (wolffian) ducts are well established. At this time the paired müllerian (paramesonephric) ducts begin their development. These structures are formed by an invagination of the celomic epithelium adjacent to that investing each developing ovary. The müllerian ducts are intimately related to the mesonephric ducts, and their normal formation appears in fact to be dependent on the presence of the mesonephros.

As the müllerian ducts grow caudally, they approach the midline where the distal portions fuse. Shortly after this fusion, the apposed medial duct walls disappear, bringing the two lumina into continuity to form a single cavity. Further downward growth of the fused müllerian structures (now termed the uterovaginal primordium) brings them into contact with the urogenital sinus. At this stage both the mesonephric ducts and the müllerian ducts are present in the fetus.

### Female Differentiation

The differentiation of the indifferent internal genitalia into male or female structures depends on whether the fetus possesses ovaries or testes. In the male fetus, the Leydig cells and the Sertoli cells in the developing testes secrete testosterone and a nonsteroidal müllerian inhibiting substance. The net effect of this secretory activity is to ensure the persistence, differentiation, and growth of the mesonephric ducts to form the male genital system and the regression of the müllerian system. In the absence of a secreting testis (e.g., in a normal female fetus with ovaries or in a fetus with nonfunctioning gonads) the müllerian structures persist, whereas the mesonephric ducts regress. The nonfused portions of the müllerian ducts form the fallopian tubes; the fused segments develop into the uterus and probably the upper third of the vagina. Incomplete fusion of the caudal portion of the müllerian ducts results in a spectrum of uterovaginal abnormalities (9).

By the 21st week, the uterus and vagina are well formed. In contrast to the adult cervix, the cervix of the prenatal uterus is disproportionately large and makes up two thirds of the length of the organ. The second half of gestation is marked by uterine growth; from the 28th week to birth, a period of approximately 10 weeks, the fetal uterus doubles in size. However, the earlier cervicocorpus disproportion is maintained into childhood.

## GROSS ANATOMY

### Premenarchal Uterus and Fallopian Tubes

#### *Neonatal Period*

At birth the uterus averages about 4 cm in length, and its bulk and shape are dominated by its disproportionately large cervix (the cervicofundal ratio is approximately 3–5:1) (Fig. 2). The impact of the maternal hormonal environment is reflected in the markedly thickened rugal vaginal mucosa typically present at birth and, to a certain extent, in the histologic appearance of the endometrium, which is most often proliferative or weakly secretory. Maternal estrogen also results in cervical squamous cell maturation with glycogen storage. These mucosal changes regress shortly after birth (10–15).

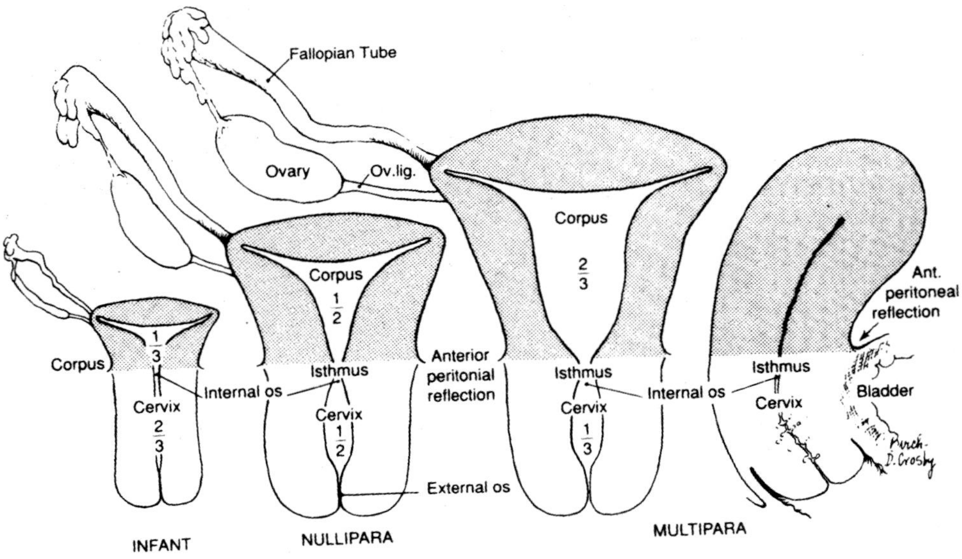


**FIG. 2.** Drawings illustrating comparative sizes of prepubertal, mature nonparous, and parous uteri. The relative proportions of uterine corpus and cervix are seen to change with age and parity. Frontal and sagittal sections are presented. (After Ranice W. Crosby.) Reprinted with permission (342).

### *Infancy*

Uterine growth continues into the second year of life, at which time it reaches a plateau that persists until the premenarchal growth spurt at about 9 years of age. Until approximately the 13th year, the cervix continues to account for greater than half of the uterine length.

## Adult Uterus and Fallopian Tubes

### *General Relations and Attachments*

The uterus is located anterior to the rectum and posterior to the bladder (Fig. 3). It is covered anteriorly and posteriorly by a reflection of pelvic peritoneum that continues laterally to form the anterior and posterior leaves of the broad ligament. The posterior peritoneal reflection forms the uterine wall of the pouch of Douglas and covers a longer segment of the uterine isthmus than does the anterior peritoneal reflection. The tentlike broad ligaments house the major uterine vessels and the efferent lymphatic trunks; they also contain the fallopian tubes at their apices. Each ovary is attached to the ipsilateral uterine cornu by the utero-ovarian ligament, which is situated posterolateral and inferior to the uterine attachment of the fallopian tubes. The round ligaments arise anterolateral and inferior to the attachment of the fallopian tubes and pass anteriorly to insert into the canal of Nuck. These anatomic relations are of obvious importance to the surgeon but also of value to the pathologist because they often enable proper orientation of the hysterectomy specimen. The anterior surface of the uterus is distinguished by its longer "bare" region (i.e., lacking peritoneum) and the anteriorly directed stump of the round ligament. The posterior surface is more extensively covered by peritoneum, and the utero-ovarian ligament is attached to the posterior cornual aspect of the uterus. The uterus is anchored to its surroundings by a number of connective tissue bands; notable among them are the cardinal, uterosacral, and pubocervical ligaments (16–19).

## Gross Anatomic Features of the Uterus

The adult nulliparous uterus is a hollow, pear-shaped muscular organ weighing 40 to 80 g and measuring approximately 7 to 8 cm along its long axis, 5.0 cm at its broadest extent (cornu to cornu), and 2.5 cm in anteroposterior dimension. These measurements vary considerably as a function of age, phase of the menstrual cycle, and parity. In general, high parity and youth are positively correlated with increasing uterine size (20). The adult uterus consists of an

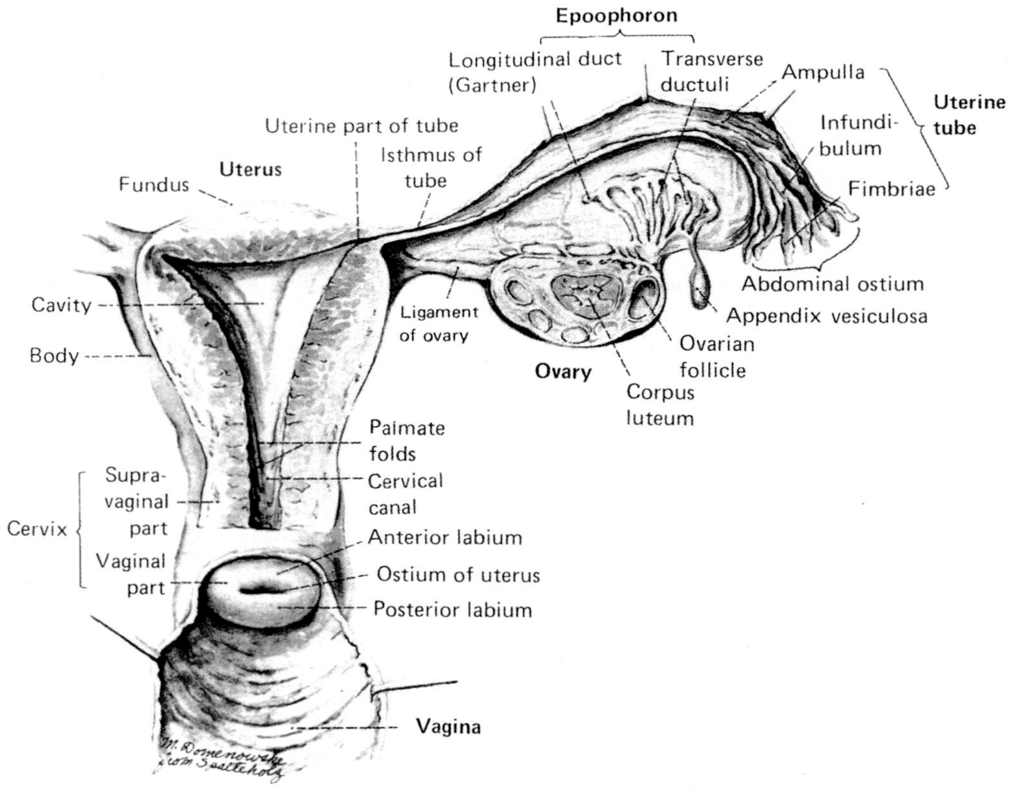


**FIG. 3.** The normal internal female genitalia. Reprinted with permission (343).

expanded body, the corpus, and a smaller cervix. That portion of the corpus cephalad to a line connecting the origin of the two fallopian tubes is called the fundus. The cornua are the two lateral regions of the fundus associated with the intramural portion of the fallopian tubes. The remainder of the corpus tapers from the fundus into the isthmus or the lower uterine segment, which shares histologic features with both of the uterine segments that it bridges: the uterine corpus and the endocervix. The existence of an anatomically and functionally significant lower uterine segment has been disputed by some authorities (21). The uterine cavity has the approximate configuration of the uterus, but its internal dimensions are much smaller, reflecting the substantial thickness of the uterine wall. The cavity is triangular, and the apices of this potential space are continuous, with the lumina of the fallopian tubes at the two cornua and with the endocervical canal at the internal os. The length of the cavity is approximately 6.0 cm. Again, these measurements vary considerably with the age and parity of the individual (22). The cervix is roughly cylindrical and normally measures approximately 3 to 4 cm in length (23). It is pierced through its center by the endocervical canal. Traditionally, the endocervical canal has been described as having an external os that opens onto the exocervix and an internal os that separates the endometrial canal from the endometrial cavity. Although the former is a reasonable anatomic landmark, the latter is not because grossly, the transition from endometrial cavity to endocervix is gradual, without abrupt anatomic demarcation between endocervix and endometrium. This is histologically mirrored by the gradual transition of the mucosa in this region from endocervical type to endometrial type. The mucosal surface of the endocervical canal is deeply clefted to form the plicae palmatae. The lateral connective tissue attachments of the uterus are referred to as the parametria; they contain vessels, nerves, lymphatics, and lymph nodes.

The normal myometrium consists of an outer longitudinal muscle layer, an inner circular submucosal muscle layer, and an interposed thick middle layer, richly populated by vessels and composed of randomly interdigitating fibers (24). In addition, two lateral subserosally situated longitudinal bands of distinctive muscle fibers, the fasciculus cervicoangularis, have been described (25,26). On occasion, epithelium that is histochemically and histologically similar to cervical mesonephric remnants is present within this bundle, suggesting that these structures represent the vestiges of the wolffian (mesonephric) duct. A role in electrical impulse conduction also has been postulated for these bands.

Substantial deviations from the nulliparous adult uterus naturally occur throughout adult life. The uterus undergoes small-amplitude changes in size during the menstrual cycle, attaining its greatest volume during the secretory phase (27). During pregnancy, of course, the uterus enlarges much more dramatically to accommodate the growing conceptus. This growth is due largely to combined hyperplasia and hypertrophy of the myometrium. After delivery, uterine size rapidly decreases, and over the ensuing weeks a striking resorption of connective tissue occurs that is associated with a decrease in the size of individual myocytes. However, the uterus generally does not return completely to its nulliparous size and weight. Prior pregnancy (parity) can be deduced from several gross features. The multiparous nongravid uterus tends to weigh more in consequence of its thicker and more prominently layered muscular walls; this increase in weight is proportional to the patient's parity (20). The vasculature of the multiparous uterus tends to be more prominent. The most suggestive changes of previous pregnancy, however, are seen in the cervix. The nulliparous circular small external os is transformed after pregnancy into a slit that forms prominent anterior and posterior lips. In addition, healed cervical lacerations may be pronounced, and enough endocervical tissue may reside on the exocervix to give it a red granular appearance near the os. With the waning of ovarian hormone synthesis during the menopausal years, the uterus involutes and atrophies. This is reflected by a decrease in its weight and its dimensions. On occasion the endocervical canal is almost completely obliterated. Exogenous estrogens administered during this period sometimes maintain uterine weight artificially despite the loss of ovarian hormonal support.

Parenthetically it should be noted that the increasing use of high-resolution radiographic imaging techniques has prompted a spate of in vivo studies of normal female pelvic anatomy including the cyclic variation in the appearance of the uterus (28–34). We can expect a more detailed account of normal uterine and tubal anatomic variation in the future as more of these studies are reported.

### Gross Anatomic Features of the Fallopian Tubes

The fallopian tubes are hollow epithelium-lined muscular structures 11 to 12 cm in length that run through the apex of the broad ligament to span the uterine cornu medially and the ovary laterally. Each tube is divided into four anatomic segments. The intramural segment begins at the funnel-like uppermost recess of the uterine cornu and ends where the tube emerges from the uterine wall. The course of this 8-mm, pinpoint lumened segment varies from straight to highly convoluted (35). Beyond the uterine wall the proximal tube continues for 2 to 3 cm as the isthmus, a thick-walled, narrow-calibered segment that merges into a comparatively thin-walled expanded area, the ampulla. The distal tube ends in the trumpet-shaped infundibulum whose mouth opens into the peritoneal cavity and is fringed by approximately 25 fimbria. One of these, the ovarian fimbrium, attaches to the ovary. At the time of ovulation the infundibulum forms a cap over the ovarian surface to create the ovarian bursa. The tubal mucosa and the underlying endosalpingeal stroma are thrown up into longitudinal, branching folds (the plicae) whose branches increase in complexity from the isthmus to the infundibulum. The plicae terminate in the fimbria. At the time of ovulation the fimbria sweep over the surface of the ovary to facilitate egg capture (17).

### Uterine and Tubal Vasculature

The major arterial supply of the uterus derives from the right and left uterine arteries, which arise from the corresponding hypogastric (internal iliac) arteries. The uterine artery divides into ascending and descending branches laterally at the level of the uterine isthmus. The ascending uterine artery anastomoses freely with the ovarian artery (a branch of the aorta) in the mesosalpinx, whereas the descending branch anastomoses with the vaginal arterial supply. Both the ascending and descending uterine arteries give rise to a complex network of circumferentially arranged subserosal arteries: the arcuate arteries. These in turn give rise to a series of radial arteries that penetrate the myometrium. Each of these radial vessels branches into straight and spiral arteries in the inner third of the myometrium, and these become the spiral arteries of the endometrium (36–38).

A striking characteristic of the adult intrauterine arteries is their marked tortuousity. This doubtless has to do with the variation in uterine size during reproductive life. In the postmenopausal years, striking degenerative changes may be seen in the uterine arteries, including intimal proliferation, fibrosis, and medial calcification. The severity of these changes is typically out of proportion to degenerative changes in nonuterine arteries. The venous drainage of the uterus parallels its arterial supply.

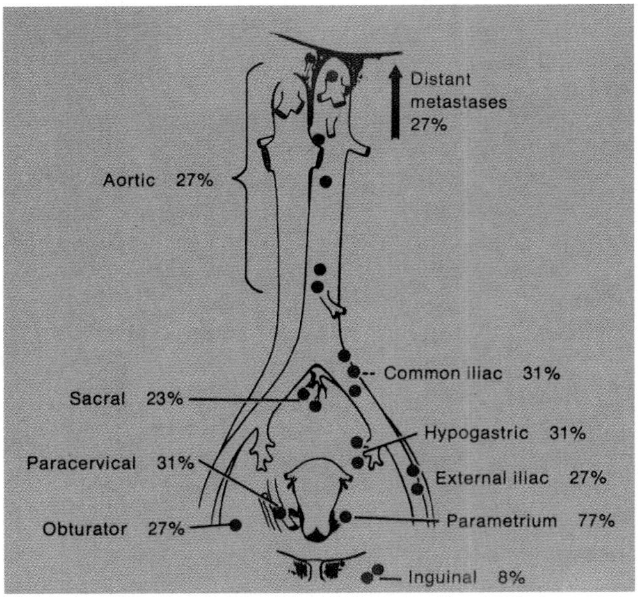


**FIG. 4.** Percentage involvement of draining lymph nodes in untreated patients with cervical cancer. Reprinted with permission (344).

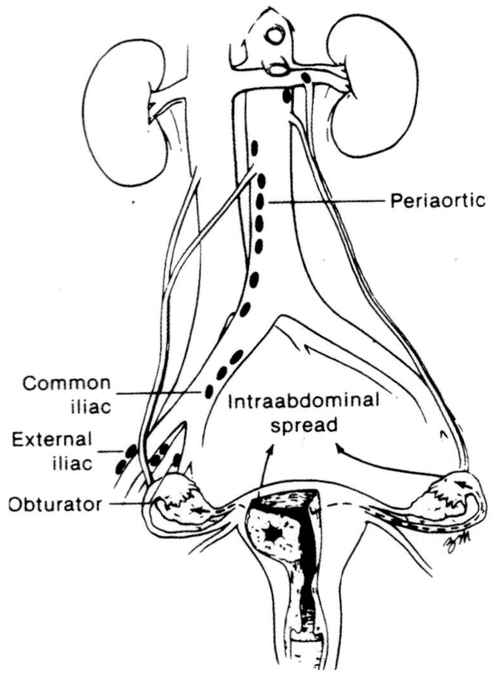


**FIG. 5.** Paths of spread available to carcinoma of the endometrium. Not only may carcinoma cells metastasize to the pelvic and periaortic lymph nodes, but they also may spread through the fallopian tube to the peritoneum or they may invade through the myometrium into the broad ligament and ovary. Reprinted with permission (345).

### Uterine and Tubal Lymphatics

Lymphatics are present in both the cervix and the corpus. In the endometrium these vessels are intimately associated with the glands of the functionalis. The myometrium and cervical stroma contain a complex labyrinth of lymphatics that course toward the subserosal plexus. The channels forming the latter ramify over the entire surface of the uterus, and the confluence of these channels forms the major efferent lymphatic trunks of the uterus. The chief interest in lymphatic drainage for the pathologist is as a guide to the dissemination of carcinoma. The major lymph node groups draining cervical and endometrial carcinoma are indicated in Figs. 4 and 5. The lymphatics of the fallopian tube drain to the lumbar and periaortic lymph nodes (39).

In both the mucosal and muscular layers, lymphatic anastomoses exist between the cervical and corpus systems, and on occasion cervical carcinomas may take advantage of this route to spread to the corpus. Whether the converse is true is unclear. Moreover, whether or not corpus carcinoma, once having invaded the cervix, then behaves like cervical carcinoma in terms of its lymphatic metastatic distribution is also unclear, even though this is a common clinical assumption. Indeed, involvement of "cervical draining nodes" by endometrial carcinoma does not necessarily imply cervical involvement. For further detail the reader is referred to specialty works and textbooks of gynecologic oncology (40–42).

## UTERINE CERVIX

The uterine cervix or "neck" is the elongate fibromuscular portion of the uterus that measures 2.5 to 3.0 cm. A part of this structure protrudes into the upper part of the vagina (vaginal part, portio vaginalis), whereas the remainder lies above the vaginal vault (supravaginal portion). The outer surface of the vaginal portion of the cervix is known variously as the ectocervix or exocervix. It is covered, at least in part, by stratified squamous epithelium that is continuous with, and histologically identical to, the mucosa of the vaginal fornices. That portion of the cervix in relation to the endocervical canal is known as the anatomic endocervix. The endocervical canal, lined for the most part by mucin-secreting epithelium that blends at one end with the squamous epithelium of the exocervix and with the epithelium of the lower uterine segment at its other end, brings the vagina into communication with the endometrial cavity. The anatomic opening of the endocervical canal onto the exocervix is known as the external os. In parous women, this most often takes on a slitlike configuration that serves to divide the exocervix into anterior and posterior lips (14, 43–51). This particular geometry is thought to be important in uterine function during gestation (52). The upper limit of the endocervical canal is known as the internal os. This is not a distinct orifice; rather, there is a gradual funnel-shaped widening of the endocervical canal and a transition from endocervical epithelium into the endometrial epithelium of the lower uterine segment. The junction of the endocervical glandular mucosa with the squamous epithelium of the exocervix is known as the squamocolumnar junction. This junction does not always lie at the external os; in fact, the squamocolumnar junction typically is located on the exocervix, where it can easily be inspected with the culposcope. This is further discussed in the section devoted to the transformation zone.

The uterine cervix obviously plays an important role in the anatomic support of the internal genitalia and plays an active role in labor and delivery, but arguably its primary role is the production of cervical mucous. Cervical mucous acts as a functional gate that prevents vaginal microorganisms from gaining access to the upper genital tract and (except for a small mid-cycle window before ovulation) denies sperm access to the uterus and fallopian tubes. At mid-cycle the chemical composition of the cervical mucous changes and its viscosity decreases. This has the effect of allowing the passage of sperm into the upper genital tract. These changes are the basis of the clinically useful Spinnbarkeit and fern tests. In addition, the cervical mucous plays an important role in removing seminal plasma constituents (preventing sperm phagocytosis) and in providing a suitable environment for sperm storage, capacitation, and migration (53).

The following discussion first focuses on the epithelium of the exocervix, the endocervix, and the transformation zone and then turns to the stroma of the cervix and the changes that occur in the cervix during pregnancy. A large body of literature reports on both the transmission and scanning electron microscope features of the cervix, which are not reviewed here (45,49,54–57).

### Epithelium of the Exocervix

The squamous epithelium covering the exocervix is normally noncornified, and it grows, matures, and accumulates glycogen in its upper layers in response to circulating estrogens, most notably estradiol (Fig. 6). Because low blood levels of estrogen are the rule during childhood and the postmenopausal years, the squamous cells of the cervix do not proliferate or mature, and glycogen is not stored in the upper layers of the epithelium during these periods unless estrogen is made available as a result of therapy or functioning ovarian tumors (58). In the immediate postnatal period, the squamous epithelium of the newborn cervix is fully mature due to maternal estrogen, but the epithelium quickly becomes atrophic and glycogen disappears as estrogen levels decrease.

The estrogenically stimulated cervical squamous epithelium of the sexually mature woman can be divided into three layers: the basal/parabasal cell layer, the midzone layer (or stratum spongiosum), and the superficial layer (Fig. 6). The basal cell layer is composed of cells with scant cytoplasm and oval to cuboidal nuclei with dense chromatin. These cells are usually mitotically inactive, do not take up tritiated thymidine on radioautography, and do not mark immunohistochemically with proliferation markers (e.g., Ki-67 and PCNA [proliferating cell nuclear antigen] (59). The cells immediately above the basal layer comprise the lower portion of the midzone layer and are known as parabasal cells, a term

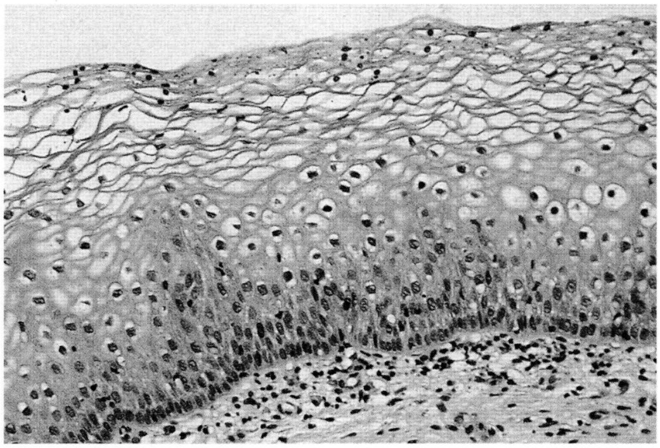

**FIG. 6.** Mature squamous epithelium of the exocervix demonstrating a normal maturation sequence from basal cells to superficial cells. The cleared cytoplasm indicating glycogen storage should not be confused with koilocytosis.

often used in cytologic circles. The parabasal cells are somewhat larger than the basal cells due to their increased cytoplasm, and the nuclei have slightly less dense chromatin. In contrast to the basal layer, mitotic figures are usually present but are not abnormal or particularly numerous in the normal epithelium. This layer also exhibits uptake of tritiated thymine and displays proliferation markers (59). The midzone layer is composed of cells with even more abundant cytoplasm and somewhat smaller vesicular nuclei. These are known as intermediate cells. Glycogen accumulates in most intermediate cells, and this imparts a finely granular or clear appearance to the cytoplasm. The superficial cells contain small, rounded, regular pyknotic nuclei, and their cytoplasm is abundant and clear as a result of even greater glycogen accumulation. Keratinization occurs in both the superficial and intermediate cells and renders them flat and platelike when they are spread on a slide. The cytoplasmic clearing characteristic of normal intermediate and superficial cells is often perinuclear. Because perinuclear clearing is also a feature of cells (koilocytes) infected by papillomavirus (HPV), there is a potential for misinterpreting normal epithelial cells containing glycogen as abnormal. However, koilocytes not only feature perinuclear clearing of the cytoplasm, but their nuclei are larger, and these nuclei possess a more undulating nuclear membrane than do the nuclei found in intermediate and superficial cells (giving rise to the appearance of koilocytes sometimes described as "raisinoid" or "pruneoid"). Moreover, the nuclear chromatin of koilocytes has a ropy texture in contrast to the homogenous appearance of normal cells. The cervical squamous mucosa undergoes cyclic changes during the menstrual cycle similar to the estrogen-progesterone–induced changes in the vaginal mucosa, although the cells composing the latter are a more reliable index of hormonal status. During the luteal phase, when progesterone levels are high, there is a predominance of intermediate cells.

The exocervical epithelium in postmenopausal women (not receiving a supplement of estrogen therapy) is composed mainly of basal and parabasal cells so effected with

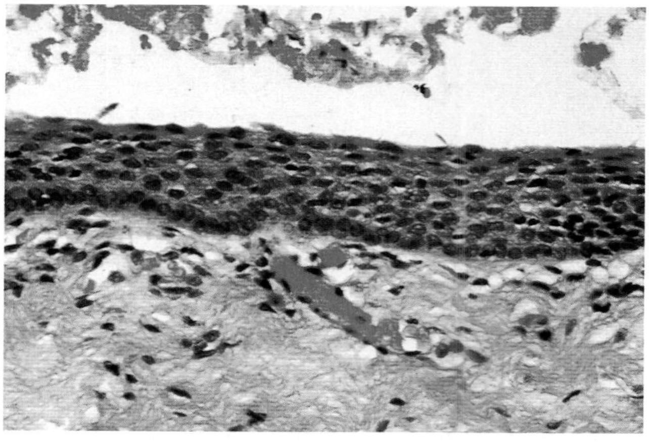

**FIG. 7.** Postmenopausal atrophy of the cervical squamous epithelium. The immature cells can resemble the cells in high-grade CIN.

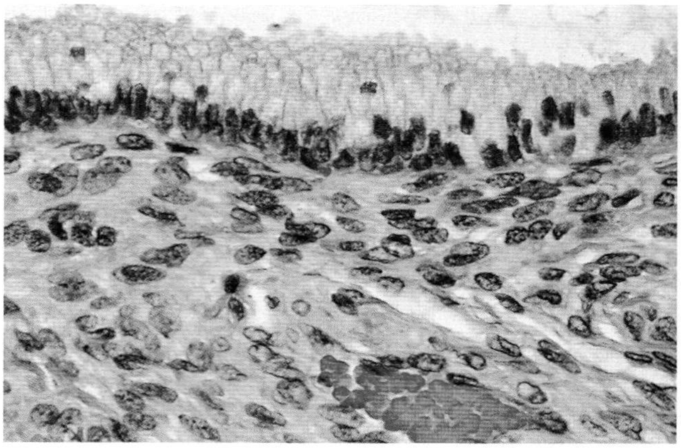

**FIG. 8.** Normal endocervical mucosa with most nuclei in the characteristic basilar location. Enlargement and rounding of these nuclei and prominent nucleoli are features that should cause a closer inspection of the endocervical glands to ensure that neoplastic transformation is not present.

scant cytoplasm and little or no cytoplasmic glycogen (Fig. 7). The cells may have the same degree of nucleus-to-cytoplasm ratio shift toward the nucleus as do the cells composing cervical intraepithelial neoplasia (CIN). Consequently, atrophic epithelium is a part of the differential diagnosis of a squamous intraepithelial lesion (SIN), and care should be taken when a diagnosis of CIN is contemplated in a postmenopausal woman. However, the basal and parabasal cells in atrophic epithelia do not demonstrate the nuclear abnormalities and high mitotic index usually seen in the cells constituting neoplastic epithelium.

Endocrine cells have been identified in the squamous epithelium of the exocervix by immunohistochemical techniques; their function is unknown, but they are thought to

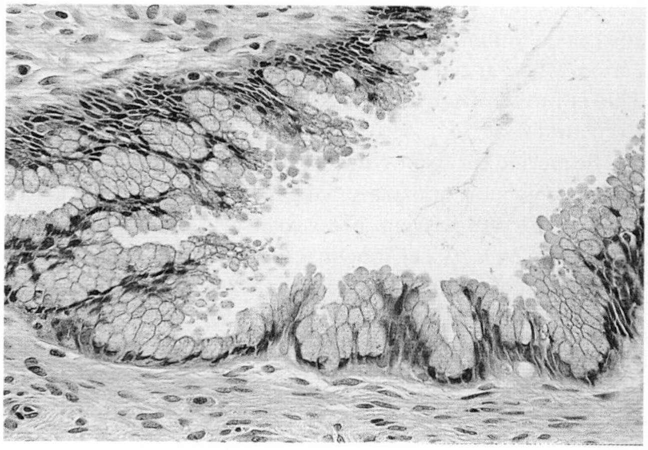

**FIG. 9.** Goblet cells in the endocervix. Not infrequently, the nuclei of mucin-containing cells are displaced to the base of the cell and compressed by cytoplasmic mucin to produce a goblet cell. The presence of goblet cells and neuroendocrine cells in the normal endocervical mucosa tends to destabilize the conventional distinction in ovarian pathology between müllerian (i.e., cervical) mucinous and intestinal mucinous differentiation.

give rise to the rare cervical carcinoid tumors (60–66). Langerhans cells also are present in the ectocervical epithelium, as well as in the transformation zone (67–71). They are involved in antigen presentation to T-lymphocytes. Melanin-containing cells have been reported in the cervical epithelium and provide a plausible cell of origin for the uncommon cervical melanoma and blue nevus (72).

**Epithelium of the Endocervix**

The anatomic endocervix extends from the external os to the internal os, but endocervical glandular epithelium is not exclusively limited to this anatomic area, particularly during the reproductive years. Rather, endocervical epithelium occupies significant regions of the anatomic exocervix during childhood and after the menarche. The movement of the endocervical epithelium out of the canal onto the exocervix is discussed in more detail below in the section devoted to the transformation zone.

The endocervix is lined by a single layer of mucin-secreting epithelium composed of cells with small, often basilar, nuclei above which is mucin-filled cytoplasm (73) (Fig. 8). Goblet cells are sometimes encountered (Fig. 9). The nuclei are generally small, elongate, and have rather dense chromatin. They tend to overlap one another. When the endocervical epithelium has been damaged and is regenerating, the nuclei may become larger and more rounded, but mitotic figures are difficult to find in non-neoplastic endocervical cells (74). If one encounters endocervical epithelium containing easily found mitotic figures, consideration should be given to the possibility of a pathologic process such as well-differentiated carcinoma or carcinoma in situ, particularly if the nuclei are enlarged and nucleoli are prominent. Nucleoli are usually not prominent in resting endocervical cells, but they may become so during regeneration, pregnancy, and neoplastic transformation.

Other types of cells may be identified in the endocervical epithelium. Ciliated cells are almost always present and can be a useful marker of a benign process when changes in the endocervical glandular epithelium raise concerns about well-differentiated adenocarcinoma. When ciliated cells are numerous, the term "ciliary metaplasia" is often used (Fig. 10A and B) (75–79). Ciliated cells can develop enlarged dense nuclei and thus come to resemble neoplastic cells. As a result, care should be taken to look for cilia before diagnosing in situ neoplastic transformation of the endocervix. Subcolumnar reserve cells that have the potential to differentiate into ciliated and mucous secretory cells have been reported to populate the endocervix, even though there is evidence that the differentiated mucous cells are capable of reproduction without the intercession of reserve cells (56,74,80,81). It is easy to confuse the lymphocytes that often migrate into the glandular epithelium with reserve cells. Endocrine cells also are present within the endocervical epithelium. Their normal function is unclear, but a generally held theory is that they give rise to the rare endocrine neoplasms such as carcinoids and neuroendocrine carcinomas that occasionally are encountered in the cervix.

The endocervical epithelium not only lines the surface of the endocervical canal, it also dips, to a variable degree, into the underlying stroma to form elongate clefts (Fig. 11A). In histologic sections, these clefts typically are cut transversely, imparting the false impression that true endocervical glands are present within the stroma. However, true glands have different epithelia lining their ductal and secretory portions. In contrast, the endocervical mucosa has a more or less uniform appearance whether it lines the surface or the deep-lying "glands." Further evidence that these are not true glands was provided in an study conducted over 30 years ago by Fluhmann (82,83). He demonstrated by means of serial sections and three-dimensional reconstructions that what appeared to be endocervical glands within the stroma are actually complex protrusions of the endocervical lining that form clefts into the underlying stroma. When the endocervical epithelium lining the stromal clefts proliferates, side channels grow out from the clefts, giving rise to a histologic pattern that even more closely suggests acini of glands (Fig. 11B). Fluhmann labeled these side channels "tunnel clusters"; we also refer to them as Fluhmann's lumens. When secretion inspissates in tunnel clusters, either because of obstruction or because of the viscosity of the secretions, it appears as bright eosinophilic material, an eye-catching pattern (see Fig. 16). Having now discharged our obligation to anatomic accuracy, we shall continue to use the terms endocervical "gland(s)" and "cleft(s)" interchangeably.

The depth to which benign endocervical glands can extend in the cervical stroma varies from cervix to cervix. They can be found as deep as 1 cm but usually are found at a depth of less than 5 mm (84–87). This anatomic variation becomes important when considering a diagnosis of "minimal deviation adenocarcinoma" (88,89). In this form of adenocarcinoma the cytologic features differ only minimally from normal endocervical epithelium, and the diagnosis depends to a large extent on the identification of abnormally shaped glands at an inappropriate depth within the cervical stroma. The trick here is to compare the depth of the glands in question with noncontroversially benign glands in the immediate neighborhood. Additionally useful in establishing a diagnosis of malignancy is a search for glands around nerves or vessels, an irregular "lobster claw" glandular configuration, and a granulation tissue stromal host response. We have not personally encountered a clinically malignant endocervical glandular proliferation that featured ciliated cells and, in our opinion, this finding argues strongly against a diagnosis of adenocarcinoma.

Endocervical cells show only minimal morphologic changes during the menstrual cycle, and even this amounts only to a shifting of the basally situated nuclei to a mid-cell position at the height of the proliferative phase. These minor cytologic changes are in contrast to the dramatic biochemical changes that occur within the endocervical cells during the menstrual cycle (53). Throughout the proliferative phase

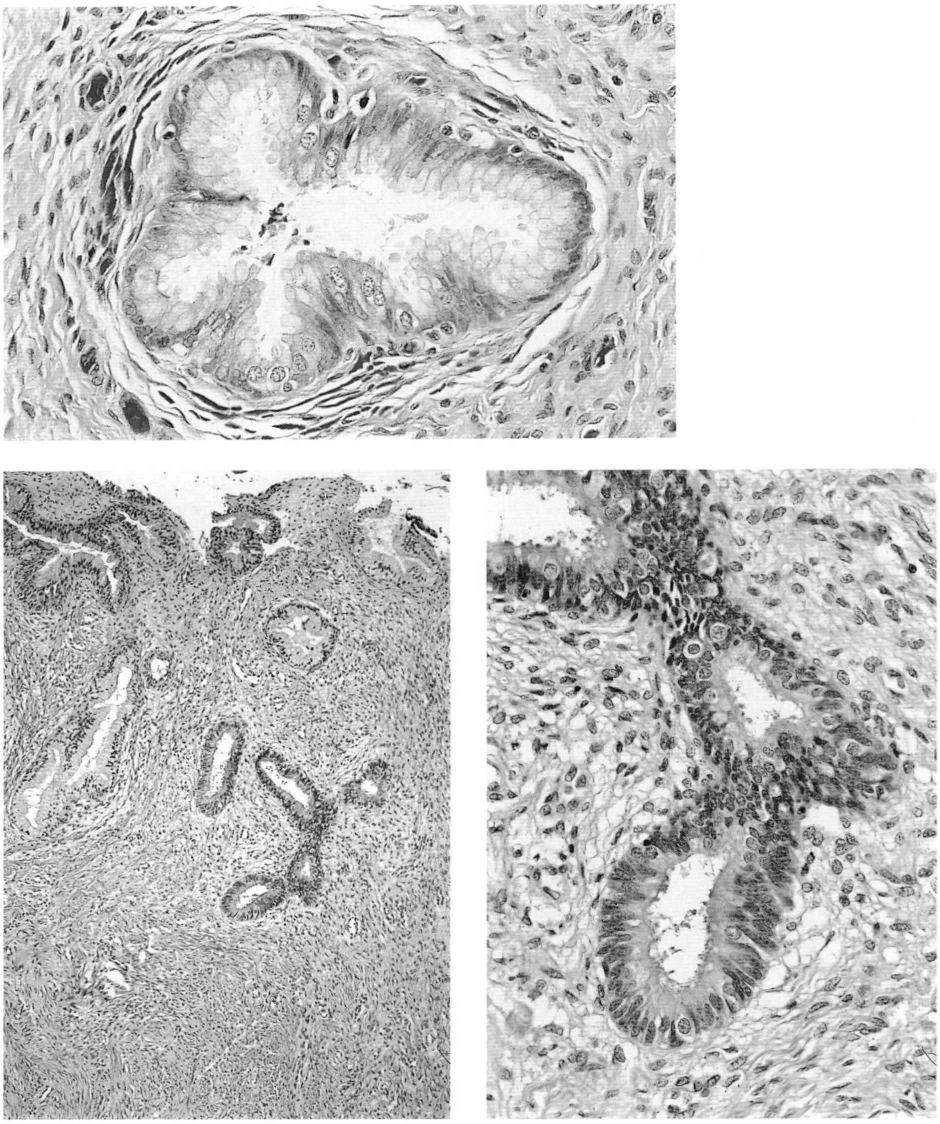

A

B,C

**FIG. 10. A:** Ciliated cells in the endocervix. The normal cervical mucinous epithelium consists of an admixture of mucin-containing cells and a smaller population of ciliated cells. The population of ciliated cells undergoes cyclic variation with the menstrual cycle. **B** and **C:** Cervical tubal metaplasia. **B:** When ciliated cells are prominent they may simulate endocervical glandular dysplasia or carcinoma in situ. At low magnification the glands feature a prominence of nuclei, a feature shared with glandular dysplasia. **C:** Higher magnification shows prominent cilia, the hallmark of ciliated cell metaplasia.

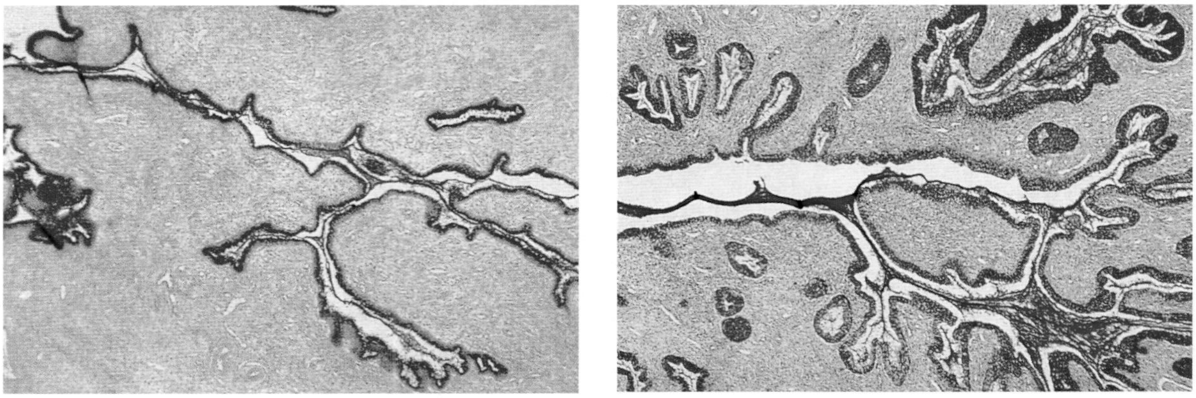

A B

**FIG. 11. A:** Tangential section of the endocervix stained with PAS to show how the gland clefts extend into the stroma and branch to form channels. **B:** When the endocervical mucosa undergoes hyperplasia and increases its surface area, as in pregnancy, the branches of the clefts proliferate and form even more collaterals (“tunnel clusters”).

of the cycle, the endocervical cells secrete a mucus of lower viscosity than at other times of the cycle. This is thought to aid penetration of the cervical canal by spermatozoa (53). When progesterone levels attain their zenith during the luteal phase, the endocervical glandular secretion becomes thick and scant. It is at this stage that the secretion may become inspissated and more visible in histologic sections. During pregnancy the number of tunnel clusters increases, and when this phenomena is extreme the term "cervical glandular hyperplasia" is often used. Pregnancy also causes the secretions of the endocervical cells to thicken and form a mucous plug that blocks the endocervical canal.

### Epithelium of the Transformation Zone

The endocervical mucosa is transient in nature (12,14,18, 46,47,90). At birth the endocervical mucosa resides on the exocervix in two thirds of infants, but it quickly moves back into the anatomic endocervical canal where in most girls it remains until near the menarche. After the onset of puberty, the endocervical mucosa again moves out onto the exocervix, usually more prominently on the anterior portion than on the posterior part (Fig. 12). The mechanism whereby endocervical mucosa changes location is apparently a mechanical one caused by swelling of the stroma of the cervical tissue in response to hormonal stimulation. As the lips of the cervix swell, they roll anteriorly and posteriorly, pulling the endocervical mucosa out of the canal onto the exocervix. The exposed endocervical tissue is often referred to as ectropion. Because the exposed endocervical mucosa appears red and ulcerated to the naked eye, it also has been interpreted as an erosion. There is, in fact, no erosion of the mucosa, rather the process is one of physiologic ectopy. After menarchial ectropion occurs there is gradual replacement of the endocervical tissue by squamous epithelium throughout the reproductive years. The area where the glandular tissue is being replaced by squamous epithelium is known as the transformation zone. The junction between the two types of epithelium is labeled the squamocolumnar junction (14,46). Two squamocolumnar junctions are usually recognized (Fig. 12B). The original squamocolumnar junction is the point where the native (original) exocervical squamous epithelium joins the endocervical glandular epithelium and is out on the exocervix during the reproductive years (90). This junction is usually sharply defined, and it is anatomically fixed. After squamous metaplasia has replaced endocervical tissue, the original squamocolumnar junction is the fusion point between the new squamous epithelium laid down in the transformation zone and the native squamous epithelium (Fig. 13). The functional squamocolumnar junction is the point of active replacement of columnar endocervical epithelium by squamous cells. This junction is often irregular and patchy, and it changes its contours and its locations during reproductive life. The functional squamocolumnar junction is usually implied when the term "squamocolumnar junction" is used without a modifier and the area between the two squamocolumnar junctions is the transformation zone. During pregnancy, particularly the first pregnancy, even more endocervical tissue moves out onto the exocervix, enlarging the area of ectopic endocervical epithelium. This phenomenon also can occur during progestogen therapy.

Because endocervical glandular epithelium is present on

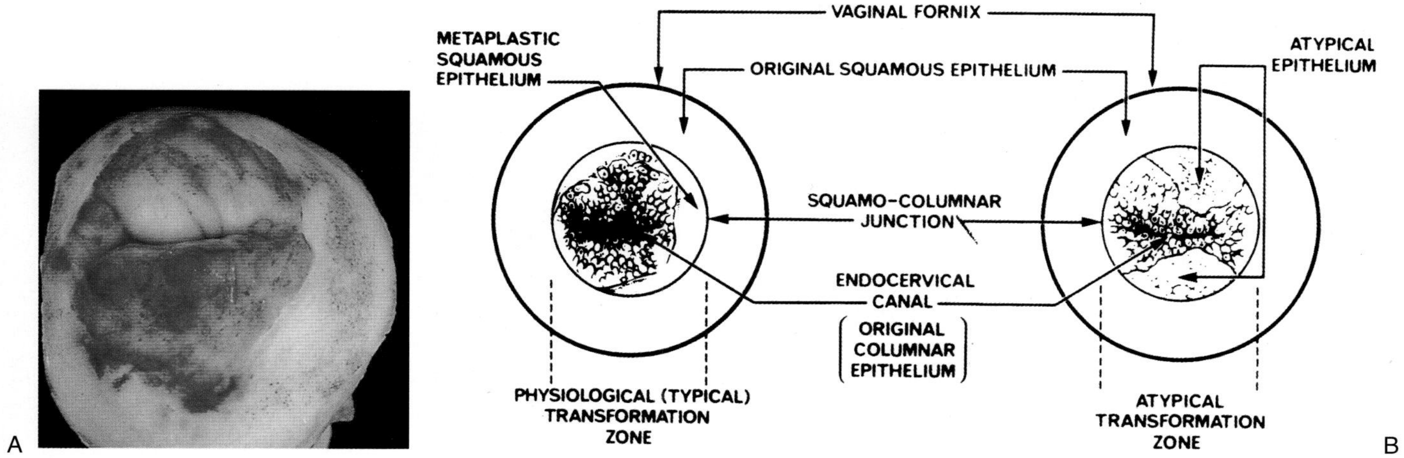


**FIG. 12. A:** Multiparous cervix during the reproductive years. Note the slitlike configuration of the external os and the erythematous endocervical tissue out on the anatomic exocervix. This endocervical tissue undergoes conversion to squamous epithelium throughout the reproductive years. The squamocolumnar junction is visible as a sharp line between the white squamous epithelium and the erythematous glandular tissue. **B:** Diagram of the cervix demonstrating the transformation zone. On the left is a normal transformation zone in which metaplastic squamous epithelium is replacing endocervical columnar epithelium. "Squamocolumnar junction" refers to the original squamocolumnar junction. On the right the metaplastic process is composed of dysplastic squamous cells and hence the process is cervical intraepithelial neoplasia. Reprinted with permission (346).

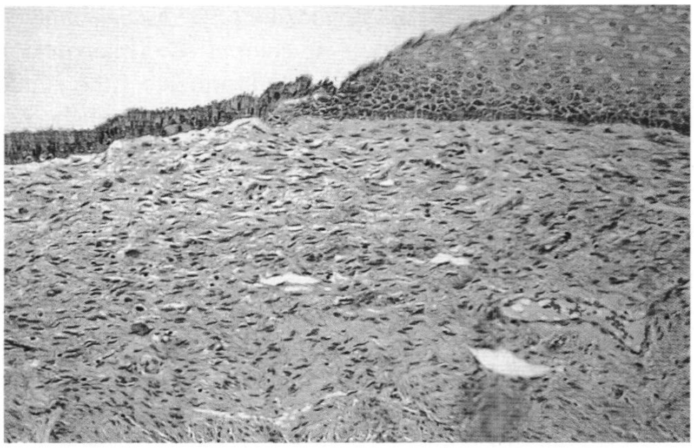

FIG. 13. Squamocolumnar junction with a distinct transition from mature squamous epithelium on the right to endocervical glandular tissue on the left. Such a sharp change can be seen at the original squamocolumnar junction as well as the junction formed by squamous epithelium with endocervical tissue in the transformation zone when squamous epithelium is mature.

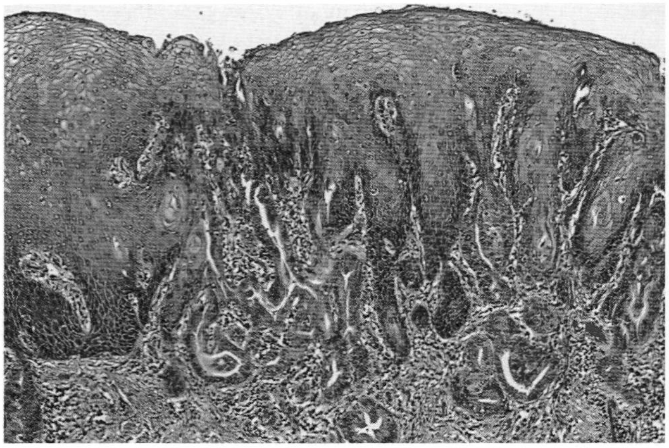

FIG. 14. Squamous epithelialization of the endocervix. Note mature squamous epithelium extending into endocervical gland clefts. This process can mimic invasive carcinoma.

the exocervix, the transformation zone can be visualized with the aid of a colposcope. This is fortunate because neoplastic change begins most commonly in the transformation zone, and neoplastic transformation is accompanied by structural alterations that can be recognized using the colposcope. The combination of cytologic preparations, colposcopic examination, biopsy, and local destruction of intraepithelial abnormalities in the transformation zone under colposcopic visualization is a powerful tool for the early detection and successful treatment of in situ neoplastic processes involving the cervix.

In the latter years of reproductive life the functional squamocolumnar junction reaches the area near the anatomic external os and, reversing its menarchal journey, begins to move up the anatomic endocervical canal. By the perimenopausal years, the squamocolumnar junction is usually concealed within the endocervical canal above the external os.

Two mechanisms are thought to be operative in transforming endocervical mucinous epithelium to squamous epithelium: (a) squamous epithelialization and (b) squamous metaplasia (5). The first involves the direct ingrowth of mature native squamous epithelium from the exocervix. This process is usually labeled "squamous epithelialization." During squamous epithelialization, mature squamous cells come to lie beneath the endocervical glandular cells. They push the endocervical cells off the basement membrane, and gradually the columnar cells degenerate and are sloughed. Squamous epithelialization initially spares the openings of the underlying endocervical glands, and at this stage the openings to the glands have the appearance of pores when examined with the colposcope. Eventually, the ingrowth of squamous epithelium involves the orifices of the glandular clefts, and then it can extend for varying distances down into the cleft spaces (Figs. 14 and 15). When this process involves the orifice, it may plug the opening, and if the mucinous epithelium below continues to secrete, a mucin-filled cyst (Nabothian cyst) or tunnel clusters filled with eosinophilic secretion result (Fig. 16). If squamous epithelialization involves the cleft and its ramifying tunnels, squamous epithelium will be surrounded by endocervical stroma. Consequently, histologic sections taken in an area of squamous epithelialization may show Nabothian cysts, mucification of tunnel clusters, and/or islands of benign squamous epithelium in the stroma beneath the surface epithelium.

When the endocervical clefts undergo squamous epithelialization, care must be taken not to confuse the deep-lying benign squamous cells with invasive carcinoma. Although the cells in squamous epithelialization may have enlarged nuclei and prominent nucleoli, they do not demonstrate the anaplasia, the pleomorphism, the chromatin abnormalities,

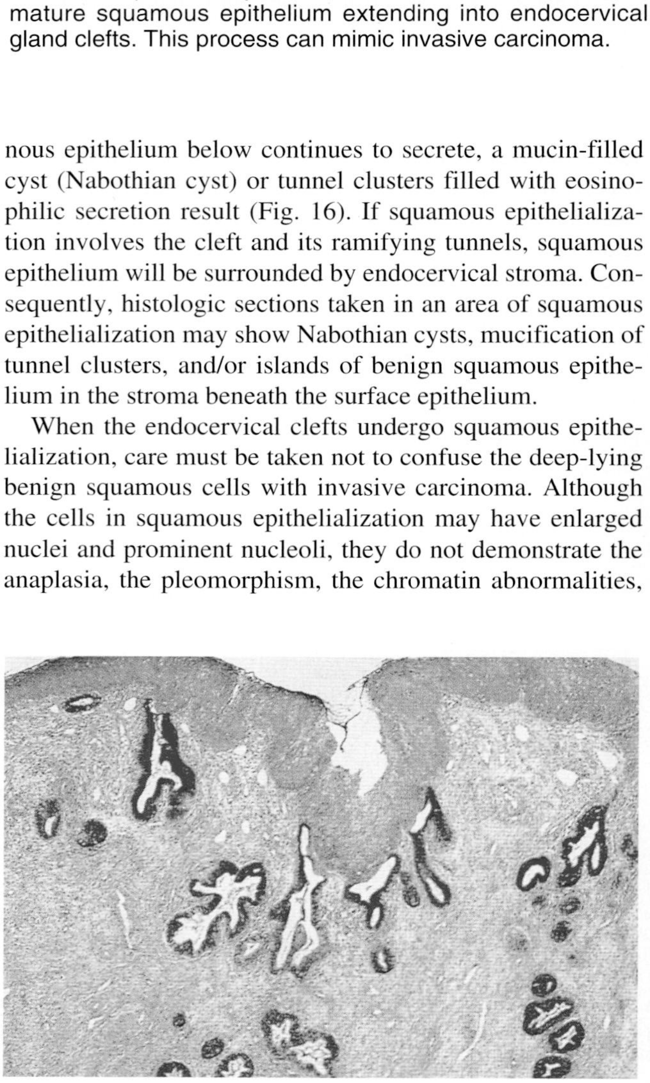

FIG. 15. Conversion to squamous epithelium in the cervix may occur more rapidly on the surface than in the clefts, causing squamous epithelium to overlie endocervical gland clefts. When the newly laid down squamous epithelium blocks the orifices of the clefts, nabothian cysts or mucification of tunnel clusters, as seen in Fig. 16, may result.

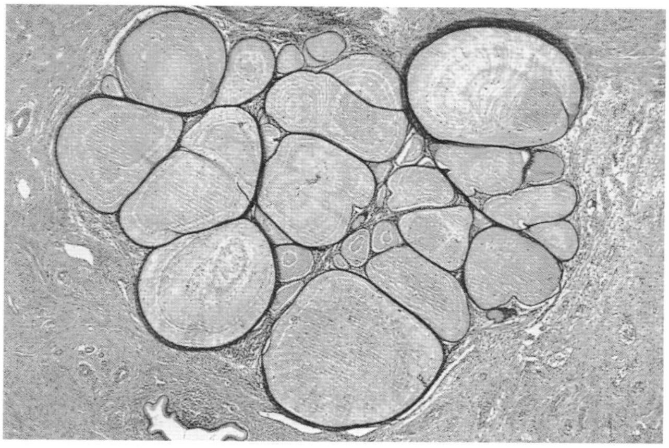

**FIG. 16.** When the newly formed squamous epithelium in the transformation zone covers the endocervical gland cleft orifices and secretion continues, the tunnel clusters fill up with secretion that may become inspissated ("mucification").

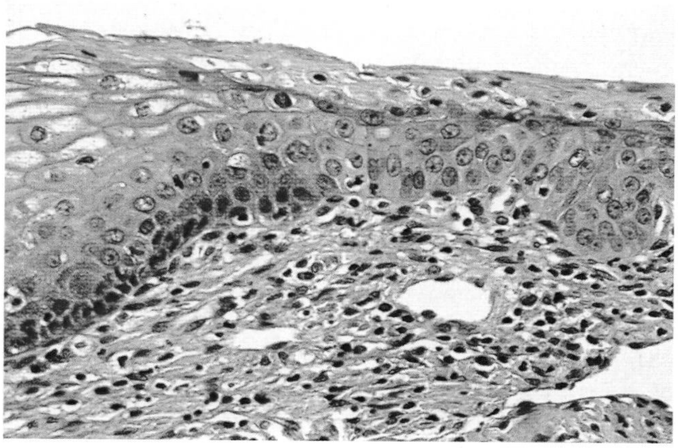

**FIG. 17.** Functional squamocolumnar junction with metaplastic epithelium on the right. Note that in this example maturation has proceeded to the parabasal cell stage with abrupt keratinization rather than the normal maturation sequence to superficial cells as seen on the left.

or the abnormal mitotic figures characteristic of invasive carcinoma. Moreover, the benign cells conform to the rounded configuration of the preexisting cleft and do not infiltrate the stroma irregularly. Typically there is no granulation tissue host response to squamous epithelialization, although chronic inflammation may be present. If squamous epithelialization involves tunnel clusters, small groups of squamous cells come to lie deep within the cervical stroma, imparting an architectural pattern that even more resembles infiltrating squamous cell carcinoma. Squamous epithelialization seems to be stimulated by chronic inflammation and local trauma, including cauterization or laser surgery.

The second mechanism thought to contribute to the conversion of endocervical mucinous epithelium to squamous epithelium entails first the proliferation of endocervical "reserve cells," and then the differentiation of these cells into squamous cells rather than mucin-producing cells (10). This process, known as squamous metaplasia or prosoplasia, can be distinguished from squamous epithelialization because, unlike the cells in squamous epithelialization, the reserve cells initially do not have squamous characteristics; rather, they appear as cuboidal cells with round nuclei growing beneath the mucinous epithelium (Fig. 17). In fact, these cuboidal cells are identical in appearance to the basal or parabasal cells of the squamous epithelium. After the reserve cells proliferate and stratify, they differentiate into squamous cells that initially have only slightly increased amounts of cytoplasm (immature squamous metaplasia). Later the cells may fully mature to glycogen-containing squamous cells indistinguishable from the superficial cells of the exocervix (Fig. 13). Confusingly, "squamous metaplasia" is commonly used as a generic term for both metaplasia and squamous epithelialization.

Immature squamous metaplastic cells without fully developed squamous characteristics or glycogen accumulation can come to occupy most or all of the thickness of an epithelium (91) (Fig. 18). Because fully mature squamous cells are not present toward the surface and because the cytoplasm of the immature cells is relatively scant and their nuclei often are elongate, immature squamous metaplasia can bear a close resemblance to intraepithelial neoplasia (dysplasia–carcinoma in situ). However, the nuclei in immature squamous metaplasia are uniform, chromatin abnormalities are minimal at most, and nuclear contours are usually smooth. Although mitotic figures may be present, in immature squamous metaplasia abnormal forms are not found. Because immature squamous metaplasia can be confused easily with carcinoma in situ and dysplasia, it is important to think of this possibility in each case where a diagnosis of intraepithelial neoplasia is contemplated (92).

Squamous metaplasia is usually patchy, giving rise to the characteristic irregularity of the functional squamocolumnar

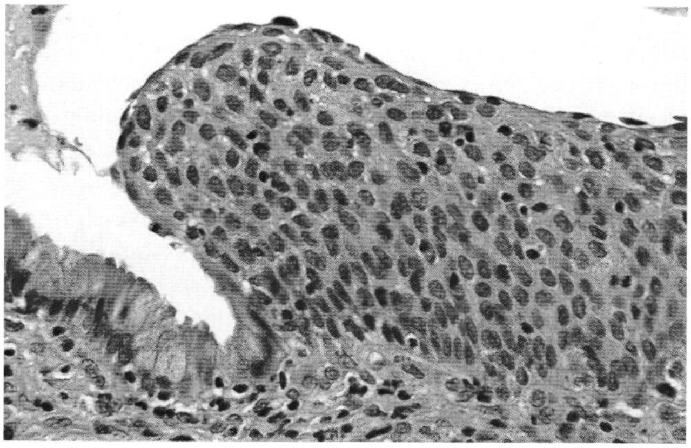

**FIG. 18.** Immature squamous metaplasia on the right. The constituent cells do not demonstrate evidence of maturation and are similar to cells normally present in the basal layer of squamous epithelium. This type of metaplasia can be confused with high-grade intraepithelial neoplasia.

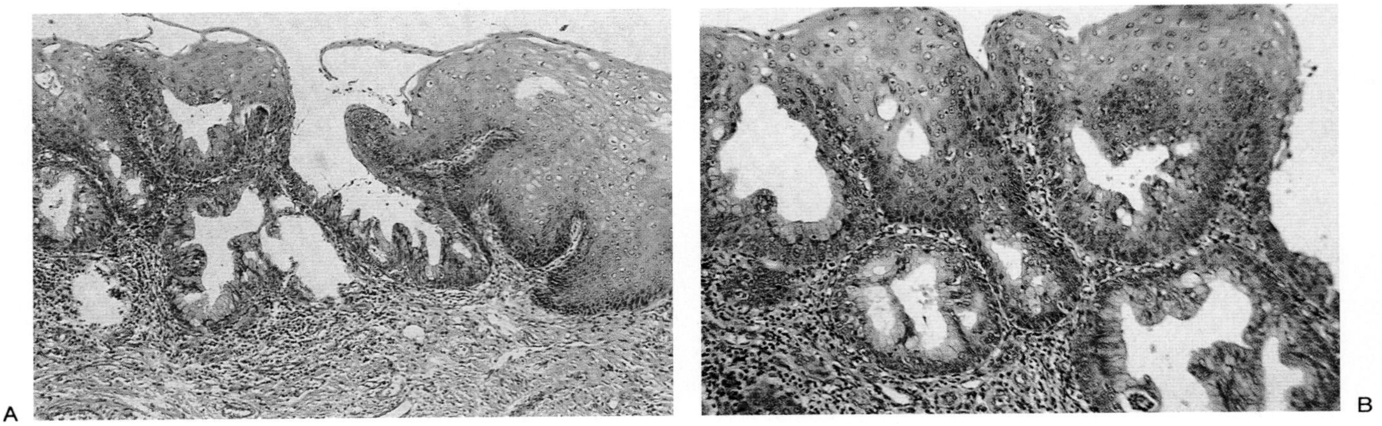


**FIG. 19. A:** Islands of metaplastic squamous epithelium in the transformation zone at the functional squamocolumnar junction. These islands will eventually coalesce. **B:** Higher power photomicrograph of the area of squamous metaplasia demonstrated in **A**.

junction (Fig. 19). As squamous metaplasia proceeds, the islands of squamous cells form bridges to other centers of metaplasia, ultimately producing a solid area of squamous epithelium.

Whatever the mechanism—either squamous epithelialization or squamous metaplasia—squamous replacement of mucinous epithelium on the exocervix is a normal process that must be distinguished from in situ and invasive neoplasms. Features that are often found in neoplasia but not in metaplasia or epithelialization are moderate to marked pleomorphism, lack of maturation sequence (this may be present in immature squamous metaplasia), irregular nuclear outlines, and abnormal mitotic figures. Nucleoli are usually inconspicuous in cervical intraepithelial neoplasia but are often prominent in metaplasia and epithelialization (a notable exception is immature squamous metaplasia).

### Cervical Stroma

In contrast to the wall of the uterine corpus, which is predominately muscular, the stroma of the exocervix is mainly fibrous tissue admixed with elastin through which run infrequent strands of smooth muscle (93–96). A large number of vessels course through the stroma. A rich capillary network interfaces with the epithelium at the stromal–epithelial junction. This interface is irregular and features fingers of connective tissue containing vessels overlain by a squamous cell mucosa of variable thickness. Much of the endocervical stroma is also fibroelastic tissue, but at the upper end of the endocervix the superficial fibrous stroma blends imperceptibly into the endometrial stroma of the lower uterine segment. Consequently, the superficial stroma of the upper endocervix and the stroma of the lower uterine segment has a hybrid endometrial–cervical appearance. This can cause localization problems when it is important to determine whether a neoplastic process in a curettage specimen involves the endometrium or the endocervix or both. We think the presence of unequivocal endometrial stroma, as determined by high cellularity (closely packed nuclei), should be present before interpreting tissue as originating from the endometrium on the basis of the stroma alone. Of course, if one type of normal glands is present, whether endocervical or endometrial, these glands can suggest the origin of the tissue, but both types of glands or even hybrid glands may be present in the transition area between the endocervix and lower uterine segment. The endocervix contains a greater number of smooth muscle fibers in its deeper stroma than does the exocervix, and in the lower uterine segment these blend into the myometrium.

Lymphocytes normally populate the endocervical stroma, and occasionally they form lymphoid nodules with or without follicular centers. Lymphoid cells in the cervix appear to be part of the mucosa-associated lymphoid system and secrete mainly immunoglobulin (Ig)A (97–101). Lymphocytes also may immigrate into the endocervical epithelium, and in this location they may take on the appearance of "cleared cells." Such cells have been misconstrued as "reserve" cells in the past. In addition, dendritic cells populate the cervix; a subset of these are Langerhans' cells involved in internalizing antigen and presenting it to T-lymphocytes in the regional lymph nodes (71,102,103). In our opinion, a diagnosis of chronic cervicitis should be withheld unless the lymphoid infiltrate is very heavy and/or lymphoid nodules are numerous. Particularly important for the diagnosis of chronic cervicitis are large numbers of plasma cells. Scattered plasma cells are normal in the cervix. Acute cervicitis is not uncommon, but true inflammatory erosion or microabscesses are rare in the cervix.

Remnants of the wolffian duct—commonly known as mesonephric rests—can be found in the endocervical stroma of the lateral portions of the cervix in about a third of women (104) (Fig. 20). Usually these are deep in the stroma, but occasionally they are found near the surface and they can even blend with the endocervical gland clefts. Mesonephric rests are tubular structures lined by a single row of cuboidal cells

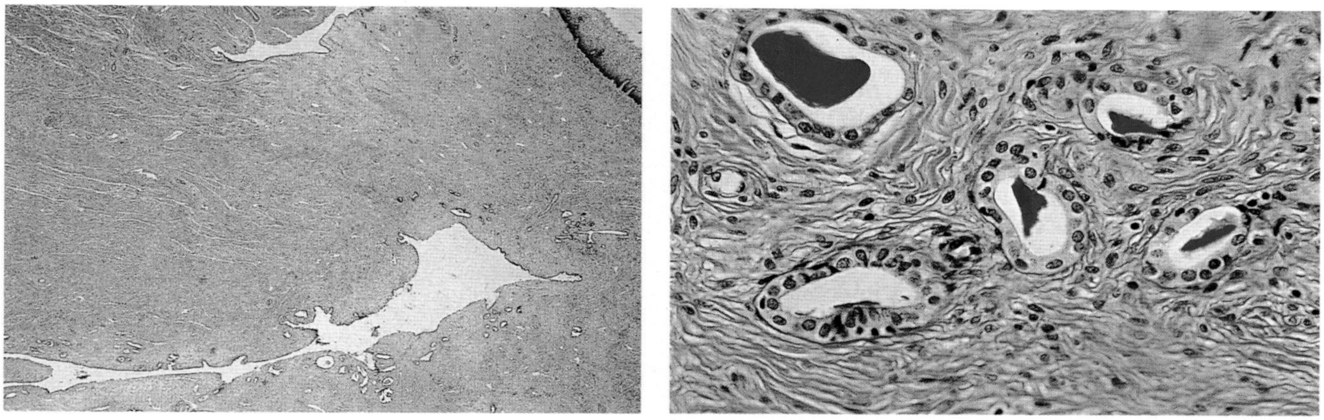

A B

**FIG. 20. A:** Mesonephric remnants in the cervix. A long cleftlike space deep in the stroma surrounded by tubules is the characteristic architectural finding. **B:** Ducts lined by bland cuboidal cells containing lumenal PAS-positive eosinophilic secretion are key features of mesonephric remnants. The blandness of the constituent cells and the organization around a central cleft are the most helpful features in distinguishing this from well-differentiated adenocarcinoma.

with a central round, cytologically bland nucleus. Typically the tubules form lumens that contain hyalin-like, eosinophilic secretions. Architecturally, there is usually a central elongate duct surrounded by smaller tubules. The combination of deep stromal location, the hyalin-like secretions, and the cuboidal cells usually serves to make identification of mesonephric rests straightforward. Even though tunnel clusters may ramify from a central cleft and contain eosinophilic secretion, they are lined by endocervical mucin-producing cells. The importance of this vestigial structure lies in its mimicry of well-differentiated adenocarcinoma. Mitotic figures are usually absent in mesonephric rests, and the chromatin of the cells is bland. Moreover, mesonephric rests do not exhibit the raggedly infiltrative growth of carcinoma even though they are located deep in the stroma. Rarely, atypical hyperplastic and neoplastic processes may involve mesonephric remnants (104).

Multinucleated giant cells rarely are found in the normal superficial endocervical stroma. These cells have enlarged and sometimes bizarre-shaped nuclei with smudged chromatin similar to those seen in vaginal polyps (105). They should not be mistaken for a neoplasm (106–109).

### Cervix During Pregnancy

During pregnancy the endocervical epithelium proliferates so that its mucus-secreting surface increases. This proliferation leads to both the formation of polypoid protrusions of endocervical epithelium into the endocervical canal and an increased number of tunnel clusters budding off preexisting clefts within the cervical stroma. The overall impression is one of an increase in the amount of endocervical tissue, and consequently this normal process is often termed "endocervical glandular hyperplasia" or when numerous small glands are packed together "microglandular hyperplasia." Identical changes can be produced by artificial progestogens. The endocervical mucus during pregnancy is thick and functions as a plug to seal off the endometrial cavity from the vagina (21,110). Arias-Stella reaction may be seen in the endocervical glandular cells (111,112). As in the endometrium, the large cells with prominent nucleoli characteristic of the Arias-Stella reaction can increase the possibility of clear cell carcinoma, but the absence of mitotic figures and the gestational setting should quickly eliminate this possibility.

The stroma of the cervix undergoes a complex series of biochemical and biomechanical changes during pregnancy and parturition that taken together are known as cervical "ripening" (113–121). The initial change seems to be extensive destruction of collagen fibers by various collagenases accompanied by the accumulation of gel-like acid mucopolysaccharides. This process causes the cervix to soften, a process that reaches its zenith immediately before parturition. As a result, the cervix is easily effaced by the presenting part of the emerging infant. Thus, the usually cylindrical cervix is transformed into a thin saccular structure. The increased fluid in the cervical stroma during pregnancy causes the cervical lips to roll further out into the vagina, everting more of the endocervical mucosa beyond the external os. Squamous epithelialization and metaplasia rapidly ensue, and at the time of delivery there is often considerable immature squamous epithelium in the transformation zone. As noted previously, the cells in immature squamous metaplasia can closely resemble those found in intraepithelial neoplasia, so caution should be exercised when examining cervical specimens taken from pregnant women.

The cervical stromal cells, particularly those near the surface of the endocervical canal, may undergo decidual change during pregnancy (Fig. 21). Cervical decidual reaction is typically patchy, and at low power this focal replacement of the cervical stroma by aggregates of epithelioid cells can resemble invasive large cell nonkeratinizing carcinoma. Awareness of this physiologic process during pregnancy and

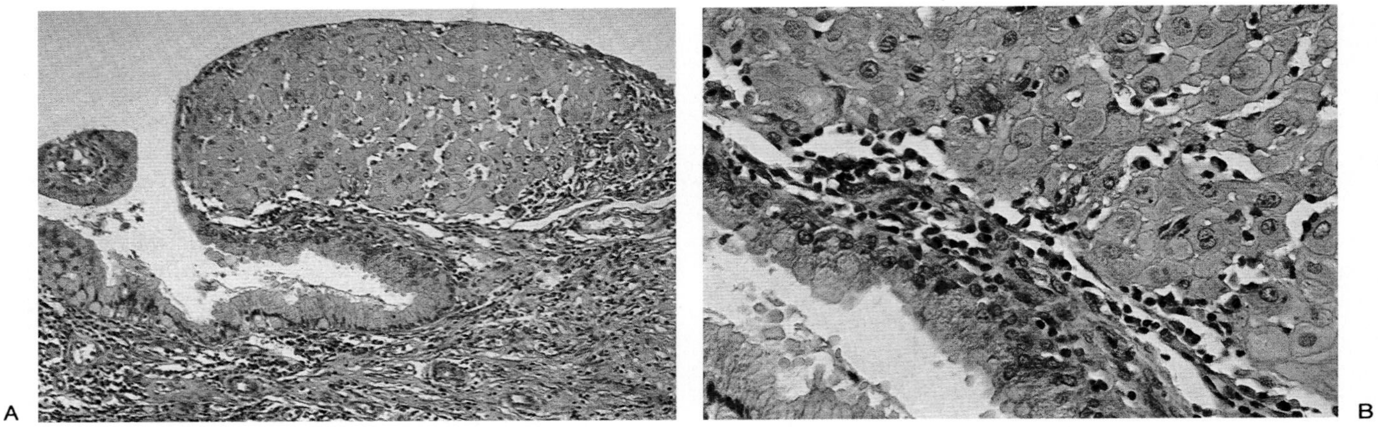

FIG. 21. A, B: Decidual reaction in the cervix. The sheetlike arrangement of the cells can mimic squamous cell carcinoma, but the nuclei are bland (see Fig. 18).

close attention to the cytologic features of the suspect cells should avoid misdiagnosis.

Normal findings in the cervix that have relevance to histopathologic differential diagnosis are presented in Table 1.

## ENDOMETRIUM

### Tissue Sampling and Associated Problems

A variety of endometrial tissue sampling techniques are available to the clinician. These techniques differ with respect to their indications, their limitations, and their associated complications (122–128).

Endometrial curettage [cervical dilation and endometrial curettage (D and C)] entails the removal of most of the uterine mucosa by scraping with a sharp curette. Under ideal circumstances, the excision is complete or nearly complete. When endometrial carcinoma is suspected clinically, a differential curettage should be performed by thoroughly curetting the endocervical canal before D and C.

Endometrial biopsy (EMB) involves the removal of a more limited sample of tissue than does the complete curettage and is performed with a smaller curette. Single strips of endometrium are usually taken from both the anterior and the posterior fundal surfaces. Even though the sample is limited, the accuracy of diagnosis approximates that of the D and C. The chief advantage of this technique is that it does not require cervical dilation (and hence does not require anesthesia). EMB thus combines convenience and low cost, with little sacrifice in diagnostic accuracy. The major limitation of EMB lies in its inherent potential to miss focal lesions, such as polyps and localized carcinomas. Accordingly, when carcinoma is suspected clinically, a negative biopsy must be followed by a complete D and C, because only this technique ensures the absence of carcinoma. When EMB is performed as part of an infertility workup, tissue should be obtained well into the presumed secretory phase, i.e., 2 to 3 days before the time of the next menstrual period as estimated by clinical and laboratory findings. Although in principle biopsy in the late luteal phase might destroy an early gestation, in practice this seems not to be the case (129–134). Increasingly hysteroscopy is being used to supplement endometrial sampling.

Three artifacts of sectioning and tissue preparation should be mentioned at this point. A frequent finding in endometrial curettings is the "telescoped" gland, which is characterized by an "inside-out" gland within the lumen of a gland with a normal configuration. This artifact is seen when an intussuscepted or telescoped gland (produced by the traumatic removal of the tissue) is cross-sectioned, and it occurs most frequently in straight glands (135). However, a similar appearance results from true intraglandular growth, as demonstrated by Hampson and Gerlis using serial sectioning and plastic model reconstructions (136). Another artifact is the result of sectioning and involves the tangential cutting of a gland to produce a "pseudo-gland-within-gland" pattern. Confusion with adenocarcinoma can be avoided by attention to cytologic detail, comparison with surrounding glands, knowledge that the gland-within-gland pattern in carcinoma is usually extensive, and awareness of this topologic problem. A third artifact involves tangential sectioning of the endometrial surface to produce pseudocystic and pseudobudded glands. Poor fixation can sometimes result in the retraction of endometrial glands from their surrounding stromal envelope. Moreover, cytoplasmic vacuolization may be a result of autolysis and can simulate early secretory vacuolated epithelium.

### Histology of the Normal Endometrium

The normal endometrium has a multiplicity of constantly changing normal patterns that depend on the nature and intensity of ovarian hormonal stimulation. The purpose of this section is to analyze the morphology of the normal non-

**TABLE 1.** *Normal findings in the cervix that have relevance to histopathologic differential diagnosis (see text for additional differential diagnostic clues) (86)*

| Finding | Diagnostic confusion | Suggestions for resolution | References where relevant |
|---|---|---|---|
| Deeply situated normal endocervical gland clefts or Nabothian cysts | Minimal deviation adenocarcinoma (MDC): | Lobster claw configuration in MDC<br>Ciliated cells in benign proliferation and almost always absent in malignant cervical glandular proliferations | (84–87) |
| Easily found mitotic figures in endocervical epithelial<br>In normal endocervical epithelium mitotic figures are rare. In metaplastic and regenerating epithelium they may be numerous but abnormal forms are not present. | Adenocarcinoma, invasive or in situ | Cytologic atypia in carcinoma<br>Compare problematic epithelium with normal epithelium elsewhere | |
| Mesonephric remnants: Mesonephric remnants, especially when florid: must be distinguished from minimal deviation adenocarcinoma. | Minimal deviation adenocarcinoma (MDC)<br>Mesonephric carcinoma | MDC has superfiical component<br>ACIS associated with MDC with high frequency | (104) |
| Decidual reaction | Large cell nonkeratinizing squamous cell carcinoma | Mitotic figures, cytologic atypia in carcinoma | |
| Arias-Stella reaction | DES-related clear cell carcinoma of the cervix/ vagina | Arias-Stella reaction usually does not feature mitotic figures which are easily found in clear cell carcinoma.<br>Maternal DES therapy was discontinued in the 1960s | (111, 112, 302) |
| Lower uterine segment vs. endocervical fragments: can make a difference when carcinoma (endocervical vs. endometrial) is found in curettings. | | Differential curettage; imaging studies. Immunohistochemistry (stain for CEA often positive in endocervical carcinoma and negative in endometrial). Are not entirely reliable in the individual case but may be helpful. | |
| Squamous metaplasia involving cervical gland clefts: | Invasive carcinoma | Assess nuclear features and evaluation for the presence or absence of infiltration | |
| Endometriosis: benign endometrial glands and stroma | Adenocarinoma: When stroma inconspicuous<br>Endometrial stromal sarcoma when glands inconspicuous<br>Adenosarcoma: look for stromal mitotic figures | Think of the possibility of endometriosis.<br>Look for the missing component in additional levels<br>Cytologic atypia is usually minimal in endometriosis | (327, 328) |
| Squamous epithelialization involving gland clefts: | (Micro)invasive carcinoma. | Look for nuclear atypia, abnormal mitotic figures, ragged infiltration. | |
| Microglandular adenosis and endocervical glandular hyperplasia: | Adenocarcinoma | Prominent nucleoli and abnormal division figures are features of carcinoma. Easily found mitotic figures almost always are a carcinoma feature. | (329, 330) |
| Immature squamous metaplasia: | High-grade SIL: may mimic because nuclei of the cells are large and cytoplasm is relatively scant. | Look for nucleoli (often present in metaplasia, but often inconspicuous in CIN) and abnormal mitotic figures and abnormal chromatin patterns. | |
| Glycogen storage in superficial squamous cells: | Koilocytosis (HPV infection). | Koilocytic nuclei: 1) enlarged, 2) irregular nuclear membranes, 3) dense ropy chromatin. | |
| Tubal metaplasia: Endocervical epithelium lined by prominent and numerous ciliated cells may suggest adenocarcinoma in situ or endometrioid carcinoma | Cervical adenocarcinoma in situ | Numerous mitotic figures and abnormal mitotic figures are features of CIL not luteal metaplasia. Look for ciliated cells; if numerous the process is almost surely benign. | (75–79) |
| Multinucleated stromal giant cells: these may be a normal finding; probably myofibroblastic cells | Neoplasm, particularly sarcoma.<br>Granulomatous inflammation | Look for abnormal mitotic figures, high cellularity, and granulomas. | |

gravid endometrium in some detail from three points of view. First, we discuss regional variations, then the individual components of the endometrium; finally, using this background, we describe the temporal variations in the histology of the endometrium that occur throughout life.

### *Regional Variations*

The uterine lining can be divided into two regions on the basis of its morphology: the mucosa of the lower uterine segment and the mucosa of the corpus proper. The mucosa of

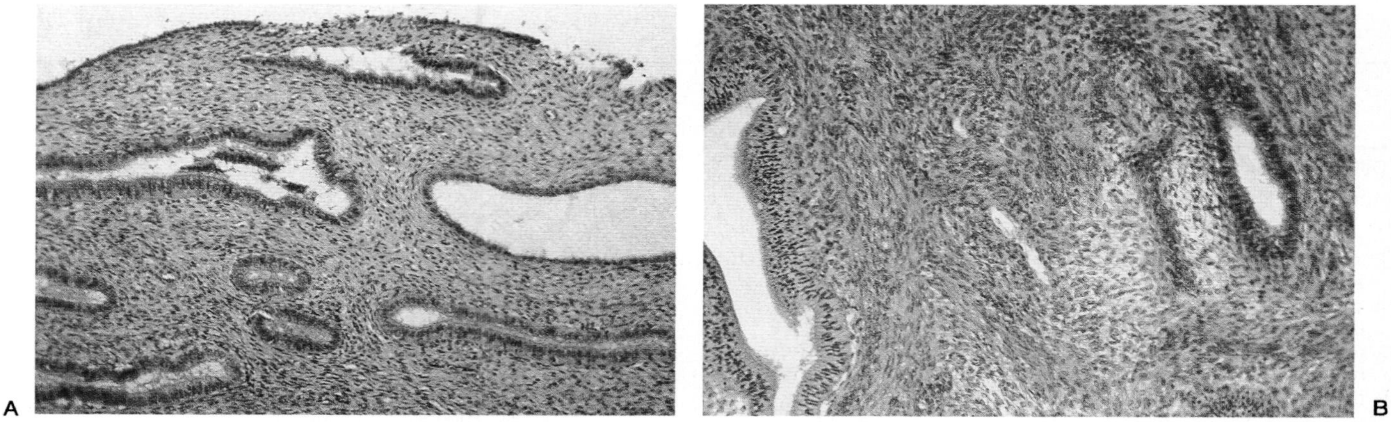

FIG. 22. The lower uterine segment contains stroma and glands that are either hybrid between those seen in the endocervix and those in the fundus or a mixture of endometrial and endocervical glands and stroma. **A:** The stroma is fibrous appearing but more cellular than that typically found in the endocervix. **B:** An endometrial gland and an endocervical gland are found next to each other in this area of the lower uterine cervix.

the lower uterine segment (isthmus) is in general thinner than the fundal mucosa (137). The glands and stroma tend to be only sluggishly responsive to hormonal stimulation, and in consequence this portion of the endometrium most often lags behind the rest of the endometrium in its development. The morphologic transition from endocervical mucosa to lower uterine segment mucosa is gradual, and in fact the hybrid endocervical–endometrial appearance of both the glands and the stroma of the lower uterine segment serves to identify this zone in endometrial curettings (Fig. 22).

The major portion of the uterine lining, the corpus mucosa proper, is normally fully responsive to hormonal stimulation.

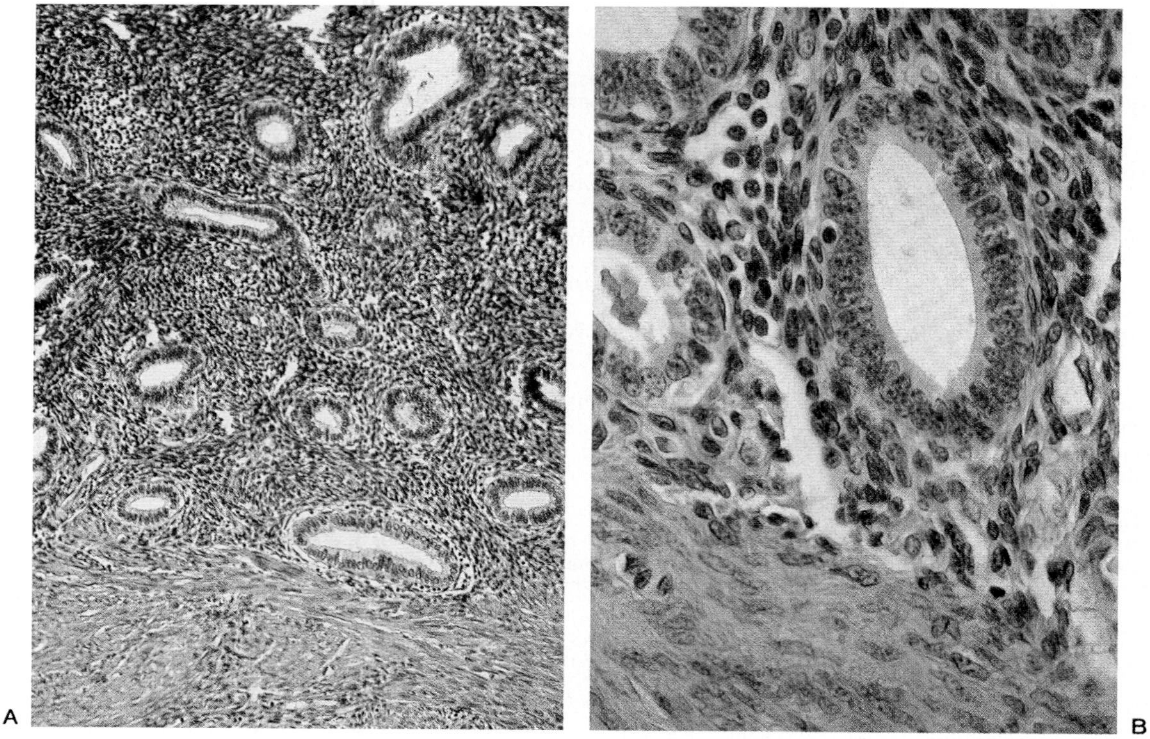

FIG. 23. **A, B:** The basalis of the endometrium is demonstrated. Throughout the menstrual cycle the basalis maintains a weakly proliferative appearance. As a result, dating of endometrium should be performed on fragments containing surface epithelium.

Two layers can be readily identified within the endometrium throughout this region: the lowermost is labeled the basalis and the overlying one the functionalis. The basalis is that zone of weakly proliferative glands and associated dense-spindled stroma immediately adjacent to the myometrium (Fig. 23). Characteristically, the junction of the basalis and myometrium is irregular, and smooth muscle and endometrial stroma interdigitate and blend together at this point (Fig. 24). When florid, this irregularity may give the false impression that endometrial tissue is pathologically isolated within the myometrium. This deception is particularly important when evaluating the presence or absence of superficial myometrial invasion in patients with endometrial adenocarcinoma. Of less importance is the confusion it creates in the diagnosis of adenomyosis. The basalis, despite its unimpressive, inactive, and undifferentiated appearance, plays a crucial role in the endometrial economy because it constitutes the "reserve cell layer" of the endometrium. After the bulk of the overlying functionalis is shed during menstruation, or after the functionalis is removed by curettage, the basalis and the residual deep functionalis are responsible for regenerating the endometrium (138). The remaining surface epithelium of the lower uterine segment also participates in this regeneration (139,140).

The appearance of the basalis is relatively constant throughout the menstrual cycle. Specifically, the glands usually appear weakly proliferative; that is, they possess pseudostratified elongate nuclei, rare mitotic figures, and dense intensely basophilic chromatin. Most importantly, they lack secretory change (Fig. 23), and the stroma is spindled and nondecidualized. A notable exception to this generalization is the basalis during the latter half of pregnancy, which usually exhibits secretory glandular changes and stromal decidualization (141). The importance of recognizing the basalis of the endometrium lies in not mistaking it for the functionalis in a curettage specimen. This confusion would result in an erroneous impression that this weakly proliferative appearance represented the fully developed state of the functionalis.

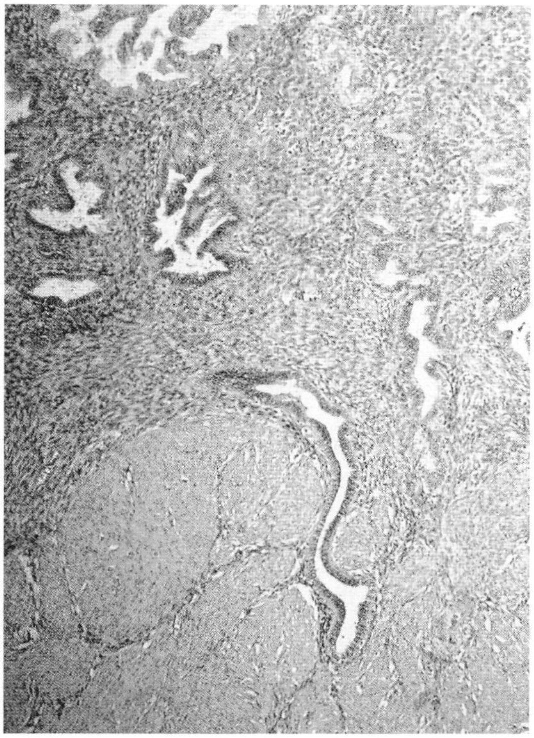

**FIG. 24.** This is an example of an irregular endometrial–myometrial junction. This phenomenon is important to think about when determining whether or not adenocarcinoma is superficially invading the myometrium.

It is the functionalis that exhibits the protean changes so characteristic of the normal endometrium. This layer has been traditionally divided into two strata—the compactum and the spongiosum—based on the morphologic appearances of each during the late secretory phase of the menstrual cycle and during pregnancy. Unless otherwise specified, the term "endometrium" refers to the functionalis in the subsequent discussion.

### *Individual Components of the Endometrium*

The normal endometrium consists of both epithelial (surface and glandular) and mesenchymal (stromal and vascular) elements, which during reproductive years first synchronously proliferate, then differentiate, and finally disintegrate at roughly monthly intervals.

#### *Epithelial Elements*

The endometrial glandular and surface epithelia are both composed of four morphologically distinct cells, two of which are functional variants of the same cell.

*Proliferative and Basalis-Type Cells.* The basalis-type cells and the proliferative cells of the functionalis are morphologically similar. These cells both have high nucleus-to-cytoplasm ratios and elongate sausage-shaped nuclei with dense chromatin and inconspicuous nucleoli. The cytoplasm is scant and generally basophilic to amphophilic (see Fig. 33). Mitotic figures are common in the cells that compose the glands of the functionalis during the proliferative phase. When proliferative cells are the predominant cell type composing the epithelium (as in the proliferative endometrium), the nuclei appear pseudostratified. The electron microscopic appearance of proliferative cells is not distinctive.

*Secretory Cells.* The characteristic cytoplasmic differentiation of the endometrial epithelial cell is nonmucinous secretion. Shortly after ovulation, secretory products accumulate in a subnuclear location in the proliferative cells; these products gradually shift to a supranuclear position and are ultimately discharged into the glandular lumens. This sequence of changes results in two easily recognizable secretory cell types: vacuolated and nonvacuolated secretory cells (see Figs. 35B and 36C). Although vacuolated cells may have a nucleus similar to those seen in proliferative phase cells, the nonvacuolated secretory cells possess nuclei that are distinct from those seen in the undifferentiated proliferative phase cells. In contrast to the dense intensely basophilic elongate nuclei of the proliferative cells, the nuclei of the nonvacuolated secretory cells are rounded and vesicular, they have uniformly dispersed chromatin, and occasionally nucleoli become prominent. The nonvacuolated secretory cells have uniform, moderately dense eosinophilic cytoplasm and often a frayed luminal border (see Fig. 36C).

Another type of secretory cell is encountered, one that closely resembles the secretory cell of the fallopian tube. This cell has an elongate nucleus with coarse chromatin, a moderate amount of densely eosinophilic cytoplasm, and a rounded luminal bleb similar to those found in apocrine glands. These cells are common in the surface epithelium and occasionally may line an entire endometrial gland. Some of these cells may in fact represent "exhausted" ciliated cells.

*Ciliated Cells.* The ciliated cells of the endometrium have received little emphasis in the past. However, they are consistently present in endometrial specimens and presumably represent one line of differentiation open to the basalis-type cell. These cells are more prominent near the uterine isthmus and during the proliferative phase (142–144).

Ciliated cells have distinctive round, smoothly contoured vesicular nuclei containing finely stippled chromatin (Fig. 25). Although the nuclear features remain relatively unchanged throughout cell development, the configuration and location of ciliated cells vary as a function of the stage of ciliogenesis. The earliest identifiable ciliated cells are situated adjacent to the basal lamina of the gland and are roughly pyramidal in shape. They possess distinctively clear cytoplasm with central round nuclei. A rounded cytoplasmic zone containing eosinophilic fibrillary material can be identified with routine stains. This zone corresponds to the intracytoplasmic cilia seen with the electron microscope. When the growing ciliated cells reach the luminal surface, the cilia are exposed to the glandular lumen. Initially the luminal surface of the ciliated cell is concave, but as the cell continues its development, this surface becomes convex, and ultimately the cilia may pinch off as a merocrine secretion. During this stage the cell has a characteristic fusiform-to-pear shape. Ciliated cells can come to predominate the cellular population of glands, and when they do the term "ciliary metaplasia" has been used.

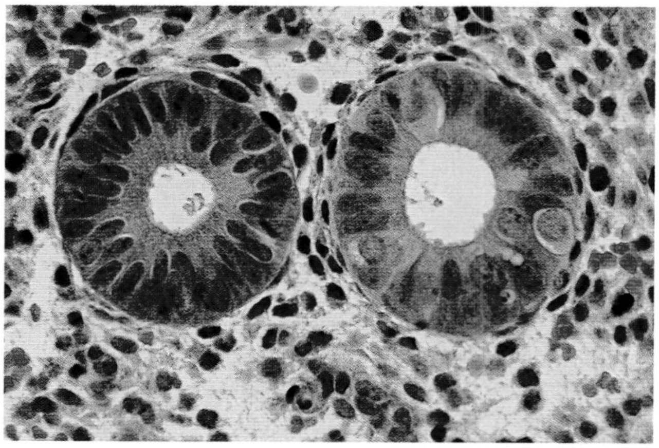

**FIG. 25.** Proliferative phase glands with ciliated cells in the gland at the right. The round cell with clear cytoplasm at the 3:00 o'clock position has the characteristic appearance of ciliated cells before they have extruded their cilia into the glandular lumen. The other ciliated cells have a pyramidal shape.

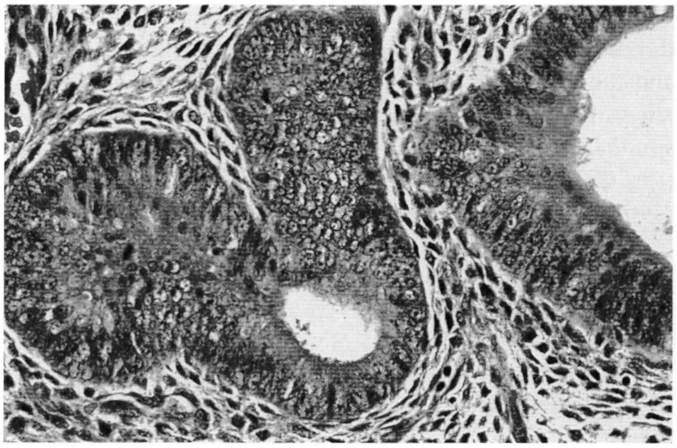

**FIG. 26.** Proliferative phase glands and stroma. Note the elongate shape of the stromal cell nuclei.

*The Gland as a Whole.* The normal endometrial gland is lined by the aforementioned cells arranged in a nonstratified cuboidal-to-columnar epithelium, which during the proliferative phase deceptively appears to be stratified (i.e., it is pseudostratified). During the early proliferative phase, the glands are straight and have narrow lumens (Fig. 26). Beginning in the midproliferative period and lasting throughout the rest of the cycle, the glands exhibit increasing degrees of coiling, but not branching. This culminates in the serrated saw-toothed appearance of the glands in the late secretory and menstrual endometrium. The surface epithelium is composed predominantly of apocrine-like secretory cells and ciliated cells, and has a relatively constant appearance throughout the cycle.

### *Mesenchymal Elements*

*Cellular Elements.* The endometrial stromal cell is the predominant cellular component of the stroma, and its appearance varies greatly with the stage of the menstrual cycle. During the early proliferative phase these cells have scant indistinct cytoplasm and dense oval-to-fusiform nuclei (Fig. 27). This undifferentiated appearance is reflected ultrastructurally in the paucity of cytoplasmic organelles. As the menstrual cycle proceeds, the stromal cells become more elongate and acquire more cytoplasm. During the late proliferative phase and well into the secretory phase, electron microscopy shows increasing amounts of rough endoplasmic reticulum and both intra- and extracytoplasmic col-

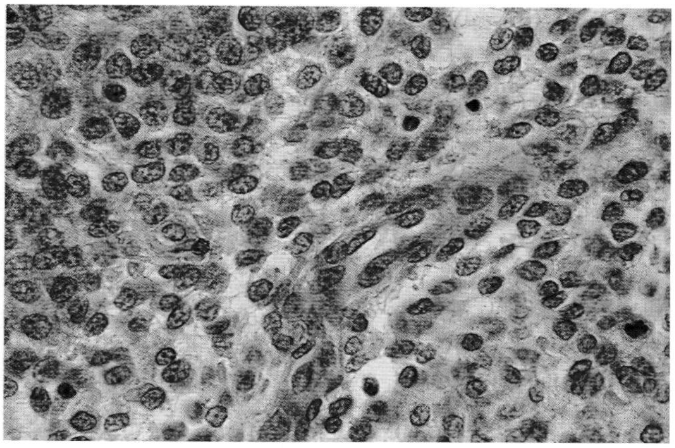

**FIG. 27.** The proliferative phase endometrial stromal cells have scant, hard-to-discern cytoplasm and round nuclei.

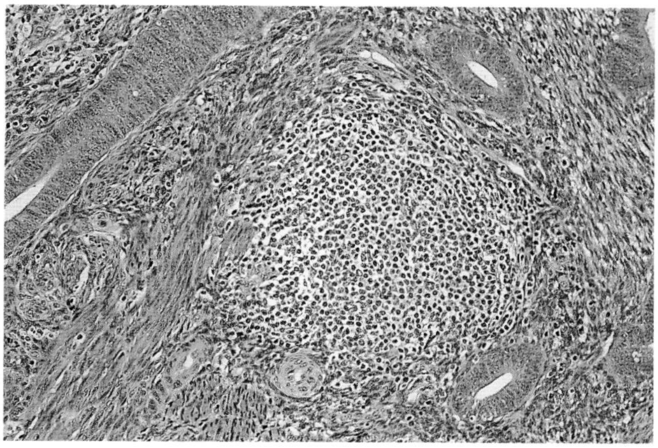

**FIG. 29.** Lymphoid follicle. Scattered lymphoid follicles may be encountered in clinically normal women with otherwise unremarkable endometrium. When present in large numbers and when associated with plasma cells, this finding is pathologic.

lagen. Toward the end of the secretory phase, the stromal cells in the perivascular region become rounded, acquire more cytoplasm, and develop vesicular nuclei with occasionally prominent nucleoli. Cytoplasmic borders become generalized and fully developed so that the entire endometrial stroma is transformed into sheets of cells with sharp and distinct cytoplasmic borders, abundant cytoplasm, and centrally placed vesicular nuclei (Fig. 28). This unique müllerian stromal transformation is called decidualization when fully developed (e.g., during pregnancy) and predecidualization when partially developed (e.g., during the late secretory phase of the menstrual cycle) (145). Ultrastructurally, the abundant cytoplasm of the decidual cell is populated by dilated rough endoplasmic reticulum, Golgi apparatus, and distinctly small mitochondria. Decidual cells form basal lamina and have complex intercellular interdigitations and tight junctions. Decidual cells appear to be capable of phagocytosis and are thought to play a role dismantling the collagen scaffolding at the implantation site (146). Early studies raised the possibility that decidual cells were bone marrow derived because of their expression of CD13 and CD10 (145). However, more recent studies dispute this notion (147–149). A second prominent cellular constituent, particularly in the late secretory phase, is the stromal granulocyte. Early ultrastructural and histochemical studies suggested that a subset of these granulocytic cells was distinct from the marrow-derived granulocytes, and it was thought that such cells were responsible for relaxin production and were histogenetically related to the endometrial stromal cell (150–156). In recent years with the use of modern immunohistochemical techniques it has become apparent that the stromal granulocytes are hematolymphoid cells and represent either a subpopulation of T-lymphocytes or macrophages (149,157–160). The ordinary neutrophil is typically present in the normal menstrual and immediately premenstrual endometrium.

Frequently cells with bean-shaped nuclei and abundant vacuolated lipid-containing cytoplasm are present in the stroma of endometria stimulated by estrogen. These have

A

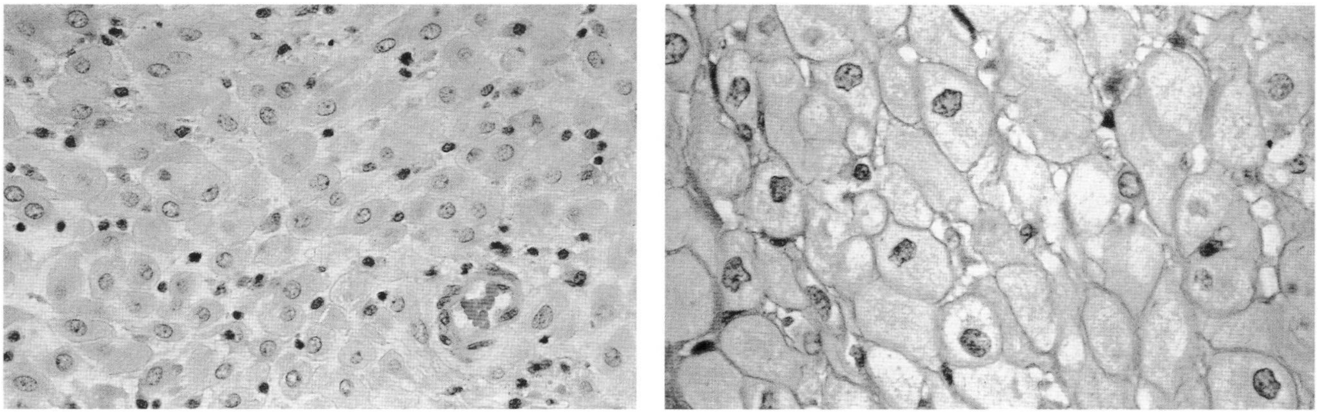

B

**FIG. 28. A, B:** These photomicrographs demonstrate decidual reaction during pregnancy. The cells have abundant cytoplasm and sharp cell margins.

been termed stromal foam cells, and their origin has been disputed (Fig. 29). Dallenbach-Hellweg believes them to be of stromal rather than histiocytic origin (153,161). Lymphocytes are normal constituents of the endometrial stroma and may aggregate to form lymphoid follicles (101,162–165). Lymphoid aggregates, when present, are usually in the basalis (Fig. 30). It has traditionally been held that plasma cells are abnormal. Certainly this is plausible when large numbers are present, although the pathologic significance of scattered plasma cells is unknown. The endometrial stromal cells elaborate a reticulin framework that becomes progressively denser as the endometrium develops during the menstrual cycle, so that by the late secretory phase each stromal cell is enmeshed in reticulin. This framework undergoes dissolution during menstruation. The stromal intercellular space is also rich in high-molecular-weight mucopolysaccharides during the mid-proliferative and late secretory phase.

*Vascular Elements.* The endometrial vasculature exhibits a unique adaptability throughout the reproductive years; it is centrally involved in menstruation and is responsible for forming a successful interface with the fetal circulation. The spiral arterioles of the endometrium are the primary site of these activities (166–169).

The radial arteries of the endometrium derive from the myometrial arcuate system. As the radial arteries course toward the uterine cavity they give off basal branches and then continue as endometrial spiral arteries. The basal arteries are unresponsive to steroid hormones, whereas the spiral arteries respond to varying hormone levels both by proliferation and, during the luteal phase of the menstrual cycle, by intermittent contraction.

In the early proliferative phase the sprouting spiral arteries are thin-walled and straight. As the proliferative phase proceeds, they, along with the glands, become coiled and their walls increase in thickness. During the luteal phase this growth continues. If implantation fails to occur, declining steroid levels are accompanied by longer and longer periods of vascular contraction. This results in ischemic necrosis of the functionalis and its subsequent sloughing.

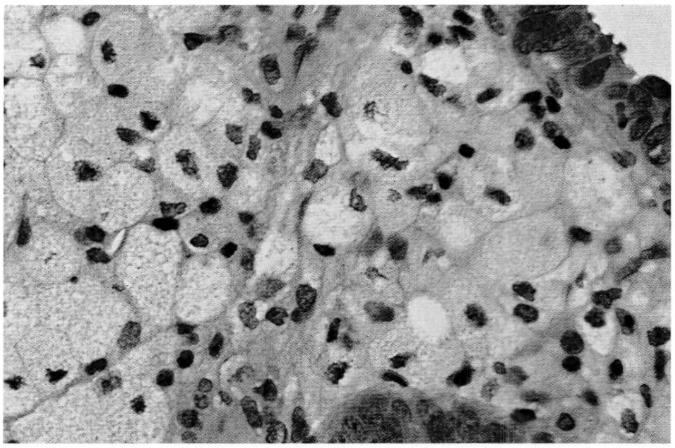

**FIG. 30.** Lymphoid follicle. Scattered lymphoid follicles may be encountered in clinically normal women with otherwise unremarkable endometrium. When present in large numbers and when associated with plasma cells, this finding is pathologic.

*Ultrastructural Features: Immunoperoxidase Studies and Biochemical Studies*

Both transmission and scanning electron microscopic study of the endometrium has produced an immense body of literature (124,128,170–173). Despite its scientific interest and the high aesthetic quality of many of the electron micrographs, little of this literature is currently of diagnostic relevance to the surgical pathologist. Mention should be made of two distinctive ultrastructural features found in the early secretory glandular cell: the giant mitochondrion complex (174–176) and the nucleolar channel system (177,178). These two features seem to be the earliest postovulatory morphologic change in the endometrial glandular cell.

The cytokeratins of the endometrium have been reviewed recently (179). There is a large and growing body of literature concerning the secretory products of the endometrium, a topic beyond the scope of this chapter. These studies have recently been reviewed (126,180–183)

### *Temporal Variations*

Unlike morphologically unchanging epithelia, such as vagina or gastrointestinal mucosa, that have an essentially constant appearance throughout the cell's lifetime, the endometrium undergoes dramatic temporal morphologic changes. The changes are cyclic and particularly striking during the reproductive years. These changes can be conveniently considered under six headings: newborn, premenarchal, perimenarchal, reproductive, perimenopausal, and postmenopausal years (126,184,185).

*Newborn*

The genitalia of the newborn girl respond to the high levels of circulating maternal and placental steroids by a transient burst of precocious development. The endometrium may be well developed and have either a proliferative or, less commonly, a secretory appearance. Within 2 weeks these changes have regressed, and the long hormonal quiescence of the premenarchal years begins. This quiescent period is characterized by a thin endometrium populated by inactive glands set within a spindled inactive stroma. Rarely, estrogen-secreting lesions of the ovary (follicular cysts, gonadal stromal tumors) may cause abnormal endometrial growth, with resulting abnormal bleeding as part of the syndrome of precocious pseudopuberty. The endometrium under these circumstances is proliferative or hyperplastic. That this phenomenon occurs suggests that the inactive appearance of the normal endometrium during this period results from an absence of hormonal stimulation rather than from transient end-organ unresponsiveness (8).

*Menarche*

The onset of uterine bleeding (menarche) is one of the many changes that signal the maturation of the reproductive system. In the United States this usually occurs between 12 and 15 years of age. Characteristically, the perimenarchal period is marked by greater variability in the length of individual cycles than is seen in the reproductive years and by the occurrence of anovulatory cycles (185). Disordered proliferative endometria are commonly encountered in this setting (see section Disordered Proliferative Endometrium).

*Reproductive Years*

The reproductive years are characterized by regularly occurring, roughly monthly, cycles, the end of which is signaled by menstrual bleeding (186,187). The dominant ovarian steroid secreted during the first half of the menstrual cycle is estradiol (E2), which induces endometrial proliferation. The second half of the cycle (beginning after ovulation) is hormonally dominated by both progesterone and estradiol, and this combination of hormones induces endometrial glandular secretion and stromal predecidualization. With the withdrawal of corpus luteum steroidal support, the endometrium is shed, setting the stage for the next cycle. These regularly recurring cycles may be interrupted by pregnancies, but after the termination of pregnancy, cycling is soon restored.

The biochemistry of the steroid molecules and their receptors that are responsible for the remarkable morphologic changes of the menstrual cycle have been the subject of intense study over the past decade (188–195). Steroid molecules are hydrophobic and easily diffuse through cell membranes and freely enter all cells. The endometrium, vaginal mucosa, and other steroid-sensitive tissues are target organs by virtue of the presence of high-affinity, high-specificity, low-capacity saturable receptors for E2 and progesterone. Although initially thought to reside in the cytoplasm, it now appears that both E2 and progesterone receptors are in the nucleus (193). These receptors are absent in nonresponsive cells. A detailed description of hormone receptors is beyond the scope of this chapter, but several excellent reviews on the topic have been published (196–200). In broad terms, the steroid molecule combines with the appropriate receptor, and the steroid–receptor complex becomes associated with a nonhistone nucleoprotein. The net effect of this linkage is to alter both qualitatively and quantitatively DNA-dependent RNA transcription. The consequence is an altered profile of protein biosynthesis. Furthermore, the unique response of a particular target cell type depends on what specific growth and differentiation program is initiated by the steroidal signal. The endometrium is a major target organ for this continual barrage of steroidal information, and it responds by undergoing the dramatic morphologic alterations that constitute the normal menstrual cycle. A number of studies have chronicled the time of appearance and location of estrogen receptors and progesterone receptors in the cycling endometrium (201–204). Increasingly it is being appreciated that the endometrium itself is the site of production of a variety of nonsteroidal products important to its function. The best documented of these are prostaglandins and prolactin (126,182,205–210).

***Morphology of the Normal Menstrual Cycle Endometrium***

The first day of the menstrual cycle has conventionally been identified as the first day of menstrual flow. Menses usually lasts for less than 5 days and is followed by the endometrial proliferative phase, the length of which exhibits great variation (9–20 days), but on average it lasts for 10 days. After ovulation, the coordinated and highly predictable series of stromal and glandular changes characteristic of the secretory (luteal) phase takes place. The traditional view is that the length of this phase is constant (14 days), and it is this alleged constancy that provides the basis for endometrial dating. The conventional endometrial dating features are presented in the ensuing paragraphs. Problems with this account and a discussion of the clinical relevance of endometrial dating are then taken up (Figs. 31 and 32, Table 2) (125,126,211–218).

*Proliferative Endometrial Phase (Ovarian Follicular Phase)*

The endometrium responds to rising estrogen levels by synchronous proliferation of glands, stroma, and vessels. During the first third of the proliferative phase (early proliferative), the rate of growth of all three of these elements is coordinated, and as a consequence both vessels and glands are noncoiled. After a few days the growth of both glands and vessels outstrips that of the stroma; as a result, these tubular structures become coiled (mid- and late proliferative) (Fig. 33).

In early proliferation the glands are either straight or demonstrate early coiling and are lined by pseudostratified columnar cells with high nucleus-to-cytoplasm ratios and dense chromatin (Fig. 34). Mitotic figures are almost always easy to find. These cells are present throughout the proliferative phase and even into early secretion. After about 10 to 11 days, irregular subnuclear vacuoles begin to appear. During the last 2 days mitotic activity decreases, glandular coiling becomes more prominent, and vacuoles are easily found.

The interval period is the 48 hours between ovulation and the presence of uniformly vacuolated indicative of postovulatory day 2. Mitotic figures are present during this period, and the cells retain their proliferative nuclear features.

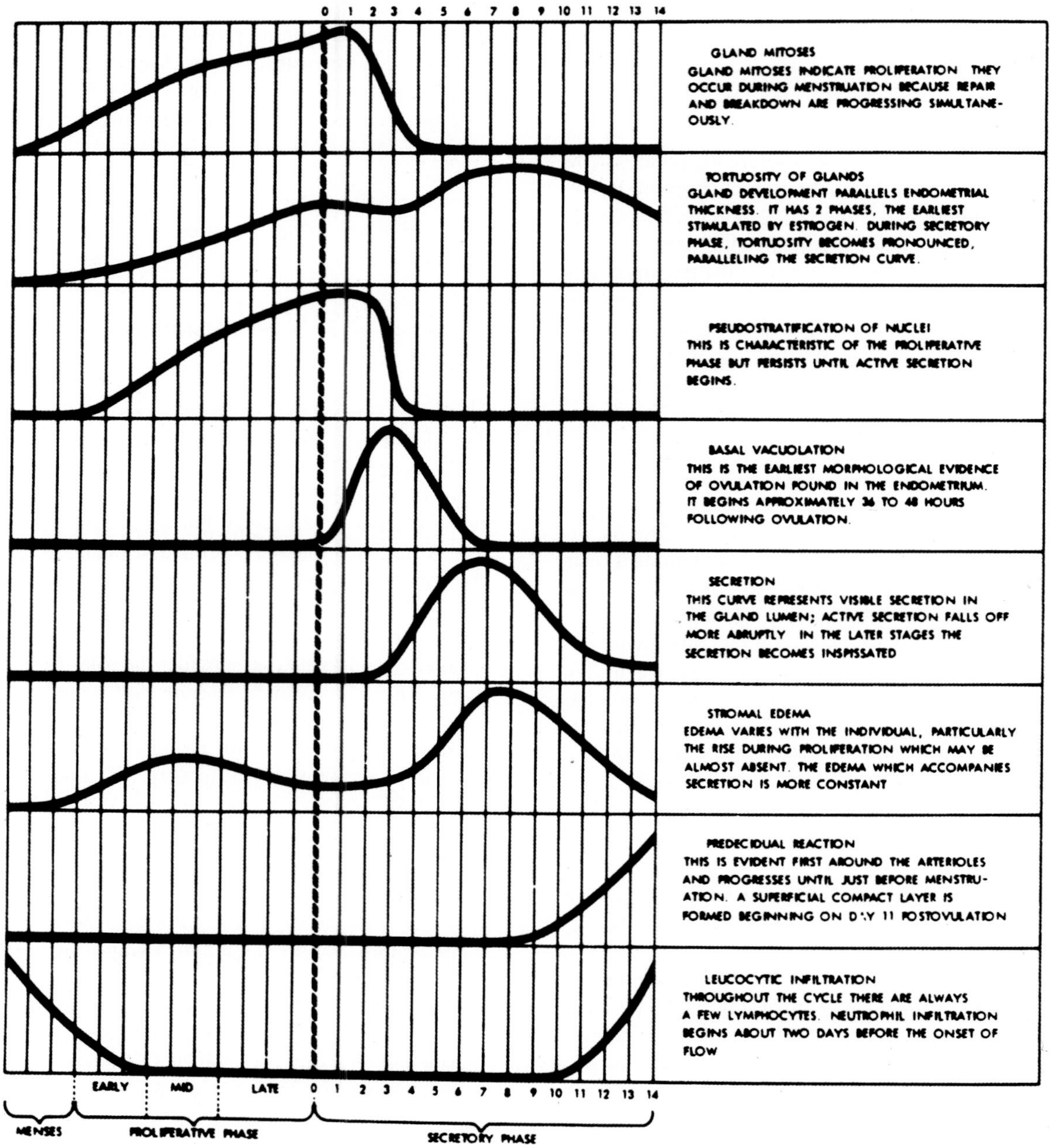


**FIG. 31.** Approximate qualitative changes in eight morphologic criteria found to be most useful in dating human endometrium. Reprinted with permission (347).

*Endometrial Secretory Phase (Ovarian Luteal Phase)*

Ovulation is mediated by the luteinizing hormone (LH) surge, a synchronous burst of LH and follicle-stimulating hormone secretion that peaks on the 14th day of the ideal 28-day cycle. Ovulation occurs roughly 10 to 12 hours after this peak. The length of time from the last menstrual period to the day of ovulation for an individual woman is the length of her follicular phase. This surge of pituitary hormones initiates a complex series of events that results in the expulsion of the oocyte from the developed tertiary follicle and the transformation of the follicle into a corpus luteum. As a consequence of this transformation, the biosynthetic profile of the follicle changes, and both estradiol and large quantities of progesterone, are secreted. The biosynthetic lifetime of the corpus luteum defines the ovarian luteal phase that corresponds to endometrial secretory development. Both ovarian and endometrial luteal phases last 14 days on the average, but this can be variable (219).

The endometrium, which has proliferated and has been primed by estrogen, responds to the simultaneous stimulation of estrogen and progesterone by differentiating in a dis-

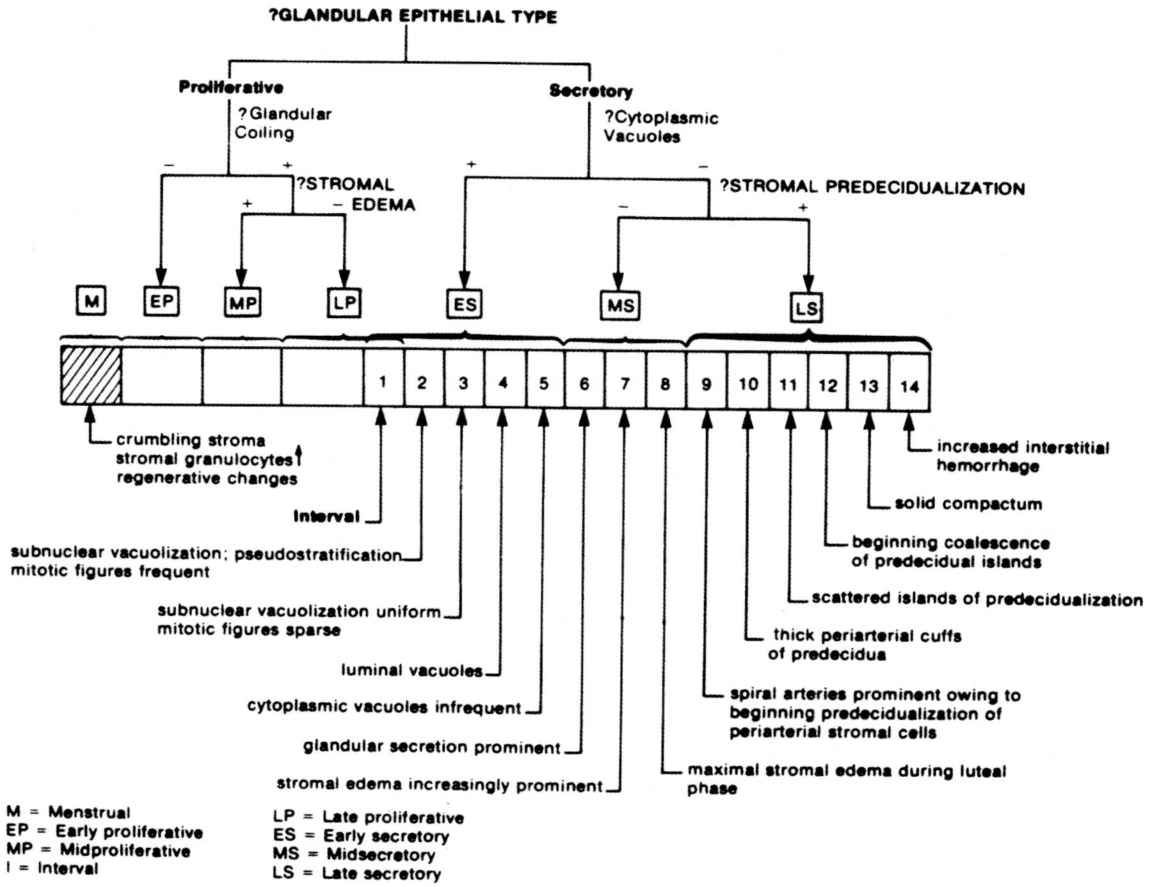


**FIG. 32.** Decision tree for endometrial dating. Reprinted with permission (348).

tinctive fashion. The morphologic changes can be divided into four periods: interval, early secretory, mid-secretory, and late secretory. The first 24 to 36 hours of the secretory phase are morphologically silent because the endometrium for the most part retains its late proliferative appearance, although scattered nonuniform subnuclear vacuoles may appear. This morphologically indeterminate endometrium is termed "interval." The first unequivocal light microscopic indication that ovulation has occurred is the presence of uniform subnuclear vacuoles involving more than 50% of the endometrial glands. Over the next few days these vacuoles shift from a subnuclear to a supranuclear location. By the fifth postovulatory day, most of the secretion has been discharged into the gland lumen. The morphologic hallmark then of the early secretory phase (postovulatory days 2 to 5) is the vacuolated gland (Fig. 35).

The mid-secretory phase lasts from postovulatory days (PODs) 5 to 9 and is characterized by nonvacuolated, prominently coiled secretory glands set within a spindled edematous stroma. Luminal secretion is most prominent during this period, and the overall appearance is one of glandular crowding (220). The secretory cells usually have round somewhat vesicular nuclei. This serves to separate them from the nuclei found in early secretory phase cells (Fig. 36). The distinctive feature of the late secretory endometrium (PODs 10–14) is stromal predecidualization. This diagnostic stromal change is heralded by an increased prominence of the spiral arteries. By the 10th postovulatory day cuffs of predecidual cells are present around these arteries, initially involving the part of the vessel adjacent to the surface of the endometrium (Fig. 37). Subsequently, islands of predecidual cells appear in the superficial compactum. By POD 13 these islands become confluent. The extent of predecidualization is roughly paralleled by the degree of stromal infiltration by stromal granulocytes, although recently some investigators have suggested that the intensity of this infiltration is more closely correlated with the time of onset of menses (221). The appearance of the glands during the late secretory phase is not significantly different from their appearance during the mid-secretory phase. They are lined by nonvacuolated secretory cells with round vesicular nuclei, and during the later days of this period the glands typically have the saw-toothed appearance sometimes referred to as secretory exhaustion. As the late secretory phase progresses, increasing numbers of dense granular subnuclear bodies accumulate within stromal macrophages and within the epithelial cells themselves. Many of these granules have the histochemical reactions and ultrastructural appearance of nuclear fragments (222).

**TABLE 2.** *Decision tree for endometrial dating*

What type of gland is present?

A. Proliferative Gland (Early proliferative, midproliferative, late proliferative, interval)
  - Is the gland straight or coiled?
    - *Straight:* Early proliferative
    - *Coiled:* Midproliferative, late proliferative, interval
  - Is there stromal edema:
    - *Yes:* Midproliferative
    - *No:* Late proliferative, interval
  - Are there scattered subnuclear vacuoles present, but with less than 50 per cent of the glands exhibiting uniform subnuclear vacuolization?
    - *No:* Late proliferative
    - *Yes:* Interval—consistent with but not diagnostic of POD 1

B. Secretory Gland-Vacuolated (Early secretory)
  - *POD 2:* Subnuclear vacuolization uniformly present, leading to exaggerated nuclear pseudostratification: mitotic figures frequent (>50% of the glands exhibit uniform subnuclear vacuolization)
  - *POD 3:* Subnuclear vacuoles and nuclei uniformly aligned; scattered mitotic figures
  - *POD 4:* Vacuoles assume luminal position; mitotic figures rare
  - *POD 5:* Vacoules infrequent; secretion in lumen of gland, nonvacuolated cells have nonvacuolated secretory appearance

C. Secretory Gland-Nonvacuolated (Midsecretory, late secretory, menstrual)
  - Is there stromal predecidualization?
    - *No:* Midsecretory
      - *POD 6:* Secretion prominent
      - *POD 7:* Beginning stromal edema
      - *POD 8:* Maximal stromal edema
    - *Yes:* Late secretory, menstrual
  - Is there crumbling of the stroma?
    - *No:* Late secretory
      - *POD 9:* Spiral arteries first prominent
      - *POD 10:* Thick periarterial cuffs of predecidua
      - *POD 11:* Islands of predecidua in superficial compactum
      - *POD 12:* Beginning coalescence of islands of predecidua
      - *POD 13:* Confluence of surface islands; stromal granulocytes prominent
      - *POD 14:* Extravasation of red cells in stroma; prominence of stromal granulocytes
    - *Yes:* Menstrual
      - Crumbling stroma, hemorrhage
      - Intravascular fibrin thrombi
      - Stromal granulocytes prominent
      - Polymorphs present
      - Late menstrual: Regenerative changes prominent

An algorithmic approach to endometrial dating. This diagram presupposes that the diagnostician is examining a *normal* endometrium that has not been obtained during a cycle of conception. From ref. 348.

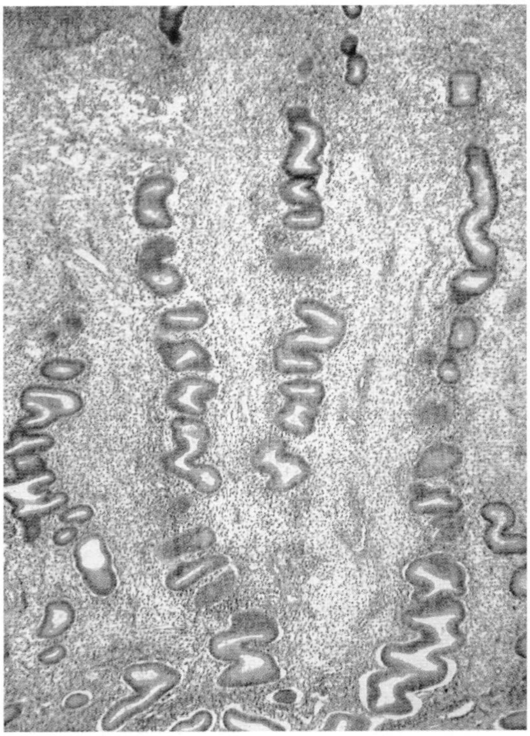

**FIG. 33.** Mid-proliferative endometrium. Note the early coiling and synchronously developed glands.

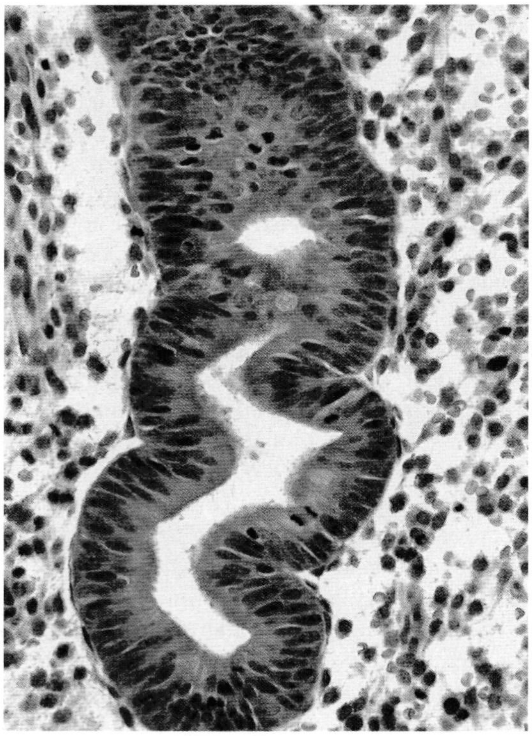

**FIG. 34.** High-power view of a proliferative phase gland. The constituent cells are pseudostratified, and the elongate glandular nuclei have dense chromatin.

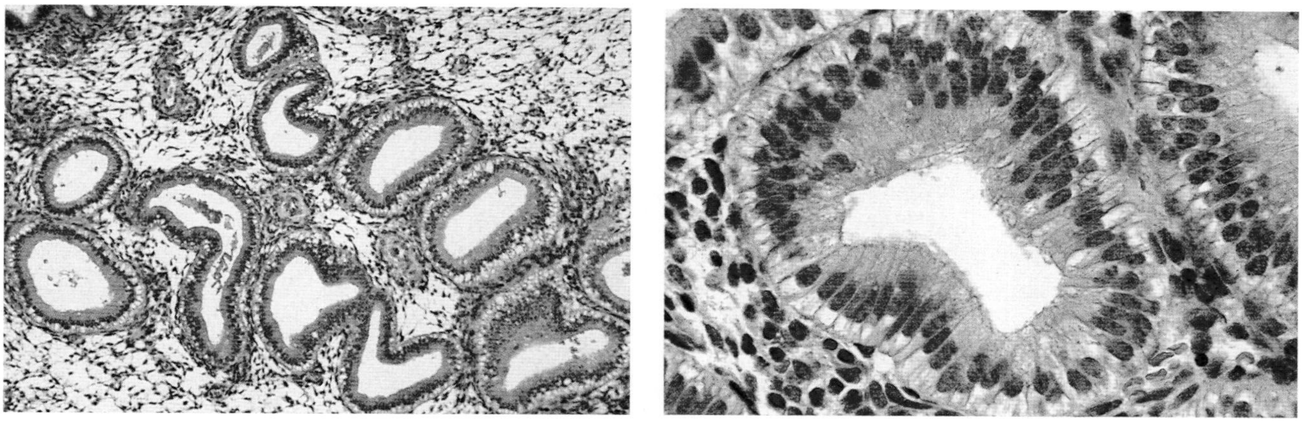
A B

**FIG. 35. A, B:** Early secretory endometrium with subnuclear vacuoles. The nuclei retain the dense chromatin of the proliferative phase. Cytoplasmic vacuoles are the most useful marker of the first third of the secretory phase.

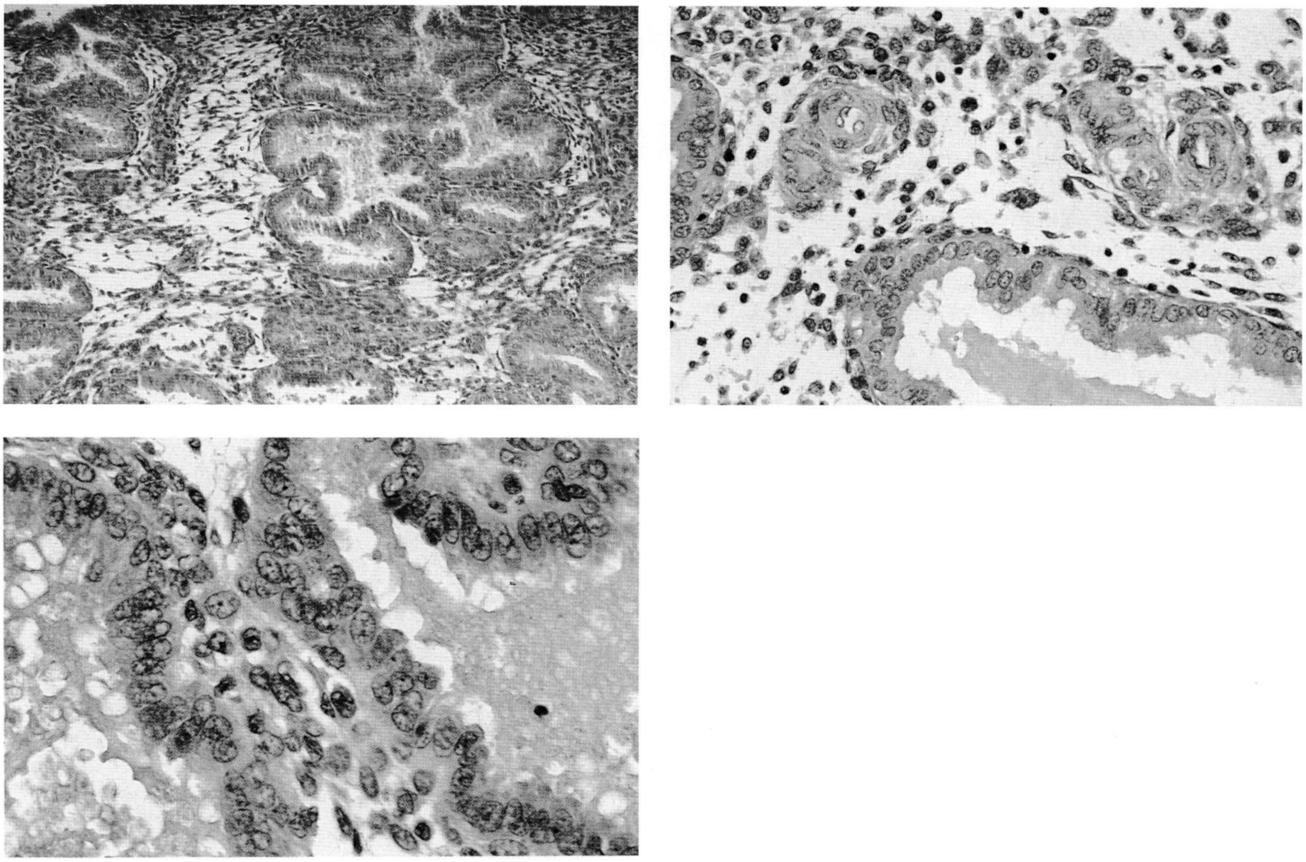
A B C

**FIG. 36.** Mid-secretory endometrium. The hallmarks of this period can be seen in these three photomicrographs. At low magnification (**A**), extreme glandular coiling and stromal edema are apparent. At a somewhat higher magnification (**B**), the coiled spiral arteries are seen within an edematous stroma. Perivascular predecidual reaction has not occurred. At yet higher magnification (**C**), the round vesicular nuclei of the mid-secretory endometrium are apparent (contrast with proliferative phase nuclei in Fig. 26).

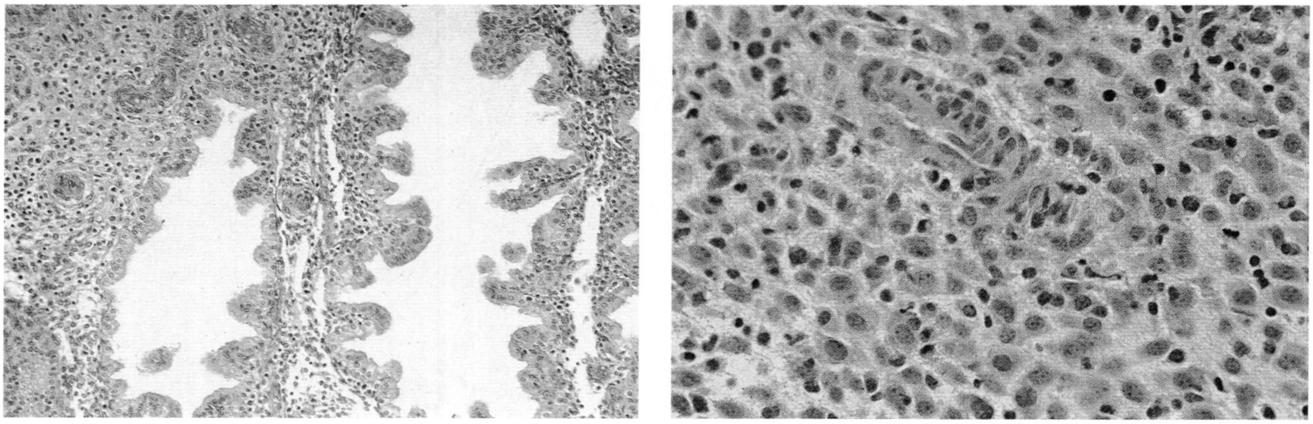


**FIG. 37.** Late secretory endometrium. At low magnification (**A**), the serrated appearance of the gland reflects their coiled state. The stroma cells have undergone predecidual reaction (**B**). Predecidual reaction begins around the spiral arteries, and this reaction serves to distinguish mid-secretory endometria from late secretory endometria.

*Menstruation*

*Menstrual Phase (cycle days 1–4).* The abrupt withdrawal of both estrogen and progesterone accompanying the demise of the corpus luteum initiates menstrual bleeding. The endometrium on the first day of menstrual bleeding (cycle day 1) is thin and compact. It is composed of the basalis and—relative to the fully developed secretory endometrium—a substantially shrunken, dense functionalis. The basalis maintains the relatively constant histologic appearance it has throughout the endometrial cycle. The shrinkage of the functionalis is largely due to "deflation" consequent on the withdrawal of interstitial fluid. Microscopically the picture in the functionalis is dominated early in this period by disruption and dissolution of the premenstrual endometrium. Features include interstitial hemorrhage, fragmentation of stroma, disruption of vessels, neutrophil infiltration, and necrosis (Fig. 38). The extent of functionalis loss during menstruation is a matter of some controversy. Some believe that the entire functionalis is lost during this process (128), whereas others believe that substantial amounts of the functionalis are remodeled and retained (139,140,213,223–225).

There is rapid onset of endometrial repair during this time. Numerous studies have demonstrated the outgrowth of epithelium from the stumps of the disrupted endometrial glands and ingrowth from the intact areas of the cornual and isthmic endometrium. This process begins during the 2nd or 3rd day and is completed by the 4th or 5th day. This early repair phase is thought by some to be estrogen independent. In normal women, almost 50% of menstrual blood loss occurs on the first day.

Much has been written speculating on the mechanism of menstruation. Initial vasoconstriction and vascular stasis undoubtedly play a role, and prostaglandins (particularly prostaglandin $F_{2a}$) increasingly are thought to be involved in this process. In nonprimate animals in which endometrial remodeling serves the function of primate menstrual shedding, lysosome-mediated destruction of individual cells plays a prominent role. Fragmented cell constituents including nuclei are phagocytosed by macrophages, which can be seen migrating through the remodeled epithelium. Evidence that this mechanism also may be at work in menstruation is pro-

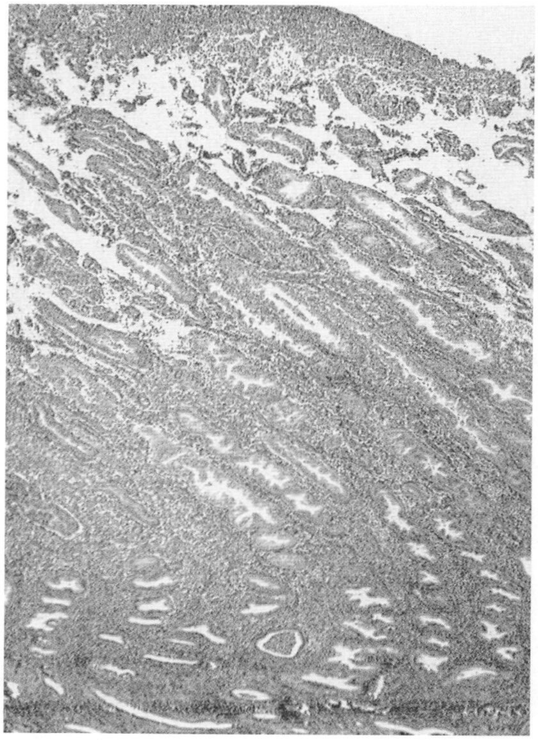

**FIG. 38.** A low-power view of a menstrual endometrium showing the unresponsive basalis in the lower part of the photomicrograph and the functionalis disintegrating near the surface.

vided by the finding of macrophages containing apoptotic bodies in premenstrual and menstrual endometria (222). These cells are identical to those seen in the germinal centers of lymph nodes, where they go by the name "tingible body macrophages." In the endometrium these macrophages serve as useful diagnostic markers of imminent endometrial dissolution.

Hemostatic mechanisms are obviously important in the controlled hemorrhage of normal menstruation. A delicate balance must exist between those mechanisms that promote blood flow and effect the removal of some part of the functionalis and those mechanisms that arrest the hemorrhage after this process is complete. A detailed discussion of this complex issue is beyond the expertise of the authors, the patience of the readers, and the scope of this monograph. The interested reader is referred to several comprehensive reviews on this evolving topic (223,226). Recently much attention has been directed to the important role of prostaglandins in this process. Prostaglandins have diverse and multiple effects on vascular smooth muscle and platelet function, and a wide variety of prostaglandins with competing effects are present in menstrual fluid. The relative amounts of different species of prostaglandins vary in normally menstruating patients as compared with those with dysfunctional uterine bleeding (DUB). Of additional interest is the notion that prostaglandins are probably the culprits involved in producing the uterine discomfort (dysmenorrhea) experienced by some menstruating women.

In summary, the successful removal of the last cycle's endometrial functionalis and the expeditious staunching of the associated hemorrhage depends on three factors: the synchronous removal of all parts of the functionalis from isthmus to cornua; the construction of a relatively compact endometrium with an anatomic plane of cleavage separating the shedding endometrium from the endometrium that will remain; and, finally, the presence of a suitably developed vasculature that can play its important role in initiating and concluding menstruation. As we shall see, DUB is a result of the failure of one or more of these anatomic ingredients .

The imminent dissolution of the endometrium is first suggested by the appearance of stromal hemorrhage and increased numbers of stromal leukocytes. Subsequently the functionalis undergoes shrinkage, and then its constituent glands and stroma fragment and crumble. Fibrin thrombi appear in vessels and within the stroma. As the stroma disintegrates, the endometrial glands are randomly arranged and may come to lie close to one another. The degenerative atypia of these glands, the necrotic background, and the close approximation of glands may suggest a diagnosis of malignancy (Fig. 39). The general strategy of not making a

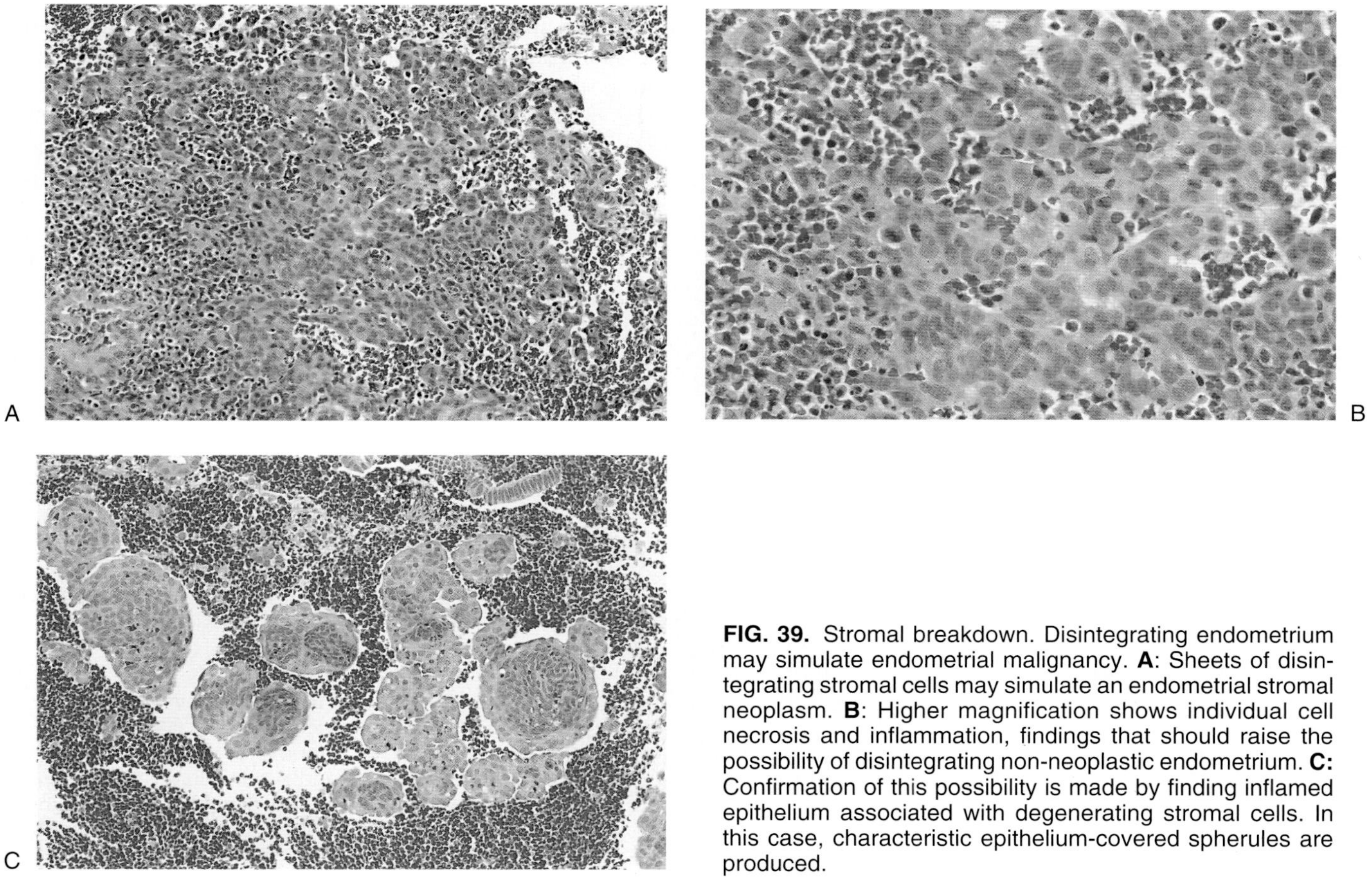


**FIG. 39.** Stromal breakdown. Disintegrating endometrium may simulate endometrial malignancy. **A**: Sheets of disintegrating stromal cells may simulate an endometrial stromal neoplasm. **B**: Higher magnification shows individual cell necrosis and inflammation, findings that should raise the possibility of disintegrating non-neoplastic endometrium. **C:** Confirmation of this possibility is made by finding inflamed epithelium associated with degenerating stromal cells. In this case, characteristic epithelium-covered spherules are produced.

diagnosis of malignancy in the absence of well-preserved tissue should prevent such a mistake.

*Regeneration Phase.* The first 5 days of the cycle feature early hormone-independent regenerative changes that gradually merge into the pattern of the early proliferative endometrium (224,227–229).

*Endometrial Morphology During the Luteal Phase of the Cycle of Conception*

If implantation of a blastocyst occurs, it will be during the midsecretory phase (PODs 6–8), and this event is associated with a resurgence of glandular secretion and a persistence of stromal edema. After this time, biopsy findings will feature prominent glandular secretion (which in a nongravid cycle would have subsided), stromal edema, and stromal predecidualization (Fig. 40) (230,231).

The developing predecidua is gradually converted to decidua after POD 14 of the luteal phase of conception. This transformation is complete by the end of the first month of gestation. The fully developed decidual reaction is distinctive. Almost all of the endometrial stroma is converted into pavementlike sheets of epithelioid cells with prominent cytoplasmic margins and central vesicular nuclei (Fig. 28). In the superficial portion of the functionalis, the glands are compressed and their lining becomes flattened and endothelium-like. This compact sheetlike zone, the zona compactum, overlies saw-toothed scalloped glands that continue to exhibit secretory features. This latter area is termed the zona spongiosum. Many of the glands in the spongiosum are lined by cells with enlarged nuclei that often have atypical nuclear features approaching those of the Arias-Stella reaction (Fig. 41). Scattered stromal granulocytes are often present. Decidual cells may exhibit a marked degree of nuclear pleomorphism and cytologic atypia. This is particularly prominent in the region of the implantation site. In addition, this region is also routinely infiltrated by trophoblastic cells, which normally have a bizarre cytologic appearance. The infiltration of decidua and the underlying myometrium by trophoblasts has been termed "syncytial metritis," not a particularly felicitous label because the process has little to do with inflammation (Fig. 42). Accordingly, the current term for this process is "implantation site reaction" and is diagnostic of intrauterine pregnancy (232). Both placental site reaction and decidual atypia may incorrectly suggest malignancy, but confusion with adenocarcinoma is avoided by noting the secretory setting of these findings as well as the clinical history (233). Although a fully developed decidual reaction is a constant feature of intrauterine pregnancy, it is by no means a diagnostic finding. An identical decidual reaction may be seen in extrauterine (ectopic) pregnancy and gestational trophoblastic disease; it also can be produced by progestational agents or can be associated with persistence of the corpus luteum unassociated with pregnancy (e.g., corpus luteum cyst).

Previous intrauterine pregnancy is strongly suggested in the postpartum endometrium by the presence of cuffs of hyalinized decidua around sclerotic ectatic spiral arteries. The decidual cells composing this cuff often have hyperchromatic smudged and degenerate nuclei, and the vessels are often thrombosed. These findings have been referred to as subinvolution of the placental site and can be responsible for postpartum hemorrhage (234,235). This presumably occurs because these severely altered vessels are incapable of contraction. With time the foci of hyalinization shrink and the nuclei may disappear, leaving a small pink scar resem-

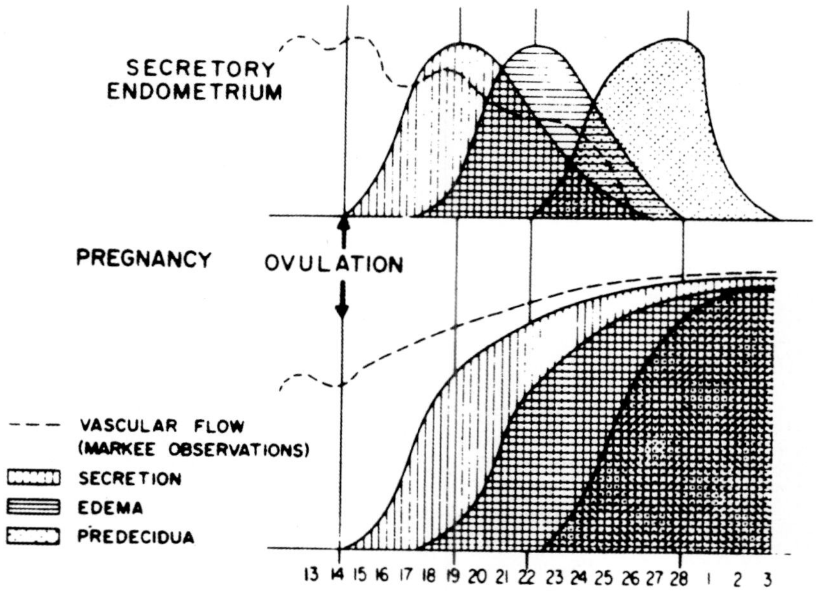


**FIG. 40.** The transition from secretory to gestational endometrium is shown. The simultaneous occurrence of intense secretion, edema, and predecidual reaction and maintained vascular flow characterizes the early endometrial gestational responses. Reprinted with permission (349).

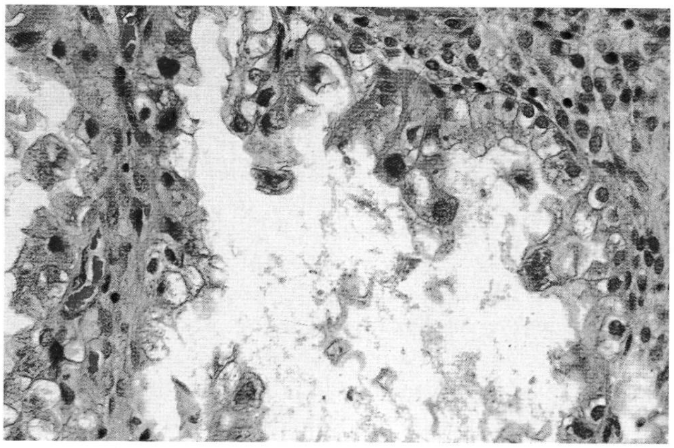

**FIG. 41.** Secretory endometrium during pregnancy. This gland is lined by cells with enlarged dense nuclei characteristic of the Arias-Stella reaction.

bling an ovarian corpus atreticum. These distinctive foci have been referred to as pregnancy plaques, and they may persist in the basalis for many years. A similar lesion featuring intermediate trophoblast has been termed placental site nodule or placental site plaque (234).

Hyperprogestational states (particularly pregnancy) are sometimes associated with the distinctive glandular change to which Arias-Stella first drew attention in 1954 and that now bears his name (236–240). Most commonly this change is encountered in endometrial glands, but on occasion it may be present in foci of endometriosis or adenomyosis, in endocervical glands, in fallopian tube epithelium, or in the glands within polyps. The Arias-Stella phenomenon characteristically involves a focus of tightly packed glands whose extreme coiling and collapse throw the lining epithelium into prominent papillary folds. This epithelium is composed of cells exhibiting marked nuclear pleomorphism and hyperchromatism. The nuclei typically have a smudged appearance. The cell cytoplasm may be strikingly hypervacuolated and cleared (clear cells) or densely eosinophilic (dark cells) (Fig. 41). One or the other cell type may predominate from area to area. Occasionally the eosinophilic cells may line the glands in a hobnail fashion. Mitotic figures are only rarely present. Elsewhere the endometrium usually exhibits the other changes one would anticipate with progestational stimulation, such as secretory glands and a stromal decidual reaction.

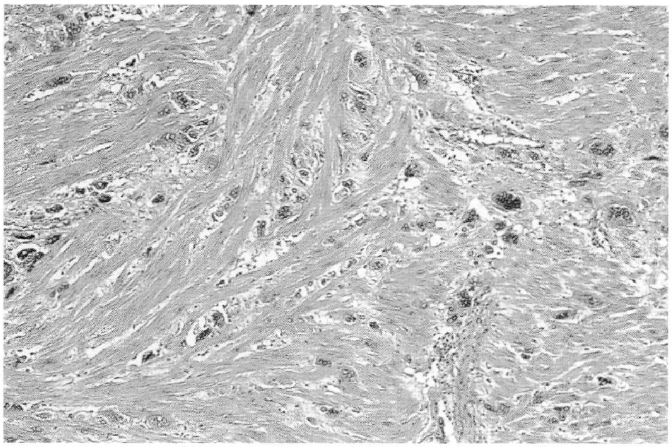

**FIG. 42.** Myometrium beneath an implantation site containing infiltrating trophoblasts. This must not be misinterpreted as evidence of malignancy.

Less striking degrees of nuclear hyperchromasia, nuclear pleomorphism, and cytoplasmic vacuolization are, in our experience, constant features of the secretory glands of every pregnancy. The Arias-Stella reaction appears to represent the extreme end of the morphologic spectrum of the glandular epithelial changes seen in all pregnancies.

Ultrastructurally, the clear cells of the Arias-Stella gland usually contain abundant glycogen that may be demonstrated with periodic acid-Schiff (PAS) stain. The densely eosinophilic cells (dark cells) contain a variety of organelles, including abundant rough endoplasmic reticulum and mitochondria (241).

An endometrial Arias-Stella change may be present in a variety of clinical settings, including normal intrauterine pregnancy, extrauterine pregnancy, gestational trophoblastic disease, and persistent corpus luteum (239,242). In a retrospective review of patient's coded as having Arias-Stella reaction, 16% had an extrauterine gestation. It also may be produced by the administration of ovulation-inducing drugs or progestational agents (236,237).

Because of the marked nuclear atypia of the epithelium lining the closely packed glands, the Arias-Stella phenomenon can be confused with adenocarcinoma, particularly with the architectural and cytologic features of clear cell carcinoma. This difficulty largely can be avoided by remembering that the Arias-Stella phenomenon occurs in a secretory setting; that is, more conventional secretory glands and decidualized or predecidualized stroma are usually found elsewhere in the specimen and the patient is premenopausal. Moreover, glandular mitotic figures tend not to be a prominent feature, although they may occasionally be encountered (243). Clear cell carcinoma (like any carcinoma) is fundamentally a proliferative process, and the constituent cells not only possess malignant features but also exhibit mitotic activity. Most importantly, clear cell carcinoma of the endometrium develops almost exclusively in postmenopausal women.

Occasionally in a gestational setting glandular nuclei may exhibit marked nuclear clearing reminiscent of herpetic infections (Fig. 43) (244).

### *Endometrial Vasculature*

The transition from the endometrium of early gestation to that of fully developed pregnancy is marked by the accelerated development of the endometrial vasculature, resulting

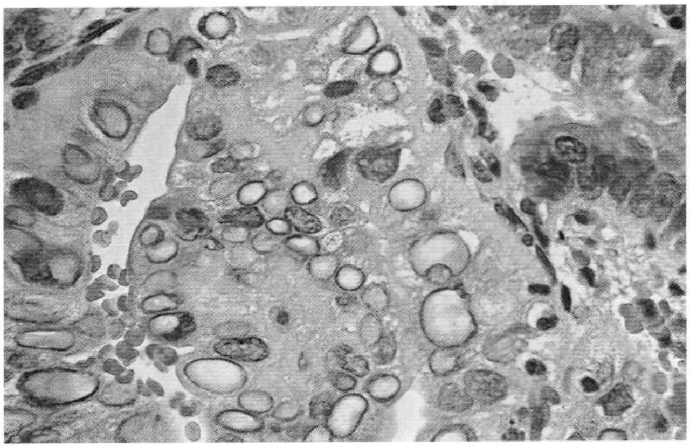

FIG. 43. Nuclear clearing of the glandular cells in the endometrium may be seen in a gestational setting. This change should not be misconstrued as evidence of herpes virus infection.

in increased thickness of the spiral arteries, as reflected in their mean cross-sectional diameter (168,245).

*Perimenopausal and Postmenopausal Years*

With the waning of hormonal function in the fifth decade of life, a woman enters the perimenopause, during which time uterine bleeding characteristically again becomes erratic, and the length of time between bleeding episodes lengthens. Thus, both the perimenopause and the perimenarche may be marked by erratic ovarian function and consequent dysfunctional (abnormal) uterine bleeding.

The end of ovarian follicular development and ovulation results in cessation of the menstrual periods and the menopause. Thereafter, the uterus enters a second inactive period, and the endometrial, glandular epithelium, as in the premenarchal years, is typically atrophic. However, the glandular architecture and thickness of the endometrium may vary considerably. Several different patterns may be seen in the peri- and postmenopausal endometrium, which are described in the following sections.

*Atrophic Endometrium*

Atrophic epithelium is nonstratified and composed of a single layer of flattened to cuboidal cells. Mitotic figures are not present, the nucleus-to-cytoplasm ratio is high, and there is usually no specific cytoplasmic differentiation, although cilia may be present occasionally. The defining and only constant feature of atrophic endometria is the atrophic epithelial lining of its constituent glands, which may have any configuration, including cystic dilatation and glandular crowding. The stroma is spindled and is neither predecidualized nor decidualized. The nuclei may be densely pyknotic (as in postmenopausal endometria or endometrial polyps) or plump (as in endometria associated with oral contraceptives). Stromal disintegration may be present (Fig. 44) (246–248).

Atrophic endometria can occur in a variety of clinical settings. It is the normal state during the premenarchal and later postmenopausal years. During the reproductive years, atrophic patterns may be seen in association with premature ovarian failure or, more commonly, in patients taking oral contraceptives.

*Weakly Proliferative Endometrium*

Weakly proliferative epithelium is nonstratified, although some degree of nuclear pseudostratification may be present, and its constituent cells are thin (pencil shape). This epithelium differs from the normal proliferative epithelium in the paucity of mitotic figures, the greater density of the nuclear chromatin, and, in the usual case, the overall lack of organization of the glands. The glands may be of any configuration, but the glands-to-stroma ratio is almost always near unity or there can be a slight stromal predominance. The stroma is spindled; stromal cell nuclei may be densely pyknotic or plump.

The morphologic variability of the weakly proliferative endometrium parallels that of the atrophic endometrium. The difference between them is solely based on the appearance of the epithelial cells: weakly proliferative rather than flattened or cuboidal. The clinical settings in which these two endometria occur overlap considerably. It is conceptually convenient to regard the weakly proliferative endometrium as lying on a continuum between normal and atrophic endometrium; the weakly proliferative patterns may then be conceived of as representing a transition between normal proliferation and atrophy. Weakly proliferative endometria are most often encountered in patients in the peri- or postmenopausal years whose endometria appear to be weakly

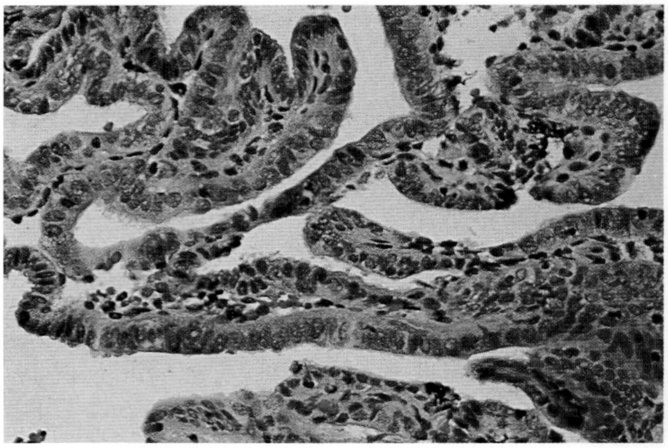

FIG. 44. Endometrial atrophy as seen in an endometrial sampling. On occasion, atrophic surface epithelium may be removed in coiled masses and simulate hyperplasia because the glands are closely approximated. Reprinted with permission (350).

supported by low levels of endogenous or exogenous estrogen. This pattern is normal in the hormonally hyporesponsive lower uterine segment of the normally cycling premenopausal women.

*Disordered Proliferative Endometrium*

We regard "disordered proliferation" as the morphologic bridge between normal proliferation and hyperplasia. It is the endometrial pattern encountered in women with sporadic anovulatory cycles and thus is most commonly encountered in the perimenopausal and perimenarchal years. It is also commonly seen in women receiving estrogen therapy. Disordered proliferation differs from normal proliferation by virtue of a loss of synchrony of glandular development so that some glands are tubular, whereas others are cystically dilated or have complex shapes. Budding may be present so that there may be a shift in the glands-to-stroma ratio in favor of the glands, but this shift is never marked. When glandular predominance is so marked that the proliferation is almost all glands, a diagnosis of hyperplasia is warranted (Fig. 45).

We think that disordered proliferation (in the sense above) represents the response of a normal endometrium to sporadic unopposed estrogen stimulation. There is no evidence that this pattern is a marker for an increased risk for the subsequent development of endometrial carcinoma. Because the term "hyperplasia" connotes to many clinicians such an increased risk, we part company with those pathologists who include this pattern in the hyperplasia group.

Histologically, the variously shaped glands are lined by normal proliferative cells with elongate dense nuclei that are most often pseudostratified. Mitotic figures are usually present and may be numerous. Stromal cells are spindled with plump nuclei.

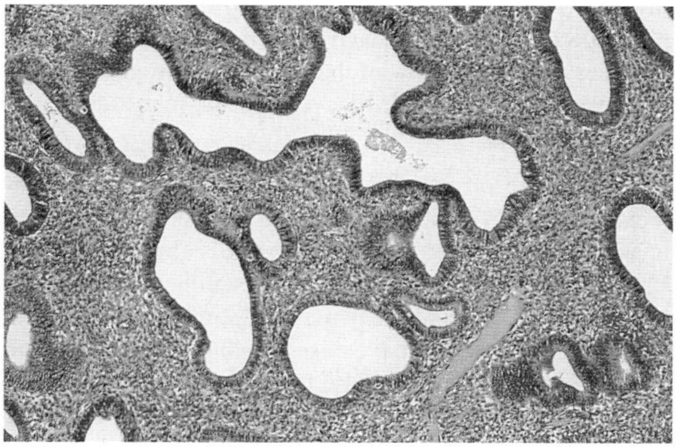

**FIG. 45.** Disordered proliferation is the result of anovulatory cycles and is normal during the perimenopausal years. It is often found in the endometrium of women receiving estrogen therapy. Disordered proliferation is characterized by nonsynchronous growth of the glands including budding, but the glands-to-stroma ratio is unity or with a slight glandular predominance. This pattern of endometrial growth serves as a bridge between normal proliferation and hyperplasia.

### Relevance of Endometrial Dating to Diagnostic Surgical Pathologists

The particulars of the normal menstrual cycle are chiefly important for the interpretation of the EMB performed for infertility (249). In women being evaluated for infertility, the three clinical questions of major interest are as follows:

*Clinical question 1:* Is there an intrinsic abnormality of the endometrium that might explain the couple's infertility (e.g., endometrial polyps, submucous leiomyomata, endometritis hyperplasia, carcinoma)? Much of this information is provided by hysterosalpingogram, hysteroscopy, and laparoscopy—increasingly routine procedures for the workup of the infertility patient (250–253).

*Clinical question 2:* If the endometrium is normal, does the morphology of the endometrium provide evidence that the patient ovulated in the biopsy cycle? This amounts to deciding whether the endometrium is secretory. The answer to this question is also relevant for the patient undergoing EMB for abnormal bleeding in the reproductive years; the approach to the therapy of DUB depends on whether such bleeding is ovulatory (secretory pattern of some sort) or anovulatory (nonsecretory pattern of some sort).

*Clinical question 3:* If the endometrium is secretory, is it appropriately developed for the patient's chronologic dates. The only importance of this observation is that, under certain circumstances, the establishment of endometrial maturational delay warrants the diagnosis of luteal phase deficiency (LPD), a relatively uncommon condition that is thought by some to be responsible for infertility and correctable using a variety of therapies. As discussed below, LPD is defined in terms of a greater than 3-day disparity between the woman's chronologic date of ovulation and her endometrial morphologic date when this disparity occurs more than sporadically.

Thus, after determining that the endometrium is normal, an essential part of the evaluation of the EMB of the infertility patient is to assign the endometrium a morphologic date (211,215,254–256). The following provides a brief review of normal endometrial histology.

In evaluating the endometrium, it is important to carefully distinguish between the morphologic postovulatory date assigned to a morphologically normal endometrium and the chronologic postovulatory date. The morphologic date is a summary characterization of the histologic development of the endometrium based on an assessment of glandular and stromal features. Endometrial development is characterized either in terms of conventional light microscopic features or, in recent years (and in research settings), with more sophisticated and reproducible morphometric semiquantitated features. The morphologic findings may be summarized either in terms of postovulatory days, cycle days, or phases. For example, the morphologic pattern associated with a particular "standard" postovulatory day is assigned the number of that day; e.g., POD 12 refers to the pattern seen on POD 12 of the "standard" cycle. Equivalently, this morphologic information can be conveyed using cycle day or phase (e.g., late secretory). The precise details of the morphologic patterns corresponding to standard cycle dates are presented in Table 2 and Figs. 31 and 32.

The chronologic date is an estimate of when the patient actually ovulated and does not use any information about the morphologic appearance of the endometrium (257,258). Chronologic dates are established in a variety of more or less indirect ways. Before the availability of hormonal assays, the two methods used for assessing chronologic dates were the analysis of the basal body temperature chart (the nadir marks the time of ovulation) and back-dating from the first day of the menstrual period after the EMB, i.e., the next menstrual period. The next menstrual period technique makes no assumption about the length of the follicular phase but does assume that the luteal phase is 14 days in length. When this method is used, the biopsy cannot be interpreted in relation to the patient's cycle until the date of her next menstrual period is known. Both of these methods for determining chronologic dates have come under attack in recent years, and a number of replacements have been suggested. The current standard for the estimate of the time of ovulation is ultrasonic visualization of the disappearance of the dominant follicle. This method is not used in the routine workup of infertility patients, but is reserved for either research settings or in the course of egg harvesting for in vitro fertilization therapy. Measurement of the time of the preovulatory LH peak, the LH surge, is now possible with home kits (259).

Over the past 15 years, work in a number of laboratories has drawn into question much of the conventional wisdom about the normal menstrual cycle. Much of that wisdom was accumulated before assays were available to chart the cyclic changes of serum gonadotropins and steroids and before techniques were available to establish the woman's chronologic date (260).

Recent observations relevant to the evaluation of the EMB for infertility are listed as follows:

1. The luteal phase of the normally fertile and normally cycling woman is of variable length (212,218,261–264). Landgren et al. (262) studied 68 normally menstruating women of proven fertility and confirmed that the follicular phase was highly variable (9–23 days). Surprisingly, the luteal phase, which was long thought to have a relatively fixed length of 14 days, in fact varied from 8 to 17 days. Slightly less than half of the women studied had a luteal phase length of 14 to 15 days. The importance of this observation is that many women who are otherwise normal have sporadic or even sequential luteal phases that are more than 2 days shorter than the ideal 14 days. The term "short luteal phase" has been suggested for patients whose luteal phase is no longer than 11 days and is regarded by many as a type of LPD. These observations have been confirmed by many workers.

2. Conventional Noyes' dating has low reproducibility (217,265,266). That the interobserver agreement for conventional histologic dating of the endometrium using the criteria of Noyes et al. is poor has been known for some time. Noyes and Haman reported that two observers agreed on the same morphologic date 29% of the time, were within one day of each other in 63% of cases, and were within 2 days of one another in 82% of cases (267). These results have been duplicated in more recent studies (217,266,268,269). As a consequence, the results of endometrial dating should be reported as a range of 2 days to reflect this variability. Morphometric dating is more reproducible than Noyes' dating and, although providing insight into the development of the normal endometrium and insight into those deviations from normal that would warrant the label "luteal phase defect," is of little practical clinical value at this time (212,217,218,265,266).

3. Endometrial morphology is more highly correlated with LH surge than the next menstrual period (263,266,270,271). As a consequence of this observation, there is a growing tendency to use as the point of reference the mid-cycle surge of LH (which sets ovulation into motion 10 to 12 hours after the LH peak) rather than the first day of menstrual flow (272).

4. The correlation of endometrial pattern (whether assessed morphometrically or using Noyes' criteria) with the LH surge is the highest during those portions of the follicular phase and the luteal phase that straddle the day of the LH surge. Johannisson et al. undertook a morphometric analysis of the endometrial biopsies of 90 apparently reproductively normal women and noted that the morphology of the endometrium was remarkably uniform among women during the period 3 days before the LH surge and 8 days after (212,218). Thus, substantial variability is present in normal women during the late luteal phase of the cycle, the usual time recommended for obtaining an EMB. Similar results have been reported by the Sheffield group (217,273). Thus, it seems that the timing of the EMB in an infertility patient involves a trade-off between precision (first half of luteal phase better than second half) and relevance (second half provides one with a view of the cumulative progesterone effect over the duration of the cycle). Most investigators opt for relevance.

All of these observations expose the considerable problems involved in deciding whether a secretory endometrium is appropriately developed for a woman's chronologic date. Importantly, these problems tend to destabilize the definition of LPD. For these and other reasons, some investigators in infertility management have raised doubts about the wisdom of incorporating the EMB into the initial workup of the infertile couple. There are better ways of (a) ruling out structural disease of the uterus (hysterosalpingogram, hysteroscopy, laparoscopy) and (b) establishing that cycles are ovulatory (e.g., noting that cycles are regular and obtaining a mid-luteal progesterone level); and (c) the diagnosis of LPD may not be worth the effort and expense of the EMB except in a small, select subset of patients (257,274–278).

These skeptical observations notwithstanding, pathologists are still expected to assign morphologic dates to cycling endometria and (for the biopsies of infertility patients) to correlate that date with some estimate of the patient's chronologic date. When information about ovulation in the current cycle is not available, the chronologic date can be estimated by back dating. However, it must be cautioned that back dating (using the next menstrual period method) has been found by most investigators to be inadequate for assessing the presence of corpus luteum defects (271). It is important to emphasize that the morphologic changes occurring from day to day are continuous, resulting in overlapping morphologic patterns that in most observers' view precludes reliably assigning postovulatory morphologic dates more closely than within a 48-hour interval anchored on one's best guess at the true morphologic date (e.g., "the endometrium looks most like the POD 10 pattern but my next choice of pattern would be POD 11"; diagnosis, POD 10–11) (279,280).

Deciding whether a woman has ovulated by examining an EMB taken in what is presumed to be her late luteal phase is usually a trivial matter; the presence of a late secretory endometrium means ovulation. Deciding whether ovulation has occurred in the early luteal phase is more problematic. The characteristic light microscopic postovulatory secretory changes in the endometrium lag behind actual ovulation by at least 1 day. A biopsy on POD 2 will show spotty, nonuniform subnuclear vacuolization (interval pattern). Such vacuolization may be seen in late proliferative endometria as well as in other types of nonsecretory endometria and is, for this reason, not diagnostic of ovulation. Because of the ambiguous morphologic picture in the early postovulatory period, endometrial biopsies are usually obtained well into the presumed luteal phase of the cycle, preferably on PODs 11 to 13. We require uniform subnuclear vacuolization in 50% of the glands before diagnosing the earliest morphologic evidence of ovulation; this usually is present by POD 3.

Accurate endometrial dating requires attention to a number of details (211). Dating features should be sought only in fragments of endometrial functionalis, which are lined by surface epithelium; fragments of basalis and lower uterine segment should be ignored. The assigned date should be of the most developed area and should be based on features near the surface epithelium (the "egg's eye view" of Noyes) (211).

The preconditions for assigning a morphologic date to an endometrium are described as follows. Assigning a date to an EMB is obviously not possible in the absence of an adequate specimen, in a noncycling endometrium (e.g., nonsecretory pattern other than proliferative), in a patient being treated with medication that alters the morphology of the endometrium, or in an endometrium that is inflamed or that houses an intrauterine device. Thus, a precondition for applying the dating criteria is that one is dealing with a roughly normal endometrial pattern. Scanning power examination should establish the presence of pattern uniformity (apart from the expected variation due to sectioning randomly oriented fragments and normal out of phase curettage inhabitants such as fragments of the lower uterine segment, cervical epithelium, and stratum basalis), the absence of significant budding and branching of glands, and the absence of necrosis and inflammation. Examination at higher power should exclude the presence of significant epithelial nuclear atypia and the absence of significant numbers of stromal plasma cells

A checklist for the contents of the pathology report of endometrial biopsies is provided in Table 3.

**TABLE 3.** *The contents of the pathology report for an infertility endometrial biopsy*

| |
|---|
| Statement of the adequacy of the biopsy |
| Suggest rebiopsy if: |
| Sample is inadequate |
| The endometrium is disintegrating and not clearly menstrual (i.e., postovulatory) |
| The endometrium is disintegrating, postovulatory but otherwise undatable and the main concern is with the adequacy of the luteal phase |
| Statement about evidence of ovulation |
| Statement about pattern uniformity |
| An estimate of the endometrium's morphologic date (2-day interval) |
| Correlation with information about the chronological date (time of LH surge or basal body temperature shift) |
| Statement about presence or absence of "organic disease" |
| Inflammation |
| Endometrial polyps |
| Submucous leiomyomas |

From ref. 331.

### Endometrial–Myometrial Junction

The endometrial–myometrial junction is normally irregular, a phenomenon that must be kept in mind when assessing the presence or absence of myoinvasion by endometrial adenocarcinoma and in diagnosing superficial adenomyosis (Fig. 24).

### Apoptosis

The role of programmed cell death or apoptosis in the remodeling of the endometrium was mentioned earlier in this chapter (222). Apoptosis and its hormonal control in both human and animal endometrium is an area of active investigation by a number of groups.

Withdrawal of progesterone in the rabbit endometrium correlates with the development of apoptosis (281–285).

Bcl-2 is a protooncogene initially described in the (14;18) translocation in follicular lymphoma. It has been shown to prolong cell survival by preventing apoptosis. Gompel et al. studied Bcl-2 expression immunohistochemically in the nor-

**TABLE 4.** *Normal findings in the endometrium that have relevance to histopathologic differential diagnosis (see text for additional differential diagnostic clues)*

| Finding | Diagnostic confusion | Suggestions for resolution | References |
|---|---|---|---|
| "Glands within glands" this can occur from trauma of D&C (telescoping) and tangential cutting | Hyperplasia: Rolled up carpet effect may simulate the architectural complexity of hyperplasia or carcinoma | This artifact is usually only focal and often at the periphery or otherwise normal fragments of functionalis. Check that epithelium is identical to architecturally normal glands in the sample. | (249) |
| Strips of normal surface epithelium<br>Commonly obtained seen with atrophic endometrium | Hyperplasia/Carcinoma: Rolled up carpet effect may simulate the architectural complexity of hyperplasia or carcinoma | In contrast to hyperplasia and carcinoma, the rolled up atrophic endometrium is cytologically bland and mitotically inactive. | (249) |
| Lower uterine segment | Dating problem: The glands respond weakly at best to hormones and the stroma is often fibrous<br>Adenocarcinoma: Cervical involvement by adenocarcinoma (see Table 1) | Look for mucinous epithelial component. Unless the sample is inadequate for dating the endometrium, there will be other fragments around with an appearance more typical of functionalis. | |
| Normal basalis | Dating problem: The glands respond weakly at best to hormones and the stroma is inactive | When assigning a morphologic date to an endometrial fragment, use only glands in close approximation to surface epithelium | |
| Ciliated cells | Adenocarcinoma: Intraepithelial ciliated cells have rounded pear-shaped contours and open rounded nuclei with nucleoli | Look for cilia.<br>Endometria containing ciliated cells have a polymophous appearance; the cytologic features are uniform within each subpopulation of cells. | (249) |
| Foam cells | Endometritis<br>Foam cells are commonly encountered in hyperestrogenic settings and are thought to be one differentiated form of endometrial stromal cells | Look for plasma cells to establish a diagnosis of chronic endometritis. Macrophages with foamy cytoplasm may occur in the endometrium as a component of a chronic inflammatory process. Commonly seen as a reaction to a foreign body or to keratin (e.g. in setting of proliferations shedding keratin). | |
| Arias-Stella reaction | Adenocarcinoma: Particularly clear cell carcinoma | Clear cell carcinoma is most frequent in postmenopausal women.<br>Arias-Stella reaction usually does not feature mitotic figures which are almost always easily found in clear cell carcinoma. | (236, 238, 242, 243, 302) |
| Implantation site | Gestational trophoblastic disease: Early gestations may mimic choriocarcinoma. The often bizarre shapes of trophoblastic cells may raise the possibility of choriocarcinoma a molar gestation, or PSTT | Clinical history to establish time course of gestation.<br>Insistence on a bilaminar pattern of cytotrophoblast alternating with syncytiotrophoblast for choriocarcinoma, villi are not present in choriocarcinoma. PSTT features. | |
| | Clinically relevant endometritis: Chronic endometritis is a normal finding in the implantation site | The implantation site used to be called "syncytiometritis." This term for the infiltration of intermediate trophoblast into the endometrium and myometrium has been abandoned. Clinically relevant endo-myometritis can occur but is only rarely diagnosed initially on endometrial samplings. The vast majority of cases of "chronic endometritis" seen in practice represent a clinically insignificant "physiologic" finding. | |
| Irregular endometrial-myometrial junction | Adenomyosis: Glands and stroma surrounded by smooth muscle | Associated smooth muscle hypertrophy is a common feature of adenomyosis and not irregular junctions. Superficial myometrial location of suspected foci favors irregular junctions. | (249) |
| | Myoinvasive adenocarcinoma: The irregular junction, when expanded by hyperplasia or carcinoma, often simulates myoinvasive carcinoma. Tangential sectioning often reinforces this impression | Absence of stromal host response that is usual in myoinvasive carcinoma. Presence of endometrial stroma or normal glands means irregular junction (or adenomyosis). | |
| Menstrual endometrium | Adenocarcinoma: "Cytologic atypia" produced by degenerating, poorly preserved glandular elements<br>Stromal neoplasm: Degenerating stroma may produce pattern resembling endometrial stromal sarcoma with or without sex cord elements | Obtain history; menstrual fragments have degenerating not neoplastic nuclei. | |

*(continued)*

**TABLE 4.** *Continued.*

| Finding | Diagnostic confusion | Suggestions for resolution | References |
|---|---|---|---|
| Lymphoid nodules | Endometritis | The presence of scattered lymphoid nodules does not correlate with significant clinical disease. Large numbers of lymphoid nodules and germinal centers are usually associated with the conventional sine qua non of "chronic endometritis," the plasma cell. | |
| Stromal "granulocytes" | Acute or chronic endometritis | "Stromal granulocytes" are a normal feature of the late secretory endometrium and serve as one of the original Noyes dating criteria. In the fullness of time it has been established that these "granulocytes" are subpopulations of lymphocytes (see text).<br>Clinically significant inflammation (of the type encountered in patients with established salpingitis) features the presence of easily found plasma cells and is usually accompanied by acute inflammation and necrosis of the surface epithelium.<br>Not infrequently, endometrial stromal cells or normal lymphoid constituents may have somewhat eccentric nuclei and amphophilic cytoplasm that mimics that of a plasma cell. This is usually a problem with one or two scattered cells in a fragment. Plasma cells have to be easily found before they amount to anything clinically. | (212, 333–335) (336) |
| Pseudo-herpes inclusions<br>Nuclear ground glass appearance to nuclei of epithelial cells in gestational setting and with progestogen therapy | Herpes endometritis | Herpes endometritis is rare; obtain history.<br>Immunohistochemistry may be helpful. | (244) |

mal endometrium (286). They found that Bcl-2 predominated in glandular cells and reached a maximum at the end of the follicular phase but disappeared at the onset of secretory activity. These results strongly suggest hormone-dependent regulation of Bcl-2 expression.

The role of tumor necrosis factor-alpha (TNF-$\alpha$) in the induction of apoptosis was explored by Tabibzadeh et al (287). They found that the TNF receptor as well as Fas protein were expressed in endometrial epithelium throughout the entire menstrual cycle and were most prominent in the basalis. They concluded that endometrial epithelium, by expressing receptors for TNF-$\alpha$ and Fas protein can respond to ligands that regulate apoptosis.

Normal findings in the endometrium that have relevance to histopathologic differential diagnosis are shown in Table 4.

## MYOMETRIUM

The bulk of the myometrium comprises smooth muscle cells, but an important contribution is made by extracellular components such as collagen and elastin. The smooth muscle within the corpus is more concentrated relative to collagen and elastin than the muscle in either the cervix or the lower uterine segment. This distribution of muscle is consistent with the passive role of the cervix during parturition; the uterine contents propelled by fundal contractions are thought to passively dilate a cervix previously softened by the action of collagenase. The uterine smooth muscle cells are spindled, with blunt-ended fusiform nuclei. The volume of their cytoplasm depends on whether the patient is pregnant (288–291). The cells range in length from 20 $\mu$m in the nongravid state to 600 $\mu$m in the term uterus (292). Scattered normal mitotic figures may be encountered, particularly during the secretory phase of the endometrial cycle (293). Characteristic ultrastructural features of smooth muscle include (a) numerous dense, 60- to 80-A myofilaments without cross striations, which almost fill the cytoplasm; (b) small round dense bodies along the trajectory of the filaments; (c) dense plaques arranged along the inner aspect of the plasma membrane; and (d) plasma membrane–related vesicles that may play a role in ionized calcium movement across the plasma membrane during contraction (292). In addition, there is the usual complement of cytoplasmic organelles, including smooth and rough endoplasmic reticulum, mitochondria, and a Golgi apparatus. Typically these organelles arrange themselves around the nucleus, which often has an irregular shape. These ultrastructural features reflect the dual function of the uterine myocyte: muscular contraction and collagen and elastin synthesis. The ultrastructural appearance varies with the levels of circulating steroidal hormones. In particular, estrogen appears to sharply increase myocyte protein synthesis. This correlates morphologically in an increased volume of rough endoplasmic reticulum and increased num-

**TABLE 5.** *Comparison of differentiated features for endometrial stromal cells and smooth muscle cells (From ref. 332)*

| Technique | Endometrial stromal cell | Usual smooth muscle cell | Epithelioid smooth muscle cells | Endometrial stroma with epithelioid and/or glandular areas |
|---|---|---|---|---|
| Lightmicroscopy<br>Architectural features | Haphazardly arranged cells resembling normal proliferative phase endometrial stromal cells | Cells arranged in looping intersecting fascicles | Rounded or polygonal cells with moderate amount of cytoplasm | Biphasic pattern<br>Stromal component (featuring cellular endometrial stroma or fibroblastic stroma)<br>+ Epithelioid component<br>{• Travecular epithelial pattern<br>or<br>• nests<br>or<br>• insular pattern<br>or<br>• Sertoli-like tubular pattern<br>or<br>• glands} |
| | Complex plexiform vascular pattern | Vascular component not complex | Foci of neoplasm often exhibit standard smooth muscle features | When the entire neoplasm has this biphasic appearance the term 'uterine tumour resembling ovarian sex cord tumours' has been used<br>When the change is focal within what is otherwise an endometrial stromal neoplasm (either stromal nodule or endometrial stromal sarcoma) the endometrial stromal diagnosis is supplemented with 'with epithelioid or glandular areas' (Clement & Scully, 1988) |
| | Hyaline sometimes abundant with a tendency to be glassy | | | |
| Cytological features<br>Nucleus | Blunt, fusiform, uniform, bland | Elongate, cigar-shaped | Round, crumpled | Small, round and regular nuclei<br>• Minimal nuclear pleomorphism<br>• Only rare mitotic figures |
| Cytoplasm | Scanty (on H & E and trichrome) | Moderate amount (on H & E and trichrome), typically fibrillar | Cytoplasm may be clear around the nucleus, clear at the periphery of the cell, or entirely clear<br>Glycogen (+), in slightly over half of cases<br>PAS with diastase (−)<br>Lipid (−) except for slight positivity in some | Scanty cytoplasm<br>or<br>may have abundant eosinophilic or foamy (lipid-rich) cytoplasm |
| Ultra-structure | Endometrial stromal cells are undifferentiated mesenchymal cells | | Clear cell pattern<br>• Multiple cytolysosomes composed of vesicular membranous material<br>• Intracytoplasmic glycogen<br>• Smooth muscle myofilaments with dense bodies<br>• Mazur suspects this EM profile is a reflection of sublethal cell injury | • No resemblance to either granulosa cell tumors or Sertoli-Leydig cell tumors<br>• Smooth muscle features<br>• Epithelial features |

*(continued)*

**TABLE 5.** *Continued.*

| Technique | Endometrial stromal cell | Usual smooth muscle cell | Epithelioid smooth muscle cells | Endometrial stroma with epithelioid and/or glandular areas |
|---|---|---|---|---|
| Ultra-structure (*cont.*) | | | | |
| | No myofilaments or dense bodies in the typical case (the more ambiguous the lightmicroscopic appearance, the greater the tendency to acquire smooth muscle features)<br>Intercellular collagen | Abundant, 6.0–8.0 nm, longitudinally arranged myofilaments parallel to long axis of cell; some filaments at oblique angles to these<br>Marginal spindle-shaped to oval dense bodies adjacent to plasmalemma (plaques) or along the trajectory of the filaments | *Plexiform pattern*<br>Smooth muscle features | |
| | No micropinocytotic vesicles in the usual case<br>Complex cytoplasmic processes<br>No basal lamina | Micropinocytotic vesicles adjacent to plasma membrane<br>Occasional cilia<br>Interrupted basal lamina around individual cells (these features are variably present in tumors) | | |
| Ultra-structural references: | Komorowski et al, 1970; Akhtar et al, 1975; Fekete & Vellios, 1984 | Ferenczy et al, 1971; Morales et al, 1975; Mazur & Askin, 1978; Fujii et al, 1989; Fujii et al, 1990 | Goodhue et al, 1974; Nunez-Alonso & Battifora, 1979; Kaminski & Tavassoli, 1984; Mazur & Priest, 1986 | Tang et al, 1979; Fekete et al, 1985; Kantelip et al, 1986; McCluggage et al, 1993 |
| Immunohisto-chemistry | Normal endometrial stromal cells are reported to express vimentin, desmin and muscle actin; they are negative for cytokeratin and EMA; endometrial stromal sarcoma cells are reported to express desmin, vimentin, muscle actin, and less commonly cytokeratin; EMA has been negative with rare exceptions | Essentially the same immunohistochemical profile as normal endometrial stromal cells except normal smooth muscle cells may express cytokeratin; AE1 is positive in 20%, desmin in 90%, and CD34 in 30%, EMA positive in close to 50% of cases | AE1 is positive in 40% of cases, desmin is positive in 80%, and CD34 in 10% | Epithelioid areas<br>• Muscle specific actin (HHF-35) positive<br>• Vimentin positive<br>• Cytokeratin positive |
| Immunohisto-chemistry references: | Abrams et al, 1989; Dabbs et al, 1989; Binder et al, 1991; Devaney & Tavassoli, 1991; Farhood & Abrams, 1991; Franquemont et al, 1991 | Brown et al, 1987; Norton et al, 1987; Azumi et al, 1988; Gown et al, 1988; Miettinen, 1988; Ramaekers et al, 1988; Dabbs et al, 1989; Devaney & Tavassoli, 1991 | Devaney & Tavassoli 1991; Rizeq et al, 1993 | Balaton et al, 1986; Sullinger & Scully, 1989; Lillemoe et al, 1991; McCluggage et al, 1993 |

bers of cytoplasmic contractile elements. The biochemistry and electrophysiology of the myometrium have been extensively reviewed (290,294,295). The histologic and ultrastructural appearance of smooth muscle cells differ substantially from those of the endometrial stromal cell. These differences are set out in Table 5. However, it should be noted that cells with a hybrid smooth muscle–stromal phenotype occur normally at the endometrial–myometrial junction and that this phenotypic ambiguity is sometimes expressed by spindle cell neoplasms of the uterine corpus (296). Some uterine smooth muscle cells have been shown to express some classes of keratins (297–300).

**Pregnancy-related Changes**

To accommodate the growing fetus and to prepare for its role in fetal expulsion, the uterus undergoes a 20-fold increase in size and weight during pregnancy both by hyper-

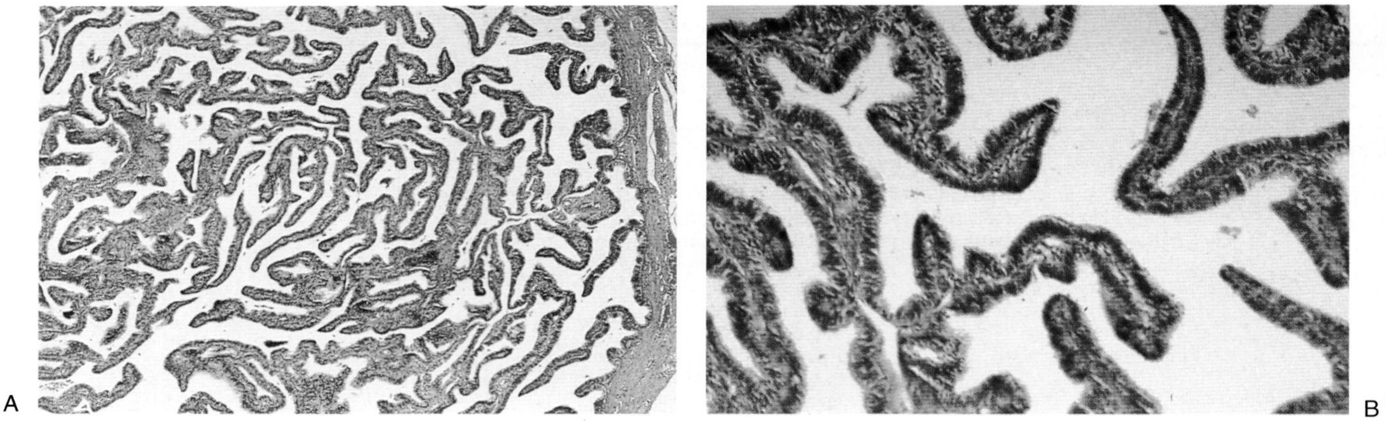

FIG. 46. **A, B:** Ampulla of the fallopian tube. Note the long slender plicae or folds resting on the muscularis.

trophy and to a much lesser extent by hyperplasia. Normal mitotic figures are often increased and may be present in large numbers. Uterine growth during pregnancy appears to be largely promoted by estradiol, whereas progesterone probably functions to inhibit uterine contractions during gestation. The light microscopic appearance of the hypertrophied uterine smooth muscle cells of pregnancy is distinctive. They are enlarged and have abundant, rather glassy cytoplasm and vesicular elongate nuclei with occasionally prominent nucleoli. Changes occur in the ultrastructural appearance of the smooth muscle cells as well. In addition to an increase in size and the number of myofilaments, there is a striking increase in the number of gap junctions (301,302). These establish the contact between cells required for the coordinated uterine contractions that expel the term infant (303). These myometrial changes are closely coordinated with the dramatic structural changes of cervical "ripening" required for cervical effacement (see section Uterine Cervix). In the postpartum period, the uterus undergoes an extraordinary 85% reduction in weight within 3 weeks of delivery (24). This weight loss is primarily due to a reduction in individual cell volume rather than a reduction in cell number. In addition, a large amount of collagen is degraded over this brief period. Complete return of the uterus to the nulliparous weight does not occur if gestation has proceeded beyond the second trimester.

## THE FALLOPIAN TUBE

### Histology of the Fallopian Tube

The fallopian tube is lined by a nonstratified epithelium that is separated from the endosalpingeal stroma by a basement membrane. Each of the tubal segments is lined by a mixture of three basic cell types: ciliated cells, secretory cells, and intercalated (peg) cells (Fig. 46). In recent years it has become apparent that the peg cell is, in reality, a stage in the cyclic variation during the menstrual cycle of the secretory cell (304). The relative number of these cells differs in each of the anatomic regions of the tube. In addition, many investigators believe that the numbers of the three types of cells within each of these anatomic regions undergo regular variations throughout the menstrual cycle (305–309). Ciliated cells are most prominent at the ovarian (distal) end of the tube—particularly in the fimbrial mucosa—and predominate during mid-cycle; their numbers diminish progressively to achieve a nadir at the time of menstruation (Fig. 47). In a gestational cycle the number of cilia continue to decrease. Ciliary movement rather than muscular contractions is chiefly responsible for the movement of the egg toward the site of fertilization: the ampulloisthmic junction.

Secretory cells are most prominent toward the uterine end of the tube and undergo cyclic changes in cell height and appearance, reflecting their elaboration, accumulation, and discharge of oviduct secretions as the menstrual cycle proceeds. Most often they have ovoid somewhat dense nuclei, and they may contain an apical vacuole (Fig. 48). The oviduct fluid secreted by these cells serves many important functions and has been the subject of a review (310).

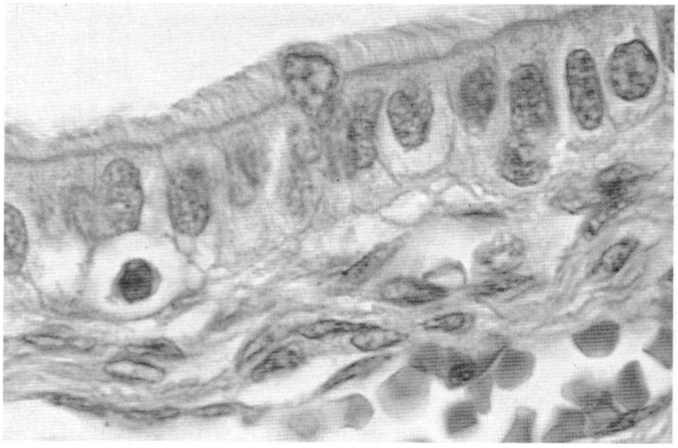

**FIG. 47.** This high-power photomicrograph of tubal epithelium shows numerous ciliated cells with a compressed secretory cell nucleus above the level of the ciliated cells. The cell with clear cytoplasm is probably a lymphocyte.

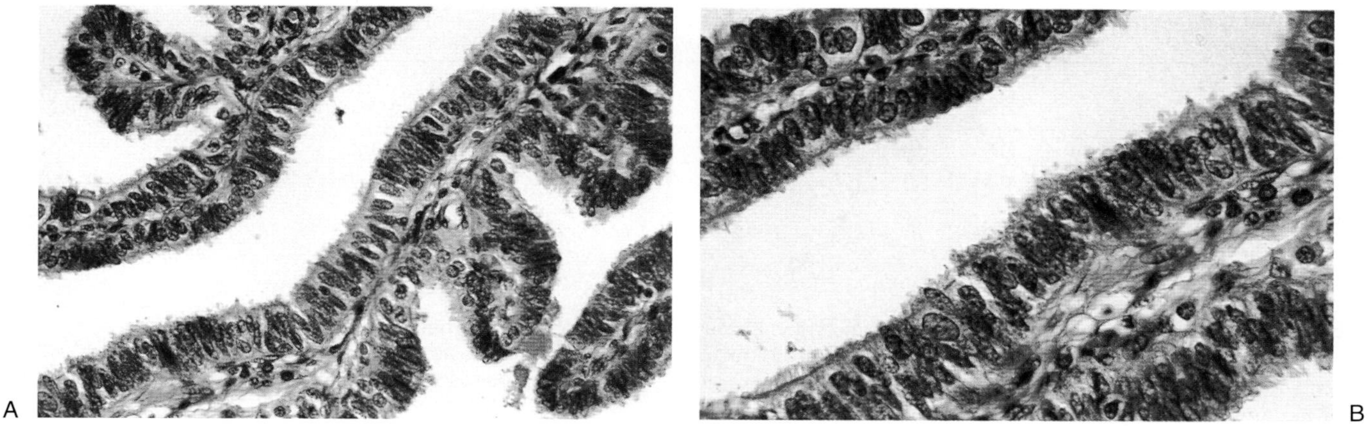

**FIG. 48. A, B:** In this area the tubal epithelial cells are crowded, a pattern that is common in the fallopian tube when ciliated cells are not numerous.

Intercalated cells have been thought to represent either effete secretory cells or some type of reserve cells. They have a thin dense nucleus and little cytoplasm. Endocrine cells have been noted in the fallopian tube; their function is as mysterious here as it is in the uterus (311). The "basal cells" reported in the early literature have been shown to be lymphocytes, which may represent a tubal component of a mucosa-associated lymphoid system (27,312–315). Scattered lymphocytes and occasional lymphoid follicles should be considered to be within normal limits and constitute part of the mucosa-associated lymphoid system (316).

Ciliogenesis is promoted by estradiol and deciliation by progesterone. Prolonged exposure to progestogens (whether endogenously as in pregnancy or exogenously) or withdrawal of estrogen (as in the postmenopausal years) leads to epithelial atrophy. Postmenopausal estrogen administration leads to regrowth of cilia.

Mitotic figures are rarely seen in the fallopian tube epithelium, so no cyclic regeneration occurs as in the endometrium. Both the transmission and scanning electron microscopic appearance of the normal tubal mucosa have been extensively documented over the past two decades. Of interest to the diagnostic pathologist are the abnormalities of ciliogenesis found in patients with Kartagener's syndrome (317).

### *Myosalpinx*

The myosalpinx is composed of an inner circular layer and an outer longitudinal layer. The isthmus near the uterotubal junction also possesses an inner longitudinal layer.

### Physiology

The details of the physiology of the tube are beyond the scope of this chapter; interested readers are referred to recent reviews (307,318). Unresolved mysteries include how the sperm moved so rapidly from the vagina to the ampulla (in some cases within 5 minutes) and how the tube manages to orchestrate fertilization so that spermatozoa moving toward the ovary and an egg moving away from the ovary meet in the right part of the fallopian tube.

### Fallopian Tube in Pregnancy

The fallopian tube has already played its part when the fertilized ovum implants in the endometrium. It is now inactive throughout the gestational period. A muted version of endometrial decidual change often occurs in the endosalpingeal stroma during the latter part of pregnancy, while the epithelium of the fallopian tube undergoes atrophy (Fig. 49). The fallopian tube is the most common site of ectopic gestation. A review of physiologic factors in its development has been presented (319). Morphologic changes in the fallopian tube can be produced by birth control pills and of course tubal ligation (320–322).

Normal findings in the fallopian tubes that have relevance to histopathologic diagnosis can be found in Table 6.

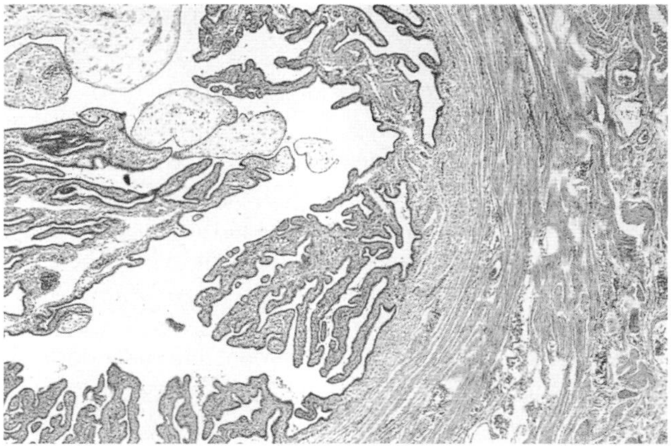

**FIG. 49. A, B:** Fallopian tube containing decidual cells. The stromal cells of the plicae frequently undergo decidual change during pregnancy.

**TABLE 6.** *Normal findings in the fallopian tube and uterine serosa that have relevance to histopathologic differential diagnosis (see text for additional differential diagnostic clues)*

| Finding | Diagnostic confusion | Suggestions for resolution | References when relevant |
|---|---|---|---|
| Decidual reaction (usually encountered in post-partum tubal ligation specimens but may also be seen in the tubes of patients on progestational agents) | Do not misinterpret as carcinoma | Nuclei are bland in decidua. | (337, 338) |
| Endosalpingiosis | Distinguish from endometriosis and ovarian tumor of low malignant potential (borderline tumors) | Look for endometrial stroma to confirm diagnosis of endometriosis; look for complex papillae with micropapillae to confirm diagnosis of serous LMP implant. | |
| Crowded cells and dense nuclei | Carcinoma in situ | Carcinoma in situ features prominent nucleoli and abnormal mitotic figures. Nuclear atypia and glandular complexity can be significant in chronic salpingitis. | |
| Mucinous and eosinophilic metaplasia (may be associated with Peutz-Jeghers' syndrome) | Carcinoma | Metaplasia lacks the architectural complexity, the nuclear atypia and the mitotic activity of carcinoma. | (339, 340) |
| Squamous metaplasia | Carcinoma | Metaplasia lacks the architectural complexity, the nuclear atypia and the mitotic activity of carcinoma. | |
| Walthard cell rests | | | |

### Paraovarian and Paratubal Structures

The broad ligament and environs are populated by a variety of tubular and cystic structures with the propensity to form clinically or surgically noticeable cysts (37,39). These are indicated in Fig. 50. Many are lined by müllerian-type epithelium. Walthard rests are universal findings over the serosal surface of the fallopian tubes. They are lined by transitional-type epithelium. A more or less constant finding in sections that include the peritubal soft tissue are the tortuous remnants of the mesonephric ducts. These are lined by cuboidal epithelium and possess a fibromyovascular cuff.

## APPENDIX: GENERAL REFERENCES

A chronicle of the changing concepts of the uterus through the ages is provided by Ramsey (323), and a fascinating discussion of the role of preconceptions in filtering the "facts" of uterine anatomy is provided by Laqueur (324). There has been recent interesting speculation on the evolutionary purposes of menstruation (325,326).

Several extensive treatises on reproductive endocrinology have been published or revised in recent years:

Adashi EY, Rock JA, Rosenwaks Z. *Reproductive endocrinology, surgery, and technology.* Philadelphia: Lippincott-Raven; 1996.
Ferin M, Jewelewicz R, Warren M. *The menstrual cycle.* New York: Oxford University Press; 1993.
Speroff L, Glass RH, Kase NG. *Clinical gynecologic endocrinology and infertility.* 5th ed. Baltimore: Williams & Wilkins; 1994.
Yen SSC, Jaffe RB. *Reproductive endocrinology: physiology, pathophysiology and clinical management.* 3rd ed. Philadelphia: WB Saunders; 1991.

Two monographs devoted exclusively to the biology of the uterus are listed as follows:

Chard T, Grudzinskas JG. *The uterus.* New York: Cambridge; 1994.
Wynn RM, Jollie WP. *Biology of the uterus.* 2nd ed. New York: Plenum; 1989.

More general treatments of the territory surveyed in this chapter with more emphasis on basic science issues and less emphasis on practical surgical pathology diagnostics are listed as follows.

### Uterine Cervix

Ferenczy A, Wright TC. Anatomy and histology of the cervix. In: Kurman RJ, ed. *Blaustein's pathology of the female genital tract.* 4th ed. New York: Springer-Verlag; 1994:185–201.
Singer A. Anatomy of the cervix and physiological changes in cervical epithelium. In: Fox H, Wells M, eds. *Haines and Taylor obstetrical and gynaecological pathology.* 4th ed. Vol. 1. New York: Churchill Livingstone; 1995:225–248..

### Uterine Endometrium and Myometrium

More I. The normal human endometrium. In: Fox H, Wells M, eds. *Haines and Taylor obstetrical and gynaecological pathology.* 4th ed. Vol. 1. New York: Churchill Livingstone; 1995:365–382.

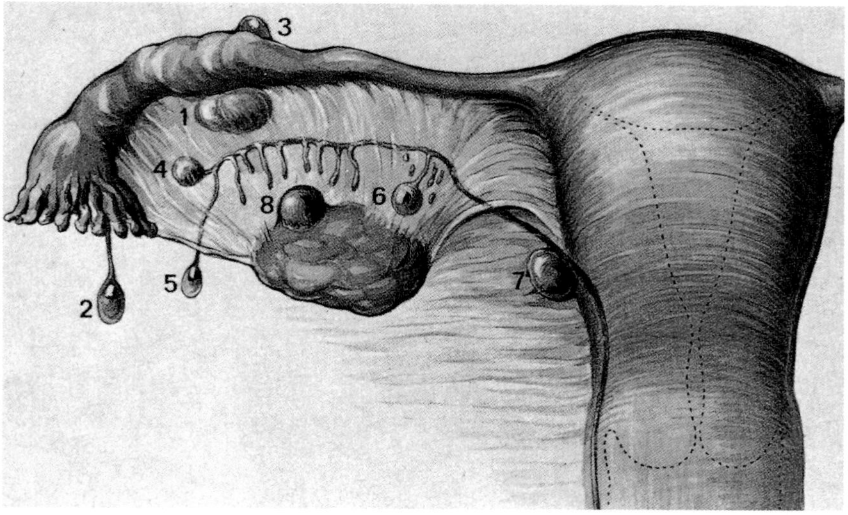


**FIG. 50.** Topography of various cysts encountered in the female internal genitalia. 1, Parovarian cyst of paramesonephric origin (type I); 2, hydatid cyst of Morgagni (paramesonephric origin); 3, subserosal müllerian cyst (paramesonephric origin); 4, parovarian cyst of mesonephric origin (type II); 5, Kobelt's cyst (appendix vesiculosa); 6, cyst of the paroophoron; 7, duct cyst; 8, cyst of the rete ovarii. Reprinted with permission (351).

Ferenczy A. Anatomy and histology of the uterine corpus. In: Kurman RJ, ed. *Blaustein's pathology of the female genital tract.* 4th ed. New York: Springer-Verlag; 1994:327–366.

Warren M, Li T, Klentzeris L. Cell biology of the endometrium: histology, cell types and menstrual changes. In: Chard T, Grudzinskas J, eds. *The uterus.* New York: Cambridge; 1994:94–124.

Giudice LC, Ferenczy A. The endometrial cycle. In: Adashi EY, Rock JA, Rosenwaks Z, eds. *Reproductive endocrinology, surgery, and technology.* 1st ed. Vol. 1. Philadelphia: Lippincott-Raven; 1996:272–300.

Ferenczy A, Bergeron C. Histology of the human endometrium: from birth to senescence. In: Bulletti C, Gurpide E, eds. *The primate endometrium, annals of the New York Academy of Sciences.* New York: New York Academy of Sciences; 1991: 6–27.

Ferenczy A, Guralnick M. Endometrial microstructure: structure–function relationships throughout the menstrual cycle. *Semin Reprod Endocrinol* 1983;1:205.

## Normal Gestational Findings

Silverberg SG, Kurman RJ. Tumors of the uterine corpus and gestational trophoblastic disease. In: Rosai J, ed. *Atlas of tumor pathology.* Vol. 3. Washington, DC: AFIP; 1992.

## Fallopian Tube

Honore L. Pathology of the fallopian tube and broad ligament. In: Fox H, Wells M, eds. *Haines and Taylor obstetrical and gynaecological pathology.* 4th ed. Vol. 1. New York: Churchill Livingstone; 1995:623–671.

Brenner RM, Slayden OD. The fallopian tube cycle. In: Adashi EY, Rock JA, Rosenwaks Z, eds. *Reproductive endocrinology, surgery, and technology.* Vol. 1. Philadelphia: Lippincott-Raven; 1996:326–339.

## REFERENCES

1. Lauchlan SC. Metaplasias and neoplasias of müllerian epithelium. *Histopathology* 1984;8:543–557.
2. Cunha GR, Lung B. The importance of stroma in morphogenesis and functional activity of urogenital epithelium. *In Vitro* 1979;15:50–71.
3. Gray SW, Skandalakis JE. *Embryology for surgeons: the embryological basis for the treatment of congenital defects.* Philadelphia: WB Saunders; 1972:633–664.
4. McLean JM. Embryology and anatomy of the female genital tract. In: Fox H, Wells M, eds. *Haines and Taylor obstetrical and gynaecological pathology.* 4th ed. Vol. 1. New York: Churchill Livingstone; 1995:1–40.
5. Moore KL. *The developing human. Clinically oriented embryology.* 3rd ed. Philadelphia: WB Saunders; 1982:207–221.
6. O'Rahilly R. Prenatal human development. In: Wynn RM, Jollie WP, eds. *Biology of the uterus.* 2nd ed. New York: Plenum; 1989:35–56.
7. Gondos B. Development of the reproductive organs. *Ann Clin Lab Sci* 1985;15:363–373.
8. Ramsey EM. Development of the human uterus and relevance to the adult condition. In: Chard T, Grudzinskas J, ed. *The uterus.* New York: Cambridge; 1994:41–53.
9. Patton GW, Kistner RW. *Atlas of infertility surgery.* 2nd ed. Boston: Little, Brown; 1984
10. Forsberg JG. Cervicovaginal epithelium: its origin and development. *Am J Obstet Gynecol* 1973;115:1025–1043.
11. Nussbaum AR, Sanders RC, Jones MD. Neonatal uterine morphology as seen on real-time US. *Radiology* 1986;160:641–643.
12. Pixley E. Basic morphology of the prepuberal and youthful cervix: topographic and histologic features. *J Reprod Med* 1976;16:221–230.
13. Pryse-Davies J. The development, structure and function of the female pelvic organs in childhood. *Clin Obstet Gynecol* 1974;1:483–508.
14. Singer A. Anatomy of the cervix and physiological changes in cervical epithelium. In: Fox H, Wells M, ed. *Haines and Taylor obstetrical and gynaecological pathology.* 4th ed. Vol. 1. New York: Churchill Livingstone; 1995:225–248.
15. Haber HP, Mayer EI. Ultrasound evaluation of uterine and ovarian size from birth to puberty [see comments]. *Pediatr Radiol* 1994;24:11–13.
16. Blandau RJ. Comparative aspects of tubal anatomy and physiology as they relate to reconstructive procedures. *J Reprod Med* 1978;21:7–15.
17. Eddy CA, Pauerstein CJ. Anatomy and physiology of the fallopian tube. *Clin Obstet Gynecol* 1980;23:1177–1193.
18. Singer A. The uterine cervix from adolescence to the menopause. *Br J Obstet Gynaecol* 1975;82:81–99.
19. Warwick R, Williams PL. *Gray's anatomy.* 35th ed. Philadelphia: WB Saunders; 1973:1356–1359.
20. Langlois PL. The size of the normal uterus. *J Reprod Med* 1970; 4:220–228.
21. Calder AA. The cervix during pregnancy. In: Chard T, Grudzinskas J, ed. *The uterus.* New York: Cambridge; 1994:288–307.
22. Kurz KH, Tadesse E, Haspels AA. In vivo measurements of uterine cavities in 795 women of fertile age. *Contraception* 1984;29:495–510.
23. Zemlyn S. The length of the uterine cervix and its significance. *JCU* 1981;9:267–269.
24. Finn CA, Porter DG. *The uterus. Reproductive biology handbooks.* Vol. 1. Acton, MA: Publishing Sciences Group; 1975.
25. Tóth S, Toth A. Undescribed muscle bundle of the human uterus: fasciculus cervicoangularis. *Am J Obstet Gynecol* 1974;118:979–984.
26. Toth A. Studies on the muscular structure of the human uterus. II. Fasciculi cervicoangulares: vestigial or functional remnant of the mesonephric duct? *Obstet Gynecol* 1977;49:190–196.

27. Hricak H. MRI of the female pelvis: a review. *AJR* 1986;146: 1115–1122.
28. Cullinan JA, Fleischer AC, Kepple DM, Arnold AL. Sonohysterography: a technique for endometrial evaluation. *Radiographics* 1995;15: 501–514.
29. de Souza NM, Hawley IC, Schwieso JE, Gilderdale DJ, Soutter WP. The uterine cervix on in vitro and in vivo MR images: a study of zonal anatomy and vascularity using an enveloping cervical coil. *AJR* 1994; 163:607–612.
30. de Ziegler D, Bouchard P. Understanding endometrial physiology and menstrual disorders in the 1990s. *Curr Opin Obstet Gynecol* 1993; 5:378–388.
31. Scoutt LM, Flynn SD, Luthringer DJ, McCauley TR, McCarthy SM. Junctional zone of the uterus: correlation of MR imaging and histologic examination of hysterectomy specimens. *Radiology* 1991;179: 403–407.
32. Scoutt LM, McCauley TR, Flynn SD, Luthringer DJ, McCarthy SM. Zonal anatomy of the cervix: correlation of MR imaging and histologic examination of hysterectomy specimens. *Radiology* 1993;186: 159–162.
33. Mogavero G, Sheth S, Hamper UM. Endovaginal sonography of the nongravid uterus. *Radiographics* 1993;13:969–981.
34. Hricak H. Current trends in MR imaging of the female pelvis. *Radiographics* 1993;13:913–919.
35. Merchant RN, Prabhu SR, Chougale A. Uterotubal junction—morphology and clinical aspects. *Int J Fertil* 1983;28:199–205.
36. Ramsey EM. Vascular anatomy. In: Wynn RM, Jollie WP, ed. *Biology of the uterus.* 2nd ed. New York: Plenum; 1989:58–68.
37. Wydrzynski M. Anatomical principles of microsurgery of the tubal arteries. *Anat Clin* 1985;7:233–236.
38. Greiss FC Jr, Rose JC. Vascular physiology of the nonpregnant uterus. In: Wynn R, Jollie W, eds. *Biology of the uterus.* 2nd ed. New York: Plenum; 1989:69–88.
39. Blackwell PM, Fraser IS. Superficial lymphatics in the functional zone of normal human endometrium. *Microvasc Res* 1981;21: 142–152.
40. DiSaia PJ, Creasman WT. *Clinical gynecologic oncology.* 4th ed. St. Louis: Mosby Year Book; 1993
41. Morrow CP, Curtin JP, Townsend DE. *Synopsis of gynecologic oncology.* 4th ed. New York: Churchill Livingstone; 1993
42. Plentl AA, Friedman EA. *Lymphatic system of the female genitalia. The morphologic basis of oncologic diagnosis and therapy.* Philadelphia: WB Saunders; 1971
43. Conrad JT, Ueland K. Physical characteristics of the cervix. *Clin Obstet Gynecol* 1983;26:27–36.
44. Danforth DN. The morphology of the human cervix. *Clin Obstet Gynecol* 1983;26:7–13.
45. Feldman D, Romney SL, Edgcomb J, Valentine T. Ultrastructure of normal, metaplastic, and abnormal human uterine cervix: use of montages to study the topographical relationship of epithelial cells. *Am J Obstet Gynecol* 1984;150:573–688.
46. Ferenczy A, Wright TC. Anatomy and histology of the cervix. In: Kurman RJ, ed. *Blaustein's pathology of the female genital tract.* 4th ed. New York: Springer-Verlag; 1994:185–201.
47. Krantz KE. The anatomy of the human cervix, gross and microscopic. In: Blandau R, Moghissi K, eds. *The biology of the cervix.* Chicago: University of Chicago Press; 1973:57–59.
48. Graham CE. Functional microanatomy of the primate uterine cervix. In: Greep R, Astwood E, eds. *Handbook of physiology. Female reproductive system.* Baltimore: Williams & Wilkins; 1973:1–24.
49. Friedrich ER. The normal morphology and ultrastructure of the cervix. In: Blandau R, Moghissi K, eds. *The biology of the cervix.* Chicago: University of Chicago Press; 1973:79–102.
50. Hafez ES. Structural and ultrastructural parameters of the uterine cervix. *Obstet Gynecol Surv* 1982;37:507–516.
51. Shearman RP. Clinical Reproductive Endocrinology. In: Shearman R, ed. *Clinical reproductive endocrinology.* New York: Churchill Livingstone; 1985.
52. Aspden RM. The importance of a slit-like lumen cross-section for the mechanical function of the cervix. *Br J Obstet Gynaecol* 1987;94: 915–916.
53. Gorodeski GI. The cervical cycle. In: Adashi EY, Rock JA, Rosenwaks Z, ed. *Reproductive endocrinology, surgery, and technology.* 1st ed. Vol. I. Philadelphia: Lippincott-Raven; 1996:302–324.
54. Ferenczy A, Richart RM. *Female reproductive system: dynamics of scan and transmission electron microscopy.* New York: Wiley; 1974.
55. Chretien FC, Gernigon C, David G, Psychoyos A. The ultrastructure of human cervical mucus under scanning electron microscopy. *Fertil Steril* 1973;24:746–757.
56. Gould PR, Barter RA, Papadimitriou JM. An ultrastructural, cytochemical, and autoradiographic study of the mucous membrane of the human cervical canal with reference to subcolumnar basal cells. *Am J Pathol* 1979;95:1–16.
57. Sekiba K, Okuda H, Fukui H, Ishii Y, Kawaoka K, Fujimori T. A scanning electron microscope study of the fine angioarchitecture of the uterine cervix using a newly established cast formation technique. *Obstet Gynecol Surv* 1979;34:823–826.
58. Madile BM. The cervical epithelium from fetal age to adolescence. *Obstet Gynecol* 1976;47:536–539.
59. Konishi I, Fujii S, Nonogaki H, Nanbu Y, Iwai T, Mori T. Immunohistochemical analysis of estrogen receptors, progesterone receptors, Ki-67 antigen, and human papillomavirus DNA in normal and neoplastic epithelium of the uterine cervix. *Cancer* 1991;68:1340–1350.
60. Albores-Saavedra J, Rodriguez-Martinez HA, Larraza-Hernandez O. Carcinoid tumors of the cervix. *Pathol Annu* 1979;14:273–291.
61. Fetissof F, Berger G, Dubois MP, et al. Endocrine cells in the female genital tract. *Histopathology* 1985;9:133–145.
62. Fetissof F, Dubois MP, Heitz PU, Lansac J, Arbeille Brassart B, Jobard P. Endocrine cells in the female genital tract. *Int J Gynecol Pathol* 1986;5:75–87.
63. Fetissof F, Arbeille B, Boivin F, Sam Giao M, Henrion C, Lansac J. Endocrine cells in ectocervical epithelium. An immunohistochemical and ultrastructural analysis. *Virchows Arch [A]* 1987;411:293–298.
64. Fetissof F, Serres G, Arbeille B, de Muret A, Sam Giao M, Lansac J. Argyrophilic cells and ectocervical epithelium. *Int J Gynecol Pathol* 1991;10:177–190.
65. Fetissof F, Heitzman A, Machet MC, Lansac J. Unusual endocervical lesions with endocrine cells. *Pathol Res Pract* 1993;189:928–939.
66. Scully RE, Aguirre P, DeLellis RA. Argyrophilia, serotonin, and peptide hormones in the female genital tract and its tumors. *Int J Gynecol Pathol* 1984;3:51–70.
67. Figueroa CD, Caorsi I. Ultrastructural and morphometric study of the Langerhans cell in the normal human exocervix. *J Anat* 1980;131:669–682.
68. Morris HH, Gatter KC, Stein H, Mason DY. Langerhans' cells in human cervical epithelium: an immunohistological study. *Br J Obstet Gynaecol* 1983;90:400–411.
69. Morelli AE, di Paola G, Fainboim L. Density and distribution of Langerhans cells in the human uterine cervix. *Arch Gynecol Obstet* 1992;252:65–71.
70. Hussain LA, Kelly CG, Fellowes R, et al. Expression and gene transcript of Fc receptors for IgG, HLA class II antigens and Langerhans cells in human cervico-vaginal epithelium. *Clin Exp Immunol* 1992; 90:530–538.
71. Miller CJ, McChesney M, Moore PF. Langerhans cells, macrophages and lymphocyte subsets in the cervix and vagina of rhesus macaques. *Lab Invest* 1992;67:628–634.
72. Osamura RY, Watanabe K, Oh M. Melanin-containing cells in the uterine cervix: histochemical and electron-microscopic studies of two cases. *Am J Clin Pathol* 1980;74:239–242.
73. Laguens RP, Lagrutta J, Koch OR, Quijano F. Fine structure of human endocervical epithelium. *Am J Obstet Gynecol* 1967;98:773–780.
74. Hiersche HD, Nagl W. Regeneration of secretory epithelium in the human endocervix. *Arch Gynecol* 1980;229:83–90.
75. Suh KS, Silverberg SG. Tubal metaplasia of the uterine cervix. *Int J Gynecol Pathol* 1990;9:122–128.
76. Novotny DB, Maygarden SJ, Johnson DE, Frable WJ. Tubal metaplasia. A frequent potential pitfall in the cytologic diagnosis of endocervical glandular dysplasia on cervical smears. *Acta Cytol* 1992;36: 1–10.
77. Pacey F, Ayer B, Greenberg M. The cytologic diagnosis of adenocarcinoma in situ of the cervix uteri and related lesions. III. Pitfalls in diagnosis. *Acta Cytol* 1988;32:325–330.
78. Jonasson JG, Wang HH, Antonioli DA, Ducatman BS. Tubal metaplasia of the uterine cervix: a prevalence study in patients with gynecologic pathologic findings. *Int J Gynecol Pathol* 1992;11:89–95.
79. Ismail SM. Cone biopsy causes cervical endometriosis and tubo-endometrioid metaplasia. *Histopathology* 1991;18:107–114.

80. Odor DL. The question of "basal" cells in oviductal and endocervical epithelium. *Fertil Steril* 1974;25:1047–1062.
81. Peters WM. Nature of "basal" and "reserve" cells in oviductal and cervical epithelium in man. *J Clin Pathol* 1986;39:306–312.
82. Fluhmann CF. The nature of development of the so-called glands of the cervix. *Am J Obstet Gynecol* 1957;74:753–768.
83. Fluhmann CF. *The cervix uteri and its diseases.* Philadelphia: WB Saunders; 1961
84. Anderson MC, Hartley RB. Cervical crypt involvement by intraepithelial neoplasia. *Obstet Gynecol* 1980;55:546–550.
85. Teshima S, Shimosato Y, Kishi K, Kasamatsu T, Ohmi K, Uei Y. Early stage adenocarcinoma of the uterine cervix. Histopathologic analysis with consideration of histogenesis. *Cancer* 1985;56:167–172.
86. Young RH, Clement PB. Pseudoneoplastic glandular lesions of the uterine cervix. *Semin Diagn Pathol* 1991;8:234–249.
87. Clement PB, Young RH. Deep nabothian cysts of the uterine cervix. A possible source of confusion with minimal-deviation adenocarcinoma (adenoma malignum). *Int J Gynecol Pathol* 1989;8:340–348.
88. Bertrand M, Lickrish GM, Colgan TJ. The anatomic distribution of cervical adenocarcinoma in situ: implications for treatment. *Am J Obstet Gynecol* 1987;157:21–25.
89. Gilks CB, Reid PE, Clement PB, Owen DA. Histochemical changes in cervical mucus-secreting epithelium during the normal menstrual cycle. *Fertil Steril* 1989;51:286–291.
90. McDonnell JM, Emens JM, Jordan JA. The congenital cervicovaginal transformation zone in sexually active young women. *Br J Obstet Gynaecol* 1984;91:580–584.
91. Crum CP, Egawa K, Fu YS, et al. Atypical immature metaplasia (AIM). A subset of human papilloma virus infection of the cervix. *Cancer* 1983;51:2214–2219.
92. Richart RM. Cervical intraepithelial neoplasia. In: Sommers S, ed. *Pathology annual.* New York: Appleton-Century Crofts; 1973: 301–328.
93. Aspden R. M. Collagen organisation in the cervix and its relation to mechanical function. *Coll Rel Res* 1988;8:103–112.
94. Kiwi R, Neuman MR, Merkatz IR, Selim MA, Lysikiewicz A. Determination of the elastic properties of the cervix. *Obstet Gynecol* 1988; 71:568–574.
95. Leppert PC, Cerreta JM, Mandl I. Orientation of elastic fibers in the human cervix. *Am J Obstet Gynecol* 1986;155:219–224.
96. Leppert PC, Yu SY. Three-dimensional structures of uterine elastic fibers: scanning electron microscopic studies. *Connect Tissue Res* 1991;27:15–31.
97. Bienenstock J, Befus AD. Mucosal immunology. *Immunology* 1980; 41:249–270.
98. Edwards JN, Morris HB. Langerhans' cells and lymphocyte subsets in the female genital tract. *Br J Obstet Gynaecol* 1985;92:974–982.
99. Ernst PB. Immunity in mucosal tissues. In: Stites D, Stobo J, Wells J, eds. *Basic and clinical immunology.* Norwalk, CT: Appleton & Lange; 1987:159–166.
100. Green FH, Rebello R, Fox H. Proceedings: a study of the secretory immune system of the female genital-tract. *J Med Microbiol* 1975; 8:xviii.
101. Rebello R, Green FH, Fox H. A study of the secretory immune system of the female genital tract. *Br J Obstet Gynaecol* 1975;82:812–816.
102. Roncalli M, Sideri M, Gie P, Servida E. Immunophenotypic analysis of the transformation zone of human cervix. *Lab Invest* 1988;58: 141–149.
103. Hughes RG, Norval M, Howie SE. Expression of major histocompatibility class II antigens by Langerhans' cells in cervical intraepithelial neoplasia. *J Clin Pathol* 1988;41:253–259.
104. Ferry JA, Scully RE. Mesonephric remnants, hyperplasia, and neoplasia in the uterine cervix. A study of 49 cases. *Am J Surg Pathol* 1990; 14:1100–1111.
105. Norris HJ, Taylor HB. Polyps of the vagina. A benign lesion resembling sarcoma botryoides. *Cancer* 1966;19:227–232.
106. Clement PB. Multinucleated stromal giant cells of the uterine cervix. *Arch Pathol Lab Med* 1985;109:200–202.
107. Metze K, Andrade LA. Atypical stromal giant cells of cervix uteri—evidence of Schwann cell origin [see comments]. *Pathol Res Pract* 1991;187:1031–1035.
108. Abdul Karim FW, Cohen RE. Atypical stromal cells of lower female genital tract. *Histopathology* 1990;17:249–253.
109. Elliott GB, Elliott JD. Superficial stromal reactions of lower genital tract. *Arch Pathol* 1973;95:100–101.
110. Ledger WL, Anderson AB. The influence of steroid hormones on the uterine cervix during pregnancy. *J Steroid Biochem* 1987;27: 1029–1034.
111. Cove H. The Arias-Stella reaction occurring in the endocervix in pregnancy: recognition and comparison with an adenocarcinoma of the endocervix. *Am J Surg Pathol* 1979;3:567–568.
112. Schneider V. Arias-Stella reaction of the endocervix: frequency and location. *Acta Cytol* 1981;25:224–228.
113. Bouyer J, Papiernik E, Dreyfus J, Collin D, Winisdoerffer B, Gueguen S. Maturation signs of the cervix and prediction of preterm birth. *Obstet Gynecol* 1986;68:209–214.
114. Ekman G, Malmstrom A, Uldbjerg N, Ulmsten U. Cervical collagen: an important regulator of cervical function in term labor. *Obstet Gynecol* 1986;67:633–636.
115. Fuchs U, Seeger H, Voelter W, Lippert TH. Immunoreactive relaxin in human cervico-vaginal secretion. *Arch Gynecol Obstet* 1988;243: 37–39.
116. Minamoto T, Arai K, Hirakawa S, Nagai Y. Immunohistochemical studies on collagen types in the uterine cervix in pregnant and non-pregnant states. *Am J Obstet Gynecol* 1987;156:138–144.
117. Uldbjerg N, Ulmsten U, Ekman G. The ripening of the human uterine cervix in terms of connective tissue biochemistry. *Clin Obstet Gynecol* 1983;26:14–26.
118. Huszar G. Biology and biochemistry of myometrial contractility and cervical maturation. *Semin Perinatol* 1981;5:216–235.
119. Huszar G, Naftolin F. The myometrium and uterine cervix in normal and preterm labor. *N Engl J Med* 1984;311:571–581.
120. Osmers R, Rath W, Adelmann Grill BC, et al. Origin of cervical collagenase during parturition. *Am J Obstet Gynecol* 1992;166: 1455–1460.
121. Granstrom LM, Ekman GE, Malmstrom A, Ulmsten U, Woessner JF Jr. Serum collagenase levels in relation to the state of the human cervix during pregnancy and labor. *Am J Obstet Gynecol* 1992;167: 1284–1288.
122. Ferenczy A. Anatomy and histology of the uterine corpus. In: Kurman RJ, ed. *Blaustein's pathology of the female genital tract.* 4th ed. New York: Springer-Verlag; 1994:327–366.
123. More IAR. The normal human endometrium. In: Fox H, Wells M, eds. *Haines and Taylor obstetrical and gynaecological pathology.* 4th ed. vol. 1. New York: Churchill Livingstone; 1995:365–382.
124. Warren MA, Li TC, Klentzeris LD. Cell biology of the endometrium: histology, cell types and menstrual changes. In: Chard T, Grudzinskas J, eds. *The uterus.* New York: Cambridge; 1994: 94–124.
125. Wynn RM. The human endometrium: cyclic and gestational changes. In: Wynn R, Jollie W, eds. *Biology of the uterus.* 2nd ed. New York: Plenum; 1989:289–332.
126. Giudice LC, Ferenczy A. The endometrial cycle. In: Adashi EY, Rock JA, Rosenwaks Z, eds. *Reproductive endocrinology, surgery, and technology.* 1st ed. Vol. I. Philadelphia: Lippincott-Raven; 1996:272–300.
127. Ferenczy A, Bergeron C. Histology of the human endometrium: from birth to senescence. In: Bulletti C, Gurpide E, eds. *The primate endometrium, annals of the New York Academy of Sciences.* New York: New York Academy of Sciences; 1991:6–27.
128. Ferenczy A, Guralnick M. Endometrial microstructure: structure-function relationships throughout the menstrual cycle. *Semin Reprod Endocrinol* 1983;1:205.
129. Hill GA, Herbert CM 3d, Parker RA, Wentz AC. Comparison of late luteal phase endometrial biopsies using the Novak curette or PIPELLE endometrial suction curette. *Obstet Gynecol* 1989;73:443–445.
130. Arronet GH, Bergquist CA, Parekh MC, Latour JP, Marshall KG. Evaluation of endometrial biopsy in the cycle of conception. *Int J Fertil* 1973;18:220–225.
131. Buxton CL, Olson LE. Endometrial biopsy inadvertently taken during conception cycle. *Am J Obstet Gynecol* 1969;105:702–706.
132. Karow WG, Gentry WC, Skeels RF, Payne SA. Endometrial biopsy in the luteal phase of the cycle of conception. *Fertil Steril* 1971;22: 482–495.
133. Rosenfeld DL, Garcia CR. Endometrial biopsy in the cycle of conception. *Fertil Steril* 1975;26:1088–1093.
134. Sulewski JM, Ward SP, McGaffic W. Endometrial biopsy during a cycle of conception. *Fertil Steril* 1980;34:548–551.
135. Von Numers C. On the traumatic effect of curettage on the endometrial biopsy with special reference to so-called invagination pictures and the "crumbling endometrium." *Acta Obstet Gynecol (Scand)* 1949;28:305–313.

136. Hampson F, Gerlis LM. Some form variations in endometrial tubules. *J Obstet Gynaecol Br Emp* 1954;61:744–749.
137. Sorvari TE, Laakso L. Histochemical investigation of epithelial mucosubstances in the uterine isthmus. *Obstet Gynecol* 1970;36:76–81.
138. McLennan CE, Rydell AH. Extent of endometrial shedding during normal menstruation. *Obstet Gynecol* 1965;26:605–621.
139. Ferenczy A. Studies on the cytodynamics of human endometrial regeneration. I. Scanning electron microscopy. *Am J Obstet Gynecol* 1976;124:64–74.
140. Ferenczy A. Studies on the cytodynamics of human endometrial regeneration. II. Transmission electron microscopy and histochemistry. *Am J Obstet Gynecol* 1976;124:582–595.
141. Sandberg EC, Cohn F. Adenomyosis in the gravid uterus at term. *Am J Obstet Gynecol* 1962;84:1457–1465.
142. Denholm RB, More IA. Atypical cilia of the human endometrial epithelium. *J Anat* 1980;131(Pt 2):309–315.
143. Masterton R, Armstrong EM, More IA. The cyclical variation in the percentage of ciliated cells in the normal human endometrium. *J Reprod Fertil* 1975;42:537–540.
144. Schueller EF. Ciliated epithelia of the human uterine mucosa. *Obstet Gynecol* 1968;31:215–223.
145. Kearns M, Lala PK. Life history of decidual cells: a review. *Am J Reprod Immunol* 1983;3:78–82.
146. Lawn AM, Wilson EW, Finn CA. The ultrastructure of human decidual and predecidual cells. *J Reprod Fertil* 1971;26:85–90.
147. Imai K, Maeda M, Fujiwara H, et al. Human endometrial stromal cells and decidual cells express cluster of differentiation (CD) 13 antigen/aminopeptidase N and CD10 antigen/neutral endopeptidase. *Biol Reprod* 1992;46:328–334.
148. Fowlis DJ, Ansell JD. Evidence that decidual cells are not derived from bone marrow. *Transplantation* 1985;39:445–446.
149. Kamat BR, Isaacson PG. The immunocytochemical distribution of leukocytic subpopulations in human endometrium. *Am J Pathol* 1987; 127:66–73.
150. Bryant-Greenwood GD. The human relaxins: consensus and dissent. *Mol Cell Endocrinol* 1991;79:C125–132.
151. Bryant-Greenwood GD. Relaxin as a new hormone. *Endocr Rev* 1982; 3:62–90.
152. Cardell RR Jr, Hisaw FL, Dawson AB. The fine structure of granular cells in the uterine endometrium of the rhesus monkey (Macaca mulatta) with a discussion of the possible function of these cells in relaxin secretion. *Am J Anat* 1969;124:307–339.
153. Dallenbach-Hellweg G. *Histopathology of the endometrium.* 3rd ed. New York: Springer-Verlag; 1981
154. Dallenbach-Hellweg G, Battista JV, Dallenbach FD. Immunohistological and histochemical localization of relaxin in the metrial gland of the pregnant rat. *Am J Anat* 1965;117:433–450.
155. Weiss G. Relaxin. *Annu Rev Physiol* 1984;46:43–52.
156. Yki-Jarvinen H, Wahlstrom T, Seppala M. Immunohistochemical demonstration of relaxin in gynecologic tumors. *Cancer* 1983;52: 2077–2080.
157. Bulmer JN, Lunny DP, Hagin SV. Immunohistochemical characterization of stromal leucocytes in nonpregnant human endometrium. *Am J Reprod Immunol Microbiol* 1988;17:83–90.
158. Bulmer JN, Sunderland CA. Bone-marrow origin of endometrial granulocytes in the early human placental bed. *J Reprod Immunol* 1983; 5:383–387.
159. Marshall RJ, Jones DB. An immunohistochemical study of lymphoid tissue in human endometrium. *Int J Gynecol Pathol* 1988;7:225–235.
160. Press MF, King WJ. Distribution of peroxidase and granulocytes in the human uterus. *Lab Invest* 1986;54:188–203.
161. Dallenbach FD, Rudolph HG. Foam cells and estrogen activity of the human endometrium. *Arch Gynakol* 1974;217:335–347.
162. King A, Wellings V, Gardner L, Loke YW. Immunocytochemical characterization of the unusual large granular lymphocytes in human endometrium throughout the menstrual cycle. *Hum Immunol* 1989;24: 195–205.
163. Morris H, Edwards J, Tiltman A, Emms M. Endometrial lymphoid tissue: an immunohistological study. *J Clin Pathol* 1985;38:644–652.
164. Sen DK, Fox H. The lymphoid tissue of the endometrium. *Gynaecologia* 1967;163:371–378.
165. Tabibzadeh S. Proliferative activity of lymphoid cells in human endometrium throughout the menstrual cycle. *J Clin Endocrinol Metab* 1990;70:437–443.
166. Farrer-Brown G, Beilby JO, Rowles PM. Microvasculature of the uterus. An injection method of study. *Obstet Gynecol* 1970;35:21–30.
167. Ramsey EM. Anatomy of the uterus. In: Chard T, Grudzinskas J, eds. *The uterus.* New York: Cambridge University Press; 1994:18–40.
168. Burchell RC, Creed F, Rasoulpour M, Whitcomb M. Vascular anatomy of the human uterus and pregnancy wastage. *Br J Obstet Gynaecol* 1978;85:698–706.
169. Ramsey EM. Vascular anatomy. In: Wynn RM, ed. *Biology of the uterus.* New York: Plenum; 1977:59–76.
170. Diplock J, Robertson WB. The ultrastructure of the endometrial stromal cell. *J Pathol* 1971;104:i.
171. Ferenczy A, Richart RM. Scanning and transmission electron microscopy of the human endometrial surface epithelium. *J Clin Endocrinol Metab* 1973;36:999–1008.
172. Fechner RE, Bossart MI, Spjut HJ. Ultrastructure of endometrial stromal foam cells. *Am J Clin Pathol* 1979;72:628–633.
173. Philipp E. Symposium on scanning electron microscopy of fertility and infertility, Eighth World Congress of Fertility and Sterility, Buenos Aires, Argentina, November 1974. Normal endocervical endothelium. *J Reprod Med* 1975;14:188–191.
174. Armstrong EM, More IA, McSeveney D, Carty M. The giant mitochondrion-endoplasmic reticulum unit of the human endometrial glandular cell. *J Anat* 1973;116:375–383.
175. Coaker T, Downie T, More IA. Complex giant mitochondria in the human endometrial glandular cell: serial sectioning, high-voltage electron microscopic, and three-dimensional reconstruction studies. *J Ultrastruct Res* 1982;78:283–291.
176. Dockery P, Rogers AW. The effects of steroids on the fine structure of the endometrium. *Baillieres Clin Obstet Gynaecol* 1989;3:227–248.
177. More IA, McSeveney D. The three dimensional structure of the nucleolar channel system in the endometrial glandular cell: serial sectioning and high voltage electron microscopic studies. *J Anat* 1980; 130:673–682.
178. More IA, Armstrong EM. Proceedings: the nuclear channel system of the human endometrial glandular cell. *J Clin Pathol* 1973;26:984.
179. Moll R, Levy R, Czernobilsky B, Hohlweg-Majert P, Dallenbach-Hellweg G, Franke WW. Cytokeratins of normal epithelia and some neoplasms of the female genital tract. *Lab Invest* 1983;49:599–610.
180. Aplin JD. Cellular biochemistry of the endometrium. 2nd ed. In: Wynn RM, Jollie WP, eds. *Biology of the uterus.* New York: Plenum; 1989:89–130.
181. Aplin JD. Products of endometrial differentiation. In: Chard T, Grudzinskas J, eds. *The uterus.* New York: Cambridge; 1994: 125–147.
182. Giudice LC. Growth factors and growth modulators in human uterine endometrium: their potential relevance to reproductive medicine. *Fertil Steril* 1994;61:1–17.
183. Seppala M, Julkunen M, Riittinen L, Koistinen R. Endometrial proteins: a reappraisal. *Hum Reprod* 1992;1:31–38.
184. Speroff L, Glass RH, Kase NG. *Clinical gynecologic endocrinology and infertility.* 5th ed. Baltimore: Williams & Wilkins; 1994.
185. Treloar AE, Boynton RE, Behn BG, Brown BW. Variation of the human menstrual cycle through reproductive life. *Int J Fertil* 1970;12: 77–126.
186. Fritz MA, Speroff L. The endocrinology of the menstrual cycle: the interaction of folliculogenesis and neuroendocrine mechanisms. *Fertil Steril* 1982;38:509–529.
187. Hodgen GD. Neuroendocrinology of the normal menstrual cycle. *J Reprod Med* 1989;34(suppl):68–75.
188. Kenigsberg D, Hodgen GD. Physiology of the menstrual cycle and ovarian function: clinical correlates and implications. In: eds? *Gynecology: principles and practice*, 1st ed. New York: Macmillan; 1987.
189. Marshall JC, Kelch RP. Gonadotropin-releasing hormone: role of pulsatile secretion in the regulation of reproduction. *N Engl J Med* 1986; 315:1459–1468.
190. Yen SSC. The human menstrual cycle. In: Yen SSC, Jaffe RB, eds. *Reproductive endocrinology: physiology, pathophysiology and clinical management*, 2nd ed. Philadelphia: WB Saunders; 1986.
191. Hodgen GD. The dominant ovarian follicle. *Fertil Steril* 1982;38: 281–300.
192. Alberts B, Bray D, Lewis J, Raff M, Roberts K, Watson JD. Cell signaling. In: Alberts B, Bray D, Lewis J, Raff M, Roberts K, Watson J, eds. *Molecular biology of the cell.* 3rd ed. New York: Garland; 1994: 721–785.

193. Clark JH, Schrader WT, O'Malley BW. Mechanisms of action of steroid hormones. In: Wilson J, Forster D, eds. *Williams' textbook of endocrinology.* 8th ed. Philadelphia: WB Saunders; 1992:35–90.
194. Carlstedt-Duke J, Wright A, Gottlicher M, Okret S, Gustafsson J. Molecular mechanisms of hormone action: regulation of target cell function by the steroid hormone receptor supergene family. In: Felig P, Baxter J, Frohman L, eds. *Endocrinology and metabolism.* 3rd ed. New York: McGraw-Hill; 1995:169–199.
195. Leavitt WW. Cell biology of the endometrium. In: Wynn RM, Jollie WP, eds. *Biology of the uterus.* 2nd ed. New York: Plenum; 1989: 131–174.
196. Bayard F, Damilano S, Robel P, Baulieu EE. Cytoplasmic and nuclear estradiol and progesterone receptors in human endometrium. *J Clin Endocrinol Metab* 1978;46:635–648.
197. Bergeron C, Ferenczy A, Shyamala G. Distribution of estrogen receptors in various cell types of normal, hyperplastic, and neoplastic human endometrial tissues. *Lab Invest* 1988;58:338–345.
198. Evans RM. The steroid and thyroid hormone receptor superfamily. *Science* 1988;240:889–895.
199. Gehring U. Steroid hormone receptors: biochemistry, genetics, and molecular biology. *Trends Biochem Sci* 1987;12:399–402.
200. Katzenellenbogen BS. Dynamics of steroid hormone receptor action. *Annu Rev Physiol* 1980;42:17–35.
201. Abel MH, Kelly RW. Metabolism of prostaglandins by the nonpregnant human uterus. *J Clin Endocrinol Metab* 1983;56:678–685.
202. Bergeron C, Ferenczy A, Toft DO, Schneider W, Shyamala G. Immunocytochemical study of progesterone receptors in the human endometrium during the menstrual cycle. *Lab Invest* 1988;59:862–869.
203. Press MF, NousekGoebl N, King WJ, Herbst AL, Greene GL. Immunohistochemical assessment of estrogen receptor distribution in the human endometrium throughout the menstrual cycle. *Lab Invest* 1984; 51:495–503.
204. Van der Walt LA, Sanfilippo JS, Siegel JE, Wittliff JL. Estrogen and progestin receptors in human uterus: reference ranges of clinical conditions. *Clin Physiol Biochem* 1986;4:217–228.
205. Bigazzi M. Specific endocrine function of human decidua. *Semin Reprod Endocrinol* 1983;1:343.
206. Daly DC, Maslar IA, Riddick DH. Prolactin production during in vitro decidualization of proliferative endometrium. *Am J Obstet Gynecol* 1983;145:672–678.
207. Healy DL, Hodgen GD. The endocrinology of human endometrium. *Obstet Gynecol Surv* 1983;38:509–530.
208. Jansen RPRS, Johannisson E. Endocrine response in the female genital tract. In: Shearman R, ed. *Clinical reproductive endocrinology.* New York: Churchill Livingstone; 1985:109–164.
209. Riddick DH, Daly DC, Walters CA. The uterus as an endocrine compartment. *Clin Perinatol* 1983;10:627–639.
210. Riddick DH, Daly DC. Decidual prolactin production in human gestation. *Semin Perinatol* 1982;6:229–237.
211. Noyes RW. Normal phases of the endometrium. In: Hertig A, Norris H, Abell M, eds. *The Uterus.* Baltimore: Williams & Wilkins; 1973: 110–135.
212. Johannisson E, Parker RA, Landgren BM, Diczfalusy E. Morphometric analysis of the human endometrium in relation to peripheral hormone levels. *Fertil Steril* 1982;38:564–571.
213. Ferenczy A, Bertrand G, Gelfand MM. Proliferation kinetics of human endometrium during the normal menstrual cycle. *Am J Obstet Gynecol* 1979;133:859–867.
214. Ferenczy A. How to date the endometrial cycle. *Contemp Obstet Gynecol* 1981;18:115–133.
215. Noyes RW, Hertig AT, Rock J. Dating the endometrial biopsy. *Fertil Steril* 1950;1:3–25.
216. Strauss JF III, Gurpide E. The endometrium: regulation and dysfunction. In: Yen S, Jaffe R, eds. *Reproductive endocrinology: Physiology, pathophysiology and clinical management.* 3rd ed. Philadelphia: WB Saunders; 1991:309–356.
217. Li TC, Dockery P, Rogers AW, Cooke ID. How precise is histologic dating of endometrium using the standard dating criteria? *Fertil Steril* 1989;51:759–763.
218. Johannisson E, Landgren BM, Rohr HP, Diczfalusy E. Endometrial morphology and peripheral hormone levels in women with regular menstrual cycles. *Fertil Steril* 1987;48:401–408.
219. Wolf DP, Blasco L, Khan MA, Litt M. Human cervical mucus. IV. Viscoelasticity and sperm penetrability during the ovulatory menstrual cycle. *Fertil Steril* 1978;30:163–169.
220. Milwidsky A, Palti Z, Gutman A. Glycogen metabolism of the human endometrium. *J Clin Endocrinol Metab* 1980;51:765–770.
221. Daly DC, Tohan N, Doney TJ, Maslar IA, Riddick DH. The significance of lymphocytic-leukocytic infiltrates in interpreting late luteal phase endometrial biopsies. *Fertil Steril* 1982;37:786–791.
222. Hopwood D, Levison DA. Atrophy and apoptosis in the cyclical human endometrium. *J Pathol* 1976;119:159–166.
223. Christiaens GC, Sixma JJ, Haspels AA. Hemostasis in menstrual endometrium: a review. *Obstet Gynecol Surv* 1982;37:281–303.
224. Ferenczy A, Bertrand G, Gelfand MM. Studies on the cytodynamics of human endometrial regeneration. III. In vitro short-term incubation historadioautography. *Am J Obstet Gynecol* 1979;134:297–304.
225. Wilborn WH, Flowers CE Jr. Cellular mechanisms for endometrial conservation during menstrual bleeding. *Semin Reprod Endocrinol* 1984;2:307–341.
226. Baird DT, Michie EA. *Mechanisms of menstrual bleeding.* Vol. 5. New York: Raven Press; 1985.
227. Ferenczy A. Regeneration of the human endometrium. In: Fenoglio C, Wolff M, eds. *Progress in surgical pathology.* New York: Masson; 1980:157–173.
228. Johannisson E, Fournier K, Riotton G. Regeneration of the human endometrium and presence of inflammatory cells following diagnostic curettage. *Acta Obstet Gynecol Scand* 1981;60:451–457.
229. McLennan CE. Endometrial regeneration after curettage. *Am J Obstet Gynecol* 1969;104:185–194.
230. Parr MB, Parr EL. The implantation reaction. In: Wynn RM, Jollie WP, eds. *Biology of the uterus.* 2nd ed. New York: Plenum Press; 1989:233–288.
231. Hertig AT. Gestational hyperplasia of endometrium: a morphologic correlation of ova, endometrium, and corpora lutea during early pregnancy. *Lab Invest* 1964;13:1153–1191.
232. O'Connor DM, Kurman RJ. Intermediate trophoblast in uterine curettings in the diagnosis of ectopic pregnancy. *Obstet Gynecol* 1988;72: 665–670.
233. Finn CA. The implantation reaction. In: Wynn RM, Jollie WP, eds. *Biology of the uterus.* New York: Plenum Press, 1977:245–308.
234. Young RH, Kurman RJ, Scully RE. Placental site nodules and plaques. A clinicopathologic analysis of 20 cases. *Am J Surg Pathol* 1990;14:1001–1009.
235. Ober WB, Grady HG. Sub-involution of the placental site. *Bull NY Acad Med* 1961;37:713–730.
236. Arias-Stella J. Atypical endometrial changes produced by chorionic tissue. *Hum Pathol* 1972;3:450–453.
237. Arias-Stella J. Gestational endometrium. In: Hertig A, Norris H, Abell M, eds. *The Uterus.* Baltimore: Williams & Wilkins, 1973: 185–212.
238. Fienberg R, Lloyd HE. The Arias-Stella reaction in early normal pregnancy—an involutional phenomenon. The ovary–placenta changeover as a possible cause. *Hum Pathol* 1974;5:183–190.
239. Kjer JJ, Eldon K. The diagnostic value of the Arias-Stella phenomenon. *Zentralbl Gynakol* 1982;104:753–756.
240. Wagner D, Richart RM. Polyploidy in the human endometrium with the Arias-Stella reaction. *Arch Pathol* 1968;85:475–480.
241. Thrasher TV, Richart RM. Ultrastructure of the Arias-Stella reaction. *Am J Obstet Gynecol* 1972;112:113–120.
242. Silverberg SG. Arias-Stella phenomenon in spontaneous and therapeutic abortion. *Am J Obstet Gynecol* 1972;112:777–780.
243. Arias-Stella J Jr, Arias-Velasquez A, Arias-Stella J. Normal and abnormal mitoses in the atypical endometrial change associated with chorionic tissue effect. *Am J Surg Pathol* 1994;18:694–701. [Erratum in *Am J Surg Pathol* 1994; 18:968.]
244. Mazur MT, Hendrickson MR, Kempson RL. Optically clear nuclei. An alteration of endometrial epithelium in the presence of trophoblast. *Am J Surg Pathol* 1983;7:415–423.
245. Lichtig C, Deutch M, Brandes J. Vascular changes of endometrium in early pregnancy. *Am J Clin Pathol* 1984;81:702–707.
246. Archer DF, McIntyre Seltman K, Wilborn WW Jr, et al. Endometrial morphology in asymptomatic postmenopausal women. *Am J Obstet Gynecol* 1991;165:317–322.
247. Choo YC, Mak KC, Hsu C, Wong TS, Ma HK. Postmenopausal uterine bleeding of nonorganic cause. *Obstet Gynecol* 1985;66:225–228.
248. Meyer WC, Malkasian GD, Dockerty MB, Decker DG. Postmenopausal bleeding from atrophic endometrium. *Obstet Gynecol* 1971;38: 731–738.
249. Hendrickson MR, Kempson RL. The uterine corpus. In: Sternberg S, ed. *Diagnostic surgical pathology.* 2nd ed. New York: Raven; 1994: 2091–2193.

250. Corson SL. Operative hysteroscopy for infertility. *Clin Obstet Gynecol* 1992;35:229–241.
251. Valle RF. Hysteroscopy. *Curr Opin Obstet Gynecol* 1991;3:422–426.
252. Gutmann JN. Imaging in the evaluation of female infertility. *J Reprod Med* 1992;37:54–61.
253. March CM. Hysteroscopy. *J Reprod Med* 1992;37:293–311.
254. Dallenbach-Hellweg G. *Histopathology of the endometrium.* 4th ed. New York: Springer-Verlag; 1987.
255. Speroff L, Glass RH, Kase NG. *Clinical gynecologic endocrinology and infertility.* 4rd ed. Baltimore: Williams & Wilkins; 1989.
256. Robertson WB. A reappraisal of the endometrium in infertility. *Clin Obstet Gynaecol* 1984;11:209–226.
257. Collins JA. Diagnostic assessment of the ovulatory process. *Semin Reprod Endocrinol* 1990;8:145–155.
258. Pillet MC, Wu TF, Adamson GD, Subak LL, Lamb EJ. Improved prediction of postovulatory day using temperature recording, endometrial biopsy, and serum progesterone. *Fertil Steril* 1990;53:614–619.
259. Martinez AR, Voorhorst FJ, Schoemaker J. Reliability of urinary LH testing for planning of endometrial biopsies. *Eur J Obstet Gynecol Reprod Biol* 1992;43:137–142.
260. McNeely MJ, Soules MR. The diagnosis of luteal phase deficiency: a critical review [see comments]. *Fertil Steril* 1988;50:1–15.
261. Lenton EA, Landgren BM, Sexton L. Normal variation in the length of the luteal phase of the menstrual cycle: identification of the short luteal phase. *Br J Obstet Gynecol* 1984;91:685.
262. Landgren BM, Unden AL, Diczfalusy E. Hormonal profile of the cycle in 68 normally menstruating women. *Acta Endocrinol (Copenh)* 1980;94:89–98.
263. Davis OK, Berkeley AS, Naus GJ, Cholst IN, Freedman KS. The incidence of luteal phase defect in normal, fertile women, determined by serial endometrial biopsies [see comments]. *Fertil Steril* 1989;51: 582–586.
264. Grunfeld L, Sandler B, Fox J, Boyd C, Kaplan P, Navot D. Luteal phase deficiency after completely normal follicular and periovulatory phases. *Fertil Steril* 1989;52:919–923.
265. Li TC, Rogers AW, Dockery P, Lenton EA, Cooke ID. A new method of histologic dating of human endometrium in the luteal phase. *Fertil Steril* 1988;50:52–60.
266. Li TC, Rogers A, Lenton E, Dockery P, Cooke I. A comparison between two methods of chronological dating of human endometrial biopsies during the luteal phasse, and their correlation with histologic dating. *Fertil Steril* 1987;48:928.
267. Noyes RW, Haman JO. Accuracy of endometrial dating. *Fertil Steril* 1953;4:504–517.
268. Gibson M, Badger GJ, Byrn F, Lee KR, Korson R, Trainer TD. Error in histologic dating of secretory endometrium: variance component analysis. *Fertil Steril* 1991;56:242–247.
269. Scott RT, Snyder RR, Strickland DM, et al. The effect of interobserver variation in dating endometrial histology on the diagnosis of luteal phase defects. *Fertil Steril* 1988;50:888–892.
270. Kim-Björklund T, Landgren BM, Hamberger L, Johannisson E. Comparative morphometric study of the endometrium, the fallopian tube, and the corpus luteum during the postovulatory phase in normally menstruating women. *Fertil Steril* 1991;56:842–850.
271. Shoupe D, Mishell DR Jr, Lacarra M, et al. Correlation of endometrial maturation with four methods of estimating day of ovulation. *Obstet Gynecol* 1989;73:88–92.
272. Koninckx PR, Goddeeris PG, Lauweryns JM, De Hertogh RC, Brosens IA. Accuracy of endometrial biopsy dating in relation to the midcycle luteinizing hormone peak. *Obstet Gynecol Surv* 1977;32: 613–615.
273. Li TC, Lenton EA, Dockery P, Rogers AW, Cooke ID. The relation between daily salivary progesterone profile and endometrial development in the luteal phase of fertile and infertile women. *Br J Obstet Gynaecol* 1989;96:445–453.
274. Collins JA. Diagnostic assessment of the infertile female partner. *Curr Probl Obstet Gynecol Fertil* 1988;11:1–42.
275. Collins JA. Diagnostic assessment of the infertile male partner. *Curr Probl Obstet Gynecol Fertil* 1987;10:173–224.
276. Davidson BJ, Thrasher TV, Seraj IM. An analysis of endometrial biopsies performed for infertility. *Fertil Steril* 1987;48:770–774.
277. Van Bogaert LJ, Maldague P, Staquet JP. Endometrial biopsy interpretation. Shortcomings and problems in current gynecologic practice. *Obstet Gynecol* 1978;51:25–28.
278. Thompson DW. The role of histologic assessment of endometrium and cytohormonal applications in the diagnosis and treatment of infertility. *Curr Opin Obstet Gynecol* 1990;2:863–868.
279. Wentz AC. Luteal phase inadequacy. In: Behrman S, Kistner R, Patton GJ, ed. *Progress in infertility.* Boston: Little, Brown; 1988: 405–462.
280. Koninckx PR, Goddeeris PG, Lauweryns JM, de Hertogh RC, Brosens IA. Accuracy of endometrial biopsy dating in relation to the midcycle luteinizing hormone peak. *Fertil Steril* 1977;28:443–445.
281. Rotello RJ, Lieberman RC, Lepoff RB, Gerschenson LE. Characterization of uterine epithelium apoptotic cell death kinetics and regulation by progesterone and RU 486. *Am J Pathol* 1992;140:449–456.
282. Rotello RJ, Lieberman RC, Purchio AF, Gerschenson LE. Coordinated regulation of apoptosis and cell proliferation by transforming growth factor beta 1 in cultured uterine epithelial cells. *Proc Natl Acad Sci U S A* 1991;88:3412–3415.
283. Rotello RJ, Hocker MB, Gerschenson LE. Biochemical evidence for programmed cell death in rabbit uterine epithelium. *Am J Pathol* 1989; 134:491–495.
284. Gerschenson LE, Rotello RJ. Apoptosis: a different type of cell death. *FASEB J* 1992;6:2450–2455.
285. Gerschenson LE, Rotello RJ. Apoptosis and cell proliferation are terms of the growth equation. In: Tomei L, Cope F, eds. *Apoptosis: the cell molecular basis of cell death.* New York: Cold Spring Harbor Laboratory Press; 1991:175–192.
286. Gompel A, Sabourin JC, Martin A, et al. Bcl-2 expression in normal endometrium during the menstrual cycle. *Am J Pathol* 1994;144: 1195–1202.
287. Tabibzadeh S, Zupi E, Babaknia A, Liu R, Marconi D, Romanini C. Site and menstrual cycle–dependent expression of proteins of the tumour necrosis factor (TNF) receptor family, and BCL-2 oncoprotein and phase-specific production of TNF alpha in human endometrium. *Hum Reprod* 1995;10:277–286.
288. Garfield RE, Yallampalli C. Structure and function of uterine muscle. In: Chard T, Grudzinskas J, eds. *The uterus.* New York: Cambridge; 1994:54–93.
289. Cole WC, Garfield RE. Ultrastructure of the myometrium. In: Wynn RM, Jollie WP, eds. *Biology of the uterus.* 2nd ed. New York: Plenum; 1989:455–504.
290. Kao CY. Electrophysiological properties of uterine smooth muscle. In: Wynn RM, Jollie WP, eds. *Biology of the uterus.* 2nd ed. New York: Plenum; 1989:403–454.
291. Huszar G, Walsh MP. Biochemistry of the myometrium and cervix. In: Wynn RM, Jollie WP, eds. *Biology of the uterus.* 2nd ed. New York: Plenum; 1989:355–402.
292. Schoenberg CF. The contractile mechanism and ultrastructure of the myometrium. In: Wynn RM, ed. *Biology of the uterus.* New York: Plenum; 1977:497–544.
293. Kawaguchi K, Fujii S, Konishi I, Nanbu Y, Nonogaki H, Mori T. Mitotic activity in uterine leiomyomas during the menstrual cycle. *Am J Obstet Gynecol* 1989;160:637–641.
294. Hamoir G. *Biochemistry of the myometrium.* In: Wynn RM, ed. *Biology of the uterus.* New York: Plenum; 1977:377–421.
295. Marshall JM. The physiology of the myometrium. In: Hertig AT, Norris HJ, Abell MR, eds. *The uterus.* Baltimore: Williams & Wilkins; 1973:89–109.
296. Bird CC, Willis RA. The production of smooth muscle by the endometrial stroma of the adult human uterus. *J Pathol Bacteriol* 1965; 90:75–81.
297. Azumi N, Sheibani K, Battifora H. Keratin-like immunoreactivity in leiomyosarcomas, uterine leiomyomas, and normal myometrium by multiple antikeratin antibodies [Abstract]. *Lab Invest* 1988;58:6.
298. Brown DC, Theaker JM, Banks PM, Gatter KC, Mason DY. Cytokeratin expression in smooth muscle and smooth muscle tumours. *Histopathology* 1987;11:477–486.
299. Langloss JM, Kurman RJ, Bratthauer GL, et al. Expression of keratin by normal and neoplastic smooth muscle cells of the human uterus. 1990.
300. Norton AJ, Thomas JA, Isaacson PG. Cytokeratin-specific monoclonal antibodies are reactive with tumours of smooth muscle derivation. An immunocytochemical and biochemical study using antibodies to intermediate filament cytoskeletal proteins. *Histopathology* 1987;11:487–499.
301. Silverberg SG, Kurman RJ. Tumors of the uterine corpus and gestational trophoblastic disease. In: Rosai J, ed. *Atlas of tumor pathology.* Vol. 3. Washington, DC: AFIP; 1992.

302. Clement PB, Young RH, Scully RE. Nontrophoblastic pathology of the female genital tract and peritoneum associated with pregnancy. *Semin Diagn Pathol* 1989;6:372–406.
303. Garfield RE, Hayashi RH. Appearance of gap junctions in the myometrium of women during labor. *Am J Obstet Gynecol* 1981;140: 254–260.
304. Brenner RM, Slayden OD. The fallopian tube cycle. In: Adashi EY, Rock JA, Rosenwaks Z, eds. *Reproductive endocrinology, surgery, and technology.* 1st ed. Vol. I. Philadelphia: Lippincott-Raven; 1996: 326–339.
305. Bonilla Musoles F, Ferrer Barriendos J, Pellicer A. Cyclical changes in the epithelium of the fallopian tube. Studies with scanner electron microscopy (SEM). *Clin Exp Obstet Gynecol* 1983;10:79–86.
306. Donnez J, Casanas Roux F, Caprasse J, Ferin J, Thomas K. Cyclic changes in ciliation, cell height, and mitotic activity in human tubal epithelium during reproductive life. *Fertil Steril* 1985;43:554–559.
307. Jansen RP. Endocrine response in the fallopian tube. *Endocr Rev* 1984;5:525–551.
308. Lindenbaum ES, Peretz BA, Beach D. Menstrual-cycle–dependent and –independent features of the human fallopian tube fimbrial epithelium: an ultrastructural and cytochemical study. *Gynecol Obstet Invest* 1983;16:76–85.
309. Verhage HG, Bareither ML, Jaffe RC, Akbar M. Cyclic changes in ciliation, secretion and cell height of the oviductal epithelium in women. *Am J Anat* 1979;156:505–521.
310. Leese HJ. The formation and function of oviduct fluid. *J Reprod Fertil* 1988;82:843–856.
311. Sivridis E, Buckley CH, Fox H. Argyrophil cells in normal, hyperplastic, and neoplastic endometrium. *J Clin Pathol* 1984;37:378–381.
312. Constant O, Cooke J, Parsons CA. Reformatted computed tomography of the female pelvis: normal anatomy. *Br J Obstet Gynaecol* 1989; 96:1047–1053.
313. de Castro A, Yebra C, Aznar F, et al. Measurement of the endometrial cavity length using Wing Sound I. *Adv Contracept* 1987;3:133–137.
314. Geppert M, Geppert J, Bohle A. On the lympho-epithelial relationships in the human oviduct. *Virchows Arch [A]* 1977;373:133–142.
315. Morris H, Emms M, Visser T, Timme A. Lymphoid tissue of the normal fallopian tube—a form of mucosal-associated lymphoid tissue (MALT)? *Int J Gynecol Pathol* 1986;5:11–22.
316. Kutteh WH, Blackwell RE, Gore H, Kutteh CC, Carr BR, Mestecky J. Secretory immune system of the female reproductive tract. II. Local immune system in normal and infected fallopian tube. *Fertil Steril* 1990;54:51–55.
317. Lurie M, Tur Kaspa I, Weill S, Katz I, Rabinovici J, Goldenberg S. Ciliary ultrastructure of respiratory and fallopian tube epithelium in a sterile woman with Kartagener's syndrome. A quantitative estimation. *Chest* 1989;95:578–581.
318. Lindblom B, Wilhelmsson L, Wikland M, Hamberger L, Wiqvist N. Prostaglandins and oviductal function. *Acta Obstet Gynecol Scand Suppl* 1983;113:43–46.
319. Pulkkinen MO, Talo A. Tubal physiologic consideration in ectopic pregnancy. *Clin Obstet Gynecol* 1987;30:164–172.
320. Donnez J, Casanas Roux F, Ferin J. Macroscopic and microscopic studies of fallopian tube after laparoscopic sterilization. *Contraception* 1979;20:497–509.
321. Donnez J, Casanas Roux F, Ferin J, Thomas K. Tubal polyps, epithelial inclusions, and endometriosis after tubal sterilization. *Fertil Steril* 1984;41:564–568.
322. Mills SE, Fechner RE. Stromal and epithelial changes in the fallopian tube following hormonal therapy. *Hum Pathol* 1980;11:583–585.
323. Ramsey EM. Concepts of the uterus: a historical perspective. In: Chard T, Grudzinskas J, eds. *The uterus.* New York: Cambridge; 1994:1–17.
324. Laqueur T. *Making sex: body and gender from the Greeks to Freud.* Cambridge, MA: Harvard University Press; 1990.
325. Profet M. Menstruation as a defense against pathogens transported by sperm. *Q Rev Biol* 1993;68:335–386.
326. Strassmann BI. The evolution of endometrial cycles in menstruation. *Q Rev Biol* 1996;71:181–220.
327. Clement PB, Young RH, Scully RE. Stromal endometriosis of the uterine cervix. A variant of endometriosis that may simulate a sarcoma. *Am J Surg Pathol* 1990;14:449–455.
328. Clement PB. Pathology of endometriosis. *Pathol Annu* 1990; 1:245–295.
329. Young RH, Scully RE. Atypical forms of microglandular hyperplasia of the cervix simulating carcinoma. A report of five cases and review of the literature. *Am J Surg Pathol* 1989;13:50–56.
330. Leslie KO, Silverberg SG. Microglandular hyperplasia of the cervix: unusual clinical and pathological presentations and their differential diagnosis. *Pathol Annu* 1982;:95–114.
331. Hendrickson MR, Kempson RL. The uterine corpus. In: Sternberg S, ed. *Diagnostic surgical pathology.* 2nd ed. New York: Raven Press; 1994:2103.
332. Hendrickson MR, Kempson RL. Pure mesenchymal neoplasms of the uterine corpus. In: Fox H, ed. *Obstetrical and gynaecological pathology.* New York: Churchill-Livingstone; 1995:519–586.
333. Poropatich C, Rojas M, Silverberg SG. Polymorphonuclear leukocytes in the endometrium during the normal menstrual cycle. *Int J Gynecol Pathol* 1987;6:230–234.
334. Winkler B, Crum CP. Chlamydia trachomatis infection of the female genital tract. Pathogenetic and clinicopathologic correlations. *Pathol Annu* 1987;22(Pt 1):193–223.
335. Jones RB, Mammel JB, Shepard MK, Fisher RR. Recovery of chlamydia trachomatis from the endometrium of women at risk for chlamydial infection. *Am J Obstet Gynecol* 1986;155:35–39.
336. Kiviat NB, WolnerHanssen P, Eschenbach DA, et al. Endometrial histopathology in patients with culture-proved upper genital tract infection and laparoscopically diagnosed acute salpingitis. *Am J Surg Pathol* 1990;14:167–175.
337. Green LK, Kott ML. Histopathologic findings in ectopic tubal pregnancy. *Int J Gynecol Pathol* 1989;8:255–262.
338. Mills SE, Fechner RE. Stromal and epithelial changes in the fallopian tube following hormonal therapy. *Hum Pathol* 1980;11(suppl): 583–585.
339. Fetissof F, Berger G, Dubois MP, Philippe A, Lansac J, Jobard P. Female genital tract and Peutz-Jeghers syndrome: an immunohistochemical study. *Int J Gynecol Pathol* 1985;4:219–229.
340. Saffos RO, Rhatigan RM, Scully RE. Metaplastic papillary tumor of the fallopian tube—a distinctive lesion of pregnancy. *Am J Clin Pathol* 1980;74:232–236.
341. Ramsey EM. Embryology and developmental defects of the female reproductive tract. In: Danforth D, Scott J, eds. *Obstetrics and gynecology.* 5th ed. New York: JB Lippincott; 1986:106–119.
342. Ramsey EM. Anatomy of the uterus. In: Chard T, Grudzinskas J, eds. *The uterus.* New York: Cambridge University Press; 1994:23.
343. Crafts RC, Krieger HP. Gross anatomy of the female reproductive tract, pituitary, and hypothalamus. In: Danforth D, Scott J, eds. *Obstetrics and gynecology.* Philadelphia: JB Lippincott; 1986:64.
344. Henriksen E. The lymphatic spread of carcinoma of the cervix and the body of the uterus. A study of 420 necropsies. *Am J Obstet Gynecol* 1949;58:924.
345. DiSaia PJ, Creasman WT. *Clinical gynecologic oncology.* 3rd ed. St. Louis: CV Mosby; 1989:176.
346. Fox H, ed. *Haines and Taylor obstetrical and gynaecological pathology.* Vol. 1. New York: Churchill Livingstone; 1987:221.
347. Noyes RW. Normal phases of the endometrium. In: Hertig A, Norris H, Abell M, eds. *The uterus.* Baltimore: Williams & Wilkins; 1973: 112.
348. Hendrickson MR, Kempson RL. *Surgical pathology of the uterine corpus.* Philadelphia: WB Saunders; 1980:85.
349. Arias-Stella J. Gestational endometrium. In: Hertig A, Norris H, Abell M, eds. *The uterus.* Baltimore: Williams & Wilkins; 1973:191.
350. Hendrickson MR, Kempson RL. The uterine corpus. In: Sternberg S, ed. *Diagnostic surgical pathology.* 2nd ed. New York: Raven Press; 1994:2114.
351. Janovski NA. *Ovarian tumors.* Vol. 4. Major problems in obstetrics and gynecology. Philadelphia: WB Saunders; 1973:191.

*Histology for Pathologists, second edition,*
Edited by Stephen S. Sternberg.
Lippincott-Raven Publishers, Philadelphia


# CHAPTER 40

# Histology of the Ovary

Philip B. Clement



## EMBRYOLOGY

Approximately 5 weeks after fertilization, a thickening of the coelomic epithelium (mesothelium) along the medial and ventral borders of the mesonephros results in the formation of the genital ridge. The gonadal anlage forms as a result of continued proliferation of this epithelium and the subjacent mesenchyme (1). Simultaneously, primordial germ cells migrate to the gonad from the yolk sac endoderm, reaching the genital ridge during the 5th and 6th weeks of embryonic life (2). These cells (oogonia) undergo mitotic activity and become most numerous at mid-gestation; two thirds of them will undergo atresia by term (1,3). At 12 to 15 weeks' gestation, the oogonia begin meiosis and arrest in meiotic prophase. At this stage they are referred to as primary oocytes (3–5).

At 2 months, the primitive gonad is recognizable as an ovary because, in contrast to the testis, it has remained basically unaltered. At 7 to 9 weeks' gestation, the outer zone of the ovary has enlarged to form the definitive cortex, which consists of confluent sheets of primitive germ cells admixed haphazardly with a smaller number of smaller pregranulosa cells (4,6). Vascular connective tissue septa at 12 to 15 weeks begin to radiate from the medullary mesenchyme into the inner portion of the cortex and extend into the superficial part of the cortex by 20 weeks (5,6). The cortex thereby becomes divided into cellular groups composed of oocytes and pregranulosa cells (sex cords). Simultaneously, the pregranulosa cells begin to surround individual germ cells to form primordial follicles. Folliculogenesis begins in the inner part

P. B. Clement: Departments of Pathology, Vancouver Hospital and Health Sciences Centre, and the University of British Columbia, Vancouver, Canada.

of the cortex at 14 to 20 weeks' gestation (2,3,5,7) and gradually extends to the outer cortex by the early neonatal period (8). The occasional follicles that mature into preantral and antral follicles in late gestation become surrounded by a condensation of mesenchymal cells that become the theca interna (4,7). The rete ovarii is present in the hilus as early as 12 weeks (5).

The origin of the gonadal sex cords (pregranulosa cells in the ovary and Sertoli cells in the testis) is controversial. Some investigators (2,4,8,9) believe that they are derived from the coelomic epithelium, whereas others (10) favor an origin from the mesenchyme. Still others (11,12) believe that the gonadal blastema is too undifferentiated to classify as either epithelial or mesenchymal. More recent observations indicate that the sex cords are likely of mesonephric origin (13–16). Satoh (14) found that rudimentary cordlike structures arise from coelomic epithelial cells but disappear before contributing to the formation of the definitive sex cords, which are derived from cells that originate from the mesonephros.

## GROSS ANATOMY

The ovaries are paired pelvic organs that lie on either side of the uterus close to the lateral pelvic wall, behind the broad ligament and anterior to the rectum. Each ovary is attached (a) along its anterior (hilar) margin to the posterior aspect of the broad ligament by a double fold of peritoneum, the mesovarium; (b) at its medial pole to the ipsilateral uterine cornu by the ovarian (or utero-ovarian) ligament; and (c) from the superior aspect of its lateral pole to the lateral pelvic wall by the infundibulopelvic (or suspensory) ligament. The location of the ovary posterior to the broad ligament and a similar relationship of the ovarian ligament to the ipsilateral fallopian tube aids in the determination of the laterality of a salpingo-oophorectomy specimen.

### Prepubertal Ovaries

The ovary in the newborn is a tan, elongated, and flattened structure that lies above the true pelvis. It sometimes has a lobulated appearance with irregular edges (Fig. 1A). It has approximate dimensions of $1.3 \times 0.5 \times 0.3$ cm, and a weight of less than 0.3 g (17–20). Throughout infancy and childhood, the ovary enlarges, increases in weight 30-fold, and changes in shape so that by the time of puberty it has reached the size, weight, and shape of the adult ovary and lies within the true pelvis (18–20). Inspection of the external and cut surfaces, particularly during the first few months of life and at puberty, may reveal prominent cystic follicles (21) similar to those seen in polycystic ovary disease (Fig. 1B).

### Adult Ovaries

Adult ovaries are ovoid, approximately 3.0 to 5 cm by 1.5 to 3.0 cm by 0.6 to 1.5 cm, and weigh 5 to 8 g. However, their size and weight vary considerably depending on their content of follicular derivatives. They have a pink–white exterior, which in early reproductive life is usually smooth (Fig. 1C) but thereafter becomes increasingly convoluted. Three ill-defined zones are discernible on the cut surface, an outer cortex, an inner medulla, and the hilus. Follicular structures (cystic follicles, yellow corpora lutea, white corpora albicantia) are typically visible in the cortex and medulla.

### Postmenopausal Ovaries

After the menopause, the ovaries typically shrink to a size approximately one half that seen in the reproductive era. However, their size varies considerably with the number of ovarian stromal cells and unresorbed corpora albicantia (19,22). Most postmenopausal ovaries have a shrunken, gyriform, external appearance (Fig. 1D), whereas some are more smooth and uniform. They have a firm consistency and a predominantly solid, pale cut surface, although occasional cysts measuring several millimeters in diameter (inclusion cysts) may be discernible within the cortex. Small white scars (corpora albicantia) are typically present within the medulla. Thick-walled blood vessels may be appreciable within the medulla and hilus.

## BLOOD SUPPLY

The ovarian artery, a branch of the aorta, courses along the infundibulopelvic ligament and the mesovarial border of the ovary, where it anastomoses with the ovarian branch of the uterine artery. Approximately 10 arterial branches from this arcade penetrate the ovarian hilus, becoming markedly coiled and branched as they course through the medulla (23,24). These helicine arteries possess, along their length, longitudinal ridges of intimal smooth muscle (23). At the corticomedullary junction, the medullary arteries and arterioles form a plexus from which smaller, straight cortical arterioles arise and penetrate the cortex in a radial fashion, perpendicular to the ovarian surface. The cortical arterioles branch and anastomose several times forming sets of interconnected vascular arcades (24). These arcades give rise to capillaries that form dense networks within the theca layers of the ovarian follicles. The intraovarian veins accompany the arteries, becoming large and tortuous in the medulla. They form a plexus in the hilus that drains into the ovarian veins; the latter traverse the mesovarium and course along the infundibulopelvic ligament (23,24). The ovarian veins also anastomose with tributaries of the uterine veins. The left and right ovarian veins drain into the left renal vein and the inferior vena cava, respectively.

In postmenopausal women, the medullary blood vessels may appear particularly numerous and closely packed (Fig. 2) and should not be mistaken for a hemangioma on histologic examination. In addition, many of the same vessels may be calcified or have thickened walls and narrowed lumina due to medial deposition of a hyaline, amyloid-like material.

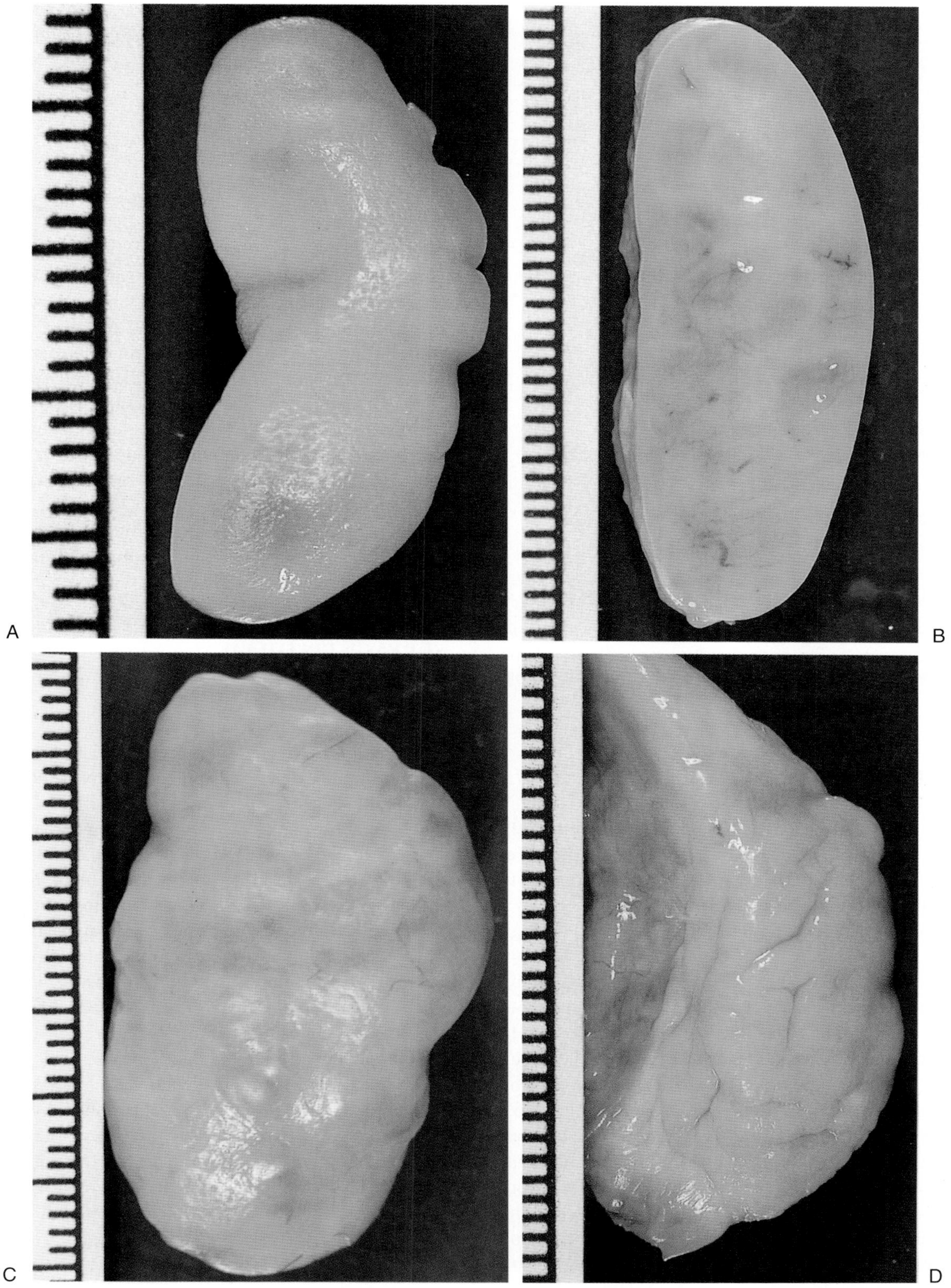


**FIG. 1.** Gross appearance of ovary. **A:** Newborn, external aspect. **B:** Pubertal (age 15 years), cut surface. Note the elongate shape and multiple cystic follicles. **C:** Adult (age 30 years), external aspect. **D:** Postmenopausal, external aspect. Note the shrunken, gyriform appearance.

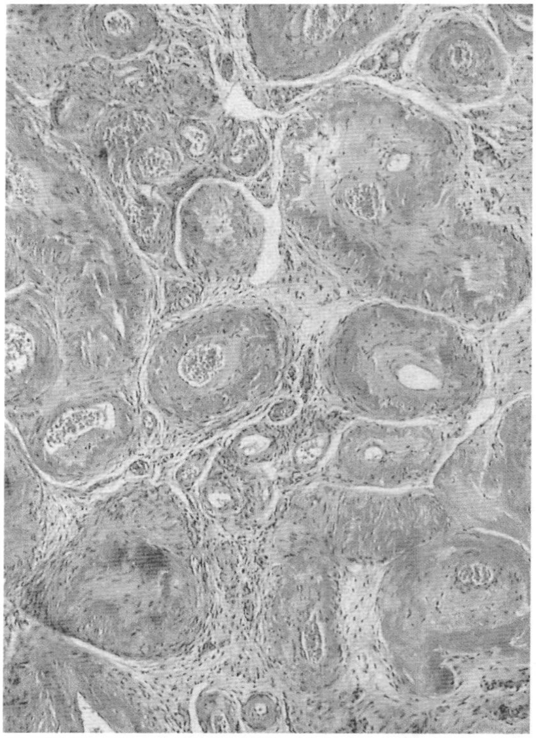

**FIG. 2.** Numerous crowded thick-walled blood vessels within ovarian medulla of postmenopausal woman. Some of the vessels have an eosinophilic amyloid–like material within their walls.

## LYMPHATICS

The lymphatics of the ovary originate predominantly within the theca layers of the follicles. The granulosa layer of a maturing follicle is devoid of lymphatics, in contrast to its counterpart within the corpus luteum, which possesses a rich supply of lymphatics (25). The lymphatics pass through the ovarian stroma, independent of blood vessels, to drain into larger trunks that form a plexus at the hilus (25). Within the hilus, the lymphatics and blood vessels converge, with the former coiled around veins in a helicoid fashion. Four to eight efferent channels pass into the mesovarium, where they converge to form the subovarian plexus, which is joined by branches from the fallopian tube and uterine fundus (25). Leaving the plexus, the drainage trunks diminish in number and size, passing along the free border of the infundibulopelvic ligament enmeshed with the ovarian veins. From there they accompany the ovarian vessels, juxtaposed to the psoas muscle, and drain into the upper para-aortic lymph nodes at the level of the lower pole of the kidney (19,25,26). The major lymphatic drainage of the ovary is therefore in a cephaloid direction toward the para-aortic nodes. However, accessory channels may bypass the subovarian plexus, passing through the broad ligament to the internal iliac, external iliac, and interaortic lymph nodes, or, in some females, via the round ligament to the iliac and inguinal lymph nodes (19,25,26). When the pelvic and para-aortic lymph nodes are extensively replaced by tumor, retrograde lymphatic flow may represent a rare mechanism of tumor spread to the ovaries (19).

## NERVE SUPPLY

The nerve supply of the ovary arises from a sympathetic plexus that is enmeshed with the ovarian vessels in the infundibulopelvic ligament (27). Nerve fibers, which are predominantly nonmyelinated, accompany the ovarian artery, entering the ovary at the hilus. Delicate terminal fibers, many surrounding small arteries and arterioles, penetrate the medulla and cortex to terminate as plexi surrounding the follicles (27,28). Adrenergic nerve fibers and terminals have been shown to be in close contact with smooth muscle cells in the cortical stroma and theca externa. The physiologic significance of ovarian sympathetic innervation is not clear, although it has been suggested that it may play a role in follicular maturation, follicular rupture, or both (27,29,30). In addition, catecholamines can stimulate progesterone production by the ovarian follicles and androgen production by the ovarian stroma in vitro (31).

## SURFACE EPITHELIUM

### Histology

The ovary is covered by a single, focally pseudostratified layer of modified peritoneal cells that constitute the surface epithelium. The cells vary from flat to cuboidal to columnar, and several types may be seen in different areas of the same ovary (Fig. 3). The surface cells are separated from the underlying stroma by a distinct basement membrane. This epithelium is extremely fragile and is almost always denuded in oophorectomy specimens because of undesirable rubbing of the surface by the surgeon and the pathologist, as well as lack of prompt fixation resulting in drying. Preserved epithelium is often confined to areas protected by surface adhesions or lining sulci (19).

Histochemical studies have demonstrated glycogen, as well as acid and neutral mucopolysaccharides, within surface epithelial cells (32,33). Seventeen-beta hydroxysteroid dehydrogenase activity, absent in extraovarian mesothelial cells, also has been demonstrated (32). Immunohistochemical methods have shown positivity for cytokeratin, Ber-EP4, desmoplakin, vimentin, transforming growth factor-alpha, and receptors for estrogen, progesterone, and epidermal growth factor (34–41).

Epithelial inclusion glands (EIGs) arise from cortical invaginations of the surface epithelium that have lost their connection with the surface. Larger examples, epithelial inclusion cysts (EICs), may be recognized on macroscopic examination; a diameter of 1 cm has been suggested as a dividing line between an EIC and the smallest cystadenoma

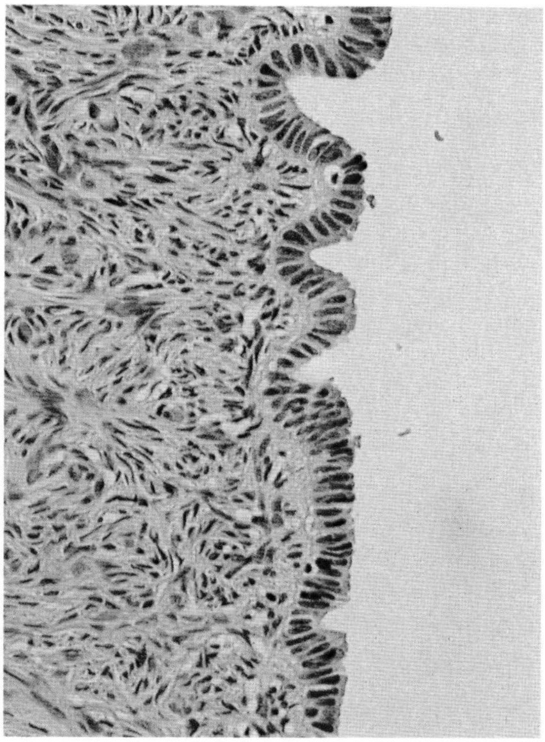

**FIG. 3.** Ovarian surface epithelium composed of a single layer of columnar cells.

(19). EIGs have been identified on microscopic examination of ovaries from all age groups, including fetuses, infants, and adolescents (42,43). Inclusion glands and cysts (EIGCs) become more numerous with age, and are common incidental findings in late reproductive and postmenopausal age groups. They are typically multiple, scattered singly or in small clusters throughout the superficial cortex (Fig. 4); less commonly, extension into the deeper cortical or medullary stroma may occur. EIGCs are typically lined by a single layer of ciliated columnar cells mimicking tubal (endosalpingeal) epithelium; psammoma bodies within their lumina or the adjacent stroma are occasionally present. Similar glands, with or without associated psammoma bodies, encountered on the ovarian surface, within periovarian adhesions, and elsewhere on the pelvic peritoneum and omentum, are designated "endosalpingiosis" (44,45). Less frequently, EIGCs may be lined by other müllerian cell types (endometrioid, mucinous) or nonspecific columnar or flattened cells (46,47).

EIGCs are probably the site of origin of most cystic surface epithelial tumors (48). One study (49) found that EIGCs were more common in ovaries contralateral to a unilateral ovarian carcinoma and that they were more often lined by serous epithelium than in age-matched control patients without ovarian carcinoma. Dysplastic changes also have been described within EIGCs (48). The histogenetic relationship between the ovarian surface epithelium, EIGCs, and tumors of epithelial type is reflected by the immunohistochemical demonstration of antigens associated with ovarian epithelial tumors within the normal surface epithelial cells (CA125, CA19-9, MH99) and within the cells lining EIGs [CA125, CA19-9, carcinoembrionic antigen, human chorionic gonadotropin (hCG), placental lactogen, alpha-2 glycoprotein, beta-1 glycoprotein, placental alkaline phosphatase, and human milk fat globule protein] (50–55). Hyperplasia and metaplasia of the surface epithelium and of that within EIGs are more common in women with polycystic ovarian disease and endometrial carcinoma (56), suggesting a possible hormonal basis for these changes.

Urothelial differentiation is also within the metaplastic potential of the ovarian surface epithelium and pelvic peritoneum. Such differentiation typically takes the form of Walthard nests of transitional cells, a common microscopic finding within the serosa or the immediately subjacent stroma of the fallopian tube, mesosalpinx, and mesovarium; less commonly they may be similarly located within the ovarian hilus (Fig. 5) (57–60). The larger nests frequently become cystic and may be lined by columnar mucinous cells. Brenner tumors also are characterized by urothelial differentiation; as many as half of those encountered by the pathologist are of microscopic size (19).

Hyperplastic mesothelial cells, usually a response to chronic pelvic inflammation, may involve the surface of the ovary and focally replace the ovarian surface epithelium. Florid examples exhibiting tubulopapillary (Fig. 6) and

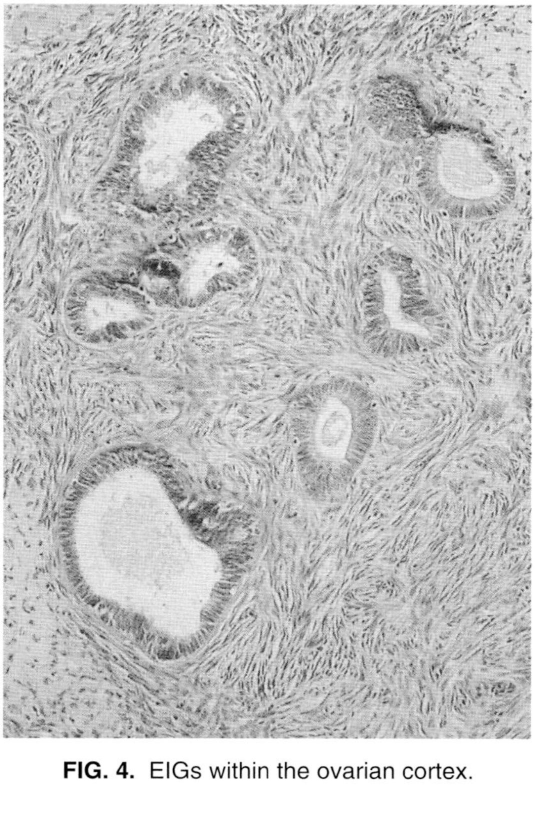

**FIG. 4.** EIGs within the ovarian cortex.

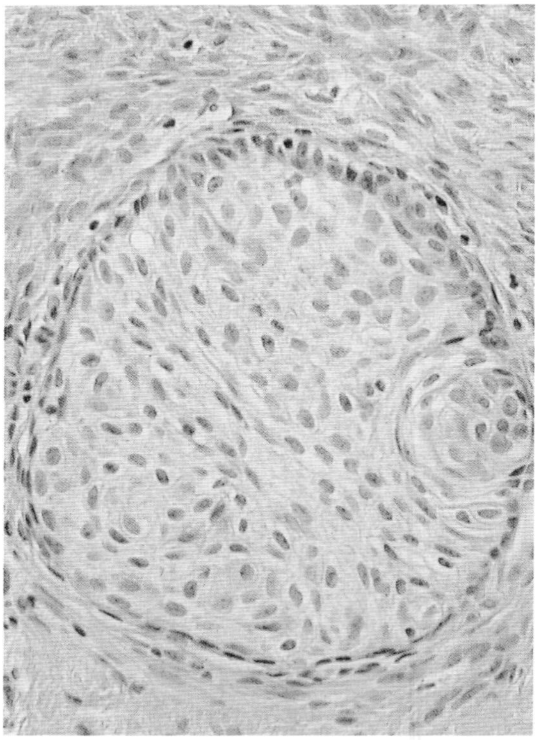

**FIG. 5.** Walthard nest within ovarian hilus abutting the medullary stroma.

pseudoinfiltrative patterns, as well as varying degrees of nuclear atypia, must be distinguished from a malignant mesothelioma or a primary ovarian or metastatic carcinoma.

## Ultrastructure

The ultrastructural appearance of the ovarian surface epithelium is similar to that of the extraovarian peritoneum (61–63). On scanning and transmission electron microscopy, the cell surfaces have dome-shaped apices covered by numerous, often branching, microvilli, occasional single cilia, and pinocytotic vesicles (Fig. 7). The cytoplasm contains abundant polysomes, free ribosomes, abundant mitochondria, and bundles of intermediate filaments and tonofilaments. Lipid droplets are sometimes present in the basal cytoplasm. The nuclei have indented nuclear membranes and peripheral nucleoli. Straight or convoluted lateral plasma membranes are reinforced by luminal junctional complexes, scattered desmosomes, and desmosome–tonofilament complexes. The membranes may be widely separated in areas creating dilated intercellular spaces (62). A well-developed basal lamina separates the surface epithelium from the underlying stroma.

# STROMA

## Histology

Because the cortical and medullary stroma is continuous and similar in appearance, the boundary between these two zones is ill defined and arbitrary. The spindle-shaped stromal cells, which have scanty cytoplasm, are typically arranged in whorls or a storiform pattern (Fig. 8). Fine cytoplasmic lipid droplets may be appreciable with special stains, especially in the late reproductive and postmenopausal age groups (64). Immunohistochemical stains show cytoplasmic vimentin, actin, and desmin (34,36,37,65–67). Stromal cells are separated by a dense reticulum network (Fig. 8 inset) and a variable amount of collagen, which is most abundant in the superficial cortex. Although the latter is frequently referred to as the tunica albuginea, it lacks the densely collagenous, almost acellular appearance and sharp delineation of the tunica albuginea of the testis.

A variety of other cells may be found within the ovarian stroma, most of which are probably derived from cells of the fibroblastic type (19). Luteinized stromal cells, which lie in the stroma at a distance from the follicles, are found singly or in small nests, most often in the medulla. They are characterized by a polygonal shape, abundant eosinophilic to clear cytoplasm containing variable amounts of lipid, a central round nucleus, and a prominent nucleolus (Fig. 9). Cytoplasmic immunoreactivity for testosterone has been described (68). The numbers of luteinized stromal cells increase during pregnancy and after the menopause, probably secondary to elevated levels of circulating gonadotropins during these periods (22,64). In one autopsy study, luteinized stromal cells were demonstrated after diligent searching in 13% of women under 55 years of age and in one third of women over that age; the frequency of their detection increased with increasing degrees of stromal prolifera-

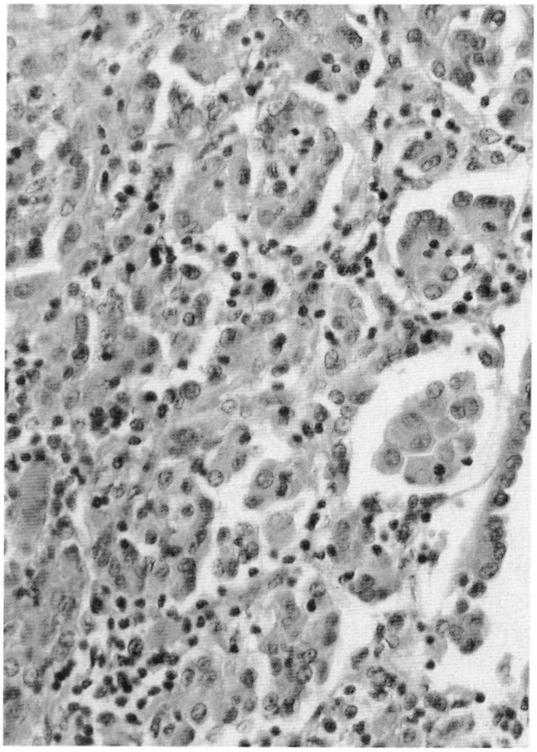

**FIG. 6.** Hyperplastic mesothelial cells on the ovarian surface. Note the admixed inflammatory cells.

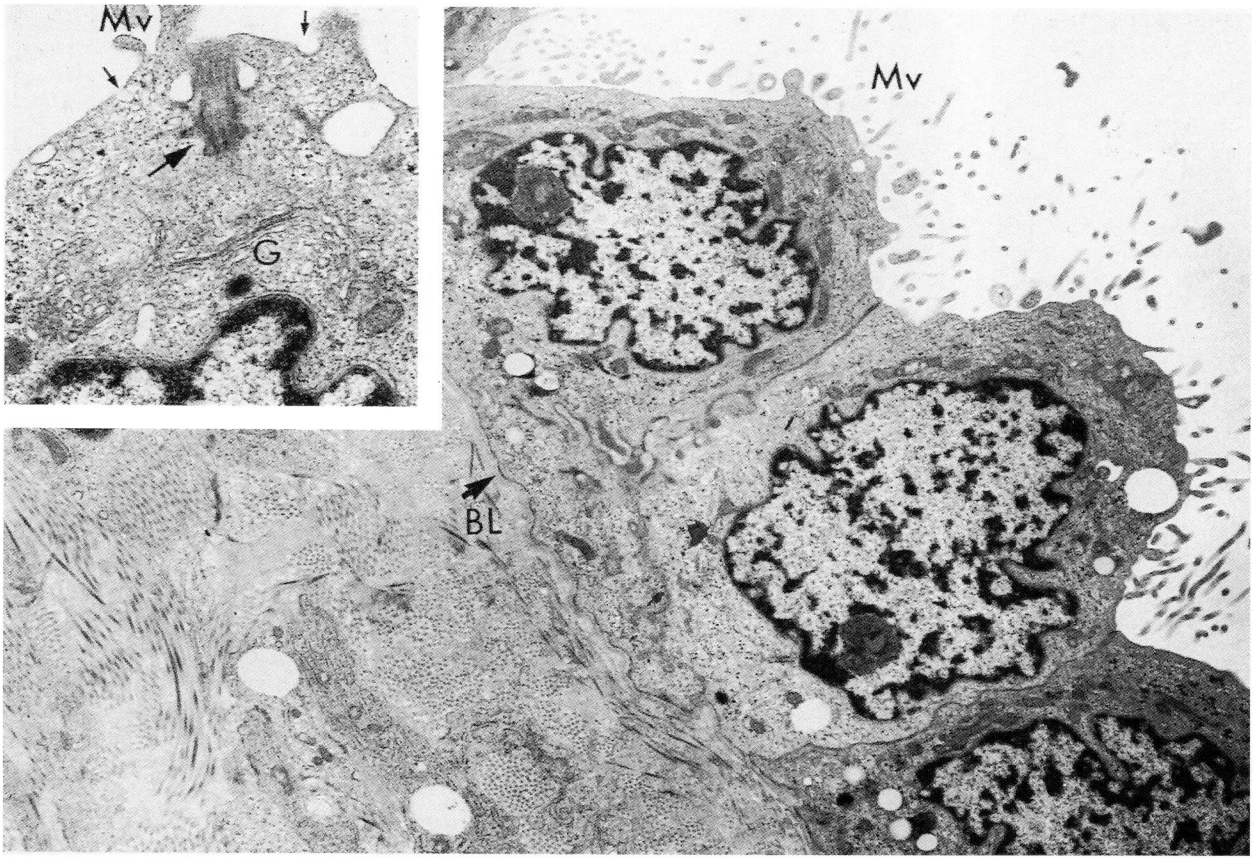


**FIG. 7.** Electron micrograph of ovarian surface epithelium. The cells have numerous microvilli (Mv) and well-developed organelles in a perinuclear location. The nuclei have indented membranes and peripheral nucleoli. The lateral plasma membranes are reinforced by luminal junctional complexes and scattered desmosomes but are occasionally widely separated, producing dilated intercellular spaces. A well-defined basal lamina (BL) separates the cells from the underlying stroma (original magnification ×**6,400**). **Inset:** The surface microvilli are associated with micropinocytotic vesicles (*short arrows*) and occasional single cilia (*long arrow*). Note the Golgi complex (G) (original magnification ×**22,000**). Reprinted with permission (62).

tion (22). More exhaustive sampling might indicate that luteinized stromal cells may be a normal finding in the ovary, particularly in later life. In this age group, the presence of luteinized cells is not usually associated with clinical evidence of a hormonal disturbance. In some older women, but more often in younger patients, however, more striking degrees of stromal luteinization (stromal hyperthecosis) are frequently associated with androgenic and estrogenic manifestations. Occasionally in such cases, nodules of luteinized stromal cells may be appreciable on low-power microscopic examination (nodular hyperthecosis).

Enzymatically active stromal cells (EASCs) are characterized by their oxidative and other enzymatic activity (19,64,69–71). The frequency of their detection and their numbers increase with age, occurring in over 80% of postmenopausal women, typically in the medulla (69,70). Some EASCs correspond to luteinized stromal cells, but most cannot be distinguished from neighboring, nonreactive stromal cells in routine histologic preparations (19,69).

Decidual cells may occur singly, as small nodules, as confluent sheets within the stroma of the superficial cortex, or within periovarian adhesions (Fig. 10). The appearance of the decidual cells is usually identical to eutopic decidua, but occasional examples may exhibit cytologic atypia potentially mimicking metastatic carcinoma on histologic examination (19,72–77). A network of distended capillaries and a sprinkling of lymphocytes are typically present within the decidual foci. A decidual reaction within the ovary is almost always a response of the ovarian stromal cells to elevated circulating or local levels of progesterone; progesterone receptors have been identified in the ovarian stromal cells (38). The process is seen most commonly in pregnancy, occurring as early as the 9th week of gestation, and by term is present in all ovaries. Less commonly it may occur in association with trophoblastic disease, in patients treated with progestagens, in the vicinity of a corpus luteum, or in association with hormonally active, hyperplastic, or neoplastic ovarian lesions (19,22,72,74). Prior pelvic irradiation may be a predisposing factor by increasing the sensitivity of the stromal cells to hormonal stimulation (74). Foci of ovarian decidua have been occasionally described in both pre- and postmenopausal women with no obvious cause (22,74).

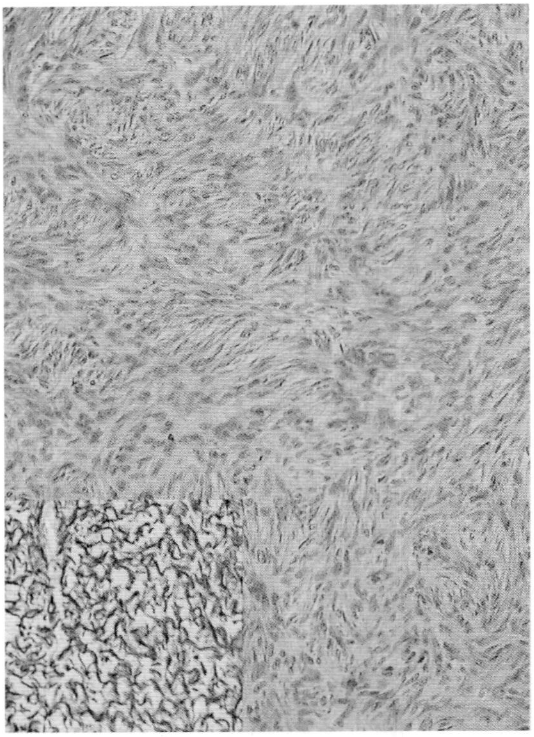

**FIG. 8.** Ovarian stroma composed of whorls of plump spindle cells of fibroblastic type. **Inset:** Note the dense reticulum network (reticulin stain).

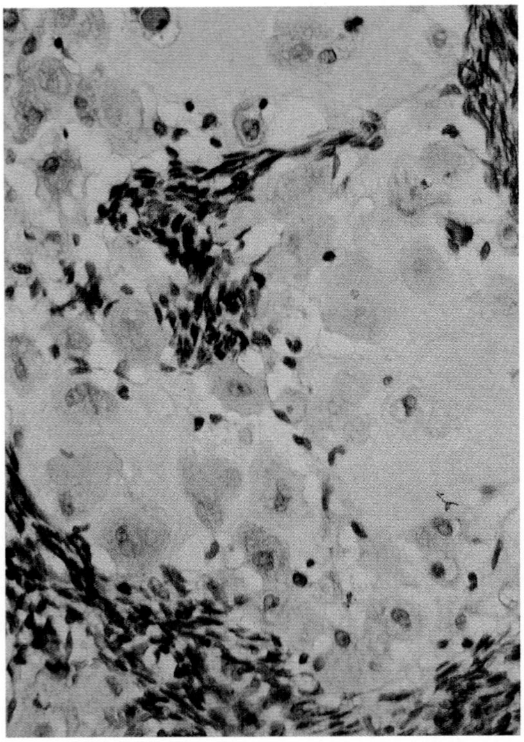

**FIG. 10.** A nest of decidual cells within the ovarian stroma.

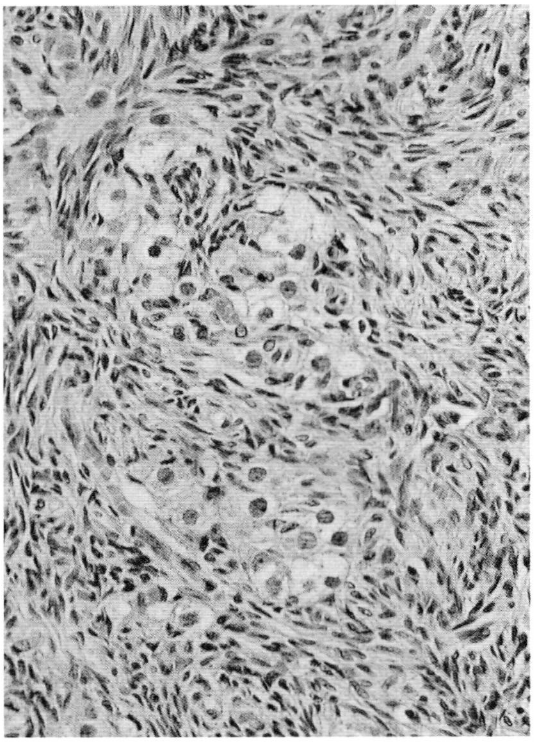

**FIG. 9.** Luteinized stromal cells.

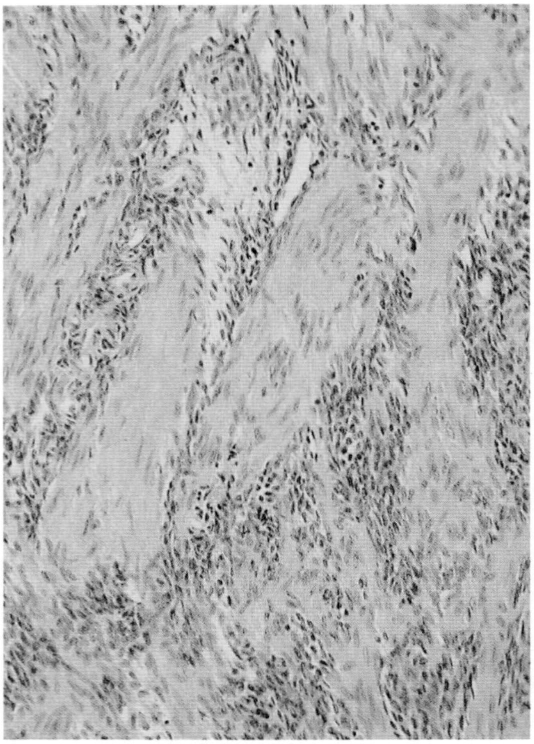

**FIG. 11.** Smooth muscle cells within the ovarian stroma.

Bundles of smooth muscle may be seen within otherwise unremarkable ovarian stroma (Fig. 11), within hyperplastic ovarian stroma such as that typically associated with stromal hyperthecosis or sclerocystic ovaries (78), and within the stroma surrounding non-neoplastic and neoplastic cysts (79). Nests of cells resembling endometrial stromal cells (stromal endometriosis) occur within the ovarian stroma, usually in the absence of typical endometriosis (Fig. 12) (80,81). Foci of mature fat cells may be encountered as an incidental histologic finding within the subcapsular ovarian stroma (82,83); a possible association with obesity was noted in one study (83). Reinke crystal–containing Leydig cells, presumably representing transformed stromal cells, may occur rarely, typically associated with stromal hyperthecosis or within the non-neoplastic stroma in or adjacent to an ovarian neoplasm (84–86). So-called neuroendocrine or amine precursor uptake and decarboxylation (APUD) type cells have been demonstrated within the ovarian stroma in approximately 6% of normal women in one study (87). The cells occur in small groups in the corticomedullary stromal junction and exhibit argyrophilia and argentaffinity. Their clinical significance and hormonal function, if any, is unknown, but it has been suggested that they may represent the cell of origin of rare primary ovarian carcinoid tumors not associated with teratomatous or mucinous elements (87).

### *Aging Changes*

Although there is typically a gradual increase in its volume from the fourth to the seventh decades of life (88), the ovarian stroma in postmenopausal women exhibits a wide spectrum of appearances (22,70,88). At one extreme there is stromal atrophy manifested by a thin cortex and minimal amounts of medullary stroma (Fig. 13). At the other extreme there is marked stromal proliferation warranting the designation "stromal hyperplasia." However, most postmenopausal subjects exhibit varying degrees of nodular or diffuse proliferation of the cortical and medullary stromal cells that lie between these two extremes (Fig. 14) (22,70), making the normal appearance difficult to define.

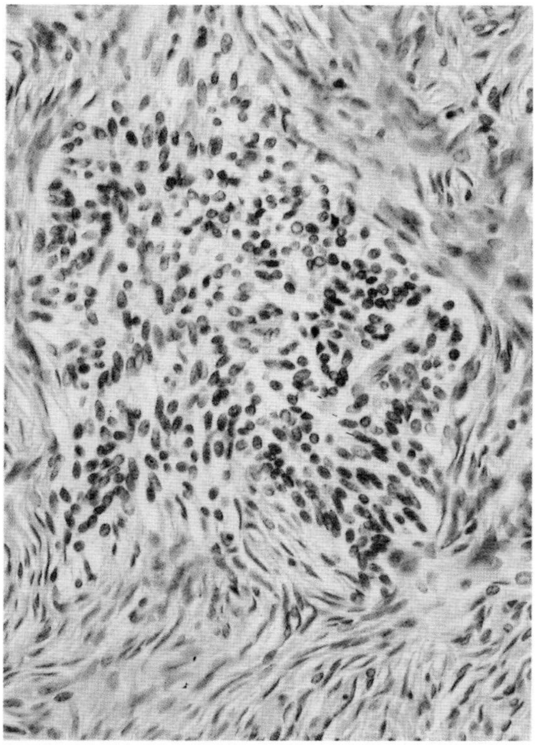

**FIG. 12.** Focus of endometrial stromal cells (stromal endometriosis) within the ovarian cortex.

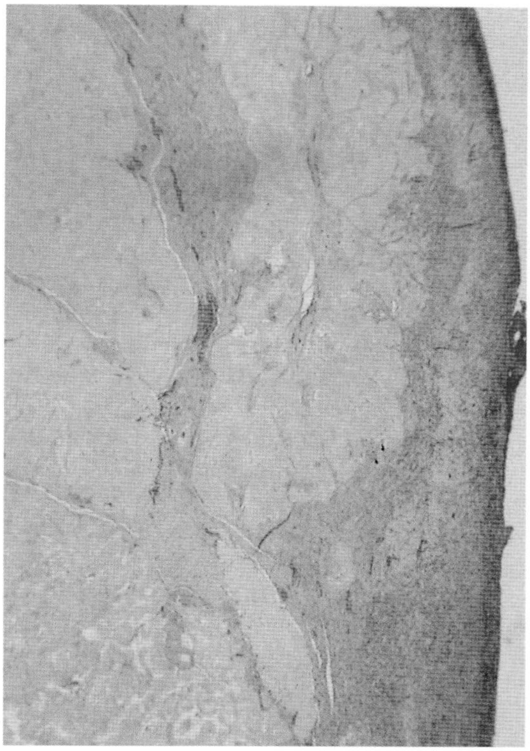

**FIG. 13.** Atrophic postmenopausal ovary. The cortex is thin, and multiple corpora albicantia are present within the medulla.

Broad irregular areas of cortical fibrosis may be encountered in peri- and postmenopausal ovaries (22). When well circumscribed, these foci resemble a small fibroma, but this designation is applied to lesions 1 cm or greater in diameter (19). A similar size limit could be used to distinguish between the foci of surface stromal papillarity commonly encountered in this age group (Fig. 15) and serous surface papillomas. Cortical "granulomas" are common incidental microscopic findings in the late reproductive and postmenopausal age groups, having been demonstrated in up to 45% of women over 40 years of age (22,80,81,89–91). They consist of spherical circumscribed aggregates of epithelioid cells, lymphocytes, and, occasionally, multinucleated giant cells; anisotropic fat crystals also may occur (Fig. 16). Cortical granulomas and the spherical, cloudlike, hyaline scars (Fig. 17) present within the superficial cortical stroma of almost all postmenopausal ovaries are of uncertain histogene-

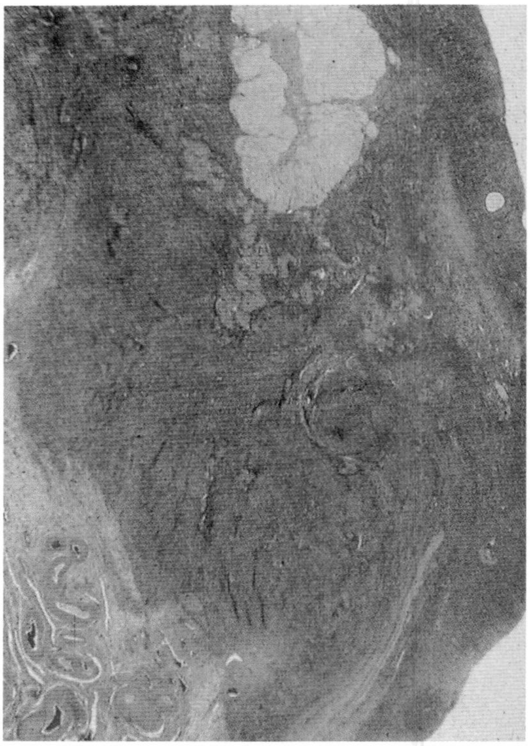

**FIG. 14.** Postmenopausal ovary with a moderate degree of stromal proliferation.

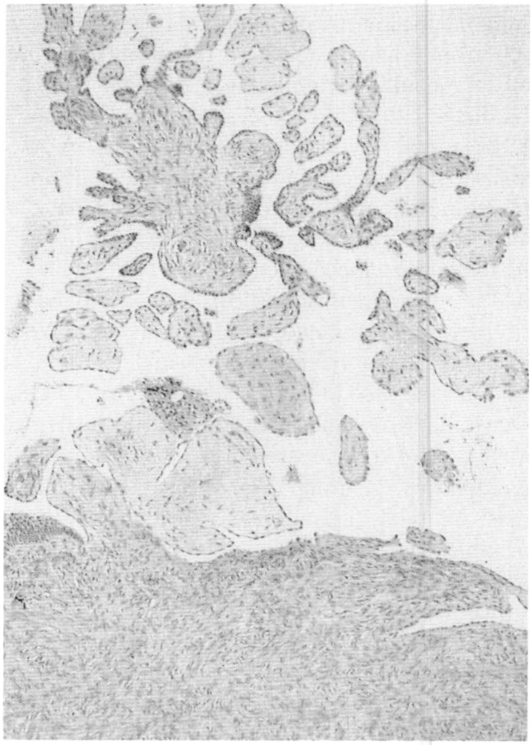

**FIG. 15.** Papillary stromal projections from the ovarian surface.

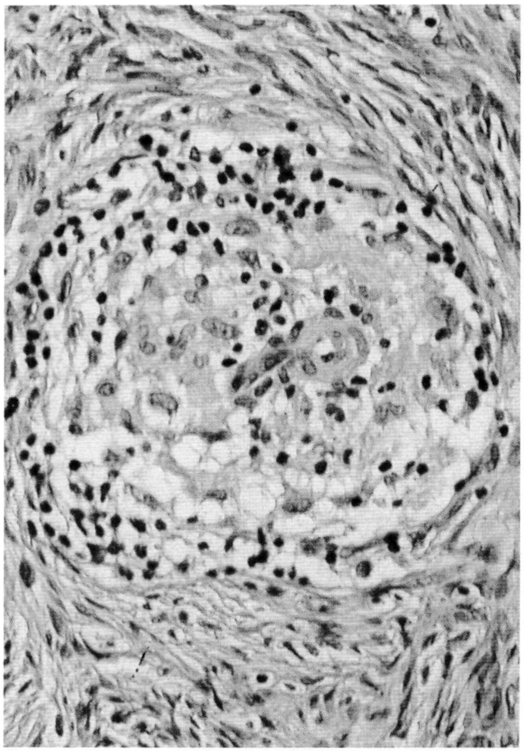

**FIG. 16.** Cortical granuloma.

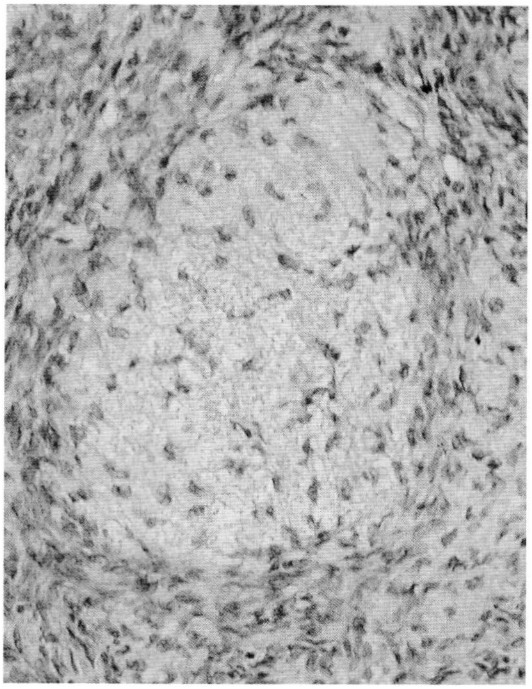

**FIG. 17.** Hyaline scar.

sis. It has been suggested that they may represent regressed foci of stromal endometriosis, ectopic decidua, or luteinized stromal cells.

### Ultrastructure

Typical ovarian stromal cells have slender spindle-shaped nuclei and complex cytoplasmic processes (62,70). Their scant cytoplasm is rich in organelles required for collagen synthesis, including free ribosomes and mitochondria. Tropocollagen, concentrated at the periphery of the cytoplasm, is deposited in the extracellular space and eventually converted to collagen (Fig. 18). Rows of micropinocytotic vesicles occur along the plasma membrane, and desmosome-like attachments may be found between the cells (70). Luteinized stromal cells have abundant cytoplasm containing lipid droplets and steroidogenic organelles, including smooth endoplasmic reticulum (ER), mitochondria with tubular cristae, and Golgi bodies (62,70,71,92). Some cells have ultrastructural features that are intermediate between those of fibroblasts and luteinized cells (62,70). Argyrophilic stromal cells have electron-dense, membrane-bound, 300- to 750-nm cytoplasmic granules (87).

### Hormonal Aspects

Numerous studies have demonstrated the steroidogenic potential and the gonadotropin responsiveness of the ovarian stroma in both pre- and postmenopausal women (93–105). In vitro incubation of ovarian stromal tissue indicates that its principal steroid product is androstenedione, in addition to smaller quantities of testosterone and dehydroepiandrosterone (106). In vitro production of androgens is enhanced by hCG, pituitary gonadotropins, and insulin, consistent with the presence of receptors for these hormones within the stromal cells (68,71,107). To what extent the ovarian stroma contributes to the androgen pool in normal premenopausal women is unknown, but it is likely that it is the source of small amounts of testosterone. With cessation of follicular activity at the time of the menopause, the ovarian stroma becomes, together with the adrenal glands, the major source of androgens. Testosterone and androstenedione are the major androgens secreted by the ovarian stroma in postmenopausal women (93–95,97,105), and in vitro and in vivo studies have shown that ovaries with stromal hyperplasia secrete more androstenedione, estrone, and estradiol (E2) than do nonhyperplastic ovaries (98,100). However, approximately 80% of the circulating levels of androstenedione in postmenopausal women is of adrenal origin (94). Despite a cessation of follicular synthesis of E2 in postmenopausal subjects, small amounts of this hormone are present in the circulation, probably derived from the adrenal glands by peripheral conversion of estrone (94,108) and from the ovarian stroma itself (93,95,109). Estrone, however, becomes the major circulating estrogen after the menopause, derived predominantly from the peripheral aromatization of androstenedione that occurs in fat, muscle, liver, kidney, brain, and adrenals

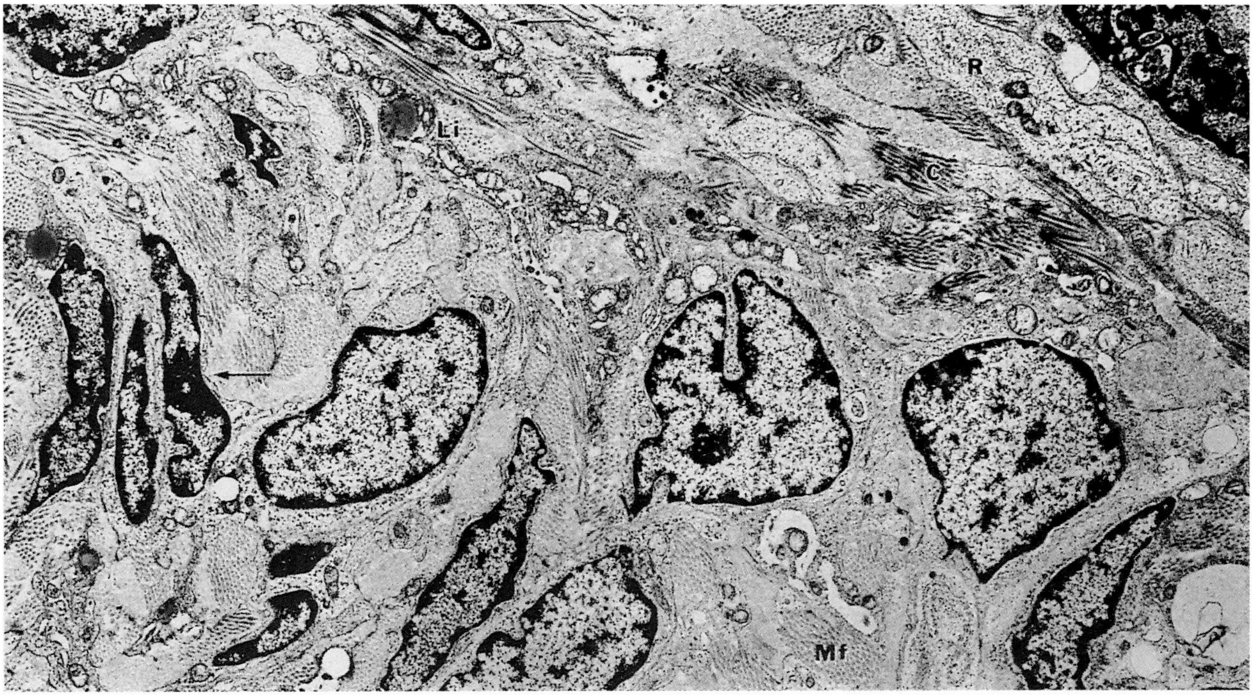


**FIG. 18.** Electron micrograph of ovarian stromal cells. The cells are fibroblastic in type. C, collagen fibers; Mf, tropocollagen; R, free ribosomes; Li, lipid inclusions; *upper arrow*, perinuclear clustering of mitochondria (original magnification ×**3,000**). Reprinted with permission (198).

(94,109,110). Increased aromatization in postmenopausal women, likely due to high levels of endogenous luteinizing hormone (LH) in these subjects, leads to a twofold increase in the daily production rate of estrone compared with that in premenopausal women; aromatization is also higher in obese subjects. In some postmenopausal women, sufficient estrogen is elaborated by this mechanism to prevent the clinical manifestations of estrogen withdrawal and to play a role in the genesis of endometrial carcinoma (88,94). An association between the degree of stromal proliferation and postmenopausal endometrial adenocarcinoma has been noted (88), and the ovarian stroma in postmenopausal women with endometrial adenocarcinoma produces more androgens in vitro than that of control subjects without endometrial cancer (111). The variations that exist in the ovarian steroid hormone output from one postmenopausal woman to another may correspond to similar variations in the morphologic appearance of the stroma in this age group, although no correlative functional and structural studies have been performed.

## PRIMORDIAL FOLLICLES

### Histology

The approximately 400,000 primordial follicles present at the time of birth fill the ovarian cortex (Fig. 19). After this period, their numbers decrease progressively through the processes of atresia and folliculogenesis until their eventual disappearance, which marks the end of the menopause. Rare

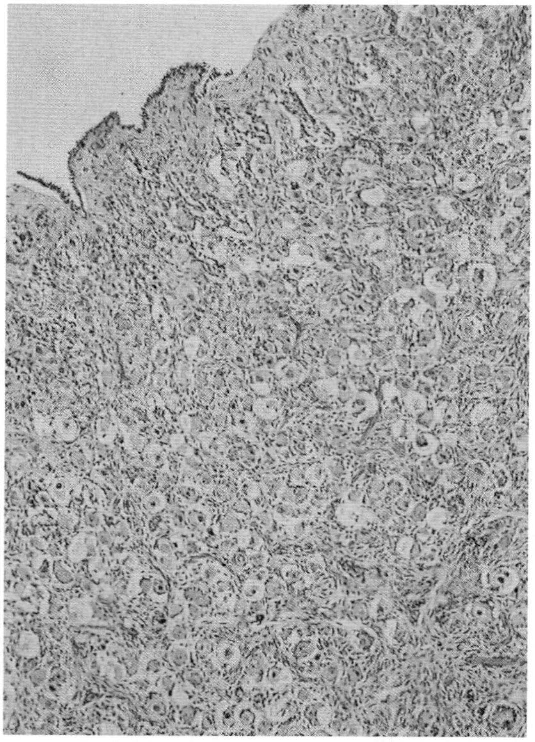

**FIG. 19.** Newborn ovary. Multiple primordial follicles fill the ovarian cortex.

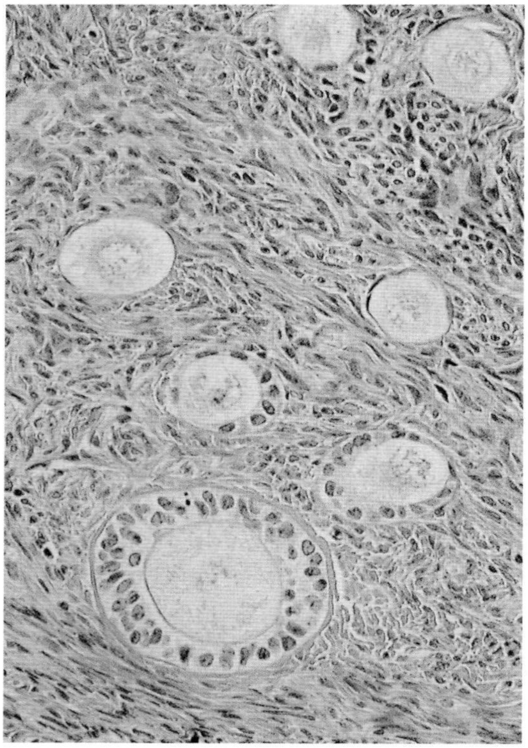

**FIG. 20.** Primordial follicles (four at top) and primary follicles (three at bottom).

follicles may persist for several years after the cessation of menses, however, accounting for sporadic ovulation and occasional episodes of postmenopausal bleeding (112).

In the reproductive era, primordial follicles are found scattered irregularly in clusters throughout a narrow band in the superficial cortex. They consist of a primary oocyte, measuring 40 to 70 $\mu$m in diameter, surrounded by a single layer of flattened, mitotically inactive granulosa cells resting on a thin basal lamina (Fig. 20). Rare primordial (and maturing) follicles may contain multiple oocytes, particularly in individuals younger than 20 years of age (20,113–115). The oocyte is arrested at the dictyate stage of meiotic prophase at the time of birth, entering an interphase period until follicular maturation before ovulation or degeneration of the oocyte during atresia (116). The large spherical nucleus of the oocyte has finely granular, uniformly dispersed chromatin and one or more dense, threadlike nucleoli (116); rare oocytes may have multiple nuclei (114,115). Within the cytoplasm of the oocyte is a paranuclear, eosinophilic, crescent-shaped zone representing a complex of interelated organelles, so-called Balbiani's vitelline body (BVB) (117,118). Within the vitelline body is a dark spot (the centrosome) surrounded by a halo, which in turn is flanked by darker, periodic acid-Schiff (PAS)-positive, granular zones rich in mitochondria (117,118). The cytoplasm of the oocyte lacks the abundant glycogen and the high alkaline phosphatase activity characteristic of the primordial germ cells and the oogonia of the embryonic gonad (19).

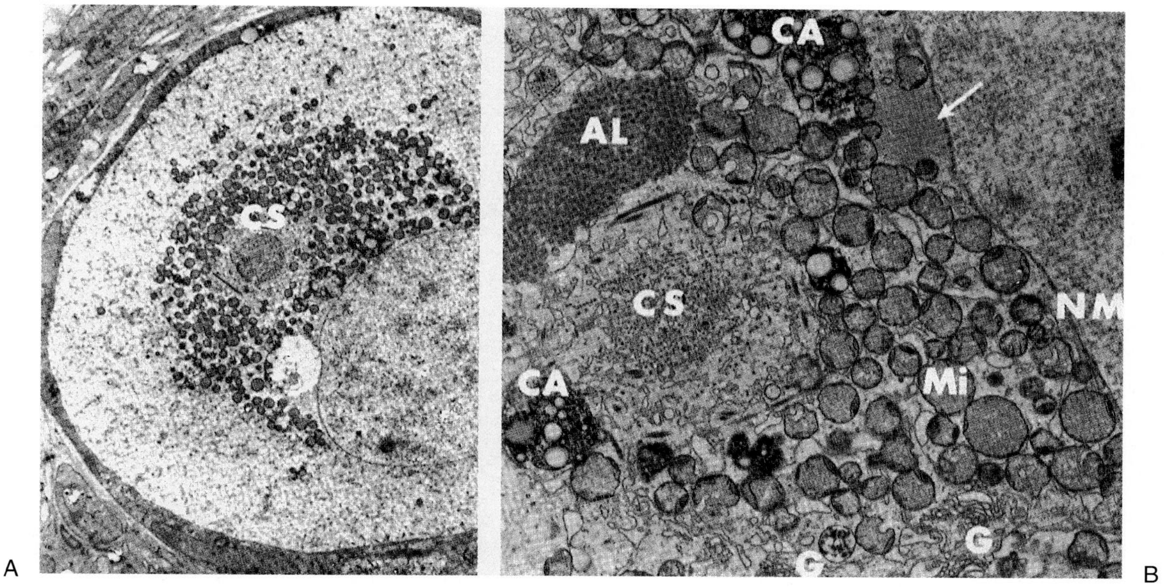


**FIG. 21.** Electron micrograph of a primordial follicle. **A:** Balbiani's vitelline body consists of a juxtanuclear centrosome (CS) surrounded by a condensation of mitochondria, Golgi complexes, ER, and lysosomes (original magnification ×2,400). **B:** Detailed view of Balbiani's vitelline body. A cluster of closely packed spiral fibrils (*arrow*) is attached to the nuclear envelope (NM). The centrosome (CS) is composed of dense granules, some arranged periodically on fine fibers, and small vesicles, with a peripheral zone of ER and dense fibers. Surrounding the centrosome are masses of mitochondria (Mi) and compound aggregates (CA). A stack of annulate lamellae (AL) is seen tangentially. Note the prominent ER in close association with multiple Golgi complexes (G) at the periphery of the vitelline body. Reprinted with permission (117).

### Ultrastructure

The granulosa cells of the primordial follicle have sparse organelles, occasional desmosomal attachments with each other, and microvillous projections that attach to the oocyte through tight apposition (62). Within the oocyte, the juxtanuclear centrosome of BVB (Fig. 21) consists of dense granules, closely packed vesicles, and dense fibers that form a basketlike structure at the periphery of the centrosome (Fig. 21B) (117,118). The centrosome is surrounded by a zone of smooth ER, which represents the halo seen by light microscopy. More peripherally and constituting the rest of BVB are a concentration of most of the oocyte's organelles, including multiple Golgi complexes, prominent compound aggregates, numerous mitochondria intimately associated with sparsely granular ER, and annulate lamellae (Fig. 21B) (117,118). The latter structures, which may be attached or immediately adjacent to the nucleus or free within BVB, are constantly present in primary oocytes and other rapidly growing embryonal or neoplastic cells. They are arranged in stacks or concentric arrangements of up to 100 parallel, smooth, paired membranes, which delineate greatly flattened cisternal spaces 30 to 50 $\mu$m wide. At regularly spaced intervals, the paired membranes of each lamellar unit become fused with one another (116). When the lamellae are sectioned along a tangential plane, the sites of apposition of the membranes are seen as regularly spaced annuli 100 nm in diameter. At their periphery they are connected to the granular ER (117). The paired membranes of the annulate lamellae mimic the two leaflets of the nuclear membrane, and it is likely that they are formed from its outer leaflet (62,116,117). Their function is not known with certainty, but it has been suggested that they may have a role in nucleocytoplasmic exchange of substances related to metabolic activity or the transfer of genetic information (62,117).

In some oocytes, Golgi bodies, ER, and mitochondria also may be found outside the vitelline body, closely applied to the entire circumference of the nucleus (117). Similarly, microtubules present throughout the oocyte cytoplasm are most prevalent around the circumference of the nuclear membrane. Bundles of spiral filaments occasionally abut the nuclear membrane (Fig. 21B) or are seen in the more peripheral cytoplasm (118). A variety of different vacuoles also may be seen in the peripheral cytoplasm, some containing multiple small vesicles (117).

## MATURING FOLLICLES

### Histology and Ultrastructure

#### *Folliculogenesis*

Folliculogenesis refers to the continuous process occurring throughout reproductive life whereby cohorts of primordial follicles undergo maturation during each menstrual cycle. Follicular maturation begins during the luteal phase and continues throughout the follicular phase of the next cycle. Each month only one such follicle, the preovulatory (or dominant) follicle, achieves complete maturation, culminating in the release of the oocyte (ovulation). The other follicles that have begun the maturational process undergo atresia at earlier stages of their development. Folliculogenesis and atresia also occur prenatally, throughout childhood, and during pregnancy, although maturing follicles rarely reach the preovulatory follicle stage during these periods (20,119–127).

The first morphologic evidence of follicular maturation is the assumption of a cuboidal to columnar shape by the surrounding layer of granulosa cells accompanied by enlargement of the oocyte (primary follicle) (Fig. 20). Mitotic activity in the granulosa cells results in their stratification and three to five concentric layers around the oocyte (secondary or preantral follicle) (Fig. 22). At this stage an eosinophilic, PAS-positive, homogeneous, acellular layer, the zona pellucida, appears, encasing the oocyte. Its formation is usually attributed to the granulosa cells, but the oocyte also may play a role. At the end of its development, the zona pellucida is a membrane 20 to 25 $\mu$m thick and rich in acid mucopolysaccharides and glycoprotein (Figs. 22–25) (62). Preantral follicles measure 50 to 400 $\mu$m in diameter, and as they increase in size, they migrate into the deeper cortex and medulla. Simultaneously, the surrounding ovarian stromal cells become specialized into several layers of theca interna cells and an outer, ill-defined layer of theca externa cells. Secretion of mucopolysaccharide-rich fluid by the granulosa cells results in their separation by fluid-filled clefts. The latter eventually coalesce to form a single large cavity or antrum lined by several layers of granulosa cells (tertiary, antral, or vesicular follicle). The first evidence of antrum formation occurs in follicles measuring 200 to 400 $\mu$m in diameter, after which the follicles progressively enlarge due to continued fluid secretion into the antrum. Concurrently, the oocyte enlarges to its definitive size and assumes an eccentric position at one pole of the follicle. At this site the granulosa cells proliferate to form the cumulus oophorus, which, containing the oocyte in its center, protrudes into the antrum (mature or Graafian follicle) (Fig. 23).

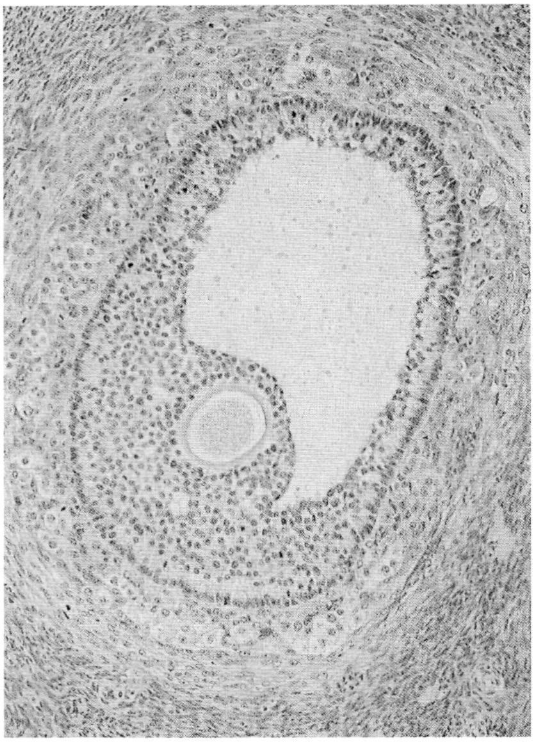

**FIG. 23.** Mature follicle. Oocyte within cumulus oophorous projects into antrum. The theca layers are well developed.

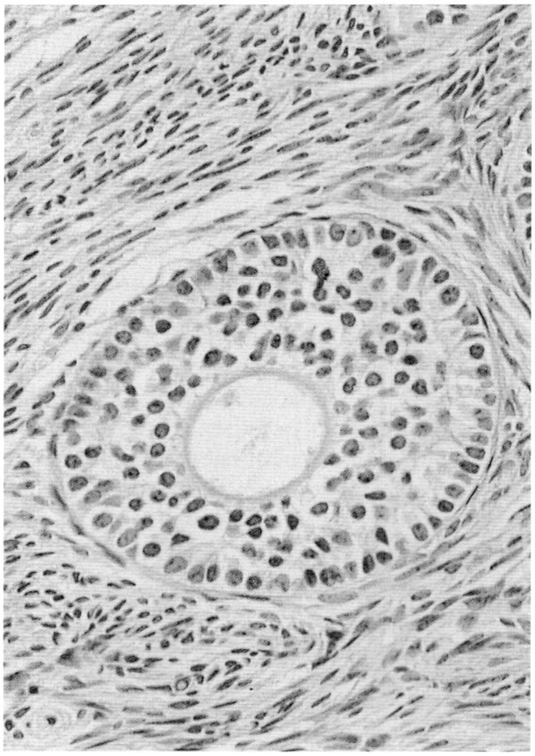

**FIG. 22.** Preantral follicle. Several layers of granulosa cells surround the oocyte. A theca interna layer is not yet apparent.

### *Ovulation*

During each cycle, only a small number of mature follicles (fewer than four per ovary) reach a diameter of 4 to 5 mm by the mid- to late luteal phase; one of them becomes the preovulatory follicle of the subsequent cycle (128,129). Late in follicular growth, the oocyte, its surrounding zona pellucida, and a single layer of radially disposed, columnar granulosa cells (the corona radiata) detach from the cumulus oophorus and float in the antral fluid. The preovulatory follicle shortly before ovulation reaches a diameter of 15 to 25 mm (29,129). It partially protrudes from the ovarian surface at a point that

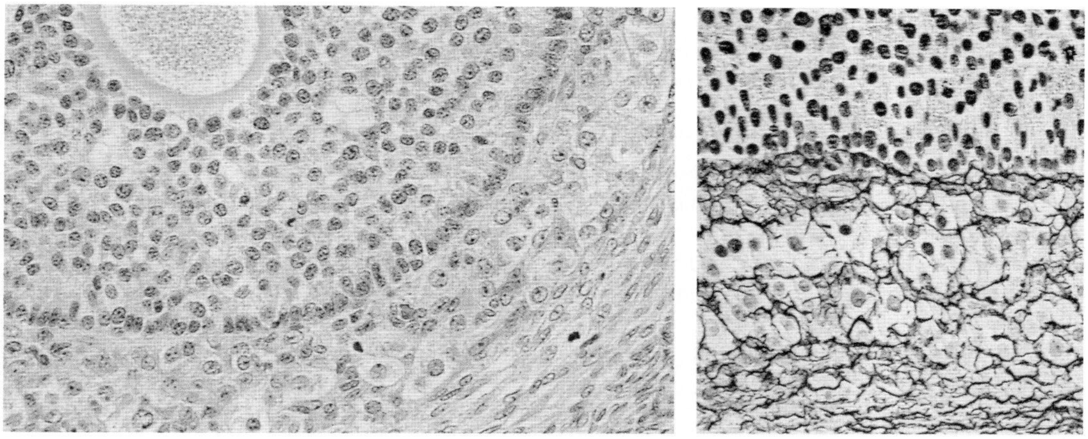


**FIG. 24. A:** Mature follicle, high-power view. The granulosa layer, which contains several Call-Exner bodies, abuts the zona pellucida of the oocyte. The granulosa layer is surrounded by a layer of luteinized theca interna cells. Note the mitotic figures in granulosa and theca cells. **B:** There is a reticulum network in the theca interna layer but an absence of reticulin in the granulosa layer.

represents the eventual rupture point, or stigma. Here the overlying surface epithelial cells exhibit progressive flattening, degeneration, and desquamation (29). The stroma in this area becomes attenuated and almost avascular, with degeneration of the stromal cells, fragmentation of collagen fibers, and an accumulation of intercellular fluid (29). These surface epithelial and stromal changes that immediately precede ovulation may be secondary to local ischemia and release of proteolytic enzymes and prostaglandins into the stroma (29). The preovulatory follicle then ruptures, possibly secondary to contraction of the perifollicular smooth muscle cells, with liberation of the follicular fluid and oocyte (with its sur-

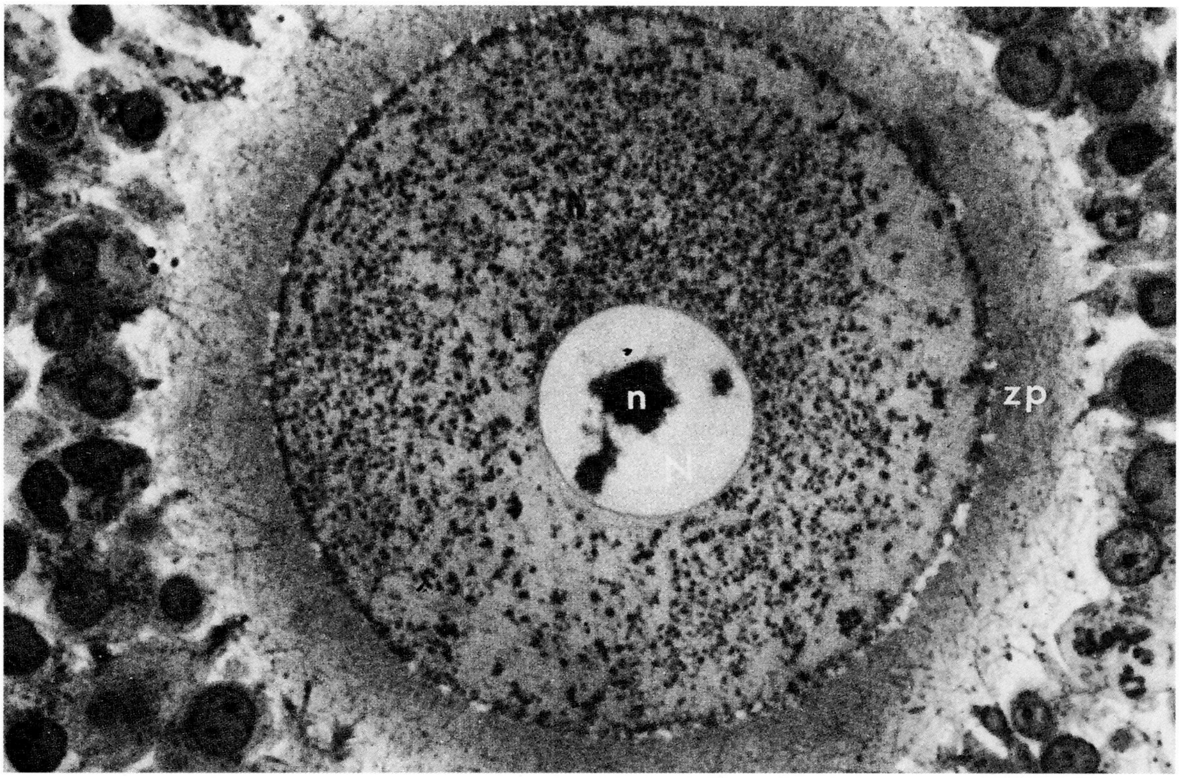


**FIG. 25.** Maturing oocyte. Note the uniform distribution of the organelles and the row of dense granules in the cytoplasm immediately subjacent to the plasma membrane of the oocyte. A continuous zona pellucida (zp) surrounds the oocyte and separates it from the granulosa cells. Numerous cytoplasmic processes of the granulosa cells are visible within the zona pellucida. N, nucleus; n, nucleolus. Thick section, $OsO_4$ fixed, Epon-embedded, toluidine blue stain. Reprinted with permission (116).

rounding layers) into the peritoneal cavity. After ovulation, the stigma is occluded by a mass of coagulated follicular fluid, fibrin, blood, granulosa, and connective tissue cells; it is eventually converted to scar tissue.

Shortly before ovulation, the oocyte within the ovulatory follicle enters telophase of the first meiotic division. Chromosomal reduction occurs by migration of one half the oocyte chromosomes into a portion of the oocyte cytoplasm, which separates from the cell as the first polar body. The first meiotic division begun in fetal life is now complete, and the oocyte is now designated the secondary oocyte. Immediately after expulsion of the first polar body, the secondary oocyte enters the second meiotic division, arresting at metaphase until fertilization occurs.

### *Granulosa Layer*

Granulosa cells are almost entirely formed from their embryonic precursors by the time of birth (19). Those within maturing and mature follicles are polyhedral cells 5 to 7 μm in diameter. Cells resting on the basement membrane are often columnar in shape. They have pale, scant cytoplasm, indistinct cell borders, and small, round to oval, hyperchromatic nuclei that typically lack nuclear grooves (Fig. 24A) (130). Mitotic figures within granulosa cells are usually numerous in maturing follicles, decreasing in numbers before ovulation. Until the onset of luteinization several hours before ovulation, cytoplasmic lipid is absent (or sparse), as are steroidogenic histochemical patterns (131,132). The cytoplasm of granulosa cells of primary, secondary, and mature follicles are immunoreactive for cytokeratin, vimentin, and desmoplakin (34,36,37).

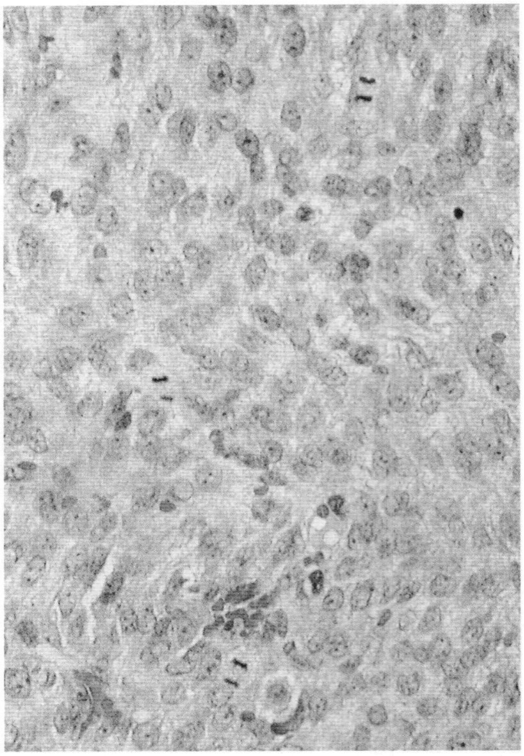

**FIG. 26.** Theca externa of mature follicle composed of plump spindle cells. Note the mitotic figures.

The granulosa cells typically surround small cavities, Call-Exner bodies (Fig. 24A), which have a distinctive appearance, representing one of the most specific features of granulosa cells, both normal and neoplastic. Call-Exner bodies are delimited from the granulosa cells by a basal lamina, and typically contain a deeply eosinophilic, PAS-positive, filamentous material consisting of excess basal lamina (19,23,62). Unlike the theca layers, the granulosa layer of the maturing and Graafian follicles is avascular and devoid of a reticulum framework (Fig. 24B).

Mitochondria with lamelliform cristae, granular ER, free ribosomes, and Golgi bodies gradually increase in abundance within the granulosa cells of maturing follicles (23). These ultrastructural features suggest active protein synthesis. Histochemical and ultrastructural features (abundant smooth ER and mitochondria with tubular cristae) indicative of steroid biosynthesis are absent until shortly before ovulation (64,69,131–134). The granulosa cells of follicles of varying stages contain adherent junctions, gap junctions, and desmosomes between adjacent granulosa cells (36,62,116). The slender cytoplasmic extensions of the granulosa cells of the corona radiata that traverse the zona pellucida have gap junctions and puncta adhaerentia with the plasma membrane of the oocyte (Fig. 25) (36,62,116).

### *Theca Layers*

In contrast to granulosa cells, theca cells differentiate continuously from the stromal cells at the periphery of developing follicles from fetal life until the termination of the menopause (19). The thecal component of the antral follicle is characterized by a well-developed theca interna and a less well defined theca externa.

The theca interna layer is three or four cells in thickness and lies external to the granulosa layer (Fig. 24A), from which it is separated by a basement membrane. Unlike the granulosa cells of the developing and mature follicles, the theca interna cells typically have a luteinized or partially luteinized appearance (Fig. 24A) and exhibit steroidogenic histochemical patterns (19,64,131–133). Luteinization of the theca interna of maturing follicles is particularly prominent during pregnancy. The round to polygonal cells are 12 to 20 μm in diameter and have abundant, eosinophilic to clear, vacuolated cytoplasm containing variable amounts of lipid; a central, round, vesicular nucleus typically contains a single, prominent nucleolus (Fig. 24A). The cells differ from granulosa cells but resemble stromal cells in being immunoreactive for vimentin but not cytokeratin (37). Mitotic figures are typically present with the theca cells of maturing follicles. The layer contains a rich vascular plexus consisting of dilated capillaries, as well as a dense reticulum that surrounds each cell (Fig. 24B). Tangential sections through the theca interna may result in seemingly isolated nodules of luteinized theca cells that may occasionally be misinterpreted as foci of stromal luteinization.

The theca externa is an ill-defined layer of variable thickness that surrounds the theca interna and merges almost imperceptibly with the adjacent ovarian stroma. It is composed of circumferentially arranged collagen bundles, blood and lymphatic vessels, and plump spindle cells that lack steroidogenic histochemical features (135). The spindle cells of the theca externa are typically highly mitotic and have been misinterpreted as early fibrosarcoma, particularly when only the edge of the follicle is seen microscopically (Fig. 26).

Ultrastructural examination of theca interna cells shows the organelles to be associated with steroidogenesis, similar to those within granulosa-lutein cells. The theca externa cells, some of which exhibit smooth muscle differentiation, lack such organelles (136).

### Hormonal Aspects

The initiation of folliculogenesis and early preantral follicular development are independent of gonadotropin influence, whereas the later stages of follicular maturation are under gonadotropin control. As a small antral follicle develops into a preovulatory follicle, the sequence of endocrine events within its antral fluid differs from most, if not all, other antral follicles in the same ovary (137,138). The early stages of this development are reflected by increasing concentrations of follicle-stimulating hormone (FSH) receptors and intrafollicular FSH within the preovulatory follicle (137–140). There is a concomitant increase in E2 receptors within the granulosa cells and the E2 level within the follicular fluid. The latter reaches peak concentration (10,000 times the circulating level) during the mid- to late proliferative phase (137–139) when plasma FSH decreases to a basal level. At this stage the preovulatory follicle is self-sustaining, continuing to mature under the influence of intrafollicular FSH and E2 (102). During the late proliferative phase, plasma LH rises and LH receptors within the granulosa cells of the preovulatory follicle, but not other follicles, become apparent (140). In contrast, LH receptors are present within the theca cells of all follicles throughout the follicular phase (140). Eden et al. found concentrations of insulin-like growth factor (IGF1) to be significantly higher in the follicular fluid of preovulatory follicles than in their matched cohorts and suggested that IGF1 may have a role in the selection of the dominant follicle (141).

Whereas circulating E2 is likely derived from both the granulosa cells and the LH-stimulated theca cells, intrafollicular E2 is derived almost exclusively from the granulosa cells by both de novo synthesis and by FSH-dependent aromatization of theca-derived androstenedione (102,142). Aromatase activity is highest in the preovulatory follicle, thereby maintaining a high E2:androstenedione ratio (137,138,143). In contrast, follicles that will undergo atresia are FSH and aromatase deficient and have high androstenedione:E2 ratios within their intrafollicular fluid. High circulating estrogen levels initiate a preovulatory surge of plasma LH (144,145), which induces luteinization of the granulosa cells, an increase in intrafollicular progesterone concentration, and a small preovulatory rise in circulating progesterone (137,138,146). The rising plasma progesterone level and the peaking estrogen level further augment the LH surge and initiate a smaller increase in FSH, triggering ovulation. The latter has been estimated to occur 36 to 38 hours after the onset of the LH surge, 24 to 36 hours after the E2 peak, and 10 to 12 hours after the LH peak (146).

The ovarian follicles also produce nonsteroidal hormones. Inhibin, a glycoprotein synthesized by the granulosa cells, is secreted into the follicular fluid and ovarian venous effluent in amounts that correlate with steroid levels (146–148). Inhibin, which is predominantly under the control of LH (149), reduces, by negative feedback, FSH secretion from the hypothalamic–pituitary unit. High concentrations of prorenin are present within the fluid of mature follicles (150), and their granulosa cells, as well as theca and stromal cells, are immunoreactive for renin and angiotensin II (151). The function, if any, of the renin–angiotensin system within the ovary is currently unknown.

## CORPUS LUTEUM OF MENSTRUATION

After ovulation on the 14th day of the typical 28-day menstrual cycle, and in the absence of fertilization, the collapsed ovulatory follicle becomes the corpus luteum of menstruation (CLM). When mature, the CLM is a 1.5- to 2.5-cm, round, yellow structure with festooned contours and a cystic center filled with a gray, focally hemorrhagic coagulum.

### Histology

During the 14 days after ovulation, the CLM undergoes an orderly sequence of histologic changes, which allows an approximate estimation of its age. Corner has described these stages in detail, using endometrial histology and menstrual data to establish the age of the CLM (152,153). A subsequent study that correlated the histologic date of the CLM (using Corner's criteria) with the interval between the LH peak and the biopsy of the CLM, determined that the use of the histology of the CLM for retrospective timing of ovulation is subject to an error of variable magnitude due to the unequal duration of each stage as well as considerable individual variation (154).

In contrast to the granulosa cells of the maturing and preovulatory follicles, the luteinized granulosa cells of the mature CLM (granulosa-lutein cells) are large (30 to 35 $\mu$m) polygonal cells with abundant, pale eosinophilic cytoplasm that may contain numerous small lipid droplets (Figs. 27 and 28) (135). The spherical nucleus contains one or two large nucleoli. The histochemical pattern of these cells varies with the age of the CLM but is generally typical of steroid hor-

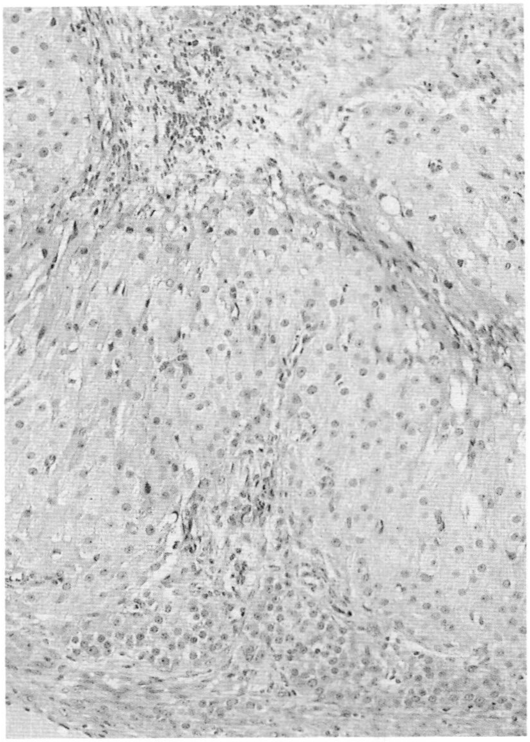

**FIG. 27.** Mature corpus luteum of menstruation. The lining is composed of a thick layer of large granulosa-lutein cells and an outer, thinner layer of smaller theca-lutein cells. The cavity (*top*) contains erythrocytes and fibrin.

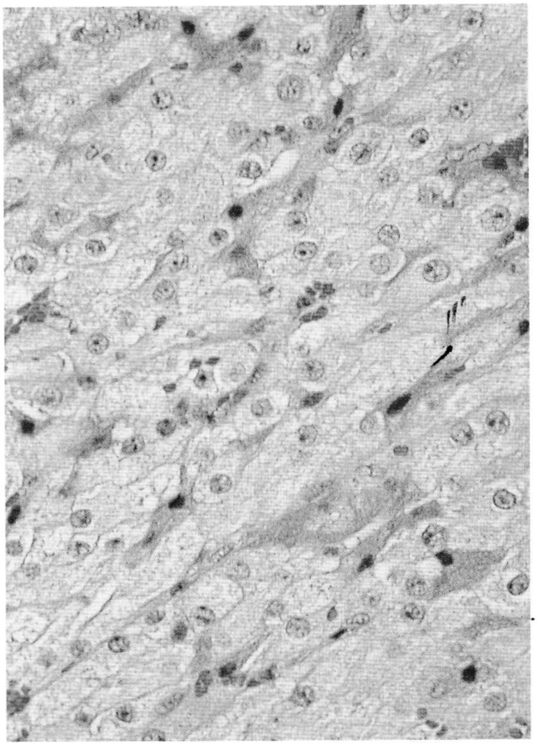

**FIG. 28.** Mature corpus luteum of menstruation. K cells with darkly staining cytoplasm and pyknotic nuclei are interspersed between granulosa-lutein cells.

mone-producing cells (64,132,133,155). The cytoplasm of luteinized granulosa cells contains vimentin but, in contrast to granulosa cells of maturing and mature follicles, little or no cytokeratin (36).

The theca interna forms an irregular and often interrupted layer several cells in thickness around the circumference of the CLM (Fig. 27) and ensheaths the vascular septa that extend into its center (135). When these septa are cut in cross section, triangular nests of theca cells appear at intervals throughout the granulosa layer. In all but the earliest stages of the CLM, the theca-lutein cells are approximately half the size of the granulosa-lutein cells. They contain a round to oval nucleus with a single prominent nucleolus. Their less abundant, more darkly staining cytoplasm contains lipid droplets, which are usually larger than those in the granulosa-lutein cells, and exhibits steroidogenic histochemical patterns (132).

A third type of cell, the so-called K cell present in small numbers within the theca interna of the mature follicle, appears in greater numbers within the granulosa layer of the early CLM (130). K cells persist until menstruation, at which time they degenerate. They are characterized by a stellate shape, a deeply eosinophilic cytoplasm, and an irregular, hyperchromatic, or pyknotic nucleus (Fig. 28). The cytoplasm is uniformly sudanophilic due to the presence of phospholipid (130). K cells lack the histochemical patterns of

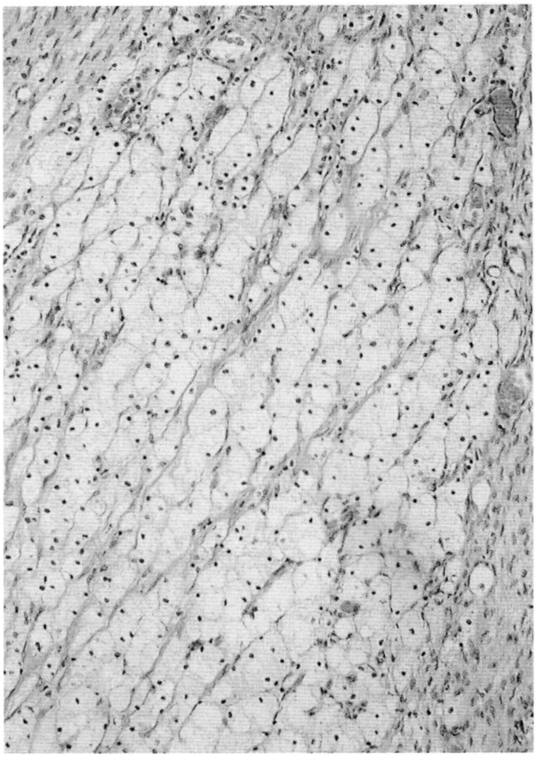

**FIG. 29.** Degenerating corpus luteum of menstruation. Granulosa-lutein cells have pyknotic nuclei and abundant cytoplasmic lipid.

steroidogenic cells and have been shown to be T-lymphocytes (156).

During the maturation of the CLM, capillaries originating from the theca interna layer penetrate the granulosa layer and reach the central cavity. Fibroblasts that accompany the vessels form an increasingly dense reticulum network within the granulosa layer as well as an inner fibrous layer that lines the central cavity (Fig. 27) (33).

Involutional changes begin on the 8th or 9th day after ovulation (152). The granulosa-lutein cells decrease in size, develop pyknotic nuclei, and accumulate abundant cytoplasmic lipid (Fig. 29). There is a decrease in histochemical staining of enzymes associated with steroid biosynthesis and an increase in hydrolytic enzymes (133). Eventually the cells undergo dissolution and are phagocytosed (157). There is progressive fibrosis and shrinkage over a period of several months and eventual conversion to a corpus albicans.

### Ultrastructure

At the ultrastructural level, luteinization is characterized by a gradually increasing content of steroidogenic organelles, specifically smooth ER and abundant mitochondria with tubular cristae (Fig. 30) (135,157–160). The smooth ER exhibits a characteristic regional modification in the form of a folded membrane complex consisting of highly folded, radiating, tubular cisternae that communicate and interdigitate with adjacent cisternae (159). Well-developed, dispersed, and perinuclear Golgi bodies, free and bound ribosomes, lipid droplets, and lipofuschin pigment also are seen (Fig. 30) (135,157–160). The cells are separated by a narrow space of variable width, but occasionally the outer leaflets of their plasma membranes become closely apposed and reinforced by desmosomal and pentalaminar tight junctional complexes (135,157,160). Nearly all the cells have a free surface which borders on a broad pericapillary space from which they are separated by an interrupted basal lamina (135). Many irregular microvillous cytoplasmic extensions project into these pericapillary, as well as the intercellular, spaces (Fig. 30) (62,135,157,159). Occasional interdigitation of these microvilli has been noted between adjacent cells to form intercellular channels (159). Underlying the microvilli is a narrow zone of cytoplasm filled with a network of filaments that also extend into the microvilli (135).

Theca-lutein cells are similar ultrastructurally to granulosa-lutein cells except for the presence of localized perinuclear Golgi bodies and the absence of folded membrane complexes, microvilli, and a network of fine filaments (135,159). The varying degrees of cell density appreciable on histologic examination also are seen at the ultrastructural

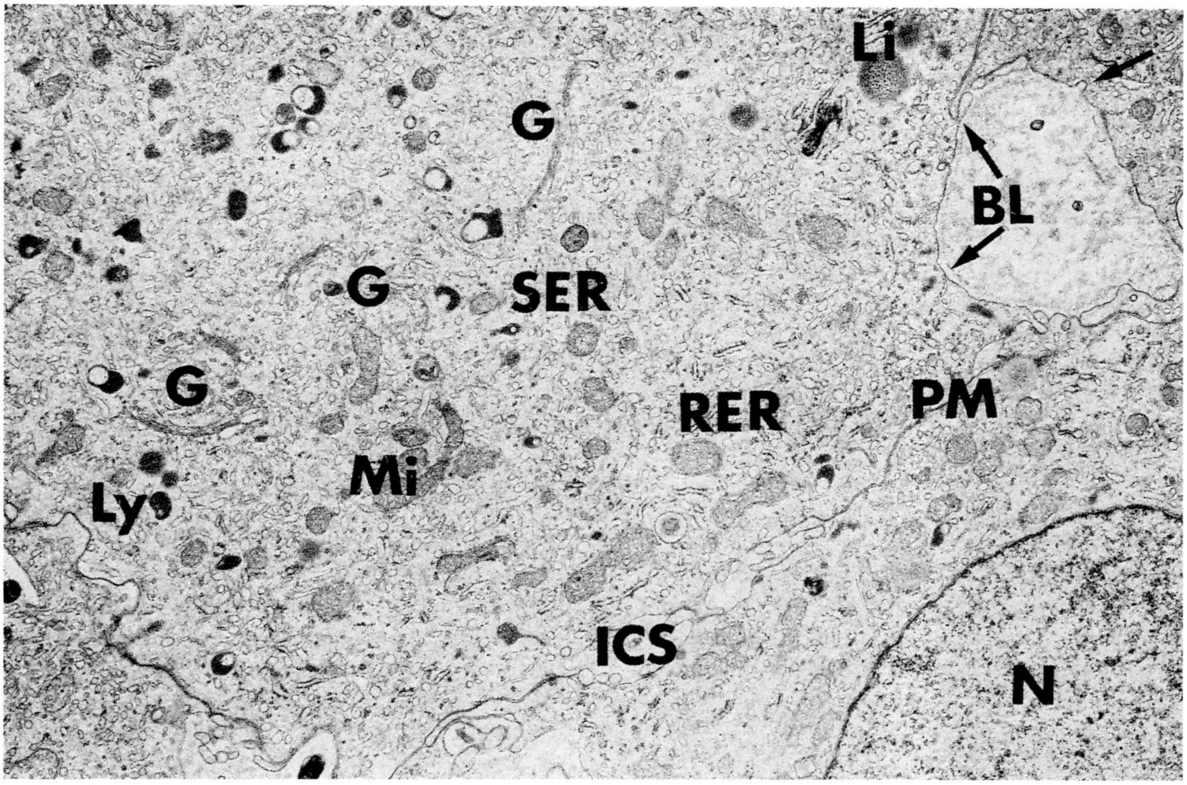


**FIG. 30.** Electron micrograph of granulosa-lutein cell of a mature corpus luteum of menstruation. Note the abundant smooth ER (SER), mitochondria (Mi), Golgi complex (G), rough ER (RER), lipid droplets (Li), and intercellular space (ICS). BL, basal lamina; N, nucleus of granulosa-lutein cells; Ly, lysosomes; PM, plasma membrane; *arrow*, micropinocytotic vesicle (original magnification ×**3,600**). Reprinted with permission (62).

level and may represent an artifact of fixation (135). The theca externa layer of the CLM does not differ significantly from that of the graafian follicle.

The lutein cells of the degenerating CLM exhibit disorganization and fragmentation of the smooth ER, alterations of the mitochondria, and an increase in cytolysosomes (62). Lipid droplets are increased and irregular in size and show increased osmiophilia (157).

### Hormonal Aspects

The formation and function of the CLM is under the control of LH, reflected by the high content of LH receptors within the granulosa-lutein cells (140,146). Receptors for FSH (140) and growth hormone (158) also have been identified in the corpus luteum, although their roles in luteal function are unknown. Although progesterone is the major steroid formed in vivo and in vitro by the CLM, it also synthesizes, both in vitro and in vivo, estrone and E2, as well as androgens, mostly androstenedione (161).

After ovulation, LH, FSH, and E2 levels decrease, but the LH concentration is sufficient to maintain the CLM, producing a mid-luteal peak in progesterone and E2 concentration. If fertilization does not occur, the increased levels of progesterone and estrogen through negative feedback result in a decrease of LH and FSH to basal levels, a reduction in LH and FSH receptors within the CLM, and a marked decline in progesterone and E2 synthesis after the 22nd day of the cycle (139,140,146,162,163). These changes are reflected by the morphologic involution of the CLM and the onset of menses. Luteolysis appears to be estrogen related, possibly secondary to an estrogen-induced reduction in LH receptors or by enhancement of the luteolytic action of prostaglandins synthesized by the CLM (146,164). A nonsteroidal LH receptor–binding inhibitor, which increases in concentration during the luteal phase, also may play a role (146).

## CORPUS LUTEUM OF PREGNANCY

### Gross Appearance

On gross inspection, the corpus luteum of pregnancy (CLP) may be indistinguishable from the CLM but is usually larger and bright yellow in contrast to the orange–yellow of the late CLM (165). The larger size, which may account for up to one half the ovarian volume, is due primarily to the presence of a central cystic cavity filled with fluid or a coagulum composed of fibrin and blood (76,125,166). However, the cavity size can be highly variable. If the central cyst results in a corpus luteum measuring over 3 cm in diameter, the CLP (or less commonly a corpus luteum of menstruation) is designated a corpus luteum cyst, or if less than this size, a cystic corpus luteum. When the cavity of CLP is large, typically in the first trimester, the wall may lose its convolutions, becoming stretched and attenuated to the extent that it may consist focally of only the inner fibrous layer (126). Obliteration of the cavity usually begins by the 5th month and is typically completed by term (126). The CLP thus gradually decreases in size, and by the last trimester it is not a conspicuous structure. During the puerperium, the CLP undergoes involution and conversion to a corpus albicans.

### Histology

The CLP, in contrast to the CLM, does not mature in an orderly sequence that allows an estimation of its age; however, early and late stages are recognizable on histologic examination.

#### *Granulosa Layer*

The first morphologic evidence within the corpus luteum that conception has occurred is the absence of the regressive changes that normally appear in the CLM on the 8th or 9th days. Instead, the granulosa-lutein cells enlarge, reaching their maximum size of 50 to 60 $\mu$m by 8 to 9 weeks' gestation. They assume a round or polyhedral shape with abundant eosinophilic cytoplasm, round to oval, vesicular nuclei, and one or two prominent nucleoli (126) (Fig. 31A). The granulosa cells of the early CLP are characterized by cytoplasmic vacuoles that initially are minute but eventually increase in size to occupy almost the entire cell, often with displacement and flattening of the nucleus (Fig. 31A). The vacuoles tend to diminish in number and size as gestation progresses and usually disappear after the 4th month (126). Fine, diffusely scattered, cytoplasmic lipid droplets are also commonly seen within the cells, particularly in early CLP. With increasing age of the corpus luteum, the droplets become fewer and larger (126).

Eosinophilic colloid or hyaline droplets within the granulosa cells of a CLP, which can be identified as early as 15 days after ovulation (19), are almost diagnostic of pregnancy; however, they may occur rarely within a CLM (126). These inclusions initially appear as small, round or irregular, often multiple, droplets but eventually enlarge, possibly by fusion of smaller droplets, into one or several large bodies that may fill the entire cell (Fig. 31A). They become more numerous as gestation progresses (166), although by term their numbers decrease as they undergo calcification, which continues into the puerperium (Fig. 31B) (126,166). It is likely that these calcified bodies eventually are resorbed because they are not a feature of corpora albicantia (126).

K cells identical to those within the CLM are typically found in the granulosa layer of the early CLP. They are most numerous in the 2nd, 3rd, and 4th months of gestation, after which time they are rarely encountered (125,126,166).

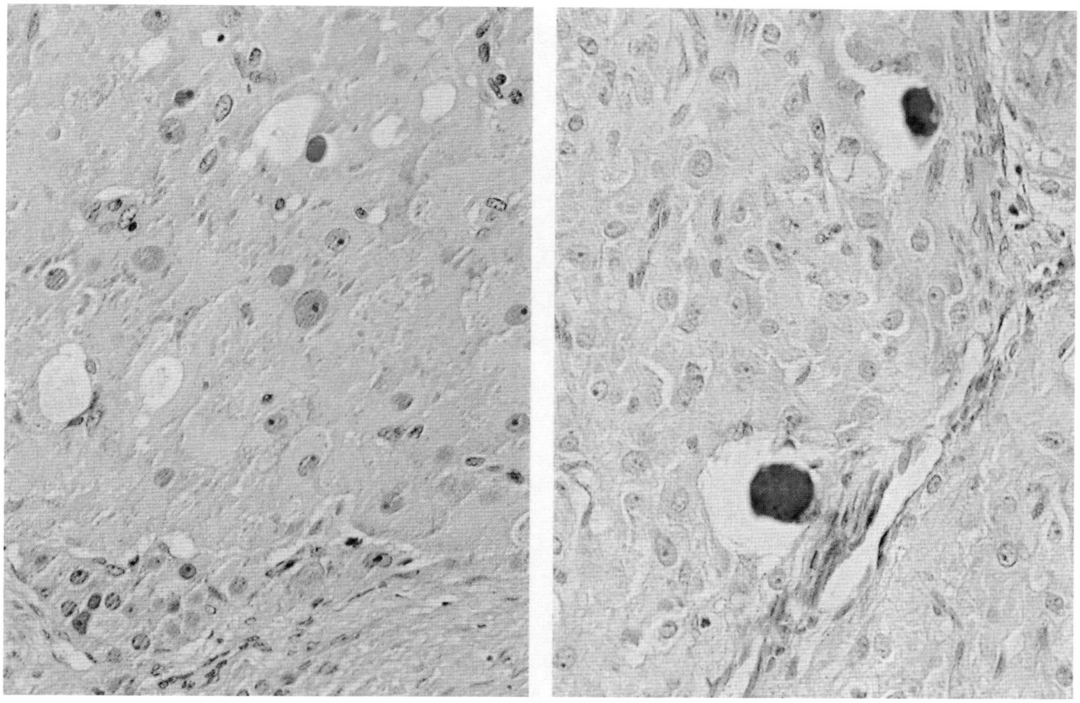

A B

**FIG. 31.** Corpus luteum of pregnancy. **A:** Note the granulosa-lutein cells with large irregular vacuoles and densely eosinophilic hyaline body. Nests of theca cells are seen at bottom left. **B:** Focal calcification within a late corpus luteum of pregnancy.

### *Theca Layer*

The theca interna is thickest in the early CLP, at which time it resembles its counterpart in the CLM, surrounding the granulosa-lutein layer and forming triangular, vascular septa that extend into the latter. In the CLP, the theca cells are polyhedral or round and approximately one fourth the size of the granulosa-lutein cells (Fig. 31A). Their cytoplasm is more darkly staining and granular than in the latter, and typically nonvacuolated. Their nuclei are central, round, and more hyperchromatic than those of the granulosa cells; one or two prominent nucleoli are usually present. The characteristic colloid inclusions seen within the granulosa cells are absent or rare within the theca cells (126). Occasional K cells may be seen in early pregnancy but in smaller numbers than in the granulosa layer (130,166). After the 4th month, the theca interna and its trabeculae become much thinner as the theca cells become smaller and fewer in number, with darker, more irregular, oblong to spindle-shaped nuclei, so that they resemble fibroblasts (166). By term, the theca interna layer has almost completely disappeared.

### *Connective Tissue*

As in the mature CLM, the central cystic cavity is typically lined by a layer of fibrous tissue, composed of variable numbers of fibroblasts, collagen and reticulin fibers, and blood vessels (126). Its thickness is highly variable, not only within the same CLP, but also from one CLP to another and from one phase of pregnancy to another (166). As noted, in some CLPs with large cystic cavities, the granulosa layer is focally absent, and its wall is formed entirely by this fibrous layer. As gestation advances, the central cyst or coagulum is eventually obliterated by connective tissue that may exhibit focal hyalinization and calcification (125).

Reticulin staining shows a pattern similar to that of the mature CLM, i.e., a dense pattern within the theca interna and inner fibrous layer, and a sparser framework within the granulosa layer (126). In the early CLP, many, often large, vessels are present in the theca externa and interna, which give origin to smaller vessels that penetrate the granulosa and inner fibrous layers. In the late CLP, the vessels develop sclerotic walls with luminal narrowing or obliteration (126,166). The amount of connective tissue around the vessels increases in proportion to the decreasing vascularization and regression of the theca interna layer (166).

## Ultrastructure

The ultrastructural appearance of the CLP is similar to that of the CLP and remains intact throughout pregnancy despite a reduction in its metabolic activity (167–169). The increased cell volume of the granulosa cells in the CLP is reflected by increased smooth ER, which exhibits many folded membrane complexes. There is also an increase in rough ER, which is localized in stacks and characteristic concentric whorls not usually seen in the CLM (159,168). Electron dense, membrane-bound, 150- to 200-nm granules are closely associated with the cisternae of the rough ER. Mitochondria, including large spherical mitochondria not seen in the CLM, are typically highly variable in their size, shape, and internal structure (159,168). The colloid or hyaline inclusions consist of homogeneous electron-opaque material that may surround occasional needle-shaped crystals (Fig. 32). They typically have no relationship to any organelle, although occasional smaller hyaline bodies are surrounded by rough ER. The vacuoles seen by light microscopy are lined by attenuated microvilli and contain an electron-translucent material (167). Unlike the CLM, extensive bundles of microfilaments are typically encountered throughout the cytoplasm in most lutein cells and become more prominent as pregnancy progresses (167,168). Collagen fibrils are encountered more frequently in the intercellular and perivascular spaces of the term CLP compared with the CLM (168).

### Hormone Aspects

After fertilization, placental hCG stimulates progesterone production by the granulosa-lutein cells. Progesterone concentration within the postovulatory corpus luteum increases sixfold, whereas the E2 level decreases to 10% of that within the preovulatory follicle (137,138). hCG alone cannot maintain progesterone secretion from the CLP for more than a few days, and the regulation of progesterone secretion beyond that time is unknown. Progesterone production by the CLP begins to decline by the end of the 2nd month of gestation as its production is largely assumed by the placenta. However, in vivo and in vitro studies indicate that the CLP continues to produce progesterone throughout the remainder of gestation, albeit in reduced amounts, consistent with the maintenance of its structural integrity until term (124,167, 168,170,171). It is not known if progesterone derived from the CLP has a biologic role during this period or is redundant because of the massive progesterone production by the placenta (161,172). There is a rapid decline in function during the puerperium, reflecting decreasing hCG levels during this period.

Relaxin, a polypeptide hormone, is also produced during gestation and the puerperium by the CLP, probably under the control of hCG (172–175). The concentration of relaxin in ovarian vein plasma during pregnancy correlates with progesterone levels. The placenta and uterus also have been suggested as additional, but less important, sources for this hormone. Its reported actions include cervical dilatation and softening, inhibition of uterine contractions, and relaxation of the pubic symphysis and other pelvic joints (172–175). Immunoreactivity for renin and angiotensin II, similar to that noted within the preovulatory follicle (see above), has been demonstrated within the CLP (151), consistent with the observation that prorenin, likely of ovarian origin, increases 10-fold in pregnant women soon after conception (150).

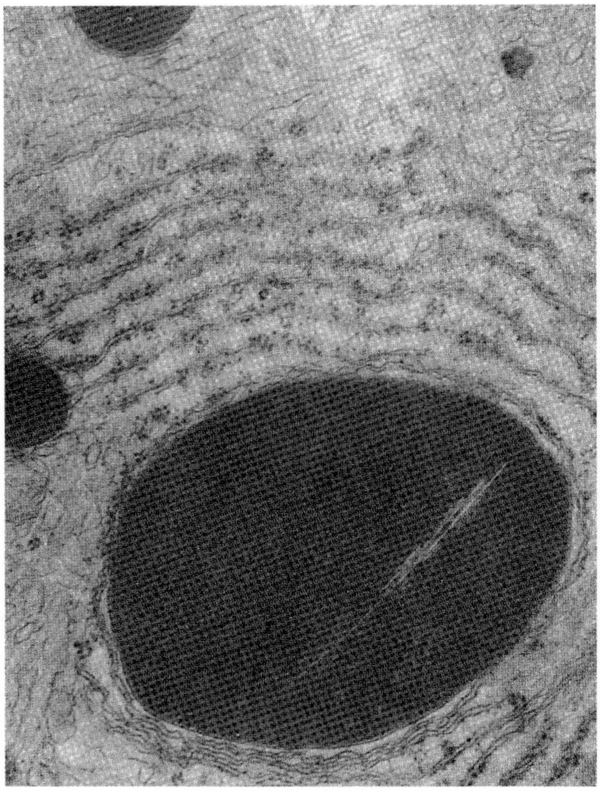

**FIG. 32.** Hyaline bodies within a lutein cell from a corpus luteum of pregnancy consisting of homogeneous, electron-opaque material. Note the needle-shaped cleft within the largest hyaline body. Some smaller hyaline bodies are surrounded by granular ER (original magnifiction ×**22,000**). Reprinted with permission (157).

## CORPUS ALBICANS

The regressing CLM is invaded by connective tissue that gradually converts it to a scar, the corpus albicans. The degenerating corpus luteum and the young corpus albicans may contain macrophages laden with ceroid and hemosiderin pigment (177). The mature corpus albicans is a well-circumscribed structure with convoluted borders composed almost entirely of densely packed collagen fibers with occasional admixed fibroblasts (Figs. 13 and 33). Focal calcification and ossification may be occasionally encountered. Most corpora albicantia are eventually resorbed and replaced by ovarian stroma (19,176). Persistent corpora albicantia are typically found in the medulla of postmenopausal women (Fig. 13), suggesting that this resorption process decelerates or terminates before the menopause.

## ATRETIC FOLLICLES

### Histology

Of the original 400,000 primordial follicles present at birth, approximately 400 mature to ovulation. The remaining

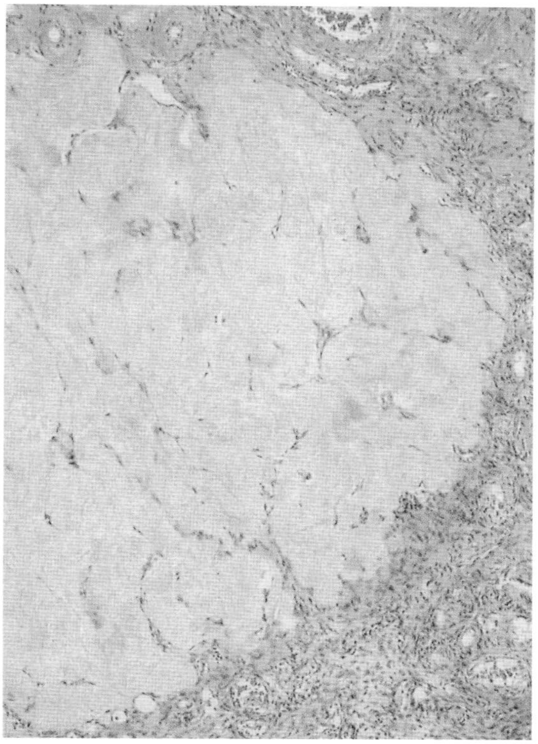

**FIG. 33.** Corpus albicans.

99.9% undergo atresia, which begins before birth and continues throughout reproductive life, but is most intense immediately after birth and during puberty and pregnancy (119–123,125,127). Factors that initiate atresia and determine which follicles will ultimately undergo atresia are unknown. The atretic process varies with the stage of follicular maturation that has been reached. Atresia of early follicles (primordial and preantral) begins with degeneration of the oocyte manifested by nuclear changes (chromatin condensation, pyknosis, fragmentation) and cytoplasmic vacuolation. Degeneration of the granulosa cells soon follows, and the follicle disappears without a trace. In contrast, atresia of follicles that have reached the antral stage of development is more complex and variable but ultimately leads to obliterative atresia and the formation of a scar, the corpus fibrosum (23). The earliest evidence of this process is mitotic inactivity of the granulosa cells and a decrease in their numbers, manifested by thinning and focal exfoliation of the granulosa layer. Some follicles may persist for an indefinite period of time at this stage as atretic cystic follicles (Fig. 34); those that exceed 3 cm are designated follicular cysts. Atretic cystic follicles and follicular cysts may persist for a number of years after the menopause (178,179). Atretic follicles are ultimately invaded by vascular connective tissue that eventually fills the central cavity (Fig. 35). The oocyte may persist for an indefinite period of time but eventually degenerates.

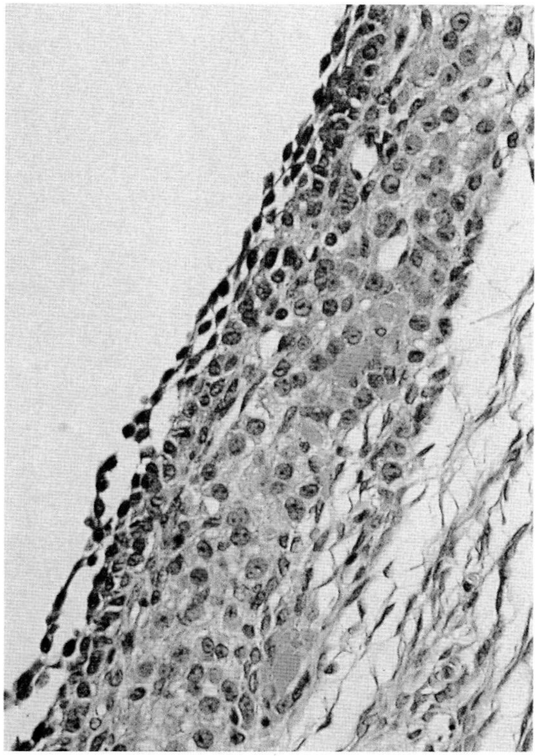

**FIG. 34.** Lining of atretic cystic follicle composed of a thin inner layer of small, exfoliating granulosa cells and an outer, luteinized theca interna layer.

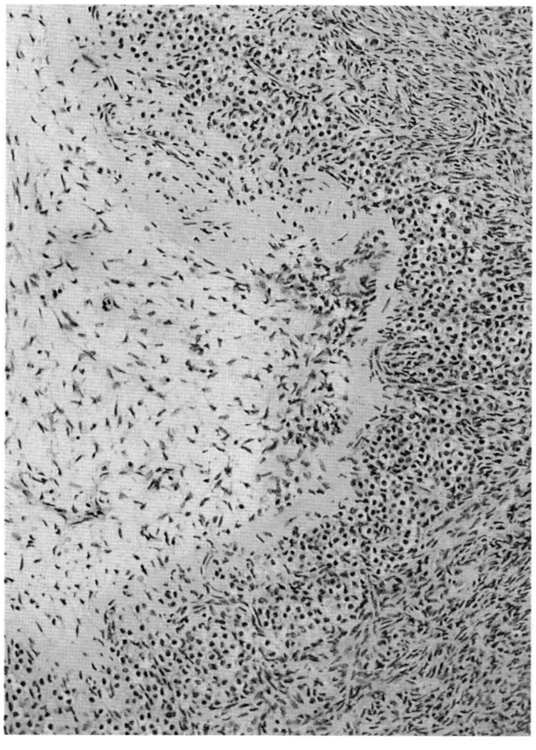

**FIG. 35.** Atretic cystic follicle undergoing obliterative atresia. Loose connective tissue is replacing the central cavity. The wavy basement membrane (glassy membrane) is thickened and hyalinized. A prominent layer of luteinized theca interna is evident.

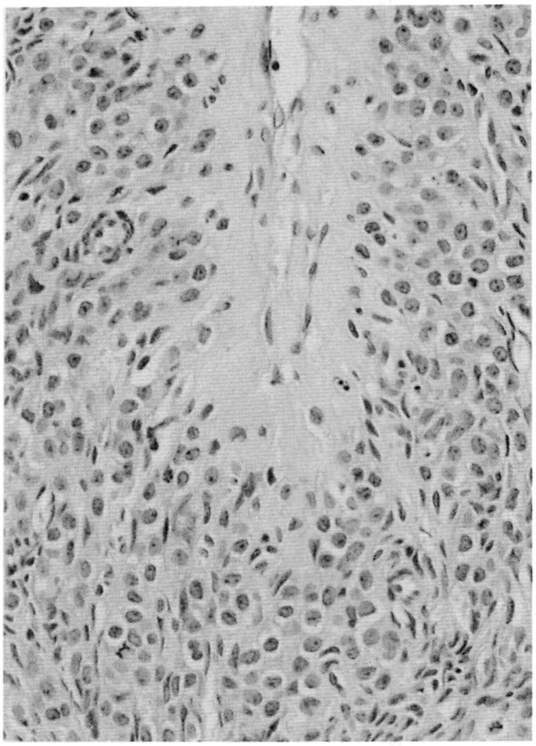

**FIG. 36.** Edge of follicle in late stage of obliterative atresia. Hyalinized fibrous tissue occupies the central cavity and extends into the persistent luteinized theca interna layer.

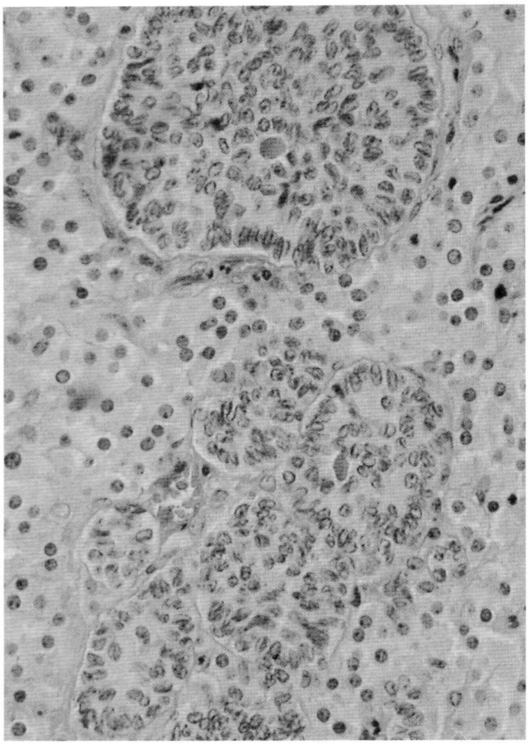

**FIG. 37.** Atretic follicle in pregnancy. Within the center of the follicle is a proliferation of persistent granulosa cells surrounded by luteinized theca interna cells.

Concurrent with these changes, the basement membrane between the granulosa and theca interna layers becomes transformed into a thick, wavy, eosinophilic, hyalinized band, the so-called glassy membrane (Figs. 35 and 36). The theca interna layer typically persists, often with prominent luteinization (Figs. 35 and 36) until the late stages of atresia, at which time cords and nests of theca cells become surrounded by proliferating connective tissue (Fig. 36). Luteinization of both theca and granulosa layers is particularly striking in atretic follicles during infancy and childhood (180) and pregnancy (Fig. 37) (126). Microscopic proliferations of persistent granulosa cells within the centers of atretic follicles of pregnant, and less commonly nonpregnant women, may mimic small granulosa cell tumors (Fig. 37) or, rarely, Sertoli cell tumors (181). Similarly, structures resembling microscopic gonadoblastomas and sex cord tumors with annular tubules have been identified within atretic follicles in up to 35% of normal fetuses and infants (115,182,183). There is no evidence to suggest that any of these tumorlike proliferations represent early stages of neoplasia (115,181).

Continued shrinkage and hyalinization of an atretic follicle produces a serpiginous strand of hyaline tissue, the corpus fibrosum or atreticum (Fig. 38). Like corpora albicantia, most corpora fibrosa are probably resorbed by the ovarian stroma.

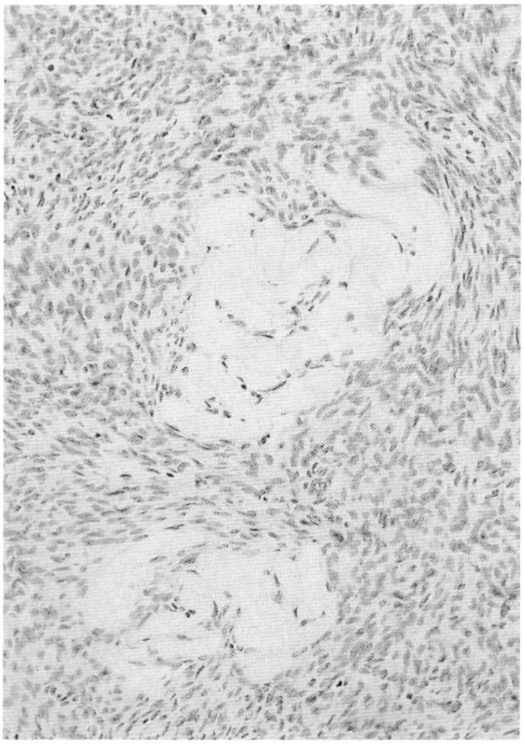

**FIG. 38.** Two corpora fibrosa.

### Hormonal Aspects

In contrast to preovulatory follicles, the microenvironment of follicles undergoing atresia is predominantly androgenic, with high concentrations of intrafollicular androstenedione and low concentrations of FSH and E2 (17,103, 137,138,184). As noted, these follicles are deficient in granulosa cells, and the residual granulosa cells do not respond to FSH in vitro (129); the levels of both FSH receptors and LH receptors are lower than in nonatretic follicles (140). Oocytes from atretic follicles are unable to complete the first meiotic division (129). It is likely that an androgenic intrafollicular milieu is the major factor that halts follicular growth and initiates atresia of that follicle.

## HILUS CELLS

### Histology

Ovarian hilus cells, morphologically identical to testicular Leydig cells (with the exception of a female chromatin pattern), are present during fetal life but not during childhood. They reappear at the time of puberty and are demonstrable in all postmenopausal women (185–187). Their number and location can be highly variable, and their numbers increase during pregnancy, with increasing age after the menopause, and with increasing degrees of ovarian stromal proliferation and stromal luteinization (22). Mild hilus cell hyperplasia is a relatively common incidental histologic finding in postmenopausal women (19,70).

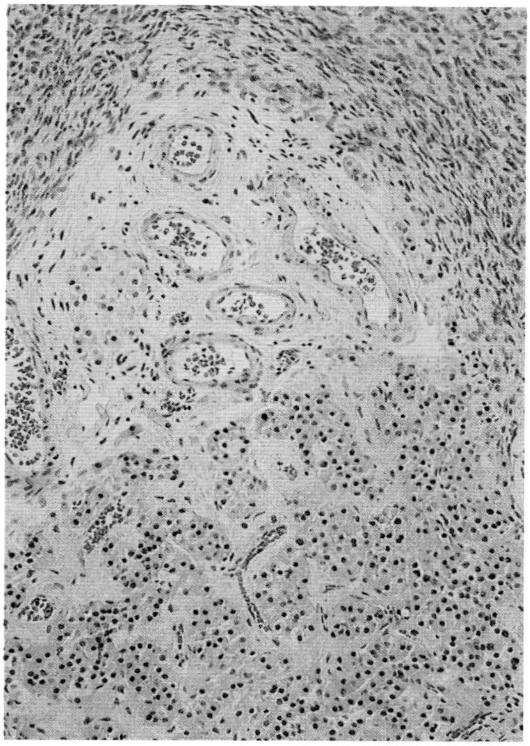

**FIG. 40.** Nest of hilus cells with admixed small blood vessels abutting medullary stroma (*top*).

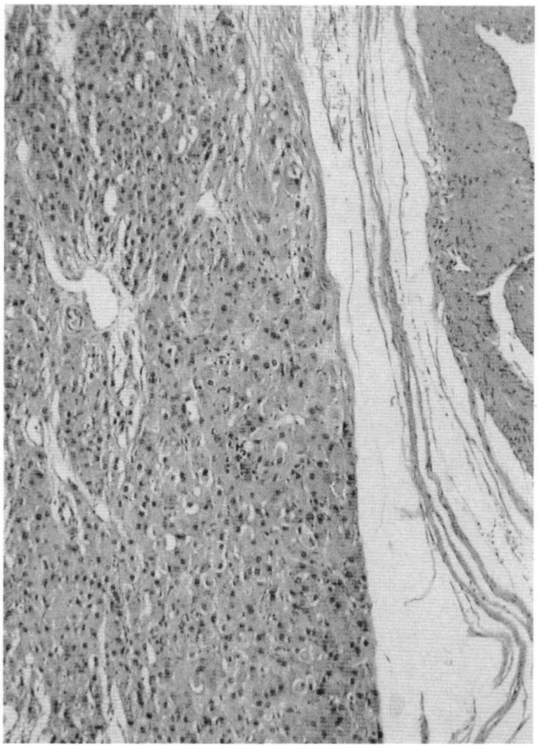

**FIG. 39.** Nest of hilus cells adjacent to large vessel within the ovarian hilus.

Hilus cell aggregates of variable size and shape are typically found in the ovarian hilus and adjacent mesovarium (Figs. 39 and 40). They are more numerous in the lateral and medial poles of the hilus and near the junction of the ovarian ligament with the ovary, typically lying close to the junction of the hilus with the medullary stroma (Fig. 40) (185). The aggregates are closely associated with large hilar veins and lymphatic sinusoids and may form nodular protrusions into their lumina (185). Hilus cells characteristically ensheath, or less commonly lie within, nonmedullated nerves (Fig. 41), and occasionally surround the rete ovarii (185). Nests also may be present within the medullary stroma near the hilus, probably representing extensions of the hilus into the medulla, and as previously noted, cells of the hilus type also may occur rarely within the ovarian stroma at a distance from the hilus (stromal Leydig cells). Hilus cells also may be encountered rarely in the perisalpinx and fimbrial endosalpinx (188).

Hilus cell nests are unencapsulated, typically lying within loose connective tissue, or rarely ovarian-type stroma, within the hilus (85). The cells measure 15 to 25 $\mu$m in diameter, are round to oval and less commonly elongate, with abundant eosinophilic cytoplasm and a spherical vesicular nucleus that contains one or two prominent nucleoli (Fig. 42). Hilus cells, particularly in postmenopausal women, may

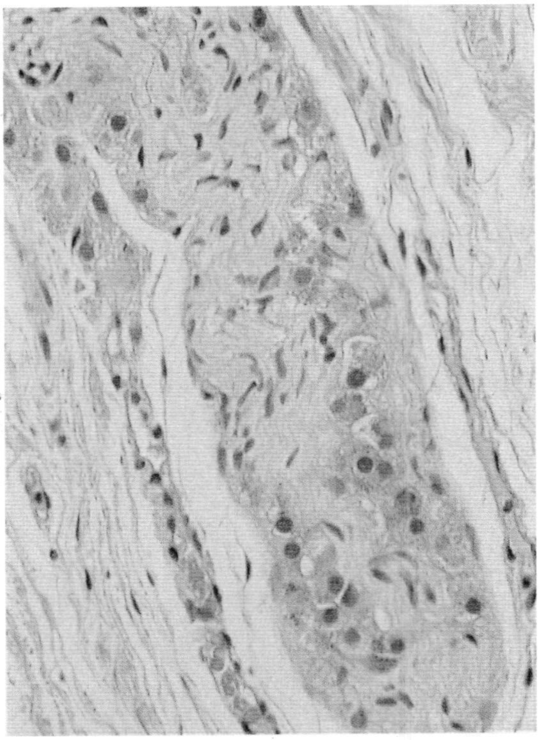

**FIG. 41.** Perineural and intraneural hilus cells. Note the fine brown lipochrome pigment within the hilus cells.

have bizarre shapes and contain hyperchromatic, pleomorphic nuclei.

Hilus cells contain specific crystals of Reinke, which are homogenous, eosinophilic, nonrefractile, rod-shaped structures 10 to 35 $\mu$m in length with blunt, but occasionally tapered, ends (Fig. 42). The crystals typically lie in a parallel or stacked arrangement within a cell and often are surrounded by a clear halo; occasionally they appear to extend through or overlie cell membranes. The crystals are unevenly distributed and are typically present in only a minority of cells; frequently they are not identified (189). Their visualization may be facilitated by the use of Masson's trichrome and iron hematoxylin methods, which stain them magenta and black, respectively. Additionally, the crystals fluoresce yellow when hematoxylin and eosin–stained sections are viewed under ultraviolet light (190).

Also present within hilus cells, often in greater numbers than crystals, are spherical or ellipsoidal hyaline structures that have an otherwise identical appearance to crystals and probably represent their precursors. Elongated erythrocytes compressed within capillaries should not be confused with crystals and crystal precursors. The cytoplasm of Leydig cells also may contain perinuclear eosinophilic granules, peripheral lipid vacuoles, and golden brown lipochrome pigment (Fig. 41). Delicate collagen fibrils surround each cell. Typically admixed with the hilus cells are fibroblasts and cells intermediate in appearance between the two cell types (191). The hilus cells and intermediate cells have intimate attachments to nerves, including true synaptic connections, suggesting that hilus cells may originate from hilar fibroblasts, possibly under the inductive influence of hilar nerves (185,191).

Hilus cells should be distinguished from adrenal cortical rests. The latter are extremely rare in the ovary (192) but are found in the mesovarium and occasionally within the ovarian hilus in approximately one quarter of women (193). Their histologic appearance mimics that of the normal adrenal cortex, with most of the cells containing numerous lipid vacuoles.

### Ultrastructure

Hilus cells have a steroidogenic ultrastructure consisting of prominent smooth ER and mitochondria with tubular cristae, as well as well-developed Golgi bodies, large lysosomes, and osmiophilic lipid inclusions (191). Reinke crystals have a true crystalline appearance composed of dense parallel hexagonal microtubules with a mean thickness of 12 nm separated by clear spaces 15 nm wide producing the appearance of woven fabric (Fig. 43) (191). The crystals are typically oriented in many directions in the same cell. They appear to be formed by progressive association of precrys-

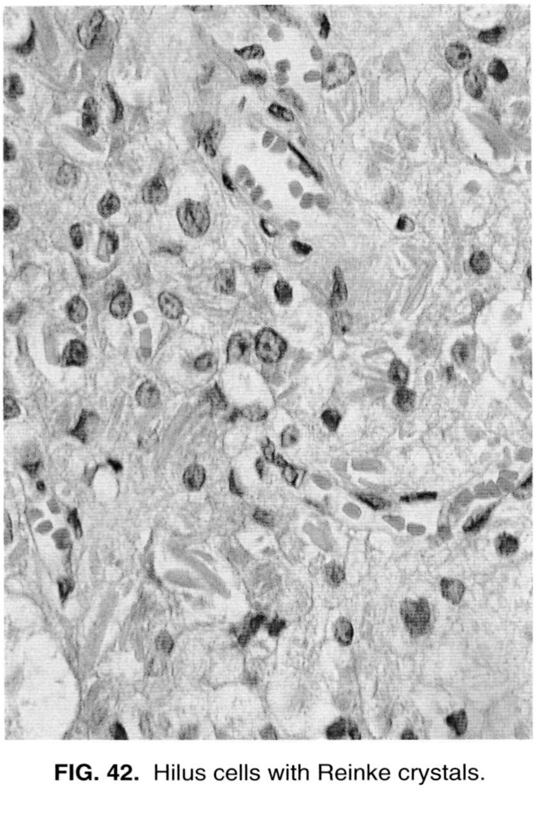

**FIG. 42.** Hilus cells with Reinke crystals.

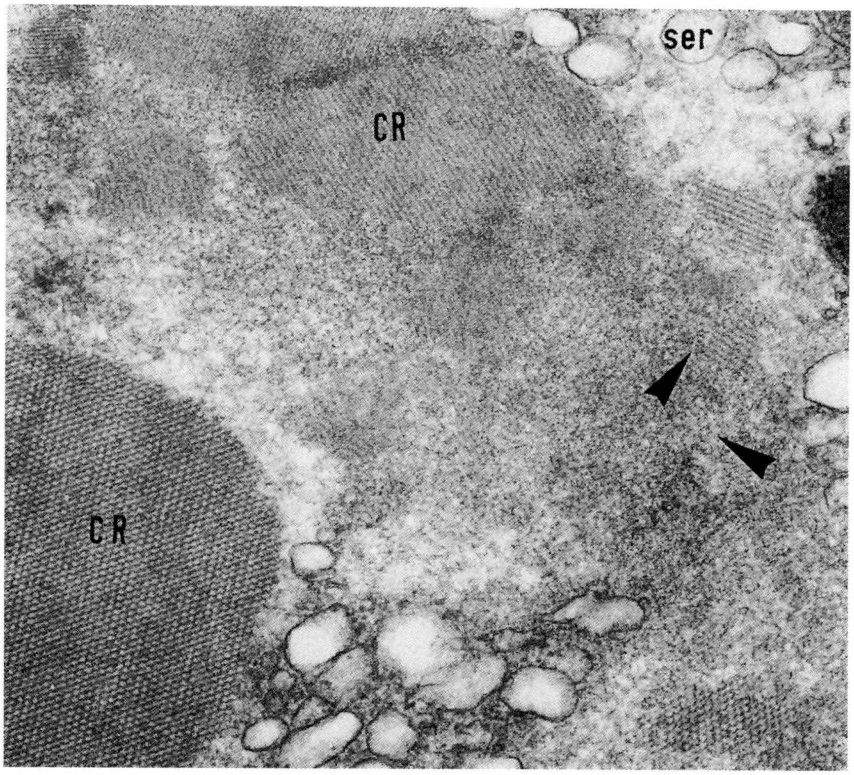


**FIG. 43.** Reinke crystals with hexagonal internal pattern (CR) formed by association of precrystalline units (*arrowheads*). ser, smooth ER (original magnification ×**25,000**). Reprinted with permission (191).

talline units each of which is composed of bundles of four or five parallel filaments (Fig. 43).

Typically found admixed with hilus cells are fibroblasts and cells intermediate in ultrastructural appearance between the two cell types (191). Hilus cells and more commonly, the intermediate cells, have intimate attachments to nerves in the form of simple membranous contacts, invaginations of axon terminals into hilus cells, or surface membrane thickenings resembling a true synapse (191). These findings suggest that hilus cells most likely originate from hilar fibroblasts, possibly under the inductive influence of hilar nerves (69,191).

### Hormonal Aspects

The light and electron microscopic morphology and enzyme content of hilus cells are those of steroid hormone–producing cells, although to what extent hilus cells contribute to the steroid hormone pool in normal females is unknown (19,33,185). In vitro incubation studies indicate that the major steroid produced by ovarian hilus cells is androstenedione and that it is produced in amounts higher than that produced from ovarian stroma (194). Lesser amounts of E2 and progesterone are also produced in vitro. Hilus cells are responsive in vivo to both exogenous and endogenous hCG stimulation, manifested by an increase in cell size, mitotic activity, and cell numbers (186).

## RETE OVARII

The rete ovarii, the ovarian analogue of the rete testis, is present in the hilus of all ovaries. It consists of a network of irregular clefts, tubules, cysts, and intraluminal papillae, lined by an epithelium that varies from flat to cuboidal to columnar (Fig. 44) (195,196). Solid cords of similar cells also may be seen. Characteristically, the rete is surrounded by a cuff of spindle cell stroma similar to, but discontinuous from, the ovarian stroma (Fig. 44).

The cytoplasm of the cells of the rete is immunoreactive for cytokeratin, vimentin, and desmoplakin (36,37). Ultrastructural examination has shown two types of cells, one ciliated and the other nonciliated, with apical microvilli (36). The cytoplasm contains many mitochondria, a moderate amount of rough ER, many free polyribosomes, and some glycogen. Numerous desmosomes with associated tonofilament bundles connect adjacent cells. The basal lamina is well defined.

The rete juxtaposes and may communicate with mesonephric tubules within the mesovarium (196). Rare hilar cysts originate from the rete (196), and small tumorlike proliferations of the rete have been referred to as rete adenomas (196,197). The transitional cell metaplasia that has been encountered in the rete epithelium (195) may account for the occasional small hilar Brenner tumors that have been contiguous with and possibly derived from the rete (195).

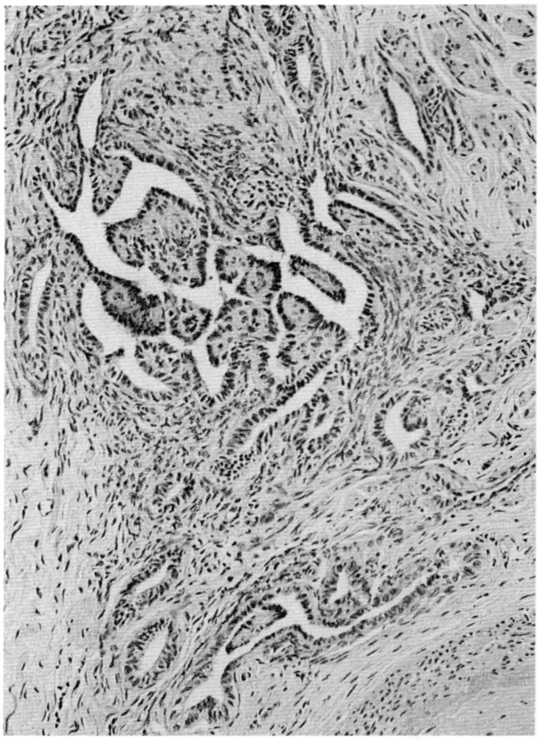

**FIG. 44.** Rete ovarii.

## REFERENCES


1. Baker TG, O WS. Development of the ovary and oogenesis. *Clin Obstet Gynaecol* 1976:3:3–26.
2. Minh H, Smadja A, Herve De Sigalony JP, Orcel L. Etude histologique de la gonade a differenciation ovarienne au cours de l'organogenese. *Arch Anat Cytol Pathol* 1989;37:201–207.
3. Gondos B, Bhiraleus P, Hobel CJ. Ultrastructural observations on germ cells in human fetal ovaries. *Am J Obstet Gynecol* 1971;110: 644–652.
4. Gondos B. Cellular interrelationships in the human fetal ovary and testis. *Prog Clin Biol Res* 1981;59B:373–381.
5. Konishi I, Fujii S, Okamura H, Parmley T, Mori T. Development of interstitial cells and ovigerous cords in the human fetal ovary: an ultrastructural study. *J Anat* 1986;148:121–135.
6. Gondos B. Surface epithelium of the developing ovary. Possible correlation with ovarian neoplasia. *Am J Pathol* 1975;81:303–320.
7. Rabinovici J, Jaffe RB. Development and regulation of growth and differentiated function in human and subhuman primate fetal gonads. *Endocr Rev* 1990;11:532–557.
8. Van Wagenen G, Simpson ME. *Embryology of the ovary and testis, Homo sapiens and Macaca mulatta.* New Haven, CT: Yale University Press; 1965.
9. Fukuda O, Miyayama Y, Fujimoto T, Okamura H. Electron microscopic study of gonadal development in early human embryos. *Prog Clin Biol Res* 1989;296:23–29.
10. Pinkerton JHM, McKay DG, Adams EC, Hertig AT. Development of the human ovary—a study using histochemical techniques. *Obstet Gynecol* 1961;18:152–181.
11. Gruenwald P. The development of the sex cords in the gonads of man and mammals. *Am J Anat* 1942;70:359–389.
12. Jirasek JE. Development of the genital system in human embryos and fetuses. In: *Development of the genital system and male pseudohermaphroditism.* Baltimore: Johns Hopkins Press; 1971:3–41.
13. Byskov AG. Differentiation of mammalian embryonic gonad. *Physiol Rev* 1986;66:71–117.
14. Satoh M. Histogenesis and organogenesis of the gonad in human embryos. *J Anat* 1991;177:85–107.
15. Wartenberg H. The influence of the mesonephric blastoma on gonadal development and sexual differentiation. In: Byskov AG, Peters H, eds. *Development and function of reproductive organs.* Amsterdam: Excerpta Medica; 1981:3–12.
16. Wartenberg H. Development of the early human ovary and role of the mesonephros in the differentiation of the cortex. *Anat Embryol* 1982; 165:253–280.
17. Nicosia SV. Morphological changes of the human ovary throughout life. In: Serra GB, ed. *The ovary*. New York: Raven Press; 1983:57–81.
18. Pryse-Davies J. The development, structure and function of the female pelvic organs in childhood. *Clin Obstet Gynaecol* 1974;1:483–508.
19. Scully RE. Tumors of the ovary and maldeveloped gonads. In: *Atlas of tumor pathology.* Second series, fascicle 16. Washington, DC: Armed Forces Institute of Pathology; 1979.
20. Valdes-Dapena MA. The normal ovary of childhood. *Ann N Y Acad Sci* 1967;142:597–613.
21. Merrill JA. The morphology of the prepubertal ovary: relationship to the polycystic ovary syndrome. *South Med J* 1963;56:225–231.
22. Boss JH, Scully RE, Wegner KH, Cohen RB. Structural variations in the adult ovary—clinical significance. *Obstet Gynecol* 1965;25: 747–763.
23. Bloom W, Fawcett DW. *A textbook of histology*. 10th ed. Philadelphia: WB Saunders; 1975.
24. Reeves G. Specific stroma in the cortex and medulla of the ovary. Cell types and vascular supply in relation to follicular apparatus and ovulation. *Obstet Gynecol* 1971;37:832–844.
25. Plentl AA, Friedman EA. *Lymphatic system of the female genitalia.* Philadelphia: WB Saunders; 1971.
26. Eichner E, Bove ER. In vivo studies on the lymphatic drainage of the human ovary. *Obstet Gynecol* 1954;3:287–297.
27. Jacobowitz D, Wallach EE. Histochemical and chemical studies of the autonomic innervation of the ovary. *Endocrinology* 1967;81: 1132–1139.
28. Owman C, Rosengren E, Sjoberg N. Adrenergic innervation of the human female reproductive organs: a histochemical and chemical investigation. *Obstet Gynecol* 1967;30:763–773.
29. Balboni GC. Structural changes: ovulation and luteal phase. In: Serra GB, ed. *The ovary*. New York: Raven Press; 1983:123–141.
30. Mohsin S. The sympathetic innervation of the mammalian ovary. A review of pharmacological and histochemical studies. *Clin Exp Pharmacol Physiol* 1979;6:335–354.
31. Dyer CA, Erickson GF. Norepinephrine amplifies human chorionic gonadotropin–stimulated androgen biosynthesis by ovarian theca-interstitial cells. *Endocrinology* 1985;116:1645–1652.
32. Blaustein A, Lee H. Surface cells of the ovary and pelvic peritoneum: a histochemical and ultrastructural comparison. *Gynecol Oncol* 1979; 8:34–43.
33. McKay DG, Pinkerton JHM, Hertig AT, Danziger S. The adult human ovary: a histochemical study. *Obstet Gynecol* 1961;18:13–39.
34. Miettinen M, Lehto V, Virtanen I. Expression of intermediate filaments in normal ovaries and ovarian epithelial, sex cord–stromal, and germinal tumors. *Int J Gynecol Pathol* 1983;2:64–71.
35. Czernobilsky B, Moll R, Franke WW, Dallenbach-Hellweg G, Hohlweg-Majert P. Intermediate filaments of normal and neoplastic tissues of the female genital tract with emphasis on problems of differential tumor diagnosis. *Pathol Res Pract* 1984;179:31–37.
36. Czernobilsky B, Moll R, Levy R, Franke WW. Co-expression of cytokeratin and vimentin filaments in mesothelial, granulosa and rete ovarii cells of the human ovary. *Eur J Cell Biol* 1985:37:175–190.
37. Benjamin E, Law S, Bobrow LG. Intermediate filaments cytokeratin and vimentin in ovarian sex cord–stromal tumours with correlative studies in adult and fetal ovaries. *J Pathol* 1987;152:253–263.
38. Isola J, Kallioniemi O-P, Korte J-M, et al. Steroid receptors and Ki-67 reactivity in ovarian cancer and in normal ovary: correlation with DNA flow cytometry, biochemical receptor assay, and patient survival. *J Pathol* 1990;162:295–301.
39. Rodriguez GC, Berchuk A, Whitaker RS, Schlossman D, Clarke-Pearson DL, Bast RC Jr. Epidermal growth factor receptor expression in normal ovarian epithelium and ovarian cancer. II. Relationship between receptor expression and response to epidermal growth factor. *Am J Obstet Gynecol* 1991;164:745–750.
40. Jindal SK, Snoey DM, Lobb DK, Dorrington JH. Transforming growth factor alpha localization and role in surface epithelium of nor-

mal human ovaries and in ovarian carcinoma lines. *Gynecol Oncol* 1994;53:17–23.
41. Latza U, Niedobitek G, Schwarting R, Nekarda H, Stein H. Ber-EP4: new monoclonal antibody which distinguishes epithelia from mesothelia. *J Clin Pathol* 1990;43:213–219.
42. Blaustein A. Surface cells and inclusion cysts in fetal ovaries. *Gynecol Oncol* 1981;12:222–233.
43. Blaustein A, Kantius M, Kaganowicz A, Pervez N, Wells JK. Inclusions in ovaries of females aged day 1–30 years. *Int J Gynecol Pathol* 1982;1:145–153.
44. Sidaway MK, Silverberg SG. Endosalpingiosis in female peritoneal washings: a diagnostic pitfall. *Int J Gynecol Pathol* 1987;6:340–346.
45. Zinsser KR, Wheeler JE. Endosalpingiosis in the omentum. A study of autopsy and surgical material. *Am J Surg Pathol* 1982;6:109–117.
46. Mulligan RM. A survey of epithelial inclusions in the ovarian cortex of 470 patients. *J Surg Oncol* 1976;8:61–66.
47. Von Numers C. Observations on metaplastic changes in the germinal epithelium of the ovary and on the aetiology of ovarian endometriosis. *Acta Obstet Gynecol Scand* 1965;44:107–116.
48. Scully RE. Ovary. In: Henson DE, Albores-Saavedra J, eds. *The pathology of incipient neoplasia*. Vol. 28. Major problems in pathology. Philadelphia: WB Saunders; 1993:283–300.
49. Mittal KR, Zeleniuch-Jacquotte A, Cooper JL, Demopoulos RI. Contralateral ovary in unilateral ovarian carcinoma: a search for preneoplastic lesions. *Int J Gynecol Pathol* 1993;12:59–63.
50. Blaustein A, Kaganowicz A, Wells J. Tumor markers in inclusion cysts of the ovary. *Cancer* 1982;49:722–726.
51. Charpin C, Bhan AK, Zurawski VR Jr, Scully RE. Carcinoembryonic antigen (CEA) and carbohydrate determinant 19-9 (CA 19-9) localization in 121 primary and metastatic ovarian tumors: an immunohistochemical study with the use of monoclonal antibodies. *Int J Gynecol Pathol* 1982;1:231–245.
52. Cordon-Cardo C, Mattes MJ, Melamed MR, Lewis JL Jr, Old LJ, Lloyd KO. Immunopathologic analysis of a panel of mouse monoclonal antibodies reacting with human ovarian carcinomas and other human tumors. *Int J Gynecol Pathol* 1985;4:121–130.
53. Kabawat SE, Bast RC Jr, Bhan AK, Welch WR, Knapp RC, Colvin RB. Tissue distribution of coelomic-epithelium–related antigen recognized by the monoclonal antibody OC125. *Int J Gynecol Pathol* 1983;2:275–285.
54. Nouwen EJ, Pollet DE, Schelstraete JB, et al. Human placental alkaline phosphatase in benign and malignant ovarian neoplasia. *Cancer Res* 1985;45:892–902.
55. Nouwen EJ, Hendrix PG, Dauwe S, Eerdekens MW, De Broe ME. Tumor markers in the human ovary and its neoplasms. A comparative immunohistochemical study. *Am J Pathol* 1987;126:230–242.
56. Resta L, Scordari MD, Colucci GA, et al. Morphological changes of the ovarian surface epithelium in ovarian polycystic disease or endometrial carcinoma and a control group. *Eur J Gynaecol Oncol* 1989; 10:39–41.
57. Bransilver BR. Ferenczy A, Richart RM. Brenner tumors and Walthard cell nests. *Arch Pathol Lab Med* 1974;98:76–86.
58. Danforth DN. Cytologic relationship of Walthard cell rest to Brenner tumor of ovary and the pseudomucinous cystadenoma. *Am J Obstet Gynecol* 1942;43:984–996.
59. Roth LM. The Brenner tumor and the Walthard cell nest. An electron microscopic study. *Lab Invest* 1974;31:15–23.
60. Teoh TB. The structure and development of Walthard nests. *J Pathol* 1953;66:433–439.
61. Papadaki L, Beilby JOW. The fine structure of the surface epithelium of the human ovary. *J Cell Sci* 1971;8:445–465.
62. Ferenczy A, Richart RM. *Female reproductive system: dynamics of scan and transmission electron microscopy*. New York: Wiley & Sons; 1974.
63. Blaustein A. Peritoneal mesothelium and ovarian surface epithelial cells—shared characteristics. *Int J Gynecol Pathol* 1984;3:361–375.
64. Feinberg R, Cohen RB. A comparative histochemical study of the ovarian stromal lipid band, stromal theca cell, and normal ovarian follicular apparatus. *Am J Obstet Gynecol* 1965;92:958–969.
65. Czernobilsky B, Shezen E, Lifschitz-Mercer B, et al. Alpha smooth muscle actin (alpha-SM actin) in normal human ovaries, in ovarian stromal hyperplasia and in ovarian neoplasms. *Virchows Arch [B]* 1989;57:55–61.
66. Lastarria D, Sachdev RK, Babury RA, Yu HM, Nuovo GJ. Immunohistochemical analysis for desmin in normal and neoplastic ovarian stromal tissue. *Arch Pathol Lab Med* 1990;114:502–505.
67. Shaw JA, Dabbs DJ, Geisinger KR. Sclerosing stromal tumor of the ovary: an ultrastructural and immunohistochemical analysis with histogenetic considerations. *Ultrastruct Pathol* 1992;16:363–377.
68. Nagamani M, Hannigan EV, Van Dinh T, Stuart CA. Hyperinsulinemia and stromal luteinization of the ovaries in postmenopausal women with endometrial cancer. *J Clin Endocrinol Metab* 1988;67:144–148.
69. Scully RE, Cohen RB. Oxidative-enzyme activity in normal and pathologic human ovaries. *Obstet Gynecol* 1964;24:667–681.
70. Loubet R, Loubet A, Leboutet M-J. The ovarian stroma after the menopause: activity and ageing. In: de Brux J, Gautray J-P, eds. *Clinical pathology of the ovary*. Boston: MTP Press; 1984:119–141.
71. Nakano R, Shima K, Yamoto M, Kobayashi M, Nishimori K, Hiraoka J. Binding sites for gonadotropins in human postmenopausal ovaries. *Obstet Gynecol* 1989;73:196–200.
72. Bassis ML. Pseudodeciduosis. *Am J Obstet Gynecol* 1956;72: 1029–1037.
73. Israel SL, Rubenstone A, Meranze DR. The ovary at term. I. Decidua-like reaction and surface cell proliferation. *Obstet Gynecol* 1954; 3:399–407.
74. Ober WB, Grady HG, Schoenbucher AK. Ectopic ovarian decidua without pregnancy. *Am J Pathol* 1957;33:199–217.
75. Bersch W, Alexy E, Heuser HP, Staemmler HJ. Ectopic decidua formation in the ovary (so-called deciduoma). *Virchows Arch [A]* 1973; 360:173–177.
76. Starup J, Visfeldt J. Ovarian morphology in early and late human pregnancy. *Acta Obstet Gynecol Scand* 1974;53:211–218.
77. Herr JC, Heidger PM Jr, Scott JR, Anderson JW, Curet LB, Mossman HW. Decidual cells in the human ovary at term. I. Incidence, gross anatomy and ultrastructural features of merocrine secretion. *Am J Anat* 1978;152:7–28.
78. Hughesdon PE. Morphology and morphogenesis of the Stein-Leventhal and of so-called "hyperthecosis." *Obstet Gynecol Surv* 1982;37: 59–77.
79. Scully RE. Smooth-muscle differentiation in genital tract disorders [Editorial]. *Arch Pathol Lab Med* 1981;105:505–507.
80. Hughesdon PE. The origin and development of benign stromatosis of the ovary. *Br J Obstet Gynaecol* 1972;79:348–359.
81. Hughesdon PE. The endometrial identity of benign stromatosis of the ovary and its relation to other forms of endometriosis. *J Pathol* 1976; 119:201–209.
82. Hart WR, Abell MR. Adipose prosoplasia of ovary. *Am J Obstet Gynecol* 1970;106:929–930.
83. Honore LH, O'Hara KE. Subcapsular adipocytic infiltration of the human ovary: a clinicopathological study of eight cases. *Eur J Obstet Gynaecol Reprod Biol* 1980;10:13–20.
84. Sternberg WH, Roth LM. Ovarian stromal tumors containing Leydig cells. I. Stromal-Leydig cell tumor and non-neoplastic transformation of ovarian stroma to Leydig cells. *Cancer* 1973;32:940–951.
85. Zhang J, Young RH, Arseneau J, Scully RE. Ovarian stromal tumors containing lutein or Leydig cells (luteinized thecomas and stromal Leydig cell tumors)—a clinicopathological analysis of fifty cases. *Int J Gynecol Pathol* 1982;1:270–285.
86. Rutgers JL, Scully RE. Functioning ovarian tumors with peripheral steroid cell proliferation: a report of twenty-four cases. *Int J Gynecol Pathol* 1986;5:319–337.
87. Hidvegi D, Cibils LA, Sorensen K, Hidvegi I. Ultrastructural and histochemical observations of neuroendocrine granules in nonneoplastic ovaries. *Am J Obstet Gynecol* 1982;143:590–594.
88. Snowden JA, Harkin PJR, Thornton JG, Wells M. Morphometric assessment of ovarian stromal proliferation—a clinicopathological study. *Histopathology* 1989;14:369–379.
89. Bigelow B. Comparison of ovarian and endometrial morphology spanning the menopause. *Obstet Gynecol* 1958;11:487–513.
90. Roddick JW Jr, Greene RR. Relation of ovarian stromal hyperplasia to endometrial carcinoma. *Am J Obstet Gynecol* 1957;73:843–852.
91. Woll E, Hertig AT, Smith GVS, Johnson LC. The ovary in endometrial carcinoma. *Am J Obstet Gynecol* 1948;56:617–633.
92. Laffargue P, Adechy-Benkoel L, Valette C. Ultrastructure du stroma ovarien. *Ann Anat Pathol* 1968;13:381–401.
93. Aiman J, Fornery JP, Parker R Jr. Secretion of androgens and estrogens by normal and neoplastic ovaries in postmenopausal women. *Obstet Gynecol* 1986;68:1–5.
94. Chang RJ, Judd HL. The ovary after menopause. *Clin Obstet Gynaecol* 1981;24:181–191.
95. Dennefors BL, Janson PO, Knutsson F, Hamberger L. Steroid pro-

duction and responsiveness to gonadotropin in isolated stromal tissue of human postmenopausal ovaries. *Am J Obstet Gynecol* 1980;136: 997–1002.
96. Greenblatt RB, Colle ML, Mahesh VB. Ovarian and adrenal steroid production in the postmenopausal woman. *Obstet Gynecol* 1976;47: 383–387.
97. Judd HL, Judd GE, Lucas WE, Yen SSC. Endocrine function of the postmenopausal ovary: concentration of androgens and estrogens in ovarian and peripheral vein blood. *J Clin Endocrinol Metab* 1974;39: 1020–1024.
98. Judd HL, Lucas WE, Yen SSC. Effect of oophorecomy on circulating testosterone and androstenedione levels in patients with endometrial carcinoma. *Am J Obstet Gynecol* 1974;118:793–798.
99. Longcope C, Hunter R, Franz C. Steroid secretion by the postmenopausal ovary. *Am J Obstet Gynecol* 1980;138:564–568.
100. Lucisano A, Russo N, Acampora MG, et al. Ovarian and peripheral androgen and oestrogen levels in post-menopausal women: correlations with ovarian histology. *Maturitas* 1986;8:57–65.
101. Mattingly RF, Huang WY. Steroidogenesis of the menopause and postmenopausal ovary. *Am J Obstet Gynecol* 1969;103:679–693.
102. McNatty KP, Makris A, DeGrazia C, Osathanondh R, Ryan KJ. The production of progesterone, androgens, and estrogens by granulosa cells, thecal tissue, and stromal tissue from human ovaries in vitro. *J Clin Endocrinol Metab* 1979;49:687–699.
103. McNatty KP, Smith DM, Makris A, et al. The intraovarian sites of androgen and estrogen formation in women with normal and hyperandrogenic ovaries as judged by in vitro experiments. *J Clin Endocrinol Metab* 1980;50:755–763.
104. Plotz EJ, Wiener M, Stein AA, Hahn BD. Enzymatic activities related to steroidogenesis in postmenopausal ovaries of patients with and without endometrial carcinoma. *Am J Obstet Gynecol* 1967;99: 182–197.
105. Vermeulen A. The hormonal activity of the postmenopausal ovary. *J Clin Endocrinol Metab* 1976;42:247–253.
106. Rice BF, Savard K. Steroid hormone formation in the human ovary: IV. Ovarian stromal compartment; formation of radioactive steroids from acetate-1-$_{14}$C and action of gonadotropins. *J Clin Endocrinol* 1966;26:593–609.
107. Barbieri RL, Makris A, Randall RW, Daniels G, Kistner RW, Ryan KJ. Insulin stimulates androgen accumulation in incubations of ovarian stroma obtained from women with hyperandrogenism. *J Clin Endocrinol Metab* 1986;62:904–910.
108. Reed MJ, Beranek PA, Ghilchik MW, James VHT. Conversion of estrone to estradiol and estradiol to estrone in postmenopausal women. *Obstet Gynecol* 1985;66:361–365.
109. Longcope C. Metabolic clearance and blood production rates of estrogens in postmenopausal women. *Am J Obstet Gynecol* 1971;111: 778–781.
110. Grodin JM, Siiteri PK, MacDonald PC. Source of estrogen production in postmenopausal women. *J Clin Endocrinol Metab* 1973;36: 207–214.
111. Nagamani M, Stuart CA, Doherty MG. Increased steroid production by the ovarian stromal tissue of postmenopausal women with endometrial cancer. *J Clin Endocrinol Metab* 1992;74:172–176.
112. Dawood MY, Strongin M, Kramer EE, Wieche R. Recent ovulation in a postmenopausal woman. *Int J Gynaecol Obstet* 1980;18:192–194.
113. Sherrer CW, Gerson B, Woodruff JD. The incidence and significance of polynuclear follicles. *Am J Obstet Gynecol* 1977;128:6–12.
114. Gougeon A. Frequent occurrence of multiovular follicles and multinuclear oocytes in the adult human ovary. *Fertil Steril* 1981;35: 417–422.
115. Manivel JC, Dehner LP, Burke B. Ovarian tumorlike structures, biovular follicles, and binucleated oocytes in children: their frequency and possible pathologic significance. *Pediatr Pathol* 1988;8:282–292.
116. Baca M, Zamboni L. The fine structure of the human follicular oocyte. *J Ultrastruct Res* 1967;19:354–381.
117. Hertig AT. The primary human oocyte: some observations on the fine structure of Balbiani's vitelline body and the origin of the annulate lamellae. *Am J Anat* 1968;122:107–138.
118. Hertig AT, Adams EC. Studies on the human oocyte and its follicle. I. Ultrastructural and histochemical observations on the primordial follicle stage. *J Cell Biol* 1967;34:647–675.
119. Curtis EM. Normal ovarian histology in infancy and childhood. *Obstet Gynecol* 1962;19:444–454.
120. Dekel N, David MP, Yedwab GA, Kraicer PF. Follicular development during late pregnancy. *Int J Fertil* 1977;22:24–29.
121. Govan ADT. Ovarian follicular activity in late pregnancy. *J Endocrinol* 1970;48:235–241.
122. Himelstein-Braw R, Byskov AG, Peters H, Faber M. Follicular atresia in the infant human ovary. *J Reprod Fertil* 1976;46:55–59.
123. Maqueo M, Goldzieher JW. Hormone-induced alterations of ovarian morphology. *Fertil Steril* 1966;17:676–683.
124. Mikhail G, Allen WM. Ovarian function in human pregnancy. *Am J Obstet Gynecol* 1967;99:308–312.
125. Nelson WW, Greene RR. The human ovary in pregnancy. *Int Abstr Surg* 1953;97:1–23.
126. Nelson WW, Greene RR. Some observations on the histology of the human ovary during pregnancy. *Am J Obstet Gynecol* 1958;76:66–89.
127. Peters H, Himelstein-Braw R, Faber M. The normal development of the ovary in childhood. *Acta Endocrinol* 1976;82:617–630.
128. McNatty KP, Hillier SG, Van Den Boogaard AMJ, Trimbos-Kemper TCM, Reichert LE Jr. Van Hall EV. Follicular development during the luteal phase of the human menstrual cycle. *J Clin Endocrinol Metab* 1983;56:1022–1031.
129. McNatty KP, Smith DM, Makris A, Osathanondh R, Ryan KJ. The microenvironment of the human antral follicle: interrelationships among the steroid levels in antral fluid, the population of granulosa cells, and the status of the oocyte in vivo and in vitro. *J Clin Endocrinol Metab* 1979;49:851–860.
130. White RF, Hertig AT, Rock J, Adams E. Histological and histochemical observations on the corpus luteum of human pregnancy with special reference to corpora lutea associated with early normal and abnormal ova. *Contrib Embryol* 1951;34:55–74.
131. Jones GES, Goldberg B, Woodruff JD. Histochemistry as a guide for interpretation of cell function. *Am J Obstet Gynecol* 1968;100:76–83.
132. Sasano H, Mori T, Sasano N, Nagura H, Mason JI. Immunolocalization of 3beta-hydroxysteroid dehydrogenase in human ovary. *J Reprod Fertil* 1990;89:743–751.
133. Deane HW, Lobel BL, Romney SL. Enzymic histochemistry of normal human ovaries of the menstrual cycle, pregnancy, and the early puerperium. *Am J Obstet Gynecol* 1962;83:281–294.
134. Mestwardt W, Muller O, Brandau H. Structural analysis of granulosa cells from human ovaries in correlation with function. In: Channing CP, Marsh JM, Sadler WA, eds. *Ovarian follicular and corpus luteum function. Advances in experimental medicine and biology*. Vol. 112. New York: Plenum; 1978.
135. Gillim SW, Christensen AK, McLennan CE. Fine structure of the human menstrual corpus luteum at its stage of maximum secretory activity. *Am J Anat* 1969;126:409–428.
136. Okamura H, Virutamasen P, Wright KH, Wallach EE. Ovarian smooth muscle in the human being, rabbit, and cat. *Am J Obstet Gynecol* 1972;112:183–191.
137. McNatty KP. Follicular determinants of corpus luteum function in the human ovary. In: Channing CP, Marsh JM, Sadler WA, eds. *Ovarian follicular and corpus luteum function. Advances in experimental medicine and biology*. Vol. 112. New York: Plenum; 1978:465–477.
138. McNatty KP. Cyclic changes in antral fluid hormone concentrations in humans. *Clin Endocrinol Metab* 1978;7:577–600.
139. Erickson GF. Normal ovarian function. *Clin Obstet Gynecol* 1978;21: 31–52.
140. Shima K, Kitayama S, Nakano R. Gonadotropin binding sites in human ovarian follicles and corpora lutea during the menstrual cycle. *Obstet Gynecol* 1987;69:800–806.
141. Eden JA, Carter GD, Jones J, Alaghband-Zadeh J. Insulin-like growth factor 1 as an intra-ovarian hormone—an integrated hypothesis and review. *Aust N Z J Obstet Gynaecol* 1989;29:30–37.
142. McNatty KP, Makris A, DeGrazia C, Osathanondh R, Ryan KJ. The production of progesterone, androgens, and estrogens by human granulosa cells in vitro and in vivo. *J Steroid Biochem* 1979;11:775–799.
143. Hillier SG. Intrafollicular paracrine function of ovarian androgen. *J Steroid Biochem* 1987;27:351–357.
144. Pauerstein CJ, Eddy CA, Croxatto HD, Hess R, Siler-Khodr TM, Croxatto HB. Temporal relationships of estrogen, progesterone, and luteinizing hormone levels to ovulation in women and infrahuman primates. *Am J Obstet Gynecol* 1978;130:876–886.
145. Yussman MA, Taymor ML. Serum levels of follicle stimulating hormone and luteinizing hormone and of plasma progesterone related to ovulation by corpus luteum biopsy. *J Clin Endocrinol* 1970;30: 396–399.
146. Futterweit W. *Polycystic ovarian disease. Clinical perspectives in obstetrics and gynecology*. New York: Springer-Verlag; 1985.

147. Tanabe K, Gagliano P, Channing CP, et al. Levels of inhibin-F activity and steroids in human follicular fluid from normal women and women with polycystic ovarian disease. *J Clin Endocrinol Metab* 1983;57:24–31.
148. Tsonis CG, Messinis IE, Templeton AA, McNeilly AS, Baird DT. Gonadotropic stimulation of inhibin secretion by the human ovary during the follicular and early luteal phase of the cycle. *J Clin Endocrinol Metab* 1988;66:915–921.
149. McLachlan RI, Cohen NL, Vale WW, et al. The importance of luteinizing hormone in the control of inhibin and progesterone secretion by the human corpus luteum. *J Clin Endocrinol Metab* 1989;68: 1078–1085.
150. Sealey JE, Glorioso N, Itskovitz J, Laragh JH. Prorenin as a reproductive hormone. New form of the renin system. *Am J Med* 1986;81: 1041–1046.
151. Palumbo A, Jones C, Lightman A, Carcangiu ML, DeCherney AH, Naftolin F. Immunohistochemical localization of renin and angiotensin II in human ovaries. *Am J Obstet Gynecol* 1989;160:8–14.
152. Corner GW Jr. The histological dating of the human corpus luteum of menstruation. *Am J Anat* 1956;98:377–401.
153. Visfeldt J, Starup J. Dating of the human corpus luteum of menstruation using histological parameters. *Acta Pathol Microbiol Scand* 1974; 82:137–144.
154. Croxatto H, Ortiz M, Croxatto HB. Correlation between histologic dating of human corpus luteum and the luteinizing hormone peak-biopsy interval. *Am J Obstet Gynecol* 1980;136:667–670.
155. Wiley CA, Esterly JR. Observations on the human corpus luteum: histochemical changes during development and involution. *Am J Obstet Gynecol* 1976;125:514–519.
156. Hameed A, Fox WM, Kurman RJ, Hruban RH, Podack ER. Perforin expression in human cell–mediated luteolysis. *Int J Gynecol Pathol* 1995;14:151–157.
157. Adams EC, Hertig AT. Studies on the human corpus luteum. I. Observations on the ultrastructure of development and regression of the luteal cells during the menstrual cycle. *J Cell Biol* 1969;41:696–715.
158. Tamura M, Sasano H, Suzuki T, et al. Immunohistochemical localization of growth hormone receptor in cyclic human ovaries. *Hum Reprod* 1994;9:2259–2262.
159. Crisp TM, Dessouky DA, Denys FR. The fine structure of the human corpus luteum of early pregnancy and during the progestational phase of the menstrual cycle. *Am J Anat* 1970;127:37–70.
160. Green JA, Maqueo M. Ultrastructure of the human ovary. I. The luteal cell during the menstrual cycle. *Am J Obstet Gynecol* 1965;92: 946–957.
161. LeMaire WJ, Conly PW, Moffett A, Spellacy WN, Cleveland WW, Savard K. Function of the human corpus luteum during the puerperium: its maintenance by exogenous human chorionic gonadotropin. *Am J Obstet Gynecol* 1971;110:612–618.
162. Centola GM. Structural changes: follicular development and hormonal requirements. In: Serra GB, ed. *The ovary*. New York: Raven Press; 1983:95–111.
163. Rao CV. Receptors for gonadotropins in human ovaries. In: *Recent advances in fertility research.* Part A: Developments in reproductive endocrinology. New York: Alan R. Liss; 1982:123–135.
164. Vijayakumar R, Walters WAW. Ovarian stromal and luteal tissue prostaglandins, 17beta-estradiol, and progesterone in relation to the phases of the menstrual cycle in women. *Am J Obstet Gynecol* 1987; 156:947–951.
165. Hertig AT. Gestational hyperplasia of endometrium. A morphologic correlation of ova, endometrium, and corpora lutea during early pregnancy. *Lab Invest* 1964;13:1153–1191.
166. Visfeldt J, Starup J. Histology of the human corpus luteum of early and late pregnancy. *Acta Pathol Microbiol Scand* 1975;83:669–677.
167. Adams EC, Hertig AT. Studies on the human corpus luteum. II. Observations on the ultrastructure of luteal cells during pregnancy. *J Cell Biol* 1969;41:716–735.
168. Green JA, Garcilazo JA, Maqueo M. Ultrastructure of the human ovary. II. The luteal cell at term. *Am J Obstet Gynecol* 1967;99: 855–863.
169. Pedersen PH, Larsen JF. The ultrastructure of the human granulosa lutein cell of the first trimester of gestation. *Acta Endocrinol* 1968;58: 481–496.
170. LeMaire WJ, Rice BF, Savard K. Steroid hormone formation in the human ovary. V. Synthesis of progesterone in vitro in corpora lutea during the reproductive cycle. *J Clin Endocrinol Metab* 1968;28: 1249–1256.
171. Weiss G, Rifkin I. Progesterone and estrogen secretion by puerperal human ovaries. *Obstet Gynecol* 1975;46:557–559.
172. Weiss G, O'Byrne EM, Hochman JA, Goldsmith LT, Rifkin I, Steinetz BG. Secretion of progesterone and relaxin by the human corpus luteum at midpregnancy and at term. *Obstet Gynecol* 1977;50: 679–681.
173. Weiss G, O'Byrne EM, Steinetz BG. Relaxin: a product of the human corpus luteum of pregnancy. *Science* 1976;194:948–949.
174. Schmidt CL, Black VH, Sarosi P, Weiss G. Progesterone and relaxin secretion in relation to the ultrastructure of human luteal cells in culture: effects of human chorionic gonadotropin. *Am J Obstet Gynecol* 1986;155:1209–1219.
175. Quagliarello J, Goldsmith L, Steinetz B, Lustig DS, Weiss G. Induction of relaxin secretion in nonpregnant women by human chorionic gonadotropin. *J Clin Endocrinol Metab* 1980;51:74–77
176. Reagan JW. Ceroid pigment in the human ovary. *Am J Obstet Gynecol* 1950;59:433–436.
177. Joel RV, Foraker AG. Fate of the corpus albicans: a morphologic approach. *Am J Obstet Gynecol* 1960;80:314–316.
178. Centola GM. Structural changes: atresia. In: Serra GB, ed. *The ovary*. New York: Raven Press; 1983:113–122.
179. Strickler R, Kelly RW, Askin FB. Postmenopausal ovarian follicle cyst: an unusual cause of estrogen excess. *Int J Gynecol Pathol* 1984; 3:318–322.
180. Kraus FT, Neubecker RD. Luteinization of the ovarian theca in infants and children. *Am J Clin Pathol* 1962;37:389–397.
181. Clement PB, Young RH, Scully RE. Ovarian granulosa cell proliferations of pregnancy: a report of nine cases. *Hum Pathol* 1988;19: 657–662.
182. Kedzia H. Gonadoblastoma: structures and background of development. *Am J Obstet Gynecol* 1983;147:81–85.
183. Safneck JR, DeSa DJ. Structures mimicking sex cord stromal tumours and gonadoblastomas in the ovaries of normal infants and children. *Histopathology* 1986;10:909–920.
184. Bomsel-Helmreich O, Gougeon A, Thebault A, et al. Healthy and atretic human follicles in the preovulatory phase: differences in evolution of follicular morphology and steroid content of follicular fluid. *J Clin Endocrinol Metab* 1979;48:686–694.
185. Sternberg WH. The morphology, androgenic function, hyperplasia, and tumors of the human ovarian hilus cells. *Am J Pathol* 1949;25: 493–521.
186. Sternberg WH, Segaloff A, Gaskill CJ. Influence of chorionic gonadotropin on human ovarian hilus cells (Leydig-like cells). *J Clin Endocrinol Metab* 1953;13:139–153.
187. Merrill JA. Ovarian hilus cells. *Am J Obstet Gynecol* 1959;78: 1258–1271.
188. Honore LH, O'Hara KE. Ovarian hilus cell heterotopia. *Obstet Gynecol* 1979;53:361–464.
189. Janko AB. Sandberg EC. Histochemical evidence for the protein nature of the Reinke crystalloid. *Obstet Gynecol* 1970;35:493–503.
190. Schmidt WA. Eosin-induced fluorescence of Reinke crystals. *Int J Gynecol Pathol* 1986;5:88–89.
191. Laffargue P, Benkoel L, Laffargue F, Casanova P, Chamlian A. Ultrastructural and enzyme histochemical study of ovarian hilar cells in women and their relationships with sympathetic nerves. *Hum Pathol* 1978;9:649–659.
192. Symonds DA, Driscoll SG. An adrenal cortical rest within the fetal ovary: report of a case. *Am J Clin Pathol* 1973;60:562–564.
193. Falls JL. Accessory adrenal cortex in the broad ligament. Incidence and significance. *Cancer* 1955;8:143–150.
194. Dennefors BL, Janson PO, Hamberger L, Knutsson F. Hilus cells from human postmenopausal ovaries: gonadotrophin sensitivity, steroid and cyclic AMP production. *Acta Obstet Gynecol Scand* 1982;61: 413–416.
195. Sauromo H. Development, occurrence, function, and pathology of the rete ovarii. *Acta Obstet Gynecol Scand* 1954(suppl);33:29–66.
196. Rutgers JL, Scully RE. Cysts (cystadenomas) and tumors of the rete ovarii. *Int J Gynecol Pathol* 1988;7:330–342.
197. Gardner GH, Greene RR, Peckham B. Tumors of the broad ligament. *Am J Obstet Gynecol* 1957;73:536–555.

*Histology for Pathologists, second edition,*
Edited by Stephen S. Sternberg.
Lippincott-Raven Publishers, Philadelphia
© 1997.

# CHAPTER 41

# Placenta

Steven H. Lewis and Kurt Benirschke



The placenta is a remarkable organ that, with the exception of a few pathologists and clinicians, has received little attention. It is fortuitous for those interested in the placenta that the medicolegal aspects of placentation have brought this organ to the forefront, making discussions and reports on its complex anatomic, pathologic, and physiologic aspects more commonplace. The placenta may be pivotal in adjudicating the etiology of "bad babies" (1,2). An objective, thorough, well-documented analysis also can provide important data for maternal and neonatal care.

These complex considerations cannot be addressed without a thorough understanding of the normal structure of the placenta, and it is to this end that this chapter is devoted. Pathologic entities are discussed to better demonstrate normal anatomy and histology. Because the placenta is a misunderstood organ, it is beneficial for the practicing pathologist to observe the contrast between normal and abnormal to better understand and demonstrate both normal anatomy and histology. For more encyclopedic and complete discussions regarding placental pathology, the reader is directed elsewhere (1,2). It is easiest and most appropriate to describe the principal structural components of the placenta in a compartmentalized manner. These consist of the umbilical cord, the membranes (amnion and chorion), the villous parenchyma, and the maternal decidual tissue.

## ROUTINE STORAGE, EXAMINATION, AND PROCESSING

After obstetric delivery, placentas may be stored at 4°C in a refrigerator before examination. The period of time for this storage generally should not exceed 1 week. Placentas should not be frozen before evaluation because the gross examination is rendered difficult and histologic features are obscured. For refrigeration, suitable containers include cardboard buckets or styrofoam storage cups. It has been advocated by some to immediately fix the placenta in 10% buffered formalin for later examination (3). It should be

S. H. Lewis: Department of Obstetrics and Gynecology, Indian River Memorial Hospital; the Doctors' Clinic, Vero Beach, Florida; Department of Pathology and Obstetrics and Gynecology, University of South Florida, Tampa, Florida 33620.

K. Benirschke: Department of Pathology and Reproductive Medicine, University of California at San Diego, and University Medical Center, San Diego, California 92103.

noted that when this method of processing is used, placental weights increase by a factor of approximately 10% (4).

It should be underscored that although assessment of the placenta is considered in the pathologist's domain, it is the obstetrician who first visualizes the specimen. An educated clinician may facilitate proper submission and aid the pathologist by providing appropriate clinical information and recognize abnormalities that will lead to submission and processing. It has been our experience that through routine seminars, the obstetrician may learn to understand and identify which placentas are most important for review. Labor and delivery suites should have a list of appropriate clinical and pathologic entities that require pathologic examination of the placenta (5). Most institutions do not perform histologic evaluation of all placentas from all deliveries. However, many institutions at least examine all placentas grossly and submit tissues for histologic study from those placentas for which perinatal pathology is suspect. In our two institutions, histologic examination is performed on approximately 10% to 20% of all delivered placentas.

The gross morphologic assessment of the placenta should be approached in a thorough, routine fashion. Our procedure for the gross assessment and sectioning of placentas is illustrated in Table 1.

The placenta is removed from its container and its shape described. It is usually discoid, but additional lobes may be present. It is next convenient to note the location of insertion of the umbilical cord, describe its length and diameter, note irregularities in its contour and texture, describe its color, and note the number of vessels it contains. The cord is then amputated at its base, and representative sections are immersed in fixative.

Attention is next directed to the membranes (amnion and chorion), which are inspected for completeness. Usually, the placenta is delivered vaginally with the membranes surrounding the placental maternal surface ("Schultze"). The membranes are then manually reflected to their normal anatomic position and the smallest distance from the point of rupture to the placental disk (the narrowest width of membranes) is measured. When this measurement equals zero (after vaginal delivery), a low-lying or marginal placenta previa is implicated. The membranes are then assessed for their color, transparency, sheen, and surface irregularities, as well as for the presence of membranous vessels or accessory lobes. The membranes are then removed from the placental disk margin, keeping track of the point of rupture. This point is grasped with a toothed forceps and rolled in a concentric fashion to produce a "membrane roll". With the membranes rolled in such a fashion, the point of rupture can be identified histologically. The presence of inflammatory cells confined to this region suggests early mild chorioamnionitis. Representative sections are immersed in fixative. The fetal surface of the placenta is next examined. Chorionic vascular thrombi, if present, and nodules or irregularities of the amnion are noted. The maternal surface of the placenta is then inspected, and any blood clot that has settled in the storage container with the dependent portions of the organ is removed. Areas of blood clot that are adherent or discolored brown (indicating chronicity) and depressing the maternal surface are considered indicative of retroplacental hemorrhage (clinically designated as abruptio). Should this be noted, the dimensions or percentage of the maternal surface involvement are recorded. The organ is next weighed free of its cord and associated membranes. The average weight of the term placenta is approximately 400 to 600 g. Placental weight varies with neonatal weight and normal weights have been reviewed for all gestational ages (1). The average dimensions of the term placenta are approximately 18 × 16 × 2.3 cm.

The villous parenchyma is then inspected by sectioning the placenta at 1- to 2-cm intervals looking for irregularities in the parenchyma that indicate infarction, thrombi, or other pathologic entities. There are normally 16 to 20 cotyledonous units that do not have distinct functional correlates. An absent cotyledon may indicate a portion of retained placenta in utero. Representative sections of abnormal areas are blocked out, and areas of normal-appearing parenchyma (usually three) are placed into fixative along with the already sectioned membrane roll and umbilical cord.

The fixation of the materials for study is routine. We prefer to fix tissues in Bouin's solution for a period of 24 h before trimming and submission for final processing. This process of fixation allows for excellent tissue penetration and ease of sectioning. In addition, it provides superior cytologic detail. The drawbacks to the Bouin's fixation are twofold. One is that if certain special studies are of interest (i.e., immunohistochemistry and in situ hybridization), Bouin's fixation may interfere with antigen–antibody reactions or nucleic acid hybridization. This problem may be eliminated by fixing tissues desired for such studies in Bouin's solution for only a limited period of time. For small uterine cervix biopsies, it has been shown that Bouin's fixation for less than 8 h produces good results with in situ hybridization (6). The second problem with Bouin's fixation is that if in the final preparation lithium carbonate is omitted, increased extraneous pigment formation occurs.

Pathologists are accustomed to using 10% buffered formalin solution for the processing of most tissues, and this is not contraindicated in the processing of placentas. We find that when using formalin, the period of time required to create sufficient tissue hardness for proper sectioning delays processing and histologic resolution is somewhat inferior to that obtained with Bouin's fixation. It is our procedure to stain tissue sections with hematoxylin and eosin (H & E) or hematoxylin-phloxine and saffron (HPS). Other standard special stains may be used for the detection of specific infectious agents, secretory activity, or structural composition; [silver stains, periodic acid-Schiff (PAS), Masson's trichrome, etc.]. Furthermore, a host of immunohistochemical stains have been used to elucidate functions of specific placental cell types.

**TABLE 1.** *Recording format*[a]

| | |
|---|---|
| | **Unit No:** |
| | **Name:** |
| | **Date of Birth:** **Sex:** |
| | **Location:** |
| | **Path. No:** |
| | Date of Delivery:<br>Date Received:<br>Physician:<br>Baby's Unit No: |
| **Previous Specimens:** | |

**SPECIMEN:** Placenta

**CLINICAL INFORMATION:** (Circle and fill in pertinent information)

| | | |
|---|---|---|
| NSVD C-section | GA: ______ wk | DM class ______ |
| Chorioamnionitis | Preeclampsia | Fetal distress |
| Newborn wt. ______ grams | 5 min Apgar <7 | Other: ______ |

**GROSS DESCRIPTION:**

| | | |
|---|---|---|
| Cord: | __ × __ cm | Insertion: |
| | # pieces: ______ | Vessel #: ______ |
| Membranes: | complete/incomplete | Narrowest width: ______ cm |
| | clear/opaque | Meconium: old/recent/none |
| | vascular thrombi: present/none | Calcification: present/none |
| Parenchyma: | red/pale/friable | Abruptio: ______ % |
| | Infarct: ______ % | Weight: ______ grams |
| Dimensions: | __ × __ × __ cm | |
| Other: | | |

**MICROSCOPIC DESCRIPTION:** (__) slides evaluated.

**DIAGNOSIS(ES):**

Umbilical cord:

Membranes:

Villi:

Decidua:

Reviewed by:

**Date Dictated:**
**Date Typed:**
**Print Date:**

[a] This format is easily converted to a computerized final report that includes final microscopic diagnoses.

## UMBILICAL CORD

### Embryology

Specific embryologic considerations are germane to the understanding of the normal umbilical cord structure, including its frequent possession of embryologic remnants. The open region on the ventral surface of the developing embryo diminishes in size and then forms the early umbilicus. Through this structure extend both the yolk stalk and the body stalk, as well as the allantois. This cylindrical structure elongates, and its surface becomes covered by the expanding amnion. This is a single-layered epithelium on a layer of connective tissue. Therefore, the developing umbilical cord

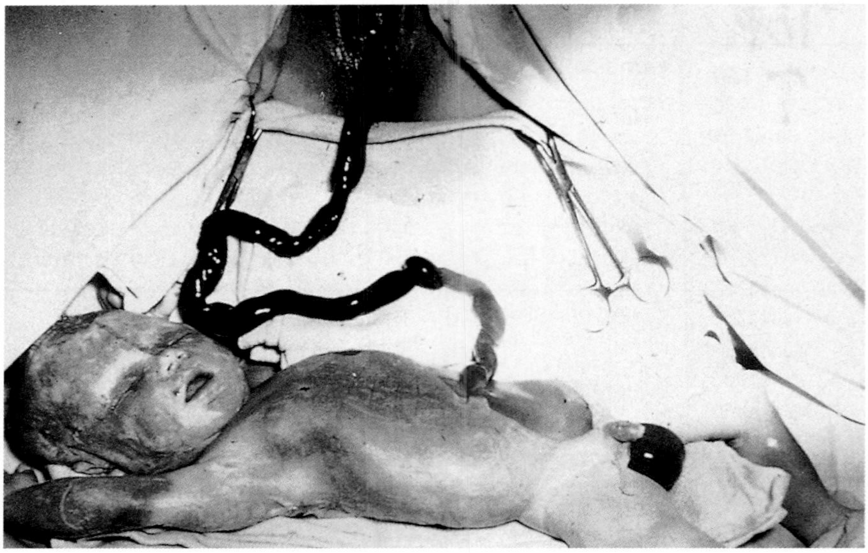

**FIG. 1.** True knot, in this case, resulted in intrauterine fetal death. [Reprinted with permission (1).]

contains the yolk stalk, a pair of vitelline blood vessels, the allantois, and the allantoic blood vessels (two arteries and one vein) and is covered by amnionic epithelium. These anatomic relationships explain the presence of the omphalomesenteric duct (the connection between developing endoderm and the yolk sac) and the allantoic duct (which has its communication in early gestation with the urachus) within sections of proximal (fetal) umbilical cord.

### Gross Morphology

The gross anatomic features of the umbilical cord that are of importance are the location of its insertion in the placental disk, its length, and the number of vessels. The presence of true knots (Fig. 1) may be considered normal when there is no adverse outcome, yet this occurrence may lead to fetal demise when the knot is tight. The presence of vascular tortuosities (false knots) is common and rarely of clinical significance (Fig. 2). The finding of meconium staining and the presence of surface plaques are definitely abnormal and are described below.

The normal umbilical cord is pearly white and somewhat translucent. The length of the umbilical cord has great significance, principally when it is excessively long or excessively short. Cord length has been shown to vary with gestational age, and measurements indicate that the cord elongates as gestation proceeds. At approximately 20 weeks' gestational age, the average cord length is 32 cm (7). The normal length of the umbilical cord at term has been determined to be, on average, between 55 and 65 cm (1,7–9) (Fig. 3). The literature contains many articles that relate the significance of abnormal cord lengths with both in utero fetal activity and neonatal outcome. The reader is referred to an extensive review of the subject (1).

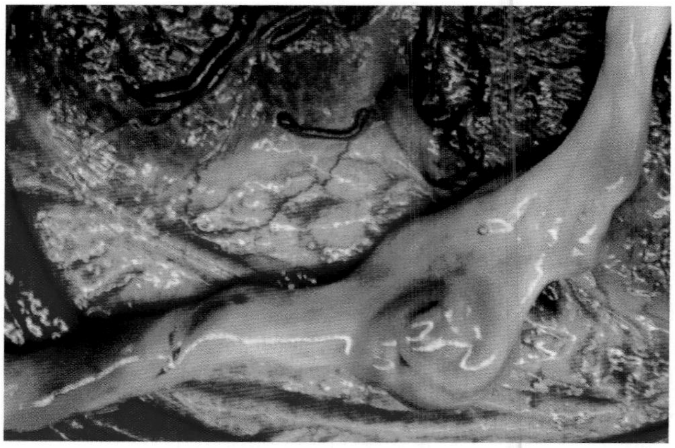

**FIG. 2.** False knot. Note the unrelated abnormal membranous vessels connecting placental lobes.

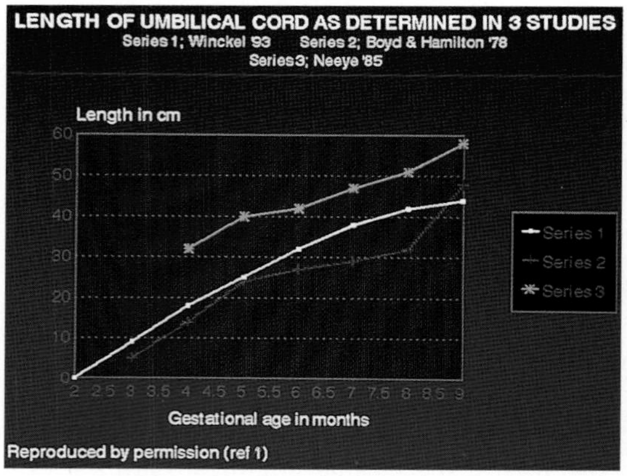


**FIG. 3.** Normal cord length dimensions associated with changes in gestational age. [Reprinted with permission (1).]

## Histology

Histologic examination of the umbilical cord shows several distinct layers. On the surface is a well-defined single layer of amnionic epithelium. The epithelium is squamoid and, in the region of fetal cord insertion, often becomes multilayered and closely resembles its epidermal contiguity. Electron microscopy studies performed on cord amnionic cells have suggested that the epithelium is responsible for fluid equilibrium activities (10). True squamous metaplasia of the umbilical cord is considered a normal variant, and ultrastructural studies of this epithelium have shown morphologic similarities between this epithelium and the fetal epidermis (11).

Deep to the amnionic epithelium that comprises the surface of the cord is the substance of Wharton's jelly. This material largely is composed of mucopolysaccharides (hyaluronic acid and chondroitin sulfate). Ultrastructural examination of this material shows the presence of delicate interlacing microfibrils and sparse collagen. Mast cells are prominent. Their frequency is increased in the near periphery of the cord vasculature (12). In this same region and in the cord in general, macrophages are rarely identified.

Embedded within the substance of Wharton's jelly are the

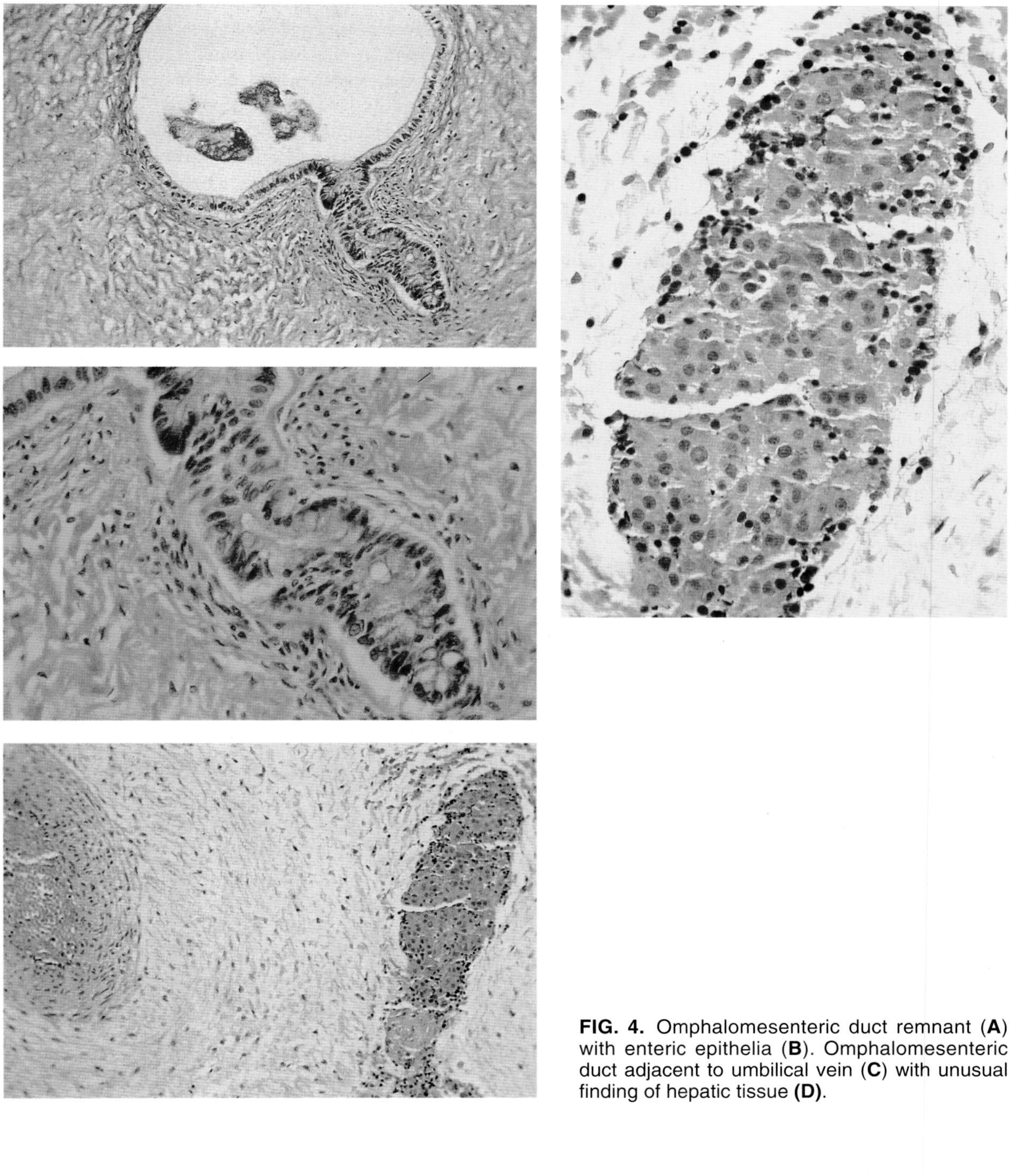

A B C D

**FIG. 4.** Omphalomesenteric duct remnant (**A**) with enteric epithelia (**B**). Omphalomesenteric duct adjacent to umbilical vein (**C**) with unusual finding of hepatic tissue **(D)**.

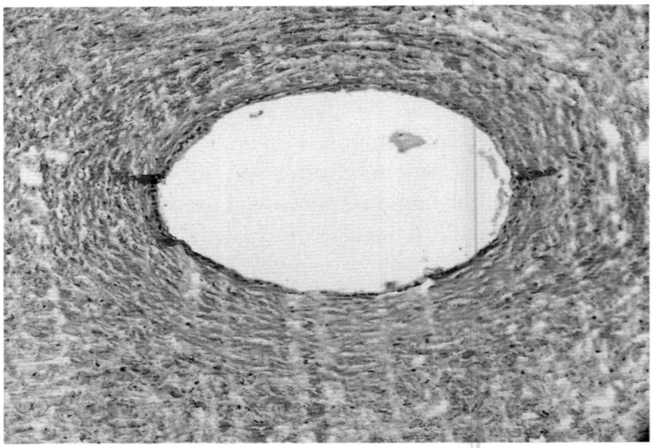

**FIG. 5.** Allantoic duct remnant hematoxylin and eosin (H&E stain).

umbilical vessels. There have been considerable interest and discussion focused on the identification of vasa vasorum and vascular neuronal innervation. Although the vasculature of the umbilical cord is of a considerable caliber, there are no vasa vasorum or lymphatic channels present in this structure. Studies investigating vascular innervation have concluded that no nerves are present within the umbilical cord. This has been borne out by electron microscopic studies (13). Occasionally, however, autonomic nerves are identified using acetylcholinesterase thiocholine techniques in the proximal (fetal) end of the cord (14). Such findings are compatible with the persistence of peripheral vagal neuronal elements associated with the ductus venosus, which are entrapped in the proximal portion of the umbilical cord. Certainly any neuronal vestiges found within the umbilical cord are best considered as remnants, and to date there has been no demonstration of their functional significance (15).

Because the yolk sac connects to the primitive midgut through the body stalk in early development, vestiges of this epithelium-lined duct are common in the umbilical cord. The persistence of the omphalomesenteric duct is characterized by a tubular structure present within Wharton's jelly and lined by a single layer of low cuboidal to columnar, mucin-secreting epithelium (Fig. 4). Remnants of the duct may form cystic structures that contain a variety of endodermally derived epithelia, including pancreatic, intestinal (small and large), and gastric components. Such findings are rarely of any clinical significance, although secretory products of gastric origin resulted in umbilical vascular ulceration, hemorrhage, and fetal death in a case report described by Blanc and Allan (16).

The allantois differentiates as a protuberance from the yolk sac into the body stalk and is essential for the development of the umbilical vessels. This structure is incorporated into the anterior aspect of the hindgut, where it communicates with the urachus. Remnants of the allantoic duct are often found in sections of proximal umbilical cords. Its intimate relationship with the formation of umbilical vessels explains its presence between the two umbilical arteries, when it is identified. These remnants rarely have clinical significance. The lining of this tract is often devoid of a lumen and consists of aggregates of epithelial cells with a variety of epithelia represented (transitional, bladder, and yolk sac–derived endodermally classified cells) (Fig. 5).

The vasculature of the umbilical cord is composed of two arteries and a single vein. The arteries possess no internal elastic lamina and have a double-layered muscular wall. Each of these muscular layers is composed of a network of interlacing smooth muscle bundles. The vein does have an inner elastic lamina. As noted, no vasa vasorum are present. Remnants of the vitelline vasculature in the proximal portion of the cord sometimes may be observed in sections taken from this region. The umbilical vein, which generally has a larger diameter, possesses a thinner muscular coat consisting of a single layer of circular smooth muscle (Fig. 6).

Of further interest, distinguishing umbilical vasculature from other systemic vessels, is that no true vascular adventitia is found. Near the placental insertion, it is common to identify anastomotic channels between the two umbilical arteries (17,18) (Fig. 7).

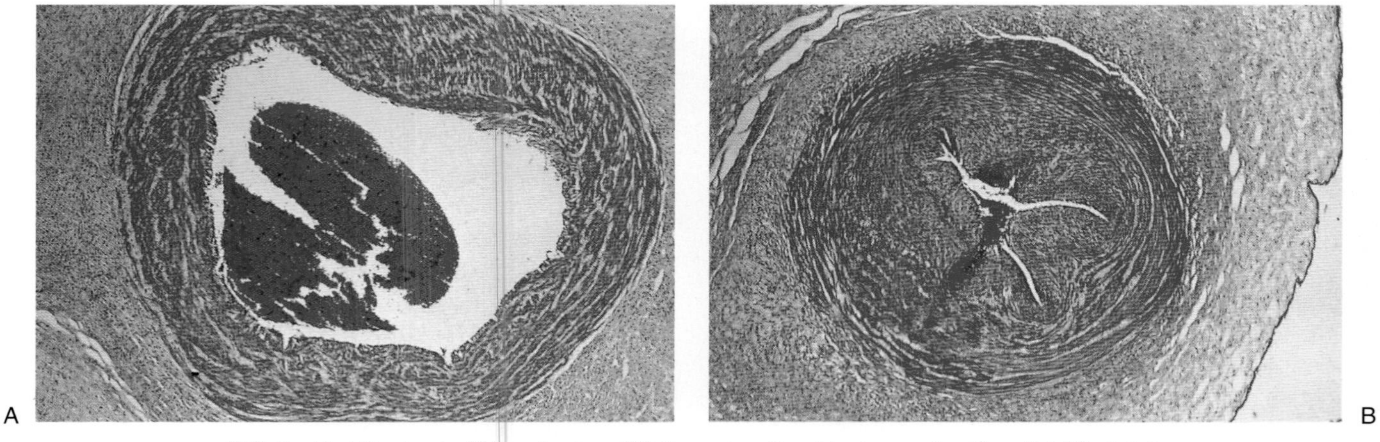


**FIG. 6.** Umbilical vein (**A**) and artery (**B**) [hematoxylin-phloxine and saffron (HPS) stain].

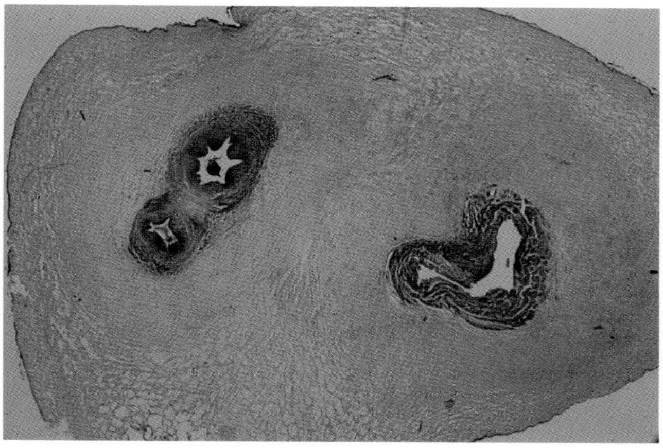

**FIG. 7.** Normal proximal anastomosis of umbilical arteries rendering the appearance of a single umbilical artery.

Transverse serial sections confirm that two umbilical arteries spiral in parallel around the umbilical vein. Often, multiple twists in the cord occur. The proposed origin of this spiraling has been extensively discussed; however, its true functional significance and origin remain to be definitively elucidated (1).

### Pathologic Alterations

Distinguishing normal anatomy from pathologic entities is the essence of proper understanding of the normal anatomy and histology of the umbilical cord. Most pathology of the cord may be seen in the gross sense. Histology is confirmatory. A tight knot with notching indicating stricture associated with proximal vascular dilatation may result in fetal death. Interestingly, although true knots occur frequently and are associated with long cords, adverse outcomes are rare events; therefore, in most instances a true knot can be considered a normal variant. The absence of an umbilical artery is a well-established observation and easy to identify grossly or in histologic sections (Fig. 8). This phenomenon has been found in approximately 1% of neonates. The association of this finding with congenital anomalies is well known, and these malformations often take the form of urinary tract malformations.

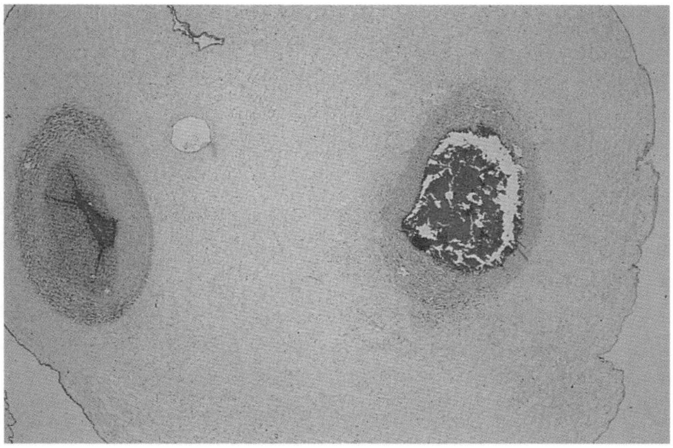

**FIG. 8.** Single umbilical artery (HSP stain).

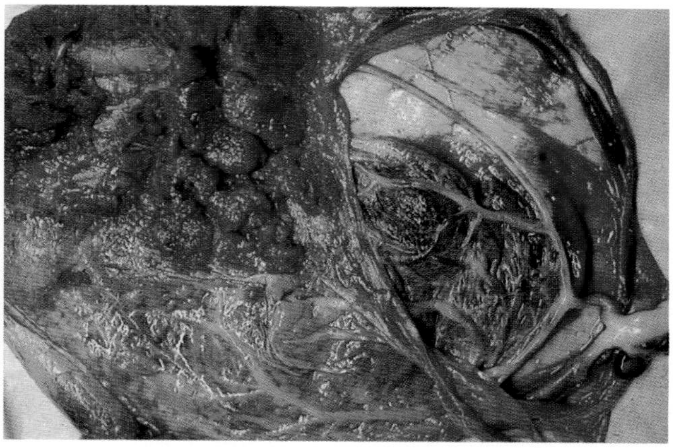

**FIG. 9.** Velamentous insertion of umbilical cord. Umbilical vessels insert in membranes adjacent to the chorionic plate. In this case the fetus exsanguinated after amniotomy and rupture of membranous vessels.

Persistence of a second (right) umbilical vein is an unusual phenomenon. The pathologist is cautioned in this regard. It is not unusual to find histologic sections identifying more than three vessels in an umbilical cord. This finding is related to commonly identified tortuosities. These tortuosities have been termed "false knots" (Fig. 2) and have little clinical significance. An exception is that these vessels rarely may be prone to thrombosis.

The presence of thrombotic material in the vasculature of the umbilical cord is truly pathologic. The process may be related to the genesis of a single umbilical artery when it occurs in early gestation. Abnormal umbilical insertions may cause thrombosis.

Velamentous cord insertions are abnormal and are charac-

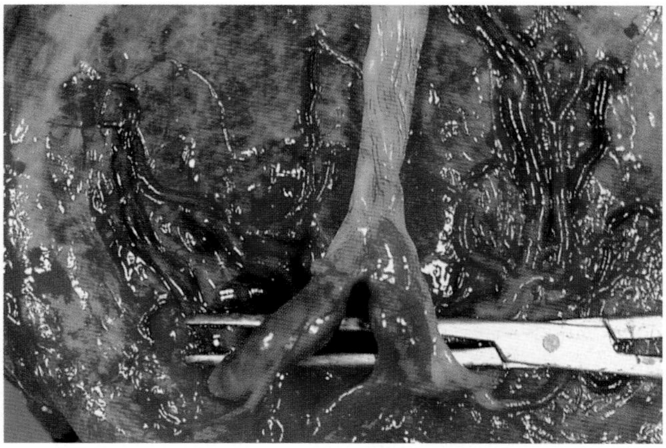

**FIG. 10.** Furcate insertion of umbilical cord. Umbilical cord vessels insert into placental substance individually (UA, *left*; UA and UV, *right*) not surrounded by Wharton's jelly.

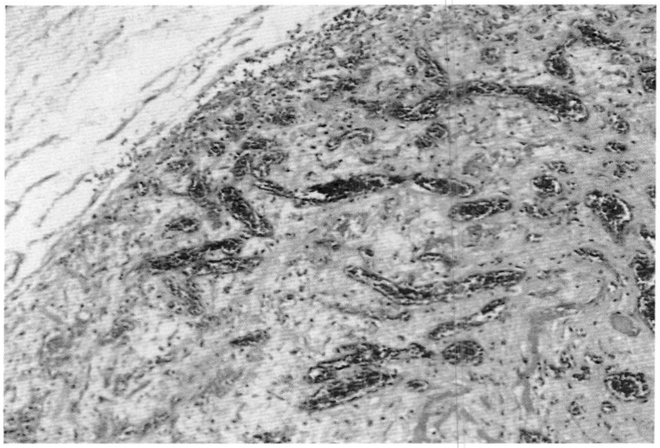

**FIG. 11.** Dilated vascular lumina of umbilical cord hemangioma (HPS stain).

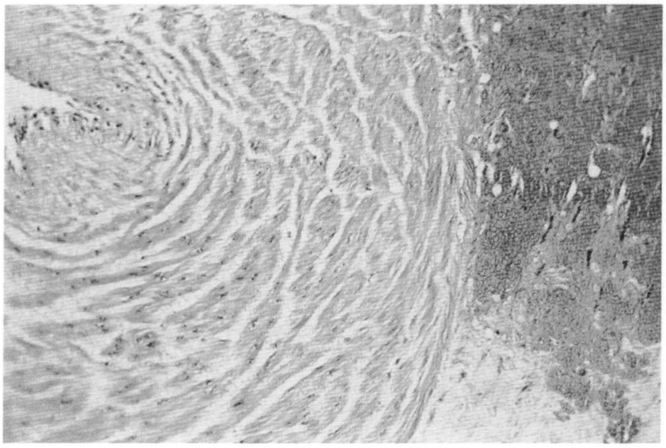

**FIG. 13.** Perivascular hemorrhage located adjacent to umbilical artery found in the region of a cord clamp (HPS stain).

terized by the presence of the umbilical vasculature implanting in the placental membranes as opposed to the usual implantation over the placental disk (Fig. 9). These vessels course independently within the chorion and are unguarded by the protective substance of the umbilical cord (Wharton's jelly). Thrombosis thus results from pressure on those vessels by fetal parts, and these vessels are subject to injury at the time of spontaneous or, more commonly, artificial membrane rupture.

Other abnormalities and pathologic findings of the umbilical cord (certainly to be distinguished from normal morphology and histology) that are of clinical importance are umbilical cord vascular rupture, complete absence of Wharton's jelly (Fig. 10), and neoplasms of the umbilical cord [hemangioma (Fig. 11) and teratoma, both unusual findings].

Most significant when considering normal histologic changes in the umbilical cord is the presence of hemorrhagic material in the perivascular region, which would suggest umbilical cord vascular rupture. Although true cord hematomas do occur on occasion (Fig. 12), the presence of hemorrhage in this region is common and generally attributed to the mode of delivery of the placenta, with traction or clamping of the umbilical cord producing this artifactual finding (Fig. 13).

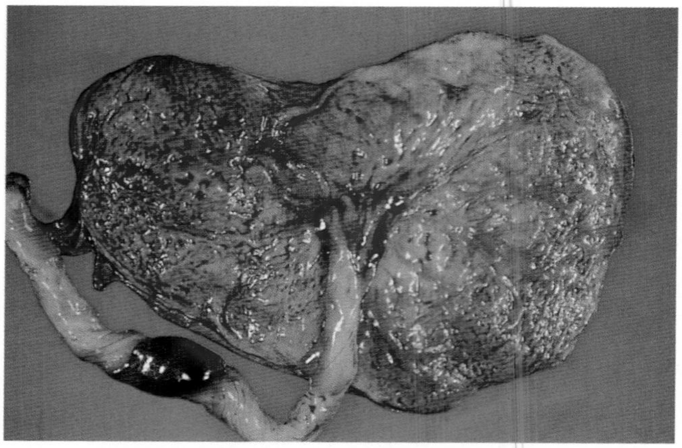

**FIG. 12.** Hematoma of umbilical cord. This placenta was delivered by cesarean section and there was no traction or clamping of this segment of cord.

Umbilical torsion and stricture are associated with excessive fetal movement and focal absence of Wharton jelly, respectively. Both are associated with adverse outcomes (1). In the former, the normal twist or coiling of the cord becomes excessive. There is an association with long cords. The latter is less well understood but may at times be a function of torsion (Fig. 14). Additionally, excessive coiling has been associated with increased fetal activity, cocaine use, abnormal fetal heart rate tracings and preterm deliveries (19). Nascent dimensions of cord width are therefore germane. There is little literature that actually defines the dimensions of normal cords, although published data correlate abnormalities associated with fat and thin cords (7,7a) (Fig. 15).

Another definitively pathologic entity that must be distinguished from normal histology is the presence of leukocytes within the cord substance. Such findings are indicative of funisitis and are the result of inflammatory response to infectious antigens and recruitment through inflammatory pathways (Fig. 16). When the process is prominent (severe) and with calcifications, the term *necrotizing funisitis* is applicable. Such severe pathology is indicative of chronic inflammation and may be seen in syphilis as well as other infections (1) (Fig. 17). The identification of fungal elements about the umbilical cord are often difficult to discern from an overgrowth storage phenomenon. In this regard, the difficulty lies in the usual absence of associated inflammatory infiltrate. The cord, when involved, has white surface plaques. Fungal elements (i.e., *Candida albicans*) may be identified merely with hematoxylin and eosin stains, although special

A
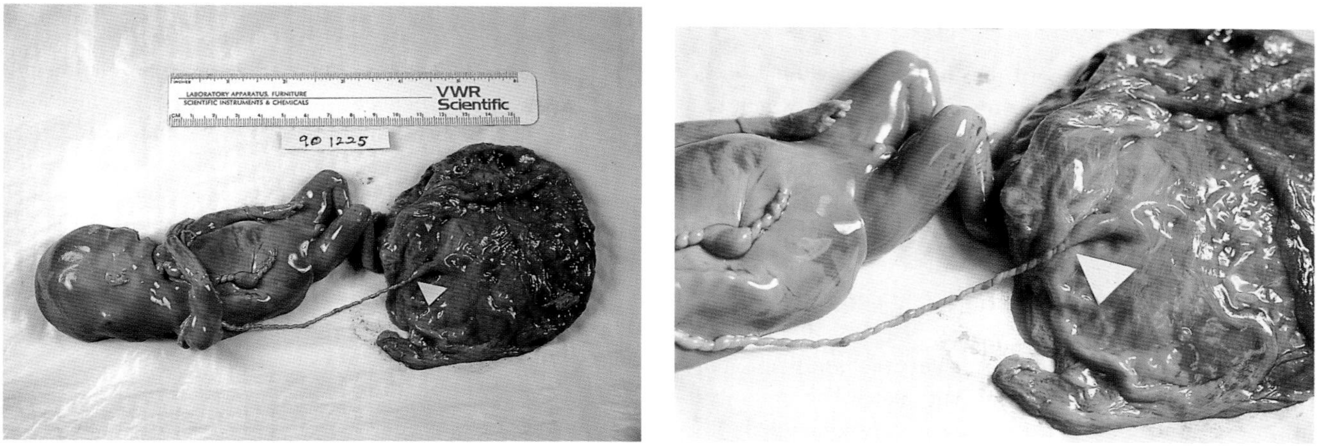

B

**FIG. 14.** Excessive spiraling (**A**) leading to torsion (**B**) and stricture resulting in fetal death.

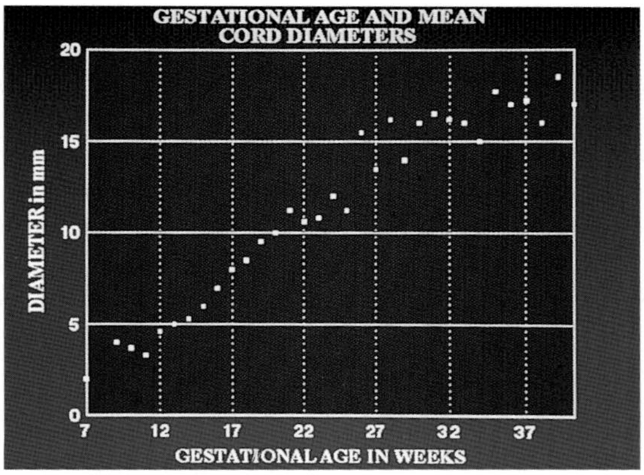


**FIG. 15.** Mean cord width (as determined by ultrasound 2 cm from umbilical insertion) versus advancing gestational age ($n = 100$, $p < 0.05$). [Reprinted with permission (7a).]

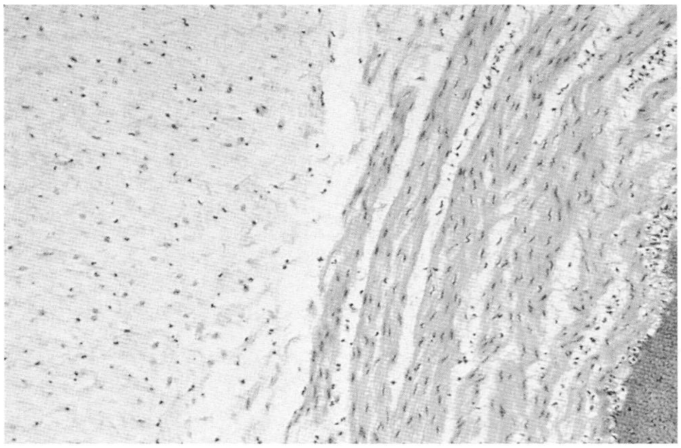

**FIG. 16.** Acute funisitis. Polymorphonuclear leukocytes are present within the umbilical vein muscularis and adjacent Wharton's jelly.

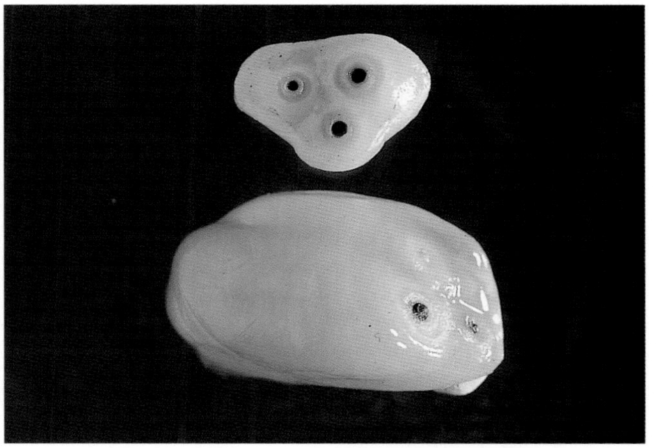

**FIG. 17.** Necrotizing funisitis with intense perivascular malformations associated with calcification (peripheral white circular bands) may be seen in the gross.

stains for fungi can be helpful when such pathology is suspect (1).

Last, a finding in the cord that is notably pathologic is meconium-induced medial destruction (Fig. 18), which results from direct meconium toxicity and necrobiosis of vascular media (20). Associated vascular spasm and medial degeneration may adversely affect hemodynamics in the cord and chorionic vasculature.

## RAMIFICATION OF CHORIONIC VASCULATURE

At this point it is convenient to discuss the ramification of the umbilical vessels in the chorionic plate. The umbilical cord inserts in a central or eccentric fashion. Although abnormal insertion at the margin (Battledore) and in the membranes (velamentous) comprises a small portion of cord insertions, both should be considered pathologic and not normal variants insofar as they have been attributed to adverse outcomes when extensively analyzed (21).

The pattern of vascular ramification within the chorion is described as either magistral (characterized by large-diameter vessels, radially diminishing in caliber to the periphery of the placenta) or disperse (characterized by multiple small vessels emanating directly from the cord insertion site). It is of interest that in the chorionic vasculature, no distinction can be made between branches of the umbilical vein and umbilical arteries using histologic criteria (in counterdistinction to the aforementioned description of differentiation between vein and artery in the umbilical cord). The only means of identifying which vessels are branches of arteries and which are veins is by noting their gross anatomic distribution. Arteries always cross over veins when observed from the fetal surface (Fig. 19). The notation of such vascular relationships is of extreme significance when considering vascular anastomoses, as may be seen in some twin pregnancies (22).

The primary branches of the umbilical vasculature that course through the chorionic plate periodically dive beneath this stratum to establish the circulation of primary vascular ramifications ending in the terminal villi.

## PATHOLOGIC ALTERATIONS OF THE CHORIONIC VASCULATURE

Abnormalities in the chorionic vasculature are similar to those found in the umbilical cord, the most significant being thrombosis of a chorionic vessel. During the gross examination of placentas so affected, the presence of thrombotic material may readily be identified by noting dilated vessels containing firm thrombotic substance. On the other hand, vascular thrombi may be more subtle and their appearance characterized only by the presence of faintly highlighted linear white streaks that parallel the peripheral margin of vessels involved (Fig. 20). These findings can be confirmed histologically.

The presence of polymorphonuclear leukocytes migrating from the chorionic vasculature and from the umbilical vasculature is pathognomonic of chorionitis and umbilical cord funisitis, respectively. Findings of chorionitis are histologically similar to those aforementioned in acute funisitis (Fig. 16).

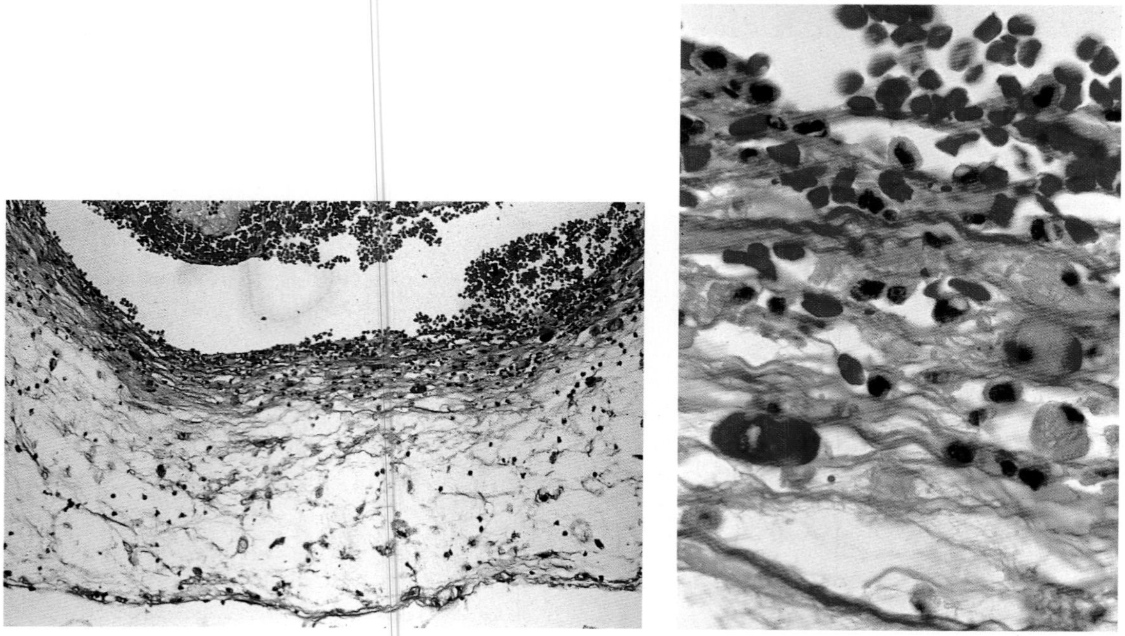

A B

**FIG. 18.** Globular degenerated necrobiotic medial cells so effected by meconium. The process is focal and contrasts with adjacent normal myocytes. Luna Ishak stain (**A**). Intensified magnification for delineation (**B**) [Reprinted with permission (20).]

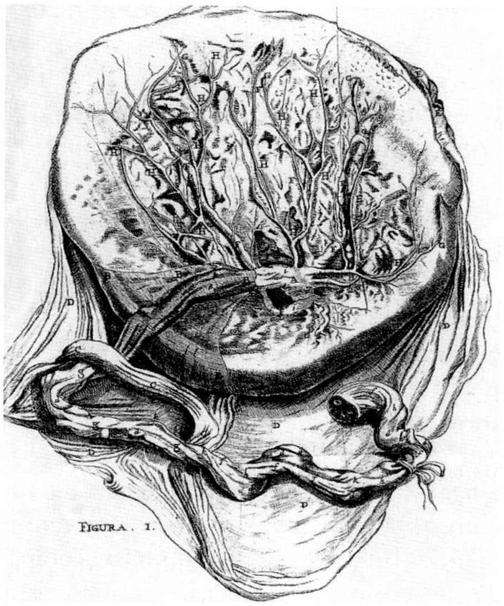


**FIG. 19.** As early as the 1600s, Nicholas Hoboken recognized that chorionic arteries (H) overlie veins, and this was beautifully depicted in his painstaking drawings. These are the earliest accurate drawings of the human placenta known to exist.

## MEMBRANES

### Embryology

The placental membranes consist of the amnion and chorion. The amnion, which constitutes the innermost aspect of the embryonic cavity, develops from the margin of the embryonic disk. As the embryonic disk begins to take the form of a tube, the amnionic periphery also folds inward and its attachment to the ventral body is defined. The amnionic cavity subsequently develops by the process of cavitation. Elongation of the body stalk coincides with embryonic prolapse into the amnionic compartment. As development proceeds, the resultant cavity expands, and by 12 weeks from the last menstrual period the amniotic cavity completely occupies the chorionic sac. At this point, fusion occurs with the chorionic wall. This event is commonly identified by clinicians via routine ultrasonographic analysis of advancing gestations. At this gestational age, the potential space between the chorion and amnion is visibly obliterated. The amnionic cavity remains filled with amnionic fluid, which by the end of gestation amounts to approximately 1 L.

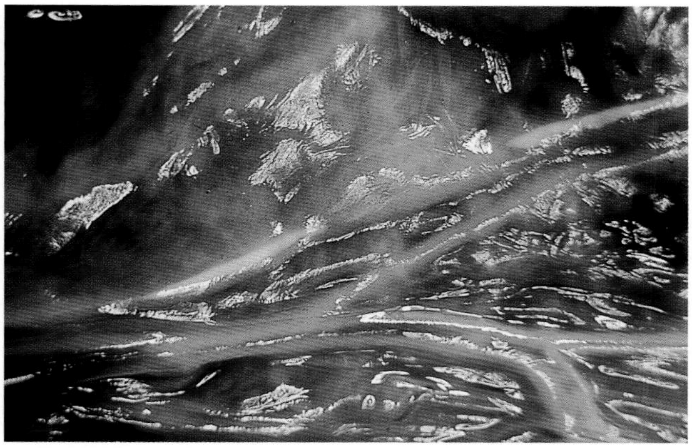

**FIG. 20.** Chorionic vascular thrombosis characterized by a linear streak paralleling the vascular course (in this case a chorionic vein). [Reprinted with permission (1).]

The chorion forms the base for the peripherally radiating villi and serves to encapsulate the embryo and developing amnion. As the early implantation embryo develops, the embryonic tissues (the trophoblast and its mesodermal investments) continue to expand in a spherical fashion. The inner aspect of the condensation of mesoderm, which forms the inner capsular structure deep to the peripheral trophoblast, is also termed the chorion. In the region that becomes the placental disk proper, chorionic villi continue to develop beneath these structures, and the placenta proper or the chorion frondosum is defined. The region of the chorion that covers the expanded amnionic cavity forms what has been termed the chorionic laeve. This constitutes the reflected membranes and is discerned from the membranous covering of the chorionic plate. Chorionic villi in the region of the laeve (which delimits the sac containing amnionic fluid) atrophy by pressure, although remnants of villous tissue may be found in association with this structure. In the region of the chorion frondosum, the fetal blood vessels invest the chorionic plate. Such vessels only occur in the chorion; the amnion is an avascular structure.

### Amnion and Chorion

#### *Gross Morphology*

The fetal membranes have a particular and characteristic appearance in normal deliveries. The sac, when viewed from the fetal surface, is clear and often has a bluish hue, and the amnion is devoid of vasculature. Remnants of atrophied vasculature may be seen in the overlying chorion and appear as filamentous streaks. The chorionic plate also has a characteristic blue sheen and, as described previously, the distribution of chorionic vessels has a characteristic appearance. The membranes of the chorionic plate are distinguished from the laeve as described above. It is not infrequent to find a peripheral nodule on the surface of the disk membranes. This normal nodule is the remnant of the fetal yolk sac (Fig. 21).

#### *Gross Morphologic Alterations*

Although chorionic vessels are normal in the chorion of the chorionic plate overlying the disk, the persistence of functional vasculature in the chorion laeve is aberrant and equates to membranous vessels. These vessels may connect lobes of placenta or relate to the membranous insertion of the umbilical cord (velamentous insertion as described above).

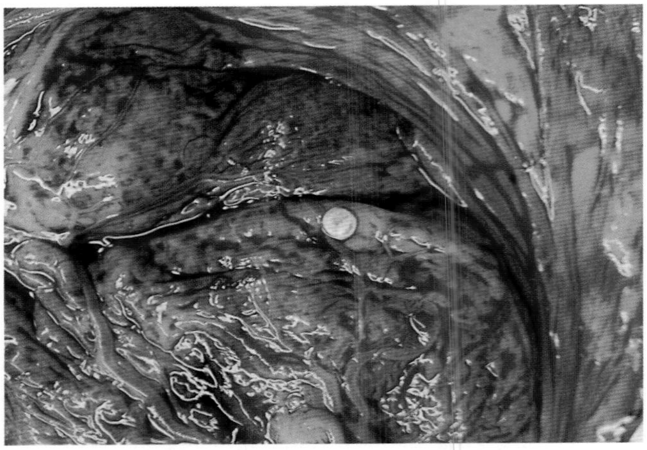

**FIG. 21.** White nodule is the residua of the fetal yolk sac.

On occasion, the chorionic plate may possess a ring of fibrin that forms a concentric ridge between the insertion of the cord and the margin of the placental disk. This fibrin ring, which lies deep to the amnion, is indicative of an extrachorial placentation. Such a placentation is characterized by two forms: the circumvallate placentation and the circumarginate placentation. In the former, the membranes are reflected upon themselves at the ridge of the fibrin deposition. They then cover the remaining margin of the placental disk in a loose fashion (Fig. 22). In the circumarginate placenta, the ring of fibrin is present over the chorion, and the overlying amnion is not reflected upon itself at this fibrinous ring (Fig. 23). The amnion thus extends to the margin of the placental disk, and its departure to form the amnionic sac occurs at this margin. It is currently felt that this fibrinous ring represents placental migration in conjunction with an enlarging uterus during the second trimester (so-called trophotropism) (1).

The common occurrence of squamous metaplasia on the amnionic surface can be identified grossly by its characteristic appearance. It is a normal finding unless its presence is extensive. Immersion of the placental membranes in water generally defines this area by its failure to become moist as opposed to the normal surrounding amnion. Thus, these areas are more clearly defined. In pathologic conditions, metaplasia in these regions may be pronounced, and large plaques and nodules may form (Fig. 24). These nodules are distinguished from the truly pathologic condition of amnion nodosum by their failure to be easily denuded from the surface of the amnion by slight mechanical pressure.

A

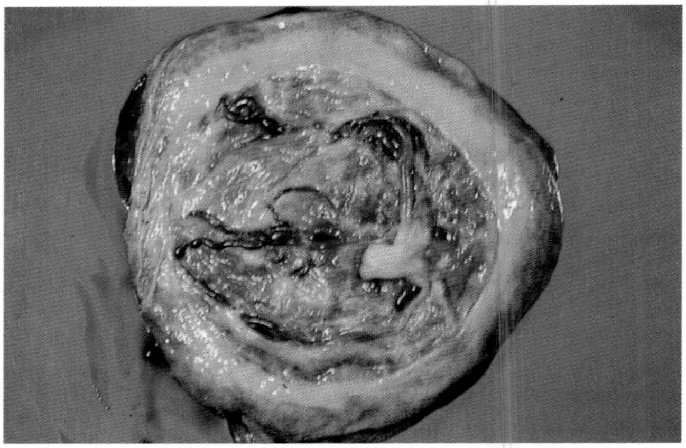

B

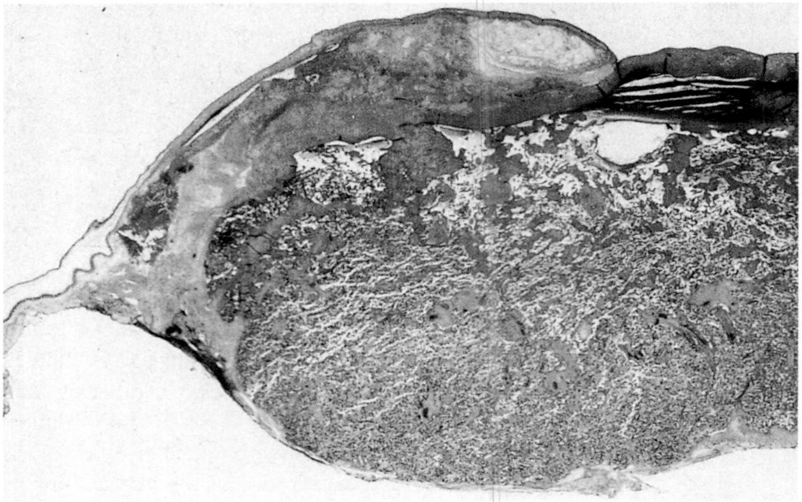

**FIG. 22. A:** Circumvallate placenta. **B:** Note loose association of amnion peripheral to marginal subamnionic fibrin deposition. [Reprinted with permission (1).]

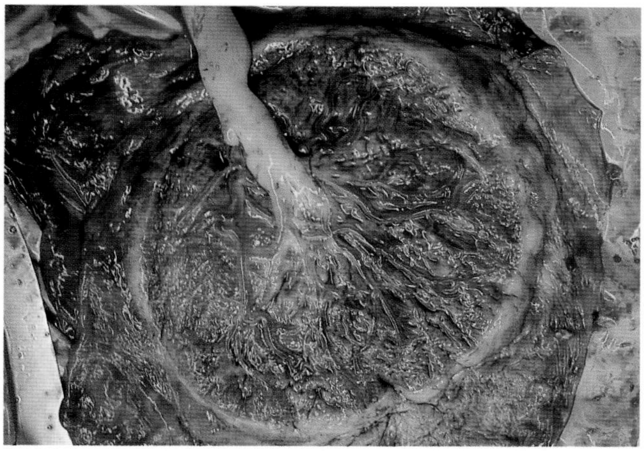

**FIG. 23.** Circummarginate placenta. Note the close association of amnion to the disk peripheral to the fibrin ring.

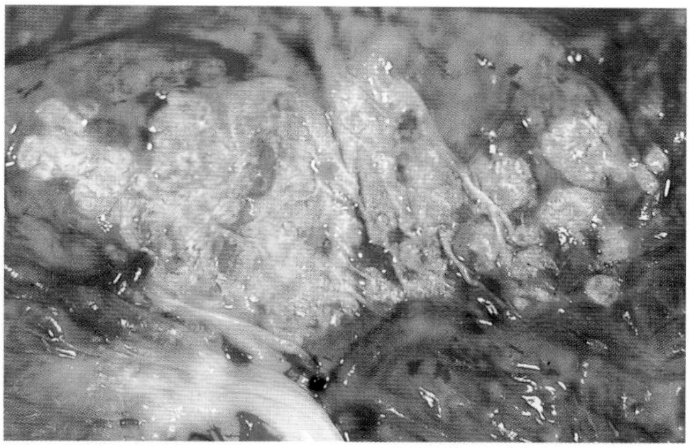

**FIG. 24.** Extensive squamous metaplasia on the amnionic surface from a fetus with an encephalocele. It is believed that irritation from the encephalocele in this region produced the extensive metaplasia.

The presence of amnion nodosum is characterized in the gross sense by the presence of multiple small papules on the amnionic surface (Fig. 25). The clinical history is suggestive, and oligohydramnios characterizes these gestations. The small papules are easily removed from the amnionic surface by excoriation, and their substances are confirmed histologically by the presence of debris and degenerated squames. The origin of these cells is fetal epidermal, and their presence on the amnionic surface is related to apposition of this membrane and fetal skin in conditions where there is diminished amnionic fluid.

Amnionic bands are rare. The condition is responsible for in utero fetal part amputation and trauma and is a phenomenon that occurs in approximately one in 10,000 births. The occurrence is important because it demonstrates potential difficulties from abnormal amnionic membrane development. The precise mechanism is not known in most cases, but rupture of the amnion (most probably in the first trimester) allows the fetus to enter the chorionic sac. The remnants of amnion form the substance of the resulting amnionic bands. At term these placentas have highly opaque chorionic surfaces that reflect hyperplasia of this uncovered layer. The remaining amnionic epithelium is densely adherent to the umbilical cord from which it cannot be stripped. Only small amounts of amnion are present, which distinguishes this condition from artifactual disruption of the amnion from the chorionic plate during the delivery process (1,23,24). Occasionally, an abnormal "web" will be present at the base of the cord insertion, and this may limit normal cord movement (5) (Fig. 26).

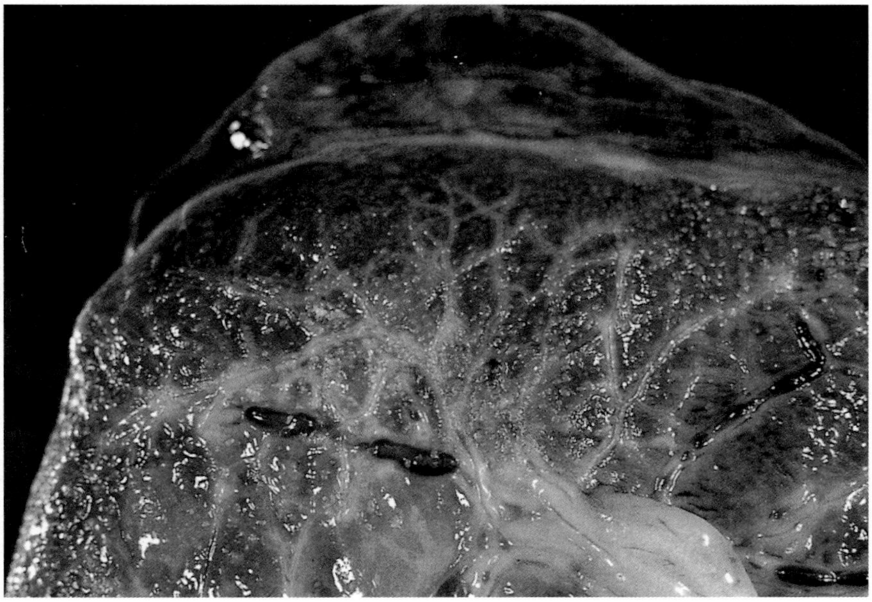

**FIG. 25.** Multiple papules of amnion nodosum stipple the amnionic surface of this placenta from a gestation characterized by oligohydramnios.

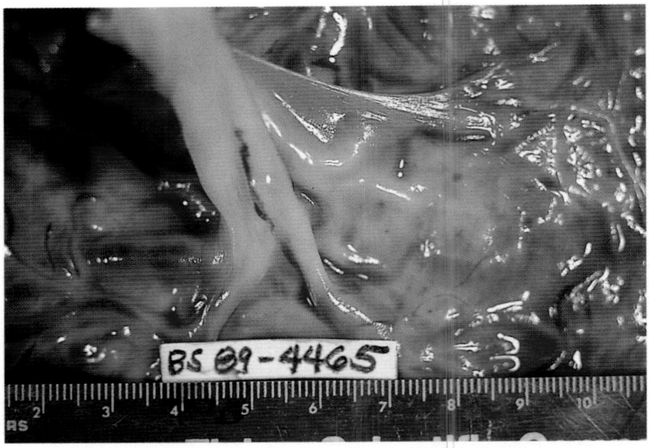

**FIG. 26.** Amniotic web partially immobilizes the cord by limiting its movement at the cord base.

### *Amnion Histology*

The amnion, the innermost layer of the amnionic cavity, is lined by a single layer of epithelial cells that resides on a basement membrane. The basement membrane is attached to an underlying thin layer of connective tissue (25) (Fig. 27). The amnion, although adjacent to the chorion, is not truly fused to it and may be separated with minimum effort. This juxtaposition of the two membranous layers occurs at 12 weeks' gestational age (26) (Fig. 28). Before this time, as the amnion develops, it is separated from the chorion by the so-called magma reticulare, which is a viscous and thixotropic gelatinous fluid. Stellate mesenchymal cells may be found within this subtance. These cells also have epithelial characteristics and have been stained immunohistochemically and found to be cytokeratin and vimentin positive (27).

The epithelial cell layer of the amnion is composed of one distinct cytologic type (28). The epithelium is a single layer, squamoid to cuboidal, and devoid of secretory activity. Ultrastructural studies show extensive microvillous projections (29). Multiple vesicular structures have been identified at the base of these epithelia. It has been postulated that these vesicles represent pinocytotic activity (10). This observation is important because, as stated earlier, the amnion possesses no vasculature. This also pertains to its mesenchymal component. Therefore, the cytologic components of this layer gain their nutrition from adjacent amnionic fluid, which in turn is rich in nutrients from transudation (from fetal vasculature) and fetal excretory products. In early gestation, this nutrition is derived from the magma reticulare. Channels that have also been considered responsible for fluid transmission (30) are felt to be the residua of epithelial cell loss. A postulate relating to cell loss may invoke a newly revitalized theoretical discussion (initiated by Virchow) that describes "apoptosis" as a form of programmed cell death. Such epithelial loss or "cell death by suicide" also has been noted in placental components, including the wall of the yolk sac and in the endothelium of umbilical veins. Further investigation in these areas may enhance understanding of developmental biology and with refinement may be used for addressing future methodologies for the treatment of neoplasia (31,32).

Amnionic epithelial cells are attached to one another by desmosomes in freeze-fracture experiments (33). Furthermore, the amnionic epithelium attaches to the underlying basement membrane by hemidesmosomes (34).

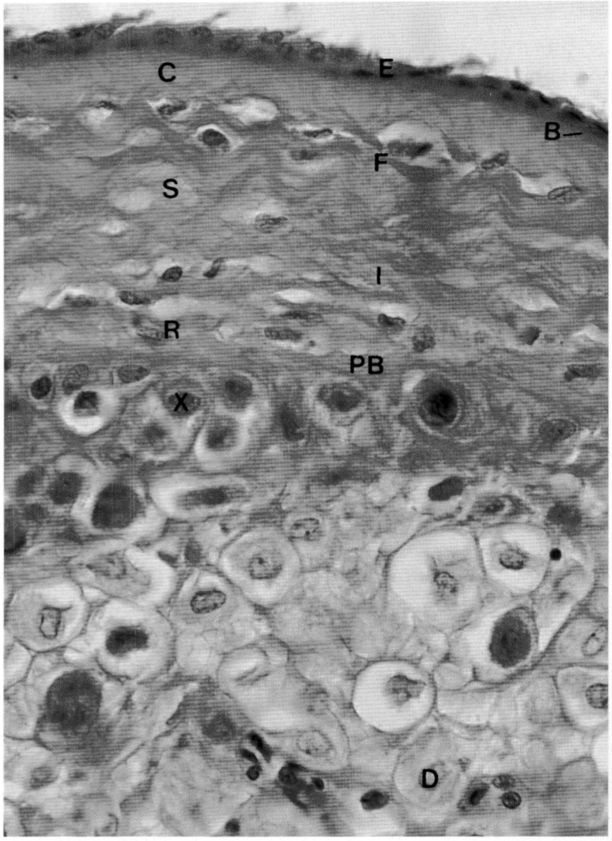


**FIG. 27.** Flattened to cuboidal amnionic epithelial cells (E) adhere to their basement membrane (B). Beneath this is the compact layer of the amnion (C), which is acellular and may form a barrier to PMNs. The compact layer is rarely affected by edema and is probably the strongest amnionic layer. A fibroblastic layer (F) lies beneath the compact layer, and macrophages may be found. A spongy layer (S) relatively devoid of fibroblasts separates the amnion from the chorion, although the two may merge imperceptibly. Often, an artifactual separation may be present near the plane of true fusion. The amnion usually measures from 0.2 to 0.5 mm in thickness (1). The most superficial layer of chorion is usually an incomplete cellular zone (I) that overlies a thick reticular layer (R). This layer is composed of fibroblasts and macrophages. Beneath the reticular layer is a pseudo–basement membrane (PB) overlying trophoblastic X cells (X) and then maternal decidua (D) (HPS stain).

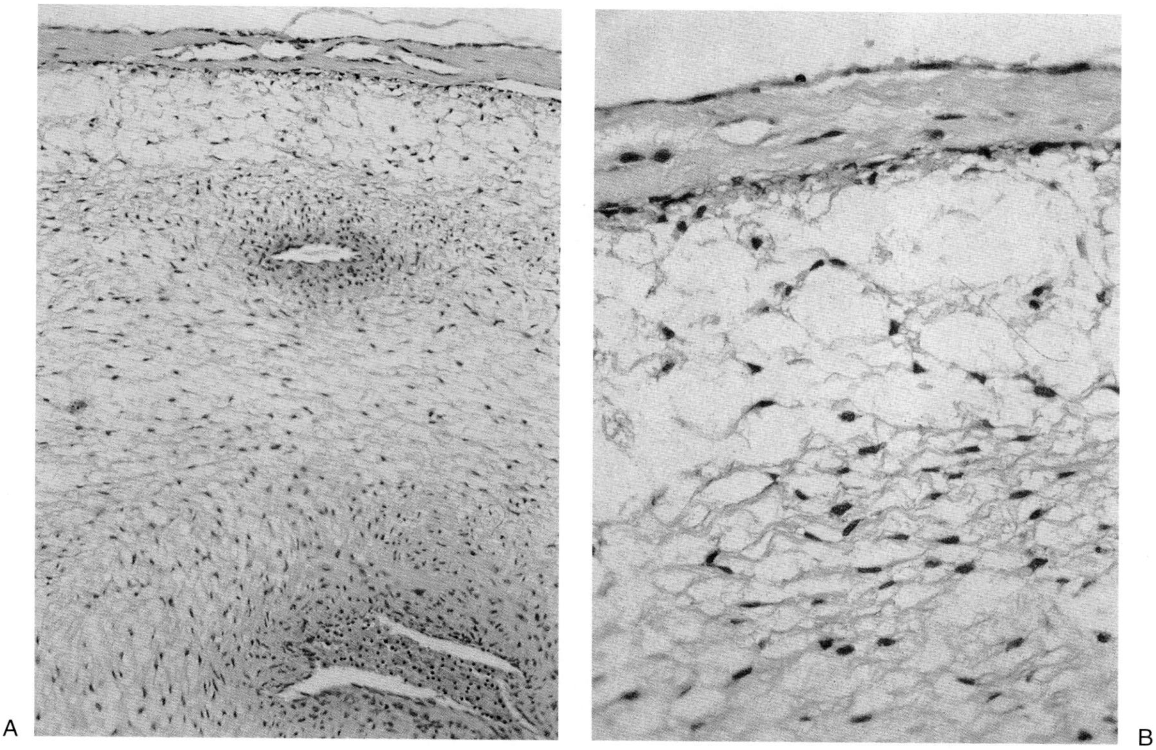

**FIG. 28.** The separation between amnion and chorion is more apparent in early gestations as seen in this section from the chorionic plate of a 10- to 12-week placenta. The amnion is readily distinguished from the underlying chorion, which contains the easily identifiable chorionic vessels. Mesynchymal components are prominent (H&E stain).

Amnionic epithelial cells divide by mitosis (35). On occasion, multinucleated cells are identified. Morphometry studies have demonstrated that polyploid cells exist in this layer (36). Other karyotypic anomalies occur, and amniocentesis for chromosomal defects may yield false-positive results when these amnionic cells contaminate preparations (37).

Although the epithelium of the amnion does not actively secrete, lipid droplets have been noted within these cells, an observation that correlates with increasing gestational age (35,38,39). Glycogen also has been found within amnionic cells.

Squamous metaplasia is a common occurrence in the amnionic epithelium, especially near the insertion of the umbilical cord (Fig. 29). This epithelium may become keratinized, and keratohyaline granules can be identified. Although this appears to result from irritation of the amnionic epithelial surface, these changes can be found in more than half of all term placentas (1).

Beneath the basement membrane of the amnionic epithelium, an additional component of the amnion is identified. This layer principally is divided into a compact and a fibroblastic region. The connective tissue within this region may harbor macrophages, which have been identified within the first trimester of pregnancy (40).

### *Amnion Histopathology*

Histologic abnormalities of the amnion are heralded by an abnormal gross appearance. For example, membranes that are stained green may reflect deposition of meconium. Amnionic membranes that are white may be indicative of poly-

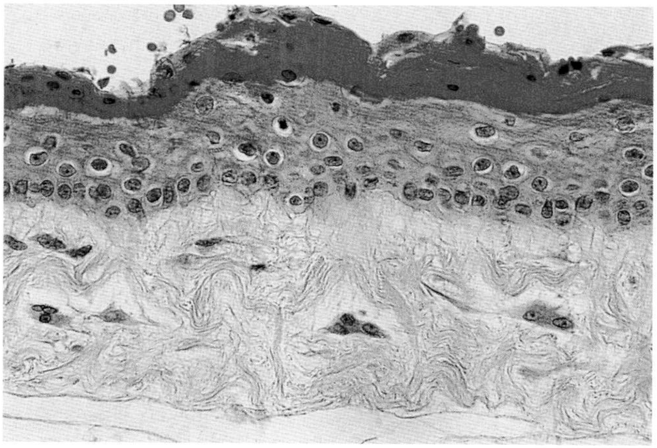

**FIG. 29.** Squamous metaplasia of the amnion with hyperkeratosis (HPS stain).

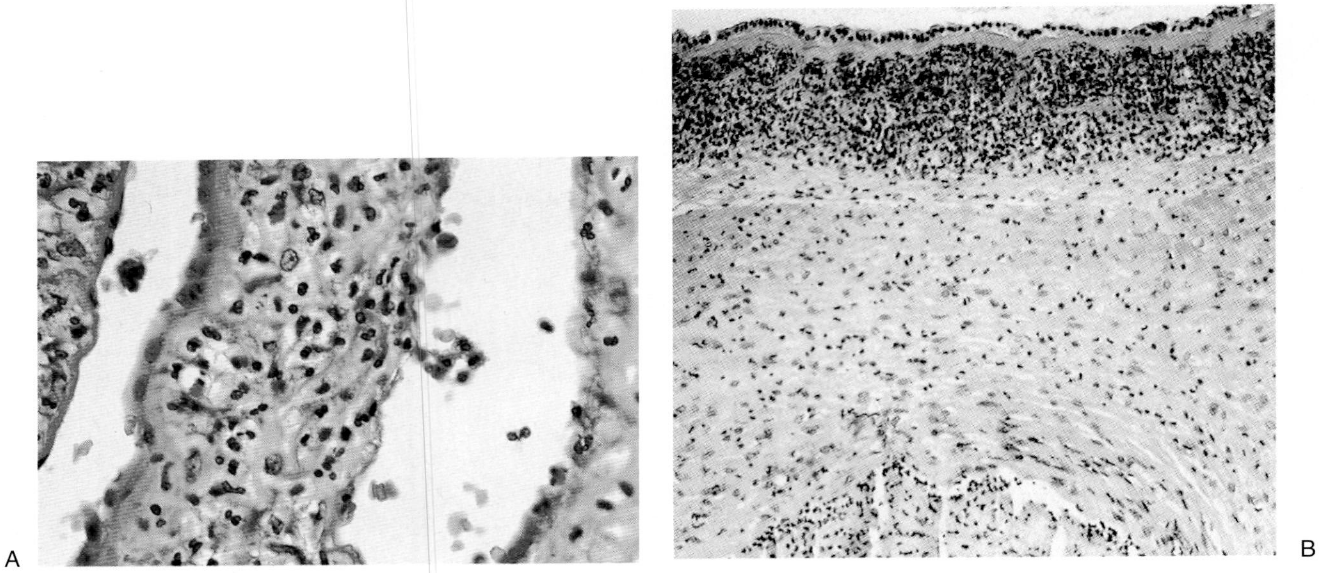

FIG. 30. Acute chorioamnionitis in membrane roll (**A**) (HPS stain) and in chorionic plate (**B**) (H&E stain).

morphonuclear leukocyte infiltration and acute chorioamnionitis (25) (Fig. 30).

Abnormalities of amnionic epithelial cells, although suggested by gross examination, can be confirmed by histologic assessment. Abnormalities that reflect degenerative changes are characterized by the presence of vacuolated cytoplasm and elongation to columnar forms. A rather rare and unusual finding associated with gastroschisis carries a pathognomonic histologic aberrancy of the amnion whereby amnionic epithelial cells contain innumerable vacuoles (1) (Fig. 31).

Amnionic epithelial degeneration (Fig. 32) is characteristic when meconium is present. Such findings may be confirmed when macrophages, present within the amnionic layer, contain meconium (a coarse brown pigment), which does not stain for iron (Fig. 33). On the other hand, hemosiderin deposition may be found within the amnionic layer in macrophages, and this can be confirmed by the use of iron stains (i.e., Prussian blue).

Although there are no true tumors of the amnion, occasional cysts representing edema may be identified. Although they may be striking in their gross appearance, it must be rec-

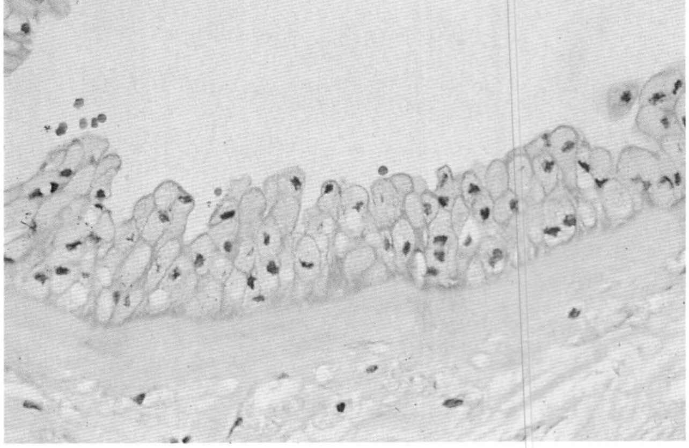

**FIG. 31.** Unusual vacuolated elongated amnionic epithelial cells pathognomonic of gastroschisis. The pathophysiology is uncertain (H&E).

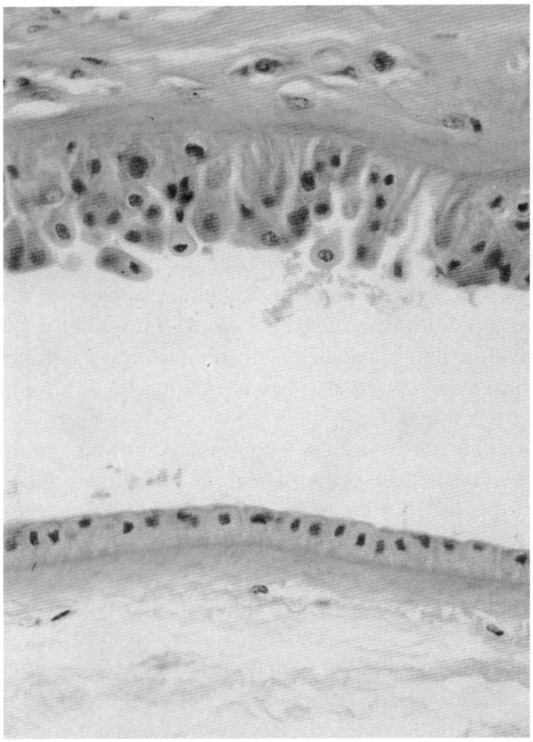

**FIG. 32.** A twisted membrane roll with amnionic epithelial degeneration (*above*) and normal amnionic epithelium (*below*) (HPS stain).

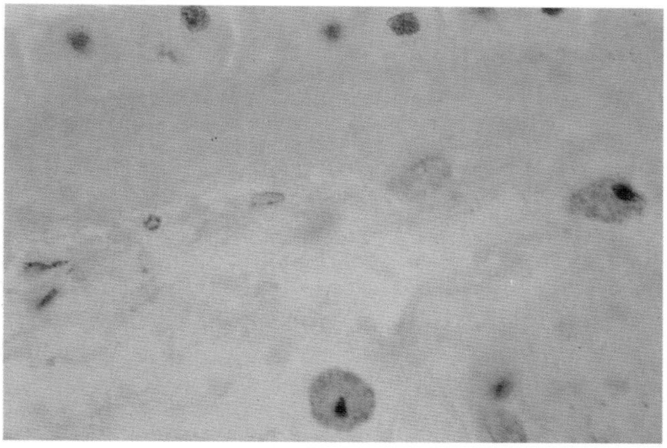

**FIG. 33.** Amnionic epithelial degeneration overlies pigment-laden macrophages containing meconium (HPS stain).

ognized that no clinical significance can be identified. Occasional cysts of ectodermal and mesodermal tissue have been identified deep to the amnionic layer, but such findings are not considered true neoplasms. Teratomas have been described (41). These lesions probably represent degenerative acardiac twins (1), but the lack of directed differentiation from pluripotential stem cells could account for the former.

The papules of amnion nodosum are clearly pathologic and reflect, in most cases, decreased amnionic fluid. In such instances, vernix (desquamated epithelia from the fetus) forms minute nodules on the amnionic surface in this characteristic fashion (Fig. 34). The lesions are composed of acellular debris and remnants of cells (42). The material within these papules is PAS and alcian blue positive.

### *Chorion Hist ology*

The chorion is composed of a connective tissue membrane that carries the fetal vasculature. Its inner aspect is bounded by the outer layer of the amnion, and the outer aspect is directly associated with the trophoblastic villi that sprout from its surface. There are two distinct aspects of the chorion: the chorion frondosum and the chorion laeve. The chorion of the reflected membranes (chorion laeve) is composed of an inner cellular layer, a "reticular'' layer, a "pseudo-basement membrane,'' and an outer trophoblastic layer (43) (Fig. 27). The precise origin of the mesenchymal component of the chorion is not clear, but it is believed that this connective tissue is derived from the primitive streak and not the trophoblast (44,45) (Fig. 28). Electron microscopy studies have shown the connective tissue cells adjacent to the amnion to be rich in endoplasmic reticulum (46,47). Macrophages and degenerative endothelial cells also have been described as part of the cytologic makeup of this layer (47). Acid mucopolysaccharides are prominent within the connective tissue matrix of the chorion (48). Although present in other regions of the placenta, type VI collagen is a prominent constituent of the chorionic layer (49). The chorion frondosum is similarly constituted but contains functional chorionic vessels and is bordered deeply by functional villi.

### *Chorion Histopathology*

Pathology of the chorionic vasculature (described above in the context of its umbilical cord continuity) includes chorionitis and thromboses. The fetal chorionic vessels allow permeation of polymorphonuclear cells (PMNs) in response to intraamnionic bacterial antigens. Maternal PMNs also may be seen in the chorion laeve. In both cases, the amnion is later affected (Fig. 30).

Chorionic cysts, which do not truly arise from the chorion proper, are derived from trophoblastic cytologic components (X cells). Multiple cysts may be present, bulging the fetal surface of the disk. These may appear terribly abnormal but in fact carry no significance in the form of true pathology (Fig. 35). These cysts, which are commonly found in the chorionic plate and within placental septa, are discussed further below.

## MULTIPLE GESTATION

The normal relationship of the placental membranes are germane to the understanding of twin or multiple-gestation placentations. These relationships are described briefly, but

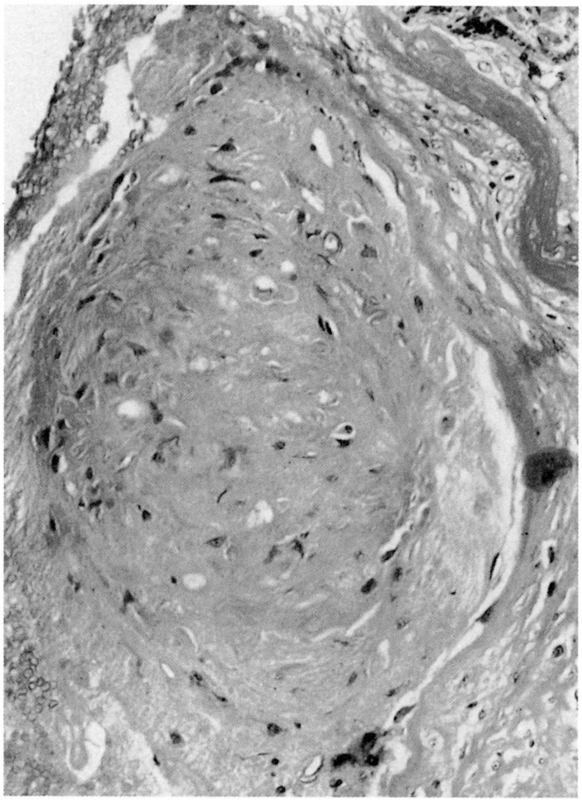

**FIG. 34.** Amnion nodosum (H&E stain).

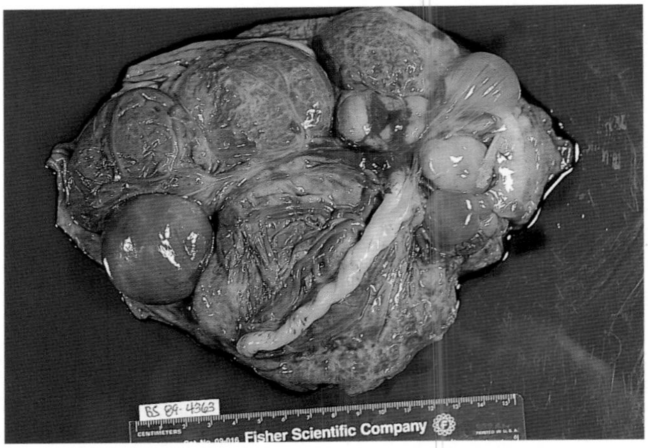


**FIG. 35.** Multiple normal chorionic cysts.

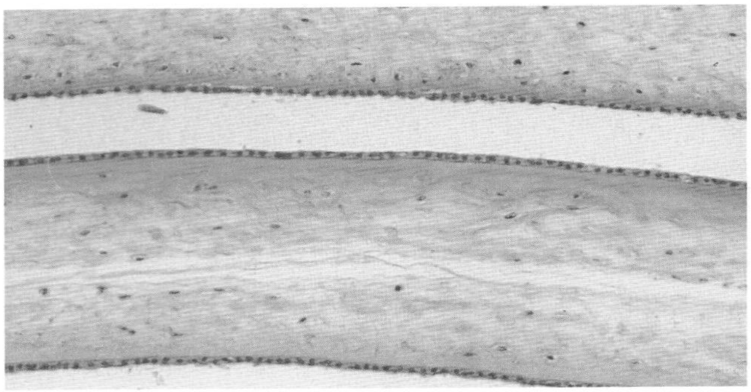

**FIG. 36.** Intervening membrane from diamnionic monochorionic twin placenta. Note the absence of an intervening chorionic layer (HPS stain).

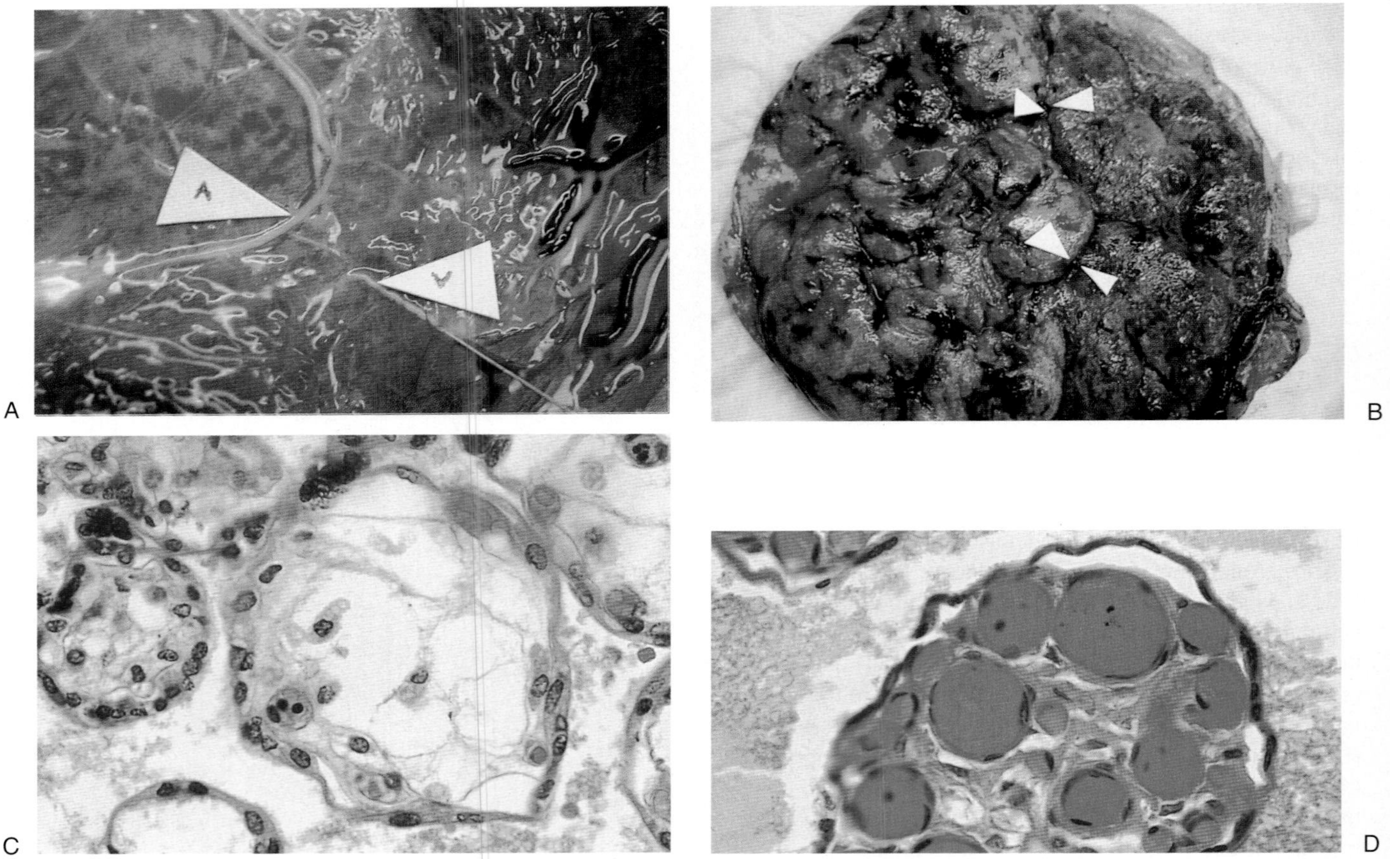


**FIG. 37. A:** Twin–twin anastomosis characterized by artery-to-vein transfusion. **B:** Note pale anemic and edematous parenchyma of donor (*left*) and dark congested parenchyma of recipient (*right*). The *arrowheads* mark the vascular equator along the maternal surface. **C:** Villi from the anemic twin are edematous with abundant macrophages, and vascular spaces contain nucleated hematologic precursors denoting high-output failure and increased red cell production, respectively. **D:** Villi from plethoric twin are markedly congested (HPS stain). Characteristic "classic" twin–twin transfusion outcomes may not always occur. Although one twin may be smaller, hemoglobin may be increased in a paradoxical fashion suggesting shifts in flow before analysis (1).

for a more complete discussion of twinning and associated pathological conditions, readers are referred to an extensive and detailed review of the topic (1).

The majority of twin placentas (incidences show a dependence on geographic location and ethnic background) are dizygotic. The dizygotic twin placenta has a variety of presentations: separate placentas or fused placentas. In the latter, the intervening membrane should be studied to distinguish dichorionic from monochorionic twin placentas. The intervening membrane of about 70% of monozygotic twin placentas is devoid of a chorion, and the term "diamnionic–monochorionic" (DiMo) is applicable (Fig. 36). All DiMo placentas are monozygotic. In these gestations (DiMo), the shared chorion invests only the chorionic plate and is not present in the intervening membrane. In DiMo placentas, shared vascular districts between placentas are possible, and vein-to-vein and artery-to-artery anastomoses are the most common. Artery-to-vein anastomoses are relatively infrequent and are the etiology of the twin–twin transfusion syndrome (Fig. 37).

The diamnionic–dichorionic (DiDi) placenta is distinguished morphologically by examining the intervening membrane and noting the presence of two fused chorions beneath the two amnionic layers (Fig. 38). Most of these placentas are dizygotic; however, approximately 30% of DiDi twin placentas result from monozygotic twin implantations and are the result of splitting within 3 days of fertilization. Vascular anastomoses are reportable.

The complete absence of an intervening membrane (monoamnionic–monochorionic) in a twin gestation is also diagnostic of monozygotic twins. There, splitting of the embryo occurs later in gestation (at approximately 7 days of age), and although twin–twin transfusions can occur, these are less common than in DiMo placentations. The significant pathologic problems from these placentations result from cord entanglements, and fetal death is common. Even later separations result in fused twin fetuses (Siamese twins).

## VILLI

### Embryology

After formation of the blastocyst, the trophectoderm gives rise to extraembryonic trophoblastic villi. The organization of the inner cell mass gives rise to the embryo proper. The trophoblastic derivatives of the early implantation embryo are best characterized by discussing their structures and cell types. The trophoblastic villus forms the functional unit of the placenta. In the first trimester, trophoblastic villi are composed of an outer syncytiotrophoblastic layer and an inner cytotrophoblastic layer encompassing villous mesenchyme in which the fetal vasculature differentiates. Although the majority of the villus is surrounded by the characteristic two-cell layers, a polarity to the villi can be identified and their basal implantation regions are composed

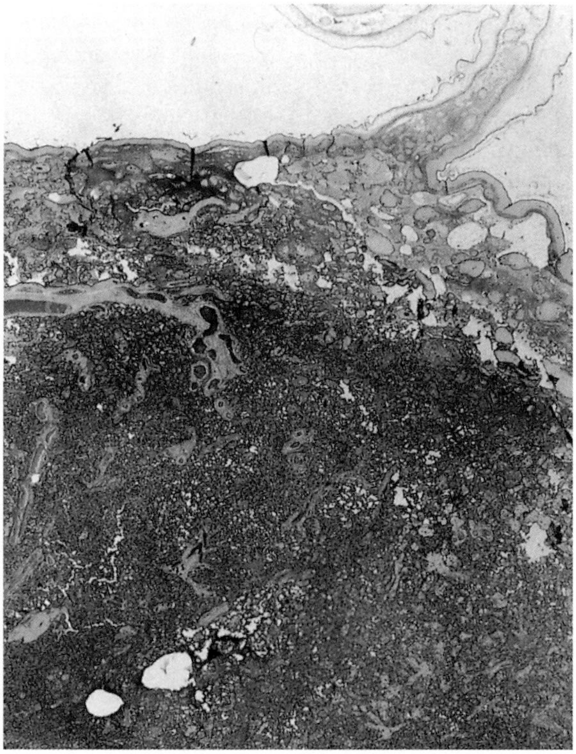
A

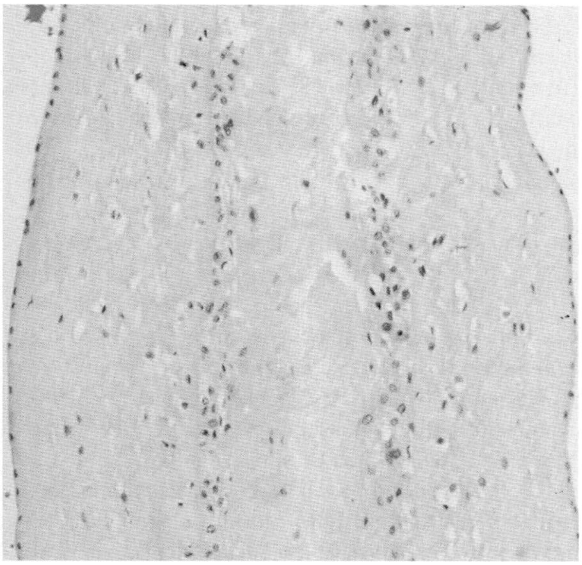
B

**FIG. 38. A:** Diamnionic–dichorionic intervening membrane, site of fushion at chorionic plate ("T zone") (H&E stain). **B:** Note the more cellular intervening chorion separating the two layers of amnion (A) (HPS stain).

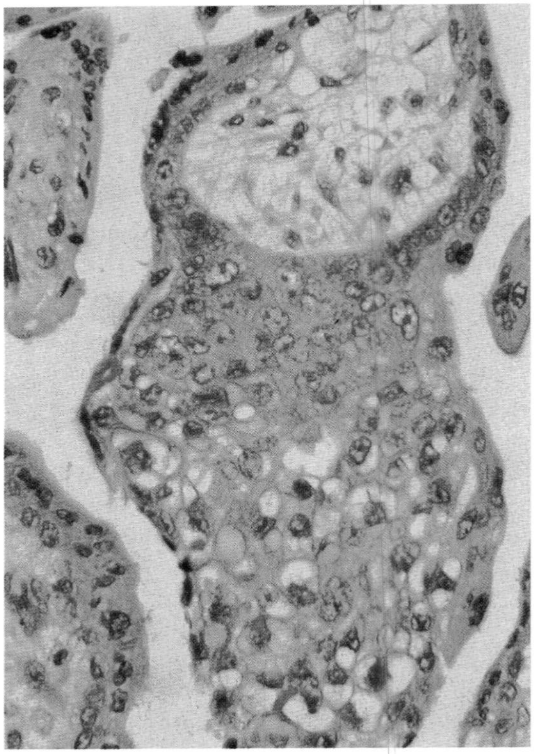

**FIG. 39.** Polar trophoblastic proliferation comprising trophoblastic cell column. Many vacuolated X cells are identified (H&E stain).

of additional trophoblastic constituents, which make up the trophoblastic cell columns (Fig. 39). Cytotrophoblast gives rise to syncytiotrophoblast. The origin of X cells (which contribute to the trophoblastic cell columns and "percolate" into the maternal decidua along with syncytiotrophoblast) is less clearly understood.

As gestation progresses, the characteristic elements of the trophoblastic villus, as described from the early implantation, differentiate and develop to form a more functionally efficient unit. This occurs with gradual diminution in the size of peripheral branching villi. The tertiary villi, which stem from secondary villi, which in turn are derived from major stem villi, have a characteristic appearance (Fig. 40). The previously noted two-cell layer is less apparent, and the cytotrophoblast becomes much more difficult to identify. The overlying syncytiotrophoblast of the villus thins so that a syncytiovascular membrane forms the villous interface with the maternal intervillous blood. Deep to the trophoblast lies a basement membrane (also present in earlier villi), which in turn surrounds the villous mesenchyme. Deep to the villous mesenchyme, fetal blood courses within capillaries lined by endothelial cells supported on a basement membrane. These are the constituents of the "syncytial vascular membrane" separating fetal from maternal blood across which transport of essential nutrients and waste products must occur.

The course of development also impacts on the mesenchyme. Early in development, when villi have a pronounced double trophoblastic cell layer, the mesenchyme is prominent. The cytologic constituents of this region alter with development. Before 6 weeks from the last menstrual period, capillary lumina are not readily identified (Fig. 41). After this point, the development of vascularization within villous tissue becomes more pronounced. The vasculature is derived from branches of the stem vessels that connect with the vasculature of the chorionic plate. By about 8 weeks' gestational age (from the last menstrual period), only nucleated hematologic precursors are evident within these villous capillary spaces (Fig. 42). Many of these primitive blood cell precursors have their origin within the yolk sac. As gestational age progresses, there is a decrease in the number of nucleated hematologic precursors, such that between 10 and 12 weeks' gestational age (from the last menstrual period) only approximately 10% of these blood cells are nucleated. The near absence of nucleated hematologic precursors after 12 weeks is readily apparent in histologic sections (Fig. 43). Surrounding the early villous vasculature, the villous mesenchyme is also prominent early in gestation. The mesenchymal structural units (primitive fibroblastic cells) form about 50% of the cells in this region. The remainder of cells are composed of members of the macrophage family. These cells bear antigens that characterize them as such (CD4, LeuM3, and a variety of other macrophage markers can be identified) (50).

The villous macrophages or so-called Hofbauer cells lose their prominence as gestation proceeds. The maturing tertiary villus, although it possesses this cell type, has fewer of them at term. The function of Hofbauer cells, although not completely understood, is important in water regulation activities, the transport of various nutrients and waste, and villous homeostasis. This cell type also may be important to immune regulatory functions as an intermediate in the processing of infectious agents that are blood borne.

Chorionic villi may be useful in prenatal diagnosis. Karyotype analysis may be assessed at 10 to 12 weeks' gestational age through chorionic villus sampling (CVS). It should be noted that although early diagnosis is often preferable (to later amniocentesis), several concerns exist. There have been controversies regarding limb reduction abnormalities, but the vast majority of evidence does not confirm this adverse event, especially in "experienced hands." Of genuine concern, CVS is not useful in the diagnosis of neural tube defects (amniotic fluid for alpha fetoprotein determination is required) and fragile X syndrome, which also requires amniotic fluid due to alterations in methylation patterns found in trophoblast as compared with fetal squames (51).

### Gross Morphology

The villous parenchyma is discoid and occupies the space beneath the chorionic plate. The substance of the parenchyma is red and "beefy." On sectioning, it appears ho-

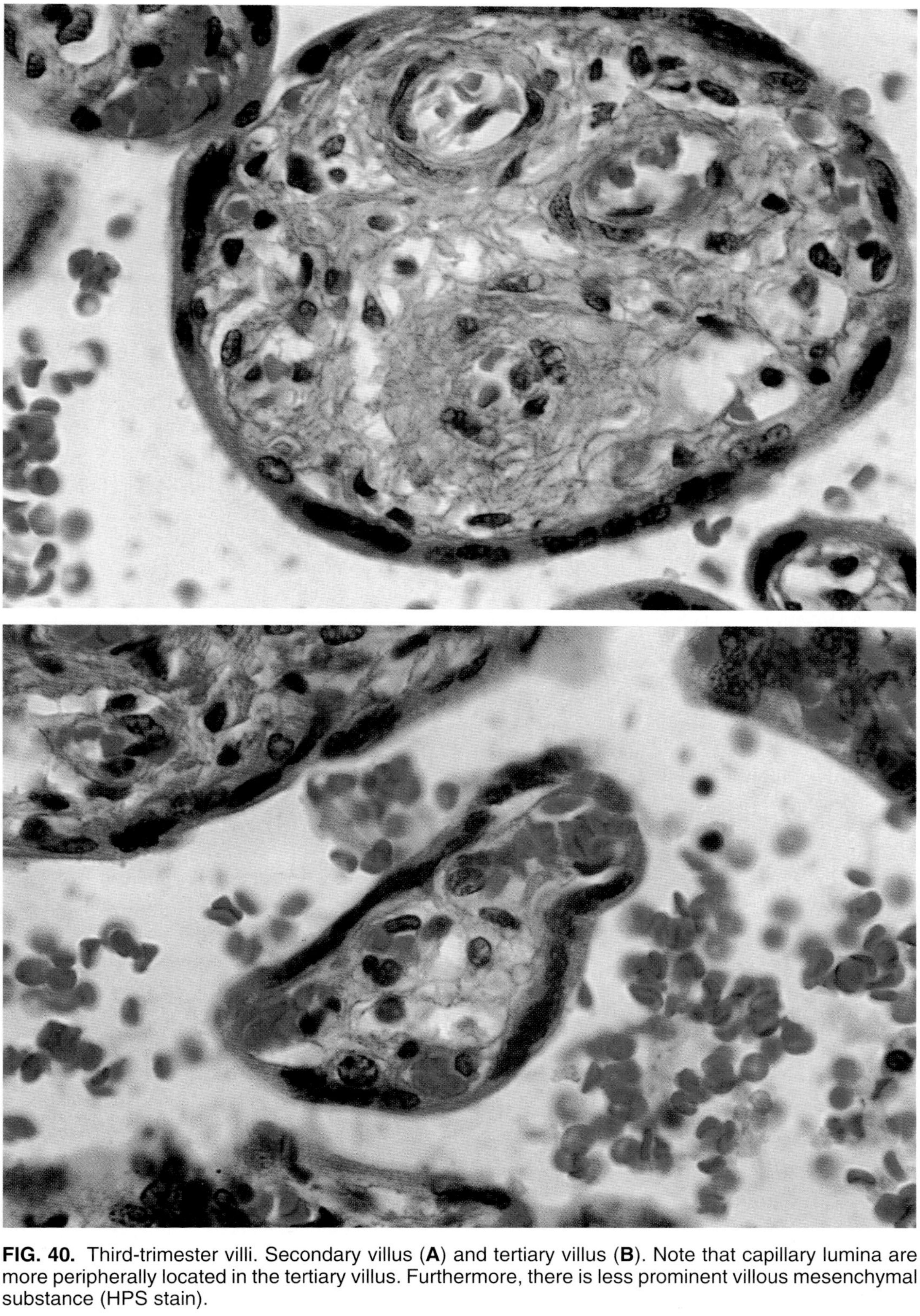

A

B

**FIG. 40.** Third-trimester villi. Secondary villus (**A**) and tertiary villus (**B**). Note that capillary lumina are more peripherally located in the tertiary villus. Furthermore, there is less prominent villous mesenchymal substance (HPS stain).

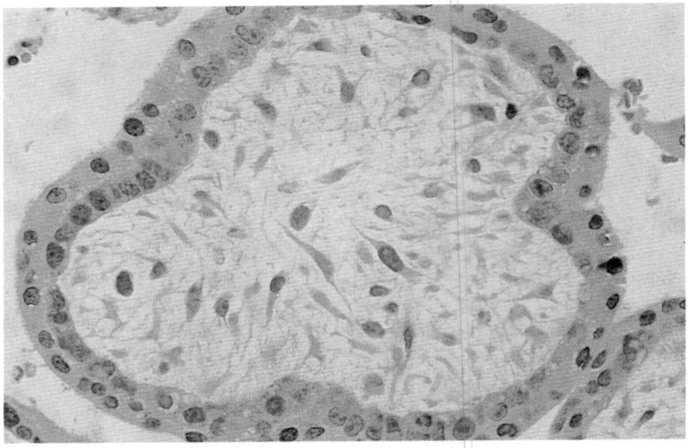

**FIG. 41.** Villus from gestation of less than 6 weeks. No capillary lumina are present and no embryonic erythropoiesis is identified (H&E stain).

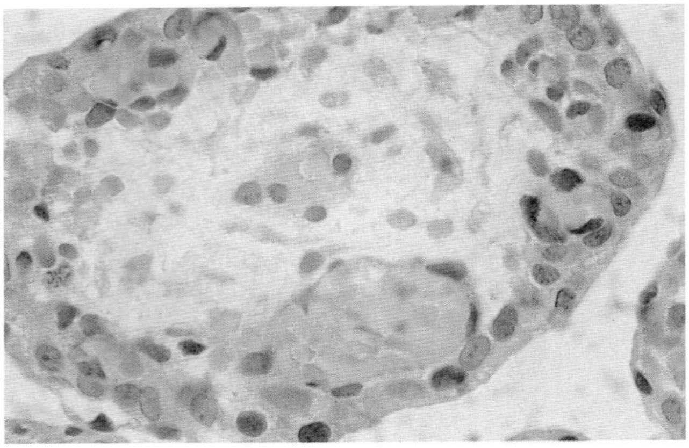

**FIG. 43.** Near absence of nucleated hematologic precursors within villous capillaries after 12 weeks' gestation (H&E stain).

mogeneous in contour and texture. Irregularities within the substance denote abnormalities within the villous parenchyma. Many abnormalities so identified are common, and in most instances, due to their frequent occurrence, they should be considered as normal varients (unless they are unduly prominent). Such entities include infarcts and perivillous fibrin deposition.

In addition to the perivillous fibrin deposition, other fibrinous depositions are common and are generally considered normal within the placenta. The so-called Langhans' stria, located below the chorionic plate, is probably related to alterations of materal intervillous blood flow. By virtue of its distance from the decidual vasculature, it tends to be more static.

Nitabuch's fibrin is present between the floor of the placenta and the maternal decidua. This layer was once believed to prevent allograft rejection, but now the precise nature and functional significance of this fibrin deposition are not clear.

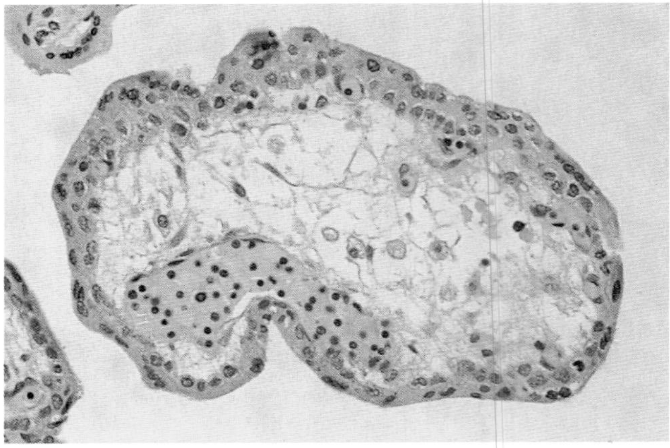

**FIG. 42.** Trophoblastic villus at 8 weeks' gestation. Note only nucleated hematologic precursors present within villous capillary spaces (H&E stain).

On occasion, the placental parenchyma have spherical defects (usually 1 to 2 cm in greatest dimension), which represent so-called jet lesions. These cleared areas within the villous parenchyma represent pressure heads from maternal decidual vascular flow. It is not uncommon to histologically identify a small zone of acute infarction peripheral to these lesions.

Calcification is a common phenomenon in the mature placenta. Calcification has been used to diagnose placental maturity by ultrasonographic evaluation during pregnancy. Third-trimester gestations have an increase in the amount of calcium present in the placenta, and when calcifications are prominent, placentas are considered grade 3. A mature placenta detected by ultrasound does not necessarily denote fetal maturity. The appearance of calcium deposition in the gross sense is that of fine, pinhead-sized deposits of yellow–white, gritty material. Calcification of the placenta is a normal physiologic response to development and aging (52,53).

### Gross Morphologic Alterations

Many placentas normally have some degree of infarction. When infarction roughly exceeds 10% to 15% of the placental surface, or when it is more central than peripheral, this should be considered pathologic. Infarcts are characterized grossly as either acute or "old." Acute infarcts are pale, poorly demarcated regions that are slightly granular on palpation. "Old" infarcts are white, often triangular, and they too are granular (Fig. 44).

Infarcts evaluated grossly are distinguished from perivillous fibrin deposition. Upon palpation, infarcts are granular and firm. Perivillous fibrin, on the other hand, tends to be nodular and smooth. Further distinctions are made histologically, and these are described in detail below.

Intervillous thrombi also may be identified during the

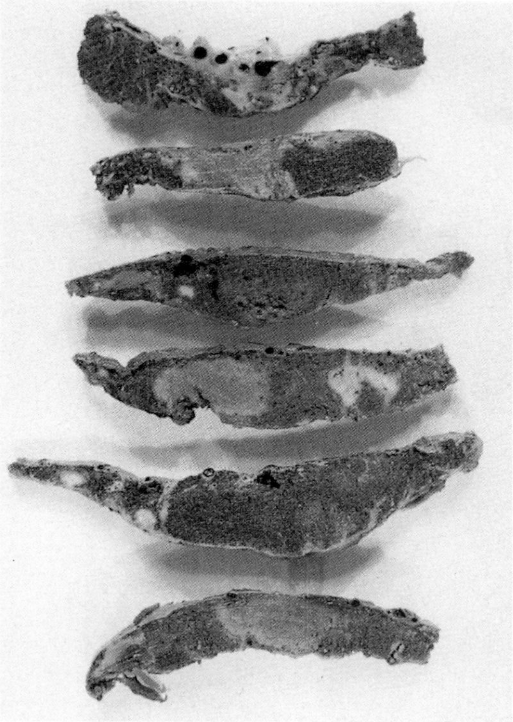

**FIG. 44.** Multiple old infarcts from a hypertensive pregnancy.

gross examination of the placenta. These triangular or diamond-shaped lesions within the placenta may consist of soft gelatinous red to white (depending on age of lesion) aggregates of collected blood. The lamellations of fibrin within this thrombotic material may be observed grossly. It is this aspect, as well as the gelatinous soft makeup of this material, that distinguishes these lesions from infarcts and perivillous fibrin deposition upon gross examination.

## Histology

The histologic variations in placental architecture are largely dependent on the developmental state at which observations are made. The histology of the individual cell types involved directly in villous implantation is now described.

X cells, also termed intermediate trophoblasts, are major constituents of the cell columns that form the deepest structural components of the implantation site. These cytologic components of trophoblastic origin are unique with respect to other trophoblastic derivatives (syncytiotrophoblasts and cytotrophoblasts). X cells are secretorily distinct and produce human placental lactogen and major basic protein, and are electron microscopically distinct insofar as they contain large numbers of mitochondria with tubular cristae (54–56). Similar cell types are identified along with the chorion laeve (Fig. 45), and these cells have been characterized histologically as being eosinophilic or vacuolated; it was suggested that they represent two distinct subpopulations in this region (57). In the implantation site, these cells are morphologically distinguished from decidual elements in that their cytoplasm is generally darker and they are occasionally multinucleated. Furthermore, these cells tend to be more vacuolated then their neighboring decidual cells. Difficulty in distinguishing these cell types has resulted in some problem with the diagnosis of intrauterine pregnancy when these are the only trophoblastic cells present in currettage specimens. In the absence of villi, most pathologists confirm their diagnosis of intrauterine pregnancy (and hence generally exclude the possibility of a tubal pregnancy) based on the presence of multinucleated trophoblastic derivatives, which are more readily distinguished from the surrounding decidua. Should difficulty arise with morphologic assessment of the true nature of the uninuclear cells in question, immunohistochemical localization of human placental lactogen within X cells is helpful (58). This cell type is of important immunologic interest because it may be responsible for the synthesis of fibronectin (1). An excess of immature intermediate trophoblasts has been associated with preeclampsia and eclampsia (59).

An interesting normal finding within the placenta is the so-called chorionic cyst. These cysts occur in placental septae and are composed largely of decidua and X cells. The cysts are entirely lined by X cells. As noted above, such cysts also may be seen in in the chorionic plate (Fig. 35). On sectioning, gelatinous fluid may be present, and the major constituent of this fluid is one of the substances produced by X cells: major basic protein. The function of these cysts is not known. They should not be considered pathologic when present (1).

The syncytiotrophoblast, the outer cell layer, possesses a brush border. Microvilli that constitute this border are felt to be involved in pinocytotic activity. Vacuoles within the cytoplasm of these cells are indicative of the absorptive and secretory activities of the syncytiotrophoblast. Syncytiotrophoblasts are composed of pyknotic (often multiple) nuclei that are hyperchromatic. In addition of the multiple vesicles present within this cell type, ultrastructural examinations show a cytoplasm that is rich in endoplasmic reticulum, mitochondria, lipid droplets, and Golgi bodies (60).

The cytotrophoblastic nuclei are more round and open. Tritiated thymidine incorportion experiments have shown that uptake and incorporation are confined to the cytotrophoblastic layer and not the syncytiotrophoblastic layer (61). On occasion, cytotrophoblasts may possess mitotic figures (Fig. 46). Ultrastructurally, the cytotrophoblast has fewer organelles than does the syncytiotrophoblast. Most prominent are large mitochondria, which may be numerous.

Human placental lactogen may be localized within X cells and syncytiotrophoblasts. Human chorionic gonadotropin can be identified within syncytiotrophoblast cells, but not within cytotrophoblast cells (54,62).

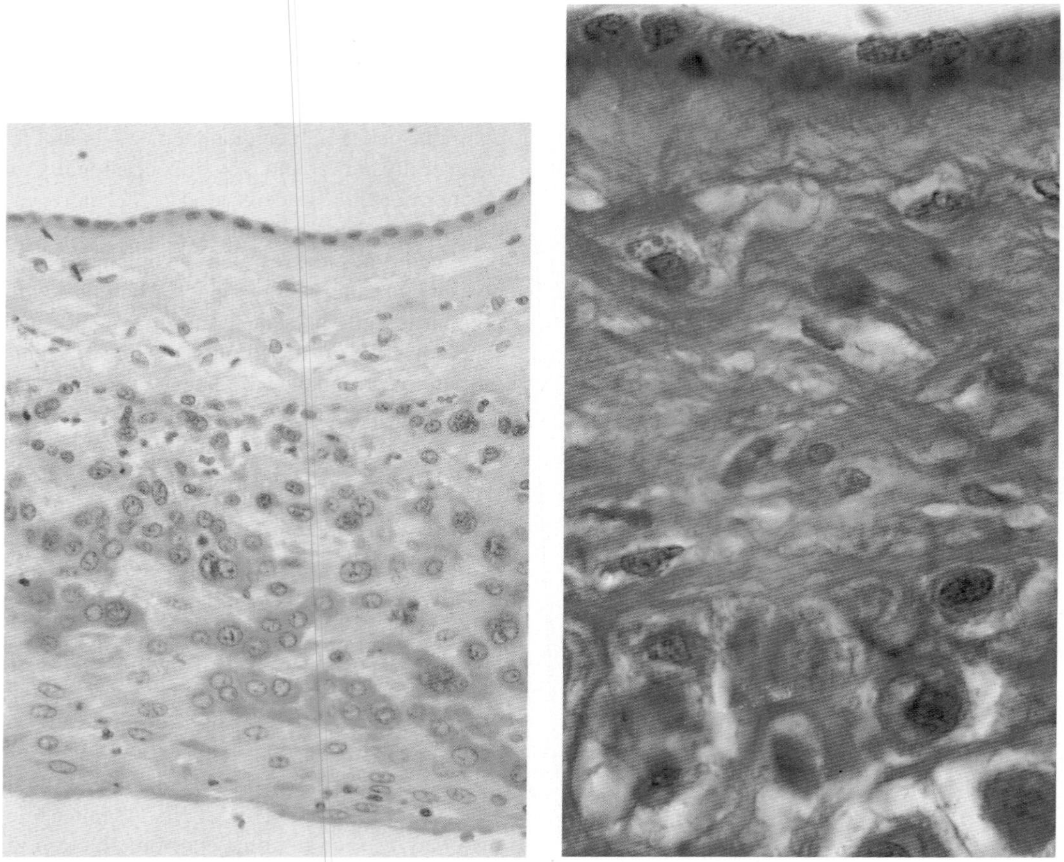

A B

**FIG. 45.** Prominent nonvacuolated X cells within the decidua of the chorionic laeve. Note their darker cytoplasm and occasional multinucleation (**A**) and vacuolated X cells deep in the chorion (**B**) (HPS stain).

**Histopathology**

Various pathologic entities, which may be identified within the villous parenchyma at the histologic level, serve to better illustrate the normal histology of the placenta.

Infarcts, which are common in the placental substance, have a characteristic gross appearance. Acute infarcts are characterized histologically by the presence of faint staining villi, which are aggregated, compressed, or agglutinated to one another and have interspersed polymorphonuclear leukocytes within the intervillous space (Fig. 47). (As described below, it is crucial to distinguish this inflammation from that which occurs in an intravellous fashion). Earlier forms of infarction may be characterized by the presence of villous agglutination and congestion, with lysis of intervillous maternal blood (Fig. 48). In very advanced ("old") infarcts, complete absence of villous architecture is noted and a fuzzy outline of remaining villous constituents can be identified (Fig. 49). No viable staining cells are identified, and an acute inflammatory infiltrate may persist. The placenta rarely undergoes "organization" or fibrosis. When acute infarcts resolve and become "old," fibroblasts are generally lacking. It is for this reason that organization is not a term applied to the placenta. Classic organization as might apply to other organ systems undergoing ischemic change does not occur. The variance probably relates to the two distinct vascular supplies (maternal and fetal). Disturbance in maternal flow results in placental infarction.

Infarcts are distinguished from perivillous fibrin deposition histologically in that regions of the latter contain cytotrophoblastic nuclear remnants that are often prominent (Fig. 50). Intervillous thrombi are identified histologically by the presence of lamellated thrombotic material displacing neighboring villi (Fig. 51).

Other abnormalities of the villous parenchyma include villous edema, where edema fluid displaces intravillous cytologic architecture; it is considered pathologic, especially in premature gestations (Fig. 52) and has been reported as a cause of fetal ischemia. Its etiology is not clear (21). Tenney-Parker change is characteristic of placentas from preeclamptic gestations. This change is characterized by increased syncytial knotting on villi (Fig. 53). These syncytial knots are best considered failed adaptive responses to low oxygen tension within the intervillous space. As noted above, increased

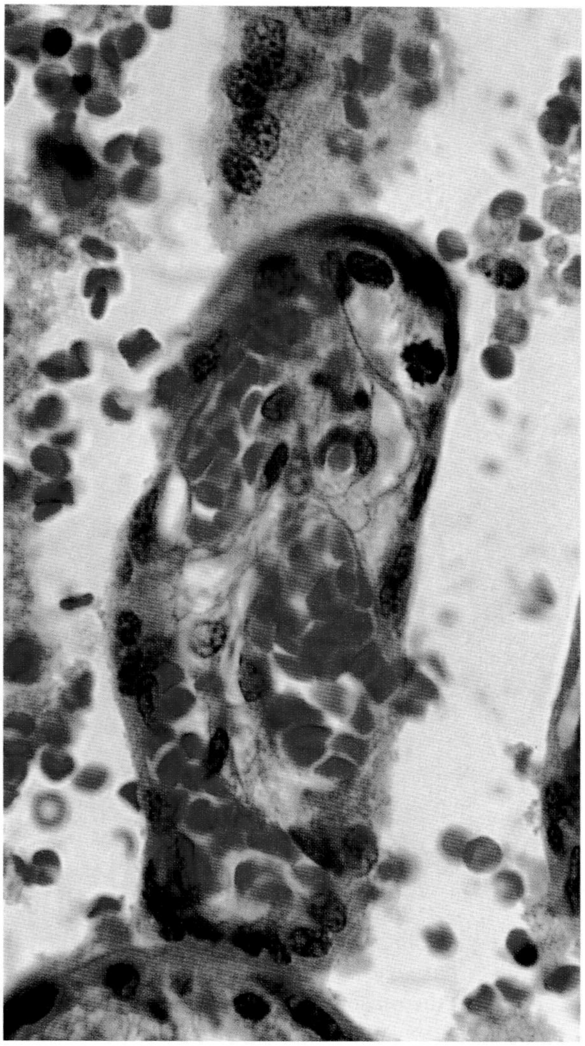

FIG. 46. Sparse cytotrophoblast with rare mitotic figure in terminal villus from a third-trimester placenta (HPS stain).

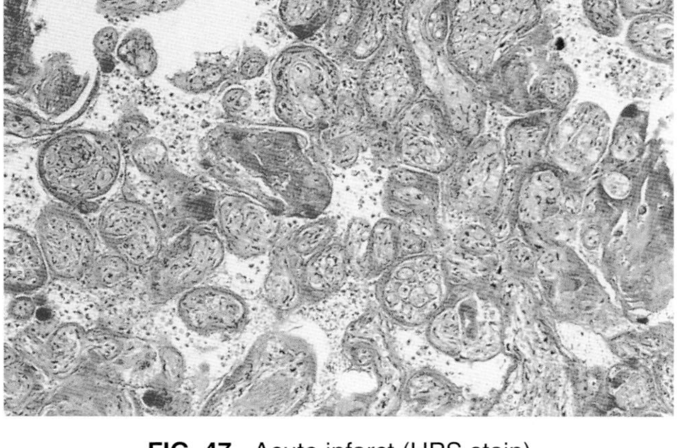

FIG. 47. Acute infarct (HPS stain).

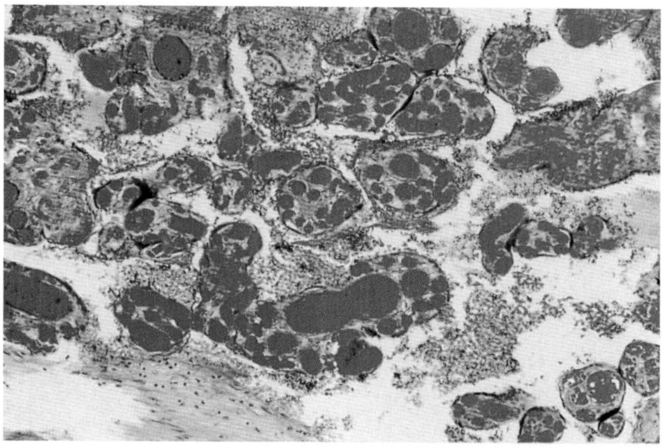

FIG. 48. Villous vascular congestion may indicate early infarction or need to be more closely examined to exclude chorangiosis (HPS stain).

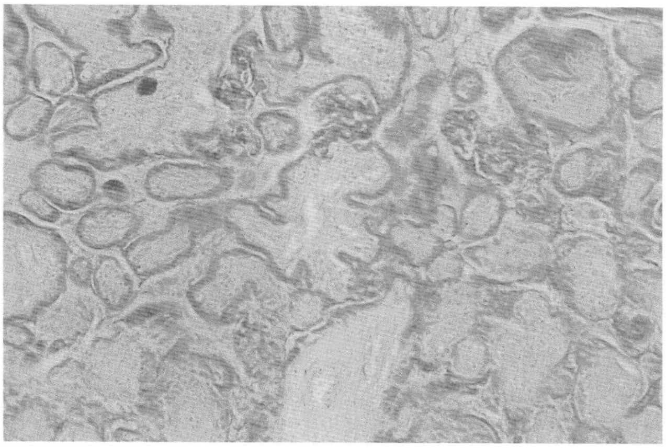

FIG. 49. "Old" infarct (HPS stain).

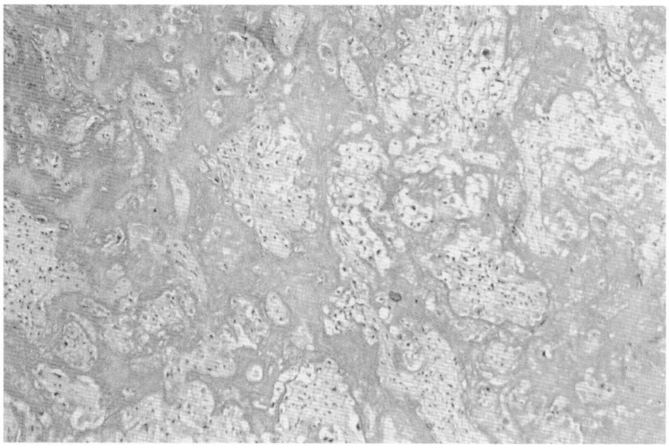

FIG. 50. Increased perivillous fibrin. Note trophoblastic nuclear remnants encased in fibrin (HPS stain).

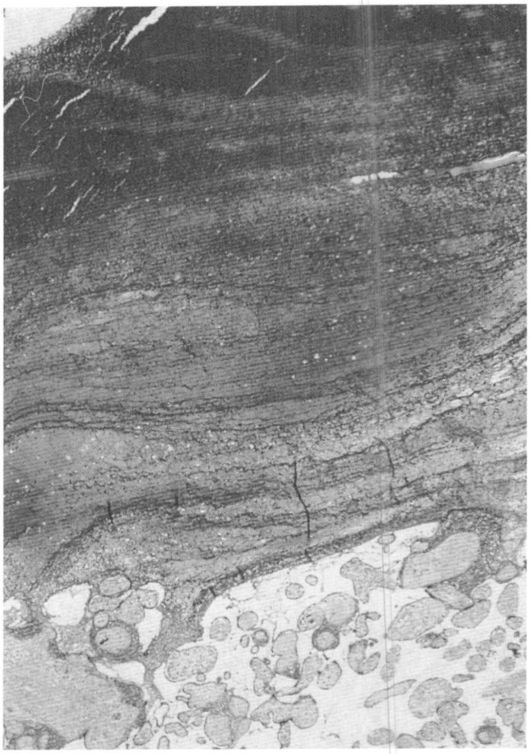

**FIG. 51.** Intervillous thrombus. Note lamellated lines of Zahn (HPS stain).

intermediate trophoblasts also may be seen (59). Infarcts are not uncommon (1), and in preeclamptic/eclamptic gestations, decidual vasculopathy is also encountered and is discussed below.

Unusual appearances of villous vasculature take three unrelated forms. First, villous vasculature may be congested (Fig. 48), and this may have no pathologic significance or may be indicative of early infarction. Second, increased numbers of villous capillaries, so-called chorangiosis, has been considered to be indicative of chronic hypoxic changes. The definition is precise, and in histologic terms three criteria (10 vessels/10 villi/10 fields at 10×) need to be met (63). Third, abnormal proliferations of villous vessels which form histologically hemangiomatous nodules, are termed chorioangiomas when present in the placenta (Fig. 54). These lesions have pathologic significance when prominent and may result in high-output cardiac failure in the fetus or microangiopathic hemolytic phenomena.

Dysmaturity of villi is also considered pathologic. Villi that show the characteristic two-cell layer of the first-trimester implantation, when present in third-trimester placentas, are indicative of abnormal developmental events. This change has been noted to occur in mothers who are diabetic.

Nucleated red blood cells are common in very early gestations, but as gestation proceeds, and especially in the third trimester, nucleated red blood cells should not be present.

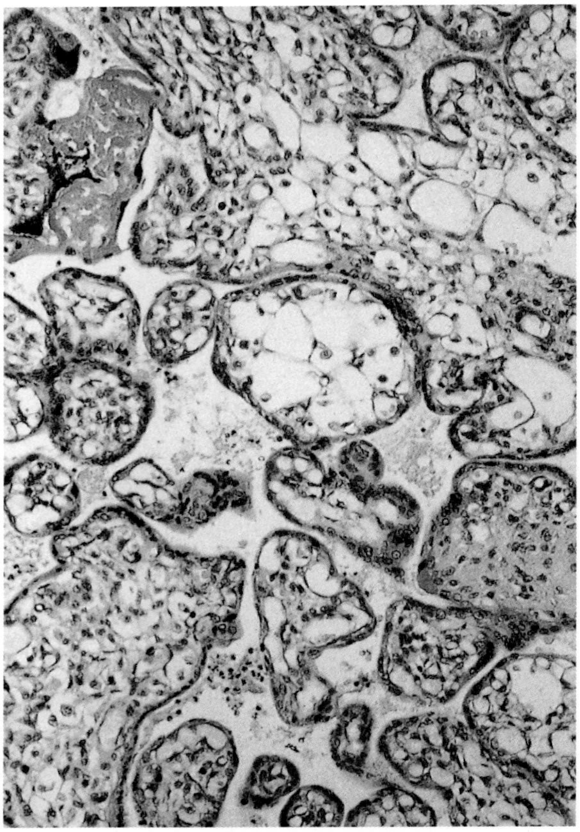

**FIG. 52.** Focal edema (H&E stain).

When present, fetal anemia with increased erythroid production should be suspected. Additionally, recent investigations have addressed the presence of nucleated red blood cells (in advanced-gestation placentas), correlating such findings with erythropoietin secretion by the fetus and concomitant fetal hypoxia (1) (Fig. 55).

In patients with sickle cell disease, it is not unusual to find sickling of maternal erythrocytes within the intervillous

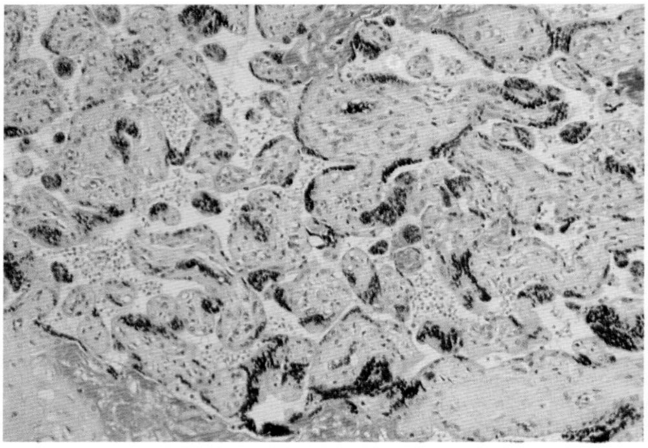

**FIG. 53.** Increased syncytial knots in a hypertensive pregnancy (HPS stain).

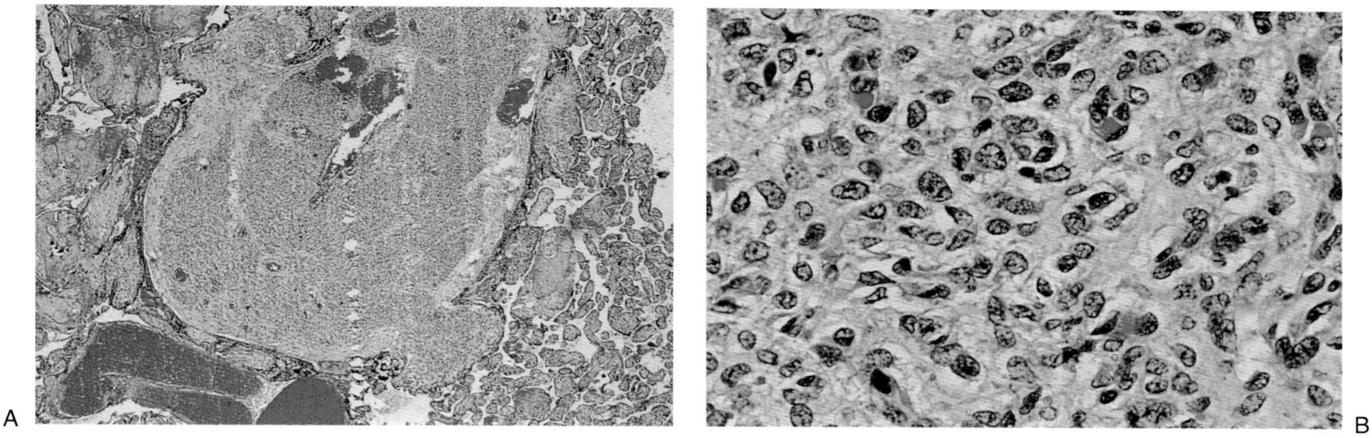

**FIG. 54.** Chorioangioma (**A**) characterized by hemangiomatous proliferation (**B**) (HPS stain).

spaces. This is promoted by diminished oxygen tension in the setting of abnormal maternal hemoglobin S. It is wise to correlate histopathologic findings with clinical status in that it has been reported that hypoxia during and after placental separation causes sickling (64) (Fig. 56).

Inflammatory changes within villi are probably one of the most interesting aspects of placental pathology. These inflammatory changes herald the presence of infectious disease agents in many cases. The presence of syphilis and cytomegalovirus (CMV) should be considered when infiltrates of lymphocytes and plasma cells are found within trophoblastic villi. Special stains may be confirmatory. It is important to distinguish this chronic inflammation from that of the acute inflammatory infiltrate (surrounding villi) associated with acute infarction. An acute inflammatory infiltrate within villi may suggest *Listeria* infection with extensive microabscess formation throughout the placenta. This often can be seen in the gross sense as innumerable white dots. The odor has been characterized as "sweet" (1). In many instances, inflammatory changes within the villi are limited to an increase in the villous cellularity (increased Hofbauer cells), and no specific infectious disease agent can be identified. Increased numbers of inflammatory cells (without plasma cells) also signify chronic villitis; however, in most instances when this occurs, no infectious disease organism can be identified. These inflammatory changes within the placenta have been termed "villitis of unknown etiology" (63,65) (Fig. 57). The infiltrate has been identified as maternal in origin (66).

The absence of inflammation does not always coincide with the absence of infection. For example, in parvovirus B19 infection, hydropic villi and the presence of villous vascular nucleated red blood cells (occasionally with "smudged" amphophilic intranuclear inclusion bodies) may herald the presence of severe congenital infection even in the setting of absence of maternal symptoms (1) (Fig. 58).

Confounding the topic of placental and neonatal infection is the entity of "histologically silent villitis." In this regard, not only may there be absent inflammatory responses, but placentas appear entirely histologically normal. Only special molecular studies will detect antigens and nucleic acids indicating the presence of infectious materials (67) (Fig. 59).

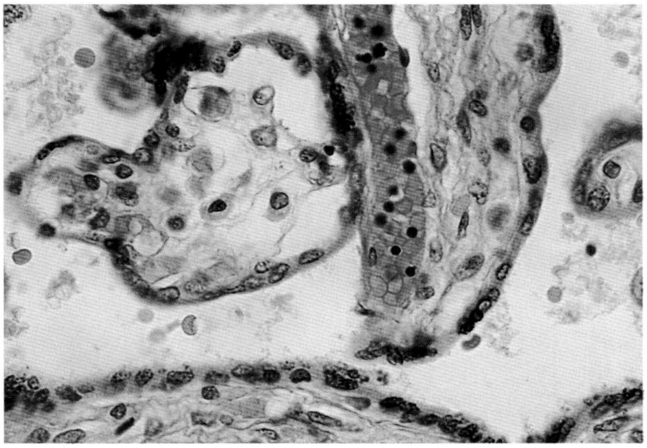

**FIG. 55.** Fetal nucleated red blood cells are abnormal at term. There is associated focal villous edema (H&E stain).

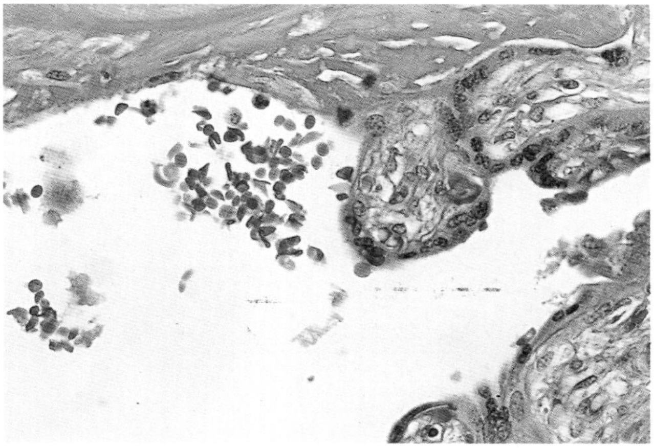

**FIG. 56.** Intervillous maternal red cell sickling in patient with sickle cell disease (H&E stain).

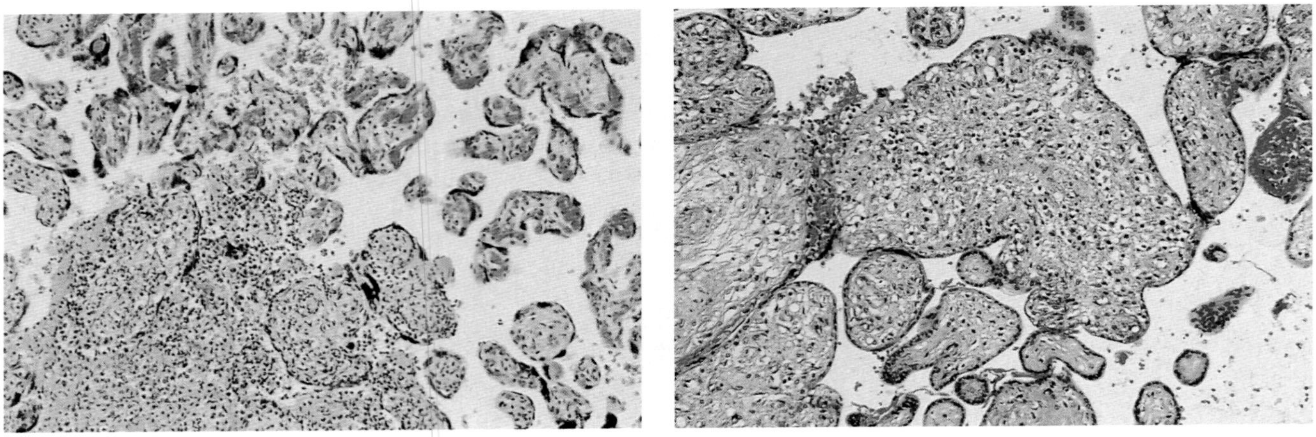
A B

**FIG. 57.** Villitis of unknown etiology (VUE) in which a chronic inflammatory infiltrate devoid of plasma cells is present (**A**) and chronic villitis due to known syphilis infection characterized by the presence of a mononuclear infiltrate containing plasma cells (**B**) (HPS stain).

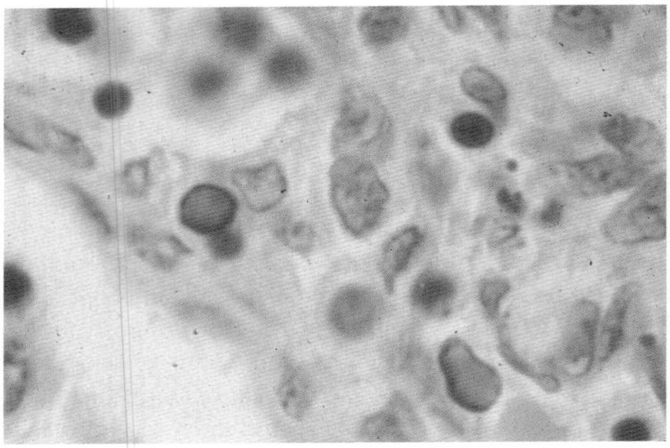

**FIG. 58.** Parvovirus B19 infection associated with villous edema and nucleated fetal red cells with characteristic inclusions (H&E).

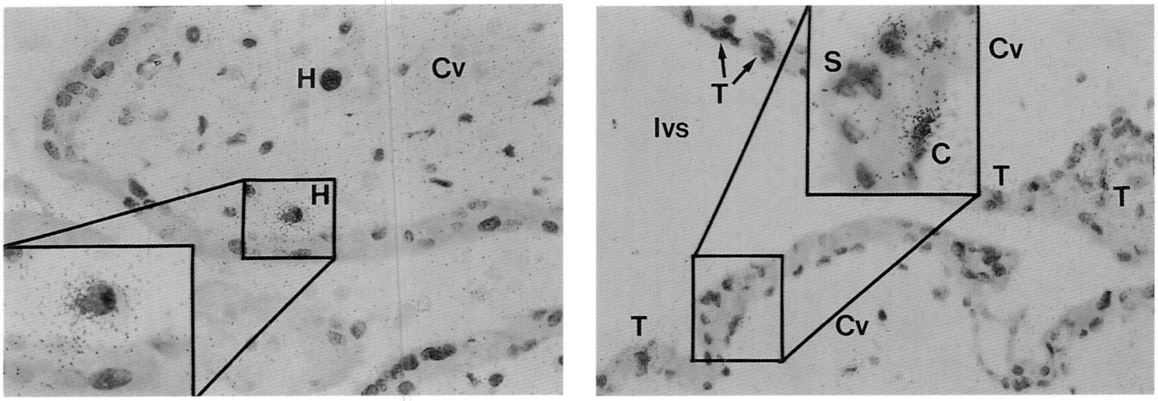

A B

**FIG. 59.** In situ hybridization with $S^{35}$ probe detects HIV-1 nucleic acids in Hofbauer (H) cells (**A**) and trophoblast (C,T) of immature villi (CV) (**B**). [Reprinted with permission (67).]

## DECIDUA

### Histology

The hypersecretory glandular epithelium of the endometrium, which is progestationally induced, affords the proper environment for implantation. At times, these hypersecretory glands may exhibit the Arias-Stella reaction in which cytologic atypia is noted (Fig. 60). In this condition, nuclei are often polyploid. However, nuclear cytoplasmic ratios remain low, distinguishing this normal finding from neoplasia. In this continued progrestational influence, endometrial glands become secretorily exhausted. The endometrial stroma has undergone its characteristic "decidualization," and decidual cells of the endometrium are characterized as epithelioid and polygonal. Their small rounded nuclei are generally situated centrally in abundant pale eosinophilic, ofen vacuolated, cytoplasm (Fig. 61). The cytoplasm is rich in glycogen and glycoproteins. In regions of decidual tissue, where trophoblastic derivatives are not present, nuclear content is diploid (68). Ultrastructural examination of the decidua shows that tight junctions separate these cells (69).

In addition to the decidual cells, an admixture of fibroblasts and lymphocytes is also identified. An additional cell type, the "granular cell," has been shown to produce relaxin (70).

The intercellular matrix contains abundant type IV collagen and laminin. Fibronectin and heparin sulfate proteins also have been identified (71). Other collagens are also present throughout the decidual matrix, and these include types I, III, and V.

Although prior reports suggested that the secretory activity of the decidua included the production of prolactin and human placental lactogen, it is known that this hormone is produced not by decidual cells but by invading trophoblastic derivatives (principally intermediate trophoblast or X cells ) (54). Much of the difficulty in studying decidual tissues and their hormonal production has resulted from the inability of

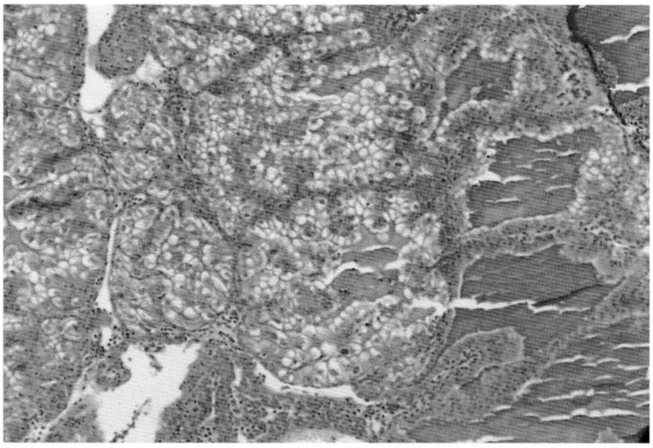

**FIG. 60.** Arias-Stella reaction (H&E stain).

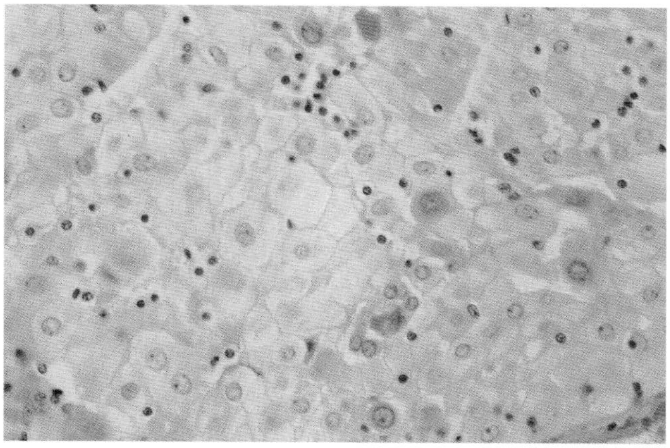

**FIG. 61.** Decidua with centrally placed open nuclei and abundant pale cytoplasm with prominent cell borders. Note sparse normal lymphocytic infiltrate and occasional X cell with cytoplasm darker than decidual cytoplasm (HPS stain).

many investigators to distinguish decidual components from invading trophoblastic contaminants (1).

The vascularization of the decidual component of the implantation site is critical to the developing gestation. The major branches of the uterine arteries extend deeply into the myometrial substance, resulting in arcuate arteries that then branch to form radial arteries. These become the spiral arterioles, the terminal components of the endometrial vasculature. These spiral vessels have been shown by injection studies to be responsible for the intervillous blood flow within cotyledonary units (72). The precise number of spiral arterioles that serve to perfuse the placenta is a debated topic. Estimates range from 25 to 300 vascular openings (73,74).

That trophoblastic cells invade the underlying decidual vasculate is a well-known phenomenon. This finding has been documented within the decidual bed, as well as in systemic maternal vascular compartments, most notably the lung (75). It is important to distinguish these decidual vascular changes from those abnormalities of the decidual vasculature that indicate pathologic conditions.

Gross inspection of the decidua is generally unrevealing, and important attributes and diagnoses are identified histologically. In through-and-through sections of the placenta disk, which includes the chorionic plate and the villous parenchyma, the underlying decidua is often denuded from the placental implantation site during the delivery process. Therefore, it is not uncommon to find sections of parenchyma devoid of decidual tissue. One region in which decidua is often prominent is on the chorion laeve. Sections of "membrane rolls," which include amnion and chorion, often include sections of adherent decidua, which represent fusion of the decidua capsularis and the decidua vera during development. In some patients in whom decidua abnormalities are suspect, decidual bed biopsies have been performed at the time of delivery. Such biopsies often reveal aberrant vascular relationships of the more proximal vascular tree (ra-

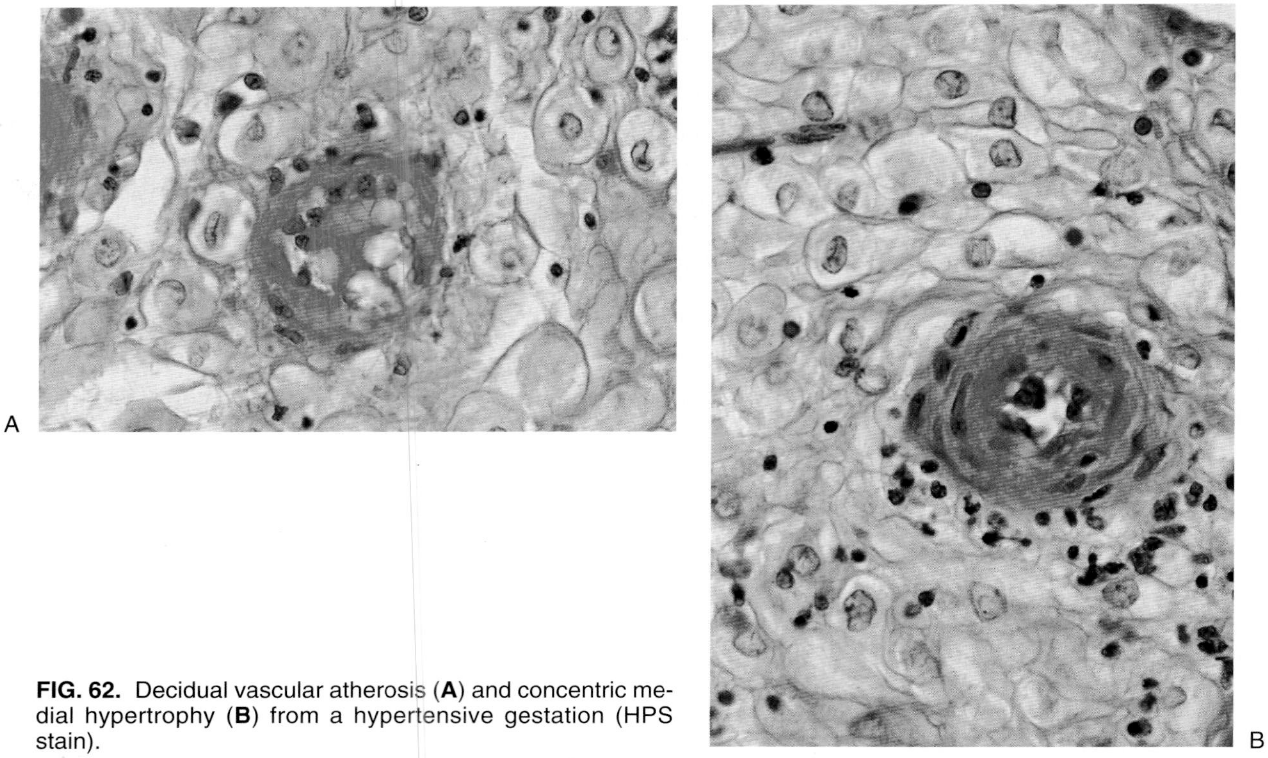

FIG. 62. Decidual vascular atherosis (A) and concentric medial hypertrophy (B) from a hypertensive gestation (HPS stain).

dial and basal arteries). The more proximal vessels are characterized by thicker vascular walls, and their arteries often have internal elastic laminae as evidenced by silver stains. The more distal arteries (the spiral arterioles) are thin walled and do not possess any internal elastic lamina.

## Histopathology

Principal among decidual pathology is the so-called atherosis of the decidual vascular bed, which is known to accompany preeclampsia and hypertensive conditions of gestation (76). These lesions are characterized by fibrinoid necrosis and hyalinization of the vascular wall along with the deposition of foamy macrophages and should be readily distinguishable from normal trophoblastic vascular invasion. Another abnormality that may characterize hypertensive pregnancies is concentric arteriolar mural hypertrophy (Fig. 62).

Bleeding (retroplacental) is responsible for premature placental separation or abruptio placenta. This has been related to two maternal conditions: increased maternal blood pressure and decidual vascular necrosis (due to vasculopathies or inflammatory-bacterial decidual infections) (Fig. 63).

When trophoblastic villi implant directly on myometrial tissue and intervening decidua is absent, the pathologic condition of placenta accreta is present (Fig. 64). This finding is more common in low implantations of the placenta, especially when prior cesarean sections have been performed. Variations in which trophoblastic villi implanted within the myometrium (placenta increta) and when implantation results in the presence of villous tissue protruding through the uterine serosal surface (placenta percreta) are more severe forms of this condition. Generally, all placental tissue cannot be removed from the uterus at delivery and severe hemor-

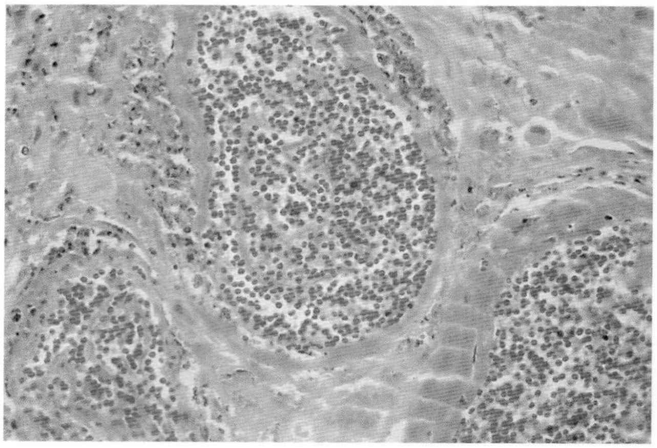

FIG. 63. Decidual vascular necrosis, in this case due to a severe acute deciduitis. Note vascular wall hyalinization and necrosis, which resulted in adjacent abruptio (H&E stain).

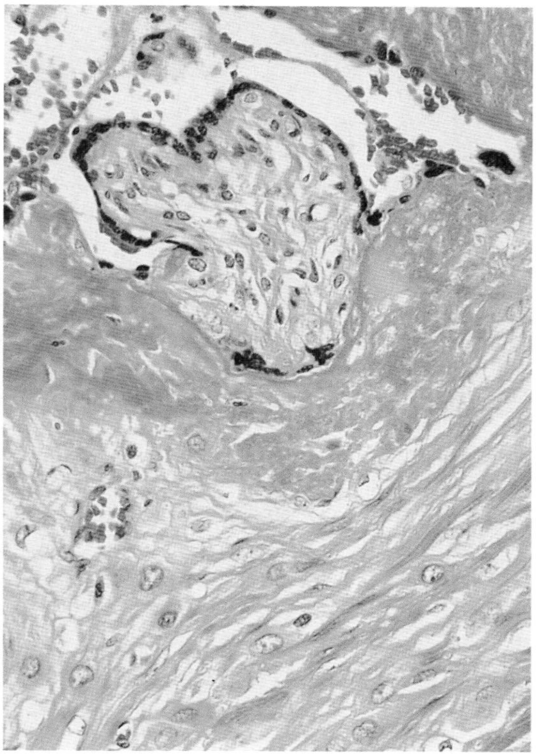

**FIG. 64.** Placenta accreta. No decidua is present between the implanting trophoblastic villi and the uterine myometrium. The presence of small amounts of fibrin does not alter the diagnosis.

rhage ensues. Heroic measures rarely save the uterus, and the condition often necessitates hysterectomy. Occasionally, accreta are confirmed by studying the decidua of the chorion laeve. Failure of resolution of villi during capsular expansion may result in myometrial implantation without intervening decidua. Also occasionally, myometrium adherent to frondosum is found without intervening decidua. In both cases the diagnosis of accreta can be made by the pathologist in the absence of the hysterectomy specimen.

The decidual bed of the delivered placenta may be infiltrated by a few polymorphonuclear leukocytes or lymphocytes. The presence of these inflammatory cells, in the absence of distinct inflammatory processes in the fetal membranes, is common. Such a finding may be physiologic but generally is indicative of infection or low-grade inflammation. However, more intense (acute) inflammatory lesions are generally associated with inflammation of the fetal membranes. When large areas of the decidual bed contains polymorphonuclear leukocytes, acute chorioamnionitis should be sought. When plasma cells are noted, syphilis and CMV should be considered.

## GESTATIONAL TROPHOBLASTIC DISEASE

Although the discussion of neoplastic trophoblastic disease is beyond the scope of this chapter, several normal or exaggerated findings of the implantation site or the placenta proper are discussed to distinguish them from more significant pathologic entities.

Degenerative changes of early trophoblastic villi are not uncommon, especially in the presence of incomplete abortus material. Trophoblastic villi from such gestations are often seen in histologic sections to be swollen (hydropic). These findings are distinguished from the gestational trophoblastic neoplasm (complete hydatidiform mole) in several aspects. Principal among these distinguishing characteristics is that no trophoblastic atypia or proliferation is present along the surface of the villi (Fig. 65). When degenerative changes have taken place and fetal components are blighted, the chorionic vasculature may be absent within the villi. However, if remnants of these vessels persist, the presence of complete hydatidiform mole is essentially not possible. The ease of identifying nucleated hematologic precursors facilitates this observation. Furthermore, should any fetal parts be identified, this too excludes the presence of complete hydatidiform mole. On the other hand, hydropic villi in the presence of fetal parts may herald genotypically abnormal gestations. This form of incomplete mole, which is rarely neoplastic, is characterized by scalloped trophoblastic borders and occasional trophoblastic island inclusions (representing tangential cuts of scalloped borders within the villous stroma) (Fig. 66).

Abundant trophoblastic derivates, prominent within the nidus of the implantation site, may from time to time need to

A
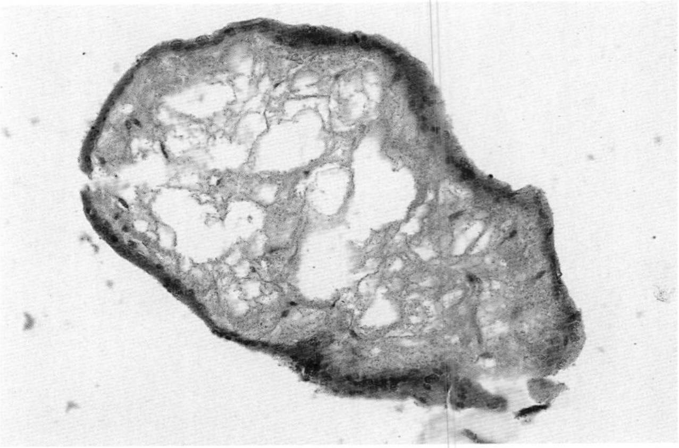

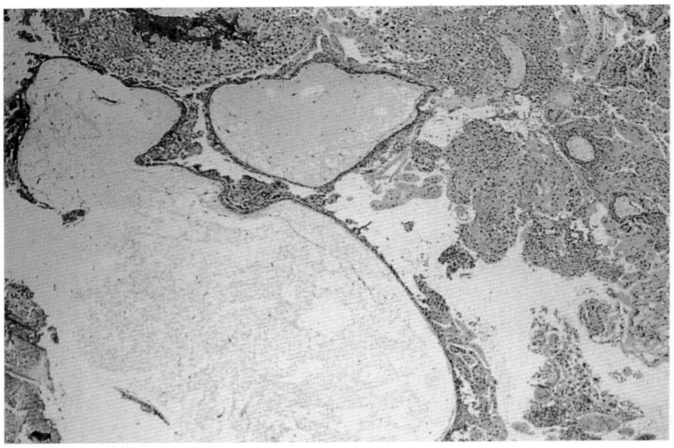
B

C
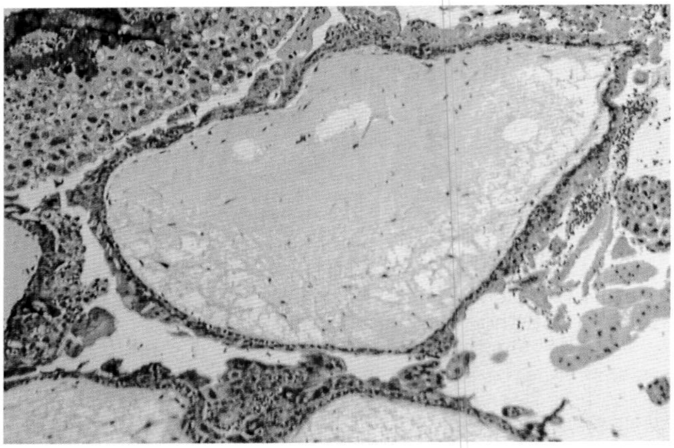

**FIG. 65.** Degenerative (nonneoplastic) focal hydropic degeneration (**A**) and (neoplastic) complete mole (**B**) with trophoblastic hyperplasia and atypia (**C**) (H&E stain).

A
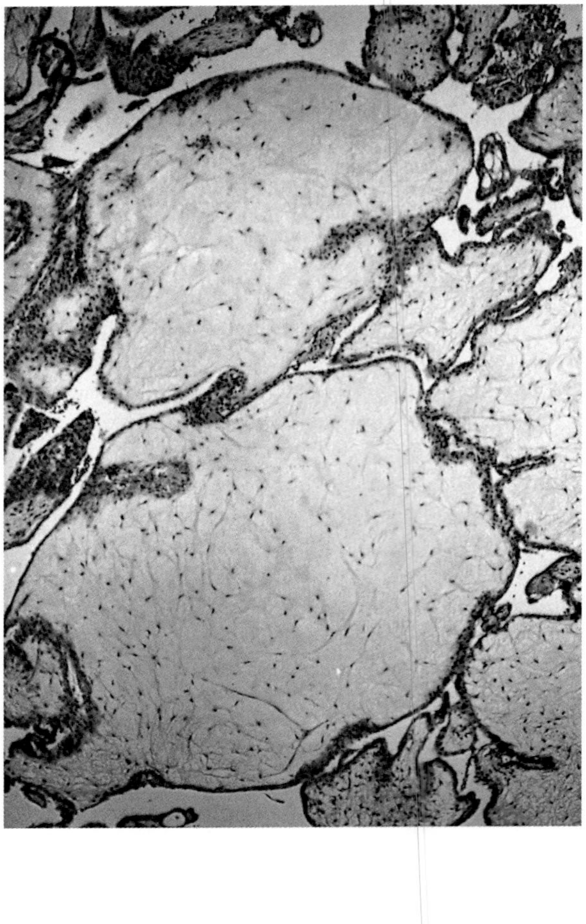

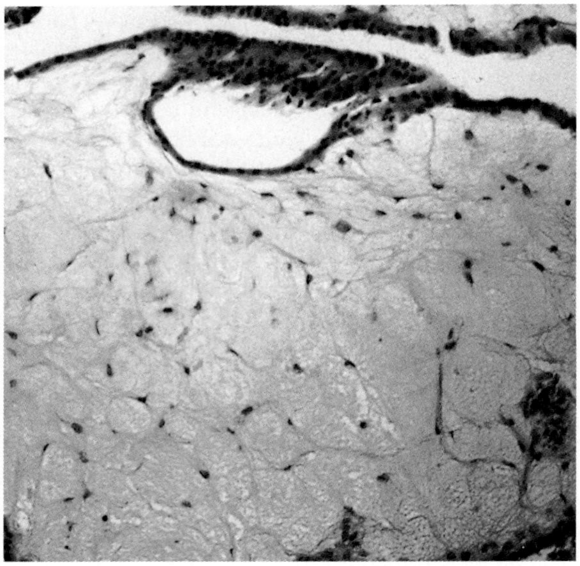
B

**FIG. 66.** Triploid incomplete mole with scalloped trophoblastic borders (**A**) and trophoblastic inclusions (**B**), which are actually tangential cuts of scalloped borders (H&E stain).

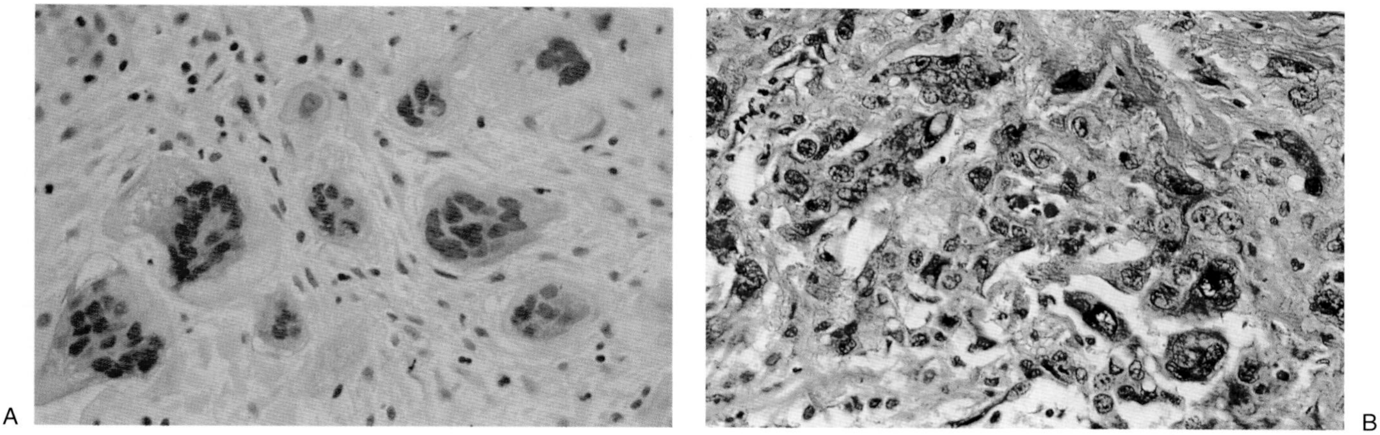

FIG. 67. Exaggerated implantation site (A) and invading choriocarcinoma (B) (H&E stain).

be distinguished from choriocarcinoma. The so-called syncytial endometritis—a poor term because it is not an inflammatory or infectious condition—refers to an exaggerated implantation site where syncytiotrophoblastic and other trophoblastic derivative counterparts are prominant (Fig. 67). In the absence of included trophoblastic villi during examination, the histologic appearance is similar to that of invading choriocarcinoma. The chief distinction is the lack of pronounced cytologic and nuclear atypia that characterizes choriocarcinoma.

Last, an unusual lesion that is neoplastic is the placental site trophoblastic tumor. This neplasm is composed solely of X cells [or, as described by Kurman et al. (54), intermediate trophoblasts] (Fig. 68).

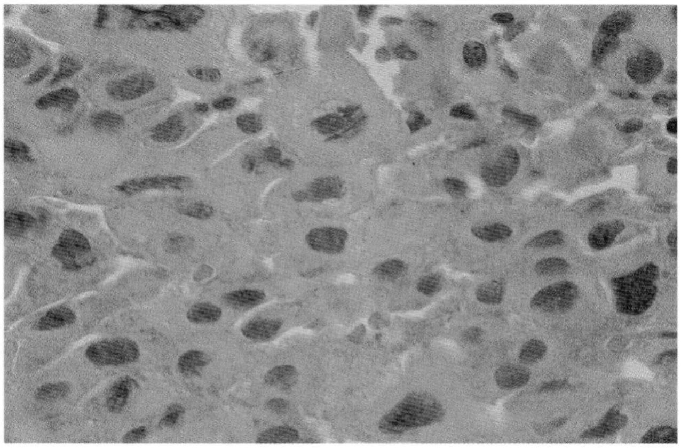

FIG. 68. Placental site trophoblastic tumor (H&E stain).

## ACKNOWLEDGMENT

We thank Jacque Walker for diligent preparation of the manuscript.

## REFERENCES

1. Benirschke K, Kaufmann P. *The pathology of the human placenta, 3rd ed.* New York: Springer-Verlag; 1995.
2. Perrin EVDK, ed. *Pathology of the placenta.* New York: Churchill Livingstone; 1984.
3. Bartholomew RA, Colvin ED, Grimes WH, Fish JS, Lester WM, Galloway WH. Criteria by which toxemia of pregnancy may be diagnosed from unlabeled formalin-fixed placenta. *Am J Obstet Gynecol* 1961;82:277–290.
4. Schremmer BN. Gewichtsveränderungen verschiedener Gewebe nach Formalinfixierung. *Frank Z Pathol* 1967;77:299–305.
5. The examination of the placenta on patient care and risk management. *Arch Pathol* 1991;115.
6. Nuovo G, Richart RM. Buffered formalin is the superior fixative for the detection of HPV DNA by *in situ* hybridization analysis. *Am J Pathol* 1989;34:837–842.
7. Naeye RL. Umbilical cord length: clinical significance. *J Pediatr* 1985;107:278–281.

7a. Lewis SH, Starr C. Cord width. *In Utero* (Unpublished).

8. Grosser O. *Frühentwicklung, Eihautbildung und Placentation des Menschen und der Säugetiere.* Munich: JF Bergman; 1927.
9. Gardiner JP. The umbilical cord; normal length; length in cord complications; etiology and frequency of coiling. *Surg Gynecol Obstet* 1922;34:252–256.
10. Wynn RM, French GL. Comparative ultrastructure of the mammalian amnion. *Obstet Gynecol* 1968;31:759–774.
11. Hoyes AD. Ultrastructure of the epithelium of the human umbilical cord. *J Anat* 1969;105:145–162.
12. Moore RD. Mast cells of the human umbilical cord. *Am J Pathol* 1956;32:1179–1183.
13. Nadkarni BB. Innervation of the human umbilical artery: an electron-microscope study. *Am J Obstet Gynecol* 1970;107:303–312.
14. Ellison JP. The nerves of the umbilical cord in man and the rat. *Am J Obstet Gynecol* 1984;148:219–220.
15. Lauweryns JM, deBruyn M, Peuskens J, Bourgeois N. Absence of intrinsic innervation of the human placenta. *Experientia* 1969;25:432.
16. Blanc WA, Allan GW. Intrafunicular ulceration of the persistent omphalomesenteric duct with intra-amniotic hemorrhage and fetal death. *Am J Obstet Gynecol* 1961;82:1392–1396.

17. Priman J. A note on the anastomosis of the umbilical arteries. *Anat Rec* 1959;134:1–5.
18. Arts NFT. Investigations on the vascular system of the placenta. Part 1. General introduction and the fetal vascular system. *Am J Obstet Gynecol* 1961;82:147–168.
19. Jagpal R, Ebert GA, Kappy, KA. Adverse perinatal outcome with an abnormal umbilical coiling index. *Obstet Gynecol* 1995;85:523–578.
20. Altshuler G, Hyde S. Meconium-induced vasocontraction: a potential cause of cerebral and other hypoprofusion and of poor pregnancy outcome. *J Child Neurol* 1989;4:137–142.
21. Naeye RL. *Disorders of the placenta, fetus and neonate. Diagnosis and clinical significance.* St. Louis: Mosby Year Book; 1992.
22. Vonthobitien N. *Anatomia Suc Undina Human.* 1668.
23. Garza A, Cordero JR, Mulinare J. Epidemiology of the early amnion rupture spectrum of defects. *Am J Dis Child* 1988;142:541–544.
24. Torpin R. *Fetal malformations caused by amnion rupture during gestation.* Springfield, IL: Charles C Thomas; 1969.
25. Danforth DM, Hull RW. The microscopic anatomy of the fetal membranes with particular reference to the detailed structure of amnion rupture during gestation. *Am J Obstet Gynecol* 1958;75:536–550.
26. Boyd JD, Hamilton WJ. *The human placenta.* Cambridge, MA: Heffer & Sons, 1970.
27. Michael H, Ulbright TM, Brodhecker C. Magma reticulare-like differentiation in yolk sac tumor and its pluripotential nature [Abstract]. *Mod Pathol* 1988;1:63.
28. King BF. Developmental changes in the fine structure of rhesus monkey amnion. *Am J Anat* 1980:157:285–307.
29. Mukaida T, Yoshida K, Kikyokawa T, Soma H. Surface structure of the placental membranes. *J Clin Electron Microsc* 1977;10:447–448.
30. Bourne GL. The microscopic anatomy of the human amnion and chorion. *Am J. Obstet Gynecol* 1960;79:1070–1073.
31. Majno G, Joris I. Review apoptosis oncosis and necrosis and overview of cell death. *Am J Pathol* 1995;146:3–15.
32. Tsukada T, Eguchi K, Migita K, Nagataki S. Transforming growth factor beta-1 induces apoptotic cell death in cultured human umbilical vein endothelial cells with down regulated expression of BCL-2. *Biochem Biophys Res Commun* 1995:210:1076–1082.
33. Bartels H, Wang T. Intercellular junctions in the human fetal membranes. *Anat Embryol* 1983;166:103–120.
34. Robinson HL, Anhalt GJ, Patel HP, Takahashi Y, Labib RS, Diaz LA. Pemphigus and pemphigoid antigens are expressed in human amnion epithelium. *J Invest Dermatol* 1984;83:234–237.
35. Schwarzacher HG, Klinger HP. Die Entstehung mehrkerniger Zellen durch Amitose in Amnionepithel des Menschen und die Aufteilung des chromosomalen Materials auf deren einzelne Kerne. *Z Zellforsch* 1963; 60:741–754.
36. Schindler PD. Nuclear deoxyribonucleic acid (DNA) content, nuclear size and cell size in the human amnion epithelium. *Acta Anat* 1985;44: 273–285.
37. Kalousek DK, Fill FD. Chromosomal mosaicism confined to the placenta in human conceptions. *Science* 1983;221:665–667.
38. Bautzmann H, Hertenstein C. Zur Histogenese und Histologie des meschlichen fetalen und Neugeborenen-Amnion. *Z Zellforsch* 1957;45: 589–611.
39. Schmidt W. Struktur und Funktion des Amnionepithels von Menschen und Huhn. *Z Zellforsch* 1963;61:642–660.
40. Schwarzacher HG. Beitrag zur Histogenese des menschlichen Amnion. *Acta Anat* 1960;43:303–311.
41. Nickell KA, Stocker JT. Placental teratoma: a case report. *Pediatr Pathol* 1987;7:645–650.
42. Salazar H, Kanbour AI, Pardo M. Amnion nodosum. Ultrastructure and histopathogenesis. *Arch Pathol* 1974;98:39–46.
43. Bourne GL. *The human amnion and chorion.* London: Lloyd-Luke; 1962.
44. Luckett P. The origin of extraembryonic mesoderm in the early human and rhesus monkey embryos. *Anat Rec* 1971;169:369–370.
45. Rossant J, Croy BA. Genetic identification of tissue of origin of cellular populations within the mouse placenta. *J Embryol Exp Morphol* 1985;86:177–189.
46. Hoyes AD. Ultrastructure of the human mesenchymal layers of the human chorion in early pregnancy. *Am J Obstet Gynecol* 1970;106: 557–566.
47. Hoyes AD. Ultrastructure of the mesenchymal layers of the human chorion laeve. *J Anat* 1971;109:17–30.
48. Sala MA, Matheus M. Histochemical study of the fetal membranes in the human term pregnancy. *Gegenbaurs Morphol Jahrb* 1984;130: 699–705.
49. Hessle H. Engvall E. Type VI collagen. *J Biol Chem* 1984;259: 3955–3961.
50. Goldstein J. Braverman M. Salafia C, Buckley P. The phenotype of human placental macrophages and its variation with gestational age. *Am J Pathol* 1988;133:648–659.
51. American College of Obstetricians and Gynecologist. A106 Committee Opinion (Committee on Genetics) Chorionic Villus Sampling 1995; no. 160.
52. Pitkin RM, Reynolds WA, Williams GA, Hargis GK. Calcium metabolism in normal pregnancy: a longitudinal study. *Am J Obstet Gynecol* 1979;133:781–790.
53. Tsang RC, Donovan EF, Steichen JJ. Calcium physiology and pathology in the neonate. *Pediatr Clin North Am* 1976;23:611–626.
54. Kurman RJ, Main CS, Chen H-C. Intermediate trophoblast: a distinctive form of trophoblast with specific morphological, biochemical and functional features. *Placenta* 1984;5:349–370.
55. Wasmoen TL, Benirschke K, Gleich GJ. Demonstration of immunoreactive eosinophil granule major basic protein in the plasma and placentae of non-human primates. *Placenta* 1987;8:283–292.
56. Wynn RM. Cytotrophoblastic specializations: an ultrastructural study of the human placenta. *Am J Obstet Gynecol* 1972;114:339–355.
57. Yeh I-T, O'Connor DM, Kurman RJ. Vacuolated cytotrophoblast: a subpopulation of trophoblast in the chorion laeve. *Placenta* 1989;10: 429–438.
58. O'Connor DM, Kurman RJ. Utilization of intermediate trophoblast in the diagnosis of an *in utero* gestation in endometrial curettings without chorionic villi [Abstract]. *Mod Pathol* 1988;1:68.
59. Redline RW, Patterson P. Preeclampsia is associated with an excess of proliferative immature intermediate trophoblast. *Hum Pathol* 1995;26: 594–600.
60. Wislocki GB, Dempsey EW. Electron microscopy of the human placenta. *Anat Rec* 1995;123:133.
61. Richart RM. Studies of placental morphogenesis: I. Radioautrographic studies of human placenta utilizing tritiated thymidine. *Proc Soc Exp Biol Med* 1961;106:829.
62. Pierce GB Jr. Midgley AR Jr. The origin and function of human syncytiotrophoblastic giant cells. *Am J Pathol* 1963;43:153.
63. Altshuler G. Placental infection and inflammation. In: Perrin EVDK, ed. *Pathology of the placenta.* New York: Churchill Livingstone; 1984.
64. Fujikura T, Froehlich L. Diagnosis of sickling by placental examination. *Am J Obstet Gynecol* 1968;100:1122–1124.
65. Knox WF, Fox H. Villitis of unknown aetiology: its incidence and significance on placentae from a British population. *Placenta* 1984;5: 395–402.
66. Redline RW, Patterson P. Villitis of unknown etiology is associated with major infiltration of fetal tissue by maternal inflammatory cells. *Am J Pathol* 1993;473–479.
67. Lewis SH, Reynolds-Kohler C, Faulks HE, Nelson JA. HIV-1 trophoblastic and villous Hofbauer cells, and hematologic precursors in 8-week fetuses. *Lancet* 1990;355:565–568.
68. Sachs H. Quantitativ histochemische Untersuchung des Endometrium in der Schwangerschaft und der Placenta (Cytophotometrische Messungen). *Arch Gynecol* 1968;205:93–104.
69. Lawn AM, Wilson EW, Finn CA. The ultrastructure of human decidual and predecidual cells. *J Reprod Fertil* 1971;26:85–90.
70. Dallenbach FD, Dallenbach-Hellweg G. Immunohistologische Untersuchungen zur Lokalisation des Relaxins in menschlicher Placenta und Decidua. *Virchows Arch [A]* 1964;337:301–316.
71. Wewer UM, Faber M, Liotta LA, Albrechtsen R. Immunochemical and ultrastructural assessment of the nature of pericellular basement membrane of human decidual cells. *Lab Invest* 1985;53:624–633.
72. Freese UE. The uteroplacental vascular relationship in the human. *Am J Obstet Gynecol* 1968;101:8–16.
73. Borell U, Fernstrom I, Ohlson L, Wiqvist N. Effect of uterine contractions on the uteroplacental blood flow at term. *Am J Obstet Gynecol* 1965;93:44–57.
74. Haller U. Beitrag zur Morphologic der Utero-Placentagefässe. *Arch Gynecol* 1968;205:185–202.
75. Attwood HD, Park WW. Embolism to the lung by trophoblast. *J Obstet Gynecol Br Commonwealth* 1961;68:611–617.
76. Hertig AT. Vascular pathology in hypertensive albuminuric toxemias of pregnancy. *Clinic* 1945;4:602–614.

# Male Genital System

*Histology for Pathologists, second edition,*
Edited by Stephen S. Sternberg.
Lippincott-Raven Publishers, Philadelphia


# CHAPTER 42

# Prostate

John E. McNeal



## EMBRYOLOGY AND DEVELOPMENT OF THE PROSTATE

The prostate appears in early embryonic development as a condensation of mesenchyme along the course of the pelvic urethra. By 9 weeks of embryonic life, a number of features that are characteristic of adult contour and location are evident (Fig. 1). The mesenchymal condensation is most dense along the posterior (rectal) aspect of the urethra and distal (apical) to its mid-point. This is the only region where highly condensed mesenchyme is in immediate contact with urethral lining epithelium, and only here is the urethra lined by a tall columnar epithelium (1). Between its mid-point and the bladder neck, the proximal urethral segment shows a sharp anterior angulation. However, the strip of highly condensed mesenchyme continues directly proximally to a dome-shaped base, leaving a gap between prostatic mesenchyme and proximal urethra.

The ejaculatory ducts penetrate the mesenchyme toward the future verumontanum, which is located at the urethral mid-point. This is wolffian duct tissue, but its stroma is indistinguishable from the remaining prostatic mesenchyme, which is mainly derived from the urogenital sinus (2). However, that portion of the mesenchyme that surrounds the ejaculatory ducts and expands proximally to occupy nearly the entire prostate base is distinguishable in the adult as the central zone, which is probably also derived from the wolffian duct, as are the seminal vesicles (1). In this concept, the prostate is of dual embryonic derivation.

At about 10 weeks, epithelial buds begin to branch mainly posteriorly and laterally from the posterior and perhaps the lateral walls of the distal urethral segment into the condensed mesenchyme. Recent computer reconstructions of serially sectioned specimens have shown that the branching pattern that is established initially is identical to that described for the adult later in this chapter (3).

This developmental program is activated by androgen secreted by the fetal testis. However, the eventual size of the neonatal prostate—less than 1 cm in diameter—is predetermined by the stroma as a programmed number of stromal cell divisions, after which the stroma ceases to have further inductive influence on the branching duct system.

The prostate is not again exposed to hormonal stimulation until puberty, and it grows at a slow rate, reaching less than 2 cm in diameter by that time. During this period, the ducts and acini are lined by epithelium, which undergoes little change from the neonatal period. Gland spaces are lined by cells that are crowded with multilayered dark nuclei (Fig. 2). There is a superficial resemblance to adult postinflammatory atrophy, but the histologic features are quite different.

The pubertal growth acceleration and maturation of the prostate gland appears not to be complete until at least 20 years of age. The average prostate by this time measures about 4.5 cm in width, 3.5 to 4.0 cm in length, and 3 cm in thickness. In most men over 50 years of age, there is focal resumption of growth as benign nodular hyperplasia (BPH). This process increases the thickness of the gland prominantly and its length least; in massive BPH, however, the prostate becomes nearly spherical, with a diameter of 6 cm or more. Dissections show that BPH represents enlargement of only a single tiny region of the gland. In fact, the normal mass of the glandular portion of the prostate after subtraction of the BPH-prone region remains at nearly constant mean

J. E. McNeal: Department of Urology, Stanford University School of Medicine, Stanford, California 94305.

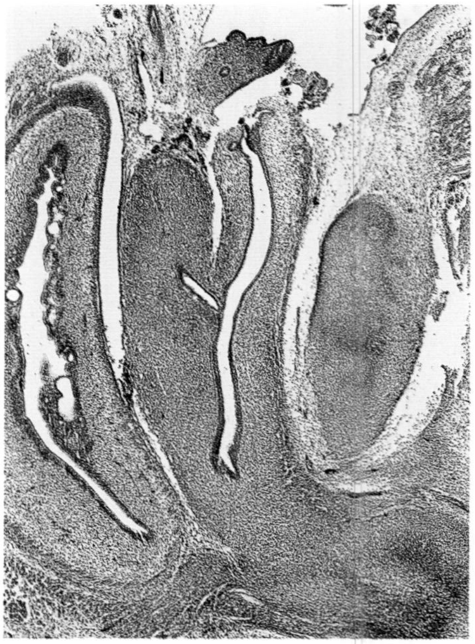

FIG. 1. Embryonic prostate, age 9 weeks, in the sagittal plane of the pelvis. Urethra (narrow central lumen) is angulated to right at mid-point where ejaculatory duct approaches from above left. Vertical strip of highly condensed prostate mesenchyme contacts posterior urethral wall only distal to ejaculatory ducts. Prostate is flanked by rectum on left and pubis on right. Duct buds have not yet formed.

volume until 70 years of age or more. However, the range about the mean increases in men more than 50 years of age, suggesting that the normal, non-BPH glandular prostate may continue enlarging into old age rather than undergoing atrophy.

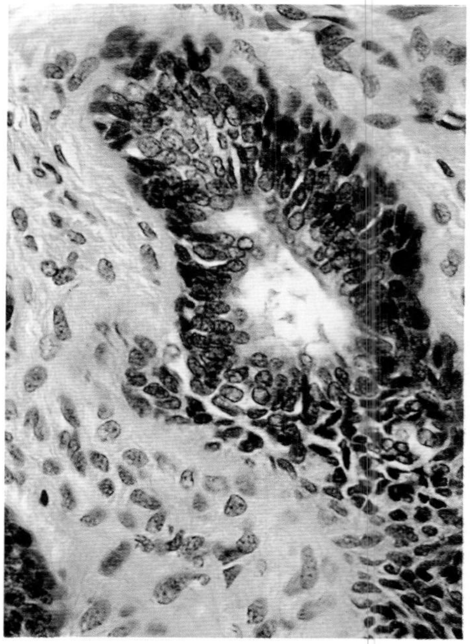

FIG. 2. Prepubertal prostatic duct lined by epithelium with multiple layers of nuclei and showing no cytoplasmic differentiation.

## GENERAL RELATIONSHIPS: THE GLANDULAR PROSTATE

The human prostate gland is a composite organ, made up of several glandular and nonglandular components. These different tissues are tightly fused together within a common capsule so that gross dissections are difficult and unreliable. Anatomic features are best demonstrated by examination of cut sections in carefully selected planes (4,5). The nonglandular tissue of the prostate is concentrated anteromedially and is responsible for much of the anterior convexity of the organ. The contour of the glandular prostate approximates a disk with lateral wings that fold anteriorly to partially encircle the nonglandular tissue. There are four distinct glandular regions, each of which arises from a different segment of the prostatic urethra.

The urethra is a primary reference point for describing anatomic relationships. These relationships are best visualized in a sagittal plane of section (Fig. 3). The prostatic urethra is divided into proximal and distal segments of approximately equal length by an abrupt anterior angulation of its posterior wall at the mid-point between prostate apex and bladder neck (1,6). The angle of deviation is roughly 35°, but it is quite variable and is greater in men with nodular hyperplasia. The base of the verumontanum protrudes from the posterior urethral wall at the point of angulation. The verumontanum bulges into the urethral lumen along its posterior wall for about half the length of the distal segment and tapers distally to form the crista urethralis.

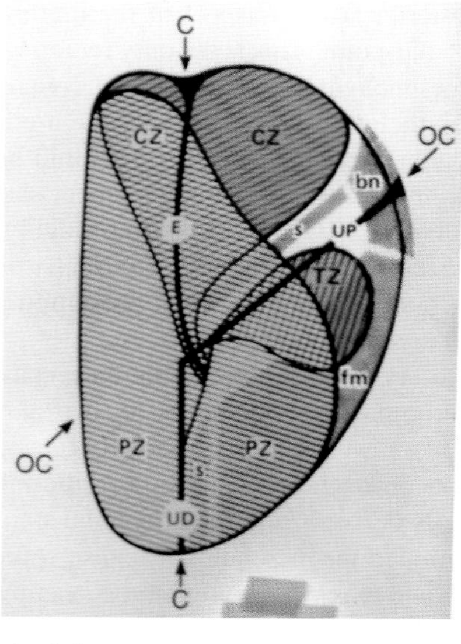


FIG. 3. Sagittal diagrams of distal prostatic urethral segment (UD), proximal urethral segment (UP), and ejaculatory ducts (E) showing their relationships to a sagittal section of the anteromedial nonglandular tissues [bladder neck (bn), anterior fibromuscular stroma (fm), preprostatic sphincter (s), distal striated sphincter (s)]. These structures are shown in relation to a three-dimensional representation of the glandular prostate [central zone (CZ), peripheral zone (PZ), transition zone (TZ)]. Coronal plane (C) of Fig. 4 and oblique coronal plane (OC) of Fig. 5 are indicated by arrows.

The distal urethral segment receives the ejaculatory ducts and the ducts of about 95% of the glandular prostate; it is, therefore, the only segment that is primarily involved in ejaculatory function. The ejaculatory ducts extend proximally from the verumontanum to the base of the prostate, following a course that is nearly a direct extension of the long axis of the distal urethral segment, although usually offset a few millimeters posteriorly.

A coronal plane of section along the course of the ejaculatory ducts and distal urethral segment provides the best demonstration of the anatomic relationships between the two major regions of the glandular prostate (7) (Fig. 4). The peripheral zone comprises about 70% of the mass of the normal glandular prostate. Its ducts exit from the posterolateral recesses of the urethral wall along a double row extending from the base of the verumontanum to the prostate apex. The ducts extend mainly laterally in the coronal plane, with major branches that curve anteriorly and minor branches that curve posteriorly (Fig. 4). The central zone comprises about 25% of the glandular prostate mass. Its ducts arise in a small focus on the convexity of the verumontanum and immediately surrounding the ejaculatory duct orifices. The ducts branch directly toward the base of the prostate along the course of the ejaculatory ducts, fanning out mainly in the coronal plane to form a conical structure that is flattened in anteroposterior dimension. The base of the cone comprises almost the entire base of the prostate. The most lateral central zone ducts run parallel to the most proximal peripheral zone ducts, separated only by a narrow band of stroma.

The proximal segment of the prostatic urethra is best visualized in an oblique coronal plane of section running along its long axis from the base of the verumontanum to the bladder neck (Fig. 5). The proximal urethral segment is related to only about 5% of the prostatic glandular tissue, and almost all of this is represented by the transition zone (8). This zone consists of two independent small lobes whose ducts leave the posterolateral recesses of the urethral wall at a single point, just proximal to the point of urethral angulation and at the lower border of the preprostatic sphincter. The sphincter is a sleeve of smooth muscle fibers surrounding the proximal urethral segment (6,8) (Fig. 6). The main ducts of the transition zone extend laterally around the distal border of the sphincter and curve sharply anteriorly, arborizing toward the bladder neck immediately external to the preprostatic sphincter. Main duct branches fan out laterally and ventrally toward the apex but not dorsally above the plane of the urethra. The most medial ducts and acini of the transition zone curve medially to penetrate into the sphincter (Fig. 6).

The periurethral gland region is only a fraction of the size of the transition zone. It consists of tiny ducts and abortive acinar systems scattered along the length of the proximal

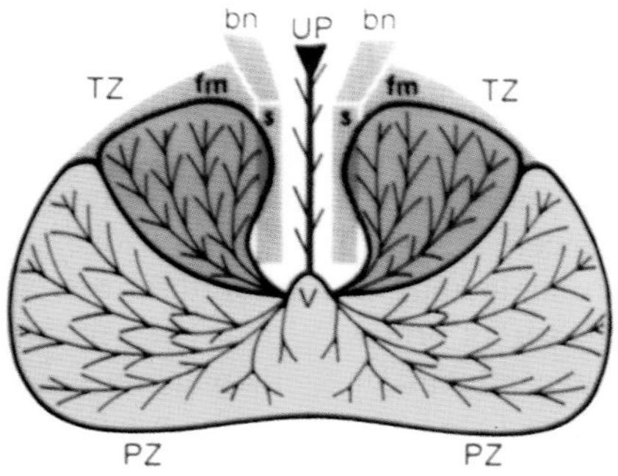


**FIG. 5.** Oblique coronal section diagram of prostate showing location of peripheral zone (PZ) and transition zone (TZ) in relation to proximal urethral segment (UP), verumontanum (V), preprostatic sphincter (S), bladder neck (bn), and periurethral region with periurethral glands. Branching pattern of prostatic ducts is indicated: the medial transition zone ducts penetrate into the sphincter.

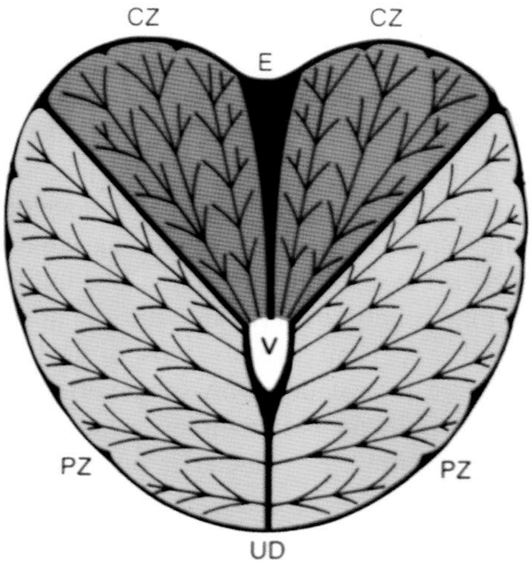


**FIG. 4.** Coronal section diagram of prostate showing location of central zone (CZ) and peripheral zone (PZ) in relation to distal urethral segment (UD), verumontanum (V), and ejaculatory ducts (E). Branching pattern of prostatic ducts is indicated; subsidiary ducts provide uniform density of acini along entire main duct course.

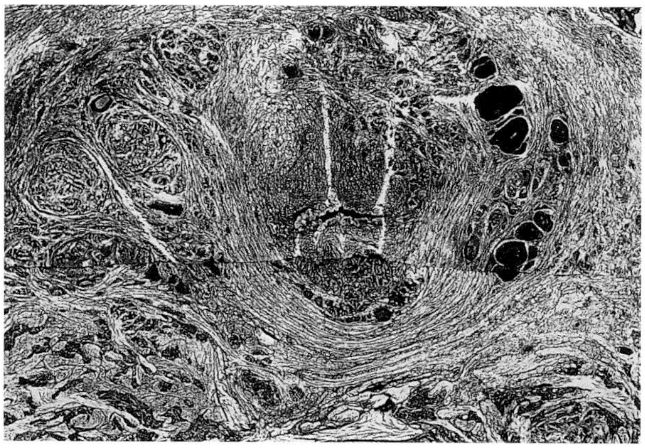

**FIG. 6.** Preprostatic sphincter in section transverse to long axis of proximal urethral segment. Sphincter is most compact dorsal to urethra (*below*) and separates periurethral tissue (*dark central area*) from central zone glands (*bottom*, right, and left). Laterally, transition zone glands are embedded in the sphincter. They show cystic change on right and nodule formation on left.

urethral segment and arborizing exclusively inside the confines of the preprostatic sphincter. These glands lie within the longitudinal periurethral smooth muscle stroma.

The peripheral zone is the most susceptible region to inflammation (7) and is the site of origin of most carcinomas (9). Some cancers arise in the transition zone, and most tumors found incidentally at transurethral resection (TUR) represent this site of origin (10,11). The central zone is resistant to both carcinoma and inflammation.

The transition zone and periurethral region are the exclusive sites of origin of BPH (8). Most cases consist almost entirely of transition zone enlargement, so-called lateral lobe hyperplasia. BPH in the periurethral region seldom attains significant mass, except as the occasional mid-line dorsal nodule at the bladder neck protruding into the bladder lumen. The above anatomic descriptions have gained acceptance over the past 10 years, replacing a number of previous anatomic models that suffered from less accurate descriptions of morphologic detail (12).

## GENERAL RELATIONSHIPS: NONGLANDULAR TISSUE

The nonglandular tissues of the prostate are the preprostatic sphincter, striated sphincter, anterior fibromuscular stroma, and prostatic capsule. The nerves and vascular supply are also included in this section.

The preprostatic sphincter consists of precisely parallel, compact ring fibers forming a cylinder whose proximal end abuts against the detrusor muscle surrounding the urethra at the bladder neck. The coarsely interwoven, somewhat randomly arranged smooth muscle bundles of the detrusor contrast sharply with the uniform arrangement of the sphincter fibers, but there is no boundary between the two structures.

The preprostatic sphincter is thought to function during ejaculation to prevent retrograde flow of seminal fluid from the distal urethral segment. It also may have resting tone that maintains closure of the proximal urethral segment (6). Dorsal to the urethra, the sphincter is compact but laterally its fibers spread apart and mingle with the small ducts and acini of the medial transition zone (Fig. 6) (8). Anterior and ventral to the urethra, its fibers do not form identifiable complete rings but blend with the tissue of the anterior fibromuscular stroma.

The anterior fibromuscular stroma is an apron of tissue that extends downward from the bladder neck over the anteromedial surface of the prostate, narrowing to join the urethra at the prostate apex (8) (Figs. 3 and 7). Its lateral margins blend with the prostate capsule along the line where the capsule covers the most anteriorly projecting border of the peripheral zone (Fig. 5). Its deep surface is in contact with the preprostatic sphincter and transition zone proximally and with the striated sphincter distally. It is composed of large compact bundles of smooth muscle cells that are similar to those of the bladder neck and blend with them at its proximal extent. The smooth muscle fibers are more random in orientation than those of the bladder neck, but they tend to be aligned more or less vertically. They are often separated by bands of dense fibrous tissue.

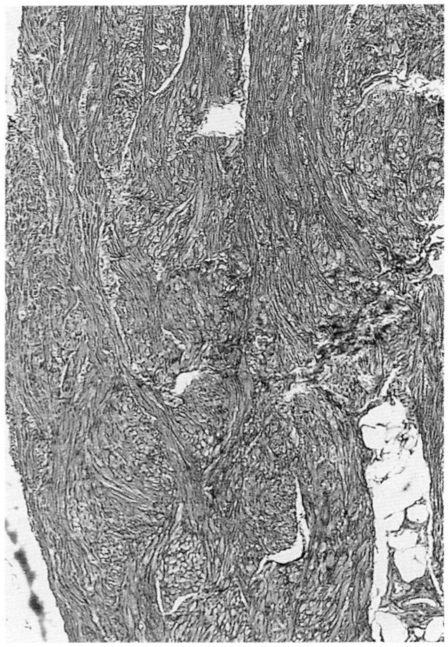

**FIG. 7.** Texture of anterior fibromuscular stroma in an area with little fibrous component. Muscle bundles are coarse and interwoven (trichrome stain).

The anterior fibromuscular stroma is distinguished from the capsule of the prostate by its thickness, its coarse interwoven muscle bundles, and its rough external surface. Microscopically its external aspect shows interdigitation of the muscle bundles along its surface with the adipose tissue of the space of Retzius.

Between the verumontanum and the prostate apex, there is a striated sphincter of small, uniform, compactly arranged striated muscle fibers. It is best developed near the apex and is continuous with the external sphincter below the prostate apex (6,14). The sphincter is incomplete posterolaterally, where its semicircular fibers anchor into the anterior glandular tissue of the peripheral zone rather than encircling the posterior aspect of the urethra. Its degree of development and precise anatomic relationships are variable between prostates. Near the apex in some prostates, individual striated fibers may penetrate deeply into the glandular tissue of the peripheral zone. Consequently, most of the length of the prostatic urethra is provided with sphincteric muscle. The distal striated sphincter is incomplete posteriorly, and the proximal smooth muscle sphincter is probably incomplete anteriorly.

The prostatic capsule envelopes most of the external surface of the prostate, and the terminal acini of the central zone and peripheral zone abut on the capsule. The terminal acini of the transition zone abut on the anterior fibromuscular stroma, and the periurethral glands never reach the prostate surface (8,11). At the prostate apex, there is a defect in the capsule anteriorly and anterolaterally. Here the most distal fibers of the anterior fibromuscular stroma and the striated sphincter together often mingle with the prostatic glandular tissue anterolateral to the urethra, and the relative extent of these three tissue components may vary considerably between prostates. Hence, if carcinoma at the prostate apex invades anteriorly, it may occasionally be difficult to determine whether it has invaded beyond the boundary of the gland. However, around most of the circumference of the apex, the capsule is complete up to the border of the periurethral stroma, where the urethra penetrates the prostate surface. Even with extensive BPH, a thin compressed rim of peripheral zone tissue enclosed by capsule usually still forms the apical prostate boundary except anterior and anterolateral to the urethra.

The capsule of the prostate ideally consists of an inner layer of smooth muscle fibers, mainly oriented transversely, and an outer collagenous membrane. However, the relative and absolute amounts of fibrous and muscle tissue and their arrangement vary considerably from area to area (Fig. 8) (15,16). At the inner capsular border, transverse smooth muscle blends with periacinar smooth muscle, and clear separation between them cannot be identified either microscopically or by gross dissection. The distance from terminal acinus to prostate surface is variable even between different regions within a single prostate, and the proportion and arrangement of collagenous tissue is inconstant except for the most superficial layer, which appears to form a thin continuous collagenous membrane over the prostate surface. Consequently, the prostate capsule cannot be regarded as a well-defined anatomic structure with constant features, except for its external surface. In evaluating capsule penetration by prostatic carcinoma, there are no reliable landmarks for determining the depth of capsule invasion. However, it has been proposed that only complete penetration with perforation through the capsule surface may be related to prognosis in prostatic carcinoma (16,17). Hence, penetration of cancer into the capsule without perforation is not of clinical importance.

Over the medial half of the posterior (rectal) surface of the prostate, the thickness of the capsule is increased by its fusion to Denonvilliers' fascia (Figs. 9 and 10). This is a thin, compact collagenous membrane whose smooth posterior surface rests directly against the muscle of the rectal wall (18). The capsule is typically fused to the inner aspect of the fascia, obliterating any trace of its original surface except for occasional remnants of an interposed adipose layer that embryonically covered the anterior aspect of the fascia. In the

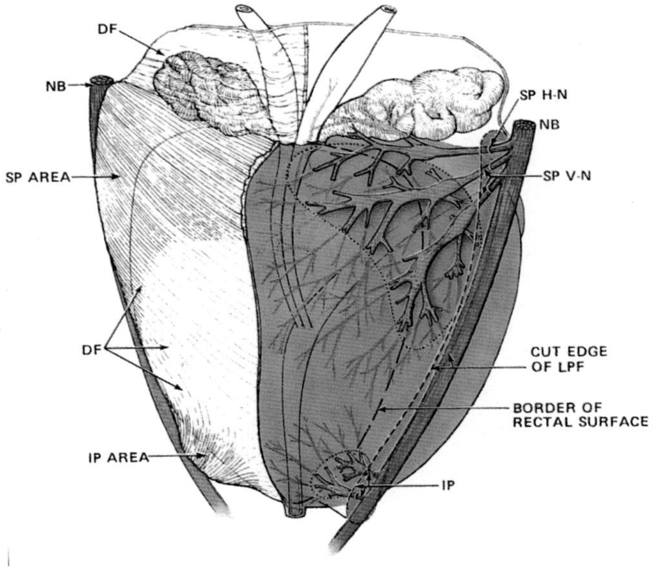


**FIG. 9.** Distribution of nerve branches to prostate, right posterolateral view. Nerves within the neurovascular bundle (NB) (red) branch to supply the prostate (brown) in a large superior pedicle (SP) at the prostate base and a small inferior pedicle (IP) at the prostate apex. Nerve branches (orange) leave the lateral pelvic fascia (not shown) to travel in Denonvilliers' fascia (DF), which has been cut away from the right half of the prostate. Nerve branches from the superior pedicle fan out over a large pedicle area. A small horizontal subdivision (H-N) crosses the base to mid-line; a large vertical subdivision (V-N) fans out extensively over the prostate surface as far distally as mid-prostate. Branches continue their course within the prostate after penetration into the capsule within a large nerve penetration area (green). A small inferior pedicle has a limited ramification and nerve penetration area (green).

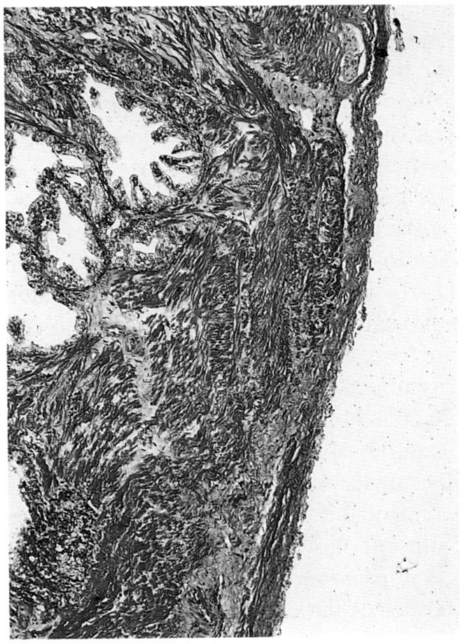

**FIG. 8.** Prostate capsule consists of a layer of mainly transverse smooth muscle bundles (red), which is of variable thickness and blends with periacinar smooth muscle bundles at the capsule's poorly defined inner aspect (*left*). Collagen fibers (blue) are always present and usually concentrated in a thin compact membrane at the external capsular border (*right*) (trichrome stain).

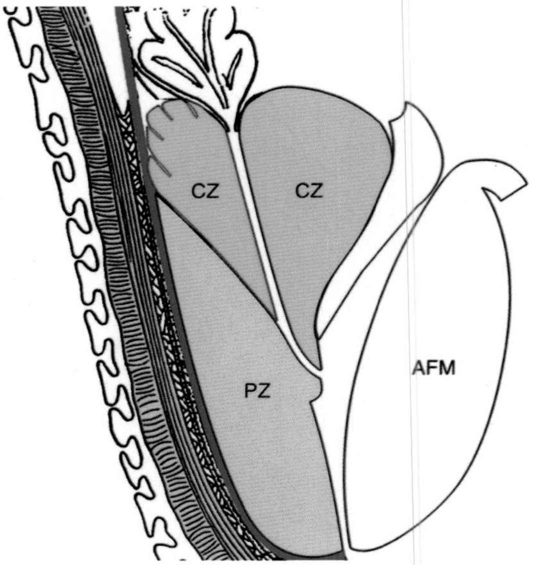


**FIG. 10.** Relationships of Denonvilliers' fascia (narrow red band) to sagittal plane of prostate (yellow and orange) on right and to rectal smooth muscle (brown) on left.

adult there remain only scattered microscopic islands of fat, usually forming a layer that is only one adipose cell thick.

Smooth muscle fibers are found to a variable extent in Denonvilliers' fascia, but they usually course vertically, in contrast to the transverse muscle fibers of the adherent capsule. In some prostates, the smooth muscle of Denonvilliers' fascia is gathered into a thick, flattened vertical band at the midline, where it easily may be mistaken in a radical prostatectomy specimen for muscle of the rectal wall. This is an important distinction because carcinoma invading such a longitudinal muscle bundle may still be confined within the prostate and should not be considered to have invaded the rectum. Wherever the capsule and fascia are fused, it is the surface of the fascia rather than the capsule surface that presents a barrier to the spread of carcinoma.

Superiorly, Denonvilliers' fascia extends above the prostate to cover the posterior surface of the seminal vesicles, but it is only loosely adherent to them (Figs. 9 and 10). Laterally the fascia leaves the posterior capsule where the prostate surface begins to deviate anteriorly, and it continues in a coronal plane to anchor against the pelvic sidewalls. So the prostate and seminal vesicles are suspended along the anterior aspect of this fascial membrane as the uterus is suspended from the broad ligament in the female. This can be demonstrated in the radical prostatectomy specimen after surgery for carcinoma. If the specimen is picked up at the right and left superior margins, its posterior aspect is a smooth-surfaced triangular membrane whose apex coincides with the prostate apex and whose base is a transverse line above the seminal vesicles. Any surgical defect in the fascia potentially compromises the complete resection of the tumor because tears in the fascia tend to extend through the adherent capsule and into the gland.

Where Denonvilliers' fascia separates from the prostate capsule posterolaterally, the space between them is filled with adipose tissue in a thick layer between the anterior aspect of the fascia and the posterolateral capsular surface of the prostate. The autonomic nerves from the pelvic plexus to the seminal vesicles, prostate, and corpora cavernosa of the penis travel in this fatty layer. The nerves, along with the blood vessels to the prostate, originate from the paired neurovascular bundles that course vertically along the pelvic sidewalls just anterior to the junction of Denonvilliers' fascia with the pelvis (Fig. 9) (19). Most of the nerve branches to the prostate leave the neurovascular bundle at a single level just above the prostate base and course medially as the superior pedicle. These nerve branches fan out to penetrate the superior pedicle insertion area of the capsule, which is centered at the lateral aspect of the prostate base posteriorly (19,20). The insertion area does not usually extend far onto the rectal surface but extends toward the prostate apex as far as the midprostate. Some nerve trunks travel medially across the prostate base, sending branches into the central zone, but the majority of nerve branches fan out distally and penetrate the capsule at an oblique angle.

Most examples of capsule penetration by cancer represent tumor extension through the capsule along perineural spaces (20). Because of the oblique retrograde nerve pathway toward the prostate base, perforation though the full capsule thickness is most commonly located near or even above the superior border of the cancer within the gland. Because of the boundaries of the superior pedicle insertion area plus the additional thickness of Denonvilliers' fascia overlying the capsule posteromedially, penetration of cancer directly through the rectal surface of the prostate is uncommon.

Before supplying the corpora cavernosa, nerve branches

leave the neurovascular bundle at the prostate apex in the very small inferior pedicle and penetrate the capsule directly in a small apical insertion area located laterally and posterolaterally (20). Here the distance from neurovascular bundle to prostate capsule is narrowed to only a few millimeters. The prostate apex is the most common location for positive surgical margins at radical prostatectomy. This may result from capsule penetration along inferior pedicle nerves by cancers that are located near the apex, but it most commonly results from inadvertent surgical incision into the prostate. In this area the surgeon is most concerned to stay close to the prostate capsule in order to spare the nerves involved in erectile function (21,22).

Arterial branches follow the nerve branches from the neurovascular bundle; they spread over the prostate surface and penetrate the capsule to extend directly inward toward the distal urethral segment between the radiating duct systems of the central zone and peripheral zone (23,24). A major arterial branch enters the prostate at each side of the bladder neck and runs toward the verumontanum parallel to the course of the proximal urethral segment. It supplies the periurethral region and medial transition zone. TUR regularly obliterates this arterial branch and all the tissue supplied by it (23).

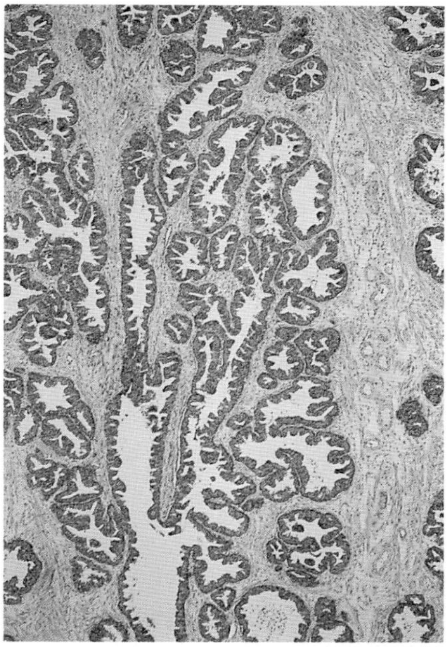

**FIG. 11.** Ducts and acini of peripheral zone, immunostained with antibody to PSA and showing uniform distribution of protein throughout cytoplasm of all ducts and acini.

## ARCHITECTURE OF THE GLANDULAR PROSTATE

The biologic role of the prostate calls for the slow accumulation and occasional rapid expulsion of small volumes of fluid. These requirements are optimally met by a muscular organ having a large storage capacity and low secretory capacity. In such an organ the functionally different specialization of ducts and acini found in organs of high secretory capacity, such as the pancreas, would appear to be of limited value. Accordingly, the prostatic ducts are morphologically identical to the acini except for their geometry, and both appear to function as distensible secretory reservoirs. Within each prostate zone, the entire duct–acinar system, except for the main ducts near the urethra, is lined by columnar secretory cells of identical appearance between ducts and acini. Immunohistochemical staining for prostate-specific antigen (PSA) and prostatic acid phosphatase (PAP) shows uniform granular staining of all ductal and acinar cells (Fig. 11). In view of these considerations, there is probably no functional duct–acinar distinction in the prostate, and it is unlikely that there is any morphologic or biologic distinction between carcinomas of ductal versus acinar origin.

The main ducts of the prostate originate at the urethra and terminate near the capsule, except for the main transition zone ducts, which terminate at the anterior fibromuscular stroma (4,7,8) (Figs. 4 and 5). Because ducts and acini within each zone have comparable caliber, spacing, and histologic appearance, ducts and acini cannot reliably be distinguished microscopically except in sections cut along the ductal long axis. Hence, abnormalities of architectural pattern are identified in routine sections mainly by deviations from normal size and spacing of glandular units.

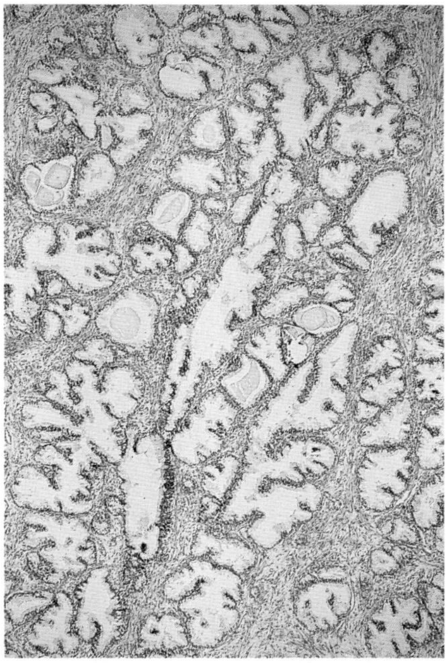

**FIG. 12.** Subsidiary duct and branches in peripheral zone terminating in small, rounded acini with undulating borders. Ducts and acini have similar calibers and histologic appearances.

The main excretory duct orifices of the peripheral zone arise from the urethral wall about every 2 mm along a double lateral line extending the full 1.5 cm length of the distal urethral segment. About every 2 mm along the course of each main excretory duct from urethra to capsule a cluster of three or four subsidiary ducts arise. They branch at angles of about 15° and extend only a short distance, rebranching and giving rise to groups of acini (Fig. 12). Hence, acini tend to be distributed with nearly uniform density along the course of the main duct between urethra and capsule, except that no acini are found immediately adjacent to the urethra. Conversely, for a few millimeters beneath the capsule all glands are acinar. The architecture in the transition zone is similar to the peripheral zone. However, there is more extensive arborization because the main ducts arise from the urethra in a small focus.

The duct origins of the transition zone and periurethral glands from the proximal urethral segment represent a proximal continuation of the double lateral line of the peripheral zone duct origins along the distal urethral segment. However, periurethral ducts also originate anteriorly and posteriorly. This accounts for the presentation of periurethral gland BPH as a dorsal midline bladder neck mass, whereas the lateral locations of transition zone BPH masses reflect the constant location of their main ducts (8).

In the peripheral zone and transition zone, ducts and acini are usually 0.15 to 0.3 mm in diameter and have simple rounded contours that are not perfectly circular because of prominent undulations of the epithelial border (5,7). The undulations mainly reflect the presence of corrugations of the wall, which presumably provide for expansion of the lumina as secretory reservoirs. An important criterion for the diagnosis of many highly differentiated prostatic carcinomas is their tendency toward precisely round or oval glandular contours (25,26), reflecting a loss of reservoir function.

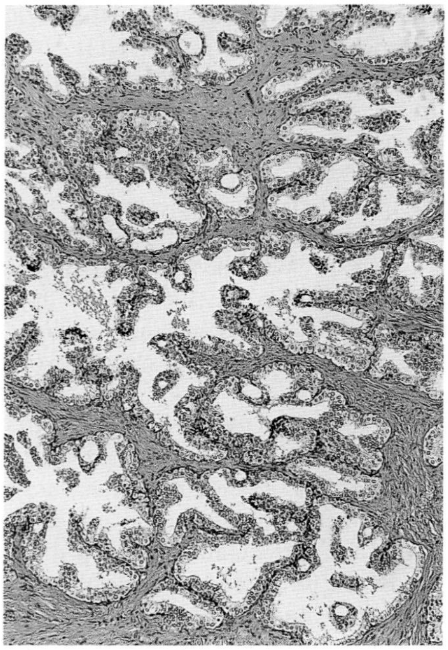

**FIG. 14.** Large central zone acini just beneath prostate base seen in transverse plane of section. Intraluminal ridges are prominent. Tiny cavities within epithelial strip are lacunae.

Central zone ducts and acini are distinctively larger than those of the peripheral zone and transition zone: up to 0.6 mm in diameter or larger (Fig. 13). Unlike the peripheral zone, both ducts and acini of the central zone become pro-

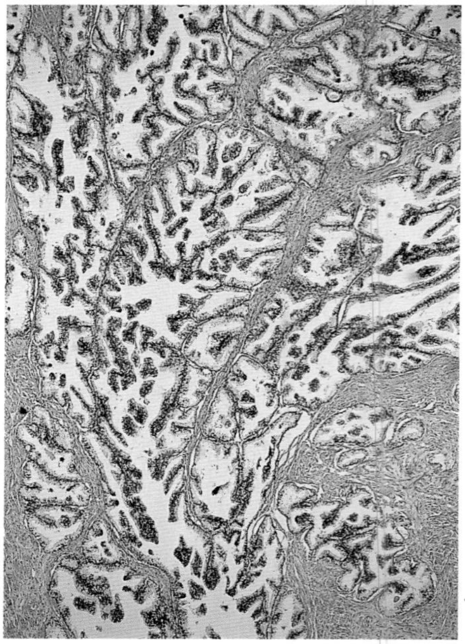

**FIG. 13.** Subsidiary ducts and acini in the central zone form a compact lobule with flattened gland borders and prominent intraluminal ridges.

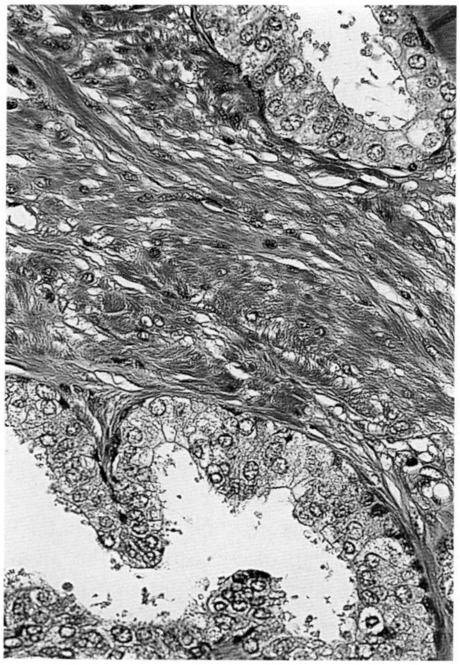

**FIG. 15.** Central zone acini at lobule border surrounded by compact muscular stroma. Secretory cells are irregularly arranged with large nuclei at different levels and granular, variably dark cytoplasm. Basal cells are visible.

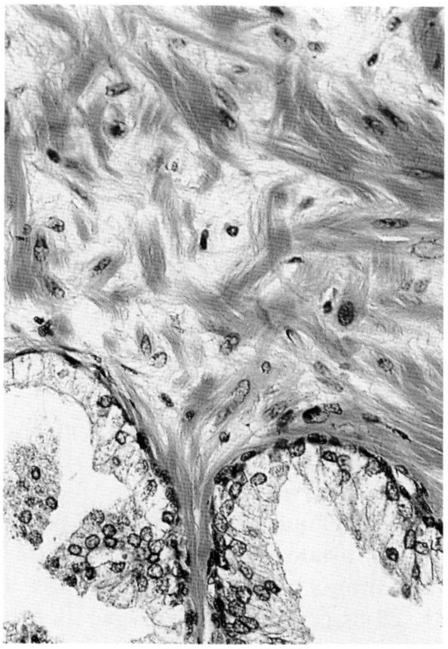

**FIG. 16.** Peripheral zone acini set in loosely woven fibromuscular stroma. Secretory cells are more regular than in central zone, with smaller basal nuclei and pale cytoplasm. Basal cells are visible.

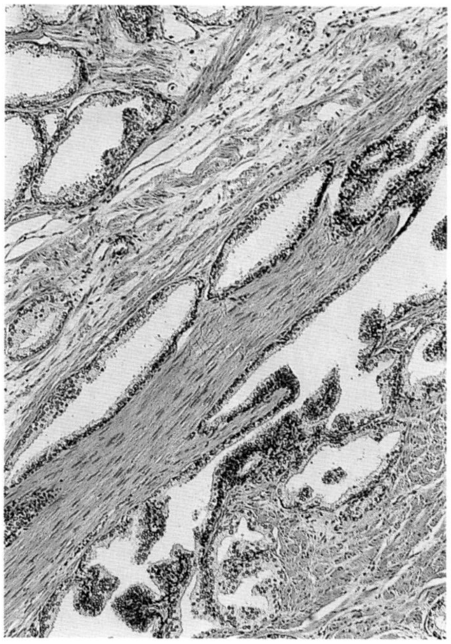

**FIG. 17.** Border between the peripheral zone (*above*) and transition zone shows contrast in stromal texture and band of smooth muscle at zone boundary. Glandular histology is similar between zones.

gressively larger toward the capsule at the prostate base (Fig. 14), where they often exceed 1 mm in diameter. There is also a gradient of increasing density of acini toward the base. Both of these gradients reflect the great expansion of central zone cross-sectional area from a small focus on the verumontanum to almost the entire prostate base. Near the urethra, the central zone ducts have few branches and lack distinctive histologic features. Hence, they may not be recognizable in transverse planes of section near the base of the verumontanum. Acini are clustered into lobules around a central subsidiary duct, which is distinguishable from the acini in cross section only by its central location. Ducts and acini are polygonal in contour. Many of the corrugations in their walls are exaggerated into distinctive intraluminal ridges with stromal cores, which partially subdivide acini (Figs. 13 and 14).

Glandular subdivisions within a given duct branch in the central zone are separated by narrow bands of distinctively compact smooth muscle fibers (Fig. 15), whereas broader bands separate different branches. The normal overall ratio of epithelium to stroma here (lumens excluded) is roughly 2. The epithelial/stromal ratio of the peripheral zone and transition zone is close to 1. In the peripheral zone, the more abundant stroma is loosely woven, with randomly arranged muscle bundles separated by indistinct spaces containing loose, finely fibrillar collagenous tissue (Fig. 16). Between the glandular spaces in a given duct branch, stroma is as abundant as between different branches.

There is an abrupt contrast in stromal morphology that delineates the boundary between central zone and peripheral zone and a similar contrast between peripheral zone and transition zone (11) (Fig. 17). The transition zone stroma is composed of compact interlacing smooth muscle bundles (Fig. 18). This stromal density contrasts sharply with the adjacent loose peripheral zone stroma, but it blends with the stromas of the preprostatic sphincter and anterior fibromus-

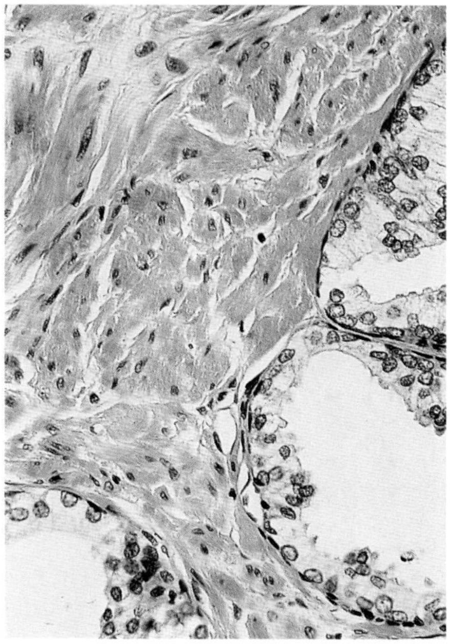

**FIG. 18.** Transition zone acini set in a compact stroma composed of interlacing, coarse, smooth muscle bundles. Acinar histology is identical to peripheral zone. Basal cells are visible.

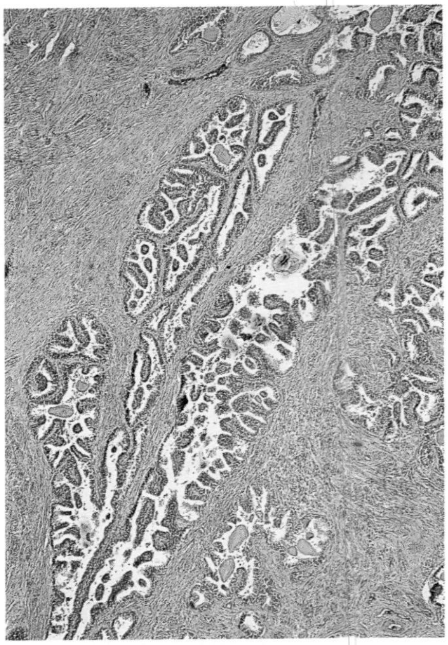

**FIG. 19.** Diffuse atrophy of aging in central zone with shrunken simplified glands and reduced luminal area.

cular stroma. Stromal distinctions are less evident in older prostates and may be obliterated by disease.

Atrophy in the prostate related to aging and presumably due to androgen withdrawal is a fairly consistent finding only in men more than 70 years of age (27,28) but even then is not universal. There is no explanation for a great range of variation in the rate of involution seen between individuals under 70 years of age, but severe debilitating disease can produce advanced atrophy even in young men (7).

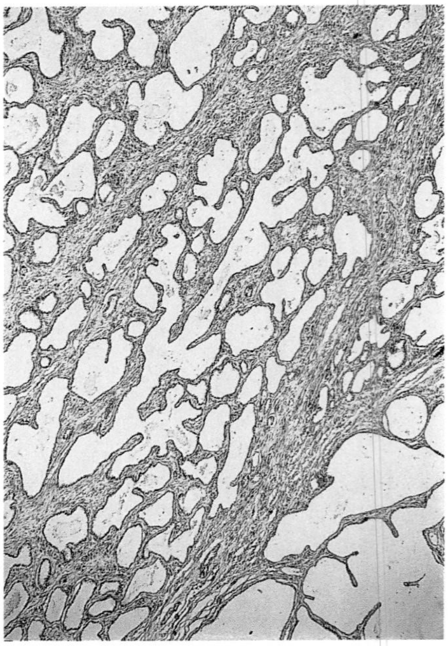

**FIG. 20.** Advanced diffuse atrophy of aging in peripheral zone with ducts and acini of normal caliber and markedly flattened epithelium. A focus of cystic atrophy is seen at lower right.

Atrophy due to aging is characteristically diffuse. In its advanced stage, reduced secretory cell volume is usually accompanied by markedly reduced or absent staining for PSA and PAP. Nuclei are small and densely staining, and cytoplasm is scant. In the central zone, architecture is dramatically altered. Intraluminal ridges are often lost, and the normally polygonal ducts and acini collapse into a stellate outline with reduced luminal area (Fig. 19). In the peripheral zone and transition zone, there is no change in architecture, or gland lumina may be somewhat enlarged (Fig. 20).

## EPITHELIAL COMPARTMENTS OF THE PROSTATE

As with other glandular organs, the secretory cells throughout the prostate are separated from the basement membrane and stroma by a layer of basal cells. These cells are markedly elongated and flattened parallel to the basement membrane and have slender, filiform dark nuclei and usually little or no discernible cytoplasm (29) (Figs. 15,16,18). They are typically quite inconspicuous, and in routine preparations the basal cell envelope may appear incomplete or even absent around individual ducts or acini. However, immunohistochemical staining for basal cell–specific keratin usually shows the envelope to be complete even where no basal cells are identified with routine stains (30). This stain is consistently negative in the cells of invasive malignant glands (31).

Basal cells are not myoepithelial cells analogous to those of the breast because by electron microscopy they do not contain muscle filaments (29). Logically, myoepithelial cells would appear to be functionally superfluous in a muscular organ (29). Basal cells have been found to be the proliferative compartment of the prostate epithelium, normally dividing and maturing into secretory cells (32–34). Using immunostaining for proliferating cell nuclear antigen as a marker for cycling cells, roughly 1% of basal cells and 0.1% of secretory cells were labeled in each zone, and there was no difference between ducts and acini. Eighty-three percent of all labeled cells were basal cells, even though they comprised only 30% of the total epithelial cell population (34).

In all zones of the prostate, the epithelium contains a small population of isolated, randomly scattered endocrine–paracrine cells (35) that are rich in serotonin-containing granules and contain neuron-specific enolase. Subpopulations of these cells also contain a variety of peptide hormones such as somatostatin, calcitonin, and bombesin. They rest on the basal cell layer between secretory cells but do not typically appear to extend to the lumen or may send a narrow apical extension to the lumen. They often have laterally spreading dendritic processes (Fig. 21). They are not reliably identifiable microscopically except with immunohistochemical and other special stains. Their specific role in prostate biology is unknown, but they presumably have paracrine function, perhaps in response to neural stimulation. Like similar cells in the lung and other organs, they occasionally

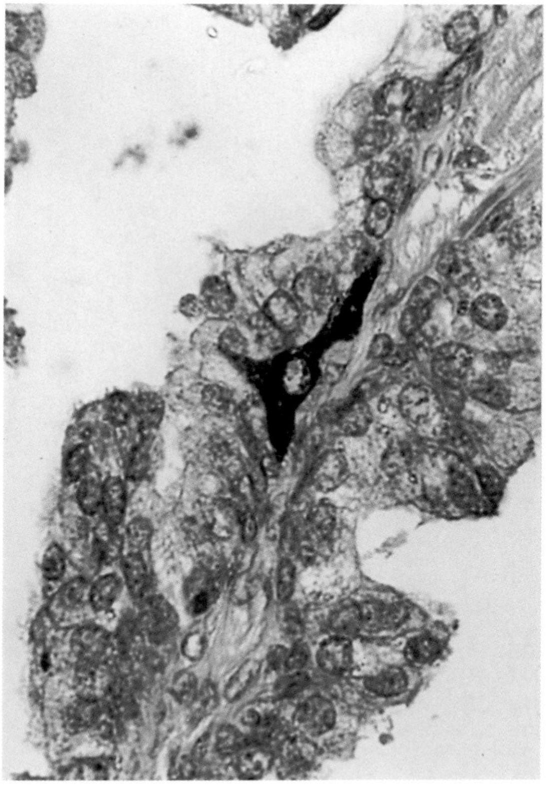

**FIG. 21.** Cytologic features of serotonin-containing cells showing the basal location between secretory cells and lateral dendritic processes, with no apparent luminal contact (immunoperoxidase stain with serotonin antibody).

give rise to small cell carcinomas, which do not contain PSA or PAP (36). Not infrequently, however, small cell carcinoma arises as a variant morphologic pattern within adenocarcinomas that elsewhere contain PSA and PAP; peptide hormones are found only in the small cell component (36). Hence, the status of these cells as an independent lineage is doubtful in the prostate.

The secretory cells of the prostate contribute a wide variety of products to the seminal plasma. PSA and PAP are produced by the secretory cells of the ducts and acini of all zones. Pepsinogen II (37) and tissue plasminogen activator (38) are normally produced only in the ducts and acini of the central zone. Lactoferrin is also exclusively a secretory product of the central zone, except in areas of inflammation where both the cells and secretions anywhere in the prostate may produce this substance (39). Lectin staining for cell membrane carbohydrates also shows significant differences between the two zones (40). It has been suggested that the central zone may be specialized for the production of enzymes whose substrates are secreted by the peripheral zone (38), but probable substrates have not been identified. In fact, no secretory product has so far been identified which is produced exclusively by the peripheral zone or transition zone.

The cytoplasm of the normal secretory cell in all zones is similar in appearance and is dominated by the universal abundance of uniform small clear secretory vacuoles. By

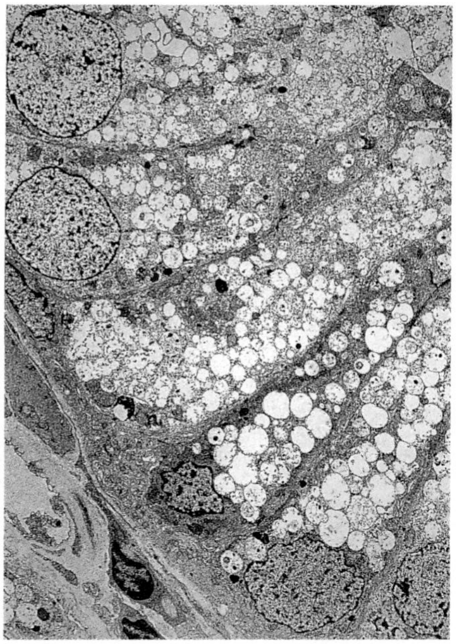

**FIG. 22.** Electron photomicrograph of normal peripheral zone, showing abundance of closely packed small, clear vacoules of roughly uniform diameter. Nuclei are often at base of cell.

electron microscopy, vacuoles in peripheral zone and transition zone cytoplasm are packed at nearly maximum density (41) (Fig. 22), whereas in the central zone a more abundant dense cytoplasm is associated with a somewhat wider spacing and lower vacuole density (Fig. 23). Because the secretory vacuoles appear empty by routine microscopy, periph-

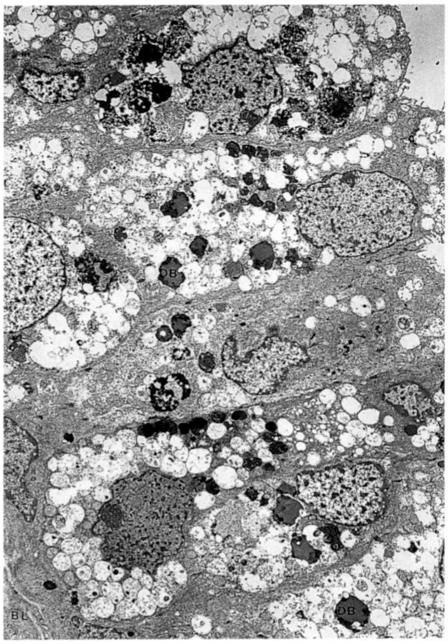

**FIG. 23.** Electron photomicrograph of central zone, showing more heterogeneous distribution of clear vacuoles with focally lower density. Epithelium appears more disordered, with nuclei at multiple levels.

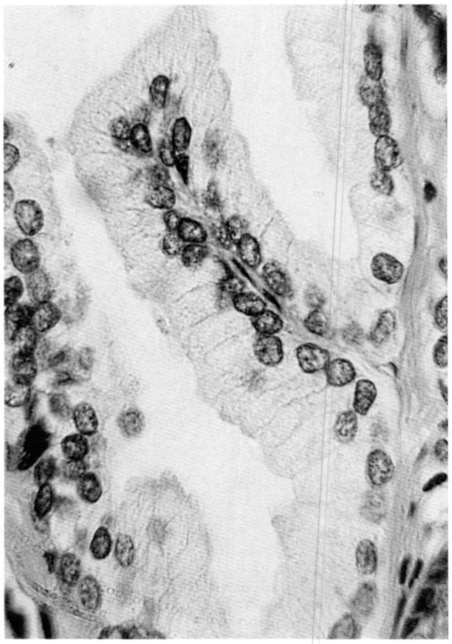

**FIG. 24.** Peripheral zone epithelium showing clear cells whose cytoplasm is barely discernable as composed of a sheet of small empty vacuoles with delicate pale partitions.

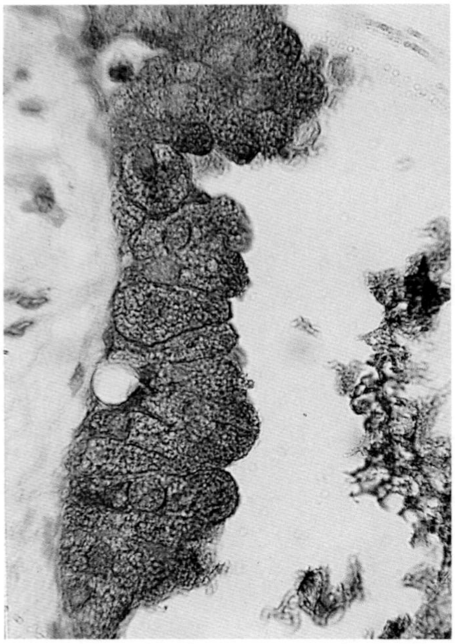

**FIG. 25.** Peripheral zone epithelium immunostained with antibody to PSA. Protein is concentrated in a reticulated pattern which spares vacuole lumens and accentuates portions of vacuole partitions.

eral zone and transition zone cells are pale to clear, and central zone cells are typically somewhat darker.

However, the appearance of normal cell cytoplasm on tissue sections is strongly influenced by staining technique and by the type of fixative used. In the peripheral zone and transition zone, light hematoxylin and eosin (H&E) staining after formalin fixation shows that normal cells are "clear cells" in which a faint network of pale-staining cytoplasmic partitions between vacuoles can be visualized with careful scrutiny under high magnification (Fig. 24). Only an occasional cell shows complete outlines that define numerous intact vacuoles, but immunostaining with PSA or PAP on the same tissue sharply outlines all the cytoplasmic vacuolar partitions and shows no evidence of protein within the vacuoles (Fig. 25). Denser H&E staining not only darkens the partitions but also produces a paler diffuse staining throughout the cytoplasm, which obscures both the clear cell appearance and the visualization of the vacuoles. Regardless of staining, ductal cells are indistinguishable from acinar cells, and central zone cells are distinctive by their somewhat darker cytoplasmic staining (Fig. 26).

The contents of the apparently empty vacuoles consist partly of lipid, as judged by interpretation of fat stains on fresh frozen sections, but there is also a nonlipid component. With H&E staining after fixation in glutaraldehyde or the commercial fixative Ultrim (American Histology Reagent Co., Stockton, CA, U.S.A.), the clear vacuoles are replaced by brightly staining red granules. The nature of the stained product is unknown, but the circumstances of its demonstration suggest that it may be a low-molecular-weight alkaline substance such as spermine. Using these alternate fixatives, immunostaining for protein such as PSA or PAP is still negative within vacuole lumens.

Vacuoles are usually reduced or absent in the cytoplasm in dysplasia (prostatic intraepithelial neoplasia) (41) (Fig. 27) and in most invasive carcinomas of Gleason grade 3 or

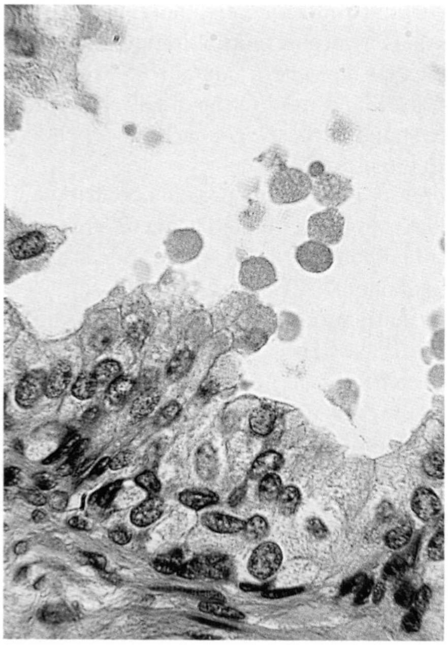

**FIG. 26.** Central zone epithelium with dark cytoplasmic staining in an area of active apocrine secretion. Clear vacuoles are absent from apocrine secretion. Nuclei appear crowded and disordered, lying at different levels.

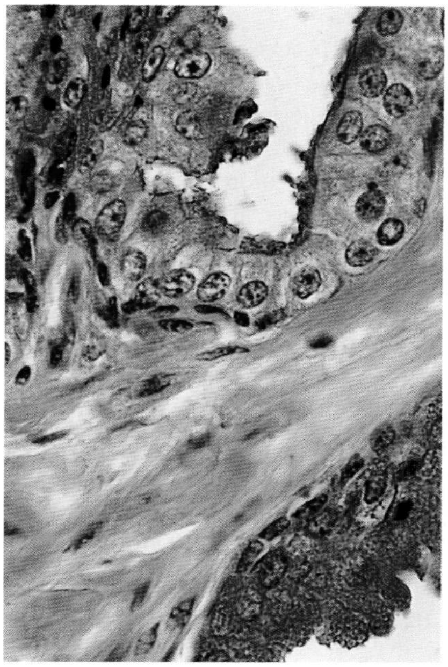

**FIG. 27.** Peripheral zone epithelium in dysplasia (prostatic intraepithelial neoplasia) at top of field, contrasted with normal epithelium (*below*) using heavy immunostaining with prostatic acid phosphatase antibody. Dysplasia cytoplasm is dark because of absent, clear vacuoles, and PAP staining is also nearly absent. Nuclei differ from normal central zone and are hyperchromatic with prominent nucleoli.

higher. In Gleason grades 1 and 2 cancer, as well as some areas in grade 3 cancer, cytoplasmic vacuoles are retained, and these tumors have been referred to as clear cell carcinomas.

The secretory lining of peripheral zone glands conveys an orderly appearance, with a single layer of columnar cells having basally oriented nuclei. But in most glands, the epithelial row shows considerable random variation between neighboring cells in the ratio of cell height-to-width and in apparent cell volume. Nuclear location also varies from the basal cell aspect to the mid-portion of the cell. The luminal cell border is consequently often uneven, and its roughness is accentuated by frequent cells whose luminal aspect is irregular and frayed (Fig. 28).

These deviations from uniformity and the resulting slightly untidy pattern of the normal epithelial strip appear intimately related to secretory function. Cytokeratin immunostaining of secretory cells shows that the cytoskeleton does not extend as far as the luminal aspect of each cell (Fig. 28); it usually terminates somewhat above the midportion of the cell level in a sharp transverse line whose level from cell to cell defines a more uniform thickness of the epithelial row than the full thickness that is stained by H&E. All of the cell contents toward the lumen from this transverse line appear to represent an isolated apocrine secretion compartment having diminished or absent cytoskeleton. As much as one third of total height of some cells may belong to this apocrine compartment. Lumenward from the terminal line of the keratin cytoskeleton, neighboring cells may lose their adhesion and are sometimes separated by a narrow cleft. The indistinct luminal aspect of some cells appears to represent disintegration of this apical portion of the cell in situ. Release of contents of apocrine secretion into the lumen by fragmentation while still attached to the cell is the characteristic mode of peripheral zone and transition zone secretions; release of intact apocrine sacs from the underlying cell is rarely seen.

The morphologic appearance of normal peripheral zone epithelium is closely mimicked by only that minority of clear cell well-differentiated carcinomas that retain abundant cytoplasmic clear vacuoles, often Gleason's grades 1 and 2 (25,26). However, these malignant cells usually differ in having a sharply defined luminal plasma membrane that lies at the same height between epithelial cells and traces an even transverse line around the gland perimeter (Fig. 29). Thus, the fragmenting apocrine compartment is usually absent, and correspondingly the cytoskeleton as visualized by keratin immunostaining fills the entire cytoplasm. Also, these malignant clear cells are of more nearly equal dimensions and contours than their benign counterparts, and nuclei are more strictly localized at the cell base. In dysplasia (Fig. 27), and in most grade 3 carcinomas, secretory vacuoles are much reduced or absent; cell cytoplasm is correspondingly dark (41).

Central zone epithelium by contrast shows an accentuation of the mild disorder of cell arrangement of the peripheral zone/transition zone (Fig. 30). Here the epithelium is variably thickened by prominent cell crowding. Nuclei,

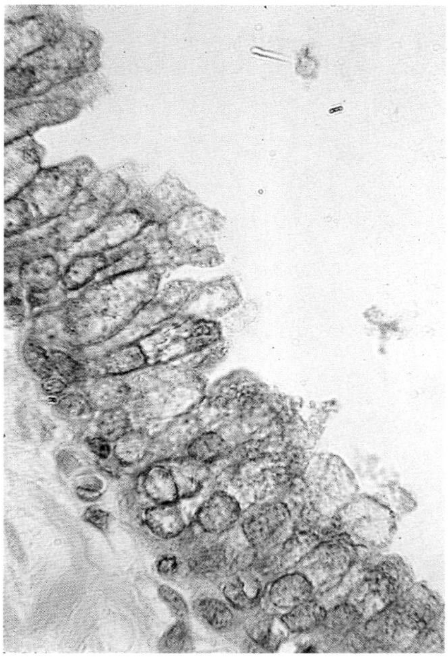

**FIG. 28.** Peripheral zone epithelium immunostained with antibody to secretory cell cytokeratin. Normal epithelial cells appear quite variable in size and shape, and some nuclei are displaced from cell base. Cytokeratin is accentuated toward luminal border, but at lower right and upper middle, clusters of cells have attached apocrine compartment lumenward, which have no cytokeratin staining and accentuate the irregularity of luminal epithelial border.

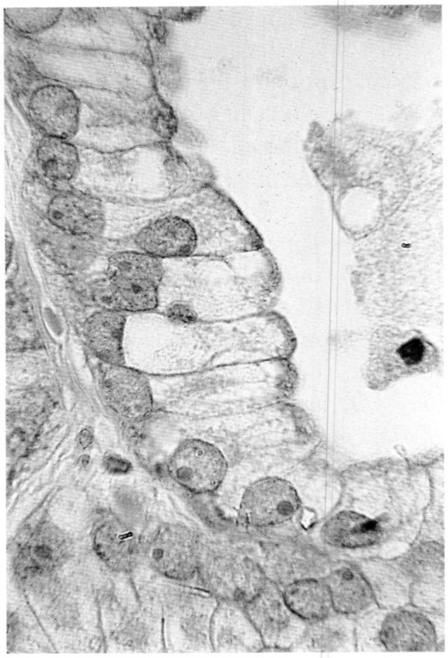

**FIG. 29.** Clear cell carcinoma immunostained with antibody to secretory cell cytokeratin shows stronger cytokeratin accentuation at a luminal epithelial border, which is more even than in Fig. 28 and lacks the apocrine secretory compartment. Cells are larger and more uniform than in Fig. 28, with more basally located nuclei.

which are usually larger than in the peripheral zone, are often displaced further from the cell base than in the peripheral zone and may give the illusion of stratification in more crowded areas. Cell height is often widely variable, and because the luminal cell border usually is intact rather than disintegrating, irregular protrusion of cell apices into the lumen is prominent. Apocrine secretion in the central zone may be identical to that in the peripheral zone, but often it is characterized by intact spherical sacs in the gland lumen containing no vacuoles and staining more densely than the parent cell. They tend to remain intact after secretion as dense luminal spheres (Fig. 26).

The dark cytoplasm, thickened variable epithelium, and complex architecture in the central zone may be misinterpreted as atypical hyperplasia or dysplasia on needle biopsies. However, the distinctive histologic features plus the absence of nuclear size variability, hyperchromosia, and loss of polarity rule against dysplasia. The central zone is not often sampled by needle biopsies because its maximum extent is mainly restricted close to the prostate base.

Unique specialized secretory structures called lacunae are also common in the central zone (39). These are tiny round lumens that appear to lie entirely within the epithelial cell layer, isolated from the main duct–acinar lumen system (Figs. 14, 30, and 31). A complete layer of flattened epithelial cells is seen to surround each lacuna, but these lacunar cells have no apparent contact with stroma. They only abut onto surrounding secretory cells. Lacunae are a specialized apparatus for lactoferrin production and storage, as demonstrated by immunohistochemical staining.

The central zone appears to represent a separate glandular organ within the prostate capsule. Aside from its unique morphologic features, its ducts arise from the urethra separately from the double lateral line of the remainder of the prostate. In addition, its ducts are in close anatomic proxim-

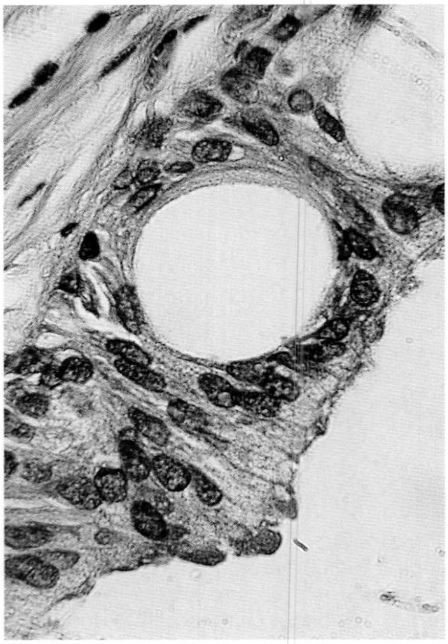

**FIG. 30.** Central zone epithelium showing increased thickness relative to peripheral zone, with darker cytoplasm and larger, stratified nuclei. Two lacunae are present.

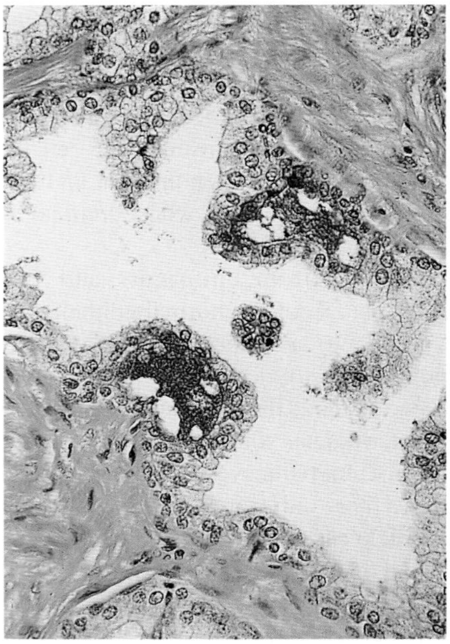

**FIG. 31.** Central zone gland immunostained with antibody to lactoferrin. Lacunae on both sides of lumen are densely stained, but cell cytoplasm is negative.

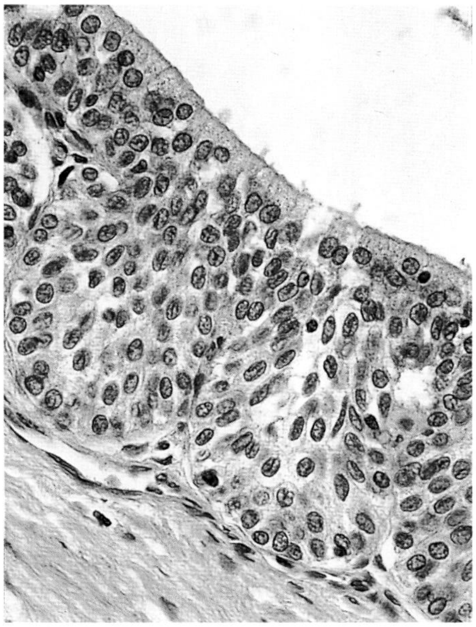

**FIG. 32.** Epithelial lining of main peripheral zone duct near urethra is identical to lining of prostatic urethra. Multilayered transitional epithelium is surmounted by a single layer of luminal secretory cells.

ity to the ejaculatory ducts and seminal vesicles. It has been suggested that the central zone may arise embryonically as an intrusion of wolffian duct stroma around the ejaculatory ducts into an organ that is otherwise of urogenital sinus origin (7). Pepsinogen II (37) and lactoferrin (39) are secreted by both central zone and seminal vesicle but are not found under normal conditions in peripheral zone or transition zone.

The transitional epithelium, which lines the prostatic urethra and extends for a variable distance into the main prostatic ducts, differs histologically from that which lines the bladder and is also distinguishable from the lining of the female urethra (1). The transitional epithelial cells of the prostatic urethra and main ducts have scant cytoplasm with no evidence of maturation toward luminal umbrella cells. Instead, the luminal surface is lined by a single layer of columnar secretory cells that resemble the secretory epithelium of the peripheral zone (Fig. 32) and are positive with immunohistochemical stains for PSA and PAP. The extent of transitional epithelium lining the normal main prostatic ducts in proximity to the urethra is extremely variable; in occasional prostates it is nearly absent.

## DEVIATIONS FROM NORMAL HISTOLOGY

Beyond the age of 30 years, many prostates begin to show a variety of focal deviations from normal morphology (4,7,27,28). Their prevalence, extent, and severity progressively increase with age so that most prostates by the seventh decade of life are quite heterogeneous in histologic composition. Although these deviant histologic patterns seldom have clinical significance, their distinction from adenocarcinoma or BPH is sometimes difficult.

Early morphologic studies concluded that focal atrophy in the prostate was a manifestation of aging and was seen as early as 40 years of age. In fact, focal atrophy in the prostate is almost always the consequence of previous inflammation rather than aging (4,7,28). The number and extent of atrophic foci tend to be greater in older men, but their histologic appearance is identical to that of isolated foci found as early as 30 years of age. The histologic features are identical to those produced by chronic bacterial prostatitis, but no etiologic agent has been identified in the vast majority of cases, most of which appear to be asymptomatic.

Postinflammatory atrophy is an extremely common lesion and is mainly a disease of the peripheral zone, where its distribution is sharply segmental along the ramifications of a duct branch (4,7). It is characterized by a marked shrinkage of ducts and acini with periglandular fibrosis and variable distortion of architecture (Figs. 33 and 34). Glandular units may be drawn together into clusters or spread out into a pattern suggesting invasive carcinoma. In addition to the presence of tiny distorted glands, the resemblance to cancer is further increased by the fact that nuclei may remain relatively large with occasional small nucleoli.

In contrast to carcinoma, cell cytoplasm is usually much reduced in volume, and evidence of the original duct–acinar architecture often can be detected. Furthermore, there is usually residual inflammation, with scattered round cells in the adjacent stroma. Finally, there is sometimes an admixture of glands showing the earlier active phase of the process, with

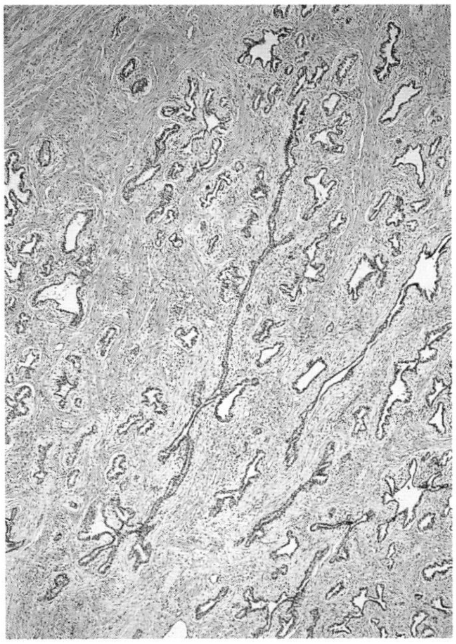

**FIG. 33.** Focus of postinflammatory atrophy in peripheral zone. Duct–acinar architecture is apparent but distorted by marked gland shrinkage, with reduced luminal area and perigland fibrosis.

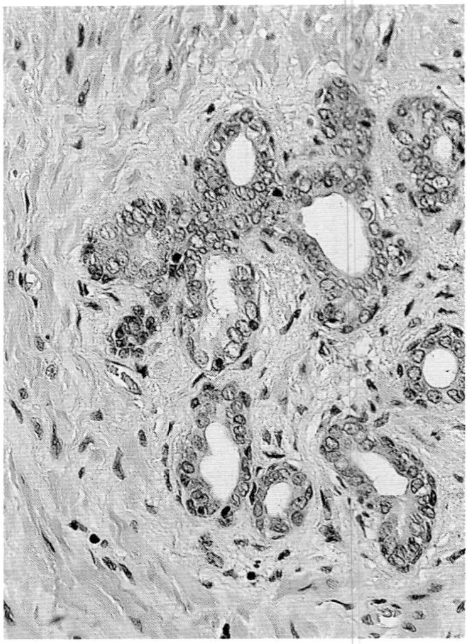

**FIG. 34.** Tiny distorted glands of postinflammatory atrophy. Irregular contour and large nuclei mimic carcinoma, but cytoplasm is scant, and there are periglandular collagenous rings.

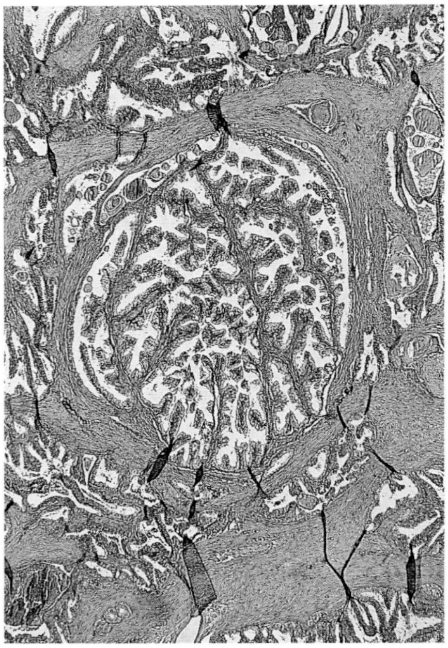

**FIG. 36.** Small BPH nodule with increase of epithelial/stromal ratio to roughly 2 and surrounded by normal transition zone with epithelial/stromal ratio far below 1.

prominent periductal and periacinar chronic inflammatory infiltrate and less prominent gland shrinkage.

Cystic atrophy is another common focal lesion that is typically found in the peripheral zone and is segmental in distri-

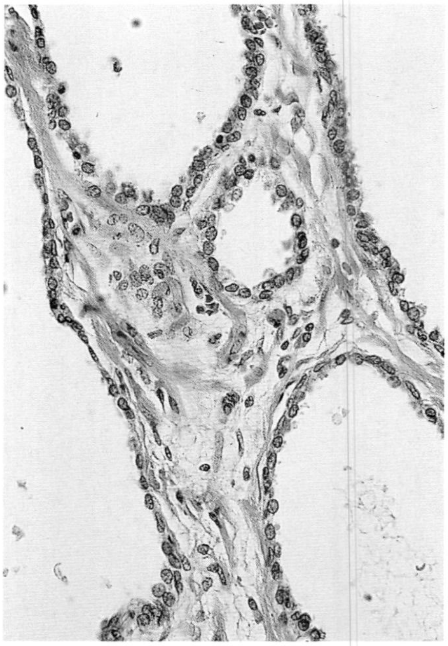

**FIG. 35.** Cystic atrophy in peripheral zone. Enlarged glands have flattened epithelium but are not spherical, suggesting nearly normal luminal pressure. Stroma shows prominent reduction in smooth muscle concentration.

bution. The markedly enlarged acini with flattened epithelium and the segmental distribution suggest an obstructive cause (Fig. 35). However, obstruction is not typically demonstrable, and the stroma between glands is usually attenuated rather than compressed by luminal expansion. This suggests that stromal atrophy may be the main pathogenetic event.

The histologic hallmark of BPH is the expansile nodule, produced by the budding and branching of newly formed duct–acinar structures (Fig. 36), by the focal proliferation of stroma, or by a combination of both elements (4,5,8,42). It mainly affects the transition zone, with occasional contribution from the puriurethral region. Individual BPH nodules rarely become larger than 1.6 cm in greatest diameter, and in any prostate median nodule diameter is almost always less than 8 mm. An exception is produced in massive BPH by secondary nodule enlargement due to cystic dilatation of component glands.

Grossly BPH is usually recognized as a globular mass replacing each transition zone and composed of numerous individual nodules embedded within a diffusely hyperplastic transition zone tissue (Fig. 36). Only the nodular component is recognizable histologically as a deviation from normal pattern; internodular tissue, even when increased in amount, is not distinguishable microscopically from normal transition zone.

The enlargement of transition zone BPH produces a characteristic progressive deformity of overall prostate contour (Fig. 37). The tissue lateral and posterior to the prostatic urethra (central zone and peripheral zone) is relatively unyield-

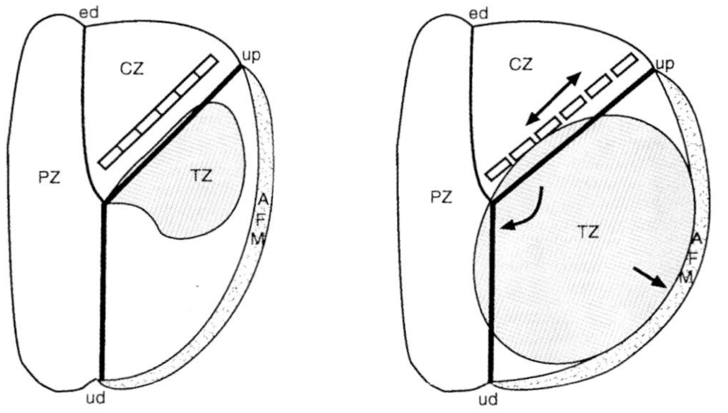


**FIG. 37.** Sagittal diagrams of prostate showing main features of deformity produced by transition zone BPH. Transition zone is bounded by distal urethral segment, proximal urethral segment, and anterior fibromuscular stroma (see Fig. 3). Only the last leg of this triangular compartment yields easily to the pressure of transition zone expansion. Increased angulation and lengthening of urethra produce a more spherical compartment with increased capacity. Arrows indicate main features of deformity.

ing, and expansion is directed anteriorly and toward the apex at the selective expense of stretching and thinning of the anterior fibromuscular stroma. This produces a predominant increase in the thickness (anteroposterior dimension) of the gland. The anterolateral wings of the peripheral zone where they taper to join the anterior fibromuscular stroma (Fig. 5) are compressed and thinned concomitant with increase of overall prostate width. But posterior and lateral peripheral zones are not significantly thinned except in massive BPH.

The central zone is the least compressed region, but it is pulled forward over the BPH mass, accompanied by characteristic lengthening of the proximal urethral segment. As the urethra lengthens, its angulation at the midpoint increases, sometimes approaching 90° (Fig. 38). Increased angulation produces a more globular anteroapical compartment, which accommodates a larger BPH mass. The mucosa of the lateral urethral walls is compressed between the two opposed transition zone masses, and its surface area is stretched to a larger expanse as the transition zone masses expand.

Basal cell hyperplasia is most often seen as a secondary change in BPH nodules or inflammatory foci (33). The basal cells of ducts and acini become rounded with oval nuclei, and they form a multilayered lining that stains for basal cell–specific cytokeration (Fig. 39). There is typically a single luminal row of columnar secretory cells that stain positive for PSA.

In BPH, basal cell hyperplasia is common at the margin of nodule infarcts, where it presumably represents a reaction to ischemia. Consistent with this proposal is the finding of smooth muscle atrophy and replacement by fibroblastic stroma in these areas. Much more commonly, basal cell hyperplasia is found in BPH nodules without frank infarction (Fig. 40), but the almost invariable presence of fibroblastic stroma and smooth muscle atrophy suggest that ischemia may be etiologic here also. Gland shrinkage also usually accompanies these foci (Fig. 41) and may suggest a superficial resemblance to carcinoma.

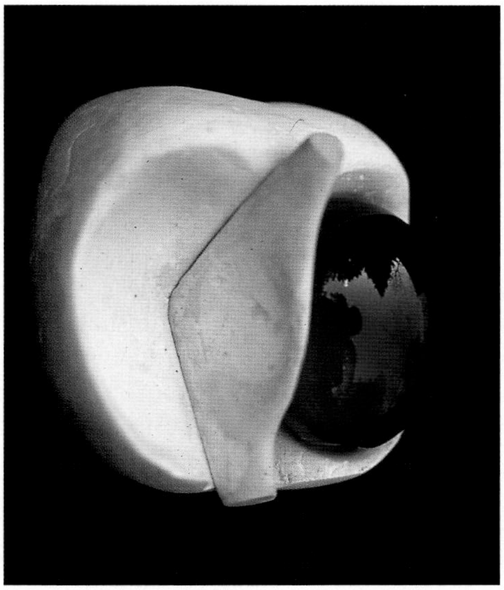

**FIG. 38.** Model of prostate with severe BPH seen in 3/4 frontal view. Transition zone mass on far side (blue) shows growth mainly anterior and toward apex. BPH mass has been removed on near side showing concavity in peripheral zone caused mainly by stretching and thinning of anterolateral margin. Urethra shows prominent increased angulation, with anterior stretching of lateral walls between BPH masses.

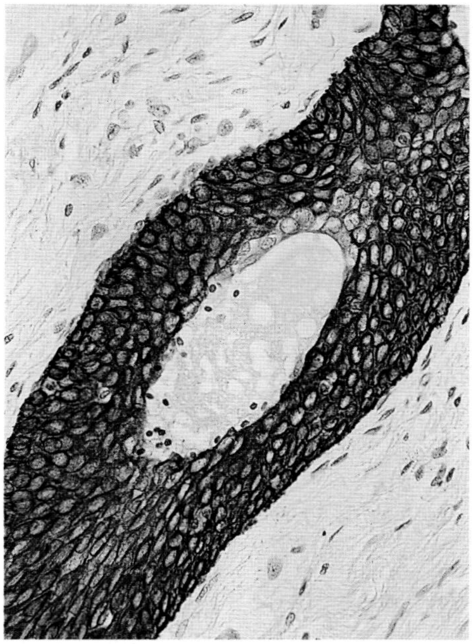

**FIG. 39.** Prostatic duct with basal cell hyperplasia immunostained with antibody to basal cell–specific cytokeratin. Basal cells create multiple layers, but single luminal layer is secretory and remains unstained.

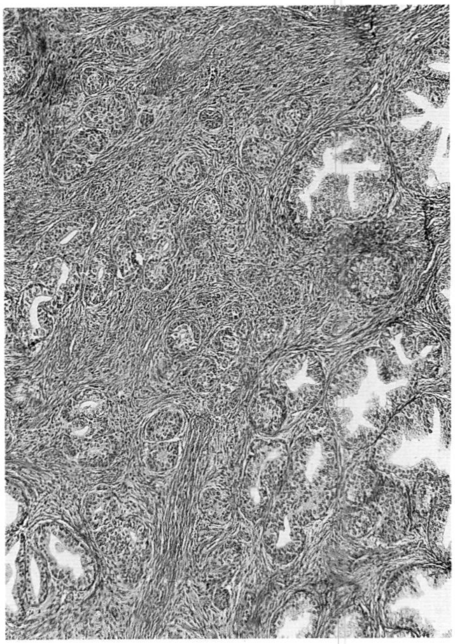

**FIG. 40.** Basal cell hyperplasia focus within a BPH nodule. Affected glands are reduced in size with indistinct lumina, and there is replacement of muscular stroma by cellular collagen (trichrome stain).

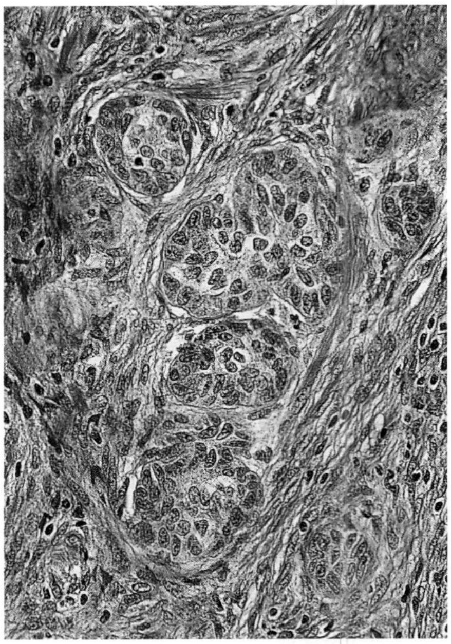

**FIG. 41.** Basal cell hyperplasia, as in Fig. 40. Tiny glands suggest carcinoma, but there are two distinct cell populations with central secretory cells even where no lumen is seen. Cellular fibrous stroma is oriented concentrically around glands (trichrome stain).

## EVALUATION OF RADICAL PROSTATECTOMY SPECIMENS

Normal morphologic features can be difficult to evaluate in the age group in which radical prostatectomy is usually performed. Landmarks are often obscured or distorted by retrogressive changes with aging or inflammation, whereas some prostates retain the normal appearance of the third decade of life, and some show increased glandular epithelial activity with or without atypia. Not infrequently, the morphologic appearance of any zone seems unrelated to the changes in other zones. Difficulties of interpretation are compounded when all sections are cut in the same plane rather than different planes designed for optimum visualization of each zone.

Transverse planes of section, perpendicular to the rectal surface are the most common type of routine prostate sectioning, partly because they are the easiest to cut. They are also nearly parallel to the plane of many ultrasound and magnetic resonance images. They show much the same relationships as the oblique coronal planes except that the urethra is never seen along its long axis. It is important to review the expected appearance of transverse planes at different levels because of the considerable differences encountered.

Transverse sections distal to the base of the verumontanum demonstrate the transition zone at most levels of section toward the apex in most men over 50 years of age, even when there are few nodules to signify BPH (8,42). Diffuse transition zone enlargement accompanying nodule development is nearly universal with age, and expansion is mainly anterior and toward the apex. The boundary between the transition zone and peripheral zone is often visualized more clearly by ultrasound imaging than by histologic study. Microscopically the difference in texture of the stroma between the two zones is the most important evidence for the location of the boundary between them, but it may not be apparent at all points. Often there is a band of compact smooth muscle fibers aligned along the boundary and paralleled by the course of a major duct or duct branch (Fig. 17). Recognition of a combination of features may be needed to accurately localize the boundary, and often these features are better appreciated with the hand lens than the microscope. If properly localized, the boundary usually approximates the same size and location on both sides of the prostate and at several levels. In normal prostates of men under 50 years of age the transition zone may be easily recognized on only a single section near the level of the base of the verumontanum.

The boundary of the transition zone with the peripheral zone seldom extends closer than 1.0 cm to the posterior (rectal) prostate surface. If there has been a previous TUR, the resection cavity usually extends mainly anteriorly from the posterior urethral wall. Significantly, the TUR often spares the lateral portion of the transition zone, sometimes with residual nodules, and the transition zone boundary remains intact.

Proximal to the base of the verumontanum, only one or two sections still show a transition zone unless there is a large mass of BPH tissue. The ejaculatory ducts now appear on these proximal sections, with the utricle between them. The dorsal, compact transverse portion of the preprostatic sphincter may be seen just anterior to the ejaculatory ducts. The sphincter and urethral lumen progress more anteriorly at each level of section cephalad until they reach the anterior tissue border at the bladder neck.

The bladder neck lies a variable number of sections below (apical to) the highest transverse section cut at the prostate base (Fig. 42). The central zone may not be apparent histologically until the bladder neck level of section or higher. It usually appears suddenly between two levels of section separated by only 3 mm. This is because the central zone is an inverted flared cone whose apical region near the verumontanum consists predominantly of main duct branches that cannot be readily distinguished from those of other zones. At the transverse level where it is first recognizable, the anterior portion of the central zone may lie directly above the area occupied by the transition zone in the section just one level below, and the transition zone is usually no longer visible. The central zone has a more distinctive histologic appearance in sections toward the base because of the rather abrupt increase in size and number of branches (Fig. 42). The most basal section is usually almost entirely composed of central zone and consists mostly of acini that are distinctively large, polygonal, and closely packed (14).

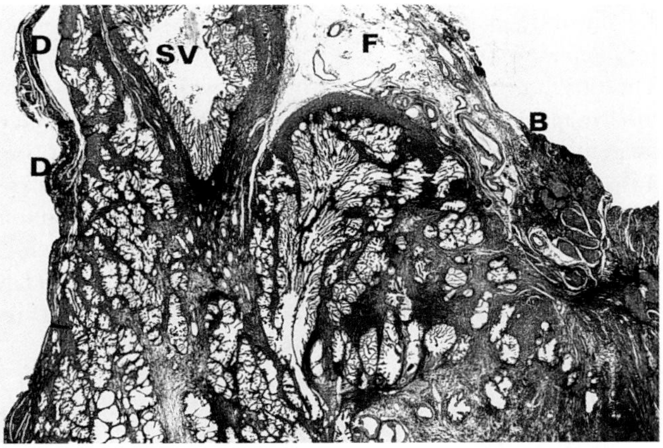


**FIG. 42.** Parasagittal section of prostate base located almost at mid-line. Bladder neck smooth muscle above the level of bladder neck lumen is seen as small dark patch (B) at far right. At top center a layer of fat (F) covers the dome-shaped surface of the anterior central zone. The seminal vesicle (SV) enters the prostate, splitting the central zone. All glandular tissue within is central zone. At center, one main duct is seen in profile as it flares out toward base, generating elaborate acinar structures. Behind seminal vesicle, posterior central zone extends more cephalad as a narrow plate. Denonvilliers' fascia (D) is not adherent behind seminal vesicles but blends with capsule below.

As the seminal vesicles leave the prostate base, they extend laterally along its surface (Fig. 9). Often there is no capsule between the two organs, at least for the medial centimeter or more of the seminal vesicle. The degree of fusion between the two muscular walls is variable between prostates, but there is frequently no boundary whatever between the two organs medially, and only one millimeter of common muscular wall may separate the most basal central zone gland lumen from the seminal vesicle lumen.

The origin of the ejaculatory ducts at the junction of seminal vesicles and vas deferens is surrounded by central zone glandular tissue and usually situated so that about two thirds of the central zone mass is anterior to the ejaculatory ducts. However, it is quite common for the ejaculatory ducts to be situated more posteriorly; occasionally they enter the prostate on the rectal surface and entirely posterior to the central zone.

The most basal transverse section of prostate usually has some bladder neck muscular wall at its anterior extent (Fig. 42). Behind this muscle is a strip of fat that lies between the seminal vesicles and the bladder and rests on top of the most anterior aspect of the central zone. That portion of the central zone anterior to the ejaculatory ducts usually terminates at a lower level than the posterior portion, and the latter extends further cephalad as a thin plate between seminal vesicles and Denonvilliers' fascia (Fig. 42). The strip of fat contains the large nerve trunks extending medially from the autonomic ganglia of the superior pedicle, which is situated lateral to the central zone at this level. When cancer penetrates the capsule at the prostate base, it is often seen within the fatty strip between bladder neck and central zone. Less often it is associated with the nerves and ganglia of the superior pedicle lateral to the gland. Occasionally cancer extends above the prostate base posteriorly within the layers of Denonvillier's fascia. In large cancers, these three routes of extension—anteriorly, laterally, and posteriorly—often fuse with cancer in the seminal vesicle to produce a confluent mass of tumor above the prostate base.

At the apex of the prostate, sections should be taken as serial parasagittal subsections of a 6-mm thick block (Fig. 43). This procedural modification sacrifices the transverse sectioning of the last level, which would lie 3 mm above the apex. However, it creates the advantage of showing the apical prostate tissue in planes that are more nearly perpendicular to the apical capsule surfaces, so that penetration of cancer can be more easily evaluated. In this area where positive surgical margins are relatively common, and capsule layers may be indistinct, such an advantage is important. Anterior to the urethra and for a narrow span anterolaterally, there is no capsule but only the distal end of the anterior fibromuscular stroma. Here there is a variable admixture of glands, striated muscle and smooth muscle, and evaluation of capsule penetration is difficult. However, this is an area where adequate surgical resection is particularly difficult, and a positive margin may occasionally be created by transection

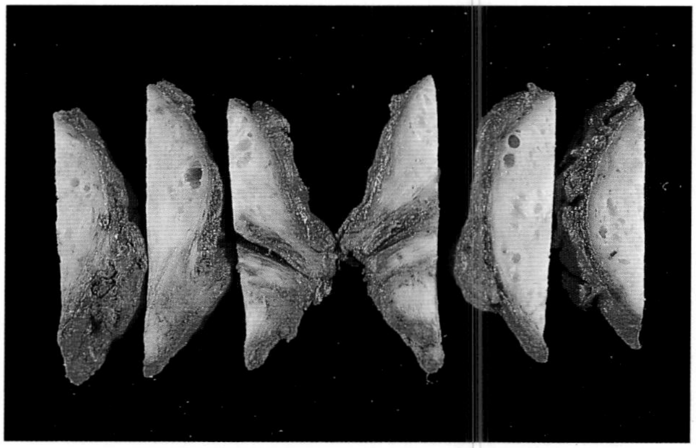

**FIG. 43.** Apex of prostate seen grossly after 6-mm thick apical block has been subsectioned parasagittally at 3-mm intervals. Orientation of sections and localization of lesions are easily demonstrated, and cuts through capsule are nearly perpendicular to apical surface.

of a small anterior cancer that was incidental, whereas the clinically detected cancer was elsewhere and has been successfully removed.

## CONSIDERATIONS IN TRANSURETHRAL RESECTION AND NEEDLE BIOPSY SPECIMENS

Tissue distortion by heat coagulation near the edges of TUR chips can create important diagnostic problems that occasionally may be insurmountable. Basal cell hyperplasia, adenomatous hyperplasia, inflammatory atrophy, and fragments of BPH nodules with small glands may be indistinguishable from carcinoma. Loss of nuclear detail occurs to a greater depth into the chip than obvious cell distortion. Hence, small foci of cancer may be more difficult to diagnose because of the artifactual absence of nucleoli. Gleason has indicated that the identification of occasional nucleoli larger than 1 $\mu$m in diameter is an important criterion for distinguishing well-differentiated cancer from adenosis (26).

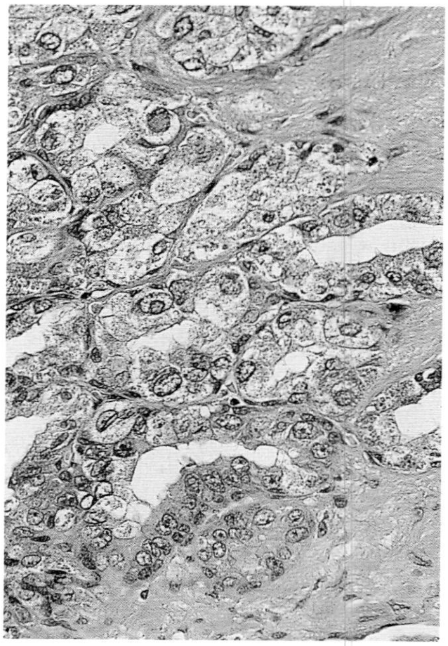

**FIG. 44.** Benign tubular envaginations from the wall of the intraprostatic seminal vesicle showing architectural and cytologic features that suggest carcinoma. Note the characteristic yellow–brown cytoplasmic granules.

The same problems are seen in needle biopsies, where the artifact is presumably due to compression rather than heat. The presence of artifact is usually limited to loss of nuclear detail and is more subtle because areas of severe tissue distortion are not often represented.

The regions of the prostate sampled by TUR and by needle biopsy tend to be quite different. Most needle biopsies represent peripheral zone tissue. Unless a special effort is made, the needle seldom reaches the central zone or the more anterior portions of the transition zone.

In the majority of cases, TUR specimens consist of transition zone tissue, urethral and periurethral tissues, bladder neck fragments, and anterior fibromuscular stroma (42). The preprostatic sphincter is always present but usually not identifiable. Occasionally, fragments of the proximal end of the striated sphincter are present. Our study of radical prostatectomy specimens post-TUR has shown that the resection usually does not extend beyond the transition zone boundary into the central or peripheral zones and usually not all the transition zone tissue has been removed (42).

Occasionally, peripheral zone or central zone tissue may be sampled at TUR. Central zone fragments show distinctive architectural and cytologic features described above. They are not infrequently accompanied by fragments of ejaculatory duct, intraprostatic vas deferens, and/or seminal vesicle. The tiny tubular outgrowths from the walls of these structures may be misinterpreted as adenocarcinoma when seen in tangential sections that do not reveal the main lumen (Fig. 44). This impression may be further encouraged by the frequent presence of enlarged dark nuclei of bizarre contour. The presence of golden brown cytoplasmic granules, which may be few and inconspicuous, helps to establish the true diagnosis. Uniform negative staining for PSA and PAP are confirmatory.

## REFERENCES


1. McNeal JE. Developmental and comparative anatomy of the prostate. In: Grayhack J, Wilson J, Scherbenske M, eds. *Benign prostatic hyperplasia.* DHEW publication no. (NIH)76-1113. Washington, DC: Department of Health, Education and Welfare; 1976:1–10.
2. Cunha GR, Donjacour AA. Mesenchymal–epithelial interactions in the growth development of the prostate. In: Leportt, Ratcliff TL, eds. *Urologic Oncology.* Boston: Kluwer Academic; 1989:159–175.
3. Timms BG, Mohs TV, Didioh JA. Ductal budding and branching patterns in the developing prostate. *J Urol* 1994;151:1427–1432.
4. McNeal JE, Stamey TA, Hodge KK. The prostate gland: morphology, pathology, ultrasound anatomy. *Monogr Urol* 1988;9:36–54.
5. McNeal JE. Anatomy of the prostate and morphogenesis of BPH. *Prog Clin Biol Res* 1984;145:27–53.

6. McNeal JE. The prostate and prostatic urethra: a morphologic synthesis. *J Urol* 1972;107:1008–1016.
7. McNeal JE. Regional morphology and pathology of the prostate. *Am J Clin Pathol* 1968;49:347–357.
8. McNeal JE. Origin and evolution of benign prostatic enlargement. *Invest Urol* 1978;15:340–345.
9. McNeal JE. Origin and development of carcinoma in the prostate. *Cancer* 1969;23:24–34.
10. McNeal JE, Price H, Redwine EA, Freiha FS, Stamey TA. Stage A versus stage B adenocarcinoma of the prostate: morphologic comparison and biologic significance. *J Urol* 1988;139:61–65.
11. McNeal JE, Redwine EA, Freiha FS, Stamey TA. Zonal distribution of prostatic adenocarcinoma: correlation with histologic patterns and direction spread. *Am J Surg Pathol* 1988;12:897–906.
12. Villers A, Steg A, Boccon–Gibod L. Anatomy of the prostate: review of different models. *Eur Urol* 1991;20:261–268.
13. Blacklock NJ. Anatomical factors in prostatitis. *Br J Urol* 1947;46:47–54.
14. Myers RP, Goellner JR, Cahill DR. Prostate shape, external striated urethral sphincter and radical prostatectomy: the apical dissection. *J Urol* 1987;138:543–550.
15. Ayala AG, Rae YR, Babaian R, Troncoso P, Grignon DJ. The prostatic capsule: does it exist?: its importance in the staging and treatment of prostatic carcinoma. *Am J Surg Pathol* 1989;13:21–27.
16. McNeal JE, Villers A, Redwine EA, Freiha FS, Stamey TA. Capsular penetration in prostate cancer: significance for natural history and treatment. *Am J Surg Pathol* 1990;14:240–247.
17. McNeal JE, Bostwick DG, Kindrachuk RA, Redwine EA, Freiha FS, Stamey TA. Patterns of progression in prostate cancer. *Lancet* 1986;1:60–63.
18. Villers A, McNeal EA, Freiha FS, Boccon-Cibod L, Stamey TA. Invasion of Denonvilliers' fascia in radical prostatectomy specimens. *J Urol* 1993;149:793–798.
19. Lepor H, Gregerman M, Crosby R, Mostofi FK, Walsh PC. Precise localization of the autonomic nerves from the pelvic plexus to the corpora cavernosa: a detailed anatomical study of the adult male prostate. *J Urol* 1985;133:207–212.
20. Villers A, McNeal JE, Redwine EA, Freiha FS, Stamey TA. The role of perineural space invasion in the local spread of prostatic adenocarcinoma. *J Urol* 1989;142:763–768.
21. Catalona WJ, Dresner SM. Nerve-sparing radical prostatectomy: extraprostatic tumor extension and preservation of erectile function. *J Urol* 1985;134:1149–1151.
22. Eggleston JC, Walsh PC. Radical prostatectomy with preservation of sexual function: pathologic findings in the first 100 cases. *J Urol* 1985;134:1146–1148.
23. Flocks RH. Arterial distribution within the prostate gland: its role in transurethral prostatic resection. In: Nesbit RM, ed. *Transurethral prostatectomy.* Springfield, IL: Charles C. Thomas; 1943:3–11.
24. Clegg EV. The vascular arrangements within the human prostate gland. *Br J Urol* 1956;28:428–435.
25. Gleason DF. Histologic grading and staging of prostatic carcinoma. In: Tannenbaum M, ed. *Urologic pathology: the prostate.* Philadelphia: Lea & Febiger; 1977:171–197.
26. Gleason DF. Atypical hyperplasia, benign hyperplasia and well differentiated adenocarcinoma of the prostate. *Am J Surg Pathol* 1985;9(suppl):53–67.
27. McNeal JE. Age-related changes in the prostatic epithelium associated with carcinoma. In: Griffiths K, Pierrepoint CG, eds. *Some aspects of the aetiology and biochemistry of prostatic cancer.* Cardiff, Wales: Tenovus; 1970:23–32.
28. McNeal JE. Aging and the prostate. In: Brocklehurst JC, ed. *Urology in the elderly.* Edinburgh: Churchill Livingstone; 1984:193–202.
29. Mao P, Angrist A. The fine structure of the basal cell of the human prostate. *Lab Invest* 1966;15:1768–1782.
30. Brawer MK, Peehl DM, Stamey TA, Bostwick DG. Keratin immunoreactivity in the benign and neoplastic human prostate. *Cancer Res* 1985;45:3663–3667.
31. Bostwick DG, Brawer MK. Prostatic intra-epithelial neoplasia and early invasion in prostate cancer. *Cancer* 1987;59:788–794.
32. Dermer GB. Basal cell proliferation in benign prostatic hyperplasia. *Cancer* 1978;41:1857–1862.
33. Cleary KR, Choi HY, Ayala AG. Basal cell hyperplasia of the prostate. *Am J Clin Pathol* 1983;80:850–854.
34. McNeal JE, Haillot O, Yemoto C. Cell proliferation in dysplasia of the prostate: analysis by PCNA immunostaining. *Prostate* 1995;27:258–268.
35. diSant' Agnese A. Neuroendocrine differentiation in prostatic carcinoma. *Cancer* 1995;75:1850–1859.
36. Ro JY, Tetu B, Ayala AG, Ordonez NG. Small cell carcinoma of the prostate: II. Immunohistochemical and electron microscopic studies of 18 cases. *Cancer* 1987;59:977–982.
37. Reese JH, McNeal JE, Redwine EA, Samloff IM, Stamey TA. Differential distribution of pepsinogen II between the zones of the human prostate and the seminal vesicle. *J Urol* 1986;136:1148–1152.
38. Reese JH, McNeal JE, Redwine EA, Stamey TA, Freiha FS. Tissue type plasminogen activator as a marker for functional zones within the human prostate gland. *Prostate* 1988;12:47–53.
39. Reese JH, McNeal JE, Goldenberg L, Redwine EA, Sellers RG. Distribution of lacteroferrin in the normal and inflamed human prostate: an immunohistochemical study. *Prostate* 1992;20:73–85.
40. McNeal JE, Leav I, Alroy J, Skutelsky E. Differential lectin staining of central and peripheral zones of the prostate and alterations in dysplasia. *Am J Clin Pathol* 1988;89:41–48.
41. de Vries CR, McNeal JE, Pensch K. The prostatic epithelial cell in dysplasia: an ultrastructural perspective. *Prostate* 1992;21:209–221.
42. Price H, McNeal JE, Stamey TA. Evolving patterns of tissue composition in benign prostatic hyperplasia as a function of specimen size. *Hum Pathol* 1990;578–585.

*Histology for Pathologists, second edition,*
Edited by Stephen S. Sternberg.
Lippincott-Raven Publishers, Philadelphia


# CHAPTER 43

# Testis and Excretory Duct System

Thomas D. Trainer



The adult testes are paired organs that lie within the scrotum suspended by the spermatic cord (Fig. 1). The average weight of each is 15 to 19 g, the right usually being 10% heavier than the left (1). The scrotal covering layers are skin, dartos muscle and Colles' fascia, an external spermatic fascia, and the parietal layer of the tunica vaginalis (Fig. 2). The dartos muscle, of the nonstriated type, is closely attached to the overlying skin but glides freely over the underlying loose fascial layer.

## SUPPORTING STRUCTURES

The supporting structures of the testis consist of a tough capsule, the posterior portion of which is called the mediastinum, and a number of fibrous septa that divide the testis into approximately 250 lobules or compartments. The mediastinum contains blood vessels, nerves, lymphatics, and the mediastinal portion of the rete testis. The capsule has three distinctive layers: the outer serosa or tunica vaginalis, the thick, collagenous tunica albuginea, and the inner tunica vasculosa. The tunica vaginalis consists of a flattened layer of mesothelial cells overlying a well-developed basement membrane. The tunica albuginea is composed of a layer of collagen fibers, within which are embedded fibroblasts, myocytes, mast cells, nerve fibers, and nerve endings resembling Meissner's corpuscles. The myocytes, found primarily in the posterior aspect of the testis, undergo regular contractions and cause a transient increase in intratesticular pressure. The tunica vasculosa, a loose connective tissue layer containing blood vessels and lymphatics, sends septa into the testicular parenchyma to form the individual lobules. Blood vessels passing through the tunica do so in an oblique plane, which may or may not have some significance with respect to blood flow within the testis. It is well known that the pulse pressure in the testicular parenchyma is extraordinarily low. The tunica varies greatly in thickness with age, averaging 300 μm at birth, decreasing to 230 μm at age 6 years, and increasing to 380 μm in early puberty. The thickness in young adults is 400 to 450 μm and progressively increases to 900 to 950 μm in men over 65 years of age (2,3).

T. D. Trainer: Department of Pathology, University of Vermont College of Medicine, Burlington, Vermont 05405.

## SEMINIFEROUS TUBULES

Each lobule of the testis contains one to four seminiferous tubules (Fig. 1). The individual tubule is a highly convoluted, closed loop structure with numerous communications between the arms of the loop but without any blind endings or branches. Each arm of the loop empties into the septal portion of the rete testis, although infrequently, seminiferous tubules may empty directly into the mediastinal rete. The total length of seminiferous tubules in each testis has been estimated between 299 and 981 m, with an average around 540 m (4). The average tubule diameter in young adults is 180

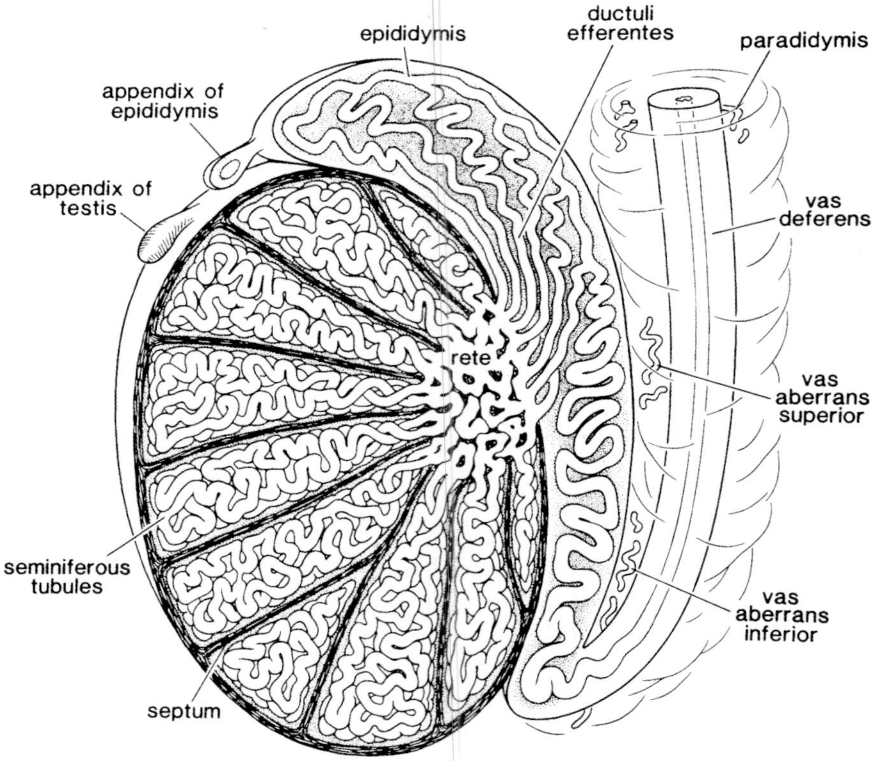


**FIG. 1.** Diagrammatic view of testis, epididymis, and portion of vas deferens.

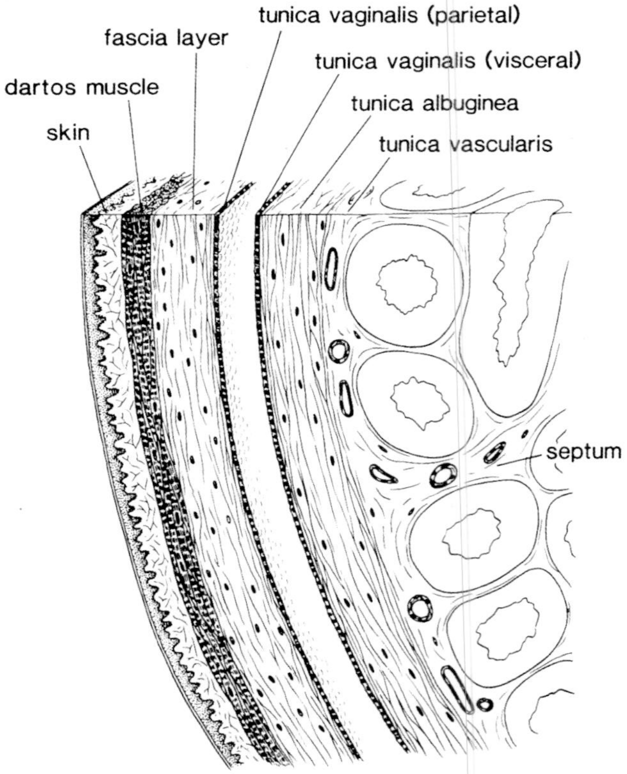


**FIG. 2.** Scrotal covering layers and capsule of testis.

μm (±30). The usual open testicular biopsy may encompass tubules from up to five lobules along with portions of the intervening septa. It is important not to interpret the latter as foci of interstitial fibrosis. The seminiferous tubules are composed of Sertoli cells and germ cells in varying stages of differentiation. Each tubule has a distinctive basement membrane and a thin lamina propria (Fig. 3).

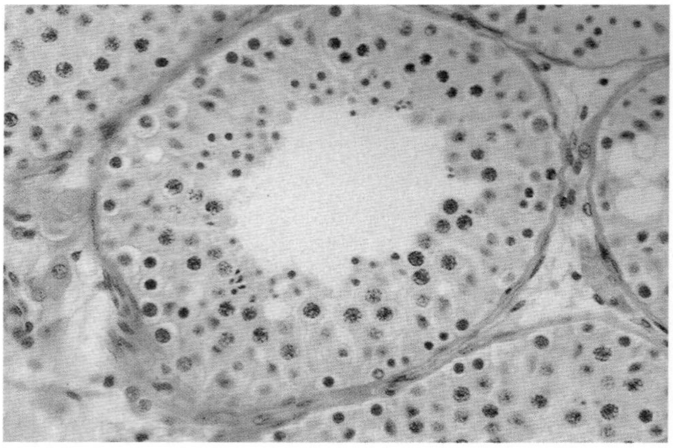

**FIG. 3.** Seminiferous tubule and interstitium: a cross-sectional view of the seminiferous tubule. Germ cell maturation is variable around the tubule, a normal finding.

## SERTOLI CELLS

Sertoli cells in the normal adult testis are nondividing cells, which are relatively inconspicuous on a cross section of the seminiferous tubule and comprise about 10% to 15% of the tubular cellular elements. These columnar cells lie on the basement membrane of the tubule and send cytoplasmic extensions around the germ cell elements. Sertoli cell nuclei are irregularly shaped, highly folded, and contain a prominent nucleolus, which permits easy separation of these cells from the germ cell elements (Fig. 4). The Sertoli cell nucleus is basally oriented within the tubule, lying just central to the nuclei of the spermatogonia. The cytoplasm may contain lipid vacuoles and/or granular eosinophilic material. Much of the phagocytosed material represents remnants of the residual bodies of the spermatid or degenerated earlier germ cell forms. Adult Sertoli cells contain vimentin as intermediate filaments, whereas embryonic and prepubertal Sertoli cells also contain low-molecular-weight cytokeratins 8, 18, and 19 (5). The transient appearance of cytokeratins is of interest in view of the report of a malignant Sertoli cell tumor containing both cytokeratins and vimentin (6). Low-molecular-weight cytokeratins also occasionally may be identified in atrophic tubules of the adult testis (7).

Both Sertoli cells and Leydig cells contain the hormones inhibin and activin, both of which play important roles as feedback regulators of follicle-stimulating hormone and modulators of testicular autocrine and paracrine function (8). The presence of inhibin, as demonstrated with a monoclonal antibody directed against the inhibin alpha subunit, has been shown to be a useful marker for granulosa cell tumors in females and undoubtedly will serve that same function for sex cord tumors in the male (9). Also present in the cytoplasm are the crystalloids of Charcot-Böttcher (10). These bundles of filamentous structures, located primarily in the basal portion of mature Sertoli cells, are best seen by ultrastructural examination but occasionally are large enough to be seen by light microscopic studies (Fig. 5). Ultrastructurally they appear to merge with vimentin-labeled intermediate filaments, both of which are increased in the cryptorchid testes and the Sertoli cell-only syndrome (5).

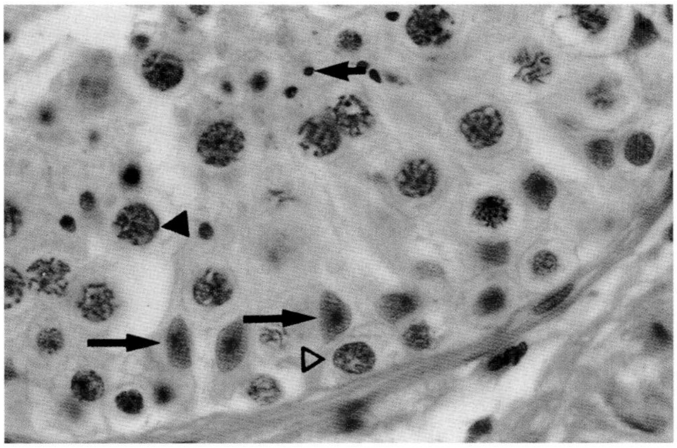

**FIG. 4.** Seminiferous tubule with Sertoli cells (*large arrows*), spermatogonia (△), primary spermatocytes (▲), and spermatids (*small arrow*).

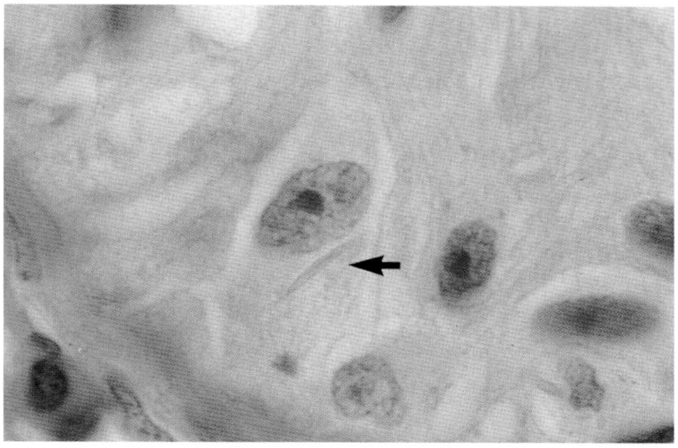

**FIG. 5.** Sertoli cell with intracytoplasmic Charcot-Böttcher crystalloids (*arrow*) from a patient with germ cell aplasia. Note the prominent nucleolus and slightly wrinkled nuclear membrane.

The Sertoli cell cytoplasm forms a meshwork closely surrounding the developing germ cells. At puberty, a tight junction complex forms between adjacent Sertoli cells, dividing the tubule into basal and adluminal compartments; the former contains spermatogonia and preleptotene spermatocytes and the latter holds the remaining primary spermatocytes, secondary spermatocytes, and spermatids. A transient, intermediate compartment is formed by adjacent Sertoli cells as germ cells move from the basal compartment to the adluminal compartment. A tight junction complex forms behind the germ cells to seal off the intercellular space, thereby ensuring the integrity of the Sertoli cell barrier (11). This junction forms the major blood–testis barrier, preventing access of blood-borne constituents to the adluminal compartment except through the Sertoli cell cytoplasm. Still unclear is the mechanism that serves to promote the movement of germ cells from the basal compartment to the adluminal compartment.

Other cell connections between adjacent Sertoli cells include gap junctions, desmosomes (rarely), and ectoplasm specialization sites (12). Intercellular junction like structures also have been described between Sertoli cells and germ cells, presumably serving as the conduit by which the Sertoli cell plays a role in the regulation of spermatogenesis.

In addition to their phagocytic capacity and role in modulating spermatogenesis, the Sertoli cell is active in the synthesis of a wide variety of proteins and other substances, including transferrin, growth factor, ceruloplasm, testibumin, activin, and inhibin. In embryonic life, Sertoli cells are thought to produce a nonsteroidal substance, müllerian inhibitory factor, which suppresses development of the müllerian duct system. In the prepubertal state, the Sertoli cell also supplies a substance that suppresses meiotic division of the gametes. This regulatory process does not apply to those germ cells that have failed in embryonic life to reach the gonad (13). The Sertoli cell contains a large amount of steroid-binding protein that serves to transport testosterone to the tubule lumen for use by the epithelial cells of the rete testis and the remaining portion of the excretory duct (14).

## GERM CELLS

Germ cells are derived from tissues in the yolk sac and migrate in early embryonic life to the gonadal ridge (15). Deviations in this migration route account for the appearance in abnormal locations of tumors derived from these cells (Fig. 6). The germ cell elements comprise the bulk of the cells seen in the adult seminiferous tubule (Figs. 3 and 4). Maturation in humans covers a period of 70 ± 4 days (16), with no evidence that this time requirement is altered by age or pathologic states. The undifferentiated spermatogonia in the basal compartment undergo proliferation and renewal; some of them give rise to primary spermatocytes, heralding the first meiotic division of spermatogenesis. The earliest of the primary spermatocytes, the preleptotene forms, are also located in the basal compartment. The preleptotene spermatocytes are then moved by an unknown signal into the adluminal compartment, where they sequentially become leptotene, zygotene, pachytene, and diplotene primary spermatocytes, this phase of the cycle involving a period of 24 days (17). The classification of primary spermatocytes is based on the alteration of the nuclear chromatin pattern (18). After this relatively long period of gametogenesis, the first meiotic division occurs with the formation of secondary spermatocytes. These cells have an extremely short half-life and soon undergo the second meiotic division to form haploid spermatids, which are then converted into spermatozoa through a series of complex steps of metamorphosis (Fig. 7).

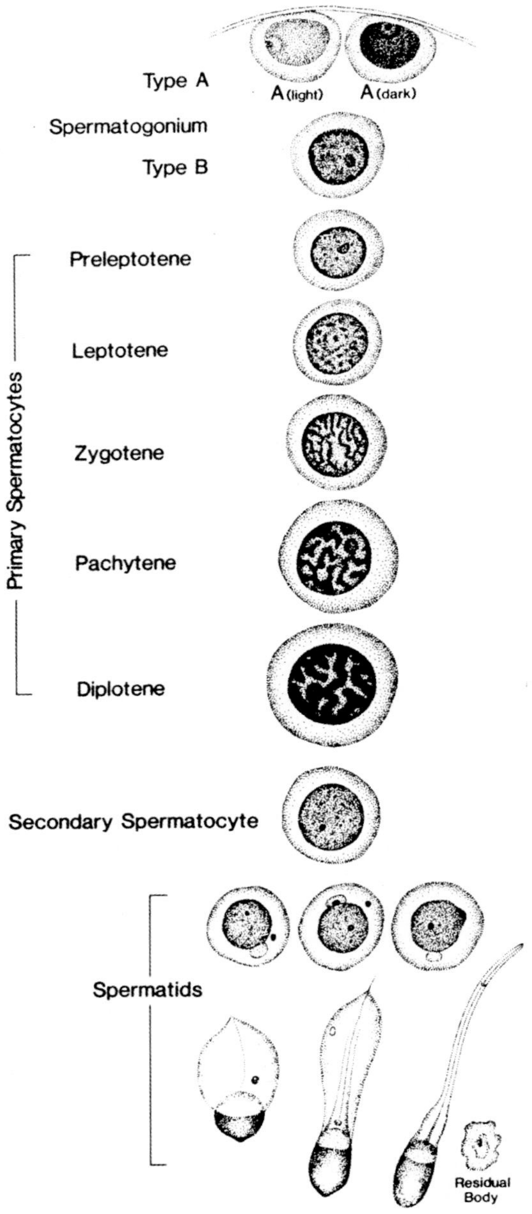


**FIG. 7.** Steps in spermatogenesis.

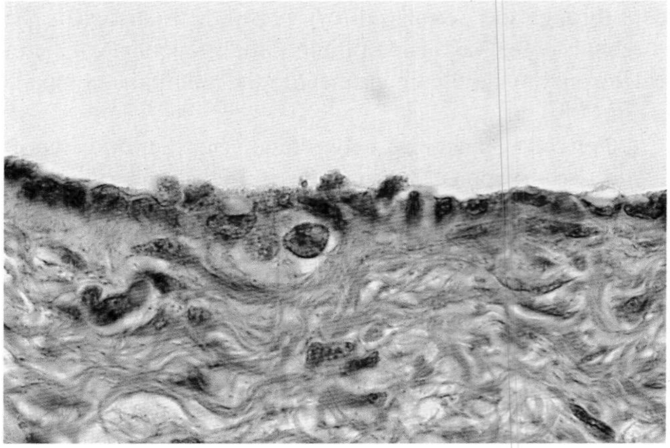

**FIG. 6.** Germ cells located immediately beneath the mesothelial lining cells of the process vaginalis of a 16-week fetus.

Until spermatozoa are formed, all progeny of a spermatogonium are connected together by a narrow cytoplasmic bridge that allows for sharing of cytoplasmic organelles and permits simultaneous maturation of interconnected cells. Of interest is the lack of these intercellular connections in seminomas and intratubular germ cell neoplasm, but their occasional presence is spermatocytic seminomas (19). A failure of cell separation is reflected in the tubular lumen and seminal fluid by the presence of multinucleated spermatids or multiheaded spermatozoa. In the late spermatid phase, excess cytoplasm is discarded by the spermatid and is phagocytosed by the enveloping Sertoli cells. The sloughing of germ cells into the seminiferous tubule lumen and the presence of immature and abnormal forms observed in patients with varicocele and other pathologic states suggest a failure of Sertoli cell regulation of this maturation process. One must take care to separate this pathologic sloughing process from the artifactual sloughing that frequently occurs in open biopsy specimens (Fig. 8).

Maturation of germ cells proceeds in an ordered, nonrandom fashion along the length of the seminiferous tubule. Groups of evolving germ cells of one level of development tend to be found in association with developing germ cells of another level of development at any point along the tubule. Clermont (18) described 14 cell association patterns in the rat testis and six such cell associations in humans. In the rat, a given cross section of seminiferous tubule shows only one cell association around the circumference of the tubule, whereas in humans up to three cell associations may be seen in a tubule cross section. Recently, this arrangement of cell clusters has been shown to form an overlapping helical pattern along the length of the tubule, the helices being contracted conically toward the lumen of the tubule (20,21). Of practical importance is the need to recognize that not all stages of differentiation of germ cells may be seen in any one cross-sectional view of a seminiferous tubule. Mature spermatozoa and late spermatids may be seen in one portion of a tubule cross section, and the opposite wall may show maturation only to the early spermatid level (Fig. 3). It has been recognized for many years that not all spermatogonia or spermatocytes progress to become spermatozoa and that degenerative changes in these precursor cells can be seen regularly in the seminiferous tubules (22). Studies in rats have demonstrated apoptotic activity in germ cells of developing animals, a process that is under the influence of gonadotropins and that can be accelerated by hypophysectomy in rats 16 to 28 days of age (23). Adult rats rendered gonadotropin deficient by the administration of a gonadotropin-releasing hormone antagonist also demonstrate germ cell apoptosis, involving both preleptotene and pachytene spermatocytes as well as spermatids. Furthermore, the apoptotic changes under these conditions occur at specific stages of germ cell maturation. In contrast, the control animals demonstrate apoptosis primarily of spermatogonia rather than of later cell forms (24). This normal physiologic process should not be mistaken for maturation arrest.

The germ cell elements can be recognized with relative ease and one should be able to distinguish spermatogonia, primary spermatocytes, secondary spermatocytes, and spermatids (25). Spermatogonia are located in the basal compartment of the seminiferous tubule, part of the cell being in contact with the tubule basement membrane. Their nuclei have a relatively dense, homogeneous chromatin pattern and contain an easily identifiable nucleolus (Fig. 9). Within the cytoplasm in a perinuclear location are the crystalloids of Lubarsch. These structures, measuring up to 6 $\mu$m in length, may be found in adults and infants as early as the 5th postnatal week. They are composed of a mixture of parallel arrays of fibrils 80 to 150 Å thick and ribosome-like granules (26). The leptotene spermatocytes are characterized by a change in the chromatin pattern into a filamentous structure with a fine-beaded arrangement. Zygotene spermatocytes have an even coarser granularity of the chromosome filaments, and there is a tendency for the chromatin material to gather eccentrically within the nucleus. Pachytene and diplotene spermatocytes are the most easily recognized of the primary spermatocytes because of their large size and their prominent nucleus containing thick, short chromatin filaments (Fig. 9). Secondary spermatocytes, having an extremely short half-life, make up only a small minority of the cells seen in a cross section of the tubule. Their nuclei, substantially smaller than the primary spermatocytes, have a finely granular chromatin pattern. These cells differ only slightly from the very early spermatids (Figs. 4 and 9). The latter have a heavily stained granular pattern to the nucleus and, if the plane of section is appropriate, a slight depression

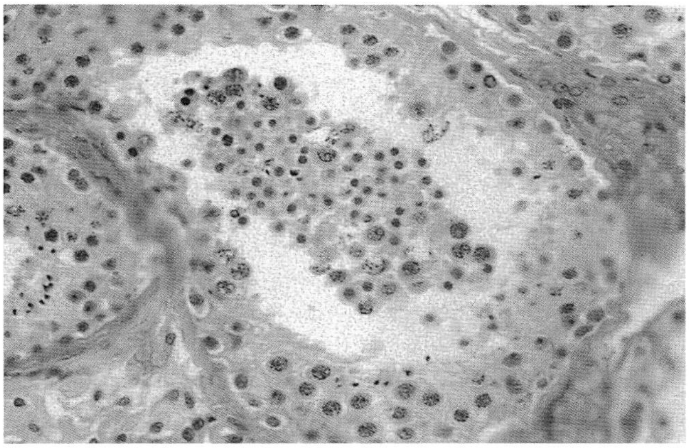

**FIG. 8.** Seminiferous tubule with artifactual sloughing of germ cell elements into tubule lumen.

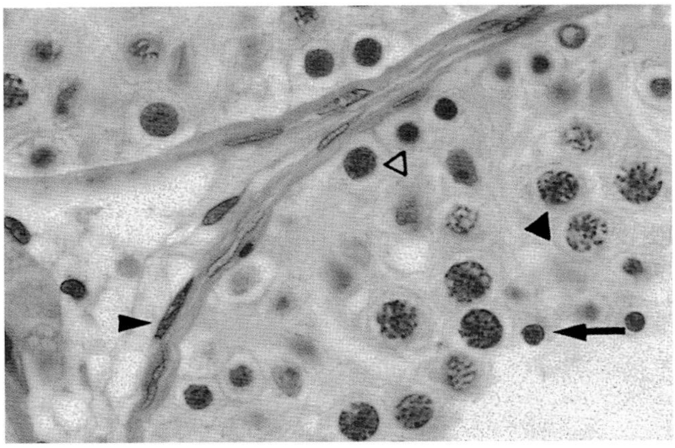

**FIG. 9.** Portion of seminiferous tubule showing spermatogonia (△), pachytene primary spermatocyte (▲), early spermatid (*small arrow*), and fibromyocyte of tunica propria (*arrowhead*).

on the surface of the cell, representing the beginning of the acrosome. The late spermatid form is characterized by a change in the nucleus, first to an oval shape with highly condensed chromatin material, then to an elongated form, and eventually assuming the configuration of a mature spermatozoon.

Elaborate methods have been developed for quantitatively assessing the germ cell elements and the relationship of spermatogenesis to seminal fluid sperm density (27–30). The method of Johnson (28) applies a score of 1 to 10 for each tubule cross section examined. The criteria are as follows: 10, complete spermatogenesis and perfect tubules; 9, many spermatozoa present but disorganized spermatogenesis; 8, only a few spermatozoa present; 7, no spermatozoa but many spermatids present; 6, only a few spermatids present; 5, no spermatozoa or spermatids present but many spermatocytes present; 4, only a few spermatocytes present; 3, only spermatogonia present; 2, no germ cells present; 1, no germ cells or Sertoli cells present. The mean score count should be at least 8.90 with an average of 9.38, and 60% or more of the tubules should score at 10.

Two relatively simple methods are helpful to the surgical pathologist. The first method (31) involves establishing a germ cell:Sertoli cell ratio by counting at least 30 tubule cross sections. This ratio is relatively constant at approximately 13:1 in young healthy men. An average of 12 Sertoli cells per tubule cross section is considered normal, and approximately half the germ cell elements within the tubule should be in the spermatid stage. A reasonably good assessment of the presence or absence of hypospermatogenesis or maturation arrest can be made with this technique. An assumption is made that the Sertoli cell population is stable throughout adult life (see Aging Testis).

A second method involves counting spermatids per tubule cross section (32). Only the mature spermatids, that is, those with oval nuclei and dark, densely stained chromatin, are counted. Excellent correlations have been made with seminal fluid sperm counts. A spermatid/tubule cross section count of 45 corresponds to a seminal fluid sperm count of 85 $\times$ $10^6$/ml. Spermatid/tubule counts of 40, 20, and 6 to 10 correspond to sperm counts of 45, 10, and 3 $\times$ $10^6$/ml, respectively. A minimum of 20 tubules must be counted.

## INTERSTITIUM

The interstitium of the testis accounts for 25% to 30% of the testicular mass. It can be divided loosely into intertubular and peritubular regions. Within the former are Leydig cells, blood vessels, lymphatics, nerves, macrophages, and mast cells. The macrophages are often found in close association with Leydig cells (33), where the two cells form complex cell–cell interdigitations. There is increasing evidence for an important paracrine role for macrophages in Leydig cell function (34). Surrounding each seminiferous tubule in a sheathlike fashion are the lamina propria and an intervening homogeneous basement membrane, which together measure 0.3 to 0.4 $\mu$m in width. Ultrastructurally, the basement membrane is multilayered with frequent splitting and knobby thickenings. These knobs are intimately associated with the basal portion of Sertoli cells. The lamina propria consists of an inner zone of collagen fibers and an outer zone of spindle-shaped myofibroblasts (Fig. 9). These cells have the capacity to produce collagen and other extracellular fibrils and also have contractile ability, a function that is probably important in the movement of spermatozoa toward the rete testis. They stain intensely for actin and desmin but only focally for vimentin, findings that are reversed in tubules that have undergone sclerosis (35,36). Elastic fibers first appear at puberty in the outermost layer of the lamina propria (37). There is a striking absence of elastic fibers in the sclerotic tubules in patients with Klinefelter's syndrome in contrast to their abundance in patients with postpubertal tubular sclerosis of multiple causes.

A common finding in patients with oligozoospermia or azoospermia due to primary testicular failure is the accumulation of eosinophilic acellular material in the lamina propria. This material is an admixture of increased collagen fibers, elastic fibrils, and basement membrane–like material (38). The peritubular tissue of patients with hypogonadotropic hypogonadism is underdeveloped, having only a single layer of myoid cells and a few collagen fibers and intermyoid fibrils. In contrast, there is a large accumulation of collagen in the lamina propria of patients with cryptorchidism. This change, which is quite obvious by light microscopic examination at puberty, can be demonstrated by ultrastructural studies as early as 2 years of age (26).

## LEYDIG CELLS

Leydig cells are found singly and in clusters within the interstitium of the testis; some lie in intimate association with capillaries, whereas others lie close to the peritubular myofibrocytes (Fig. 10). They also may be seen in the tunica albuginea, epididymis, spermatic cord, and, quite commonly, mediastinum of the testis. They are often located in intimate association with large nerve fibers (Fig. 11) (39) and have been seen in the fetus as well as the adult (see Gubernaculum). Ultrastructural studies show evidence of indirect and direct innervation of Leydig cells in children and adults but not in the fetus (40). Intratubular Leydig cells are not found in the normal testis but may be seen in sclerosed tubules or those in the Sertoli cell–only syndrome (41). The single nucleus of the cell is round and vesicular, with one to two eccentrically located nucleoli. Occasional binucleated cells are present. The cytoplasm is usually abundant and stains intensely with acid dyes. Lipid droplets and lipofuscin pigment are found in the cytoplasm, first appearing at the time of puberty. The pigment becomes more prominent in the aging testis. Mitotic division of adult Leydig cells has only rarely been encountered (42). The characteristic intracytoplasmic (infrequently intranuclear) Reinke crystalloids, seen exclusively in humans and the wild bush rat, are present only in

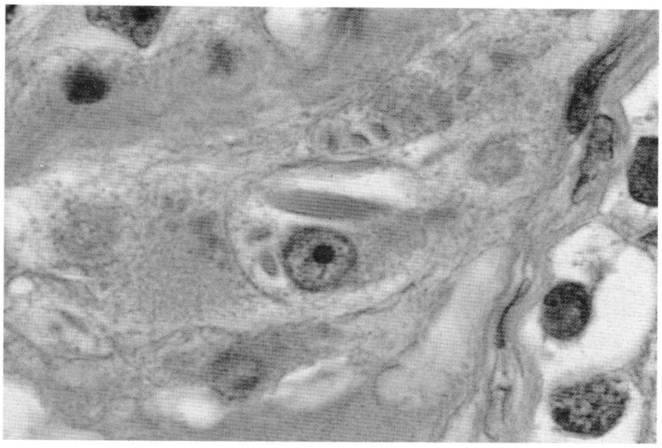

**FIG. 10.** Leydig cells in interstitium of testis. An eosinophilic crystalloid of Reinke and abundant lipofuscin are prominent features in the cytoplasm of the Leydig cell in the center of this field.

the postpubertal state (Fig. 10). Their presence is highly variable in the normal testis, and they are frequently absent in Leydig cell tumors. The ultrastructural appearance is that of a hexagonal prism, giving them a honeycombed appearance. The nature of the material is still unknown, although it is presumed to represent a protein product of the cell (43).

Quantitation of Leydig cells has been a parameter difficult to assess. Several indices have been used: mean Leydig cell number per seminiferous tubule; mean number of Leydig cells per Leydig cell cluster; mean number of Leydig cell clusters per seminiferous tubule; mean number of Leydig cell clusters per seminiferous tubules; Leydig cell:Sertoli cell ratio; and ratio of Leydig cell area to seminiferous tubule area (44). Heller et al. (45), using the Leydig cell:Sertoli cell ratio, found a value of 0.39 and a range of 0.19 to 0.72. In that same study, they also determined the average number of Sertoli cells per tubular cross section to be $10.03 \pm 0.6$. They made an assumption that the Sertoli cell population was stable in their calculation of the Leydig cell population. As a rule, normal adults should have approximately five Leydig cells for each tubular cross section.

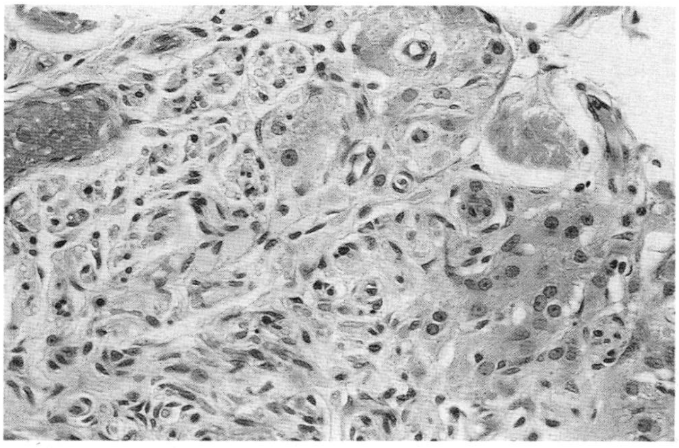

**FIG. 11.** Leydig cells in intimate association with a nerve in the hilus of the testis.

Leydig cells, in addition to their responsibility for testosterone production, contain a number of marker substances that suggest a neuroendocrine function. These include oxytocin, proopiomelanocortin, neural cell adhesion molecules, substance P, and B-endorphin. The production of these substances undoubtedly indicates an important paracrine function that Leydig cells share with Sertoli cells, peritubular cells, macrophages, and nerves. Immunocytochemical staining indicates the presence of synaptophysin, chromogranin A-B, neuron-specific enolase, neurofilament proteins, and S100 but not vimentin or desmin. Electron microscopic studies show dense core vesicles measuring 100 to 300 nm in diameter (46). Glial fibrillary acid protein (GFAP) reactivity of Leydig cells also has been demonstrated, particularly in those cells found in intimate association with capillaries (47).

## VASCULAR SUPPLY

The blood supply to the testis is derived primarily from the internal spermatic artery with a smaller contribution from the branches of the vasal portion of the internal vesicle artery. The testicular artery is highly coiled and extremely long relative to its diameter and has a low-pulse pressure as it enters the testis (48). The artery plays an important role in thermal regulation via countercurrent heat exchange with the veins of the pampiniform plexus. The combination of this vascular heat exchange and the heat lost via the thin scrotal covering layers serves to maintain the testicular temperature 2°C below body temperature. Arterial branches of the testicular artery arborize over the surface of the testis, penetrate the capsule, and pass in a centripetal fashion within the septa to the mediastinum, where they form a dense cluster. Only a few branches enter the lobules from these centripetal arteries. From the mediastinum, the small arterial segments then pass in a centrifugal fashion within the parenchyma where they branch into arterioles and capillaries. The veins run either centrifugally or centripetally to the capsule or mediastinum, respectively, and eventually anastomose posteriorly to form the pampiniform plexus of the testicular vein. Biopsy specimens of the testis of patients with varicoceles often show a striking sclerosis of vascular walls (49). These changes appear to involve both arteries and veins. The significance of these vascular alterations with respect to seminiferous tubule function in patients with varicoceles is uncertain.

At puberty, there is an extensive development of the intratesticular microvascular architecture, the most notable features being a marked coiling of the arteries and a great expansion of the peritubular capillary network. Unlike other capillaries of the systemic system, the testicular capillary walls have a prominent basement membrane and an incomplete outer layer of pericytes (50). Arteriovenous anastomoses occur in two locations: beneath the tunica albuginea between branches of the centripetal artery and vein, and deep within the parenchyma between branches of the centrifugal artery and vein. The role of these anastomoses is unknown.

The microvasculature of the testis resembles more that of the brain than the systemic capillary system. Both brain and testis capillaries are continuous and nonfenestrated with few vesicles and long intercellular junction profiles. They both have a glucose transporter system and a P-glycoprotein, which may inhibit transport of lipophilic substances. Unlike the brain, the capillaries of the testis lack a transferrin and do have some expanded clefts at cell junctions, suggesting a greater degree of permeability of these vessels. The findings strongly support an additional blood–testis barrier, which probably complements the well-known barrier provided by the Sertoli cells in segregating the germ cell population (47).

The capillary network appears to have a very structured arrangement with respect to the Leydig cells and the seminiferous tubules. The postarterial capillaries ramify around and within the Leydig cell–macrophage clusters and then penetrate the tunica propria of the seminiferous tubules. Not all areas of the tubule wall appear to be supplied with this elaborate network, and the reason for this is still unclear. The capillaries then reenter the loose interstitium as postcapillary venules, where they receive other capillaries coming from the Leydig cell clusters (51). The intralobular veins then enter the septa, where they move either to the mediastinum or to the tunica vasculosa.

There is a remarkable species-to-species variation in the distribution of lymphatic channels in the testis (52). Lymphatics in the rat testis are intimately associated with Leydig cells and also form a complex network in the tunica propria about the seminiferous tubules. In humans, ill-defined lymphatic spaces are found in the interstitium adjacent to Leydig cell clusters, but a peritubular lymphatic network is lacking. The lymphatic channels drain into the septa and thence to either the capsule or the mediastinum, where they join on the posterior aspect of the testis. They then anastomose with lymphatic channels from the epididymis and enter the spermatic cord.

## FETAL AND PREPUBERTAL TESTIS

The fetal testis becomes recognizable at 7 to 8 weeks of gestation, at which time primitive testicular cords become evident. By the 9th week the cords contain primordial germ cells, referred to as gonocytes, as well as supporting stromal cells destined to be Sertoli cells. The gonocytes are mitotically active during the next 4 to 5 weeks and are characterized by the presence of intracytoplasmic glycogen and a cell surface–located alkaline phosphatase, which cross reacts with antibodies raised against placental alkaline phosphatase. This enzyme, known as placental-like alkaline phosphatase, is rapidly lost from the normal gonocytes by 12 to 15 weeks but is retained by neoplastic germ cells, a finding that serves the surgical pathologist in identifying in situ and invasive germ cell neoplasms of the prepubertal and adult testis (53). Early fetal germ cells also express reactions to the monoclonal antibody TRA-1-60, which recognizes a mucinlike cell surface glycoprotein, and to the monoclonal antibody M2A, which recognizes an uncharacterized cell surface carbohydrate. These markers also disappear from germ cells early in the second trimester of fetal life and are reexpressed postnatally in germ cell tumors (54).

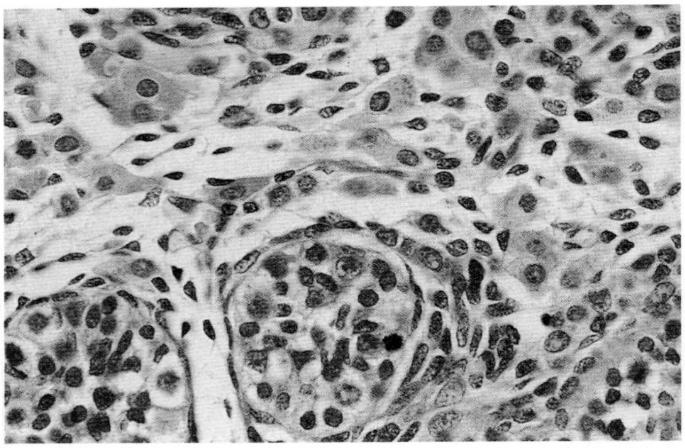

**FIG. 12.** Fetal testis of 20 weeks' gestation, with numerous Leydig cells throughout the interstitium.

At 20 weeks of fetal life the testis is characterized by abundant, well-developed Leydig cells filling the interstitium (Fig. 12). The seminiferous tubules are solidly filled and measure 45 to 50 $\mu$m in diameter. The fetal tubules contain Sertoli cells and primordial germ cells, referred to as gonocytes (Fig. 13).

The gonocyte is randomly distributed through the seminiferous tubule and is easily identified by its large nucleus with a granular and chunky chromatin pattern (Fig. 13). Shortly before and after birth, the germ cells migrate to the periphery of the tubule and take on the features of spermato-

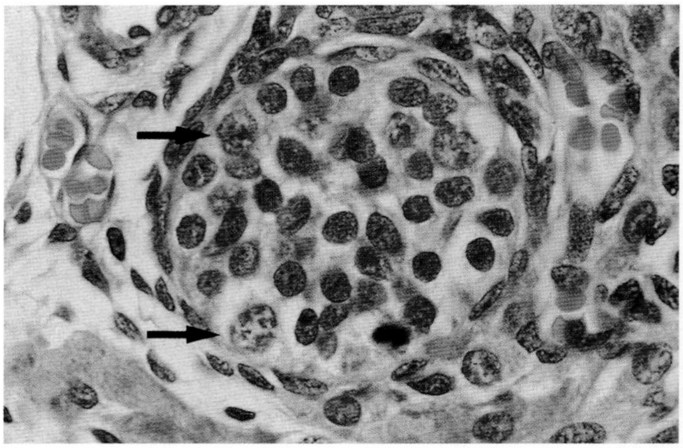

**FIG. 13.** Same sample as shown in Fig. 12. Note the mitotic figure, probably of a Sertoli cell. Larger cells (*arrows*) are undifferentiated germ cells. The remaining cells are immature Sertoli cells.

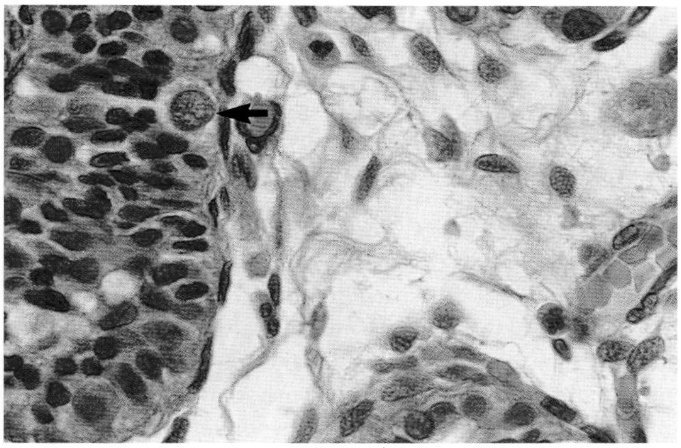

**FIG. 14.** Testis of 11-month-old child. A spermatogonium is present adjacent to the basement membrane (*arrow*). The interstitium contains undifferentiated spindle cells.

gonia (Fig. 14). The latter have nuclei that are the largest of the cells in the immature tubule and have their basal cell wall opposed to the tubule basement membrane. In addition to spermatogonia, early prespermatocytes can now be identified. Unlike spermatogonia, these cells have no connection with the tubule basement membrane and remain in the middle of the tubule surrounded by Sertoli cells. On average one to two germ cells should be seen per tubule cross section between birth and the 4th year of life, and this number should double during the 5th through 8th years. Several studies have demonstrated a marked diminution in the number of germ cells in the prepubertal cryptorchid testis (Fig. 15) and a less predictable decrease of germ cells in the truly ectopic testis (26,55).

The fetal seminiferous tubules lack lumens and average 45 to 50 $\mu$m in diameter through the latter half of fetal life (56). The postnatal tubules slowly increase in size to reach a prepubertal diameter of 64 $\mu$m (range 43–70), at which time lumens begin to appear (57).

Fetal Sertoli cells outnumber germ cells in a ratio of 7:1 (56) and undergo active mitotic division during this period. Unlike its adult counterpart, the immature Sertoli cell has an oval to round nucleus and an inconspicuous nucleolus (Fig. 13).

Early studies had suggested that the Sertoli cell is mitotically inactive after birth, but stereologic studies indicate their number increases from 260 million late in fetal life, to 1,500 million between 3 months and 10 years, and to 3,700 million in the adult testis (58). Sertoli cells average 30 per tubule cross section in the fetal testis after 20 weeks, increase to 42 at the 4th postnatal month, decrease to 26 per cross section at age 13 years, and to 12 to 15 in the adult testis (26,56). At puberty there is a fivefold increase in Sertoli cell volume, and Charcot-Böttcher crystalloids appear for the first time. Commonly in the cryptorchid testis are found nodules or "congeries" of immature Sertoli cells (Fig. 16). These collections are often multiple and usually microscopic in size (59).

The early prepubertal lamina propria is relatively undeveloped and is separated from the tubules by a thin basement membrane that lacks the knoblike thickening and splitting of the adult testis. The collagen fiber layer is relatively thin, and only one or two spindle-shaped cells are seen in the outer portion of the lamina propria.

Leydig cells are first recognizable by the 8th week of fetal life and become prominent in the fetal testis at 15 to 20 weeks of gestation (Fig. 12), after which there is a progressive decline in their relative number. Although a few cells with the characteristics of mature Leydig cells still may be seen up until the age of 1 year, most of the cells assume the shape of undifferentiated fibroblasts (Fig. 14) and a lesser number have a slightly plump nucleus and a relatively prominent nucleolus. Ultrastructural studies have demonstrated that 63% of the fusiform cells in the interstitium are primitive intratubular fibroblasts, 28% are peritubular fibroblasts, and 9% represent Leydig cell precursors (60). Af-

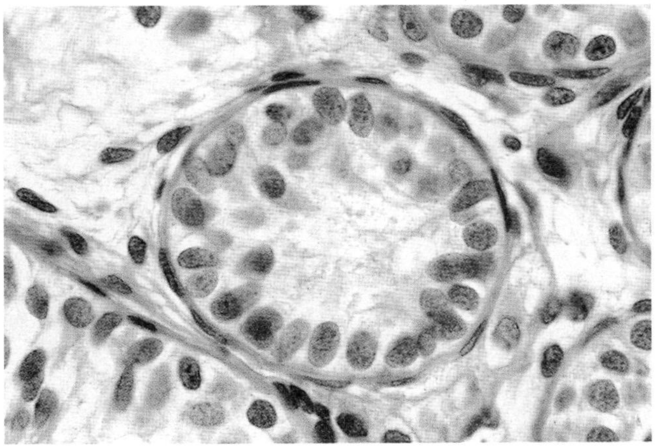

**FIG. 15.** Thirteen-year-old prepubertal boy with bilateral cryptorchidism. Mature Leydig cells are absent in the interstitium. The tubules lack a lumen. The Sertoli cells are immature, and germ cells are absent.

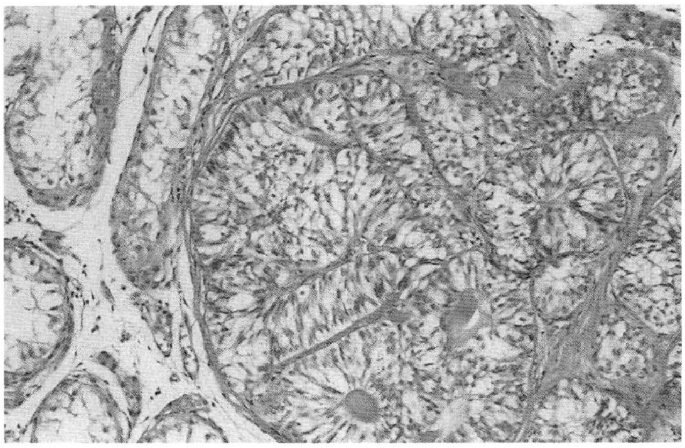

**FIG. 16.** Sertoli cell collections or congeries. The tubules are composed of immature Sertoli cells and lack both germ cells and lumina.

ter 7 years of age, the precursor Leydig cells progressively differentiate and eventually take on the appearance of adult Leydig cells shortly before and during puberty. Still unclear is whether adult Leydig cells are derived from dedifferentiated fetal Leydig cells or from the primitive fibroblast cell population, but the evidence favors the former (61). Blood vessels and lymphatic channels are relatively inconspicuous until just before puberty.

## AGING TESTIS

There is a general consensus that a decline in testicular function occurs with advancing age (1). These physiologic changes are matched by involutional changes in the testicular parenchyma, including hypospermatogenesis, peritubular fibrosis, and hyalinization of the seminiferous tubules. A few sclerosed tubules are found occasionally in the normal adult testis (62), but larger, focal, or diffuse areas of sclerosis are distinctly pathologic. Abnormal sperm maturation, sloughing of germ cells into the tubule lumen, degeneration of germ cell elements, and Sertoli cell lipid accumulation and cytoplasmic vacuolization are frequent findings. Of interest have been studies (63,64) of elderly men in whom concomitant chronic illness was excluded whose testicular weights were not significantly different from young adults.

Interstitial changes are highly variable in the aging testis. Peritubular sclerosis and hyalinization may be pronounced. Thickening of the intratubular arterial walls with hyalinization, sometimes seen in otherwise normal testes, is found in over 90% of testes in which there are large zones of tubular fibrosis. The capillary bed in the aged testis becomes sparse and poorly organized (65). These vascular changes probably play a causal role in the peritubular sclerosis and tubular hyalinization.

Substantial controversy exists regarding the Leydig cell population in the aging testis, different reports indicating an increase (66), no change (67), or a decline (68,69) in their number. According to Neaves et al. (70), Leydig cell numbers and size both progressively decline with advancing age, the total Leydig cell population decreasing by 50% during the first 30 years of adult life. The production of testosterone by Leydig cells is relatively maintained despite a loss of total Leydig cell mass, probably because of the large reserve of these cells in the adult testis. When the Leydig cell mass decreases to a certain threshold point, daily sperm production is depressed. The aged Leydig cell contains large amounts of lipofuscin pigment and numerous vacuoles within the cytoplasm.

There is also a decline in the number of mitochondria and a decrease in smooth endoplasmic reticulin (71). Earlier studies indicated that the Sertoli cell population was stable throughout the postpubertal years (72,73). However, Johnson et al. (74) found that men 20 to 48 years of age had significantly more Sertoli cells per tubule cross section than did men 50 to 85 years of age, and there was a relatively constant relationship between Sertoli cells and germ cells in both age groups. Furthermore, these investigators suggested that the decline in spermatozoa production in the elderly may be due to a decrease in Sertoli cell function and mass.

## RETE TESTES

The rete testis, a network of channels at the hilus of the testis, receives the luminal contents of the seminiferous tubules (Fig. 1). It is divided into three components: the septal portion containing the tubulae rete, the mediastinal or tunica rete, and the extratesticular portion also known as the bullae retis (75). The tubulae rete are short tubules 0.5 to 1.0 mm in length found within the interlobular septa of the testis and serve to connect the two ends of the seminiferous tubule loop to the mediastinum testis. There are approximately 1,500 entrances of seminiferous tubules into the rete; a few tubules may enter the mediastinal rete directly without intervening tubulae rete. The mediastinal rete is a cavernous network of interconnecting channels that exits from the testis to form several dilated, vesicular channels or antechamber-like structures called the bullae retis. These structures, measuring up to 3.0 mm in width, anastomose together to form the ductuli efferentia.

The rete epithelium is a simple squamous or low columnar type (Fig. 17), the luminal surface of which is studded with microvilli. Each cell contains a single, central flagellum that is inconspicuous on light microscopic examination. The epithelium sits on a relatively thick basal lamina, beneath which are a few fibroblasts and myoid cells intermixed with collagen and elastic fibers to form the rete wall. Traversing the mediastinum and the extratesticular rete are epithelium-covered columns or strands called chordae retis. These columns, often appearing as islands on a cross section of the rete testis (Fig. 18), vary greatly in length (15–100 $\mu$m) and thickness (5–40 $\mu$m) and serve to connect opposing walls of the chambers. The cytoplasm of the rete epithelium contains keratin and vimentin intermediate filaments, the former be-

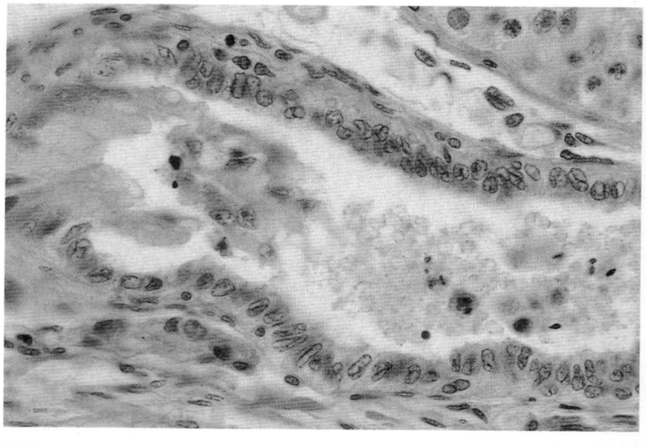

**FIG. 17.** Junction of septal rete testis and terminal end of seminiferous tubule. Note the Sertoli cells "pouting" into lumen of rete. Rete epithelium is a low columnar type.

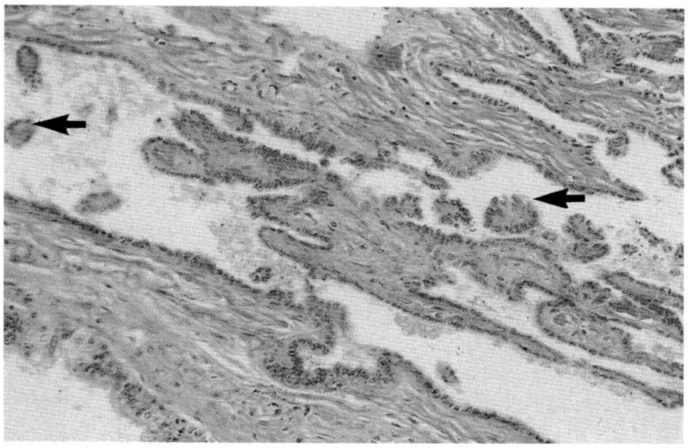

**FIG. 18.** Rete testis, mediastinal portion, with irregular cavernous channels and cross sections of intratubular chordae (*arrows*).

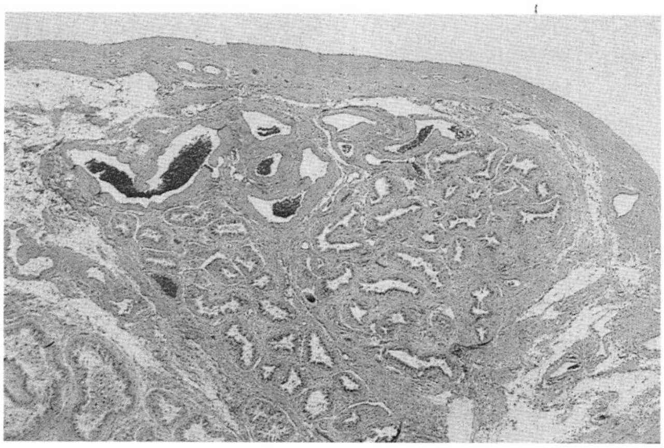

**FIG. 19.** Head of epididymis, showing cross sections of distal portions of ductuli efferentia and epididymis (*lower left*).

ing located primarily in the apical portion of the cell and the latter being found in the basal region. The keratins are primarily of low-molecular-weight, can be first identified at the 10th week of fetal life, and precede the appearance of vimentin by 2 to 3 weeks (76). One would expect coexpression of these two intermediate filaments in the rare carcinoma of the rete or in hyperplasia of the rete. However, a report of nine cases of hyperplasia of the rete testis showed strong keratin and epithelial membrane antigen staining but a negative reaction to vimentin (77).

The rete serves multiple functions: (a) as a mixing chamber for the contents of the seminiferous tubules, (b) as a pressure gradient between the seminiferous tubules and the epididymis, (c) as a possible source of as yet unknown components of the seminal fluid (78), and (d) as a reabsorptive site of proteins from the luminal contents (79).

## DUCTULI EFFERENTIA

The ductuli efferentia consist of 12 to 15 tubules that arise from the extratesticular rete testis (Fig. 1). They are involved primarily in resorption of fluid (80) and do not appear to store spermatozoa for any length of time. These tubules aggregate to form a significant portion of the caput of the epididymis proper (Fig. 19). The cells of the efferent ductules are composed of ciliated and nonciliated columnar cells, basal cells, and scattered intraepithelial lymphocytes, giving the epithelium a pseudostratified appearance (Fig. 20). Coexpression of low-molecular-weight cytokeratins and vimentin as well as epithelial membrane antigen is evident within the epithelial cytoplasm (76).

Scattered giant epithelial cells with irregular, hyperchromatic nuclei may be encountered (81). These appear first as a fusion of nuclei from adjacent cells to form a multinucleated cell; subsequently, aggregation and condensation of the nuclei occur to form irregular, hyperchromatic nuclear masses that often bulge into the lumina. They resemble the epithelial changes seen in the seminal vesicles.

The epithelium sits on a thick basement membrane, surrounding which is a coat of smooth muscle cells and fibroblasts as well as a few scattered macrophages. Intraluminal macrophages are rarely seen except when distal duct obstruction exists, at which time macrophages may be found actively phagocytizing spermatozoa.

## EPIDIDYMIS

The epididymis, a highly coiled, tubular structure of 4 to 5 m (82) in length, can be divided anatomically into caput, corpus, and cauda portions (Fig. 1). The epididymis plays an important role in (a) sperm transport, (b) sperm maturation, including the acquisition of motility, (c) sperm concentration, and (d) sperm storage. The average sperm transit time through the epididymis in humans is 12 days (83). The trans-

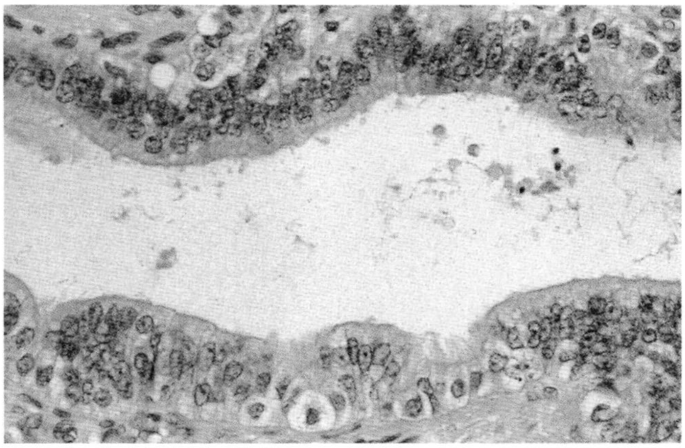

**FIG. 20.** Epithelium of ductus efferent. The columnar epithelial cells are mixed with basal cells and occasional intraepithelial lymphocytes, giving the epithelium a pseudostratified appearance.

port mechanism is by way of muscle contractions of the thick, muscular coat that surrounds the epididymal tubules. There is extensive reabsorption of intraluminal fluid, particularly in the caput portion of the epididymis. Most of the sperm are stored in the caudal segment until ejaculation occurs, and it is in this location in humans that sperm maturation takes place (84). In humans, the cauda is a relatively small reservoir, explaining the rapid decline in seminal fluid sperm counts in men having frequent ejaculations. Many spermatozoa apparently undergo senescence and degeneration in the cauda via an unknown mechanism.

The epithelium of the epididymis consists of tall columnar or principal cells, basal cells, clear cells, tall slender or apical cells rich in mitochondria (apical mitochondria-rich cells), and scattered intraepithelial lymphocytes and macrophages (85). The principal cells, comprising over 95% of the columnar cells, have straight stereocilia (Fig. 21), which in the caput are tall and nearly obliterate the lumen but become progressively shorter as the cauda is reached. The principal cells stain strongly for vimentin, epithelial membrane antigen (EMA), and acid phosphatase and modestly for cytokeratins AE1/AE3. The intensity of the vimentin staining progressively declines in the cauda section (86). The mitochondria-rich apical cells, located primarily in the caput, show intense staining for cytokeratins and less intense reactivity for vimentin (85). The basal cells also stain strongly for cytokeratins and recently have been shown to have immunocytochemical markers that suggest a macrophage-like role (87). Any of the epididymal cells may contain lipofuscin pigment, which tends to be more prominent in the caput segment and is particularly evident when there is obstruction of the epididymis (88).

Intranuclear, eosinophilic, periodic acid-Schiff–positive and diastase-resistant inclusions (Fig. 22), measuring 1 to 14 $\mu$m, are found in the columnar cells of the adult epididymis as well as throughout the vas and seminal vesicles. Electron microscopic examination shows the electron-dense globules to be enclosed by a single membrane and to lack any features suggesting viral structures (89). They are most common in the distal epididymis and adjacent vas and least common in the ampulla of the vas and seminal vesicles. With one exception, they have been described exclusively in the postpubertal state. The exception was in a 4-year-old child with macrogenitosomia praecox (90).

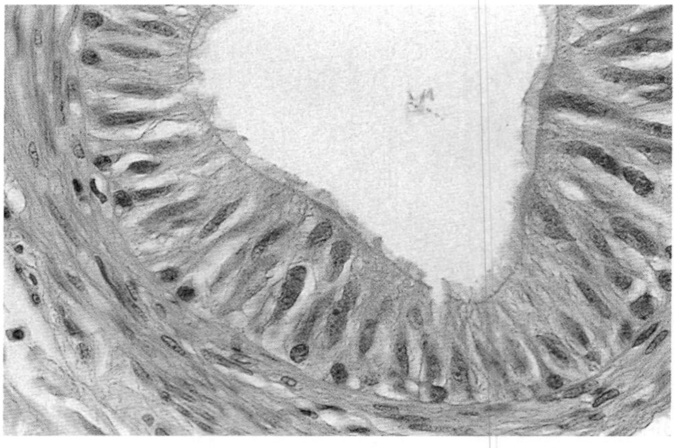

FIG. 21. Epithelium of epididymis. Compare the tall columnar cells of the epididymis with the pseudostratified cells of the ductus efferent. A few intraepithelial lymphocytes are present. The stereocilia are somewhat short, indicating the caudal segment. A layer of muscle cells forms the wall.

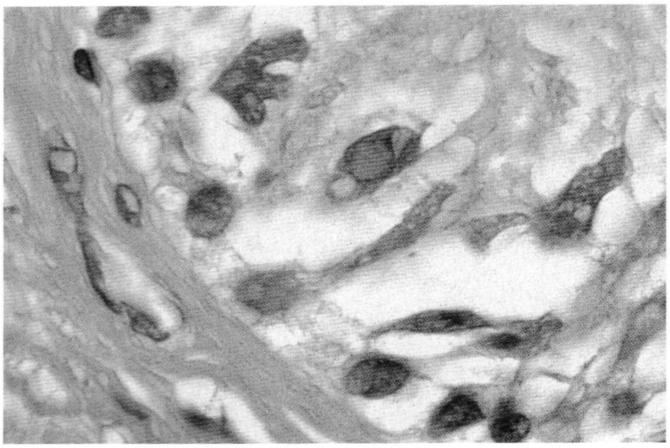

FIG. 22. Intranuclear inclusions present in the epithelium of the epididymis. Similar inclusions are found in the epithelium of the vas deferens.

The epididymis is supported by a thick basement membrane, surrounding which is a well-defined muscular coat. The latter plays an important role in sperm movement through the epididymis. Mast cells are found throughout the connective tissue of the epididymis in a pattern similar to that seen in the tunica and interstitium of the testis (91), being numerous in infancy, decreasing in childhood, and then increasing at the time of puberty. A progressive decline in numbers occurs in adulthood.

## DUCTUS (VAS) DEFERENS

The ductus (vas) deferens, a tubular structure arising from the caudal portion of the epididymis, measures 30 to 40 cm in length. The distal 4 to 7 cm portion is enlarged to form the ampulla. The latter joins the excretory duct of the seminal vesicle to form the ejaculatory duct (Fig. 23). The adult vas is lined by a pseudostratified, columnar epithelium, composed of columnar cells and basal cells by light microscopic examination. Ultrastructural studies show four different cell types: principal cells, pencil or peg cells, mitochondria-enriched cells, and basal cells. The luminal surface of the columnar cell (92) is lined by tall stereocilia throughout most of the vas. These stereocilia are substantially shorter and sparser in the ampullary region. Prominent intranuclear inclusions as described above in the epididymis may be seen (89). In addition, occasional lipid-positive vacuoles are present within the cytoplasm. The epithelium of the vas is

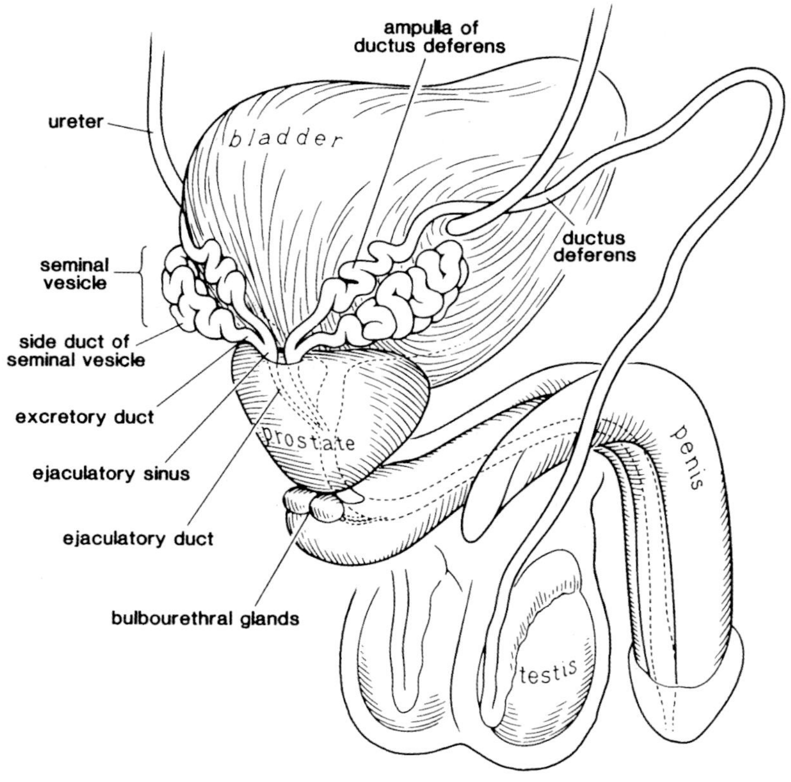


**FIG. 23.** Diagram of excretory duct system from the vas to the ejaculatory ducts.

thrown into folds, which are relatively simple in the proximal vas (Fig. 24) but become much more complex in the ampullary segment (Fig. 25). The ampulla has highly complex infoldings and many outpocketings or diverticula that reach into the muscle coat. Beneath the epithelium of the vas is a loose, connective tissue stroma that, after puberty, contains a well-defined, circumferentially oriented layer of elastic fibers (93). These fibers, lacking in infants and children, become frayed and fragmented in the aged vas. The muscle coat is an extraordinary thick structure with inner and outer longitudinal coats and a middle oblique or circular zone. The entire muscle mass progressively decreases as one approaches the ampulla, although the inner longitudinal layer becomes somewhat thicker as one progresses distally (92). The epithelium in the ampulla contains significant amounts of lipofuscin pigment and rather closely resembles the epithelium seen in the seminal vesicles. Active phagocytosis of degenerated spermatozoa has been demonstrated in the ampullary region of a number of mammalian species (94).

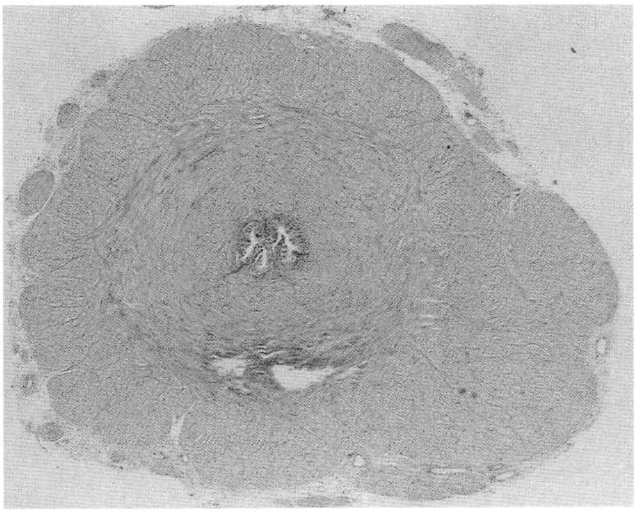

**FIG. 24.** Proximal vas deferens. This cross section shows a thick muscle coat, tiny lumen, and slightly folded mucosa.

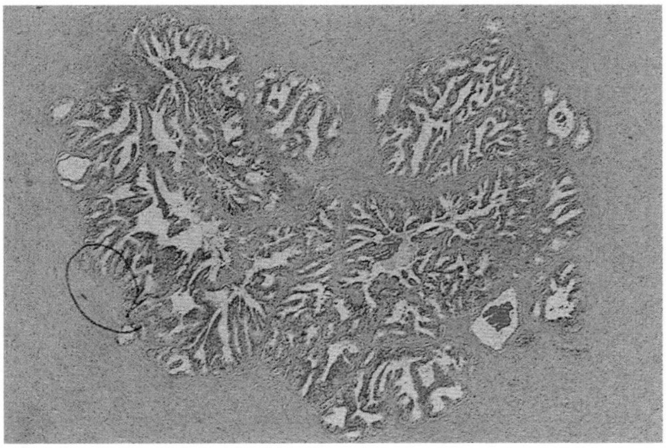

**FIG. 25.** Ampullary region of vas deferens. Note the complex folding and outpouching of the mucosa into the muscular coat.

## SEMINAL VESICLES

The seminal vesicles are paired, highly coiled, tubular structures lying posterolateral to the base of the bladder and in a parallel path with the ampulla of the vas deferens (Fig. 23). Each vesicle measures 3.5 to 7.5 cm in length and 1.2 to 2.4 cm in thickness in the adult. The main duct, which is duplicated in approximately 10% of individuals, measures 10 to 15 cm in length when unraveled. Six to eight first-order side ducts extend off the main duct, and from these are derived several secondary side ducts. The upper part of the main duct is bent backward in a hooklike fashion. A short excretory duct combines with the ampulla of the vas to form the ejaculatory duct (Fig. 23). The wall of the seminal vesicle has a thin external longitudinal and a thicker internal circular muscle layer. The mucosal folds, relatively simple and shallow in infancy and childhood, become highly complex and alveolus-like in the reproductive years (Fig. 26) and are blunted in the aged vesicle. The lumen may contain a few sloughed epithelial cells and debris. Spermatozoa refluxed from the ejaculatory duct occasionally may be present, although they are not normally stored within the seminal vesicles.

The vesicle epithelium is composed of columnar and basal cells. The former have short microvilli projecting from the surface. Ultrastructurally, the columnar cells contain abundant mitochondria and rough endoplasmic reticulum, dilated cisternae, and a prominent Golgi apparatus (95). The cytoplasm characteristically contains a large amount of lipofuscin pigment, a feature important in recognizing these cells obtained by needle biopsy or aspiration cytology studies of the prostate. Similar lipofuscin pigment is found in the ampulla of the vas deferens and in the epithelium of the ejaculatory ducts.

An unusual feature of the seminal vesicular epithelium is the presence of peculiar, monstrous epithelial cells (Fig. 27).

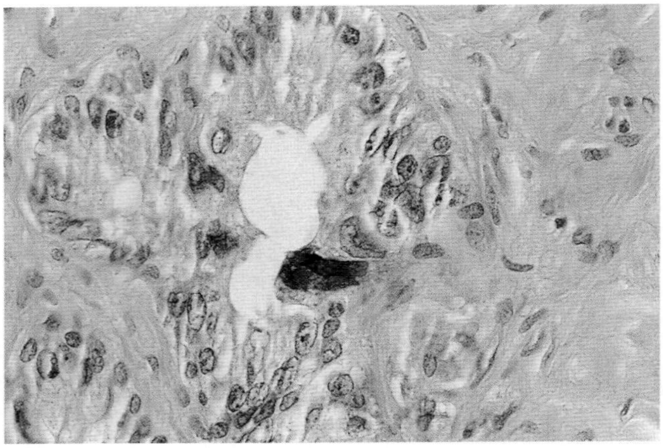

**FIG. 27.** Seminal vesicle epithelium. Tall columnar cells line the lumen. A single hyperchromatic "monster" cell is present. These cells should not be mistaken for malignant cells.

These cells have enlarged, hyperchromatic, and often grossly misshapen nuclei and prominent nucleoli. These cells are found in approximately three quarters of adult seminal vesicles and are somewhat more frequently encountered in older individuals. They are not seen in infants or children. Their genesis is unknown but may be related to endocrine influences, similar to the Arias-Stella cells seen in gestational endometrium. Because these cells may be encountered in both needle biopsy and aspiration biopsy specimens, the surgical pathologist must be alert to avoid identifying them as malignant cells (81). The presence of lipofuscin in the cytoplasm is a helpful clue, but sometimes this pigment may be inconspicuous.

Also encountered in the muscle portion of the seminal vesicle are hyaline globules (Fig. 28) thought to represent degenerating smooth muscle cells. They also may be seen occasionally in the muscular coat of the vas and within the prostatic parenchyma (96).

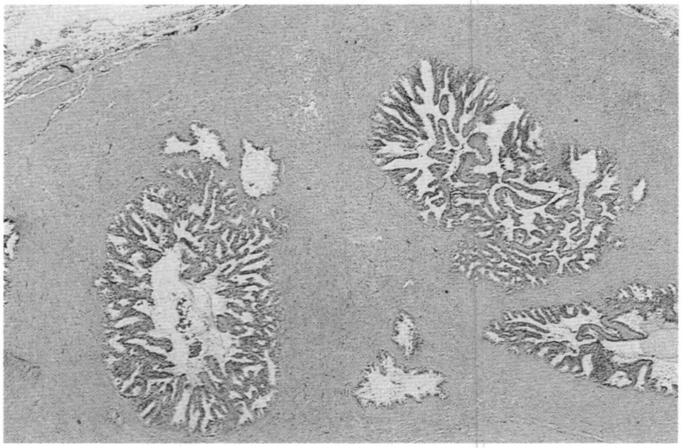

**FIG. 26.** Seminal vesicle: alveolar-like arrangement of mucosal folds and cross sections of side ducts.

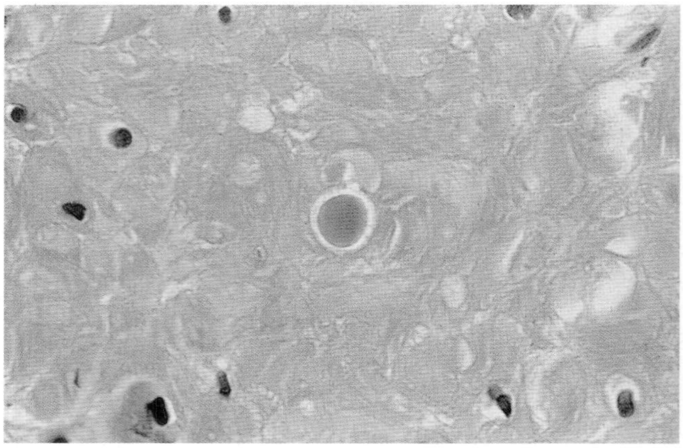

**FIG. 28.** Muscle coat of seminal vesicle: hyaline globule, probably representing a degenerated smooth muscle cell.

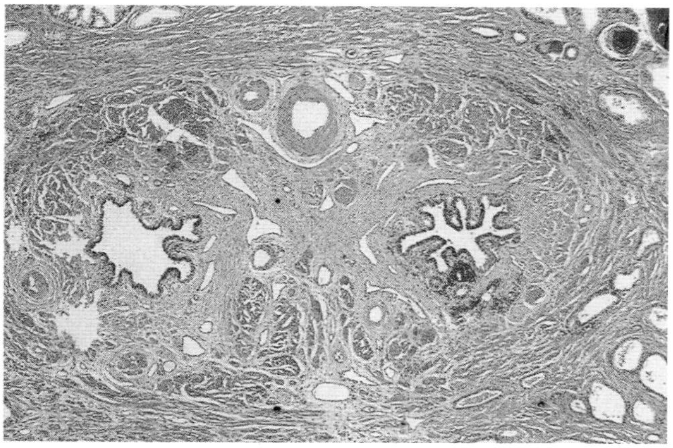

FIG. 29. Paired ejaculatory ducts within the prostatic parenchyma. This section is adjacent to the verumontanum of the prostatic urethra.

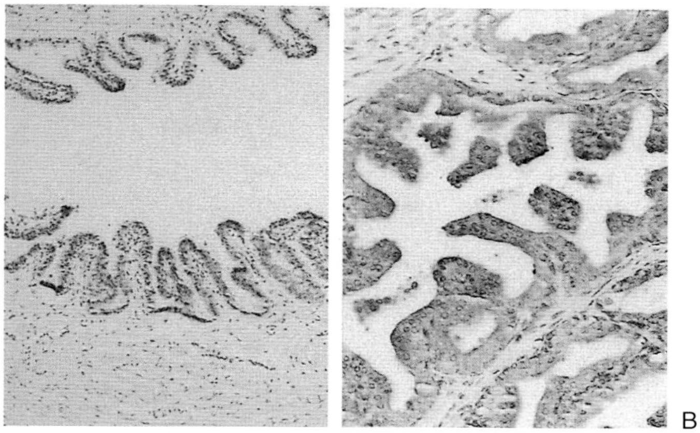

FIG. 31. Ejaculatory duct (**A**) and prostatic tissue (**B**). Prostate-specific antigen immunoperoxidase stain. This section is taken from the posterior aspect of the prostate just after the ejaculatory ducts penetrate the prostatic capsule.

## EJACULATORY DUCTS

The ejaculatory ducts are short (1.5 cm) paired ducts, arising from the confluence of the excretory duct of the seminal vesicle and the ampulla of the vas, that quickly converge and enter the prostate. They run through the prostatic parenchyma in a course parallel to and slightly posterior to the distal prostatic urethra (97) and enter the posterior aspect of the distal prostatic urethra at the verumontanum (Fig. 29). The outer portion of the ejaculatory ducts have a thin muscle coat that progressively becomes more attenuated as the ducts pass through the prostate. The epithelium of the ejaculatory ducts resembles that of the ampulla of the vas (Fig. 30). It is not uncommon to have within a needle biopsy of the prostate a portion of one or both of these ducts, making it imperative that the surgical pathologist be aware of the characteristics of these cells. The presence of lipofuscin pigment in the cytoplasm gives a clue to the cell origin. Immunoperoxidase stains for prostate-specific antigen demonstrate a sharp contrast between the positive-staining prostatic parenchyma and the negative-stained cells of the intraprostatic ejaculatory ducts (Fig. 31).

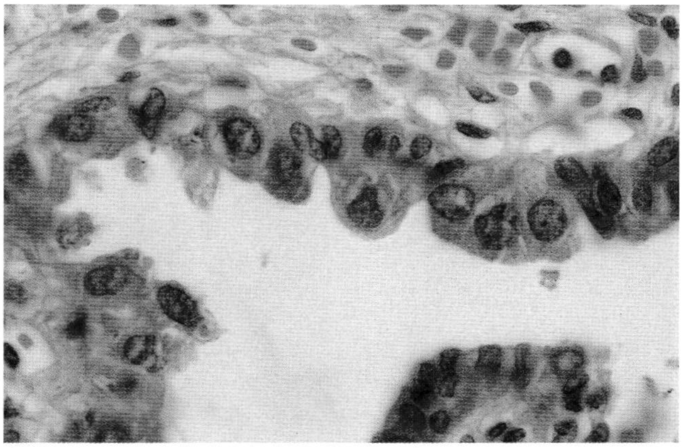

FIG. 30. Epithelium of prostatic portion of ejaculatory duct. This epithelium may be encountered in a needle biopsy or aspiration biopsy of the prostate and should not be misinterpreted as malignant.

## TESTICULAR APPENDAGES

The four testicular appendages are the appendix testis (hydatid of Morgagni), appendix epididymis, vas aberrans (organ of Haller), and paradidymis (organ of Giraldes) (Fig. 1).

The appendix testis, a remnant of the cranial portion of the müllerian duct, is attached to the tunica vaginalis on the anterosuperior aspect of the testis just below the head of the epididymis. Occasionally, it is attached to both the testis and the epididymis. It is most often pedunculated, oval, or fan shaped and measures 0.5 to 2.5 cm in greatest dimension (Fig. 32) (98). It is occasionally represented by only a slight roughening or a calcified thickening of the tunica vaginalis. Over 90% of individuals have an appendix testis, and two thirds of them have an appendix testis bilaterally. The appendix is covered by a columnar, usually nonciliated epithelium (Fig. 33). Rarely, the epithelium is cuboidal or focally stratified. The latter is particularly common near the base of the appendix. The structure has a highly vascular fibrous core, containing variable numbers of smooth muscle cells. The appendix is often associated with small, simple or branched tubules within the adjacent tunica vaginalis, at the epididymis–testis junction, or along the lateral aspect of the body of the epididymis. Rarely, a macroscopic cyst may be present. Because of its pedunculated structure, the appendix testis may become twisted, causing hemorrhagic infarction (99) and producing severe testicular pain.

The appendix epididymis (Fig. 34), a remnant of the most

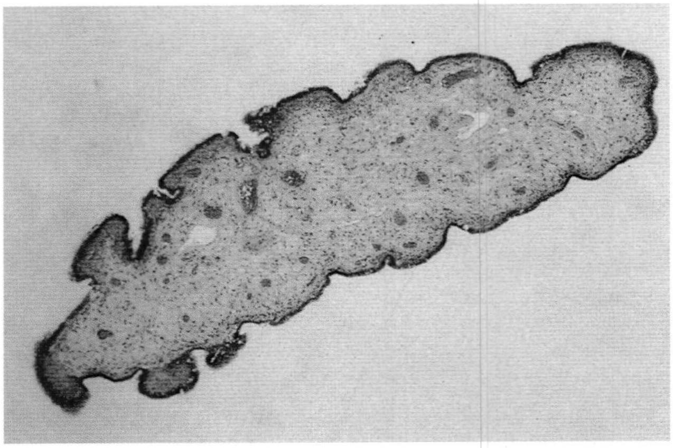

**FIG. 32.** Appendix testis. This specimen was an incidental finding in a surgically removed testis. It was pedunculated and measures 0.9 cm in greatest length.

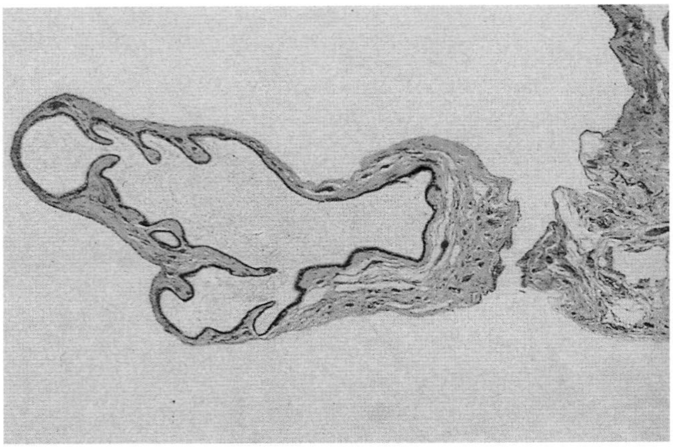

**FIG. 34.** Appendix epididymis. A pedunculated cystic structure is attached to the head of the epididymis.

cranial portion of the mesonephric duct, is present in approximately 25% of testes (100). It is almost invariably cystic, the vesicle lumen being filled with secretions derived from the columnar epithelial cells lining the cyst (Fig. 35). The external surface is covered by a flattened layer of serosal cells. Because it may be pedunculated, it is also subject to torsion and infarction.

The other appendicular structures are derived from remnants of the mesonephric tubules and are variably encountered, usually as microscopic incidental findings. These are the vas aberrans inferior, the vas aberrans superior, and the paradidymis. They all have similar histologic features, with a low columnar epithelium lining a small cystic space and a thin muscular coat. Some investigators collectively refer to these structures as the paradidymis (101). The vas aberrans inferior is a tubular structure (Fig. 36) that uncoiled may measure from 3.5 to 35.0 cm in length. It is located near the junction of the vas and the caudal portion of the epididymis and may or may not communicate with either the epididymis or the vas.

The vas aberrans superior is a small collection of tubules located near the head or body of the epididymis. It may communicate with the epididymis or the rete testis. Remnants of the vas aberrans may be the origin of epididymal cysts seen sporadically in isolated individuals, in patients whose mothers had been treated with diethylstilbestrol (102), or in patients with von Hippel-Lindau disease (103).

The paradidymis is represented by one or more tubules embedded in the spermatic cord, adjacent to the vas deferens, and near the head of the epididymis. These tubules may be encountered in a section of the wall of an inguinal hernia sac and should not be mistaken for a portion of the vas deferens (104). Rarely they may form small cysts in the spermatic cord (105).

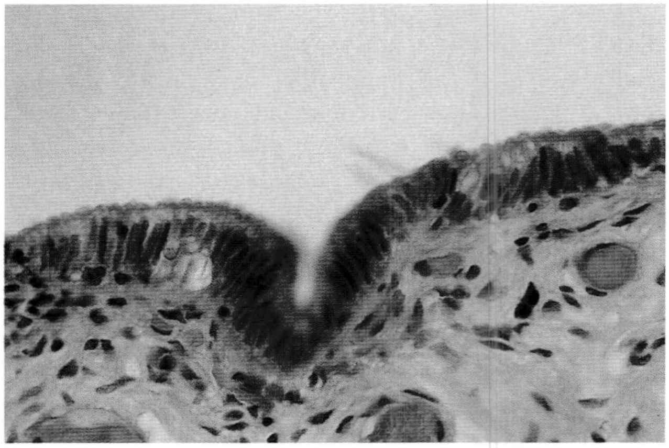

**FIG. 33.** Appendix testis with covering of low columnar, nonciliated epithelium.

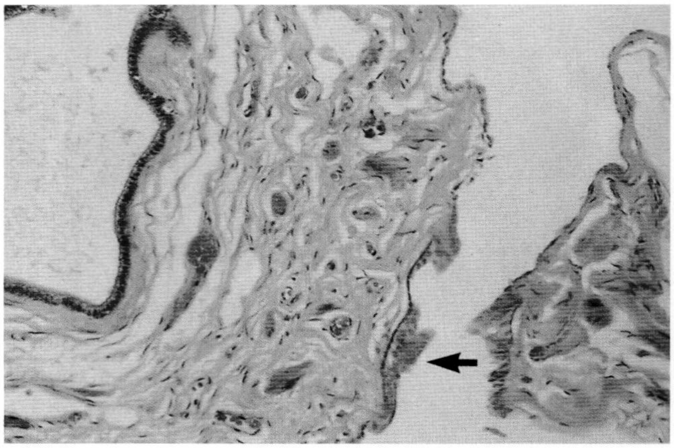

**FIG. 35.** Appendix epididymis. Low columnar epithelium lines cystic space. Outer covering of simple squamous epithelium has become stratified at the point of attachment to the head of the epididymis (*arrow*).

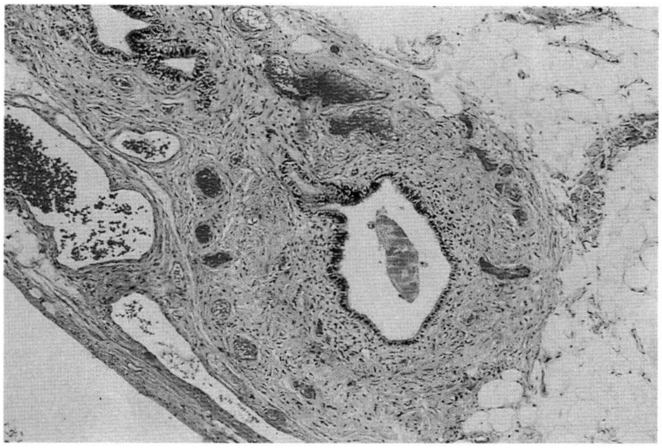

**FIG. 36.** Vas aberrans inferior. A tubular structure is found near the caudal portion of the epididymis.

## GUBERNACULUM

The gubernaculum has been the center of attention with respect to the descent of the testis since it was first described by John Hunter in 1762 and its specific role is still being debated (106). In the fetus this cylindrical, gelatinous structure is attached cranially to the testis and epididymis (Fig. 37) and caudally to the anterior abdominal wall at the site of the inguinal canal. Just before the descent of the testis through the inguinal canal, the gubernaculum increases in net weight disproportionately to the testis, supporting the theory that this structure plays a crucial role in this phase of the passage of the testis into the scrotum.

Histologically the fetal gubernaculum is composed of a loose undifferentiated mesenchymal tissue similar to Wharton's jelly. Large amounts of glycosoaminoglycans fill the extracellular space and separate the individual spindle cells. At the periphery of the gubernaculum where it attaches to the inguinal wall a few striated muscle cells can be identified. These fibers are derived from the developing cremasteric muscle. The cranial portion of the early fetal gubernaculum is completely devoid of striated muscle. After the testis descends into the scrotum, the gubernaculum undergoes degenerative changes, loses much of the intercellular matrix and becomes infiltrated by blood vessels, collagen fibers, and striated muscle.

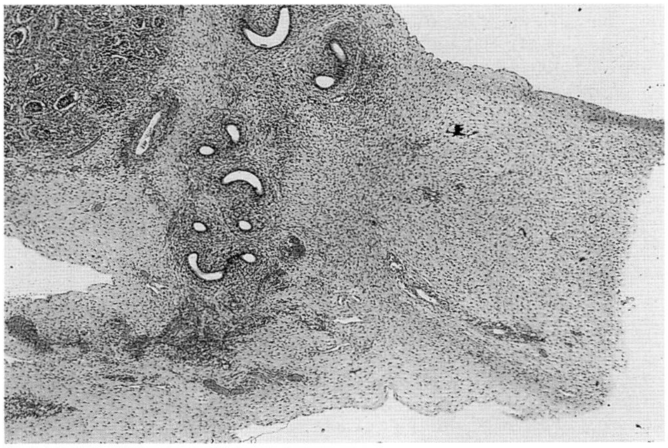

**FIG. 37.** Gubernaculum, cranial attachment to epididymis and testis. Fetus, 26 weeks.

## REFERENCES


1. Handelsman DJ, Stara S. Testicular size: the effects of aging, malnutrition, and illness. *J Androl* 1985;6:144–151.
2. Sosnik H. Studies of the participation of the tunica albuginea and rete testis (TA and RT) in the quantitative structure of human testis. *Gegenbaurs Morphol Jahrb* 1985;131:347–356.
3. Vilar O. Histology of the human testis from the neonatal period to adolescence. *Adv Exp Med Biol* 1970;10:95–111.
4. Lennox B, Ahmad RN, Mack WS. A method for determining the relative total length of the tubules in the testis. *J Pathol* 1970;102: 229–238.
5. Aumüller G, Schulze C, Viebahn C. Intermediate filaments in Sertoli cells. *Microsc Res Tech* 1992;20:50–72.
6. Nielsen K, Jacobsen GK. Malignant Sertoli cell tumor of the testis: an immunohistochemical study and a review of the literature. *APMIS* 1988;96:755–760.
7. Stosick P, Kasper M, Karsten U. Expression of cytokeratin 8 and 18 in human Sertoli cells of immature and atrophic seminiferous tubules. *Differentiation* 1990;43:66–70.
8. Vliegen M, Schlatt S, Weinbauer G. Bergmann M, Groome N, Nieschlag E. Localization of inhibin/activin in subunits in the testis of adult nonhuman primates and men. *Cell Tissue Res* 1993;273: 261–268.
9. Flemming P, Wellmann A, Maschek H, Lang H, Georgïi A. Monoclonal antibodies against inhibin represents key markers of adult granulosa cell tumors of the ovary even in their metastases. *Am J Surg Pathol* 1995;19:927–933.
10. Schulze C. Sertoli cells and Leydig cells in man. *Adv Anat Embryol Cell Biol* 1984.;88:1–104.
11. Dym M. The fine structure of the monkey (Macaca) Sertoli cell and its role in maintaining the blood–testis barrier. *Anat Rec* 1973;175: 639–656.
12. Russell LD, Peterson RN. Sertoli cell junctions: morphological and functional correlates. *Int Rev Cytol* 1985;94:177–211.
13. McLaren A. Studies on mouse germ cells inside and outside the gonad. *J Exp Zool* 1983;228:167–171.
14. Ritzen EM, Hansson V, French FS. The Sertoli cell. In: Burger H, de Kretser DM, eds. *The testis.* New York: Raven Press; 1981:171–194.
15. Witschi E. Migration of the germ cells of human embryos from the yolk sac to the primitive gonadal fold. *Carnegi Inst Wash Contrib Embryol* 1948;209:67–80.
16. Heller CG, Clermont Y. Kinetics of the germinal epithelium in man. *Rec Prog Horm Res* 1964;20:545–571.
17. Kerr, JB, de Kretser DM. The cytology of the human testis. In: Burger H, de Kretser DM, eds. *The testis.* New York: Raven Press; 1981: 141–169.
18. Clermont Y. Kinetics of spermatogenesis in mammals: seminiferous epithelium cycle and spermatogonial renewal. *Physiol Rev* 1972;52: 198–236.
19. Gondos B. Ultrastructure of developing and malignant germ cells. *Eur Urol* 1993;23:68–75.
20. Schulze W, Rehder U. Organization and morphogenesis of the human seminiferous epithelium. *Cell Tissue Res* 1984;237:395–407.
21. Schulze W, Riemer M, Rehder U, Hohne K. Computer-aided three-dimensional reconstructions of the arrangement of primary spermatocytes in human seminiferous tubules. *Cell Tissue Res* 1986;244:1–8.
22. Bartke A. [Editorial]. Apoptosis of male germ cells, a generalized or a cell type-specific phenomenon? *Endocrinology* 1995;136:3–4.
23. Billig H, Furata I, Rivier C, Tapanainen J, Parvinen M, Hsueh A. Apoptosis in testis germ cells: developmental changes in gonadotropin dependence and localization to selective tubule stages. *Endocrinology* 1995;136:5–12.
24. Hikim A, Wang C, Leung A, Swerdloff R. Involvement of apoptosis

in the induction of germ cell degeneration in adult rats after gonadotropin-releasing hormone antagonist treatment. *Endocrinology* 1995;136:2270–2775.
25. Trainer TD. Histology of the normal testis. *Am J Surg Pathol* 1987;11: 167–171.
26. Hadziselimovic F. Ultrastructure of normal and cryptorchid testes development. *Adv Anat Embryol Cell Biol* 1977;53:47–50.
27. Johnson L, Petty CS, Neaves WB. The relationship of biopsy evaluations and testicular measurements to over-all daily sperm production in human testes. *Fertil Steril* 1980;34:36–40.
28. Johnson SG. Testicular biopsy score count—a method for registration of spermatogenesis in human testis: normal values and results in 335 hypogonadal males. *Hormones* 1970;1:2–25.
29. Weissbach L, Ibach B. Quantitative parameters for light microscopic assessment of the tubuli seminiferi. *Fertil Steril* 1976;27:836–847.
30. Zuckerman Z, Rodriguez-Rigau L, Weiss D, Chowdhury AK, Smith KD, Steinberger E. Quantitative analysis of the seminiferous epithelium in human testicular biopsies, and the relation of spermatogenesis to sperm density. *Fertil Steril* 1978;30:448–455.
31. Skakkebaek NE, Heller CG. Quantification of human seminiferous epithelium. *J Reprod Fertil* 1973;32:379–389.
32. Silber SJ, Rodriguez-Rigau LJ. Quantitative analysis of testicular biopsy: determination of partial obstruction and prediction of sperm count after surgery for obstruction. *Fertil Steril* 1981;36:480–485.
33. Miller SC, Bowman BM, Kowland HG. Structure, cytochemistry, endocytic activity and immunoglobulin (Fc) receptors of rat testicular interstitial-tissue macrophages. *Am J Anat* 1983;168:1–13.
34. Hutson J. Testicular macrophages. *Int Rev Cytol* 1994;149:99–143.
35. Santamaria L, Martin R, Nistal M, Paniagua R. The peritubular myoid cell in the testis from men with varicocele: an ultrastructural, immunohistochemical and quantitative study. *Histopathology* 1992;21: 423–433.
36. Martin R, Santamaria L, Nistal M, Fraile B, Paniagua R. The peritubular myofibroblast in the testis from normal men and men with Klinefelter's syndrome. A quantitative, ultrastructural, and immunohistochemical study. *J Pathol* 1992;168:59–66.
37. DeMenczes AP. Elastic tissue in the limiting membrane of the human seminiferous tubule. *Am J Anat* 1977;150:349–374.
38. de Kretser DM, Kerr JB, Paulsen CA. The peritubular tissue in the normal and pathological human testis: an ultrastructural study. *Biol Reprod* 1975;12:317–324.
39. Nistal M, Paniagua R. Histogenesis of human extraparenchymal Leydig cells. *Acta Anat* 1979;105:188–197.
40. Prince F. Ultrastructural evidence of indirect and direct autonomic innervation of human Leydig cells: comparison of neonatal, childhood and pubertal ages. *Cell Tissue Res* 1992;269:383–390.
41. Regadera J, Codesal J, Paniagua R, Gonzalez-Peramato P, Nistal M. Immunohistochemical and quantitative study of interstitial and intratubular Leydig cells in normal men, cryptorchidism and Klinefelter's syndrome. *J Pathol* 1991:164:299–306.
42. Amat P, Paniagua R, Nistal M, Martin A. Mitosis in adult human Leydig cells. *Cell Tissue Res* 1986;243:219–221.
43. Naguno T, Ohtsuki I. Reinvestigation of the fine structure of Reinke crystal in the human testicular interstitial cell. *J Cell Biol* 1971;51: 148–160.
44. Weiss DB, Rodriguez-Rigau L, Smith KD, Chowdhury A, Steinberger E. Quantitation of Leydig cells in testicular biopsies of oligospermic men with varicocele. *Fertil Steril* 1978;30:305–312.
45. Heller CG, Lalli MF, Pearson JE, Leach DR. A method for the quantification of Leydig cells in man. *J Reprod Fertil* 1971;25:177–184.
46. Davidoff M, Schulze W, Midderidoff R, Hostein A. The Leydig cell of the human testis—a new member of the diffuse endocrine system. *Cell Tissue Res* 1993;271:429–439.
47. Holash J, Harik S. Barrier properties of the testis microvessels. *Proc Natl Acad Sci U S A* 1993;90:11069–11073.
48. Kormano M, Suoranta H, Reijonen K. Blood supply to testis and excurrent ducts. In: Raspe G, ed. *Advances in the biosciences.* Vol. 10. Oxford, England: Pergamon Press; 1972:72–83.
49. Andres T, Trainer T, Lapenas D. Small vessel alterations in the testes of infertile men with varicocele. *Am J Clin Pathol* 1981;76:378–384.
50. Fawcett DW, Leak LV, Heidger PM. Electron microscopic observations on the structural components of the blood–testis barrier. *J Reprod Fertil* 1979;22(suppl 10):105–122.
51. Ergüns S, Stingl S, Holstein A. Microvasculature of the human testis in correlation to Leydig cells and seminiferous tubules. *Andrologia* 1994;26:255–262.
52. Fawcett DW, Neaves WB, Flores MN. Comparative observations on intertubular lymphatics and the organization of the interstitial tissue of the mammalian testis. *Biol Reprod* 1973;9:500–532.
53. Hofmann M, Millan J. Developmental expression of alkaline phosphatase genes; reexpression in germ cell tumors and in vitro immortalized germ cells. *Eur Urol* 1993;23:38–45.
54. Jorgensen N, Rajpert-De Meyts E, Graem H, Müller J. Giwercman A, Skakkebaek N. Expression of immunological markers for testicular carcinoma in situ by normal human fetal cells. *Lab Invest* 1995;72: 223–231.
55. Nistal M, Paniagua R, Queizan A. Histological lesions in undescended ectopic obstructed testis. *Fertil Steril* 1985;43:455–462.
56. Waters B, Trainer T. The development of the fetal testis. *Pediatr Pathol Lab Med* 1996 (in press).
57. Muller J, Skakkebaek NE. Quantification of germ cells and seminiferous tubules by stereological examination of testicles from 50 boys who suffered sudden death. *Int J Androl* 1983;6:143–156.
58. Cortes D, Müller J, Skakkebaek NE. Proliferation of Sertoli cells during development of the human testis assessed by stereological methods. *Int J Androl* 1987;10:589–596.
59. Symington T, Cameron K. Endocrine and genetic lesions. In: Pugh CB, ed. *Pathology of the testis.* Oxford, England: Blackwell Scientific; 1976:259–303.
60. Prince FP. Ultrastructure of immature Leydig cells in the human prebubertal testis. *Anat Rec* 1984;209:165–176.
61. Nistal M, Paniagua R, Regadera J, Santamaria L, Amal P. A quantitative morphological study of human Leydig cells from birth to adulthood. *Cell Tissue Res* 1986;246:229–236.
62. Paniagua R, Nistal M, Amat P, Rodriguez M, Agustin M. Seminiferous tubule involution in elderly men. *Biol Reprod* 1987;36:939–947.
63. Johnson L, Petty CS, Neaves WB. Influence of age on sperm production and testicular weights in men. *J Reprod Fertil* 1984;70:211–218.
64. Neaves WB, Johnson L, Porter J, Parker RC, Petty CS. Leydig cell numbers, daily sperm count production, and serum gonadotropin levels in aging men. *J Clin Endocrinol Metab* 1984;59:756–763.
65. Suoranta H. Changes in the small blood vessels of the adult human testis in relation to age and to some pathological conditions. *Virchows Arch [A]* 1971;352:165–181.
66. Kothari LK, Gupta AS. Effect of ageing on the volume, structure and total Leydig cell content of the human testis. *Int J Fertil* 1974;19: 140–146.
67. Sokal Z. Morphology of the human testis in various periods of life. *Folia Morphol* 1964;23:102–111.
68. Sargent JW, McDonald JR. A method for the quantitative estimate of Leydig cells in the human testis. *Proc Staff Meetings Mayo Clin* 1948; 23:249–254.
69. Kaler LW, Neaves WB. Attrition of the human Leydig cell population with advancing age. *Anat Rec* 1978;192:513–518.
70. Neaves WB, Johnson L, Petty C. Seminiferous tubules and daily sperm production in older adult men with varied numbers of Leydig cells. *Biol Reprod* 1987;36:301–308.
71. Paniagua R, Nistal M, Saez F, Fraile B. The ultrastructure of the aging human testis. *J Electron Microsc Tech* 1991;19:241–260.
72. Rowley MJ, Heller CG. Quantitation of the cells of the seminiferous epithelium of the human testis employing the Sertoli cell as a constant. *Z Zellforsch Mikrosh Anat* 1971;115:461–472.
73. Steinberger A, Steinberger E. Replication pattern of Sertoli cells in maturing rat testis in vivo and organ culture. *Biol Reprod* 1971; 4:84–87.
74. Johnson L, Zane RS, Petty CS, Neaves WB. Quantification of the human Sertoli cell population: its distribution, relation to germ cell numbers, and age-related decline. *Biol Reprod* 1984;31:785–795.
75. Roosen-Runge EC, Holstein AF. The human rete testis. *Cell Tissue Res* 1978;189:409–433.
76. Dinges H, Zatloukal K, Schmid C, Mair S, Wirnsherger G. Co-expression of cytokeratin and vimentin filaments in rete testis and epididymis. *Virchows Arch [A]* 1991;418:119–127.
77. Hartwick RY, Ro J, Srigley J, Ondoñez N, Ayul A. Adenomatous hyperplasia of the rete testis: a clinicopathological study of nine cases. *Am J Surg Pathol* 1991;15:350–357.
78. Setchel PB. Secretions of the testis and epididymis. *J Reprod Fertil* 1974;37:165–177.

79. Hinton BT, Keefer DA. Evidence for protein absorption from the lumen of the seminiferous tubule and rete of the rat testis. *Cell Tissue Res* 1983;230:367–375.
80. Hermo L, Morales C. Endocytosis in nonciliated epithelial cells of the ductuli efferentes in the rat. *Am J Anat* 1984;171:59–74.
81. Kuo T, Gomez LG. Monstrous epithelial cells in human epididymis and seminal vesicles: a pseudomalignant change. *Am J Surg Pathol* 1981;5:483–490.
82. Maneely RB. Epididymal structure and function. A historical and critical review. *Acta Zool* 1959;40:1–21.
83. Rowley MJ, Teshima F, Heller CB. Duration of transit of spermatozoa through the human male ductular system. *Fertil Steril* 1970;21: 390–395.
84. Hinrichsen MJ, Blagaier JA. Evidence supporting the existence of sperm maturation in the human epididymis. *J Reprod Fertil* 1980;60: 291–294.
85. Regardera J, Cobo P, Paniagua R, Martinez-Garcia F, Placios J, Nistal M. Immunohistochemical and semiquantitative study of the apical mitochondria-rich cells of the human prebubertal and adult epididymis. *J Anat* 1993;183:507–514.
86. Kasper M, Stosick P. Immunohistochemical investigation of different cytokeratins and vimentin in the human epididymis from the fetal period up to adulthood. *Cell Tissue Res* 1989;257:661–664.
87. Yeung C, Nashan D, Sorg C, et al. Basal cells of the human epididymis—antigenic and ultrastuctural similarities to tissue-fixed macrophages. *Biol Reprod* 1994;50:917–926.
88. Rajalakshmi B, Kumar K, Kapur M, Pal P. Ultrastructural changes in the efferent duct and epididymis of men with obstructive infertility. *Anat Rec* 1993;237:199–207.
89. Madara JL, Haggitt RC, Federman M. Intranuclear inclusions of the human vas deferens. *Arch Pathol Lab Med* 1978;102:648–650.
90. Gilmour JR. Intranuclear inclusions in the epithelium of the human male genital tract. *Lancet* 1937;1:373–375.
91. Nistal M, Santamaria L, Paniagua R. Mast cells in the human testis and epididymis from birth to adulthood. *Acta Anat* 1984;119: 155–160.
92. Paniagua R, Regadera J, Nistal M, Abaurrea MA. Histological, histochemical and ultrastructural variations along the length of the human vas deferens before and after puberty. *Acta Anat* 1981;111:190–203.
93. Paniagua R, Regadera J, Nistal M, Santamaria L. Elastic fibres of the human ductus deferens. *J Anat* 1983;137:467–476.
94. Murakami M, Nishida T, Shiromoto M, Inokuchi T. Scanning and transmission electron microscopic study of the ampullary region of the dog vas deferens, with special reference to epithelial phagocytosis of spermatozoa and latex beads. *Anat Anz* 1986;162:289–296.
95. Riva A. Fine structure of human seminal vesicle epithelium. *J Anat* 1967;102:71–86.
96. Kovi J, Jackson MA, Akberzie ME. Unusual smooth muscle change in the prostate. *Arch Pathol Lab Med* 1979;103:204–205.
97. McNeal JE. Normal histology of the prostate. *Am J Surg Pathol* 1988; 12:634–640.
98. Sundarasivarao D. The müllerian vestiges and benign epithelial tumors of the epididymis. *J Pathos Bacterial* 1953;LEVI:417–432.
99. Skoglund RW, McRoberts JW, Ragde H. Torsion of testicular appendages: presentation of 43 new cases and a collective review. *J Urol* 1970;104:598–600.
100. Rolnick D, Kawanoue S, Szanto P, Bush IM. Anatomical incidence of testicular appendages. *J Urol* 1988;100:755–756.
101. Sadler TW. *Langman's medical embryology.* 5th ed. Baltimore: Williams & Wilkins; 1985:264.
102. Whitehead ED, Leiter E. Genital abnormalities and abnormal semen analysis in male patients exposed to diethylstilbesterol in utero. *J Urol* 1981;125:47–51.
103. Bernstein J, Gardner KD Jr. Renal cystic disease and renal dysplasia. In: Walsh PC, Gittes RF, Permutter AD, Stamey TA, eds. *Campbells urology.* Vol. 2. Philadelphia: WB Saunders; 1986:1760–1803.
104. Popek E. Embryonal remnants in inguinal hernia sacs. *Hum Pathol* 1990;21:339–349.
105. Wollin M, Marshall F, Fink M, Malhotra R, Diamond D. Aberrant epididymal tissue: a significant clinical entity. *J Urol* 1987;138: 1247–1250.
106. Heyns C. The gubernaculum during testicular descent in the human fetus. *J Anat* 1987;153:93–112.

*Histology for Pathologists, second edition,*
Edited by Stephen S. Sternberg.
Lippincott-Raven Publishers, Philadelphia


# CHAPTER 44

# Penis

José Barreto, Carmelo Caballero, and Antonio Cubilla



The penis is a special organ where different types of tissues converge. This diversity is reflected in the various diseases affecting this anatomic site. Urologists are the most commonly consulted physicians for penile disorders, but significant pathologic processes often need to be discussed, diagnosed, or treated by internists, dermatologists, pediatricians, pathologists, oncologic surgeons, radiotherapists, clinical oncologists, plastic surgeons, or laser specialists. The old methods of visual physical examination are now supplemented by studies of cavernosography, ultrasonography, angiography, peniscopy (1,2), or cross sections or longitudinal sections of computed tomography (CT), magnetic resonance imaging (MRI), or complex physiologic dynamic studies of erectile tissue (3–6). Deeply located, mysterious, and not totally understood structures such as Cowper's, Littre's, and Tyson's glands (7,8), Morgagni's lacunae, Buck's fascia, albuginea, dartos, and polsters are now being questioned or precisely identified by these new methods or by more objective morphologic evaluation (3,9).

The interest in the pathology of penile cancer, still frequent in certain parts of the world (10,11), is being renewed and emphasizes the need for adequate gross and microscopic descriptions of anatomic compartments of the organ to understand better the biology of the cancer, predict prognosis, and plan for proper treatment (12). The recent interest and advancement of knowledge of viral diseases such as bowenoid papulosis (13), human papillomavirus–related female uterine cervical lesions (14,15), the corresponding alterations of penile surface epithelium of their sexual partners (16,17), the question of potency and methods for achieving adequate erections (18,19), penile prostheses, and the transsexual surgery revolution (20) have created the need for a more detailed knowledge of the anatomy of the penis.

## GROSS ANATOMY

Three cylindrical, firmly adherent, tubular erectile tissues are the basic constituents of the penis. The foreskin and penis proper are the two principal components; the latter is subdivided into the glans, coronal sulcus, and corpus or shaft. The conically shaped glans, covered by a pink smooth mucous membrane, is the distal portion of the organ and shows in its central and ventral region the meatus urethralis. The erectile and spongy corpus spongiosum is the central and main tissue of the glans. Within the corpus spongiosum we find the distal two-thirds of the urethra (Fig. 1). In fact, the corpus spongiosum originates its anteroposterior course in the urethral bulb, just at the point where the urethra leaves its membranous portion, always surrounding the urethra and terminating as a conical cup over the anterior end of the penis. The base of this conus is an elevated rim or border, the corona, occupying 80% of the head of the glans. The diameter of the corona is superior to that of the corpus. Behind the corona we find the coronal sulcus (Fig. 2), with length and disposition identical to that of the corona. The mucous membrane of the glans continues to cover this region as well as the inner surface of the foreskin. The penile shaft or corpus of the penis is composed of two corpora cavernosa. This

J. Barreto and C. Caballero: Department of Pathology, Hospital del Cancer, Capiata, Paraguay.
A. Cubilla: Department of Pathology, Facultad de Ciencias Médicas, Asunción, Paraguay.

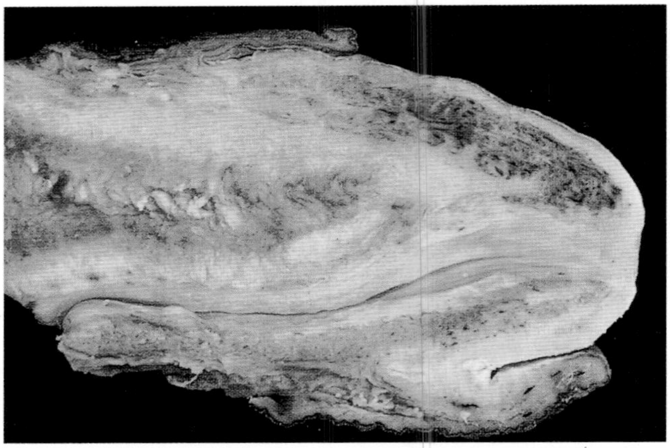

A

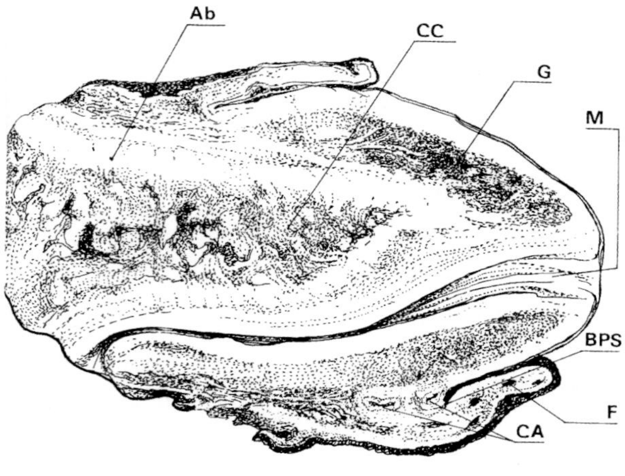


B

**FIG. 1.** Partial penectomy specimen from a 55-year-old man with a small in situ and infiltrating epidermoid carcinoma (CA) located in the balanopreputial sulcus (BPS). Longitudinal section of distal end of the penis shows the glans (G), urethral meatus (M), foreskin (F), and anterior end of the corpora cavernosa (CC). The albuginea (Ab) is also seen.

wide net of vascular spaces is surrounded by a thick, firm, resistant, fibrous covering called the albuginea. Both corpora cavernosa are inserted in the ischiopubic bone from where they converge to fuse up and above at the level of the inferior portion of the pubic symphysis. From this point the corpora cavernosa firmly adhere to each other with wide vascular communications. The corpus spongiosum and central urethra are located in the concave space of both corpora cavernosa. All these structures are covered by a thin, delicate, and elastic skin. Beneath the dermis there is a smooth discontinuous muscle layer called the dartos. Between the albuginea and the dartos there is a highly elastic tubelike sheath encasing all three corpora cavernosa and spongiosum, designated as Buck's fascia (Fig. 2). This fascia separates the penis into its dorsal (corpora cavernosa) and ventral (corpus spongiosum) portions as can be seen via CT or MRI (3). Vascular structures and peripheral nerves run within this fibrous and elastic tissue. The skin slides over this fascia. The foreskin is the prolongation of the shaft's skin and normally covers most of the glans, reflecting beyond itself and transforming into a mucosal inner surface. This mucous membrane covers the coronal sulcus as well as the surface of the glans (Fig. 3).

## Arteries

The arteries of the penis are branches of the internal pudenda, which is a branch of the iliac. There are two systems: the dorsal and the cavernous arteries. The dorsal arteries are located from the base of the penis near and on both sides of the dorsal profunda vein within Buck's fascia and in the superior groove formed by the corpora cavernosa (Fig. 4).

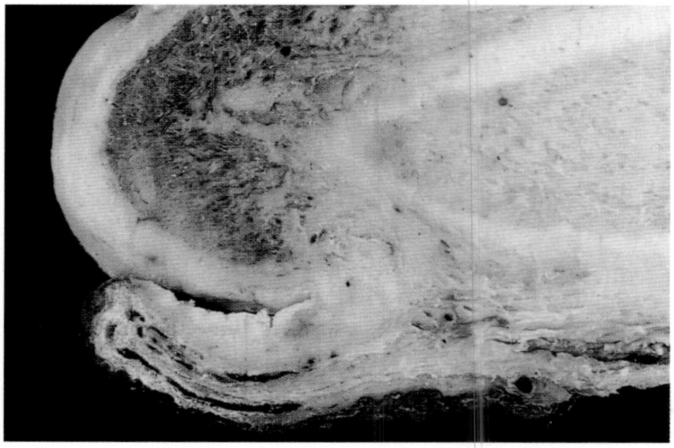

A

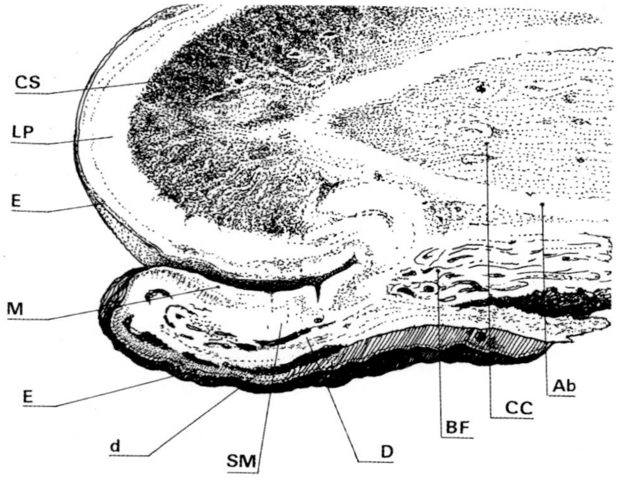


B

**FIG. 2.** A section parallel to that shown in Fig. 1 of the glans epithelium (E), lamina propria (LP), and corpus spongiosum (CS). Note all five foreskin layers: epidermis (E), dermis (d), dartos (D), submucosa (SM), and mucosa (M). The corpus cavernosum (CC) shows the thick albuginea (Ab). Buck's fascia (BF) is also seen.

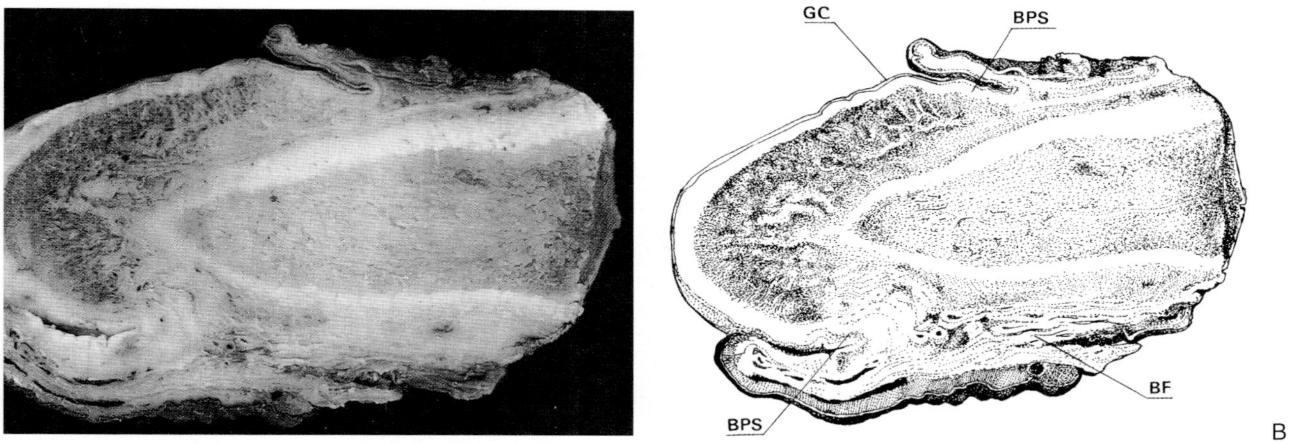


**FIG. 3.** In another section of the same specimen the Buck's fascia (BF) is better noted ending at the level of the balanopreputial sulcus (BPS). The glans corona (GC) is also seen.

Small-caliber branches, or circumflex arteries, irrigate the corpora cavernosa and the periurethral corpus spongiosum. They also perforate the albuginea to reach the corpora. The terminal branches irrigate the glans, and collateral branches are the skin nutrients. Cavernous arteries penetrate the corpora cavernosa at the site where the corpora join, and they run longitudinally near the central septum, which divides the corpora. From the cavernous arteries originate the vasa vasorum, small arteries that irrigate the erectile tissues. The helicine branches also originate from the cavernous arteries, and they are responsible for filling the vascular spaces during the process of erection (21,22).

## Veins

The superficial veins are irregularly distributed and easily noted under the skin. They end in the superficial dorsal vein; this vascular structure runs straight from the foreskin to the base of the penis. It drains the foreskin venous blood and the skin and is located in the space between the dermis and Buck's fascia. The deeper venous system, whose axis is the deep dorsal vein, runs along the superficial dorsal vein but in a plane separated by the Buck's fascia. The circumflex veins originate in the periurethral corpus spongiosum and terminate in the deep dorsal vein system. Similarly, there are veins originating in the corpora cavernosa that, after forming a small plexus at the base of the penis, terminate in the internal pudenda vein.

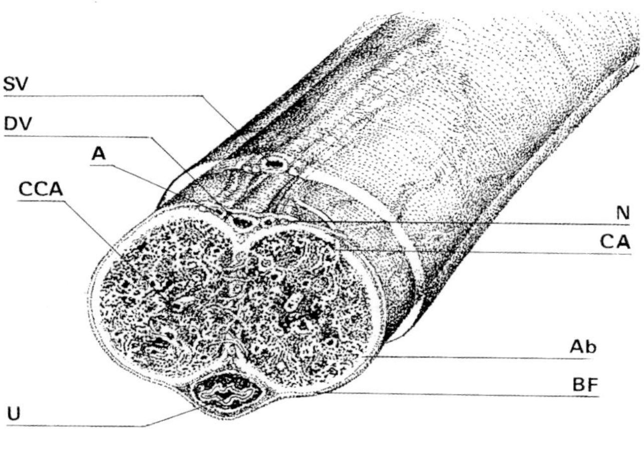


**FIG. 4.** Cross section of the penis. Diagram showing the location of arteries (A), nerves (N), superficial dorsal vein (SV), deep dorsal vein (DV), circumflex artery (CA), and cavernous artery (CCA). The Buck's fascia (BF), albuginea (Ab), and urethra (U) are also noted.

## Lymphatics

The lymphatics of the foreskin spring from a network that covers its internal and external surfaces; they arise from the lateral aspect and converge dorsally with the skin of the shaft lymphatics to form four to 10 vessels that run toward the pubis; here they diverge to drain into the right and left superficial inguinal lymph nodes. The lymphatics draining the glands form a rich network that, beginning in the lamina propia, course toward the frenulum where they coalesce with two or three trunks from the distal urethra to form several collecting trunks following the coronal sulcus. A collar of lymphatics entirely surrounds the corona, forming two or three trunks that run along the dorsal surface of the penis deep to the fascia along together with the deep dorsal vein. At the presymphyseal region they form a rich anastomosing plexus draining into superficial and deep inguinal lymph nodes (23). The lymphatics of the urethra, corpus spongiosum, and corpora cavernosa run toward the ventral surface of the body of the penis, reaching the raphe and the dorsum, where they run with the dorsal vein ending in the superficial and deep inguinal lymph nodes.

## Nerves

The nerves originate in the sacral and lumbar plexuses. Peripheral nerves run along the arteries. Dorsal nerves are located external to the arteries, giving circumflex branches to the corpora cavernosa. The terminal branches end in the glans and foreskin.

## MICROSCOPIC ANATOMY

### Glans

#### *Epithelium*

The glans is covered in the uncircumsized male by a thin, nonkeratinized, stratified squamous epithelium five- to six-cell layers thick. After circumcision the epithelium becomes keratinized. Under various pathologic conditions a thin granular layer with some keratinization can be present. The superficial cells contain no glycogen (Fig. 5).

In inflammatory conditions and adjacent to neoplastic processes it is not uncommon to find acanthosis or nonspecific squamous cell hyperplasia of the prickle cell layer. Dysplasia or carcinoma in situ are also lesions noted in this layer (24). A common interesting type of squamous carcinoma originating in this layer is the surface spreading carcinoma. An extensive centrifugal spread of carcinoma in situ surrounds an invasive focus, usually involving the glans, sulcus, or foreskin. There is a suggestion of a whole field (squamous mucosa of glans, sulcus, and foreskin) prone to malignant transformation. From the point of view of a surgical pathologist's histology, this area should be considered as one tissue compartment (25).

In some patients with or without circumcision, small pigmented lesions in the glans can be noted. They correspond usually to benign common lentigos (26) or junctional nevi. In the corona of the glans (mainly in its dorsal aspect) of sexually active individuals, small pediculated 1- to 2-mm lesions are commonly seen; they are painless, either isolated or multiple, and lined in orderly fashion. Histologically they are covered by keratinized squamous epithelium with a fibrous tissue stalk and are called hirsutoid papillomas or papillomatosis corona penis or glandis (27–29) (Fig. 6).

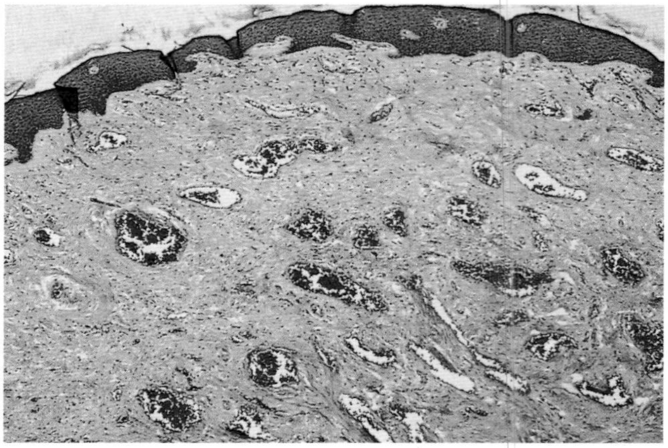

**FIG. 5.** The three layers of the glans are noted: nonkeratinized stratified mucosa, lamina propria, and corpus spongiosum.

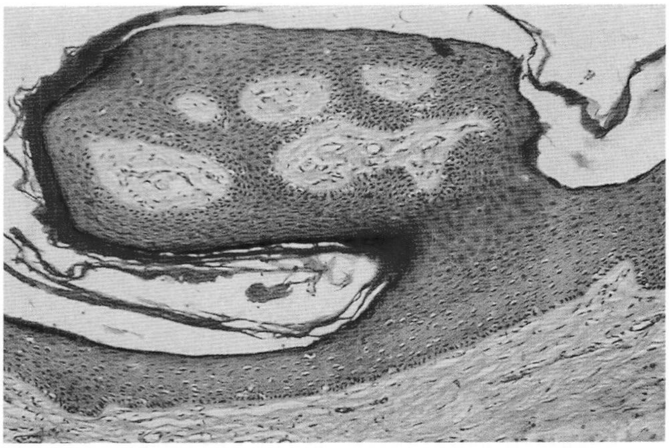

**FIG. 6.** Glans corona with a small papilloma, a common finding. This structure is covered by keratinized stratified squamous epithelium.

The normal papillae, round and wide, may become atrophic or even disappear in cases of fibrosis of the lamina propria and in balanitis xerotica obliterans. Rarely, embryologically misplaced mucus-producing cells can be noted in the glans epithelium, in the perimeatal region. They may be the source of the adenosquamous carcinoma of the glans penis. No adnexal or glandular structures are noted in the glans.

#### *Lamina Propria*

Lamina propia or chorion is the prolongation of the loose connective tissue of the foreskin submucosa or lamina propria, forming a sort of aponeurosis encasing and separating the corpus spongiosum from the glans epithelium. It measures approximately 2 to 3 mm in depth. This loose connective fibrous tissue is somewhat similar to the connective tissue of the corpus spongiosum, although it is more compact and contains fewer peripheral nerve bundles than the erectile structure. The transition between lamina propria and corpus spongiosum is sometimes difficult to determine at higher or medium magnifications. However, at low power or even after a careful gross inspection or with a magnifying lens, this delimitation is evident and follows a line corresponding to the geographic limit of the extension of venous sinuses of the corpus spongiosum (Fig. 5). The thickness of the lamina propria varies from 1 mm at the glans corona to 2.5 mm near the meatus (Fig. 1).

We did not observe while using routine stains any specialized nerve ending in the lamina propria such as Meissner or Golgi-Manzoni bodies, as previous reports have noted (30,31).

#### *Corpus Spongiosum*

Corpus spongiosum is the principal tissue component of the glans penis and is composed of specialized venous sinuses. These vascular spaces of variable caliber are lined by endothelial cells and are surrounded by a thin layer of smooth muscle fibers. These fibers coalesce in various extraluminal parts of the vessels to form the subendothelial cushions or polsters. The vascular spaces are widely interconnected with each other because of the branching structure and are continuous with the general venous system. These cavities are larger near the surface, whereas toward the axis of the urethra they are short and narrow (32). It is a unique and discrete vascular space with numerous collaterals (Fig. 7). Contrary to the corpora cavernosa, the interstitial fibrous connective tissue is more abundant in the corpus spongiosum. It is a loose fibrous tissue containing many nerve endings and lymphatic vessels. In this erectile tissue we find, although in fewer numbers, the usual type of blood vessels. The corpus spongiosum surrounding the urethra forms the urethral bulb, which is surrounded by the albuginea, which invaginates as a septum and can be noted via MRI (3).

### Coronal Sulcus

The coronal sulcus is a narrow and circumferential cul de sac located behind the glans corona. It is found in both lateral and dorsal aspects of the penis, but not in the ventral region, which is occupied by the frenulum, a mucosal fold that fixes the foreskin to the inferior portion of the glans, just below the urethral meatus. There are three histologic layers: (a) the epithelium or squamous mucosa, identical to the glans epithelium; (b) a thin lamina propria or corion, which is a prolongation of the foreskin and glans lamina propria; and (c) the point of insertion of smooth muscle fibers coming from the penile body or dartos (Fig. 8).

The coronal sulcus has been reported as the most frequent site of so-called Tyson's glands (31,33–38), described as modified sebaceous glands and reported as responsible for smegma production. Smegma represents epithelial debris and secretions collected in this space (39). There has been some question about the existence of the Tyson's glands (39,40). Several studies with numerous tissue sections failed to demonstrate these glands (39,41,42). We could not find Tyson's glands in a pathologic study of 65 sectioned penises removed for carcinoma of the penis. Apparently the original descriptions by Tyson (43) were based on an animal study that could not be confirmed in humans. After circumcision, occasionally some sebaceous glands can be found in the mucosa adjacent to the skin. They are probably skin sebaceous glands misplaced after surgery.

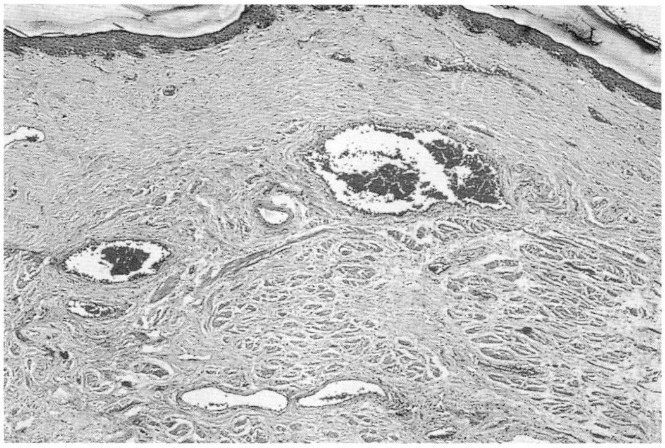

**FIG. 8.** A low-power view of coronal sulcus. Histologic components of both glans and peneal body are present. This specimen from a circumcised person shows the mucosa at top, lamina propria below, then dartos, or smooth muscle layer and Buck's fascia.

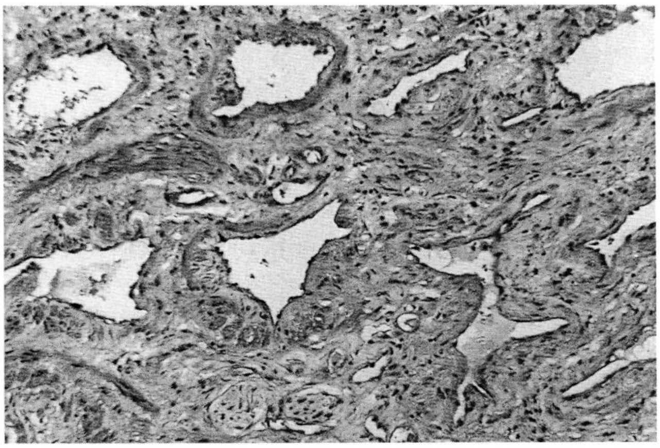

**FIG. 7.** Glans: higher view of the corpus spongiosum. The vascular spaces are irregularly shaped and are lined by endothelial cells. A fairly organized longitudinal smooth muscle layer is noted around the vessels. Some isolated branches of smooth muscle fibers can be seen. There are also some small peripheral nerves branches. Interstitial connective tissue is more abundant than in corpora cavernosa.

### Foreskin (or Prepuce)

Most newborn males show an unretracted foreskin at the time of delivery (44). The meatus is not seen unless some retractive manipulation is done. During this period there exists a certain adherence between the glans and the preputial inner surfaces, but the phenomenon gradually decreases with aging. When boys reach the age of 5 to 6 years the foreskin can be completely retracted beyond the level of the glans corona, but in some cases this can be done only at puberty. Circumcision, a type of surgery known to mankind as early as 12,000 B.C. and practiced for religious or tribal rites by, among others, Egyptians, Jews, Muslims, and Aztecs (45,46), has been practiced and recommended in more recent years for hygienic reasons and to prevent penile cancer. However, in 1975 the American Academy of Pediatrics no longer backed this recommendation (47,48). Recently some people are again proposing circumcision because the mucosal inner surface of the foreskin from newborns shows a propensity to be colonized by fimbriated bacteria and the subsequent occurrence of serious urinary tract infection (47). For this reason it has been postulated that the prepuce could be a mistake of nature (48). In adult populations, the variable length of the foreskin has motivated some studies, especially those related to the relation of length and amount of smegma in the balanopreputial sulcus (46,49,50).

Congenital phimosis is found in 4% of boys 6 to 17 years of age, but with a diminishing incidence in later years, from 8% in the 6- to 7-year-old group to 1% in the 16- to 17-year-old group (49). In nonphimotic boys, where the preputial space can be inspected, smegma is present in 5% of the cases. Production of smegma appears to increase in quantity in the 16- to 17-year-old group (49). Because of the prominent vascular network, the prepuce can be used by plastic surgeons to correct hypospadias.

There are five layers in the histologic evaluation of the foreskin:

1. The epidermis, which is similar to the one described earlier.
2. The dermis, which is the typical skin dermis showing some Vater-Pacinian bodies. Few sebaceous and sweat glands are noted, and they are not present beyond the dartos.
3. The dartos, which is a smooth muscle fiber layer and is the central axis of the foreskin. Similar to the penile body dartos, the smooth muscle fibers vary in their disposition. At the level of the edge of the foreskin, the fibers are transversely arranged to form a sphincter to close this edge over the anterior end of the glans. There are numerous nerve endings in close association with the smooth muscle fibers. Nerve bundle density in the foreskin was noted to be highest in the ventral preputial tissue (mean 17.9 bundles/nm) as opposed to lateral (8.6/nm) or dorsal (6.2/nm) (51).
4. The lamina propria or corion is similar to the glans lamina propria but contains more elastic fibers. There are no sebaceous or sweat gland-type glandular structures.
5. The mucosa, which is identical to and a prolongation of the common squamous mucosa of the glans and coronal sulcus, except that the basal layer shows a progressive pigmentation toward the free edge of the foreskin, where it reaches the skin epidermis (Fig. 9).

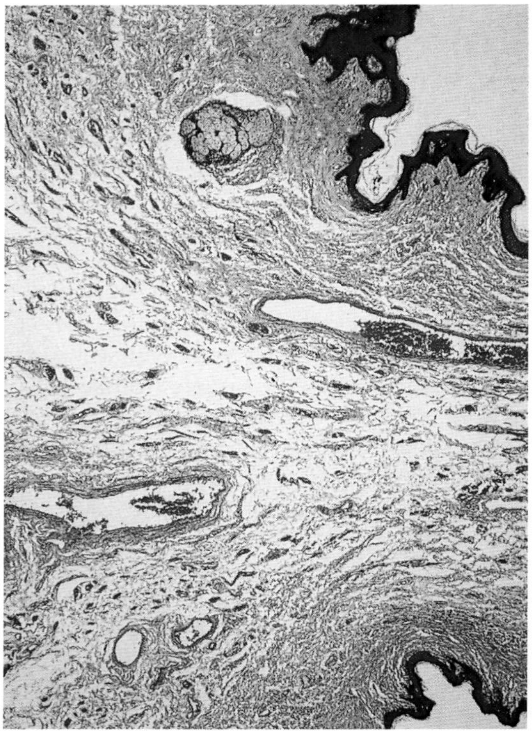

**FIG. 9.** Foreskin. Full-thickness of prepuce shows all five layers: keratinized stratified squamous epithelium, dermis with sebaceous glands, dartos, submucosa, and squamous mucosa.

### Penile Body or Shaft

The skin is rugged and elastic. It shows a thin epidermis composed of a few cell layers and minimal keratinization. The epidermal papillae are thin and deep. The basal layer is hyperpigmented. There are hair follicles in the dermis in only the proximal half of the penile body. They are scanty and contain no piloerector muscle. There are a few sebaceous glands, not related to hair follicles. There are also poorly developed sweat glands.

The penile dartos is composed of a discontinuous layer of smooth muscle fibers, variably arranged in transverse and longitudinal branches, separated from each other by fibrous connective tissue. At the level of the balanopreputial sulcus are some fibers, but others run farther to become the preputial dartos. The penile dartos, similar to scrotal smooth muscle fibers, produces a retraction of genital structures when the exterior temperature falls. The penile dartos is the skin equivalent of the penile hypodermis, but without adipose tissue. Buck's fascia is a fibroelastic continuous membrane that encases the corpora cavernosa and the corpus spongiosum. The yellow color is related to the numerous elastic fibers present in the fascia. Most blood vessels and nerves of the penis run within Buck's fascia. Its flexibility allows the skin to slide over the penile body. Some investigators point to Buck's fascia as the site of origin of Peyronie's disease (52). It is thinner than albuginea.

The tunica albuginea is a thick sheath of partially hyalinized collagen fibers covering both the corpora cavernosa and corpus spongiosum. It variably terminates in a V-shaped pattern within the coronal sulcus, at the level of coronal sulcus or behind it. The tunica albuginea enveloping the corpora cavernosa is thicker than that enveloping the corpus spongiosum as seen via MRI (3). In the flaccid state it measures 2 to 3 mm in thickness. It is composed mainly of collagen fibers arranged longitudinally in the external branches and in a circular fashion in the inner portion (31). The outer layer, which appears to determine the variation in the thickness and strength of the tunica, is absent in the ventral portion of the corpus spongiosum, transforming this portion of tunica in a vulnerable area to perforation. This anatomic aspect proba-

A 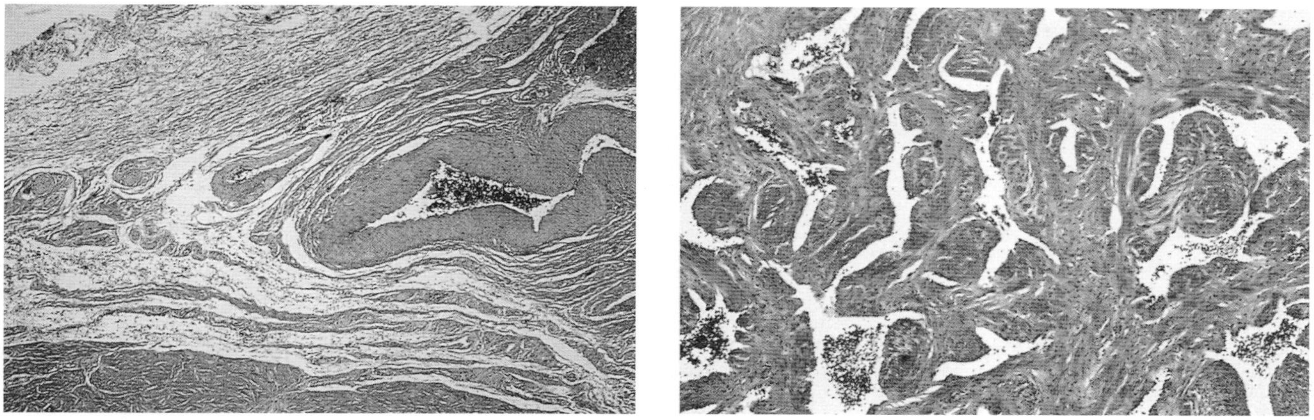 B

**FIG. 10.** Penile body. **A:** The outer layer corresponds to Buck's fascia containing nerves and vessels. Below it is the thin connective tissue of albuginea. In the central portion is the corpus spongiosum. **B:** There are numerous vascular spaces with irregularly shaped lumina, lined by endothelial cells and surrounded by smooth muscle layer. Note the thin smooth muscle layer arranged as subendothelial "polsters" or cushions.

bly explains why most prostheses tend to extrude in this area (53). The collagen fibers are wavy in the flaccid state and become straight during erection. The tunica albuginea forms an incomplete fibrous septum separating both corpora cavernosa. The fibers are arranged in such a way so as to permit some elasticity necessary for erection. Elastic fibers are rare, however. In the erect state it can become very thin (0.5 mm) and somewhat fragile. This structure is poorly vascular, with only a few branches of circumflex vessels crossing the albuginea as demostrated by factor VIII and CD34 antibody staining. The tunica albuginea surrounding the urethral corpus spongiosum is much thinner than the one around the corpora cavernosa, showing also more elastic fibers at this level. The tunica albuginea is probably the real barrier to infiltration of epidermoid carcinoma. Previously Buck's fascia was considered the barrier to the spread of the cancer (54). In some unusual cases of Fournier's gangrene (55), an infection of the lower urinary tract can spread to the corpus spongiosum. Eventually the tunica albuginea may be penetrated, and with involvement of Buck's fascia (Fig. 10) the infection can rapidly spread to the dartos and directly extend to Colles' scrotal fascia and Scarpa's fascia of the anterior abdominal wall. The infection can spread to the buttocks, thigh, and ischiorectal space (56).

The corpora cavernosa are the main anatomic structures used during erection. They consist of numerous vascular spaces with wide and irregularly shaped lumina, lined by endothelial cells and surrounded, like the erectile tissues in the corpus spongiosum, by a thin smooth muscle layer (Fig. 11). There is a highly structured criss-crossing of interconnected fibers and spaces that are tensed as the cylinder expands during erection (18,57). This creates an internal strength and rigidity that is far greater than that possible in a hollow tube filled to equivalent pressure. This specialized network appears to be necessary for erection (57). The interconnection between the venous sinuses is so wide that if a contrast is injected at one point, both corpora cavernosa can be immediately and completely visualized. The venous sinuses are wider in the central area than in the periphery. In the flaccid state the vascular spaces are 1-mm slits that increase several times in diameter with erection. The main difference between the corpora cavernosa and corpus spongiosum is that in the latter the interstitial connective tissue is abundant, whereas it is scanty in the former.

A progressive increase of collagen fibers and decrease of smooth muscle and elastic fiber may be seen over the course of time (58). High concentrations of vasoactive intestinal peptides (VIPs) were detected by immunocytochemistry and radioimmunoassay in the erectile tissue of 30 surgical specimens obtained after gender reassignment operation (20). In diabetic patients a complete absence of VIPs in nerves is noted (59). Corpora cavernosum endothelial cells synthetize

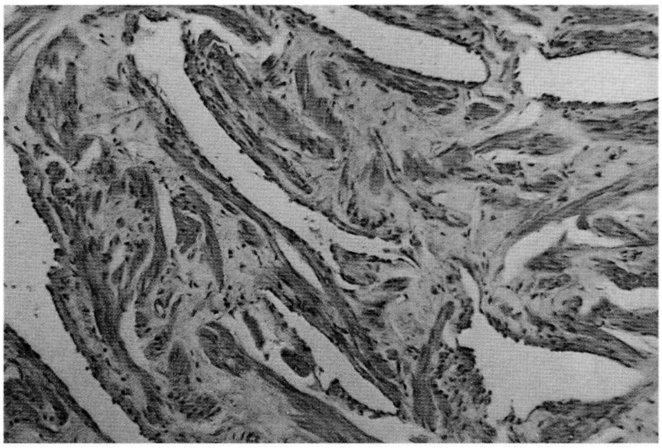

**FIG. 11.** Corpus cavernosum. There are numerous elongated vascular channels. Smooth muscle fibers around vessels and mainly in the interstitial space are arranged in a disorderly manner. Connective tissue is not abundant.

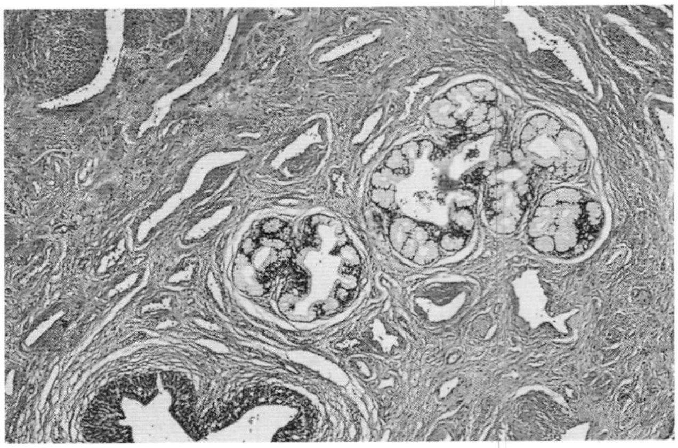

**FIG. 12.** Cross section of penile urethra. Note the stellate-shaped mucosa with stratified ciliated cylindric epithelium. There is a basal membrane separating it from lamina propria, composed of connective tissue and capillaries. Note Littre's mucous glands.

and release endothelin and nitric oxide; the former is a potent vasoconstrictor peptide and the latter a relaxing factor.

There is no connection between the erectile tissues of the corpus spongiosum and the corpora cavernosa vascular systems.

## Urethra

The penile urethra is in close relationship to the corpus spongiosum, which forms a protective cylindrical sheath around it. A stellate shape can be noted in cross section of the penile urethra owing to the folds of epithelium and lamina propria.

There is much variation in the composition of the urethral epithelium. Near the navicular fossa the epithelium can be stratified squamous or stratified columnar ciliated. The latter

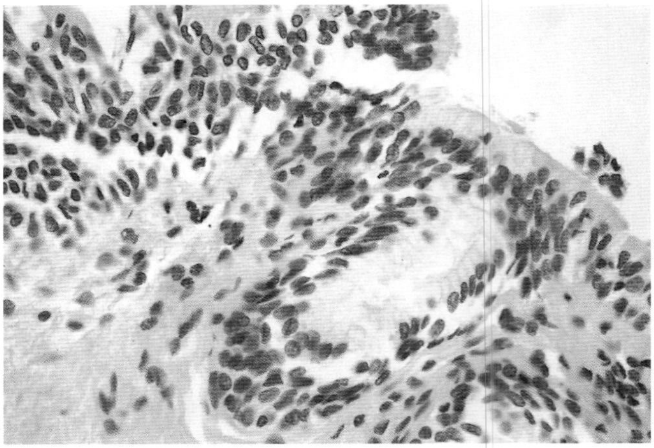

**FIG. 13.** Penile urethra. In this section an intraepithelial glandular structure is present.

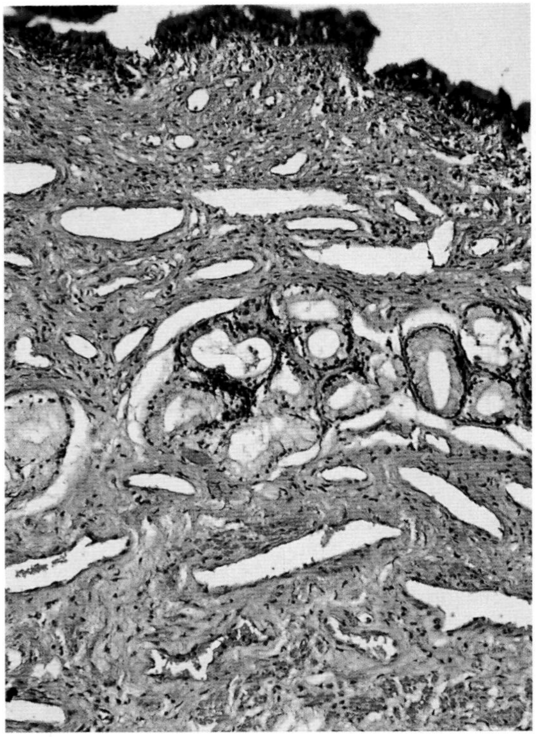

**FIG. 14.** Penile urethra. Below urethral epithelium and deep in the region between the lamina propria and corpus spongiosum is a cluster of tubular and acinar Littre's mucous glands.

is noted in most of the penile and bulbomembranous urethra, with vertically elongated nuclei perpendicular to the basement membrane (Fig. 12). The cytoplasm is slightly eosinophilic.

Occasional chromogranin-positive cells may be found close to the basal membrane by immunohistochemical

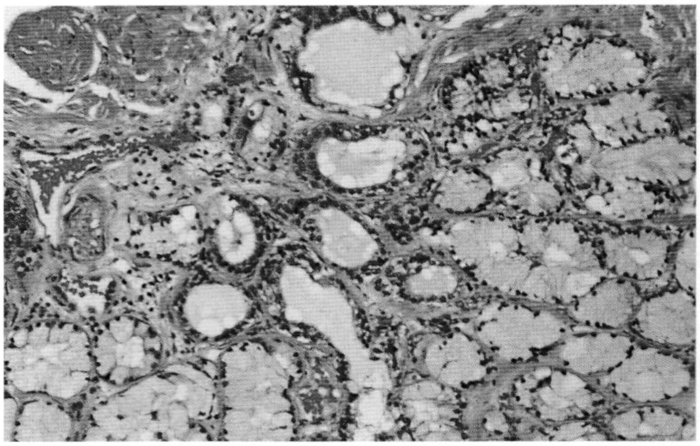

**FIG. 15.** Cowper's gland. Specimen taken from autopsy showing acinous–mucous structures, which are located deeply in the membranous urethra. (Courtesy Dr. Victor Reuter, Memorial Sloan-Kettering Cancer Center.)

stains. The intraepithelial glands, which are clusters of one-layer, cylindrical mucous glands with clear cytoplasm, can be noted within the epithelium (Fig. 13). We have recently noted a case of low-grade mucoepidermoid carcinoma that probably originated in these glands.

Under pathologic conditions and even in the normal urethra it is common to observe squamous metaplasia of the urethral epithelium. This variegated composition is reflected in the different tumor types found in the urethra. Squamous carcinoma is noted mainly in the penile urethra, adenocarcinoma and epidermoid cancers are noted mainly in the bulbomembranous segment (most common site for tumor origin), and transitional carcinomas are noted mainly in the proximal prostatic urethra. The urethral lamina propria is a thin layer of loose fibrous and elastic tissue. Littre's glands are tubuloacinous mucous structures. They are located along the full length of the corpus spongiosum, in close relation with erectile tissue (Fig. 14).

Littre's glands end in the urethra at the level of the intraepithelial lacunae. Some cysts have been described as originating in the parameatal Littre's glands (8). Inflammation of Littre's glands can clinically simulate a tumor (60). The Cowper's or bulbourethral glands are two small structures deeply located at the level of the membranous (or bulbous) urethra where they end, through two small ducts (7). They are mucous–acinous structures (Fig. 15). The clear cells of these glands can be confused with prostatic carcinoma in a core needle biopsy specimen.

# APPENDIX

Sites of origin of common penile disorders:

A. Glans
  - Squamous mucosa
    - Various inflammatory disorders
    - Hyperkeratosis, acanthosis, papillomatosis
    - Papilloma
    - Papillomatosis corona glandis
    - Herpes vesicles, condyloma
    - Bowenoid papulosis (13)
    - Dysplasia
    - Queyrat's erythroplasia
    - Buschke-Löewenstein tumor (61)
    - Squamous carcinoma
    - Lentigo, junctional nevi
    - Malignant melanoma (62)
  - Lamina propria
  - Various venereal and nonspecific inflammatory disorders
    - Syphilitic hard chancre
    - Soft (Ducrey) chancre
    - Granuloma inguinale
    - Fusospirochetosis
    - Balanitis xerotica obliterans (or lichen sclerosus et atrophicus)
    - Infiltrating squamous carcinoma
    - Infiltrating melanoma
  - Corpus spongiosum
    - Hemangioma
    - Leiomyoma
    - Neurofibroma (63)
    - Fibrosarcoma
    - Kaposi's sarcoma
    - Angiosarcoma
    - Leiomyosarcoma
    - Metastatic carcinoma

B. Balanopreputial sulcus
  - Same processes as described in the glans penis, epithelium, and lamina propria

C. Foreskin
  - Squamous mucosa and lamina propria: identical lesions as in glans
  - Epidermis and dermis: any type of lesion observed in the skin. Neoplastic lesions include basal cell carcinoma, epidermoid carcinoma, Bowen's disease (associated with 20% to 30% of visceral cancers), melanomas, and granular cell tumors

D. Penile body
  - Skin: similar to epidermis and dermis
  - Dermis
    - Paraffinomas
    - Tancho's nodules (64)
    - Necrotizing granulomas in penile base
  - Dartos
    - Torsion of the penis (65)
    - Fournier's gangrene
  - Buck's fascia
    - Peyronie's disease (fibromatosis)
    - Congenital torsion (66)
  - Corpora cavernosa
    - Coumarin necrosis (67)
    - Abscess (68)
    - Priapism, primary and secondary (69)
    - Metastatic carcinoma

## REFERENCES


1. Fitzpatrick T. The corpus cavernosum intercommunicating venous drainage system. *J Urol* 1975;113:494–496.
2. Boon ME, Schneider A, Hogewoning CJA, Van Der Kwast TH, Bolhuis P, Lambrecht PK. Penile studies and heterosexual partners. Peniscopy, cytology, histology and immunocytochemistry. *Cancer* 1988;61: 1652–1659.
3. Hricak H, Marotti M, Gilbert TJ, Lue T, Wetzel LH, Tanagho E. Normal penile anatomy and abnormal penile condition: evaluation with MR imaging. *Radiology* 1988;169:683–690.
4. Leport H, Gregerman M, Ranice C, Mostofi FK, Walsh PC. Precise localization of the autonomic nerves from the pelvic plexus to the corpora cavernosa: a detailed study of the adult male pelvis. *J Urol* 1985;133: 207–212.
5. Lue TF, Zeineh SJ, Schmidt RA, Tanagho EA. Neuroanatomy of penile erection: its relevance to iatrogenic impotence. *J Urol* 1984;131: 273–279.
6. Melman A, Henry D. The possible role of catecholamines of the corpora in penile erection. *J Urol* 1979;121:419–421.
7. Bourne CW, Kilcoyne RF, Kraenzler EJ. Prominent lateral mucosal folds in the bulbous urethra. *J Urol* 1981;126:326–330.
8. Shiraki IW. Parameatal cysts of the glans penis: a report of 9 cases. *J Urol* 1975;114:544–548.
9. Benson SG, Mc Connell JA, Schmists WA. Penile polsters: functional structures or atherosclerotic changes? *J Urol* 1981;125:800–803.
10. Dodge OG, Linsell CA. Carcinoma of the penis in Uganda and Kenya Africans. *Cancer* 1963;16:1255–1263.
11. Riveros M, Lebron R. Geographical pathology of cancer of the penis. *Cancer* 1963;16:798–811.
12. Cubilla AL, Caballero C, Barreto J, Riveros M. Factores patológicos relacionados con met stasis inguinal en el carcinoma epidermoide del glande peneal. In: *Anales de la Facultad de Ciencias Medicas*. Asunción, Paraguay: Facultad de Ciencias Médicas, 1991.
13. Wade TR, Kopf AW, Ackerman BA. Bowenoid papulosis of the penis. *Cancer* 1978;42;1890–1903.
14. Boon ME, Susanti I, Tasche MJA, Kok LP. Human papillomavirus (HPV) associated male and female genital carcinomas in a Hindu population. The male as vector and victim. *Cancer* 1989;64:559– 565.
15. Reeves WC, Brinton LA, García M, et al. Human papillomavirus infection and cervical cancer in Latin America. *N Engl J Med* 1989;320: 1437–1441.
16. Barrasso R, De Brux J, Croissant O, Orth G. High prevalence of papillomaviruses associated intraepithelial penile neoplasia in sexual partners of women with cervical intraepithelial neoplasia. *N Engl J Med* 1987;317:916–923.
17. Krebs HB, Schneider V. Human papillomavirus-associated lesions of the penis: colposcopy, cytology and histology. *Obstet Gynecol* 1987; 70:299–304.
18. Goldstein AMB, Meehan JP, Zakhary R, Buckley PA, Rogers FA. New observations on microarchitecture of corpora cavernosa in man and possible relationship to mechanisms of erection. *Urology* 1982;20: 259–266.
19. Krane RJ, Goldstein I, Saenz de Tejada I. Impotence. *N Engl J Med* 1989;321:1648–1659.
20. Polak JM, Gu J, Mina S, Bloom SR. Vipergic nerves in the penis. *Lancet* 1981;2:217–219.
21. Breza J, Aboseif SR, Owis BR, Lue TF, Tanagho EA. Detailed anatomy of penile neurovascular structures: surgical significance. *J Urol* 1989; 141:437–443.
22. Krane RJ. Sexual function and disfunction. In: Walsh PC, Gittes R, Perlmutter AD, Stamey TA, eds. *Campbell's urology*. Vol. 1, 5th ed. Philadelphia: WB Saunders; 1986:700–735.
23. Cunéo B, Marcille M: Note sur les lymphatiques du gland. *Bull Soc Anat Paris* 1901;76:671–674.
24. Mcaninch JW, Moore CA. Precancerous penile lesions in young men. *J Urol* 1970;104:287–290.
25. Cubilla AL, Barreto J. Pathological types of cancer of the penis. A whole section study [Abstract]. *Mod Pathol* 1988;1:2.
26. Leicht S, Younberg G, Díaz-Miranda C. Atypical penile maculas. *Arch Dermatol* 1988;124:1267–1270.
27. Hyman AB, Brownstein MH. "Tyson's glands." Ectopic and papillomatosis penis. *Arch Dermatol* 1969;99:31–36.
28. Tanenbaum MH, Becker SW. Papillae of the corona of the glans penis. *J Urol* 1965;93:391–395.
29. Winer JH, Winer LH. Hirsutoid papillomas of the coronal margin of the glans penis. *J Urol* 1955:74:375–378.
30. Cormack DH. *Histología de Ham*. 9th ed. Mexico: Herla; 1988:823.
31. Fawcett DW. *"Tratado de histología" de Bloom-Fawcett*. 11th ed. Mexico: Interamericana; 1989:853.
32. Stein AW. The histology and physiology of the penis. *N Y Med J* 1872; 595–606.
33. Bouchet A, Cuilleret J. *Anatomía descriptiva, topanatomía humana*. Vol. IV. 9th ed. Barcelona: Salvat; 1952:1105.
34. Kölliker A. Auber die tysonischen drüsen des menschen. *Anat Anzeiger* 1897; XIII:7.
35. Poirier P, Charpy A. Traité d'anatomie humaine. Paris: Masson et cie, 1901:183.
36. Saalfeld E. Ueber die Tyson'schen drüsen. *Arch Mikr Anat* 1899:212–218.
37. Tandler J, Dömeny P. Ueber Tyson'schen drüsen. *Wiener Klin Wochen* 1898;23:555–556.
38. Testut L, Latarjet A. *Tratado de anatomía Humana*, vol IV, 9th ed. Barcelona: Salvat, 1952:1105.
39. Parkash S, Jekayumar S, Subramayan K, Chaudhuri S. Human subpreputial collection: its nature and formation. *J Urol* 1973;110: 211–212.
40. Keith A, Shillitoe A. The preputial or odoriferous glands of man. *Lancet* 1904;1:146–148.
41. Shabad AL. Penile cancer. Some epidemiological data from the USSR and experimental data with special references to precancerous lesions. *Rev Inst Nac Cancer (Mexico)* 1964;15:310– 314.
42. Sprunk H. Ueber die vermeintlichen Tyson'schen drauusen [Dissertation]. University of Königsberg, Germany, 1897.
43. Tyson E. Orangoutang or the anatomy of the pygmie compared with that of a monkey, an ape and a man. University of London, 1699.
44. Ben-Ari J, Merlob P, Mimouni F, Reissner SH. Characteristic of the male genitalia in the newborn. *J Urol* 1985;134:521–522.
45. Arellano-Arroyo A. La cirugía entre los aztecas [Thesis]. Facultad de Medicina, Universidad Nacional Autonoma de Mexico, Ciudad de Mexico, Mexico, 1962.
46. Riveros M. Cancer del pene. Artes Gráficas Zamphirópolos *Asuncion* 1968:170.
47. Fussell EN, Kaak MB, Charry R, Roberts JA. Adherence of bacteria to human foreskin. *J Urol* 1988;140:997–1001.
48. Winberg J, Bollgren I, Gothefors L, Herthelius M, Tullus K. The prepuce: a mistake of nature? Lancet 1989;1:598–599.
49. Oster J. Further fate of the foreskin: incidence of preputial adhesions, phimosis and smegma among Danish school boys. *Arch Dis Child* 1968;43:200–203.
50. Winder SL, Licklider SD. The question of circumcision. *Cancer* 1960; 13:442–445.
51. Modwing R, Valderrama E. Immunohistochemical analysis of nerve distributions pattern within preputial tissues [Abstract]. *J Urol* 1989; 141(suppl 1):489.
52. Mostofi FK, Davis C Jr. Male reproductive system and prostate. In: Kissane JM, ed. *Anderson's pathology*. Vol. 1. 8th ed. St. Louis: CV Mosby; 1985:791.
53. Hsu GL, Brock G, Martínez Pineiro L, et al. Anatomy and strength of the tunica albuginea: its relevance to penile prosthesis extrusion. *J Urol* 1994;151:1205–1208.
54. Oota K. Cancer of the penis in Japan. *Rev Inst Nac Cancer (Mexico)* 1964;15:289–292.
55. Fournier AJ. Gangrene foudroyante de la verge. *Sem Med* 1883;3:345.
56. Spirnack PJ. Fournier's gangrene: report of 20 patients. *J Urol* 1984; 131:289–291.
57. Zinner NR, Sterling AM, Coleman RV, Ritter RC. The role of internal structure in human penile rigidity [Abstract]. *J Urol* 1989;141(suppl 1):221.
58. Fontana D, Rolle L, Lacivita A, et al. Modificazioni anatomo-funzionali dei corpi caverniosi nell'anziano. *Arch Ital Urol Androl* 1993;65: 483–486.
59. Lincoln J, Crowe R, Beacklay F, Pryor JP, Lumley JSP, Burnstock G. Changes in the vipergic, cholinergic and adrenergic innervations of human penile tissue in diabetic and non-diabetic impotent males. *J Urol* 1987;137:1053–1059.
60. Krowitt LN, Schechterman L. Inflammation of the periurethral glands of Littre simulating tumor. *J Urol* 1977;118:685.
61. Buschke A, Loewënstein L. Üeber carcinomauahnliche condylomata acuminata des penis. *Klin Wochenschr* 1925;36:1726–1728.

62. Begun FP, Grossman HB, Diokno AC, Sogani PC. Malignant melanoma of the male genitalia and male urethra. *J Urol* 1984;132:123–125.
63. Dwosh J, Mininberg DT, Schlossberg S, Peterson P. Neurofibroma involving the penis in a child. *J Urol* 1984;132:988–989.
64. Gilmore JAI, Weingad DA, Burgdorf WHC. Penile nodules in Southeast Asian men. *Arch Dermatol* 1983;119:446–447.
65. Redman JF. Torsion of the penis. *J Urol* 1983;130:316–318.
66. Corriere JN Jr. Involvement of Buck's fascia in congenital torsion of the penis. *J Urol* 1981;126:410–411.
67. Barkley C, Badalament RA, Metz EN, Nesbitt J, Drago JR. Coumarin's necrosis of the penis. *J Urol* 1989;141:946–948.
68. Sater AA, Vandrendis M. Abscess of corpus cavernosum. *J Urol* 1989;141:949.
69. Altebarmakian VM, Rabinowitz R, Rana SR, Ettinger LV. Transvascular cavernosum—spongiosum shunt for leukemic priapism in childhood. *J Urol* 1980;123:287–288.

# Endocrine System

*Histology for Pathologists, second edition,*
Edited by Stephen S. Sternberg.
Lippincott-Raven Publishers, Philadelphia


CHAPTER 45

# Pituitary and Sellar Region

P. J. Pernicone, Bernd W. Scheithauer, E. Horvath, and K. Kovacs



## EMBRYOLOGY

To fully appreciate the anatomy of the pituitary (hypophysis), an understanding of its embryogenesis is essential. The gland consists of an anterior lobe (adenohypophysis), a posterior lobe (neurohypophysis), and an intermediate zone (Fig. 1). The development of each differs significantly.

The adenohypophysis or anterior lobe has its origin in a thickening of stomodeal ectoderm (1–4). During the 3rd week of gestation, this thickened plate invaginates in a cephalad direction to form Rathke's pouch, all the while retaining its connection to the stomodeum via a narrow stalk. In the 6th week the stalk becomes so attenuated that the pouch loses its stomodeal attachment as it comes into contact with the infundibulum. Interestingly, a remnant of the pharyngohypophyseal stalk, demonstrable in fetuses and occasionally encountered in adults, comprises the pharyngeal pituitary (5,6). Located in the midline, beneath the muco-periosteum of the nasopharynx, it extends from the posterior border of the vomer along the sphenoid bone. Although the full spectrum of pituitary hormones may be demonstrated in pharyngeal pituitaries, they are rarely the seat of medical or surgical disease.

Rare developmental malformations of the pituitary gland, including ectopic pituitary gland and pituitary dystopia, have been reported (7,8).

Cellular proliferation in the anterior wall of Rathke's pouch gives rise to the pars distalis, the principal portion of the anterior lobe. In addition, a tonguelike extension of the pars distalis, the pars tuberalis, grows upward to partially surround the anterior surface of the infundibulum. The posterior portion of Rathke's pouch gives rise to what in humans is a thin segment of pituitary, the pars intermedia or intermediate lobe. In this zone microcystic remnants of Rathke's pouch containing colloidlike material are commonly seen (Fig. 1). Gross cystic dilatation of such remnants is common, but infrequently produces clinically significant intermediate lobe or Rathke's cleft cysts.

The neurohypophysis develops from a neuroectodermal bud first noticeable in the floor of the diencephalon at 4 weeks' gestation (1,3). Two weeks later, the outgrowth grows ventrally to abut the posterior portion of Rathke's pouch. This specialized portion of the nervous system comprises magnocellular nuclei, their axons within the median eminence and infundibular stalk, and their terminations in the pars nervosa (posterior lobe). Oxytocin and vasopressin, as well as their carrier proteins, the neurophysins, are detectable in supraoptic and paraventricular nuclei at 19 weeks and in the posterior lobe at 23 weeks (9).

As early as 7 to 8 weeks' gestation the portal system begins to develop. Although by 12 weeks both the median eminence and the anterior lobe are vascularized, the circulation of the hypothalamic–pituitary portal system is not completed until 18 to 20 weeks (9).

By using immunohistochemical stains, the times of appearance of the various hormone-producing cells of the adenohypophysis have been determined. Somatotrophs and corticotrophs appear first between 5 and 12 weeks, followed by thyrotrophs and gonadotrophs at 12 to 13 weeks. Finally, lactotrophs appear between 13 and 16 weeks (9–11).

P. J. Pernicone and B. W. Scheithauer: Department of Laboratory Medicine and Pathology, Mayo Clinic, Rochester, Minnesota 55905.
E. Horvath and K. Kovacs: Department of Pathology, St. Michael's Hospital, Toronto, Ontario, M5B 1W8 Canada.

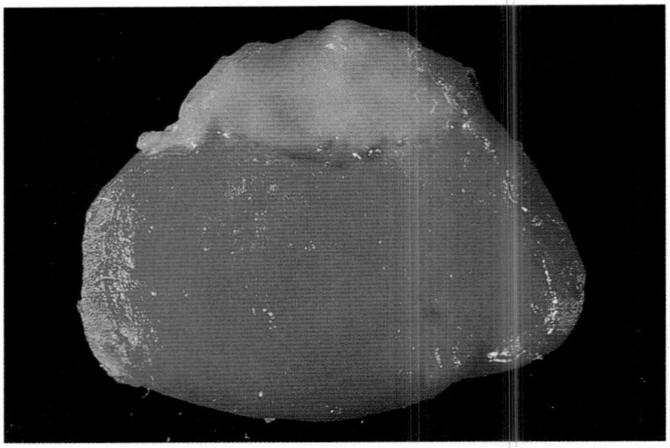

**FIG. 1.** Normal unfixed adult pituitary gland cut in the horizontal plane. The posterior lobe is located at the top of the field. A few intermediate lobe cysts are present. The deep red color of the anterior lobe is a reflection of its extensive vascularity.

The hypothalamus develops from a swelling in the diencephalon. Although hypothalamic nuclei as well as the supraopticohypophyseal tract are demonstrable at 8 weeks' gestation, unmyelinated axons, growing ventrally from the magnocellular (supraoptic and paraventricular) nuclei, do not reach the posterior lobe until 6 months.

By 12 weeks, a number of cartilaginous plates have fused to form the cartilaginous neurocranium (1). The body of the sphenoid bone and the sella turcica result from fusion of hypophyseal cartilage plates located on either side of the developing pituitary. The sella is well formed by 7 weeks and matures through a process of enchondral ossification.

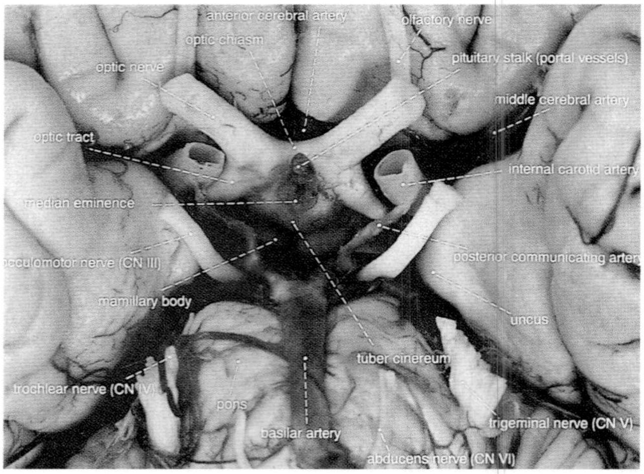


**FIG. 2.** Ventral surface of normal brain showing the pituitary stalk and surrounding structures. The pituitary gland has been removed. The proximity of the optic chiasm to the pituitary is the basis for the visual field deficits accompanying suprasellar extension of pituitary adenomas. Visible along the posterior aspect of the stalk are tributaries of the portal system.

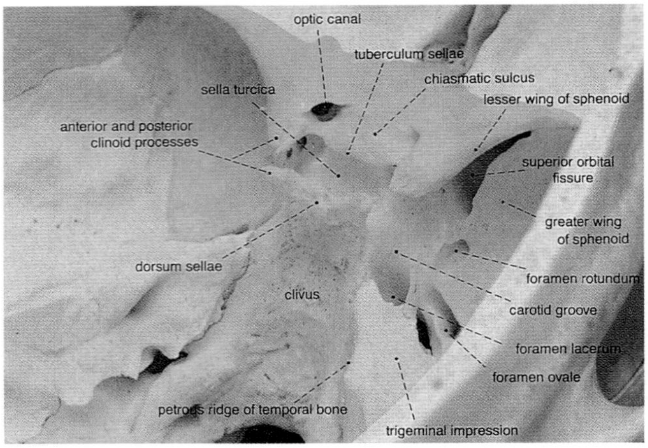


**FIG. 3.** Oblique view of the normal skull base; the various skull bones are indicated in color. The sella turcica is centrally located with several foramina nearby. The foramen spinosum is not visible in this view. Yellow, sphenoid; pink, occipital; light blue, temporal; green, parietal; white, frontal.

## GROSS ANATOMY

### Bony Sella

The pituitary gland is centrally situated at the base of the brain, where it lies safely nestled in the sella, a saddle-shaped concavity within the sphenoid bone (Figs. 2–4). It is attached to the hypothalamus by both the pituitary stalk and a tenuous vascular network (Figs. 5–7). By virtue of its location, the pituitary gland has many important anatomic relations (12–14). Anterior to the sella, the sphenoid bone forms a midline slope, the tuberculum sella, as well as a transverse indentation, the chiasmal sulcus, so named for the overlying optic chiasm (Figs. 3 and 4). The optic canals, which transmit the optic nerves, lie anterolateral to the sulcus, whereas the optic tracts are posterolateral. In view of the pituitary's proximity to the optic apparatus, pituitary lesions that extend

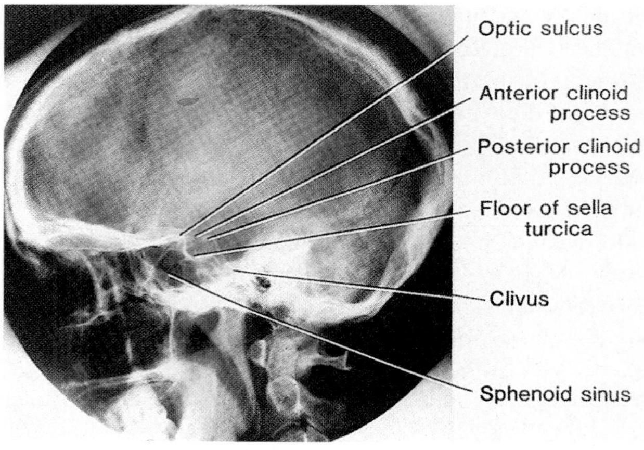


**FIG. 4.** This normal lateral skull radiograph shows the central location of the sella turcica and surrounding bony anatomy.

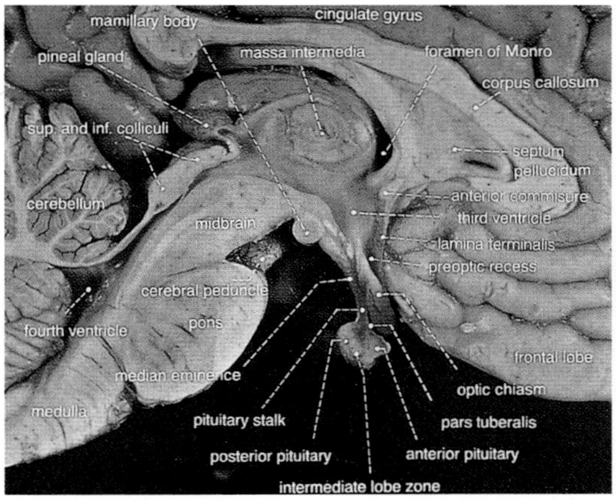


**FIG. 5.** Midline sagittal section through the brain at the level of the pituitary stalk and pituitary gland, showing the sella and pituitary gland with surrounding structures including hypothalamus, third ventricle, optic chiasm, and sphenoid sinus.

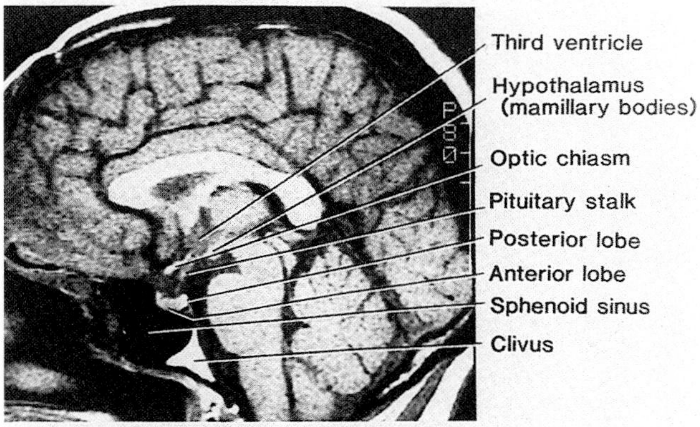


**FIG. 7.** Magnetic resonance imaging (MRI) sagittal view of the brain at the level of the pituitary stalk and gland. The clarity of the pituitary gland, stalk, hypothalamus, and optic chiasm is remarkable, making MRI an excellent imaging modality for the assessment of pituitary lesions. One advantage of MRI over CT is the absence of bony artifact with MRI.

superiorly may cause significant visual field deficits (Figs. 2 and 5–11). Specifically, compression of decussating fibers in the chiasm produces bitemporal hemianopsia, whereas compromise of an optic tract leads to homonymous hemianopsia. Further suprasellar extension may cause hypothalamic dysfunction and hydrocephalus.

The floor of the sella forms a portion of the roof of the sphenoid air sinus, a fortuitous relationship that permits ready surgical access (15) (Figs. 4 and 6–12). Indeed, the transsphenoidal approach to the pituitary initially involves mobilization of the nasal septal cartilage followed by resection of a portion of the ethmoid plate. A sublabial incision is then made, and the sphenoid speculum is placed in the septal space, permitting direct visualization of the anterior wall of the sphenoid sinus. Upon breaking through the anterior sphenoid wall, the sella may be seen bulging into the roof of the sinus. A septated sphenoid sinus may affect the surgeon's orientation at surgery (Figs. 8 and 9). The pituitary is then exposed by traversing the bony sellar floor and incising the dural investment around the gland.

The sloping anterior sellar wall terminates in posterolateral projections, the anterior clinoid processes (Figs. 3 and 4). Posterior to the sella, the sphenoid bone continues as the dorsum sellae, anterolateral portions of which form the posterior clinoid processes (Figs. 3 and 4). Posterior to the dor-

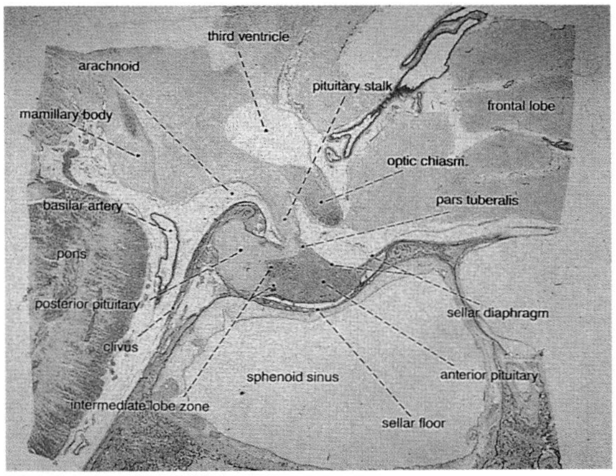


**FIG. 6.** Sagittal whole-mount section of normal pituitary gland and surrounding structures. The anterior and posterior lobes are clearly delineated. The pars tuberalis is the thin tongue-shaped portion of anterior lobe that extends for a short distance up the stalk. This diagram illustrates the proximity of the optic chiasm to the pituitary. Superior extension of a pituitary tumor may compress the optic chiasm with resultant visual field deficits, whereas downward extension may fill the sphenoid sinus (Luxol-fast blue–PAS).

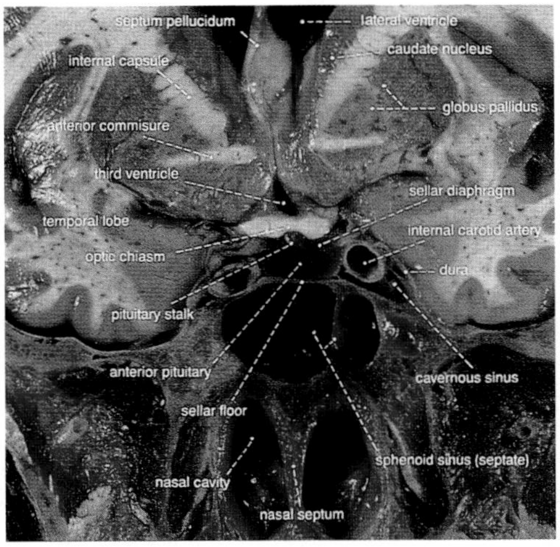


**FIG. 8.** Coronal section of the head at the level of the pituitary stalk and gland. This photograph clearly illustrates the intimate relationships between the cavernous sinuses, the sphenoid sinus, and the pituitary gland. Invasive adenomas may extend laterally into one or both cavernous sinuses or inferiorly into the sphenoid sinus. Note the proximity of the optic chiasm to the pituitary.

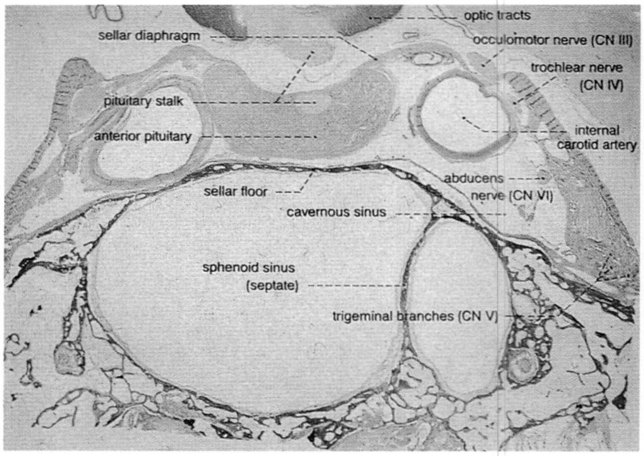


**FIG. 9.** Coronal whole-mount view of the normal pituitary gland and surrounding structures. Note the location of cranial nerves III, IV, VI, and branches of the Vth nerve within the cavernous sinuses, a relationship explaining the occurrence of cranial nerve palsy in association with invasive pituitary adenomas. This section also illustrates the proximity of the internal carotid arteries to the pituitary gland (Luxol-fast blue–PAS).

sum sellae lies the downward-sloping clivus, notorious as the site of predilection of chordomas (Figs. 3, 4, 6, and 7). A number of neurovascular foramina are situated in the sellar region; by name and contents from anterior to posterior, they include the foramen rotundum (maxillary nerves), ovale (mandibular nerves), spinosum (middle meningeal arteries), and lacerum (internal carotid arteries) (Fig. 3).

## Meninges

The physical relationship of the meninges to the pituitary and sella is unusual in that the pituitary lacks a leptomeningeal investment. Periosteal dura lines the sella turcica, whereas the dura proper covers the lateral aspects of the cavernous sinuses and forms the sellar diaphragm. The diaphragm is usually thin at the center and thick at its periphery and possesses a variably sized central aperture through which the pituitary stalk passes (12). Leptomeninges do encircle the stalk but, somewhat below the level of the sellar diaphragm, they reflect back upon themselves to form a circumferential trough, the infradiaphragmatic hypophyseal cistern. This arrangement explains not only the development of meningiomas about the stalk, but also the rare occurrence of intrasellar examples.

In some individuals, the leptomeninges exhibit an important anatomic variation. It consists of extension or herniation of the arachnoid through an inordinately large diaphragmatic opening. In one study the incidence of an intrasellar arachnoidocele was found to exceed 20% (16). In such cases, transsphenoidal surgery may result in persistent cere-

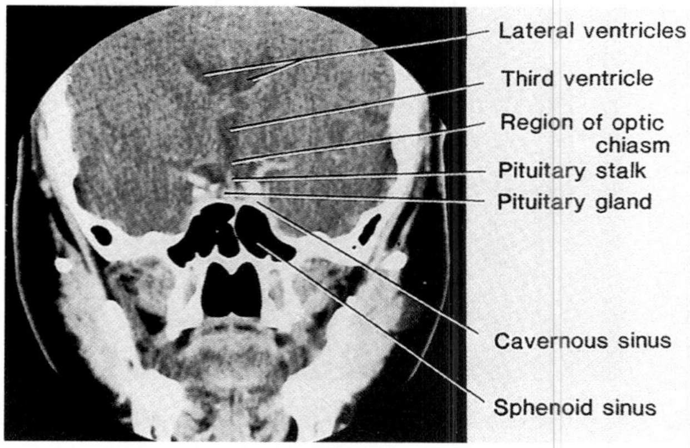


**FIG. 10.** A computed tomographic (CT) coronal view of the normal skull and brain at the level of the pituitary stalk and gland. CT scan is a good imaging modality for assessing the pituitary gland; however, radiologists often encounter problems with bony artifact. For this reason, MRI is superior.

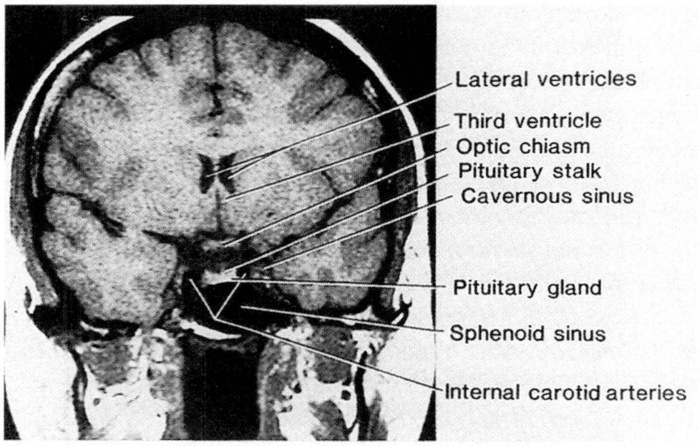


**FIG. 11.** Coronal MRI of the skull and brain at the level of the pituitary stalk and gland.

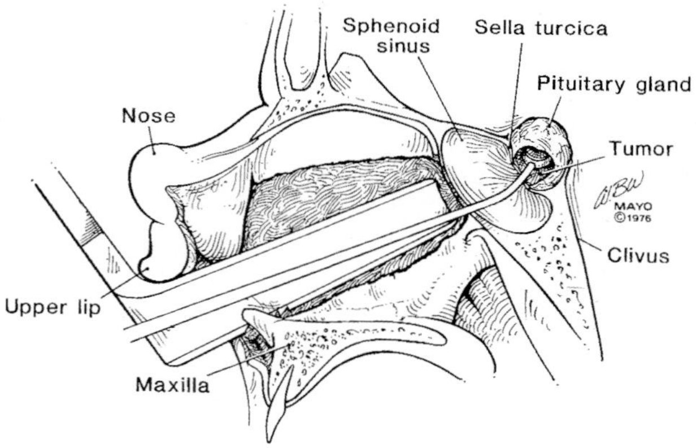


**FIG. 12.** Transsphenoidal approach to the pituitary gland. After mobilizing the nasal septal cartilage and resecting a portion of ethmoid plate, a sublabial incision is made, and a sphenoid speculum is placed. Next, the floor of the sphenoid sinus and the floor of the sella turcica are traversed. Finally, the dural investment of the pituitary gland is incised, and the gland is exposed. This diagram illustrates a curette in place for removal of a pituitary adenoma.

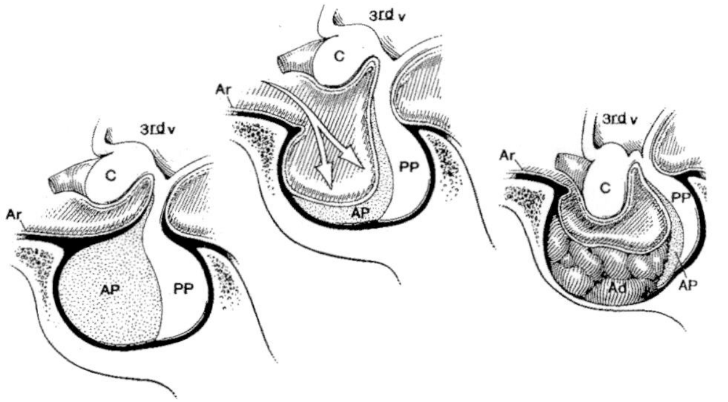


**FIG. 13.** Illustration of normal as well as variants of the empty sella. The normal pituitary-sellar relationships are illustrated on the *left.* The leptomeninges cover the stalk and sellar diaphragm but do not extend into the sella. In primary empty sella syndrome (*middle*) an excessively large diaphragmatic orifice permits herniation of leptomeninges into the sella. Prolonged CSF pressure compresses the gland against the sellar floor. Secondary empty sella may result from infarction of a pituitary adenoma (*right*), infarction of the pituitary gland, and surgical or radioablation of the gland.

brospinal fluid (CSF) rhinorrhea due to inadvertent violation of the subarachnoid space. With prolonged exertion of even normal CSF pressure, enlargement of such arachnoidoceles may produce sellar enlargement and pituitary compression, the gland being reduced to a thin crescent on the posterior sellar floor (Figs. 13 and 14). The condition, dubbed empty sella syndrome, shows a distinct predilection for obese females. Its anatomic manifestations are fully expressed in as many as 5.5% of autopsies (17,18). Compression of the gland and traction deformation of the pituitary stalk may cause mild to moderate hypopituitarism and hyperprolactinemia, respectively.

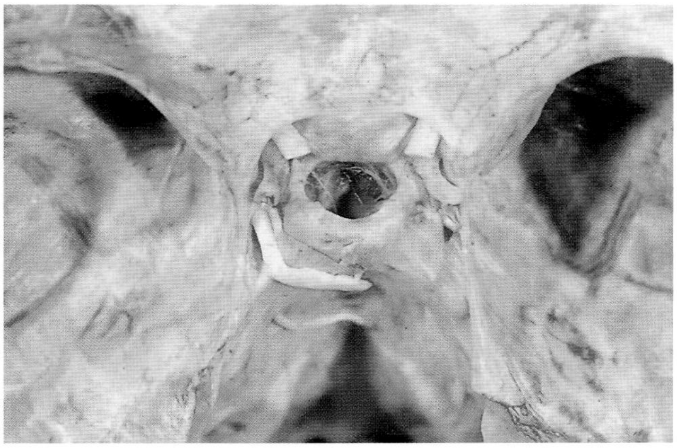

**FIG. 14.** Superior view of the skull base, demonstrating an incidentally encountered primary empty sella. Normally in this view the upper surface of the pituitary gland would be visible through the diaphragmatic aperture, but here the sella appears empty. Only rarely is primary empty sella syndrome symptomatic. This specimen is from a 57-year-old obese diabetic woman.

### Vasculature

Vascular structures of major surgical significance abound in the sellar region. Elegant in design but anatomically complex, the paired cavernous sinuses are situated on either side of the sella and, in part, lie lateral and superior to the sphenoid sinuses (Figs. 8–11). Each cavernous sinus is partially invested by dura of the middle fossa, as well as by thin bony walls of the sphenoid sinus. Venous drainage to the sinuses comes from a number of sources, including the eye (superior ophthalmic vein), the brain (inferior and middle cerebral veins), and the sphenoparietal sinus. Communication between right and left cavernous sinuses takes place through intercavernous sinuses bordering the anterior and posterior aspects of the sella (19). The complex thus forms a venous ring around the sella and its contents. Additional intercavernous sinuses are located along the ventral surface of the pituitary. The cavernous sinuses proper are more than simply a confluence of venous channels. Rather, they represent extradural cavities that, in addition to their content of venous sinuses, contain a number of vital neurovascular structures (20,21). These include the cavernous segments of the internal carotid arteries, as well as segments of cranial nerves III (occulomotor), IV (trochlear), V (trigeminal), and VI (abducens) (Figs. 8 and 9). Delicate areolar tissue fills the interstices between venous channels, arteries, and nerves. The location of the horizontal portions of the internal carotid arteries within the cavernous sinuses varies, not only from person to person but from left to right. As a result, and to the frustration of the surgeon, the carotids may lie immediately adjacent to the sella, in which case they pose a surgical hazard (16) (Figs. 8 and 9). Furthermore, the anterior portions of the carotids may indent the sphenoid bone and thus be separated from the cavity itself by as little as 1 mm of bone (12). Several branches of the internal carotid artery arise within the cavernous sinus, including the meningohypophyseal trunk, the largest intracavernous branch, the artery of the inferior cavernous sinus, and small capsular branches (20,21). The meningohypophyseal trunk gives rise to several vessels, one of which, the inferior hypophyseal artery, supplies the posterior or neural lobe and the pituitary capsule.

Given their location, the cavernous sinuses may be directly involved by pituitary tumors. For example, extension of an invasive adenoma into the cavernous sinuses not infrequently produces neuropathies of cranial nerves III through VI (Fig. 9).

The principal arterial supply of the pituitary originates in two branches of the internal carotid vessels: the superior and inferior hypophyseal arteries (22,23) (Fig. 15). A single superior hypophyseal artery springs from each carotid shortly after its entry into the cranial cavity and promptly divides into posterior and anterior branches, each of which anastomoses with the corresponding branch from the opposite side to form an arterial ring around the upper pituitary stalk. The anterior branches give rise to trabecular or loral arteries, which descend on the upper surface of the anterior lobe,

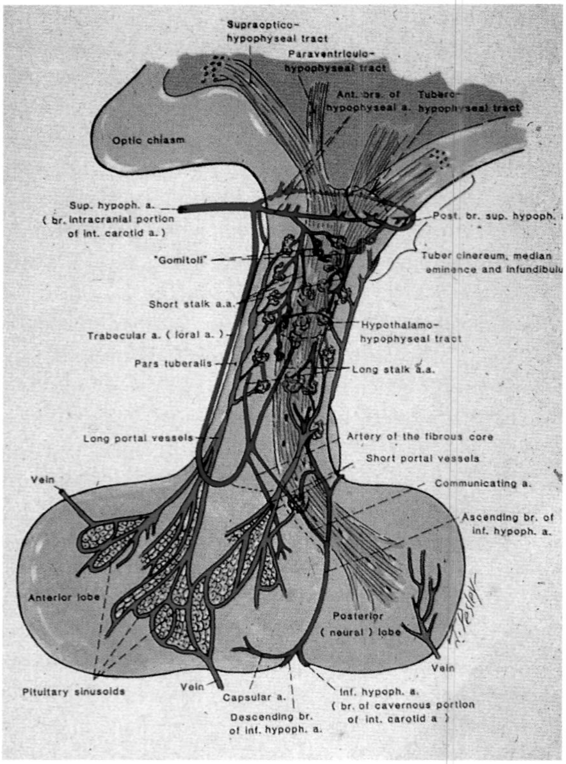


**FIG. 15.** Diagrammatic representation of the vasculature of the pituitary gland. The superior and inferior hypophyseal arteries and branches of the internal carotid arteries comprise the major blood supply of the gland. Small terminal branches of the superior and inferior hypophyseal arteries give rise to tangled capillary loops termed gomitoli, which drain into portal vessels. The latter traverse the length of the stalk and terminate as a capillary bed in the anteior lobe. The anterior pituitary thus receives the majority of its blood supply not from arteries but from the portal system. The portal system forms a vital link between the hypothalamus and the pituitary gland.

course toward the pituitary stalk, and terminate in long stalk arteries along the pars tuberalis. In their brief course along the anterior lobe, trabecular arteries each give rise to a small artery of the fibrous core (22). The posterior and anterior branches of the superior hypophyseal arteries are also the source of short stalk arteries, which penetrate the superior aspect of the pituitary stalk to run upward or downward within it. In contrast to the superior hypophyseal arteries, the inferior branches originate from the meningohypophyseal trunks within the cavernous sinuses; they contact the inferolateral portions of the gland and bifurcate into medial and lateral branches that anastomose with their opposite counterparts to form an arterial circle about the posterior lobe. Thus, branches of the inferior hypophyseal arteries supply primarily the posterior lobe and lower portion of the stalk, contributing only small capsular branches to the periphery of the anterior lobe (24). Although many of the arterial branches in the pituitary stalk and infundibulum form arterioles and capillaries, some give rise to unique vascular complexes termed gomitoli (Figs. 15 and 16). Transliterated, these balls of

A

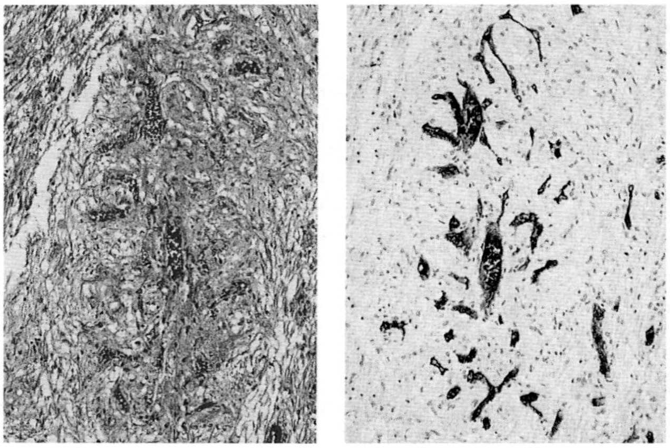

B

**FIG. 16.** Gomitoli, tortuous capillary loops surrounding a central arteriole in the upper portion of the pituitary stalk (**A**) (H&E, original magnification ×100). The complex vascularity of the gomitoli is highlighted by staining with *Ulex europeus* lectin (**B**) (immunostain, original magnification ×100).

thread consist of a central artery surrounded by a glomeruloid tangle of capillaries. The transition from central arteries to the capillaries is via short specialized arterioles endowed with thick smooth muscle sphincters that serve to regulate blood flow. The jumble of periarteriolar capillaries drains into an extensive pampiniform network, the portal system, which enshrouds the stalk (Figs. 2 and 15).

The hypophyseal portal system, the crucial link between hypothalamus and pituitary, takes its origin from the capillary plexus of the median eminence and stalk, which itself is derived from terminal ramifications of the superior and inferior hypophyseal arteries (25) (Fig. 17). The capillary plexus in the median eminence and superior stalk, the site of uptake of hypophysiotrophic factors, drains into the long portal ves-

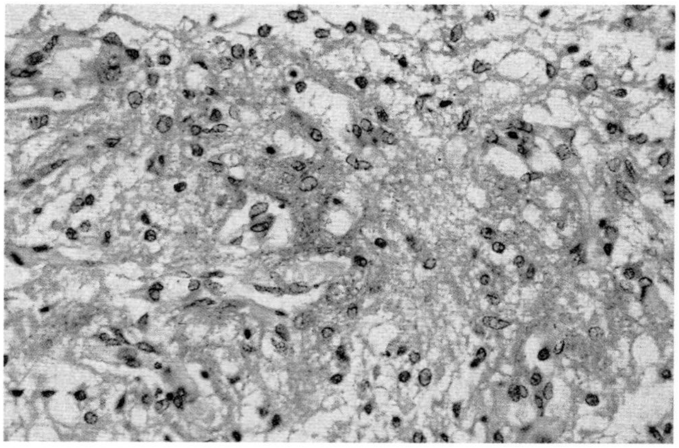

**FIG. 17.** Region of the median eminence showing staining of intra-axonal accumulations of corticotropin releasing hormone (CRH). The median eminence represents the first portion of the portal system. Here, nerve terminals of the hypothalamohypophyseal tract deposit releasing and inhibiting hormones into the system for transport to the anterior lobe (immunostain, original magnification ×100).

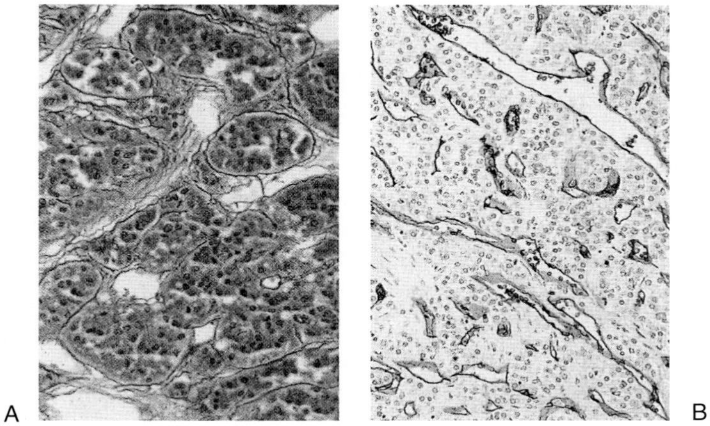


**FIG. 18. A:** The intricate capillary and connective tissue network outlined in reticulin stain. The reticulin stain is invaluable in the evaluation of pituitary adenomas, which are largely devoid of reticulin, whereas the surrounding normal gland retains it (Gomori reticulin, original magnification ×100). **B:** The capillary endothelium of the the anterior lobe capillary network stains strongly for *Ulex europeus* lectin (immunostain ×100).

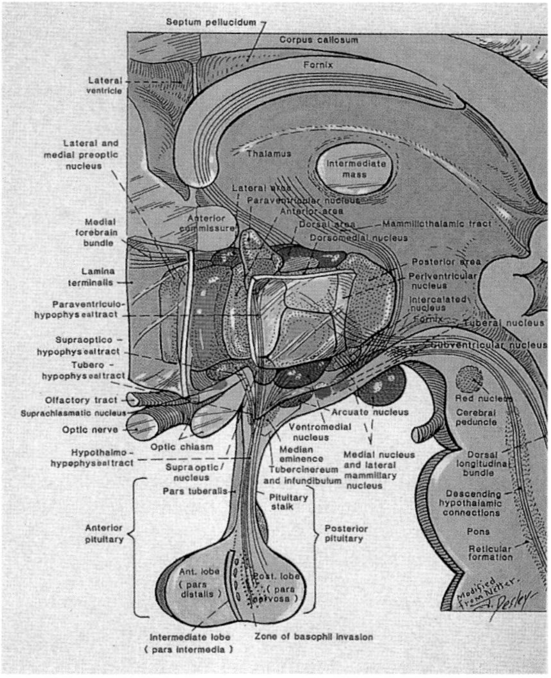


**FIG. 19.** A diagrammatic representation of the hypothalamic nuclei, showing the supraopticohypophyseal and paraventriculohypophyseal tracts, as well as the tuberohypophyseal tract. The former carry vasopressin and oxytocin along axons to the posterior lobe, whereas the latter carries hypothalamic releasing and inhibiting hormones to the median eminence, where they enter the portal system for transport to the anterior lobe.

sels that course along the surface of the stalk to supply the majority (90%) of the anterior lobe, whereas the smaller capillary plexus in the lower stalk gives rise to the short portal vessels that descend into its central portion, including that bordering the posterior lobe (24,25). Distally, the portal system communicates with a delicate capillary network in the anterior lobe, one that carries hypophysiotrophic factors into the pituitary and conveys anterior lobe hormones to the general circulation (Fig. 18).

Venous outflow of the pituitary is via collecting vessels that drain into the subhypophyseal sinus, cavernous sinus, and superior circular sinus (23).

There is considerable variability in the vascular anatomy of the pituitary. Aside from a minor direct arterial supply via capsular branches of the inferior hypophyseal arteries, the majority of the anterior lobe's circulation is venous, originating from the portal vessels (22,23). In contrast to that of the anterior lobe, the blood supply of the posterior lobe is direct and arterial, an arrangement that explains the predilection of metastatic carcinomas for the neural lobe.

## Hypothalamus

Although considered the master gland, the pituitary is known to be under significant hypothalamic control. In fact, it and the hypothalamus form a complex neurohormonal circuit, the most vital element of the endocrine orchestra.

Weighing approximately 5 g and forming the walls and floor of the inferior third ventricle, the hypothalamus lies above the pituitary to which it is connected by the pituitary stalk (Figs. 5–7, 19, and 20). As the name suggests, the hypothalamus lies inferior to the thalamus. Although at first glance it appears poorly demarcated, the hypothalamus is bordered anteriorly by the anterior commissure, lamina terminalis, and optic chiasm, posteriorly and superiorly by the midbrain tegmentum and mamillary bodies, dorsally by the hypothalamic sulcus, and laterally by subthalamic nuclei

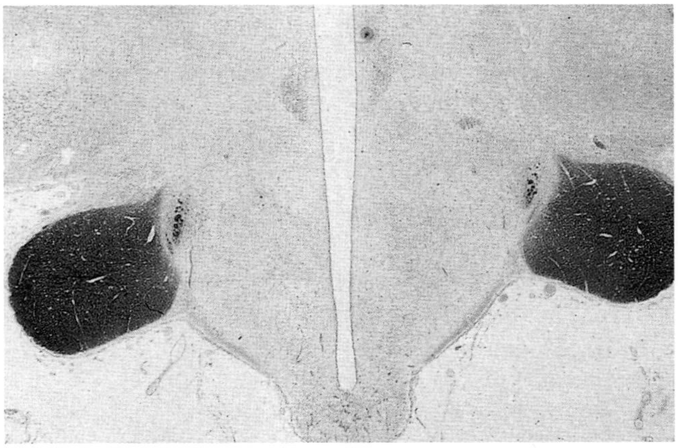

**FIG. 20.** Coronal whole-mount section through the hypothalamus and third ventricle. The paraventricular nuclei are visible as darkly staining areas beneath the ependyma of the third ventricle (*upper field*), whereas the supraoptic nuclei lie above the heavily myelinated optic tracts. The arcuate nucleus lies inferior to the base of the third ventricle (Cresyl violet).

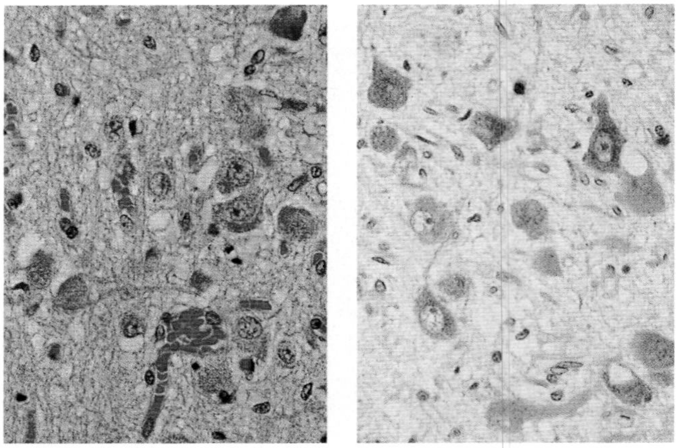

A B

**FIG. 21.** The paraventricular nucleus of the hypothalamus. **A:** Its high degree of vascularity is a characteristic of magnocellular nuclei (H&E, original magnification ×100). **B:** The nerve cell bodies stain positively for vasopressin (immunostain, original magnification ×100).

(26,27). The region consists of several ill-defined but functionally related neuronal groups termed nuclei (Figs. 19–22). Afferent and efferent connections bring these nuclei into contact with nearby as well as remote portions of the central nervous system, including other diencephalic structures, the cerebrum, brain stem, and spinal cord. In our attempt to develop a working knowledge of the hypothalamic–pituitary axis, here we concentrate primarily on two distinct hypothalamohypophyseal secretory systems. One consists of the supraoptic and paraventricular nuclei and their projections to the posterior lobe (supraopticohypophyseal and paraventriculohypophyseal tracts); the other is composed mainly of nuclei of the tuberal region, the funnel-shaped floor of the third ventricle, and their processes terminating in the median eminence (tuberohypophyseal tract) (Fig. 19).

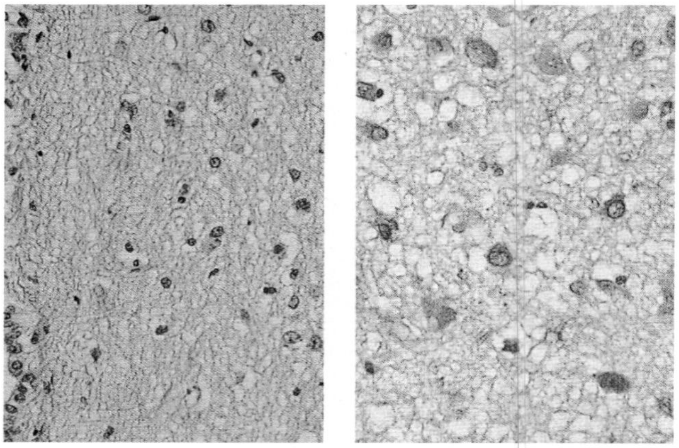

A B

**FIG. 22.** Periventricular nucleus. **A:** Lying beneath the ependyma of the third ventricle, this ill-defined nucleus is composed of small nerve cell bodies (H&E, original magnification ×63). **B:** Its constituent neurons stain for CRH, a tropic hormone that exerts its effect on corticotrophs in the anterior lobe (immunostain, original magnification ×100).

The supraoptic nuclei are located superior to the optic tracts, whereas the wedge-shaped paraventricular nuclei lie ventromedial to the fornix and abut the walls of the third ventricle (Fig. 20). Due to their predominant composition of large neurons measuring up to 25 m, these nuclei are termed magnocellular (Fig. 21). Each contains vasopressin- and oxytocin-producing neurons, but only one hormone is produced by a given neuron. Their axons form the supraopticohypophyseal and paraventriculohypophyseal tracts, which carry vasopressin and oxytocin, the two so-called neurohypophyseal hormones, as well as their respective carrier proteins, the neurophysins, to the posterior lobe of the pituitary gland. Oxytocin and vasopressin, both nonapeptides, are synthesized as 20-kDa prohormones, which include in their structure the cysteine-rich neurophysin carrier proteins. The precursor molecules are packaged into secretory granules within the Golgi apparatus and transported by axoplasmic flow within unmyelinated axons to nerve terminals in the posterior lobe. Here they are released by a process of calcium-dependent exocytosis (28). Large intra-axonal accumulations of these hormones, Herring bodies, are often visible by light microscopy as round, granular structures that appear eosinophilic on hematoxylin and eosin (H&E) sections (Fig. 23). In transit from the hypothalamus to the posterior lobe, prohormones undergo extensive processing and cleavage to form the final products, vasopressin and oxytocin. Although they differ by only two amino acids, oxytocin exhibits virtually no antidiuretic activity, and vasopressin has negligible oxytocic effect. Oxytocin mediates the milk let-down reflex by stimulating contraction of myoepithelial cells surrounding terminal mammary lobules. In addition, it serves a role in parturition, binding and facilitating contraction in the final stages of parturition. Interestingly,

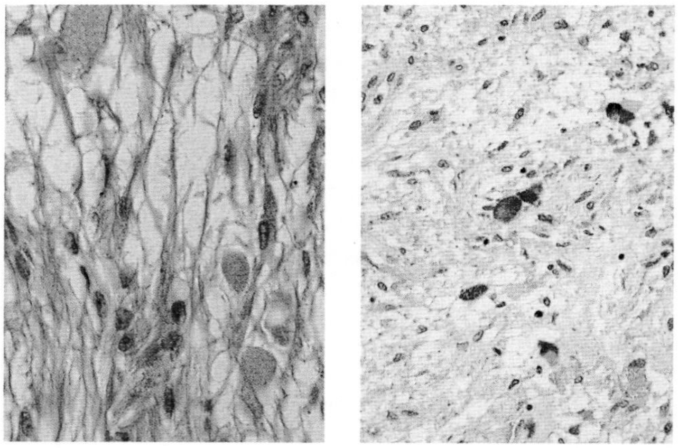

A B

**FIG. 23.** Pituitary stalk. Axonal swellings termed Herring bodies characterize its axons. **A:** One is in the upper and two are in the lower portions of the field. They are characterized by their ovoid shape and granular character on H&E. Herring bodies represent intra-axonal accumulations of oxytocin- and vasopressin-containing granules en route to the posterior lobe (H&E, original magnification ×100). **B:** Herring bodies staining for vasopressin (VP) (immunostain, original magnification ×100).

**TABLE 1.** *Hypothalamic hormones: their effect on pituitary hormone secretion*

| Affected pituitary hormone | Hypothalamic hormone: Stimulatory | Hypothalamic hormone: Inhibitory |
|---|---|---|
| Growth hormone (GH) | Growth hormone releasing hormone (GHRH, somatoliberin, somatocrinin) | Somatostatin |
| Prolactin (PRL) | Thyrotropin releasing hormone (TRH)<br>Vasoactive intestinal peptide (VIP) | Dopamine (?Prolactin-inhibiting factor, PIF) |
| Adrenocorticotropin (ACTH) | Corticotropin releasing factor (CRH, corticoliberin) | ? |
| Follicle-stimulating hormone (FSH)<br>Luteinizing hormone (LH) | Gonadotropin releasing hormone (GnRH) | ? |
| Thyroid-stimulating hormone (TSH) | Thyrotropin releasing hormone (TRH) | ? |

the initiation of labor is not dependent on oxytocin. The major physiologic role of vasopressin (antidiuretic hormone) is the formation of hypertonic urine. Acting via cyclic adenosine monophosphate, vasopressin increases the water permeability of renal collecting ducts, allowing the hypotonic intraductal fluid to equilibrate with the hypertonic fluid in the medullary interstitium. The results are concentrated urine and conservation of body water. Damage to the neurohypophysis from head trauma, surgery, inflammatory processes (e.g., sarcoidosis), or neoplasms may destroy vasopressin-producing neurons and cause diabetes insipidus. Patients with diabetes insipidus may excrete greater than 40 L of inappropriately dilute urine in a single day. Additional hormones and neuropeptides have been identified in the neurohypophysis; these include somatostatin, thyrotropin-releasing hormone (TRH), gonadotropin releasing hormone (GnRH), melanocyte-stimulating hormone, substance P, histamine, serotonin, dopamine, corticotropin-like intermediate lobe peptide (CLIP), and beta-lipotropin ($\beta$-LPH) (26). The functions of these substances within the posterior lobe are unknown.

The second component of the hypothalamohypophyseal system is the tuberoinfundibular tract. Its fibers originate in a number of hypothalamic nuclei lying within the walls of the inferior third ventricle and tuberal region (26) (Figs. 19, 20, and 22). Products of these nuclei, targeted for the anterior pituitary, consist of releasing and inhibiting hormones. Unlike the magnocellular neurons of the supraoptic and paraventricular nuclei, these are small, hence the term parvicellular neurons (Fig. 22). Their processes project to the median eminence, a highly vascular zone, located in the posterior proximal portion of the pituitary stalk. Here the hypophysiotrophic factors are released into the first portion of the portal system for transport to the anterior lobe. Ultra-

**TABLE 2.** *Major hypothalamic hormones: their composition and localization*

| Hormone | Composition | Hypothalamic sites | Extrahypothalamic sites |
|---|---|---|---|
| Growth hormone releasing hormone (GHRH, somatoliberin, somatocrinin) | 40 and 44 Amino acids | Arcuate nucleus | ? |
| Thyrotroin releasing hormone (TRH) | 3 Amino acids | Widely distributed in CNS with concentration in ventromedial, dorsal, and paraventricular nuclei, particularly on left | Brain and spinal cord, fetal pancreatic islet cells, gut neuroendocrine cells |
| Gonadotropin releasing hormone (GnRH, gonadoliberin) | 10 Amino acids | Widespread distribution with concentration in the arcuate, ventromedial, dorsal, and paraventricular nuclei | Brain (limbic system), breast (lactation), placenta |
| Corticotropin releasing hormone (CRH, corticoliberin) | 41 Amino acids | Periventricular, medial paraventricular nuclei | Brain (cerebral cortex, limbic system, brain stem, spinal cord) |
| Somatostatin | 14 Amino acids | Periventricular nucleus, paraventricular nuclei (paravicellular neurons), arcuate nuclei | Brain, retina, peripheral nervous system, pancreatic islet cells, gut neuroendocrine cells, thyroid, placenta |
| Dopamine | Catecholamine | Arcuate nucleus | Brain, GI tract |
| Vasopressin (VP, ADH) | 9 Amino acids | Paraventricular, supraoptic nuclei | Brain |
| Oxytocin (OT) | 9 Amino acids | Paraventricular, supraoptic nuclei | Brain |

A, B

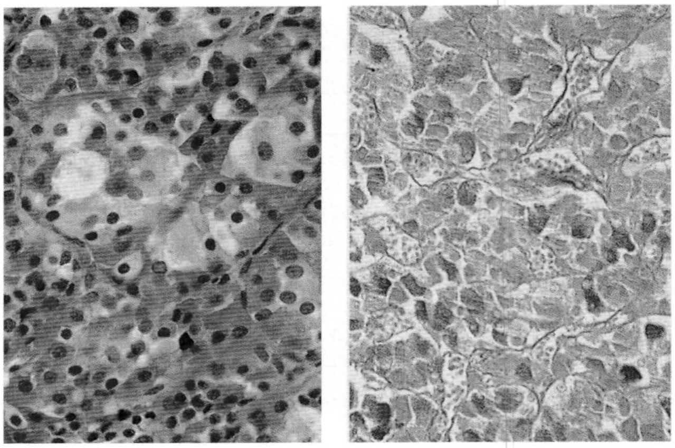

**FIG. 24.** Anterior lobe. **A:** An H&E-stained section shows chromophobic, acidophilic, and basophilic cells. Acidophils are most numerous in the lateral wings, whereas basophils are found in greatest number in the central or mucoid wedge. **B:** PAS–orange G stains acidophils orange and basophils blue, whereas chromophobes appear gray or lack staining.

A

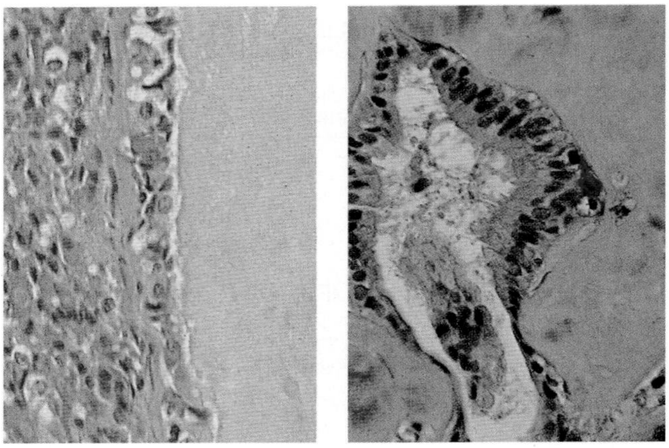

B

**FIG. 26.** Intermediate lobe remnant. Such cysts are lined by a single layer of cuboidal to columnar epithelium that may be nonciliated, ciliated, mucin-producing, or granulated. **A:** The cyst contains an eosinophilic colloid (H&E, original magnification ×100). **B:** Intermediate lobe cells may stain for pituitary hormones, in this case PRL (immunostain, original magnification ×100).

structurally, the median eminence consists of closely packed nerve terminals containing membrane-bound neurosecretory granules. Because the terminals lie in close proximity to the fenestrated capillaries that form the origin of the portal system, the overall anatomic arrangement permits ready entry of releasing and inhibiting hormones and perhaps other modulators into the portal system and hence the anterior lobe. The sites of synthesis of the various hypothalamic hormones, their characteristics, and target cells are summarized in Tables 1 and 2.

### Adenohypophysis

Grossly, the pituitary is a tan to brown, bean-shaped structure varying in weight from 500 to 700 mg (Fig. 1). An average-sized gland of 600 mg measures about 13 × 10 × 6 mm. Generally, the weight of the female pituitary is greater than that of the male (29). Among females, the gland is smaller in nulliparas than in multiparas. In pregnancy the gland enlarges significantly (up to 30%) due primarily to prolactin (PRL) cell hyperplasia (29,30). The anterior lobe comprises 80% of the pituitary and includes the pars distalis, intermedia, and tuberalis. As a functional unit, the neurohypophysis consists of the infundibulum, pituitary stalk, and posterior lobe. The body and stalk of the gland are surrounded by a delicate capsule derived from the meninges (31). Staining characteristics roughly divide the pars distalis into a central mucoid wedge and two lateral wings, zones best visualized in coronal and horizontal sections.

By light microscopy, the cells of the anterior lobe show

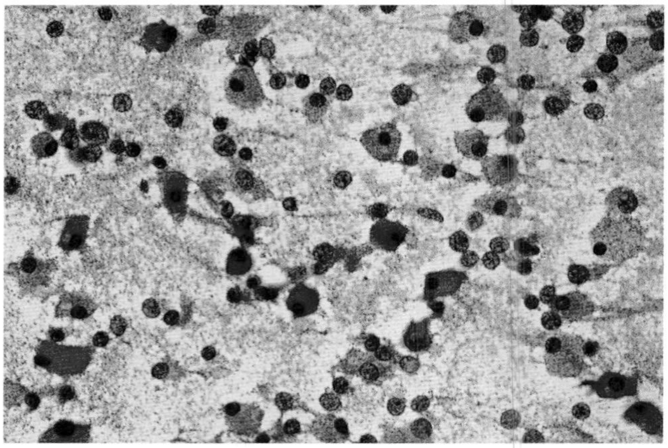

**FIG. 25.** H&E-stained cytologic smear of the normal anterior lobe, demonstrating acidophils, chromophobes, and basophils. Delicate nuclei, inconspicuous nucleoli, and variable cytoplasmic staining characterize normal cells and permit their distinction from adenoma cells.

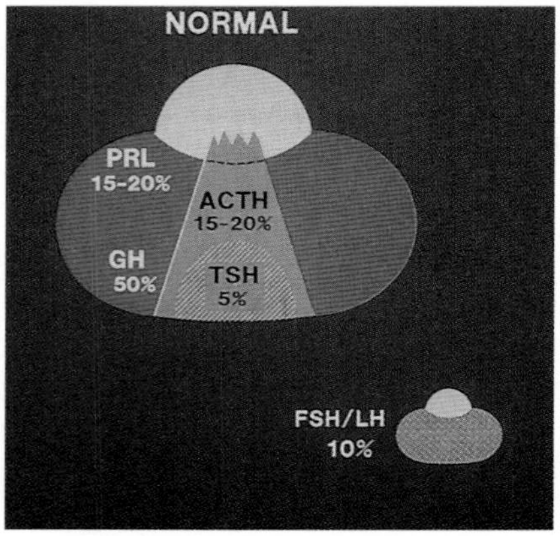


**FIG. 27.** Preferential localization and relative frequency of functional anterior lobe cell types in the normal pituitary gland. Note that gonadotrophs (LH/FSH cells), represented in the small gland (*lower right*), are distributed diffusely and show no preferential localization.

variation, not only in size and shape but also in their histochemical staining characteristics (Figs. 24 and 25). They are arranged in nests and cords bounded by an interlacing capillary network that is best seen on reticulin stain (Fig. 18). This architectural pattern, altered in hyperplasia and conspicuously absent in adenomas, is of considerable diagnostic significance. The pars intermedia, poorly developed in humans, consists in large part of epithelium-lined spaces containing periodic acid-Schiff (PAS)-positive colloid; the constituent cells are ciliated, goblet, and endocrine; the last show variable immunoreactivity for pituitary hormones (32) (Fig. 26). Incidental Rathke's cleft remnants, the vast majority of which are microscopic in size, are present in 30% of sellar and 15% of pharyngeal pituitaries (33). Of sellar examples, 80% occur in the intermediate lobe, the remainder in relation to the pars tuberalis.

In H&E-stained sections, three principal cell types are identified in the normal anterior lobe: acidophils (40%), basophils (10%), and chromophobes (50%) (Figs. 24 and 25). The designations reflect their staining affinities for acidic and basic dyes, with the chromophobic cells lacking affinity for either. These reactivities form the basis of an outdated classification of pituitary cells that, although convenient, offers little in specifying their hormone content or endocrine function. On the other hand, recent advances in immunohistochemistry permit morphologic and functional correlation (Fig. 27). Numerous cells in the central or mucoid wedge are basophilic and stain strongly via the PAS method. Such cells are adrenocorticotropin (ACTH) and glycoprotein hormone (LH, FSH, TSH) producing. In contrast, most cells in the lateral wings are acidophilic and are engaged either in growth hormone (GH) or, less frequently, in PRL production. The essential morphologic features of the five principal cell types and the biochemical characteristics of the six hormones of the anterior pituitary are summarized in Table 3. Their ultrastructural features are presented in Table 4.

Somatotrophs or GH cells occur in greatest density in the lateral wings and comprise approximately 50% of all adenohypophyseal cells. They are medium-sized, ovoid cells with round, centrally located nuclei, relatively prominent nucleoli, and abundant acidophilic granules (Figs. 28 and 29).

The product of GH cells has far-reaching effects despite the fact that the substance has no specific target organ. Working through mediators of hepatic origin called somatomedins (IGF-1), GH functions as the major promotor of growth. Its release from the anterior lobe is under the control of the two hypothalamic hormones, growth hormone releasing hormone (GHRH) and the inhibitory hormone somatostatin. Although GH exhibits a diurnal pattern of secretion with relatively stable basal levels, superimposed surges in GH output are noted, particularly 1 hour after the onset of sleep. Hypersecretion of GH in children causes gigantism, whereas its overproduction in adults leads to acromegaly.

Lactotrophs or PRL cells comprise approximately 20% of anterior pituitary cells and are concentrated in the posterior portions of the lateral wings. Histologically, they appear either acidophilic (densely granulated) or chromophobic (sparsely granulated). Densely granulated lactotrophs are

**TABLE 3.** *The normal anterior pituitary: morphologic and functional features of secretory cells*

| Cell | Product | Serum level (males/females) | Location | Percentage of cells | Histochemical staining[a] | Immunoperoxidase staining |
|---|---|---|---|---|---|---|
| Somatotroph[b] | Growth hormone (GH); 21,000 dalton polypeptide | 0 to 5 ng/ml/ 0 to 10 ng/ml | Lateral wings | 50 | Acidophilic; PAS (−) | GH |
| Lactotroph[b] | Prolactin (PRL); 23,500 dalton polypeptide | 0 to 20 ng/ml/ 0 to 23 ng/ml | Resting cells—generalized; secreting cells—posterolateral wings | 15 to 20 | Acidophilic/PAS (−) Herlant's eythrosin and Brooke's carmoisine (+) | PRL |
| Corticotroph | Adrenocorticotrophic hormone (ACTH); 4,507 dalton polypeptide | <60 pg/ml | Mucoid wedge | 15 to 20 | Basophilic; PAS and lead hematoxylin (+) | ACTH, $\beta$-LPH, MSH, endorphin, enkephalin |
| Gonadotroph | Follicle stimulating and luteinizing hormone (FSH/LH); 35,100 and 28,260 dalton glycoproteins | <22 IU/liter/ <20 IU/liter FSH[d] <4–24 IU/liter/ <30 IU/liter LH[e] | Generalized | 10 | Basophilic; PAS, lead hematoxylin, aldehyde fuchsin, and aldehyde thionine (+) | FSH and LH[c] |
| Thyrotroph | Thyrotrophic hormone (TSH); 28,000 dalton glycoprotein | 0.4 to 6 milli IU/ liter | Anterior mucoid wedge | ~5 | Same as for gonadotroph | TSH |

[a] The tinctorial characteristics of normal pituitary cells depend on adequate cytoplasmic granulae storage. If sparsely granulated, cells otherwise functional may appear nonreactive or "chromophobic."
[b] Rare acidophilic stem cells (presumed somatotroph and lactotroph precursor cells producing both GH and PRL) are present in the normal pituitary.
[c] Many gonadotrophs are capable of producing both FSH and LH, although immunohistochemical and ultrastructural evidence suggests that some gonadotrophs may produce only one hormone.
[d] Value given for females is non-midcycle value. Midcycle, <40 IU/liter; postmenopausal, 40 to 160 IU/liter.
[e] Value given for females is non-midcycle value. Midcycle, 30 to 150 IU/liter; postmenopausal, 30 to 120 IU/liter.

**TABLE 4.** *The normal pituitary; ultrastructural features*

| Cell | Granularity | Cell size and shape | Nucleus | Cytoplasm | Golgi complex | Rough endoplasmic reticulum | Granules |
|---|---|---|---|---|---|---|---|
| Somatotroph | | | | | | | |
| Densely granulated (resting phase) | +++, ++++ | Medium, spherical-oval | Spherical and central, with prominent nucleoli | Lucent | + | + | Abundant; dense, spherical; closely apposed limiting membrane; no exocytoses; 350 to 600 nm (range 250 to 600 nm) |
| Sparsely granulated (secretory phase) | +, ++ | Medium, spherical-oval | Irregular | Lucent | +++ | +++ Peripherally disposed | Sparse; dense, spherical; closely apposed limiting membrane; no exocytoses; 350 to 600 nm (range 250 to 600 nm) |
| Lactotroph | | | | | | | |
| Densely granulated (resting phase) | +++, ++++ | Large, polyhedral-elongate | Oval-elongate | Lucent | + | ++ Peripherally disposed | Abundant; dense, spherical-oval, irregular; 500 to 800 nm; occasional exocytoses |
| Sparsely granulated (secretory phase) | +, ++ | Medium, polyhedral-elongate | Oval | Lucent | +++, ++++ Juxtanuclear | ++++ "Nebenkern" formation | Sparse; dense, irregular; 200 to 350 nm; frequent normal and misplaced exocytoses |
| Corticotroph | ++, +++ | Medium, oval-polygonal | Spherical, eccentric | Electron-dense; cytoplasmic type I microfilaments; large lysosomes ("enigmatic bodies") | ++ | ++, +++ Dispersed, slightly dilated | Variable density, spherical—irregular; 300 to 350 nm (range 250 to 700 nm, rarely 1,000 nm); frequently peripheral; no exocytoses |
| Gonadotroph | ++ | Medium, oval | Spherical, eccentric | Lucent | ++, +++ Prominent, globular | ++, +++ Stacked or dispersed and slightly dilated | Dense, spherical; 250 to 400 nm; no exocytoses |
| Thyrotroph | +, ++ | Medium, polygonal | Spherical, eccentric | Lucent; scattered lysosomes | ++, +++ Globular, with numerous vesicles | +++ Short dispersed profiles | Dense, spherical; frequently peripheral; 150 nm; no exocytoses |

Follicle cells: hypogranulated adenohypophyseal cells surrounding degenerated cells. Follicle cells are bound by typical junctional complexes.

thought to represent a storage phase, whereas sparsely granulated cells are engaged in active secretion. The more numerous chromophobic cells, located predominantly in the posterior lateral wings, possess elongate processes and, despite an abundance of endoplasmic reticulum and well-developed Golgi complexes, contain relatively few cytoplasmic granules (Figs. 30 and 31, and Table 4). A recognized, but as yet unexplained, feature of PRL cells is their tendency to encircle or embrace gonadotrophs, likely an expression of an intimate physiologic relationship (Fig. 30). The existence of mammosomatotrophs, cells engaged in PRL and GH production and possessing unique ultrastructural features, attests to the existence of a histogenetic relationship between PRL and GH cells.

With the exception of pregnancy and lactation, there is no significant difference in PRL cell number between males and females. The doubling in volume of the pituitary during pregnancy is due to striking hyperplasia as well as hypertrophy of chromophobic lactotrophs, termed pregnancy cells. They persist until shortly after delivery or the termination of lactation (29,30). PRL cell hyperplasia also may accompany estrogen administration as well as hypothyroidism (34).

PRL secretion is primarily under the inhibitory control of dopamine, the principal hypothalamic PRL-inhibitory factor (PIF). A fragment of GnRH also has been shown to inhibit PRL release, whereas TRH and VIP are known to stimulate PRL release. Any space-occupying sellar or parasellar mass (e.g., pituitary adenoma, Rathke's cleft cyst, craniopharyngioma, or glioma) that compresses the pituitary stalk impedes PIF delivery to the anterior lobe, causing hyperprolactinemia, a phenomenon termed stalk effect. The most striking example of stalk effect is the hyperprolactinemia that follows surgical transection of the stalk, a practice now obsolete but once used in the past for the treatment of metastatic breast cancer (35).

The function of PRL is to stimulate the formation of ca-

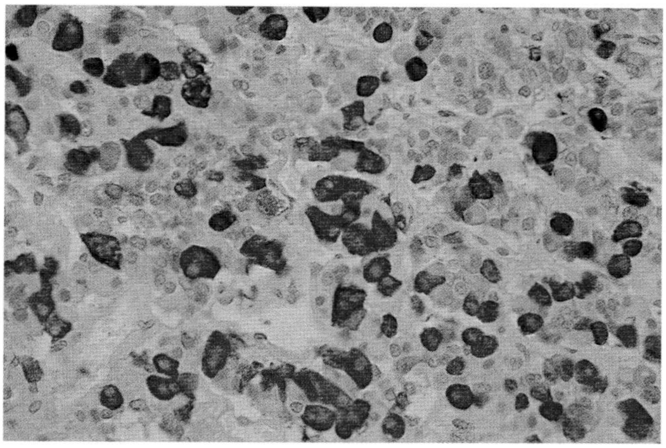

**FIG. 28.** Adenohypophysis stained for GH. Somatotrophs, medium-sized ovoid cells with abundant cytoplasm, comprise 50% of anterior lobe cells. The strong staining reaction is a reflection of the numerous secretory granules present at the ultrastructural level (see Fig. 29) (immunostain, original magnification ×100).

sein, lactalbumin, lipids, and carbohydrates, all essential components of breast milk. During pregnancy, high levels of estrogen, progesterone, placental lactogen, and PRL induce acinar development and promote milk formation. As previously noted, milk secretion is under the control of oxytocin, a potent stimulator of myoepithelial cell contraction in breast tissue.

Corticotrophs or ACTH cells comprise 15% to 20% of adenohypophyseal cells and are most numerous in the mid- and posterior portions of the mucoid wedge (Fig. 27). Histologically, ACTH cells are polygonal, medium to large sized, and amphophilic (Fig. 32). Strong PAS positivity is due to a carbohydrate moiety contained in proopiomelanocortin (POMC), the precursor molecule of ACTH. In immunostained preparations, corticotrophs may be shown to contain not only ACTH but $\beta$-LPH, melanocyte-stimulating hormone (MSH), endorphin, enkephalin, and other POMC derivatives. One intriguing characteristic of these cells is an unstained region adjacent to the nucleus, the enigmatic body (32,36) (Figs. 32–34). This spherical structure, with its clear center and surrounding dark-staining rim, corresponds ultrastructurally to one or several partially empty membrane-

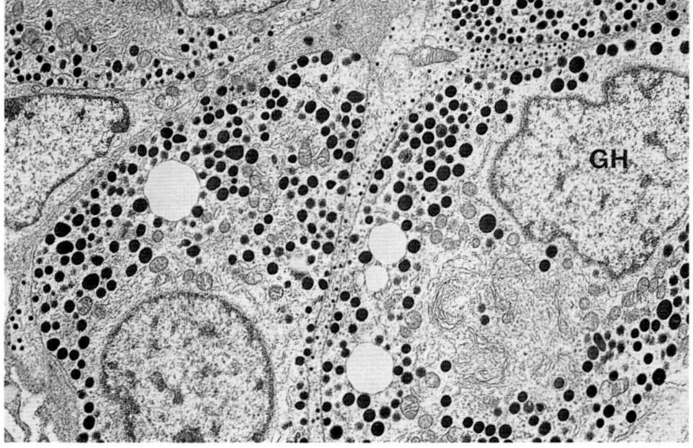


**FIG. 29.** Densely granulated GH cells showing prominent Golgi and numerous 200- to 500-nm secretory granules (original magnification ×11,700).

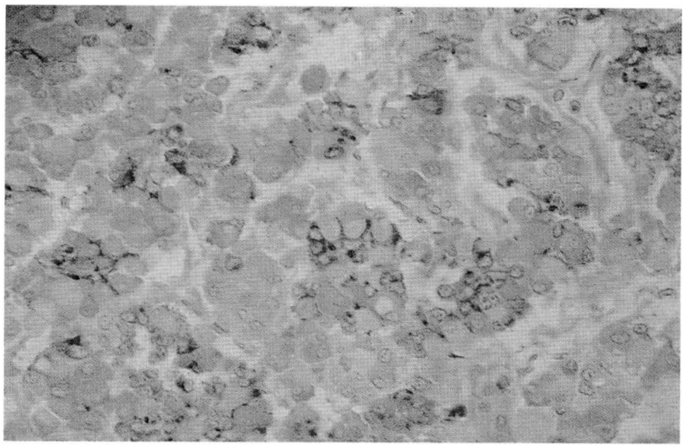

**FIG. 30.** Adenohypophysis stained for PRL. Lactotrophs comprise 15% to 20% of anterior lobe cells. The majority are sparsely granulated angular cells with processes that may wrap around adjacent cells. In the center of the field several PRL cell processes are seen to embrace adjacent gonadotrophs. Many lactotrophs in this field show paranuclear staining, a pattern corresonding to PRL in the Golgi apparatus. A densely granulated lactotroph is present in the upper portion of the field (immunostain, original magnification ×100).

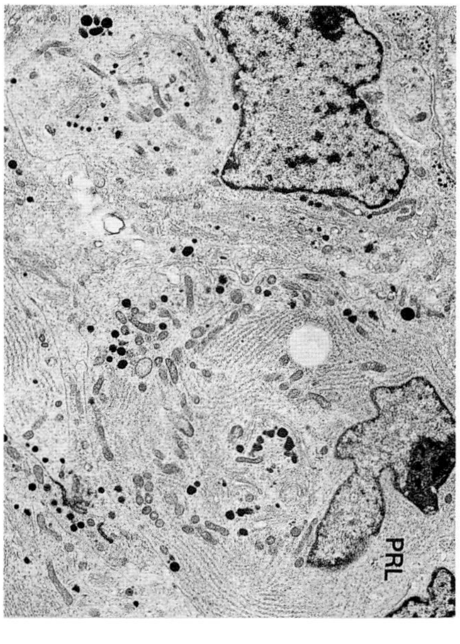


**FIG. 31.** Sparsely granulated PRL cell. Note the abundant cisternae of rough endoplasmic reticulum and the prominent Golgi complex containing pleomorphic developing granules. Mature PRL granules range in size from 200 to 350 nm (original magnification ×8,700).

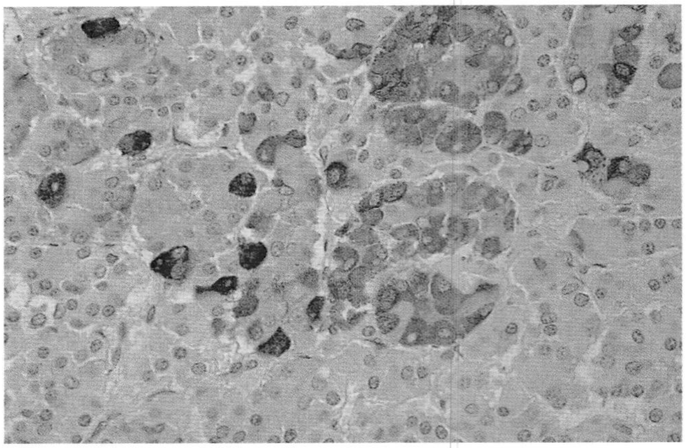

**FIG. 32.** Adenohypophysis stained for ACTH. Corticotrophs comprise about 15% to 20% of anterior lobe cells and are mainly located in the mucoid wedge. They are ovoid to polyhedral. Many have an unstained region near the nucleus, representing a massive PAS-positive lysosome once termed the enigmatic body. Note the clustering of cells, a characteristic feature of corticotrophs (immunostain, original magnification ×100).

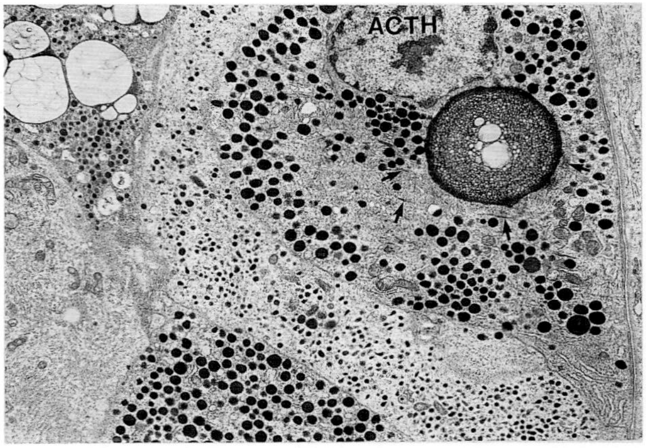


**FIG. 34.** Normal corticotroph. The cell contains the typical large lysosome (enigmatic body) and spherical to slightly pleomorphic and variably electron-dense secretory granules measuring 150 to 450 nm. Bundles of type I microfilaments (*arrows*) are a regular feature of ACTH cells. The adjacent cells with small granules are likely TSH cells (original magnification, ×8,250).

bound vacuoles, specialized lysosomal structures, the significance of which is unclear. Perinuclear bundles of cytokeratin filaments are also a characteristic feature of ACTH cells (see Table 4 for ultrastructural features). Under conditions of glucocorticoid excess, either exogenous or intrinsic, corticotrophs accumulate type I microfilaments as a manifestation of Crooke's hyaline change (Figs. 35–37).

ACTH, the principal product of corticotrophs and the main POMC derivative, stimulates secretion of glucocorticoids, mineralocorticoids, and androgens from the adrenal cortices. In addition, it enhances protein synthesis in the adrenal glands, an effect that may manifest grossly as cortical hyperplasia. Aside from these functions, ACTH plays a critical role in both the transport of amino acids and glucose into muscle as well as the stimulation of insulin release from the pancreas. Excess secretion of ACTH, such as occurs in Cushing's disease, leads to stereotypic abnormalities including truncal obesity, hypertension, diabetes mellitus, amenorrhea, hirsutism, muscle atrophy, striae, impaired wound healing, and mental status changes. Hyperpigmentation also may occur in this setting and is due to the effects of MSH, also a POMC derivative.

Thyrotrophs or TSH cells are located primarily in the anterior part of the mucoid wedge and comprise only 5% of adenohypophyseal cells (37). They are medium sized and angular or elongate. Like corticotrophs, normal TSH cells stain with basic dyes and are PAS positive (Figs. 38 and 39) (see Table 4 for ultrastructural features).

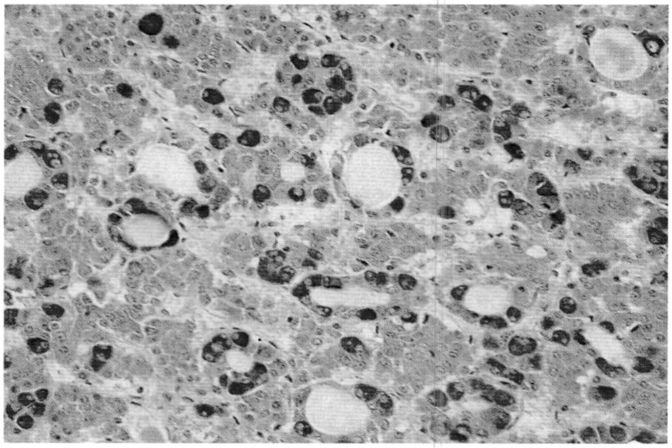

**FIG. 33.** Follicles in the anterior pituitary. Several well-formed follicles are seen to stain, in large part, for ACTH. Corticotroph cells frequently contribute to follicle formation (immunostain, original magnification ×63).

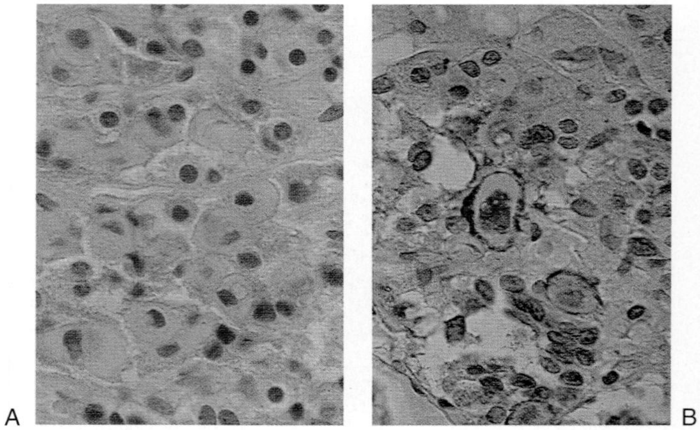


**FIG. 35.** Crooke's hyaline change. **A:** Crooke's cells are characterized by a conspicuous eosinophilic perinuclear ring consisting of cytokeratin (H&E, original magnification ×100). **B:** ACTH stains show central displacement of the nucleus and organelles by filament accumulation (immunostain, original magnification ×100).

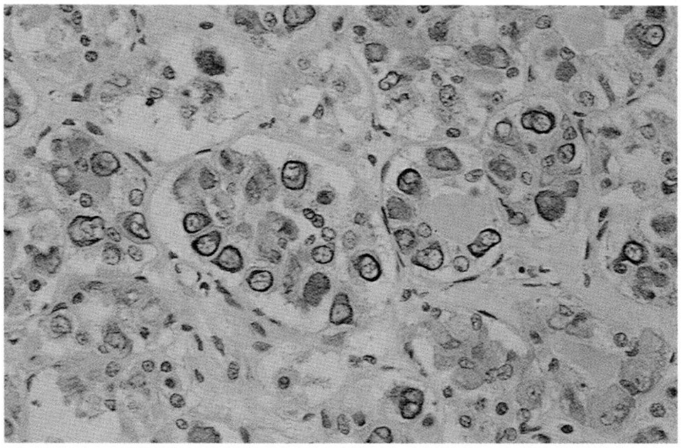

**FIG. 36.** Crooke's cells staining for MAB Leu-5, a monoclonal panepithelial antibody. The cytokeratin filaments show strong reactivity (immunostain, original magnification ×100).

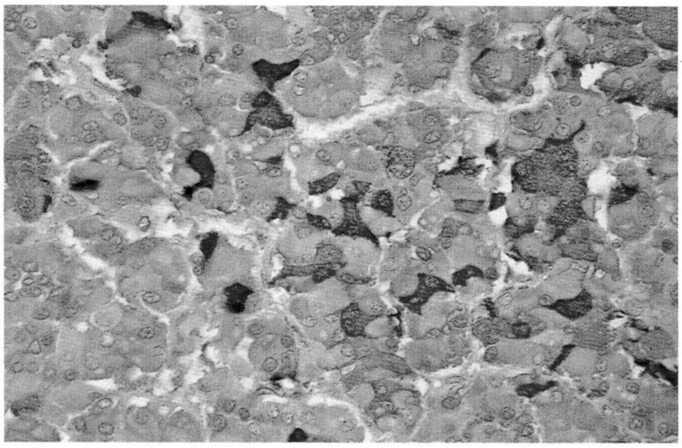

**FIG. 38.** Anterior pituitary stained for TSH. Thyrotrophs are medium-sized angulated cells with some demonstrating elongate processes. They comprise only about 5% of anterior lobe secretory cells and show strong immunoreactivity (immunostain, original magnification ×100).

TSH, a glycoprotein hormone, binds to thyroid cells, inducing RNA and protein synthesis and thereby the production of thyroglobulin and thyroid hormones. In the setting of primary hypothyroidism, thyrotrophs undergo hypertrophy and hyperplasia (34). When excessive, the response may produce sufficient hypertrophy of the pituitary gland to mimic adenoma. Pituitary adenomas that elaborate TSH are rare; most occur in the setting of hypothyroidism (32), although a minority result in hyperthyroidism.

Gonadotrophs, or FSH and LH cells, comprise 10% of the pars distalis, show a strong affinity for both basic and PAS stains, and generally are evenly distributed throughout the anterior lobe. Immunohistochemical and ultrastructural studies have shown that FSH and LH may be produced in isolation or by the same cell (38) (Figs. 40 and 41) (see Table 4 for ultrastructural features).

LH and FSH play a distinct but essential role in the reproductive physiology of males and females. In the female, LH is required for ovulation and follicular luteinization. In males, it stimulates interstitial Leydig cells to produce testosterone. FSH promotes follicular development in the female, whereas in the male it induces Sertoli cells to produce an androgen-binding protein.

The pars tuberalis, an upward extension of the anterior lobe along the pituitary stalk, is composed of normal acini of pituitary cells scattered among surface portal vessels. These cells often show immunoreactivity for ACTH, FSH, LH, and alpha subunit (Figs. 42 and 43). Although in functional terms they may or may not differ from similar cells in the pars distalis, these cells do show a distinct tendency to undergo squamous metaplasia (39).

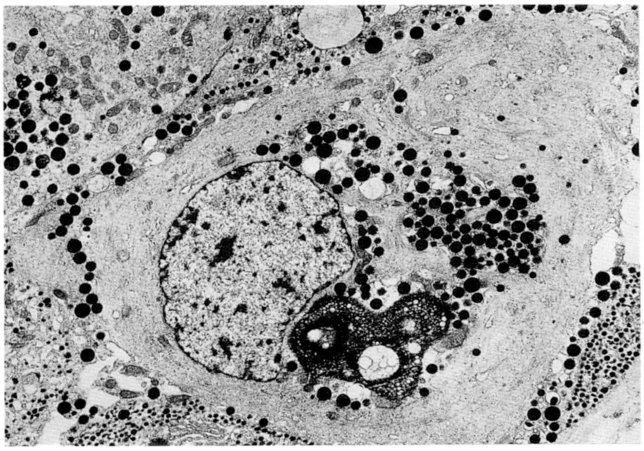

**FIG. 37.** Crooke's cell. This electron micrograph of the pituitary adjacent to a corticotroph cell adenoma displays massive accumulation of cytokeratin filament. Secretory granules are displaced to the perinuclear zone or to the periphery of the cytoplasm. Note the large lysosome (enigmatic body) in the lower portion of the field (original magnification, ×6,720).

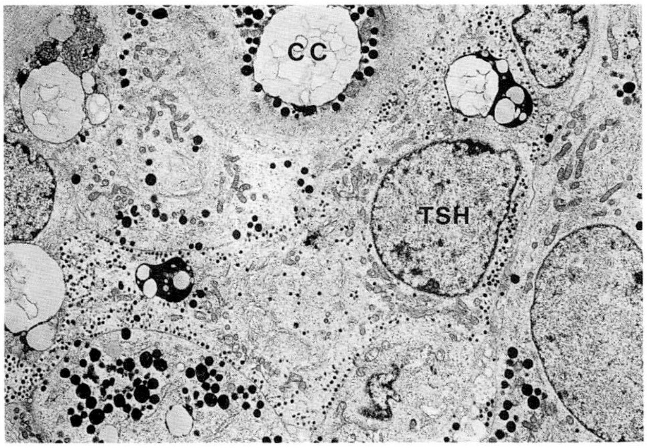


**FIG. 39.** TSH cell. This micrograph of the normal anterior pituitary shows the characteristic elongate thyrotrophs, the large lysosomes frequently observed in cells of this type, and small (150-nm) peripherally located secretory granules. Part of a Crooke's cell (CC) is also shown (original magnification ×5,300).

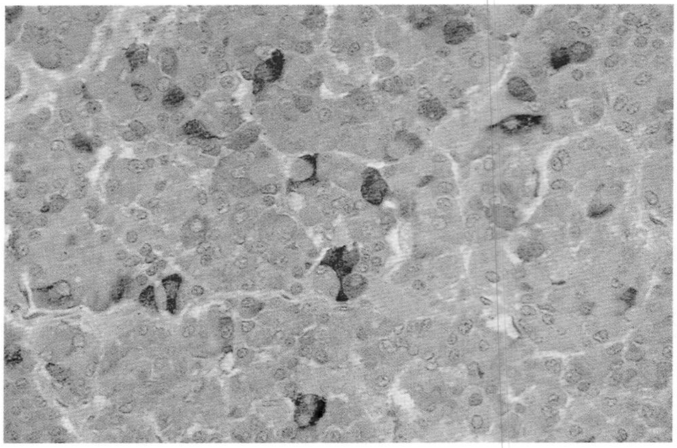

**FIG. 40.** Anterior pituitary stained for FSH. Gonadotrophs manufacture both LH and FSH. The paucity of strongly staining cells in this field reflects the fact that only 10% of anterior lobe secretory cells are gonadotrophs (immunostain, original magnification ×100).

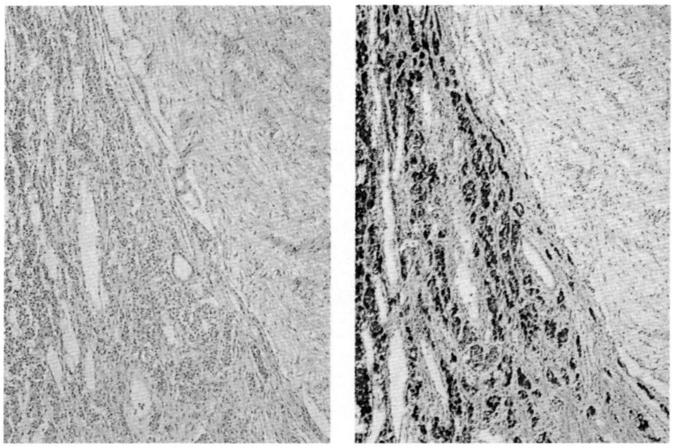

A B

**FIG. 42.** Anterior pituitary, pars tuberalis. **A:** H&E-stained section showing secretory cells of the pars tuberalis (*lower left*) clustered along the surface of the pituitary stalk (*upper right*) (H&E original magnification ×63). **B:** The same section stained for FSH shows prominent staining in pars tuberalis cells, the majority of which are gonadotrophs. Occasional ACTH-positive cells are also encountered (immunostain, original magnification ×63).

Follicles are not an uncommon feature of the normal anterior pituitary. Their functional constituent cells, termed follicular cells, appear to be derived in large part from various secretory cells. Ultrastructurally, they are often poorly granulated or agranular and linked by apical junctional complexes. Within follicular lumina, one often finds cellular debris. The stimulus for follicle formation is therefore thought to be damage or rupture of anterior lobe secretory cells (40) (Figs. 44–46).

The folliculostellate cell, an unusual cell type of indeterminate nature, comprises less than 5% of the anterior lobe cells (41). They are scattered about the anterior lobe, contribute to the formation of anterior lobe follicles and cysts of the intermediate lobe, and in some cases are present in adenomas. They are readily identified by their reactivity for S-100 protein, a substance not present in the other anterior lobe cells. Glial fibrillary acidic protein and vimentin reactivity have been identified by some. The physiologic role of folliculostellate cells, if any, is unclear, though they may serve a role in regulation of hormone secretion. Their configuration as well as their content of small numbers of secretory granules suggest they may be derived from ordinary secretory cells (41) (Fig. 46). The relationship of follicle cells to folliculostellate cells remains unsettled.

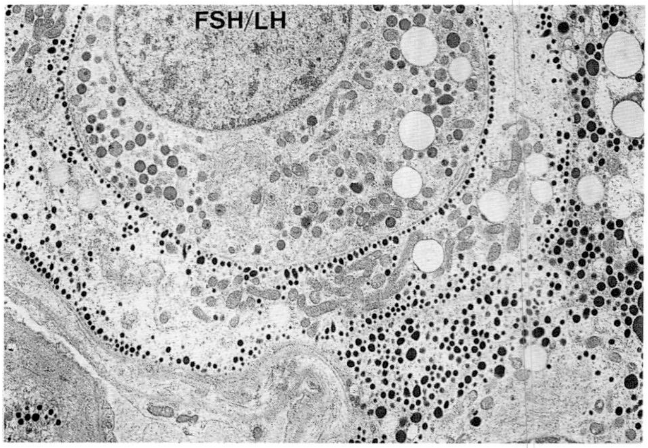


**FIG. 41.** Normal gonadotroph (FSH/LH) cell. The dull, low-contrast appearance of the cell is typical of gonadotrophs. Their spherical and slightly irregular secretory granules are characteristic; they have variable electron density and measure 250 to 400 nm. The cell process surrounding the gonadotroph likely belongs to a thyrotroph (original magnification ×8,250).

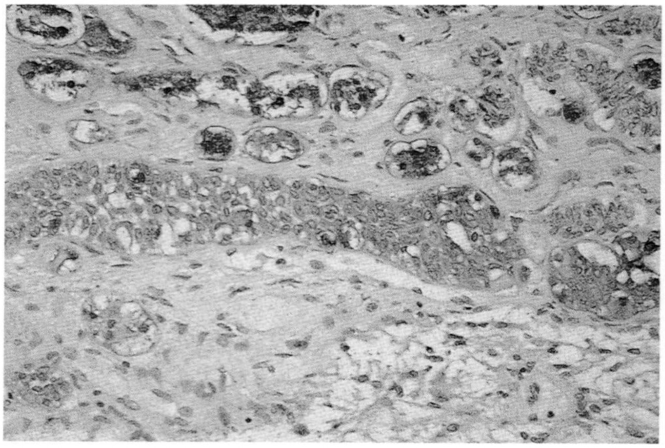

**FIG. 43.** Anterior pituitary, pars tuberalis. Squamous metaplasia of secretory cells is a common feature of this portion of the gland. Staining for FSH within squamous cells in the midportion of the field illustrates this phenomenon (immunostain, original magnification ×63).

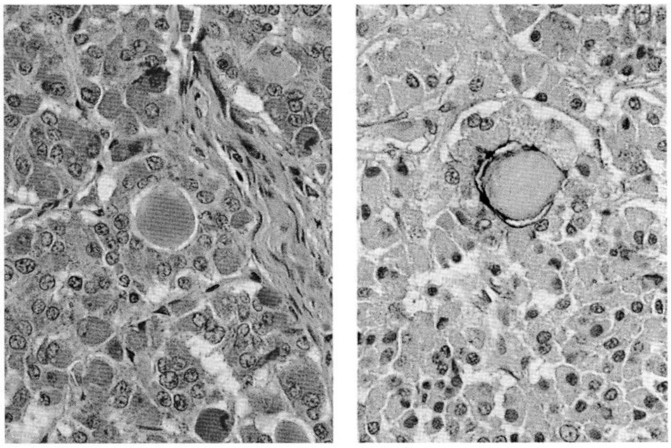

A B

**FIG. 44.** Anterior pituitary, follicle formation. **A:** Follicles, some containing a small quantity of colloidlike material, are commonly found in the anterior lobe (H&E, original magnification ×100). **B:** Follicles show prominent apical staining for epithelial membrane antigen (EMA) (immunostain, original magnification × 100).

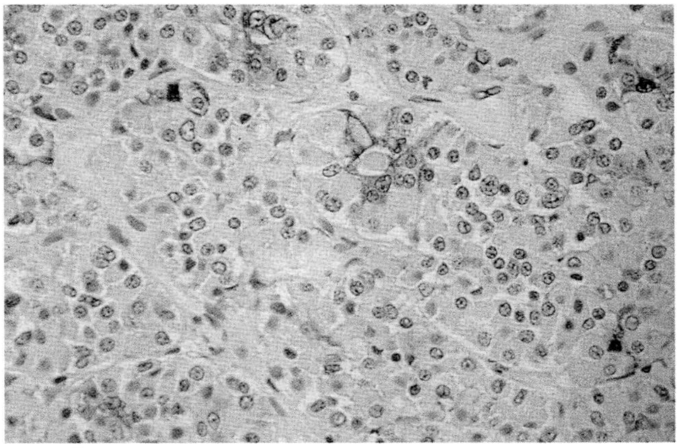

**FIG. 46.** Anterior lobe folliculostellate cells. A follicle in the upper portion of the field shows such cells staining for S-100 protein. Folliculostellate cells comprise less than 5% of anterior lobe cells and are scattered throughout the pituitary, including the intermediate lobe zone. Such cells also stain for GFAP and vimentin (immunostain, original magnification ×100).

### *Variation in Normal Morphology*

A number of normal histologic variations in the pituitary gland may mimic clinically significant lesions. Examples include squamous cell nests in the pars tuberalis, basophil invasion of the posterior lobe, granular cell clusters and tumorlettes of the stalk and neurohypophysis, and salivary gland rests.

Squamous cell nests show a definite predilection for the pars tuberalis; they have been found in up to 24% of autopsy cases, occur more commonly in elderly patients, and show no sex predilection (42). They arise through a process of metaplastic transformation from adenohypophyseal cells, as evidenced by simultaneous expression of keratin and pituitary hormones, most often FSH, LH, or ACTH (39) (Fig. 43). Once thought to be precursors of craniopharyngioma, the two lesions are now considered unrelated. Because squamous metaplasia also may accompany foci of ischemic infarction in the anterior lobe, it appears to be an inherent property of pituitary secretory cells.

Basophil invasion, a finding more common in males and the elderly, may at first glance mimic an adenoma. It consists of corticotrophic basophils extending from the pars intermedia into the neurohypophysis (Figs. 47 and 48). Although, like ordinary corticotrophs, these basophilic cells are im-

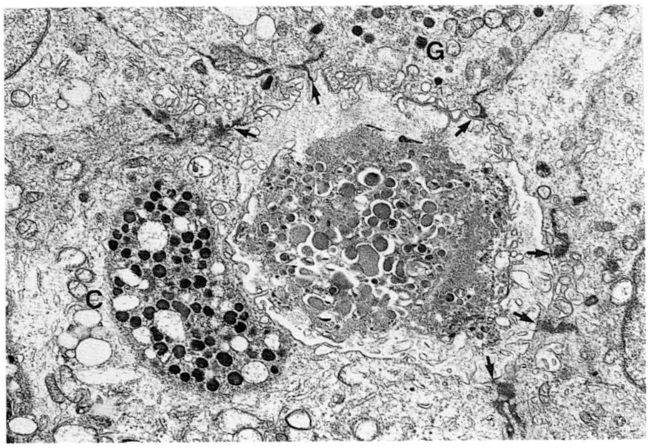


**FIG. 45.** Electron micrograph of a pituitary follicle. This young follicle contains cell debris within its lumen. The gonadotroph (G), but not the corticotroph (C), is part of this follicle. Follicles are composed of granulated adenohypophyseal cells that, through the formation of junctional complexes (*terminal bars, arrows*), surround damaged adenohypophyseal cells (original magnification ×12,600).

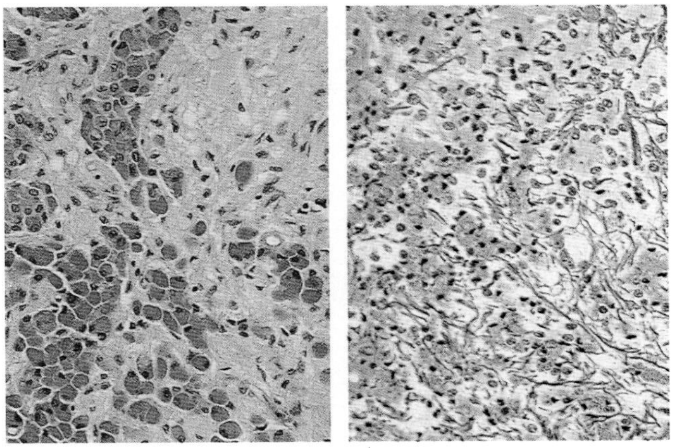

A B

**FIG. 47.** Basophil invasion. **A:** This subpopulation of corticotroph cells appears to infiltrate the substance of the posterior lobe (H&E, original magnification ×63). **B:** The invading cells are seen to lie among the axons of the posterior lobe (Bodian, original magnification ×63).

A 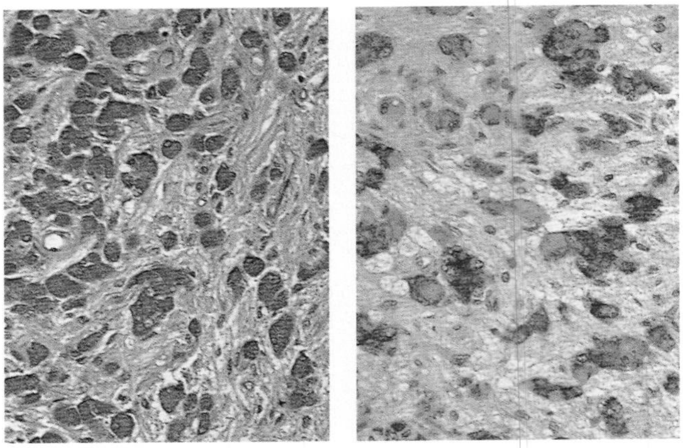 B

**FIG. 48.** Basophil invasion. **A:** PAS, original magnification ×63. **B:** ACTH, original magnification ×63.

munoreactive for ACTH, $\beta$-LPH, endorphins, and other POMC derivatives, they contain few cytokeratin filaments and are less susceptible to Crooke's hyalinization in response to hypercortisolism (32).

Salivary gland rests appear as tubular glands upon the surface or in the substance of the neurohypophysis, often just posterior to the pars intermedia (Fig. 49). They are composed of a single layer of cuboidal to columnar epithelium with basally oriented nuclei and finely granular, strongly PAS-positive cytoplasm. Salivary gland rests are often oncocytic; their ultrastructural features include well-developed rough endoplasmic reticulum, secretory droplets, microvilli, and desmosomes, all of which support the contention that they are indeed salivary glands (43).

Granular cell nests or tumorlettes, most located in the stalk or posterior lobe, are found in about 6% of autopsy pituitaries and are more common among the elderly (44). Varying from scattered cells to compact tumorlike nodules, they are composed of plump cells with granular acidophilic and strongly PAS-positive cytoplasm and relatively small nuclei (Fig. 50). Only rarely do granular cells form clinically significant tumors (45).

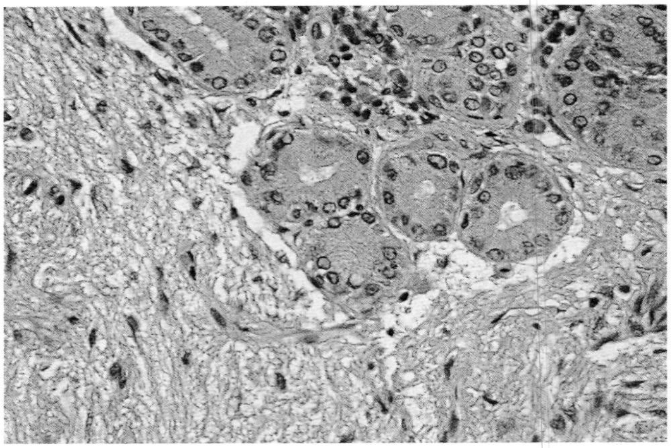

**FIG. 49.** Salivary gland rest in the posterior lobe. The glands are composed of a single layer of cuboidal to columnar epithelium with basally oriented nuclei and granular PAS-positive cytoplasm. Salivary gland rests are encountered both on the surface of or within the posterior lobe, where it abuts the intermediate lobe zone (H&E, original magnification ×63).

Apoptosis remains to be studied in the human pituitary gland. Data regarding the occurrence of apoptosis in the pituitary gland is based primarily on animal studies, assessing the affect of estrogen withdrawal and dopamine agonist administration on stimulated PRL cells (46). Resultant involution of PRL cells results in the formation of apoptotic bodies. Phagocytosis of the latter is one function of folliculostellate cells. The contribution of apoptosis in the involution of PRL cells after pregnancy or after estrogen administration, as well as its possible role in bromocriptine therapy of human prolactinomas, remains to be studied.

### *Age-Related Changes*

The cytology of the pituitary varies with age. For instance, the late fetal or term pituitary gland shows PRL cell hyperplasia, no doubt a reflection of high maternal estrogen levels. Also, when compared with the adult pituitary, the prepubertal gland shows gonadotrophic cells to be poorly developed. In adults the pituitary undergoes several changes with increasing age (47,48).

With few exceptions, the main one being pregnancy, the gland weight remains stable throughout life, decreasing only slightly in the elderly due to anterior lobe atrophy. Pregnancy results in a doubling of the size of the pituitary due to gradual increase in large chromophobic PRL cells ("preg-

A 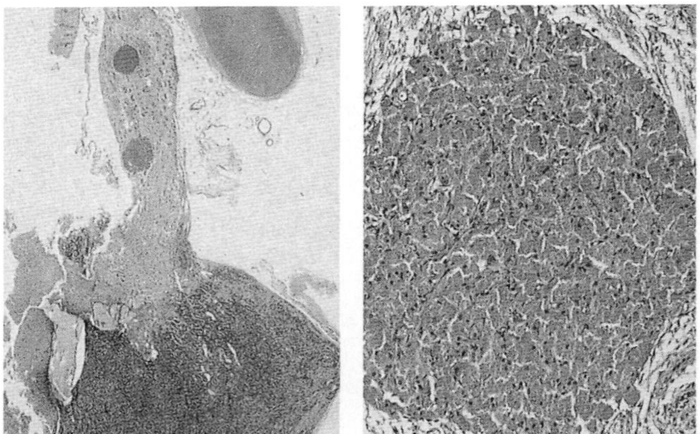 B

**FIG. 50.** Pituitary stalk, granular cell tumorlettes. **A:** Low-power view of the stalk shows two tumorlettes. The optic chiasm is at the upper portion of the field; the anterior lobe is at the lower portion of the field (H&E, original magnification ×20). **B:** High-power view of a granular cell tumorlette. Such nodules are composed of pituicytes, modified glial cells, with abundant lysosome-rich eosinophilic cytoplasm. Tumorlettes, as well as individual granular cells, also a common finding, are of no clinical significance (H&E, original magnification ×100).

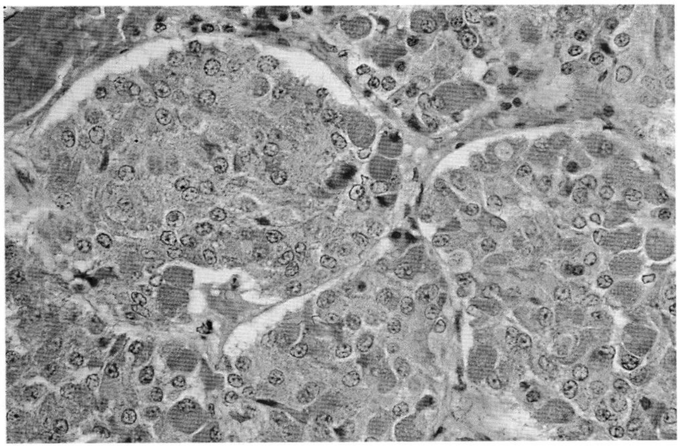

**FIG. 51.** The pituitary in a pregnancy features abundant pale chromophobic PRL cells (pregnancy cells) (H&E, original magnification ×100).

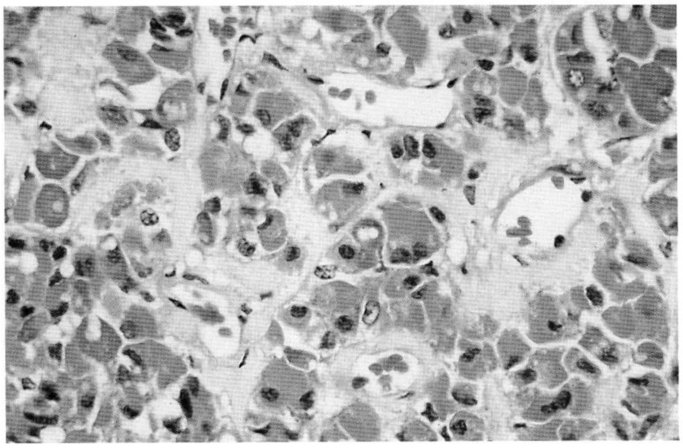

**FIG. 52.** Perivascular fibrosis is a common feature of the aging pituitary (H&E, original magnification ×100).

nancy cells") (49,50) (Fig. 51). The increase in PRL-producing cells during pregnancy results not only from proliferation of PRL cells but also from recruitment of GH cells to PRL production. This increase in PRL-producing cells, in large part a hyperplasia, gradually disappears within months after delivery or abortion. The process is often incomplete; hence, the pituitaries of multiparas are larger than those of women never pregnant. Pregnancy also results in a significant decrease of gonadotropin immunoreactivity, a reflection of the production of gonadotropic hormones by the placenta. The effects of age on the cellular contents of several pituitary hormones has been studied. Specifically, both GH and PRL cells have been shown to undergo no significant decrease in number, granularity, distribution, or immunoreactivity with increasing age (51,52). ACTH and TSH cells also appear to be unaffected by age, but no data are available regarding the effects of senescence on FSH and LH cells. Small foci of lymphocytes, usually in the intermediate lobe, are present in about 40% of adult pituitaries but are conspicuously absent in newborns and very young children (47).

Fibrosis is the most frequent age-related change in elderly patients. It is generally perivascular in distribution (Fig. 52) but is on occasion patchy, suggesting a remote microinfarct. A study of amyloid in the pituitary gland has recently been reported (53). Interstitial deposits were seen in 80% in autopsy-derived anterior pituitaries. Immunohistochemically, these reacted for antiamyloid lambda light chain and amyloid P component. The mean volume percentage of such deposits is approximately 0.5% of the anterior lobe. The occurrence of amyloid and its degree of deposition was related not only to patient age but also to the prevalence of chronic obstructive pulmonary disease and to non–insulin-dependent diabetes mellitus.

### *Artifacts*

Mechanical trauma at surgery or autopsy may induce cellular changes in the adenohypophysis. Most important is hyperchromasia and apparent loss of cytoplasm resulting in what appear to be "small cells." Such cells should not be mistaken for metastatic carcinoma or lymphoma.

### Neurohypophysis

The posterior lobe, a ventral extension of the central nervous system, is the site of release of the hypothalamic hormones oxytocin and vasopressin. Its cellular elements consist of unmyelinated axons originating from the supraoptic and paraventricular nuclei and, to a lesser extent, from cholinergic neurons of the hypothalamus, an extensive vascular network, as well as specialized glial cells termed pituicytes (Fig. 53). The latter, the most numerous cells of the neurohypophysis, are immunoreactive for glial fibrillary acidic protein (GFAP), an intermediate filament characteris-

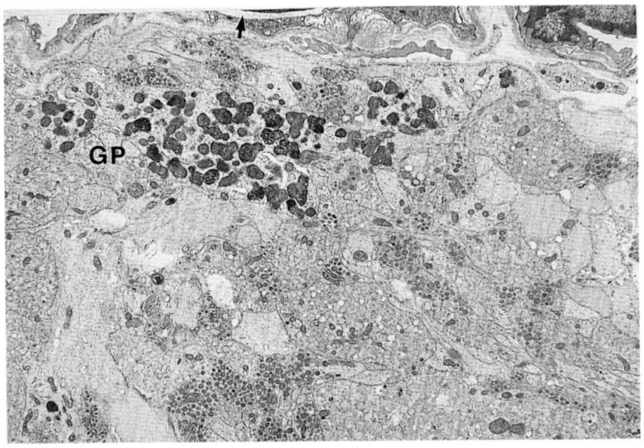


**FIG. 53.** Pituitary, posterior lobe. **A:** The fibrillary texture results from the large number of pituicytes, glial cells indigenous to the posterior lobe (H&E, original magnification ×100). **B:** Axonal fibers emanating from neurons in the hypothalamic magnocellular nuclei are plainly seen on Bodian stain (Bodian, original magnification ×100).

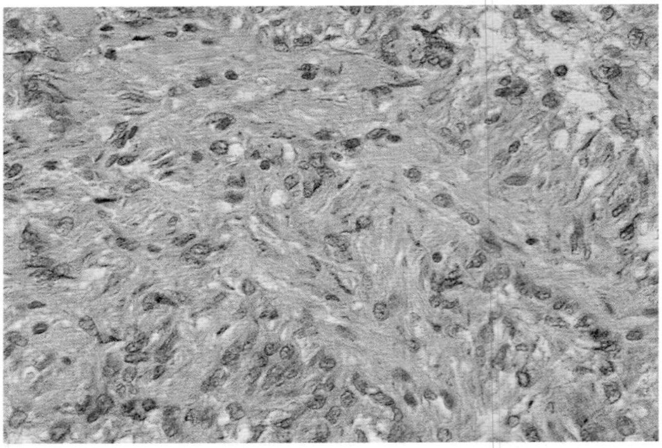

**FIG. 54.** Posterior lobe. Pituicytes stain positively for glial fibrillary acid protein (GFAP) (GFAP, original magnification ×100).

tic of astrocytes, as well as S-100 protein and vimentin (Fig. 54). Neurosecretory fibers are closely associated with pituicytes, their axons often being ensheathed by them (Fig. 55). Histologically, the axons of the posterior lobe are readily identified using silver stains. Focal axonal dilatations, known as Herring bodies, represent intra-axonal accumulations of posterior lobe hormones (Fig. 23). At the ultrastructural level, the unmyelinated axons appear as delicate fibers, measuring 0.05 to 1.0 $\mu$m in diameter, which contain longitudinal arrays of microtubules and neurofilaments. Two types of neurosecretory axon, A and B, have been described based on the morphology of their neurosecretory granules. Type A fibers, far more numerous than type B, contain 100- to 300-nm oxytocin and vasopressin granules, whereas type B fibers, likely aminergic in nature, contain granules ranging from 50 to 100 nm (54).

Pituicytes, the glial cells of the neurohypophysis, exist in five principal forms: major, dark, ependymal, oncocytic, and granular (55). Their morphologic diversity, ranging from astrocytic to ependymal, is thought to be a reflection of their physiologic role, which as yet is unclear. The most important function of the neurohypophysis is the transfer of hormonal substances from neurosecretory granules to the intravascular space. The complex anatomy of the neuronal, vascular, and perivascular compartments forms the basis for this elaborate process. Beginning at the neuronal side, neurohormonal factors appear to be released into minute channels that traverse the outermost or abluminal basement membrane of vessels to communicate with the perivascular space. They then traverse the inner or luminal basement membrane and endothelium in order to gain access to the vascular space (56) (Fig. 55).

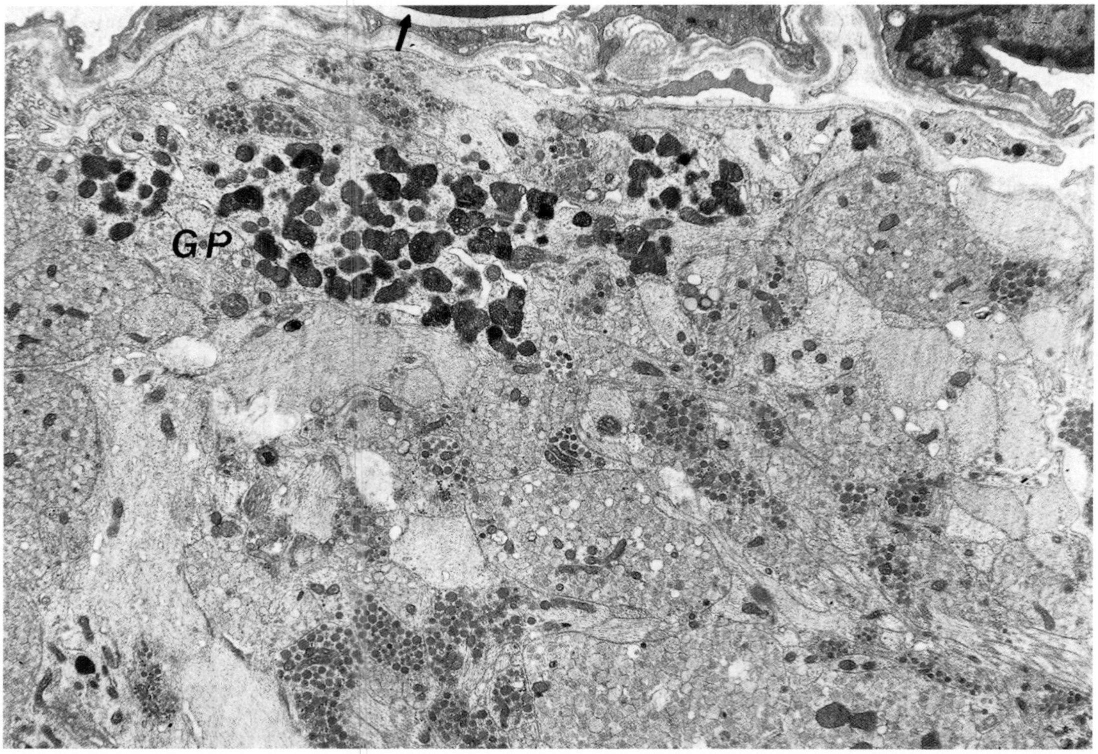


**FIG. 55.** Pituitary, posterior lobe. This electron micrograph shows axonal processes containing neurosecretory granules of varying electron density. A granular pituicyte (GP) containing numerous prominent lysosomes lies in close proximity to the intravascular space (*arrow*). The intravascular space is bounded by fenestrated endothelial cells as seen here. Outside the endothelium lies the perivascular space, a region containing a variety of cells types (not shown here), including pericytes, histiocytes, fibroblasts, and mast cells (original magnification, ×6,200).

## DIFFERENTIAL DIAGNOSIS

The principal consideration in differential diagnosis of pituitary lesions is the distinction of normal pituitary tissue from adenoma. The most conspicuous architectural feature of the adenohypophysis is the arrangement of its cells in acini that, depending on orientation of section, vary from round to oval or somewhat elongate. The acini are surrounded, usually completely, by a delicate, PAS- or reticulin-positive capillary network. In contrast, pituitary adenomas lack this uniform acinar architecture, showing only scant reticulin to be limited to scattered vessels. Although most normal pituitary acini are heterogeneous in their cellular content, thus permitting the distinction of normal from adenomatous tissue on H&E alone, some parts of the pituitary contain largely a single cell type and appear fairly monomorphous. For instance, eosinophilic GH cells are present in large number in the lateral means. On the other hand, occasional adenomas composed of mixed cell populations, often ones associated with acromegaly, superficially resemble normal adenohypophysis. As a result, the distinction of normal from adenomatous tissue may be more easily achieved by PAS and reticulin staining than by immunohistochemistry alone.

A limited biopsy of the pituitary may occasionally include intermediate zone cysts, normal derivatives of Rathke's cleft. Correlation with radiologic and operative data usually obviates confusion with Rathke's cleft cyst. As a rule, clinically significant cysts are readily evident on neuroimaging and are identified as sizeable cysts by the experienced surgeon.

As previously noted above, adenohypophyseal cells may undergo squamous metaplasia, particularly in the pars tuberalis. This location is only occasionally sampled in surgical specimens. Scant in extent, intimately associated with adenohypophyseal cells, and cytologically benign, they are unlikely to be confused with either cysts (epidermoid cysts, dermoid cysts) or with neoplasms (craniopharyngioma of adamantinomatous or papillary type, squamous carcinoma). In very small number, cytologic benign lymphocytes are seen in the intermediate zone of the normal pituitary in 10% of autopsied subjects (57). Unassociated with endocrine disease, such cells are readily distinguished from the far more widespread and dense infiltrates of lymphocytic hypophysitis or abscess.

A limited biopsy of the neurohypophysis can readily be mistaken for glioma in that the vast majority of its nucleated cells are specialized astrocytes (pituicytes). Unlike pilocytic astrocytomas, the tumor most closely mimicked by posterior pituitary tissue, the neurohypophysis contains large numbers of axons terminating on vessels. Of these axons, some possess PAS-positive swellings (Herring bodies). Secondary involvement of the pituitary by more ordinary diffuse astrocytomas is exceedingly rare.

## REFERENCES


1. Moore KL. The nervous system. In: Wonsiewicz M, ed. *The developing human.* Philadelphia: WB Saunders; 1988:364–401.
2. Conklin JL. The development of the human fetal adenohypophysis. *Anat Rec* 1968;160:79–92.
3. Sabshin JK. The pituitary gland—anatomy and embryology. In: Goodrich I, Lee KJ, eds. *The pituitary, clinical aspects of normal and abnormal function.* Amsterdam: Elsevier Science; 1987:19–27.
4. Falin LI. The development of human hypophysis and differentiation of cells of its anterior lobe during embryonic life. *Acta Anat* 1961;44: 188–205.
5. Boyd JD. Observations on the human pharyngeal hypophysis. *J Endocrinol* 1956;14:66–77.
6. McGrath P. Aspects of the human pharyngeal hypophysis in normal and anencephalic fetuses and neonates and their possible significance in the mechanism of its control. *J Anat* 1978;127:65–81.
7. Colohan ART, Grady MS, Bonnin JM, Thorner MO, Kovacs K, Jane JA. Ectopic pituitary gland simulating a suprasellar tumor. *Neurosurgery* 1987;20:43–48.
8. Lennox B, Russell DS. Dystopia of the neurohypophysis: two cases. *J Pathol Bacteriol* 1951;63:485–490.
9. Asa SL, Kovacs K. Functional morphology of the human fetal pituitary. *Pathol Annu* 1984;19:275–315.
10. Dubois PM, Begeot M. Immunocytological localization of LH, FSH, TSH and their subunits in the pituitary of normal and anencephalic human fetuses. *Cell Tissue Res* 1978;191:249–265.
11. Begeot M, Dubois MP, Dubois, PM. Growth hormone and ACTH in the pituitary of normal and anencephalic human fetuses; immunocytochemical evidence for hypothalamic influences during development. *Neuroendocrinology* 1977;24:208–220.
12. Renn WH, Rhoton AL. Microsurgical anatomy of the sellar region. *J Neurosurg* 1975;43:288–298.
13. Lang J. Anatomy of the midline. *Acta Neurochir Suppl* 1985;35:6–22.
14. Osteology. In: Williams PL, Warwick R, eds. *Gray's anatomy.* 36th ed. Philadelphia: WB Saunders; 1980:230–418.
15. Kern EB, Laws ER. The rationale and technique of selective transsphenoidal microsurgery for the removal of pituitary tumors. In: Laws ER, Randall RV, Kern EB, Abboud CF, eds. *Management of pituitary adenomas and related lesions with emphasis on transsphenoidal microsurgery.* New York: Appleton-Century-Crofts; 1982:219–244.
16. Bergland RM, Bronson SR, Torack RM. Anatomical variations in the pituitary gland and adjacent structures in 225 human autopsy cases. *J Neurosurg* 1968;28:93–99.
17. Berke JP, Buxton LF, Kokmen E. The empty sella. *Neurology* 1975;25: 1137–1143.
18. Kaufman B, Chamberlain WB. The ubiquitous empty sella turcica. *Acta Radiol* 1972;13:413–425.
19. Kaplan HA, Browder J, Krieger AJ. Intercavernous connections of the cavernous sinuses. *J Neurosurg* 1976;45:166–168.
20. McGrath P. The cavernous sinus: an anatomical survey. *Aust N Z J Surg* 1977;47:601–613.
21. Harris FS, Rhoton AL. Anatomy of the cavernous sinus. *J Neurosurg* 1976;45:169–180.
22. Stanfield JP. The blood supply of the human pituitary gland. *J Anat* 1960;94:257–273.
23. Xuereb GP, Prichard MM, Daniel PM. The arterial supply and venous drainage of the human hypophysis cerebri. *Q J Exp Physiol* 1954;39: 199–217.
24. Gorczyca W, Hardy J. Arterial supply of the human anterior pituitary gland. *Neurosurgery* 1987;20:369–377.
25. Xuereb GP, Prichard MM, Daniel PM. The hypophyseal portal system of vessels in man. *Q J Exp Physiol* 1954;39:219–229.
26. Scheithauer BW. *The hypothalamus and neurohypophysis.* Boston: Blackwell; 1990.
27. Pansky B, Allen DJ. *Review of neuroscience.* New York: Macmillan; 1980.
28. Brownstein MJ, Russell JT, Gainer H. Synthesis, transport, and release of posterior pituitary hormones. *Science* 1980;207:373–378.
29. Scheithauer BW, Sano T, Kovacs K, Young WF Jr, Ryan N, Randall RV. The pituitary gland in pregnancy. *Mayo Clin Proc* 1990;65: 461–474.

30. Goluboff LG, Ezrin C. Effect of pregnancy on the somatotroph and the prolactin cell of the human adenohypophysis. *J Clin Endocrinol* 1969; 29:1533–1538.
31. Ciric I. On the origin and nature of the pituitary gland capsule. *J Neurosurg* 1977;46:596–600.
32. Kovacs K, Horvath E. *Tumors of the pituitary gland.* Washington, DC: Armed Forces Institute of Pathology; 1986.
33. McGrath P. Cysts of sellar and pharyngeal hypophyses. *Pathology* 1971;3:123–131.
34. Scheithauer BW, Kovacs K, Raymond RV, Ryan N. Pituitary gland in hypothyroidism. *Arch Pathol Lab Med* 1985;109:499–504.
35. Turkington RW, Underwood LE, Van Wyk JJ. Elevated serum prolactin levels after pituitary-stalk section in man. *N Engl J Med* 1971; 285:707–710.
36. Horvath E, Ilse G, Kovacs K. Enigmatic bodies in human corticotroph cells. *Acta Anat* 1977;98:427–433.
37. Phifer RF, Spicer SS. Immunohistochemical and histologic demonstration of thyrotropic cells of the human adenohypophysis. *J Clin Endocrinol Metab* 1973;36:1210–1221.
38. Phifer RF, Midgley AR, Spicer SS. Immunohistologic and histologic evidence that follicle-stimulating hormone and luteinizing hormone are present in the same cell type in the human pars tuberalis. *J Clin Endocrinol Metab* 1973;36:125–141.
39. Asa SL, Kovacs K, Bilbao JM. The pars tuberalis of the human pituitary. *Virchows Arch [A]* 1983;399:49–59.
40. Horvath E, Kovacs K, Penz G, Ezrin C. Origin, possible funciton and fate of follicular cells in the anterior lobe of the human pituitary. *Am J Pathol* 1974;77:199–212.
41. Mai KT, Lach B, Gregor A. Folliculo-stellate cells in pituitary. (in press).
42. Luse SA, Kernohan JW. Squamous nests of the pituitary gland. *Cancer* 1955;8:623–628.
43. Schochet SS, McCormick WF, Halmi NS. Salivary gland rests in the human pituitary. *Arch Pathol* 1974;98:193–200.
44. Luse SA, Kernohan JW. Granular-cell tumors of the stalk and posterior lobe of the pituitary gland. *Cancer* 1955;8:616–622.
45. Liwnicz BH, Liwnicz RG, Huff SJ, McBride BH, Tew JM. Giant granular cell tumor of the suprasellar area: immunocytochemical and electron microscopic studies. *Neurosurgery* 1984;15:246–251.
46. Drewett N, Jacobi JM, Willgoss DA, Lloyd HM. Apoptosis in the anterior pituitary gland of the rat: studies with estrogen and bromocriptine. *Neuroendocrinology* 1993;57:89–95.
47. Shanklin WM. Age changes in the histology of the human pituitary. *Acta Anat* 1953;19:290–304.
48. Sano T, Kovacs K, Scheithauer BW, Young WF Jr. Aging in the human pituitary. *Mayo Clin Proc* 1993;68:971–977.
49. Scheithauer BW, Sano T, Kovacs K, et al. The pituitary gland in pregnancy: a clinicopathologic and immunohistochemical study of 69 cases. *Mayo Clin Proc* 1990;65:461–474.
50. Stefaneanu L, Kovacs K, Lloyd R, Scheithauer BW, Sano T, Young WF Jr. Pituitary lactotrophs and somatotrophs in pregnancy: a correlative in situ hybridization and immunocytochemical study. *Virchows Arch [B]* 1992;62:291–296.
51. Calderon L, Ryan N, Kovacs K. Human pituitary growth hormone cells in old age. *Gerontology* 1978;24:441–447.
52. Kovacs K, Ryan N, Horvath E, Penz G, Ezrin C. Prolactin cells of the human pituitary gland in old age. *J Gerontol* 1977;32:534–540.
53. Röcken C, Saeger Fleege JC, Linke RP. Interstitial amyloid deposits in the pituitary gland. *Arch Pathol Lab Med* 1995;119:1055–1060.
54. Seyama S, Pearl GS, Takei Y. Ultrastructural study of the human neurohypophysis. I. Neurosecretory axons and their dilatations in the pars nervosa. *Cell Tissue Res* 1980;205:253–271.
55. Takei Y, Seyama S, Pearl GS, Tindall GT. Ultrastructural study of the human neurohypophysis. II. Cellular elements of neuronal parenchyma, the pituicytes. *Cell Tissue Res* 1980;205:273–287.
56. Seyama S, Pearl GS, Takei Y. Ultrastructural study of the human neurohypophysis. III. Vascular and perivascular structures. *Cell Tissue Res* 1980;206:291–302.
57. Shanklin WM. Lymphocytes and lymphoid tissue in the human pituitary. *Anat Rec* 1951;111:177–191.

*Histology for Pathologists, second edition,*
Edited by Stephen S. Sternberg.
Lippincott-Raven Publishers, Philadelphia
© 1997.

# CHAPTER 46

# Thyroid

Maria Luisa Carcangiu



## EMBRYOLOGY

The human thyroid is formed from a median anlage and two lateral anlagen. The median anlage develops in the floor of the primitive pharynx at the foramen cecum (a dimplelike depression at the base of the tongue) from a median ductlike invagination that grows caudally. This formation, known as the thyroglossal duct, contains at its base the developing thyroid gland, which is at first spherical but later, when approaching its final site in front of the trachea at about 7 weeks of gestation, becomes bilobed (1). During this downward migration, the thyroglossal duct undergoes atrophy, leaving as a vestige the pyramidal lobe in about 40% of individuals. Faulty downward migration of the medial anlage or persistence of parts of the thyroglossal duct gives rise to ectopic thyroid tissue, thyroglossal duct cysts, and cervical fistulae.

M. L. Carcangiu: Department of Pathology, Yale University School of Medicine, New Haven, Connecticut 06520.

The initially solid thyroid anlage begins to form cords and plates of follicular cells during the 9th week of gestation. Small follicles appear by the 10th week. Inside these primitive follicles, a finely granular material begins to collect which by the 20th week acquires the morphologic features of colloid. By week 14 there are well-developed follicles lined by follicular cells that contain thyroglobulin (TGB)-positive colloid in their lumen (Fig. 1A, B). Labeled amino acid studies have suggested that TGB synthesis actually begins at a much earlier stage, when the thyroid is still a solid mass at the base of the tongue and long before lumen formation and colloid secretion can be detected morphologically (2,3).

The two lateral anlagen of the thyroid derive from the ultimobranchial bodies (UBBs), which in turn originate from the IVth–Vth branchial pouch complex. UBBs, while still connected to the pharynx, start their migration downward on each side of the neck together with the parathyroid IV primordium. At 7 to 8 weeks they separate from the pharynx and the parathyroid. Their lumens become obliterated by proliferating cells, so that they appear as solid masses that

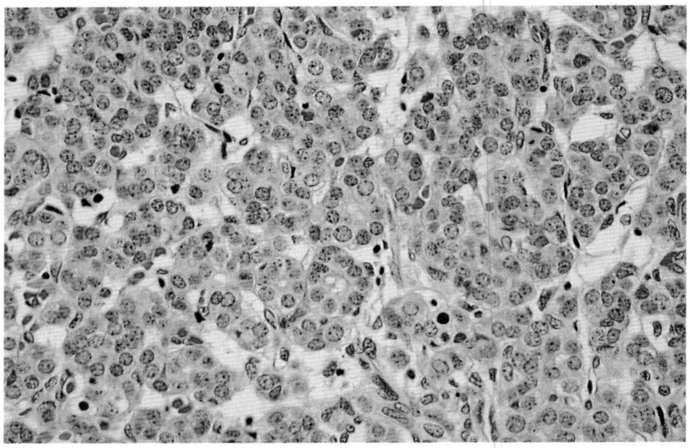
A

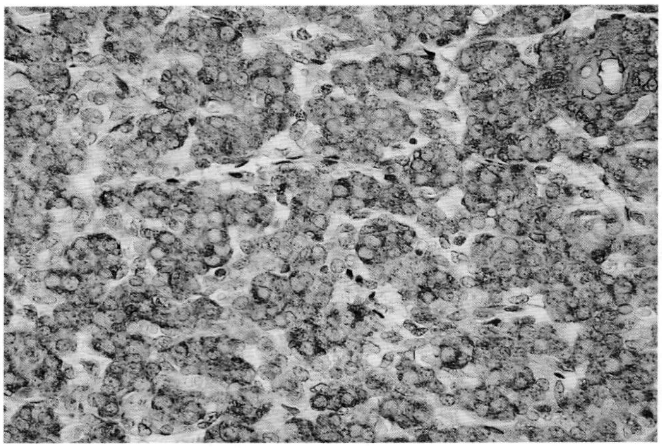
B

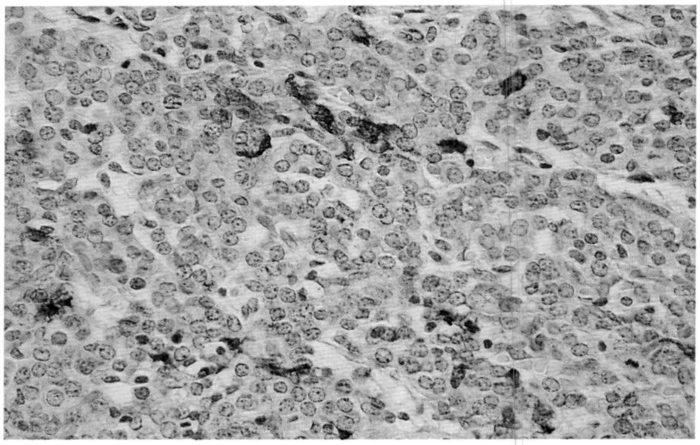
C

**FIG. 1.** Developing thyroid gland in a 14 weeks fetus. **A:** Rare primitive follicles are seen within a mostly solid proliferation. **B:** The cytoplasm of the follicular cells and the material contained in the lumen of the primitive follicles are immunoreactive for TGB. **C:** C cells, as seen in a CT immunostain preparation, are scattered within follicles.

fuse with the dorsolateral aspects of the median thyroid anlage and become incorporated into the developing lateral lobes (4).

After its fusion with the medial thyroid, the UBB divides into a central thick-walled stratified epithelial cyst and a peripheral component composed of cell groups dispersed among the follicles: the C cells (5,6) (Fig. 1C). In postnatal life, the central epithelial cyst largely disappears, its occasional remnants corresponding to the so-called solid cell nests (SCNs).

C cells are thought to derive from the neural crest and to migrate to the UBBs before the incorporation of the latter in the thyroid (7–10). Evidence for a relationship between UBBs and C cells comes from several sources:

1. Patients with DiGeorge syndrome, characterized by complete or partial absence of derivatives of the IIIrd and IVth–Vth pouch complexes, have C cells in their thyroid in only 25% of cases (11,12).
2. C cells are completely absent in thyroglossal duct remnants and cysts, as well as in lingual thyroid (13).
3. In the adult thyroid gland, C cells and follicles carrying such cells in their walls are especially numerous in the vicinity of the UBB remnants (13).

There is some controversy as to whether the role of UBBs in thyroid development is limited to the production of C cells as already described or whether they also contribute to the follicular cell population. Williams et al. (14) described five cases of maldescent of the medial thyroid anlage in which cystic structures were present in the lateral neck in the region of the upper parathyroids. Four of these cystic structures contained intercystic glandular nodules composed of solid areas of irregularly distributed cells that stained positively for calcitonin (CT) and CT gene–related peptide; these cells were intermixed with follicular structures that were immunoreactive for thyroglobin. On the basis of these observations, the investigators concluded that the UBB contributes both C cells and follicular cells to the thyroid gland, and they speculated on the possible role of UBB-derived cells in the genesis of so-called intermediate or mixed medullary and follicular carcinomas. Contradicting this hypothesis is the observation that in humans with thyroid nondescent (or unilateral aplasia) there are no recognizable thyroid follicles in the usual locations (15).

The fetal thyroid gland develops rapidly until the 4th month of intrauterine growth (crown–rump length 18 mm). After birth the thyroid growth rate parallels that of the body, reaching the normal adult weight at around 15 years of age.

## GROSS ANATOMY

The normal adult thyroid has a shape reminiscent of a butterfly, with two bulky lateral lobes connected by a thin isthmus. Each lateral lobe is 2 to 2.5 cm wide, 5 to 6 cm long, and 2 cm deep. Their upper and lower extremities (one having a pointed shape and the other featuring blunt contours) are referred to as upper and lower thyroid poles, respectively. One lobe may be larger than the other, and the isthmus may be exceptionally wide. The pyramidal lobe, a vestige of the thyroglossal duct, is found in about 40% of thyroids; it appears as a narrow projection of thyroid tissue that extends upward from the isthmus to lie on the surface of the thyroid cartilage.

The thyroid gland is located in the midportion of the neck, where it is attached to the anterior trachea by loose connective tissue. The two lateral lobes surround the ventral and lateral aspects of the larynx and trachea, reaching the lower halves of the thyroid cartilage and covering the second, third, and fourth tracheal rings.

The normal weight of the adult thyroid is 15 to 25 g in nongoitrous areas. However, there are significant individual variations, most of them related to gender, age, corporal weight, hormonal status, functional status of the gland, and iodine intake (16). In women, the thyroid volume is known to increase during the secretory phase of the menstrual cycle (17).

A thin fibrous capsule invests the thyroid. Connected to this capsule are numerous fibrous septa that penetrate the thyroid parenchyma and divide it into lobules (so-called thyromeres). The microscopic integrity of the capsule was assessed in a study on 138 thyroid glands from autopsies of adults (age 20–40 years) by Komorowski and Hanson (18). Although grossly all of these capsules seemed complete, microscopically they were focally incomplete in 62% of the cases. Furthermore, thyroid follicles were found within the thyroid capsule in 14% of cases and in the pericapsular connective tissue in 88%. In the latter location, they were mostly seen as nodular aggregates.

The color of the normal thyroid is red–brown. A phenomenon exceptionally seen in normal thyroid glands of elderly individuals is the accumulation in the follicular cells of a melanin-like pigment that imparts to the gland a characteristic coal black stain, easily apparent on gross examination. These changes are qualitatively identical to those seen in more florid form in thyroids of patients on chronic minocycline therapy (19–21).

Nodularity of thyroid parenchyme is identified grossly in about 10% of thyroids of endocrinologically normal individuals (22).

The blood supply of the thyroid gland derives primarily from the inferior thyroid artery (which originates from the thyrocervical trunk of the subclavian artery) and the superior thyroid artery (which arises from the external carotid). A thyroidea ima artery also may be present, which widely varies in size from a small vessel to one the size of the inferior thyroid artery. The superior and medial thyroid veins and the inferior vein drain (via a venous plexus in the thyroid capsule) into the internal jugular and the brachiocephalic vein, respectively (23,24).

An intricate lymphatic network permeates the thyroid gland, encircling the follicles and connecting the two lateral lobes through the isthmus. It empties into subcapsular channels, which in turn give rise to collecting trunks within the thyroid capsule in close proximity to the veins. The lymph vessels draining the superior portion of the thyroid lobes and isthmus collect into the internal jugular lymph nodes, whereas those draining the inferior portion of the gland collect into the pre- and paratracheal and prelaryngeal lymph nodes. The pretracheal lymph node situated close to the isthmus is also known as the delphian node (25). Other lymph node stations are the recurrent laryngeal nerve chain and the retropharyngeal and retroesophageal groups. The anterosuperior mediastinal nodes are secondary to the recurrent laryngeal nerve chain and pretracheal groups; however, injection studies have shown that dye injected into the thyroid isthmus can drain directly into the mediastinal nodes (26).

Some correlations exist between the site of a thyroid tumor within a given lobe and the location of the initial lymph node metastasis. However, the degree of anastomosing between these various nodal groups is such that any of them can be found to be the site of disease regardless of the precise location of the primary tumor.

Vasomotor nonmedullated postganglionic neural fibers originating from the superior and midline cervical sympathetic ganglia influence indirectly the secretory activity of the thyroid gland through their action on the blood vessels. In addition, adrenergic receptors in follicular cells and a network of adrenergic fibers ending near the follicular basement membrane have been demonstrated (27). It has therefore been hypothesized that thyroid secretion is regulated both by direct neural signals and by indirect vascular nerve signals (28–30). A role for direct neural influences in the secretion of CT and other C cell–derived hormones is supported by the demonstration in chickens of a rich cholinergic network encircling the C cells (31).

Small paraganglia are normally present close to the thyroid and are occasionally found beneath the thyroid capsule; their presence explains the rare occurrence of peri- and intrathyroidal paragangliomas.

## MICROSCOPIC ANATOMY

The fundamental unit of the thyroid is the follicle, a round to slightly oval structure lined by a single layer of epithelial cells resting on a basement membrane (Fig. 2A). The lumen of the follicle contains colloid, a viscous material that is mostly composed by proteins secreted by the follicular cells including TGB. The follicles, which are separated from each other by a loose fibroconnective tissue, have an average diameter of 200 $\mu$m. Their size may vary even within the same gland depending on the functional status of the thyroid and the age of the individual. Variations in the shape of follicles exist, but elongated follicles are a feature of hyperplastic or neoplastic conditions or are the result of compression adjacent to an expansile mass (Fig. 2B).

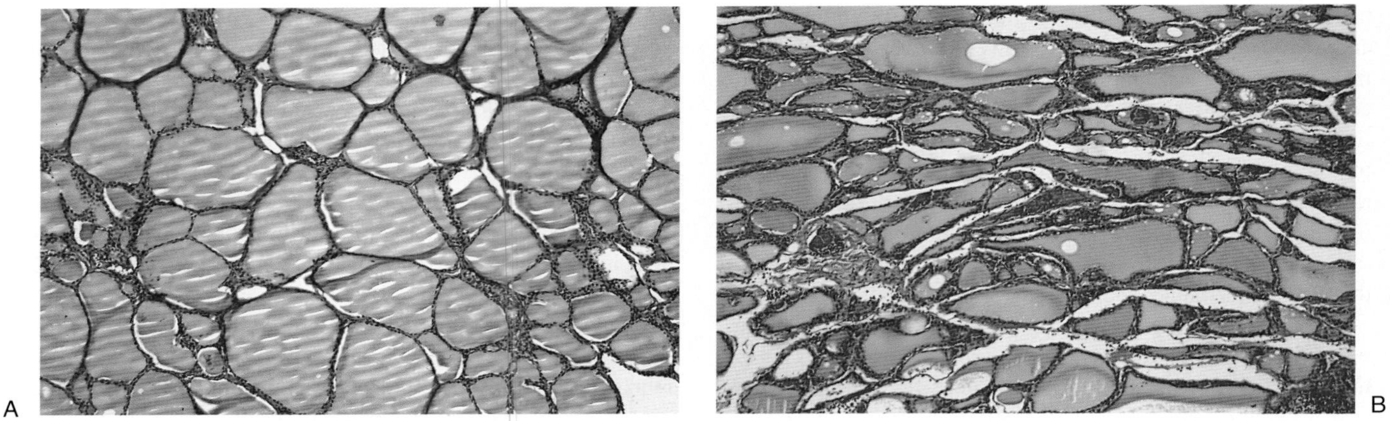

**FIG. 2. A:** Low-power view of normal adult thyroid gland. The follicles have a round to oval shape. **B:** Elongated follicles as a result of compression are seen in the vicinity of an adenoma (not shown in this picture.)

The colloid, which is pale eosinophilic in the actively secreting gland, acquires a deeply eosinophilic staining quality in resting follicles. In some follicles the colloid may have an amphophilic or basophilic staining quality, probably the result of an increase in the amount of acidic groups in the TGB molecule (Fig. 3). In the most advanced expression of this phenomenon, the intraluminal material acquires a distinct mucinlike appearance.

The glycoproteic material present within the follicles stains for periodic acid-Schiff (PAS) and alcian blue and is immunoreactive for TGB. A row of small vacuoles is seen at the interface between follicular epithelium and the colloid in actively functioning glands; these are referred to as resorption vacuoles. In addition, it is not unusual to find a large round or oval clear space within the colloid; this often appears empty but it may contain a crystalline material.

Another morphologic variation of the colloid is represented by collections of round basophilic corpuscles clustering at one pole of the follicle.

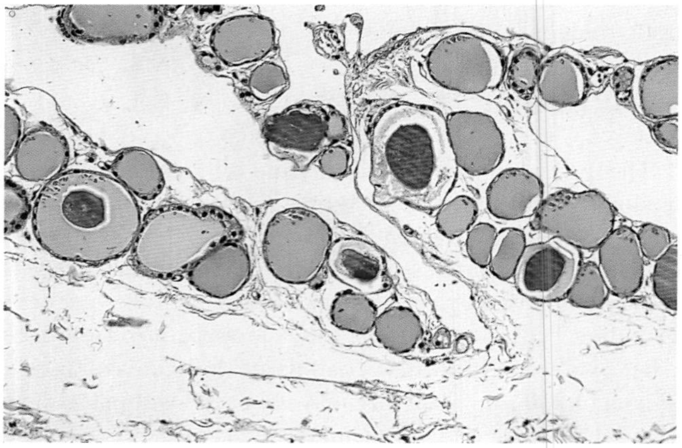

**FIG. 3.** The colloid accumulated in these follicles exhibits different densities and tintorial qualities, the latter ranging from acidophilic to basophilic.

The epithelial glandular cells lining the follicle are known as follicular cells or thyrocytes; among them, there is a second cellular component known as C cells.

## FOLLICULAR CELL

### Light Microscopy

The cells lining the follicles—follicular cells or thyrocytes—show variations in their shape and size according to the functional status of the gland. Three major types, expressions of a morphologic continuum, are described: flattened (endothelioid), cuboidal, and columnar (cylindrical) (Fig. 4A). Flattened cells are relatively inactive. Cuboidal cells (their height equaling their width) are the most numerous and their major function is to secrete colloid. The rarer columnar cells resorb the TGB-containing colloid, liberate the active hormones, and excrete these hormones into blood vessels.

Functional polarity is apparent at the level of the follicle and the follicular cell. A single follicle may have flattened cells on one side and cuboidal or low columnar cells on the other (Fig. 4B), the most florid expression of this phenomenon being the Sanderson's polster.

At the cellular level, all follicular cells manifest a definite polarity, resting with their bases on the basement membrane and having the apexes directed toward the lumen of the follicle. Size and position of the nucleus and some components of the cytoplasm may vary considerably. In the resting thyroid, the nucleus is round or oval, is located toward the center of the cell, and usually contains one nucleolus that is eccentrically located. Its chromatin may be finely granular or clumped. In actively secreting cells, the nucleus is enlarged; because of the mostly apical enlargement of the cytoplasm, it acquires a basal position. The cytoplasm is usually weakly eosinophilic; only exceptionally in an otherwise normal thy-

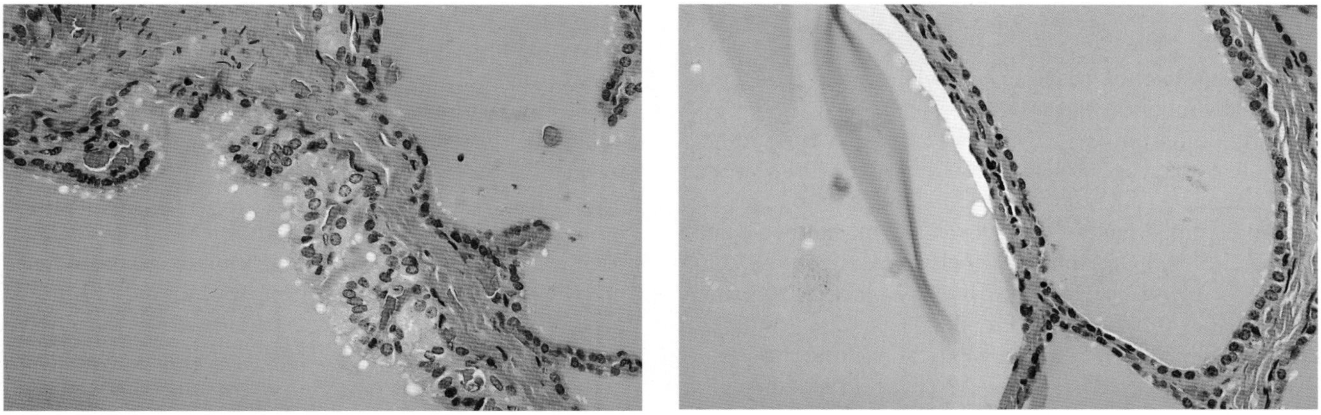

A B

**FIG. 4. A:** The epithelium of one follicle is low cuboidal and relatively inactive. The adjacent follicle shows a taller epithelium and reabsorption vacuoles. **B:** The epithelium of the same follicle is flattened on one side and cuboidal on the other, as an expression of functional polarization.

roid does it appear granular and intensely eosinophilic, i.e. oncocytic (so-called Hurthle cells). Occasionally, it is seen to contain a golden brown pigment of lipofuscin type (Fig. 5A), which should be distinguished from the melanin-like pigment already mentioned (Fig. 5B).

### Electron Microscopy

Ultrastructurally, the follicular cells are arranged in a single layer around the colloid and rest on a basement membrane, approximately 35 to 40 nm in thickness, that separate them from the interstitial stroma. Microvilli emanate from the surface of the cells, their number being increased and their length greater in actively functioning cells. Cell membranes of adjacent cells interdigitate in a complex fashion and are joined by junctional complexes toward the apex (32,33). The cytoplasm contains variable amounts of endoplasmic reticulum, mitochondria of usually small size, and lysosomes. When the number of mitochondria is highly increased, the cell acquires at the light microscopic level an intensely eosinophilic granular cytoplasmic appearance (corresponding to the above mentioned Hurthle cells).

Ultrastructural changes related to hormone production are further discussed in the Microscopic Anatomy section.

### Immunohistochemistry

Immunohistochemically, both the cytoplasm of the follicular cells and the intraluminal colloid are positive for TGB (with mono- and polyclonal antibodies), T3, and T4 (34,35). Follicular cells are also immunoreactive for low-molecular-weight keratin, epithelial membrane antigen (EMA), and occasionally for vimentin (36–40). Estrogen and progesterone receptors also have been detected (41–43). The basement membrane on which the follicles rest is immunoreactive for laminin and type IV collagen (44).

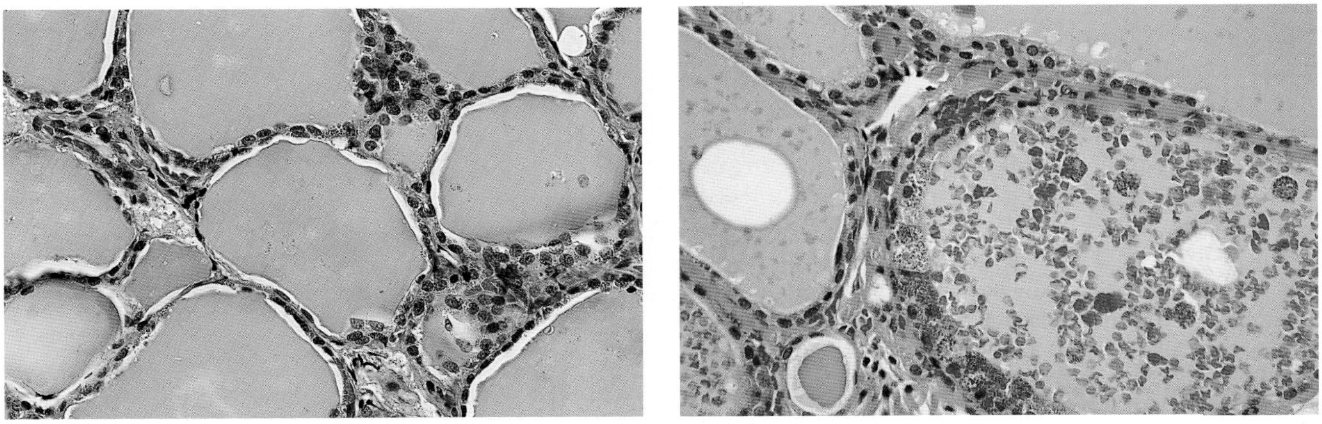

A B

**FIG. 5. A:** Lipofuscin in the cytoplasm of the follicular cells. **B:** Granular black pigment in the follicular epithelium and colloid of the thyroid of a 73-year-old patient who was not on mynocycline therapy.

## Physiology

The main function of the thyroid gland is the production of thyroid hormones, the most important being thyroxin (T4) and triiodothyronine (T3). These hormones regulate metabolism, increase protein synthesis in every tissue of the body, and increase $O_2$ consumption. Thyroid hormones are particularly important for body development and for the normal maturation of the central and peripheral nervous system.

Steps in thyroid hormone biosynthesis include ingestion of iodine ions from water and food, concentration of the iodide within the thyroid, and organification of iodide to iodine. This last step is dependent on the action of iodide peroxidase, which oxidates the iodine ion to a highly reactive form of iodine, which in turn binds to tyrosine. The results are monoiodotyrosine (MIT) when one iodine molecule is attached, or diiodotyrosine (DIT) when two iodine molecules are attached. The iodotyrosine residues are condensed to form the biologically active thyroid hormones thyroxin (T4) and triiodotyronine (T3). Thyroxin results from the coupling of two molecules of DIT, and triiodotyronine from the coupling of one molecule of MIT with a molecule of DIT (30).

Thyroid hormones are stored in TGB, a large protein with numerous iodinated tyrosine residues, including biologically active T4 and T3. TGB is collected at the center of the thyroid follicles and is the main constituent of colloid.

Ultrastructural studies have correlated the morphologic changes that accompany thyroid hormone production and secretion. The synthesis of TGB begins in the endoplasmic reticulum and continues in the Golgi apparatus, where the end sugars of the carbohydrate site are incorporated; it is then packaged in small apical microvesicles, the contents of which are discharged into the follicular lumen after fusion of the vesicle membranes with the luminal side of the plasma membrane.

Resorption of TGB takes place through cytoplasmic pseudopodia (streamers) that engulf minute portions of colloid, which are then drawn into the cell in the form of membrane-bound colloid droplets. These subsequently fuse with lysosomes, and their content is digested by the lysosomal enzymes (45–49). T3 and T4 diffuse in the blood stream, where they are transported primarily by the specific carrier protein, thyroxin-binding globulin (TBG). TBG normally transports more than 70% of thyroid hormones. Approximately 20% of circulating thyroid hormones is carried by transthyretin (prealbumin) and albumin (50). Only a small portion of circulating thyroid hormones (approximately 0.05% of T3 and 0.015% of T4) is unbound and, therefore, biologically active. Free, circulating, biologically active T3 and T4 are in equilibrium with the hormones bound to the carrier proteins. The amount of circulating T4 is much larger than that of T3; however, T3 is about four times more active biologically; as a result, the final contribution of T3 to the biologic activity of thyroid hormones equals that of T4 (51).

Thyroid biosynthetic and secretory activities are controlled by the level of thyroid stimulating hormone (TSH), a glycoprotein synthesized and secreted by the anterior pituitary gland (52). TSH binds to a specific receptor located on the external surface of follicular thyroid cells, and by activating the adenylate-cyclase pathway regulates the complex mechanism responsible for T3 and T4 synthesis (53). TSH release is in turn regulated by a tripeptide secreted by the hypothalamus, thyrotropin releasing hormone (TRH). TSH and TRH release are regulated by the circulating levels of free T3 and T4, via a negative feedback on the pituitary and hypothalamus (low levels of free T3 and T4 stimulate the release of TSH and TRH). In contrast, TSH and TRH releases are inhibited by high levels of circulating free T3 and T4 (52–54).

## Apoptosis

The role of apoptosis in thyroid homeostasis has not been studied in detail. Dremier et al. (55), using as a model primary cultures of dog thyroid cells, were able to trigger morphologic changes characteristic of apoptotic death by various manipulations, suggesting that thyrocytes are endowed with a constitutive apoptosis program.

## Microscopic Variations

### *Sanderson's Polster*

A characteristic structure, present in the usual thyroid but accentuated in hyperplastic conditions, is the so-called Sanderson's polster. This refers to an aggregate of small follicles lined by flattened epithelium and covered by an undulating layer of columnar epithelium that is seen bulging into the lumina of larger follicles (Fig. 6). This perfectly benign and to some extent physiologic change needs to be distinguished from papillary microcarcinoma.

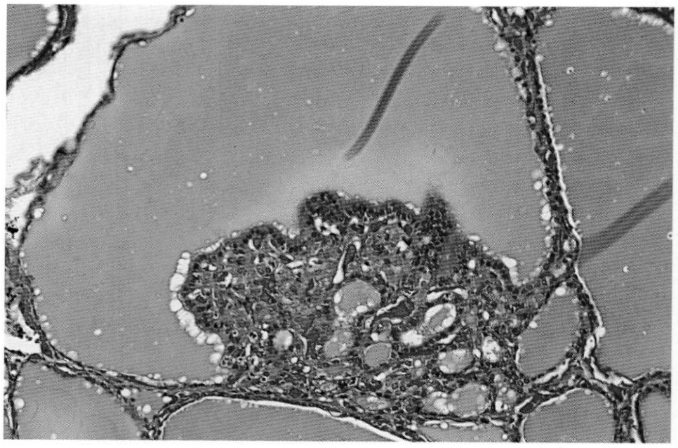

**FIG. 6.** Sanderson's polster protruding into the lumen of a follicle.

### *Granulomas*

Granulomas are a relatively common finding in otherwise normal surgically resected thyroids and in autoptic material. Both foreign material and colloid may elicit this process. Talc or suture are the most frequent cause of formation of granulomas in completion thyroidectomy specimens. Larger foreign body granulomas sometimes simulating a thyroid nodule have been reported in thyroids of patients who underwent laryngeal injection of Polytef (polytetrafluoroethylene) (56,57). This material may migrate through the lymphatics into adjacent tissues, where it may start the inflammatory process.

Rarely interstitial granulomas are seen as a reaction to oxalate crystals that have been released by broken follicles (58).

Granulomatous lesions originated by the rupture of follicles and their invasion by macrophages and leukocytes as a reaction to the extruded colloid are a common incidental finding in surgically resected thyroids. Carney et al. (59) referred to this process as palpation thyroiditis (and also as multifocal granulomatous folliculitis) and attributed it to the minor trauma resulting from physical examination. Support for this interpretation comes from the observation that the number and size of the granulomas is related to the intensity of the palpation (59) and the fact that similar changes have been described in individuals engaged in martial arts (so-called martial-arts thyroiditis) (60).

Grossly, a gland affected by palpation thyroiditis appears normal or shows tiny foci of hemorrhage. Histologically multiple small granulomas centered in a disrupted follicle and composed by histiocytes, lymphocytes, and plasma cells are seen scattered in the thyroid gland (Fig. 7A). Some of the histiocytes are foamy, and others have the appearance of multinucleated giant cells. The appearance depends on the stage of the process, a common picture being a cluster of foamy macrophages hanging from the follicular epithelium into the lumen (Fig. 7B). Necrosis, hemosiderin, and iron deposition are seen only rarely. Sometimes up to four or five follicles are involved in a single granuloma. Immunohistochemically, most of the lymphocytes are T cells; among the plasma cells, K-positive cells predominate (61).

Palpation thyroiditis seems to represent a variation in the theme of colloidophagy, a process described many years ago and characterized by a granulomatous reaction to colloid in follicles allegedly undergoing spontaneous rupture in thyroids affected by goiter or thyroiditis (62).

Palpation thyroiditis needs to be distinguished from interstitial giant cell thyroiditis (in which the granulomas are centered not in the follicles but in the interstitium), necrotizing granulomas following surgical procedures (similar to those more commonly seen in bladder and prostate and characterized by a central area of necrosis surrounded by a palisading of epithelioid cells) (63), and aggregates of C cells (which are immunoreactive for CT) (64).

### *Crystals*

Anisotropic crystals of calcium oxalate may be present within the colloid in normal adult thyroid glands. They may be seen in ordinary light, but are more easily identified under polarized light (Fig. 8). Their shape varies from rhomboid to irregular plaques and their size shows wide variations (65).

In autoptic studies they have been found with a frequency of up to 85% of thyroids examined (66). Their number appears to increase with age; this, together with the observation that the crystals have been found more frequently in colloid with low positivity for TGB, has prompted the suggestion that they result from variations in colloid and calcium concentration in the gland secondary to a low functional state of the thyroid (65–67).

In one study the number of crystals was markedly elevated in glands with subacute thyroiditis, where they were found in

A B

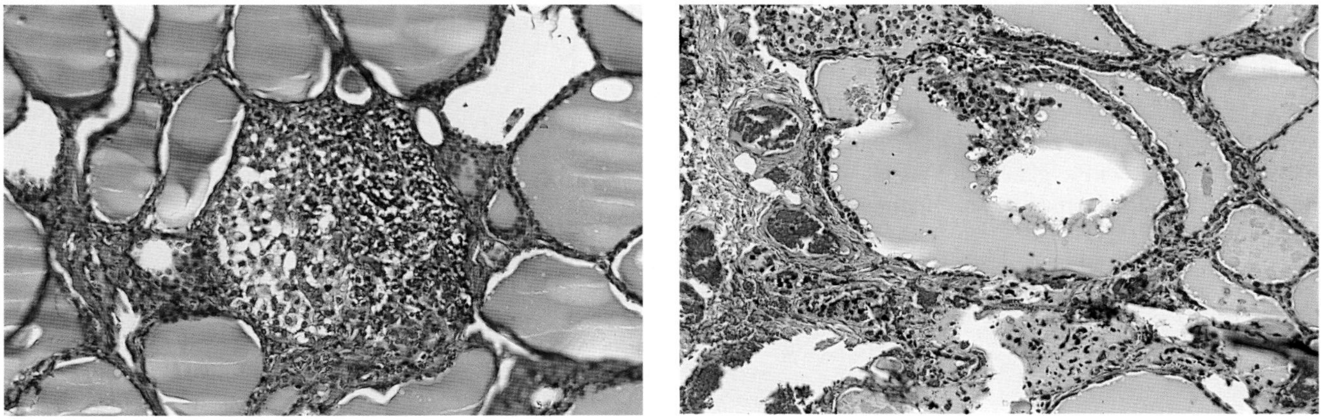

**FIG. 7.** Palpation thyroiditis. **A:** This thyroid follicle is replaced by thyrocytes, lymphocytes, and plasma cells. A strip of follicular epithelium is seen in the center. **B:** In this case the follicle is only partially involved. Inflammatory cells and desquamated follicular cells protrude into the lumen.

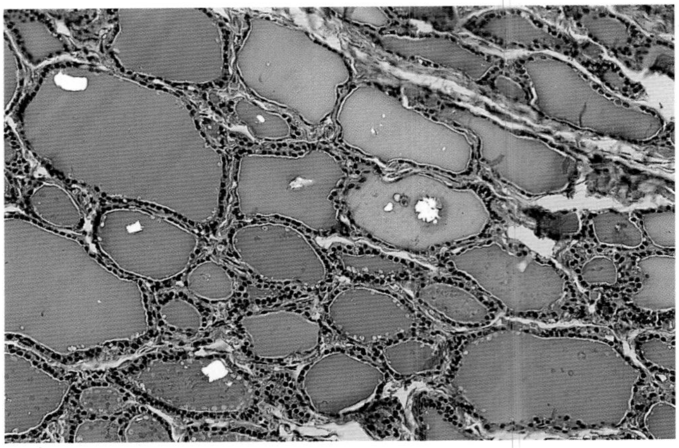

**FIG. 8.** Multiple birefringent calcium oxalate crystals are seen in the lumina of normal thyroid follicles (polarized light).

the giant cells, in remnants of colloid, and in the thyroid stroma. In the same study crystals were identified only rarely in thyroids with chronic thyroiditis or glandular hyperplasia (68).

Oxalate crystals in the thyroid are also seen in large number in patients undergoing dialysis for renal failure. In this setting, the thyroid is just another site of oxalate deposition, together with the kidney, myocardium, and other sites (69). Rarely crystals released by follicular breakdown may elicit a granulomatous reaction in the nearby thyroid stroma (58).

### *Squamous Metaplasia*

Benign squamous cells occur as an expression of squamous metaplasia of follicular cells in various benign and malignant thyroid lesions and under exceptional circumstances in an otherwise normal thyroid (70–72). They need to be distinguished from transversally cut follicles and from the SCNs of UBB derivation. It also should be mentioned that squamous epithelium is regularly observed as a component of the epithelium of thyroglossal duct cysts.

## C CELLS

C cells (parafollicular cells) represent a minor component of the thyroid gland. It has been estimated that they comprise not more that 0.1% of the glandular mass. They have a neuroendocrine function, being responsible for the production of the peptide hormone CT. The term "C cell" was introduced by Pearse (73) to underline their role in secreting and storing this hormone. More recently, other hormones have been found to be produced by C cells, but only in small quantity and not in every cell.

### Light Microscopy

C cells are identified only with difficulty in sections stained with hematoxylin and eosin, where they appear polygonal and with a granular weakly eosinophilic cytoplasm that is larger and paler than that of follicular cells. The nucleus is round to oval, pale, with a centrally located nucleolus.

C cells are located, individually or in small groups, within thyroid follicles. Specifically, most are found at the periphery of the follicular wall (hence the adjective parafollicular), within its basement membrane and without contact with the follicular lumen. Occasional C cells have prominent cytoplasmic processes that extend beyond the adjacent follicular cells. In normal adults and neonates, C cells are restricted to the midupper and upper thirds of the lateral lobes of the thyroid, in the area where UBBs (from which they derive) fuse with the thyroid median anlage. The number of C cells varies with the development of the gland, being more numerous in early age. In one study, up to 100 C cells per low-power field were demonstrated in neonates and children, whereas in adults only a maximum of 10 cells per low-power field were counted (74). In another study, no difference in the number of C cells was found between young and middle-aged groups, but in the elderly the number of such cells was variable, with groups of up to 20 or more cells sometimes being observed (75). However, no statistically significant differences among the various age groups in adults were demonstrated. Other studies have since confirmed that normal adult thyroid glands may contain numerous C cells, sometimes in the form of small nodules (18,76) (Fig. 9). Gibson et al. (76) suggested that such clusters of C cells, in the absence of disturbances in calcium metabolism and of a family history of medullary carcinoma, do not constitute a precursor of medullary carcinoma but may be instead the expression of either a partial failure of embryonic C-cell migration and dispersion within the gland or of age-related hyperplasia. It needs to be mentioned that C-cell hyperplasia of presumed reactive nature has been observed in the immediate periphery of nonmedullary thyroid neoplasms (77,78), in association with lymphocytic thyroiditis (79–81), and in secondary

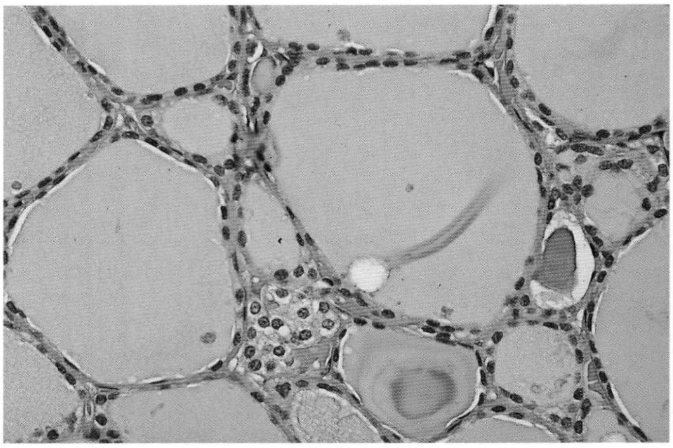

**FIG. 9.** Clusters of C cells in the thyroid of an elderly individual with no known clinical or laboratory evidence of calcium disturbance.

hyperparathyroidism (82). As already mentioned, C cells tend to aggregate in the vicinity of SCNs.

### Electron Microscopy

Electron microscopy has shown that C cells occupy an intrafollicular (rather than interfollicular) position, and that they are separated from the thyroid interstitium by the follicular basal lamina. The presence of C cells in the interfollicular stroma has never been convincingly demonstrated ultrastructurally (83).

The main ultrastructural characteristic of C cells is the presence of secretory granules, which range in diameter from 60 to 550 nm (84). Two main types of granules have been identified. Type I granules have an average diameter of 280 nm and a moderately electron-dense, finely granular content which is closely applied to the limiting membranes of the granules. Type II granules are smaller (average diameter of 130 nm) with a more electron-dense content, which are separated from the limiting membranes by a small but distinct electron-lucent space. Most normal C cells are filled with type I secretory granules, with no or few type II granules. Immunocytochemical studies performed at the ultrastructural level have shown that both type I and II secretory granules contain immunoreactive CT (85).

### Histochemistry and Immunohistochemistry

In sections stained with argyrophil techniques such as the Grimelius reaction, the cytoplasm of the C cell is characterized by the deposition of fine silver-positive granules (84). Lead hematoxylin also stains the cytoplasm of C cells selectively (86). These methods, widely used in the past for the identification of C cells, have been largely replaced by the use of immunohistochemical techniques using polyclonal or monoclonal antibodies to CT (Fig. 10) (84,85,87,88). In addition to CT, C cells also contain katacalcin and the CT gene–related peptide (CGRP). Messengers RNAs (mRNAs) encoding both CT and CGRP also have been demonstrated in normal C cells via in situ hybridization techniques (89).

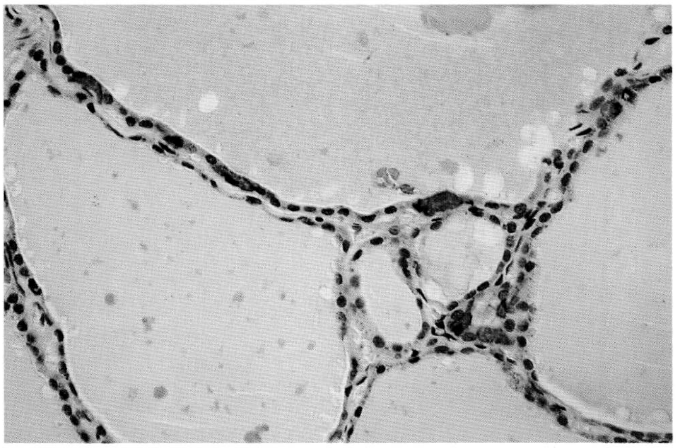

**FIG. 10.** Immunoperoxidase stain for CT demonstrates C cells within follicles, arranged either individually or in small groups.

As already mentioned, a small proportion of CT-positive cells are also positive for other neuropeptides. These include somatostatin (78,90–92), bombesin (93,94), substance P (95), and helodermin (96). Normal C cells are also positive for a variety of generic neuroendocrine markers, such as neuron-specific enolase, chromogranin, and synaptophysin (97). They are negative for neurofilament proteins but typically contain low-molecular-weight cytokeratins. It is possible that neuroendocrine cells other than C cells exist in the thyroid (92) and that they represent the cell of origin of the rare thyroid "neuroendocrine carcinomas" having histologic and immunohistochemical features different from those of medullary carcinoma.

### Physiology

CT is a 32–amino acid peptide whose main function is the regulation of the level of calcium in the plasma by a feedback mechanism. This is brought about by the inhibition of osteoclastic activity. When calcium plasma levels are increased, CT is released from the thyroid. CT also acts in the kidney to enhance the production of vitamin D.

The major physiological role of CT is most likely the protection of the skeleton during periods of calcium stress such as growth, pregnancy and lactation (98). However, absence of CT is not associated with hypercalcemia, nor does a marked excess of the hormone (as seen in patients with medullary thyroid carcinoma) produce hypocalcemia. In addition to calcium, both gastrin and cholecystokinin induce the secretion of CT, as does the chronic administration of estrogenic hormones.

The CT gene is located on the short arm of chromosome 11 and consists of six axons that encode katacalcin (C-terminal flanking peptide) and CGRP (98–100). The primary transcript of the CT gene gives rise to two different mRNAs by tissue-specific alternative splicing events, leading to the production of CT and CGRP mRNAs. The CT-CGRP gene is expressed both in thyroid and nervous tissues, but CT is produced in large quantities only in the thyroid.

In normal male adults, basal CT levels range from 3 to 36 pg/ml (0.9 to 10.5 pmol/L). Plasma levels in females range from 3 to 17 pg/ml (0.9 to 5.0 pmol/L). Normal values after pentagastrin stimulation are less than 106 pg/ml (30.9 pmol/L) for males and less than 29 pg/ml (8.5 pmol/L) for females.

Katacalcin, the C-terminal flanking peptide of CT, is a 21–amino acid peptide that is cosecreted with CT in equimolar amounts (100). Its function, however, is unknown. CGRP is a 37–amino acid peptide that is an extremely potent vasodilator and also serves a neuromodulator or neurotransmitter function (98).

## STROMA

### Lymphocytes

In thyroids surgically resected because of a mass, it is not uncommon to observe in the interstitium of the normal portion of the gland a few collections of lymphocytes, sometimes admixed with rare plasma cells. Simple chronic thyroiditis and focal lymphocytic thyroiditis are the names given to this process that most likely does not represent a nosologic entity but rather the epiphenomenon of etiologically different conditions. Similar changes may in fact be seen in the proximity of neoplasms, in thyroids of patients taking lithium, or in individuals who have received low-dose external radiotherapy (101).

### Fibrous Tissue

The usually thin fibrous septa that separate the thyroid lobules may exhibit microscopic variations. In a study on normal thyroids collected at autopsy from young adults, Komorowski and Hanson (18) found that 8% of the thyroid glands showed extensive fibrosis. According to their description, dense and largely acellular collagen fibers divided the thyroid into small nodules, giving it an appearance akin to micronodular cirrhosis of liver.

Another change that may occur in the interstitium, albeit rarely, is so-called multifocal sclerosing thyroiditis. It is characterized histologically by numerous microscopic foci of stellate-shaped fibrosis composed of cellular fibroblastic tissue frequently entrapping few thyroid follicles in the center. Even if at low power the individual lesions appear similar to those of papillary microcarcinoma, the epithelial component of such lesions lack the cytoarchitectural features of a papillary neoplasm (Fig. 11A and B). Furthermore, the number of lesions in multifocal sclerosing thyroiditis greatly exceeds that seen in papillary microcarcinoma. The etiology and pathogenesis of this process are not known.

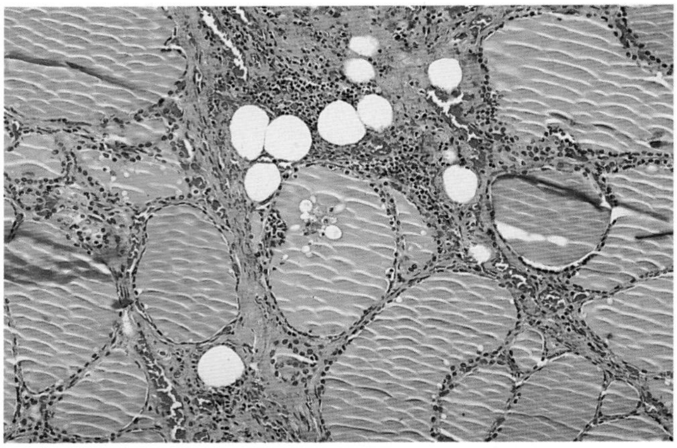

FIG. 12. Adipose metaplasia of thyroid stroma. Mature adipocytes are seen between follicles.

### Fat, Muscle, and Cartilage

Thyroid stroma may undergo adipose metaplasia, resulting in the presence of islands of mature adipose tissue between follicles (Fig. 12). Mature fat also occasionally may be seen in proximity to the thyroid gland capsule, its presence in this location most likely resulting from the close relationship of fat and thyroid tissue during fetal life (102).

A localized intrathyroid deposit of adipose tissue 1.8 × 1.8 × 2.7 cm in size, mimicking because of its nodularity and size a follicular adenoma, has been described by Morizumi et al. (103).

Other tissues that grow in close proximity to the thyroid gland during their development and that can be found within the capsule of adults are cartilage and muscle. Most in-

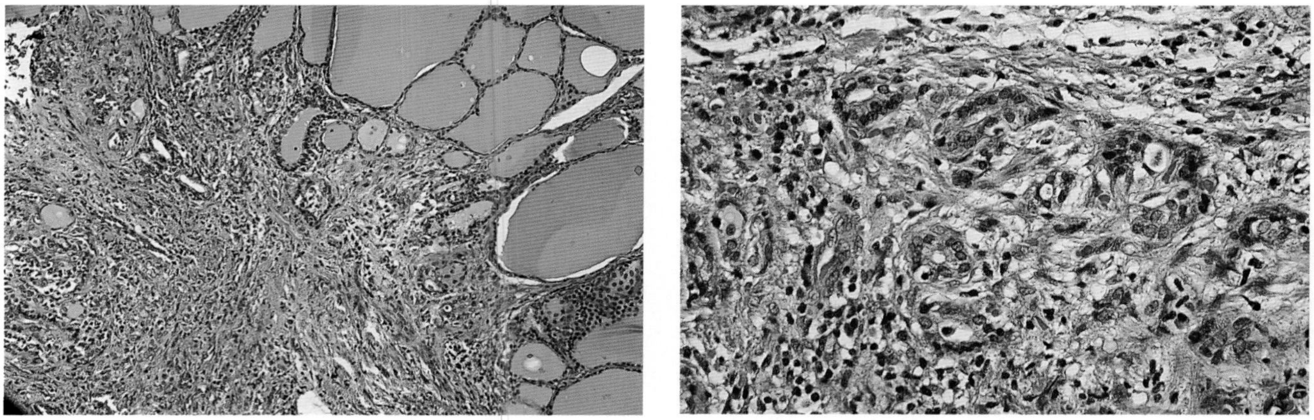

A B

FIG. 11. A: Multifocal sclerosing thyroiditis. On low power, the appearance resembles that of a papillary microcarcinoma. B: At higher power, the follicles entrapped in the fibrosis are irregularly shaped but do not show any of the cytologic features of papillary carcinoma.

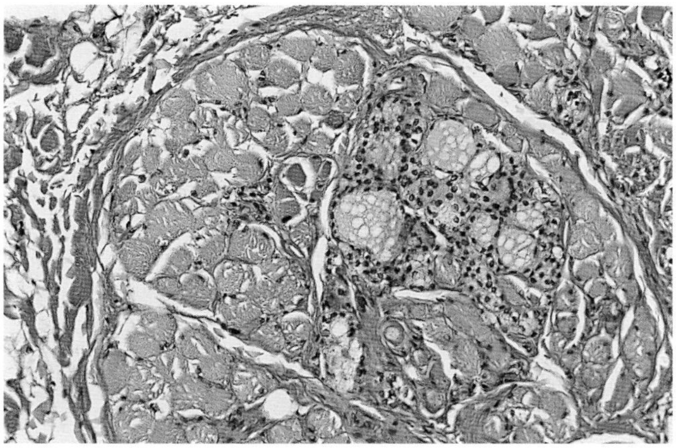

**FIG. 13. A:** Clusters of thyroid tissue intimately admixed with bundles of skeletal muscle adjacent to the thyroid gland.

trathyroidal islands of mature cartilage probably represent remnants of the branchial pouch apparatus (14,104).

In one study striated muscle was found within the thyroid parenchyma of 19 glands, usually in the region of the isthmus or in the pyramidal lobe of the gland (18). Conversely, in 10 specimens thyroid follicles were found within fascicles of strap muscle from the same areas (Fig. 13). Follicles entrapped in perithyroidal skeletal muscle are more easily identifiable when they undergo hyperplastic changes (105).

### Calcium

Dystrophic calcifications may be seen in normal thyroid of old age, particularly in relation to vessels. They can easily be distinguished from psammoma bodies because of the lack of laminations and the irregularity of their contours.

Psammoma bodies have been rarely described in benign thyroid lesions but not in normal thyroid (106–108). Finding psammoma bodies in an otherwise normal thyroid or in a cervical lymph node should always prompt a careful search for an occult papillary carcinoma (Fig. 14).

## BRANCHIAL POUCH–DERIVED AND OTHER ECTOPIC TISSUES

### Solid Ultimobranchial Body Remnants (Solid Cell Nests)

So-called solid cell nests are clusters of epithelial cells interspersed among the follicles. Because they may exhibit squamous differentiation, they have sometimes been misinterpreted in the past as foci of squamous metaplasia in follicles (72). However a UBB origin for what in retrospect are clearly the same formations had already been suggested by Erdheim in 1904 (109) and Getzowa in 1907 (110), following their demonstration of clusters of epithelial cells with solid or rarely cystic appearance in individuals with thyroid aplasia. Additional evidence along these lines was provided by the demonstration of marked similarities of human SCNs with the normal UBB of the rat and the hyperplastic or neoplastic UBB remnants in bulls (111–113).

SCNs are relatively common in normal thyroid, the probability of finding them increasing with the number of sections examined. In one study SCNs were found in only 3% of routinely examined thyroids but in as many as 61% of specimens when the gland was blocked serially at 2- to 3-mm intervals (114). For unknown reasons SCNs are more common in males than in females. Most SCNs measure an average 0.1 mm in diameter, but occasionally they can reach 2 mm. They may be single or multiple. They are usually within the stroma and more or less demarcated by the adjacent thyroid follicles. Adipose tissue and cartilage may be present in their vicinity (115) (Fig. 15). Most SCNs are found along the central axis of the middle and upper third of the lateral lobes (i.e., in the same area where C cells usually occur); this constitutes additional proof for their origin from

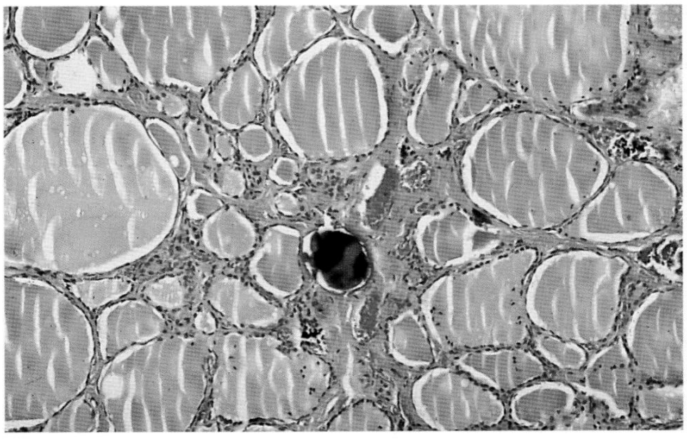

**FIG. 14.** Psammoma body in non-neoplastic thyroid tissue adjacent to a papillary carcinoma (not shown in the picture).

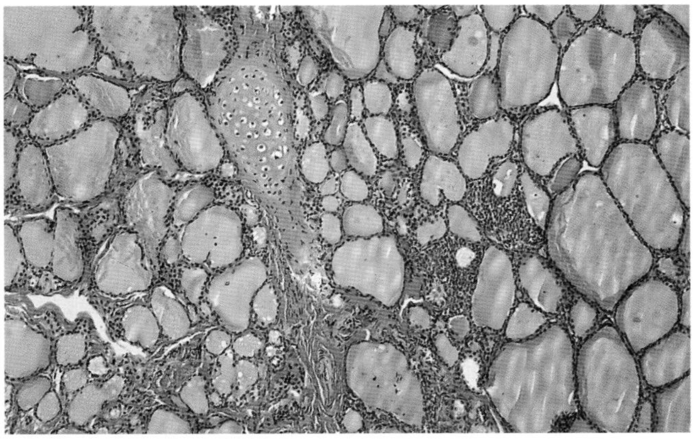

**FIG. 15.** Cartilage island is seen in the proximity of SCNs.

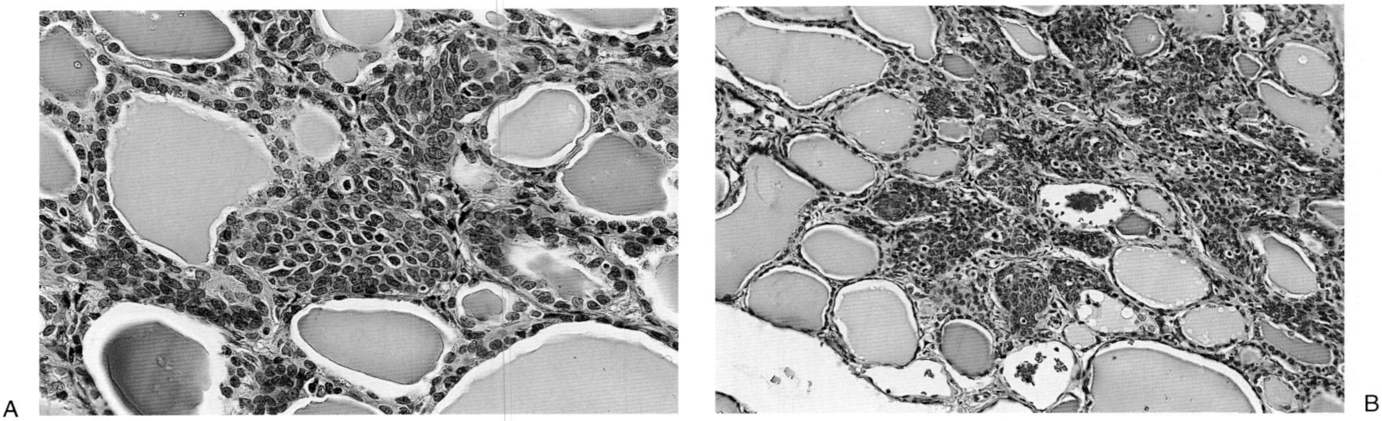

FIG. 16. A: SCN in normal thyroid. Note the uniform appearance of the epithelial cells. B: Low-power view shows the multilobed shape often exhibited by groups of SCNs.

the UBB, as it does the fact that the number of C cells is increased in the vicinity of SCNs (115,116).

SCNs have a round to oval shape and sometimes feature a palisaded edge (Fig. 16A). They are often grouped in clusters featuring a multilobed shape on low-power examination (Fig. 16B). They have a dual cell population. The predominant component is made up of cells of polygonal to oval shape, elongated nuclei with finely granular chromatin, and acidophilic cytoplasm. Some of these cells show clear-cut squamous differentiation. Immunohistochemically, they are reactive for keratins and/or carcinoembryonic antigen, and ultrastructurally they feature bundles of tonofilaments (117–122). The second cell population, numerically less conspicuous, is characterized at the light microscopic level by clear cytoplasm and round nuclei, at the ultrastructural level by dense-core secretory granules, and at the immunohistochemical level by immunoreactivity to CT (115, 117–119). All of these features are indicative of a C-cell nature for this population and constitute a further link between SCNs and the UBBs. Cystic cavities containing acid mucin are frequently observed in association with SCNs (see next section). A variation in the theme is represented by the admixture of SCNs (pure or admixed with a cystic component) with groups of small follicles lined by low cuboidal TGB-immunoreactive epithelium, forming the so-called mixed follicles (Fig. 17). The fact that a similar admixture is seen in mixed medullary-follicular carcinomas has led some investigators to suggest that these rare tumors may arise from uncommitted stem cells of the UBBs that have the potential to differentiate into C cells, follicular cells, or both (123).

SCNs need to be distinguished from collections of C cells, follicles with squamous metaplasia, and tangential sections of normal follicles (Fig. 18).

### Cystic Ultimobranchial Body Remnants

UBB remnants also may take the form of cysts. These occur most commonly in the soft tissues of the neck adjacent to the thyroid. Indeed, it is possible that some of the clinically evident branchial pouch cysts located in close proximity to the thyroid gland and sometimes confused clinically with thyroid lesions or lymph nodes are of UBB origin.

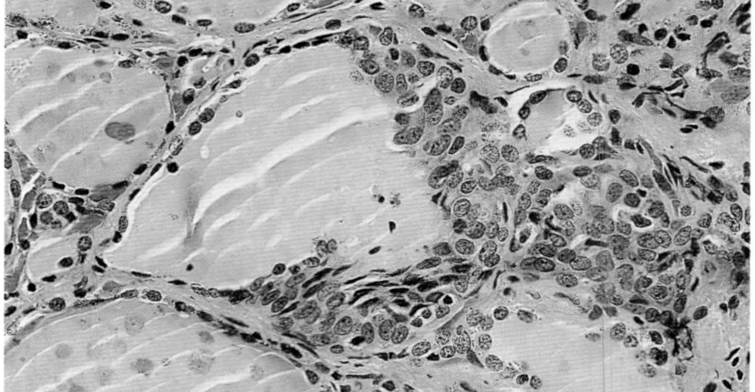

FIG. 17. So-called mixed follicle. An SCN merges with a follicle lined by a flattened epithelium with colloid in the lumen.

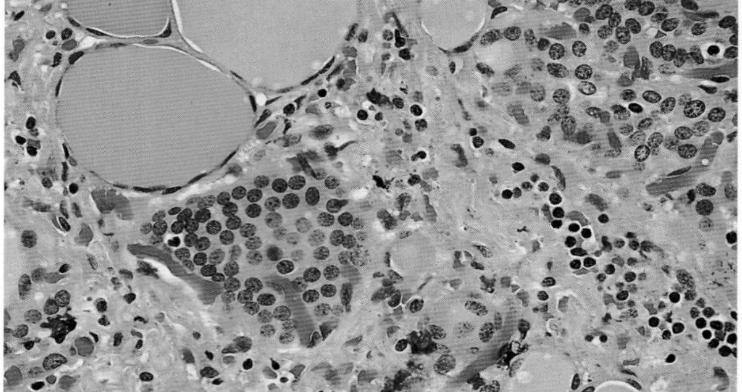

FIG. 18. Tangential cut of a follicle. This should not be misinterpreted as an SCN.

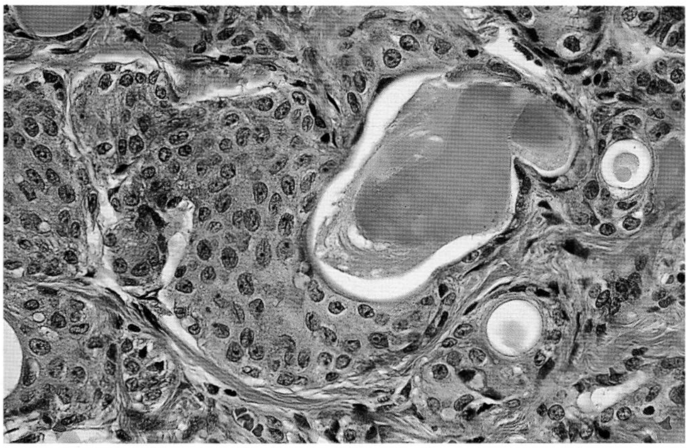

**FIG. 19.** SCN with associated cystic formation. A dense eosinophilic material fills the lumen of the cyst.

These cysts also may develop within the thyroid itself (124). In the latter instance, they may occur by themselves, may be adjacent to SCNs, or may be intimately admixed with them (Fig. 19). These cysts are lined most frequently by a flattened multilayered epithelium of squamous type, and less commonly by a ciliated columnar epithelium (Fig. 20); they often contain clumps of eosinophilic material in their lumen. They are especially common in neonates and also are probably the source for the gross cystic formations occasionally seen accompanying Hashimoto's thyroiditis (125, 126).

**Parathyroid Tissue**

The development of the parathyroid glands and thymus from the branchial pouches in close proximity to the thyroid gland explains why these organs occasionally may be found adjacent to the thyroid capsule or even within the thyroid itself (Fig. 21).

True intrathyroidal parathyroid glands in adults are rare. However, in a study where 58 human fetal thyroid glands obtained at autopsy were systematically studied for the presence of intrathyroidal parathyroid tissue, the latter was found in 13 thyroid lobes from 12 fetuses (22.4%). It was located subcapsularly in nine of 58 cases (15.5%), and it was lying deep in thyroid tissue in four (68%) (127). These intra- and perithyroidal parathyroid structures can be affected by primary or secondary chief cell hyperplasia, adenoma, or carcinoma and represent an often overlooked cause of surgical failure in primary hyperparathyroidism (128).

**Thymic Tissue**

Most of the thymus derives embryologically from the third branchial pouch, together with the lower pair of parathyroid glands. There is also a small and inconstant portion that derives from the fourth branchial pouch together with the upper pair of parathyroid glands and the UBB, which form the lateral thyroid anlage. It is from the latter source that the islands of thymic tissue occasionally found in or around the thyroid are thought to derive (Fig. 22) (129). The fact that ectopic thymic tissue is observed more frequently in neonates and infants supports this hypothesis. Harach and Vujanic (130) searched systematically for the presence of intrathyroid tissue in 58 thyroid glands obtained at autopsy from fetuses with proven retrosternal thymus. Subcapsular thymic tissue was found in two cases (3.4%) and intrathyroid thymic tissue in one (1.7%). An entire thymic gland within the thyroid of an infant has been described by Neill (131). Mizukami et al. (132) reported thymic tissue in the interlobular septum of the thyroid of a patient with Graves disease. Damiani et al. (133) found thymic rests in 1.4% of more than 2,000 of the adult thyroid glands that they examined.

Ectopic thymic tissue may show cystic changes and present clinically as a cystic neck mass. It also may be the source of peri- and intrathyroidal thymomas (134).

A

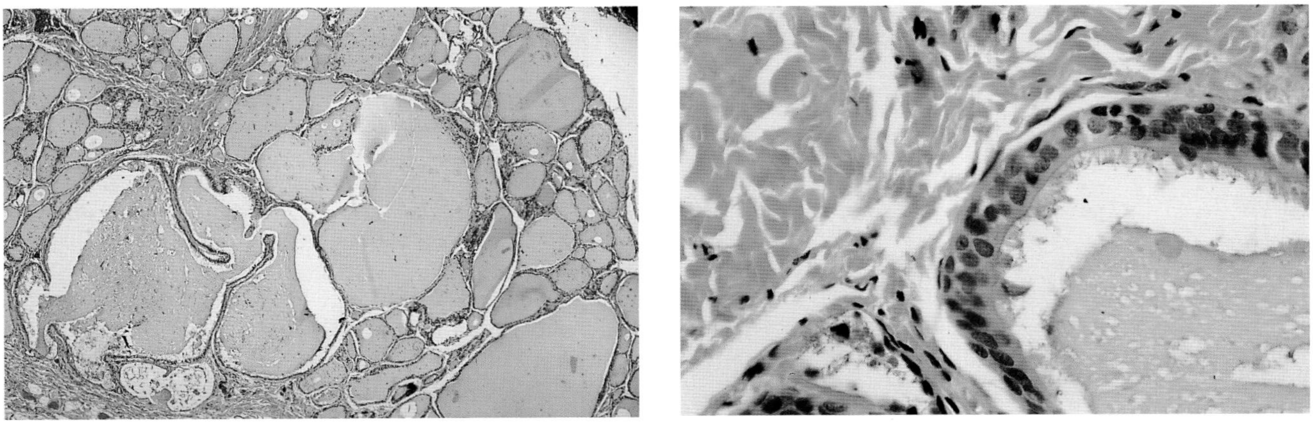

B

**FIG. 20. A:** Intrathyroidal cyst of probable branchial pouch derivation. **B:** Higher-power view showing ciliated epithelium.

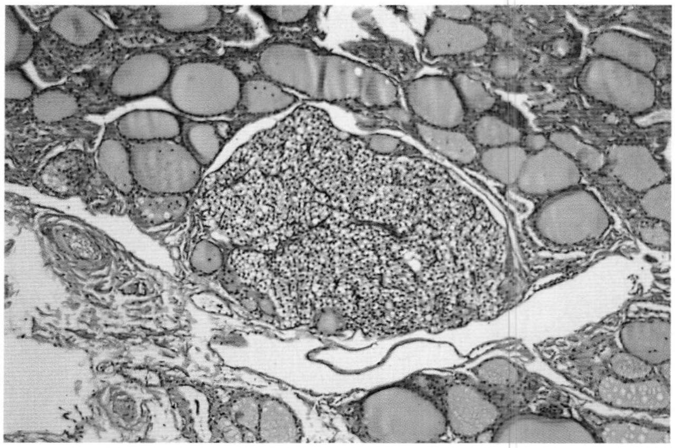

**FIG. 21.** Parathyroid gland entirely located within thyroid.

### Salivary Gland–Type Tissue

Rarely salivary gland–type tissue has been found within the thyroid. Most of the reported cases have been seen in association with a benign thyroid condition, such as multinodular goiter (135).

## THYROID TISSUE IN ABNORMAL LOCATIONS

The presence of non-neoplastic thyroid tissue outside the normal anatomical confines of the gland may be caused by a variety of mechanisms, ranging from congenital abnormalities to acquired processes. Their main practical interest resides in the fact that lack of knowledge of their occurrence may lead to a mistaken diagnosis of metastatic thyroid carcinoma.

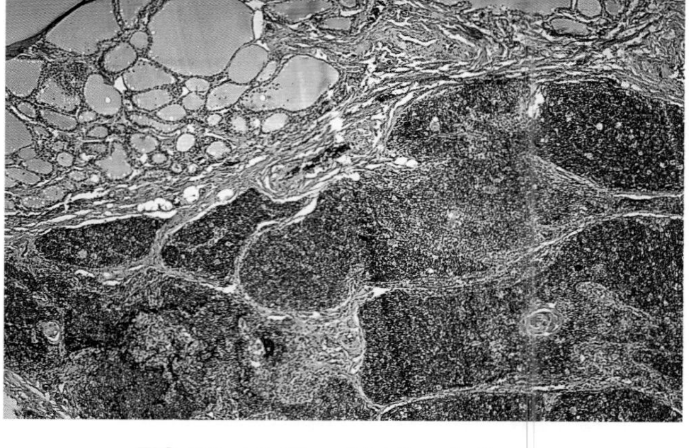

**FIG. 22.** Intrathyroidal thymic tissue.

### In Midline Structures (Ectopic Thyroid)

Ectopic thyroid is derived from abnormalities in migration patterns of the medial anlage and is therefore more commonly found in the neck in a midline position, at any point in the normal pathway of descent of the thyroglossal duct from the foramen cecum to the lower neck (136–139). In most cases the ectopy is partial, clinically insignificant, and discovered accidentally. The base of the tongue (lingual thyroid) and the hyoid bone and its surroundings (as a component of a thyroglossal cyst) are the most common sites. The opposite phenomenon is represented by exaggerated descent of the median anlage into the mediastinum, which may lead to location of thyroid tissue substernally in the preaortic area, in the pericardial cavity, and in the substance of the heart (140–144). However, the majority of mediastinal goiters represent a dislocation downward of normal glands that have been pulled down by the hyperplastic changes that occurred in them.

Lingual thyroid is a relatively common incidental microscopic finding. The follicles appear normal but because of their intimate relationship with the surrounding skeletal muscle they may raise the differential diagnosis with carcinoma (145). Sauk et al. (146) and Baughman et al. (147) found thyroid tissue in the tongue in 10% of individuals examined at autopsy, with the sex distribution being equal. The tongue is the most common location of ectopic thyroid tissue in the rare cases of total ectopy (148). In this condition ectopic glands are prone to functional insufficiency, frequently followed by compensatory hyperplasia, which may be the cause of dyspnea or dysphagia. Acute hypothyroidism may follow the removal of this ectopic tissue (149).

The other site where ectopic thyroid tissue is found more commonly is the wall of thyroglossal cysts. It appears in the form of small groups of follicles and is present in 25% to 65% of cysts examined histologically, its frequency being related to the number of sections submitted for histologic examination (149). The medial location and the presence of thyroid tissue in the wall distinguish thyroglossal duct cysts from the rarer branchial pouch cysts. Ectopic thyroid derived from abnormalities in migration of the medial anlage typically does not contain C cells. In one study of median anlage anomalies including 23 cases of thyroglossal cysts with adjacent thyroid tissue and one case of lingual thyroid, not a single C cell was found in either the thyroid tissue or the epithelium lining the cysts (13).

Only rarely can thyroid tissue be found in locations outside its place of embryonic development. These locations include larynx, trachea, esophagus, diaphragm, gallbladder, common bile duct, retroperitoneum, vagina, sella turcica, and inguinal region (150–155).

### In Pericapsular Soft Tissues and Skeletal Muscles

As already discussed, the presence of thyroid tissue in these locations is not a rare event. It most likely results from the intimate relationship of the thyroid gland with the mesodermal structures of the neck during development.

### In the Lateral Neck

This phenomenon, frequently referred to as lateral aberrant thyroid, has different pathogeneses. It has been suggested that surgery and trauma may cause implantation of thyroid tissue in the lateral neck. Typically when this is the case, a few nodules of normal-appearing thyroid tissue, always of microscopic size and frequently surrounded by a fibrous capsule, are seen in the lateral neck close to the cervical lymph nodes (156–158). History of previous trauma or surgery on the neck, the presence of suture material (in cases of previous surgery), and the benign appearance of the dislocated thyroid tissue are useful in distinguishing them from metastatic carcinoma. It has to be kept in mind that the latter may appear deceptively benign on microscopic examination. Spontaneous separation of thyroid tissue with subsequent implant in the lateral neck may occur in nodular goiter or Hashimoto's thyroiditis (159,160). In both of these conditions, nodules of thyroid tissue extrude and separate from the surface of the gland and deposit in the extrathyroidal soft tissue, where they may acquire an autonomous blood supply (so-called parasitic nodules). The differential diagnosis with metastatic lymph nodes may be very problematic, especially in the presence of Hashimoto's thyroiditis.

### In Cervical Lymph Nodes

Normal-appearing thyroid tissue in medially located cervical lymph nodes is rarely the result of a developmental anomaly (161). Where this is the case, a few microscopic nests of benign-looking follicles are seen in the marginal sinus of the lymph node (Fig. 23). The follicular cells that compose them should lack all of the cytologic features typical of papillary carcinoma (162). Psammoma bodies and papillae should also be absent. Numerous sections are sometimes needed to rule out a metastasis from a papillary microcarcinoma, which is by far the most frequent cause of thyroid tissue in cervical nodes.

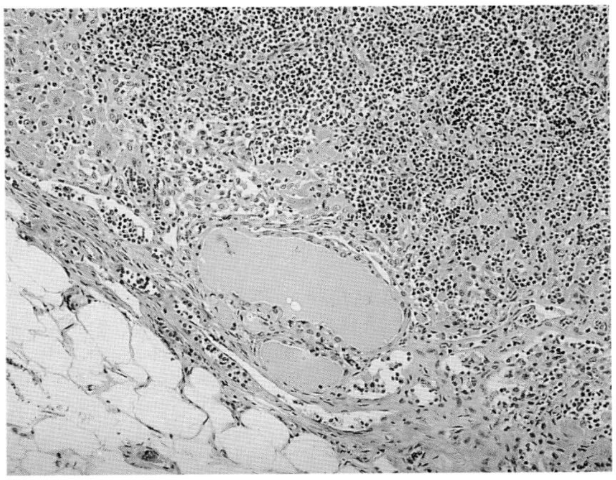

**FIG. 23.** A group of benign-appearing thyroid follicles is seen close to the marginal sinus of a cervical lymph node. This patient did not have a carcinoma in the thyroid gland.

## REFERENCES


1. Hoyes AD, Kershaw DR. Anatomy and development of the thyroid gland. *Ear Nose Throat J* 1985;64:318–333.
2. Shepard TH. Onset of function in the human fetal thyroid: biochemical and radioautographic studies from organ culture. *J Clin Endocrinol Metab* 1967;27:945–958.
3. Gitlin D, Biasucci A. Ontogenesis of immunoreactive thyroglobulin in the human conceptus. *J Clin Endocrinol Metab* 1969;29:849–853.
4. Norris EH. The parathyroid glands and the lateral thyroid in man: their morphogenesis, histogenesis, topographic anatomy and prenatal growth. *Contrib Embryol Carnegie Inst* 1937;159:249–294.
5. Chan AO, Conen PE. Ultrastructural observations on cytodifferentiation of parafollicular cells in the human fetal thyroid. *Lab Invest* 1971; 25:249–259.
6. Sugiyama S. The embryology of the human thyroid gland including ultimobranchial body and others related. *Ergeb Anat Entwicklungsgesch* 1971;44:6–110.
7. LeDourain NM, Teillet MA. The migration of neural crest cells to the wall of the digestive tract in the avian embryo. *J Embryol Exp Morphol* 1973;30:31–48.
8. LeDouarin N, Fontain J, LeLievre C. New studies on the neural crest origin of the avian ultimobranchial glandular cells—interspecific combinations and cytochemical characterization of C cells based on the uptake of biogenic amine precursors. *Histochemistry* 1974;38: 297–305.
9. Nadiz J, Weber E, Hedinger C. C cells in vestiges of the ultimobranchial body in human thyroid glands. *Virchows Arch [A]* 1978;27: 189–191.
10. Ito M, Kameda Y, Tagawa T. An ultrastructural study of the cysts in chicken ultimobranchial glands, with special reference to C cells. *Cell Tissue Res* 1986;246:39–44.
11. Conley ME, Beckwith MD, Mancer JFK, Tenckoff L. The spectrum of the DiGeorge syndrome. *J Pediatr* 1979;94:883–890.
12. Burke BA, Johnson D, Gilbert EF, Drut RM, Ludwig J, Wick MR. Thyrocalcitonin containing cells in the DiGeorge anomaly. *Hum Pathol* 1987;18:355–360.
13. Ljungberg O. *Biopsy pathology of the thyroid and parathyroid*. London: Chapman & Hall; 1992.
14. Williams ED, Toyn CE, Harach HR. The ultimobranchial gland and congenital thyroid abnormalities in man. *J Pathol* 1989;159:135–141.
15. Harada T, Nishikawa Y, Ito K. Aplasia of one thyroid lobe. *Am J Surg* 1972;124:617–619.
16. Hegedus L, Perrild H, Poulsen LR, et al. The determination of thyroid volume by ultrasound and its relationship to body weight, age and sex in normal subjects. *J Clin Endocrin Metab* 1983;56:260–263.
17. Hegedus L, Karstrup S, Rasmussen N. Evidence of cyclic alterations of thyroid size during the menstrual cycle in healthy women. *Am J Obstet Gynecol* 1986;155:142–145.
18. Komorowski RA, Hanson GA. Occult thyroid pathology in the young adult: an autopsy study of 138 patients without clinical thyroid disease. *Hum Pathol* 1988;19:689–696.
19. Gordon G, Sparano BM, Kramer AW, Kelly RG, Iatropoulos MJ. Thyroid gland pigmentation and minocycline therapy. *Am J Pathol* 1984;117:98–109.
20. Alexander CB, Herrera GA, Jaffe K, Yu H. Black thyroid: clinical manifestations, ultrastructural findings, and possible mechanisms. *Hum Pathol* 1985;16:72–78.
21. Landas SK, Schelper RL, Tio FO, Turner JW, Moore KC, Bennett-Gray J. Black thyroid syndrome: exaggeration of a normal process? *Am J Clin Pathol* 1986;85:411–418.
22. Brown RA, Al-Moussa M, Beck JS. Histometry of normal thyroid in man. *J Clin Pathol* 1986;39:475–482.

23. Imada M, Kurosimi M, Fujita H. Three dimensional imaging of blood vessels in thyroids from normal and levothyroxine sodium-treated rats. *Arch Histol Jpn* 1986;49:359–367.
24. Imada M, Kurosimi M, Fujita H. Three dimensional aspects of blood vessels in thyroids from normal, low iodine diet–treated, TSH-treated and PTU-treated rats. *Cell Tissue Res* 1986;245:291–296.
25. Feind C. The head and neck. In: Haagensen CD, Feind C, Herter FP, Slanetz CA, Weinberg JA, eds. *The lymphatics in cancer*. Philadelphia: WB Saunders; 1972:59–123.
26. Crile G Jr. The fallacy of the conventional radical neck dissection for papillary carcinoma of the thyroid. *Ann Surg* 1957;145:317–320.
27. Uchiyama Y, Murakami G, Ohno Y. The fine structure of nerve endings on rat thyroid follicular cells. *Cell Tissue Res* 1985;242:457–460.
28. Melander A, Ericson LD, Sundler F, Ingbar SH. Sympathetic innervation of the mouse thyroid and its significance in thyroid hormone secretion. *Endocrinology* 1974;94:959–966.
29. Tice LW, Creveling CR. Electron microscopic identification of adrenergic nerve endings on thyroid epithelial cells. *Endocrinology* 1975; 97:1123–1129.
30. Ingbar SH. The thyroid gland. In: Wilson JD, Foster DW, eds. *Williams textbook of endocrinology*. 7th ed. Philadelphia: WB Saunders; 1985:682–815.
31. Kameda Y, Okamoto K, Ito M, Tagawa T. Innervation of the C-cells of chicken ultimobranchial glands studied by immunohistochemistry, fluorescence microscopy, and electron microscopy. *Am J Anat* 1988; 182:353–368.
32. Heimann P. Ultrastructure of human thyroid. A study of normal thyroid, untreated and treated diffuse goitre. *Acta Endocrinol* 1966; 53(suppl 110):1–102.
33. Klinck GH, Oertel JE, Winship TH. Ultrastructure of normal human thyroid. *Lab Invest* 1970;22:2–22.
34. Kurata A, Ohta K, Mine M, et al. Monoclonal antihuman thyroglobulin antibodies. *J Clin Endocrinol Metab* 1984;59:573–579.
35. Permanetter W, Nathrath WBJ, Lohrs U. Immunohistochemical analysis of thyroglobulin and keratin in benign and malignant thyroid tumors. *Virchows Arch [A]* 1982;398:221–228.
36. Miettinen M, Franssila K, Lehto VP, Paasivuo O, Virtanen I. Expression of intermediate filament proteins in thyroid gland and thyroid tumors. *Lab Invest* 1984;50:262–269.
37. Buley ID, Gatter KC, Heryet A, Mason DY. Expression of intermediate filament proteins in normal and diseased thyroid glands. *J Clin Pathol* 1987;40:136–142.
38. Dockhorn-Dworniczak B, Franke WW, Schroder S, Czernobilsky B, Gould VE, Bocker W. Patterns of expression of cytoskeletal proteins in human thyroid gland and thyroid carcinomas. *Differentiation* 1987; 35:53–71.
39. Stanta G, Carcangiu ML, Rosai J. The biochemical and immunohistochemical profile of thyroid neoplasms. *Pathol Annu* 1988;23: 129–157.
40. Viale G, Dell Orto P, Coggi G, Gambacorta M. Coexpression of cytokeratins and vimentin in normal and diseased thyroid glands: lack of diagnostic utility of vimentin immunostaining. *Am J Surg Pathol* 1989;13:1034–1040.
41. Clark O, Gerend PL, Davis M, Goretski PE, Hoffman PG. Estrogen and thyroid-stimulating hormone (TSH) receptors in neoplastic and nonneoplastic human thyroid tissue. *J Surg Res* 1985;38:89–96.
42. Bur M, Shiraki W, Masood S. Estrogen and progesterone receptor detection in neoplastic and non-neoplastic thyroid tissues. *Mod Pathol* 1993;6:469–472.
43. Prinz RA, Sandberg L, Chandhuri PK. Androgen receptors in human thyroid tissue *Surgery* 1984;96:996–1000.
44. Miettinen M, Virtanen I. Expression of laminin in thyroid gland and thyroid pathology. An Immunohistologic study. *Int J Cancer* 1984;34: 27–30.
45. Deiss WP, Peake RL. The mechanism of thyroid hormone secretion. *Ann Intern Med* 1968;69:881–890.
46. Green WL. The physiology of the thyroid gland and its hormones. In: Green WL, ed. *The thyroid*. New York: Elsevier; 1987:1–46.
47. Bjorkman U, Ekholm R, Elmqvist LG, Ericson LE, Melander A, Smeds S. Induced unidirectional transport of protein into the thyroid follicular lumen. *Endocrinology* 1974;95:1506–1517.
48. Ericson LE, Engstrom G. Quantitative electron microscopic studies on exocytes and endocytosis in the thyroid follicle cell. *Endocrinology* 1978;103:883–892.
49. Ide M. Immunoelectron microscopic localization of thyroglobulin in the human thyoid gland. *Acta Pathol Jpn* 1984;34:575–584.
50. Sterling K. Thyroid hormone action at the cell level. *N Engl J Med* 1979;300:117–123.
51. Liddle GW, Liddle RA, Endrocrinology. In: Smith LH, Thier SO, eds. *Pathophysiology*. Philadelphia: WB Saunders; 1981.
52. Larsen PR. Thyroid–pituitary interaction. *N Engl J Med* 1982;306: 23–32.
53. Pittman JA. Thyrotropin-releasing hormone. *Adv Intern Med* 1974;19: 303–325.
54. Wilber JF. Thyrotropin releasing hormone: secretion and actions. *Annu Rev Med* 1973;24:353–364.
55. Dremier S, Golstein J, Mosselmans R, Dumont JE, Galand P, Robaye B. Apoptosis in dog thyroid cells. *Biochem Biophys Res Commun* 1994;200:52–58.
56. Walsh FM, Castelli JB. Polytef granuloma clinically simulating carcinoma of the thyroid. *Arch Otolaryngol* 1975;101:262–263.
57. Sanfilippo F, Shelburne J. Analysis of a Polytef granuloma mimicking a cold thyroid nodule 17 months after laryngeal injection. *Ultrastruct Pathol* 1980;1:471–475.
58. Chaplin AJ. Histopathological occurrence and characterization of calcium oxalate: a review. *J Clin Pathol* 1977;30:800–811.
59. Carney JA, Moore SB, Northcutt RC, Wooler LB, Stillwell GK. Palpation thyroiditis (multifocal granulomatous folliculitis). *Am J Clin Pathol* 1975;64:639–647.
60. Blum M, Schloss MF. Martial-arts thyroiditis. *N Engl J Med* 1984; 311:199–200.
61. Harach R, Jasani B. Thyroid multifocal granulomatous folliculitis (palpation thyroiditis): an immunocytochemical study. *Endocr Pathol* 1993;4:105–109.
62. Hellwig, CA. Colloidophagy in the human thyroid gland. *Science* 1951;113:725–726.
63. Manson C, Cross P, De Sousa B. Post-operative necrotizing granulomas of the thyroid. *Histopathology* 1992;21:392–394.
64. Harach HR. Palpation thyroiditis resembling C cell hyperplasia. *Pathol Res Pract* 1993;189:488–490.
65. Richter MN, McCarty KS. Anisotropic crystals in the human thyroid gland. *Am J Pathol* 1954;30:545–553.
66. Katoh R, Suzuki K, Hemmi A, Kawaoi A. Nature and significance of calcium oxalate crystals in normal human thyroid gland. *Virchows Arch [A]* 1993;422:301–306.
67. Reid JD, Choi CH, Oldroyd NO. Calcium oxalate crystals in the thyroid: their identification, prevalence, origin, and possible significance. *Am J Clin Pathol* 1987;87:443–454.
68. Gross S. Granulomatous thyroiditis with anisotropic crystalline material. *Arch Pathol* 1955;59:412–417.
69. Fayemi AO, Ali M, Braun EV. Oxalosis in hemodialysis patients. *Arch Pathol Lab Med* 1979;103:58–62.
70. Klinck G, Menk K. Squamous cells in the human thyroid. *Milit Surgeon* 1951;109:406–414.
71. Harcourt-Webster JN. Squamous epithelium in the human thyroid gland. *J Clin Pathol* 1966;19:384–388.
72. LiVolsi VA, Merino MJ. Squamous cells in the human thyroid gland. *Am J Surg Pathol* 1978;2:133–140.
73. Pearse AGE. The cytochemistry of the thyroid C-cells and their relationship to calcitonin. *Proc R Soc Lond [Biol]* 1966;164:478–487.
74. Wolfe HJ, DeLellis RA, Voelkel EF, Tahjian AH Jr. Distribution of calcitonin-containing cells in the normal neonatal human thyroid gland: a correlation of morphology with peptide content. *J Clin Endocrinol Metab* 1975;41:1076–1081.
75. O Toole K, Fenoglio-Preisler C, Pushparaj N. Endocrine changes associated with the human aging process: III. Effect of age on the number of calcitonin immunoreactive cells in the thyroid gland. *Hum Pathol* 1985;16:991–1000.
76. Gibson WCH, Peng T-Ch, Croker BP. Age-associated C-cell hyperplasia in the human thyroid. *Am J Pathol* 1982;106:388–393.
77. Albores-Saavedra J, Gorraez de la Mora T, de la Torre-Rendon F, Gould E. Mixed medullary-papillary carcinoma of the thyroid. A previously unrecognized variant of thyroid carcinoma. *Hum Pathol* 1990; 21:1151–1155.
78. Scopsi L, DiPalma S, Ferrari C, Holst JJ, Rehfeld JF, Rilke F. C-cell hyperplasia accompanying thyroid diseases other than medullary carcinoma: an immunohistochemical study by means of antibody to calcitonin and somatostatin. *Mod Pathol* 1991;4:297–304.
79. Libbey NP, Nowakowski KJ, Tucci JR. C-cell hyperplasia of the thyroid in a patient with goitrous hypothyroidism and Hashimoto's thyroiditis. *Am J Surg Pathol* 1989;13:71–77.

80. Biddinger PW, Brennan MF, Rosen PP. Symptomatic C-cell hyperplasia associated with chronic lymphocytic thyroiditis. *Am J Surg Pathol* 1991;15:599–604.
81. Guyetant S, Wion-Barbot N, Rousselet MC, Franc B, Bigorgne JC, Saint-Andre JP. C-cell hyperplasia associated with chronic lymphocytic thyroiditis. A retrospective quantitative study of 112 cases. *Hum Pathol* 1994;25:514–521.
82. Tomita T, Millard DM. C-cell hyperplasia in secondary hyperparathyroidism. *Histopathol* 1992;21:469–474.
83. Teitelbaum SL, Moore KE, Shieber W. Parafollicular cells in the normal human thyroid. *Nature* 1971;230:334–335.
84. DeLellis RA, Wolfe HJ. The pathobiology of the human calcitonin (C)-cell: a review. *Pathol Annu* 1981;16:25–52.
85. DeLellis RA, Nunnemacher G, Wolfe HJ. C-cell hyperplasia. An ultrastructural analysis. *Lab Invest* 1977;36:237–248.
86. Pearse AGE. Common cytochemical and ultrastructural characteristics of cells producing polypeptide hormones (the APUD series) and their relevance to thyroid and ultimobranchial C-cells and calcitonin. *Proc R Soc Lond [Biol]* 1968;170:71–80.
87. Bussolati G, Pearse AGE. Immunofluorescent localization of calcitonin in the C cells of the pig and dog thyroid. *J Endocrinol* 1967;37: 205–209.
88. McMillan PJ, Hooker WM, Defots LJ. Distribution of calcitonin-containing cells in the human thyroid. *Am J Anat* 1974;140:73–80.
89. Zajac JD, Penschow J, Mason T, Tregear G, Coghlan J, Martin TJ. Identification of calcitonin and calcitonin gene–related peptide messenger ribonucleic acid in medullary thyroid carcinoma by hybridization histochemistry. *J Clin Endocrinol Metab* 1986;62:1037–1043.
90. Van Norden S, Polak JM, Pearse AGE. Single cellular origin of somatostatin and calcitonin in the rat thyroid gland. *Histochemistry* 1977;53:243–247.
91. Yamada Y, Ito S, Matsubara Y, Kobayashi S. Immunohistochemical demonstration of somatostatin-containing cells in the human, dog and rat thyroid. *Tohoku J Exp Med* 1977;122:87–92.
92. Kusumoto Y. Calcitonin and somatostatin are localized in different cells in canine thyroid gland. *Biomed Res* 1980;1:237–241.
93. Kameya T, Bessho T, Tsumuraya M, et al. Production of gastrin releasing peptide by medullary carcinoma of the thyroid. *Virchows Arch [A]* 1983;401:99–108.
94. Sunday ME, Wolfe HJ, Roos BA, Chin WW, Spindel ER. Gastrin-releasing peptide gene expression in developing hyperplastic and neoplastic human thyroid C-cells. *Endocrinology* 1988;122: 1551–1558.
95. Kakudo K, Vacca LL. Immunohistochemical study of substance P-like immunoreactivity in human thyroid and medullary carcinoma of the thyroid. *J Submicrosc Cytol* 1983;15:563–568.
96. Sundler F, Robberecht P, Yanaihara N, et al. Is helodermin produced by medullary thyroid carcinoma cells and normal C-cells? Immunocytochemical evidence *Regul Pept* 1988;20:83–89.
97. DeLellis RA. Endocrine tumors. In: Calvin RB, Bhan AR, McCluskey RT, eds. *Diagnostic immunopathology.* New York: Raven Press; 1988.
98. MacIntyre I. Calcitonin, physiology, biosynthesis, secretion, metabolism, and mode of action. In:DeGroot LJ, ed. *Endocrinology.* Vol. 2. Philadelphia: WB Saunders; 1989:892–901.
99. Amara SG, Jonas V, Rosenfeld MG, Ong SG, Evans RM. Alternative RNA processing in calcitonin gene expression generates mRNAs encoding different polypeptide products. *Nature* 1982;298:240–244.
100. Ali-Rachedi A, Varndell IM, Facer P, et al. Immunocytochemical localization of katacalcin, a calcium-lowering hormone cleaved from the human calcitonin precursor. *J Clin Endocrinol Metab* 1983;57: 680–682.
101. Kantozoglou T, Mambo N. The histopathologic features of lithium-associated thyroiditis. *Hum Pathol* 1983;14:737–739.
102. Carpenter GR, Emery JL. Inclusions in the human thyroid. *J Anat* 1976;122:77–89.
103. Morizumi H, Sano T, Tsuyuguchi M, Yoshinari T, Morimoto S. Localized adiposity of the thyroid, clinically mimicking an adenoma. *Endocr Pathol* 1991;2:226–229.
104. Finkle HI, Goldman RL. Heterotopic cartilage in the thyroid. *Arch Pathol* 1973;95:48–49.
105. Gardner WR. Unusual relationships between thyroid gland and skeletal muscle in infants. *Cancer* 1956;4:681–691.
106. Klinck GH, Winship T. Psammoma bodies and thyroid cancer. *Cancer* 1959;12:656–662.
107. Batsakis JG, Nishiyama RH, Rich CR. Microlithiasis (calcospherites) and carcinoma of the thyroid gland. *Arch Pathol* 1960;69:493–498.
108. Dugan JM, Atkinson BF, Avitabile A, Schimmel M, LiVolsi VA. Psammoma bodies in fine needle aspirate of the thyroid in lymphocytic thyroiditis. *Acta Cytol* 1987;31:330–334.
109. Erdheim J. I. Uber Schilddrusenaplasie. II. Geschwulste des Ductus Thyreoglossus. III. Uber einige menschliche Kiemenderivate. *Beitr Pathol Anat* 1904;35:366–433.
110. Getzowa S. Zur Kenntnis des postbranchialen Korpers und der branchialen Kanalchen des Menschen. *Virchows Arch [A]* 1907;88: 181–235.
111. Calvert R, Isler H. Fine structure of a third epithelial component of the thyroid gland of the rat. *Anat Rec* 1970;168:23–41.
112. Black HE, Capen CC, Young DM. Ultimobranchial thyroid neoplasms in bulls. *Cancer* 1973;32:865–878.
113. Ljungberg O, Nilsson PO. Hyperplastic and neoplastic changes in ultimobranchial remnants and in parafollicular (C) cells in bulls:a histologic and immunohistochemical study. *Vet Pathol* 1985;22:95–103.
114. Harach HR. Solid cell nests of the human thyroid in early stages of postnatal life. Systematic study. *Acta Anat* 1986;127:262–264.
115. Janzer RC, Weber E, Hedinger CHR. The relation between solid cell nests and C cells of the thyroid gland. *Cell Tissue Res* 1979;197: 295–312.
116. Chan JKC, Tse CCH. Solid cell nest–associated C-cells. Another possible explanation for "C-cell hyperplasia" adjacent to follicular cell tumors. *Hum Pathol* 1989;20:498.
117. Nadig J, Weber E, Hedinger C. C-cells in vestiges of the ultimobranchial body in human thyroid glands. *Virchows Arch [B]* 1978;27: 189–191.
118. Harach HR. Histological markers of solid cell nests of the thyroid. With some emphasis on their expression in thyroid ultimobranchial-related tumors. *Acta Anat* 1985;124:111–116.
119. Autelitano F, Santeusanio G, DiTondo U, Costantino AM, Renda F, Autelitano M. Immunohistochemical study of solid cell nests of the thyroid gland found from an autopsy study. *Cancer* 1987;59:477–483.
120. Cameselle-Teijeiro J, Varela-Duran J, Sambade C, Villanueva JP, Varela-Nunez R, Sobrinho-Simoes M. Solid cell nests of the thyroid: light microscopy and immunohistochemical profile. *Hum Pathol* 1994;25:684–693.
121. Mizukami Y, Nonomura A, Michigishi T, et al. Solid cell nests of the thyroid. A histologic and immunohistochemical study. *Am J Clin Pathol* 1994;101:186–191.
122. Yamaoka Y. Solid cell nest (SCN) of the human thyroid gland. *Acta Pathol Jpn* 1973;23:493–506.
123. Ljungberg O, Nilsson PO. Intermediate thyroid carcinoma in humans and ultimobranchial tumors in bulls: a comparative morphological and immunohistochemical study. *Endocr Pathol* 1991;2:24–39.
124. Beckner ME, Shultz JJ, Richardson T. Solid and cystic ultimobranchial body remnants in the thyroid. *Arch Pathol Lab Med* 1990; 114:1040–1052.
125. Louis DN, Vickery AL Jr, Rosai J, Wang CA. Multiple branchial cleft–like cysts in Hashimoto's thyroiditis. *Am J Surg Pathol* 1989;13: 45–49.
126. Apel RL, Asa SL, Chalvardjian A, LiVolsi VA. Intrathyroidal lymphoepithelial cysts of probable branchial origin. *Hum Pathol* 1994;25: 1238–1242.
127. Harach HR, Vujanic GM. Intrathyroidal parathyroid. *Pediatr Pathol* 1993;13:71–74.
128. Spiegel AM, Marx SJ, Doppman JL, et al. Intrathyroidal parathyroid adenoma or hyperplasia. An occasionally overlooked cause of surgical failure in primary hyperparathyroidism. *JAMA* 1975;234: 1029–1033.
129. LiVolsi V. Branchial and thymic remnants in the thyroid and cervical region: an explanation for unusual tumors and microscopic curiosities. *Endocr Pathol* 1993;4:115–119.
130. Harach HR, Vujanic GM. Intrathyroidal thymic tissue: an autopsy study in fetuses with some emphasis on pathological implications. *Pediatr Pathol* 1993;13:431–434.
131. Neill J. Intrathyroid thymoma. *Am J Surg Pathol* 1986;10:660–661.
132. Mizukami Y, Nonomura A, Michigishi T, Noguchi M, Nakamura S. Ectopic thymic tissue in the thyroid gland. *Endocr Pathol* 1993; 4:162–164.
133. Damiani S, Filotico M, Eusebi V. Carcinoma of the thyroid showing thymoma-like features. *Virchows Arch [A]* 1991;418:463–466.
134. Miyauchi A, Kuma K, Matsuzuka F, et al. Intrathyroidal epithelial

thymoma: an entity distinct from squamous cell carcinoma of the thyroid. *World J Surg* 1985;9:128–135.
135. Cameselle-Teijeiro J, Varela-Duran J. Intrathyroid salivary gland–type tissue in multinodular goiter. *Virchows Arch* 1994;425:331–334.
136. Guimaraes SB, Uceda JE, Lynn HB, Thyroglossal duct remnants in infants and children. *Mayo Clin Proc* 1972;47:117–120.
137. Ellis P, Van Norstrand AW. The applied anatomy of thyroglossal tract remnants. *Laryngoscope* 1977;87:765–770.
138. Larochelle D, Arcand P, Belzile M, Gagnon NB. Ectopic thyroid tissue—a review of the literature. *J Otolaryngol* 1979;8:523–530.
139. Allard RH. The thyroglossal cyst. *Head Neck Surg* 1982;5:134–146.
140. De Andrade MA. A review of 128 cases of post mediastinal goiter. *World J Surg* 1977;1:789–797.
141. de Sauza FM, Smith PE. Retrosternal goiter. *J Otolaryngol* 1983;12: 393–396.
142. Kantelip B, Lusson JR, deRiberolles C, Lamaison D, Bailly P. Intracardiac ectopic thyroid. *Hum Pathol* 1986;17:1293–1296.
143. Pollice L, Caneso G. Struma cordis. *Arch Pathol Lab Med* 1986;110: 452–453.
144. Shemin RJ, Marsh JD, Schoen FJ. Benign intracardiac thyroid mass causing right ventricular outflow tract obstruction. *Am J Cardiol* 1985;56:828–829.
145. Wapshaw H. Lingual thyroid. *Br J Surg* 1974;30:160–165.
146. Sauk JJ Jr. Ectopic lingual thyroid. *J Pathol* 1970;102:239–243.
147. Baughman RA, Gainsville MSD. Lingual thyroid and lingual thyroglossal tract remnants. *Oral Surg* 1972;34:781–799.
148. Ulrich HF. Lingual thyroid. *Ann Surg* 1932;95:503–507.
149. LiVolsi VA, Perzin KH, Savetsy L. Carcinoma arising in median ectopic thyroid (including thyroglossal duct tissue). *Cancer* 1974;34: 1303–1315.
150. Bone RC, Biller HF, Irwin TM. Intralaryngotracheal thyroid. *Ann Otol Rhinol Laryngol* 1972;81:424–428.
151. Donegan JO, Wood MD. Intratracheal thyroid—familial occurrence. *Laryngoscope* 1985;95:6–8.
152. Kaplan M. Kauli R, Lubin E, Grunebaum M, Laron Z. Ectopic thyroid tissue. A clinical study of 30 children and review. *J Pediatr* 1978;92: 205–209.
153. Kurman RJ, Prabha AC. Thyroid and parathyroid glands in the vaginal wall. *Am J Clin Pathol* 1973;59:503–507.
154. Reuchti C, Balli-Antunes H, Gerber HA. Follicular tumor in the sellar region without primary cancer of the thyroid. Heterotopic carcinoma? *Am J Clin Pathol* 1987;87:776–780.
155. Rahn J. Uber eine eigenartige. Heterotopic von Schilddrusengewebe. *Zentralbl Allg Pathol* 1958;99:80–86.
156. Block MA, Wylie JH, Patton RB, Miller JM. Does benign thyroid tissue occur in the lateral part of the neck? *Am J Surg* 1966;112:476–481.
157. Klopp CT, Kirson SM. Therapeutic problems with ectopic non-cancerous follicular thyroid tissue in the neck: 18 case reports according to etiological factors. *Ann Surg* 1966;163:653–664.
158. Moses DC, Thompson NW, Nishiyama RH, Sisson JC. Ectopic thyroid tissue in the neck. Benign or maligant. *Cancer* 1976;38:361–365.
159. Hathaway BM. Innocuous accessory thyroid nodules. *Arch Surg* 1965;90:222–227.
160. Sisson JC, Schmidt RW, Beierwaltes WH. Sequestered nodular goiter. *N Engl J Med* 1964;270:927–932.
161. Meyer JS, Steinberg LS. Microscopically benign thyroid follicles in cervical lymph nodes. Serial section study of lymph node inclusions and entire thyroid gland in 5 cases. *Cancer* 1969;24:302–211.
162. Frantz VK, Forsythe R, Hanford JM, Rogers WM. Lateral aberrant thyroids. *Ann Surg* 1942;115;161–183.

*Histology for Pathologists, second edition,*
Edited by Stephen S. Sternberg.
Lippincott-Raven Publishers, Philadelphia
© 1997.

# CHAPTER 47

# Parathyroid Glands

Sanford I. Roth and Graziella M. Abu-Jawdeh



The surgical pathology of the parathyroid glands largely involves interpretation of their histology in patients with hyperfunction due to neoplastic or primary hyperplastic processes, that is, primary hyperparathyroidism (1–5). Secondary hyperparathyroidism, in contrast, is a consequence of stimulation of parathyroid gland growth and hormone secretion by hypocalcemia due to diseases of other organs, such as renal insufficiency or malabsorption (6–8). This results in a secondary hyperplasia, histologically indistinguishable but clinically easily distinguishable from primary hyperplasia. Because other disorders, such as hypoparathyroidism, pseudohypoparathyroidism, and familial hypocalciuric hypercalcemia (9), are not treated surgically and neonatal severe hyperparathyroidism (9) is rare, the parathyroid glands are rarely available for examination in these diseases. In order to adequately interpret the pathology of the parathyroid glands, the surgical pathologist must have a thorough knowledge and understanding of calcium metabolism, the biochemistry of the parathyroid glands, the differential diagnosis and pathobiology of parathyroid disease, and the normal and pathologic anatomy of the glands (10). This chapter presents the normal histology of the parathyroid glands, the alterations of the glands that occur with age, and a brief discussion of calcium metabolism.

## HISTORICAL REVIEW

In 1850 Professor Richard Owen (11), before the Royal College in London, first described the parathyroid glands in the Indian rhinoceros as "a small, compact yellow glandular body . . . attached to the thyroid at the point where the veins emerge." Interestingly this paper (11) was not published for twelve years after its presentation. Remak (12) in 1855 and Virchow (13) in 1863 described similar glands in cats and humans, respectively. However, it was not until 1880 that the anatomy and histology of the parathyroid glands of several species, including humans, were clearly established by a medical student, Ivor Sandström (14,15). He demonstrated that the glands, which he named "glandulae parathyroidae," were structures separate from the thyroid. He used this terminology to suggest the physical, as well as the possible embryologic, relationship to the thyroid. Kohn (16,17) proposed the term *Epithelköperchen* after he demonstrated by animal experiments that the glands originated independently from the thyroid. However, this terminology has survived only in the German literature.

## EMBRYOLOGY

The parathyroid glands arise as diverticula of the endoderm of the third and fourth branchial pouches (18–21). They make their first appearance as bilateral localized proliferations along the anterodorsal surface of pouch III and the lateral portion of the dorsal extremity of pouch IV during the 5th week of gestation (9-mm embryo). The glands are thus referred to as parathyroid III or parathyroid IV, depending on their pouch of origin (the singular is used because of the symmetrical growth). Parathyroid III, along with the thymus, forms as the third pouch separates from the pharynx. At this stage parathyroid III lies cephalad and lateral to parathyroid IV, and the two are separated by the medial thyroid. Differential growth rates of the thymus and the adjacent structures determine the final position the glands occupy after birth.

S. I. Roth: Department of Pathology, Northwestern University Medical School, Chicago, Illinois 60611.
G. M. Abu-Jawdeh: Department of Pathology, Beth Israel Hospital and Harvard Medical School, Boston Massachusetts 02115.

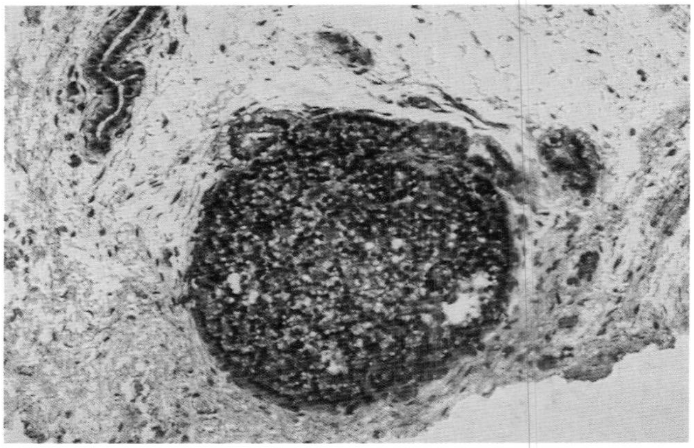

**FIG. 1.** An embryonic parathyroid gland still attached to the remnant of the branchial pouch. The chief cells are closely packed and uniform. No stroma is visible.

The thymus, the most lateral of these structures, attaches to the pericardium and comes to lie largely in the thorax. The attached parathyroid III also develops a more caudad position as the more medial structures grow cephalad. In the 18 mm embryo, when parathyroid III is at the level of the lower pole of the thyroid, it usually separates from the thymus, forming the lower parathyroid gland. Variations in the level at which this separation takes place are frequent and account for the marked anatomic variations in the final position of the adult glands. Parathyroid IV and the lateral thyroid (the ultimobranchial or postbranchial body) derive from the caudal part of the fourth branchial pouch (Fig. 1). Together they form a bilobate complex and, as they separate, parathyroid IV acquires its adult position as the upper gland, near the intersection of the recurrent laryngeal nerve and the medial thyroid artery. Due to its medial position, closer association with midline structures, and shorter embryonic migrations, parathyroid IV has a more constant location and is usually cephalad to parathyroid III. Although an ectodermal origin of the glands has been suggested (22,23), the consensus is that the glands arise from the endodermal region of the branchial pouch. Studies suggest that the parathyroid glands are functioning even in the embryo (Fig. 2) (24–29), possibly as early as 14 weeks (Roth, *unpublished data*).

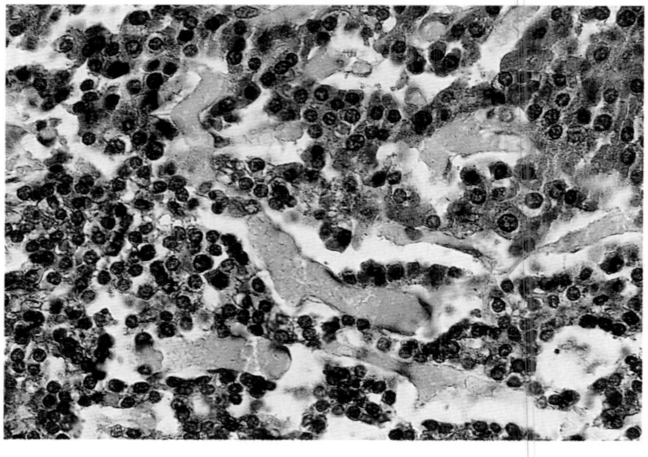

**FIG. 2.** Immunohistochemical stain demonstrating PTH in the gland of a 20-week fetus.

## CALCIUM AND PARATHYROID METABOLISM

Calcium is one of the most closely controlled ions in mammals. The serum level of ionized calcium ($Ca^{2+}$) is maintained within the limits of laboratory error in most individuals. The serum calcium concentration ([$Ca^{+}$]) is commonly measured as the total calcium, although it is the ionized calcium that is meaningful. In humans approximately 50% of the total serum calcium is bound, primarily to albumin, but also to chelating agents such as citrate. The serum [$Ca^{2+}$] is regulated through five organs: the parathyroid glands, the C cells of the thyroid (probably of minimal importance in humans), the bones, the kidneys, and the gastrointestinal tract (30). In humans the two primary hormones responsible for control of [$Ca^{2+}$] are the parathyroid hormone (PTH) and the metabolites of vitamin D, primarily $1\alpha$,25 $(OH)_2$ vitamin D (31).

Acute control of the serum [$Ca^{2+}$] is the primary responsibility of PTH (31). PTH operates through a cell surface receptor, primarily found in the proximal convoluted tubule of the kidney and the osteoblasts of the bone. PTH acts to increase the serum calcium. It promotes tubular reabsorption of calcium in the kidney, increases the activity of the $1\alpha$ vitamin D hydroxylase [thus increasing the synthesis of the active form of vitamin D ($1\alpha$,25 $(OH)_2$ vitamin D) and increasing bone resorption and gastrointestinal calcium transport]. The effect on bone requires the osteoblasts and the osteoclast precursors (see Chapter 5), which have PTH receptors. These cells produce paracrine factors that stimulate osteoclastic bone resorption because the osteoclasts lack PTH receptors. PTH also operates through the osteocytes, resulting is osteocytic osteolysis of the perilacunar bone.

The most active metabolite of vitamin D, $1\alpha$,25 $(OH)_2$ vitamin D, increases calcium resorption from the gastrointestinal tract and acts in synergy with PTH to increase bone resorption (32). $1\alpha$,25 $(OH)_2$ vitamin D also acts as a negative feedback on PTH synthesis and secretion. This action is mediated by inhibiting translation of prepro-PTH messenger through a vitamin D–responsive element related to an upstream promotor of the PTH gene (33).

PTH synthesis and secretion are controlled by the ambient [$Ca^{2+}$]. Increased ambient [$Ca^{2+}$] decreases PTH synthesis and secretion and intracellular [$Ca^{2+}$], whereas decreased serum [$Ca^{2+}$] increases PTH synthesis and secretion. This is in contrast to other organs, where increased intracellular [$Ca^{2+}$] increases hormone synthesis and secretion, whereas decreased [$Ca^{2+}$] decreases synthesis and secretion.

Recently a calcium ion–sensing cell surface receptor has been identified (34,35). This receptor is a member of the superfamily of guanine-nucleotide-regulatory G proteins. The gene for this receptor is located on the long arm of chromosome 3 (34,35). The receptor has been identified on the cell membrane of the parathyroid glands and is thought to be responsible for mediating the effect of calcium on the synthesis and secretion of PTH, much as vitamin D acts through its receptor.

Mutations of the calcium receptor gene have been identified in familial hypocalciuric hypercalcemia and severe neonatal hyperparathyroidism (34,36–38). These heterozygous and homozygous mutations result in inactivation of the receptor. The chief cell is thus stimulated to hypersecrete. In some cases of hypoparathyroidism, hyperactivity mutations have been identified in this gene (39), resulting in decreased synthesis and secretion of PTH.

Paracrine control of PTH secretion has been demonstrated in tissue culture, with decreasing cell density resulting in decreasing hormone secretion (40). Chromogranin A, which is cosecreted with PTH and its proteolytic products pancreastatin and parastatin, also inhibit PTH secretion (41–43).

## NUMBER AND LOCATION

Ninety percent to 97% of patients have four parathyroid glands (44–50). However, the number varies between two and 12 glands (44,45). The incidence of supernumerary glands in adults varies between 2% and 6.5% (50). Supernumerary glands are most commonly intrathymic and are thought to result from embryonic division of one or more glands (Fig. 3). Their presence is one of the factors responsible for persistent hyperparathyroidism after surgical therapy of primary hyperplasia of the parathyroids (50,51) and must be distinguished from other causes of recurrent or persistent hyperparathyroidism such as parathyroid carcinoma and parathyromatosis (52). It is probably rare for there to be less than four glands in the absence of other abnormalities such as thymic aplasia. Because studies of the number of glands are based on autopsy material, we feel that most of the cases with fewer than four glands are due to failure to locate aberrant glands in unusual locations. Despite the known variation in the adult position of the parathyroid glands (17,27–29,34), there is a definite pattern in their anatomic distribution, which is related to their embryonic derivation (Fig. 4). The most common location of the upper (parathyroid IV) glands (77%) is at the cricothyroid junction posteriorly or just above the intersection of the recurrent laryngeal nerve and inferior thyroid artery (70%) (46). The second most common location is behind the upper pole of the thyroid (22%) (46), in which case the glands are often within the surgical capsule of the thyroid (Fig. 5). Other uncommon locations include a more caudal position by the inferior thyroid artery, a

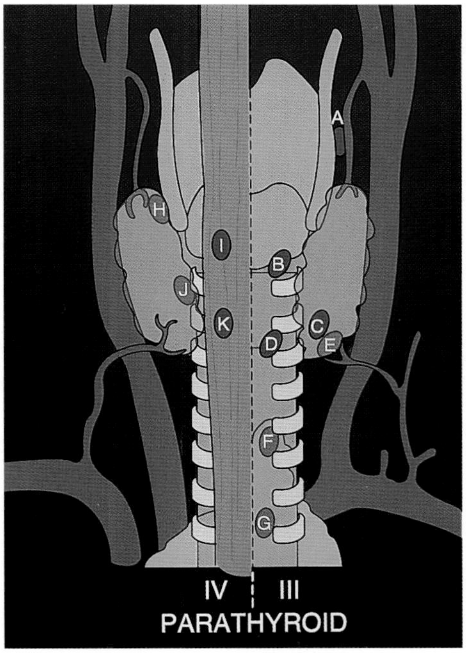


FIG. 4. Diagram demonstrating the location of the parathyroid glands. [Modified with permission (44) and reprinted with permission (9).]

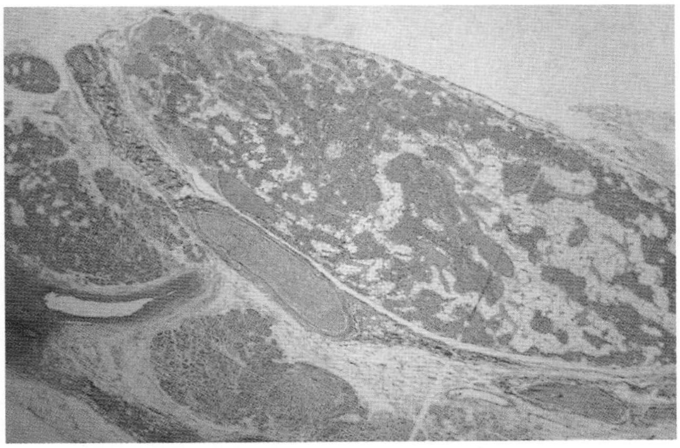

FIG. 3. Parathyroid glands of a newborn, divided into several portions by the vascular bundle and recurrent laryngeal nerve.

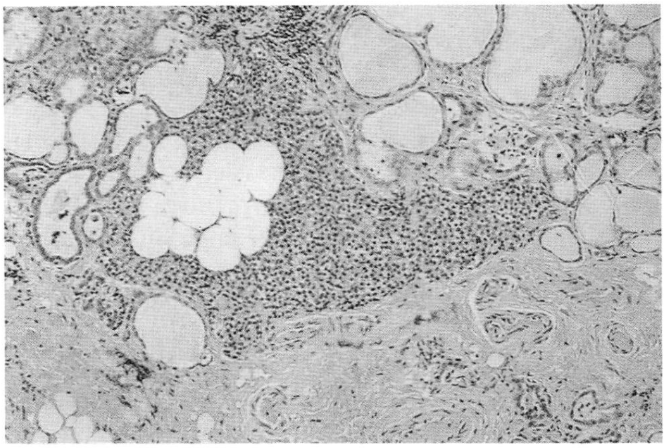

FIG. 5. A parathyroid gland of a young adult just below the thyroid gland capsule in the thyroid parenchyma. A large accumulation of adipocytes is present within the parathyroid. Only chief cells are seen within the parathyroid.

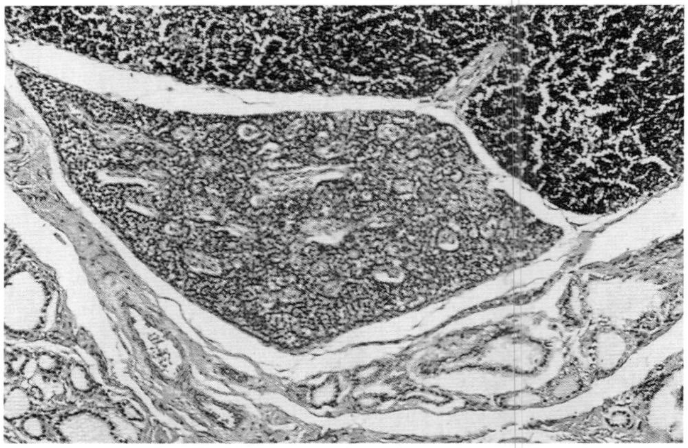

**FIG. 6.** A fetal thyroid (33 weeks' gestation) located between the thymus and lower pole of the thyroid (*bottom*). A small amount of stroma surrounds the vessels. The gland is composed of pure tightly packed chief cells.

retropharyngeal or retroesophageal position, and rarely within the thyroid parenchyma (Fig. 5).

The lower parathyroid glands (parathyroid III) have a more diverse distribution but are most commonly located between the lower pole of the thyroid and the thymus (Fig. 6). They can occur as high in the neck as the hyoid bone, however, or as low as the pericardium (53,54). In 42% to 61% of the cases they are located on either side of the lower thyroid or in a juxtathyroidal location. Another common location is the "thymic tongue" or "cervical extension of the thymus." Uncommon locations are the mediastinal thymus and the anterior mediastinum (46–50). Ectopic intravagal parathyroid tissue has been reported (55). The gland locations are symmetrical in 80% of patients.

## SIZE AND SHAPE

Each adult gland measures 3 to 6 mm in length, 2 to 4 mm in width, and 0.5 to 2.0 mm in thickness (Fig. 7). Its shape varies because it is molded by the adjacent structures. The glands are a flattened, ovoid pancake with "sharp" edges. They are yellow to orange–tan, depending on the amount of stromal fat, number of oxyphil cells, and degree of vascularity (4). The glands are soft and malleable, although they may show a marked increase in firmness, swelling, and a dark red color if surgical manipulation causes intraglandular hemorrhage. Abnormal glands are usually more bulbous, with rounded edges, and have a firmer consistency and a darker red–tan color (4).

Gland weight and parenchymal cell content are important parameters used in the histopathologic assessment of the parathyroid gland (56–65), and all parathyroid glands or part of glands removed at surgery must be carefully measured and weighed to the nearest milligram. The total parathyroid weight gradually increases throughout embryonic life, reaching a mean total of 5 to 9 mg at the postpartum age of 3 months (61,62). This is followed by a steep linear increase in total parathyroid weight until the third or fourth decade of life, when it levels off at a mean of 120 ± 3.5 mg in men and 142 ± 5.2 mg in women (4). The mean weight per gland is 31.1 mg in men and 29.8 mg in women (63). The lower parathyroid glands are larger then the upper glands (61,64). The parenchymal cell content of the glands is extremely variable and difficult to evaluate. It is reported to average 74% of the weight of the gland in adults (49). It is a somewhat better indicator of gland function than gland weight alone but requires careful morphometric analysis in conjunction with careful evaluation of the total gland weight. The average parenchymal weight per gland is 21.6 mg for men and 18.2 mg for women (63), whereas the mean total parenchymal weight for four glands is 82.0 ± 2.6 mg for men and 88.9 ± 3.9 mg for women (60,61). The total gland weight has been reported to be higher in blacks than in whites (65). The total (8) and parenchymal (64) gland weight are inversely related to serum calcium concentration in patients with secondary hyperparathyroidism. In these patients a direct relationship has been found between the total gland weight and the serum phosphorus and renal function as expressed by serum urea nitrogen (8).

## HISTOLOGY

The normal parathyroid gland has a thin fibrous capsule that separates it from adjacent tissue (Figs. 8 and 9), which, except for those glands embedded in the thyroid or its capsule, is adipose tissue or thymus. At the vascular pole, an artery and vein are present, surrounded by fibrous tissue.

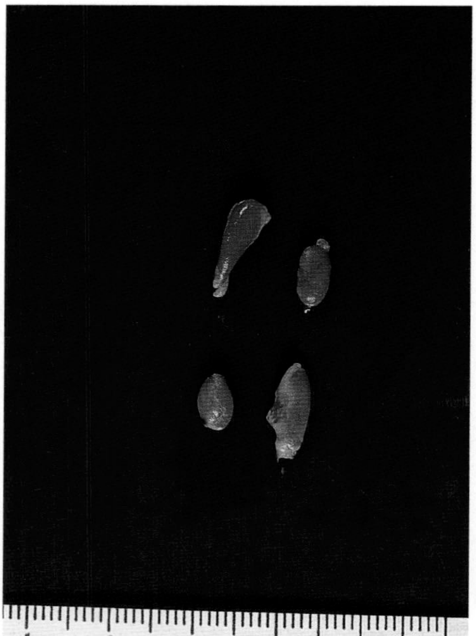

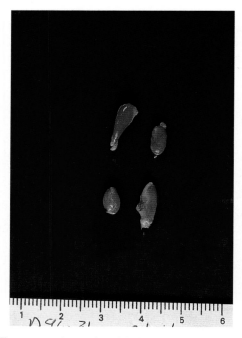


**FIG. 7.** Four normal parathyroid glands removed at autopsy from a 53-year-old man.

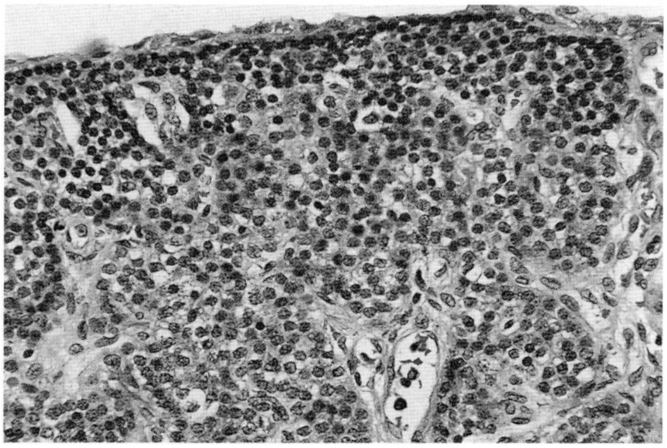

**FIG. 8.** A parathyroid gland from a 7.5-month-old girl. The chief cells are the only cell type seen and are arranged in sheets, between the large vascular channels. The capillaries can be seen between individual chief cells. The chief cells show central regular nuclei and a clear amphophilic cytoplasm. A thin fibrous capsule separates the gland from the stoma.

These branch into smaller arteries and veins, which form a complex readily visible in the capsule. The capsular arteries and veins are connected by arterioles, capillaries, and venules located in the fibrous septa between the parenchymal cells (65). This capillary network abuts every chief cell. Due to the rich capillary network, the cut surface bleeds readily, providing an easy way for the surgeon to distinguish the parathyroid from lymph nodes, adipose tissue, thymus, and thyroid, which do not show such prominent bleeding from their cut surfaces. The capillary endothelial lining cells have pores or fenestrations resembling those seen in other endocrine glands (66,67). Dense bodies, Weibel-Palade bodies, pinocytotic vesicles, tight junctions, or zonulae occludens are constituents of the parathyroid capillary endothelium. Two interconnecting plexuses of lymphatic capillaries in the capsule surround the parathyroid glands. From the inner plexus, loops of lymphatics dip into the gland parenchyma, whereas the efferent lymphatics arise from the outer plexus via special lymphatics or those of the thyroid (68). The interstitial space is limited by the basement membranes of the chief cells and capillaries and contains collagen bundles and elastic fibers (66). Nerve bundles in close proximity to chief cells suggest autonomic innervation (69–72). In the rabbit the nerves have been shown to originate in the medulla oblongata, the dorsal nucleus of the vagus, and the vagus nerve (69,72).

In infants and children the interstitium consists only of the capillary network and the extracellular space. Little collagen is present (Fig. 8). With age there is focal-increasing collagenization of the perivascular stroma, forming delicate fibrous septa in adult glands, imparting to them a somewhat lobulated appearance. Surrounding the capillaries and lymphatics are interstitial cells that consist of fibroblasts, pericytes, mast cells, and a few lymphocytes. Adipocytes are sparse in the stroma of infants and children. Stromal fat cells begin to appear late in the first decade of life and increase throughout life. At puberty, especially in women, there is an increased rate of accumulation of adipocytes. Stromal fat cells increase in number with increasing age, reaching a maximum in the third to fifth decades of life. There is a marked variation in the amount and distribution of stromal fat within a single gland, between glands in the same individual, and among individuals of the same age (Figs. 8–15). Recent studies (60,73,74) confirmed the initial reports of Gilmour (19) that in adults adipocytes occupy an average of 50% of the stromal volume rather than of the total parathyroid volume. Women have a higher percentage of stromal fat than do men. The stromal fat is affected by the same factors that affect total body fat, for example, nutrition, chronic illness (such as malignancy), and genetics. These variations make interpretation of the level of parathyroid function difficult to assess on the basis of the stromal fat. In normal glands the stromal fat appears to "compress" the surrounding

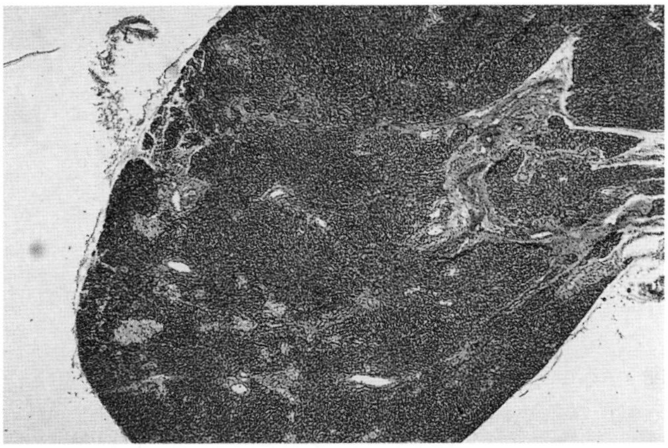

**FIG. 9.** A parathyroid from a 27-year-old woman showing only sheets of chief cells and no stromal fat. The vascular pole can be seen at the right margin of the micrograph. A thin fibrous capsule is seen.

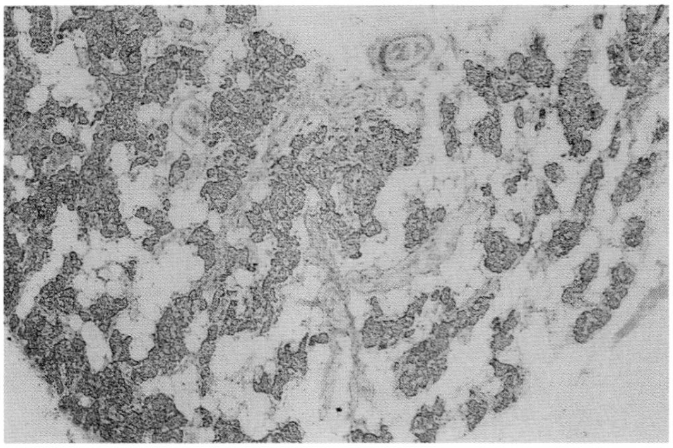

**FIG. 10.** Photomicrograph of a parathyroid from a 39-year-old man. There is abundant stromal fat separating the cords of chief cells.

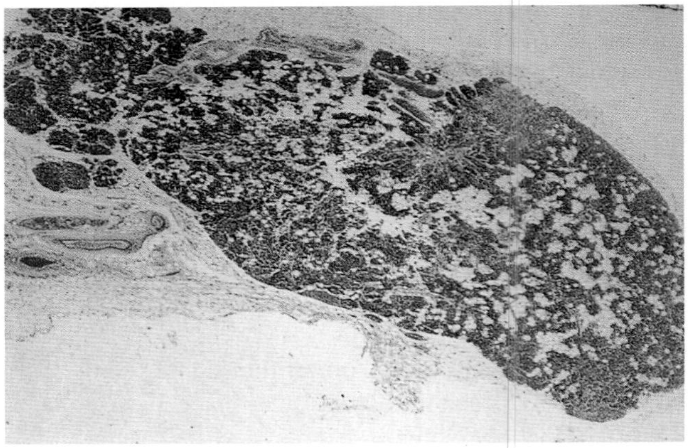

**FIG. 11.** A parathyroid from a 69-year-old woman. There is a moderate amount of stromal fat, largely concentrated in the center of the gland. A few small oxyphil nodules can be seen in the parenchyma.

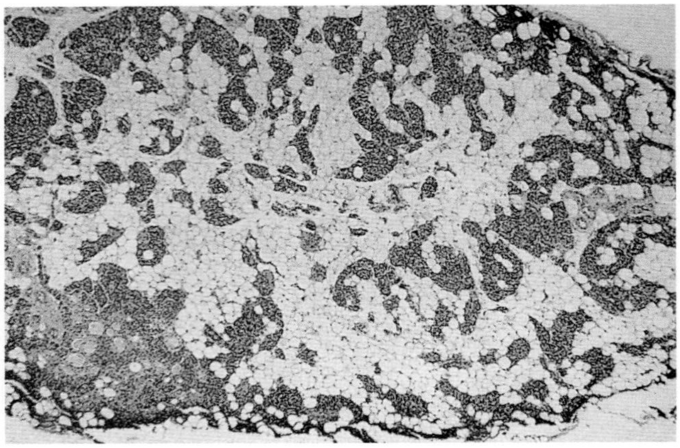

**FIG. 13.** A parathyroid from a 77-year-old man. There is abundant stromal fat.

parenchyma, whereas in hyperplastic or adenomatous glands the fat cells appear scattered among the parenchymal cells. In the fourth decade there is a relative decrease in parenchymal adipocytes. Alterations in body fat caused by diet, malignancy, or disease may affect the amount of stromal fat in the glands.

Each parenchymal cell is separated from the stroma by a prominent basement membrane. The parenchymal cells are arranged in irregular sheets without prominent stroma in infants and prepubertal children. In infants and young children only one type of cell is present, the chief cell. The chief cells of the newborn and infantile parathyroid gland are small and regular, measuring 6 to 8 $\mu$m in diameter (Fig. 16). The chief cell membranes are poorly demarcated, and the cytoplasm is amphophilic, relatively lucent, and occasionally vacuolated. Intracellular fat in the chief cells is low compared with the adult gland, with only 30% to 40% of the chief cells of children containing large intracellular fat droplets on fat stains (75). The nuclei are often molded and overlap. The nuclei are centrally located, with uniform chromatin and small, inconspicuous nucleoli.

In the adult, the parenchymal cells are arranged in solid nests, rounded or lobulated masses and trabeculae, or a combination of these (Figs. 8–17). A pseudofollicular pattern also has been described in normal glands (Fig. 18) (76–78). Ultrastructural evidence indicates that follicle formation in the parathyroid is the result of a proliferation of parenchymal cells, with ischemic necrosis and degeneration of those cells separated from their blood supply by other parenchymal cells.

These pseudofollicles are usually filled with cellular debris and a pink eosinophilic homogeneous material resembling the colloid seen in thyroid follicles (Fig. 18) (76). This material contains glycoproteins as evidenced by the positive periodic acid-Schiff (PAS) reaction and PTH as evidenced by immunostaining. Several investigators have further reported that it stains with Congo red and shows the apple-green birefringence characteristic of amyloid (77). A similar

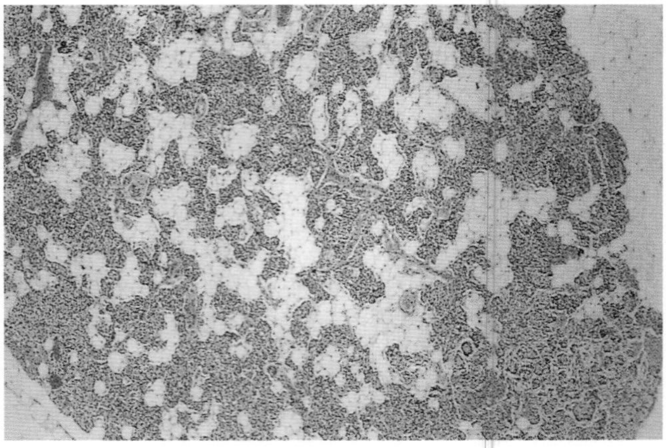

**FIG. 12.** A parathyroid from a 76-year-old man. There is a moderate amount of stromal fat, largely in the center of the gland. Small oxyphil nodules are present.

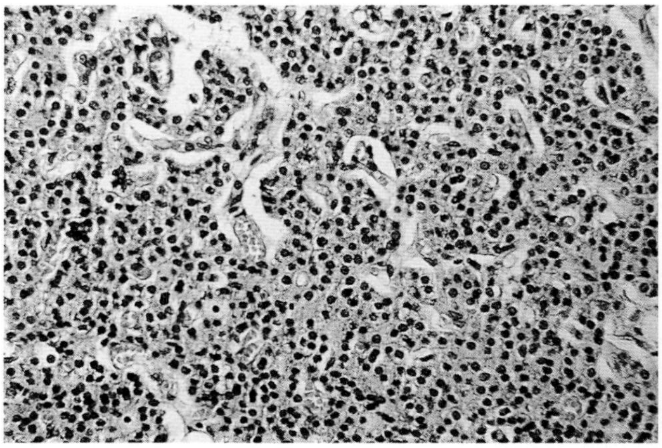

**FIG. 14.** A normal parathyroid from a 70-year-old woman showing almost no stromal fat or oxyphil cells.

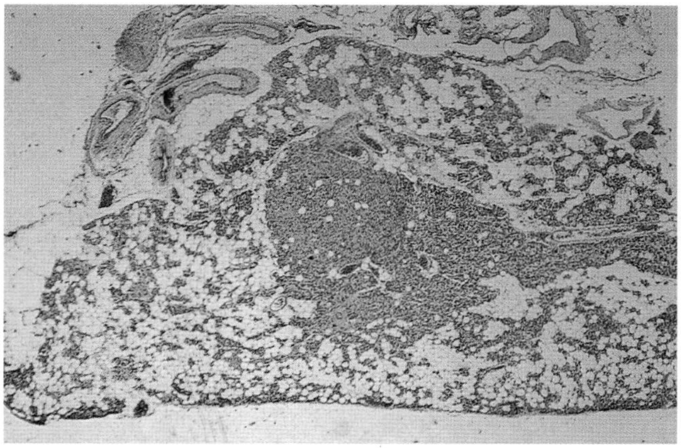

**FIG. 15.** A parathyroid gland of a 77-year-old man. The stroma is almost completely replaced by adipocytes. There is a large oxyphil nodule in the center of the gland.

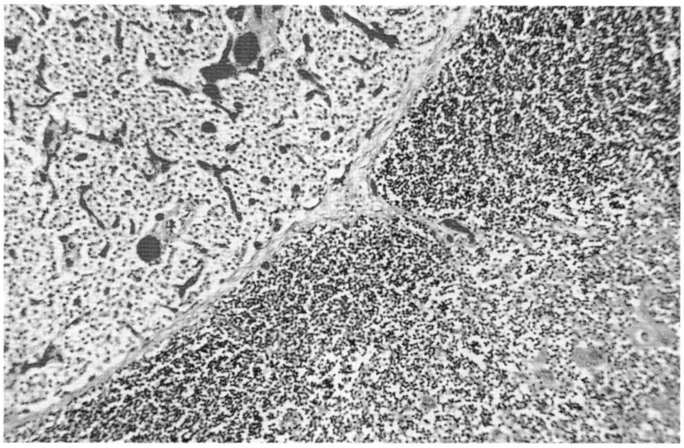

**FIG. 17.** Sheets of parathyroid chief cells showing amphophilic clear cytoplasm, adjacent to the thymus. The prominent vascularity of the gland is visible.

finding has been reported in the follicles of pathologic parathyroid glands (78,79). Cinti et al. (76) were unable to confirm either the presence of amyloid or glycoproteins in the follicles of a series of normal parathyroids removed at the time of thyroidectomy. However, electron microscopy of follicles in a pathologic parathyroid gland did demonstrate fibrils closely resembling those of amyloid in pseudofollicles (75).

There are two types of parenchymal cells recognized by light microscopy in the adult normal parathyroid gland. These are the chief cells (Figs. 15, 18–20), in their active and inactive forms, and the oxyphil cell (Figs. 15, 18–20) (16,80, 81). In adults the chief cells are arranged in sheets, cords, trabeculae, and small nodules. They are spherical and measure 8 to 12 $\mu$m in diameter. The cell borders are poorly defined. The cytoplasm is amphophilic or faintly eosinophilic, with 70% to 80% of the chief cells containing large prominent fat droplets (Fig. 21) (4,14), corresponding to the lipid bodies seen in the resting chief cells by electron microscopy (82). It is of interest that these lipid droplets were first recognized in human chief cells by Sandström (14,15), although he did not appreciate their significance. By ordinary light microscopy, the active chief cell may be difficult to identify. The inactive chief cell may be recognized by the vacuolated clear appearance of the cytoplasm that is filled with lipid, glycogen, and lysosomes (82–85). Deposition of silver particles on the secretory granules is responsible for the argyrophil reaction seen in normal parathyroid glands using the Grimelius silver nitrate stain (82,86–88). The granules correspond to the location of PTH (Fig. 22) (89–93) and chromogranin (Fig. 23) (90). Differences in the parathyroid and chromogranin content of the chief cells indicate a variation in the secretory granule content and supports the presence of a secretory cycle in the parathyroid chief cell. The nuclei are round, centrally located, have a sharp nuclear outline, even chromatin, and small rare nucleoli (4,75).

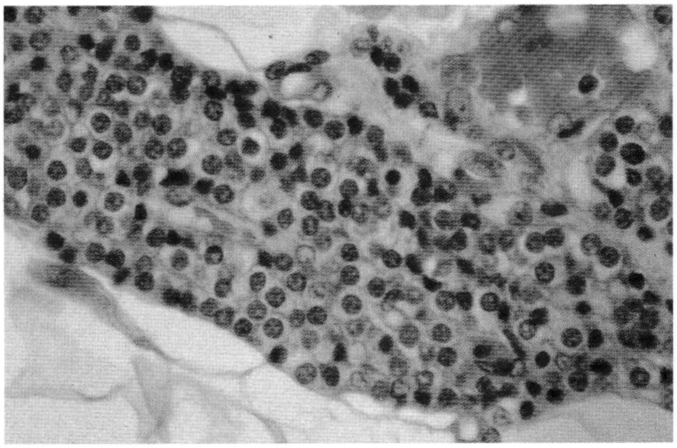

**FIG. 16.** Sheets of chief cells in a newborn. The stroma has little collagen and is outside the large sheet. The cell membranes are poorly demarcated. The cytoplasm is eosinophilic.

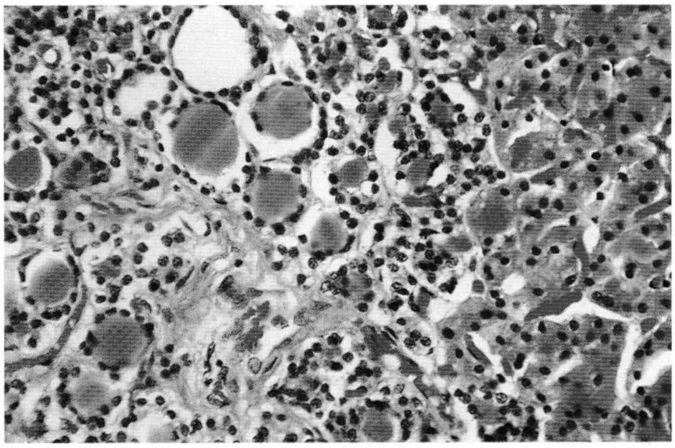

**FIG. 18.** Numerous pseudofollicles in a normal parathyroid of a 58-year-old white man. Lining the pseudofollicles are chief cells. At the right of the micrograph is the edge of an oxyphil nodule.

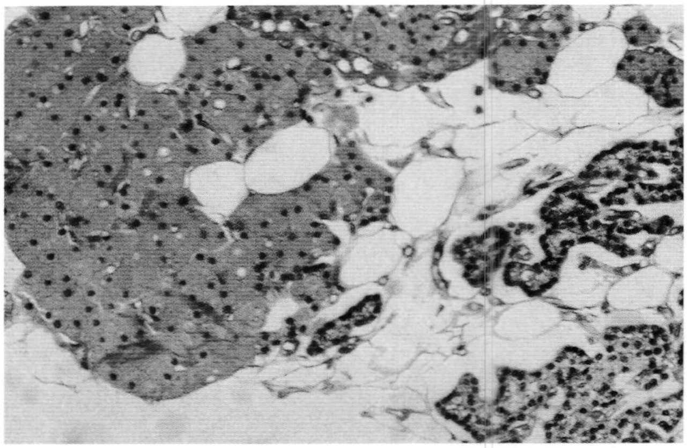

**FIG. 19.** Nests and cords of oxyphil cells and chief cells among the adipocytes of the stroma.

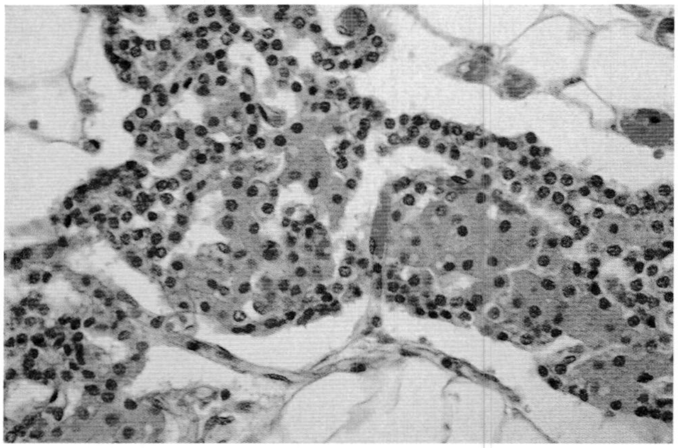

**FIG. 20.** Trabecula of parathyroid showing mixture of oxyphil and chief cells.

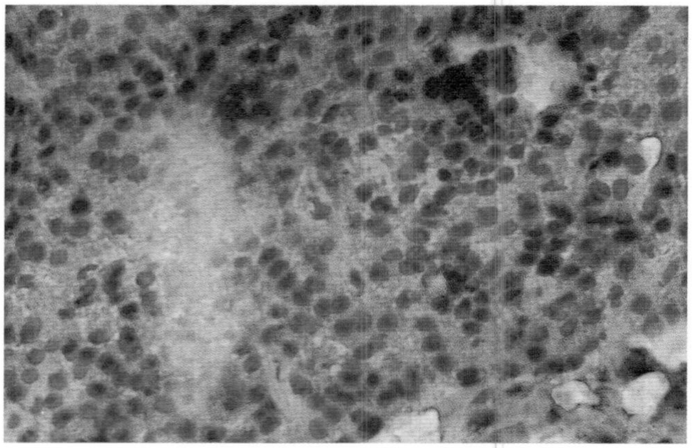

**FIG. 21.** Chief cells with intracytoplasmic lipid droplets (Sudan IV and hematoxylin).

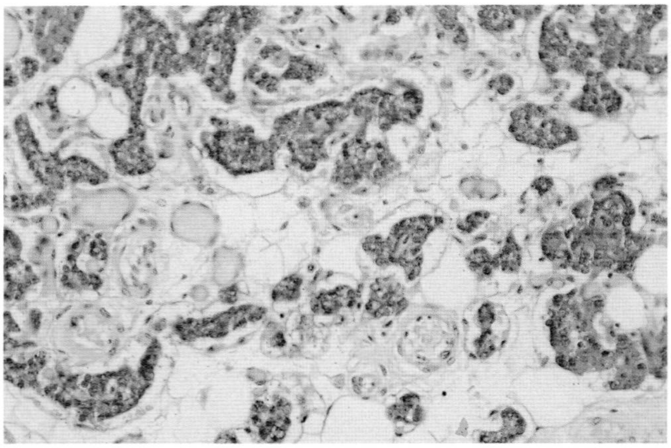

**FIG. 22.** Chief cells showing abundant PTH in the parathyroid gland. Note the marked variation in the amount of hormone in various chief cells. (Immunoperoxidase stain for PTH, hematoxylin counterstain).

Ultrastructural features of the chief cell correlate with its functional activity (82–84,91–97). The chief cell, considered the basic functional unit of the parathyroid gland, is responsible for the production and secretion of PTH and, in turn, in the maintenance of the homeostasis of ionized calcium (98–101). To achieve this, each individual chief cell undergoes a secretory cycle (82–84,91–95) (Fig. 24) similar to that of the follicle of the thyroid. Each chief cell is polarized with the Golgi apparatus and granular endoplasmic reticulum farthest from the basement membrane–lined perivascular surface (102).

The resting phase, which corresponds to the inactive chief cell, is characterized by accumulation of glycogen and large lipid bodies that correspond to the lipid seen by light microscopy (Fig. 21). The rest of the cell organelles, the Golgi apparatus, the granular endoplasmic reticulum, and secretory granules are small and inconspicuous. This is best seen in the chronically suppressed cell in atrophic parathyroid

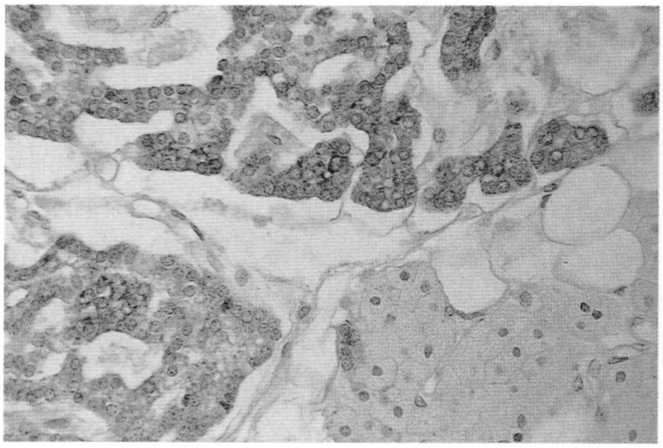

**FIG. 23.** Parathyroid gland showing abundant chromogranin in the chief cells. The chief cells have different amounts of chromogranin. The oxyphil cells are free of chromogranin.

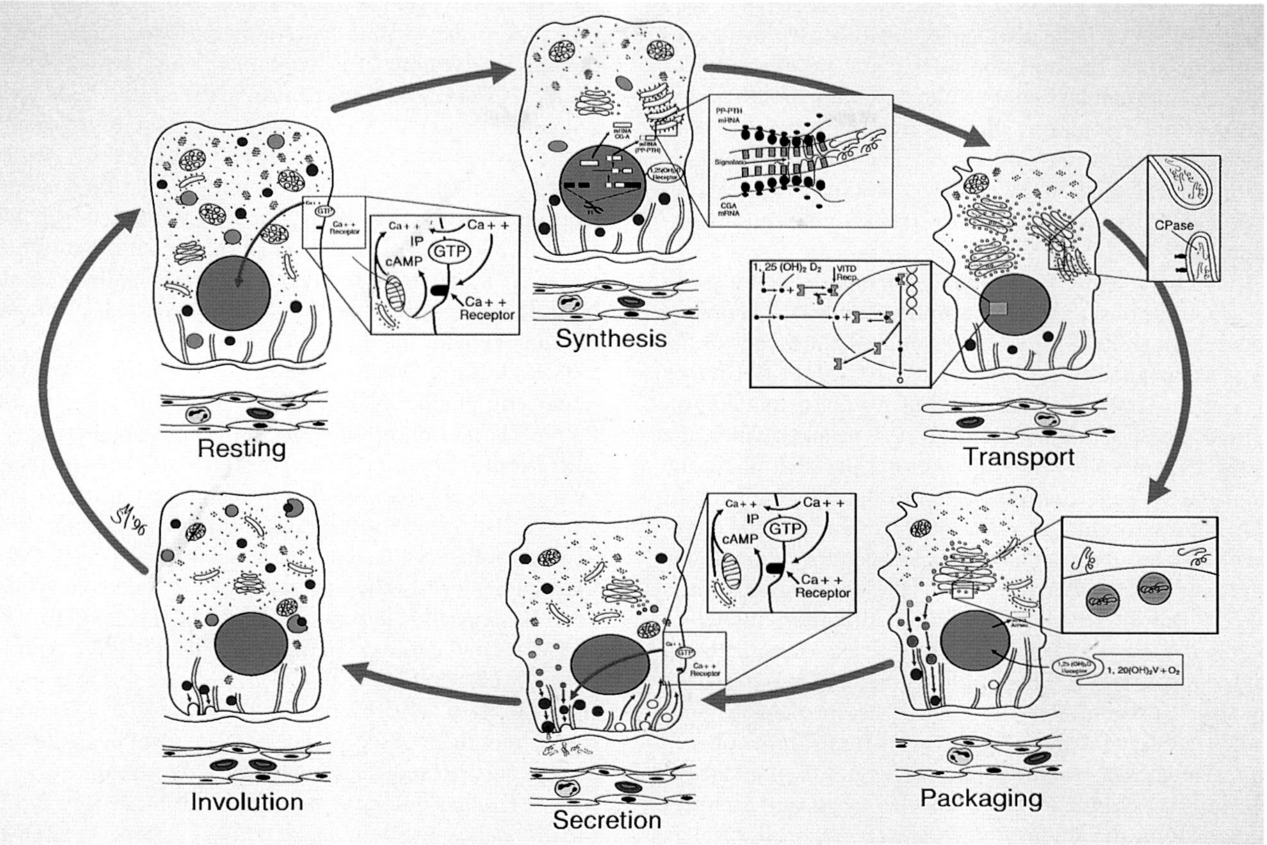


**FIG. 24.** Diagram of the secretory cycle of the parathyroid chief cells. Although this is a continuum, typical stages have been recognized ultrastructurally. During the resting phase the cells are rich in glycogen and lipid bodies, with dispersion of the granular endoplasmic reticulum (GER) and free ribosomes. Dense-core secretory granules are relatively uncommon and scattered throughout the cytoplasm. Rare lysosomes are seen. The Golgi apparatus is small and inconspicuous, with few vesicles and vacuoles. The cell membranes are relatively straight with few interdigitations. At the end of the resting phase presumably due to decreased cytoplasmic [$Ca^{2+}$] and release of vitamin D metabolite from the upstream promotor site, the cell begins the process of PTH synthesis. As the synthetic phase begins, transcription of the gene for PTH begins with production of the complimentary RNA for prepro-PTH and presumably accompanied by a similar transcription of chromogranin. The mRNA is produced by removal of the introns and splicing of the exons. The mRNA moves to the granular endoplasmic reticulum, which aggregates [the perinuclear body of Pappenheimer and Wilens (48)]. This is accompanied by aggregation of the free ribosomes to polysomes. The preprohormone crosses into the lumen of the GER, where the preportion of the molecule is removed by a ligase. Other alterations include depletion of the dense-core granules, lysosomes, glycogen, and lipid bodies. The cell membrane increases in tortuosity, probably due to loss of cytoplasmic volume. The synthesis and secretion of hormone is halted, presumably by the action of 1$\alpha$,25 dihydroxyvitamin D on the upstream promotor region of PTH and the cytosolic [$Ca^{2+}$]. In the transport phase, the hormone, supposedly accompanied by chromogranin, is transported through the cisternae of the GER to the Golgi apparatus as the pro segment is removed by a "clipase." The hormone is conveyed to the Golgi vesicles. Further depletion of lipid bodies, glycogen, and secretory granules occurs, and the cisternae of the GER disperse. In the packaging phase the hormone is bundled along with chromogranin into dense-core granules, and the Golgi apparatus begins its involution. Secretion occurs as the dense-core granules containing PTH and chromogranin move along the microtubules, fuse with the cell membrane, and release the hormone into the pericapillary extracellular space. Depending on the ambient [$Ca^{2+}$], the granules are rapidly passed along the microtubules and secreted (low [$Ca^{2+}$]) or left free in the cytoplasm (high [$Ca^{2+}$]), to be destroyed by lysosomes or to be secreted at a later time. The Golgi continues to decrease in size and complexity. The free ribosomes disaggregate. The cells begin to involute toward the resting phase with gradual loss of secretory granules and further involution of the Golgi apparatus. The cells begin to accumulate glycogen and lipid bodies and approach the resting phase. Lysosomes containing acid phosphatase accumulate in the cells. These presumably serve to destroy excess hormone and unsecreted secretory granules. [Modified with permission (9).]

glands (82–84,91,94,96,97). During this stage, lysosomes (103) as well as variable numbers of small dense-core secretory granules are present, the latter being peripherally located. Sacs of granular endoplasmic reticulum are dispersed throughout the cytoplasm, whereas free ribosomes are only partially aggregated into polysomes. The Golgi apparatus is small and inconspicuous, with few vacuoles and prosecretory granules. The cell membranes are straight with few interdigitations (66).

The synthetic phase is marked by the parallel aggregation of the cisternae of rough granular endoplasmic reticulum and is noted at the light microscopic level by the presence of the body of Pappenheimer and Wilens (82,104). Free ribosomes aggregate into polysomes. It is during this phase that prepro-PTH and chromogranin (82,96) are synthesized within the granular endoplasmic reticulum. During the next phase the prohormone is split and transferred to the Golgi apparatus, which begins to enlarge with increases in smooth membranes, vesicles and vacuoles, and prosecretory granules of different electron densities. As the packaging phase emerges, the granular endoplasmic reticulum disperses throughout the cytoplasm, and larger dense-core secretory granules appear by the Golgi region, gradually moving to the periphery. PTH and chromogranin A are present in these granules, as demonstrated by ultrastructural immunohistochemical studies, as well as in the aggregates of granular endoplasmic reticulum (90,91). As the secretory granules progress along the microtubules toward the cell surface, there is an involution of the Golgi apparatus; acid phosphatase appears at the secretory face and eventually is transferred into large lysosomes (103). Separation of the secretory granules from the microtubules into the cytoplasm could account for the second compartment of PTH storage postulated by Cohn and MacGregor (98). The cell cytoplasm in the synthetic and secretory phases becomes depleted of glycogen and lipid bodies. During the last phase there is margination of the lysosomes and secretory granules, fusion of the plasma membrane with that of the secretory granules, and emptying of the products into the extracellular space. The membranes of the secretory granules and lysosomes are probably recycled (105). Shannon and Roth (103) and Hashizume et al. (106) demonstrated that the stored parathyroid secretory granules fuse with lysosomes which provide a mechanism for intracellular degradation of PTH. The chief cell returns to the resting phase with a resultant accumulation of glycogen and complex lipid bodies, which are the best indicators of the resting or functionally suppressed cell. In chronically suppressed normal glands adjacent to a hyperfunctioning adenoma, 90% to 95% of the chief cells are inactive. In comparison, the normal adult gland has 70% to 80% of the chief cells in the resting phase, and the normal prepubertal gland has 30% to 40% in the resting phase (75,83).

Correlative morphologic studies in normal, adenomatous, and hyperplastic glands have shown that the intracellular content of fat in the chief cells is inversely related to its endocrine activity and is a better indicator of hormonal function than is the stromal fat. An increased cytoplasmic lipid content is a feature of a functionally suppressed chief cell (82,83,107–112), whereas hormonally active cells of adenoma and hyperplasia are largely in the active stages of hormone synthesis and secretion and thus are fat depleted. Based on this fact, evaluation of intracellular fat content has been demonstrated to be useful in differentiating between normal, adenomatous, and hyperplastic parathyroid glands (103–112). Care must be taken in interpreting these fat stains because some areas of adenomas and hyperplasias may contain intracellular fat (113–116).

Cell culture studies (117,118) using a sequential hemolytic plaque assay confirm the cyclical secretion of both PTH and chromogranin A by individual parathyroid cells. Roth and Raisz (96) demonstrated that the ambient ionized [$Ca^{2+}$] controls the length of the resting phase of the chief cell cycle. Proliferation of parathyroid chief cells is also controlled by the ambient ionized [$Ca^{2+}$] (119). Molecular studies (120) have shown that the mechanism of this control may be via depression of cyclins D1 and D2.

The second cell type in the adult gland is the oxyphil cell (Figs. 9, 12, 15, 17, 19, and 25). These are felt to be derived from the chief cells (62,121–124), although the stimulus for the development of oxyphil cells has not yet been identified. Before puberty, only extremely rare oxyphil cells are present in the glands. Beginning at puberty and increasing throughout life, increasing numbers of these cells appear (121). They are distributed among the chief cells as individual cells, sheets, and small or large nodules (4,75), indicating that there is both a continual transformation (Figs. 19, 20, and 24) from the chief cells and clonal proliferation of the oxyphil cells (122). Rarely, these nodules enlarge enough to be visible grossly. When this happens it is not possible to differentiate these presumably nonfunctioning oxyphil nodules from functioning oxyphil adenomas (4).

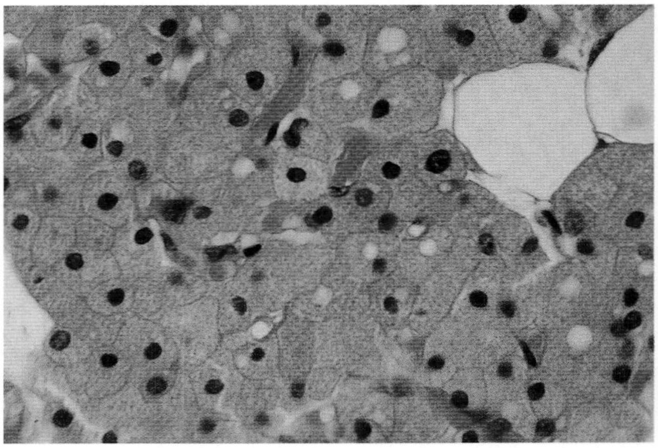

**FIG. 25.** Oxyphil cells of the parathyroid in an 80-year-old woman. The centrally located, variably sized, pyknotic nuclei are seen within the granular eosinophilic cytoplasm. The cell membranes and the vascular channels are easily visible.

Oxyphil cells in multiple organs, including abnormal parathyroid glands, have been demonstrated to contain decreased cytochrome oxidase (125). Previous studies (126) manifested decreased concentrations of mitochondrial enzymes when measured against the amount of mitochondrial protein. This is in contrast to histochemical studies showing marked increases in mitochondrial enzymes (127–129). These studies, along with the fact that oxyphil cells increase with age, suggest that there is a mitochondropathy, which may lead to the proliferation of the mitochondria within the cells. PTH-related peptide has been described in oxyphil cells (130), although its function is not clear.

The oxyphil cell measures 12 to 20 $\mu$m in diameter and has a clearly demarcated cell membrane, a pyknotic nucleus, and abundant eosinophilic granular cytoplasm (Fig. 25), rich in mitochondria and resembling the Hürthle cells of the thyroid or the oncocytes of other endocrine organs (121–124). Ultrastructurally, their cytoplasm is completely filled with mitochondria, often with a bizarre shape and size, as well as occasional lysosomes and lipofuscin granules (82). Their function is unknown; however, the oxyphil cells in normal glands do not seem to contain the organelles responsible for PTH synthesis and secretion [i.e., granular endoplasmic reticulum, Golgi apparatuses, and secretory granules (81, 82)], as indicated by electron microscopy and the absence of PTH and chromogranin (Fig. 23). However, cases of functioning oxyphil cell adenomas (131) and chief cell hyperplasias (83) have been reported. Protein secretory and synthetic organelles have been demonstrated in these tumor cells.

Transitional oxyphil cells may be recognized by light microscopy by the decreased density of their cytoplasmic eosinophilia. By electron microscopy these cells have lesser numbers of mitochondria and some of the organelles associated with PTH synthesis and secretion, such as granular endoplasmic reticulum, Golgi apparatuses, and dense-core secretory granules. Both forms of oxyphil cells contain sparse amounts of lipid droplets (112,113).

The use of pure histologic criteria in the estimation of the functional or hormonal activity of the gland and in the differentiation between normal, hyperplastic, and adenomatous glands is difficult. The gland size and weight, the shape, and the relative proportion of stromal adipocytes and chief cells are all important criteria in making these distinctions. Account must be taken of the number of oxyphil cells because in normal glands, but not adenomas or primary hyperplastic glands, oxyphil cells are nonfunctional. We have found that the appraisal of these elements, along with the patient's clinical history, and evaluation of cellular cytology and intracellular fat content of the chief cells all must be carefully considered in arriving at a proper pathologic diagnosis.

## REFERENCES


1. Mallette LE. Review: Primary hyperparathyroidism, an update: incidence, etiology, diagnosis, and treatment. *Am J Med Sci* 1987;293: 239–249.
2. Cope O. Hyperparathyroidism: diagnosis and management. *Am J Surg* 1960;99:394–403.
3. Aurbach GD, Potts JT Jr. The parathyroids. *Adv Metab Dis* 1964; 1:45–93.
4. Castleman B, Roth SI. Tumors of the parathyroid glands. In: *Atlas of tumor pathology*. Series 2, part 2. Washington DC: Armed Forces Institute of Pathology; 1978:1–94.
5. O'Malley BW, Kohler PO. Hypoparathyroidism. *Postgrad Med* 1968; 44:71–75,182–186.
6. Hanley DA, Sherwood LM. Secondary hyperparathyroidism in chronic renal failure. *Med Clin North Am* 1978;62:1319–1339.
7. Katz AI, Hampers CL, Merrill JP. Secondary hyperparathyroidism and renal osteodystrophy in chronic renal failure. Analysis of 195 patients, with observation on the effects of chronic dialysis, kidney transplantation and subtotal parathyroidectomy. *Medicine* 1969;48: 333–374.
8. Roth SI, Marshall RB. Pathology and ultrastructure of the human parathyroid glands in chronic renal failure. *Arch Intern Med* 1969; 124:397–407.
9. Roth SI. Parathyroid glands. In: Damjanov I, Linder J, eds. *Anderson's pathology*. 10th ed. St. Louis: Mosby-Year Book; 1966: 1980–2007.
10. Roth SI, Wang C-A, Potts JT Jr. The team approach to primary hyperparathyroidism. *Hum Pathol* 1975;6:645–648.
11. Owen R. On the anatomy of the Indian rhinoceros (Rh. unicornis, L). *Trans Zool Soc (Lond)* 1862;4:31–58.
12. Remak R. *Untersuchungen über die Entwickelung der Wierbelthiere*. Berlin: Reimer; 1855:3–40,122–124.
13. Virchow R. *Die krankhaften Geswültste*. Vol. 3. Berlin: Hirschwald; 1863:13.
14. Sandström I. Om en ny Körtel hos menniskan och ätskilliga däggdjur. *Ups Lakaref Forsch* 1880;15:441–471.
15. Seipel CM. An English translation of Sandström's "Glandulae Parathyroideae" with biographical notes by Professor J August Hammar. *Bull Inst Hist Med* 1938;6:179–222.
16. Kohn A. Studien über die Schilddrüse. *Arch Mikrosk Anat Entwicklungsmech* 1895;44:366–422.
17. Kohn A. Die Epithelkörperchen. *Ergeb Anat Entwicklungsgeshch* 1899;9:194–252.
18. Welsh DA. Concerning the parathyroid glands: a critical anatomical and experimental study. *J Anat Physiol* 1898;32:292–307.
19. Gilmour JR. The embryology of the parathyroid glands, the thymus, and certain associated rudiments. *J Pathol Bacteriol* 1937;45: 507–522.
20. Weller GL. Development of the thyroid, parathyroid and thymus glands in man. *Contrib Embryol* 1933;24:93–138.
21. Norris EH. The parathyroid glands and the lateral thyroid in man: their morphogenesis, histogenesis, topographic anatomy and prenatal growth. *Contrib Embryol* 1937;26:247–294.
22. Pearse AGE, Takor TT. Neuroendocrine embryology and the APUD concept. *Clin Endocrinol* 1976;5(suppl):229–244.
23. Medrida-Velasco JA. Experimental study of the origin of the parathyroid glands. *Acta Anat* 1991;141:163–169.
24. Norris EH. Anatomical evidence of prenatal function of the human parathyroid glands. *Anat Rec* 1946;96:129–142.
25. Nakagami K, Yamazaki Y, Tsunoda Y. An electron microscopic study of the human fetal parathyroid gland. *Zellforschung* 1968;85:89–95.
26. Ishizaki N, Shoumura S, Emura S, et al. Ultrastructure of the parathyroid gland of the mouse fetus after calcium chloride or ethylenediamine tetraacetic acid administration. *Acta Anat* 1989;135:164–170.
27. Leroyer-Alizon E, David L, Anast CS, Dubois PM. Immunocytological evidence for parathyroid hormone in human fetal parathyroid glands. *J Clin Endocrinol Metab* 1981;52:513–516.
28. Scothorne RJ. Functional capacity of fetal parathyroid glands with reference to their clinical use as homografts. *Ann N Y Acad Sci* 1964;120: 669–676.
29. MacIsaac RJ, Heath JH, Rodda CP, Moseley JM, Care AD, Martin TJ. Role of the fetal parathyroid glands and parathyroid-related protein in the regulation of placental transport of calcium, magnesium and inorganic phosphate. *Reprod Fertil Dev* 1991;3:447–457.
30. Brown EM. Homeostatic mechanisms regulating extracellular and intracellular calcium metabolism. In: Bilezikian JP, Levine MA, Marcus R, eds. *The parathyroids*. New York: Raven Press; 1994:15–54.
31. Kronenberg HM, Bringhurst FR, Segre GV, Potts JT Jr. Parathyroid hormone biosynthesis and metabolism. In: Bilezikian JP, Levine MA, Marcus R. eds. *The parathyroids*. New York: Raven Press; 1994: 125–137.

32. Henry HL, Normal AW. Metabolism of vitamin D. In: Coe FL, Favus MJ, eds. *Disorders of bone and mineral metabolism.* New York: Raven Press; 1992:149–162.
33. Silver J. Regulation of parathyroid hormone synthesis and secretion. In: Coe FL, Favus MJ, eds. *Disorders of bone and mineral metabolism.* New York: Raven Press; 1992:83–106.
34. Brown EM, Pollack M, Seidman CE, et al. Calcium-ion–sensing cell-surface receptors. *N Engl J Med* 1995;333:234–240.
35. Brown EM, Pollak M, Chou YH, Seidman CE, Seidman JG, Herbert SC. The cloning of extracellular $Ca^{++}$-sensing receptors from parathyroid and kidney: molecular mechanisms of extracellular $Ca^{++}$-sensing. *J Nutr* 1995;125(suppl 7):1965–1979.
36. Pollak MR, Chou YH, Marx SJ, et al. Familial hypocalciuric hypercalcemia and neonatal severe hyperparathyroidism. Effects of mutant gene dosage on phenotype. *J Clin Invest* 1994;93:1108–1112.
37. Chou YH, Pollak MR, Brandi ML, et al. Mutations in the human $Ca^{++}$-sensing-receptor gene that cause familial hypocalciuric hypercalcemia. *Am J Hum Genet* 1995;56:1075–1079.
38. Pollak MR, Brown EM, Chou YH, et al. Mutations in the human $Ca^{++}$-sensing receptor gene cause familial hypocalciuric hypercalcemia and neonatal severe hyperparathyroidism. *Cell* 1992;75: 1297–1303.
39. Pollak MR, Brown EM, Estep HL, et al. Autosomal dominant hypocalcaemia caused by a $Ca^{++}$-sensing receptor gene mutation. *Nat Genet* 1994;8:303–307.
40. Sun F, Maercklein P, Fitzpatrick LA. Paracrine interactions among parathyroid cells: effect of cell density on cell secretion. *J Bone Min Res* 1994;9:971–976.
41. Cohn DV, Fasciotto BH, Reese BK, Zhang JX. Chromogranin A: a novel regulator of parathyroid gland secretion. *J Nutr* 1995;125(suppl 7):2015–2019.
42. Zhang JX, Fasciotto BH Darling DS, Cohn DV. Pancreastatin, a chromogranin A–derived peptide, inhibits transcription of the parathyroid hormone and chromogranin A genes and decreases the stability of the respective messenger ribonucleic acids in parathyroid cells in culture. *Endocrinology* 1994;134:1310–1316.
43. Fasciotto BH, Trauss CA, Greeley GH, Cohn DV. Parastatin (porcine chromogranin A347–419), a novel chromogranin A–derived peptide, inhibits parathyroid cell secretion. *Endocrinology* 1994;133:461–466.
44. Gilmour JR. Gross anatomy of parathyroid glands. *J Pathol Bacteriol* 1938;46:133–149.
45. Vail AD, Coller FC. The number and location of parathyroid glands recovered from 202 routine autopsies. *Mo Med* 1966;63:347–350.
46. Wang C-A. The anatomic basis of parathyroid surgery. *Ann Surg* 1976;183:271–275.
47. Alveryd A. Parathyroid glands in thyroid surgery. *Acta Chir Scand Suppl* 1968;389:1–120.
48. Åkerström G, Malmaeus J, Bergström R. Surgical anatomy of human parathyroid glands. *Surgery* 1984;95:14–21.
49. Grimelius L, Åkerström G, Johansson H, Bergström R. Anatomy and histopathology of human parathyroid glands. *Pathol Annu* 1981;16: 1–24.
50. Hooghe L, Kinnaert P, Van Geertruyden J. Surgical anatomy of hyperparathyroidism. *Acta Chir Belg* 1992:92;1–9.
51. Edis AJ, Purnell DC, van Heerden JA. The undescended "parathymus." An occasional cause of failed neck exploration for hyperparathyroidism. *Ann Surg* 1979;190:64–68.
52. Fitko R, Roth SI, Hines JR, Roxe DM, Cahill E. Parathyromatosis in hyperparathyroidism. *Hum Pathol* 1990;21:234–237.
53. Halstead W, Evans H. The parathyroid glandules. Their blood supply and their preservation in operation upon the thyroid gland. *Ann Surg* 1907;46:489–506.
54. Brewer LA III. The occurrence of parathyroid tissue within the thymus: report of four cases. *Endocrinol Bull Assoc Study Int Secret* 1930;18:393–408.
55. Lack EE, Delay S, Linnoila RI. Ectopic parathyroid tissue within the vagus nerve. *Arch Pathol Lab Med* 1988;112:304–306.
56. Åkerström G, Grimelius L, Johansson H, Lundqvist H. Estimation of the parenchymal-cell content of the parathyroid gland, using density-gradient columns. *Acta Pathol Microbiol Scand* 1977;85:555–557.
57. Åkerström G, Grimelius L, Johansson H, Pertoft H, Lundqvist H. Estimation of the parathyroid parenchymal cell mass by density gradients. *Am J Pathol* 1980;99:685–694.
58. Åkerström G, Grimelius L, Johansson H, Lundqvist H, Pertoft H, Bergström R. The parenchymal cell mass in normal human parathyroid glands. *Acta Pathol Microbiol Scand* 1981;89:367–375.
59. Grimelius L, Åkerström G, Johansson H, Lundqvist H. Estimation of parenchymal cell content of human parathyroid glands using the image analyzing computer technique. *Am J Pathol* 1978;93:793–800.
60. Dufour DR, Wilkerson SY. The normal parathyroid revisited: percentage of stromal fat. *Hum Pathol* 1982;13:717–721.
61. Gilmour JR, Martin WJ. The weight of the parathyroid glands. *J Pathol* 1937;44:431–462.
62. Roth SI. Recent advances in parathyroid gland pathology. *Am J Med* 1971;50:612–622.
63. Dufour DR, Wilkerson SY. Factors related to parathyroid weight in normal persons. *Arch Pathol Lab Med* 1983;107:167–172.
64. Matsushita H, Hara M, Shishiba Y, Nakazawa H. An evaluation of the size of the parathyroid glands. *Endocrinol Jpn* 1984;31:127–131.
65. Ghandur-Mnaymneh L, Cassady J, Hajianpour MA, Paz J, Reiss E. The parathyroid gland in health and disease. *Am J Pathol* 1986;125: 292–299.
66. Thiele J. Human parathyroid gland: a freeze fracture and thin section study. In: Grundmann E, Kirsten WH, eds. *Current topics in pathology.* Vol. 65. Berlin: Springer-Verlag; 1977:31–80.
67. Mazzocchi G, Meneghelli V, Frasson F. The human parathyroid glands: an optical and electron microscopic study. *Lo Sperimentale* 1967;117:383–447.
68. Balashev VN, Ignashkina MS. Lymphatic system of parathyroid glands in man. *Prob Endokrinol Gormonoterapii* 1964;10:52–53.
69. Altenähr E. Electron microscopical evidence for innervation of chief cells in human parathyroid gland. *Experientia* 1971;27:1077.
70. Yeghiayan E, Rojo-Ortega JM, Genest J. Parathyroid vessel innervation: an ultrastructural study. *J Anat* 1972;112:137–142.
71. Isono H, Shoumura S. Effects of vagotomy on the ultrastructure of the parathyroid gland of the rabbit. *Acta Anat* 1980;108:273–280.
72. Shoumura S, Iwasaki Y, Ishizaki N, et al. Origin of autonomic nerve fibers innervating the parathyroid gland in the rabbit. *Acta Anat* 1983; 115:9–295.
73. Saffos RO, Rhatigan RM, Urgulu S. The normal parathyroid and the borderline with early hyperplasia: a light microscopic study. *Histopathology* 1984;8:407–422.
74. Dekker A, Dunsford HA, Geyer SJ. The normal parathyroid gland at autopsy: the significance of stromal fat in adult patients. *J Pathol* 1979;128:127–132.
75. Roth SI. The parathyroid gland. In: Silverberg SG, ed. *Principles and practice of surgical pathology.* Vol. 2, 2nd ed. New York: Churchill Livingstone; 1989:1923–1955.
76. Cinti S, Balercia G, Zingaretti MC, Amati S, Osculati F. The normal human parathyroid gland: a histochemical and ultrastructural study with particular reference to follicular structures. *J Submicrosc Cytol* 1983;15:661–679.
77. Anderson TJ, Ewen SWB. Amyloid in normal and pathological parathyroid glands. *J Clin Pathol* 1974;27:656–663.
78. Lieberman A, DeLellis RA. Intrafollicular amyloid in normal parathyroid glands. *Arch Pathol* 1973;95:422–423.
79. Leedham PW, Pollock DJ. Intrafollicular amyloid in primary hyperparathyroidism. *J Clin Pathol* 1970;23:811–817.
80. Gilmour JR. The normal histology of the parathyroid glands. *J Pathol Bacteriol* 1939;48:187–222.
81. Roth SI, Olen E, Hansen L. The eosinophilic cells of the parathyroid (oxyphil cells), salivary (oncocytes), and thyroid (Hürthle cells) glands. *Lab Invest* 1962;11:933–941.
82. Munger BL, Roth SI. The cytology of the normal parathyroid glands of man and Virginia deer. *J Cell Biol* 1963;16:379–400.
83. Roth SI, Munger BL. The cytology of the adenomatous, atrophic and hyperplastic parathyroid glands of man. A light and electron microscopic study. *Virchows Arch [A]* 1962;335:389–410.
84. Roth SI, Capen CC. Ultrastructural and functional correlations of the parathyroid gland. In: Richter GW, Epstein MA, eds. *International review of experimental pathology.* Vol. 161. New York: Academic Press; 1974:13–221.
85. Capen CC, Roth SI. Ultrastructural and functional relationships of normal and pathologic parathyroid cells. In: Ioachim HL, ed. *Pathobiology annual.* Vol. 3. New York: Appleton-Century-Crofts; 1973: 129–175.
86. Frigerio B, Capella C, Wilander E, Grimelius L. Argyrophil reaction in parathyroid glands. *Acta Pathol Microbiol Immunol Scand* 1982; 90:323–326.
87. Weymouth RJ, Baker BL. The presence of argyrophilic granules in the parenchymal cells of the parathyroid glands. *Anat Rec* 1954;119: 519–527.

88. Weymouth RJ. The cytology of the parathyroid glands of the rat after bilateral nephrectomy, administration of parathyroid hormone and hypophysectomy. *Anat Rec* 1957;127:509–527.
89. Futrell JM, Roth SI, Su SPC, Habener JF, Segre GV, Potts JT Jr. Immunocytochemical localization of parathyroid hormone in bovine parathyroid glands and human parathyroid adenomas. *Am J Pathol* 1979;94:615–622.
90. Ravazzola M, Orci L, Habener JF, Potts JT Jr. Parathyroid secretory protein: immunocytochemical localization within cells that contain parathyroid hormone. *Lancet* 1978;2:371–372.
91. Stork PJ, Herteaux C, Frazier R, et al. Expression and distribution of parathyroid hormone messenger RNA in pathological conditions of the parathyroid [Abstract]. *Lab Invest* 1989;60:92.
92. Stork PJ, Herteaux C, Frazier R, Kronenberg H, Wolfe HJ. Expression and distribution of parathyroid hormone messenger RNA in pathological conditions of the parathyroid. *Diagn Mol Pathol* (in press).
93. Kendall CH, Potter L, Brown R. Jasani B, Pringle JH, Lauder I. In situ correlation of synthesis and storage of parathormone in parathyroid gland disease. *J Pathol* 1993;169:61–66.
94. Thiele J. The human parathyroid chief cell—a model for a polypeptide hormone producing endocrine unit as revealed by various functional and pathological conditions. A thin section and freeze-fracture study. *J Submicrosc Cytol* 1986;18:205–220.
95. Thiele J, Kärner J, Fischer R. Ultrastructural morphometry on human parathyroid tissue. Morphological and functional implications. *J Submicrosc Cytol* 1988;20:491–500.
96. Roth SI, Raisz LG. The course and reversibility of the calcium effect on the ultrastructure of the rat parathyroid gland in organ culture. *Lab Invest* 1966;15:1187–1211.
97. Altenähr E. Ultrastructural pathology of parathyroid glands. *Curr Top Pathol* 1972;56:1–54.
98. Cohn DV, MacGregor RR. The biosynthesis, intracellular processing, and secretion of parathormone. *Endocr Rev* 1981;2:1–26.
99. Habener JF, Rosenblatt M, Potts JT. Parathyroid hormone: biochemical aspects of biosynthesis, secretion, action and metabolism. *Physiol Rev* 1984;64:958–1053.
100. MacCallum WG, Voegtlin C. On the relation of the parathyroid gland to calcium metabolism and to tetany. *J Exp Med* 1909;11:118–151.
101. Patt HM, Luckhardt AB. Relationship of a low blood calcium to parathyroid secretion. *Endocrinology* 1942;31:384–392.
102. Svensson O, Wernerson A, Reinholt FP. The parathyroid glands in the rat as seen by ultrathin step and serial sectioning. *Bone Min* 1989; 6:237–248.
103. Shannon WA, Roth SI. Ultrastructural study of acid phosphatase activity in normal, adenomatous and hyperplastic (chief cell type) human parathyroid glands. *Am J Pathol* 1974;77:493–506.
104. Pappenheimer AM, Wilens SL. Enlargement of the parathyroid glands in renal disease. *Am J Pathol* 1935;11:73–91.
105. Wild P, Schraner EM, Eggenberger E. Quantitative aspects of membrane shifts in rat parathyroid cells initiated by decrease in serum calcium. *Biol Cell* 1984;50:263–272.
106. Hashizume Y, Waguri S, Watanabe T, Kominami E, Uchiyama Y. cysteine proteinases in rat parathyroid cells with special reference to their correlation with parathyroid hormone (PTH) in storage granules. *J Histochem Cytochem* 1993:41;273–282.
107. Roth SI, Gallagher MJ. The rapid identification of "normal" parathyroid glands by the presence of intracellular fat. *Am J Pathol* 1976;84: 521–528.
108. Sasano H, Geelhoed GW, Silverberg SG. Intraoperative cytologic evaluation of lipid in the diagnosis of parathyroid adenoma. *Am J Surg Pathol* 1988;12:282–286.
109. Ljungberg O, Tibblin S. Preoperative fat staining of frozen sections in primary hyperparathyroidism. *Am J Pathol* 1979;95:633–642.
110. King DT, Hirose FM. Chief cell intracytoplasmic fat used to evaluate parathyroid disease by frozen section. *Arch Pathol Lab Med* 1979; 103:609–612.
111. Bondeson A-G, Bondeson L, Ljungberg O, Tibblin S. Fat staining in parathyroid disease—diagnostic value and impact on surgical strategy: clinicopathologic analysis of 191 cases. *Hum Pathol* 1985;16: 1255–1263.
112. Monchik JM, Farrugia R, Teplitz C, Teplitz J, Brown S. Parathyroid surgery: the role of chief cell intracellular fat staining with osmium carmine in the intraoperative management of patients with primary hyperparathyroidism. *Surgery* 1983;94:877–886.
113. Alpern HD, Roth SI, Olson JE. Intracellular lipid droplets in functioning transitional parathyroid oxyphil adenomas. A caveat. *Arch Surg* 1990;125:410–411.
114. Chen KTK. Fat stain in hyperparathyroidism. *Am J Surg Pathol* 1982; 6:191–192.
115. Kasdon EJ, Cohen RB, Rosen S, Silen W. Surgical pathology of hyperparathyroidism: usefulness of fat stain and problems in interpretation. *Am J Surg Pathol* 1981;5:381–384.
116. Dekker A, Watson CG, Barnes EL Jr. The pathologic assessment of primary hyperparathyroidism and its impact on therapy. A prospective evaluation of 50 cases with oil-red-O stain. *Ann Surg* 1979;190: 671–675.
117. Ritchie CK, Cohn DV, Maercklein PB, Fitzpatrick LA. Individual parathyroid cells exhibit cyclic secretion of parathyroid hormone and chromogranin-A (as measured by a novel sequential hemolytic plaque assay). *Endocrinology* 1992;131:2638–2642.
118. Fitzpatrick LA. Heterogeneous secretory response of parathyroid cells. *Rec Prog Horm Res* 1993;48:471–475.
119. Lee MJ, Roth SI. Effect of calcium and magnesium on deoxyribonucleic acid synthesis in rat parathyroid glands in vitro. *Lab Invest* 1975; 33:72–79.
120. Bianchi S, Fabiani S, Muratori M, et al. Calcium modulates the cyclin D1 expression in a rat parathyroid cell line. *Biochem Biophys Res Commun* 1994;204:691–700.
121. Hamperl H. Über das Vorkommen von Onkocyten in verschiedenen Organen und ihren Geschwülsten (Mundspeicheldrüsen, Bauschpeicheldrüse, Epithelkörperchen, Hypophyse, Schilddrüse, Eileiter). *Virchows Arch [A]* 1936;298:327–375.
122. Hamperl H. Onkocyten und Onkocytome. *Virchows Arch* 1962;335: 452–483.
123. Tremblay G. The oncocytes. *Methods Achiev Exp Pathol* 1969; 4:121–140.
124. Christie AC. The parathyroid oxyphil cells. *J Clin Pathol* 1967;20: 591–602.
125. Müller-Höcker J. Random cytochrome-C-oxidase deficiency of oxyphil cell nodules in the parathyroid gland. A mitochondrial cytopathy related to cell ageing? *Pathol Res Pract* 1992;188:701–706.
126. Tandler B, Hoppel CL. *Mitochondria.* New York: Academic Press; 1972:1–59.
127. Balogh K Jr, Cohen RB. Oxidative enzymes in the epithelial cells of normal and pathologic human parathyroid glands: a histochemical study. *Lab Invest* 1961;10:354–360.
128. Fischer R. Über den histochemischen Nachwies oxydativer Enzyme in Onkocyten verschiedener Organe. *Virchows Arch [A]* 1961;334: 445–452.
129. Tremblay G, Cartier GE. Histochemical study of oxidative enzymes in the human parathyroid. *Endocrinology* 1961;69:658–661.
130. Kitazawa R, Kitazawa S, Fukase M, et al. The expression or parathyroid hormone–related protein (PTHrP) in parathyroid: histochemistry and in situ hybridization. *Histochemistry* 1992:98;211–215.
131. Wolpert HR, Vickery AL Jr, Wang C-A. Functioning oxyphil cell adenomas of the parathyroid gland. *Am J Surg Pathol* 1967;20;591–602.

*Histology for Pathologists, second edition,*
Edited by Stephen S. Sternberg.
Lippincott-Raven Publishers, Philadelphia


# CHAPTER 48

# Adrenal Gland

J. Aidan Carney



The paired adrenal glands are a composite of two endocrine organs—one steroid producing, the other catecholamine producing—that are located in the retroperitoneum, superomedial to the kidneys. The two organs have a different embryonic origin, histology, and function.

## ANATOMY

The main portions of the adrenal gland are easily recognized on the fresh or formalin-fixed cut surface (Fig. 1). Externally, a relatively thick yellow layer is applied to a narrow dark brown band that abuts on a solid, pearly gray interior. The former two zones correspond histologically to the zona fasciculata and zona reticularis of the cortex, and the latter to the medulla of the organ.

The anatomic location of the human adrenal glands that sandwiches them between several organs is responsible for their particular shape: pyramidal on the right and crescent shaped on the left. The depression and ridge (crest) on the posterior surfaces (Fig. 2) result from their close relationship to the kidneys. When a kidney is congenitally absent, the corresponding adrenal is round and the characteristic longitudinal ridge on the posterior surface is missing (1).

## EVOLUTION

The anatomic relationship of the adrenal cortex to the medulla that exists in mammals is not found in lower animals. In the shark, for example, the cortex and medulla are topographically completely separate; in amphibians, the two structures are in close contact; in birds, they are intermingled. Only in mammals does the intimate proximity seen among the human adrenal cortex and medulla occur. In a prototypic mammal (e.g., the rat), the medulla forms a central core that is uniformly surrounded by the cortex. The distribution of the two zones in the human adrenal is different.

J. A. Carney: Emeritus, Department of Laboratory Medicine and Pathology, Mayo Clinic and Mayo Foundation, Rochester, Minnesota 55905.

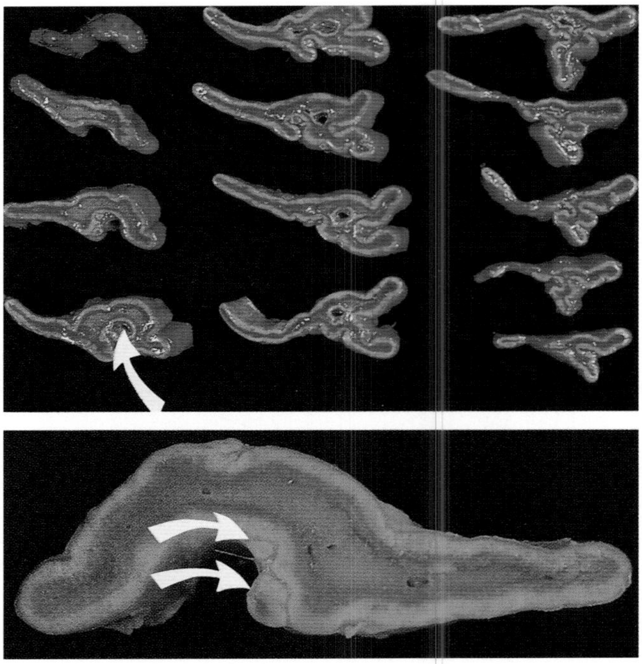

A

B

**FIG. 1.** Normal adrenal gland. **A:** Fresh gland sliced from head (*upper left*) through body (*center*) to tail (*lower right*). The yellow cortex and pearly gray medulla are visible in the head (*left*). Yellow zona fasciculata surrounds dark brown zona reticularis in the tail (*right*), where medulla is absent. The gland can be identified as the left adrenal because the adrenal vein runs in a well-developed groove on the surface of the gland at the junction of the head and body (*arrow*). Invaginated cortex surrounds the central vein in the interior of the body. **B:** Slice of formalin-fixed adrenal gland showing, from exterior inward, cortical zona fasciculata (yellow), zona reticularis (brown), and medulla (gray). The cortex is about 1 mm in thickness. Dilated tributaries of the central vein are seen in the medulla. The adrenal vein has been removed from its groove. Accessory cortex is present (*arrows*).

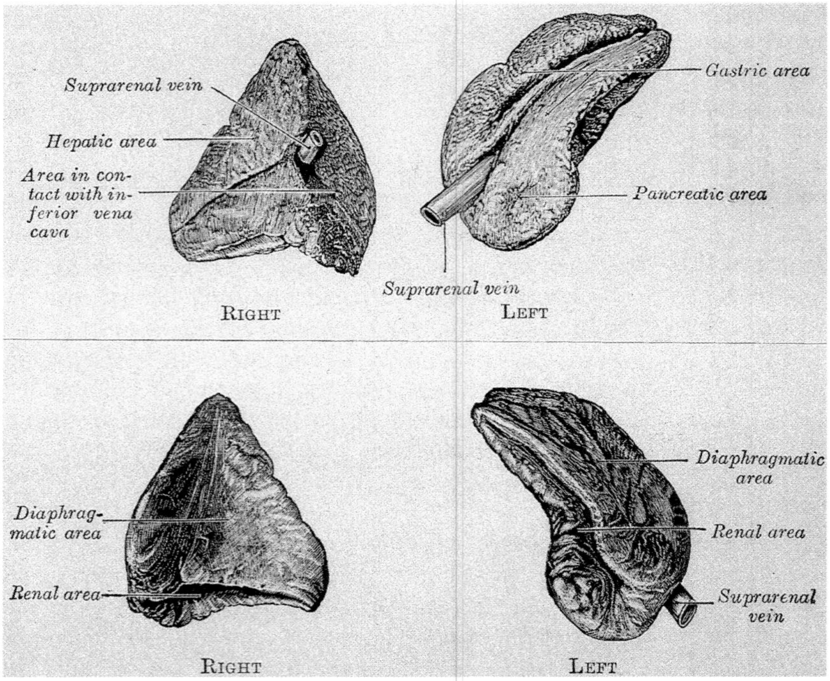


**FIG. 2.** External appearance of anterior (*above*) and posterior aspects (*below*) of right and left adrenal glands. The right gland is pyramidal, and the left is crescent shaped. The right adrenal vein is short. The left vein is longer and lies in a groove on the anterior surface of the gland. Reprinted with permission (15).

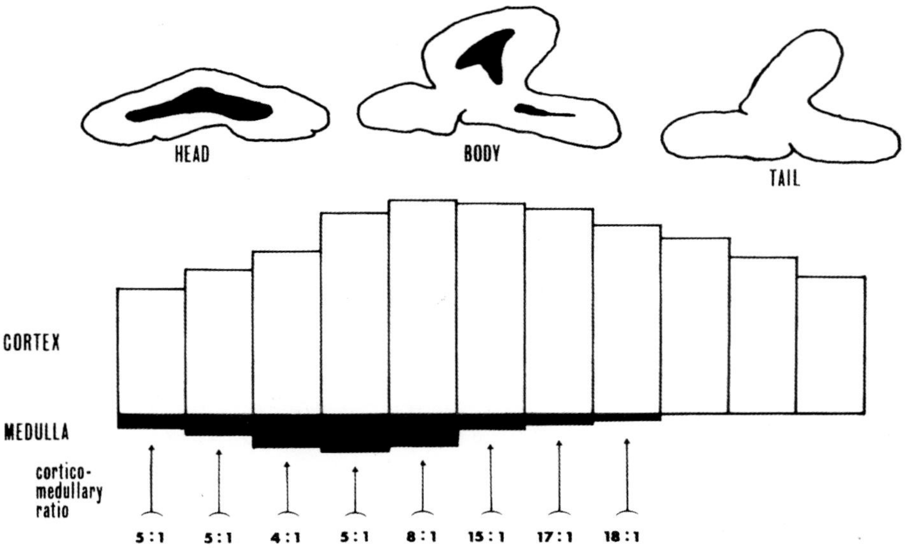


**FIG. 3.** Diagrammatic illustration of the distribution of medulla (black) in the head, body, and tail of the adrenal gland (*above*) and corresponding corticomedullary ratios (*below*). Reprinted with permission (3).

In the human adrenal (Fig. 3), most of the medulla is in the head of the gland (medial), some occurs in the body, and there is usually none in the tail (lateral) (3). Two bands of cortex applied one to the other form the alae of the glands.

## DEVELOPMENT

### Cortex

The adrenal cortex is of mesodermal origin. Its primordia appear at the 9-mm embryo stage (6th week of gestation) as bilateral cellular aggregations (Fig. 4) at the mesenteric root, medial to the developing gonad and anterior to the kidney (mesonephros) (4,5). These primordia are composed of two groups of mesenchymal cells, one destined to be the precursor of the transitory provisional or fetal cortex, the other to become the adrenal capsule and its supporting connective tissue framework (5). By the 7th week of gestation, the primordia have become more defined, have separated from the coelomic lining, and include polyhedral cells with eosinophilic, lipid-poor cytoplasm. These cells increase in size and proliferate rapidly, forming a series of parallel columns and cords of cells that ultimately compose the bulk of the provisional cortex. External to this dominant mass, a thin subcapsular rim of smaller cells (the precursor of the permanent or adult cortex) appears (Fig. 5). These cells are arranged in nests and arches that cap the columns of deeper cells. They have hyperchromatic, closely packed, overlapping nuclei. In the cords, the nuclei are larger, more vesicular, and less hyperchromatic. There is continuous spottily distributed degeneration of the cells in the cords, and dead

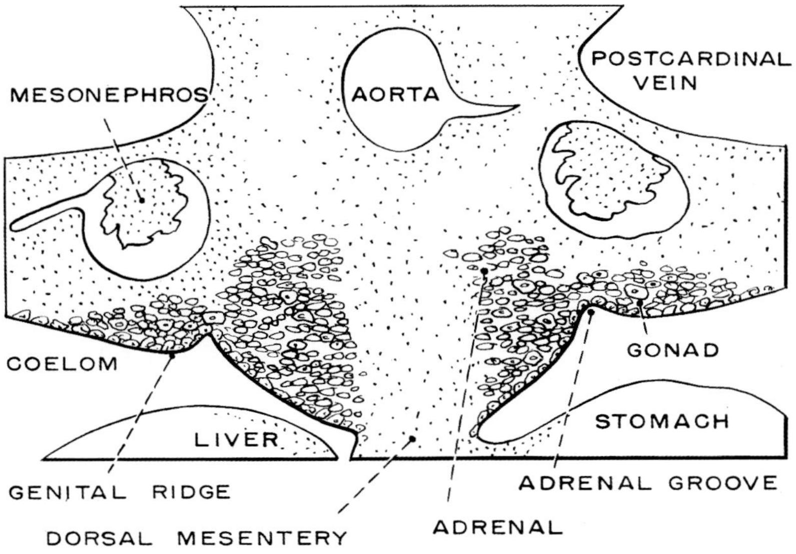


**FIG. 4.** Diagrammatic representation of a human embryo at 6 weeks' gestation showing the anatomic relationship of developing adrenal gland to coelomic cavity, gonad, and kidney (mesonephros). Reprinted with permission (16).

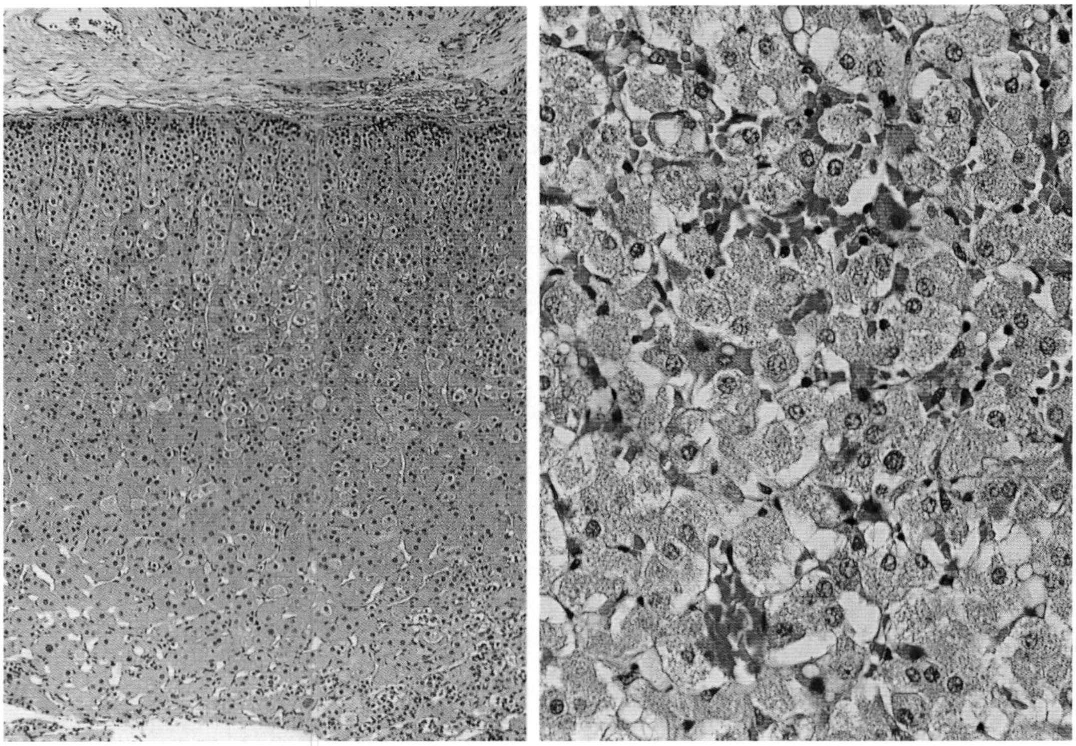

A B

**FIG. 5.** Provisional (fetal) cortex (29 weeks' gestation, stillborn infant). **A:** Cortex is dominated by large cells with eosinophilic cytoplasm in vague columns and solid sheet with prominent capillaries. Just beneath the tenuous capsule, there is a rim of smaller cells, the source of the permanent cortex. A sympathetic ganglion and a small nerve are present in the periadrenal connective tissue. **B:** Large, liverlike cells with cytoplasm that is voluminous, eosinophilic, and granular. Nuclei are vesicular with a single small nucleolus. Vascularity is prominent.

cells are continuously replaced by proliferation of cells in the narrow subcapsular band. Growth of the developing cortex is therefore centripedal (from outside inward).

At the end of gestation, the provisional cortex accounts for the bulk of the gland (Fig. 6). Within hours of birth, it becomes acutely congested and starts to degenerate. At the end of 7 to 10 days, the provisional cortex is largely disorganized and necrotic. The narrow peripheral band of cell clusters survives and becomes the source of the permanent cortex.

## Medulla

The adrenal medulla is of neuroectodermal origin (5). Precursor cells originate in the neural crest and migrate from primitive spinal ganglia (sixth thoracic to first lumbar) to form the primitive sympathetic nervous system situated dorsal to the aorta. Some cells (sympathogonia) from the sympathetic anlagen migrate farther in nerves that sprout from the sympathetic chain, and alongside large blood vessels that penetrate into the (as yet) unencapsulated fetal adrenal cortex, primarily its caudal pole (head) (very likely explaining the nonuniform distribution of medulla in the adult adrenal already mentioned). The neural cells enter the adrenal primordium as fingerlike processes and pass among the fetal cortical cells. In this manner, sympathogonia and a plexus of nerves are initially scattered among fetal cortical cells (Fig. 7). Two sets of progeny of the sympathogonia evolve: the majority, small cells with little cytoplasm and a darkly staining nucleus (neuroblasts); the minority, larger cells with a

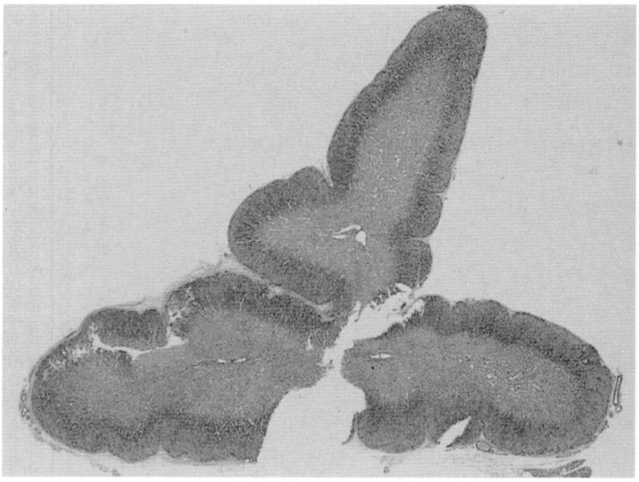

**FIG. 6.** Adrenal cortex at birth (35 weeks' gestation; infant died at 2 days). The central, degenerating, eosinophilic provisional cortex is surrounded by the developing, darkly staining outer rim of permanent cortex.

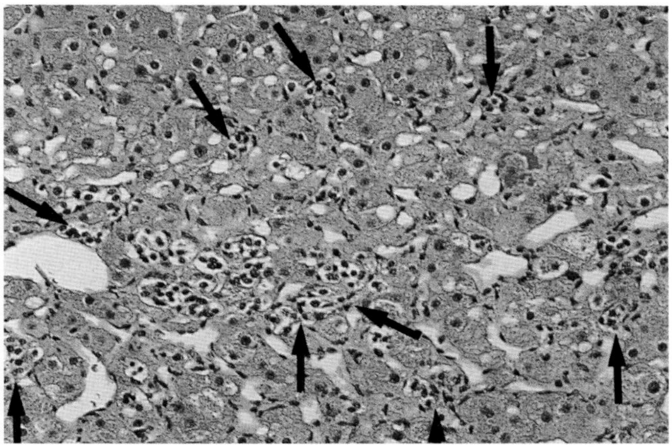

**FIG. 7.** Developing adrenal medulla (29 weeks' gestation, stillborn infant). Clusters of small medullary cells with deeply staining nuclei (*arrows*) irregularly distributed in very vascular provisional cortex. When the latter degenerates, the clusters of medullary cells survive and, lacking the support of the cortical cells, aggregate together.

vesicular nucleus and basophilic cytoplasm (pheochromoblasts). At birth, the medulla comprises a central, very thin core of these cells with offshoots stretching a short distance into the peripheral degenerating provisional cortex. The medullary cells are arranged in irregularly sized clumps containing both cell types, the larger cells now predominating. The postnatal collapse of the provisional cortex and its stroma removes the framework that supported the medullary offshoots and their associated nerve plexus in the cortex (3). With this loss of scaffolding, these structures coalesce around the central veins.

## GLAND WEIGHT AND CORTICAL THICKNESS

Although not a structural feature of the adrenal, the weight of the glands is important because assessment of the adrenal normalcy takes this feature into account. Information on truly normal adrenal weight is difficult to obtain because the organ (specifically the cortex) responds rapidly to stress by an increase in mass. Therefore, accurate normal adrenal weight can be determined only from selected autopsy material (healthy individuals who die suddenly). The combined adrenal weight in these circumstances is about 8 g (1). Exceptionally, a gland weighs as little as 2 g or as much as 6 g. Sex differences are not apparent. Formalin fixation has little effect on the gland weight.

Relative to body weight, the adrenals are actually largest at the 4th month of gestation (2). In unselected autopsy cases, the combined average weight of the glands at birth is about 20 g. By the end of the 1st week of life, this mass has decreased (as a result of involution of the provisional cortex) to about 12 g, and a further small decrease occurs during the 2nd week, such that each gland comes to weigh approximately 5 g. Total gland weight then remains constant for 2 years, then gradually rises to the adult postmortem weight of about 13 g between 15 and 20 years of age (3).

The thickness of the normal adult adrenal cortex is approximately 1 mm and ranges from about 0.7 to 1.3 mm. For accuracy, the thickness should be determined microscopically with an ocular micrometer; it is impractical to detect small alterations in the thickness using a metric scale.

## ADRENAL GLANDS FOR HISTOLOGIC STUDY

### Ideal Material

Ideally, for the reasons already mentioned, adrenal glands used for study of normal histology of the organ should be obtained from healthy patients. Results obtained from the study of glands of patients with primary adrenal disease or disorders that might affect the adrenal histology secondarily should be used with caution. Nevertheless, because the two portions of the adrenal gland, cortex and medulla, are separate functional units that apparently do not affect each other, I think that it is not unreasonable (until shown to be otherwise) to study, for example, the histology of the adrenal medulla (thinking of it as being normal) in a gland surgically removed for a clinically and biochemically nonfunctioning small adrenocortical adenoma. Similar considerations apply to the cortex.

For study of cytologic detail, material should be fresh and not autolysed and therefore obtained at surgery or shortly after death. The zona reticularis of the cortex quickly begins to show the effects of anoxia (degeneration). However, glands that are less than optimally preserved for study of the cell details are satisfactory for determination of general microanatomy of the organ. In practice, fresh (and to a variable extent "normal") adrenal is most often available at the time of radical nephrectomy, in the course of which a gland is removed with the kidney. However, many such glands are torn during the surgical procedure, limiting to some extent their use for study of normal histology. Their usefulness is also limited in that they are representative only of the gland appearance in a particular age range (middle-aged or older patients). In practice, it is difficult to get the complete range of normal adrenal specimens (fetal to aged) that would be ideal for study of normal histology.

### Actual Material

The actual tissue used for the histologic description that follows included adrenals from all the foregoing categories. Autopsy material was obtained from individuals (mostly male) who died suddenly (homicide, suicide, or traumatic injury). For some cases there was minimal or no medical history available, and the autopsy protocol and other autopsy slides could not be reviewed. Thus, the state of health of these patients and the condition of other organs could not be determined. A number of normal glands were available from patients undergoing nephrectomy. Also, opportunity was taken to study apparently normal extratumoral medulla and cortex in cases of adrenalectomy for certain primary adrenal neoplasms that were small or relatively small (adrenocortical adenomas producing aldosterone and nonfunctioning adrenocortical adenomas, and pheochromocytoma).

## HISTOLOGY

### Blood Vessels

The blood supply of the adrenal gland has been studied mostly from the anatomic point of view, often by observing the distribution of injected material in the vasculature. The tone of the subcapsular vascular plexus controls circulation through the organ. The histologic appearance of the vessels distal to the plexus suggests that the intravascular pressure in the organ is low.

### Arteries

Three separate groups of arteries—superior, middle, and inferior—arising from the inferior phrenic artery, the aorta, and the renal artery, supply each adrenal gland (Fig. 8). The main vessels divide into 50 to 60 small feeder vessels that penetrate the anterior and posterior surfaces of the glands and form a plexus beneath the capsule of the gland. The former are commonly encountered close to the capsule of the gland; in older patients, they frequently exhibit atherosclerotic changes. The subcapsular plexus, important in regulation of the circulation in the gland, as has just been indicated, is not conspicuous in routine histologic preparations.

### Intraglandular Vasculature

Capillary loops from the subcapsular plexus surround the cells of the zona glomerulosa (see later), then extend toward the interior of the organ between the columns of cells of the zona fasciculata, and ultimately open into wide interconnecting channels in the zona reticularis to form a second vascular plexus. This ends abruptly in a vascular dam at the corticomedullary junction that finally drains into the sinusoids of the medulla by a relatively few channels. The marked vascular congestion commonly seen at the corticomedullary junction of adrenal glands obtained at autopsy may be a reflection of this vascular barrier. Although the medulla receives some arterial blood supply, most of its vascular supply has already nourished the cortex.

The venous drainage of the glands from the organs occurs via a single vein that emerges from the anterior surface of each gland (Fig. 2). Inside the organs, the central adrenal vein (which ultimately becomes the adrenal vein as it leaves the organ) and its tributaries have a unique muscle coat, two to six longitudinally running muscle bundles, varying in size and eccentrically situated around the vein lumen (Fig. 9). The bundles are heavily laden with elastic fibers that extend

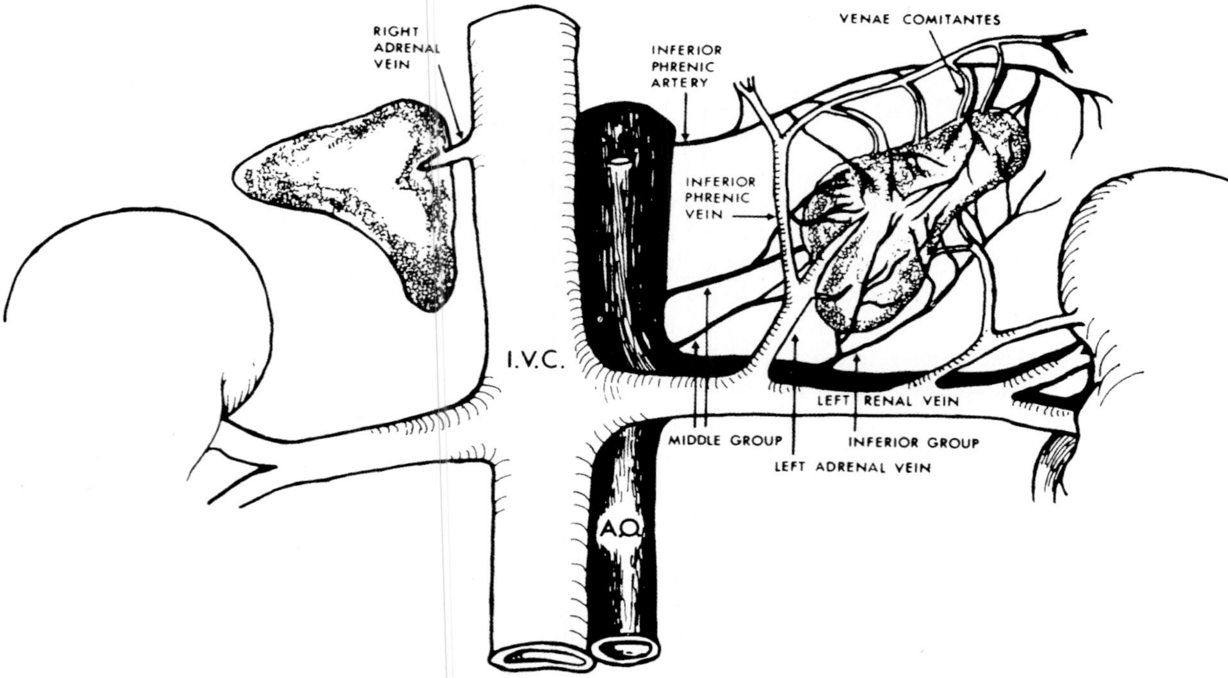


**FIG. 8.** Diagrammatic representation of the arterial supply (black) and venous drainage (light and hatched) of the left adrenal gland. Reprinted with permission (3).

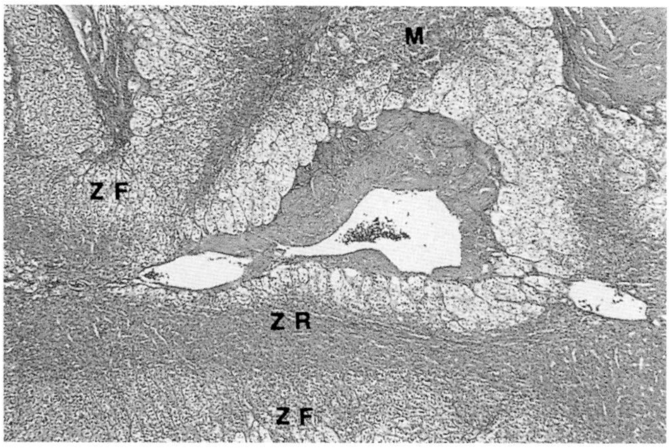


**FIG. 9.** Central adrenal vein. Low-power view of the vein surrounded by an invaginated cuff of cortical cells with clear cytoplasm (zona fasciculata type). Distribution of smooth muscle in the vein wall is uneven. The zona fasciculata (ZF) and zona reticularis (ZR) of the cortex are evident, and there is a small amount of basophilic medulla (M).

into tributaries of the larger central veins and in some instances outline clusters and trabeculae of medullary cells.

The eccentricity of the muscle bundles results in a vein wall that varies greatly in thickness and focally is devoid of muscle. In the zones where the muscle bundles are deficient (and these may be extensive), medullary cells (and sometimes cortical cells) are separated from the bloodstream by intima and a minimal amount of subintimal connective tissue only. This peculiar anatomic structure permits medullary cells or cortical cells to occasionally form polypoid endothelium-covered projections into the lumen of the central vein (Fig. 10). (This ready access of pheochromocytes to the venous lumen explains the occasional finding of an intravenous tumor plug of pheochromocytoma.) A thick cuff of invaginated cortical cells surrounds the intramedullary central vein and its larger tributaries (Fig. 10). (Development of a neoplasm in this "displaced" cortex probably explains the occasional cortical neoplasm that appears to have developed in the medulla of the organ. As explained later, there is another possible source for a cortical neoplasm in this location—from cortical cells that occur among cells of the medulla.)

### Veins

The left adrenal vein, 2 to 4 cm in length, initially lies in a groove on the anterior surface of the gland and terminates in the left renal vein (Figs. 2 and 8). The right adrenal vein is short (1–5 mm) and drains into the inferior vena cava (Figs. 2 and 8). Histologically, the extra-adrenal and immediately intra-adrenal portions of the veins have a muscular coat composed of large, similarly sized, evenly disposed smooth muscle bundles, arranged side by side—a structure found in other veins of this size.

### Nerves and Ganglia

The innervation of the adrenal gland, specifically of the medulla, emanates from the lower thoracic segments of the spinal cord and passes through the greater splanchnic nerve and the upper lumbar sympathetic ganglia via the celiac plexus. This nerve supply forms a plexus of medullated and nonmedullated nerves on the capsule of the gland, primarily on its posterior aspect. Thence, the largely preganglionic nerve fibers pass into the medulla following either the course of emerging or penetrating vessels or connective tissue trabeculae. Occasionally, a large nerve penetrates directly into the medulla. The number of nerves visible in the medulla varies greatly from case to case; some feature a perineurium, whereas others do not; frequently, they have associated ganglion cells (Fig. 11). Ganglion cells are also commonly seen singly or in clusters among the pheochromocytes (Fig. 12). The cells of the cortex do not have a nerve supply.

### Lymphatics

Injection studies have demonstrated that there is a rich plexus of lymphatic channels in the capsule of the gland (3). Lymphatics are distributed to the adventitia of the central

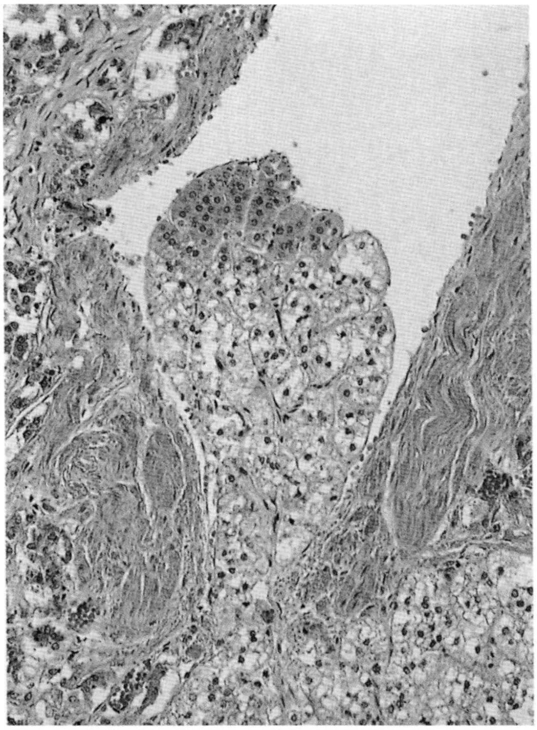

**FIG. 10.** Central adrenal vein. Intraluminal protrusion of endothelium-covered adrenocortical cells between the discontinuous muscle bundles of a tributary of the central adrenal vein.

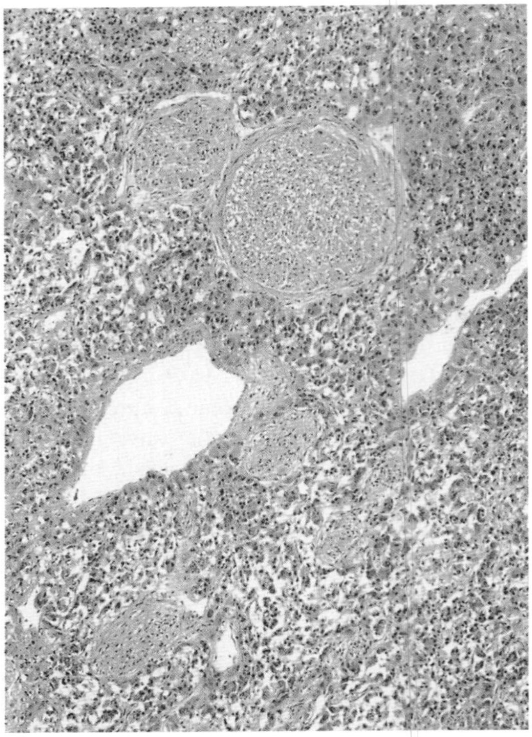

**FIG. 11.** Adrenal medulla. Unusual concentration of nerves, some with perineurium and others without.

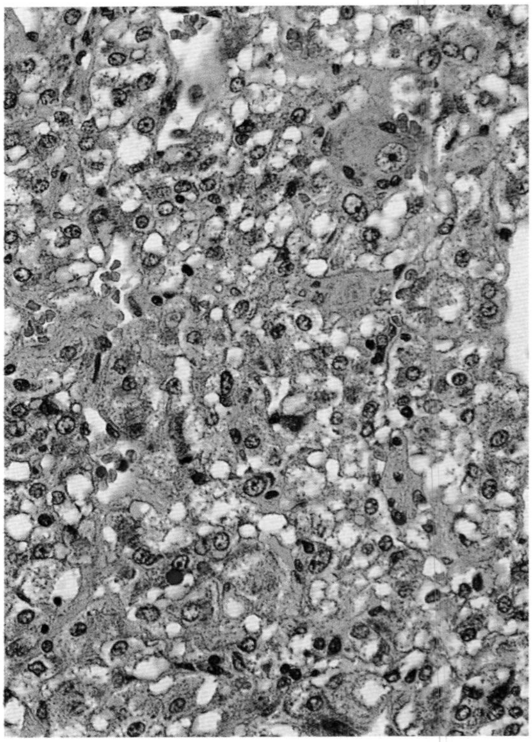

**FIG. 12.** Adrenal medulla. Sheet of medullary cells with cytoplasm that is nonhomogeneous, variably basophilic, granular, and vacuolated, resulting in a mottled appearance. A ganglion cell is present among the pheochromocytes.

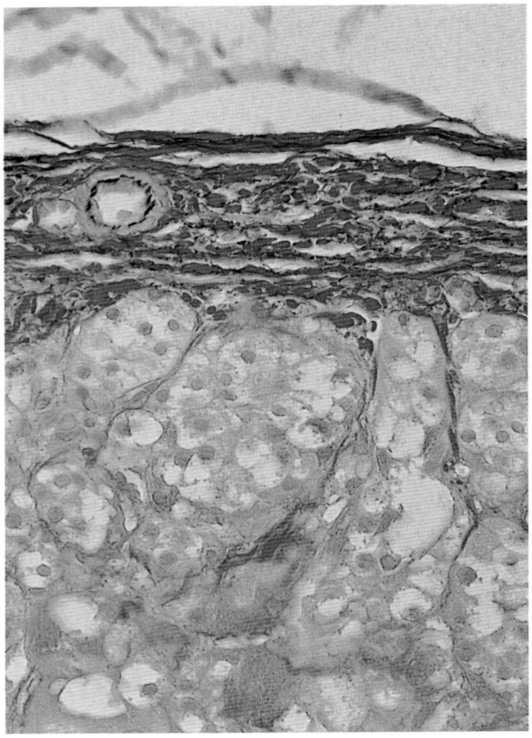

**FIG. 13.** Adrenal capsule. Elastic–van Gieson stain shows collagen bundles (red) and intermingled elastic fibers (black). A small artery is present in the capsule.

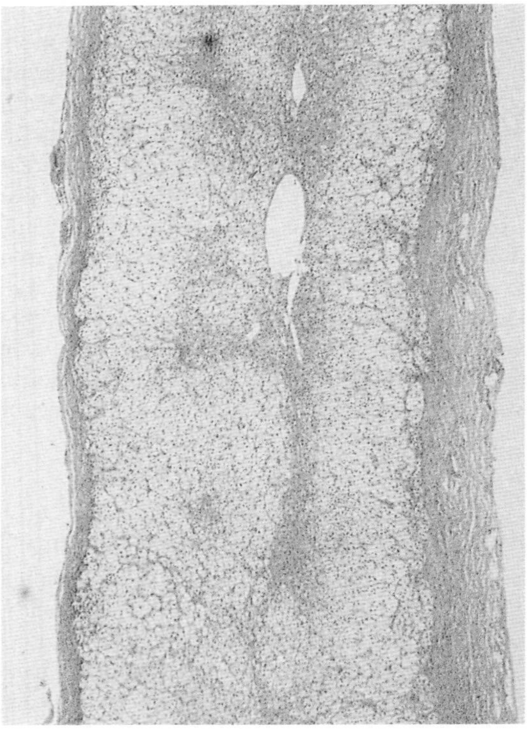

**FIG. 14.** Adrenal capsule. Fourfold variation in the thickness of the capsule, which at its maximum thickness measures 0.3 mm.

vein and its main tributaries. There is no lymphatic supply to the cortex. The lymphatics drain into aortic lymph nodes.

## Capsule

The capsule of the adrenal gland is composed of hypocellular fibrous tissue in the form of coarse, hyalinized collagen bundles and elastic fibers (Fig. 13). Usually, the capsule is thin, but it varies considerably in thickness from gland to gland and even within the same gland (Fig. 14). It is tough and hard to cut but tears easily and does not support the unfixed gland, which is limp and readily bends. The soft consistency of the fresh glands makes them difficult to section; cooling them for 15 min in a refrigerator facilitates this operation.

Because of the propinquity of development of adrenals and kidneys and the liver (on the right side), there is occasional fusion or sharing of a common capsule among the adrenal and kidney and adrenal and liver (Fig. 15). The common capsule may be deficient focally, and then parenchymal cells of two organs come into direct contact. The adrenal capsule is surrounded by adult-type fat (brown fat in the fetus and newborn) that features small arteries, veins, nerves, accessory cortex, excrescences of cortex, sympathetic ganglia, and an occasional paraganglion (Fig. 16).

The capsule is penetrated by blood vessels supplying and draining the gland, the nerves to the medulla, and lymphatic channels. In random sections of the glands, only the site of

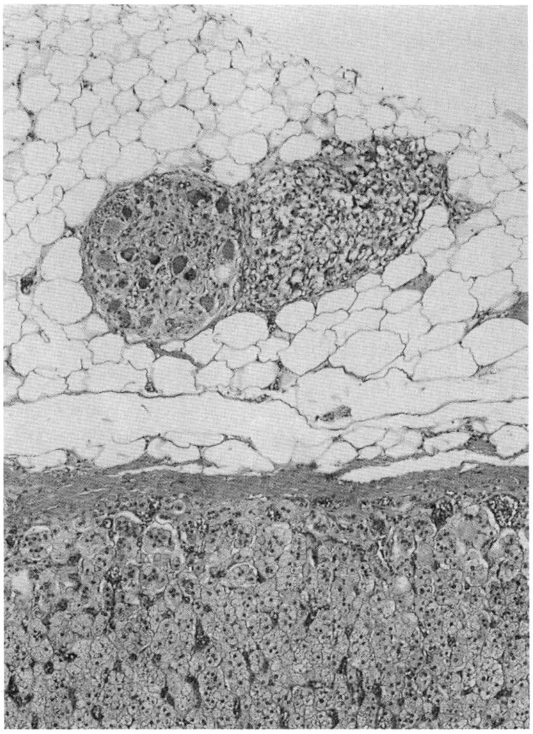

**FIG. 16.** Normal adrenal gland. Sympathetic ganglion (*above left*) and paraganglion (*above right*) in periadrenal adipose tissue. The adrenal cortex features cells with clear cytoplasm (zona fasciculata). Zona glomerulosa is not seen.

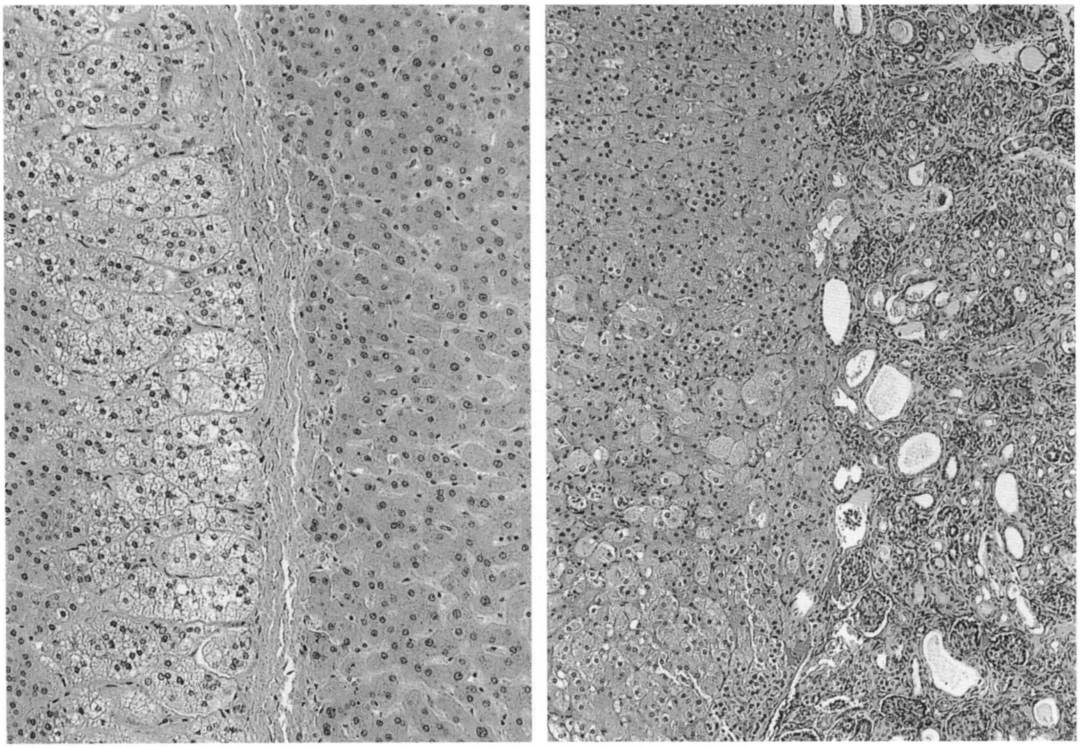

A B

**FIG. 15.** Adrenal capsule. **A:** Common capsule of adrenal (*left*) and liver (*right*). Note that a zona glomerulosa is not evident in the adrenal cortex. **B:** Absence of an adrenal (and kidney) capsule results in direct contact of adrenal cortex (provisional) and renal parenchyma.

exit of the adrenal vein is regularly encountered (because of its relatively large size); occasionally, the site of penetration of a large nerve is seen; the entry sites of the small arteries into the glands are also sometimes seen. Commonly found are narrow (occasionally wide) defects in the capsule through which the cortex protrudes into the periadrenal fat to form small nodules of cells that are sometimes delimited by a distended and attenuated adrenal capsule, sometimes not (Fig. 17). These excrescences are composed predominantly of epithelial cells with normal zonation patterns among the cells. The protrusions may contain a connective tissue component, and sometimes there is an equal mixture of cords of epithelial cells and fibrous tissue. Single rows and groups of cortical cells, small and oval or large and round, are commonly found here and there in capsular "pockets" (Fig. 18). Larger oval aggregates cause a slight depression in, and thinning of, the underlying cortex, so that the total width of the two portions of cortex—that in the capsular pocket and that normally situated—is about normal (Fig. 18).

Sometimes seen attached to the capsule are wedge-shaped foci of small, plump spindle cells with hyperchromatic nuclei. These protrude into the cortex to varying depths and are sometimes present bilaterally (Fig. 19). The cells are arranged in interlacing bundles and whorls. Largely because of their light microscopic resemblance to ovarian cortical

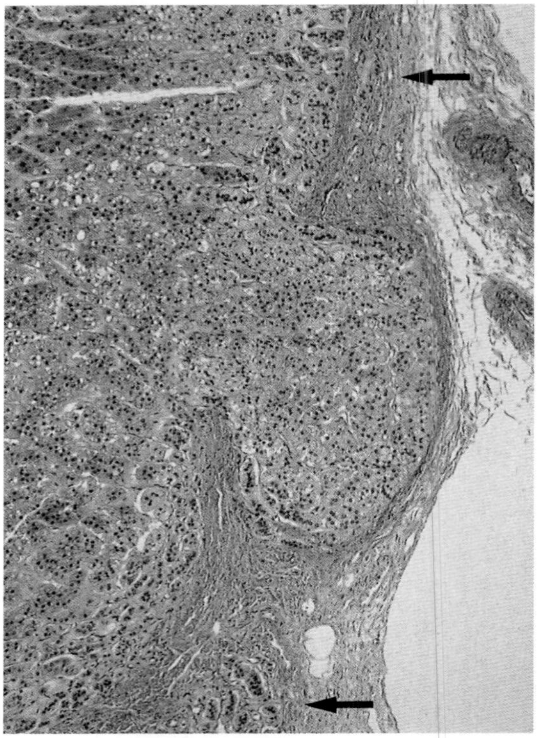

**FIG. 17.** Normal adrenal gland. Protrusion of cortical cells surrounded by attenuated capsule through a "wide" defect in the adrenal capsule. A few cortical cells in rows and small aggregates are present in the capsule (*arrows*). A suggestive zona glomerulosa is present deep to the adrenal capsule (*top*).

A

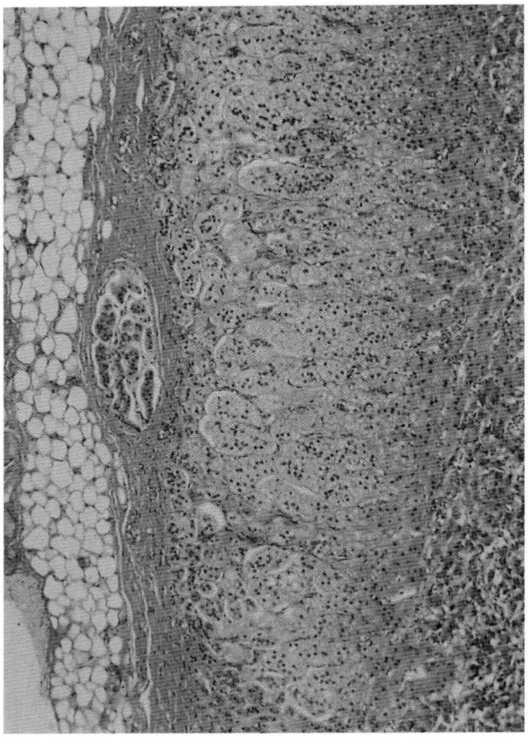

B

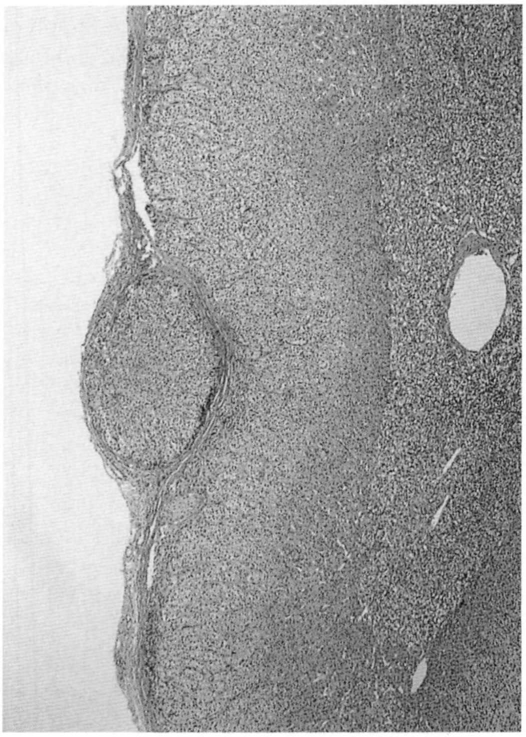

**FIG. 18.** Normal adrenal gland. **A:** Aggregate of cells with features of zona glomerulosa type in "pocket" of capsule. **B:** Cortex featuring zona fasciculata (clear cells) and zona reticularis (compact cells) envelops medulla. A larger aggregate of cortical cells with clear (peripheral) and compact cytoplasm (central) is present in a pocket in the capsule. The cortex deep to the pocket is slightly attenuated. A zona glomerulosa is not clearly visible.

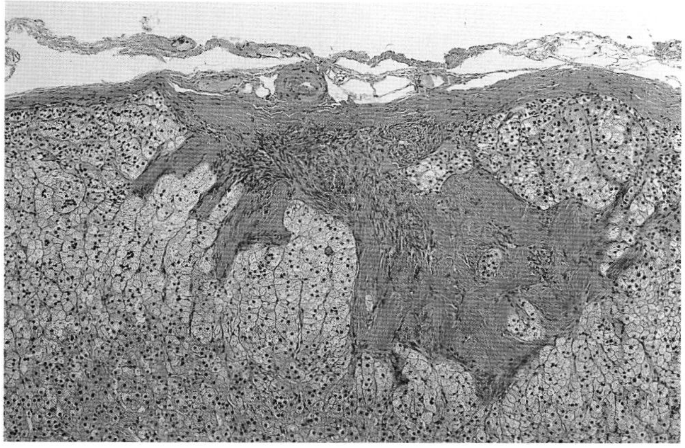

**FIG. 19.** Ovarian thecal metaplasia (63-year-old woman with a 2-cm aldosterone-producing adrenocortical adenoma). A group of packed spindle cells is attached to the adrenal capsule. Nests of cortical cells are trapped by hyalinized fibrous tissue. A poorly defined zona glomerulosa is present (*arrows*).

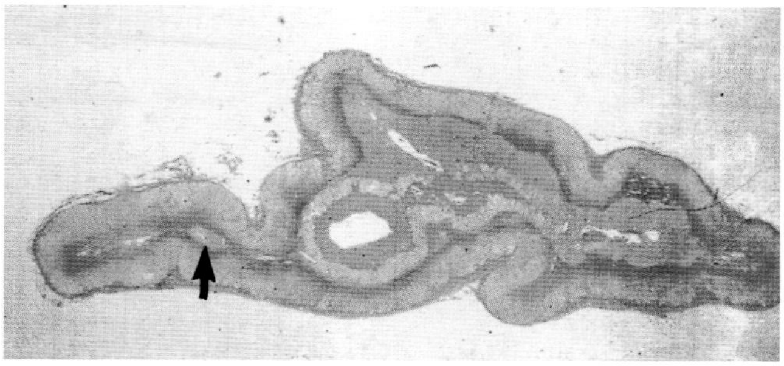

**FIG. 20.** Normal adrenal gland. A thick capsule surrounds the adrenal cortex (outer clear zona fasciculata and inner eosinophilic zona reticularis) that encloses the basophilic adrenal medulla. An area of medulla in the ala (*arrow*) is not in continuity with the main mass of medulla. The adrenal vein is surrounded by a cuff of invaginated cortex.

A

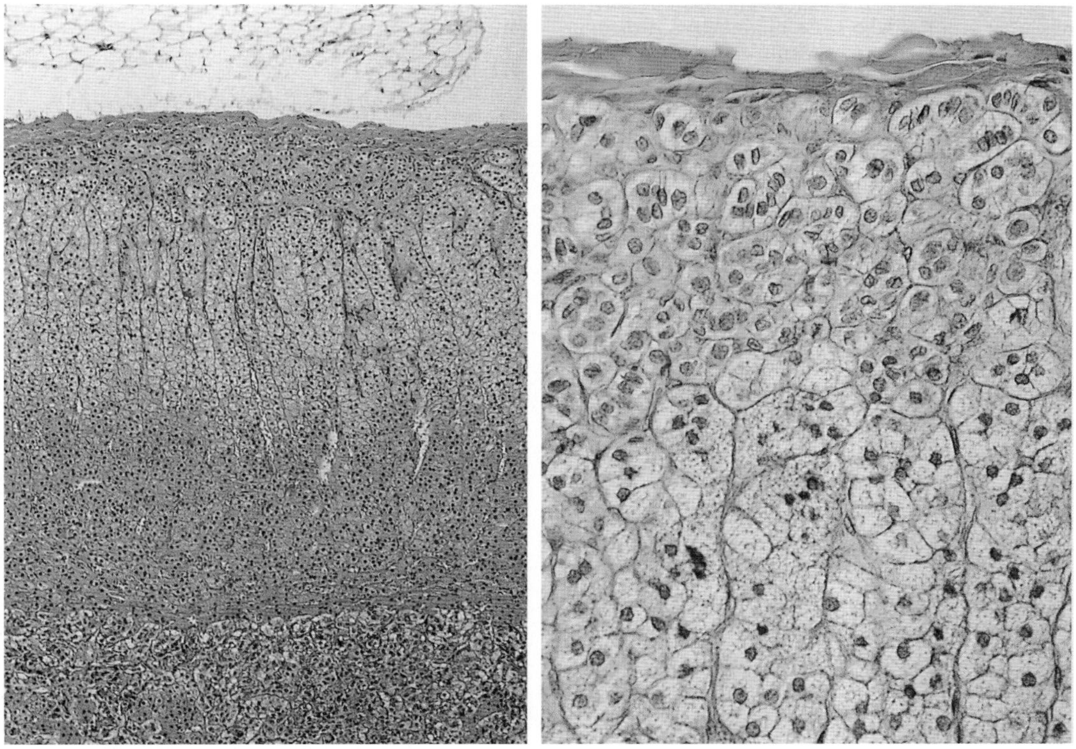

B

**FIG. 21.** Normal adrenal gland. **A:** The normal pattern of zonation of the cortex is seen (clusters of cells with stainable cytoplasm in the zona glomerulosa, columns of cells with clear cytoplasm in the zona fasciculata, and cells with acidophilic cytoplasm in the zona reticularis). There is a sharp interface between the cortex (zona reticularis) and medulla (clusters of cells with basophilic cytoplasm). **B:** Zona glomerulosa composed of packed clusters and short trabeculae of cells beneath the adrenal capsule and superficial to the columns of vacuolated cells of the zona fasciculata. The zona glomerulosa nuclei tend to be oval; those of the zona fasciculata are round.

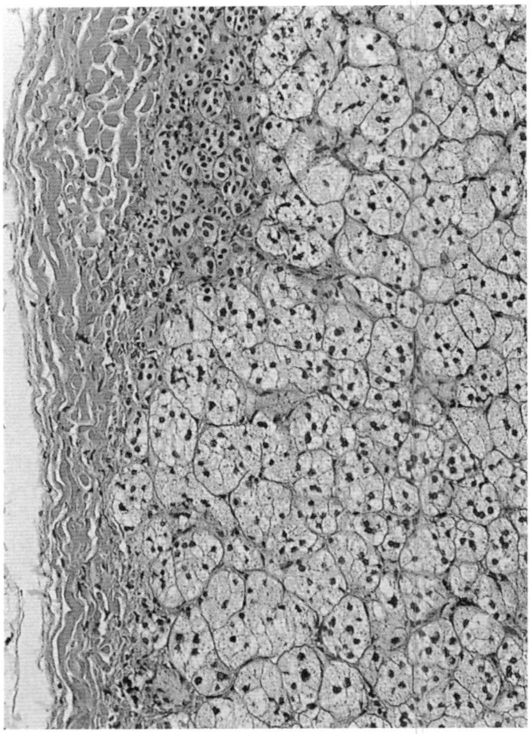

**FIG. 22.** Normal adrenal cortex with discontinuity of zona glomerulosa. Zona glomerulosa (*upper half*) composed of clusters of cells with amphophilic cytoplasm forms a distinct band beneath the capsule and is sharply demarcated from the deeper zona fasciculata with its clustered cells having clear cytoplasm. Where the zona glomerulosa is absent (*lower half*), the zona fasciculata extends to the capsule.

stroma, these aggregates have been termed "ovarian thecal metaplasia"; an alternative interpretation is that they represent areas of adrenocortical blastema that for unknown reasons have failed to mature (6–8). These foci undergo fibrosis, hyalinization, and sometimes calcification. Nests of cortical cells are occasionally found in the spindle cell proliferation, presumably entrapped. Exceptionally, the proliferations penetrate into the medulla as increasingly narrow tongues of tissue. Ovarian thecal metaplasia is said to occur in postmenopausal women, occasionally in premenopausal women, and exceptionally in old men. I have not seen it in any of the normal adrenal glands I have examined despite a good search. However, I have encountered it fairly commonly in the extratumoral cortex associated with a range of functioning adrenocortical adenomas and in adrenals removed for other pathology, cortical and medullary, always in perimenopausal or postmenopausal females. The "lesions" are generally incidental microscopic findings that were not recognized grossly.

## Cortex

Traditionally, the cortex has been divided into three areas based on light microscopy findings from the capsule inward—the zona glomerulosa, the zona fasciculata, and the zona reticularis—forming the typical zonation pattern of the adrenal cortex (Fig. 20). The functional significance of this morphologic separation is questionable, but the zona glomerulosa is the site of aldosterone production and is responsive to angiotensin and potassium, and the zona fasciculata and zona reticularis synthesize glucocorticoids and sex hormones. Cells of all zones respond to adrenocorticotrophic hormone (ACTH). Recent studies using monoclonal antibodies have shown some differential staining of the normal human cortical parenchyma (9). Division figures are rare in the normal cortex; in fact, the zone(s) of normal proliferation for replacement of effete cells is not known, although it is believed to be near the periphery of the cortex. [Under the influence of increased circulating levels of ACTH (Cushing's disease), mitotic figures may be seen in the zona fasciculata and zona reticularis, indicating that cells in the deeper areas of the cortex are also capable of proliferating.]

A number of modern techniques for studying cell proliferation and programmed cell death (apoptosis), specifically, KI-67 immunostaining and the recently developed 3′-OH nick end-labeling method, respectively, have been applied to study of the human adrenal cortex (10). Cell proliferation as indicated by KI-67 immunoreactivity occurred principally in the zona fasciculata. Cortical cells positive for nick end labeling (apoptotic) were uniformly present in the zona reticularis and in the zona glomerulosa in one third of cases. The findings suggest that cortical cells may disperse in two di-

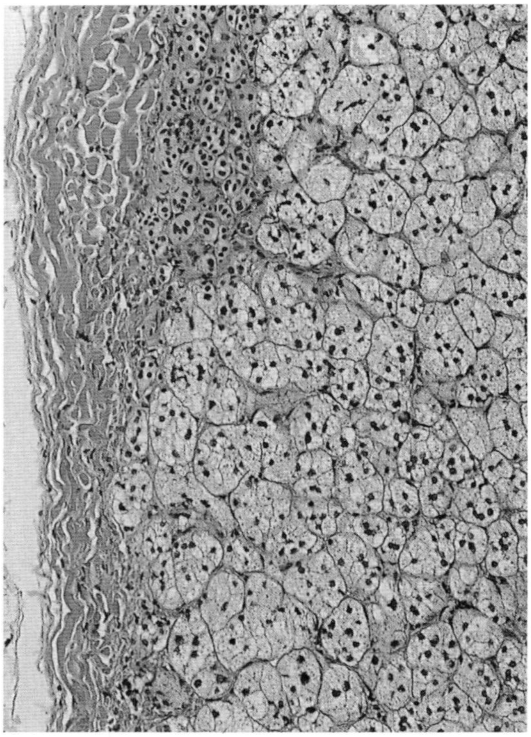

**FIG. 23.** Normal adrenal cortex. Zona fasciculata (*upper*) features two-cell wide columns of cells with clear cytoplasm, and zona reticularis (*lower*) consists of cells having acidophilic granular cytoplasm that do not form a distinct pattern. Nuclei are vesicular, and nucleoli are small.

rections, centripetally and centrifugally, from the zona fasciculata to the zona reticularis and from the zona fasciculata to the zona glomerulosa, in some cases. Biochemically, apoptosis features chromatin cleavage. Morphologically, there is shrinkage of cytoplasm, condensation, and fragmentation of nuclei and membrane blebbing. Adrenocortical cells undergoing apoptosis are believed to be phagocytosed by histiocytes and cells lining the sinusoids.

Nucleolar organizer regions, loops of ribosomal DNA that appear to be an indicator of cellular and nuclear activity, have been studied to a limited degree in the human adrenal cortex, using a silver technique and formalin-fixed paraffin-embedded tissue (11).

## Zona Glomerulosa

The zona glomerulosa is the narrow, inconstant band of cortex situated immediately beneath the capsule and superficial to the zona fasciculata (Fig. 21). Sometimes it can be identified throughout a section or over a large portion of one as a distinct rim beneath the capsule; more often it cannot. Where it is deficient, the zona fasciculata extends to the capsule (Fig. 22). The zone is often easier to identify in autopsy preparations. In routine hematoxylin and eosin (H&E) preparations, the band may merge with and be separated with difficulty from the outer cells of the zona fasciculata.

The zona glomerulosa cells are well outlined and aggregated into small clusters that are supported by a minimal amount of fibrovascular stroma (Fig. 21). The clusters occasionally merge into short trabeculae, straight, bent, or hairpin shape. The cells that tend to be columnar also occur in short cords or one-cell rows set parallel to the capsule. The cytoplasm is faintly acidophilic or amphophilic and minimally to distinctly vacuolated. The round nuclei sometimes are indistinguishable from those of the other zones of the cortex, but often they appear slightly smaller and more deeply staining. Commonly, they are ellipsoidal and elongated and display a longitudinal groove, a nuclear configuration not seen in the deeper areas of the cortex (Fig. 21). The nucleocytoplasmic ratio is high.

## Zona Fasciculata

The zona fasciculata is a broad band, more than half the thickness of the cortex, that lies between the zona glomerulosa (superficial) and the zona reticularis (deep) (Figs. 20, 21, and 23). The transition between the zones is not sharp. The zona fasciculata cells are large, have distinct cell membranes, are arranged in two-cell wide cords, with the cord axes perpendicular to capsule, and bounded laterally by par-

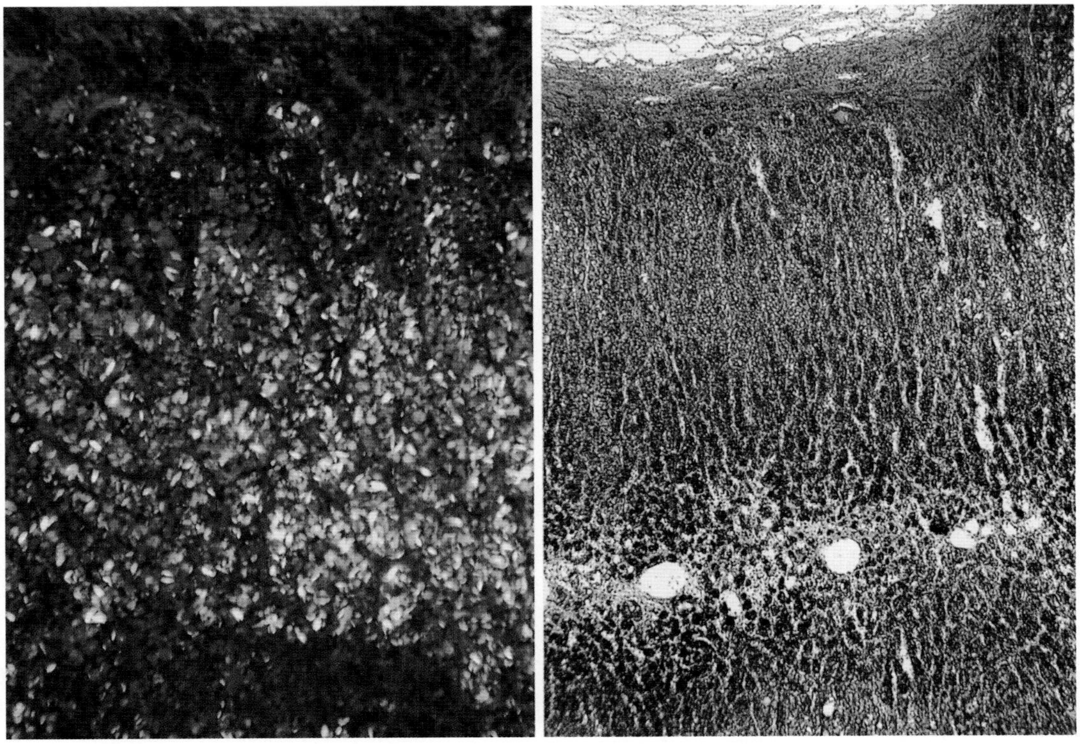


**FIG. 24.** Normal adrenal cortex. **A:** Partial polarization shows high lipid content of zona fasciculata and low content of zona glomerulosa (*above*) and zona reticularis (*below*). **B:** Fresh frozen section of adrenal cortex stained with polychrome methylene blue. One complete band of cortex and portion of another (*below*) is seen; the junction point between the two is located by the dilated sinusoidal tributaries of the central adrenal vein. Zona fasciculata cells are packed with lipid globules. There are fewer globules in the zona glomerulosa (beneath the adrenal capsule) and in the zona reticularis (on either side of the sinusoidal vessels).

allel-running capillaries. The nuclei are more vesicular and less chromatic than those of the zona glomerulosa, feature a single small nucleolus, and are central in the cells. Especially in the outer two thirds of the zone, the cells are filled with lipid (cholesterol, fatty acids, and neutral fat), much of which is birefringent (Fig. 24). Because this lipid is dissolved with the usual technical procedures, the fasciculata cells have a spongy, vacuolated, clear appearance and are often referred to as clear cells. When frozen sections are stained with a vital dye or stained for fat, the large amount of intracellular lipid can be appreciated (Fig. 24). The yellow color of the zone seen grossly is due to this high lipid content.

### Zona Reticularis

The zona reticularis lies deep to the zona fasciculata, and in the head and body of the gland abuts on the medulla (Figs. 9, 20, 21, and 23). In the tail of the gland, where there is no medulla, the zona reticularis is in contact with zona reticularis or separated from zona reticularis by venous sinusoids and connective tissue stroma. It constitutes approximately one quarter of the thickness of the cortex. Zona reticularis cells are arranged in a spongelike meshwork of gently buckled anastomosing one-cell wide rows of cells that are separated by dilated capillaries. The well-outlined cells are smaller than those of the zona fasciculata and have cytoplasm that is granular, acidophilic, and relatively lipid sparse. The cytoplasm is sometimes referred to as "compact" and the reticularis cells as "compact cells." The deepest cells adjacent to the medulla usually contain yellow lipochrome pigment (lipofuscin), diffusely distributed as coarse granules in the cytoplasm or localized in a single body (Fig. 25). The yellow pigmentation of the cytoplasm extends outward into the reticularis for a variable distance. The solid granular eosinophilic cytoplasm and the lipochrome pigment combine to produce the dark brown coloration of the zone seen on cut surface of a fresh or formalin-fixed gland.

### Accessory (Heterotopic) Adrenal

The adrenocortical primordium initially is unencapsulated and develops, as has been mentioned, close to the emerging gonad. Therefore, it is not surprising that (a) some cells of the unencapsulated adrenocortical primordium may become associated with and migrate alongside the gonad (testis or ovary) to be found postnatally distant from the adrenal in the path of gonad descent and (b) cortical cells not sequestered by adrenal capsule formation are subsequently found in the retroperitoneal fat close to the adrenal glands. In practice, accessory adrenocortical tissue is most often encountered around the adrenal glands themselves (Fig. 26); it also occurs in the inguinal region and around the ovary, fallopian tube, epididymis, and rete testis. Microscopically, accessory cortex shows normal zonation and responds to ACTH. Rarely does it contain medulla (Fig. 26).

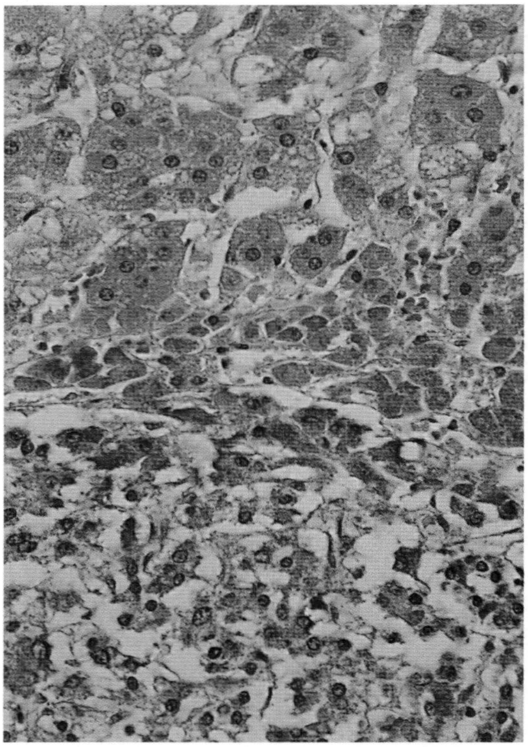

**FIG. 25.** Corticomedullary junction. The zona reticularis of the cortex (*upper*) is sharply demarcated from the medulla (*lower*). The deepest cells of the zona reticularis contain granular yellowish pigment (*lipofuscin*).

### Adrenocortical Nodules

Adrenocortical nodules, roughly spherical, uncapsulated areas of hypertrophic and hyperplastic cortical cells, are not regarded as true neoplasms. They range in size from microscopic to grossly obvious lesions (12). Before the fourth decade of life, they are rare; thereafter, they are encountered with increasing frequency. Although regarded by some as an aging phenomenon, they are not invariably found in older individuals. Usually, multiple nodules commonly consist of large, lipid-laden clear cells; some nodules are composed of clear and compact cells; a minority feature reticularis-type cells only (Fig. 27). The smallest nodules may be found at any level of the cortex, but usually they occur in the zona fasciculata. Initially, they appear to be the result of hypertrophy of contiguous cells in three or more adjacent cords. The smallest ill-defined nodules thus have the cord structure of the parent tissue. As they enlarge further due to cell proliferation, this organized appearance is lost, and larger nodules are patternless. Large nodules cause compression and distortion of the surrounding cortex.

### Medulla

The medulla is situated in the interior of the organ in the head and body of the gland, deep to the zona reticularis (Figs.

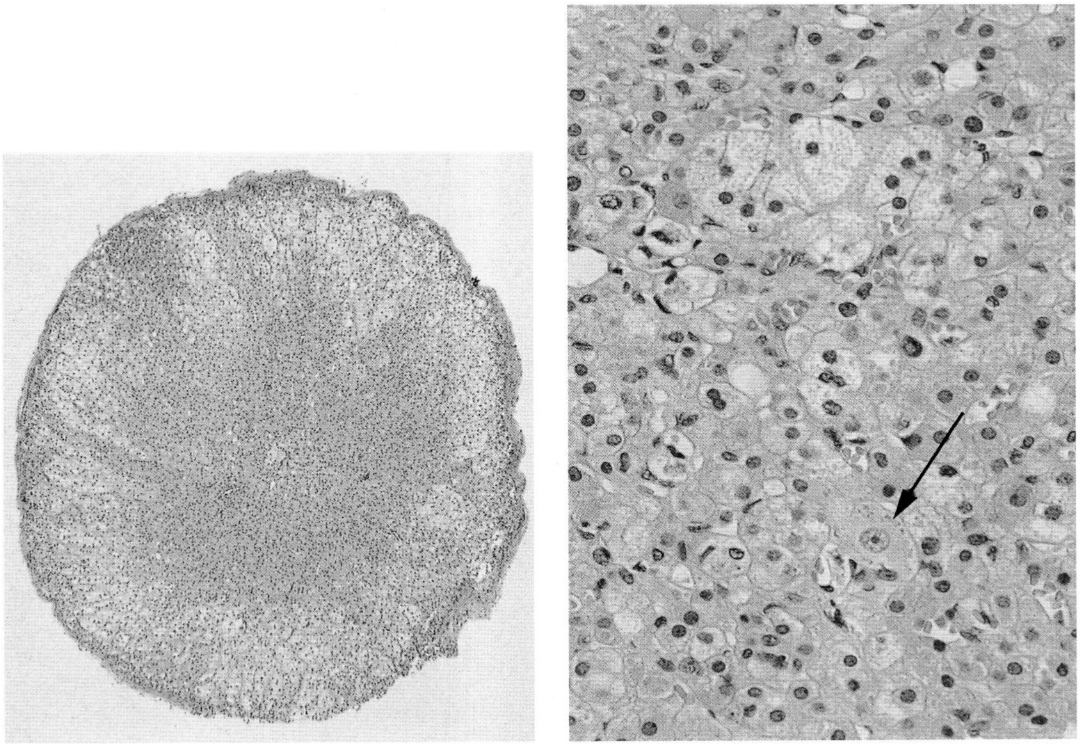

A B

**FIG. 26.** Accessory adrenal cortex in retroperitoneal fat. **A:** Normal zonation is suggested by the narrow rim of cells with clear cytoplasm that surrounds the main mass of cells with light eosinophilic cytoplasm. **B:** Ganglion cell (*arrow*) indicating presence of medulla among cortical "clear" and "compact" cells. The latter contain lipofuscin.

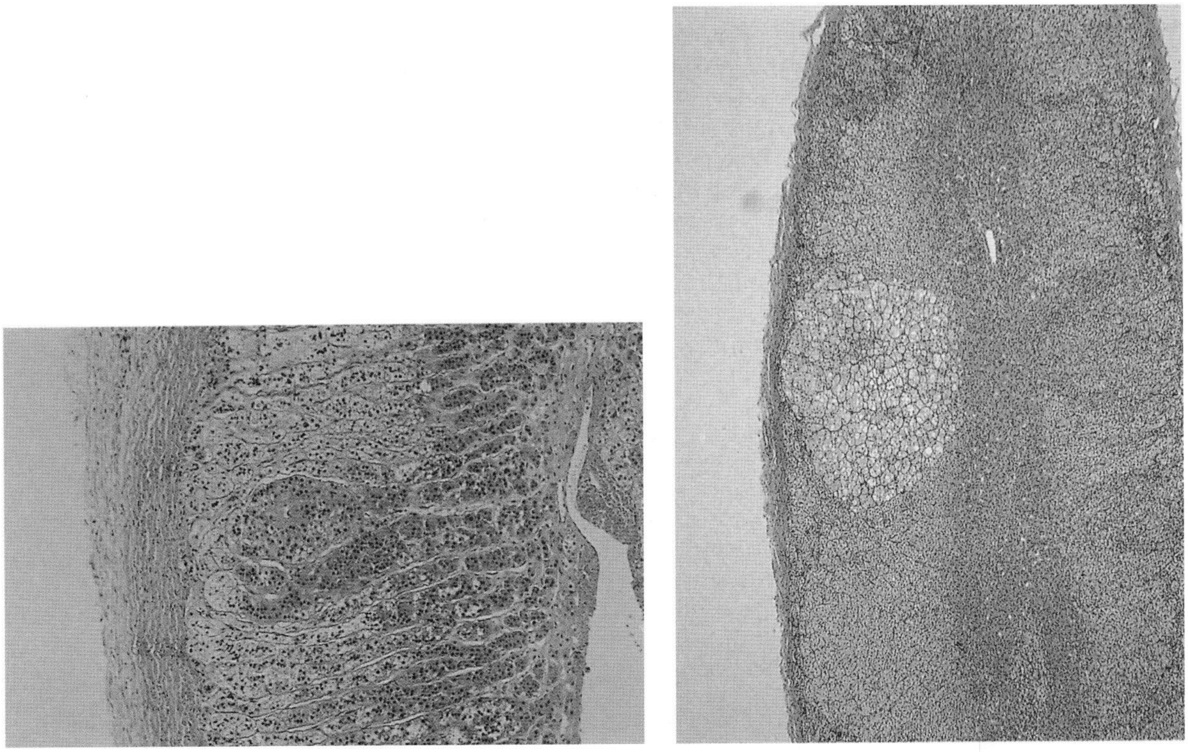

A B

**FIG. 27.** Cortical nodules (36-year-old man). **A:** Suggestive nodule in the mid-cortex. **B:** Distinct nodule composed of clear cells in outer cortex.

9 and 20). Its area and weight are one tenth those of the cortex (1,3). The medulla rarely measures more than 2 mm in thickness. Because of the different staining of cells of the two tissues—acidophilia in zona reticularis and basophilia in the medulla—the interface between cortex and medulla is readily visible on low-power microscopic examination. The junction is sharp, with no or minimal intervening connective tissue, leaving cortical and medullary cells in direct contact (Figs. 20 and 25).

The medulla extends to a variable extent into the crest of the gland (the ridge on the posterior surface) and into one or both of the alae (Fig. 20). Areas of the medulla in the alae are not necessarily in direct continuity with the main mass of the medulla around the central veins. The medulla sometimes extends into the tail of the gland. The finding of medulla in this location therefore does not automatically equate with pathologic abnormality—specifically, medullary hyperplasia. Very occasionally, a narrow tongue of medulla accompanied by a vessel or nerve or unaccompanied extends through the cortex to contact the capsule of the gland.

The medulla for practical purposes is composed of a single cell population, the pheochromocytes (medullary or chromaffin cells) (Fig. 28). Among the dominant population are scattered small groups of cortical cells and clusters and individual ganglion cells (Fig. 29). Not uncommonly, the ganglion cells feature cytoplasmic, round, lightly acidophilic, hyaline bodies, with concentrically arranged fibrillar appearance, up to 30 $\mu$m in diameter (Fig. 30). Sometimes these bodies appear to be external to the ganglionic cytoplasm but indent it; in immunostain preparations (vimentin and S-100) they are separated from it by a small amount of cytoplasm. It is unusual to observe these bodies in

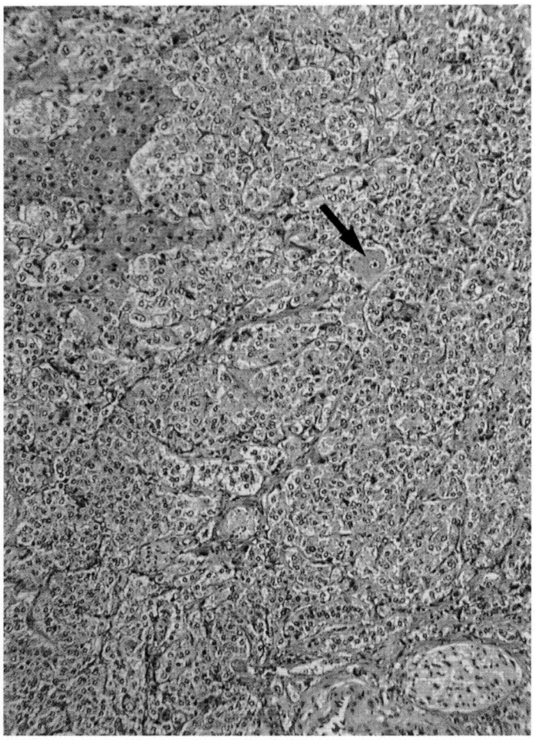

**FIG. 29.** Normal adrenal medulla. Pheochromocytes are arranged in poorly delineated clusters. An irregularly shaped group of cortical cells (upper left) and an isolated ganglion cell (*arrow*) are present.

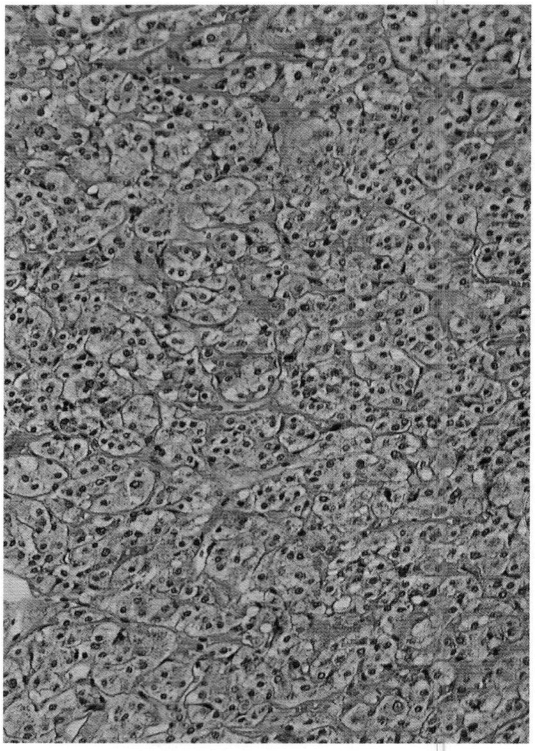

**FIG. 28.** Normal adrenal medulla. Clusters of poorly outlined cells with basophilic cytoplasm are separated by a vascularized supporting stroma. There is some variation in nuclear size and shape.

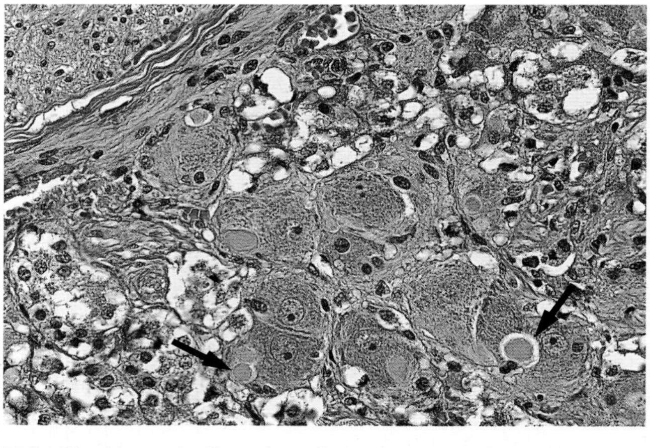

**FIG. 30.** Normal adrenal medulla. A group of ganglion cells demarcated by pheochromocytes (*upper right and lower left*) and a nerve (*upper left*). A number of the ganglion cells feature cytoplasmic acidophilic bodies, some outlined by a rim of retracted cytoplasm (*arrows*). There are two such bodies in one cell.

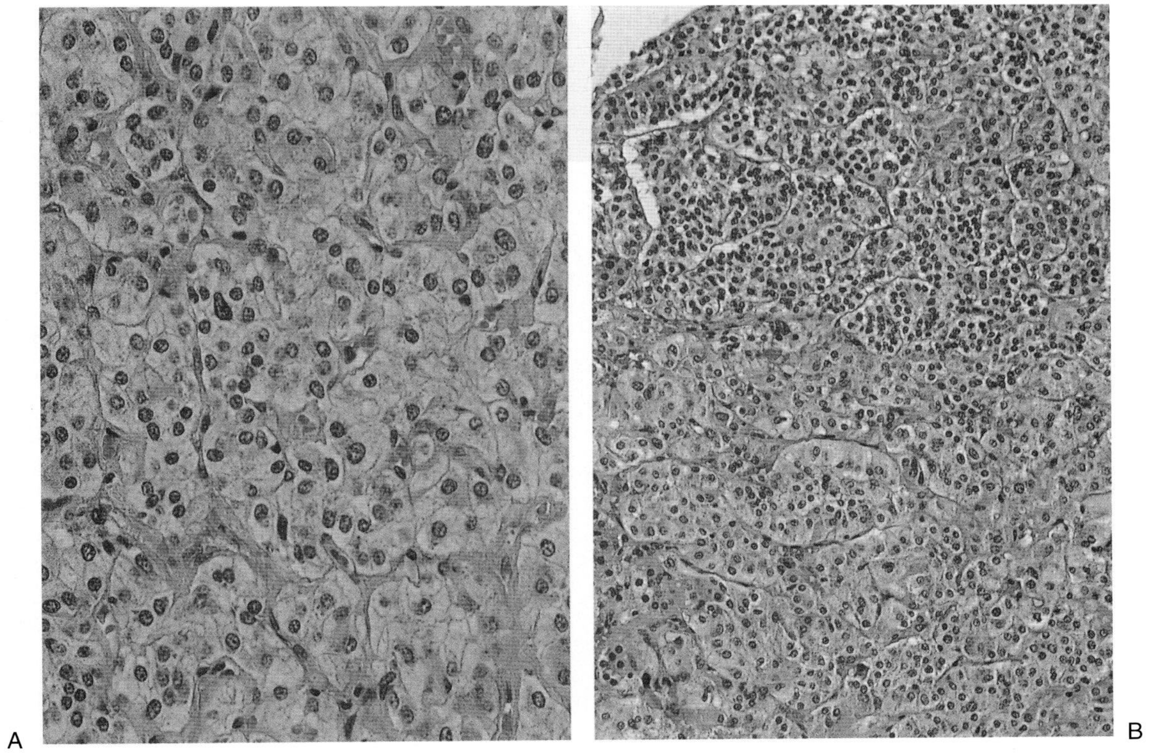

FIG. 31. Normal adrenal medulla. **A:** Pheochromocytes arranged in trabecular pattern outlined by a delicate vascular supporting stroma. **B:** Sustentacular cells identified by S-100 immunostain that also highlights two nerves.

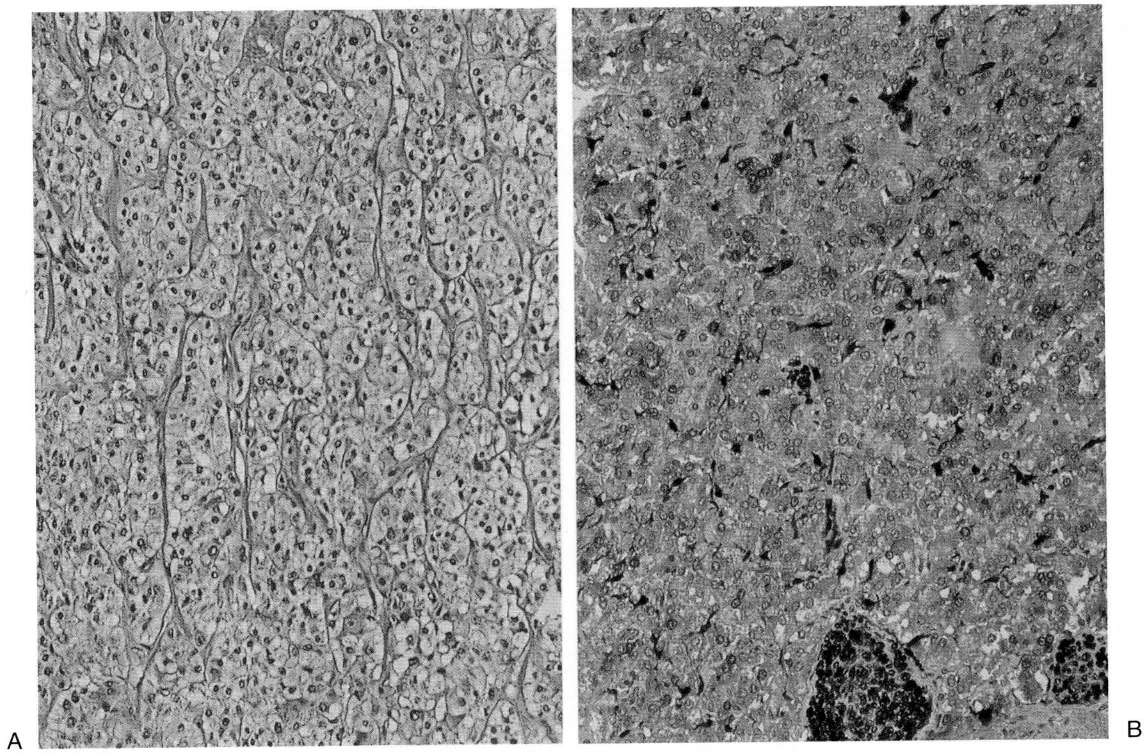

FIG. 32. Normal adrenal medulla. **A:** Pheochromocytes arranged in vague clusters. Cell outlines are visible here and there. Nuclear variation in size and shape is typical. The nuclear chromatin is coarsely clumped and often marginated at the nuclear membrane. **B:** Variation in cell size, nuclear size, and cell pattern.

ganglion cells outside the adrenal medulla. Their nature has not been investigated. The pheochromocytes are arranged in tight clusters and short trabeculae, supported by delicate fibrovascular stroma (Figs. 28 and 31). Sustentacular cells at the periphery of the clusters and trabeculae are not seen in routine histologic preparations (13) but are readily demonstrated by immunostaining for S-100 protein (Fig. 32).

The pheochromocytes are moderately large cells, polygonal to columnar, and slightly to considerably larger than cortical cells. Poorly outlined, their complete cell borders are visible only occasionally. Although the cytoplasm of most medullary cells is basophilic and finely granular and occasionally vacuolated, sometimes it is amphophilic or slightly acidophilic, and rarely is it partly basophilic and partly acidophilic. The resulting variability and unevenness of medullary cytoplasmic staining and cytoplasmic vacuolization often impart an overall mottled light and dark appearance at intermediate magnification. A rare normal cell has one or more periodic acid-Schiff (PAS)-positive cytoplasmic colloid droplets (Fig. 33). The majority of the medullary cells are roughly similar in size, but occasionally standard-sized cells merge with groups of cells that are much smaller or much larger (Fig. 31).

The nuclei of medullary cells characteristically have slight but definite variability of size, shape, and location in the cell. Most pheochromocyte nuclei are slightly larger than those of cortical cells, but nuclei that are larger and smaller than the usual ones are common. The usual nucleus has a finely or coarsely clumped chromatin pattern with a relatively clear nuclear background (Fig. 31). The chromatin tends to be peripherally disposed and separated into irregular clumps. Larger nuclei often have a prominent eosinophilic nucleolus; smaller nuclei are deeply staining. A rare cell has two or more nuclei.

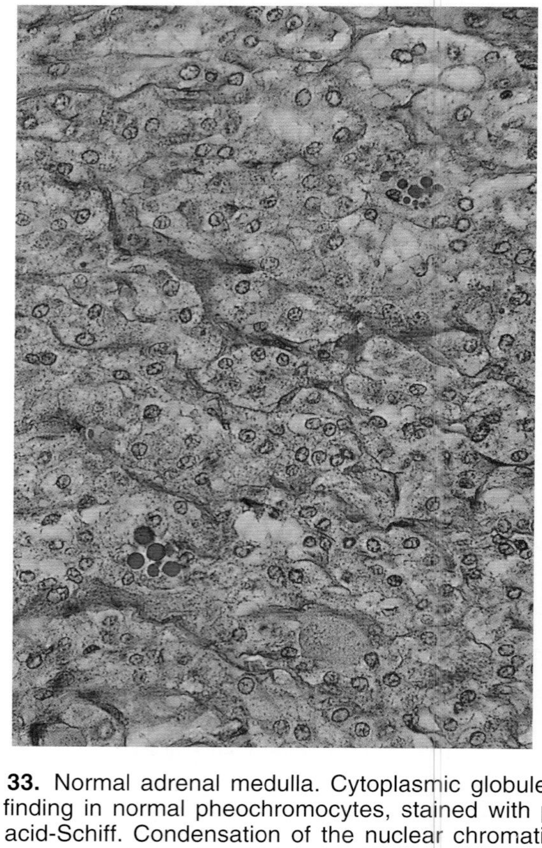

**FIG. 33.** Normal adrenal medulla. Cytoplasmic globules, a rare finding in normal pheochromocytes, stained with periodic acid-Schiff. Condensation of the nuclear chromatin at the nuclear membrane is well demonstrated.

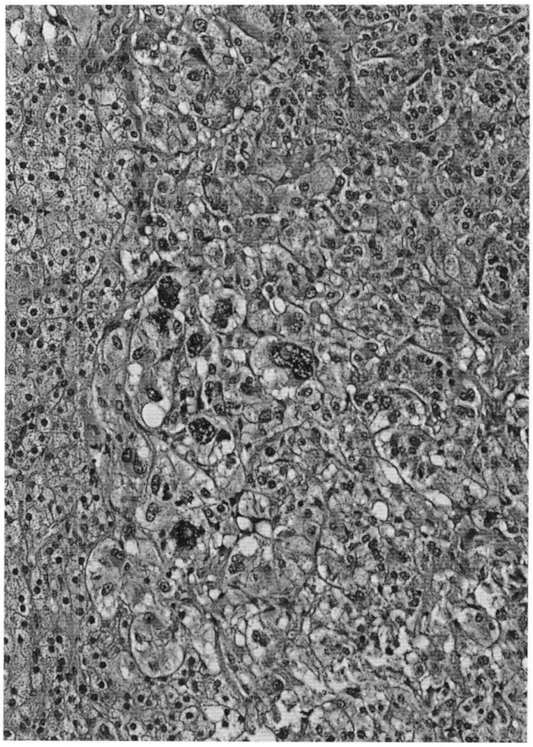

**FIG. 34.** Normal adrenal medulla. Pheochromocyte nuclear atypia at the corticomedullary junction. The number of atypical pheochromocyte nuclei crowded together here is unusual; ordinarily, the atypical nuclei are seen one to a medium-power field. The pheochromocytes have basophilic granular cytoplasm. The zona reticularis (*left*) features cells with granular eosinophilic cytoplasm and lipofuscin.

The nuclei exhibit slight but definite polymorphism. Most are spheroidal, but many are ellipsoidal, and some have other shapes. Large, intensely hyperchromatic and sometimes pleomorphic nuclei are common, usually single and located close to the corticomedullary junction (Fig. 34). The positions of the nuclei in the cells are not fixed; most are central, but some tend to be eccentric, located away from the vascular pole (Fig. 35).

The medullary cells have several distinctive histochemical reactions related to their content of secretory granules. The granules contain catecholamines, dihydroxy derivatives of tyrosine, that are converted to colored polymers by oxidizing agents such as potassium dichromate, ferric chloride, ammoniacal silver nitrate, and osmium tetroxide. The oxidized and polymerized derivatives are termed adrenochromes. This staining has been called the chromaffin reaction.

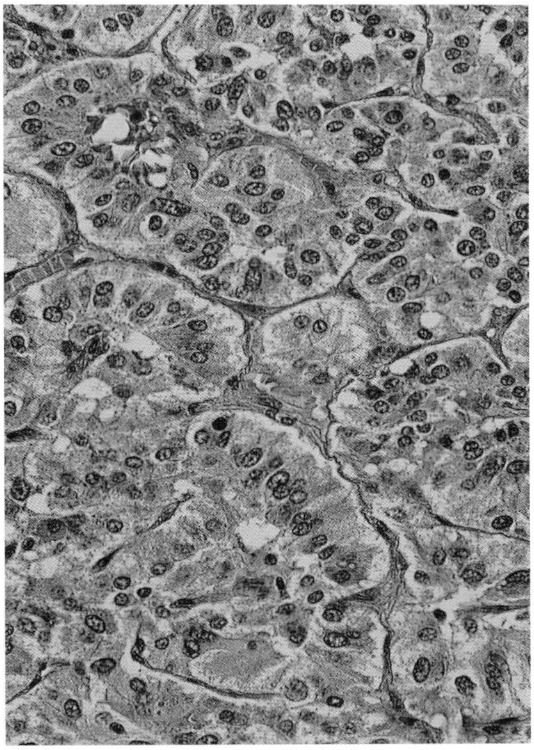

**FIG. 35.** Normal adrenal medulla. Uncommon pattern in which pheochromocytes are columnar in shape with nuclei that are ranged away from the vascular pole. The variations in size and shape of the nuclei are typical. Cytoplasmic staining is uneven and ranges from almost clear to basophilic and granular.

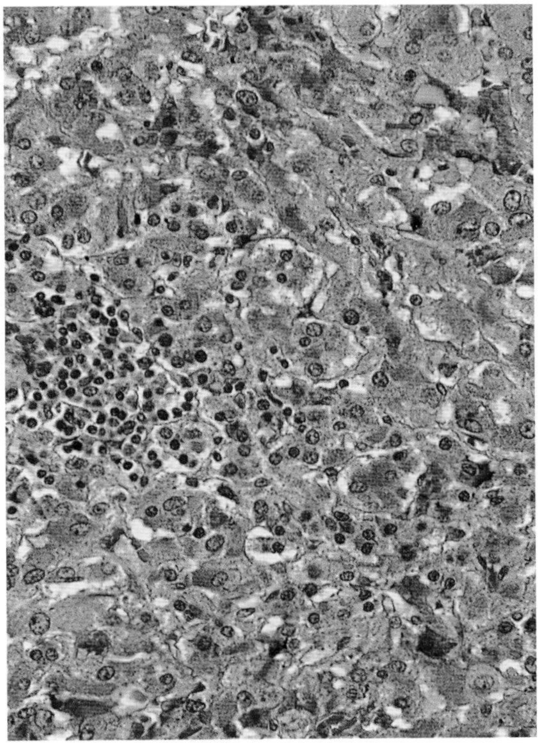

**FIG. 36.** Normal adrenal medulla. Aggregates of round cells, lymphocytes, and plasma cells are often encountered.

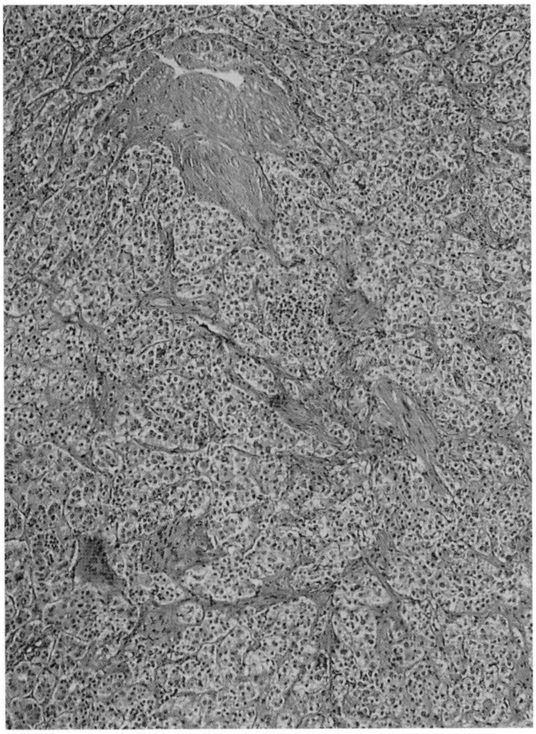

**FIG. 37.** Normal adrenal medulla. Bundles and strands of smooth muscle are derived from the smooth muscle of central veins.

Ganglion cells are scattered randomly among the pheochromocytes or in groups, often associated with a nerve (Fig. 29). Their number varies greatly from medulla to medulla; accordingly, they are found easily or not. Cortical cells also are a regular component of the medulla, found in irregularly shaped groups, sometimes in continuity with the zona reticularis, but more often not (Fig. 29).

Single or multiple small to large accumulations of round cells, plasma cells, and lymphocytes (positive for leukocyte common antigen), often paravascularly located, are common in the normal medulla (Fig. 36). They have no known significance. The delicate vascular stroma of the medulla is not conspicuous. Sometimes it is augmented focally by prolongations of the musculature of the central veins that separate groups of medullary cells (Fig. 37).

## IMMUNOCYTOCHEMISTRY

### Cortex

Cells of the normal adrenal cortex are reported to be immunoreactive against a cytokeratin cocktail and AE1 (14). In my experience, small groups of cells and isolated cells of the three zones have strong reactivity to low- and medium-molecular-weight keratin antibodies (CAM 5.2 and AE1, and MAK 6, respectively). Reactivity is greatest in the zona glomerulosa and external zona fasciculata, with some strongly reactive cells in the deep zona reticularis. The char-

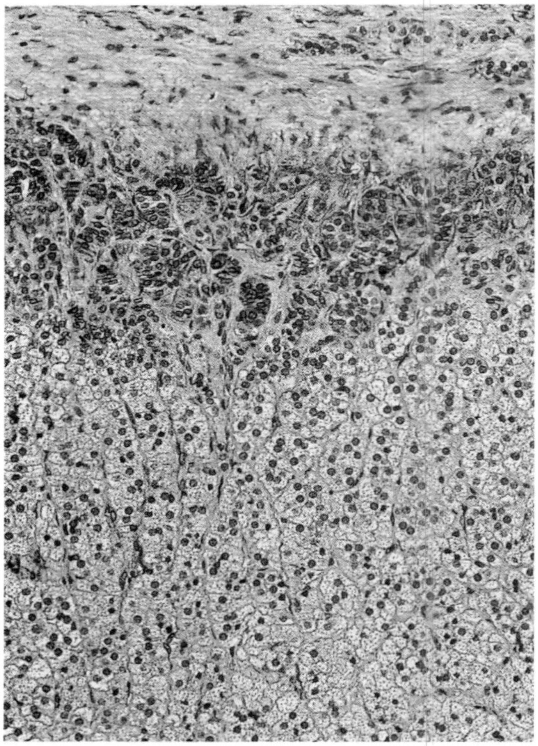

**FIG. 38.** Normal adrenal cortex. Zona glomerulosa stains positively for vimentin.

acter of the staining is variable, membranous, punctate cytoplasmic, diffuse cytoplasmic, and perinuclear, in decreasing order of frequency. There is weak staining to the keratin antibodies, often diffuse, in the zona reticularis. The zona glomerulosa is vimentin positive (Fig. 38). Cells of the three zones are variably synaptophysin positive. Cortical cells do not stain with epithelial membrane antigen, chromogranin, or S-100 antibodies.

### Medulla

Pheochromocytes stain with antibodies to chromogranin. The sustentacular cells that mantle the clusters and trabeculae of pheochromocytes are S-100 protein positive (Fig. 39), as are nerves in the medulla. Some pheochromocytes stain with S-100 antibodies.

## ULTRASTRUCTURE

### Cortex

There are ultrastructural features shared by the three layers of the cortex relating to their common function—synthesis of steroid hormones. The cells feature voluminous endoplasmic reticulum, stacks of rough endoplasmic reticulum, a well-developed Golgi apparatus, lysosomes, and many mitochondria. The distribution and internal structure of some of

A

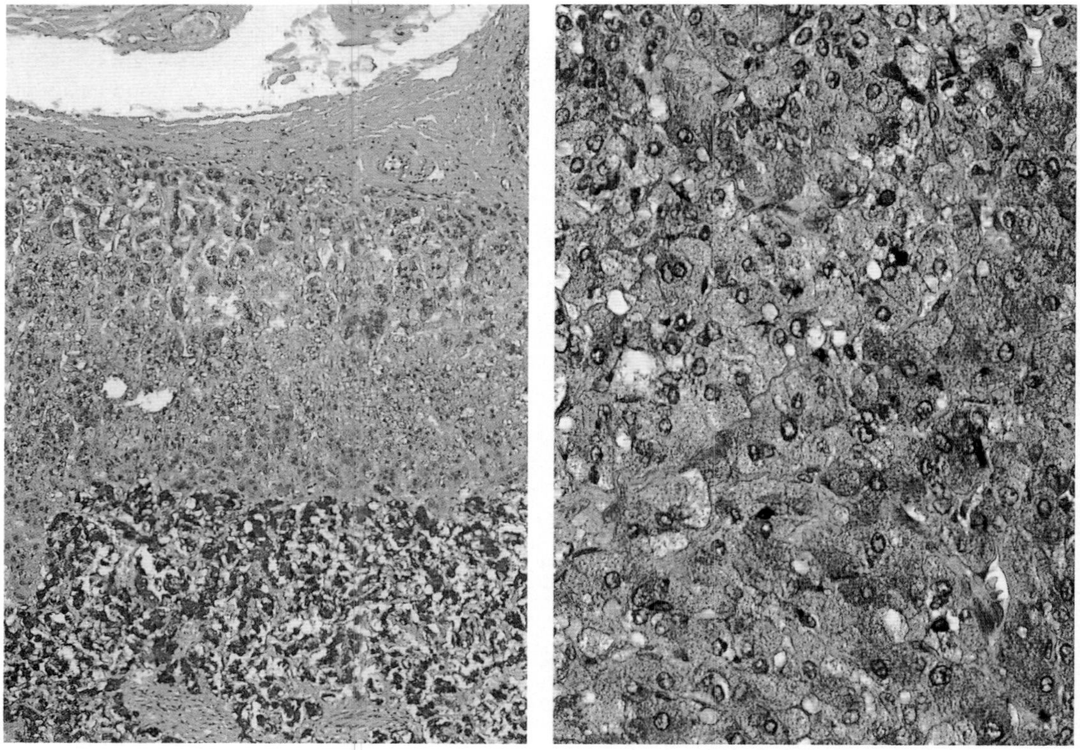

B

**FIG. 39.** Normal adrenal. **A:** Medulla (*below*) stains with chromogranin antibodies; cortex is unstained. **B:** Sustentacular cells and about one-half of the pheochromocytes are stained by S-100 protein antiserum.

the organelles (e.g., the mitochondria) vary from zone to zone. Using the electron microscope, the sometimes distinct transition seen between the zones when using the light microscope is not apparent, a gradual alteration from one organelle distribution and type to another being observed.

**Zona Glomerulosa**

Cells of the zona glomerulosa are columnar and have a round nucleus and prominent nucleolus (Fig. 40). The plasmalemma is simple except for folds and microvilli adjacent

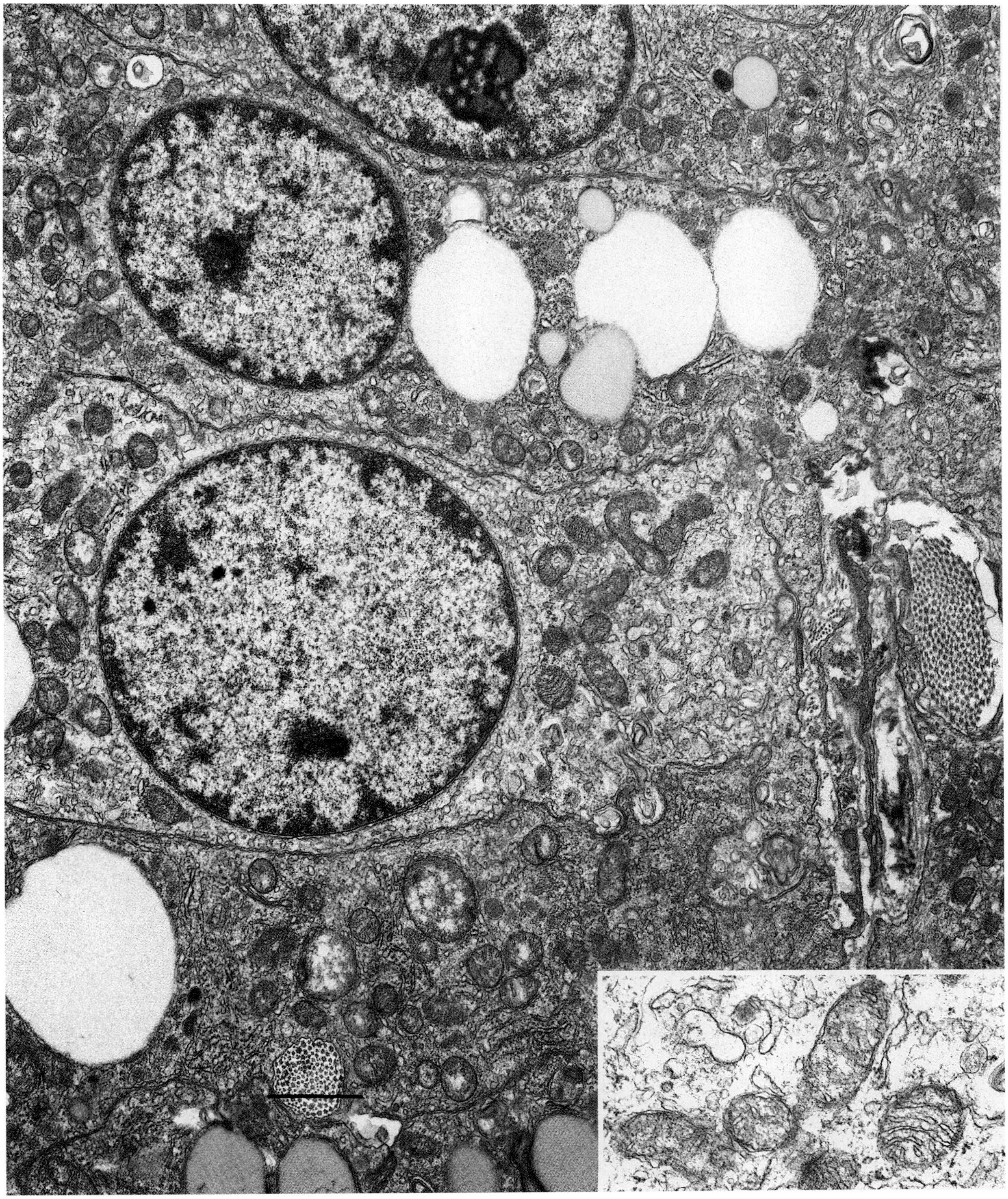

**FIG. 40.** Normal cortex. Electron micrograph of columnar zona glomerulosa cells. Cells contain some lipid. Mitochondria have lamellar pattern (*inset*). Bar = 10 $\mu$m.

to the subendothelial space, where there is also a basement lamina. The network of branching and anastomosing tubules of smooth endoplasmic reticulum is prominent. Rough endoplasmic reticulum is sparse. Mitochondria are round, oval, or elongate, with lamellar infolded cristae, resulting in a ladderlike internal structure, similar to that found in many other tissues (Fig. 40). Occasional lipid droplets are present, opaque or clear (content dissolved by processing), and often not membrane bound. The Golgi apparatus is well developed.

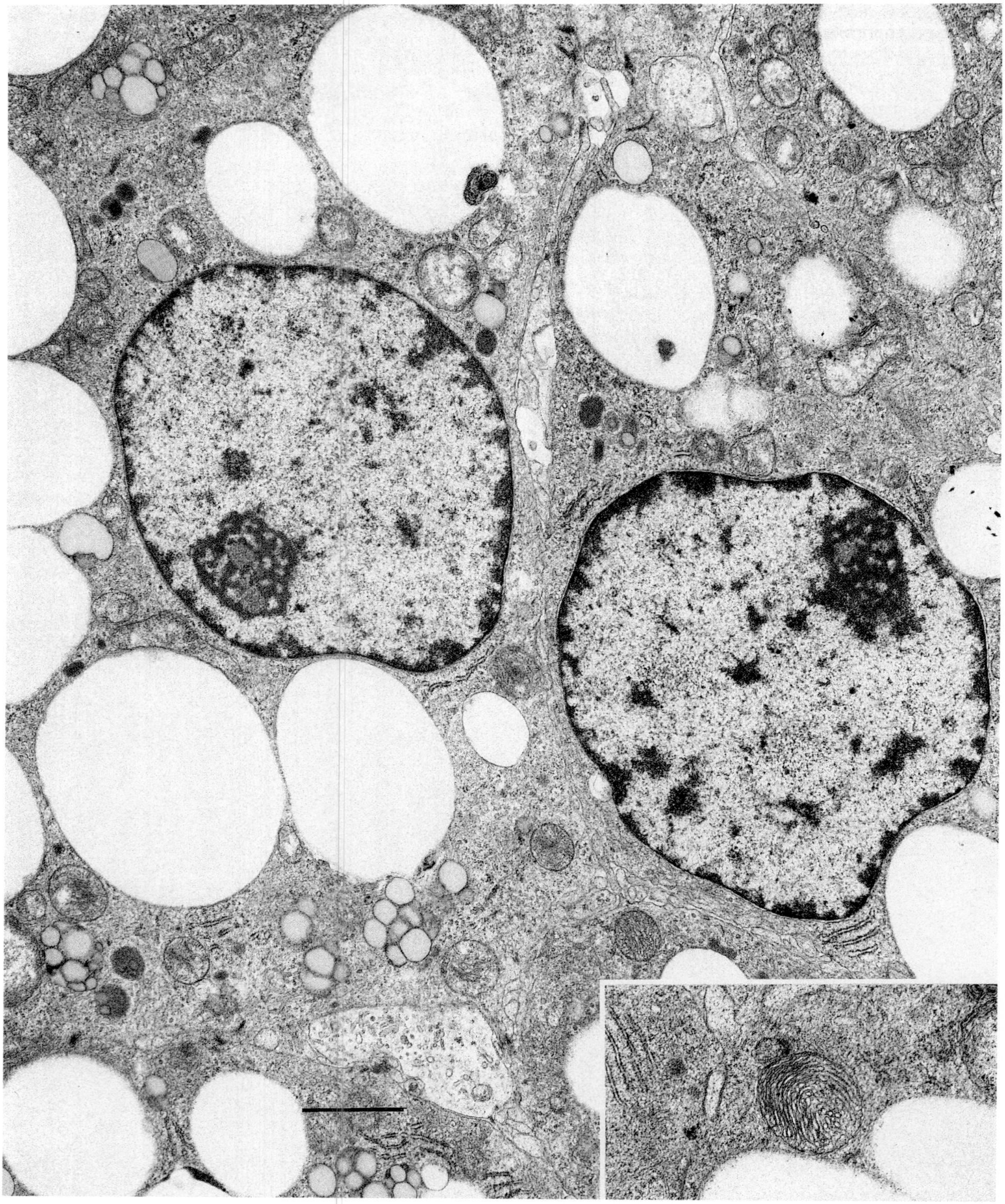

**FIG. 41.** Normal cortex. Electron micrograph of portions of four zona fasciculata cells. Lipid vacuoles are numerous and large. Mitochondria have a tubular and vesicular pattern (*inset*). Bar = 10 $\mu$m.

### Zona Fasciculata

Cells of the zona fasciculata are large, polyhedral, and have a striking amount of lipid (Fig. 41). The centrally located nucleus features peripheral condensation of chromatin. The arborizing and anastomosing tubules of the smooth endoplasmic reticulum are prominent and continuous with cisternae of rough endoplasmic reticulum. Mitochondria are large, spherical, and feature tubular cristae. Lipid droplets are large and numerous. Golgi apparatus, lysosomes, and

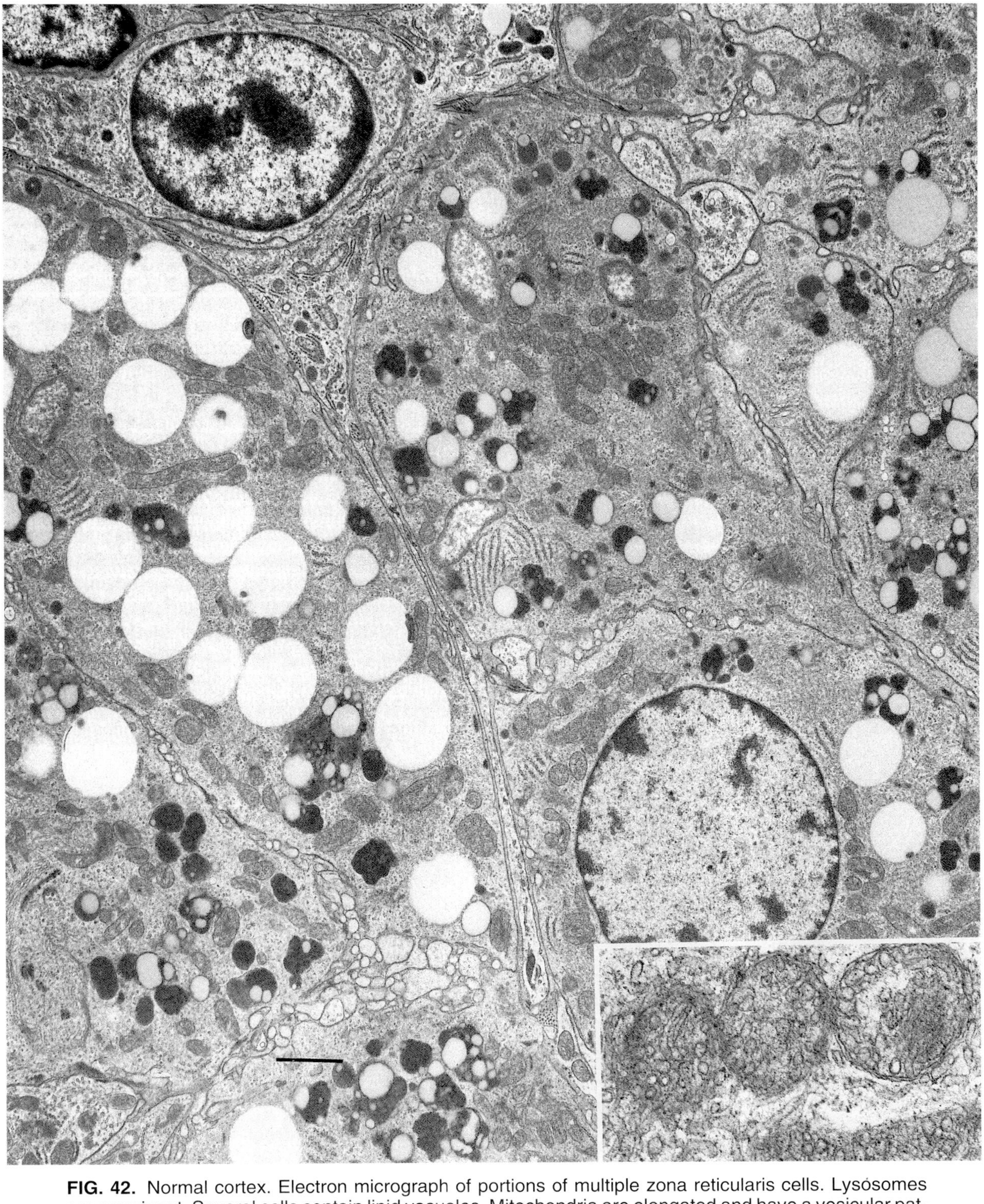

**FIG. 42.** Normal cortex. Electron micrograph of portions of multiple zona reticularis cells. Lysosomes are prominent. Several cells contain lipid vacuoles. Mitochondria are elongated and have a vesicular pattern (*inset*). Bar = 10 $\mu$m.

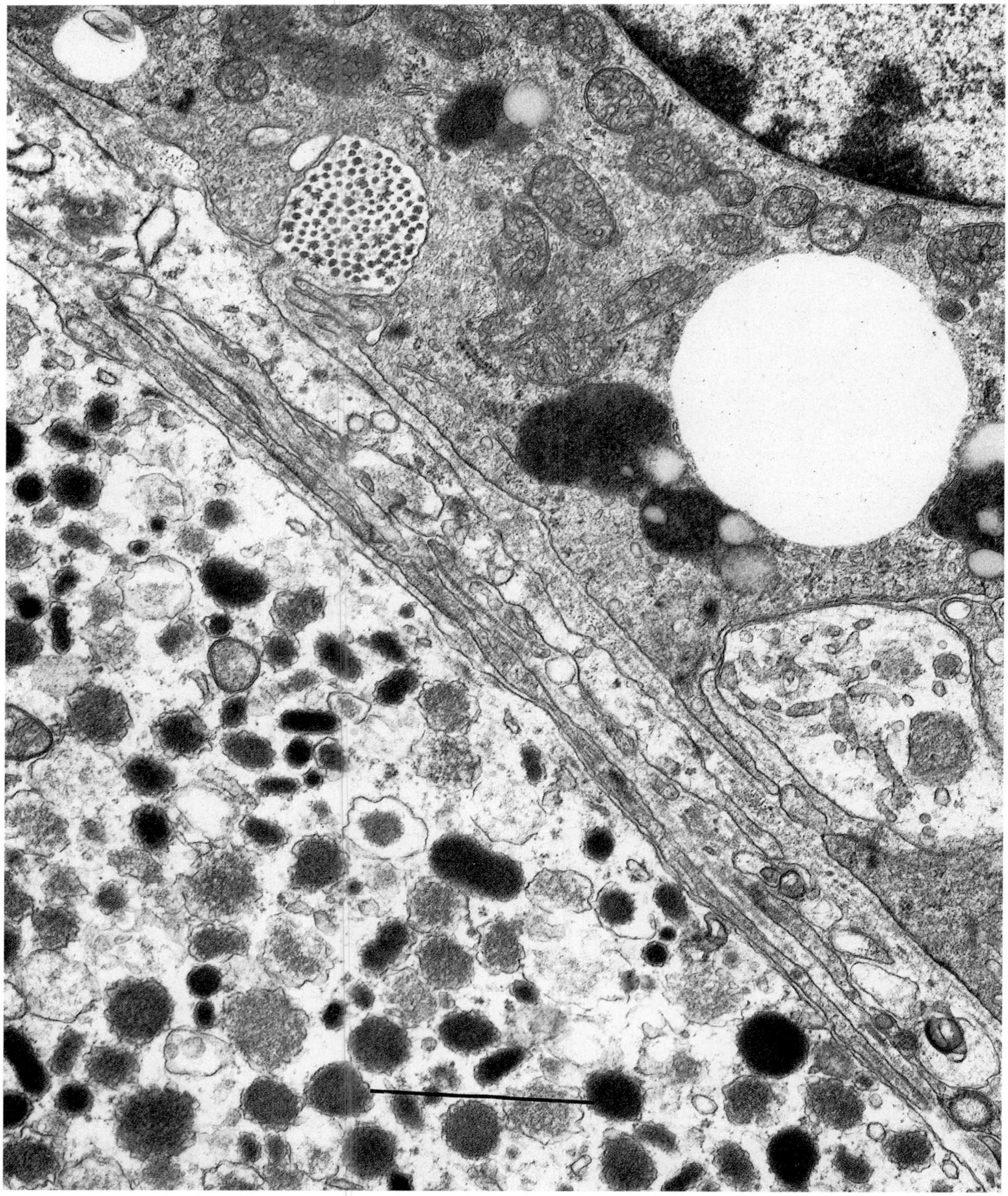

**FIG. 43.** Normal adrenal. Electron micrograph of corticomedullary junction. Microvilli of zona reticularis cells (*upper right*) are in contact with plasmalemma of pheochromocytes (*lower left*). Lysosomes are prominent in zona reticularis cells, and lipid vacuoles are also present. The pheochromocytes contain many membrane-limited granules. The content of the granules is variably electron dense and fills the majority of the sacs, findings consistent with epinephrine content. Bar = 1 $\mu$m.

lipofuscin granules are present. The latter are membrane-bound organelles with a moderately dense matrix that contains dense granules and clear lipid globules. Microvilli with associated basement lamina extend into the subendothelial space.

### Zona Reticularis

Cells of the zona reticularis exhibit many of the structures found in the zona fasciculata: smooth and rough endoplasmic reticulum, Golgi apparatus, free ribosomes, lipid droplets, and lysosomes (Fig. 42). Lipofuscin bodies are larger and more plentiful. The mitochondria tend to be more elongated and exhibit tubular and vesicular cristae that are a feature of steroid-producing cells. Glycogen is present.

### Medulla

Catecholamine-secreting cells dominate the medulla (Fig. 43). They are of two types distinguished by granule type. The polyhedral type of cells have a large round nucleus with one or two nucleoli. Microvilli are present focally on the cell surface. A large Golgi apparatus is present. A variety of organelles, mitochondria, lysosomes, vacuoles, and rough endoplasmic reticulum are distributed in the cell among the catecholamine granules. In tissue fixed in glutaraldehyde, norepinephrine granules are electron opaque, often located eccentrically within a dilated sac, and measure about 250 $\mu$m in diameter. Epinephrine granules measure about 190 $\mu$m in diameter, have a finely granular texture that is moderately dense but not opaque, and fill the enclosing membrane.

## REFERENCES


1. Quinan C, Berger AA. Observations on human adrenals with especial reference to the relative weight of the normal medulla. *Ann Intern Med* 1933;6:1180–1192.
2. Ekholm E, Niemineva K. On prenatal changes in the relative weights of the human adrenals, the thymus and the thyroid gland. *Acta Paediatr* 1950;39:67–86.
3. Symington T. *Functional pathology of the human adrenal gland.* Baltimore: Williams & Wilkins; 1969.
4. Keene MFL. Observations on the development of the human suprarenal gland. *J Anat* 1927;61:302–324.
5. Crowder RE. The development of the adrenal gland in man with special reference to origin and ultimate location of cell types and evidence in favour of the "cell migration" theory. *Carnegie Inst Contrib Embryol* 1957;251:193–210.
6. Reed RJ, Patrick JT. Nodular hyperplasia of the adrenal cortical blastema. *Bull Tulane Univ Med Faculty* 1967;26:151–157.
7. Wong T-A, Werner NE. Ovarian thecal metaplasia in the adrenal gland. *Arch Pathol* 1971;92:319–328.
8. Fidler WJ. Ovarian thecal metaplasia in adrenal glands. *Am J Clin Pathol* 1977;67:318–323.
9. Backlin C, Juhlin C, Grimelius L, Wiberg K, Hellman P, Åkerström G, Rastad J. Monoclonal antibodies recognizing normal and neoplastic human adrenal cortex. *Endocr Pathol* 1995;6:21–34.
10. Sasano H, Imatani A, Shizawa S, Suzuki T, Nagura H. Cell proliferation and apoptosis in normal and pathologic human adrenal. *Mod Pathol* 1995;8:11–17.
11. Sasano H, Saito Y, Sato I, Sasano N, Nagura H. Nucleolar organizer regions in human adrenocortical disorders. *Mod Pathol* 1990;3:591–595.
12. Dobbie JW. Adrenocortical nodular hyperplasia: the ageing adrenal. *J Pathol* 1969;99:1–18.
13. Nakajima T, Kameya T, Watanabe S, et al. S-100 protein distribution in normal and neoplastic tissues. In: DeLellis RA, ed. *Advances in immunohistochemistry.3* Masson Monogr Dian Pathol 1984;7:141–158.
14. Gaffey MJ, Traweek ST, Mills SE, et al. Cytokeratin expression in adrenocortical neoplasia: An immunohistochemical and biochemical study with implications for the differential diagnosis of adrenocortical, hepatocellular, and renal cell carcinoma. *Hum Pathol* 1992;23:144–153.
15. Goss CM, ed. *Gray's anatomy of the human body.*, 29th American ed. Philadelphia: Lea & Febiger; 1973.
16. Dahl EV, Bahn RC. Aberrant adrenal cortical tissue near the testis in human infants. *Am J Pathol* 1962;40:587.

*Histology for Pathologists, second edition,*
Edited by Stephen S. Sternberg.
Lippincott-Raven Publishers, Philadelphia
© 1997.

# CHAPTER 49

# Neuroendocrine System

Ronald A. DeLellis and Yogeshwar Dayal



The results of numerous studies over the past 50 years have established that there are many striking similarities between endocrine cells and neurons (1). Upon appropriate stimulation, both cell types release chemical messengers that react with specific receptors either in their immediate vicinities or at distant sites, and both exhibit electrical activity that increases upon release of their secretory products. Moreover, detailed biochemical and molecular studies have shown a commonality of biosynthetic products that may act as classical hormones, neurotransmitters, and paracrine or autocrine factors. Accordingly, concepts of the endocrine system have been expanded to include not only the traditional endocrine glands but also the peptidergic neurons and the system of endocrine cells that is dispersed throughout many tissues of the body. The dispersed endocrine cells, because of their striking similarities to neurons and classical endocrine cells, also have been classified as neuroendocrine cells. Although neuroendocrine cells are discussed in the context of other tissues and organs in other chapters of this volume, this chapter will provide a more general overview of this fascinating cell type.

R. A. DeLellis and Y. Dayal: Department of Pathology, Tufts University School of Medicine and New England Medical Center, Boston, Massachusetts 02111, U.S.A.

## HISTORICAL PERSPECTIVES AND NOMENCLATURE

Current concepts of the neuroendocrine system evolved directly from a series of seminal observations that were initiated more than a century ago. Heidenhain in 1870 demonstrated a population of chromaffin cells in the gastrointestinal tract and suggested that they might have an endocrine function (2). Pierre Masson (3) later showed that the intestinal chromaffin cells were also argentaffin positive, and subsequent studies by Hamperl (4) using argyrophilic staining techniques led to the identification of a second population of putative endocrine cells within the intestine and a variety of extraintestinal sites. Feyrter in 1938 suggested that the clear cells (helle Zelle) of the gastrointestinal tract formed a diffuse epithelial endocrine system ("diffuse epitheliale endokrine system") and that some of these cells might have a paracrine or local hormonal action (5,6). Similar groups of clear cells were illustrated by Frolich within the bronchial tree, and Feyrter also considered them to be a part of the diffuse epithelial endocrine system (7). Ultimately, the argentaffin, argyrophil, and clear cells were recognized as components of a diffusely distributed system of endocrine cells (8).

The modern view of the neuroendocrine cell and neurosecretory neuron stemmed directly from the observations that

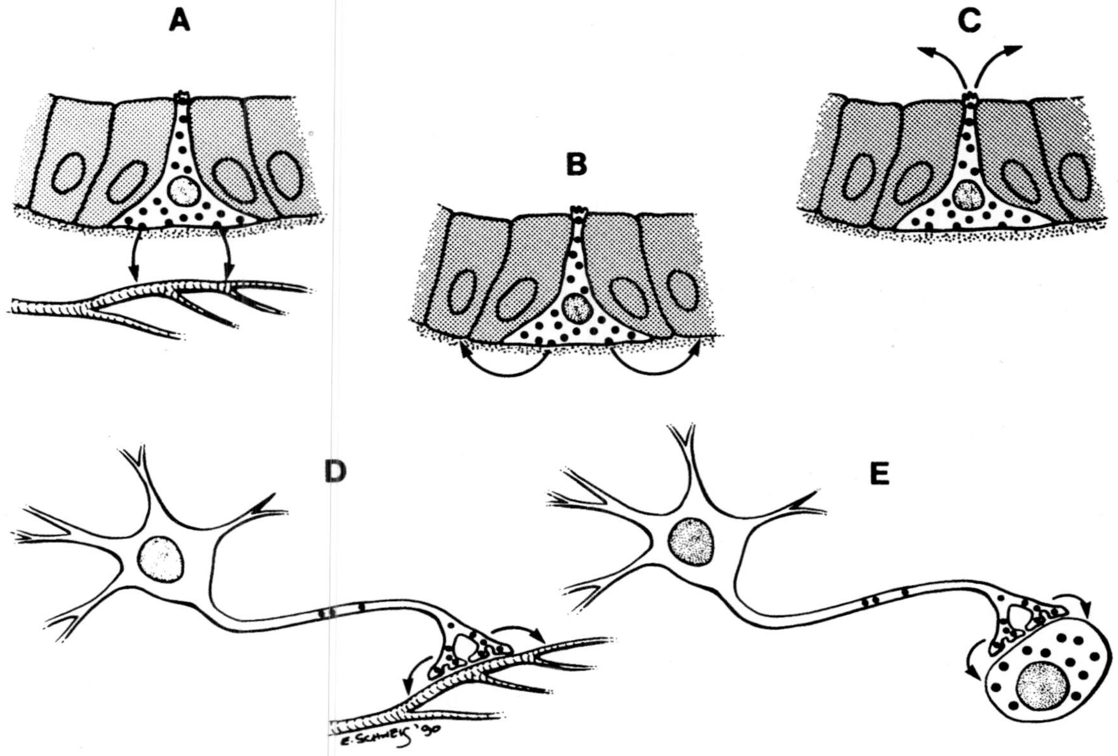


**FIG. 1.** Secretory activities of neuroendocrine cells and neurons. **A:** Neuroendocrine cells may secrete their products through the basement membranes into adjacent capillaries for interactions with target tissues at distant sites (endocrine function). **B:** Neuroendocrine cells may secrete their products locally to influence the activities of adjacent epithelial cells (paracrine function). **C:** Neuroendocrine cells may secrete their products within a glandular lumen (luminal secretion). **D:** Neurons may secrete their products into the circulation for interactions with target tissues at distant sites (neuroendocrine function). **E:** Neurons also may secrete products that serve as neurotransmitters or neuromodulators. Adapted with permission (29,40).

oxytocin and antidiuretic hormone were synthesized by hypothalamic neurons and were stored within neuronal processes in the posterior pituitary, before their release into the circulation (9). Furthermore, the discovery that hormone-releasing and -inhibiting factors were synthesized by hypothalamic neurons, transported via axonal transport to the median eminence, and secreted into the pituitary portal system for interactions with specific adenohypophyseal cell types established without doubt that neurons could function as endocrine cells (9) (Fig. 1). These cells essentially could serve as neuroendocrine transducers by converting electrical input directly into chemical or hormonal signals (10).

The discovery that the argyrophil/argentaffin cells and the cells of Feyrter's diffuse epithelial endocrine system did, indeed, have an endocrine function originated from studies conducted in the early to mid-1960s on the source of the hormone calcitonin (11,12). The thyroid glands of many species were known to contain parafollicular cells, which appeared clear in hematoxylin and eosin–stained sections and which showed varying degrees of argyrophilia or argentaffinity (13,14). With immunofluorescence techniques, the parafollicular cells were ultimately shown to be the source of calcitonin, for which they were subsequently renamed C cells (15,16). These studies also led to the discovery that certain endocrine cells shared a series of remarkable functional and morphologic similarities with neurons (15).

In addition to the presence of calcitonin, the C cells had the ability to synthesize and store catecholamines or indolylethylamines after uptake and decarboxylation of precursors of these substances (15). The latter property led to the introduction of the descriptive acronym APUD (amine precursor uptake and decarboxylation) (13). The APUD mechanism was subsequently identified in certain cells of the anterior pituitary and pancreatic islets. Cholinesterase, nonspecific esterases, $\alpha$-glycerophosphate dehydrogenase, and certain endogenous amines were also noted variably across diverse animal species and among different endocrine cell types (14) (Table 1).

In comparing the APUD cells of the thyroid, pancreas, and pituitary to cells of known neural ancestry, Pearse suggested that "the amine storing mechanism and presence of cholinesterase together point towards a common ancestral

**TABLE 1.** *Markers[a] of neuroendocrine cells*

| |
|---|
| Fluorogenic amine content |
| Amine precursor (5-hydroxytryptophan and DOPA) uptake |
| Aromatic amino acid decarboxylase |
| Nonspecific esterase or cholinesterase |
| Alpha glycerophosphate dehydrogenase |
| Peptide hormone synthesis |
| Voltage-dependent $Ca^{2+}$ or $Na^{2+}$ channels |
| Electrical excitability |
| Neuron-specific enolase |
| Chromogranins and secretogranins |
| Chromomembrin B |
| Synaptophysin and other synaptic vesicle proteins |
| Lymphoreticular antigens |
| Tetanus toxin-binding sites |
| Neural cell adhesion molecules |

[a] The first six markers in this listing were described by Pearse in the original formulation of the APUD concept; however, endogenous amine content and the capacity for amine precursor uptake and decarboxylation are present in only some members of the dispersed neuroendocrine cell system.

cell of neural origin, perhaps coming from the neural crest" (15). The list of APUD cells was then expanded to include almost all the peptide- and amine-producing cells throughout the body, including the adrenal medulla, extra-adrenal paraganglia, and parathyroid glands.

As the numbers of candidate APUD cells increased (17), it was recognized that the synthesis of regulatory peptides was a more consistent functional parameter than was synthesis of amines, and amine synthesis was ultimately dropped from the definition of these cells. In view of the many similarities between APUD cells and neurons, the essentially synonymous term "paraneuron" was introduced by Fujita and Kobayashi (18). Paraneurons, according to Fujita (19), were endocrine and sensory cells that shared structural, functional, and metabolic features with neurons and that produced substances identical with or related to neurohormones and neurotransmitters. The paraneurons also possessed neurosecretory-like granules and synapse-like vesicles, and they recognized stimuli on specific receptors and released their products via the secretory portion of the cell. Many investigators also began to apply the term "neuroendocrine cell" to these cells (17).

## EMBRYOLOGY

Embryologic data using the chick-quail chimera system have now refuted the neural crest origin of most neuroendocrine cells (20,21). Currently, the only neuroendocrine cells of proven neural crest origin are those of the adrenal medulla, extra-adrenal paraganglia, cells of the myenteric plexus and sympathetic ganglia, and the thyroid C cells (20,21); however, several studies have questioned the neural crest origin of C cells (22). The peptide- and amine-producing cells of the bronchopulmonary tract and gastroenteropancreatic axis have now been shown to be of endodermal origin.

Studies of normal, chimeric, and transgenic mice have suggested that all gut epithelial cells, including endocrine cells, originate from a single multipotential stem cell present within the base of the intestinal crypts, whereas pancreatic endocrine cells appear to originate from the ductal epithelium. However, those factors responsible for the modulation of ductal epithelium into islets of Langerhans remain largely unknown (23).

Although the neural crest origin of most neuroendocrine cells is no longer tenable, the list of neuroendocrine markers has continued to expand (Table 1). In its current context, the term "neuroendocrine" does not imply an embryologic origin from the neuroectoderm but rather implies a shared phenotype characterized by the simultaneous expression of multiple genes encoding a wide variety of neuronal and endocrine traits (24,25).

## MOLECULAR ASPECTS OF NEUROENDOCRINE CELL DEVELOPMENT

Although the precise mechanisms for the acquisition of the neuroendocrine phenotype have not been conclusively identified, recent studies suggest an important role for both positively and negatively acting transcription factors. An important class of regulatory proteins includes those with common DNA binding and dimerization domains, the basic helix-loop-helix (B-HLH) region. The genes encoding these proteins are analogous to the achaete–scute complex, which has been identified during neuronal differentiation in *Drosophila* (26). The homologous mammalial genes have been named mammalian achaete–scute homologues (MASH). These genes are expressed transiently in the embryonic rat nervous system but not in non-neuronal tissues. The human achaete–scute homologue (hASH) has been cloned from a human medullary thyroid carcinoma complimentary DNA (cDNA) library (27). Cell lines derived from human small cell carcinomas also express hASH, and the presence of this protein appears to correlate with a variety of neuroendocrine features, including l-dopa decarboxylase activity, dense-core secretory granules, and the production of polypeptide hormones. The presence of this transcription factor in small cell carcinoma cell lines suggests a role for hASH outside of the neural and neural crest–derived tissues. It is therefore likely that hASH is a regulator of neuroendocrine differentiation in cells of a variety of lineages.

Silencing factors [neuron-restrictive silencing factor (NRSF); RE-1–silencing transcription factor (REST)] that repress neuronal gene transcription in non-neuronal cells also have been identified (28,29). Chong et al. have cloned a cDNA coding REST, which mediates silencing of the type II voltage-dependent sodium channel in non-neuronal cells (29). These findings indicate that silencing factors may be

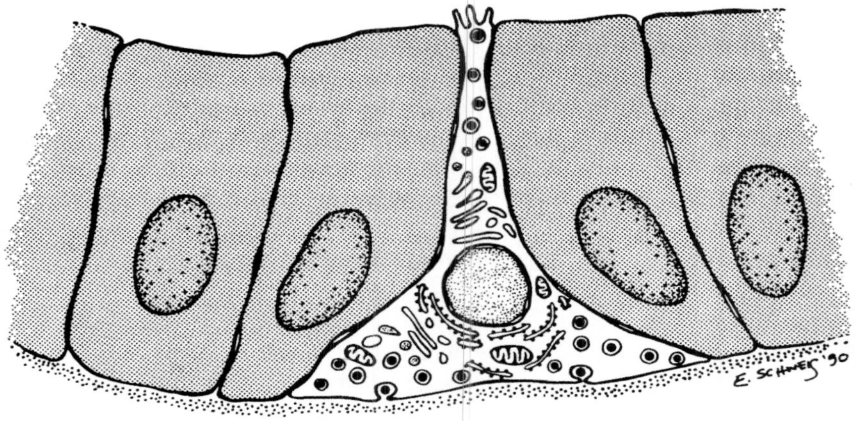

FIG. 2. Diagram of typical "opened"-type neuroendocrine cell. Secretory granules are concentrated at the basal pole of the cell. Stimulation of such a cell leads to the release of hormonal product by the process of exocytosis. The basal lamina is indicated by the stippled area. Secretory granules are also present in the apical extension of the cell.

active as master negative regulators of neuronal and neuroendocrine cell differentiation (28).

## LIGHT MICROSCOPY AND HISTOCHEMISTRY

Neuroendocrine cells are difficult to recognize in routinely prepared hematoxylin and eosin–stained sections, where they may appear as oval, pyramidal, or flask-shaped, often with clear cytoplasm (Figs. 2 and 3). In some instances, the cytoplasm may contain fine eosinophilic granules that are often difficult to resolve with usual microscopic preparations. Some neuroendocrine cell types, such as those of the intra- and extra-adrenal paraganglia and gastrointestinal tract, develop a characteristic brown to yellow coloration after primary fixation in potassium dichromate or chromic acid. This pigment results from oxidation of cellular stores of catecholamines (intra- and extra-adrenal paraganglia) or serotonin (gastrointestinal tract and other sites). In the gastrointestinal tract, the chromaffin-positive cells have also been referred to as "enterochromaffin cells" (EC).

Some neuroendocrine cells exhibit a characteristic yellow–green fluorescence after fixation in formaldehyde and other aldehyde fixatives (30) (Fig. 4). In some instances, the cells may become fluorescent only after administration of L-dihydroxyphenylalanine (DOPA) or 5-hydroxytryptophan. Formaldehyde forms highly fluorescent tetrahydroisoquinoline condensation products with catecholamines and $\beta$-carboline derivatives with tryptamines such as serotonin. Occa-

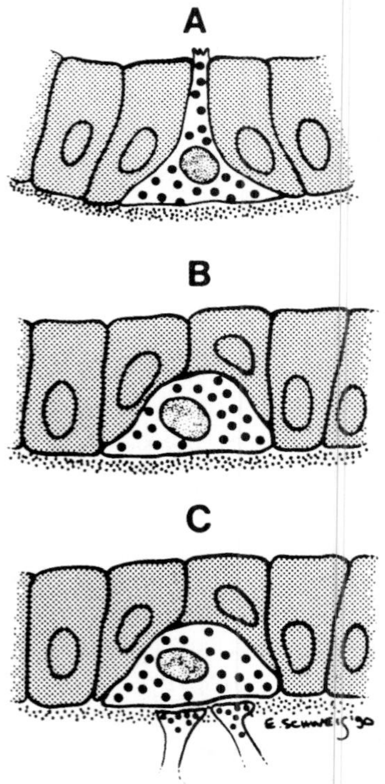


FIG. 3. Comparison of "opened" (**A**) and "closed" (**B and C**) neuroendocrine cells. **A:** Opened cells may be found within the gastrointestinal tract and other sites. **B:** Closed cells are also widely distributed. The thyroid C cells are typically of the closed type. **C:** The Merkel cells of the skin are innervated closed-type neuroendocrine cells.

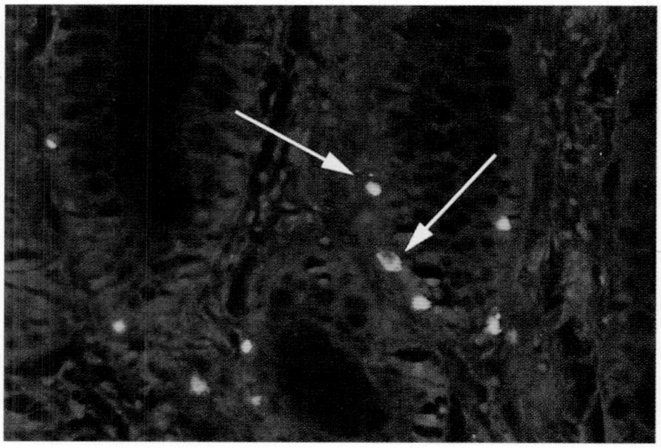

FIG. 4. Formalin-fixed rectal mucosa photographed in ultraviolet light. The strongly fluorescent cells (*arrows*) correspond to the serotonin-containing enterochromaffin-type cells.

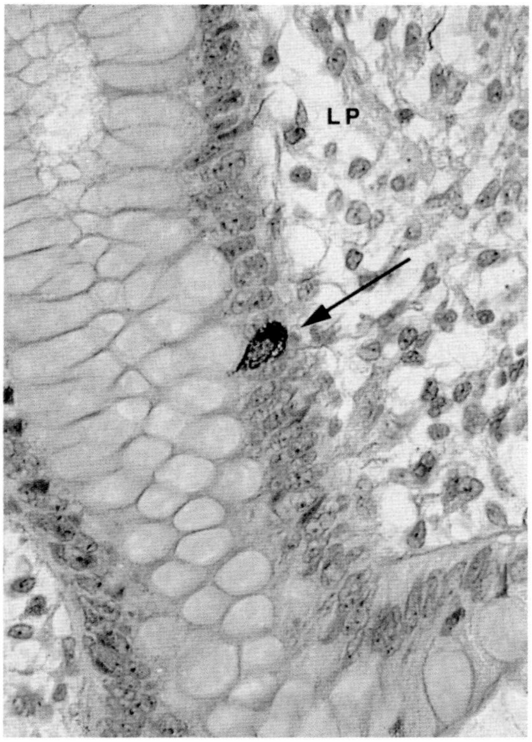


**FIG. 5.** Colonic mucosa stained for argentaffin cells with the Masson-Fontana technique and methyl green counterstain. The argentaffin cell (*arrow*) illustrated in this field is characterized by the presence of black cytoplasmic granules. LP, lamina propria.

sionally, strong fluorescence may be observed after formalin fixation and paraffin embedding. In other instances, freeze-dried tissues or fresh-frozen sections must be used for the demonstration of cellular stores of amines (30).

Some neuroendocrine cells, including those of the gastrointestinal tract, have the ability to reduce ammoniacal silver to the metallic state (3,4). Such cells are termed "argentaffin cells" (Fig. 5). In many other neuroendocrine cells, silver positivity is evident only after the addition of an exogenous reducing agent to the staining solution, and such cells are said to be argyrophilic. The chromaffin and argentaffin reactions of neuroendocrine cells in the gastrointestinal tract are due primarily to the presence of serotonin. While argentaffin cells are also argyrophilic, only a subset of argyrophil cells is argentaffin positive (31). Although the chemical basis of the argyrophil reactions (Grimelius, Churukian-Schenk, Sevier-Munger) is unknown, it is apparent that reduced silver salts have an affinity for a nonamine constituent of neuroendocrine secretory granules (32).

The argyrophil staining techniques have been used extensively for the identification of neuroendocrine cells; however, it should be recognized that these stains are nonspecific. Cellular products such as lipofuscin, glycogen, and certain proteins including $\alpha$-lactalbumin may be argyrophilic (33). Alternatively, some neuroendocrine cells are argyrophilic only with certain silver-staining sequences (Table 2).

Most neuroendocrine cells stain metachromatically with toluidine blue and coriophosphine O after acid hydrolysis of

**TABLE 2.** *Functional and morphological characteristics of gut endocrine cells*[a]

| Cell type | Hormone(s) | Granule size (nm) | Morphology/histochemistry |
|---|---|---|---|
| G | Gastrin, ACTH | 150–400 | Round, moderately dense cores; argyrophilic[b] |
| D | Somatostatin | 250–400 | Round, moderately dense cores; argyrophilic only by Hellerstrom-Hellman technique |
| IG | Gastrin | 150–220 | Round, dense; argyrophilic |
| S | Secretin | 180–220 | Round to slightly irregular; weakly argyrophilic |
| I | Cholecystokinin | 240–300 | Round with moderately dense cores; nonargyrophilic |
| K | GIP | 200–250 | Round, irregular with dense eccentric cores and less dense matrix which is argyrophilic by Sevier-Munger technique |
| N | Neurotensin | Up to 300 | Round, moderately dense; variably argyrophilic |
| L | Enteroglucagon | 250–300 | Round, moderately dense; variably argyrophilic |
| $EC_1$ | 5-HT, substance P, leu-enkephalin | 200–300 | Pleomorphic with dense cores and thin halo; argentaffinic |
| $EC_2$ | 5-HT, motilin-like, leu-enkephalin | 200–400 | Pleomorphic, round to irregular, angulated; argentaffinic |
| $EC_n$ | 5-HT, unknown | 200–300 | Elongated or oval, variably electron dense; argentaffinic |
| ECL | Histamine | | Pleomorphic, round to elongated, moderately dense contents; argyrophilic |
| $D_1$ | VIP-like | 140–200 | Round to pleomorphic granules, moderately to highly electron-dense cores with narrow halo; argyrophilic |
| P | Bombesin/GRP | 90–150 | Electron-dense cores; variably argyrophilic |
| X | Unknown | Up to 250 | Round granules, moderately dense cores; argyrophilic |

[a] From ref. 38. [b] Argyrophilia, unless otherwise stated, refers to results with the Grimelius technique.

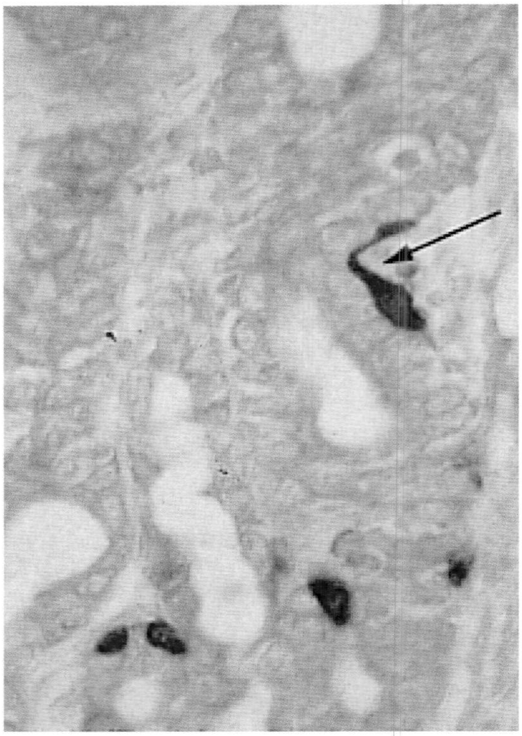

**FIG. 6.** Gastric antrum stained for somatostatin using the peroxidase–antiperoxidase technique with diaminobenzidine as the chromogen (no counterstain). A process that extends from the cell body is closely applied to the basal regions of adjacent cells (*arrow*). The somatostatin-positive cells at the lower position of this microscopic field appear to be without processes; however, the processes may be out of the plane of this section.

tissue sections (34). This property has been referred to as masked metachromasia. Acid hydrolysis not only removes DNA and RNA from the cells but also converts side chain carboxamido groups to carboxyls, which are free to react with the dyes. Both chromogranin proteins and peptide hormones are most likely responsible for the property of masked metachromasia in neuroendocrine cells (34). Lead hematoxylin also has been used for the demonstration of neuroendocrine cells (34).

Neuroendocrine cells tend to be dispersed among other cell types as single cells or as aggregates of three to four cells (Fig. 3). The basal aspects of the cells are closely applied to the subjacent epithelial basement membrane. Processes often extend from the cytoplasm to surround adjacent epithelial cells, and such neuroendocrine cells are referred to as "paracrine cells" (35,36) (Figs. 6 and 7). The products of paracrine cells are thought to be released locally where they influence the activities of adjacent endocrine and nonendocrine cells (35). The apex of the neuroendocrine cell may extend directly to the glandular lumen (opened-type cell) or may be covered by the cytoplasm of adjacent epithelial cells (Figs. 3 and 8). The latter cells are referred to as closed neuroendocrine cells (37–39) (Fig. 3). The products of opened endocrine cells may be secreted directly into the lumen of a hollow viscus. In addition, such apical processes may subserve a receptor function. Although the majority of neuroendocrine cells are not directly innervated, some cells, such as those of the skin and bronchial tree, may be innervated (Fig. 3).

In the gastrointestinal tract, scattered neuroendocrine cells are also found within the lamina propria (40) without attachment to the overlying epithelium. Such endocrine cells are typically surrounded by Schwann cells and unmyelinated nerve fibers to form an enterochromaffin cell (EC)–nerve fiber complex. The EC–nerve complexes are especially prominent in appendices with chronic inflammation and neural hyperplasia (40). Stromal endocrine cells also have been identified in the prostate gland (41).

Phylogenetic and ontogenetic studies have suggested that neurons are the earliest component of the neuroendocrine system because they are present in the most primitive organisms (coelenterates) (42). The next evolutionary step is the appearance of opened-type neuroendocrine cells in the gut, which are present in the most highly developed invertebrates. Such cells become extensively diversified in verte-

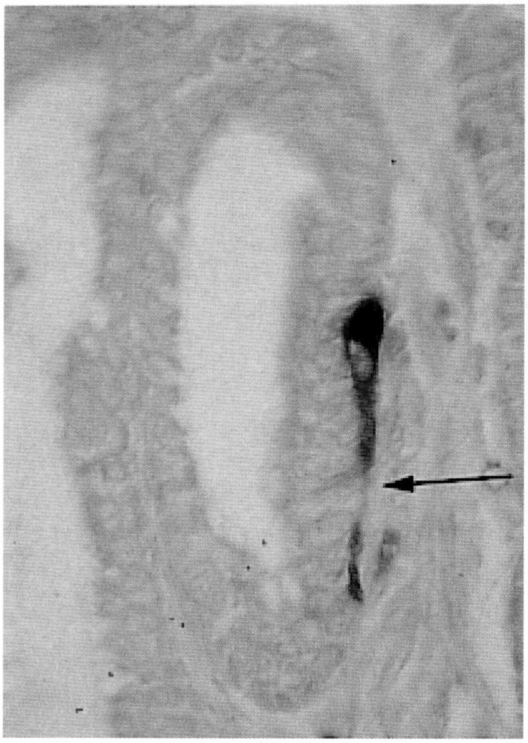

**FIG. 7.** Gastric antrum stained for somatostatin using the peroxidase–antiperoxidase technique with diaminobenzidine as the chromogen (no counterstain). The process of this somatostatin-positive cell extends along the basal portion of the gland. A portion of the process is out of the plane of section (*arrow*).

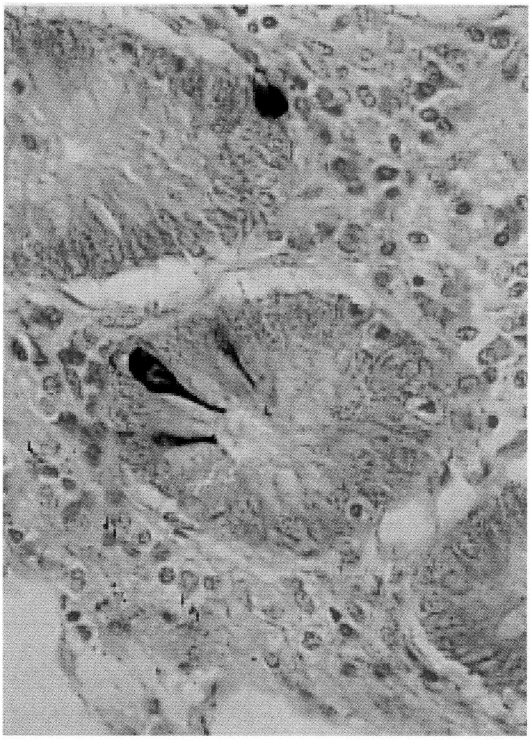

**FIG. 8.** Colonic mucosa stained for serotonin with the peroxidase–antiperoxidase technique with diaminobenzidine as the chromogen and methyl green as the counterstain. A cross section of a gland contains three opened-type endocrine cells whose apical processes extend into the lumen.

brates. The presence of gastroenteropancreatic neuroendocrine glands of classic solid type (e.g., islets of Langerhans), on the other hand, is a feature that is restricted to true vertebrates (42).

## ULTRASTRUCTURE

The most characteristic ultrastructural feature of neuroendocrine cells is the presence of membrane-bound secretory granules, which may vary from 50 to 500 nm in diameter (Figs. 9 and 10). Immunoelectron microscopic studies have shown that these granules represent storage sites of peptide and amine hormones. Granules storing different types of hormones are characterized by differences in size, density of contents, and substructure (43) (Table 2). Although most neuroendocrine secretory granules are round, others, such as those of the gastrointestinal EC and EC-like cells, are pleomorphic with elongated, reniform, round, oval, or pear-shaped forms. Secretory granules tend to be concentrated at the basal aspects of the cells in relatively close proximity to the basement membrane. Secretory granules are also prominent in cytoplasmic processes and in the apical extensions of the "opened" cells. In addition to secretory granules, many neuroendocrine cells also contain synaptic-type vesicles.

## APOPTOSIS

Apoptosis plays a critical role in the physiology of many endocrine tissues. For example, deprivation of growth factors, including thyrotropin, epidermal growth factor, and serum from cultures of thyrocytes, leads to DNA fragmentation and morphologic changes of apoptosis (44). Sasano et al. have studied the process of apoptosis in human adrenal cortex using the 3′-OH nick end-labeling or TdT-mediated deoxyuridine triphosphate-biotin nick end-labeling (TUNEL) method (45–48). With this approach, apoptotic cells were present both in the reticularis and glomerulosa, whereas proliferative cells were present primarily in the outer fasciculata. Studies of estrogen-induced prolactin cell hyperplasia in the rat have shown that withdrawal of estrogen results in increased numbers of apoptotic cells (49). This effect is enhanced by the administration of bromocriptine after estrogen withdrawal.

Although there are few published studies of apoptosis in neuroendocrine cells of the gut and other sites, this process is initiated in neurons when the concentrations of target-derived neurotrophic factors are reduced. Garcia and coworkers have demonstrated that overexpression of the *bcl*-2 proto-oncogene in cultured sympathetic neurons prevents apoptosis, which is normally induced by deprivation of nerve growth factor (50). It is likely that changes in neuroendocrine cell populations influenced by variations in trophic signals in the gastrointestinal system, pancreas, and other sites may be mediated by apoptosis. However, other mechanisms also may be operative. For example, Kaneto et al. have demonstrated that both exogenous nitrous oxide and nitrous oxide generated endogenously by interleukin (IL)-1 leads to apoptosis of isolated rat pancreatic islet cells. The action of streptozotocin appears to be mediated by a similar mechanism (51). These findings suggest that nitrous oxide–induced internucleosomal DNA cleavage is an important initial step in the destruction and dysfunction of pancreatic $\beta$ cells induced by inflammatory stimuli or by the action of streptozotocin.

## MARKERS OF NEUROENDOCRINE CELLS

Neuroendocrine cells can be identified on the basis of their contents of specific hormones (52–54), as discussed in other chapters in this volume or by the presence of nonhormonal products. The nonhormonal constituents of neuroendocrine cells include a vast array of cytoplasmic and cell membrane constituents. These products can be identified effectively via immunohistochemistry with polyclonal antisera or monoclonal antibodies. This approach is of particular importance when evaluating tissues for the presence of neuroendocrine cells when the specific hormonal product is unknown.

The chromogranins/secretogranins (Cg/Sg) represent a

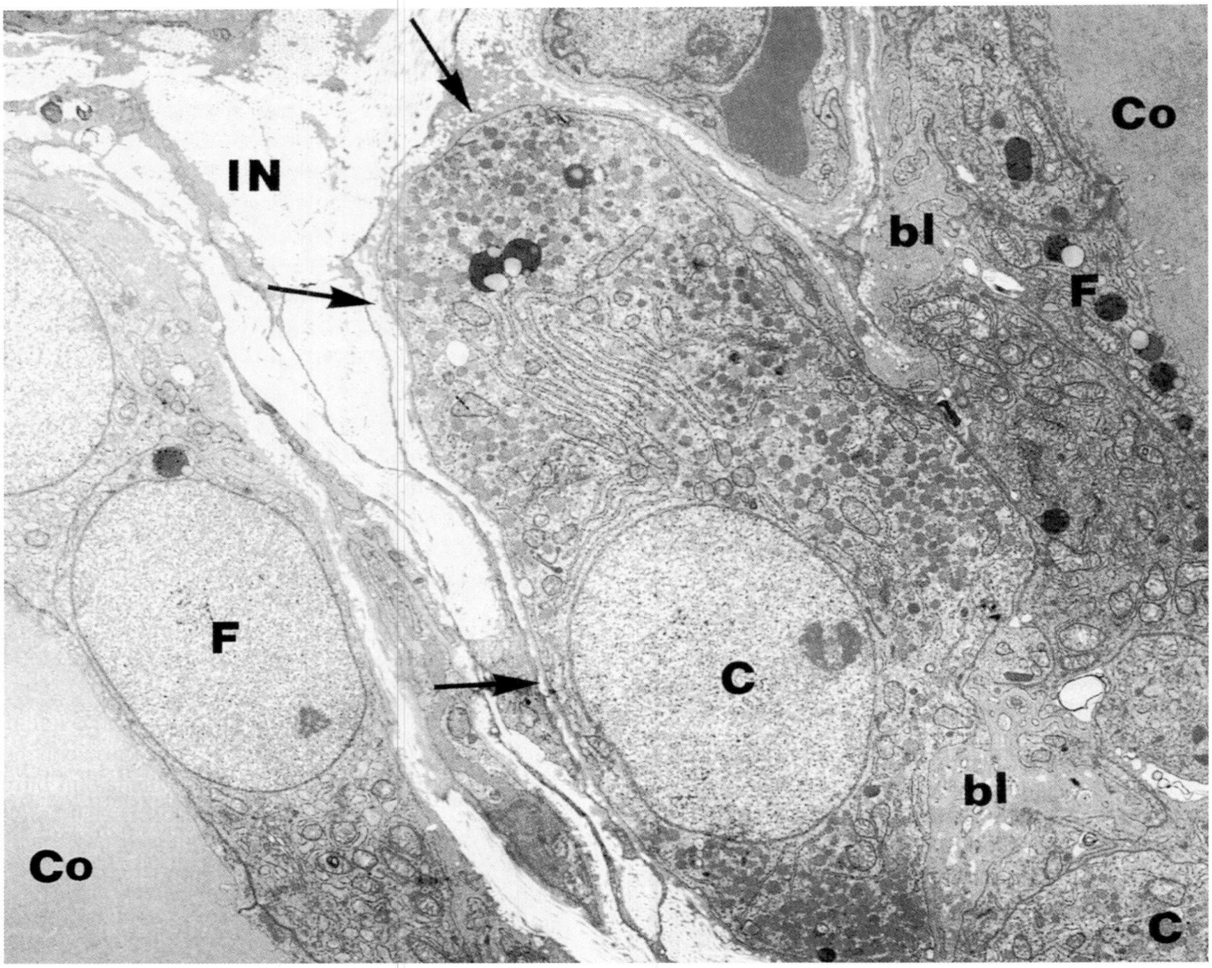


**FIG. 9.** Electron micrograph of C cell from a patient with mild C-cell hyperplasia associated with the type II MEN syndrome. The C cell is present at the base of the follicle, where it is in direct contact with the basal cytoplasm of the overlying follicular cell. The basal lamina (bl) is focally thickened at the junction of the C cell and overlying follicular cells. The C cell is separated from the interstitium by the follicular basal lamina (*arrows*). C, C cell; Co, colloid; F, follicular cell; IN, interstitium (original magnification ×**14,000**).

widely distributed family of soluble proteins that represent the predominant constituent by weight of neurosecretory granules (Table 1 and Fig. 11) (55–57). The functions of this family of proteins is unknown. It has been suggested that they represent calcium-binding proteins and that they may play important roles in the packaging and/or processing of regulatory peptides. The intact Cg/Sg proteins and their proteolytic fragments also may function as autocrine, paracrine, or endocrine hormones.

The Cg/Sg are widely distributed throughout the entire system of neuroendocrine cells and have distinctive patterns of tissue and cellular distribution (58). Although many neuroendocrine cells contain CgA, CgB, and SgII, others contain only one or two of these proteins. For example, thyroid C cells contain CgA and SgII but lack CgB. Parathyroid chief cells, on the other hand, are positive for CgA but lack SgII. The distribution of this family of proteins is reviewed in detail by Huttner et al. (58). The chromogranins are cosecreted with other granule contents, but their replenishment is differentially regulated.

Immunohistochemical studies also have demonstrated the tissue and cellular distributions of some of the biologically active proteolytic cleavage products of the Cg/Sg family. For example, both pancreastatin and chromostatin are present in most pancreatic endocrine cells, adrenal medulla, and anterior pituitary (59,60). The GAWK protein, which is derived from chromogranin B, has been localized to neuroendocrine cells in the pituitary, gastrointestinal tract, pancreas, and adrenal medulla (61).

The membranes of the small synaptic vesicles contain a complex family of proteins that include synaptophysin, synaptic vesicle–associated membrane protein (VAMP/

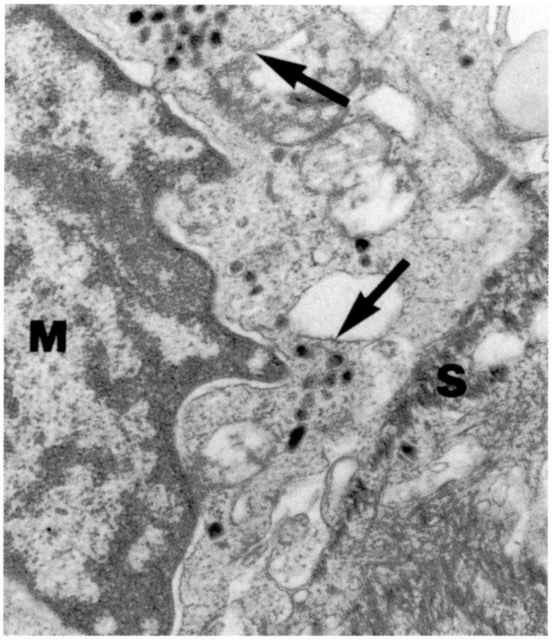


**FIG. 10.** Electron micrograph of Merkel cell. Clusters of secretory granules (*arrows*) are present within the Merkel (M) cells. S, squamous cell (original magnification ×**27,000**).

synaptobrevin), syntaxin, and synaptosome-associated protein 25 (SNAP-25), which play roles in synaptic vesicle docking, activation, fusion, and regulated exocytosis (62–66). Synaptophysin and related proteins are widely distributed in nerve terminals of the central and peripheral nervous system and are also present in neuroendocrine cells that are specialized for the regulated secretion of peptide hormones. Synaptophysin is localized in a punctate pattern in synaptic regions of neurons and has a diffuse cytoplasmic distribution in neuroendocrine cells. Ultrastructurally, synaptophysin is present in smooth-surfaced synaptic-type vesicles, but membranes of the hormone-containing secretory granules do not apparently contain this protein.

The protein gene product 9.5 (PGP 9.5) is a soluble protein with a molecular weight of 27,000 Daltons. Immunohistochemical studies have demonstrated that PGP 9.5 is present in neurons and nerve fibers at all levels of the central and peripheral nervous system. It is also present in a variety of neuroendocrine cells, except for those in the normal gastrointestinal tract (67).

Chromomembrin B (cytochrome b561), a chromaffin granule membrane, is responsible for the transport of electrons into the secretory granule matrix in order to maintain a supply of reduced ascorbic acid, which serves as an electron donor for dopamine $\beta$-hydroxylase and for amidases that modify C-terminal portions of certain neuropeptides (68). Antibodies to chromomembrin B may be useful for the identification of neuroendocrine cells that are engaged in specific functions related to catecholamine synthesis or peptide amidation (69).

A variety of different enzymes can be demonstrated by immunohistochemistry in neuroendocrine cells. Although some of the enzymes are present in most neuroendocrine cells, others have a more restricted distribution. Neuron-specific enolase has been considered as a generic marker both for neurons and neuroendocrine cells (70). The enolases are products of three independent gene loci which have been designated $\alpha$, $\beta$, and $\gamma$ (71–73). Non-neuronal enolase ($\alpha\alpha$) is present in fetal tissues, glial cells, and many nonendocrine tissues. Beta ($\beta\beta$)-enolase is present in muscle tissue, whereas hybrid enolases ($\alpha\gamma$, $\alpha\beta$) have been identified in megakaryocytes and a variety of other cell types. Neuron-specific enolase ($\gamma\gamma$) replaces non-neuronal enolase during the migration and differentiation of neurons, and it has been suggested that the appearance of neuron-specific enolase reflects the formation of synapses and the acquisition of electrical excitability. Although the sensitivity of neuron-specific enolase for the detection of neuroendocrine cells is high, its specificity is low. Seshi et al. have demonstrated a high degree of specificity with monoclonal antibodies to the form of neuron-specific enolase (74). Some of the monoclonal antibodies react predominantly with nerve fibers, whereas others react with the perikaryon exclusively or with

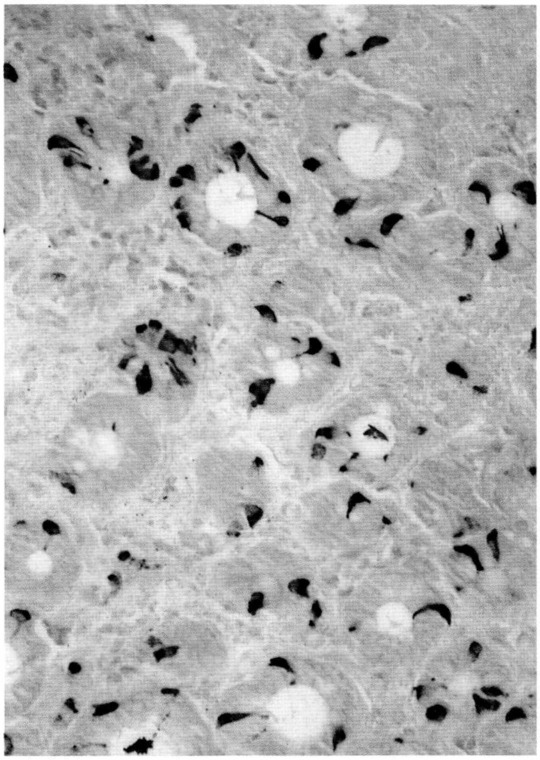

**FIG. 11.** Colonic mucosa stained with a monoclonal antibody to chromogranin A (LK2H10) via the avidin-biotin-peroxidase technique using diaminobenzidine as the chromogen and methyl green as the counterstain. This cross section is at the level of the lower third of the mucosa and shows many opened and closed neuroendocrine cells.

the perikaryon and associated nerve fibers. In contrast to the polyclonal antisera that stain a variety of non-neuronal structures, the monoclonal antibodies stain neuronal cells in a more selective fashion. Some monoclonal antibodies also react with normal adrenal medullary cells and with subsets of pancreatic islet cells.

Antibodies to catecholamine-synthesizing enzymes, including tyrosine hydroxylase, dopamine $\beta$-hydroxylase, and phenylethanolamine transferase are particularly useful for the identification of subsets of adrenal medullary and paraganglionic cells (54). In addition, these antibodies are useful for the distinction of cells that have the capacity to synthesize catecholamines from those that have the capacity for catecholamine uptake. Antibodies to histaminase are also useful for the characterization of certain neuroendocrine cells and their corresponding neoplasms (75).

The presence of certain lymphoreticular antigens in some neuroendocrine cells suggests that these proteins may serve similar functions in endocrine and lymphoid tissues (76–78). These functions might include some aspects of cell-to-cell recognition and release of secretory products (e.g., hormones and lymphokines) in response to common microenvironmental signals. The thy-1 antigen, for example, has been found in some central and peripheral neurons and in lymphocyte subsets (76). The monoclonal antibody HNK1 (CD7) recognizes epitopes in natural killer lymphocytes, myelin-associated glycoprotein, neuronal cell adhesion molecules, and a granule matrix constituent of chromaffin cells (77,78). This antibody also reacts with a subset of neuroendocrine cells in the anterior pituitary, pancreatic islets, and gastrointestinal tract (78). In addition, this antigen has been identified in Schwann cells and other nerve-supporting elements. S-100 protein, which was originally isolated from the brain, is present in cells that serve as a supporting structure in many neuroendocrine tissues, such as the adrenal medulla, paraganglia, and anterior pituitary (79).

The neural cell adhesion molecules (NCAMs) represent a family of glycoproteins that play key roles in cell binding, migration, differentiation, and proliferation (80). The NCAM family includes several major peptides that are generated by alternative splicing of RNA from a gene that is a member of the immunoglobulin super gene family. The peptide sequences that are external to the plasma membrane contain five regions that are similar to those present in immunoglobulins. The molecules are modified posttranslationally by phosphorylation, sulphation, and glycosylation. The homophilic-binding properties of NCAMs are modulated by differential expression of homopolymers of $\alpha$2,8-linked N-acetylneuraminic acid (polysialic acid).

Although initial studies had suggested that NCAM was restricted in its distribution to the brain, more recent studies indicate that it is also present in other neuroendocrine elements, including the islets of Langerhans, adenohypophysis, and adrenal medulla. Komminoth et al. have used a monoclonal antibody reactive with a long chain from of $\alpha$-2,8-linked polysialic acid that is present on NCAMs (81). They reported positive staining in cases of familial medullary thyroid carcinoma, both in the neoplastic cells and in hyperplastic C cells adjacent to the tumorous foci. Cases of primary C-cell hyperplasia unassociated with medullary thyroid carcinoma were also positively stained, whereas most normal C cells and C cells in secondary hyperplasia were nonreactive. These findings indicate that determinations of NCAMs may be helpful in distinguishing reactive proliferations of neuroendocrine cells from neoplastic and preneoplastic proliferations of these cells.

## FUNCTION OF NEUROENDOCRINE CELLS

The function of neuroendocrine cells has been established by the use of immunohistochemical techniques for the localization of specific hormones and other substances. In many instances, the use of region-specific antisera permits the localization of hormone precursors as well as mature hormones. Proinsulin immunoreactivity in the $\beta$ cells of normal pancreatic islets is present in a crescent-shaped perinuclear area that corresponds to the Golgi zone (82). Insulin, on the other hand, is present throughout the cytoplasm with a variably stained perinuclear region.

Although initial studies suggested that single neuroendocrine cells were responsible for the production of a unique hormone (one-cell, one-hormone hypothesis), more recent studies indicate that these cells are multimessenger systems (83). The peptide hormones are synthesized within the granular endoplasmic reticulum and are packaged into secretory granules by way of the Golgi region. Multiple different peptide products may be synthesized via this route in single neuroendocrine cells. Other nonpeptide hormone constituents such as catecholamines are synthesized within the cytosol and are then taken up into secretory granules (25). Any individual neuroendocrine cell can therefore vary the secretion of its products in response to different signals in normal and pathologic states.

Immunohistochemical and molecular biologic studies have led to many interesting insights into the functional interrelationships of the various components of the neuroendocrine system. For example, peptide hormones first isolated from the gastroenteropancreatic axis have been found subsequently in neurons of the central and peripheral nervous systems, where they may function as neurotransmitters or neuromodulators (10). Other peptides initially isolated from the brain have been localized to the endocrine cells of the gut, pancreas, and lung, where they may have a paracrine function (84). Furthermore, such studies have shown that the microarchitecture of endocrine organs, which may appear homogeneous in hematoxylin and eosin–stained sections, is often organized in a manner that permits paracrine interactions. The somatostatin cells of the pancreatic islets, for example, are located between the insulin and glucagon cells and typically extend short branching processes, which are in apposition to both cell types. Regulation of the secretion of insulin and glucagon may therefore be mediated by the local paracrine effects of somatostatin and by the endocrine effects of somatostatin reaching the islets by the circulation (85,86).

Neuroendocrine cells in different tissues may produce identical peptides. Somatostatin, for example, is present in certain hypothalamic neurons, pancreatic D cells, gastrointestinal D cells, bronchopulmonary endocrine cells, thymic endocrine cells, and a subset of thyroid C cells, where it is colocalized with calcitonin (85–87). Calcitonin is present in thyroid C cells, bronchopulmonary and thymic endocrine cells, and certain urogenital endocrine cells. Gastrin-releasing peptide, a 27–amino acid peptide that is the mammalian homologue of bombesin, is present in thyroid C cells, small intensely fluorescent cells of sympathetic ganglia, neuronal cells of the gastrointestinal myenteric plexus, and bronchopulmonary endocrine cells (88,89).

Neuroendocrine cells may produce multiple distinct peptides from a common precursor molecule. For example, adrenocorticotropin (ACTH) is synthesized from the large precursor molecule pro-opiomelanocortin (POMC) (90). In the adenohypophysis, POMC is processed to yield ACTH, $\beta$-lipotropin, and a 16KD N-terminal fragment. In the intermediate lobe, ACTH and $\beta$-lipotropin are processed to yield $\alpha$-MSH and $\beta$-endorphin–related peptides, respectively. Hormonal diversity in neuroendocrine cells also may result from alternate splicing pathways that produce different messenger RNAs from a single gene. Both calcitonin and the calcitonin gene–related peptide (CGRP) are produced from a primary RNA transcript that is spliced to produce two different forms of mature messenger RNA (91). More than one gene may also encode closely related peptides. In angler fish islets, for example, recombinant DNA techniques have shown two different messages for somatostatin, one of which encodes somatostatin I while the other encodes somatostatin II (92).

## DISTRIBUTION OF NEUROENDOCRINE CELLS

The histology of the adenohypophysis, parathyroid glands, intra- and extra-adrenal paraganglia, and pancreatic islets is discussed in separate chapters in this volume. The remaining sections of this chapter review the distribution of neuroendocrine cells in other tissues and organs.

### Bronchopulmonary and Upper Respiratory System

The neuroendocrine components of the lung occur singly as solitary neuroendocrine cells and in small aggregates that have been designated neuroepithelial bodies (NEBs) (93) (Fig. 12). Solitary neuroepithelial cells may be of the opened or closed type. NEBs are composed of clusters of clear to faintly eosinophilic cells that extend from the bronchial basement membrane to the lumen. NEBs are extensively innervated. Although the functions of the two neuroendocrine components are not known with certainty, NEBs most likely act as intrapulmonary chemoreceptors. Solitary neuroendocrine cells most likely subserve a paracrine function.

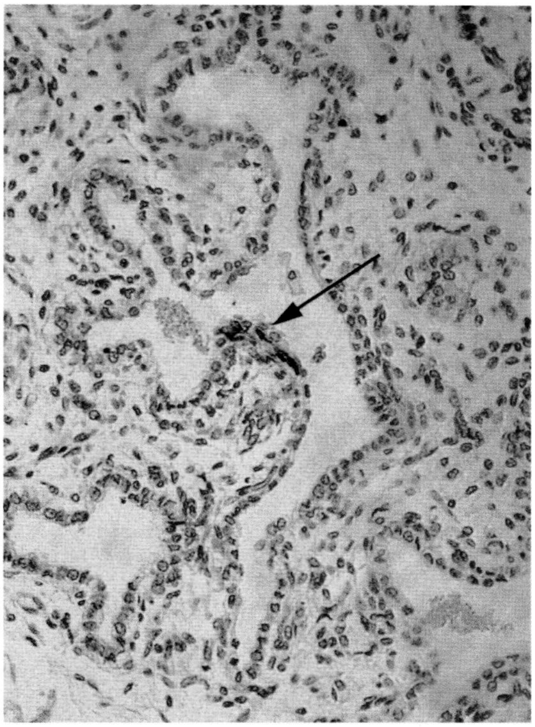

**FIG. 12.** Fetal lung stained with a monoclonal antibody to chromogranin A (LK2H10) via the avidin-biotin-peroxidase technique using diaminobenzidine as the chromogen and hematoxylin as the counterstain. A cluster of chromogranin-positive cells (*arrow*) is present just beneath the bronchial epithelium.

The secretory granules of neuroendocrine cells in the lung show considerable variation in size and density (94,95). On the basis of granule size, the bronchopulmonary neuroendocrine cells have been divided into three types. The P1 cells have granules that measure 40 to 50 nm in diameter. These cells have been noted in fetal lung. The P2 cells have granules that measure 120 to 130 nm in diameter, whereas the P3 granules measure 180 to 200 nm. The granules of Pa cells, which are found in the adult lung, measure 100 to 120 nm in diameter. Both NEBs and solitary neuroendocrine cells contain serotonin, bombesin/gastrin-releasing peptide (GRP), and calcitonin, whereas the solitary neuroendocrine cells also contain leu-enkephalin (89,93) (Fig. 13). Severely hyperplastic and dysplastic cells of the NEBs also may produce adrenocorticotropin, vasoactive intestinal peptide, and somatostatin (93). The NEBs are particularly conspicuous in fetal lung tissue but are sparse in the adult (89). The neuroendocrine components of the lung are also prominent in hypoxic conditions, including high-altitude conditions and chronic pulmonary diseases such as bronchiectasis.

Both in situ hybridization and immunohistochemical studies have shown GRP and its corresponding messenger RNA (mRNA) as early as 8 weeks of gestation in solitary neu-

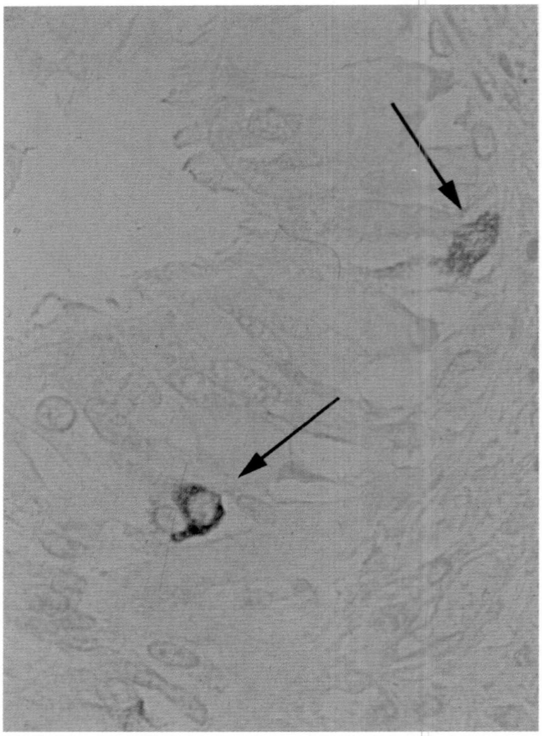

**FIG. 13.** Adult lung stained for gastrin-releasing peptide (GRP)/bombesin with an antibody to GRP with the indirect peroxidase-labeled method. Diaminobenzidine was the chromogen with methyl green counterstain. Two GRP-positive cells (*arrows*) are present within the bronchial epithelium. (Courtesy of Dr. Y. Tsutsumi, Tokai University School of Medicine, Japan.)

roendocrine cells and NEBs, primarily at branch points of bronchioles. The numbers of cells reach a peak by 16 to 30 weeks of gestation and decline at about 6 months of age. These findings suggest that GRP may be involved in the growth and development of normal lung. Increased numbers of GRP-containing cells have been found in infants with bronchopulmonary dysplasia and in children with cystic fibrosis or prolonged assisted ventilation (89).

Neuroendocrine cells, as defined by their argentaffinity or argyrophilia, are rare in the larynx. Pesce et al. were able to identify scattered argyrophil cells in only two of 43 specimens of larynx within the respiratory epithelium (96). The studies of Torre-Rendon et al. demonstrated occasional argyrophil cells both within the laryngeal squamous and respiratory epithelium (97). Argyrophil cells are also present within adjacent minor salivary glands and the epithelium of the middle ear.

### Thyroid and Thymus

In both adult and neonatal thyroid glands, the calcitonin-containing C cells are concentrated in a zone corresponding to the upper to middle thirds of the lobes along a hypothetical central axis (98). The extreme upper and lower poles, as well as the isthmus, are devoid of C cells. The C cells occupy an exclusively intrafollicular position (Figs. 9, 14, and 15). In neonates, the C cells are prominent and measure up to 40 $\mu$m in diameter. Occasional cells may show branching processes that are closely applied to the follicular basement membrane and the plasma membranes of adjacent follicular cells. Groups of up to six C cells may be present in the thyroids of neonates with up to 100 C cells per single low-power microscopic field. C cells are less numerous in adults than in neonates and appear flattened or spindle shaped. Typically, adult thyroid glands contain fewer than 50 C cells per single low-power field, although occasional normal adult glands may have a higher density of C cells. Rarely, nodules of C cells may be found in normal adult glands, as discussed in the section on aging.

Two types of secretory granule have been observed in normal as well as hyperplastic C cells (99). Type I granules have an average diameter of 280 nm, with moderately dense, finely granular contents that are closely applied to the limiting membranes of the granules. The type II granules, on the other hand, have an average diameter of 130 nm with electron-dense contents that are separated from the limiting membranes of the granules by a small but distinct electron-lucent space. Immunoelectron microscopic studies have

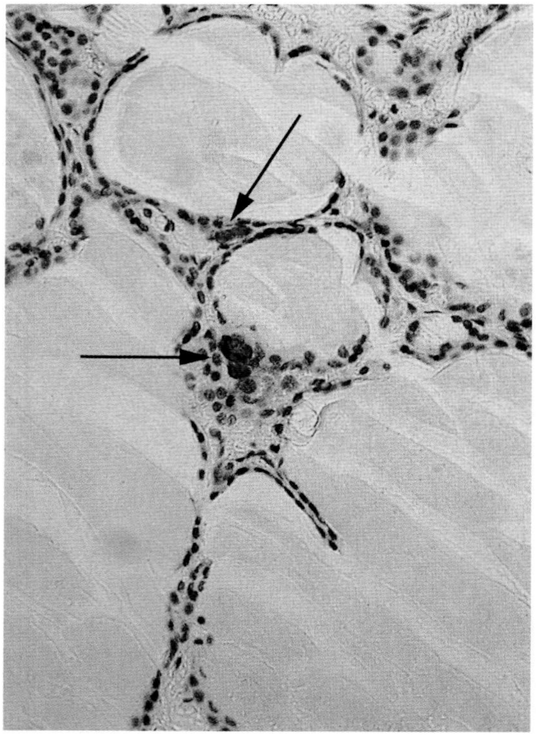

**FIG. 14.** Adult thyroid stained with a monoclonal antibody to chromogranin A (LK2H10) via the avidin-biotin-peroxidase technique using diaminobenzidine as the chromogen and hematoxylin as the counterstain. Groups of two to three C cells are present (*arrows*).

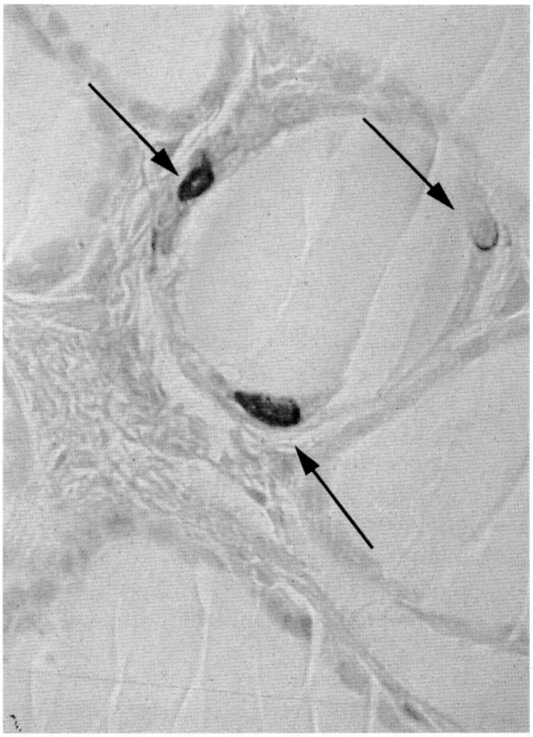

**FIG. 15.** Adult thyroid stained for calcitonin via the peroxidase–antiperoxidase technique using diaminobenzidine as the chromogen and hematoxylin as the counterstain. C cells (*arrows*) are present within the follicle as closed-type endocrine cells.

shown that both granule types contain immunoreactive calcitonin. Some of the C cells both in normal adult and in neonatal glands also contain somatostatin or bombesin/GRP (89,99,100). Approximately 70% of fetal and neonatal C cells contain GRP peptide and mRNA, whereas less than 20% of adult C cells are positive for GRP (46). It has been suggested that GRP may play a role as a thyroid growth factor analogous to its presumed role in the developing lung (89).

Although neuroendocrine cells are found commonly in the thymus glands of many animal species, these cells are sparse in human thymic tissue. In human glands, the neuroendocrine cells may be found within the perivascular connective tissue and in association with Hassall's corpuscles (101).

## Skin

The Merkel cells represent the neuroendocrine components of the skin (Fig. 9). These cells occur singly and in small clusters throughout the epidermis. Merkel cell clusters are particularly prominent in foci of specialized epithelial differentiation, such as the touch domes (102). The cells have elongate processes that surround neighboring keratinocytes. The Merkel cells are characteristically innervated by long type I myelinated fibers. Secretory granules are abundant and range from 80 to 130 nm in diameter. The granules are particularly prominent in cytoplasmic processes. Aggregates of intermediate filament proteins are predominantly of the cytokeratin type. There is considerable species variation in the content and type of peptide hormone in these cells. The most frequently encountered hormones are met-enkephalin, vasoactive intestinal peptide, and bombesin/GRP (102).

## Breast

Although clear cells have been noted in the breast by many observers, the question of whether these cells are neuroendocrine in type has engendered considerable controversy. Bussolati et al. have reported the presence of chromogranin-positive cells in a small number of normal breast samples (103). The cells were present singly or in small clusters in ductules, intralobular ducts of interlobular ducts, and between myoepithelial and epithelial cells. Occasional cell processes extended to the lumen in a manner typical of

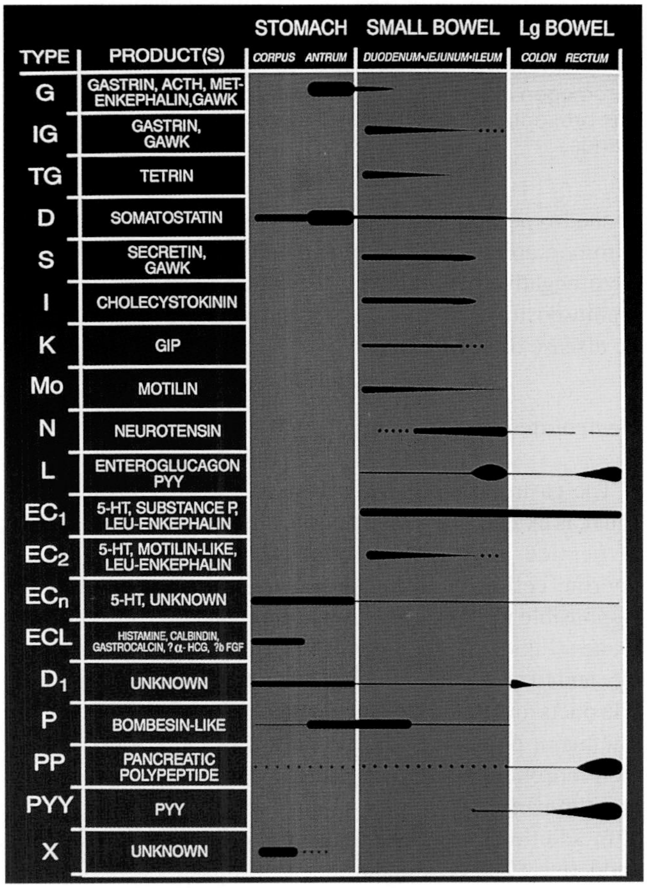


**FIG. 16.** Distribution of gastrointestinal endocrine cells. The width of the horizontal bars indicates the number of cells within different portions of the gastrointestinal tract. Reprinted with permission (38).

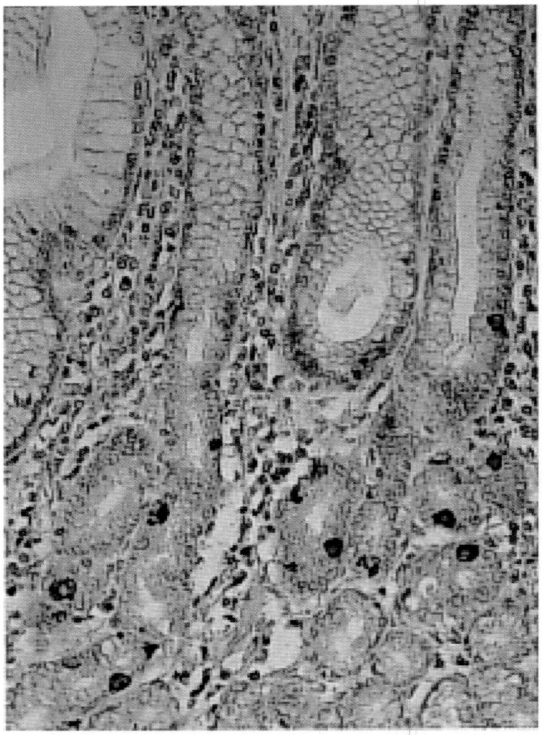

**FIG. 17.** Gastric antrum stained for gastrin using the peroxidase–antiperoxidase technique with diaminobenzidine as the chromogen and hematoxylin as the counterstain. The G cells are present primarily within the lower thirds of the gastric glands.

opened-type neuroendocrine cells. In parallel sections, the chromogranin-positive cells exhibited weak argyrophilia but were negative for a variety of peptide hormones. Chromogranin-positive cells were not identified in cases of fibrocystic disease or in papillomas.

## Gastrointestinal System

The gastrointestinal tract, from the esophagus to the anal canal, is extensively populated by a heterogeneous collection of peptide- and amine-producing neurons and neuroendocrine cells (38–40). The gut neuroendocrine cells are responsible for the production of more than 20 different hormones (Figs. 6–8, 11, 16, and 17). Cells of similar morphology and function are also present within the intraextrahepatic bile ducts and the pancreatic ductal system (Figs. 18 and 19). The major products of the gut endocrine cells, together with their morphologic characteristics and distributional patterns, are summarized in Fig. 16 and in Table 2.

In addition to their presence in mucosal and submucosal endocrine cells, peptide hormones also have been identified within submucosal glands. Brunner's glands, for example, contain neuroendocrine cells storing somatostatin, gastrin-cholecystokinin, and peptide YY. Peptidergic nerve structures containing vasoactive intestinal peptide, peptide histidine methionine, substance P, neuropeptide Y, and gastrin-releasing peptide also have been identified around Brunner's glands. All these peptides, with the exception of gastrin-releasing peptide, have been found in nerve cell bodies of the submucosal ganglia adjacent to the acini of Brunner's glands (40). These findings suggest that multiple peptides may be involved in the control of secretion from these glands.

## Urogenital System

Although argyrophil cells are not present in the adult renal parenchyma, rare argyrophilic cells have been reported in the renal pelvis. These cells may be particularly prominent in areas of glandular metaplasia. Neuroendocrine cells, as defined by their argentaffinity or argyrophilia, were first described in the urinary bladder by Feyrter (5,6). Later studies by Fetissof et al. (104) established that the endocrine cells in the urothelium were predominantly of the closed type (Fig. 20). Immunohistochemical analyses showed that the cells were positive for serotonin but did not contain peptide hormones such as ACTH, gastrin, glucagon, or somatostatin.

The neuroendocrine cells of the prostate include both opened and closed types with a predominance of the latter forms (105–107). As shown in Grimelius-stained prepara-

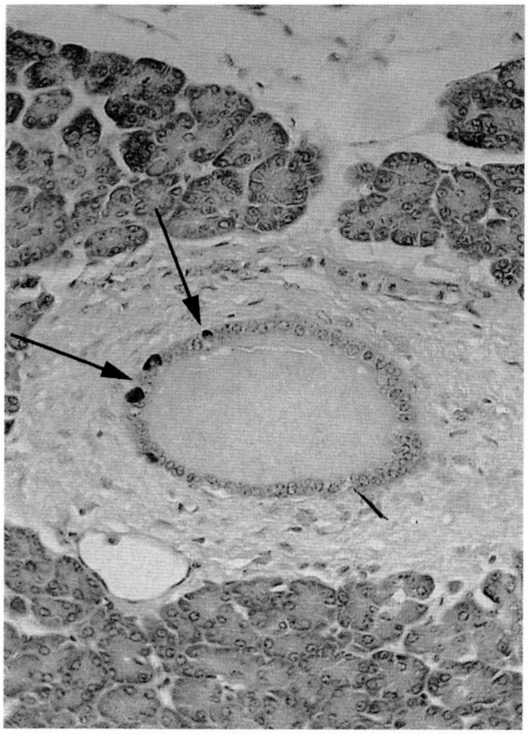

**FIG. 18.** Pancreatic duct stained with a monoclonal antibody to chromogranin A (LK2H10) via the avidin-biotin-peroxidase technique using diaminobenzidine as the chromogen and hematoxylin as the counterstain. Occasional closed-type neuroendocrine cells (*arrows*) are present within the ductal epithelium.

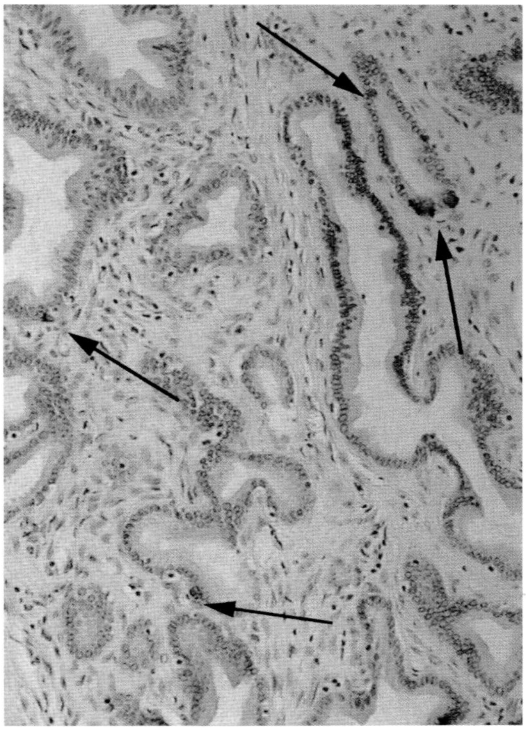

**FIG. 19.** Terminal ramifications of bile ducts stained with a monoclonal antibody to chromogranin A (LK2H10) via the avidin-biotin-peroxidase technique using diaminobenzidine as the chromogen and hematoxylin as the counterstain. Both opened and closed neuroendocrine cells (*arrows*) are present within the ductal epithelium.

tions, many of these cells have multiple dendritic processes extending between adjacent epithelial cells and occasionally abutting on other neuroendocrine cells. The neuroendocrine cells are more prominent in normal or atrophic prostate than in hyperplastic foci. Most of these cells contain serotonin,

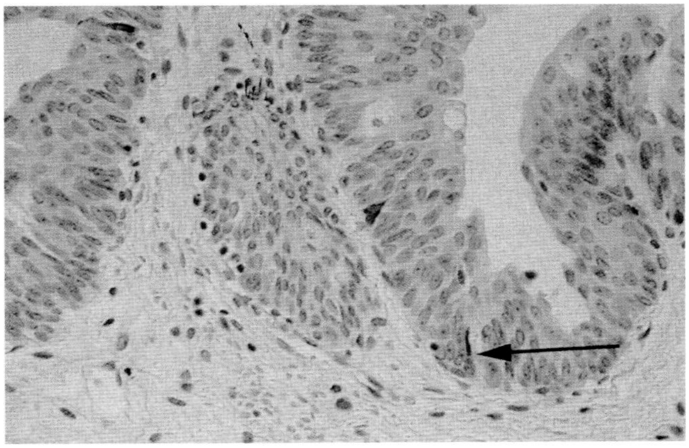

**FIG. 20.** Urinary bladder epithelium stained with a monoclonal antibody to chromogranin A (LK2H10) via the avidin-biotin-peroxidase technique using diaminobenzidine as the chromogen and hematoxylin as the counterstain. Neuroendocrine cells are present within the epithelium. A process of another neuroendocrine cell is present at the arrow.

and some also contain somatostatin. Both calcitonin and bombesin/GRP also have been observed in the normal prostate, but these hormones are present in considerably less than 5% of the neuroendocrine cells. In contrast to the anorectal canal, which is also derived from the cloaca and contains both pancreatic polypeptide and glucagon immunoreactivities, the prostatic neuroendocrine cells are negative for these peptides.

Ultrastructurally, the cells show considerable pleomorphism in granule morphology (105). The opened cells have basally oriented granules, whereas the closed cells have a more uniform distribution of granules. Prominent lamellar bodies are noted in some cells.

Neuroendocrine cells of both opened and closed types have been demonstrated in the endocervical glandular epithelium and in the exocervical squamous epithelium (108). In both sites, however, the argyrophilic cells are extremely uncommon. However, argyrophil cells have not been identified in the normal ovary, fallopian tube, or endometrium.

## AGING CHANGES

The endocrine system undoubtedly plays an important role in the aging process; however, there have been relatively few systematic studies of the effects of aging in neuroendocrine cell populations in humans. Sun et al. have demonstrated a significant age-related decline in the number and size of growth hormone–producing cells that was most marked in the transition from youth to middle age (109). Pituitary parenchymal cells also decreased in number, but there were no changes in pituitary weight. Prolactin cells, on the other hand, did not show age-related changes. Hypertrophy and relative hyperplasia of thyrotroph cells have been demonstrated in pituitaries from older individuals (110).

O'Toole et al. have studied the effects of the aging process on C-cell populations in the thyroid gland (111). Although C cells appeared to be more numerous in thyroid glands of elderly individuals, as compared with young and middle-aged individuals, the results were not statistically significant because of the large standard deviations. However, C cells more often tended to form clusters or nodules in thyroids from older individuals (112).

Age-related changes in neuroendocrine populations have been characterized in a variety of other sites, including the prostate. Cohen et al. have established that these changes in the prostate may be mediated in part by the levels of androgenic hormones (41). Although the neuroendocrine cells of the periurethral glands and prostatic ducts remain constant throughout life, those in the peripheral acini are present only when androgen levels are increased.

## SPECIAL PROCEDURES

In addition to the histochemical and immunohistochemical approaches that have been discussed throughout this chapter, molecular methodologies including in situ hybridization provide important approaches for analyzing the distribution and function of neuroendocrine cells (113,114). In contrast to immunohistochemistry, which is dependent on the peptide content of endocrine cells, in situ hybridization techniques permit the identification of cells on the basis of their content's specific mRNAs. For example, endocrine cells that are acutely stimulated or are secreting their products constitutively often produce a negative immunohistochemical signal for the particular peptide. However, studies using nucleic acid probes for the corresponding mRNAs often provide an intensely positive signal in the same cells (113). Extensive posttranslational processing and intracellular degradation of peptide products also may lead to positive hybridization signals with negative immunohistochemical reactions for the corresponding peptides. Additionally, in situ hybridization methods are of particular value for demonstrating hormone receptor mRNAs in target cells and for distinguishing de novo synthesis from uptake of hormonal peptides (113–115). The combination of in situ hybridization and immunohistochemistry has the potential for providing the maximal amount of information on the highly dynamic processes of gene transcription and translation (113,115).

The in situ hybridization method also has been combined with polymerase chain reaction (PCR) methods for demonstration of low copy number DNAs and RNAs (116,117). Detection of intracellular PCR products may be achieved indirectly by in situ hybridization using PCR product-specific probes (indirect in situ PCR) or without in situ hybridization through direct incorporation of labeled nucleotides into the PCR amplificants (direct in situ PCR). Although most protocols are designed for the demonstration of DNA, low copy RNA sequences have been demonstrated by the addition of a reverse transcriptase (RT) step to generate cDNA from RNA templates before in situ PCR. This technique, which has been called in situ RT-PCR, may be of particular value when there are fewer than 20 copies of mRNA per cell (117). This technique is of great potential value for the identification of cells with low levels of mRNA-encoding hormones, hormone receptors, cytokines, growth factors, and growth factor receptors. The technical details and potential pitfalls of these methods are discussed in detail in several recent publications (116,118,119).

## ARTEFACTS

Because neuroendocrine cells often have a clear appearance, they must be distinguished from a variety of other cell types that also may appear clear in hematoxylin and eosin–stained, formalin-fixed, paraffin-embedded sections. Cytoplasmic clearing may result from intracellular accumulations of lipids or glycogen; alternatively, this change may represent a shrinkage artefact analogous to that seen in the lacunar cells of nodular sclerosing Hodgkin's disease. For example, clear cells in the intestinal epithelium may represent lymphocytes or epithelial cells with retraction of the cytoplasm from the nucleus. In general, this type of artefact is less pronounced in tissues that have been fixed in nonaqueous fixatives. Neuroendocrine cells can be conclusively distinguished from other clear cells by the presence of neuroendocrine markers, including chromogranin proteins or synaptophysin.

Numerous artefacts may be associated with the use of immunohistochemical procedures for the demonstration of peptide hormones and nonhormonal markers. Appropriate positive and negative controls therefore must be used in conjunction with these procedures, as discussed in standard textbooks of immunohistochemistry (120). Nonspecific binding of immunoglobulins to endocrine secretory granules also may result from ionic interactions that may be suppressed to some extent by the use of buffers containing high concentrations of salt (121), as discussed in the chapter on paraganglia.

Artefacts also may occur in in situ hybridization procedures. For example, Pagani et al. have demonstrated that oligonucleotides used in in situ hybridization procedures bind to neuroendocrine cells as a result of the presence of endogenous $NH_2$ groups (122). This type of nonspecific interaction can be blocked effectively by treating the sections with acetic anhydride. Controls for standard in situ hybridization and PCR-based in situ hybridization are discussed in detail in several recent reviews (116,117,119).

## DIFFERENTIAL DIAGNOSIS

The differential diagnosis of various neuroendocrine cell populations is discussed in the chapters dealing with the specific organ systems in this volume.

## SPECIMEN HANDLING

Most histochemical and immunohistochemical procedures for the demonstration of hormones and nonhormonal constituents of neuroendocrine cells can be performed in formalin-fixed and paraffin-embedded tissues. Other fixatives, including carbodiimide, acrolein, and diethyl pyrocarbonate, also have been used in place of formalin, and these fixatives have been reported to achieve optimal fixation of low concentrations of regulatory peptides such as those occurring in peptidergic nerve fibers (123–126).

The tissue preparative techniques for in situ hybridization studies are discussed in several review articles (113,119). In general, these methods may be performed on frozen samples that are postfixed in paraformaldehyde or in formalin-fixed samples that have been embedded in paraffin.

## REFERENCES

1. Ganong WF. Neuroendocrinology. In: Greenspan FS, ed. *Basic and clinical endocrinology.* 3rd ed. Norwalk, CT: Appleton & Lange; 1991:66–78.
2. Heidenhain R. Untersuchangen uber den Bau der Labridusen. *Arch Mikrosk Anat Entwicklungsmech* 1870;6:368–406.

3. Masson P. La glande endocrine de l'intestin chez l'homme. *Acad Sci (Paris)* 1914;158:57–61.
4. Hamperl H. Was sind argentaffine Zellen? *Virchows Arch [A]* 1932; 286:811–833.
5. Feyrter F. *Uber Diffuse Endokrine Epithaliale Organe.* Leipzig, Germany: Barth; 1938.
6. Feyrter F. *Uber Die Periphheren Endokrine (Parakrine) Drusen Des Menshen.* Vienna: Maudrich; 1954.
7. Frolich F. Die "Helle Zelle" der bronchialschleinhaut und ihre beziehungen zum problem der chemoreceptoren. *Frankfurter Z Pathol* 1949;60:517–558.
8. Polak JM, Bloom SR. Peripheral localization of regulatory peptides as a clue to their function. *J Histochem Cytochem* 1980;28:918–924.
9. Scharrer B. The neurosecretory neuron in neuroendocrine regulatory mechanisms. *Am Zool* 1967;7:161–169.
10. Snyder SH. Brain peptides as neurotransmitters. *Science* 1980;209: 976–983.
11. Copp DH, Cameron EC, Cheney BA, et al. Evidence for calcitonin–a new hormone from the parathyroid that lowers blood calcium. *Endocrinology* 1962;70:638–649.
12. Pearse AGE. The cytochemistry of the thyroid C-cells and their relationship to calcitonin. *Proc R Soc Lond [Biol]* 1966;164:478–487.
13. Pearse AGE. The cytochemistry and ultrastructure of polypeptide hormone producing cells (the APUD series) and the embryologic, physiologic and pathologic implications of the concept. *J Histochem Cytochem* 1969;17:303–313.
14. Pearse AGE. 5-Hydroxytryptophan uptake by the dog thyroid C-cells and its possible significance in polypeptide hormone production. *Nature* 1966;211:598–600.
15. Pearse AGE. Common cytochemical properties of cells producing polypeptide hormones with particular reference to calcitonin and the thyroid C-cells. *Vet Rec* 1966;79:587–590.
16. Bussolati G, Pearse AGE. Immunofluorescent localization of calcitonin in the C-cells of the pig and dog thyroid. *J Endocrinol* 1967;37: 205–209.
17. Pearse AGE. The diffuse neuroendocrine system and the APUD concept: related endocrine peptides in brain, intestine, pituitary, placenta and anuran cutaneous glands. *Med Biol* 1977;55:115–125.
18. Fujita T, Kobayashi S. Current reviews on the paraneuron concept. *Trends Neurosci* 1979;2:27–30.
19. Fujita T. Present status of the paraneuron concept. *Arch Cytol Histol* 1989;52(suppl):1–8.
20. LeDouarin N, Teillet MA. The migration of neural crest cells to the wall of the digestive tract in the avian embryo. *J Embryol Exp Morphol* 1973;30:31–48.
21. LeDouarin N. *The neural crest.* Cambridge, England: Cambridge University Press; 1982.
22. Holm R, Sobrinho-Simoes M, Nesland JM, et al. Medullary thyroid carcinoma with thyroglobulin immunoreactivity. A special entity? *Lab Invest* 1987;57:258–268.
23. Vinik AI, Pittenger GL, Paulic-Renar I. Role of growth factors in pancreatic endocrine cells. *Endocrinol Metab Clin North Am* 1993;22: 875–887.
24. DeLellis RA, Dayal Y, Tischler AS, Lee AK, Wolfe HJ. Multiple endocrine neoplasia syndromes: cellular origins and interrelationships. *Int Rev Exp Pathol* 1986;28:163–215.
25. Tischler AS. The dispersed neuroendocrine cells: the structure, function, regulation and effects of xenobiotics on this system. *Toxicol Pathol* 1989;17:307–316.
26. Johnson JE, Birren SJ, Anderson DJ. Two rat homologues of *Drosophila achaete–scute* specifically expressed in neuronal precursors. *Nature* 1993;356:858–861.
27. Ball DW, Azzoli CG, Baylin SB, Chi D, et al. Identification of a human achaete–scute homolog highly expressed in neuroendocrine tumors. *Proc Natl Acad Sci U S A* 1993;90:5648–5652.
28. Schoenherr CJ, Anderson DJ. The neuron-restrictive silencer factor (NRSF): a coordinate repressor of multiple neuron specific genes. *Science* 1995;267:1360–1363.
29. Chong JA, Tapia-Ramirez J, Kim S, et al. REST: a mammalian silencer protein that restricts sodium channel gene expression to neurons. *Cell* 1995;80:949–957.
30. Falck B, Owman CA. A detailed methodological description of the fluorescence method for the cellular distribution of biogenic monoamines. *Acta Univ Lund* 1965;7:5–23.
31. Grimelius L. A silver nitrate stain for A2 cells of human pancreatic islets. *Acta Soc Med Upsal* 1968;73:243–270.
32. Grimelius L, Wilander E. Silver stains in the study of endocrine cells of the gut and pancreas. *Invest Cell Pathol* 1980;3:3–12.
33. Aguirre P, Scully RE, Wolfe HJ, DeLellis RA. Endometrial carcinomas with argyrophil cells. A histochemical and immunohistochemical study. *Hum Pathol* 1984;15:210–217.
34. Cecilia M, Rost M, Rost FWD. An improved method for staining cells of the endocrine polypeptide (APUD) series by masked metachromasia. *Histochem J* 1976;8:93–98.
35. Larson LI, Golteman N, De Magistris L, et al. Somatostatin cell processes as pathways for paracrine secretion. *Science* 1979;205: 1393–1395.
36. Dockray GJ. Evolutionary relationships of the gut hormones. *Fed Proc* 1979;38:2295–2301.
37. Fujita T, Kobayashi S. The cells and hormones of the GEP endocrine system. In: Fujita T, ed. *Gastroenteropancreatic cell system.* Tokyo: Igaku-Shoin; 1973:1–16.
38. Dayal Y. Endocrine cells of the gut and their neoplasms. In: Norris HT, ed. *Pathology of the colon, small intestine and anus.* New York: Churchill Livingstone; 1983:267–300.
39. Lechago J. The endocrine cells of the digestive and respiratory systems and their pathology. In: Bloodworth JMB Jr, ed. *Endocrine pathology general and surgical.* 2nd ed. Baltimore: Williams & Wilkins; 1982:513–555.
40. Bossard A, Chery-Croze S, Cuber JC. Immunohistochemical study of peptidergic structures in Brunner's glands. *Gastroenterology* 1989; 97:1382–1388.
41. Cohen RJ, Glezerson G, Taylor LF, Grundle HAJ, Naude JH. The neuroendocrine cell population of the human prostate gland. *J Urol* 1993; 150:365–368.
42. Falkmer S. Phylogeny and ontogeny of the neuroendocrine cells of the gastrointestinal tract. *Endocrinol Metab Clin North Am* 1993;22: 731–752.
43. Gould VE, DeLellis RA. The neuroendocrine cell system: its tumors, hyperplasias and dysplasias. In: Silverberg S, ed. *Principles and practice of surgical pathology.* New York: Wiley; 1983.
44. Dremier S, Golstein J, Mosselmans R, Dumont JE, Galand T, Robaye B. Apoptosis in dog thyroid cells. *Biochem Biophys Res Commun* 1994;200:52–58.
45. Sasano H, Imatani A, Shizawa S, Suzuki T, Nagura H. Cell proliferation and apoptosis in normal and pathological human adrenal. *Mod Pathol* 1995;8:11–17.
46. Gavrieli Y, Sherman Y, Bewn-Sasson SA. Identifiction of programmed cell death in situ via specific labelling of nuclear DNA fragmentation. *J Cell Biol* 1992;119:493–501.
47. Hiraishi K, Suzuki K, Hakomori S, Adachi M, Le Y. Antigen expression is correlated with apoptosis (programmed cell death). *Glycobiology* 1993;3:381–390.
48. Sasano H. In situ end labelling and its application to the study of endocrine disease: how can we study programmed cell death in surgical pathology materials? *Endocr Pathol* 1995;6:87–89.
49. Drewett N, Jacobi JM, Willgoss DA, Lloyd HM. Apoptosis in the anterior pituitary gland of the rat: studies with estrogen and bromocriptine. *Neuroendocrinology* 1993;57:89–95.
50. Garcia I, Martinou I, Tsujimoto Y, Martinou J-C. Prevention of programmed cell death of sympathetic neurons by the *bcl*-2 proto-oncogene. *Science* 1992;258:302–304.
51. Kaneto H, Fujii J, Seo HG, Suzuki K et al. Apoptotic cell death triggered by nitric oxide in pancreatic cells. *Diabetes* 1995;44:733–738.
52. Polak JM, Bloom SR. Immunocytochemistry of regulatory peptides. In: Polak JM, Van Noorden S, eds. *Immunocytochemistry. Practical applications in pathology and biology.* Bristol, England: Wright PSG; 1983:184–211.
53. Verhofstad AAJ, Steinbusch HWM, Joosten HWJ, et al. Immunocytochemical localization of noradrenaline, adrenaline and serotonin. In: Polak JM, Van Noorden S, eds. *Immunocytochemistry. Practical applications in pathology and medicine.* Bristol, England: Wright PSG; 1983:143–168.
54. Lloyd RV. Immunohistochemical localization of catecholamines, catecholamine synthesizing enzymes and chromogranins in neuroendocrine cells and tumors. In: DeLellis RA, ed. *Advances in immunohistochemistry.* New York: Raven Press; 1988:317–340.
55. Blaschko H, Comline RS, Schneider FH, et al. Secretion of a chromaffin protein, chromogranin, from the adrenal medulla after splanchnic nerve stimulation.
56. Schober M, Fischer-Colbrie R, Schmidt KW, Bussetati G, O'Connor

DI, Winkler H. Comparison of chromogranins A, B and secretogranin II in human adrenal medulla and pheochromocytoma. *Lab Invest* 1987;57:385–391.
57. Lloyd RV, Jin L, Kulig E, Fields K. Molecular approaches for the analysis of chromogranins and secretogranins. *Diagn Mol Pathol* 1992;1:2–15.
58. Huttner WB, Gerdes H-H, Rosa P. Chromogranins/secretogranins—widespread constituents of the secretory granule matrix in endocrine cells and neurons. In: Gratzl M, Langley K, eds. *Markers for neural and endocrine cells. Molecular and cell biology, diagnostic applications.* Weinheim, Germany: VCH; 1991:93–131.
59. Kimura N, Funakoshi A, Aunis D, et al. Immunohistochemical localization of chromostatin and pancreastatin, chromogranin A derived bioactive peptides, in normal and neoplastic neuroendocrine tissues. *Endocrine Pathol* 1995;6:35–44.
60. Schmidt WE, Siegel EG, Lamberts E, et al. Pancreastatin: molecular and immunocytochemical characterization of a novel peptide in porcine and human tissues. *Endocrinology* 1988;123:1395–1404.
61. Bishop AE, Sekiya K, Salahuddin MJ, et al. The distribution of GAWK-like immunoreactivity in neuroendocrine cells of the human gut, pancreas, adrenal and pituitary glands and its colocalization with chromogranin B. *Histochemistry* 1989;90:475–483.
62. Weidenmann B, Franke WW, Kuhn C, et al. Synaptophysin: a marker protein for neuroendocrine cells and neoplasms. *Proc Natl Acad Sci U S A* 1986;83:3500–3504.
63. Gould VE, Lee I, Wiedenmann B, et al. Synaptophysin: a novel marker for neurons, certain neuroendocrine cells and their neoplasms. *Hum Pathol* 1986;17:979–983.
64. Jahn R, DeCamilli P. Membrane proteins of synaptic vesicles: markers for neurons and endocrine cells: tools for the study of neurosecretion. In: Gratzl M, Langley K, eds. *Markers for neurons and endocrine cells. Molecular, cell biology and diagnostic applications.* Weinheim, Germany: VCH; 1991:25–91.
65. Sollner T, Bennett MK, Whiteheart SW, Scheller RH, Rothman JE. A protein assembly–disassembly pathway in vitro that may correspond to sequential steps of synaptic vesicle docking, activation and fusion. *Cell* 1993;75:409–418.
66. Elferink LA, Scheller RH. Synaptic vesicle proteins and regulated exocytosis. *J Cell Sci Suppl* 1993;17:75–79.
67. Thompson RJ, Doran JF, Jackson P, Dhillon AP, Rode J. PGP 9.5—a new marker for vertebrate neurons and neuroendocrine cells. *Brain Res* 1983;278:224–228.
68. Winkler H, Westhead E. The molecular organization of adrenal chromaffin granules. *Neuroscience* 1980;5:1803–1823.
69. Njus D, Knoth J, Cook C, Kelly PM. Electron transfer across the chromaffin granule membrane. *J Cell Biol* 1983;258:27–30.
70. Schmechel D, Marangos PJ, Brightman M. Neuron specific enolase is a molecular marker for peripheral and central neuroendocrine cells. *Nature* 1978;17:834–836.
71. Lloyd RV, Warner TF. Immunohistochemistry of neuron specific enolase. In: DeLellis RA, ed. *Advances of immunohistochemistry.* New York: Masson; 1984:127–140.
72. Haimoto H, Takahashi T, Koshikawa T, et al. Immunohistochemical localization of gamma enolase in normal human tissues other than nervous and neuroendocrine tissue. *Lab Invest* 1985;52:257–263.
73. Schmechel D. Gamma subunit of the glycolytic enzyme enolase: nonspecific or neuron specific. *Lab Invest* 1985;52:239–242.
74. Seshi B, True L, Carter D, Rosai J. Immunohistochemical characterization of a set of monoclonal antibodies to human neuron specific enolase. *Am J Pathol* 1988;131:258–269.
75. Mendelsohn G. Histaminase localization in medullary thyroid carcinoma and small cell lung carcinoma. In: DeLellis RA, ed. *Diagnostic immunohistochemistry.* New York: Masson; 1981:299–312.
76. Seeger RC, Danon YL, Rayner SA, Hoover F. Definition of thy-1 on human neuroblastoma, glioma, sarcoma and teratoma cells with a monoclonal antibody. *J Immunol* 1982;128:983–989.
77. Lipinski M, Braham K, Cailland JM, et al. HNK-1 antibody detects an antigen expressed on neuroectodermal cells. *J Exp Med* 1983;158: 1775–1780.
78. Tischler AS, Mobtaker H, Mann K, et al. Anti-lymphocyte antibody leu-7 (HNK-1) recognizes a constituent of neuroendocrine granule matrix. *J Histochem Cytochem* 1986;34:1213–1216.
79. Lloyd RV, Blaivas M, Wilson BS. Distribution of chromogranin and S100 protein in normal and abnormal adrenal medullary tissue. *Arch Pathol Lab Med* 1985;109:633–635.
80. Heitz PU, Roth J, Zuber C, Komminoth P. Markers for neural and endocrine cells in pathology. In: Gratzl M, Langley K, eds. *Markers for neural and endocrine cells. Molecular and cell biology, diagnostic applications.* Weinheim, Germany: VCH; 1991:203–215.
81. Komminoth P, Roth J, Saremaslani P, et al. Polysialic acid of the neural cell adhesion molecule in the human thyroid: a marker for medullary thyroid carcinoma and primary C cell hyperplasia: an immunohistochemical study on 79 thyroid lesions. *Am J Surg Pathol* 1994;18:399–411.
82. Roth J, Kasper M, Stamm B, et al. Localization of proinsulin and insulin in human insulinoma: preliminary immunohistochemical results. *Virchows Arch [B]* 1989;56:287–292.
83. Hakanson R, Sundler F. The design of the neuroendocrine system: a unifying concept and its consequences. *Trends Pharmacol Sci* 1983; 4:41–44.
84. Pearse AGE, Polak JM, Bloom SR. The newer gut hormones. Cellular sources, physiology, pathology and clinical aspects. *Gastroenterology* 1977;72:746–761.
85. Reichlin S. Somatostatin (part 1). *N Engl J Med* 1983;309:1495–1501.
86. Reichlin S. Somatostatin (part 2). *N Engl J Med* 1983;309:1556–1563.
87. Kameda Y, Oyama H, Endoh M, Horino M. Somatostatin immunoreactive C-cells in thyroid glands from various mammalian species. *Anat Rec* 1982;204:161–170.
88. Tsutsumi Y, Osamura Y, Watanabe K, Yanaihara N. Immunohistochemical localization of gastrin releasing peptide and adrenocorticotropin releasing cells in the human lung. *Lab Invest* 1983;48: 623–632.
89. Sunday ME, Kaplan LM, Motoyama E, et al. Gastrin releasing peptide (mammalian bombesin) gene expression in health and disease. *Lab Invest* 1988;59:5–24.
90. Kruger DT. Pituitary ACTH hyperfunction: pathophysiology and clinical aspects. In: Commani F, Mueller EE, eds. *Pituitary hyperfunction: pathophysiology and clinical aspects.* New York: Raven Press; 1984:221–234.
91. Rosenfeld MG, Mermod JJ, Amara SJ, et al. Production of a novel neuropeptide encoded by the calcitonin gene via tissue specific RNA processing. *Nature* 1983;304:129–135.
92. Warren TG, Shields D. Cell free biosynthesis of somatostatin precursors: evidence for multiple forms of preprosomatostatin. *Proc Natl Acad Sci U S A* 1982;79:3729–3733.
93. Gould VE, Linnoila RI, Memoli VA, Warren WH. Neuroendocrine components of the bronchopulmonary tract: hyperplasias, dysplasias and neoplasms. *Lab Invest* 1983;49:519–537.
94. Bensch KG, Gordon GB, Miller LR. Studies on the bronchial counterpart of the Kultschitzky (argentaffin) cells and innervation of the bronchial glands. *J Ultrastruct Res* 1965;12:668–686.
95. Lauweryns JM, Peuskens JC. Neuroepithelial bodies (neuroreceptor or secretion organs?) in human infant bronchial and bronchiolar epithelium. *Anat Rec* 1972;172:471–481.
96. Pesce C, Tobia-Gallelli F, Toncini C. APUD cells of the larynx. *Acta Otolaryngol* 1984;98:158–162.
97. Torre-Rendon FE, Cisneros-Bernal E, Ochoa-Salas JA. Carcinoma indifferenciadio de cellular pequenas de la laringe. *Patologica* 1979;17: 47–57.
98. DeLellis RA, Wolfe HJ. The pathobiology of the human calcitonin (C)-cell. A review. *Pathol Annu* 1981;16:25–52.
99. DeLellis RA, Nunnemacher G, Wolfe HJ. C-cell hyperplasia: an ultrastructural analysis. *Lab Invest* 1977;36:237–248.
100. DeLellis RA, May L, Tashjian AH, Wolfe HJ. C-cell granule heterogeneity in man. An ultrastructural immunocytochemical study. *Lab Invest* 1978;38:263–269.
101. Bearman RM, Levine GD, Bensch KG. The ultrastructure of the normal human thymus. A study of 36 cases. *Anat Rec* 1978;190: 755–781.
102. Gould VE, Moll R, Moll I, et al. Neuroendocrine (Merkel) cells of the skin: hyperplasias, dysplasias and neoplasms. *Lab Invest* 1985;52: 334–353.
103. Bussolati G, Gugliotta P, Sapino A, Eusebi V, Lloyd RV. Chromogranin reactive endocrine cells in argyrophilic carcinomas (carcinoids) and normal tissue of the breast. *Am J Pathol* 1985;120: 186–192.
104. Fetissof F, Dubois MP, Arbeille-Brassart B, et al. Endocrine cells in the prostate gland, urothelium and Brenner tumors. Immunohistological and ultrastructural studies. *Virchows Arch [B]* 1985;42:53–64.
105. di Sant'Agnese PA, Jensen KD. Endocrine paracrine cells of the

prostate and prostatic urethra. An ultrastructural study. *Hum Pathol* 1984;15:1034–1041.
106. di Sant'Agnese PA, Jensen KD. Somatostatin and/or somatostatin-like immunoreactive endocrine–paracrine cells in the human prostate gland. *Arch Pathol Lab Med* 1984;108:693–696.
107. di Sant'Agnese PA. Calcitonin-like immunoreactive and bombesin-like immunoreactive endocrine paracrine cells of the human prostate. *Arch Pathol Lab Med* 1986;110:412–415.
108. Scully RE, Aguirre P, DeLellis RA. Argyrophilia, serotonin and peptide hormones in the female genital tract and its tumors. *Int Rev Gynecol Pathol* 1984;3:51–70.
109. Sun Y-K, Xi Y-P, Fenoglio CM, et al. The effect of age on the number of pituitary cells immunoreactive to growth hormone and prolactin. *Hum Pathol* 1984;15:169–180.
110. Zegarelli-Schmidt E, Yu X-R, Fenoglio-Preiser C, et al. Endocrine changes associated with the human aging process: II. Effect of age on the number and size of thyrotropin immunoreactive cells in the human pituitary. *Hum Pathol* 1985;16:277–286.
111. O'Toole K, Fenoglio-Preiser C, Pushparaj N. Endocrine changes associated with the human aging process: III. Effect of age on the number of calcitonin immunoreactive cells in the thyroid gland. *Hum Pathol* 1985;16:991–1000.
112. Gibson WC, Peng T-C, Croker BP. C cell nodules in adult human thyroid. A common autopsy finding. *Am J Clin Pathol* 1981;75:347–350.
113. DeLellis RA, Wolfe HJ. Analysis of gene expression in endocrine cells. In: Fenoglio-Preiser CM, Wilman CL, eds. *Molecular diagnostic in pathology*. Baltimore: Williams & Wilkins; 1991:299–322.
114. Lloyd RV. Introduction to molecular endocrine pathology. *Endocr Pathol* 1993;4:64–78.
115. Speel EJM, Ramaekers FCS, Hopman AHN. Cytochemical detection systems for in situ hybridization and the combination with immunohistochemistry. "Who is still afraid of red, green and blue?" *Histochem J* 1995;27:833–858.
116. Komminoth P, Long AA. In situ polymerase chain reaction. An overview of methods, applications and limitations of a new molecular technique. *Virchows Arch [B]* 1993;64:67–73.
117. Komminoth P, Long AA. In situ polymerase chain reaction and its application to the study of endocrine diseases. *Endocr Pathol* 1995; 6:167–171.
118. Sällström JF, Alemi M, Spets H, Zehbe I. Nonspecific amplification in in situ PCR by direct incorporation of reporter molecules. *Cell Vision* 1994;1:243–251.
119. Nuovo G. *PCR in situ hybridization.* New York: Raven Press; 1992.
120. Taylor CR, Cote RJ. *Immunomicroscopy: a diagnostic tool for the surgical pathologist.* 2nd ed. Philadelphia: WB Saunders; 1994: 23–28.
121. Grube D. Immunoreactivities of gastric (G-) cells. II. Non-specific binding of immunoglobulins to G cells by ionic interactions. *Histochemistry* 1980;66:149–167.
122. Pagani A, Cerrato M, Bussolati G. Nonspecific in situ hybridization reaction in neuroendocrine cells and tumors of the gastrointetinal tract using oligonucleotide probes. *Diagn Mol Pathol* 1993;2:125–130.
123. Kendall PA, Polak M, Pearse AGE. Carbodiimide fixation for immunohistochemistry. Observations on the fixation of polypeptide hormones. *Experimentia* 1971;27:1104–1106.
124. King JC, Lechan RM, Kugel G, Anthony ELP. Acrolein: a fixative for immunohistochemical localization of peptides in the central nervous system. *J Histochem Cytochem* 1983;31:62–68.
125. Pearse AGE, Polak JN, Adams C, Kendall PA. Diethyl pyrocarbonate, a vapor phase fixative for immunofluorescence studies on polypeptide hormones. *Histochem J* 1974;6:347–352.
126. Pearse AGE, Polak JM. Bifunctional reagent as vapor and liquid phase fixatives for immunohistochemistry. *Histochem J* 1975;7:179–186.

*Histology for Pathologists, second edition,*
Edited by Stephen S. Sternberg.
Lippincott-Raven Publishers, Philadelphia


# CHAPTER 50

# Paraganglia

Arthur S. Tischler



Paraganglia are anatomically dispersed neuroendocrine organs characterized by the presence of morphologically and cytochemically similar neurosecretory cells derived from the neural crest. They may be broadly divided into two groups for physiologic and pathophysiologic purposes. One of these is distributed along the prevertebral and paravertebral sympathetic chains and along sympathetic nerve branches that innervate the organs of the pelvis and retroperitoneum. The adrenal medulla is the most extensively studied and best understood example of the sympathetic paraganglia. The second group is distributed along parasympathetic nerves, predominantly cervical and thoracic branches of the glossopharyngeal and vagus nerves. The prototypical parasympathetic paraganglion is the carotid body.

## HISTORY AND NOMENCLATURE

The history of the paraganglia is among the more interesting and controversial in the recent annals of medicine. This material is addressed in detail in several excellent reviews (1–4). The concept of a unitary paraganglionic system was first proposed by Alfred Kohn at the beginning of the 20th century (5). Several earlier investigators had developed histochemical reactions that demonstrated that the adrenal medulla contained substances chemically different from those in the cortex. One of these reactions, the development of brown coloration in the presence of chromate salts, was apparently first discovered by Bertholdus Werner in 1857 (3). Kohn coined the terms "chromaffin reaction" for the color change and "chromaffin cells" for the reactive cells, which he described in several extra-adrenal locations in the retroperitoneum. He further noted that some cells in the carotid body exhibited a chromaffin reaction, confirming an earlier report by Stilling (3). Kohn believed that these carotid body cells were derived from precursors of sympathetic ganglia and were innervated by sympathetic axons, and he suggested that they were, therefore, embryologically, histochemically, and functionally comparable to retroperitoneal chromaffin cells. He proposed a new term to encompass all the tissues composed of cells that were analogous to neurons, but not neuronal: "Since the chromaffin tissue complexes form ganglion-like bodies, since their elements are derived from ganglion anlagen, since they are connected to the sympathetic nervous system and still are not genuine ganglia, I have called them paraganglia" (5; translated from German by Dr. Miguel Stadecker).

Obstacles to acceptance of Kohn's concept soon arose from DeCastro's finding that the innervation of the carotid body is primarily derived from the glossopharyngeal nerve

A. S. Tishchler: Department of Pathology, Tufts University School of Medicine, Boston, Massachusetts 02111.

(4) and from observations by many investigators that carotid body cells are usually nonchromaffin. Consequently, the paraganglion system was divided by Watzka (4) into chromaffin and nonchromaffin paraganglia, associated respectively with the sympathetic or parasympathetic nervous systems, and paraganglia of mixed type. Discovery of the chemoreceptor function of the carotid bodies created further difficulties because it implied that the nonchromaffin paraganglia served physiologically in a sensory role, in contrast to the endocrine role of the adrenal medulla and their other chromaffin counterparts. The suggestion was therefore made by Kjaergaard that the parasympathetic paraganglia be referred to by the term "chemodecton" (4) (from the Greek *dechesthaito,* receive). This name was never widely accepted, despite the earlier application by Mulligan of its counterpart, "chemodectoma," to paraganglionic tumors (4).

An additional synonym for the parasympathetic paraganglia is "glomus" (from the Latin *glomus,* ball). This term is a vestige of a 19th-century hypothesis that the carotid body is of vascular origin (4). Although it aptly describes the microscopic *Zellballen* characteristic of paraganglia, it has caused confusion because it is also applied to thermoregulatory structures in the skin and other locations (e.g., glomera cutanea and the glomus coccygeum) and to their corresponding tumors (glomus tumors or glomangiomas). These structures are modified arteriovenous anastomoses unrelated to paraganglia developmentally or functionally (6).

It is now possible to return to a unitary concept of paraganglia with a synthesis of new and old data. Paraganglionic neuroendocrine cells are probably all derived from the neural crest (7,8). All produce catecholamines or, in some cases, indolamines (7,9) detectable by more sensitive methods than the chromaffin reaction, and all in addition express multiple other neuroendocrine markers (see Chapter 17). It is now apparent that the same basic type of neuroendocrine cell may be used differently in different anatomic locations (10–13). The term "paraganglion" is useful because it connotes a constellation of generic characteristics of this type of cell and is not dependent on a single histochemical reaction. Because it was intended by Kohn to imply analogy, rather than merely proximity, to autonomic ganglia, it continues in this context to be both conceptually helpful and literally correct. In contrast, the terms "chromaffin" and "nonchromaffin" paraganglia are now confusing and should be discarded.

## SYMPATHETIC VERSUS PARASYMPATHETIC PARAGANGLIA: A CLINICOPATHOLOGIC PERSPECTIVE

Sympathetic and parasympathetic paraganglia differ dramatically from each other from a clinicopathologic standpoint, despite their similarities at the cellular level. This contrast might result from differences in the type, timing, or intensity of physiologic signals to which the two classes of paraganglia are exposed during development or in adult life. The only known clinically important pathologic changes in paraganglia are hyperplasia and neoplasia. Several generalizations concerning these proliferative lesions underscore the differences between paraganglia of the sympathetic and parasympathetic classes (14). When multiple lesions occur within families or individuals, they are, with rare exceptions, confined to one or the other class. Although both sympathetic and parasympathetic lesions produce catecholamines, clinical signs of excess catecholamine secretion are usually associated with lesions that are sympathetic, and lesions that produce significant amounts of epinephrine are almost invariably sympathetic. Lesions that occur in patients with prolonged hypoxemia or hypercapnia, on the other hand, are almost invariably parasympathetic. In addition, sympathetic paraganglia give rise to tumors of both neuronal and neuroendocrine lineage. The former (i.e., neuroblastomas, ganglioneuroblastomas, and ganglioneuromas) are common, whereas the latter (paragangliomas) are rare. Neoplasms of parasympathetic paraganglia are almost always neuroendocrine.

Despite the differences in the contexts in which they arise, sympathetic and parasympathetic paragangliomas strongly resemble each other microscopically and are often indistinguishable. They also exhibit a widely overlapping range of secretory products and other neuroendocrine markers, reflecting the similarities of the neuroendocrine cells that are their normal counterparts. A morphologic foundation for the study of paraganglionic pathology therefore requires familiarity with both systemic differences and cellular similarities.

## DISTRIBUTION OF PARAGANGLIA

Sympathetic paraganglia are found predominantly in the para-axial regions of the trunk along the prevertebral and paravertebral sympathetic chains and in connective tissue in or near the walls of the pelvic organs. In adult humans, they are especially numerous along the fibers of the inferior hypogastric plexuses leading to and entering the urogenital organs, in the wall of the urinary bladder, and among the nerve fibers of the sacral plexus (15–17) (Fig. 1). Their presence in the prostate has recently attracted attention as a potential source of diagnostic confusion (18). They are not generally known by individual names, and their precise locations are variable. Exceptions are the adrenal medulla and the organ of Zuckerkandl, located at the origin of the inferior mesenteric artery (19) (Figs. 1 and 2). The distinctive characteristic of the organ of Zuckerkandl is that it is the only extra-adrenal sympathetic paraganglion that is macroscopic. Historically, it is said to have initially been shown to Alfred Kohn as an unusual lymph node by his pupil, Emil Zuckerkandl (4,20). In its most frequent anatomic configuration, it is divided into a set of paired organs (Fig. 1), and it is therefore often referred to by the plural, "organs of Zuckerkandl" (1). Because its fragmentation and its proximity to numerous smaller paraganglia may make it difficult to identify precisely, some investigators have used the plural to encompass all preaortic

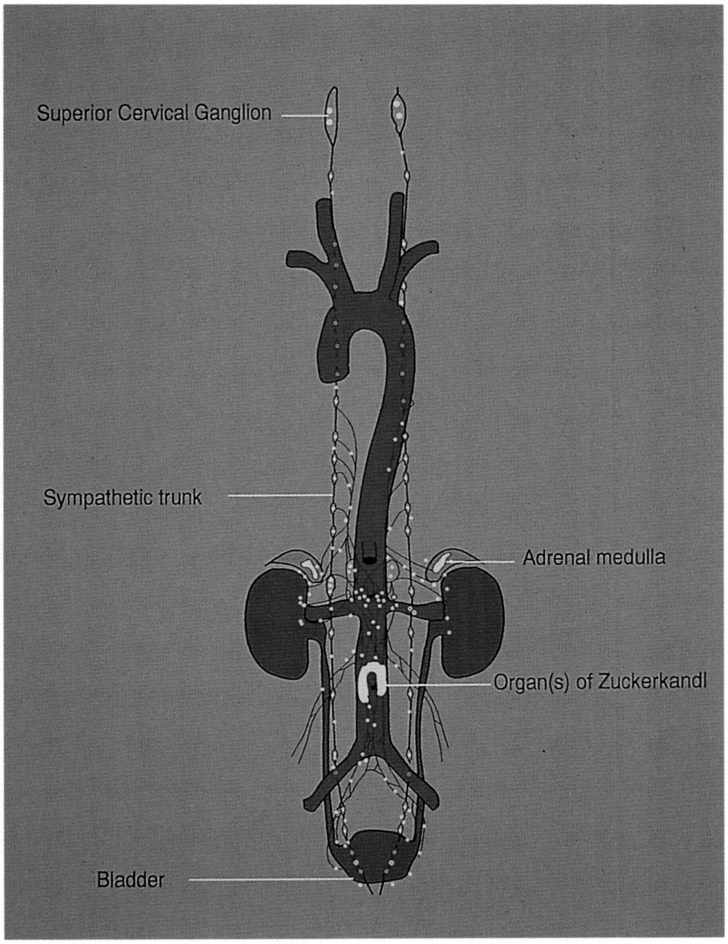


**FIG. 1.** The distribution of sympathetic paraganglia in the human fetus. Adapted with permission (1,24).

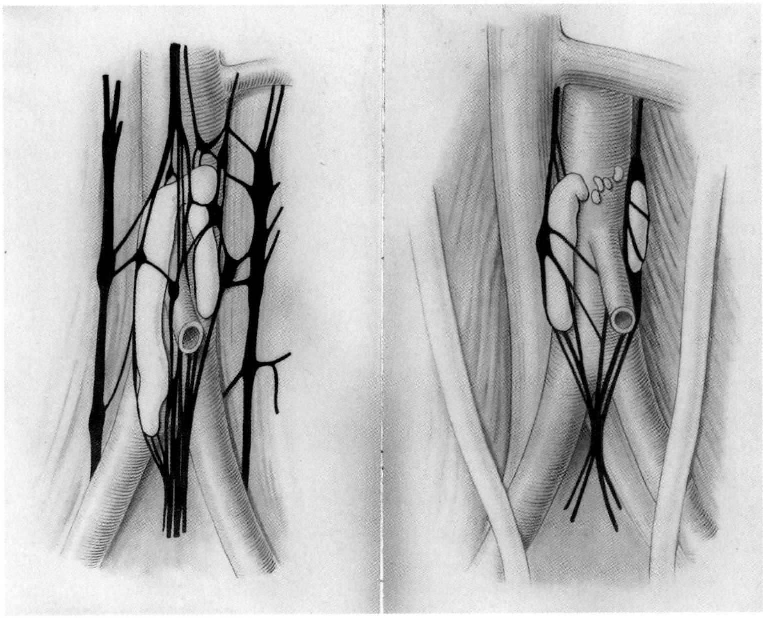

**FIG. 2.** Modified renditions of original illustrations by Zuckerkandl (19) representing the anatomic structure that bears his name. The bilobed configuration with a fragmented isthmus (*right*) is the most frequent variation. (Courtesy of Dr. E. E. Lack.)

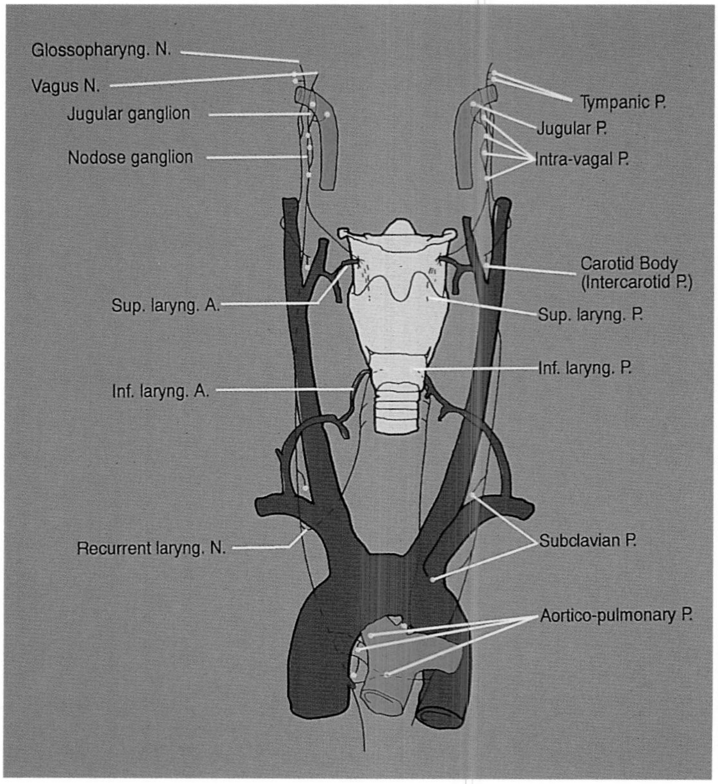


**FIG. 3.** The distribution of the principal parasympathetic paraganglia. Adapted with permission (24).

paraganglia between the inferior mesenteric artery and the aortic bifurcation (21). However, this chapter maintains the traditional, more specific, macroscopic usage.

Neuroendocrine cells are present both within and adjacent to the ganglia of the sympathetic chains. The former have been referred to in neurobiology literature as small intensely fluorescent (SIF) cells (22), intraganglionic chromaffin cells (23), or small granule-containing (SGC) cells (11,12), depending on the particular technique used to detect them. In pathology literature especially, SIF cells are often regarded as intraganglionic paraganglia (24). In anatomy literature, on the other hand, some investigators reserve the term "paraganglia" for extraganglionic sites (25).

In contrast to sympathetic paraganglia, their parasympathetic counterparts are distributed almost exclusively along the cranial and thoracic branches of the glossopharyngeal and vagus nerves (Fig. 3). With the exception of the carotid bodies, which are located between the carotid arteries just above the carotid bifurcation (Fig. 4), parasympathetic paraganglia are highly variable in both number and location (4). Their names refer to general locations, rather than to specific structures. The middle ear, for example, contains zero to 12 jugular and tympanic paraganglia, with an average of 2.8 (26). The principal paraganglia of the glossopharyngeal nerve are the tympanic paraganglia in the wall of the middle ear and the carotid bodies (4,26). Those of the vagus nerve include the jugular paraganglia in the floor of the middle ear (4,26), the superior and inferior laryngeal paraganglia (4,27), and the subclavian and aorticopulmonary or cardioaortic paraganglia near the bases of the great vessels of the heart. They sometimes also may be found in the interatrial septum (4,28). In addition, "intravagal" paraganglia are located within or adjacent to the vagal trunk in or near the nodose and jugular ganglia (4,29). These two vagal ganglia are thus the only sensory ganglia known to contain neuroendocrine

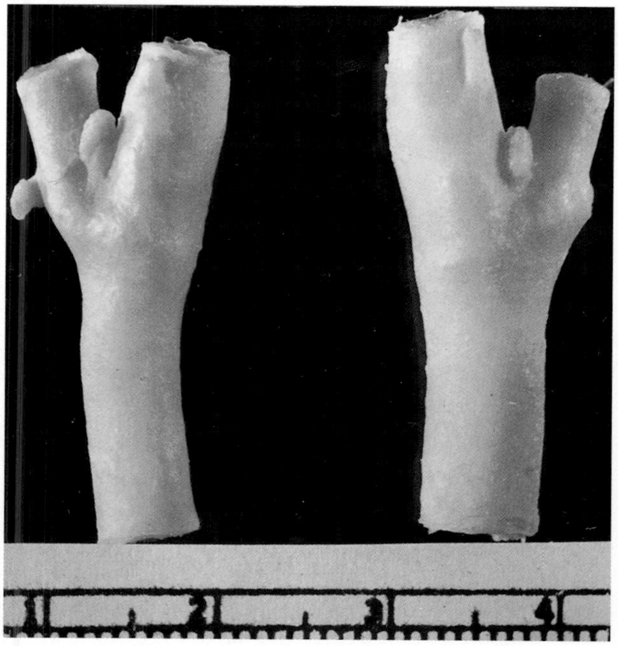

**FIG. 4.** Gross specimens from a 36-year-old woman, illustrating normal carotid bodies and their relationship to the carotid arteries. Reprinted with permission (54).

cells comparable with the SIF cells of sympathetic ganglia. These cells have been described as SIF cells in some publications (29).

Some investigators have classified the parasympathetic paraganglia as "branchiomeric" (24). This nomenclature is based on the suggestion that the branchial arches during embryogenesis are metameric, or serially homologous, structures, each with its own artery, cranial nerve branches, and associated paraganglia. The carotid body would accordingly develop in association with the glossopharyngeal nerve and the third branchial arch artery, which persists as the internal carotid. Subclavian paraganglia would develop with the vagus nerve and the fourth branchial arch artery, and so on. The evolution of this concept is reviewed elsewhere in detail (4). However, the concept does not contribute to understanding the pathophysiology of paraganglia and may cause confusion by distracting attention from the important differences between parasympathetic and sympathetic paraganglia, which may occur in close proximity to each other (e.g., the carotid bodies and the SIF cells in cervical sympathetic ganglia). It also is plagued by a number of internal inconsistencies, such as its prediction that the temporal paraganglia should be innervated by the facial nerve (4).

Knowledge of the distribution of normal paraganglionic tissue is important to pathologists because of its value in predicting the sites of origin of paragangliomas. These tumors have been reported virtually at all locations where normal paraganglia are found during fetal or adult life and tend to be most frequent in areas where paraganglionic tissue is most abundant. For example, approximately half of all sympathetic paragangliomas in children are extra-adrenal, whereas only about 10% are extra-adrenal in adults (30–32), most frequently arising in the vicinity of the organ of Zuckerkandl (see sections on "Embryologic Changes" and "Postnatal and Developmental Changes"). However, it is also important to note that paraganglia may occur in locations outside the well-established sympathetic and parasympathetic distributions, perhaps explaining the existence of paragangliomas in unusual locations. Although intravagal paraganglia in humans have been identified only in the cervical and thoracic portions of the vagus nerve (4,33), in rodents they are also present within the abdominal portions (34). It is possible that some abdominal paraganglia in humans, for example, in the gallbladder (35), may be associated with small abdominal vagus nerve branches. In scattered reports, paraganglia have been described in various sites including the orbit, mandible, and extremities. The validity of some of these reports has been questioned (4).

## EMBRYOLOGIC CHANGES

During embryogenesis, the paraganglia are first populated by small, primitive cells similar to those in the anlage of the sympathetic ganglia. These cells include precursors of neuroendocrine, neural, and glial cell lineages in adult paraganglia (36,37) (see section on "Light Microscopy"). They appear to be able to produce some catecholamines at the earliest stages of paraganglionic development (37,38) (see section on "Function"), and express cytoskeletal or other markers of immature neurons (37), or glia (36) (see section on "Special Procedures"). They are readily recognized in the paraganglia at about 7 weeks' gestation, although they first arrive somewhat earlier (1), and they are progressively superseded by larger differentiated cells. Extra-adrenal sympathetic (1) paraganglia and parasympathetic (38,39) paraganglia mature cytologically earlier than the adrenal medulla. Primitive cells usually disappear from these locations by week 25 but may persist in small numbers in the adrenal medulla until after birth (1).

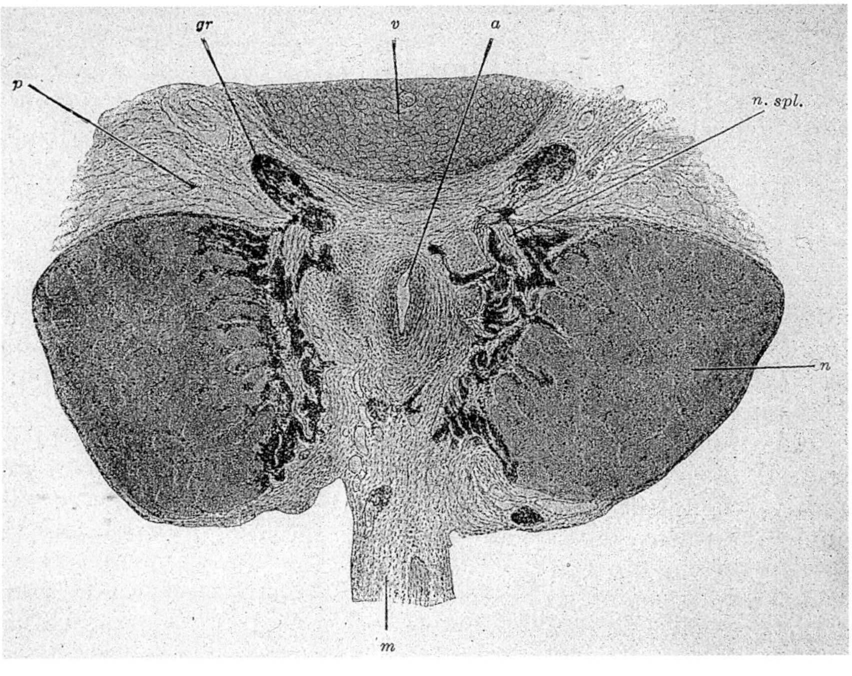


**FIG. 5.** Original illustration by Zuckerkandl of a horizontal section of a human embryo (17 mm crown–heel length) showing presumed migration of primitive sympathetic cells into the adrenal glands. The darkly stippled masses traversed by nerves are the primitive sympathetic cells. a, aorta; gr, developing sympathetic ganglia; s. spl, splanchnic nerve; v, vertebra; p, peritoneal cushion; m, mesentery; n, adrenals. Reprinted with permission (40).

Classic, descriptive, embryologic studies (40,41) show primitive sympathetic cells in large numbers around the spinal nerves and branches of the developing sympathetic trunks before the formation of the paraganglia. The cells are also described along the renal and spermatic arteries (41). The adrenal medulla is apparently colonized by invasion of primitive sympathetic cells into the cortex through the medial aspect of the capsule from the contiguous prevertebral and paravertebral sympathetic tissue (Fig. 5). The primitive sympathetic cells initially form nodular aggregates in the cortex (Fig. 6) and gradually coalesce around the central vein. They may form rosettes or pseudorosettes early in gestation (1). Chromaffin cells are identifiable among these aggregates from about week 8 on (1,42) and gradually increase in number. The centripetal pattern of migration of primitive sympathetic cells into the adrenal may result in subcapsular and intracortical chromaffin cell rests (compare with Fig. 17). Although some primitive sympathetic cells appear to penetrate the cortex along sympathetic nerve fibers, some are apparently not associated with nerve fibers (1). Innervation of the presumptive medulla by preganglionic nerve fibers does not appear to be necessary for colonization because experimental studies demonstrate that the medulla can form in adrenal primordia from 4- or 5-day chick embryos explanted to chorioallantoic membranes before the onset of innervation (1,43). Primitive cells can be observed apparently migrating to developing parasympathetic paraganglia along branches of the glossopharyngeal and vagus nerves as well as from sympathetic nerves (39). The nature, origin, and fate of these cells from different sources and their respective contributions to the mature paraganglia were vigorously debated for more than 70 years (4,39). It is of interest that both the purely morphologic studies of Kohn et al. (40) and later histochemical studies (38) suggest an origin of the neurosecretory cells of the human carotid body, the prototypical parasympathetic paraganglion, from the sympathetic progenitors of the superior cervical ganglion.

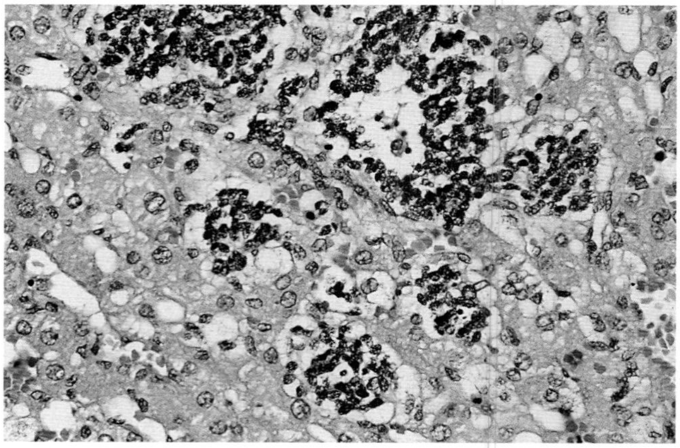

**FIG. 6.** Section of adrenal gland from a 16-week human fetus showing typical aggregates of primitive sympathetic cells that are precursors of the medulla. Pyknotic nuclei and nuclei with changes consistent with apoptosis are present within the aggregates. Many of the small cells express immunoreactive tyrosine hydroxylase, the rate-limiting enzyme in catecholamine synthesis, but do not stain for CGA or synaptophysin, which are characteristic of larger, mature or maturing chromaffin cells (37). Scattered S-100–positive cells consistent with the sustentacular cell lineage are observed at about week 20 (36).

Recognition of the primitive sympathetic cells in the adrenal medulla is particularly important to pathologists in view of the fact that their occasional abnormal persistence may account for at least some cases initially interpreted as "in situ neuroblastoma" (44,45). Nodular aggregates of these cells, up to 400 $\mu$m in greatest dimension, can be demonstrated in the adrenal glands of all fetuses between the ages of 10 and 30 weeks when the glands are thoroughly sectioned (45). Aggregates with a diameter of over 1 mm may occasionally be observed (42). Nerve fibers within human adrenals may connect intra-adrenal and extra-adrenal aggregates (45). The nodules peak in size and number between the ages of 17 and 20 weeks and then decline. Intranodular cystic degeneration is common from the age of 20 weeks onward (45). Postnatal persistence of the nodules was apparently first described by Wiesel in 1902 (40).

## POSTNATAL AND DEVELOPMENTAL CHANGES

The amount or distribution of paraganglionic tissue is known to change during development and aging. Sympathetic paraganglionic tissue in fetuses and neonates is primarily extra-adrenal, with the greatest volume in the organ of Zuckerkandl. The organ of Zuckerkandl develops maximally in humans by the age of about 3 years, when its greatest dimension may be more than 20 mm. Thereafter, the organ involutes (1,15), while the adrenal medulla enlarges until maturity. Similarly, SIF cells are present in all human sympathetic ganglia at birth but are rare in adults, where they appear concentrated in the thoracic region (1,46). Parasympathetic paraganglionic tissue also appears to decrease in some locations and to increase in others. Subclavian and intrapulmonary paraganglia, for example, have been identified in human fetuses but not in adults (4). On the other hand, the number of jugular and tympanic paraganglia apparently increases after birth (26). The carotid bodies, which are the only parasympathetic paraganglia that are macroscopic, increase in size between infancy and adult life, when they are normally about 3 mm in greatest dimension (4) (Fig. 4).

## APOPTOSIS

There have been few, if any, studies of apoptosis that are specifically focused on the paraganglia. It is generally accepted that apoptosis plays a critical role in the development of both the central and peripheral nervous systems, where excess neural progenitor cells undergo apoptotic death after failing to establish functional contacts or receive appropriate

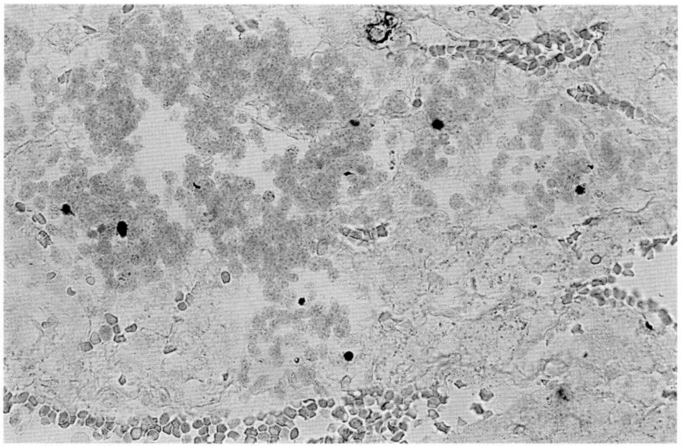

**FIG. 7.** Section of the same adrenal as in Fig. 6 showing terminal deoxynucleatidyl transferase–mediated end-labeling (49) of nuclei within a neuroblastic aggregate (black nuclei). This method, which detects fragmented DNA, can be helpful in locating apoptotic cells. (Courtesy of Dr. Salvador Diaz-Cano.)

trophic substances from target tissues (47,48). Apoptotic bodies can be identified within the aggregates of primitive sympathetic cells in the adrenal medulla (Figs. 6 and 7).

## GROSS FEATURES AND ORGAN WEIGHTS

The paraganglionic tissue of the grossly identifiable paraganglia is gray or gray–pink. Recognition of this feature is particularly important in the adrenal gland because the medulla is normally confined to the head and body of the gland but extends into the tail and alae in adrenal medullary hyperplasia (50,51). An accurate gross examination requires that the brown tissue of the cortical zona reticularis not be misidentified as medulla.

Due to the anatomic inconsistencies of the microscopic paraganglia and the organ Zuckerkandl, meaningful weights can be ascribed only to the adrenal medulla and carotid body. Extensive morphometric studies (52) have shown that the neonatal adrenal medulla accounts for approximately 0.4% of the total volume of the gland and weighs approximately 0.012 g. These values increase to 4.2% and 0.08 g at 2 years of age, 7.0% and 0.28 g between the ages of 10 and 13 years, and 9.9% and 0.46 g in adults up to the age of 40 years. After the age of 40 years, there is a small decline in medullary weight and volume. The weight of the carotid body appears to correlate more closely with body weight than with age. Lack (53) has proposed an equation to estimate carotid body weight from body weight for any age group: Combined weight of carotid bodies (mg) = 0.29 × body weight (kg) + 3.0. Standard deviations for any age group are large (54), but in normal adults the combined weight is usually less than 30 mg. The carotid body increases in size and weight in individuals living at high altitudes (55) and in patients with hypoxemia due to a variety of ailments (56–59).

## ANATOMY

All paraganglia are highly vascular, a characteristic that permits them to be localized by leakage of systemically injected dye in animal studies (60). However, the details of their blood supply are highly varied according to their location and function. For example, the adrenal medulla receives arterial blood from three arteries—the inferior phrenic artery, aorta, and renal arteries—and drains via a single adrenal vein that empties into the renal vein on the left and the aorta on the right (see Chapter 16). The carotid body receives arterial blood from one or occasionally two small arteries arising from the vicinity of the carotid bifurcation and drains via several small veins into the pharyngeal, superior laryngeal, and lingual veins (4).

The innervation of paraganglia is comparably site specific. In general, sympathetic paraganglia receive preganglionic cholinergic sympathetic innervation and variable amounts of noradrenergic and/or peptidergic innervation from intrinsic neurons, nearby sympathetic ganglia, and other sources. Most of the neuroendocrine cells in the adrenal medulla are innervated, and the innervation is complex (61). In contrast, the extra-adrenal sympathetic paraganglia are sparsely innervated (1,62), and it has been suggested that their ability to attract or maintain innervation might determine the extent to which they persist or involute at different sites (11). Parasympathetic paraganglia generally receive their innervation from branches of either the vagus or glossopharyngeal nerves but also may receive some sympathetic input. A small percentage of carotid body cells, for example, reportedly synapses with preganglionic sympathetic fibers (63). Some carotid body cells also may lack innervation (64). In addition to innervation that directly involves neuroendocrine cells, paraganglia may receive vasomotor innervation. The carotid body receives vasomotor innervation from the nearby superior cervical ganglion and from a small number of intrinsic neurons (63,65). Recent immunohistochemical studies of the human carotid body at the ultrastructural level (66) have made progress in assigning specific catecholamine and peptide neurotransmitters to nerve endings from different sources. The roles of different neurotransmitters in adrenal medullary nerve endings are also being investigated (67).

The neurovascular relationships of individual parasympathetic paraganglia have been described in great detail by several investigators (4,39). Of particular interest to pathologists are the paraganglia that give rise to glomus jugulare and glomus tympanicum paragangliomas in the floor or the wall of the middle ear. The paraganglia in the human temporal bone are distributed along the auricular branch of the vagus nerve (Arnold's nerve), and the tympanic branch of the glossopharyngeal nerve (Jacobson's nerve) (26). About 70% of paraganglia related to Arnold's nerve occur on the jugular bulb. The remainder follow the nerve through the mastoid canaliculus toward the vertical portion of the facial nerve. Paraganglia along Jacobson's nerve occur anywhere from the origin of the nerve at the petrosal ganglion (10%) to the jugular bulb (28%), tympanic canaliculus (40%), promontory of the middle ear (20%), and beyond (2%). Glomus jugulare tumors may therefore be associated with either Arnold's or Jacobson's nerve, although the former is most likely. Glomus tympanicum tumors are almost always associated with Jacobson's nerve (4).

## LIGHT MICROSCOPY

### Cell Types

Paraganglia contain two major types of cell: neuroendocrine cells and supporting cells. The former have been referred to in many publications as granule-containing cells, or chromaffin cells in sympathetic paraganglia and glomus cells, type I cells, or chief cells in parasympathetic paraganglia. The latter have been called sustentacular cells, satellite cells, supporting cells, or type II cells (4,24). In addition, there are variable numbers of connective tissue cells, vascular cells, Schwann cells, myelinated or unmyelinated nerve fibers, and intrinsic neurons. An additional commonly encountered cell type is the mast cell, which may be abundant in both ganglia and paraganglia (4,68). In hematoxylin and eosin (H&E)-stained sections, paraganglionic neuroendocrine cells are polygonal cells with amphophilic or basophilic cytoplasm and small, spherical or ovoid, pale-staining nuclei. Their identity can be confirmed by electron microscopy or argyrophil-type silver stains to demonstrate secretory granules, by fluorescence methods to demonstrate catecholamines, or by immunocytochemical stains for a variety of neuroendocrine markers (see section on "Special Procedures"). They tend to form clusters and cords, which were described as *Zellballen* and *Zellsträngen* by Alfred Kohn (4,5), and to be partially or completely surrounded by supporting cells. The latter are usually flattened, with less conspicuous cytoplasm and more deeply basophilic nuclei with coarsely clumped chromatin. They appear to be glial cells, possibly related to non–myelin-forming Schwann cells elsewhere in the peripheral nervous system (69), and can be identified by staining for S-100 protein (70). Like non–myelin-forming Schwann cells, they have been reported in some instances to also stain for glial fibrillary acidic protein (71,72). They are present in both parasympathetic (70,72) and sympathetic (71,73,74) paraganglia but are more numerous in the former, where they cause the *Zellballen* to appear more pronounced (Figs. 8–10).

### Lobular Architecture of the Carotid Body

The carotid body is architecturally distinctive in that it consists of lobules separated by connective tissue septa. Each lobule is individually reminiscent of the microscopic paraganglia that occur in other sites and is composed of nests of chief cells surrounded by other cell types. This lobular arrangement is important to pathologists because carotid body hyperplasia is generally defined as an increase in mean lobule diameter (53–57). The amount of connective tissue between lobules in the carotid body tends to increase with age. Schwann cell proliferation and axonal sprouting also may occur at the periphery of lobules (Figs. 11 and 12). One group of investigators has reported that the latter change is the pathognomonic feature of lobular hyperplasia in elderly patients with emphysema or hypertension (57). Other investigators studying specimens predominantly from patients with congenital heart disease have reported proportional proliferation of sustentacular cells and chief cells (53,54,56), whereas still others have reported chief cell hyperplasia in high-altitude dwellers (55). Lobular architecture similar to that of the carotid body is occasionally observed in other

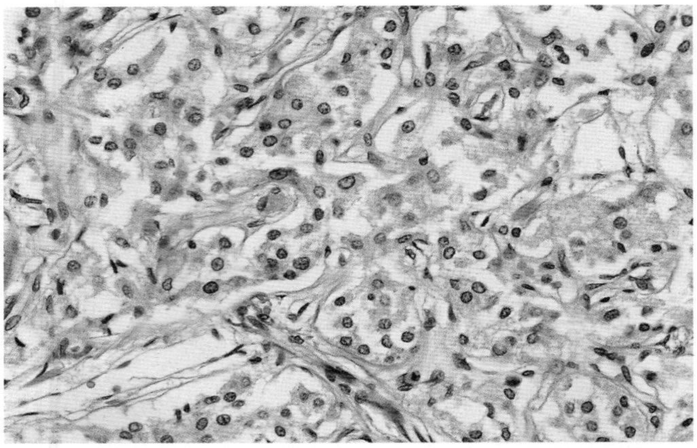

**FIG. 8.** Section of organ of Zuckerkandl from a mid-trimester human fetus, demonstrating typical cords and nests of chief cells with rounded or oval nuclei and amphophilic cytoplasm, and occasional interspersed sustentacular cells with flattened nuclei and inconspicuous cytoplasm.

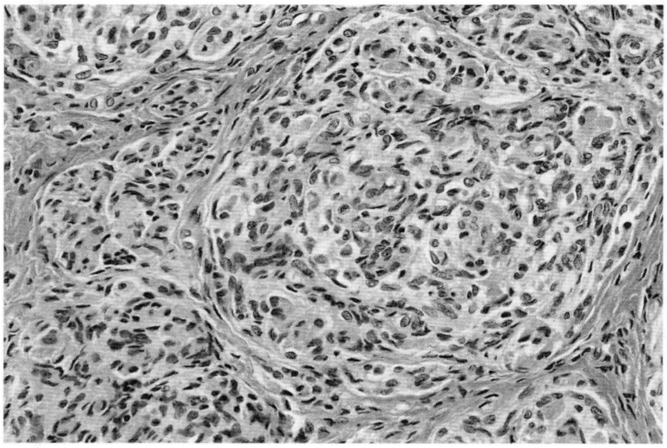

**FIG. 9.** Section of carotid body from a 6-day-old infant demonstrating a characteristically more heterogeneous cell population than in Fig. 8. Small nests of chief cells are highlighted by surrounding sustentacular cells and other cell types.

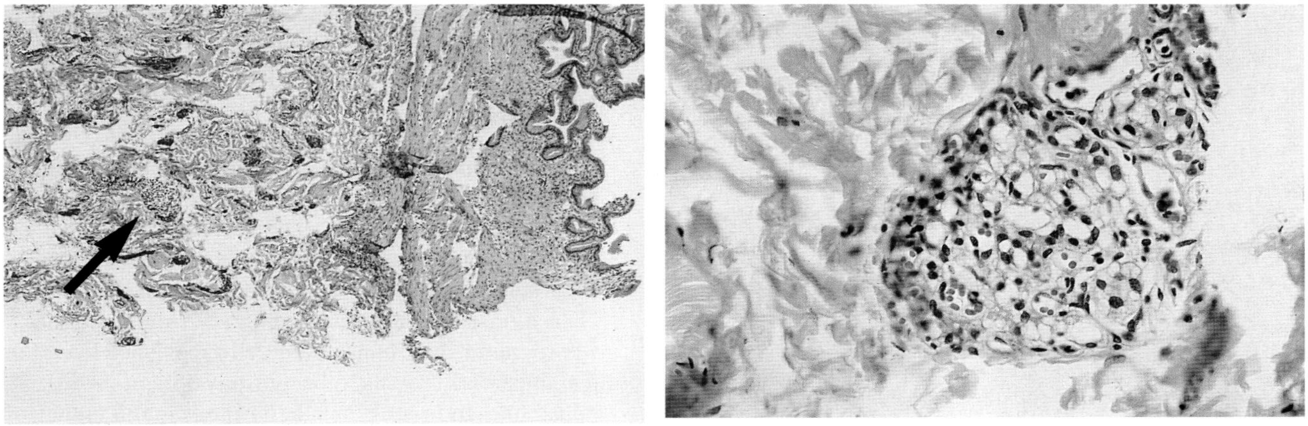

A B

**FIG. 10.** **A:** A microscopic paraganglion (small, oval, blue structure, *bottom center*) discovered as an incidental finding in the wall of the gallbladder of a 40-year-old woman. **B:** Higher magnification of the structure in (**A**), illustrating prominent capillaries and admixed cell types.

parasympathetic paraganglia, particularly if they are enlarged (54).

## ULTRASTRUCTURE

At the ultrastructural level, paraganglionic neuroendocrine cells are characterized by numerous membrane-bound granules or "dense-cored vesicles" approximately 60 to 400 nm in greatest dimension. In addition, they sometimes contain small synaptic-like vesicles, which may accumulate in clusters near the plasma membrane (22,65). Neuroendocrine secretory granules may vary in size, shape, and electron density, reflecting differences in the secretory products stored, in the functional state of individual cells, and in fixation conditions. In the rodent adrenal medulla, where epinephrine and norepinephrine are mostly stored in separate cells, fixation in glutaraldehyde and postfixation in osmium

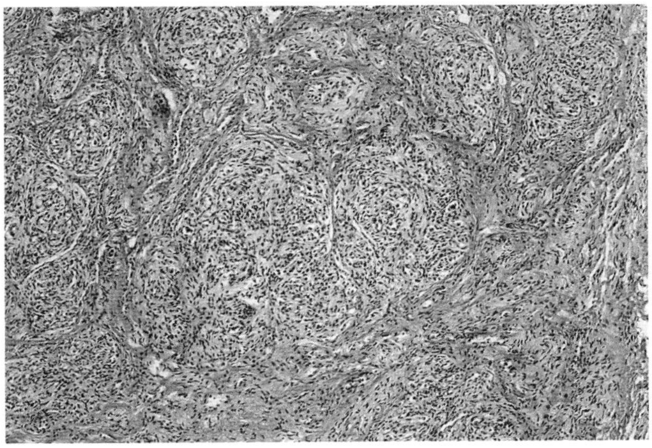

**FIG. 11.** Carotid body from a 10-day-old infant, illustrating lobules separated by connective tissue septa.

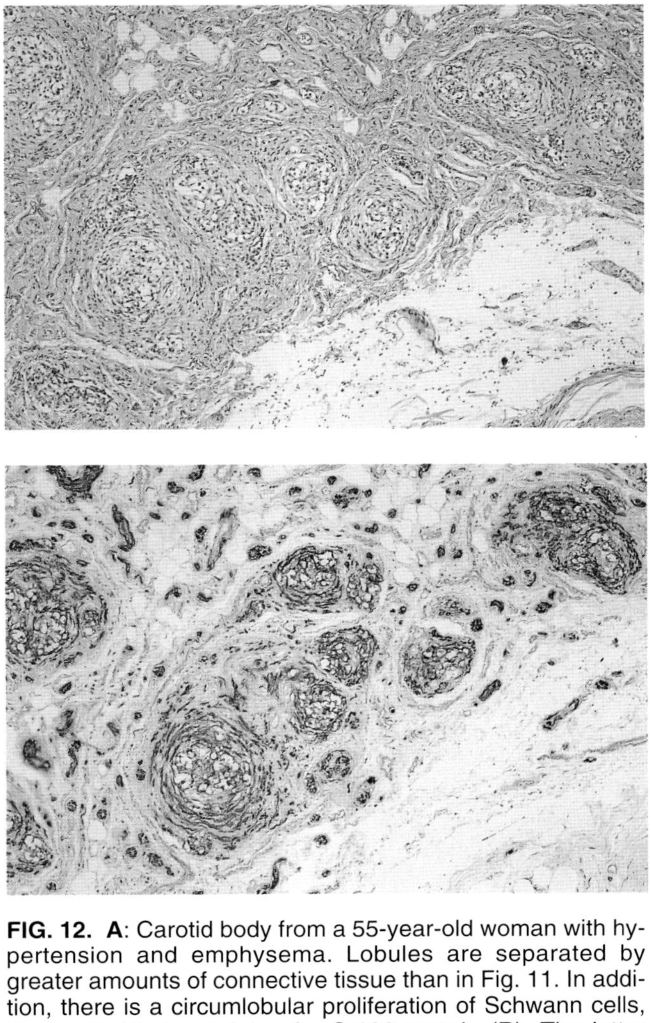

A B

**FIG. 12.** **A**: Carotid body from a 55-year-old woman with hypertension and emphysema. Lobules are separated by greater amounts of connective tissue than in Fig. 11. In addition, there is a circumlobular proliferation of Schwann cells, demonstrable by staining for S-100 protein (**B**). The latter change has been reported by some investigators to be characteristic of lobular hyperplasia in patients with hypertension (57).

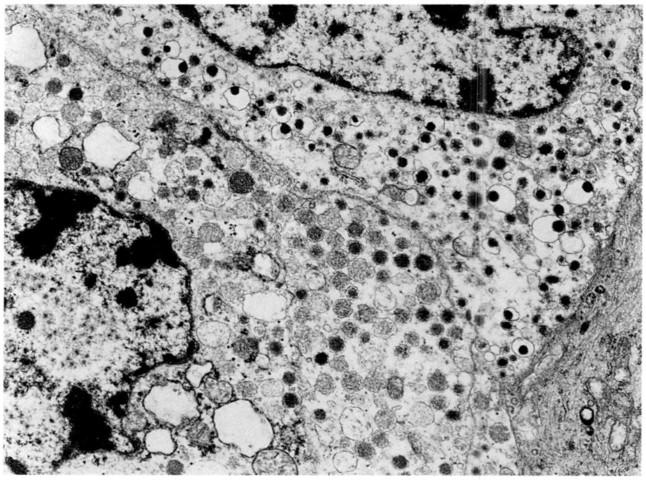

**FIG. 13.** Electron micrograph of normal human adrenal medulla fixed in glutaraldehyde and postfixed in osmium tetroxide. Portions of cells at left contain predominantly light, finely particulate epinephrine-type granules, whereas cell at right contains predominantly dark, homogeneously electron-dense norepinephrine-type granules. The eccentric location of the granule cores within their surrounding membranes is a fixation artifact most commonly observed with granules of the latter type (original magnification ×9,677). Reprinted with permission (14).

tetroxide cause granules in neuroendocrine cells to appear homogeneously electron dense, whereas those in endocrine cells are lighter and finely particulate. The mechanism for the differentiation involves formation of an insoluble reaction product between glutaraldehyde and norepinephrine, which is subsequently darkened by osmium (1,75). Because epinephrine does not similarly react with glutaraldehyde, it diffuses out of the granules, leaving behind other granule constituents that are less osmiophilic. To be successful, this method requires adequate fixation of fresh tissue. Human adrenal medullary cells occasionally exhibit homogeneous populations of endocrine- or neuroendocrine-type granules (Fig. 13) but most often have mixed granule populations (see Chapter 16, Fig. 42) (76) and synthesize both endocrine and neuroendocrine cells (77). The electron density of most granules in extra-adrenal paraganglia is comparable to that of neuroendocrine-type granules in the adrenal.

The ultrastructural organization of paraganglia and the proportions of their constituent cell types vary in different sites, apparently to suit different physiologic needs. Both sympathetic and parasympathetic paraganglia contain numerous small capillaries. In the former, portions of the surfaces of neuroendocrine cells closest to these vessels are usually separated from the capillary endothelium only by basal laminae and occasional collagen fibrils, suggesting that sympathetic paraganglia in most instances function as endocrine glands (62). In some locations, their secretory products appear to be provided for local use (10). In contrast, the neuroendocrine cells in parasympathetic paraganglia tend to be separated from the capillary lumina by sustentacular cells, pericytes, or both (Figs. 14–16). It therefore appears that a major role of their secretory products is to act directly on sensory parasympathetic nerve endings rather than to enter circulating blood (63,65,78,79).

The relationships between individual neuroendocrine cells and nerve endings in paraganglia can be defined as presynaptic, postsynaptic, or reciprocally synaptic, based on the locations of synaptic membrane densities and vesicle accumulations. In the adrenal medulla, the chromaffin cells are postsynaptic, consistent with their principal role of secreting hormones in response to neural stimulation. In contrast, nu-

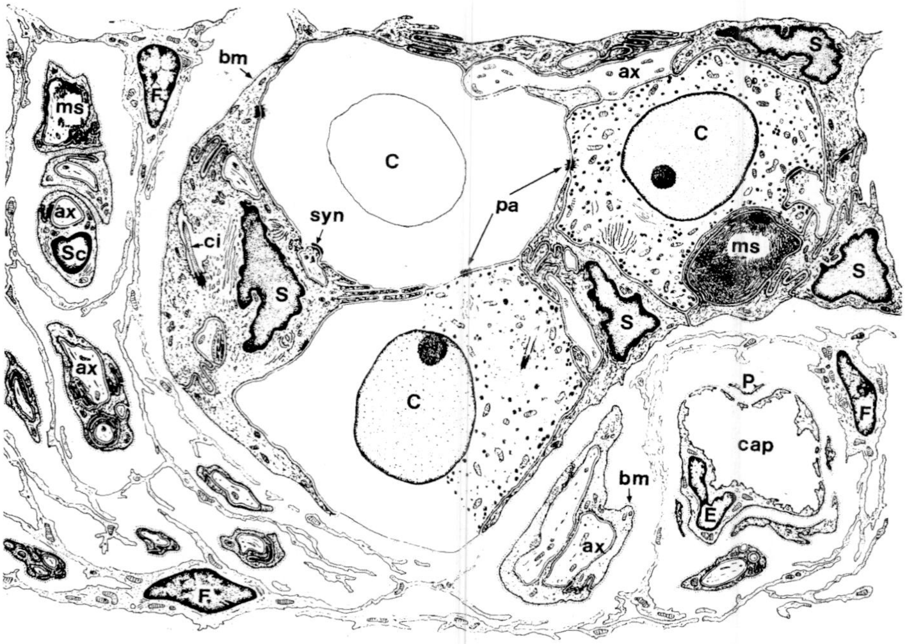


**FIG. 14.** Diagram of the architecture of the human carotid body at the periphery of a lobule. Chief cells (C) in a small nest are insulated from the lumen of a nearby capillary (cap) by sustentacular cells (S), fibroblasts (F), and pericytes (P) and form synapses (syn) with parasympathetic axons (ax). They are also joined to each other by simple "puncta adherentia" type junctions (pa). Axons surrounded by Schwann cells (Sc) are present at the periphery of the lobule. Other illustrated structures are basement membrane (bm), endothelial cells (E), cilia (ci), and mitochondrion-rich axonal dilations termed "mitochondrial sacs" (ms). Reprinted with permission (78).

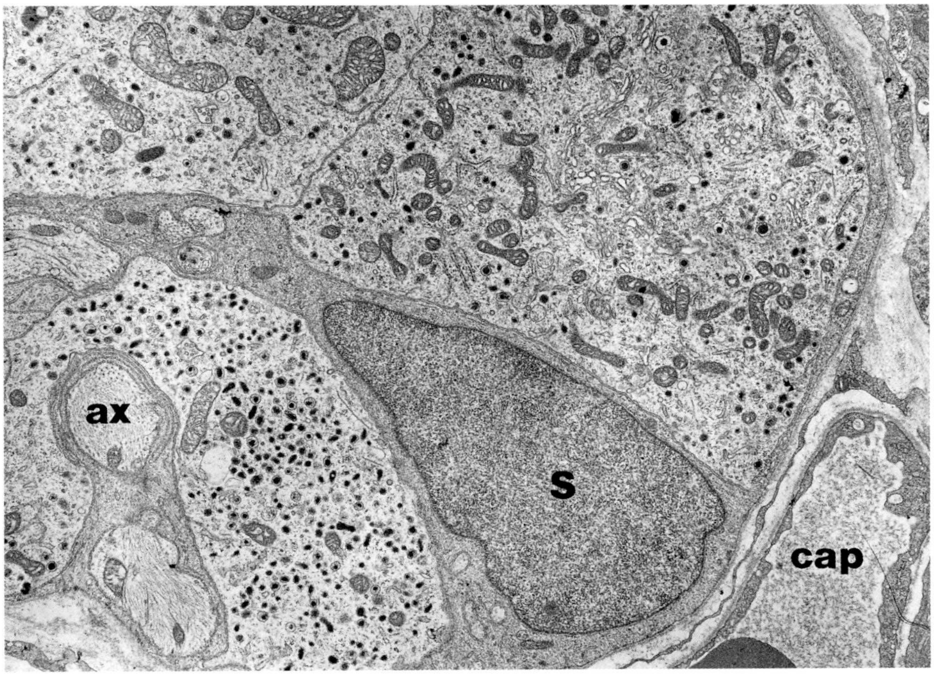


**FIG. 15.** Electron micrograph of human carotid body from an area similar to that illustrated in Fig. 14. S, sustentacular cell; cap, capillary; ax, axon (original magnification ×**8,000**). Adapted with permission (78).

merous reciprocal synapses involving nerve endings and chief cells of the carotid body are consistent with the carotid body's chemosensory functions.

Despite the above generalizations about the ultrastructural organization of sympathetic and parasympathetic paraganglia, in some instances there is overlap. This is especially apparent for SIF cells, at least in rodents, where they have been extensively studied. SIF cells are usually related to blood vessels and nerve endings comparably to other sympathetic paraganglionic cells (11). In some ganglia, however, they are insulated from the capillary lumina (11,12,22). Generally, they receive preganglionic sympathetic synapses, but

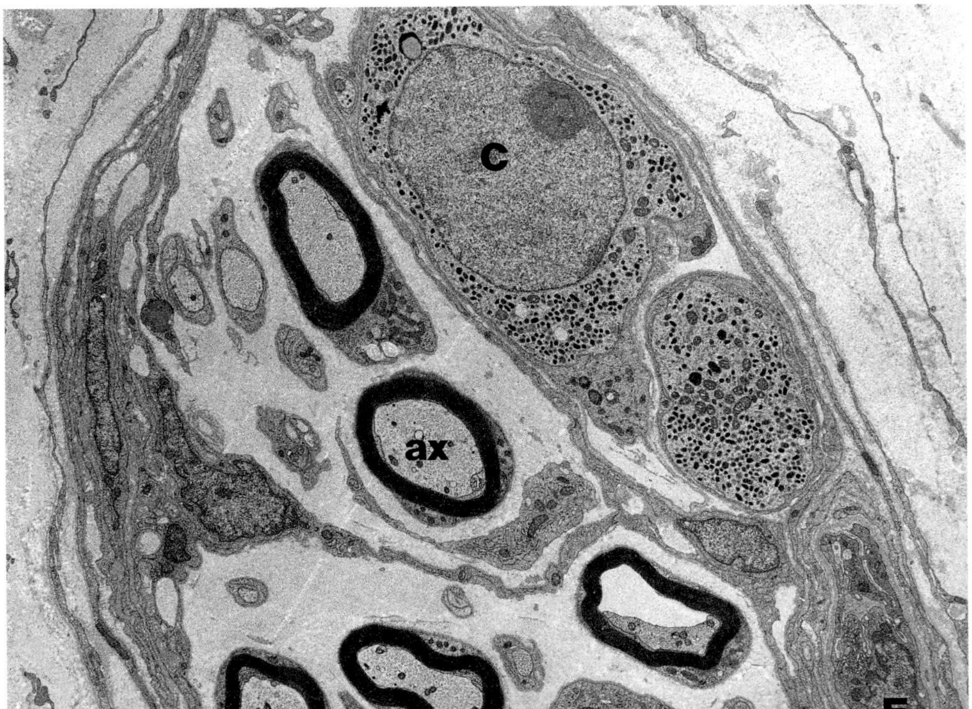


**FIG. 16.** Electron micrograph of two chief cells enclosed within the perineurium of a small myelinated nerve in the vicinity of a human carotid body. This configuration has been described for intravagal paraganglia (30,54). As in the carotid body (see Figs. 14 and 15), the chief cells are separated from the lumen of a nearby capillary (original magnification ×**5,400**). C, chief cells; E, endothelial cell; ax, axons. (Courtesy of Professor P. Böck.)

in a few locations some may apparently also provide synapses to sympathetic neurons, suggesting a role as interneurons. Some also may be involved in reciprocal synapses with their preganglionic axons, suggesting chemoreceptor functions (80). Different SIF cells within a single small cluster can have different synaptic relationships, and a single process from one SIF cell can both synapse on a neuron and be in direct contact with a capillary basal lamina (11). It is important to note that two morphologically distinct types of SIF cells have been described in rodents, accounting in part for this functional diversity. Type I SIF cells have ultrastructural features intermediate between neuroendocrine cells and neurons, whereas type II SIF cells are typical neuroendocrine cells (22). Ultrastructural studies of human SIF cells are limited. Data that are available suggest that there is only one human SIF cell type, which is neuroendocrine (2,81).

## FUNCTION

### Physiologic Roles

The physiologic role of paraganglia is to release secretory products in response to neural or chemical stimuli. These products may be used for endocrine, paracrine, neurotransmitter, or neuromodulatory functions, depending on their anatomic context. Although their secretory products are similar, sympathetic and parasympathetic paraganglia generally appear to differ in the types of stimuli to which they respond. Responses to different types of stimuli also may delineate subsets of paraganglia within the sympathetic and parasympathetic groups. However, there is also evidence suggestive of some functional overlap.

The adult adrenal medulla responds to signals that are principally neuronal. Various physiologic stressors reflexly evoke discharges of splanchnic nerve endings that synapse on chromaffin cells, causing release of secretory granules by $Ca^{2+}$-mediated exocytosis. This secretory response is accompanied by ancillary effects including activation of protooncogenes (82), activation and induction of enzymes involved in replenishing granule constituents (83,84), and possibly stimulation of chromaffin cell proliferation (85). Cellular responses to neurally derived stimulation may be modulated by chemical signals, including corticosteroids (83), growth factors (86), and hormones or neurotransmitters that increase intracellular cyclic adenosine monophosphate (84) or activate protein kinase C (86). The sparse innervation of the extra-adrenal sympathetic paraganglia (62) suggests that for them chemical signals may play a predominant role. One possible chemical signal is hypoxemia. Although adult adrenal chromaffin cells do not respond directly to hypoxemia, it has been suggested that the organ of Zuckerkandl in rabbits and humans may secrete catecholamines in response to hypoxemia during development (87,88). In other species, chemoreceptive functions also have been postulated for the immature adrenal medulla before the establishment of innervation (89) and for certain SIF cells (80,90,91).

For parasympathetic paraganglia, chemoreception is the best known function. It has been established since the 1930s that the carotid bodies and aortic paraganglia function as portions of reflex loops involving the central nervous system, whereby low $pO_2$, low pH, and high $pCO_2$ stimulate breathing (4). However, it was long debated whether the neuroendocrine cells in the carotid body are the primary receptor elements or whether their function is to modulate chemoreceptor properties intrinsic to the sensory nerve endings. Recent electrophysiologic studies of the mechanism of chemoreception in cell culture have shown that the three major chemosensory stimuli depolarize dissociated carotid body chief cells (92–94). This, in turn, may lead to influx of calcium through voltage-gated calcium channels, and calcium-dependent release of secretory products to stimulate sensory nerve endings. Other models also have been suggested. Chemoreceptor reflexes have been postulated for other parasympathetic paraganglia on the basis of their ultrastructural similarities to the carotid body or other findings (27,95), but the nature and importance of such reflexes have not been defined. It may be of interest in this regard that patients who have had their carotid bodies removed exhibit impaired ventilatory reflexes (96) and that carotid body hyperplasia occurs in association with life at high altitude (55), chronic obstructive pulmonary disease, restrictive pulmonary disease, cystic fibrosis, and cyanotic congenital heart disease (53–59). Increases in number or size of vagal paraganglia sometimes also occur but are not consistent (54). A tenfold increase in the prevalence of carotid body paragangliomas also has been reported at high altitude (97), but this association has not been established for paragangliomas at other sites.

### Secretory Products

Although studies using the chromaffin reaction suggested that catecholamines were produced by sympathetic and not by parasympathetic paraganglia (4), more sensitive methods now available indicate that they are produced by paraganglia of both classes (4,22,29). These methods include formaldehyde- (98,99) or glyoxylic acid–induced (100) fluorescence to demonstrate catecholamine stores, and immunocytochemistry to demonstrate catecholamine biosynthetic enzymes (77,101,102) (see section on "Special Procedures"). Most of the body's epinephrine production is in the adrenal medulla, where the epinephrine-to-norepinephrine ratio is approximately 4:1 (103). In contrast, over 90% of the catecholamine content of extra-adrenal sympathetic paraganglia is norepinephrine (15). Parasympathetic paraganglia produce almost no epinephrine but may produce significant quantities of dopamine (104). Serotonin has been reported in addition to catecholamines in some human paraganglia (105) and paragangliomas (14). However, it is not clear whether it represents synthesis or uptake (106).

Both sympathetic and parasympathetic paraganglia produce regulatory peptides in addition to catecholamines

(107). The most prevalent of these are enkephalins (77,102,108,109). Regulatory peptides and amines usually coexist in the same cells (102) and in the same secretory granules (108). The granules also contain numerous other constituents including chromogranin proteins (110–113), adenine nucleotides, peptide-cleaving and -amidating enzymes, dopamine beta-hydroxylase, and several glycoproteins of unknown function that are shared with neurons and other neuroendocrine cells (114,115). Peptide growth factors that might exert both autocrine and paracrine effects also may be present in some species (115,116). Together these granule constituents comprise a "secretory cocktail," the composition of which can be varied in different physiologic and pathologic states (83,114,115).

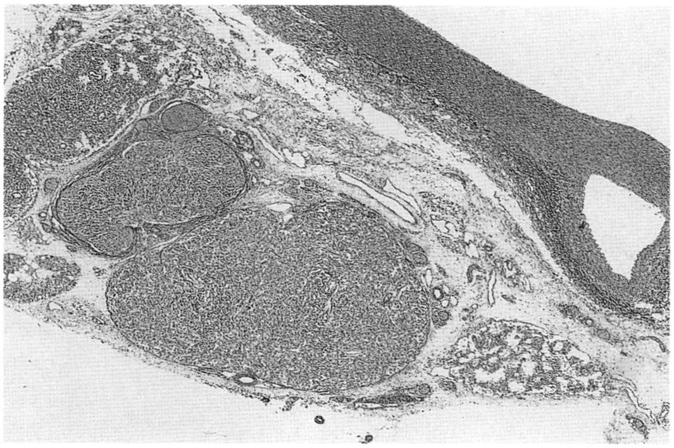

FIG. 18. Transverse section through the aorta of a mid-trimester human fetus (same specimen as in Fig. 17) at the level of the inferior mesenteric artery, demonstrating organ of Zuckerkandl and adjacent sympathetic ganglion, related as diagrammed in Fig. 2.

## SPECIAL PROCEDURES

### Immunohistochemistry

The study of normal and pathologic paraganglia has been greatly facilitated by recent advances in immunohistochemistry. Antibodies that are now commercially available permit identification and functional characterization of specific paraganglionic cell types in sections of formalin-fixed, paraffin-embedded tissue. In addition, the advent of microwave antigen retrieval (117) has both improved the quality of immunohistochemical staining (118) and eliminated some of the variability previously caused by prolonged fixation. For most purposes, immunohistochemistry can now replace previously useful but less specific or more cumbersome techniques such as silver stains, catecholamine fluorescence, and electron microscopy.

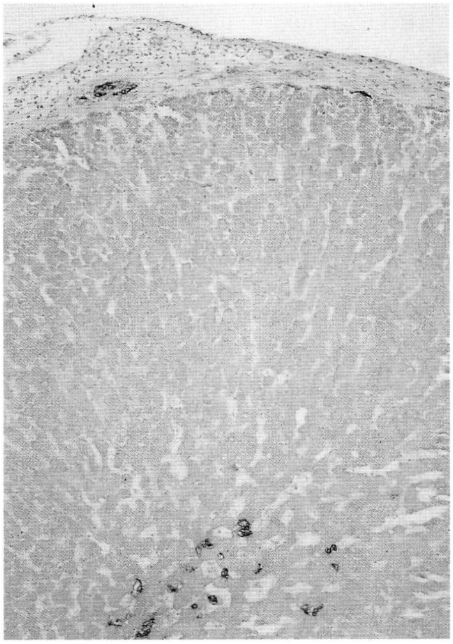

FIG. 17. Adrenal gland from a mid-trimester human fetus, stained for CGA. The medulla contains only scattered positive cells. Extra-adrenal (*upper left*) and subcapsular paraganglionic cells (*upper right*) are also identified by virtue of their immunoreactivity.

Paraganglia express a plethora of markers that are shared to varying degrees with other neural and endocrine tissues (see Chapter 17). A partial categorization includes cytoskeletal proteins, hormones and hormone-synthesizing enzymes, constituents of the secretory granule membrane, and matrix and numerous markers of unknown or poorly understood function. At least in the case of the adrenal medulla, they also express newly described proteins known as SNAPs and SNAREs (SNAP receptors) that are thought to be involved in docking of secretory granules at the cell membrane in preparation for exocytosis. These proteins include synaptobrevin, synaptotagmin, syntaxin, and SNAP-25 (119). Reagents that have been particularly valuable in histopathology are antibodies against chromogranin A (CGA), catecholamine biosynthetic enzymes, and S-100 protein (Figs. 12B and 17–29).

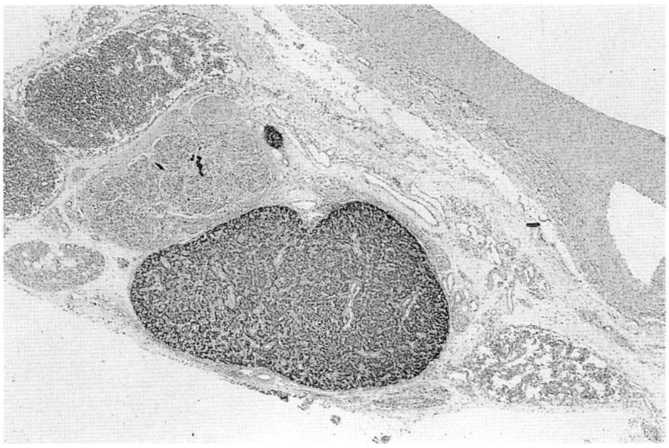

FIG. 19. Section adjacent to that shown in Fig. 18, stained for CGA. Staining is intense in the organ of Zuckerkandl and in small nests of neuroendocrine cells within and adjacent to the ganglion, but not in sympathetic neurons.

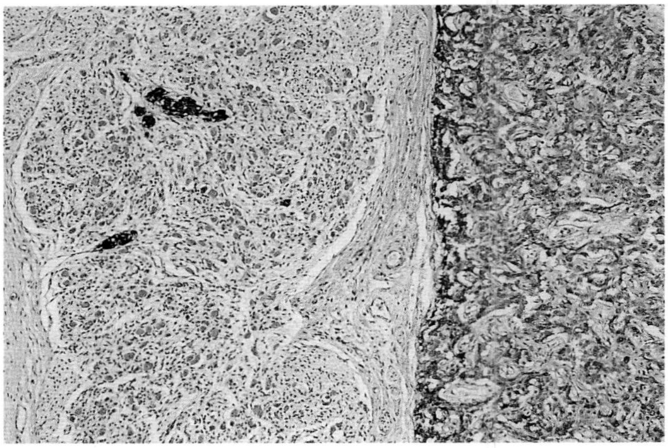

**FIG. 20.** Higher magnification of central area of section shown in Fig. 17. Organ of Zuckerkandl is on right, ganglion on left.

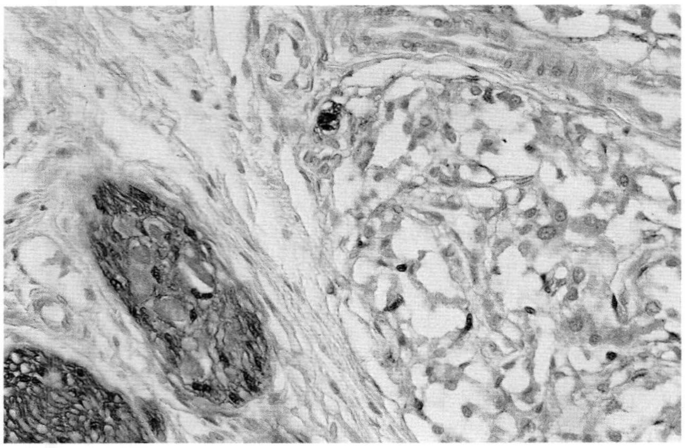

**FIG. 22.** Organ of Zuckerkandl and adjacent sympathetic ganglion (same specimen as in Figs. 17–21), stained for S-100 protein. Immunoreactivity for this antigen is typically localized in both nuclei and cytoplasm. Scattered sustentacular cells are stained in the organ of Zuckerkandl (*right*), and Schwann cells are stained in the ganglion.

CGA is an acidic protein of uncertain function that constitutes more than half the weight of many types of neuroendocrine secretory granule (110–115). It appears to be present in most or all paraganglionic neuroendocrine cells and is therefore a useful generic marker that can, in most instances, replace argyrophil-type silver stains to establish the neuroendocrine nature of particular cells or tissues in the paraganglionic system (Figs. 17–20,23,24,26). Because it is concentrated mostly in secretory granules, it may fail to stain cells that are degranulated due to low rates of synthesis, high rates of turnover, or low storage capacity. In sympathetic ganglia it can be used to conveniently discriminate SIF cells from principal sympathetic neurons, which produce chromogranins but have few perikaryal secretory granules (113) (Figs. 19, 20, and 23).

Perhaps the most important advance in decades from the standpoint of surgical pathology of the paraganglia is the availability of antibodies against the catecholamine-synthesizing enzymes tyrosine hydroxylase (TH), dopamine beta-hydroxylase (DBH), and phenylethanolamine-N-transferase (PNMT). With these reagents, it is now usually possible to infer from a paraffin section not only whether a tumor was catecholamine producing, but also what catecholamines were produced. The need for fluorescence methods that directly detect catecholamine stores but require fresh tissue is therefore, in most instances, eliminated. TH is the rate-limiting enzyme in catecholamine synthesis and is, therefore, found in all catecholamine-producing cells (Figs. 21 and 27), whereas DBH is found only in cells that produce norepinephrine, and PNMT is found only in cells that can convert norepinephrine to epinephrine. This immunocytochemical approach provides a cellular correlate to biochemical data by

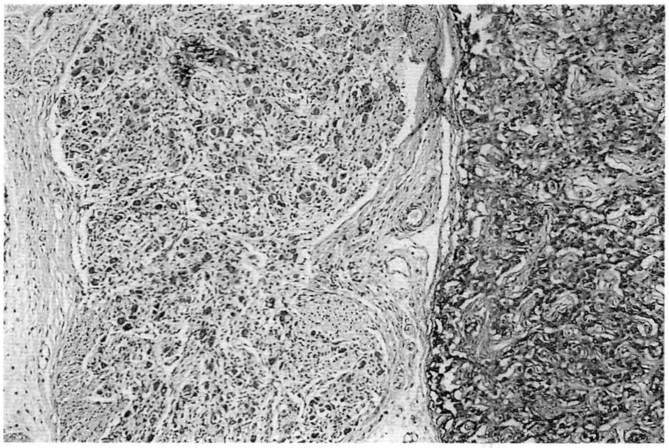

**FIG. 21.** Section adjacent to that shown in Figs. 17 to 20, stained for TH. Intense immunoreactivity is present in both sympathetic neurons and paraganglionic neuroendocrine cells.

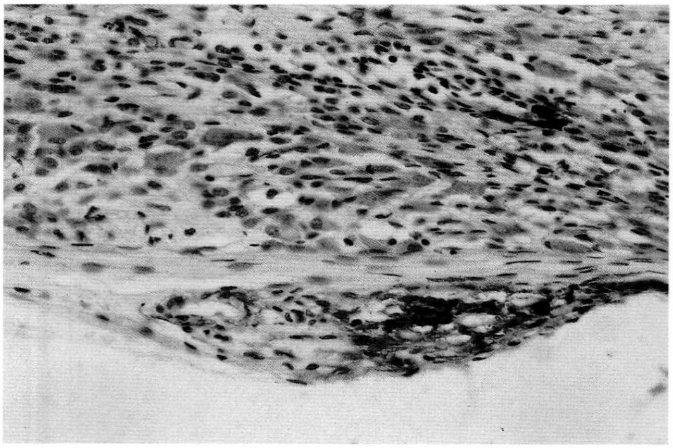

**FIG. 23.** Sympathetic ganglion from the paravertebral trunk of a mid-trimester human fetus (same specimen as in Figs. 17–20), stained for CGA. Neuroendocrine cells are identified both within and adjacent to the ganglion. CGA-positive processes, which might be derived from either neurons or neuroendocrine cells, surround a small blood vessel (*arrow*).

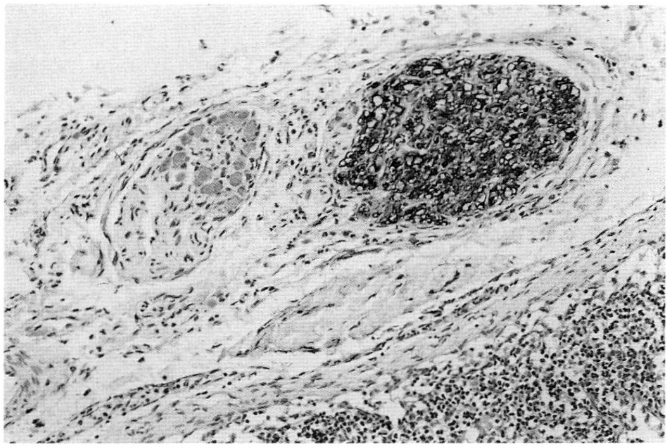

**FIG. 24.** A small retroperitoneal paraganglion similar to that in Fig. 10 and adjacent ganglion, incidentally removed along with adjacent lymph node from a 5-month-old infant during resection of a Wilms' tumor. The identity of the paraganglion was confirmed by soaking the coverslip off a routine H&E-stained histologic section and restaining for CGA. The stability and abundance of this antigen make it particularly suitable for such procedures.

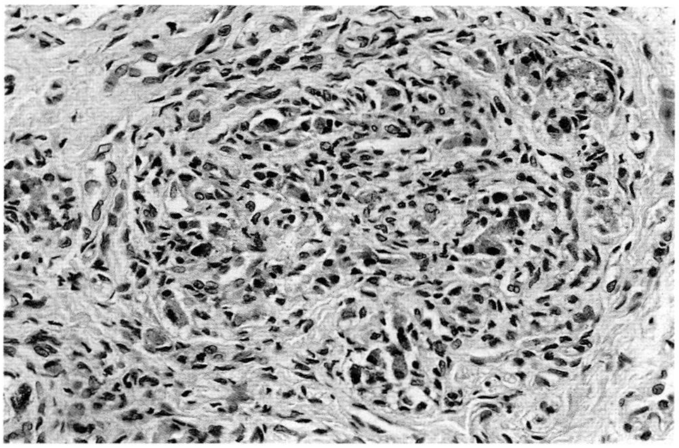

**FIG. 26.** Lobule of a carotid body stained for CGA, demonstrating nests of immunoreactive chief cells surrounded by unstained cells of other types (original magnification ×**100**).

demonstrating that only rarely do extra-adrenal paraganglionic cells stain for PNMT (102), in contrast to the adrenal medulla where the great majority of cells are stained (77) (Figs. 28 and 29). It also has been useful in demonstrating catecholamine-synthesizing ability in paragangliomas (101,120). Because TH and PNMT are cytosolic enzymes (114), staining is not dependent on storage of secretory granules. Sympathetic neurons, for example, stain strongly for TH, in contrast to their weak or absent staining for CGA (Fig. 19–21). In contrast to chromogranins, which are present in many types of neuroendocrine cells, catecholamine biosynthetic enzymes in adult humans are present only in paraganglia and neurons (101,102). In addition to their biosynthetic enzymes, catecholamines themselves may be localized by immunohistochemistry. However, the presence of catecholamines without biosynthetic enzymes under some circumstances (101) suggests that synthesis cannot be distinguished from uptake by this approach.

S-100 protein is a calcium-binding dimer consisting of alpha-alpha, alpha-beta, or beta-beta chains. Initially believed to be specific for central and peripheral nervous system glial cells, it was subsequently found to be more widely distributed (121). It nevertheless provides a useful marker in appropriate contexts. Because of their nondescript cytologic characteristics, the sustentacular cells in paraganglia have until recently been difficult to identify with certainty. The immunoreactivity of these cells for S-100 permits them to be identified in sympathetic and parasympathetic paraganglia (Figs. 12, 22, and 25). Interestingly, they also may be identi-

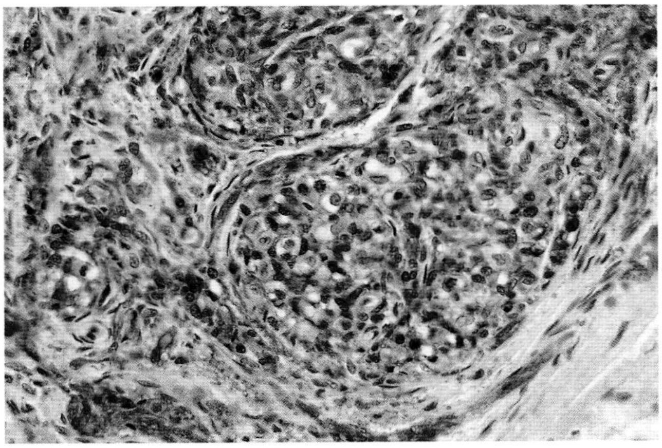

**FIG. 25.** Lobule of a carotid body from a 16-day-old infant stained for S-100 protein. In contrast to the relatively sparse S-100–positive cells in the organ of Zuckerkandl (see Fig. 22), there are numerous stained sustentacular cells within the lobule, accentuating the *Zellballen* and numerous stained Schwann cells both within and adjacent to the lobule, as diagrammed in Fig. 14.

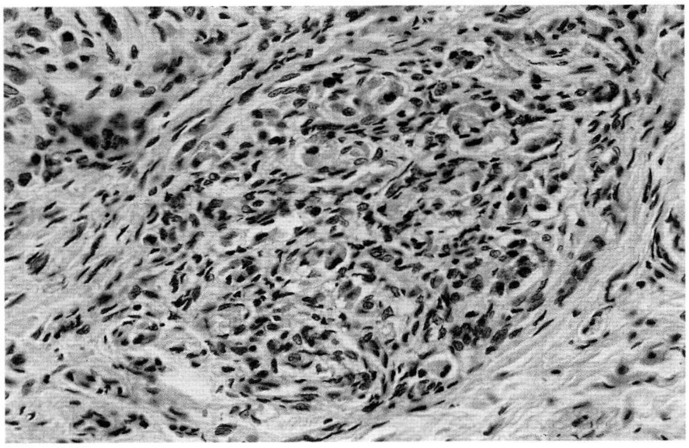

**FIG. 27.** Lobule of a carotid body stained for TH. The catecholamine-synthesizing ability of chief cells is inferred by positive staining of chief cell nests, which are surrounded by unstained cells of other types (original magnification ×**100**).

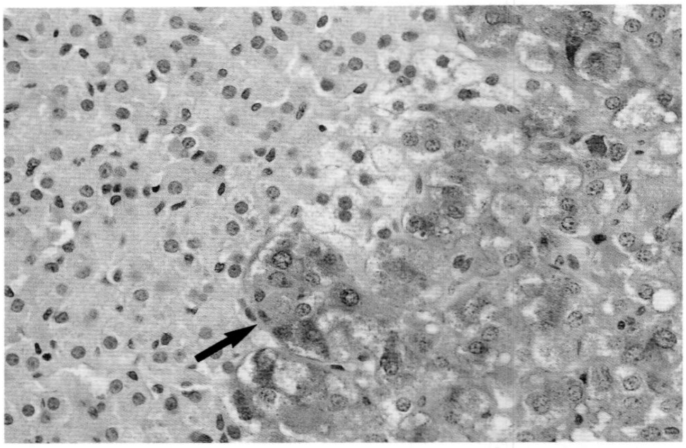

**FIG. 28.** Adult adrenal gland stained for PNMT. The ability of almost all neuroendocrine cells in the adrenal medulla to synthesize epinephrine is inferred from their positive staining. Occasional cells are unstained (*arrow*) as previously reported (77) and as suggested by the electron micrograph in Fig. 13 (original magnification ×**100**).

fied in paragangliomas (73,74), a finding that might reflect either ingrowth from nearby normal tissue or bidirectional differentiation.

### Other Special Procedures

On occasion, it may be desirable to rapidly assess catecholamine content. The situation might arise, for example, if there is an intraoperative need to determine whether tissue is or is not paraganglionic. This may be accomplished with frozen sections or touch preparations using either the formaldehyde vapor (98,99) or glyoxylic acid–induced (100) fluorescence methods. The latter is preferable because it produces nondiffusing fluorophores.

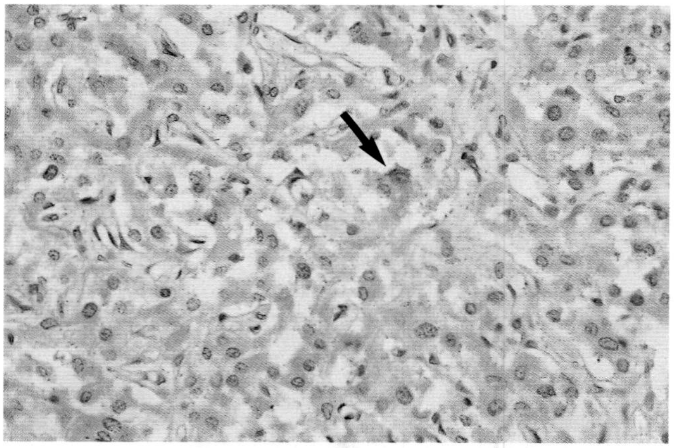

**FIG. 29.** Organ of Zuckerkandl (same specimen as in Figs. 8 and 17–23), stained for PNMT. Although all the neuroendocrine cells stain for TH and can produce catecholamines (see Fig. 21), only rare cells (*arrow*) contain immunoreactive PNMT. This finding is consistent with the limited ability of extra-adrenal paraganglia to synthesize epinephrine, the final step in the catecholamine biosynthetic pathway (original magnification ×**100**).

Several methods for identifying mutations characteristic of specific types of tumors from paraffin sections have been developed for research applications (122,123).

## GENDER DIFFERENCES

Significant gender differences in the histology of paraganglia have not been reported. However, there is some evidence for functional differences. For example, women in general appear to have slightly increased susceptibility to carotid body paragangliomas. This difference is accentuated by life at high altitude, where the tumors have a female-to-male ratio of 6:1 (124).

## AGING CHANGES

Aging changes described in human paraganglia are limited to the topographic and involutional changes described in the sections on "Distribution of Paraganglia," "Gross Features and Organ Weights," and "Lobular Architecture of the Carotid Body." Subtle histochemical changes have been described in the composition of adrenal chromaffin granules of rats (125) and also might occur in other paraganglia.

## ARTEFACTS

Important artefacts must be borne in mind in immunohistochemical studies of paraganglia are the nonspecific interactions of some, but not all, antibodies with the secretory granules of mast cells (126,127) and of certain neuroendocrine cells (128). These artefacts may be particularly troublesome because, due to their inconstancy, negative controls consisting of irrelevant antibodies or normal sera are not adequate. Adsorption controls also may not be sufficient (128). The mast cell artefact has undoubtedly resulted in erroneous published reports of neuroendocrine secretory products in nonendocrine tissues, and also could produce incorrect results in studies of paraganglia because of their sometimes high mast cell content (4).

Nonspecific binding of immunoglobulins to endocrine secretory granules appears to result from ionic interactions and may be reduced by high concentrations of salt in the buffer (128). A buffer containing 0.5 mol/L NaCl should not interfere with specific high-affinity antigen–antibody interactions and, in many instances, may even be used routinely. The mechanism of the mast cell artefact is not known (126), but in some cases the staining may be eliminated by dilution in the presence of normal serum proteins (127). In general, immunohistochemical studies should be performed with the lowest possible antibody concentration and verified, when practical, with antibodies from more than one source. Buffer composition, blocking proteins, and controls should be optimized for each antibody as discussed in many textbooks and reviews (129).

## DIFFERENTIAL DIAGNOSIS

Paraganglia must be discriminated from normal but similar-appearing nonparaganglionic structures and from a variety of malignant tumors. The ampulloglomerular organ (130), glomus coccygeum (6), and glomera cutanea (6) are thermoregulatory structures respectively located in the suboccipital and coccygeal regions and in the skin that are recognized to be unrelated to paraganglia. Lobules of fetal fat may at times appear reminiscent of paraganglia. All of these structures should be readily distinguished from paraganglia by their absence of staining for CGA, TH, or other neuroendocrine markers. Reports of paraganglia in anomalous locations (4) are also now amenable to immunohistochemical verification. Prostatic paraganglia may be misinterpreted as prostatic adenocarcinoma (18), bladder paraganglia may be confused with transitional cell carcinoma (131), and retroperitoneal paraganglia may be confused with metastatic clear cell carcinoma (132). The presence of cytologic atypia, glandular or squamous differentiation, or stromal reaction point toward a diagnosis of tumor, and questionable cases can be readily resolved by immunohistochemistry.

More problematic are cases in which paraganglia or paragangliomas must be distinguished from other normal or neoplastic neuroendocrine tissues that express many of the same markers. Knowledge of the distribution and morphology of paraganglia is essential in these cases. In addition, the presence of tyrosine hydroxylase in paragangliomas or of other site-suggestive markers in other types of tumors, for example calcitonin in medullary thyroid carcinoma, may be helpful. Tumors showing glandular or squamous differentiation are almost certainly not paraganglionic.

In the adrenal gland, developmental neuroblastic nests must be distinguished from in situ neuroblastoma (44,45). Cortical invasion, mitoses, and necrosis are all characteristic of normal cells in this instance. Ikeda et al. (42) reported that the nuclei of normal adrenal medullary progenitors are smaller on average than those of neuroblastoma cells, and this might prove to be diagnostically useful. In view of the large potential effect of fixation on nuclear size, however, the problem is more likely to be resolved using newly developed molecular techniques (122,123).

## SPECIMEN HANDLING

For most purposes, normal and pathologic paraganglionic tissue may be evaluated histologically and immunohistochemically after routine formalin fixation and paraffin embedding (see section on "Special Procedures"). In the age of microwave antigen retrieval, underfixation may create as many artifacts as the traditional problem of overfixation. Fixation of thin tissue slices overnight is usually adequate. Electron microscopy, when necessary, is optimally performed after glutaraldehyde fixation and osmium postfixation (see section on "Ultrastructure"). Catecholamines may be demonstrated in touch preparations or frozen sections using glyoxylic acid–induced fluorescence (see section on "Special Procedures").

For biochemical analysis, catecholamines may be preserved by freezing small minced tissue fragments or tissue homogenates at $-70°C$ in 0.4 mol/L perchloric acid in 1 mmol/L ethylene diamine tetra-acetic acid (84). Peptide hormones may be preserved by freezing in 1.0 mol/L acetic acid. When possible, fresh tissue should be rapidly frozen and stored in liquid nitrogen for molecular studies.

## ACKNOWLEDGMENTS

I thank Professor Peter Böck and Dr. Ernest Lack for contributing illustrative material, Dr. Harold Kozakewich for contributing tissue blocks, Laurel Ruzicka for assistance with immunocytochemical studies, Lisa Hansbury for secretarial assistance, and Dr. Ronald A. DeLellis for comments on the manuscript.

## REFERENCES

1. Coupland RE. *The natural history of the chromaffin cell.* London: Longmans Green; 1965.
2. Coupland RE. The natural history of the chromaffin cell: twenty five years on the beginning. *Arch Histol Cytol* 1989(suppl);52:331–341.
3. Carmichael SW. The history of the adrenal medulla. *Rev Neurosci* 1990;2:83–89.
4. Zak FG, Lawson W. *The paraganglionic chemoreceptor system. Physiology, pathology and clinical medicine.* New York: Springer-Verlag; 1983.
5. Kohn A. Die Paraganglien. *Arch Mikrosk Anat* 1903;52:262–365.
6. Enzinger FM, Weiss SW. *Soft tissue tumors.* 3rd ed. St. Louis: CV Mosby; 1994.
7. Pearse AGE, Polak JM, Rost FWD, Fontaine J, Lelievre, LeDouarin N. Demonstration of the neural crest origin of type I (APUD) cells in the avian carotid body using a cytochemical marker system. *Histochemie* 1973;34:191–203.
8. LeDouarin N. *The neural crest.* Cambridge, England: Cambridge University Press; 1982.
9. Hadjiconstantinou M, Potter PE, Neff NH. Trans-synaptic modulation via muscarinic receptors of serotonin-containing small intensely fluorescent cells of superior cervical ganglion. *J Neurosci* 1982; 2:1836–1839.
10. Furness JB, Sobels G. The ultrastructure of paraganglia associated with the inferior mesenteric ganglia in the guinea pig. *Cell Tissue Res* 1976;1711:123–139.
11. Matthews MR. Synaptic and other relationships of small granule-containing cells. In: Coupland RE, Fujita T, eds. *Chromaffin, enterochromaffin and related cells.* Amsterdam: Elsevier; 1976:131–146.
12. Matthews MR. Ultrastructural studies relevant to the possible functions of small granule-containing cells in the rat superior cervical ganglion. In: Eränkö O, Soinila S, Päivärinta H, eds. *Histochemistry and cell biology of autonomic neurons, SIF cells and paraneurons.* New York: Raven Press Press; 1980:77–86.
13. Mascorro JA, Yates RD. Fine structural comparisons between paraganglion cells and adrenal medullary cells in the syrian hamster. *Tex Rep Biol Med* 1973;31:520–535.
14. Tischler AS. The adrenal medulla and extra-adrenal paraganglia. In: Kovacs K, Asa SL, eds. *Functional endocrine pathology.* Cambridge, MA: Blackwell; 1990.
15. Coupland RE. The development and fate of catecholamine-secreting endocrine cells. In: Parvez H, Parvez S, eds. *Biogenic amines in development.* Amsterdam: Elsevier/North-Holland; 1980:3–28.
16. Hervonen A, Valasti A, Partanen M, Kanerva L, Vaalasti T. The paraganglia, a persisting endocrine system in man. *Am J Anat* 1976;146: 207–210.

17. Baljet B, Boekelar AB, Groen GJ. Retroperitoneal paraganglia and the peripheral autonomic nervous system in the human fetus. *Acta Morphol Neurol Scand* 1985;23:137–149.
18. Ostrowski ML, Wheeler TM. Paraganglia of the prostate. Location, frequency and differentiation from prostatic adenocarcinoma. *Am J Surg Pathol* 1994;18:412–420.
19. Zuckerkandl E. Ueber nebenorgane des sympathicus im Retroperitonealraum des menschen. *Verh Anat Ges* 1901;15:85–107.
20. Ober WB. Emil Zuckerkandl and his delightful little organ. *Path Annu* 1983;18:103–119.
21. Lack EE, Cubilla AL, Woodruff JM, Lieberman PH. Extra-adrenal paragangliomas of the retroperitoneum: a clinicopathological study of 12 tumors. *Am J Surg Pathol* 1980;4:109–120.
22. Eränkö O, Soinila S, Päivärinta H, eds. *Histochemistry and cell biology of autonomic neurons, SIF cells and paraneurons.* New York: Raven Press; 1980.
23. Kohn A. Die chromaffinen Zellen des sympathicus. *Anat Anz* 1898; 15:399–400.
24. Glenner GG, Grimley PM. Tumors of the extra-adrenal paraganglion system (including chemoreceptors). In: *Atlas of tumor pathology*. 2nd series, fascicle 9. Washington, DC: Armed Forces Institute of Pathology; 1974.
25. Helen P, Alho H, Hervonen A. Ultrastructure and histochemistry of human SIF cells and paraganglia. In: Eränkö O, Soinila S, Päivärinta H, eds. *Histochemistry and cell biology of autonomic neurons, SIF cells and paraneurons.* New York: Raven Press; 1980:149–151.
26. Guild SR. The glomus jugulare, a non-chromaffin paraganglion in man. *Ann Otol Rhinol Laryngol* 1953;62:1045–1071.
27. Dahlquist A, Carlson B, Hellstrom S. Paraganglia of the human recurrent laryngeal nerves. *Am J Otolaryngol* 1986;7:366–369.
28. Jacobowitz D. Histochemical studies of the relationship of chromaffin cells and adrenergic nerve fibers to the cardiac ganglia of several species. *J Pharmacol Exp Ther* 1967;158:227–240.
29. Grillo MA, Jacobs L, Comroe JH. A combined fluorescence histochemical and electron microscopic method for studying special monomine-containing cells (SIF cells). *J Compr Neurol* 1974;153: 1–14.
30. Melicow MM. One hundred cases of pheochromocytomas (107 tumors) at the Columbia-Presbyterian Medical Center 1926–1976. *Cancer* 1977;10:1987–2004.
31. Manger WM, Gifford RW. *Pheochromocytoma*. New York: Springer-Verlag; 1977:21,44–48.
32. Kaufman BH, Telander RL, Van Heerden JA, Zimmerman D, Sheps SG, Dawson B. Pheochromocytoma in the pediatric age group: current status. *J Pediatr Surg* 1983;18:879–884.
33. Plenat F, Leroux P, Floquet J, Floquet A. Intra- and juxtavagal paraganglia. A topographical, histochemical and ultrastructural study in the human. *Anat Rec* 1988;221:743–753.
34. Goormaghtigh N, Heymans C. On the existence of the abdominal vagal paraganglia in the adult mouse. *J Anat* 1936;71:77–90.
35. Kuo T, Anderson CB, Rosai J. Normal paraganglia in the human gallbladder. *Arch Pathol* 1974;97:46–47.
36. Cooper MJ, Hutchins GM, Israel MA. Histogenesis of the human adrenal medulla. *Am J Pathol* 1990;137:605–615.
37. Molenaar WM, Lee VM-Y, Trojanowski JQ. Early fetal acquisition of the chromaffin and neuronal immunophenotype by human adrenal medullary cells. An immunohistochemical study using monoclonal antibodies to chromogranin A, synaptophysin, tyrosine hydroxylase and neuronal cytoskeletal protein. *Exp Neurol* 1990;108:1–9.
38. Korkala O, Hervonen A. Origin and development of the catecholamine-storing cells of human fetal carotid body. *Histochemie* 1973;37:287–297.
39. Kjaergaard J. Anatomy of the carotid glands and carotid glomus-like bodies (non-chromaffin paraganglia). Copenhagen: F.A.D.L.'s Forlag; 1973.
40. Zuckerkandl E. The development of the chromaffin organs and of the suprarenal glands. In: Keibel F, Mall FP, eds. *Manual of human embryology*. Philadelphia: JB Lippincott; 1912.
41. Kuntz A The development of the sympathetic nervous system in man. *J Comp Neurol* 1920;32:173–229.
42. Ikeda Y, Lister J, Bouton JM, Buyukpamukcu M. Congenital neuroblastoma, neuroblastoma in situ and the normal fetal development of the adrenal. *J Pediatr Surg* 1981;16(suppl):636–644.
43. Willier BH. A study of the origin and differentiation of the suprarenal gland in the chick embryo by chorio-allantoic grafting. *Phys Zool* 1930;3:201–225.
44. Beckwith JB, Perrin EV. In situ neuroblastomas: a contribution to the natural history of neural crest tumors. *Am J Pathol* 1963;43: 1089–1104.
45. Turkel SB, Itabashi HH. The natural history of neuroblastic cells in the fetal adrenal gland. *Am J Pathol* 1974;225–244.
46. Coupland RE. Persistence of typical chromaffin cells in the human paravertebral sympathetic chain in the child and adult. *Am J Anat* 1979;129–196.
47. Garcia I, Martinov I, Tsujimoto Y, Martineu J-C. Prevention of programmed cell death of sympathetic neurons by the *bcl-2* proto-oncogene. *Science* 1992;258:302–304.
48. Vogel KS. Development of trophic interactions in the vertebrate peripheral nervous system. *Mol Neurobiol* 1993;7:363–382.
49. Gold R, Schmied M, Giegerich G, et al. Differentiating between cellular apoptosis and necrosis by combined use of in situ tailing and nick translation techniques. *Lab Invest* 1994;71:219–225.
50. DeLellis RA, Wolfe HJ, Gagel RF, Feldman ZT, Miller HH, Gang DL, Reichlin S. Adrenal medullary hyperplasia. *Am J Pathol* 1976;83: 177–196.
51. Carney JA, Sizemore GW, Sheps SG. Adrenal medullary disease in multiple endocrine neoplasia, type 2. *Am J Clin Pathol* 1976;66:2-79–290.
52. Kreiner E. Weight and shape of the human adrenal medulla in various age groups. *Virchows Arch [A]* 1982;397:7–15.
53. Lack EE. Carotid body hypertrophy in patients with cystic fibrosis and cyanotic congenital heart disease. *Hum Pathol* 1977;8:39–51.
54. Lack EE. Hyperplasia of vagal and carotid body paraganglia in patients with chronic hypoxemia. *Am J Pathol* 1978;91:497–516.
55. Arias-Stella J, Valcarcel J. Chief cell hyperplasia in the human carotid body at high altitudes. *Hum Pathol* 1976;7:361–373.
56. Lack EE, Perez-Atayde AR, Young JB. Carotid body hyperplasia in cystic fibrosis and cyanotic heart disease. A combined morphometric, ultrastructural and biochemical study. *Am J Pathol* 1985;119: 301–314.
57. Fitch R, Smith P, Heath D. Nerve axons in carotid body hyperplasia. *Arch Pathol Lab Med* 1985;109:234–237.
58. Smith P, Jago R, Heath D. Anatomical variation and quantitative histology of the normal and enlarged carotid body. *J Pathol* 1977;137: 287–304.
59. Heath D, Smith P, Jago R. Hyperplasia of the carotid body. *J Pathol* 1982;138:287–304.
60. McDonald DM, Blewett RW. Location and size of carotid body–like organs (paraganglia) revealed in rats by the permeability of blood vessels to Evans blue dye. *J Neurocytol* 1981;10:607–643.
61. Parker TL, Keese WK, Mohamed AA, Affwork M. The innervation of the mammalian adrenal gland. *J Anat* 1993;183:265–276.
62. Hervonen A. Development of catecholamine-storing cells in human fetal paraganglia and adrenal medulla. *Acta Physiol Scand* 1971(suppl);368:1–94.
63. McDonald DM, Mitchell RA. The innervation of glomus cells, ganglion cells and blood vessels in the rat carotid body: a quantitative ultrastructural analysis. *J Neurocytol* 1975;4:177–230.
64. Eyzaquirre C, Fidone SJ. Transduction mechanisms in carotid body: glomus cells, putative neurotransmitters and nerve endings. *Am J Physiol* 1980;138:C135–C152.
65. Verna A. Ultrastructure of the carotid body in the mammals. *Int Rev Cytol* 1979;60:271–330.
66. Kummer W, Habeck J-O. Light and electron microscopical immunohistochemical investigation of the innervation of the human carotid body. *Adv Exp Med Biol* 1993;337:67–71.
67. Holgert H, Dagerlind Å, Hökfelt T, Lagerkrant Z. Neuronal markers, peptides and enzymes in nerves and chromaffin cells of the rat adrenal medulla during postnatal development. *Brain Res Dev Brain Res* 1994;83:35–52.
68. Kraus R, Bezdicek P. The incidence of mastocytes in paraganglia. *Folia Morphol (Prague)* 1988;36:211–213.
69. Mirsky R, Jessen KR. The biology of non–myelin-forming Schwann cells. *Ann N Y Acad Sci* 1986;486:132–146.
70. Kondo H, Iwaanaga T, Nakajimi T. Immunocytochemical study on the localization of neuron-specific enolase and S-100 protein in the carotid body of rats. *Cell Tissue Res* 1982;227:291–295.
71. Korat O, Trojanowski JQ, LiVolsi VA, Merino MJ. Antigen expression in paraganglia and paragangliomas. *Surg Pathol* 1988;1:33–40.
72. Habeck J-O, Kummer W. Neuronal and neuroectodermal markers in the human carotid body in health and disease. *Adv Exp Biol Med* 1993; 337:31–35.

73. Lauriola L, Maggiano N, Sentinelli S, Michetti F, Cocchia D. Satellite cells in the normal human adrenal gland and in pheochromocytomas. *Virchows Arch [B]* 1985;49:13–21.
74. Lloyd RV, Vlaivas M, Wilson BS. Distribution of chromogranin and S-100 protein in normal and abnormal adrenal medullary tissues. *Arch Pathol Lab Med* 1985;109:633–635.
75. Coupland RE, Hopwood D. The mechanism of the differential staining reaction for adrenaline and noradrenaline storing granules in tissues fixed with glutaraldehyde. *J Anat* 1966;100:227–243.
76. Brown WJ, Barajas L, Latta H. The ultrastructure of the human adrenal medulla: with comparative studies of white rat. *Anat Rec* 1971;169:173–184.
77. Lundberg JM, Hamberger B, Schultzberg M, et al. Enkephalin and somatostatin-like immunoreactivities in human adrenal medulla and pheochromocytoma. *Proc Natl Acad Sci U S A* 1979;76:4079–4083.
78. Böck P, Stockinger L, Vyslonzil E. Die Feinstructur des glomus caroticum beim menschen. *Z Zellforsch* 1970;105:543–568.
79. Hervonen A, Korkala O. Fine structure of the carotid body of the midterm human fetus. *Z Anat Entwicklungsmech Gesch* 1972;138: 135–144.
80. Kondo H. Innervation of SIF cells in the superior cervical and nodose ganglia: an ultrastructural study with serial sections. *Biol Cell* 1977; 30:253–264.
81. Hervonen A, Alho H, Helen P, Kanerva L. Small intensely fluorescent cells of human sympathetic ganglia. *Neurosci Lett* 1979;12:97–101.
82. Greenberg ME, Zoff EB, Greene LA. Stimulation of neuronal acetylcholine receptors induces rapid gene transcription. *Science* 1986;234: 80–83.
83. Sietzen M, Schober M, Fischer-Colbrie R, Scherman D, Sperk G, Winkler H. Rat adrenal medulla. Levels of chromogranins, enkephalins, dopamine beta-hydroxylase and the amine transporter are changed by nervous activity and hypophysectomy. *Neuroscience* 1987;22:131–139.
84. Tischler AS, Perlman RL, Costopoulos D, Horwitz J. Vasoactive intestinal peptide activates tyrosine hydroxylase in normal and neoplastic chromaffin cells in culture. *Neurosci Lett* 1985;61:141–146.
85. Tischler AS, DeLellis RA, Nunnemacher G, Wolfe HJ. Acute stimulation of chromaffin cell proliferation in the adult rat adrenal medulla. *Lab Invest* 1988;58:733–735.
86. Penberthy WT, Dahmer MK. Insulin-like growth factor-I enhanced secretion is abolished in protein kinase C deficient chromaffin cells. *J Neurochem* 1994;1707–1715.
87. Brundin T. Studies on the preaortal paraganglia of newborn rabbits. *Acta Physiol Scand* 1966(suppl 70);190:1–54.
88. Hervonen A, Korkala O. The effect of hypoxia on the catecholamine content of human fetal abdominal paraganglia and adrenal medulla. *Acta Obstet Gynecol Scand* 1972;51:7–24.
89. Slotkin TA, Smith PG, Lau C, Bareis DL. Functional aspects of development of catecholamine biosynthesis and release in the sympathetic nervous system. In: Parves H, Parves S, eds. *Biogenic amines in development*. Amsterdam: North-Holland/Elsevier; 1980;28–48.
90. Dalmaz Y, Borghini N, Pequignot JM, Peyrin L. Presence of chemosensitive SIF cells in the rat sympathetic ganglia: a biochemical, immunocytochemical and pharmacological study. *Adv Exp Med Biol* 1993;337:393–399.
91. Dinger B, Wang Z-Z, Chen J, et al. Immunocytochemical and neurochemical aspects of sympathetic ganglion chemosensitivity. *Adv Exp Med Biol* 1993;337:25–30.
92. Fishman MC, Green WL, Platika D. Oxygen chemoreception by carotid body cells in culture. *Proc Natl Acad Sci U S A* 1985;82: 1448–1450.
93. Lopez-Barneo J, Lopez-Lopez JR, Urena J, Gonzalez G. Chemoreception by the carotid body K+ current modulated by $PO_2$ in type I chemoreceptor cells. *Science* 1988;241:580–582.
94. Data PG, Acker H, Lahri S, eds. In: *Neurobiology and cell physiology of chemoreception*. New York: Plenum; 1993.
95. Howe A, Pack RJ. The response of abdominal vagal fibers in the rat to changes in inspired oxygen concentration. *J Physiol* 1977;270: 37P–38P.
96. Honda Y, Myojo S, Hasegawa S, Hasegawa T, Severinghaus JW. Decreased exercise hyperpnea in patients with bilateral carotid chemoreceptor resection. *J Appl Physiol Environ Exerc Physiol* 1979;46: 908–912.
97. Saldana MJ, Salem LE, Travezan R. High altitude hypoxia and chemodectomas. *Hum Pathol* 1973;4:251–263.
98. Falck B, Hillarp NA, Thieme G, Torp A. Fluorescence of catecholamines and related compounds condensed with formaldehyde. *J Histochem Cytochem* 1962;10:348–354.
99. DeLellis RA. Formaldehyde-induced fluorescence technique for the demonstration of biogenic amines in diagnostic histopathology. *Cancer* 1971;28:1704–1710.
100. De La Torre JC. Standardization of the sucrose-potassium phosphate-glyoxylic acid histofluorescence method for tissue monamines. *Neurosci Lett* 1980;17:339–340.
101. Lloyd RV, Sisson K, Shapiro B, Verhofstad AAJ. Histochemical localization of epinephrine, norepinephrine, catecholamine-synthesizing enzymes, and chromogranin in neuroendocrine cells and tumors. *Am J Pathol* 1986;125:45–54.
102. Hervonen A, Pickel VM, John TH, et al. Immunocytochemical demonstration of catecholamine-synthesizing enzymes and neuropeptides in the catecholamine-storing cells of human fetal sympathetic nervous system. In: Enränkö O, Soinila S, Päivärinta H, eds. *Histochemistry and cell biology of autonomic neurons, SIF cells and paraneurons.* New York: Raven Press; 1980:373–578.
103. Neville AM. The adrenal medulla. In: Symington T, ed. *Functional pathology of the adrenal gland*. Baltimore: Williams & Wilkins; 1969:219–324.
104. Steele RH, Hinterberger H. Catecholamines and 5-hydroxytryptamine in the carotid body in vascular, respiratory and other diseases. *J Lab Clin Med* 1972;80:63–70.
105. Perrin DG, Chan W, Cutz E, Madapallimatam A, Sole MJ. Serotonin in the human infant carotid body. *Experimentia* 1986;42:562–564.
106. Kent C, Coupland RE. On the uptake of 5-hydroxytryptamine, 5-hydroxytryptophan and catecholamines by adrenal chromaffin cells and nerve endings. *Cell Tissue Res* 1984;236:189–195.
107. Heym C, Kummre W. *Regulatory peptides in paraganglia*. New York: Gustav Fisher Verlag; 1988.
108. Varndell IM, Tapia FJ, DeMey J, Rush RA, Bloom SR, Polak JM. Electron immunocytochemical localization of enkephalin-like material in catecholamine-containing cells of the carotid body, the adrenal medulla and in pheochromocytomas of man and other mammals. *J Histochem Cytochem* 1982;30:602–690.
109. Vaalasti A, Pelto-Huikko M, Tainio H, Hervonen A. Light and electron microscopic demonstration of enkephalin-like immunoreactivity in paraganglia of the human urinary bladder. *Cell Tissue Res* 1985; 239:683–687.
110. O'Connor DT, Burton D, Deftos W. Chromogranin A: immunohistology reveals its universal occurrence in normal polypeptide hormone–producing endocrine glands. *Life Sci* 1983;33:1657–1663.
111. Lloyd RV, Wilson BS. Specific endocrine tissue marker defined by a monoclonal antibody. *Science* 1983;222:628–630.
112. Hagn C, Schmid KW, Fischer-Colbrie R, Winkler H. Chromogranins A, B, and C in human adrenal medulla and endocrine tissues. *Lab Invest* 1985;55:405–412.
113. Fischer-Colbrie R, Lassmann H, Hagn C, Winkler H. Immunological studies on the distribution of chromogranin A and B in endocrine and nervous tissues. *Neuroscience* 1985;16:547–555.
114. Winkler H, Apps DK, Fischer-Colbrie R. The molecular function of adrenal chromaffin granules: established facts and unresolved topics. *Neuroscience* 1986;18:261–290.
115. Winkler H. The adrenal chromaffin granule: a model for large dense core vesicles of endocrine and nervous tissue. *J Anat* 1993;183: 237–252.
116. Lachmaund A, Gehrke D, Krigelstein K, Unsicker K. Trophic factors from chromaffin granules provide survival of peripheral and central nervous system neurons. *Neuroscience* 1994;62:361–370.
117. Shi S-R, Key ME, Kalra KL. Antigen retrieval in formalin-fixed, paraffin-embedded tissues: an enhancement method for immunohistochemical staining based on microwave heating of tissue sections. *J Histochem Cytochem* 1991;39:741–748.
118. Tischler AS. Triple immunohistochemical staining for bromodeoxyuridine and catecholamine biosynthetic enzymes using microwave antigen retrieval. *J Histochem Cytochem* 1995;43:1–4.
119. Söllner T, Bennett MK, Whiteheart SW, Scheller RH, Rothman JE. A protein assembly–disassembly pathway in vitro that may correspond to sequential steps of synaptic vesicle docking, activation and fusion. *Cell* 1993;75:409–418.
120. Takahashi H, Nakashima S, Kumanishi T, Ikuta F. Paragangliomas of the craniocervical region. An immunohistochemical study on tyrosine hydroxylase. *Acta Neuropathol (Berl)* 1987;73:227–232.

121. Haimoto H, Hosoda S, Kato K. Differential distribution of immunoreactive S100-alpha and S100-beta proteins in normal nonnervous human tissues. *Lab Invest* 1987;57:489–498.
122. Komminoth P, Kunz E, Hiort O, et al. Detection of *ret* proto-oncogene point mutations in paraffin-embedded pheochromocytoma specimens by nonradioactive single-strand conformation polymorphism analysis and direct sequencing. *Am J Pathol* 1994;145:922–929.
123. Leong PK, Thorner P, Yeger H, Kwan N, Zhang Z, Squire J. Detection of mycN gene amplification and deletions of chromosome 1p in neuroblastoma by in situ hybridization using routine histologic sections. *Lab Invest* 1993;69:43–50.
124. Parry DM, Li FP, Strong LC, et al. Carotid body tumors in humans: genetics and epidemiology. *J Natl Cancer Inst* 1982;68:573–578.
125. Santer RM, Hann AC. Quantitative x-ray microanalysis of adrenal medullary cells of young adult and aged rats after glutaraldehyde fixation and potassium dichromate treatment. *Histochemistry* 1993;99: 43–48.
126. Spicer SS, Spivey MA, Ito M, Schulte BA. Some ascites monoclonal antibody preparations contain contaminants that bind to selected Golgi zones or mast cells. *J Histochem Cytochem* 1994;42:213–221.
127. Simson JAV, Hintz DS, Munster AM, Spicer SS. Immunocytochemical evidence for antibody binding to mast cell granules. *Exp Mol Pathol* 1977;26:85–91.
128. Grube D. Immunoreactivities of gastrin (G-) cells. II. Nonspecific binding of immunoglobulins to G-cells by ionic interactions. *Histochemistry* 1980;66:149–167.
129. van Leeuwen F. Pitfalls in immunocytochemistry with special reference to the specificity problems in the localization of neuropeptides. *Am J Anat* 1986;175:363–377.
130. Parker WW, Valsalmis MP. The ampuloglomerular organ: an unusual neurovascular complex in the suboccipital region. *Anat Rec* 1967;159:193–198.
131. Rode J, Bentley A, Parkinson C. Paraganglial cells of urinary bladder and prostate: potential diagnostic problems. *J Clin Pathol* 1990;43: 13–16.
132. Makinen J, Nickels J. Paraganglion cells mimicking metastatic clear cell carcinoma. *Histopathology* 1979;3:459–465.

# Subject Index

Page numbers in italics indicate figures. Page numbers followed by a "t" indicate tables.

**B**

## C

**H**

**W**



**X**



**Y**



**Z**